Hunter's diseases of occupations

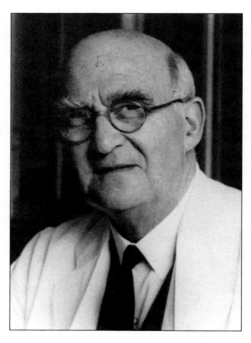

Donald Hunter CBE MD FRCP
1898–1978

Physician, The London Hospital
Senior Censor, Royal College of Physicians of London
Director, MRC Department of Research in Industrial Medicine
Founder Editor, *British Journal of Industrial Medicine*
Author, *Diseases of Occupations*

Hunter's diseases of occupations

9th edition

Edited by

Peter J Baxter MD MSc FRCP FFOM
Consultant Occupational Physician, University of Cambridge and Addenbrookes' NHS Trust Hospital, Cambridge, UK

Peter H Adams MSc PhD FRCP
Emeritus Professor, University of Manchester; formerly Professor of Medicine, University of Manchester, and Head of University Department of Medicine, Manchester Royal Infirmary; Honorary Consultant Physician, Central Manchester Health Care Trust Manchester, UK

Tar-Ching Aw MB PhD FRCP FFOM
Senior Lecturer and Consultant in Occupational Medicine, Institute of Occupational Health, University of Birmingham, Birmingham, UK

Anne Cockcroft MD DIH FRCP FFOM
Consultant in Occupational Medicine, and Director, Occupational Health and Safety Unit, Royal Free Hospital, London, UK

J Malcolm Harrington CBE MSc MD FRCP FFOM
Director of the Institute of Occupational Health, University of Birmingham, Birmingham, UK

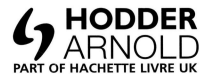

HODDER ARNOLD
PART OF HACHETTE LIVRE UK

First published in Great Britain 1955 as *Diseases of Occupations* by Edward Arnold Publishers
Sixth edition 1978
Seventh edition 1987
Eighth edition 1994
Ninth edition 2000 by
Hodder Arnold, an imprint of Hodder Education, part of Hachette Livre UK,
338 Euston Road, London NW1 3BH

www.hoddereducation.com

British Library Cataloguing in Publication Data
A catalogue record for this book is available from the British Library

Library of Congress Cataloguing-in-Publication Data
A catalog record for this book is available from the Library of Congress

ISBN: 978 0 340 67750 6

4 5 6 7 8 9 10

Commissioning Editor: Georgina Bentliff
Project Editor: Catherine Barnes
Production Editor: Julie Delf
Production Controller: Iian McWilliams
Project Manager: Jane Duncan

Typeset by Phoenix Photosetting, Chatham, Kent
Printed and bound in India

Please visit our website:
www.hoddereducation.com

6/15/09

Contents

Contributors ix

Preface xiii

PART 1 GENERAL CONSIDERATIONS

1 **The occupational history**
WR Lee, T-C Aw
3

2 **The role of laboratory techniques in the prevention and diagnosis of occupational and environmental diseases**
H Kerr Wilson, PJ Baxter
15

3 **Estimating the extent of occupational injuries and disease**
D Coggon
27

4 **Compensation schemes for industrial injuries and diseases**
J Malcolm Harrington
37

5 **Medicolegal reports and the role of the expert witness**
DM Kloss
57

PART 2 DISEASES ASSOCIATED WITH CHEMICAL AGENTS

6 **Absorption of chemicals and mechanisms of detoxification**
PG Blain
67

7 **Metals**
L Morgan, A Scott
81

8 **Gases**
PJ Baxter
123

9 **Welding, fumes and inhalation fevers**
GHG McMillan
179

10 **Pesticides and other agrochemicals**
AL Jones, AT Proudfoot
195

11 **Aliphatic chemicals**
LS Levy
221

12 **Aromatic chemicals**
T-C Aw
261

PART 3 DISEASES ASSOCIATED WITH PHYSICAL AGENTS

13 **Sound, noise and the ear**
RT Ramsden, SR Saeed
283

14   **Vibration (hand-arm and whole body)**
     PL Pelmear   307

15   **Heat and cold**
     EHN Oakley   325

16   **Raised barometric pressure**
     DH Elliott   343

17   **Flying**
     TM Gibson   361

18   **Working at high altitude**
     PJG Forster   383

19   **Ionizing radiations**
     JR Harrison, C Sharp   397

20   **Non-ionizing radiation and the eye**
     M Boulton, DH Sliney   419

21   **Extremely low frequency electric and magnetic fields**
     LI Kheifets   439

PART 4   **DISEASES RELATED TO ERGONOMIC AND MECHANICAL FACTORS**

22   **Repeated movements and repeated trauma affecting the musculoskeletal system**
     K Palmer, C Cooper   453

23   **Back pain and work**
     MIV Jayson   477

PART 5   **DISEASES ASSOCIATED WITH MICROBIOLOGICAL AGENTS**

24   **Occupation and infectious diseases**
     J Heptonstall, A Cockcroft, RMM Smith   489

25   **Genetic modification and biotechnology**
     AM Finn, AJ Scott, GM Stave   521

PART 6   **WORK AND MENTAL HEALTH**

26   **Bullying, post-traumatic stress disorder and violence in the workplace**
     M Lipsedge   539

27   **Substance abuse and the workplace**
     JD Chick   557

28   **Health and mental illness at work: clinical assessment and management**
     EL Teasdale, FH Creed   569

29   **Shift work and extended hours of work**
     G Costa, S Folkard, JM Harrington   581

PART 7   **OCCUPATIONAL LUNG DISORDERS**

30   **Imaging in occupational lung disease**
     PM Taylor   593

31   **Work and chronic air flow limitation**
     DJ Hendrick   607

32   **Byssinosis and other cotton-related diseases**
      CAC Pickering   621

33   **Occupational asthma**
      AJ Newman Taylor   633

34   **Extrinsic allergic alveolitis**
      AJ Newman Taylor   653

35   **Inorganic dusts**
      A Cockcroft, B Nemery   663

36   **Problems from indoor air in non-industrial workplaces**
      P Sherwood Burge   709

PART 8   **OCCUPATIONAL DISEASES OF THE SKIN**

37   **Occupational diseases of the skin**
      RJG Rycroft   725

PART 9   **OCCUPATIONAL CANCER**

38   **Biological mechanisms and biomarkers**
      S Venitt   741

39   **Clinical and epidemiological aspects**
      JM Harrington, P Boffetta, R Saracci   791

PART 10   **REPRODUCTION AND WORK**

40   **Workplace exposures and reproductive effects**
      SM Barlow, AD Dayan, IK Stabile   823

PART 11   **OTHER SYSTEMIC EFFECTS OF WORKPLACE EXPOSURES**

41   **Nephrotoxic effects of workplace exposures**
      GM Bell, HJ Mason   843

42   **Neurotoxic effects of workplace exposures**
      PK Thomas, MJ Aminoff   867

43   **Hepatotoxic effects of workplace exposures**
      TW Warnes, SK Jain, A Smith   881

44   **Haemopoietic effects of workplace exposures: anaemias, leukaemias and lymphomas**
      A Yardley-Jones, A Gray   901

APPENDIX
Diseases of occupations – a short history of their recognition and prevention
      T Carter
                                                                                     917

INDEX   927

Contributors

Michael J Aminoff MD FRCP
Professor of Neurology and Director of Clinical Neurophysiology Laboratories, School of Medicine, University of California, San Francisco, USA

Tar-Ching Aw MB PhD FRCP FFOM
Senior Lecturer and Consultant in Occupational Medicine, Institute of Occupational Health, University of Birmingham, Birmingham, UK

Susan M Barlow BSc PhD DipFRCPath
Consultant Toxicologist, Brighton, UK

Peter J Baxter MD MSc FRCP FFOM
Consultant Occupational Physician, University of Cambridge and Addenbrookes' NHS Trust Hospital, Cambridge, UK

Gordon M Bell BSc MB ChB FRCP(E) FRCP
Consultant Physician and Nephrologist, The Royal Liverpool University Hospitals, Liverpool, UK

Peter G Blain BMedSci MB BS PhD FIBiol FFOM FRCP
Professor of Environmental Medicine and Consultant Physician, University of Newcastle upon Tyne, Division of Environmental and Occupational Medicine, School of Health Care Sciences, The Medical School, Newcastle upon Tyne, UK

P Boffetta MD MPH
Chief, Unit of Environmental Cancer Epidemiology, International Agency for Research on Cancer, Lyon, France

Mike Boulton BSc PhD
Professor in Ocular Cell and Molecular Biology, Department of Optometry and Vision Sciences, University of Cardiff, Cardiff, UK

P Sherwood Burge MSc (OccMed) MD FRCP FFOM DIH
Consultant Physician, Birmingham Heartlands Hospital and Honorary Senior Lecturer, Institute of Occupational Health, University of Birmingham, Birmingham, UK

Tim Carter MSc FRCP FFOM
Chief Medical Adviser (Transport and Safety), Department of the Environment, Transport and the Regions, London, UK

Jonathan D Chick MA MPhil FRCPE FRCPsych
Consultant Psychiatrist, Alcohol Problems Clinic, Royal Edinburgh Hospital, Edinburgh, Scotland, UK

Anne Cockcroft MD DIH FRCP FFOM
Consultant/Senior Lecturer in Occupational Medicine and Director, Occupational Health and Safety Unit, Royal Free Hospital, London, UK

David Coggon MA PhD DM FRCP FFOM FMedSci
Professor of Occupational and Environmental Medicine, MRC Environmental Epidemiology Unit, University of Southampton, Southampton General Hospital, Southampton, UK

Cyrus Cooper MA DM FRCP
Professor of Rheumatology, MRC Clinical Scientist and Consultant Rheumatologist, MRC Environmental Epidemiology Unit, University of Southampton, Southampton General Hospital, Southampton, UK

Giovanni Costa MD
Associate Professor of Occupational Medicine, Department of Medicine and Public Health, University of Verona, Verona, Italy

Francis H Creed MD FRCPsych FRCP
Professor of Psychological Medicine, School of Psychiatry and Behavioural Sciences, University of Manchester, Manchester Royal Infirmary, Manchester, UK

Anthony D Dayan MD FRCP FRCPath FFOM FFPM FIBiol
Professor of Toxicology, St Bartholomew's and the Royal London School of Medicine and Dentistry, London, UK

David H Elliott OBE DPhil FRCP FRCPE FFOM
Shell Professorial Research Fellow in Occupational Health, Robens Institute of Health and Safety, University of Surrey, Guildford, UK

Anne M Finn MB MRCGP MFOM
Head of Occupational Health, Glaxo Wellcome Research and Development, Greenford, Middlesex, UK

Simon Folkard BSc PhD DSc
Professor of Psychology and Director of Body Rhythms and Shiftwork Centre, University College of Swansea, Swansea, UK

Peter JG Forster MD FRCP
Consultant Physician and Rheumatologist, James Paget Healthcare NHS Trust, Great Yarmouth, Norfolk and Consultant in High Altitude Medicine to the Royal Observatory, Edinburgh (Science and Engineering Research Council), UK

Air Commodore T M Gibson QHS PhD MB ChB MFOM DAvMed MRAeS RAF
Director, Medical Programmes and Plans, Ministry of Defence, Whitehall, London, UK

Atherton Gray MB ChB MD FRCPath FRCP
Consultant Haematologist, Princess Margaret Hospital, Swindon, Wiltshire, UK

J Malcolm Harrington CBE MSc MD FRCP FFOM FMedSci
Director of the Institute of Occupational Health, University of Birmingham, Birmingham, UK

John R Harrison BSc MSc MB BS FFOM
Head of Medical Division and Medical Adviser to National Radiological Protection Board, and Honorary Senior Clinical Lecturer, University of Birmingham Medical School, Birmingham, UK

David J Hendrick MD FRCP FFOM
Consultant Physician, Department of Respiratory Medicine, Royal Victoria Infirmary; Regional Unit for Occupational Lung Disease, Newcastle upon Tyne, UK

Julia Heptonstall MSc MB BS FRCP FRCPath DTM&H
Consultant Microbiologist, London, UK

Sanjiv K Jain MA MB BChir MRCP(UK)
Clinical Lecturer, Manchester Royal Infirmary, Manchester, UK

Malcolm IV Jayson MD FRCP
Professor of Rheumatology, Consultant Rheumatologist, Rheumatic Diseases Centre, University of Manchester, Salford, UK

Alison L Jones BSc MD FRCPE
Consultant Physician and Medical Toxicologist, Medical Toxicology Unit, National Poisons Information Service (London Centre), London, UK

Leeka I Kheifets PhD
Technical Executive and Business Area Manager, EMF Health Assessment and Management Environment Group, Electric Power Research Institute, Palo Alto, California, USA

Diana M Kloss LLB(Lond) LLM(Tulane)
Barrister, Gray's Inn and Senior Lecturer in Law, University of Manchester, Manchester, UK

WR Lee MD MSc FRCP FFOM
Emeritus Professor of Occupational Health, University of Manchester and formerly Consultant in Occupational Medicine, Manchester Royal Infirmary, UK and Member, Medical Appeal Tribunals, UK

Leonard S Levy BSc MSc PhD FFOM(HON)
Head of Toxicology and Risk Assessment, MRC Institute of Environment and Health, University of Leicester, Leicester, UK

Maurice Lipsedge MPhil FRCP FRCPsych FFOM
Consultant Psychiatrist, Lewisham and Guy's Mental Health Trust and Chairman, Section of Organisational Psychiatry and Psychology, Department of Psychiatry, United Medical and Dental Schools of Guy's and St Thomas's Hospitals, London, UK

Howard J Mason MSc
Principal Scientist, Health and Safety Laboratory, Research and Laboratory Services Division, Health and Safety Executive, Sheffield, UK

Grant HG McMillan MD MSc FRCP
Medical Officer in Charge, Institute of Naval Medicine, Gosport, UK

Lindsay Morgan MB BS DIH FFOM
Consultant in Occupational Health, Glynteg, Ynystawe, Swansea, UK

Benoit Nemery MD PhD
Professor, Department of Occupational Medicine and Division of Pneumology, Katholieke Universiteit Leuven, Leuven, Belgium

AJ Newman Taylor OBE FRCP FFOM
Professor of Occupational and Environmental Medicine, National Heart and Lung Institute and Consultant Physician to Royal Brompton National Heart and Lung Hospital, London, UK

E Howard N Oakley BA MB BCH MSc
Head of Survival and Thermal Medicine, The Institute of Naval Medicine, Alverstoke, Gosport, UK

Keith Palmer MA BM BCh FFOM MRCGP DRCOG
Clinical Scientist, and Honorary Consultant Occupational Physician, Medical Research Council Environmental Epidemiology Unit, University of Southampton, Southampton General Hospital, Southampton, UK

Peter L Pelmear MB BS MD FFOM DIH DPH
Formerly Consultant, St Michael's Hospital, Toronto, Canada and Associate Professor, Faculty of Medicine, University of Toronto, Canada

CAC Pickering FRCP FFOM DIH
Professor of Occupational Medicine, North West Lung Centre, Wythenshaw Hospital, Manchester, UK

Alex T Proudfoot BSc MB ChB FRCP FRCPE
Formerly Director at The Royal Infirmary NHS Trust, Scottish Poisons Information Bureau, Edinburgh, Scotland, UK

Richard T Ramsden MB ChB FRCS
Professor of Otolaryngology, Victoria University of Manchester, Manchester Royal Infirmary, Manchester, UK

Richard JG Rycroft MD FRCP FFOM DIH
Consultant Dermatologist, St John's Institute of Dermatology, St Thomas's Hospital, London and Senior Medical Inspector (Dermatology), Health and Safety Executive, London, UK

Shakeel R Saeed MB BS(Lon), FRCS(Ed), FRCS(Lon)
Consultant Otolaryngologist and Neuro-Otological Surgeon, University Department of Otolaryngology-Head and Neck Surgery, Manchester Royal Infirmary, Manchester, UK

R Saracci MD
Chief, Unit of Analytical Epidemiology, International Agency for Research on Cancer, Lyon, France

Alan Scott BSc MB MRCS FFOM
Senior Employment Medical Adviser, Field Operations Division, Health and Safety Executive, Nottingham and Clinical Assistant in Accident and Emergency Medicine, University Hospital, Nottingham, UK

Alister J Scott MB ChB MRCP MFOM
Glaxo Wellcome Research and Development, Greenford, Middlesex, UK

Chris Sharp MSc FRCP MRCGP MFOM DAvMed
Head of Medical Department, National Radiological Protection Board, Chilton, Didcot, Oxfordshire, UK

David H Sliney PhD
Program Manager, Laser/Optical Radiation Program and Commander, US Army Center for Health Promotion and Preventive Medicine, Aberdeen Proving Ground, USA

Alexander Smith BSc PhD
Principal Clinical Scientist, Liver Research Laboratories, Liver Unit, Department of Gastroenterology, Manchester Royal Infirmary, Manchester, UK

Robert MM Smith BSc PhD
Epidemiologist, Public Health Laboratory Service, Communicable Disease Surveillance Centre (Wales), Cardiff, UK

Isabel K Stabile PhD MRCOG
Medical Director, Center for Prevention and Early Intervention Policy, Florida State University, Tallahassee, Florida, USA

Gregg M Stave MD MPH
Glaxo Wellcome Research and Development, Greenford, Middlesex, UK

Paul M Taylor MB MRCP FRCR
Consultant Radiologist and Assistant Clinical Director of Radiology, Manchester Royal Infirmary, Manchester, UK

Eric L Teasdale MB ChB FRCP FFOM FRCGP FIOSH
Director of Corporate Health and Safety and Chief Medical Officer, AstraZeneca, London, UK

PK Thomas CBE DSc MD FRCP FRCPath

Emeritus Professor of Neurology, University Department of Clinical Neurosciences, Royal Free and University College Medical School, London, UK

Stanley Venitt BSc PhD

Emeritus Reader in Cancer Studies, University of London, Section of Molecular Carcinogenesis, Haddow Laboratories, Institute of Cancer Research, Sutton, Surrey and Consultant to The Institute of Cancer Research, UK

Thomas W Warnes MD FRCP

Consultant Physician, Liver Unit, Manchester Royal Infirmary, Manchester, UK

H Kerr Wilson BSc MSc PhD CBiol FIBiol

Head, Biomedical Sciences, Health and Safety Laboratory, Sheffield, UK

Anthony Yardley-Jones MB ChB PhD FFOM FRCS(Ed)

Occupational Physician, Burmah Castrol Trading Limited, Swindon, Wiltshire, UK

Preface

Much of the alleviation of conditions for the working population that we can see today has taken place in the last one hundred years. The rise of scientific medicine is even more recent and in Britain the most illustrious physician to apply the new ideas to the diseases of occupations was Donald Hunter. To recall the vision of the early editions of Hunter is to be reminded of the revolution in biomedical knowledge which has occurred in only the last 40 years and which has led to a transformation in workplace health and safety that ranks as one of the major preventive health achievements of the twentieth century.

According to the World Health Organization, however, by the beginning of the Third Millennium the global workforce will surpass three billion people and without preventive action the burden of occupational disease will escalate. Despite steady improvements in global health the future for great numbers of people is bleak, with the gaps between the rich and poor at least as wide as they were half a century ago and becoming wider still. In Britain, in the nineteenth century, the early reformers' struggle with industrialized society attacked poverty and the cruel conditions of working life that were the legacy of the Industrial Revolution. Today, we can all take pride in their humanitarian achievement, but the daily lives of millions of people around the globe are still blighted by the shadow of occupational disease and injury. Even in the most advanced industrial societies, the elimination of occupational disease remains an unattained goal.

This ninth edition of Hunter retains the same purpose as the original: to present to a wide clinical audience an up-to-date and comprehensive coverage of occupational diseases as they present in today's industrialized societies. It is a text on the clinical aspects of occupational and environmental diseases for health practitioners, for public health physicians concerned with environmental health, for consultants preparing medicolegal reports, for lawyers and for others seeking guidance on the medical consequences of work activities and industrial processes. Physicians and nurses enter the speciality of occupational health attracted by the opportunity to combine clinical medicine with epidemiological methods in preventing ill health at work and take satisfaction from making a discernible difference to people's working lives. We trust that this new edition will be an inspiration to them, as Hunter's own writings were to previous generations.

The organization of work is forever changing, with ever quickening pace, and in choosing the subject matter we have been mindful of the emergence of new influences on work-related ill-health. As well as completely revising the text, we have enlarged the coverage of this edition to include specific chapters on mental health, shift work, diagnostic imaging, chronic airflow limitation, welding, and diseases of the kidneys, liver, nervous system and the blood. We gladly acknowledge the previous contributions of Peter Elmes (Chapter 35), Tim Lee (Chapter 11) and Tony Waldron (Chapter 7), which we have been pleased to carry over to this edition. We are indebted to our expert authors for so consistently illuminating their topics for the non-specialist whilst being comprehensive, no easy task but one which has been a key to the success of previous editions. At Arnold, Georgina Bentliff and Catherine Barnes have given us invaluable and ever enthusiastic guidance, whilst Jane Duncan, Project Manager for Arnold, has most ably transformed our manuscripts for the press.

P J Baxter
P H Adams
T-C Aw
A Cockroft
J M Harrington

Part 1

General considerations

The occupational history 3
The role of laboratory techniques in the prevention
    and diagnosis of occupational and
    environmental diseases 15
Estimating the extent of occupational injuries
    and disease 27
Compensation schemes for industrial injuries
    and diseases 37
Medicolegal reports and the role of the expert witness 57

The occupational history

WR LEE, TAR-CHING AW

Why take an occupational history? 3
Effects of work on health 3
Simple questions about occupation 3
What is an occupational disease? 6

A word of caution and an ethical problem 11
The effects of disease on occupation 12
References 13

The occupational history is the most effective instrument for the proper diagnosis of occupational disease[1]

WHY TAKE AN OCCUPATIONAL HISTORY?

There are two main reasons why an occupational history may be important. First, because of the effects of work on health and second, because of the effects of health on (the capacity to) work.

A clinician will explore the first of these interactions when considering whether a patient's occupation could be either the likely cause of his illness (e.g. lead poisoning or bilateral pleural plaques) or may be one of a number of possible causes of the illness (bladder cancer, nerve deafness, asthma).

For the second of these interactions (effects of health on work), a patient's work history, in so far as it reveals his knowledge, skills and attitudes, may be important either when his fitness or suitability for a job are considered or when the question of return to work after illness or injury comes to be considered.

These two aspects of work, first as a cause of or contributor to disease and second as a place to return to after illness or injury, will be considered in turn.

EFFECTS OF WORK ON HEALTH

It is now some 300 years since Bernardino Ramazzini, Professor of Medicine at Padua, advised:[2]

> On visiting a poor home, a doctor should be satisfied to sit on a three-legged stool, in the absence of a gilt chair, and he should take time for his examination: and to the questions recommended by Hippocrates he should add one more – What is your occupation?

SIMPLE QUESTIONS ABOUT OCCUPATION

Two observations can be made on Ramazzini's classic advice to ask 'What is your occupation?' First, this is nowadays widely followed more in ritual than in thought. The short space in hospital notes opposite 'Occupation' allows a couple of words at the most and those are usually added by the admissions officer or records clerk, and they subsequently receive barely a glance from the doctor. Second, the wide variety of activities in industry and technology means that a brief occupational title rarely indicates what a worker actually does or the hazards to which he may be exposed, to say nothing about past exposures.

Medicolegal reports unfortunately sometimes reveal the ignorance of the doctor. He (or she) might feel that something should be written about 'Occupation' even if it clearly means nothing to him (or her). 'For the next 10 years he was employed as a Saggar Maker's Bottom Knocker' the doctor portentously writes without, apparently, wondering why the Saggar Maker needed his 'bottom knocked'. Or 'She has spent the last 5 years as an Alley Girl' presumably leaving it to the court to imagine (or to find out) the hazards of such a job. Why mention in a medical report the knocking of sagger makers' bottoms or hanging around alleys, unless they are relevant?*

Of course, no doctor can expect to know about every job. Some job titles are vague in that exact duties may vary considerably between individuals with similar titles in different industries or in different countries. Thus, 'labourers' not only dig holes in roads or carry bricks up ladders;

---

* For the curious: Persons who knock the bottoms into containers, known as 'saggars' in a non-mechanized pottery, might have been exposed to silica dust. 'Alley girls' worked on a production line (alley) in a soap factory. These terms are less commonly used nowadays.

they work in such diverse places as a chemical factory, a foundry or a cotton mill. The job title 'dresser' may indicate someone who treats seeds with pesticides, or assists a stage actor with costumes and cosmetics, or removes excess silica sand from metal castings, or deals with cuts and wounds in a village hospital in a developing country. Maintenance men could be exposed to a wide variety of chemicals depending on what machinery or equipment they are required to maintain. A 'stoker' used to shovel coal on board a steamship, whereas a 'stoker' in a modern power station might spend all day sitting in a white coat at a control panel. The modern day plumber, despite the antiquity of his job title, handles resins and adhesives, often with unprotected skin whilst his respiratory tract may be exposed to their fumes. He may also be exposed to asbestos fibres when working on asbestos-lagged pipes. However, it is very uncommon nowadays for him to suffer occupational lead poisoning.

So a doctor, prompted perhaps by an apparent association of symptoms with work or possibly by a remark of the patient that some workmates are similarly affected – or perhaps prompted by his own knowledge, must con-

Table 1.1 *Some occupationally related malignancies*

Condition	Industry/Occupation	Agent
Malignancies of respiratory tract		
Malignant neoplasm of nasal cavities	Woodworkers, cabinet furniture makers	Hardwood dusts
	Boot and shoe industry	Unknown
	Chromium producers, processors, users	Chromates
	Isopropyl alcohol manufacture	Unknown
	Nickel smelting and refining	Nickel
Malignant neoplasm of trachea, bronchus and lung	Asbestos industries and users	Asbestos
	Topside coke oven workers	Coke oven fumes
	Uranium and fluorspar mineworkers	Radon
	Chromium producers, processors and users	Chromates
	Nickel smelters, processors and users	Nickel
	Mustard gas manufacture	Mustard gas
	Ion exchange manufacture and ion exchange chemists	BCME (bis-chloromethyl ether)
Malignant neoplasm of larynx	Asbestos industries	Asbestos
Mesothelioma of pleura	Asbestos industries and users	Asbestos
Malignancies of urinary tract		
Malignant neoplasm of bladder	Dye manufacture	Benzidine, 1- and 2-naphthylamine, auramine, magenta, 4-aminobiphenyl
	Rubber workers	
Malignant neoplasm of kidney	Coke oven workers	Coke oven emissions
Malignancies and dyscrasias of blood formation		
Acute lymphoid leukaemia	Rubber industry	Unknown
	Exposure to ionizing radiations	Ionizing radiation
Acute myeloid leukaemia	Exposure to benzene	Benzene
	Exposure to ionizing radiations	Ionizing radiation
Erythroleukaemia	Exposure to benzene	Benzene
Aplastic anaemia	Explosives manufacture	TNT
	Exposure to benzene	Benzene
	Exposure to ionizing radiations	Ionizing radiation
Agranulocytosis or neutropenia	Exposure to benzene	Benzene
Other		
Haemangiosarcoma of liver	Vinyl chloride manufacture	Vinyl chloride monomer
Malignant neoplasm of skin (including scrotum)	Automatic lathe operators	Mineral oils
	Coke oven workers	Soots and tars
	Petroleum refinery workers	Tars
	Tar distillers	Tar distillates

Modified after Ref. 22.

sider what action he should take. His 'own knowledge' may be derived from his own experience and by reference to a check-list, such as that shown in Table 1.1. If a condition with a latent period of many years, such as occupational cancer, is suspected, then enquiries may perhaps have to extend back over the patient's lifetime.

> Informed suspicion is the principal tool for correct diagnosis of occupational disease.[1]

If job titles are not always helpful then some simple screening questions can be asked without embarking every time on an exhaustive occupational history. Such questions are:

- 'What do you work with?'[3]
- 'Do you now or did you have occupational exposure to fumes, chemicals, dust, loud noise, radiation or other toxic occupational factors?'[4]
- 'Is anyone else from work affected in the same way as you?'

Increasingly these days you may usefully ask

- 'Is there a doctor or a medical service at your place of work?'

Ask about a patient's 'work' rather than his 'job' for most of us warm to this approach, and people are pleased to explain what they do, what it entails and what they handle. It should never be forgotten that a 'tradesman' or 'craftsman' has generally had a training as long as a newly qualified hospital doctor (termed a 'senior house officer' or 'house physician' in the UK, and a 'resident', in the USA), and increasingly these days a tradesman follows some form of continuing education or refresher training (comparable in some respects with Continuing Medical Education). He frequently knows a lot about the process and about the materials he uses – including their hazards. Lord Platt's dictum, 'listen to the patient, he will tell you much' applies equally to the occupational history as it does to the clinical history. On the other hand, semi-skilled and unskilled workers generally are less knowledgeable and further information may have to be sought from the firm. Failing that, the patient's trade union or the Health and Safety Executive (in the UK) may be able to help.

When a substance produces an acute effect, direct questions should show the relation between symptoms and work; one useful line is evidence of remissions at weekends and holiday periods. Sometimes, the clinical effects may not appear until a few hours after exposure. Occupational asthma provides a good example of a disorder in which both 'immediate' and 'delayed' effects may occur (see Chapter 33, on asthma). Patients may wake up breathless at night as a result of something they have used during the day. It should be remembered that patients with non-occupational disorders may also feel better when they are away from work or on holiday.

Sensitization of the skin or respiratory tract may not appear until after several years of work with the substance concerned. However, once sensitized, the effects on re-exposure to the causative agent may be immediate or occur within hours.

Long-term effects, such as occupational cancers and some of the pneumoconioses (see Chapters 35 and 39), may take 20 or more years to develop and so the link with previous industrial exposure may be harder to substantiate, especially if the patient left the suspect job some years before.

Occasionally, evidence of significant industrial exposure or disease is discovered by chance in the course of investigations for other diseases. Thus for example, the incidental detection of pleural plaques and calcification from asbestos exposure may be detected on a chest or upper abdominal radiograph done for other clinical reasons. In these circumstances further enquiry might reveal a clear history of occupational exposure, but where this is not forthcoming the finding should prompt one to consider environmental factors.

Although the foregoing account is largely concerned with toxic hazards such as those resulting from exposure to dusts, gases or chemicals, physical workplace hazards may be approached along similar lines (it is well known, for example that the effects of overexposure to ionizing radiation may take many years to become manifest and, similarly, noise-induced hearing loss develops insidiously, generally after years of exposure). The clinician, therefore, should adapt his approach to the suspected disease and the circumstances of the patient's work. For example, the approach to the occupational history in a patient believed to be suffering from repetitive strain injury (or 'work-related upper limb disorder' as the term currently in vogue) is set out in Chapter 22.

These days, with so much self-help in home maintenance and do-it-yourself (DIY) house improvement and so much time spent on leisure pursuits which might involve toxic materials, a few questions in that direction are not misplaced (Table 1.2). A craftsman with contact dermatitis worked in a place where new adhesives had been carefully introduced. His hobby was building model aircraft at home where the hygienic controls were, perhaps, less stringent. There was ample opportunity for skin contact with the adhesives from pursuit of his hobby.

One of us (WRL) recalls a patient presenting with shortness of breath. He had been a miner for a number of years but now worked on a packing line with enzyme washing powders. At home his hobby was keeping budgerigars. A careful history dissected out these strands and investigation confirmed that exposure to enzyme washing powders at work was responsible for his symptoms.

Should the clinician consider that a fuller account of the patient's occupational history would be useful

Table 1.2 *Some examples of hazardous materials used in DIY (Do-it-yourself) activities*

Activity	Toxic materials
Painting	Various solvents; acrylic emulsions Isocyanates: epoxy resins and hardeners Paint stripper may contain methylene chloride Metal pigments e.g. lead, cadmium, arsenic (rarely cause trouble these days)
Plastics	Methyl methacrylate Isocyanates Adhesives such as acrylate glues and epoxy resins and hardeners
Woodworking	Paints, varnishes, and lacquers Solvents including toluene, xylene, acetone, white spirits, methyl ethyl ketone Adhesives e.g. epoxy resins and hardeners Wood dusts
Photography	Products likely to cause skin allergy: Hydroquinone Formaldehyde Paraphenylene diamine derivatives

some further suggestions will be found under the heading, A MORE DETAILED OCCUPATIONAL HISTORY later in this chapter.

WHAT IS AN OCCUPATIONAL DISEASE?

This is often a sterile exercise in semantics – although it may be mildly amusing. Few of us have the satisfaction of giving title to an eponymous disease but it would seem that doctors find it attractive to attach an occupational title to a disease. Changing times and advancing knowledge often serve to corrode such attachments. For example, an earlier incorrect belief was that occupational medicine was simply concerned with a list of trade diseases, ranging perhaps from Arc-Eye to Weavers' Bottom. The first, kerato-conjunctivitis from exposure to ultraviolet (B) radiation, can equally be produced by reflected ultraviolet light from large snow fields.* Weavers' Bottom was an ischial bursitis occurring in hand-loom weavers sliding from side to side all day along the bench of their broadloom. That occupation has now disappeared apart from a few heritage centres where the working hours are shorter and the work rate somewhat more leisurely.

The proclivity to attach an occupation to the name of an illness appeared in a recent description of a woman in her early 20s, admitted to hospital with pyrexia. A bone marrow trephine demonstrated Leishman–Donovan bodies:

Of course we had asked her profession, but perhaps paid it scant attention. She worked in a troop of

dancers and in such an occupation the bite of a female phlebotomus sandfly might be considered a strong occupational risk when working at night in the southern Mediterranean, where she had been employed some 10 months previously.[5]

Where the connection of occupation to disease is established it should be recorded but it is not always easy to define the relationship. For example schistosomiasis is endemic where people bathe in infested waters, but where someone's job takes them unprotected into such waters does the disease thereby become 'occupational'?

As the foregoing account indicates, very many 'occupational diseases' are simply naturally occurring diseases but having a higher incidence in people doing certain work. Thus regarded, a recent paper describes as 'occupational diseases' lobar pneumonia in welders (and other occupations with exposure to metal fume) and osteoarthrosis of the hip in farmers.[6]

Where a State offers benefit for persons who develop diseases which are considered to arise out of and in the course of their occupation, then the State must attempt to define how that relationship is to be recognized officially; this is discussed in Chapter 4.

Criteria for diagnosing occupational disease

In general, several key items of fact must be established before concluding that a patient has an occupational disease. The main criteria which should be satisfied are:

1 The *effect* – i.e. symptoms and signs must fit with what is known about the clinical features of the suspected occupational disease. The less the features match what is expected, the less likely the diagnosis.

---

* This illustrates a further difficulty. If the sufferer is an Alpine guide does he have an occupational disease? What if the sufferer is a holiday-maker in that guide's party?

2 The *exposure* must be sufficient to cause the disease. Information on exposure may be obtained from the patient's occupational history and a description of what hazards are encountered at work. Obviously, it is not sufficient to just know that there is exposure. It is essential to estimate the extent of exposure – i.e. number of substances to which the patient was exposed, intensity, frequency and duration of exposure. Sometimes, occupational hygiene or biological monitoring records may be available and these can provide the relevant details of exposure.

Interpretation of these findings for the most widely used substances often requires reference to published occupational exposure standards. In the UK, the Health and Safety Executive publishes updated standards annually in a document referred to as EH40. In the USA there are several sets of similar standards e.g. Threshold Limit Values and Biological Exposure Indices produced by the American Conference of Governmental Industrial Hygienists (ACGIH), Permissible Exposure Limits produced by the Occupational Safety and Health Administration (OSHA), and Recommended Exposure Limits from the National Institute of Occupational Safety and Health (NIOSH). In Germany, the equivalent standards are known as MAK values. There are differences between these standards, and the basis of how they are set should be understood as a prerequisite for use.

3 The *time sequence* must be correct. This includes the consideration of the appropriate latent period between exposure and effect. For occupational cancers, generally a very short time interval (say less than 5 years) between first exposure and the diagnosis of cancer suggests that exposure may not be the relevant causative agent. For occupational asthma and allergic contact dermatitis, there may be several weeks or months between first exposure and clinical manifestations. Some acute overexposures produce clinical effects immediately or within minutes of exposure e.g. hydrogen cyanide gas, or upper respiratory irritants such as sulphur dioxide, ammonia or chlorine gas (see Chapter 8).

Exposures to gases such as phosgene and nitrogen dioxide can cause a delayed onset pulmonary oedema, so the duration between exposure and effect may be several hours or 1 or 2 days.

It may appear obvious to state that for a diagnosis of occupational disease due to a specific agent, an essential requirement is that the exposure to that agent must precede the occurrence of clinical effects. However, there are situations where even though a disease has developed earlier in life, subsequent occupational exposures may trigger an episode or worsen the condition, e.g. occupational asthma or contact dermatitis.

4 Consideration must be given to the *differential diagnosis*. The examining physician should consider possible non-occupational diagnoses as well as occupational conditions. Missing an occupational disease with its possibilities for prevention is as inappropriate as labelling a condition occupational and missing out on an opportunity to provide early treatment for a non-occupational disease. An example of the former is failure to recognize contact dermatitis due to a workplace agent, and an example of the latter is assuming that a peripheral neuropathy is due to n-hexane when the patient has diabetic neuropathy. The decision on whether an illness is occupational or non-occupational is based on the balance of probability. This requires good clinical diagnostic skills and an understanding of workplace activities and exposures and their effects.

Where to obtain further information on toxic hazards

Because patients often know only the commonly used name of a chemical that they are exposed to at work, e.g. 'trike' for trichloroethylene, or 'perk' for perchloroethylene, it can be difficult for a clinician not familiar with these short names to recognize the specific chemical. Trade names are generally meaningless and often provide little help.

This, however, is becoming less of a problem because in developed countries it is generally recognized that workers should not be exposed to substances which neither they nor their employer know anything about. Unless workers have information and instructions on the substances they handle they cannot reasonably be expected to co-operate with preventive measures. In the UK, the Control of Substances Hazardous to Health (COSHH) regulations require employers to provide adequate information, instruction and training in such matters, with the result that patients may arrive at the surgery or the outpatients clinic carrying specially prepared leaflets (material safety data sheets) on chemicals, if they suspect that these may be responsible for their ill-health. Material safety data sheets (MSDS) are prepared by suppliers for users, and also for importers. A standard format for the preparation of such sheets is suggested by the Occupational Safety and Health Administration (OSHA) for suppliers in the USA, by European Community legislation in Europe, and by Worksafe Australia for those in Australia. Most MSDS contain some data on the properties of the chemical, the possible health effects, first aid treatment and safe handling and use of the chemical. There is unfortunately often some confusing variation between MSDS produced by different organizations in different countries.

The doctor can pursue enquiries on properties and toxicity of chemicals directly with the employer, preferably through the firm's occupational physician if there is one. Alternatively, he could consult a doctor from the government Factory Inspectorate or Health and Safety Inspectorate. In the UK, that would be the Employment Medical Advisory Service (EMAS), whose address and telephone number will be in the telephone directory under either Employment Medical Advisory Service or Health and Safety Executive. In the UK, section 6 of the Health and Safety at Work Act requires manufacturers, suppliers and others to provide adequate information about any measures that are necessary to protect the health and safety of the user. An employer should know therefore about any possible harmful effects (or the absence of harmful effects) of a substance used or produced on his premises. Furthermore, where such information is not available, the manufacturer or supplier may be obliged to undertake research to eliminate or minimize any risks to health and safety. Usually one can ask a patient to obtain from his workplace the name and address of the supplier.

Other factors which may be relevant

Within the framework set out above a number of other points may have to be considered:

SMOKING

Smoking affects the development of some occupational diseases. It is well known that smoking substantially increases the likelihood of an asbestos worker developing lung cancer, although not mesothelioma; it increases the likelihood of byssinosis developing in cotton workers and of lung cancer in uranium miners. Also smokers seem more likely to trigger specific IgE antibody production and are more likely to develop asthma caused by agents inhaled at work. It is less widely recognized that smoking may have a protective effect in some occupational diseases. Extrinsic allergic alveolitis is more likely to affect non-smokers than smokers (possibly by depression of alveolar macrophage phagocytic function).[7] Pneumoconiosis was said to be less likely to occur in coal miners who smoked because the increased bronchial flow of mucus carries the dust away with it, although the reverse has been argued, that decreased ciliary activity, consequent on smoking, reduces dust clearance from the lung.[8]

EXTENT OF EXPOSURE

A careful occupational history will indicate not only the materials a person has been exposed to but also the extent of his exposure. The number of weeks or years spent on the job will obviously give some idea of exposure. Similarly, in a case of acute poisoning, as from lead burning, there may be a recent history of several hours overtime in the evenings with perhaps Saturday working as well in order to get through a 'rush job'. A history of heavy manual work may suggest the possibility of increased intake of a respiratory contaminant (vapour or dust), for heavy work can increase the resting minute volume of 6 litres per minute by more than tenfold.[9,10] Not all the increased amount of vapour or dust respired, however, will necessarily be absorbed or retained.

USE OF PROTECTIVE EQUIPMENT?

The patient may have been provided with, and may claim to have used for all or part of the time, some form of respiratory protection. A careful occupational history should explore its adequacy or suitability. A 'mask' can be anything from a simple gauze pad, a filter device, to a full face respirator with an air supply from the outside. Similar considerations will apply to enquiries about protective measures for skin and eyes, e.g. whether gloves, an eyeshield or safety spectacles have been used and the length of time that they are used for that work cycle.

MAINTENANCE MEN

In many industries one group of workers whose risks are easily overlooked is the plant maintenance men, including fitters of different trades. A well designed and properly functioning plant will operate without much danger to the process workers but when things go wrong and repairs or even routine maintenance have to be carried out, maintenance workers are at risk. Such a situation is increasingly recognized in industry and is dealt with by various formal procedures, such as the 'permits to work' that are required in some chemical plants or on high voltage switchgear, or before doing so called 'hot work'. Nevertheless, some plant maintenance men, for a variety of reasons, ranging from a conscientious desire to keep the plant running through to sheer carelessness, may repeatedly expose themselves to hazardous substances. For such reasons the exposures of maintenance men are sometimes heavy and may be 'mixed' (i.e. to a variety of substances).

A similar occupational group with problems in protection against occupational hazards are contract workers. These are often employees with little training or experience in the job they are asked to perform. They may be migrant or even illegal workers who may be subject to exploitation by unscrupulous employers. Some of these duties are hazardous. Contract workers are often asked to perform a variety of tasks from day to day, usually with little information, instruction and training for those tasks.

METHOD OF HANDLING

Some examples of this are so obvious as to appear trite. A lump of lead presents a physical not a toxicological hazard but once it is converted into fume it may be inhaled and cause lead poisoning. Metallic mercury, on

Vapour pressure 0.05 mmHg at 25°C
2.4-tolylene diisocyanate

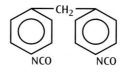

Vapour pressure 0.001 mmHg at 40°C
Diphenyl methane 4,4 diisocyanate

Figure 1.1

the other hand, has a sufficiently high vapour pressure at room temperature to cause dangerous air concentrations to develop (Chapter 7).

Both toluene diisocyanate (TDI, strictly 2,4-tolylene diisocyanate) and methylene diphenyl diisocyanate (MDI, strictly diphenyl methane 4,4 diisocyanate) (see Fig. 1.1) are well known as potent causes of occupational asthma (see Chapter 33).

However, because TDI has a much higher vapour pressure, at room temperature, than the viscous MDI, it might be expected that MDI is safer to handle. So it is, unless the process is exothermic or involves spraying. In either of those circumstances the advantage of the low vapour pressure of MDI is negated and it has been found on a number of occasions to be a potent respiratory sensitizer.

'Hazard' and 'risk' are not the same

This concept of thinking separately about the toxicity of a material and the toxic hazard of the process (or in this context of the work done by the patient) is very important. It is to be found in the distinction which is now increasingly made between 'hazard' and 'risk'.[11] 'Hazard' is the potential (even the theoretical potential) for causing harm and 'risk' is the likelihood (or the probability) that such harm will result. The term 'risk' is now sometimes extended to include consideration of the severity of effect. It is well illustrated in the (possibly apocryphal) story of the dockers who became very concerned about a chemical they were asked to handle. They learned that it could cause tinnitus, deafness and blurring of vision. Further intake would lead to restlessness, increased respiration, sometimes vomiting and ultimately, coma and death. An occupational physician called in to advise agreed that this was a true description of the toxicity, adding that in his experience dockers did not generally suffer from salicylate poisoning when handling crates packed with bottles of aspirin.[12]

Confusion over materials

Confusion sometimes occurs regarding the nature of the materials to which workers are exposed. This may arise in a number of ways:

DECOMPOSITION

From time to time things go wrong with industrial processes, causing the chemical composition or physical properties of the materials to alter and thereby materially increasing the hazard. Trichloroethylene, a widely used narcotic solvent, if overheated, may produce phosgene gas which causes pulmonary oedema. Methyl isocyanate heated above 400 °C under pressure may decompose to hydrogen cyanide:[13] $CH_3NCO \rightarrow H_2 + HCN + CO$. Cadmium plated bolts present no hazard unless cut with an oxyacetylene, oxypropane, or oxybutane torch giving rise to cadmium oxide fumes, capable of causing chemical pneumonitis.[14]

CHEMICAL NAMES

It goes without saying that the physician must be clear what substance the patient has worked with. Frequently, benzene (C_6H_6), used in industry as a solvent and known to produce narcosis, aplastic anaemia and sometimes leukaemia, is confused with benzine, which is also used as a solvent, but is a mixture of liquid hydrocarbons (generally straight chain) and without the same serious toxic effects. Another common confusion is between dioxin and dioxan (see Fig. 1.2). Dioxan (dioxane) has been used for many years as a solvent for fats and other materials. It has the expected narcotic effects of such solvents and, in very large doses, has been reported as toxic to the liver and kidneys. For dioxin see Fig. 1.4. Chlordecone (Kepone®), a pesticide known to cause spermatogenic effects in occupationally exposed males is sometimes confused with the similar-sounding dodecane – an aliphatic hydrocarbon used as a solvent. Chlordecone is no longer produced commercially, although dodecane is available and used widely.

IMPURE CHEMICALS

Even when the correct chemical name is obtained, the physician must always bear in mind that books or journals sometimes refer to the toxicity of the pure or relatively pure substance whereas, when used on a large scale industrially, chemicals will often not be pure and may well carry contaminants. For example toluene (methyl benzene), apart from narcotic properties, does not have the same serious toxic effects as benzene, mentioned above, because it is metabolized along the side chain (the methyl group) whereas benzene is metabolized on the ring, initially by the formation of an epoxide which may react with the macro-molecules of the cell. Toluene is therefore recommended, and used, as a 'safe' substitute, but commercial toluene has been known to contain up to 15% of benzene.

Other examples include the manufacture of the herbi-cide 2,4,5,-T (2,4,5-trichlorophenoxyacetic acid) during which TCDD (2,3,7,8-tetrachlorodibenzo-*p*-dioxin) may be formed (see Fig. 1.3) and choloromethyl methyl ether (CMME) which might be contaminated with bis (chloromethyl) ether (BCME) (see Fig. 1.4)

A MORE DETAILED OCCUPATIONAL HISTORY

Sometimes a clinician will require a fairly extended account of what precisely the patient does, how he does it and what tools and materials he uses and in what cir-cumstances.

It is usually helpful to adopt a systematic approach, beginning with the first job after leaving school. Spells of unemployment and periods of military service are some-times relevant and may require the same amount of detail. 'Occupation' should be interpreted in the widest sense and should include housework and voluntary ser-vice overseas. Individuals with multiple short-term jobs thereby also give some indication of their own character, abilities and circumstances.

The patient can be asked to jot down the rough details of his work history and duties before he sees you, and a

simple form (Fig. 1.5 a,b) which he can complete will often save both his time and yours.

It is easy to go through it with the patient during the consultation, correcting and amplifying what is written there. When doing this it is useful to think in terms of dates as well as the patient's age because we all tend to link some events to our age at the time and some to the year. It forms a useful cross-check. 'Blanks' – where a period is apparently omitted – need to be approached tactfully and carefully. Often they are no more than for-gotten jobs or miscalculations but occasionally they are deliberate, covering periods such as time in prison or a spell of mental illness which the patient wishes to forget or to conceal. The completed form makes a permanent record in the case notes for further reference.

HOW RELIABLE ARE OCCUPATIONAL HISTORIES?

Some readers may wonder how reliable is an occupa-tional history. In a study in Canada, extending back over the previous 13 years, the occupational histories given by male workers had a validity score (ratio of number of years for which information provided by the worker was valid to the number of years of observation) of 0.81 and there was no measurable difference in the degree of con-cordance between the first half of the 13-year period and the second half.[15] In a more recent Canadian study, extending rectrospectively over the previous 29 years, the occupational histories given by female workers were shown to have a validity score of 0.81.[16] Over this longer time span, the validity score ranged from 0.74 for 'dis-

Dioxan

Dioxin
2, 3, 7, 8 tetrachlorodibenzo-*p*-dioxin (TCDD)

Figure 1.2

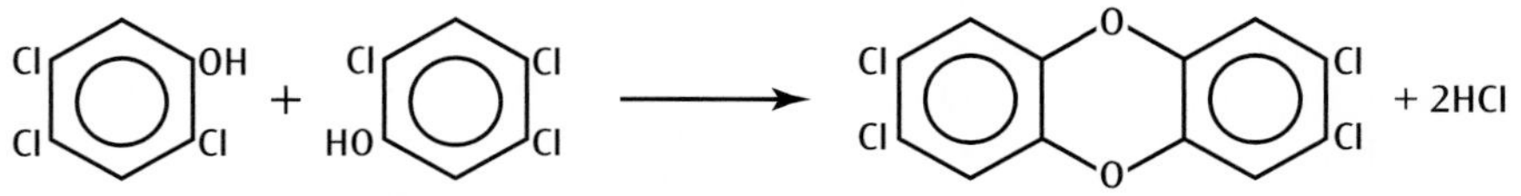

Trichlorophenol

Dioxin

+ 2HCl

Figure 1.3

$ClCH_2OCH_3$

Chloromethyl ether

$ClCH_2OCH_2Cl$

Bis(chloromethyl) ether

Figure 1.4

(a)

Name: EJ	Year of Birth: 1932	Age: 50 years	Date: 6.6.82

WORK HISTORY

Fill in the name of each job which you have had since you left school, up to the present, and put down also any periods of unemployment and service with the forces. Give the age at which you began each job and the number of years spent at it as accurately as you can.

YEARS	AGE	JOB	PERIOD
1946–1951	14	Boiler fireman at coal mine	5 years
1951–1954	19	Unemployed	3 years
1954–1973	22	Several manual labouring jobs for local council	19 years
1973–1974	41	Boiler fireman, brickworks	1 year
1974–present	42	Grog crusher	8 years

(b)

Name: JR	Year of Birth: 1925	Age: 58 years	Date: 6.9.83

WORK HISTORY

Fill in the name of each job which you have had since you left school, up to the present, and put down also any periods of unemployment and service with the forces. Give the age at which you began each job and the number of years spent at it as accurately as you can.

YEARS	AGE	JOB	PERIOD
1941–1943	16	Apprentice bricklayer	2 years
1943–1950	18	Pony driver, coal mine (Blackhall, Co Durham) Putting	7 years
1950–1952	25	Coal cutter	2 years
1952–1968	27	Went to USA–dry driller in coal mine	16 years
1968–1975	43	Labourer–building work	7 years
1975–present	50	Hospital porter	8 years to present

Figure 1.5 (a) Occupational history of a man with an unusual job at a brickworks. As a grog crusher he fed imperfect and broken refractory bricks, which contained a high proportion of silica from the kilns, into an open crushing machine which broke them down into small lumps. These were then passed to a pulverizer which converted them to a powder which was passed by conveyor belt to the mixing plant for incorporation into new bricks. Although dust extraction was in use it had been there for only 2–3 years and the operation was still very dusty. He had silicosis, from which he died. (b) This man, a hospital porter, presented with increasing breathlessness. A radiograph of his lungs showed large shadows consistent with progressive massive fibrosis of coalworkers.

tant' (i.e. earlier) employment to 0.89 for 'recent' employment.

A WORD OF CAUTION AND AN ETHICAL PROBLEM

In the present climate of complete disclosure and patients' right-to-know it might seem out of place to debate how much the patient should be told. Experience, however, suggests why some thought ought to be given to this matter. If the doctor is sure of his (or her) diagnosis, this, and its medicolegal implications should be discussed with the patient or their relatives. If, however, the doctor only *suspects* an occupational cause, then he or she must reflect carefully and consider seeking advice from others with perhaps more knowledge and experience. Like some clinical problems, many ethical dilemmas are better shared – although they must first be recognized – which means being aware that they could exist.

Patients, and their relatives, may react to the diagnosis of an occupational disease in a different way from the diagnosis of a non-occupational disease. In addition to the usual anxieties over treatment and prognosis the question of 'compensation' will often understandably come up. The term 'compensation' in the patient's thinking will cover both State Benefit and Common Law claims although he or she does not at first clearly differentiate between them (see Chapter 4).

Where there is the prospect of financial gain, attitudes may change. For example a consultant or a general practitioner, rightly wondering whether the patient's respiratory problem could be a result of their current or previous work in a cotton 'cardroom', might mention this. Such a comment can lead to an unanticipated train of events. Obviously, if it subsequently transpires that the diagnosis is correct, then the consequences regarding benefit as described in Chapter 4, will follow. But what, if after further investigation and enquiry, it transpires that the respiratory disease has no relation to the previous work? A seed has been planted by the unsuspecting doctor and, whilst the lawyers reap the harvest, the general practitioner can be left with the barren field of a disappointed and frustrated patient. People sometimes spend much fruitless time, effort and anxiety pursuing a claim based on such a chance remark. So what ought the doctor to do?

This can be a difficult ethical decision. Where there is a strong possibility of occupational cause, the doctor's duty is clear. When, however, there is only a suspicion, ought the doctor, in the best interests of the patient, to remain silent or risk starting his patient on a 'wild goose chase' with only a very small chance of success? Which is good medicine? Is it good medicine to save the patient from such a course or is it negligent to keep silent? This is but one instance of what Sieghart[17] has described as how one behaves when 'faced with a conflict between two or more moral principles to [both of] which they subscribe'. In this instance does the doctor, wittingly or unwittingly, lead the patient onto a course which might lead to some financial gain but which might lead to frustration, bitterness and disappointment after long legal wrangling?

These problems arise in clinical practice from time to time and there are, of course, no simple answers. Each case has to be judged on its merits and on the likely reaction of the patient and his or her family. Advice is dangerous, but two thoughts are offered here. First, Sieghart's thoughtful essay is worth reading in full and, second, beware advice from those doctors whose work does not bring them regularly into clinical contact with patients and who, consequently, may have apparently clear and firm but possibly wrong advice on such difficult matters. They might too readily veer towards what is 'safe' from the doctor's standpoint without giving sufficient weight to the long-term effects on the patient's total well-being. 'He jests at scars, that never felt a wound'.

THE EFFECT OF DISEASE ON OCCUPATION

Most patients are able to return directly to their own job after an illness or injury but some, because of residual disability whether temporary or permanent, are unable to return to their former work. Additionally, very many people with some impairment of function* either seek work or seek to remain at work and may ask for medical advice.

The primary purpose of a medical assessment of fitness for work is set out in the useful and authoritative book, *Fitness for Work*[18] from the Royal College of Physicians and its Faculty of Occupational Medicine. It is 'to make sure that an individual is fit to perform the task involved effectively and without risk to his own or to others' health and safety'. The main areas where such advice is needed are:

1 The patient's condition may limit, reduce or prevent him performing the job effectively (e.g. musculoskeletal conditions that limit mobility, or manipulative ability).
2 The patient's condition might be made worse by the job (e.g. excessive physical exertion in some cardiorespiratory conditions; exposure to certain allergens in asthma).
3 The patient's condition is likely to make it unsafe for him to do the job (e.g. liability to sudden unconsciousness in a hazardous situation).
4 The patient's condition is likely to make it unsafe both for him and others, whether fellow workers and/or the community (e.g. road or railway driving in someone who is liable to sudden unconsciousness or to behave abnormally).
5 The patient's condition might make it unsafe for the community (e.g. for consumers of the product, if a food-handler transmits infection).

Looking through the above list it is clear that some areas are concerned with direct risk to the patient and some relate to risks to others, either risks to the health and safety of third parties or substantial financial risks to employers. What are the ethical responsibilities of the doctor under the different circumstances? The easy – but not very helpful – answer is that it depends on the individual circumstances; but this generally fails to take the concerned doctor much further. However, the general principles are set out and briefly discussed in the chapter, 'Relationships between doctors and individuals' in the British Medical Association's *Handbook of Medical Ethics*.[19]

When he/she comes to offer advice, the doctor will find that the occupational history, described earlier in this chapter, will give a good idea of the patient's knowledge, skills and attitudes. Advice on resettlement can, therefore, be discussed more realistically. If a patient is unable to return to his own job, then knowledge of his past work experience will be useful in indicating what possible alternative work might be considered. Equally important, it might indicate what types of work are likely to be unsuitable.

For most jobs there are no clear guidelines for the level of fitness required, so the clinician can be thrown back on his own experience and judgment but, as observed earlier, no doctor can expect to know about every job. It is too dangerous to guess and the wisest course is to contact the occupational physician at the place of work or, in the UK, to contact the Health and Safety Executive's local Employment Medical Advisory Service (EMAS).

For a few occupations, such as car drivers, Large Goods Vehicle (LGV) drivers (formerly heavy goods vehicle (HGV) drivers), Passenger Carrying Vehicle (PCV) drivers (formerly Public Service Vehicle (PSV) drivers) other professional drivers and airline pilots, detailed advice has been published. In the UK, the

Medical Advisory Branch of the Driving and Vehicle Licensing Agency at Swansea will give advice to doctors about an individual patient (without requiring the patient's name and address). A most useful booklet, *Medical Aspects of Fitness to Drive*, published by the Medical Commission on Accident Prevention[20] not only indicates the medical criteria, but also discusses, albeit briefly, *why* they are important. It, therefore, provides useful background reading for a wider variety of jobs than driving. The Medical Advisory Branch of the Driver and Vehicle Licensing Agency has also produced a ready reference for medical practitioners on the current UK medical standards for fitness to drive.[21]

For other occupations, *Fitness for Work: The Medical Aspects*[18] gives authoritative guidance using as its starting points the diseases (impairments) and disabilities from which a patient might suffer. It also has appendices on the medical standards for civil aviation; divers and seafarers (the latter having since been updated in June 1988 by Merchant Shipping Notice No. M1331 issued by the Shipping Policy Directorate of the Department of Transport).

REFERENCES

1 Landrigan PJ, Baker DB. The recognition and control of occupational disease. *JAMA* 1991; **266:** 676–80.

2 Ramazzini B. *Diseases of Workers* (originally 1713). The Classics of Medicine Library. Illinois: University of Chicago Press, 1983.

3 Lee WR. What do you work with? *Br Med J* 1985; **290:** 1846–7.

4 Goldman RH, Peters JM. The occupational and environmental health history. *JAMA* 1981; **246:** 2831–6.

5 Heron RJL. Patients who changed my practice; the chance encounter. *Br Med J* 1996; **313:** 1072.

6 Coggon D. New occupational diseases. *J Roy Coll Phys Lond* 1997; **31:** 202–5.

7 Anon. Smoking, occupation and allergic lung disease. *Lancet* 1985; **i:** 965.

8 Morgan WKL, Seaton A. *Occupational Lung Diseases* 3rd edn. Philadelphia: WB Saunders Co, 1995.

9 Guyton AC. *Textbook of Medical Physiology* 9th edn. Philadelphia: WB Saunders Co, 1994.

10 Frohlich ED (ed). *Rypins' Basic Sciences Review* 16th edn. Philadelphia: JB Lippincott Co, 1993.

11 European Chemical Industry Ecology and Toxicology Centre. *Risk Assessment of Occupational Chemical Carcinogens*. Brussels: ECETOC Monograph No. 3, 1982.

12 Munn A. Health hazards to workers from industrial chemicals. *Chem Soc Rev* 1975; **4:** 82–9.

13 Blake PG, Ijadi-Maghsoodi S. Kinetics and mechanisms of the thermal decomposition of methy isocyanate. *Int J Chem Kin* 1982; **14:** 945–52.

14 Benton DC, Andrews GS, Davies HJ, Howells L, Smith GF. Acute cadmium fume poisoning. *Br J Ind Med* 1966; **23:** 292–301.

15 Baumgarten B, Siemiatycki J, Gibbs GW. Validity of work histories obtained by interview for epidemiologic purposes. *Am J Epidemiol* 1983; **118:** 583–91.

16 Brisson C, Vezina M, Bernard M and Gingras S. Validity of occupational histories obtained by interview with female workers. *Am J Ind Med* 1991; **19:** 523–30.

17 Sieghart P. Professional ethics – for whose benefit? *J Soc Occup Med* 1982; **32:** 4–14.

18 Cox RAF, Edwards FC, McCallum RI. *Fitness for Work; The Medical Aspects* 2nd edn. Oxford: Oxford Medical Publications/Royal College of Physicians, 1995.

19 British Medical Association. *Ethics Manual*. London: BMA, 1998.

20 Taylor JF (ed) *Medical Aspects of Fitness to Drive* 5th edn. London: Medical Commission on Accident Prevention/ HMSO, 1995.

21 Medical Advisory Branch, Driver and Vehicle Licensing Agency. *For Medical Practitioners: At a Glance Guide to the Current Medical Standards of Fitness to Drive*. Swansea: DVLA, 1994.

22 Rutstein DR, Mullan RJ, Todd M *et al*. Sentinel health events (occupational): a basis for physician recognition and public health surveillance. *Am J Publ Hlth* 1983; **73:** 1054–62.

2

The role of laboratory techniques in the prevention and diagnosis of occupational and environmental diseases

H KERR WILSON, PETER J BAXTER

Health surveillance and exposure assessment   15
Ethical issues   16
Interpretation of results   17
Practical considerations in biological monitoring   19

Some recent developments in biological and biological
  effect monitoring   20
Diagnosing occupational and environmental diseases   22
References   25

Laboratory techniques have an important role in the investigation and monitoring of the effects of workplace hazards on human health. Within recent years, a range of monitoring techniques has become available and is now used routinely in exposure assessment, in health surveillance and in helping to make health risk assessments. The laboratory tools available to occupational health professionals include ambient air measurements, biological monitoring of exposure and biological monitoring of effect. More recently, attention has been focused on the development of biomarkers of susceptibility. The choice of test will depend on the nature of the investigation. This chapter is primarily concerned with the practical use of biological and biological effect monitoring but reference is made to some recent developments and their likely use in occupational medicine.

Air monitoring is the measurement and assessment of external exposure to airborne workplace substances. Monitoring techniques include the use of static or personal samplers which may be used for group or individual exposure assessment. These measurements are usually used to assess compliance with an appropriate air standard, to identify emission sources or to establish the efficiency of control measures.

Biological monitoring is the measurement and assessment of workplace agents or their metabolites in biological fluids usually, blood, urine or breath of exposed workers. This procedure allows the level of internal exposure to be assessed because it reflects the total uptake by all routes of exposure including inhalation, ingestion and skin penetration.

Biological effect monitoring is the measurement and assessment of a biological effect (or response) in exposed workers. Early indicators of biological effect ideally detect potentially adverse changes before they become irreversible. These indicators are related to internal dose and are predictive of an adverse effect with increasing exposure to the workplace agent.

Biomarkers of susceptibility are those markers which indicate that an individual may be more or less susceptible to adverse effects following exposure to a particular xenobiotic. They can be used to detect inherited or acquired characteristics and would include for example, genetically determined enzyme polymorphisms.

Health surveillance is the periodic clinical examination of exposed workers designed to protect the worker's health through the early detection of adverse health effects, thereby preventing further harm.

HEALTH SURVEILLANCE AND EXPOSURE ASSESSMENT

In the clinical setting, biological monitoring is advantageous over air monitoring since it provides the physician with information about an individual worker's internal exposure, because it accounts for exposure by all routes. These exposure data can be assessed in the light of an individual's clinical history, their lifestyle and potentially confounding factors. In addition, it can give useful information on the degree of occupational hygiene being employed and the efficacy of control procedures, for example, where personal protective equipment is being used. Biological effect monitoring can be used to give an early indication of potential health problems. It normally involves measuring biochemical responses such as measuring cholinesterase activity following an acute exposure to organophosphorous pesticides or for example, urinary proteins after chronic exposure to cadmium. Exposure assessment and health surveillance are important elements in the clinical management of health risk assessment and Fig. 2.1 illustrates the relationship between these aspects and biological exposure and effect monitoring.

When a worker is exposed to a chemical or biological agent, it may enter the body through various routes. The agent may interact with cellular or molecular processes and a reversible effect may be measurable. Similarly, if the hazard is a physical one (e.g. vibration) it may have an effect on the physiological or biochemical processes. With further and prolonged exposure to the hazard it may lead to irreversibly harmful effects, ultimately resulting in a clinical condition or disease. Hence, we move from biological exposure monitoring to biological effect monitoring which runs in parallel with the progression from exposure assessment to health surveillance. At all stages in the exposure continuum, individual susceptibility factors may contribute to the development of an adverse effect and ultimately a recognizable disease. Biological monitoring is a procedure which can be used in both exposure assessment and in health surveillance.[1]

In the case of health surveillance it is used when it is possible to link the results from a biological test to an adverse health effect. Implicit in this requirement is that a no-adverse effect level can be established. It is not uncommon, however, for substances to be used in the workplace for which exposure-effect relationships cannot be defined. These circumstances do not mean however, that preventative action is not possible. The physician may consider that it would be prudent to keep exposure to as low as reasonably practicable, for example, when handling a potential carcinogen or respiratory sensitizer. In these circumstances an exposure assessment exercise involving biological monitoring may be appropriate. If it is not possible to establish a no-adverse effect level, the alternative approach of setting a hygiene-based benchmark value is recommended. This approach does not require information on dose/effect relationships. It is based on the principle of what is reasonably practicable within the context of best practice. It requires data on good occupational hygiene practice to allow comparative assessments to be made. Biological monitoring of the workforce allows an assessment to be made concerning the adequacy of control and hence the degree of risk. Thus its use in workers exposed to the potential human carcinogen, 4,4'-methylene *bis*(2-chloroaniline) (MbOCA), has demonstrated the benefit of regular biological monitoring which resulted over a period of time, in a reduction in exposure as measured by total urinary MbOCA.[2]

ETHICAL ISSUES

Since biological monitoring involves making measurements on samples taken from people, it is essential that the rights of the individual are safeguarded. Biological monitoring programmes should be discussed and agreed with employees or their representatives and an assurance given that participation or non-participation will not affect their conditions of employment. When seeking informed consent from employees, the purpose of the programme should be made clear, what samples will be required and whether

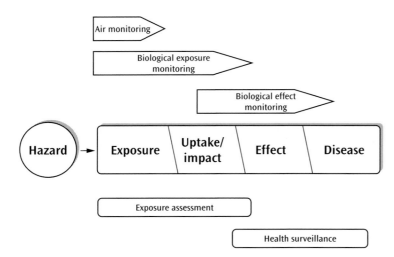

Figure 2.1 *Schematic summary of methods for monitoring exposure to a chemical.*

there are any associated risks. An indication of what action might be taken on the basis of the results and the likely benefit to the employee should be intimated. Workers need to be assured that a biological monitoring programme is under the supervision of a competent person, and that their samples will be analysed only for specified substances, to which they have consented. The results must be treated in confidence and be disclosed only to those health professionals or managers who the workers have agreed should have their results. Suitable arrangements must be put in place for feedback and the interpretation of results. In our experience these arrangements do not pose any particular problems and a well designed and executed biological monitoring programme can be an effective way of protecting workers' health.

INTERPRETATION OF RESULTS

It is axiomatic that laboratory results need to be interpreted. Ideally, the point at which intervention takes place should be derived from well designed health-based studies of exposed workers. If such data are available it may be possible to set a no-adverse effect level. However, given the vast number of substances in use at the workplace, it is unrealistic to expect that no-adverse effect levels can be set for all substances and hence alternative ways of interpreting results are necessary. One approach is to compare results obtained in the workplace with reference values set from the general unexposed population. However, this method only indicates the extent to which the workers results compare with the background levels found in the general population. It does not take into account the extent to which the results compare with other workers in the same industry or the levels one might expect in a factory where good control procedures are in operation. In recent years, this comparative approach has gained acceptance among occupational health professionals as being a practical means of monitoring and controlling exposure. It is commonly known as the 'benchmark' concept and guidance values have been set by some authorities.[3] These values are derived from studies where good working practices are employed. The approach is based on the principle of good hygiene practice and relies on what is practically achievable and is particularly useful when air monitoring does not give a reliable indication of the total exposure (e.g. skin absorption, ingestion) or where control depends on respiratory protective equipment. It is also an appropriate technique where systemic toxicity is related to long-term tissue accumulation of a substance which is not related to airborne measurements taken at a particular time (e.g. cadmium and polychlorinated biphenyls).

Biological guidance values and action levels

Some organizations have set recommended or statutory biological monitoring guidance values. The American Conference of Governmental Industrial Hygienists (ACGIH) publishes annually, a list of Biological Exposure Indices (BEI).[4] The BEIs are advisory reference values and represent the concentration of a substance which is likely to be found in the biological sample of a worker who was exposed through inhalation, to the threshold limit value. Hence, in general, the BEI is a hygiene-based equivalent value (although in some circumstances the BEI is considered to be health-based). Although BEIs do not indicate a sharp distinction between a safe or unsafe exposure, persistent values above the BEI should trigger an investigation. Deutsche Forschungsgemeinschaft (DFG) publishes an annual list of Biological Tolerance Values (Biologische Arbeitsstofftoleranzwerte, BAT).[5] A BAT is defined as the maximum permissible quantity of a substance which does not generally impair the health of a worker. In the case of carcinogens no value is set and data are given on the biological value found when a worker is exposed to a given air value. The BEI and BAT approaches reflect different philosophies in setting guidelines. The BAT definition is primarily health-based whereas the BEI is related to an equivalent hygiene limit.

In the United Kingdom the control and monitoring of lead exposure relies on the statutory measurement of blood lead. New Control of Lead at Work Regulations have introduced the concept of action levels and suspension levels.[6] However, the Health and Safety Executive (HSE) has adopted a different approach for other substances. Non-statutory biological monitoring guidance values have been set for nine substances.[3] There are two types of guidance values: health and benchmark. Health guidance values are set at a level at which there is no indication from the scientific evidence available that the substance being monitored is likely to be injurious to health. Health guidance values are therefore, health based and are equivalent in health protection terms to the United Kingdom Occupational Exposure Standards.[3] The benchmark guidance values are practicable, achievable levels set at the 90th percentile of available biological monitoring results collected from a representative sample of workplaces with good occupational hygiene practices. Table 2.1 compares some of the biological monitoring values set by HSE, ACGIH, DFG and the Finnish Institute of Occupational Health.[7] The majority of these guidance values find their use in exposure assessment because the results of the monitoring activity gives information on the uptake by the body. The published information on guidance values for biological effect monitoring is very limited. Table 2.2 lists some effect markers and recommended action levels.

Table 2.1 *Some commonly used biological monitoring tests and guidance values*

Substance	Analyte	Medium	Sampling time	BMGV (HSE 1999)	BEI (ACGIH 1998)	BAT (DFG 1998)	FIOH (1995)	Basis for action level (toxic effect)
Aluminium	Aluminium	Urine	End of shift			200 µg/litre (7.4 µmol/litre)	6 µmol/litre	Lung fibrosis
Aniline	p-Aminophenol haemoglobin conjugate	Urine, blood	End of shift End of shift		50 mg/g		500 µmol/litre	Haematotoxic
Arsenic	Arsenic	Urine	End of shift		50 µg/g (50 µmol/mol creatinine)	100 µg/litre	0.07 µmol/litre	Cancer, haemolysis
Benzene	S-phenylmercapturic acid	Urine	End of shift		25 µg/g			Bone marrow, leukaemia
Butan-2-one	Butan-2-one	Urine	End of shift	70 µmol/litre	2 mg/litre (28 µmol/litre)	5 mg/litre (70 µmol/litre)	60 µmol/litre	Respiratory, eye irritation
2-Butoxyethanol	Butoxyacetic acid	Urine	End of shift	240 mmol/mol creatinine		100 mg/litre		Haematotoxic
Cadmium	Cadmium	Urine	Random		5 µg/g		50 nmol/litre	Nephrotoxic, respiratory dysfunction
Carbon disulphide	Thiothiazolidine-4-carboxylic acid	Urine	End of shift, End of week		5 mg/g (3.5 mmol/mol creatinine)	8 mg/litre (49 µmol/litre)	2 mmol/mol-creatinine	Neurotoxic, coronary heart disease
Carbon monoxide	Carboxyhaemoglobin	Blood	End of shift		3.5%	5%	5%	Hypoxia
Chromium	Chromium	Urine	End of shift, End of week		30 µg/g (65 µmol/mol creatinine)		0.6 µmol/litre	Respiratory and skin effects (Cr VI)
Cobalt	Cobalt	Urine	End of shift, End of week		15 µg/litre		600 nmol/litre	Respiratory disease, dermatitis
N,N-Dimethyl acetamide	N-Methylacetamide	Urine	End of shift	100 mmol/mol creatinine	30 mg/g		650 µmol/litre	Hepatotoxic
Dimethylformamide	'Total' N-methylformamide	Urine	End of shift		40 mg/g (77 mmol/mol creatinine)	15 mg/litre (260 µmol/litre)	650 µmol/litre	Hepatotoxic
Dichloromethane	CoHB	Blood	End of shift			5%	5%	Hypoxia, CNS
Fluoride	Fluoride	Urine	Pre-shift		3 mg/g (18 mmol/mol creatinine)	4 mg/g (24 mmol/mol creatinine)	200 µmol/litre	Skeletal fluorosis
n-Hexane	2,5-Hexanedione	Urine	End of shift		5 mg/g (5 mmol/mol creatinine)	5 mg/litre	5 µmol/litre	Peripheral neurotoxin
Lead[a]	Lead	Blood	Random	600 µg/litre 300 µg/litre	300 µg/litre (1450 nmol/litre)	700 µg/litre 300 µg/litre (women)	2.4 µmol/litre	Renal, haem and neurological effects
Lindane	Lindane	Blood	Random	10 µg/litre		20 µg/litre		
Mercury	Mercury	Urine	Preshift, random	20 µmol/mol creatinine	35 µg/g (20 µmol/mol creatinine)	200 µg/litre (1 µmol/litre)	250 nmol/litre	Nephrotoxic CNS effects
4,4'-Methylene bis (2-chloroaniline)	'Total' MbOCA	Urine	End of shift	15 µmol/mol creatinine			30 µmol/mol	Cancer
Methylene dianiline	'Total' MDA	Urine	End of shift	50 µmol/mol creatinine			50 µmol/mol	Jaundice, cancer
4-Methylpentan-2-one	4-Methylpentan-2-one	Urine	End of shift	20 µmol/litre	2 mg/litre (20 µmol/litre)			Irritant
Styrene	Mandelic acid	Urine	End of shift		700 mg/g creatinine	600 mg/g creatinine	1.2 mmol/litre	Irritant, CNS effects
Tetrachloroethylene	Tetrachloroethylene	Blood Breath	Pre-shift		0.5 mg/litre 5 ppm	1 mg/litre	6 µmol/litre	Irritant
Trichloroethylene	Trichloroacetic acid	Urine	End of shift, end of week		100 mg/g creatinine (70 mmol/mol creatinine)	100 mg/litre	360 µmol/litre	CNS effects
Xylene	Methylhippuric acid	Urine	End of shift		1.5 g/g creatinine (900 mmol/mol creatinine)	2000 mg/litre (10.4 mmol/litre)	10 mmol/litre	CNS effects

CNS: Central nervous system
[a]Ref 6

Table 2.2 *Biological effect indicators*

Substance	Suggested analyte	Medium	Sampling time	Comments and guidance values
Cadmium	Retinol binding protein, N-acetylglucosaminidase, β2-microglobulin	Urine	Random	
Carbon monoxide	Carboxyhaemoglobin	Blood	End of shift	Values set for non-smokers range from 3.5–5%
Lead	Erythrocyte protoporphyrin 5-Aminolaevulinic acid	Blood, urine	Random	
Organophosphorus compounds	Cholinesterase inhibition	Red cell and plasma	End of shift	Need baseline sample. Action advised if >30% inhibition

PRACTICAL CONSIDERATIONS IN BIOLOGICAL MONITORING

The main steps involved in setting up a biological monitoring programme include:

- defining the purpose of the programme (health surveillance or exposure assessment);
- appointing a competent person to oversee the programme (if the programme is for health surveillance purposes a health professional should be appointed);
- selecting a valid biological monitoring strategy (a competent laboratory should be employed which operates an appropriate quality system);
- securing agreement of all concerned (maximum benefit is best achieved by involvement of employees and employer);
- and providing the workforce with feedback so that appropriate action can be taken.

It is essential that certain aspects of the detailed programme are considered before biological monitoring begins.

Choice of biological sample

The collection of non-invasive breath or urine samples which reduces the risk of the transmission of infection are preferred, provided that a validated method is available. Appropriate precautions should be taken when collecting and handling blood samples and particular attention should be paid to sending pathological specimens through the post or by courier. Each sample must be wrapped in sufficient absorbent material to absorb leakage and the package must be securely wrapped. Breath sampling for volatiles and gases is likely to become more widely used as a non-invasive alternative to blood sampling. The worker breathes out through a sampler and the final portion

of the exhalation, end-tidal or alveolar air, is captured and transferred on to a strainless steel tube packed with adsorbent material which is sent to the laboratory for analysis by gas chromatography or mass spectrometry. The alveolar air sample is in equilibrium with the blood passing through the lungs and so, like a blood sample, will reflect the total uptake by all routes of exposure to substances such as solvents.[8] This method can also be readily adapted for evaluating exposure to carbon monoxide.

Choice of analyte

The choice of analyte will depend on what information is required. If the level of exposure is being assessed then for inorganic substances such as metals, the metal itself is usually measured (e.g. cadmium). The choice for organic substances usually depends on the metabolism and kinetics of the substance (e.g. urinary mandelic acid would be chosen for styrene exposure). It is possible for some substances, to estimate the amount of substance interacting with the site of action, for example the determination of carboxyhaemoglobin following carbon monoxide exposure. Recent developments in this area for exposure assessment include the measurement of haemoglobin or DNA adducts (see below).

In the case of biological effect monitoring some knowledge of the mechanism of action will help to point towards a suitable biomarker, such as the inhibition of cholinesterase activity from organophosphorous pesticides. Further information on the chemical structure of the substance of interest will assist in the interpretation. Another example of a biological effect marker would be the determination of urinary proteins and enzymes in workers exposed to nephrotoxic substances such as lead, mecury or solvents.

Sampling time

This parameter is determined by the toxicokinetics of the compound and depends on the half-life in the body. In deciding when to sample it is helpful to know the main route of exposure (e.g. by inhalation or skin absorption). Consideration should be given to the likely exposure route since the apparent half-life of an inhaled substance will generally differ from that of the same substance which enters the body through the skin, where it is subject to a lag phase while it crosses the stratum corneum. For practical purposes the choice left to the physician is usually limited to end of shift (or work period), pre-shift on the following day or a random sample collection. Table 2.3 gives a generalized relationship between the half-life and the optimum sampling time.

Table 2.3 *Half-life of chemicals and optimum sampling time*

Half-life (hours)	Optimum sampling time
<2	Elimination too rapid to measure
Approx 2–10	End of shift or beginning of next shift
Approx 10–100	End of shift, end of week
> 100	Random (timing not critical)

Interfering factors

The interpretation of biological monitoring results requires a knowledge of possible interfering or confounding factors. For example, physiological factors including diet, sex and age can affect results. Consumption of fish may increase arsenic or mercury levels. Cadmium levels increase with age and smoking and females generally have higher erythrocyte protoporphyrin levels than males with the same blood lead concentrations. Alcohol can interfere with the metabolism of many solvents such as trichloroethylene or styrene and aspirin has been shown to affect the metabolism of xylene. Marked differences have been observed in different ethnic groups in the way in which they metabolize solvents. Consideration should also be given to the possibility that the chosen biomarker may be produced by more than one substance, for example mandelic acid is produced from both styrene and ethyl benzene and carboxyhaemoglobin is formed from both carbon monoxide and dichloromethane. Where a biomarker is produced from the substance of interest and is also produced endogenously, it is advisable to take a baseline measurement before commencing a monitoring regime. Certain pathological conditions may give rise to spurious results. When tubular disease due to cadmium exposure develops there is a disproportionate increase in urinary protein excretion when set against the cadmium exposure levels.

Creatinine correction

Urine concentration can vary widely as a result of variations in fluid intake and insensible losses, such as sweating. In hospital-based laboratory medicine this variation does not cause a problem because results can be expressed as output per 24 hours; however, in the workplace physicians are usually limited to collecting spot urine samples. It is common to make some adjustment to the analytical result to compensate for short-term concentration/dilution effects usually by adjusting for specific gravity or correcting for creatinine concentration. The use of creatinine correction has not been without criticism and in some circumstances, it might be appropriate to consider its use on an analyte by analyte basis. In general however, creatinine correction or specific gravity is advised. Creatinine correction is not advised if the creatinine value is less than 3 or more than 30 mmol/litre.

Quality assurance

Quality assurance begins with specimen collection (use of appropriate collection equipment and properly labelled samples). The sample must be appropriately transported to the laboratory (ensuring the stability and integrity of the sample). Finally, the laboratory must use a valid analytical method (reliability, accuracy and precision) and ensure the timely reporting of correct results. Physicians should satisfy themselves that the laboratory they use employs well-defined protocols, uses internal quality control samples, engages in external quality assessment schemes and that they can demonstrate internal and external quality audit. As part of the laboratory's quality management they should be able to offer information on the uncertainty or error associated with any measurement for biological monitoring as well as the reference ranges and advisory and statutory values.

SOME RECENT DEVELOPMENTS IN BIOLOGICAL AND BIOLOGICAL EFFECT MONITORING

Biological monitoring of exposure is now well established as a useful tool in occupational medicine and a wide range of tests are available. For a limited number of substances methods have been devised for biological effect monitoring. Progress is being made in a number of new areas related to exposure assessment and biomonitoring of effect (including physical hazards) and susceptibility. Although many of these developments have not yet been taken into routine use, it will be of some value to be aware of their likely development and future use.

Carcinogens and susceptibility

Most of the chemicals which are known to be human carcinogens cause damage to genomic DNA. Generally these carcinogens react covalently with DNA to form DNA adducts (e.g. benzo[a]pyrene) thereby potentially initiating the multistage process leading to cell transformation and clinical malignancy. However, only a fraction of all DNA damage will lead to mutation and several such changes are required in a cell for the cancer genotype to be acquired and for the phenotype to be manifested. Quantitative analysis of modified DNA bases is assuming increased importance as a marker of exposure to carcinogens,[9] DNA adducts of 4,4'-methylene bis(2-chloroaniline)[10] and aminobiphenyl[11] have been found in human tissues. In a recent study on coal miners exposed to diesel engine emissions, an increase in DNA adducts in white blood cells coincided with a period of intense exposure to diesel emissions.[12] Use is likely to be made of DNA adducts as indicators of exposure and as more data become available, studies may be able to show associations between the degree of adduction and likelihood of developing cancer.

Some epidemiological studies have evaluated putative associations between certain cancers and genetically based metabolic polymorphisms. These inherited polymorphisms can modify the enzymes which are involved in the activation/inactivation of known carcinogens and seem to modify the extent to which carcinogens interact with DNA in target tissues. As an example, the acetylation of aromatic amines is genetically determined. In humans, the arylamine N-acetyltransferases (NAT1 and NAT2) catalyse the acetylation of certain xenobiotics. In colorectal cancer it has been reported that fast acetylators for the NAT2 isozyme are at increased risk. Polymorphism at the NAT2 locus has been shown to be important in bladder cancer and there is general agreement that individuals with slow NAT2 activity and who are exposed to arylamines are at increased risk of bladder cancer.[13]

(For a detailed description of developments in this area see Chapter 38).

Early detection of renal effects

Numerous chemicals can cause renal failure, particularly heavy metals and some solvents. Various enzymes and proteins have been used as early indicators of renal effects. Increased excretion of albumin and transferrin serves as an indicator of glomerular damage but can also be increased when tubular reabsorption is compromised. The lysosomal enzyme N-acetyl-β-D-glucosaminidase (NAG), β2-microglobulin, alkaline phosphatase and retinol binding protein are considered useful indicators of damage to the tubular reabsorption mechanism. The test chosen will depend on the nature of the toxicant and its mode of action on the kidney.

(For a detailed description of developments in this area see Chapter 41).

Respiratory effects

Objective tests of airway inflammation and/or respiratory sensitization are useful in helping validate questionnaire data and in providing a definitive clinical diagnosis.

Recent work has shown that a range of immune cell surface markers can be used as biomarkers of immunotoxicological response. These new approaches complement existing tests such as specific IgE which can be detected in the serum of workers with a clinical history of asthma, rhinitis or conjunctivitis associated with exposure to certain chemicals or proteins. A wide range of radioallergosorbent tests (RAST) are available, including acid anhydrides, reactive dyes, environmental allergens and substances encountered in food processing and farming (Tables 2.4a, b). Whilst this approach has proved successful for many high molecular weight sensitizers, it

Table 2.4a *Allergens for which RAST is currently available*

Allergens, protein and chemical	
Green coffee bean	*Ficus* spp.
Castor bean	Latex (*Hevea brasiliensis*)
Ispaghula	Cotton seed
Silk waste	Sunflower seed
Silk (*Bombix mori*)	Chloramine T
Ethylene oxide	α-Amylase
Maleic anhydride (MA)	Pectinase
Phthalic anhydride (PA)	Trout
Tetrachlorophthalic anhydride (TCPA)	Salmon
Trimellitic anhydride (TMA)	Reactive dyes
Formaldehyde/formalin	Red spider mite (*Tetranychus urticae*)
Bacteria in cutting oils	
Pig urine	White-fly (*Trialeurodes vaporarorium*)
Cow urine	*Encarsia*
Cow dander	*Amblyseius cucermeris*
Wheat flour	*Phytoseiulus persimilis*
Rye flour	*Aspergillus* (including nitrocellulose disks for glycoprotein)
Barley flour	
Oat flour	

RAST: Radioallergosorbent tests.

Table 2.4b *Occupational allergen mixes for which RAST is available*

Occupational allergen mixes	
OA 1	Mixed anhydride (PA, TMA, TCPA, MA)
OA 2	Mixed flours
OA 3	Mixed storage mites
OA 4	Reactive dye screen

is of limited use in workers exposed to many low molecular weight chemicals. Recently, the technique of flow cytometry has been used to characterize immune cells in a number of disease states including acute asthma. Workplace exposure to toxic substances may cause changes in both the proportions of cell types and may increase their activation state. For example, workers exposed to styrene showed a modified distribution of lymphocyte subsets, with a decrease in total T-lymphocytes and an increase in natural killer (NK) cells[14] and asbestos-exposed workers showed a decrease in peripheral NK cells. Curran et al.[15] have shown activation of helper T-cells in bakers reporting work-related respiratory symptoms consistent with the changes observed in mild-to-severe asthmatics. However, workers with similar symptoms exposed to irritant chemicals did not show this pattern of phenotypic or inducible cell surface markers, reflecting an absence of airways inflammation in these workers.

In the case of workers exposed to dust which contain endotoxins, there are no objective tests to distinguish cases of asthma from non-specific respiratory symptoms. The recent development of an in vitro model of endotoxin exposure has revealed the potential of using the measurement of CD14 on monocytes as a useful biomarker of endotoxin exposure.[16] Recent studies have suggested that low molecular weight proteins might serve as peripheral biomarkers of lung toxicity.[17] Diagnosis of the irritant respiratory effect of exposure to endotoxins usually depends on the clinical and occupational history, together with the finding of a high concentration of endotoxin in the original dust involved. The Clara cell protein (CC16) found in bronchioalveolar lavage fluid or serum has been reported to be a sensitive indicator of bronchial epithelium injury. Serum CC16 was found to be decreased in several occupational groups chronically exposed to different air pollutants (silica, dust, welding fumes).

(For a detailed description of developments in this area see Chapter 33.)

Hand–arm vibration

Prolonged exposure to hand-transmitted vibration is known to cause hand-arm vibration syndrome (HAVS). This syndrome is characterized by vascular disorders causing impaired blood circulation and blanching of affected fingers and parts of the hand (vibration-induced white finger). It also gives rise to neurological and muscular damage leading to numbness and tingling in the fingers and hands and possible damage causing pain and stiffness in the hands, wrists, elbows and shoulders. The severity of these effects depends on the intensity and frequency of the vibration exposure.

Routine assessment of vibration-exposed workers is helped by using a standardized questionnaire.[18] In the

absence of symptomatology or to help evaluate the progress or regression of the disease, physiological laboratory test methods can be used, instead of reliance on clinical diagnosis, for objective assessment. In subjects with extensive exposure to vibrating hand tools, the ability to detect vibration or temperature stimuli is significantly reduced, although there may be some improvement if the employee is removed from the exposure at an early stage. The detection of vascular and neurological changes forms part of a panel of standardized objective tests.[19] These include the assessment of neurological effects by measuring the response of receptors in the fingertips to vibration stimuli (vibration perception threshold) and temperature change (thermal perception threshold). The vascular function is assessed by measuring the finger skin temperature recovery time following a cold challenge.

Pre-employment assessment by questionnaire and clinical examination will help establish a baseline from which to judge subsequent examinations. The Stockholm Workshop scales are generally used to classify symptoms. When symptoms are first reported, exposure conditions should be reviewed and the progression of symptoms should be monitored, particularly if vascular and neurological symptoms reach stage two on the Stockholm Scale. It is not advisable for workers to continue working with vibrating tools if it is likely to result in the disease progressing to Stockholm Stage 3. The objective tests in conjunction with the clinical examination will have a role in the assessment of either the progress or regression of the disease.

(For a detailed description of developments in this area see Chapter 14.)

DIAGNOSING OCCUPATIONAL AND ENVIRONMENTAL DISEASES

In a few instances the quantitative relation between internal dose and adverse health effects has been identified, for example lead and mercury in blood, cadmium in urine and carboxyhaemoglobin, and the biological variables can be considered as an indicator of health risk and hence used in diagnosis. The use of biomarkers in determining susceptibility, either inherent or acquired, still has limited use in diagnosing occupational diseases. The role of biochemical effect markers in predicting the potential health significance of exposures is also poorly defined, for example in the urinary excretion of numerous proteins, enzymes and biochemical markers in subjects exposed to nephrotoxic substances such as $\alpha1$- and $\beta2$- microglobulins, n-acetylglucosaminidase, β-galactosidase, sialic acid, retinol binding protein, thromboxane, and kallikrein[20] (see Chapter 41). Despite considerable research, the biological monitoring of mutagenic or carcinogenic substances has also been found to have limited application in determining the risk of developing occupational cancers. Tests have included mutagenic activity of urine, the thioether detoxification products (e.g. DNA adducts) and genotoxicity (e.g. the measurement of chromosomal aberrations, sister chromatid exchanges, unscheduled DNA synthesis, single strand breaks, point mutations and micronuclei in peripheral blood lymphocytes) (see Chapter 38).

Mercury (see Chapter 7)

The toxicity of mercury vapour is so well-known that exposure to mercury metal in industrial processes should nowadays be sufficiently well controlled to pose few problems to the limited number of workers involved in its use. However, inadvertent high exposure to workers can still occur through a failure in control measures, or to the general population as a result of accidental contamination of offices or homes, as well as a failure to adequately decontaminate industrial buildings before being put to other uses.[21-24]

Good assessment of the health risk in accidental exposures of this type can be made using the results of analysis of blood and urine samples from exposed adults and children. Urine levels provide a measure of low level or cumulative exposure and are usually preferred over blood levels, which are more appropriate measures after acute exposures to inorganic mercury vapour. Mild and reversible proteinuria is the most sensitive clinical indicator of mercury vapour toxicity, followed by non-specific symptoms and changes in plasma lysomal enzyme, and in more advanced cases, objective tremor and psychomotor disturbances. A potential threshold for these effects is 20 µmol/mol creatinine in the urine and 45 nmol/litre in the blood. These values equate to an airborne level of 0.020 mg/m³, the Health and Safety Executive Occupational Exposure Standard (8-hour time weighted average (TWA)).[25]

Next to nutrition, the main source of exposure to mercury in the general population is from dental amalgam.[26] Mercury vapour is released from dental amalgam fillings into the oral cavity from where it is inhaled and absorbed by the lungs. Blood and urine mercury concentrations in amalgam bearers are usually below one-tenth of the critical values described above and inside the range found in the general population, though small increases are detectable after dental procedures involving fillings.[27] However, some people have been found to have high mercury uptake from their fillings equivalent to the Occupational Exposure Limit, when removal of the fillings has been recommended.[28]

Biological monitoring for mercury using samples of hair and nail clippings is not routinely recommended because the analytic results are likely to be affected by external contamination. However, hair sampling has been used in epidemiological studies in communities to evaluate the uptake of organic mercury associated with fish consumption. Certain groups with a high fish consumption may attain a blood methyl mercury level (about 200 µg/litre corresponding to 50 µg/g of hair) associated with a low (5%) risk of neurological damage to adults. The fetus is at particular risk from organic mercury, with a 5% risk of neurological disorder in the offspring associated with a peak mercury level of 10–20 µg/g in maternal hair.[29,30]

Lead (see Chapter 7)

Severe poisoning can arise with damage to organs such as the kidney when blood concentrations exceed 100 µg/dl. Colicky intestinal pains, one of the most characteristic manifestations of lead poisoning, are rare below blood concentrations of 80 µg/dl. The risk of lead nephropathy is increased in workers with blood lead levels over 60 µg/dl. Anaemia, the clinical manifestation of the effects of lead on haem synthesis, may be seen in sensitive adults when blood levels exceed 50 µg/dl. Reversible effects on the kidneys and male reproductive organs have been described in blood concentrations over 40 µg/dl. A reduction in human peripheral nerve conduction velocity may occur with blood lead levels as low as 30 µg/dl, but this effect is also reversible.[31] Epidemiological studies in children aged 4 years and under have suggested that an increase in the blood lead concentration from 10 to 20 µg/dl is associated with an average reduction in population IQ of about two points.[32] It is important to realize that this is a statistical association, and the finding of a moderately elevated blood lead in a child, though undesirable, does not imply that the individual's mental functioning will be impaired. This association between IQ and blood lead nevertheless underlines the importance of limiting occupational and environmental exposures to women of reproductive age (lead crosses the placental barrier and can be measured in cord blood at the time of delivery).

Cadmium (see Chapter 7)

Evidence of early renal dysfunction has been reported at urine levels below 10 µmol/mol creatinine, a potential threshold for health effects. As well as urinary protein testing, the regular measurement of urinary retinol binding protein is also recommended by the UK Health and Safety Laboratory in workers with significant or increasing urinary cadmium levels.

Carbon monoxide (see Chapter 8)

Ample data exist on the relation between carboxy-haemoglobin levels and health effects[33] (Table 2.5). However, in patients with clinical poisoning the car-

Table 2.5 *The relation between carboxyhaemoglobin levels and health effects*

Blood carboxyhaemoglobin levels (%)	Observed health effects
2.5–4.0	Decreased short-term maximal exercise duration in young healthy men
2.7–5.1	Decreased exercise duration due to increased chest pain (angina) in patients with ischaemic heart disease
2.0–20.0	Equivocal effects on visual perception, audition, motor and sensorimotor performance, vigilance, and other measures of neurobehavioural performance
4.0–33.0	Decreased maximal oxygen consumption with short-term strenuous exercise in young healthy men
20–30	Throbbing headache
30–50	Dizziness, nausea, weakness, collapse
>50	Unconsciousness and death

boxyhaemoglobin level may not correlate with the severity of poisoning and should not be used alone in making decisions on clinical management.

Multiple chemical sensitivity

Multiple chemical hypersensitivity is a concept attributed to Randolph in the 1950s who was subsequently a co-founder of the Society for Clinical Ecology. A recent review[34] concluded that there is evidence to suggest that in some people exposure to chemicals can initiate a clinical response to subsequent exposures to very low doses of that chemical and structurally unrelated chemicals. However, objective evidence for the diagnosis is lacking. The condition does not fit established knowledge regarding disease processes, and various psychological and physical theories have been propounded without any experimental evidence for their backing. Some advocates of this disorder encourage testing for markers of exposure or sensitivity by

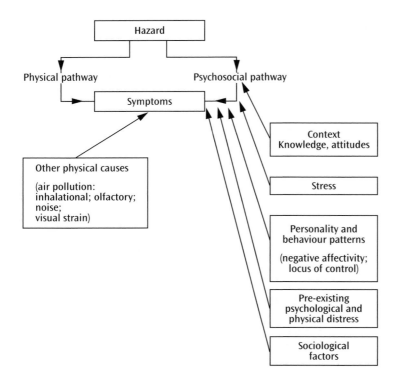

Figure 2.2 *Multifactorial approach to non-specific symptoms.*[35]

analysis of hair and other biological samples, but there is little, if any, scientific support for their approach.

Non-specific symptoms in occupational and environment syndromes

Many occupational and environmental health hazards present as an increased reporting of non-specific symptoms such as headache, backache, eye and respiratory irritation, tiredness, memory problems and poor concentration.[35] Examples include sick building syndrome, exposures to electromagnetic fields and organophosphates, acute and chronic gas exposures, as well as certain environmental incidents. An example of an environmental incident occurred in the community of Camelford, Cornwall, in 1988, when the water supply was accidentally contaminated with aluminium sulphate and residents reported symptoms of fatigue, skin rashes, gastrointestinal problems and joint pains immediately after the incident. In some people complaints of anxiety/depression and cognitive difficulties, such as memory and concentration problems, persisted. Nevertheless two separate Government enquiries failed to substantiate a link between the chronic symptoms reported and the ingestion of aluminium sulphate.[35]

A more recent review of studies of the clinical aspects of long-term, low dose exposure to organophosphates (either episodic, as in organophosphate sheep-dipping by farmers, or continual, as in professional sheep dippers), has found support for a syndrome of subtle cognitive impairment (e.g. impaired attention and reaction times), greater psychiatric morbidity and minor memory changes. However, how organophosphates might cause such effects is not known.[36]

A multifactorial approach to such symptomatology has been proposed, including the influence of psychological and social factors (Fig. 2.2). Where toxic agents are involved, the collection of blood and urine samples for measuring and validating exposure are usually only of value around the time of the incident or when occupational exposure occurred, and so biological monitoring usually has no role by the time the patient has presented with long-term symptoms.

REFERENCES

1 Health and Safety Executive. *Biological Monitoring in the Workplace, A Guide to its Practical Application to Chemical Exposure*. HSG 167. Sudbury: HSE Books, 1997.

2 Cocker J, Nutley BP, Wilson HK. Methylene bis (2-chloroaniline) (MbOCA): towards a biological monitoring guidance value. *Biomarkers* 1996; **1**: 185–9.

3 Health and Safety Executive. *Occupational Exposure Limits 1999*. EH40/99. Sudbury: HSE Books, 1999.

4 American Conference of Governmental Industrial Hygienists. *Threshold Limit Values for Chemical Substances and Physical Agents. Biological Exposure Indices*. Cincinnati, Ohio: ACGIH 1998.

5 Deutsche Forschungsgemeininschaft. *List of MAK and BAT Values 1998*. Report no. 34. Weinheim: DFG/Wiley-VCH Verlag, 1998.

6 Health and Safety Executive. *Control of Lead at Work Regulations 1998 and Approved Codes of Practice*. Sudbury: HSE Books, 1998.

7 Finnish Institute of Occupational Health. *Kemikaali-altistumisen Biomonitorointi*. Helsinki: FIOH, 1995.

8 Dyne D, Cocker J, Wilson HK. A novel device for capturing breath samples for solvent analysis. *Science Tot Environ* 1997; **199**: 83–9.

9 Farmer PB. Monitoring of human exposure to carcinogens through DNA and protein adduct determination. *Toxicol Lett* 1995; **82–83**, 757–762.

10 Kaderlik K, Talaska G, Debord DG, Osorio AM, Kadulbar FF. Methylene bis(2-chloroaniline)-DNA adduct analysis in human exfoliated cells by 32P-postlabeling. *Cancer Epidemiol Biomarkers Prev* 1993; **2**: 63–9.

11 Talaska G, Schamer M, Casetta G, Tizzani A, Vineis P. Carcinogen DNA adducts in bladder biopsies and urothelial cells: a risk exercise. *Cancer Lett* 1994; **84**: 93–7.

12 Shu-Xin Q, Leigh J, Koelmeyer H, Stacey NH. DNA adducts in coal miners: association with exposures to diesel engine emissions. *Biomarkers* 1997; **2**: 95–102.

13 Stacey M, Thygesen P, Stanley L, Matas N, Risch A, Sim E. Arylamine N-acetyltransferase as a potential biomarker in bladder cancer. *Biomarkers* 1996; **1**: 55–61.

14 Bergamaschi E, Smargiassi A, Mutti A, Franchini I, Lucchini R. Immunological changes among workers occupationally exposed to styrene. *Int Arch Occup Environ Hlth* 1995; **67**: 165–171.

15 Curran AD, Gordon SB, Morice AH, Wiley K. Expression of lymphocyte cell surface markers in workers exposed to different respiratory hazards: biomarkers of occupational respiratory disease? *Biomarkers* 1997; **2**: 367–71.

16 Swan JR, Curran AD, Beckett PN. The potential of a monocyte cell surface marker as an indicator of endotoxin exposure. *Biomarkers* 1998; **3**: 73–79.

17 Hermans C, Bernard A. Clara cell protein (CC16): characteristics and potential applications as biomarker of lung toxicity. *Biomarkers* 1996; **1**: 3–8.

18 Health and Safety Executive. *Hand–Arm Vibration*. HS(G) 88. Sudbury: HSE Books, 1994.

19 Lindsell CJ, Griffin MJ. *Standardised Diagnostic Methods for Assessing Components of Hand – Arm Vibration Syndrome*. Health and Safety Executive Contract Report. London: HSE, 1997.

20 Hoet P, Haufroid V. Biological monitoring: state of the art. *Occup Environ Med* 1997; **54**: 361–6.

21 Agocs MM, Etzel RA, Parrish RG, Paschal DC, Campagna PR *et al*. Mercury exposure from interior latex paint. *N Engl J Med* 1990; **323**: 1096–101.

22 Centers for Disease Control. Mercury exposure in a residential community – Florida, 1994. *Morbid Mortal Weekly Rep* 1995; **44**: 436–43.

23 Orloff KG, Ulirsch G, Wilder L, Block A, Fagliano J, Pasqualo J. Human exposure to elemental mercury in a contaminated residential building. *Arch Environ Hlth* 1997; **52**: 169–72.

24 Clarkson TW. Mercury – an element of mystery. *N Engl J Med* 1990; **323**: 1137–39.

25 Health and Safety Executive. *Mercury Criteria Document Summaries*. EH64, 1995 supplement. Sudbury: HSE Books, 1995.

26 International Programme on Chemical Safety (IPCS). *Inorganic mercury. Environmental Health Criteria 181*. Geneva: World Health Organization, 1991.

27 Halbach S. Amalgam tooth fillings and man's mercury burden. *Hum Exp Toxicol* 1994; **13**: 496–501.

28 Barregard L, Sällstein G, Järvolm B. People with high mercury uptake from their own dental amalgam fillings. *Occup Environ Med* 1995; **52**: 124–8.

29 International Programme on Chemical Safety (IPCS). *Mercury – environmental aspects. Environmental Health Criteria 86*. Geneva: World Health Organization, 1989.

30 International Programme on Chemical Safety (IPCS). *Methylmercury. Environmental Health Criteria 101*. Geneva: World Health Organization, 1990.

31 International Programme on Chemical Safety (IPCS). *Lead. Environmental Health Criteria 165*. Geneva: World Health Organization, 1995.

32 Department of the Environment. *Expert Panel on Air Quality Standards. Lead*. London: HMSO, 1998.

33 Department of the Environment. *Expert Panel on Air Quality Standards: Carbon monoxide*. London: HMSO, 1995.

34 Graveling RA, Pilkington A, George JPK, Butler MP, Tannahill SN. A review of multiple chemical sensitivity. *Occup Environ Med* 1999; **56**: 73–85.

35 Spurgeon A, Gompertz D, Harrington JM. Modifiers of non-specific symptoms in occupational and environmental syndromes. *Occup Environ Med* 1996; **53**: 361–6.

36 Royal College of Physicians and Royal College of Psychiatrists. *Organophosphate Sheep Dip: Clinical Aspects of Long-term Low-dose Exposure*. Report of a Joint Working Party. London: Royal College of Physicians and Royal College of Psychiatrists, 1998.

3

Estimating the extent of occupational injuries and disease

DAVID COGGON

Identification of occupational hazards to health 27
Assessing the impact of hazards 29
Conclusions 34
References 34

Reliable information about the incidence of occupational injuries and diseases is essential for the effective control of hazards in the workplace. It provides a basis for prioritizing and targeting preventive measures, and enables the outcome of such interventions to be assessed. It is also used when setting priorities for research. The starting point for estimating the frequency of occupational illness in a population is the identification of hazards.

IDENTIFICATION OF OCCUPATIONAL HAZARDS TO HEALTH

The effects of some occupational hazards are so immediate and specific that their recognition is easy. For example, no great acumen is required to appreciate that inhalation of high concentrations of sulphur dioxide causes respiratory irritation. Often, however, the relation of occupation to illness is less obvious. The disease produced may have other causes which make it common even in those with no exposure to the hazard. Thus, long-term inhalation of cadmium fumes causes emphysema, but few emphysematous patients have been significantly exposed to cadmium. Furthermore, the disease may only become apparent many years after first exposure to the hazard, and perhaps long after exposure has ceased. Pleural mesotheliomas were still being diagnosed in women who had used asbestos to make filters for wartime gas masks some 30 years after they had last carried out this work.[1] In these circumstances, recognition and confirmation of the hazard is more difficult and requires careful investigation. Information may come from clinical, epidemiological or toxicological research.

Clinical observations and investigations

Even where the link between a hazard and disease is far from obvious, the first clue to its existence has often come from clinical observations. In 1975 Doll reviewed the circumstances which had led to the discovery of 33 occupational causes of cancer, and found that 21 of them were first suspected on clinical grounds.[2] Other examples of occupational diseases that were discovered because of suspicions raised by clinicians include osteoarthritis of the hip in farmers,[3] cataract in glass manufacturers[4] and chloracne caused by certain organochlorine compounds.[5]

In the case of occupational asthma and allergic contact dermatitis, clinical observations have been important not only in providing the initial indication of an association between work and disease, but also in confirming the sensitizers that were responsible, for example by bronchial challenge, measurement of allergen-specific immunoglobulins or patch testing.

Epidemiology

There are a few notable examples of occupational hazards that have come to light incidentally in the course of epidemiological investigations. For instance, the elevated risk of bladder cancer in rubber workers was first suspected by Case during a study exploring the high incidence of bladder tumours in dye manufacturers.[2] He was reviewing the hospital records of patients in

Birmingham, chosen as a control area because it did not have a dye industry, and happened to notice that many of them had worked in a rubber factory. Subsequent investigation confirmed the association with rubber production, and showed that it resulted from the use of an anti-oxidant containing the carcinogen, 2-naphthylamine[6] (see Chapter 39).

Serendipitous discoveries of this sort have encouraged epidemiologists to search systematically for unrecognized occupational causes of disease, and various approaches have been tried. The method with the longest tradition is the analysis of occupational mortality. For example, Henry and colleagues' discovery that bladder cancer occurs excessively in coal gas manufacturers arose from a systematic analysis of deaths from bladder tumours in different occupations;[7] and more recently, routine analyses of occupational mortality have indicated a hazard of pneumonia in welders and other occupations with exposure to metal fume[8] (see Chapter 5).

Another approach has been to explore the geographical relation of mortality to industry. By combining data from a long period, say 10–20 years, it is possible to generate meaningful mortality statistics for relatively small geographical units – local authority areas in England and Wales[9] or counties in the USA.[10,11] Places where a hazardous industry employs a substantial proportion of the local population may then stand out as having high death rates from relevant diseases. This method is sufficiently sensitive to detect the effects of certain known hazards such as mesothelioma in shipbuilding and nasal cancer in furniture manufacture;[12] and at least one new hazard has come to light because of elevated death rates in a small geographic area – the increased risk of lung cancer in fluorspar miners was discovered following the observation of high mortality from the disease in a mining community in Newfoundland.[13]

Perhaps the most ambitious attempt to screen epidemiologically for unrecognized occupational hazards has been a survey carried out by Siemiatycki and colleagues in Montreal.[14] Detailed occupational histories were collected at interview from large numbers of cancer patients and from controls selected from the general population. These were then translated by a team of engineers and chemists into a list of likely chemical exposures. Associations between specific cancers and exposures were examined by comparison with the healthy controls and with other types of cancer.

Although this study generated some promising clues, it has not yet led to the firm identification of any new hazards, and in general the ability of epidemiology to reveal previously unsuspected occupational diseases has proved disappointing. A more important role of epidemiology has been in confirming the existence of hazards once suspicions have been aroused from other sources. The techniques that are most commonly used – cohort, case-control and cross-sectional studies – are described later in this chapter.

Toxicology

Toxicological research provides information about the potential of chemical, physical and biological agents to cause injury, and about the mechanisms by which such injury is produced. It includes *in vitro* studies, for example of mutagenicity and genotoxicity, as well as experiments in which known or suspected toxins are administered to animals in order to assess their acute, subacute and chronic effects.

Occasionally toxicology has provided the first indication of an occupational hazard. Fór example, the earliest evidence that vinylchloride is carcinogenic came from experiments in rats[2,15] (see Chapters 8, 43). More often, however, toxicological studies contribute to the confirmation of hazards first suspected for other reasons. Their findings often complement those from epidemiological research, helping to distinguish causal associations from those that arise spuriously through bias or confounding. Thus, the observation that bis(chloromethyl) ether was carcinogenic in rats[16] made it more plausible that the excess of lung cancer associated with occupational exposure to the compound reflected a real hazard.

Occupational clusters

The first clue to many occupational hazards has been the observation of a disease cluster. A cluster is an unusually high incidence of a disease in a defined population over a period of time during which few, if any, cases would normally be expected to occur. In a workforce of several hundred employees, the relevant period for a common complaint such as nasal stuffiness might be a few days or weeks, whereas for a rarer illness such as brain cancer a cluster could include cases diagnosed over several years.

Clusters of disease are observed quite frequently in occupational populations. Often they arise simply by chance, but occasionally they result from a hazard to which the workforce has been exposed and they provide the first clue to its existence. For example, a cluster of two cases of carcinoma of the ethmoid sinus within 1 year among the workforce of a nickel refinery was the first pointer to the carcinogenicity of nickel compounds.[2]

When an occupational cluster becomes apparent, a decision must be made whether and how far to search for a possible underlying hazard. This will depend on how suspicious the cluster appears when assessed scientifically, and also on the level of anxiety that it generates in the workforce. A first step is to establish as exactly as possible the diagnoses of the cases that make up the cluster, the time period over which their disease has occurred, and what they have in common.

This may be all that is required by way of investigation. For example, a cluster of patients with cancer may turn out to be suffering from very different types of tumour that are unlikely to share a common cause; or the patients making up a cluster may work at different locations carrying out different activities with different materials, and share nothing in common occupationally other than working for the same employer.

Where suspicion remains, a systematic search may reveal additional cases that meet criteria for inclusion in the cluster but have not already come to attention. If data on expected rates of disease are available (e.g. from national statistics of mortality or cancer incidence), it is then possible to evaluate how excessive the clustering has been. Other things being equal, the more exceptional the clustering, the greater the suspicion it provokes. In addition, further information can be sought about the cases in the cluster, including their exposure to known and suspected causes of the disease from which they suffer. Sometimes, careful assessment of their jobs identifies shared occupational exposures which could plausibly explain the cluster, and indicates a need for more formal epidemiological or toxicological investigations.

Clusters present a challenge to occupational health practitioners. If they are ignored, important opportunities for the prevention of disease may be missed. On the other hand, overinvestigation is wasteful of scarce resources.

ASSESSING THE IMPACT OF HAZARDS

Once the existence of an occupational hazard has been established, attempts can be made to assess the burden of injury or disease that it produces. Various methods are used, depending in part on the confidence with which adverse health effects can be attributed to occupation in the individual case.

Some diseases such as silicosis and asbestosis are almost always occupational in origin, and others can confidently be ascribed to occupation in individual cases on the basis of the history and clinical findings. Examples of the latter include acute injury and poisoning, where the occupational cause is usually obvious; occupational dermatitis and asthma, where the causal agent can be established from the history and by investigations such as patch testing or bronchial challenge; and diseases such as angiosarcoma of the liver in people working with vinyl chloride monomer and Raynaud's phenomenon in people using hand-held vibrating tools, where the relative risk associated with the occupational exposure is so high that when the disease occurs in an exposed person, it is almost certain that his occupation was responsible.

The impact of these types of hazard can be assessed simply by counting the relevant cases. This may be possible from information that is already collected for other purposes, such as routine statistics of mortality by cause

of death, or data on compensation for occupational injuries and diseases. Alternatively, it may be necessary to establish a register or carry out a special survey specifically to record the occurrence of cases.

Mortality statistics

Where an injury or disease is usually fatal (e.g. mesothelioma caused by asbestos), death rates provide a good index of incidence; and even if death only occurs in a minority of cases (say 20%), mortality statistics can still give some indication of how common the illness is in a population, and whether its frequency is varying over time. Most countries regularly publish statistics of mortality by cause of death. For example, Table 3.1 shows the annual numbers of deaths ascribed to asbestosis in England and Wales during 1985–94.

In most industrialized countries the death certificate also includes information about the occupation of the deceased person. For example, in Britain the last full-time occupation is recorded, and in the United States, the 'usual' occupation. This allows analysis of deaths by cause for different occupational groups. Table 3.2 shows the numbers of deaths from silicosis in England and Wales during 1979–80 and 1982–90 in selected occupations associated with exposure to silica (see Chapter 35).

Table 3.1 *Annual numbers of deaths from asbestosis in England and Wales, both sexes, 1985–94*

Year	Deaths
1985	43
1986	51
1987	43
1988	35
1989	45
1990	57
1991	59
1992	52
1993	59
1994	59

Table 3.2 *Deaths from silicosis in selected occupations, men aged 20–74, England and Wales, 1979–80 and 1982–90*

Occupation	Deaths
Miners (not coal) and quarry workers	58
Face-trained coalminers	5
Other coalminers	21
Masons and stonecutters	11
Fettlers and dressers (metal)	4
Moulders and coremakers (metal)	3
Other metal manufacturers	6

Mesothelioma is another occupational disease with high fatality. Analysis of mortality from mesothelioma in England and Wales during 1968–91 has shown a worrying increase in deaths, particularly among the generation of men who entered the workforce during the 1960s.[17] This suggests either that the statutory control limits on asbestos exposure at this time were inadequate, or that they were not satisfactorily enforced (see Chapters 35, 39). It is an example of the way in which mortality data can be used to monitor the effectiveness of regulatory controls.

The value of mortality data depends on the accuracy with which causes of death and occupations are reported on death certificates. Errors may occur because diagnoses are not sufficiently specific (e.g. a peritoneal mesothelioma is recorded as a cancer of uncertain origin), or because one disease is confused with another (e.g. a death from coal workers' pneumoconiosis is incorrectly labelled as being due to chronic obstructive lung disease). The net effect of such errors is usually an underascertainment of occupational disease rather than overascertainment, particularly in countries where deaths attributed to occupation are investigated by necropsy.

If the underascertainment of cases is small and relatively constant, it presents few problems to interpretation. Greater difficulties occur where there is a possibility that diagnostic errors have changed importantly over time. Thus, in evaluating trends in mortality from mesothelioma, it is important to consider whether recognition of the disease might have improved over the years through increased awareness among physicians and the development of better diagnostic techniques.

Inaccuracies also occur in the occupations recorded on death certificates. The information on the deceased person's job is usually supplied by a relative, and that person may not know exactly what work was done. Moreover, only one occupation is registered, while the decedent will often have worked in several different jobs over the course of his or her career. This limitation is most important for diseases such as cancer which only develop some years after first exposure to a hazard. The certified occupation may then not be the one that is relevant to the death. As with diagnostic errors, the effect of inaccurate and incomplete occupational information on death certificates is generally an underascertainment of cases attributable to work.

Compensation claims and awards

Compensation schemes are another valuable source of information on the occurrence of occupational injuries and disease. Most industrialized countries include compensation for industrial injuries in their social security provisions, and generate statistics of claims and/or awards (see Chapter 4). These data are particularly use-

ful for quantifying diseases that can be attributed to occupation with confidence in the individual case. For instance, in Sweden, insurance claims have been used to assess the frequency of occupational asthma in different occupational groups.[18]

Interpretation of data on compensation must take into account the rules under which schemes operate and the extent of their coverage. Table 3.3 shows annual numbers of new awards for occupational deafness in Britain during 1991–96. However, the British scheme excludes self-employed workers, and only pays benefit for occupational deafness that causes a hearing loss of at least 50 dB in each ear. Furthermore, even among those who are eligible to claim, uptake may not be complete. It follows that Table 3.3 underestimates the full impact of occupational deafness in Britain.

For some diseases, the rules for compensation may render data on awards virtually useless for assessing incidence. Thus, since 1983, industrial injuries benefit has only been payable to claimants in Britain when disability has been present for more than 90 days, and this has largely eliminated claims for occupational dermatitis which usually resolves more quickly. However, if interpreted with care, statistics of compensation can be extremely useful for assessing the impact of certain forms of occupational illness.

Table 3.3 *New awards of industrial injuries benefit for occupational deafness, Great Britain (England, Wales, Scotland) 1991–96*

Year	Awards
1991	5143
1992	5806
1993	4741
1994	3962
1995	3760
1996	3746

Statutory reporting schemes

To obtain better information about the occurrence of occupational diseases, some countries have enacted legislation requiring that occupational injuries and diseases be reported to a governmental agency. For example, physicians in Finland are legally obliged to report cases of occupational disease to the provincial labour protection authority, and this information is collated with that on cases notified to insurance companies to provide a national register of occupational diseases.[19]

In the USA, several states have laws requiring doctors, laboratories or other health care providers to report cases of occupational disease. However, the quality of information obtained has in the past been limited by failure to provide guidance on case definitions and inadequate training of practitioners, and this led to widespread underreporting of cases. To overcome these diffi-culties, the National Institute of Occupational Safety and Health (NIOSH) instituted an improved reporting scheme during the 1980s, initially in ten states.[20] Known as SENSOR (Sentinel Event Notification System for Occupational Risks), it relies on a network of 'sentinel providers' (individual practitioners, laboratories and/or clinics) to recognize and report selected occupational ill-nesses to surveillance centres. The disorders covered include silicosis, occupational asthma, pesticide poison-ing and lead poisoning. In states where there is no legal obligation to report the specified diseases, reporting is encouraged on a voluntary basis. Guidelines have been drawn up to help reporting practitioners, and case defi-nitions have been agreed for use in the production of summary statistics. The main purpose of SENSOR is to identify situations where interventions may benefit the health of affected workers or prevent similar disease occurring in co-workers. In addition, however, it pro-vides useful information about the frequency of the dis-orders covered by the scheme.

In Britain, the Reporting of Injuries, Diseases and Dangerous Occurrences regulations (RIDDOR) were enacted in 1985. Among other things, these require employers to report to the Health and Safety Executive all accidents at work that cause serious injuries (defined according to prescribed criteria), and all cases of a spec-ified list of diseases occurring among employees in which the employer receives a doctor's written diagnosis and the affected employee's job involves an activity listed as being associated with the disease. Unfortunately, employers do not always fulfil their obligations under this law, even for accidents in the workplace of which they are well aware. Moreover, when an employee has a specified disease, the employer will not necessarily receive the written diagnosis that would prompt a noti-fication. Nevertheless, the system does provide useful information about aspects of occupational injury that could not easily be monitored in other ways.

Voluntary reporting schemes

In addition to the statutory systems that have been described, a number of voluntary schemes have been developed for registering occupational diseases. One example is the British SWORD surveillance programme (Surveillance of work-related and occupational respiratory diseases in the UK), which was set up in 1989 to record new cases of respiratory disease caused by occupation.[21] Notifications are provided by respiratory and occupational physicians, some of whom submit returns every month and others in one randomly selected month each year. In 1995, a total of 1498 cases were reported, giving an estimated total of 2741 cases for the year once the random sampling fraction had been taken into account (Table 3.4).

Table 3.4 *Cases reported to SWORD in 1995*[21]

Disease	Cases reported	Estimated total
Allergic alveolitis	9	20
Asthma	488	851
Bronchitis/emphysema	28	50
Infectious disease	9	31
Inhalation accidents	199	353
Lung cancer	29	62
Mesothelioma	157	487
Non-malignant pleural disease	326	590
Pneumoconiosis	128	172
Other	125	125
Total	1498	2741

SWORD: Surveillance of work-related and occupational respiratory diseases.

Ascertainment by the scheme is incomplete because not all respiratory and occupational physicians partici-pate and not all patients with occupational lung dis-orders necessarily see a doctor from these specialties. Nevertheless, it provides a useful guide to the frequency of respiratory diseases caused by work and to trends in their incidence. For example, the increasing number of patients with asthma caused by sensitivity to latex over the period 1993–95 highlighted a new problem that required further investigation.[21]

The success of the SWORD scheme has led to the estab-lishment of similar systems for registering other occupa-tional diseases. These include the EPIDERM project which records occupational skin disease (reports being provided by dermatologists and occupational physicians), and another scheme known as OPRA (occupational physician reporting activity) in which occupational physicians notify occupational diseases of all kinds.

Voluntary reporting schemes have also been developed in other countries. For example, in Quebec the PROPULSE project collects information about new cases of occupational respiratory disease from chest physicians and allergists;[22] and in South Africa occupational lung dis-orders are monitored through the SORDSA programme, cases being notified by members of the South African Pulmonology Society and the South African Society of Occupational Medicine. In Taiwan, the Ministry of Health established a surveillance system in 1993 to monitor the occurrence of noise-induced hearing loss and other work-related diseases.[23]

Occasional surveys

Occasional surveys can be another useful source of information about the occurrence of occupational dis-ease. A good example is the study carried out by the Health and Safety Executive in England and Wales dur-ing 1990.[24] A nationally representative sample of adults were asked whether, in the last year, they had suffered from any illness which in their opinion was caused or made worse by their work. Further questions explored the nature of the illness and the job that was thought to be responsible. Nearly 6% of subjects reported a work-related illness, the most common being musculoskeletal conditions.

As a guide to the occurrence of occupational disease, this survey was limited by the accuracy with which those questioned ascribed their illnesses to work, and it is likely that some disorders were substantially overreported. For example, some back injuries may have been recorded as aggravated by work on the grounds that they made occupational tasks painful to perform, but this does not necessarily imply that work contributed to the injury. However, for diseases such as pneumoconiosis and occupational deafness, the information is probably more reliable. Particularly interesting was the 0.3% prevalence of persistent or recurrent morbidity arising from injuries sustained at work before the year of study. Data on this aspect of occupational injuries are not readily available from other sources. Also valuable is the information about illness attributed to stress in the workplace, again a problem not easily quantified by other methods.

Diseases that cannot confidently be ascribed to occupation in the individual case

The methods that have been described so far allow monitoring of disorders that can be ascribed to occupation with confidence in the individual case. However, many occupational diseases do not fulfil this criterion. They are statistically associated with exposure to occupational hazards, but such exposure is not essential for the disease to develop; there are no features of the individual case which distinguish disease attributable to the hazard, from disease that would have occurred anyway. For example, rates of leukaemia have been found to be elevated approximately threefold in people with moderately high occupational exposure to benzene (40–199 parts per million-years).[25] This increase in risk implies that for every three exposed workers who contract the disease, one would have developed it even without the occupational exposure, and only two acquired it because of their work. It is not possible, however, to determine which are the two-thirds of patients whose disease is occupational (see Chapter 44).

Sometimes the situation is even more complex because the disease is not an all-or-none phenomenon. Chronic obstructive pulmonary disease (COPD) is characterized by a reduction in the volume of air that can be forcibly exhaled in one second (forced expiratory volume: FEV_1), but FEV_1 in the general population is distributed continuously and unimodally, and therefore there is no threshold that unambiguously distinguishes a case of COPD from a non-case. Smoking and inhalation of coal mine dust are both causes of COPD, and are sta-

tistically associated with a reduction in FEV_1. In coal miners who smoke, the effects of the two hazards on FEV_1 appear to be additive, so that if such an individual has a low FEV_1, it is likely that his disease is partly attributable to smoking and partly to dust. However, the blame can only be apportioned on the basis of a statistical average (see Chapter 31).

Some reporting schemes ascertain not only injuries and diseases that can be ascribed to occupation with reasonable certainty, but also cases that might possibly be occupational. The value of such information will depend on the relative risk of disease that is associated with the occupational exposure. If an exposure more than doubles the risk or severity of a disease, most exposed cases will be occupational. However, if the relative risk or contribution to disease is lower, the impact of a hazard may be substantially overestimated by this approach.

To estimate more reliably the burden of such diseases that is attributable to occupation, it is necessary to compare their rates of occurrence in people with and without exposure to relevant hazards. For cancers and for diseases that are commonly fatal, routinely collected data on cancer registrations or mortality by occupation may be a useful starting point.

In Britain, analyses of occupational mortality have been published regularly since 1855.[26] Information about occupation and cause of death is gathered from death certificates in the years surrounding a national census, and related to the sizes of occupational groups as estimated from the census. To allow for the potential confounding effects of age and sex, death rates are expressed in the form of standardized mortality ratios (SMRs),* which are calculated for a broad range of occupations and causes of death.

A weakness of this method is that the sources of occupational information (death certificates and census) are different for the numerator and denominator of the mortality ratios, and this gives rise to well-documented biases in relation to certain occupational categories.[27] For example, there is a tendency to 'promote' decedents when registering their deaths, so that a man recorded as a shopkeeper at the census may be elevated to the status of company director on his death certificate. The effect is falsely to inflate SMRs for some of the more prestigious jobs.

An alternative approach which overcomes this problem is to examine proportional mortality. The proportion of deaths in an occupation that is due to a disease of interest is compared with the corresponding proportion in the general population. Again, standardization is used to take into account possible confounding effects of age and sex, the resultant statistic this time being a propor-

---

* An SMR is the ratio of the number of deaths in an occupational group from a specified cause to the number that would have been expected if the group had experienced the age- and gender-specific death rates of the general population. It is often expressed as a percentage.

tional mortality ratio (PMR). In Britain, PMRs are being used increasingly in official statistics of occupational mortality, and a parallel method has been applied to the analysis of routinely collected data on cancer registrations by occupation. Statistics of proportional mortality by occupation have also been published for the US State of Washington during the period 1950–89,[28] and for California during 1959–61.[29]

Proportional analyses avoid bias insofar as all of the occupational information comes from one source (death certificates or cancer registrations). However, care is still needed in the interpretation of findings. In particular, an occupational group can have a high PMR for a disease not only if its members are abnormally susceptible to the disorder, but also if they have unusually low mortality from other common causes.

A better study design is possible in Scandinavian countries where the existence of national identity numbers for all citizens has allowed linkage between individual census, mortality and cancer registration records. This means that mortality and cancer incidence rates can be calculated directly for occupational groups as defined at a census.

Whichever analytical method is adopted, by comparing mortality or cancer incidence in occupations exposed to a hazard with that in unexposed people, it is possible to estimate the number of cases attributable to the hazard. For example, a proportional analysis of occupational mortality for England and Wales during 1979–80 and 1982–90 found an estimated excess of 1900 deaths from chronic obstructive pulmonary disease among coal miners over the 11-year study period.[30] Like other statistics derived from occupational mortality, estimates of this sort are subject to errors from inaccurate or incomplete reporting of occupations and causes of death on death certificates. Nevertheless, they give a useful index of the relative importance of different hazards and can be valuable for assessing trends.

Where suitable data on the occurrence of a disease in different occupations are not collected routinely, information must be sought from *ad hoc* epidemiological studies. These may already have been carried out for other purposes, such as to confirm the existence of a hazard. Alternatively, they be commissioned specially to assess the amount of disease caused by a hazard. Several study designs are employed.

COHORT STUDIES

In a cohort study, subjects who have been exposed to a known or suspected hazard (the study cohort) are identified and followed over time. Their disease incidence or mortality is measured and compared with that of controls who are unexposed or exposed only at a baseline level. For example, to assess the impact of welding fume on chronic airflow obstruction, a cohort of welders and an unexposed control group might be followed up with serial measurements of respiratory function. Changes in respiratory function could then be compared between the welders and controls, with adjustment for any confounding effects of age, sex, body build and smoking habits (see Chapter 9).

Where exposure to a hazard is negligible in the population at large and the outcome of interest is mortality or cancer incidence, it may be more efficient to use published national or regional disease rates for comparison rather than follow a specially selected control group. An analysis of mortality from bladder cancer in British rubber workers first employed after 2-naphthylamine had been eliminated from the manufacturing process found no excess in comparison with national death rates, suggesting that the control measure had been effective.[31]

If a cohort study includes all the workers in a population who are exposed to a hazard, the impact of the hazard can be assessed directly. However, where only a sample of exposed workers is studied, the observed excess risk in individuals must be multiplied by the total number of exposed people in the population to obtain the required estimate. In performing such calculations allowance must be made for any differences between the levels of exposure that occur in the study sample and elsewhere. In particular, if exposure to the hazard is exceptionally high in the study cohort, there is a danger of overestimating its effect in others.

CASE-CONTROL STUDIES

In a case-control or case-referent study, patients with a disease of interest (cases) are identified, and their past exposure to suspected causes is compared with that of a control group who do not have the disease. The method has the advantage of being relatively cheap and quick, particularly for the study of rare diseases. However, there are often problems in choosing an appropriate control group and in obtaining unbiased information about past exposure.

Ideally the control group should have exposures representative of those in the population at risk of becoming cases – i.e. of those people who would have been included in the study as cases had they developed the disease. Two sources of controls are commonly used – subjects selected from the study population in a random or quasi-random manner, and patients with other diseases. Randomly selected controls would be expected to have representative patterns of exposure, but if that exposure is ascertained from memory (as it usually is), they may not recall it as reliably as the cases, who are understandably interested in finding out why they have become ill. Such differences in motivation are less likely when the controls are patients with other diseases, but then their exposures may not be representative.

Despite these difficulties, case-control investigations can be a valuable source of information on the impact of occupational disease. For example, a case-control study of hip osteoarthritis in two districts of England indicated that 28% of male cases were attributable to heavy lifting at work.[32]

CROSS-SECTIONAL STUDIES

In a cross-sectional study exposure to known or suspected hazards and the prevalence of associated disease are measured in a population at one point in time. For example, a survey of 2646 randomly selected adults aged 20–44 from five areas of Spain compared the prevalence of asthma in different occupations, and suggested that some 5% of cases were attributable to work.[33]

Care is needed in the interpretation of cross-sectional studies, particularly if the development of disease may cause some subjects to leave a study population and thus be excluded from investigation. However, the method is useful where such bias can be excluded.

CONCLUSIONS

Assessing the burden of occupational disease in a population is not always straightforward, and requires various approaches depending on the type of hazard, the adverse health outcome that it causes, and the nature of the relation between the two. All of the methods used are subject to limitations of one sort or another, and these must be taken into account when results are interpreted. Sometimes the most informative picture is obtained by collating and comparing findings from several different sources with different potentials for error. With careful evaluation, however, it is possible to obtain useful estimates of the frequency of occupational illness on which to base and monitor preventive strategies.

REFERENCES

1 Wignall BK, Fox AJ. Mortality of female gas-mask assemblers. *Br J Ind Med* 1982; **39**: 34–8.
2 Doll R. Pott and the prospects for prevention. *Br J Cancer* 1975; **32**: 263–72.
3 Coggon D, Croft P. Hip osteoarthritis in farmers: a new occupational hazard? *J Irish Coll Phys Surg* 1993; **22**: 251–2.
4 Legge TM. *Report on Cataract in Glass Workers*. London: Home Office, 1907.
5 Gawkrodger DJ. Chloracne: causation diagnosis and treatment. *J Dermatol Treat* 1991; **2**: 73–6.
6 Case RAM, Hosker ME. Tumour of the urinary bladder as an occupational disease in the rubber industry in England and Wales. *Br J Prev Soc Med* 1954; **8**: 39–50.
7 Henry SA, Kennaway EL, Kennaway NM. The incidence of cancer of the bladder and prostate in certain occupations. *J Hyg Camb* 1931; **31**: 125–37.
8 Coggon D, Inskip H, Winter P, Pannett B. Lobar pneumonia: an occupational disease in welders. *Lancet* 1994; **344**: 41–4.
9 Gardner MJ, Winter PD, Taylor CP, Acheson ED. *Atlas of Cancer Mortality in England and Wales, 1968–78*. Chichester: Wiley, 1983.
10 Mason TJ, McKay FW, Hoover R, Blot WJ, Fraumeni JF. *Atlas of Cancer Mortality for US Counties 1950–1969*. Washington: US Govt Printing Office, 1975.
11 Blot WJ, Fraumeni JF, Mason TJ, Hoover RN. Developing clues to environmental cancer: a stepwise approach with the use of cancer mortality data. *Environ Hlth Perspect* 1979; **32**: 53–8.
12 Gardner MJ, Winter PD, Acheson ED. Variations in cancer mortality among local authority areas in England and Wales: relations with environmental factors and search for causes. *Br Med J* 1982; **284**: 784–787.
13 De Villiers AJ, Windish JP. Lung cancer in a fluorspar mining community. *Br J Ind Med* 1964; **21**: 94–109.
14 Siemiatycki J, Day NE, Fabry J, Cooper JA. Discovering carcinogens in the occupational environment: a novel epidemiologic approach. *J Natl Cancer Inst* 1981; **66**: 217–25.
15 Maltoni C, Lefemine G. Carcinogenicity bioassays of vinyl chloride. I. Research plan and early results. *Environ Res* 1974; **7**: 387.
16 Van Duuren BL, Goldschmidt BM, Katz BS, Langseth L, Mercado G, Sivak A. A new type of alkylating carcinogen. *Arch Environ Hlth* 1968; **16**: 472–6.
17 Peto J, Hodgson JT, Matthews FE, Jones JR. Continuing increase in mesothelioma mortality in Britain. *Lancet* 1995; **345**: 535–9.
18 Toren K. Self-reported rate of occupational asthma in Sweden 1990–2. *Occup Environ Med* 1996; **53**: 757–61.
19 Toikkanen J, Kauppinen T, Vaaranen V, Vasama M, Jolanki R. *Occupational Diseases in Finland in 1993*. Helsinki: Finnish Institute of Occupational Health, 1993.
20 Baker EL. Sentinel event notification system for occupational risks (SENSOR): The concept. *Am J Publ Hlth* 1989; **79** (Suppl): 18–20.
21 Keynes HL, Ross DJ, McDonald JC. SWORD '95: Surveillance of work-related and occupational respiratory disease in the UK. *Occup Med* 1996; **46**: 379–81.
22 Provencher S, Labreche FP, De Guire L. Physician-based surveillance system for occupational respiratory diseases: the experience of PROPULSE, Quebec, Canada. *Occup Environ Med* 1997; **54**: 272–6.
23 Wu T-N, Liou S-H, Shen C-Y, Hsu C-C, Chao S-L, Chang P-Y. Occupational disease surveillance in Taiwan. *Lancet* 1996; **348**: 827.
24 Hodgson JT, Jones JR, Elliott RC, Osman J. *Self-reported Work-related Illness*. Sudbury: HSE Books, 1993.
25 Rinsky RA, Smith AB, Hornung R, Filloon TG, Young RJ, Okun AH, Landrigan PJ. Benzene and leukaemia, an epidemiologic risk assessment. *N Engl J Med* 1987; **316**: 1044–50.
26 Registrar General. *14th Annual Report of the Registrar*

General of Births, Deaths and Marriages in England. London:HMSO, 1855.

27 Heasman MA, Liddell FDK, Reid DD. The accuracy of occupational vital statistics. *Br J Ind Med* 1958; **15**: 141–6.

28 Milham S. *Occupational Mortality in Washington State 1950–89.* Cincinnati: The National Institute for Occupational Safety and Health (NIOSH), 1997.

29 Petersen GR, Milham S. *Occupational Mortality in the State of California 1959–1961.* Cincinnatti: The National Institute for Occupational Safety and Health (NIOSH), 1980.

30 Coggon D, Inskip H, Winter P, Pannett B. Occupational mortality of men. In: Drever F ed. *Occupational Health*: *Decennial Supplement.* London:HMSO, 1995 : 23–43.

31 Parkes HG, Veys CA, Waterhouse JAH, Peters A. Cancer mortality in the British rubber industry. *Br J Ind Med* 1982; **39**: 209–2.

32 Coggon D, Kellingray S, Inskip H, Croft P, Campbell L, Cooper C. Osteoarthritis of the hip and occupational lifting. *Am J Epidemiol* 1998; **147**: 523–8

33 Kogevinas M, Anto JM, Soriano JB, Tobias A, Burney P, Martinez Moratalla J *et al.* The risk of asthma attributable to occupational exposures: a population-based study in Spain. *Am J Respir Crit Care Med* 1996; **154**: 137–43.

4

Compensation schemes for industrial injuries and diseases

J MALCOLM HARRINGTON

Historical background	37	The future	42
The principles of compensation schemes	38	References and further reading	42
The workings of the scheme	39	Appendix 1: European schedule of occupational	
Problems of the common diseases	39	diseases	43
The European perspective	40	Appendix 2: List of prescribed diseases and occupations	
The US perspective	42	for which they are prescribed – July 1999	46

One of the important consequences of an occupational disease or injury is that the worker may be temporarily or permanently incapacitated. This in turn has obvious financial effects upon that individual, their family and indeed, the State. The State is deprived of a 'unit of production' but the affected individual, by being deprived of a livelihood, could face penury.

Compensation schemes financed by the State for such workers are in place in most developed nations as well as a number of developing countries. The purpose of this chapter is to outline the development of these schemes, the principles under which they operate and the advantages and drawbacks of a State-financed system.

As the United Kingdom was the first country to adopt a State-financed no-fault scheme, the principles and practice of such schemes will be illustrated using the British model. Schemes vary across the world but recent developments in the European Union are likely to become the driving force for future change both in this continent and elsewhere. The cost of such schemes is considerable and attempts to control this either by restrictive legislation governing who can claim or by limiting the benefits available to successful claimants are currently matters of much debate.

For the clinician, these matters are not to be ignored. There is plenty of evidence to suggest that only a fraction of those eligible to claim, do so. Research into this 'take-up' aspect of compensation suggests that at least one important factor is ignorance on the part of the affected worker that they had, indeed, suffered a compensatable disease or injury. The responsibility for ensuring that ignorance is not a factor in take-up issues falls, at least in part, on the medical practitioner whom the patient consults. This is not an obscure piece of social security law of no concern to the clinician. Knowledge of the scheme for that country and information about claimants' rights is something that should be passed by the clinician to the patient. It is part of the consultation process.

HISTORICAL BACKGROUND

In the UK up to 1897, a worker or their dependants could obtain redress for personal injury at work only if it could be shown that there was negligence or breach of statutory duty on the part of the employer. The Workman's Compensation Act 1897, however, introduced the principle that, within certain limits, an employer was responsible for compensation irrespective of their own direct or indirect negligence if it could be shown that the accident arose out of and in the course of the employment. But even during the Parliamentary debate on the second reading of the Bill, it was acknowledged that diseases could also result from employment. Consequently, a Departmental committee was set up in 1903 to review the new scheme and to give some thought to whether diseases should be included within its scope.

In 1906, six industrial diseases were listed as compensatable. They were anthrax, lead poisoning, mercury poisoning, phosphorous poisoning, arsenic poisoning and ankylostomiasis. However, because it was thought that it might be more difficult to prove a disease was occupational in origin, further clarification of the scheme followed. It soon became the norm that instead of the worker having to prove that the disease was due to the nature of employment, he or she was given the benefit of presumption that it was so due, as long as they were employed in one of the processes specified in the Act in relation to the disease 'at or immediately before' the date of the disablement. This principle of presumption remains today but it has been the source of much debate as the scheme went through various modifications by various committees over the following 40 years. In particular, the arguments (with minority reports and some acrimony) centred on presumption, the weight of evidence regarding incidence of the disease in certain occupations compared with the general population. Throughout this tortuous legal process, one principle remained centre stage: the need to have the element of *presumption* which in turn was a fundamental feature of a *no-fault* scheme.

The prescription of additional diseases followed haphazardly and piecemeal until Judge Dale was appointed in 1947 to review the burgeoning scheme. The Dale Committee pronounced on two important aspects. First, they confirmed the possibility that a prescribed disease could be common to all persons, but more common in particular occupations and, second, that the future advice on what diseases should be prescribed should come from an advisory committee of experts, with representation of employers and employee organizations – the Industrial Injuries Advisory Council (IIAC). Such recommendations for changes to the Scheme should be put by IIAC to Ministers.

The criteria for prescription was laid down in the National Insurance (Industrial Injuries) Act 1946 and has remained unchanged through subsequent Acts up to and including the latest (the Social Security Contributions and Benefits Act, 1992). The criteria are that: 'a disease or injury may be prescribed in relation to employed earners if the Minister is satisfied that:

- it ought to be treated, having regard to its causes and incidence and any other relevant considerations, as a risk of their occupation and not as a risk common to all persons;
- it is such that, in the absence of special circumstances, the attribution of a particular case to the nature of employment can be established or presumed with reasonable certainty.'

It follows from this that the scheme – which relies on presumption in the individual case – must be soundly based on good quality epidemiological evidence of an increased risk in populations. The scheme could thus be construed, by definition, as restrictive. Furthermore, such a scheme allows little room for individual proof and no room for the self-employed. These issues – which are

somewhat at odds with the proposed European schedule – will be revisited later in this chapter.

The developments outlined above have been mirrored to a large extent in most developed countries. Certainly schemes for 'workman's compensation' began in the USA in 1911 in Wisconsin and were in place in all states by 1949. For Canada the time interval for similar developments was 1913–1950. In New Zealand, the Accident Compensation scheme provides cover not just to the employed but to everyone (adults and children) who are injured, irrespective of fault and irrespective of the source or place of the accident. In the European Union, only one country, the Netherlands, has a scheme for disability benefit which does not have a separate occupational component. The remaining 14 nations have some list or other for prescribed diseases and some means or other for reviewing and adding to that list. The proposals for a harmonized list of diseases and the means of compensation are outlined later.

THE PRINCIPLES OF COMPENSATION SCHEMES

The issues of harmonizing schemes across Europe, combined with the growing costs of such schemes (in Britain, this currently amounts to £500 million per year despite cuts in eligibility for benefit) have led to much discussion about the value of having a scheme at all. Proposals for reform in Britain resulted in a position paper from IIAC on why a separate scheme is necessary. This paper puts the case for preferential treatment of those disabled by work, to counter the stance of others that disablement is disablement and that all disabled people should be treated the same.

In essence, the argument is thus: Work is necessary for society. The production of goods and services is essential for the economic and social well-being of the country and its people. Work is required of the individual. Society places upon the individual the duty of self-support. Unless that individual is too young (or old), physically incapacitated or engaged in caring responsibilities, that individual must find means of support from private sources, from another individual, or through paid work. If work is not available, social security support should be provided, so long as the individual has actively sought work. There is no right in society for a person capable of work and not prevented by other responsibilities from working, to decide not to work, or not to seek work, and yet receive support from social security benefits.

So much for the necessity of work. But work brings risks to health. Some work is acknowledged to be dangerous – even where the activity is either socially necessary or economically desirable. Efforts to reduce risk are essential but risks cannot be eliminated entirely. (If that was possible, then there would not have been nine editions of this book.) Furthermore, new processes and new substances bring new challenges to the workplace ill-health prevention programme. Therefore some jobs carry threats to health and the choice of avoiding such jobs is not available to most. The employed person, therefore, faces health risks of varying magnitude in the process of earning a living.

The consequence of all this is that some people, through no fault of their own – or even their employer – will become ill or injured through work. This form of disablement is, it is argued, special. The risks are imposed in the cause of individual and national economic goals. Ergo, the State should compensate.

If such a scheme is agreed, what are its characteristics? Ideally, they should be:

- to cover all forms of employment,
- to operate from the first day of that employment,
- to ensure that payment of benefit is speedy,
- to provide for the needs of dependants in the event of death.

In the longer term, a scheme should provide:

- a non-means tested income during incapacity sufficient to adequately support the individual and their dependants,
- for the costs of care,
- for the loss of earnings,
- for protecting pension rights and retirement income,
- for benefit for as long as it is needed.

Probably no scheme in the world does all this but it is worth stating what the ideal might be. The scheme in many countries has been eroded of late as governments seek to limit the vast sums spent on maintaining a social security system. In Britain, one particular loss recently was the decision to abolish Reduced Earnings Allowance. This was replaced by another benefit but it failed one important group of people: those who suffered a reduced income by having to change jobs to preserve their health. Classically, this applies to those who become sensitized to some agent or other, and, in order to avoid further morbidity, should avoid further exposure. The abolition of Reduced Earnings Allowance removed, at a stroke, an important preventive measure because, in practice, many workers continued their exposure to workplace allergens because they could not afford to move. The long-term effects of this will be greater morbidity and, of course, additional expense to the State health care system but, perhaps cynically, one must say, that cost is borne by a different government department.

THE WORKINGS OF THE SCHEME

Again using the UK experience as illustrative of a number of schemes, it might be of value to clinicians to fol-

low a putative case of occupational disease through the process of claiming a benefit. The scheme looks in some ways Byzantine, but part of that lies in the opportunity at several points along the line for appeal against a decision deemed unfavourable by the claimant.

The first step is the realization by the patient that they can claim at all. To claim they must be able to show that they work (or have worked in the relevant 'latent period') in a relevant occupation and, second, that they have acquired the relevant disease. The clinician's view is clearly crucial in the second part. Thereafter the patient can apply to the Benefits Agency to receive adjudication for their case. A lay officer of the Agency handles this. If all is straightforward the claim can be successful on the basis of a lay officer reading a medical report and doing some detective work on the claimant's employment history. If it is more complicated, or in doubt, a group of experts are called in to decide. Appeals by the claimant can be heard by a variety of tribunals right up to a Social Security Commissioner who reports directly to the Secretary of State and is independent of the Benefit Agency process.

The other side of the scheme is the process whereby diseases become prescribed. This is the role of the IIAC (the Chairmanship of which was, until recently, held by the author). The IIAC keeps up to date with the medical literature on occupational diseases. If a new issue arises – for example – osteoarthritis of the hip and/or knee – the Council reviews the literature and if a prima facie case exists for considering inclusion of this condition in the prescribed list, then the Council calls for written evidence by public notice. Oral evidence may also be requested from specific experts. In the end, the Council debates the evidence it has accrued through its own research subcommittee, as well as that gathered from the public call for evidence. It then writes a report to the Secretary of State, who always publishes the report, but reserves the right to accept or reject the findings. If the advice to add a disease to the list is accepted, it becomes law.

Of course, most of the obvious occupational diseases have long been prescribed; what remains is the occupational component of more common diseases and the thorny issue – yet to be grasped – of the psychosocial diseases such as stress. It would, perhaps, be useful to illustrate the problems of prescription by reviewing three recent issues – chronic bronchitis and emphysema, asthma and work-related upper limb disorders.

PROBLEMS OF THE COMMON DISEASES

Chronic bronchitis and emphysema are common conditions for which the main causative agent is undoubtedly tobacco smoke. For two decades the Council has reviewed the evidence for occupationally related bronchitis. In 1988, after much deliberation and in one of its longest reports, the Council rejected prescription for coalminers' bronchitis as it was considered to be over-shadowed in epidemiological studies by smoking (see Chapters 31, 35). The Council called for evidence on non-smoking miners and, by 1992, reports had appeared in the literature which provided sufficiently strong epidemiological evidence to recommend prescription for underground coalminers. The Council's alleged prevarication on this issue highlights the major difficulty in reviewing common diseases. To satisfy the requirements of the Act, the population-based epidemiological evidence must be sufficiently strong to enable the presumption of causality in the *individual* case. In practice, this usually means a doubling of the risk in population-based studies to afford presumption at the individual level.

Nevertheless, in the case of this very common disease, the Council asked for more than evidence of the right job and the right disease. They requested 20 years underground, evidence of dust retention on chest radiograph (1/1 on the ILO Classification) and evidence of impaired spirometry. The resulting debate on this report was heated and sustained. Claims of discrimination against short, old miners on the spirometry could be refuted. Twenty years underground could be a future problem in an industry with young miners and a high turnover. However, the chest radiograph criteria proved untenable when research emanating from the Decennial Supplement on Occupational Health (from the Office of National Statistics) showed that the pattern of mortality from chronic bronchitis and emphysema differed from that for pneumoconiosis in coal mining areas of Britain. The geology of the coal-bearing seams was a greater factor and IIAC's chest radiograph criteria could discriminate against some miners as their pneumoconiosis rates were lower than others. (By the same token, the criteria would discriminate in favour of miners in other areas but that is less of a problem in schemes whereby the spirit of the rules is to sway, if anything, in favour of the claimant.) Thus a further report followed in 1996, removing the chest radiograph criteria from the requirements.

Occupational asthma was somewhat different. Here, new, proven agents arise at a greater frequency than it is possible to cope with in practical terms of prescription. The Council thus proposed in its third report on Asthma in 1990, that an additional 'Z' category be created to cover any occupational sensitizing agent which could be shown by the claimant to be the cause of their asthma. This approach, accepted by the Secretary of State, is akin to individual proof – a process the Government has consistently opposed for years. However, the Council does not intend to extend individual proof across the board – in any case the current powers would reject it – but it will review future prescribed conditions to see if, in the particular, a case could be argued for such an approach.

So far as work-related upper limb disorders are concerned, the question of prescription is even more confusing. Early additions to the scheme such as 'writer's

cramp' and 'tendinitis' would have great difficulty in achieving prescribed disease status today (see Chapter 22). This is, of course, due to the extreme difficulty in finding good quality epidemiological studies which show a doubling of risk for specific diagnosable conditions related to specified occupations. IIAC last reviewed these conditions in 1992 and were unable to recommend any extension of the prescribed disease list except for carpal tunnel syndrome associated with the use of hand-held vibrating tools (see Chapter 14). An additional section of the report commented on the 'overwhelming clinical evidence' that many cases of carpal tunnel syndrome are of occupational origin and that they deserve compensation in an individual proof system. The government rejected this section of the report.

For some years now, the Industrial Injuries scheme in Britain has faced veiled threats to abolish it or privatize it. The arrival of a Labour government following the General Election of 1997 probably means that the scheme will survive. If it does, the IIAC will still have to come to grips with two major issues: the way to handle psychosocial illness such as stress-related diseases and the way to stay in broad agreement with developments in the European Union.

THE EUROPEAN PERSPECTIVE

There are moves afoot in various areas of the European Union towards harmonization. Occupational diseases compensation is no exception. In May 1990, the European Commission proposed a recommendation (90/326EEC) concerning the adoption of a European schedule of occupational diseases. The Commission proposed that Member States should introduce 'as soon as possible' a list of 'scientifically recognized' occupational diseases into their national laws, regulations or administrative provisions suitable for compensation and 'preventive measures'. They recommended a list for member states to consider. (This list appears as Appendix 1 and the UK list as Appendix 2 at the end of this chapter.) The Commission, however, went further. They drew up a second list which, although not carrying the force of the first list, could be considered by Member States and could provide the right for a worker to claim compensation for a disease on that list.

Additional features of the Recommendation were that national statistics on compensatable occupational diseases should be compiled and then these statistics could be used as comparators between countries. Throughout, the thrust of the proposals was to use these lists not just to compensate workers but to focus on preventive measures for such diseases. Success or failure in prevention would then be gauged over time as the numbers of claimants by disease are reviewed over the years by the Commission. At the end of 3 years (no news on this at present) the Commission would review Member States' responses 'in order to determine whether there is a need for binding legislation'.

Reviewing list 1 from the European Commission (Appendix 1) it is clear that the UK is reasonably well 'harmonized'. Approximately 50% of the European list is specifically covered in the Prescribed Diseases list. A further 25% are covered by the accident provisions and 10% more are either under active review by IIAC or the Council is considering a review. Around 15% are rejected by the UK – most of these relate to vague classifications of chemicals such as 'halogenated derivatives of aliphatic or alicyclic hydrocarbons'. The UK stance has been to review specific chemicals one by one rather than to lump a disparate and diverse group together. The only other area of contention is the European Commission's desire to see individual proof incorporated in Member States' laws. Individual proof was consistently rejected in Britain during the lifetime of the Conservative administration. The current Labour government might change this.

List 2 does, however, raise again some interesting issues for the future. Notwithstanding items such as 'dental caries associated with work in the chocolate, sugar and flour industries' (!), there are many references to agents 'not included' in list 1. This could be individual proof by another route.

On a country by country basis, it is clear that some countries already have a mixed system of specified agents and individual proof. These include Denmark, Germany and France. Some such as Italy and Spain, like the UK, use a scheduled list. The numbers on the schedule also vary between countries ranging from 52 in Greece to 91 in France (the UK has 66).

In order to aid the process of harmonization, the Commission has produced Information Notices on the Diagnosis of Occupational Diseases. The purpose of these is to agree the main features of a particular disease and the notes are designed to be used by lay adjudicators. For lead poisoning, for example, the main uses and sources of exposure are listed, followed by acute systemic effects (gastrointestinal tract, toxic encephalopathy) chronic systemic effects (haemopoietic system, gastrointestinal tract, central and peripheral nervous system, kidneys and effects on reproduction). The note concludes with biological and workplace air monitoring criteria for excessive exposure as well as the minimum duration of exposure and maximum latent period required for adverse health effects.

In order to start the process of harmonization, the European Commission has proposed that a shortlist of 30 prescribed diseases or exposures should become the basis for collecting comparable data from Member States. These are grouped together in Table 4.1.

This has clearly struck a chord in Europe as even the Dutch, who do not have a separate list of occupational diseases for disability claim purposes, have adopted the 'Euro 30' and are beginning to collect statistics on the incidence and prevalence of these conditions through their network of occupational physicians.

Outside the European Union, various schemes exist. The 'Warsaw Pact' countries, in line with the Soviet Union used to have a different system of compensation. In the Czech Republic, for example, there is a list of 83 occupational diseases. Occupational diseases in the individual must be diagnosed by a specialist working in a large State-run hospital or university hospital. If the disease is on the list, compensation is paid by the employer. It is possible to claim for a disease or injury not on the list but classified as 'other health damage caused by work.' Work-relatedness of an injury is not an acceptable label if the person concerned was under the influence of alcohol or other agents of self-abuse. Similar schemes based on the 'sanitary epidemiology' stations or on works' medical departments exist elsewhere in Eastern Europe but radical changes are underway in an effort to limit the financial burden of compensation.

Table 4.1 *Euro 30*

Chemical		Biological	Physical	
Inorganic	*Organic*		*Dusts*	*Others*
Cadmium	Carbon disulphide	Zoonoses	Asbestos[b]	Ionizing radiation
Chromium	Benzene	Viral hepatitis	Silica/silicates	Noise-induced
Mercury	Chlorine	Tuberculosis	(plus lung effects	hearing loss
Heat cataract	Aromatics		of sintered metal	Heat cataract
Manganese	Polynuclear		Co,Sn,Ba,C)	Beat conditions
Nickel	Aromatics[a]		Nerve pressure	
Lead	Isocyanates		Vibration[c]	

[a] Coal distillation
[b] Fibrogenic/carcinogenic plus: dermatitis and asthma
[c] Osteoarticular + hand–arm vibration syndrome

THE US PERSPECTIVE

In principle the means of compensating a worker for a disease or injury arising from work is similar to the European position. That is, there is 'no-fault' compensation and there are common law claim procedures for negligence. For no-fault schemes, the USA does not have a unified law as each state has its own variations on the theme. Almost all states require employers either to purchase insurance or to demonstrate that they are able to pay any claims. Where the State takes on the role of acting as the repository for employers' premiums, they tend to disburse a higher percentage of the premiums in the form of benefits then do private insurance carriers. (For a more detailed account of the American system, the reader is referred to Bodin's chapter in *Occupational Health* edited by Levy and Wegman.[1])

THE FUTURE

There is little doubt that most countries will espouse some system of no-fault compensation for workers who become ill or injured as a result of their work. Furthermore, the various schemes in Europe are likely to come closer together both in their specific listings, their means of compensation, and most importantly, in the ways these comparable listings of compensated cases can be used as a means of measuring the effectiveness of a country's efforts to prevent future illness or injury. The vexed question of the status of the self-employed remains to be answered.

What also remains to be decided is how a country will pay for the claims. Some will undoubtedly continue the most common system, that of State funding. Others, under more 'conservative' governments, are seriously reviewing whether some or all the scheme could be privatized. It is possible that industry and commerce could be made to pay for accidents. Such events are by their very nature immediate and thus the identification of the relevant employer is not difficult. The real problem would arise if there was a move to privatize the disease provisions. It is the author's view that such a scheme is untenable. Many diseases have long latent periods, and the role of an adjudicating officer is already extremely difficult in finding the relevant exposure period (and employer) for such diseases as pleural mesothelioma and noise-induced hearing loss. The relevant company may have closed down and working conditions at the time the harmful exposure is alleged to have taken place may be impossible to evaluate with any degree of certainty.

In the British case, for example, a saving of £500 million a year by privatizing the scheme is not great given the overall cost of the British social security bill which now exceeds £90 billion. Moreover, the only alternative to no-fault claims is for the worker to go to the Courts to claim negligence under the Tort System. The costs of the two systems make interesting reading. It has been estimated that the claims under the tort scheme total about £300 million per year but the administrative costs are high. For the tort scheme these amount to 45% of total expenditure compared with just over 11% for the State system of prescribed diseases and accidents. Furthermore, as the State scheme pays pensions which rise in line with inflation, the benefits to the claimant may be preferable when compared with the relatively paltry sums (often less than £1000) paid as a single sum in the event of a successful claim under Tort.

However favourable the financial arguments may be for the continuation (and extension) of State financed no-fault compensation schemes for employees, the issue at the centre of the discussion is a moral one. In a civilized society, the State has a responsibility to provide financial support for a citizen who, in the normal course of earning a living, has been temporarily or permanently disabled by their occupation.

REFERENCES AND FURTHER READING

1 Boden LI. Workers compensation. In: Levy BA, Wegman DH eds. *Occupational Health* 3rd edn. Boston: Little, Brown and Co, 1995.

2 European Commission. Information notices on diagnosis of occupational diseases. Directorate General, Employment, Industrial Relations and Social Affairs *EUR 14768 EN*. Luxembourg, 1994.

3 Department of Health and Social Security Industrial Injuries Advisory Council. *Bronchitis and Emphysema* London: HMSO: 1988, Cm 379.

4 Harrington JM. Industrial Injuries Advisory Council – its role in the benefits system. *J Soc Sec Law* 1994; **1:** 70–5.

5 Harrington JM, Newman-Taylor AJ, Coggon D. Industrial injuries compensation. *Br J Ind Med* 1991; **48:** 577–8.

6 Industrial Injuries Advisory Council. *Periodic Reports* London: HMSO, 1990; 1993.

7 Lewis R. The government's philosophy towards reform of social security: the case of industrial injury benefit. *Int Law J* 1986; **15:** 256–65.

8 Department of Social Security: Industrial Injuries Advisory Council. *Occupational Asthma* 1990, Cm 1244; *Work-Related Upper Limb Disorders* 1992, Cm; 1936; *Chronic Bronchitis and Emphysema* London: HMSO, 1996, Cm 3240.

9 Wikely N. Social security. The continuing importance of the industrial injuries compensation scheme. *Int Law J* 1994; **23:** 80–91.

Appendix 1

EUROPEAN SCHEDULE OF OCCUPATIONAL DISEASES

The diseases mentioned in this schedule must be linked directly to the occupation. The Commission will determine the criteria for recognizing each of the occupational diseases listed hereunder:

1	Diseases caused by the following chemical agents	EC No
100	Acrylonitrile	608 003 004
101	Arsenic or compounds thereof	033 002 005
102	Beryllium (glucinium) or compounds thereof	–
103.01	Carbon monoxide	006 001 002
103.02	Carbon oxychloride	–
104.01	Hydrocyanic acid	–
104.02	Cyanides and compounds thereof	006 007 005
104.03	Isocyanates	–
105	Cadmium or compounds thereof	048 001 005
106	Chromium or compounds thereof	–
107	Mercury or compounds thereof	080 001 000
108	Manganese or compounds thereof	–
109.01	Nitric acid	007 004 001
109.02	Oxides of nitrogen	007 002 000
109.03	Ammonia	007 001 005
110	Nickel or compounds thereof	–
111	Phosphorus or compounds thereof	015 001 001
112	Lead or compounds thereof	082 001 006
113.01	Oxides of sulphur	–
113.02	Sulphuric acid	016 020 008
113.03	Carbon disulphide	006 003 003
114	Vanadium or compounds thereof	–
115.01	Chlorine	017 001 007
115.02	Bromine	–
115.04	Iodine	602 005 003
115.05	Fluorine or compounds thereof	009 001 000
116	Aliphatic or alicyclic hydrocarbons derived from petroleum spirit or petrol	–
117	Halogenated derivatives of the aliphatic or alicyclic hydrocarbons	–
118	Butyl, methyl and isopropyl alchohol	–
119	Ethylene glycol, diethylene glycol, 1,4-butanediol and the nitrated derivatives of the glycols and of glycerol	–
120	Methyl ether, ethyl ether, isopropyl ether, vinyl ether, dichloroisopropyl ether, guaiscol, methyl ether and ethyl of ethylene glycol	–
121	Acetone, chloroacetone, bromoacetone, hexafluoroacetone, methyl ethyl ketone, methyl n-butyl, methyl iso-butyl ketone, diacetone alcohol, mesityl oxide, 2-methylcyclohexanone	–
122	Organophosphorous esters	–
123	Organic acids	–
124	Formaldehyde	–
125	Aliphatic nitrated derivatives	–
126.01	Benzene or counterparts thereof (the counterparts of benzene are defined by the formula: $C_n H_{2n-6}$)	601 020 008
126.02	Naphthalene or napthalene counterparts (the counterpart of naphthalene is defined by the formula: $C_n H_{2n-12}$	–
126.03	Vinyl benzene and divinylbenzene	–
127	Halogenated derivatives of the aromatic hydrocarbons	–
128.01	Phenols or counterparts of halogenated derivatives thereof	–
128.02	Naphthols or counterparts of halogenated derivatives thereof	–

Appendix 1 – *continued*

128.03	Halogenated derivatives of the alkylaryl oxides	–
128.04	Halogenated derivatives of the alkylaryl sulphonates	–
128.05	Benzoquinones	–
129.01	Aromatic amines or aromatic hydrazines or halogenated, phenolic, nitrified nitrated or sulphonated derivatives thereof	–
129.02	Aliphatic amines and halogenated derivatives thereof	–
130.01	Nitrated derivatives of aromatic hydrocarbons	–
130.02	Nitrated derivatives of phenols or their counterparts	–
131	Antimony and derivates thereof	051 003 009

2   Skin diseases caused by substances and agents not included under other headings

201   Skin diseases and skin cancers caused by:

201.01	Soot	
201.02	Tar	
201.03	Bitumen	
201.04	Pitch	
201.05	Anthracene or compounds thereof	–
201.06	Mineral and other oils	
201.07	Crude paraffin	
201.08	Carbazole or compounds thereof	–
201.09	Byproducts of the distillation of coal	
202	Occupational skin ailments caused by scientifically recognized allergy-provoking or irritative substances not included under other headings	

3   Diseases caused by the inhalation of substances and agents not included under other headings

301   Diseases of the respiratory system and cancers:

301.11   Silicosis
301.12   Silicosis combined with pulmonary tuberculosis
301.21   Asbestosis
301.22   Mesothelioma following the inhalation of asbestos dust
301.31   Pneumoconioses caused by dust silicates
302   Complication of asbestos in the form of bronchial cancer
303   Bronchopulmonary ailments caused by dusts from sintered metals
304.01   Extrinsic allergic alveolitis
304.02   Lung diseases caused by the inhalation of dusts and fibres from cotton, flax, hemp, jute, sisal and bagasse
304.03   Respiratory ailments of an allergic nature caused by the inhalation of substances consistently recognized as causing allergies and inherent to the type of work
304.04   Repiratory ailments caused by the inhalation of dust from cobalt, tin, barium and graphite
304.05   Siderosis
305.01   Cancerous diseases of the upper respiratory tract caused by dust from wood

4   Infectious and parastic diseases

401   Infectious or parasitic diseases transmitted to man by animals or remains of animals
402   Tetanus
403   Brucellosis
404   Viral hepatitis
405   Tuberculosis
406   Amoebiasis

Appendix 1 – *continued*

5	**Diseases caused by the following physical agents**
502.01	Cataracts caused by heat radiation
502.02	Conjunctival ailments following exposure to ultraviolet radiation
503	Hypoacusis or deafness caused by noise
504	Diseases caused by atmospheric compression or decompression
505.01	Osteoarticular diseases of the hands and wrists caused by mechanical vibration
505.02	Angioneurotic diseases caused by mechanical vibration
506.10	Diseases of the periarticular sacs due to pressure
506.21	Diseases due to overstraining of the tendon sheaths
506.22	Diseases due to overstraining of the peritendineum
506.23	Diseases due to overstraining of the muscular and tendonous insertions
506.30	Meniscus lesions following extended periods of work in a kneeling or squatting position
506.40	Paralysis of the nerves due to pressure
507	Miners' nystagmus
508	Diseases caused by ionizing radiation

Appendix 2

LIST OF PRESCRIBED DISEASES AND OCCUPATIONS FOR WHICH THEY ARE PRESCRIBED – JULY 1999

Prescribed disease or injury	Any occupation involving
A Conditions due to physical agents	
A1 Inflammation, ulceration or malignant disease of the skin or subcutaneous tissues or of the bones, or blood dyscrasia, or cataract, due to electromagnetic radiations other than radiant heat), or to ionizing particles	Exposure to electromagnetic radiations (other than radiant heat) or to ionizing particles.
A2 Heat cataract.	Frequent or prolonged exposure to rays from molten or red-hot material.
A3 Dysbarism, including decompression sickness, barotrauma and osteonecrosis.	Subjection to compressed or rarefied air or other respirable gases or gaseous mixtures.
A4 Cramp of the hand or forearm due to repetitive movements.	Prolonged periods of handwriting, typing or other repetitive movements of the fingers, hand or arm.
A5 Subcutaneous cellulitis of the hand.	Manual labour causing severe or prolonged friction or pressure on the hand.
A6 Bursitis or subcutaneous cellulitis arising at or about the knee due to severe or prolonged external friction or pressure at or about the knee.	Manual labour causing severe or prolonged external friction or pressure at or about the knee.
A7 Bursitis or subcutaneous cellulitis arising at or about the elbow due to severe or prolonged external friction or pressure at or about the elbow.	Manual labour causing severe or prolonged external friction or pressure at or about the elbow.
A8 Traumatic inflammation of the tendons of the hand or forearm, or of the associated tendon sheaths (tenosynovitis).	Manual labour, or frequent or repeated movements of the hand or wrist.
A9 Miners' nystagmus.	Work in or about a mine.
A10 Sensorineural hearing loss amounting to at least 50 dB in each ear, being the average of hearing losses at 1, 2 and 3 kHz frequencies and being due in the case of at least one ear to occupational noise. [Occupational deafness]	(a) the use of powered (but not hand-powered) grinding tools on cast metal (other than weld metal) or on billets or blooms, or work wholly or mainly in the immediate vicinity of those tools whilst they are being so used; or (b) the use of pneumatic percussive tools on metal, or work wholly or mainly in the immediate vicinity of those tools whilst they are being so used, or (c) the use of pneumatic percussive tools for drilling rock in quarries or underground or in mining coal or in sinking shafts or for tunnelling in civil engineering works, or work wholly or mainly in the immediate vicinity of those tools whilst they are being so used; or (ca) the use of pneumatic percussive tools on stone in quarry works, or work wholly or mainly in the immediate vicinity of those tools whilst they are being so used; or (d) work wholly or mainly in the immediate vicinity of plant (excluding power press plant) engaged in the forging (including drop stamping) of metal by means of closed or open dies or drop hammers; or

Appendix 2 – *continued*

(e) work in textile manufacturing where the work is undertaken wholly or mainly in rooms or sheds in which there are machines engaged in weaving man-made or natural (including mineral) fibres or in the high speed false twisting of fibres; or

(f) the use of, or work wholly or mainly in the immediate vicinity of, machines engaged in cutting, shaping or cleaning metal nails; or

(g) the use of, or work wholly or mainly in the immediate vicinity of, plasma spray guns engaged in the deposition of metal; or

(h) the use of, or work wholly or mainly in the immediate vicinity of, any of the following machines engaged in working of wood, that is to say: multicutter moulding machines, planing machines, automatic or semi-automatic lathes, multiple cross-cut machines, automatic shaping machines, double-end tenoning machines, vertical spindle moulding machines (including high speed routing machines), edge banding machines, bandsawing machines with a blade width of not less than 75 mm and circular sawing machines in the operation of which the blade is moved towards the material being cut; or

(i) the use of chain saws in forestry; or

(j) air arc gouging or work wholly or mainly in the immediate vicinity of air arc gouging; or

(k) the use of band saws, circular saws or cutting discs for cutting metal in the metal founding or forging industries, or work wholly or mainly in the immediate vicinity of those tools whilst they are being so used; or

(l) the use of circular saws for cutting products in the manufacture of steel, or work wholly or mainly in the immediate vicinity of those tools whilst they are being so used; or

(m) the use of burners or torches for cutting or dressing steel based products, or work wholly or mainly in the immediate vicinity of those tools whilst they are being so used; or

(n) work wholly or mainly in the immediate vicinity of skid transfer banks; or

(o) work wholly or mainly in the immediate vicinity of knock-out and shake-out grids in foundries; or

(p) mechanical bobbin cleaning or work wholly or mainly in the immediate vicinity of mechanical bobbin cleaning;

(q) the use of, or work wholly or mainly in the immediate vicinity of, vibrating metal moulding boxes in the concrete products industry; or

(r) the use of, or work wholly or mainly in the immediate vicinity of, high pressure jets of water or a mixture of water and abrasive material in the water jetting industry (including work under water); or

Appendix 2 – *continued*

(s) work in ships' engine rooms; or

(t) the use of circular saws for cutting concrete masonry blocks during manufacture, or work wholly or mainly in the immediate vicinity of those tools whilst they are being so used; or

(u) burning stone in quarries by jet channelling processes, or work wholly or mainly in the immediate vicinity of such processes; or

(v) work on gas turbines in connection with –
  (i) performance testing on test bed;
  (ii) installation testing of replacement engines in aircraft;
  (iii) acceptance testing of Armed Service fixed-wing combat planes; or

(w) the use of, or work wholly or mainly in the immediate vicinity of –
  (i) machines for automatic moulding, automatic blow moulding or automatic glass pressing and forming machines used in the manufacture of glass containers or hollow ware;
  (ii) spinning machines using compressed air to produce glass wool or mineral wool;
  (iii) continuous glass toughening furnaces.

A11 Episodic blanching, occurring throughout the year, affecting the middle or proximal phalanges or in the case of a thumb the proximal phalanx, of

(a) in the case of a person with five fingers (including thumbs) on one hand, any three

(b) in the case of a person with only four such fingers, any 2 of those fingers, or

(c) in the case of a person with less than four such fingers, any one of those fingers or, as the case may be the one remaining finger (vibration white finger).

(a) the use of hand-held chain saws in forestry; or

(b) the use of hand-held rotary tools in grinding or in or the sanding or polishing of metal, or the holding of material being ground, or metal being sanded or polished, by rotary tools;

(c) the use of hand-held percussive metal-working tools, or the holding of metal being worked upon by percussive tools, in riveting, caulking, chipping, hammering, fettling or swaging; or rotary tools

(d) the use of hand-held powered percussive drills or hand-held powered percussive hammers in mining, quarrying, demolition or on roads or footpaths, including road construction; or

(e) the holding of material being worked upon by pounding machines in shoe manufacture.

A12 Carpal tunnel syndrome

The use of hand-held vibrating tools whose internal parts vibrate so as to transmit that vibration to the hand, but excluding those which are solely powered by hand.

B Conditions due to biological agents

B1 Anthrax

Contact with animals infected with anthrax or the handling (including the loading or unloading or transport) of animal products or residues.

B2 Glanders.

Contact with equine animals or their carcases.

B3 Infection by leptospira

(a) Work in places which are, or are liable to be, infested by rats, field mice or voles, or other small mammals; or

(b) work at dog kennels or the care or handling of dogs; or

(c) contact with bovine animals or their meat products or pigs or their meat products.

Appendix 2 – *continued*

B4	Ankylostomiasis.	Work in or about a mine.
B5	Tuberculosis.	Contact with a source of tuberculous infection.

B6   Extrinsic allergic alveolitis (including farmer's lung).

Exposure to moulds or fungal spores or heterologous proteins by reason of employment in:
(a) agriculture, horticulture, forestry, cultivation of edible fungi or malt-working; or
(b) loading or unloading or handling in storage mouldy vegetable matter or edible fungi; or
(c) caring for or handling birds; or
(d) handling bagasse.

B7   Infection by organisms of the genus *Brucella*. (Brucellosis)

Contact with:
(a) animals infected by *Brucella*, or their carcasses or parts thereof, or their untreated products or
(b) laboratory specimens or vaccines of, or containing, *Brucella*.

B8   Viral hepatitis.

Contact with:
(a) human blood or human blood products; or
(b) a source of viral hepatitis.

B9   Infection by *Streptococcus suis* (rare form of meningitis from pigs)

Contact with pigs infected by *Streptococcus suis*, or with the carcasses, products or residues of pigs so infected.

B10
(a) Avian chlamydiosis.

Contact with birds infected with *Chlamydia psittaci*, or with with the remains or untreated products of such birds.

(b) Ovine chlamydiosis.

Contact with sheep infected with *Chlamydia psittaci*, or with the remains or untreated products of such sheep.

B11   Q fever.

Contact with animals, their remains or their untreated products.

B12   Orf.

Contact with sheep, goats or with the carcasses of sheep or goats.

B13   Hydatidosis.

Contact with dogs.

C   Conditions due to chemical agents

C1   Poisoning by lead or a compound of lead.

The use or handling of, and exposure to the fumes, dust or vapour of, lead or a compound of lead, or a substance containing lead.

C2   Poisoning by manganese or a compound of manganese.

The use or handling of, or exposure to the fumes, dust or vapour of, manganese or a compound of manganese, or a substance containing magnanese.

C3   Poisoning by phosphorus or an inorganic compound of phosphorus or poisoning due to the anticholinesterase or pseudo anti cholinesterase action of organic phosphorus compounds.

The use of handling of, or exposure to the fumes, dust or vapour of, phosphorus or a compound of phosphorus, or a substance containing phosphorus.

C4   Poisoning by arsenic or a compound of arsenic.

The use of handling of, or exposure to the fumes, dust or vapour of, arsenic or a compound of arsenic, or a substance containing arsenic.

C5   Poisoning by mercury or a compound of mercury.

The use of handling of, or exposure to the fumes, dust or vapour of, mercury or a compound of mercury, or a substance containing mercury.

Appendix 2 – *continued*

C6 Poisoning by carbon bisulphide.

The use or handling of, or exposure to the fumes or vapour of, carbon bisulphide or a compound of carbon bisulphide, or a substance containing carbon bisulphide.

C7 Poisoning by benzene or a homologue of benzene.

The use of handling of, or exposure to the fumes of, or vapour containing benzene or any of its homologues.

C8 Poisoning by a nitro- or amino- or chloro-derivative of benzene or of a homologue of benzene, or poisoning by nitrochlorbenzene.

The use of handling of, or exposure to the fumes of, or vapour containing a nitro- or amino- or chloro-derivative of benzene, or of a homologue of benzene, or nitrochlorbenzene.

C9 Poisoning by dinitrophenol or a homologue of dinitrophenol or by substitute dinitrophenols or by the salts of such substances.

The use of handling of, or exposure to the fumes of, or vapour containing, dinitrophenol or a homologue or substituted dinitrophenols or the salts of such substances.

C10 Poisoning by tetrachloroethane.

The use of handling of, or exposure to the fumes of, or vapour containing, tetrachloroethane.

C11 Poisoning by diethylene dioxide (dioxane).

The use or handling of, or exposure to the fumes of, or vapour containing, diethylene dioxide (dioxane).

C12 Poisoning by methyl bromide.

The use or handling of, or exposure to the fumes of or vapour containing, methyl bromide.

C13 Poisoning by chlorinated naphthalene.

The use or handling of, or exposure to the fumes of or dust or vapour containing, chlorinated naphthalene.

C14 Poisoning by nickel carbonyl.

Exposure to nickel carbonyl gas.

C15 Poisoning by oxides of nitrogen.

Exposure to oxides of nitrogen.

C16 Poisoning by *Gonioma kamassi* (African box wood).

The manipulation of *Gonioma kamassi* or any process in or incidental to the manufacture of article therefrom.

C17 Poisoning by beryllium or a compound of beryllium.

The use of handling of, or exposure to the fumes, dust or vapour of, beryllium or a compound of beryllium, or a substance containing beryllium.

C18 Poisoning by cadmium.

Exposure to cadmium dust or fumes.

C19 Poisoning by acrylamide monomer.

The use or handling of, or exposure to, acrylamide monomer.

C20 Dystrophy of the cornea (including ulceration of the corneal surface) of the eye.

(a) The use or handling of, or exposure to arsenic, tar, pitch, bitumen, mineral oil (including paraffin), soot or any compound, product or residue of any of these substances, except quinone or hydroquinone; or
(b) exposure to quinone or hydroquinone during their manufacture.

C21
(a) Localized new growth of the skin, papillomatous or keratotic (warts and scaliness).
(b) Squamous-cell carcinoma of the skin (form of skin cancer – chimney sweep's cancer).

The use or handling of, or exposure to, arsenic, tar, pitch, bitumen, mineral oil (including paraffin), soot or any compound, product or residue of any of these substances, except quinone or hydroquinone.

C22
(a) Carcinoma of the mucous membrane of the nose or associated air sinuses.
(b) Primary carcinoma of a bronchus or of a lung.

Work in a factory where nickel is produced by decomposition of a gaseous nickel compound which necessitates working in or about a building or buildings where that process or any other industrial process ancillary or incidental thereto is carried on.

Appendix 2 – *continued*

C23 **Primary neoplasm (including papilloma, carcinoma *in-situ* and invasive carcinoma) of the epithelial lining of the urinary tract (renal pelvis, ureter, bladder and urethra). (Cancer of the lining of the bladder)**

(a) Work in a building in which any of the following substances are produced for commercial purposes:
  (i) α-naphthylamine, β-naphthylamine or methylene-bis orthochloroaniline;
  (ii) diphenyl substituted by at least one nitro or primary amino group or by at least one nitro and primary amino group (including benzidine);
  (iii) any of the substances mentioned in subparagraph (ii) above if further ring substituted by halogeno, methyl or methoxy groups, but not by other groups;
  (iv) the salts of any of the substances mentioned in the subparagraphs (i) to (iii) above;
  (v) auramine or magenta; or
(b) the use or handling of any of the substances mentioned in subparagraph (a)(i) to (iv), or work in a process in which any such substance is used, handled or liberated; or
(c) the maintenance or cleaning of any plant or machinery used in any such process as is mentioned in subparagraph (b), or the cleaning of any plant or machinery used in any such process as is mentioned in subparagraph (b), or the cleaning of clothing used in any such building as is mentioned in subparagraph (a) if such clothing is cleaned within the works of which the building forms a part of in a laundry maintained and used solely in connection with such works.
(d) exposure to coal tar pitch volatiles produced in aluminium smelting involving the Soderberg process (the method of producing aluminium by electrolysis in which the anode consists of petroleum coke and mineral oil which is baked *in situ*)

C24
(a) Angiosarcoma of the liver.
(b) Osteolysis of the terminal phalanges of the fingers.
(c) Non-cirrhotic portal fibrosis.

(a) Work in or about machinery or apparatus used for the polymerization of vinyl chloride monomer, a process which, for the purposes of this provision, comprises all operations up to and including the drying of the slurry produced by the polymerization and the packaging of the dried product; or
(b) work in a building or structure in which any part of that process takes place.

C25 **Occupational vitiligo.**

The use or handling of, or exposure to, para-tertiary-butylphenol, para-tertiary-butylcatechol, paramyl-phenol, hydroquinone or the monobenzyl or monobutyl ether of hydroquinone.

C26 **Damage to the liver or kidneys due to exposure to carbon tetrachloride.**

The use of or handling of, or exposure to the fumes of, or vapour containing, carbon tetrachloride.

C27 **Damage to the liver or kidneys due to exposure to trichloromethane (chloroform).**

The use of or handling of, or exposure to the fumes of, or vapour containing, trichloromethane (chloroform).

C28 **Central nervous system dysfunction and associated gastrointestinal disorders due to exposure to chloromethane (methyl chloride)**

The use of or handling of, or exposure to the fumes of, or vapour containing chloromethane (methyl chloride).

Appendix 2 – *continued*

C29   **Peripheral neuropathy** due to exposure to *n*-hexane or methyl *n*-butyl ketone.

The use of or handling of, or exposure to the fumes of, or vapour containing, *n*-hexane or methyl *n*-butyl ketone.

C30   **Chrome dermatitis,** or ulceration of the mucous membranes or the epidermis, resulting from exposure to chromic acid, chromates or bichromates.

The use or handling of, or exposure to, chromic acid, chromates or bichromates.

D   *Miscellaneous conditions*

D1   **Pneumoconiosis** (includes silicosis and asbestosis)

(a) set out in Part II of Schedule 1 of the Social Security (Industrial Injuries) (Prescribed Diseases) Regulations 1985.

(b) specified in Regulation 2(b)(ii) of the Social Security (Industrial Injuries) (Prescribed Diseases) Regulations 1985.

D2   **Byssinosis.**

Work in any room where any process up to and including the weaving process is performed in a factory in which the spinning or manipulation of raw or waste cotton or of flax, or the weaving of cotton or flax, is carried on.

D3   **Diffuse mesothelioma** (primary neoplasm of the mesothelium of the pleura or of the pericardium or of the peritoneum) (cancer of the lining of the lung)

Exposure to asbestos, asbestos dust or any admixture of asbestos at a level above that commonly found in the environment at large.

D4   **Allergic rhinitis which is due to exposure to any of the following agents:**

   (a) isocyanates;
   (b) platinum salts;
   (c) fumes or dusts arising from the manufacture, transport or use of hardening agents (including epoxy resin curing agents) based on phthalic anhydride, tetrachlorophthalic anhydride, trimellitic anhydride or triethylene-tetramine;
   (d) fumes arising from the use of rosin as a soldering flux;
   (e) proteolytic enzymes;
   (f) animals including insects and other arthropods used for the purpose of research or education or in laboratories;
   (g) dusts arising from the sowing, cultivation, harvesting, drying, handling, milling transport or storage of barley, oats, rye, wheat or maize, or the handling, milling transport or storage of meal or flour made therefrom;
   (h) antibiotics;
   (i) cimetidine;
   (j) wood dust;
   (k) ispaghula;
   (l) castor bean dust;
   (m) ipecacuanha;
   (n) azodicarbonamide (occupational asthma);
   (o) animals including insects and other arthropods, or their larval forms, used for the purposes of pest control or fruit cultivation or the larval forms of animals used for the purposes of research, education or in laboratories;
   (p) glutaraldehyde;
   (q) persulphate salts or henna;

Exposure to any of the agents set out in column 1 of this paragraph.

Appendix 2 – *continued*

(r) crustaceans or fish or products arising from these in the food processing industry;
(s) reactive dyes;
(t) soya bean;
(u) tea dust;
(v) green coffee bean dust;
(w) fumes from stainless steel

D5 Non-infective dermatitis of external origin
(excluding dermatitis due to ionizing particles or electromagnetic radiations other than radiant heat).

Exposure to dust, liquid or vapour or any other external agent except chromic acid, chromates or bichromates capable of irritating the skin (including friction or heat but excluding ionizing particles or electromagnetic radiations other than radiant heat).

D6 Carcinoma of the nasal cavity or associated air sinuses (nasal carcinoma).

(a) Attendance for work in or about a building where wooden goods are manufactured or repaired; or
(b) attendance for work in a building used for the manufacture of footwear or components of footwear made wholly or partly of leather or fibre board; or
(c) attendance for work at a place used wholly or mainly for the repair of footwear made wholly or partly of leather or fibre board.

D7 Asthma which is due to exposure

(a) isocyanates;
(b) platinum salts;
(c) fumes or dusts arising from the manufacture, transport or use of hardening agents (including epoxy resin curing agents) based on phthalic anhydride, tetrachlorophthalic anhydride, trimellitic anhydride or triethylene-tetramine;
(d) fumes arising from the use of rosin as a soldering flux;
(e) proteolytic enzymes;
(f) animals including insects and other arthropods used for the purpose of research or education or in laboratories;
(g) dusts arising from the sowing, cultivation, harvesting, drying, handling, milling transport or storage of barley, oats, rye, wheat or maize, or the handling, milling, transport or storage of meal or flour made therefrom;
(h) antibiotics;
(i) cimetidine;
(j) wood dust;
(k) ispaghula;
(l) castor bean dust;
(m) ipecacuanha;
(n) azodicarbonamide (occupational asthma);
(o) animals including insects and other arthropods, or their larval forms, used for the purposes of pest control or fruit cultivation or the larval forms of animals used for the purposes of research, education or in laboratories;
(p) glutaraldehyde;
(q) persulphate salts or henna;

Appendix 2 – *continued*

(r) crustaceans or fish or products arising from these in the food processing industry;

(s) reactive dyes;

(t) soya bean;

(u) tea dust;

(v) green coffee bean dust;

(w) fumes from stainless steel welding;

(x) any other sensitizing agent.

D8 Primary carcinoma of the lung where there is accompanying evidence of one or both of the following:

(a) asbestosis;

(b) unilateral or bilateral diffuse pleural thickening extending to a thickness of 5 mm or more at any point within the area affected as measured by a plain chest radiograph (not being a computerized tomography scan or other form of imaging) which –

(i) in the case of unilateral diffuse pleural thickening, covers 50% or more of the area of the chest wall of the lung affected; or

(ii) in the case of bilateral diffuse pleural thickening, covers 25% or more of the combined area of the chest wall of both lungs.

(a) The working or handling of asbestos or any admixture of asbestos; or

(b) the manufacture or repair of asbestos textiles or other articles containing or composed of asbestos, or

(c) the cleaning of any machinery or plant used in any of the foregoing operations and of any chambers, fixtures and appliances for the collection of asbestos dust; or

(d) substantial exposure to the dust arising from any of the foregoing operations.

D9 Unilateral or bilateral diffuse pleural thickening extending to a thickness of 5 mm or more at any point within the area affected as measured by a plain chest radiograph (not being a computerized tomography scan or other form of imaging) which –

(i) in the case of unilateral diffuse pleural thickening, covers 50% or more of the area of the chest wall of the lung affected; or

(ii) in the case of bilateral diffuse pleural thickening, covers 25% or more of the combined area of the chest wall of both lungs.

(a) The working or handling of asbestos or any admixture of asbestos; or

(b) the manufacture or repair of asbestos textiles or other articles or other articles containing or composed of asbestos; or

(c) the cleaning of any machinery or plant used in any of the foregoing operations and of any chambers, fixtures and appliances for the collection of asbestos dust; or

(d) substantial exposure to the dust arising from any of the foregoing operations.

D10 Primary carcinoma of the lung

(a) Work underground in a tin mine; or

(b) exposure to bis(chloromethyl) ether produced during the manufacture of chloromethyl methyl ether; or

(c) exposure to zinc chromate, calcium chromate or strontium chromate in their pure forms.

D11 Primary carcinoma of the lung where there is accompanying silicosis

Exposure to silica dust in:

(a) glass or pottery manufacture

(b) tunnelling in, quarrying sandstone or granite

(c) metal ore mining

(d) slate quarrying or the manufacture of artefacts from slate

(e) clay mining

(f) using siliceous materials as abrasives

(g) stone cutting

(h) stone masonry

(i) foundary work

Appendix 2 – *continued*

D12 Chronic bronchitis or emphysema

Except in the circumstances specified in regulation 2(d),

    (a) chronic bronchitis; or

    (b) emphysema; or

    (c) both

where there is accompanying evidence of a forced expiratory volume in 1 second (measured from the position of maximum inspiration with the claimant making maximum effort) which is –

    (i) at least 1 litre below the mean value predicted in accordance with *Lung Function: Assessment and Application in Medicine* by J E Cotes, 5th edn, 1994, Oxford: Blackwell Scientific Publications Limited (ISBN 0-632-03926-9) for a person of the claimant's age, height and sex; or

    (ii) less than 1 litre.

Exposure to coal dust by reason of working underground in a coal mine for a period or periods amounting in aggregate to at least 20 years (whether before or after 5 July 1948) and any such period or periods shall include a period or periods of incapacity while engaged in such an occupation.

5

Medicolegal reports and the role of the expert witness

DIANA M KLOSS

Civil and criminal law	57	Going to court	62
The role of the doctor in providing medicolegal reports	58	The Woolf Reforms	63
The purpose of expert medical reports	60	Legal liability of the expert witness	63
The form of the expert report	61	References	64

The need for a medical opinion is a daily requirement of those who work in the field of compensation for personal injury. In disputes between employers and employees, the doctor may be asked to decide whether the employee is fit for work and, if not, whether he is likely to be able to return in the foreseeable future. Doctors also regularly appear in criminal courts to give an account of the victim's injuries or to advise on the time and cause of injury. They may be asked for an opinion on the mental state of a person accused of crime. In other areas they may be drawn into a case where relatives doubt the validity of a will signed by a testator who was allegedly incompetent, or they may become involved in child care cases. In a growing number of cases it is the doctor who stands accused of negligence and must rely on other doctors to support what he has done, or omitted to do. This chapter will centre on medicolegal reports requested by a lawyer in a case of personal injury arising out of a work-related accident or disease and will then deal with the role of the expert medical witness appearing in a court of law.

The medical expert will be confronted with a totally different regime: a world of reasonable probabilities and reasonable doubt which is foreign to his scientific training. He may sometimes be asked to give evidence that may damage his patient, and be unable to refuse. It is important that he understand a little of the legal process and of the needs of the courts.

CIVIL AND CRIMINAL LAW

Criminal law is concerned with offences against society as a whole. Prosecution is therefore brought in almost all cases by a public official (Crown Prosecution Service in England and Wales, Procurator Fiscal in Scotland). Prosecutions for offences against the criminal law of health and safety at work are brought by the Health and Safety Executive. Crimes are divided according to the seriousness of the alleged offence. The less serious crimes are tried summarily by the magistrates courts in England and Wales, the district and sheriff courts in Scotland. The most serious crimes, such as murder and rape, are tried by a judge and jury in the Crown Court in England and Wales and the High Court in Scotland. When a defendant is found guilty by the criminal court he is punished by imprisonment, fines, probation orders etc., but although the criminal courts now also have power in some cases to order compensation to the victim, this is very much secondary to the primary function of punishment. The Criminal Injuries Compensation Board awards compensation out of public funds to the victims of crimes of violence.

Civil law is concerned with the adjudication of property rights and the award of compensation to those injured by another's unlawful act. A civil action is brought by the person who has suffered injury: the claimant (formerly known as the plaintiff) in England and Wales, the pursuer in Scotland. In England cases of major importance are tried in the High Court; where less money is at stake the County Court is the proper venue.

The equivalent courts in Scotland are the Court of Session and the Sheriff Court. Jury trials are rarely found in civil actions: most cases are tried by a single judge sitting without a jury. A defendant who is found liable will most commonly be ordered to pay monetary compensation or damages. Parties to civil actions have to finance themselves, unless they qualify for legal aid or are backed by a trade union or an insurance company. The loser is ordered to pay the costs of the winner, though the party who wins in a contest with a legally aided defendant cannot as a general rule recover his costs from the legal aid fund. In recent years however, lawyers have been permitted to charge conditional fees whereby the amount of legal costs depends on the success or otherwise of the action.

In addition to the civil courts, there are a number of administrative tribunals which deal with cases in a limited area. Examples are the employment tribunals for employment disputes and the independent tribunals for disputes over entitlement to welfare benefits. Of particular interest to doctors are medical appeal tribunals whose work includes the determination of issues of medical assessment related to claims for industrial injuries benefits.

A vitally important distinction between the criminal and civil process is that in the criminal courts the prosecution must prove the defendant's guilt beyond a reasonable doubt, whereas in the civil action the burden is to prove liability on a balance of reasonable probabilities ('more likely than not').

In both civil and criminal courts the British procedure is adversarial rather than inquisitorial. Each side must call evidence to support its case. The judge acts as a referee to see fair play and to make the final decision. Experts are called by both sides, not appointed by the judge, as in the civil law system adopted in most other European countries, derived from Roman law. In the UK, the coroners' courts, which deal with sudden, accidental and unnatural deaths, exceptionally follow an inquisitorial procedure.

Membership of the European Union has added an extra dimension to English and Scottish law. Since the aim of the community at its inception was primarily to create an *economic* community, domestic laws relating to compensation for personal injury have been unaffected. In other areas, however, where laws directly or indirectly restrict competition, sweeping changes have been directed by the Council of Ministers, the legislature of the Community. Medical and other professional qualifications obtained in one Member State must be recognized in other states. The criminal law of health and safety at work and laws relating to product safety now stem mainly from Brussels, since a country which failed to achieve minimum safety standards at work or which imposed unnecessarily strict standards for consumer goods to exclude foreign imports would have an unfair advantage in an open market. Each Member State must enforce Community law through its own courts and other institutions, but a reference may be made from domestic courts to the Court of Justice of the European Communities in Luxembourg.

THE ROLE OF THE DOCTOR IN PROVIDING MEDICOLEGAL REPORTS

There are two main circumstances where a medical report might be requested:

- When a doctor has been involved in a case as an active participant and is asked to give evidence based on his knowledge of what has occurred. He may have treated the victim of a crime or accident in his surgery (office) or in hospital.
- When the doctor is asked after the event to bring his professional skill and knowledge to bear as to how an injury was caused, its effect on the person injured or the prognosis for the future. Here the doctor acts as an expert witness, not as a participant in the event being scrutinized by the court.

Doctor participants

The duty of confidentiality enshrined in the Hippocratic Oath yields to a conflicting duty to give evidence of events when called upon to do so by a court of law. Doctors, unlike lawyers, have no privilege against disclosure of their patients' secrets. A doctor who refused to obey the court's order could be punished for contempt. However, courts will sometimes rule that a doctor need not give evidence of confidential material if it is not necessary to assist the court to make a decision. The judge may be asked to peruse the relevant material in order to permit its non-disclosure.

Sometimes, a claimant will be unable to decide whether he has a cause of action at all until he has seen medical evidence. He may have been told by fellow workers that he is exhibiting classic symptoms of an occupational disease, but be unsure of the medical details of his condition or of the doctor's diagnosis. Under the Supreme Court Act 1981 he may apply to the court for an order that records be disclosed. The court has a discretion to restrict disclosure to the plaintiff's legal or medical advisers.

Until recently, the doctor or NHS Trust was free to refuse to disclose medical records and reports even to the patient himself, unless a court order was first obtained. Now, the Data Protection Acts 1984 and 1998 and the Access to Health Records Act 1990 (which came into force in November 1991) oblige the doctor to release medical records to the patient, unless disclosure would damage his physical or mental health or reveal the identity of a third party who wishes to remain anonymous.

The first statutes cover data held on computer; the second covers manually held records.

A report of this kind should begin with factual information about the doctor, his qualifications and position, and the patient. It should state how the doctor met with the patient, giving time, place and general circumstances, together with the names of any other persons present at the time. It should go on to give details of the results of the examination, and end with a summary of conclusions. At this stage the doctor may give an opinion – for example, as to the cause of the injury or the likely prognosis for the future. This evidence may be vital later when the court has to apportion blame for the accident or fix the amount of damages.

Doctor experts

Expert witnesses are called upon, not because they know anything about the *facts* of the case but because they can give an *opinion* as to a relevant issue. It is for the judge to decide whether someone is truly an expert. In medical cases formal qualifications are of course important, as is experience in the relevant specialty. Any expert report, therefore, should be prefaced with the qualifications and status of the doctor. Headed notepaper is one way of resolving this problem: a typed curriculum vitae which can be seen by the judge is a solution often used by engineering experts but not so common among doctors.

Experts may not be called to give evidence on a matter that is within the range of ordinary human experience. In *R v Turner* (1975)[1] a man was accused of killing his girlfriend under the provocation of being told of her infidelity. The trial judge refused to admit evidence from a psychiatrist that this would have had a profound emotional effect on the defendant.

In a civil action in which a claimant is suing for damages in respect of some disease or injury the claimant's lawyer will at an early stage in the proceedings commission an expert report from a doctor, who may be the doctor treating the patient and will therefore fill the dual roles of doctor participant and doctor expert, but is more likely to be someone previously unconnected with the case. A medical report must be filed with the claim when a personal injury action is commenced. If the expert's report favours the claimant's case, it will be disclosed to the other side in the hope that the defendant will settle out of court, but if it is unfavourable it will be suppressed and another doctor approached. The law is that disclosure will not be ordered of any report prepared with a view to legal proceedings, unlike the patient's medical records which, as has already been discussed, do not attract the same privilege. In *Lee v SW Thames Regional Health Authority* (1985)[2] a child with severe burns was transported from one hospital to another in an ambulance. He was found to have suffered brain damage, probably caused by lack of oxygen. The plaintiff's lawyers asked the court to order disclosure of a memorandum prepared by the ambulance crew which had been sent to the health authority with a view to obtaining legal advice on liability. It was held that the court had no power to do this: the report was privileged. However, an accident report prepared partly to make a finding as to causation and future preventive measures and partly to prepare for legal proceedings is not privileged against disclosure (*Waugh v British Rail* (1980)).[3]

If the defendant's lawyers are unhappy with the claimant's medical report, they may commission their own report from another doctor. The claimant, therefore, may have to submit to further examinations and tests, this time by a doctor who is not 'on his side'. If he unreasonably refuses, the court may decline to proceed with the action. However, he need not agree to every procedure. In *Aspinall v Sterling Mansell Ltd* (1981)[4] the court held that the plaintiff need not submit to a request to carry out patch tests in circumstances where there was a minor but real risk of dermatitis breaking out afresh. In *Prescott v Bulldog Tools* (1981),[5] an industrial deafness case, it was held reasonable for the plaintiff, who had already been examined four times by the defendant's doctors, to refuse a radiograph of the inner ear and the piercing of the ear drum with a very fine needle.

After April 1999, when new Civil Procedure Rules came into force, it is common for there to be only one expert report on which both parties rely.

From time to time the lawyers will return to the expert witness, asking him to clarify and expand his report. Accurate medical terminology must be used (the lawyers are expected to consult their medical dictionaries), but lawyers find it extremely helpful if the doctor can accompany the technical phrases with an explanation in layman's language. A diagram accompanying the report may also assist. Doctors may be intrigued to know that the leading lawyers' work on personal injury claims, *Kemp and Kemp*,[6] includes medical illustrations and a glossary of medical terms. In a case in which there is a conflict of medical evidence the doctor may later have to explain his findings in the witness-box.

What if the lawyers ask the doctor to alter what he has written? In *Noble v Robert Thompson* (1979)[7] a psychiatrist wrote a report on a depressed mother with the hope that it would assist her in gaining access to her children. The doctor wrote that access should not be enforced against the wishes of the children themselves. He refused to delete this when asked to do so and sued for his fee when the solicitors refused to pay. The judge gave judgment for the psychiatrist: 'It would be of no assistance to the courts if doctors were encouraged to abandon their professional approach and write reports designed to achieve particular objects, at the behest of the patient or anyone else'.

Once the claimant and defendant have the reports on which they intend to rely in the proceedings they must mutually disclose. As Lord Denning put it in *Naylor v Preston Area Health Authority* (1987).[8]

> The general rule is that, while a party is entitled to privacy in seeking out the 'cards' for his hand, once he has put his hand together, the litigation is to be conducted with all the cards face up on the table. Furthermore, most of the cards have to be put down well before the hearing.

If the expert is relying on published or unpublished literature, this must also be disclosed. It is in the interests of justice that each party knows the strength of the other's case early on, because this may save years of delay and legal costs. In many instances, reports can be agreed, avoiding the necessity of calling doctors at the trial.

Criminal courts also have authority to order pretrial disclosure of medical evidence (Police and Criminal Evidence Act 1984, section 81).

A novel situation arose in *W v Egdell* (1990).[9] W was detained as a patient in a secure hospital without limit of time as a potential threat to public safety after he shot and killed five people. Ten years later, he applied to a mental health review tribunal to be discharged or transferred to a regional secure unit. His responsible medical officer, who had diagnosed him as suffering from schizophrenia which could be treated by drugs, supported the application. His solicitors instructed Dr Egdell, a consultant psychiatrist, to examine W and report on his mental condition with a view to using the report to support W's application to the tribunal. In the event Dr Egdell strongly opposed the transfer. The solicitors decided that as the report was unfavourable they would not place it before the tribunal. The doctor sent a copy, in breach of confidence, to the health authority, the Secretary of State and the tribunal and the solicitors withdrew the application for the time being. It was held by the Court of Appeal as follows:

> A consultant psychiatrist who becomes aware, even in the course of a confidential relationship, of information which leads him, in exercise of what the court considers a sound professional judgment, to fear that decisions may be made on the basis of inadequate information and with a real risk of consequent danger to the public is entitled to take such steps as are reasonable in all the circumstances to communicate the grounds of his concern to the responsible authorities.

THE PURPOSE OF EXPERT MEDICAL REPORTS

It is suggested that the doctor should always keep clearly in mind what it is that must be proved to the court. In an action for damages for personal injury, for example, the claimant has to prove, on a balance of reasonable probabilities, first that the defendant was negligent or in breach of his statutory duties, second that the negligence of the defendant caused the claimant's injury and third that the claimant suffered some material injury to his physical or mental health. The amount of the damages (the legal term is quantum) will depend on the state in which the claimant is left after the accident. If a young healthy girl aged 17 years is very severely brain damaged in an accident at work caused by the negligence of her employer, and dies almost immediately her parents will receive only the statutory amount for bereavement, now £7500. But if the doctors say that she will live for another 20 years, though paralysed and insentient, she will be able to claim damages of £600 000 and more for the necessary nursing care, special accommodation and the loss of the earnings she would have made if she had not been injured. The doctors' opinion on the likely prognosis for this patient will decide the amount of damages payable. Courts cannot award periodic payments: they must fix a lump sum on the evidence available at trial, unless both parties consent to periodical payments (Damages Act 1996). They need the doctors to estimate life expectancy in round figures.

When a claimant has suffered such catastrophic injury and the damages are large, defendant insurance companies consider structured settlements. These cannot be ordered by the judge: they must be agreed between the claimant and defendant in an out-of-court settlement, which the court can then approve. A structured settlement involves the purchase of an annuity which then guarantees the claimant a sufficient income for the rest of his or her life, with no danger of damages running out if the doctors' predictions of life expectancy prove to be incorrect. The Inland Revenue has agreed that these payments will not be subject to income tax. Structured settlements, originally thought to be unavailable when the defendant was an NHS Trust, have now been used in a number of such cases.

In another case a man in his 50s is diagnosed as suffering from asbestosis due to exposure to asbestos by his employer. He is breathless and unable to work. There is a possibility that he may contract mesothelioma or lung cancer. He has been a moderate cigarette smoker all his adult life. The lawyers need from the doctor an estimate as to the percentage of disability caused by the cigarettes and a forecast of what may happen to him in future.

Because the course of disease and injury is often unpredictable in the early stages, the doctor may write in his first report that he wishes to examine the patient again after a specified period has elapsed. Settlement of the claim may be deferred, not through lawyers' delays but to allow the full extent of the damage to become apparent. When the development of a further disability such as epilepsy is possible only in the longer term the lawyers may apply for an award of provisional damages. Such a settlement allows the claimant to return for more if his medical condition deteriorates after his award of damages. However, it was held in *Willson v Ministry of Defence* (1991)[10] that the mere progression of a particular disease was not appropriate for a provisional award. The plaintiff had slipped on a polished floor at work, injuring his ankle. Medical reports a year later stated that there would be degeneration of the ankle joint, that the plaintiff would remain prone to further injuries and that there was a possibility of arthritis. It was decided that this was not a suitable case for an award of provisional damages and that damages would be awarded on a lump sum basis.

Damages are of two kinds: special damages to compensate for losses up to the date of settlement or trial, and general damages to make up for future loss. By section 22 of the Social Security Act 1989 (amended in 1997) the defendant must deduct from the damages for loss of earnings paid to the claimant in respect of an accident or injury occurring after 1 January 1989 the gross amount of any relevant Social Security benefits paid or likely to be paid to the victim. The defendant then reimburses the Secretary of State with this sum. Relevant benefits for this purpose include attendance allowance, disablement benefit, income support, incapacity benefit, disability living and working allowance and jobseeker's allowance up to the end of the period of 5 years following the accident.

Causation is a particularly difficult area in which medical evidence may be vital. In cases of occupationally induced disease, evidence of research may be more important than examination of the claimant. The rate of hearing loss of workers exposed to high levels of noise in the shipyards was a central part of the evidence in *Thompson v Smiths Shiprepairers* (1984).[11] The court decided that most of the loss had occurred in the first years of exposure at a time when employers could not reasonably be expected to guard against it – a ruling that considerably lowered the awards of damages.

THE FORM OF THE EXPERT REPORT

The report should begin with the name and qualifications of the expert, the date and circumstances of his examination. The first section should deal with the history of the disease or injury. The date of birth of the patient should always be given. In an occupational injury case the work is as important as the victim, but the lawyers will probably be asking for a separate report from an engineer on the technical aspects. In the past, lawyers were concerned about the non-admissibility of hearsay evidence, that is evidence of which the witness has no personal knowledge, but which has been reported to him. The Civil Evidence Act 1995 now permits hearsay evidence in civil proceedings, subject to safeguards.

The second section of the report should elucidate the present state of the injury. Obviously this will be made up partly of what the patient says and partly of objective examination, such as radiographs or scans. At this stage the doctor should consider whether there is any indication that the patient is inventing all or some of the symptoms and signs. Accusations of malingering should not be made lightly, however, although the patient cannot sue the doctor for defamation if he makes such an allegation. Later reports when injuries appear not to have responded to treatment may contain references to 'functional overlay' or 'compensationitis'. The law is that genuine psychological consequences of an injury do not preclude the award of damages: only if the patient is consciously inventing or exaggerating his symptoms is he not entitled to compensation. Defendant insurance companies may hire a photographer to catch such a claimant up a ladder repairing his roof when he is supposed to be in agony from a bad back. In a case in the Birmingham High Court in 1991 the court for the first time considered evidence from the Isostation B-200 which was alleged to be able to detect whether a claimant complaining of backache was faking her symptoms.

At this stage in the report the doctor should give an opinion as to the cause of the symptoms, setting out any possible alternative causes and any causes related to the conduct of the patient (e.g. obesity or cigarette smoking). As previously indicated, it is important to try to put a percentage figure on alternative causes, for example, 'the patient's smoking has contributed 50% to his reduced lung function'. To write a fully comprehensive report it is important to gain access to the patient's general practitioner and hospital records. The patient's written consent will, of course, be necessary. Some doctors follow the policy of writing a report and accompanying it with a covering letter pointing out inconsistencies or weaknesses in the patient's case. 'The patient says he has been in pain for months, but he has never visited his general practitioner during that time, nor has he been off work'. This practice is not to be encouraged. The doctor's duty to the court means that his report must be as objective as possible.

The next section should assess the effect of the disability on the patient both now and in the future. The following are important factors:

- Is there pain? Will it continue?
- Is there loss of mobility? Will it continue?
- Has the patient lost work? If still off work, how long will this continue? Will the patient be able to resume his job, or will he be permanently unfit? What job will he be able to do, if any?
- What jobs around the house is the patient unable to do? Child care? Housework? Gardening? Do-it-yourself? Will the situation improve?
- What hobbies is the patient now unable to enjoy? Will the situation improve?
- How has the disability affected the patient's general quality of life? Relationships? Enjoyment of life? What is the future likely to hold?

The report should state clearly what future complications are possible in the medical condition, if any.

Arthritis? Epilepsy? Cancer? Again, the degree of risk should be estimated and the possible time scale for example, '80% likelihood of arthritis within 5 years'. If an injury has brought forward the onset of a condition that would otherwise have remained dormant, an estimate should be made of the number of years of dormancy lost. The likely expectation of life should be given.

It is useful if the report concludes with a summary of the main points and an indication of whether and when there should be a review of the patient's condition.

A typical report from an orthopaedic surgeon on a patient who had sustained a whiplash injury in a road accident would be set out under the following headings:

- Patient details.
- History of the accident.
- Present complaints.
- On examination: clinical examination and radiographs.
- Opinion, conclusion and prognosis.

GOING TO COURT

Most actions for damages for personal injury are settled out of court. The costs of legal proceedings are such that most defendants, who are usually insurance companies, are willing to settle any claim which contains some merit. However, some claims have to be fought, because they are regarded as being without any justification or, more often, because they are in some way a test case on which other cases may depend.

The best medical expert witness from a lawyer's point of view is one who writes fair and balanced reports which he is able to defend under cross-examination. Such experts are likely to have long waiting lists. In some cases doctors give up their medical practice in order to concentrate on medicolegal work. This may eventually be counterproductive, if the other side is able to argue that the expert is out-of-date or lacks recent 'hands-on' experience.

Experts are encouraged to agree reports if this is possible. It would be unusual for two eminent doctors to have totally opposing views of a particular case. The Woolf Report on civil proceedings recommends that every attempt should be made to resolve any conflict of evidence between doctors before the trial. The court may limit the parties to one expert if that is all that is necessary.

> The basic premise of my new approach is that the expert's function is to assist the court. There should be no expert evidence at all unless it will help the court, and no more than one expert in any one speciality unless this is necessary for some real purpose ... In cases where opposing experts are involved, the court already has power to direct the parties' experts to meet,

before or after the experts have disclosed their reports, so as to identify and reduce areas of difference. Under the new rules the experts will be required (not simply authorized, as at present) to produce a report identifying matters agreed and outstanding areas of difference after such a meeting.[12]

As has been previously stated, the expert's role should be that of an independent adviser to the court. Lack of objectivity is to be avoided, especially if it arises from improper pressure by solicitors. As Lord Wilberforce said in *Whitehouse v Jordan* (1981):[13]

> It is necessary that expert evidence presented to the court should be, and should be seen to be, the independent product of the expert uninfluenced as to form or content by the exigencies of litigation.

It is not the function of the expert to comment in evidence about the parties' credibility as witnesses, merely to assess the likelihood of the truth of their story by objective criteria.

If the case does go to court, and the expert is called, certain practical points must be borne in mind. The first is that the expert must be available to give evidence, which may necessitate complicated arrangements if he or she is still in practice. Some solicitors follow the policy of subpoenaing their own witness, to be certain of his presence. Courts will be sympathetic to the needs of patients, but the doctor may have to wait for a considerable time before being called.

Obviously, an expert should try to make a good impression on the judge. Attire should be sober, and hands should be kept out of pockets and away from jewellery. When giving evidence, it is important to address the judge, not merely the advocate who is asking the questions. If there is to be reference to reports, these should be held in a paginated bundle, of which the judge and the other side should also have a copy. The expert should be positive and firm, yet reasonable, in approach and keep calm, especially under cross-examination. He should remember that counsel may attempt to cast doubt on his credibility by making him lose his temper, or contradict himself. If the expert does not understand a question, or needs time to consider it, he should ask for it to be repeated. If he does not know the answer to a question, he should say so and not be tempted to venture speculative opinions which cannot be substantiated. It may be that in the course of the proceedings the expert's opinion has changed, because new facts have come to light. If this is the case, it is vital for him to inform his barrister before giving evidence. He should never try to tell jokes or upstage the judge when in the witness box. The judge will respect expert medical qualifications, but only if he is treated with respect.

In civil proceedings, the witness is first subjected to an examination by his own counsel. Although this should be a friendly process, it is important to answer questions, rather than volunteering information. Counsel will have planned how best to elucidate the evidence he needs. This is followed by cross-examination by counsel for the other side who is, of course, likely to be more hostile, though not discourteous, since bullying a witness can be counterproductive. Finally, a re-examination is permitted to clarify points which have been raised in cross-examination, but not to repeat the original evidence.

The ultimate duty of the witness is to the court, as is that of the lawyers in the case. In *Vernon v Bosley* (No 2) (1997),[14] a father saw unsuccessful attempts to rescue his two small daughters when the car driven by their nanny plunged into a river. After the accident, his mental condition deteriorated, his business failed, and his marriage broke down. He obtained damages for post-traumatic stress disorder, and at least part of that judgment was upheld by the Court of Appeal. However, before any final order was drawn up, the defendant's counsel received anonymously in the post a copy of a judgment in family proceedings relating to the plaintiff's children, in which it was disclosed that medical experts had stated that his psychiatric health was much improved, and that he had virtually recovered. The plaintiff's lawyers knew of this before either the High Court judge or the Court of Appeal had given judgment in the personal injury proceedings, but had deliberately concealed it. It was held that the existence of the reports of the two medical experts in the family proceedings should have been disclosed to the defendant's advisers before the judge gave judgment. The case was reopened, and damages substantially reduced. Lord Justice Stuart-Smith said this:

> If a doctor whom it is proposed to call to give evidence relating to the plaintiff's expectation of life writes in any accompanying letter or subsequently that he has discovered that the plaintiff is suffering from a life-threatening disease unrelated to the accident, that letter must clearly be disclosed, if the doctor is to be called to give evidence on the question of expectation of life.

It would be the doctor's ethical duty to refuse to give evidence if he knew that a material fact was being withheld from the other side and that his evidence would therefore be misleading. As the Woolf Report concludes:

> Professional people who take on responsibilities as expert witnesses need a basic understanding of the legal system and their role within it. They also need to be able to present their evidence effectively both in written reports and orally under cross-examination. Training in presentational skills, however, should never lose sight of the fundamental point that the expert's duty is to assist the court. Otherwise it is not in the interests of justice because it may result in the truth being concealed.[15]

THE WOOLF REFORMS

New Civil Procedure Rules implementing the recommendations of Lord Woolf came into force on 26 April 1999. The aim is to simplify procedures, to make them more efficient and less dilatory, to encourage parties to settle out of court at an earlier stage and to put the Judge firmly in charge of running the case. Pre-action protocols have been created for personal injury and clinical negligence claims. A fast-track procedure has been introduced for personal injury claims for less than £15 000.

Part 35 of the Rules deals with expert evidence. The aim is to make the expert an objective witness (not a 'hired gun') whose report is addressed to the court and not to the party from whom the expert receives his instructions. It must contain a statement that the expert understands his duty to the court, has complied with that duty, and that his report is true to the best of his knowledge and belief. The expert must set out the substance of his instructions (whether written or oral) i.e. the information given to the expert by the lawyers on the basis of which he writes his report. Where there is a range of professional opinion on the matters dealt with in the report, the expert should summarize the range of opinion and give reasons for his own views.

No party may call an expert or put an expert's report in evidence without the permission of the court. The court has a duty to restrict expert evidence unless it is reasonably required to resolve the proceedings. The aim of the new rules is to encourage the parties to agree on one expert on whom both will rely. The court has power to direct that only one expert report is necessary and may select the expert if the parties cannot agree on a name. It is very likely that the parties will find that they are refused leave to call any oral expert evidence in circumstances where hitherto there would have been no opposition, especially in fast-track claims.

These major changes in the rules of civil procedure are too new to permit a comprehensive evaluation. The expert witness should note that, if he is in difficulty, he may seek guidance from the court without giving notice to any party.

LEGAL LIABILITY OF THE EXPERT WITNESS

No-one can be liable for defamation or negligence in respect of anything said in the course of judicial proceedings, which are protected by absolute privilege. In *Watson v M'Ewan*[16] the House of Lords held that this privilege also protects a witness against the consequences of statements he makes to the client and his lawyers when preparing for trial. However, a distinction needs to be made between the work of the expert witness and his work as an adviser prior to the decision to commence legal proceedings. Privilege attaches to the investigation and preparation of evidence in criminal proceedings, but apparently not to pre-action proceedings in a civil suit.

In *Hughes v Lloyds Bank plc* (1998)[17] the plaintiff was injured in a road accident. She attended her general practitioner (who had since died and was represented in court by the administrators of his estate). The general practitioner had been asked by the plaintiff to report on the severity of her injuries for the purposes of a claim for compensation. He had written that the condition was not serious, on the faith of which the plaintiff settled her claim for £600. It then became apparent that the injury was far more severe than the general practitioner had predicted. The plaintiff sued the doctor for negligence. The Court of Appeal held that he was not immune from legal proceedings. When he made his report he was not an expert witness, merely a paid adviser at a preliminary stage. If he had failed to take reasonable care he could be sued for compensation.

REFERENCES

1 [1975] 1 All ER 70
2 [1985] 2 All ER 385
3 [1980] AC 521. It should be noted that a medical report disclosed accidentally can be used by the receiving party at trial: *Pizzey v Ford Motor Co Ltd* (1993) Times 8 March.
4 [1981] 3 All ER 866
5 [1981] 3 All ER 869
6 Kemp and Kemp (eds) *The Quantum of Damages* (looseleaf). London: Sweet and Maxwell.
7 20 July 1979, unreported
8 [1987] 2 All ER 353
9 [1990] 1 All ER 835
10 [1991] 1 All ER 638
11 [1984] QB 405
12 *Access to Justice*. Final Report by Lord Woolf MR to the Lord Chancellor on the civil justice system in England and Wales. London: HMSO, 1996: 139, 140.
13 [1981] 1 WLR 246
14 [1997] 1 All ER 614
15 *op. cit.* at p. 150.
16 [1905] AC 480; Evans v London Hospital [1981] 1 W.L.R. 184; X v Bedfordshire County Council [1995] 2 AC 633.
17 [1998] PIQR 98

Part 2

Diseases associated with chemical agents

Absorption of chemicals and mechanisms of
    detoxification   67
Metals   81
Gases   123
Welding, fumes and inhalational fevers   179
Pesticides and other agrochemicals   195
Aliphatic chemicals   221
Aromatic chemicals   261

Absorption of chemicals and mechanisms of detoxification

PETER G BLAIN

Absorption and distribution of chemicals	68	Detoxification and elimination	72
Toxicokinetics	68	Summary	77
Kinetics of exposure	71	References	78

Many occupational physicians are involved in assessing the health risks associated with exposure to chemicals in the workplace. More and more this responsibility tends to include the public environment. Frequent reaction to chemicals in the environment is a necessity for any living organism and human beings are no exception. A range of complex biochemical mechanisms has evolved for protection against absorbed compounds that may be toxic. Whenever there is a risk of exposure to hazardous chemicals, it is important that the factors affecting the absorption and distribution of chemicals in the body and the processes involved in detoxification are taken into consideration. An understanding of toxicology (the study of 'poisons') is essential for occupational physicians in their role as health risk managers or when they investigate the exposure of workers to hazardous chemicals. Toxicology is growing rapidly as a science and demonstrates increasing relevance to the activities of health care professionals. A range of standard reference texts is now available.[1]

Paracelsus is credited with first recognizing the association between absorbed dose and toxicity – the dose–response relationship.[2] Whilst he undoubtedly

understood the concept of potency, his comments on the relationship of toxic effect to the amount of chemical ingested were, in fact, intended to increase consumer confidence in the safety of novel remedies that he was marketing!

The dose–response relationship is a useful indicator of the toxicity of a chemical. Toxic doses in man may range from μg to g/kg body weight and chemicals are sometimes classified according to the probable lethal human dose (Table 6.1).

In addition to intrinsic toxicity and mode of action, the dynamics of absorption, metabolism, distribution and elimination are important variables in the development of a toxic effect. Exposure in the workplace environment may be to many different chemicals and it is relevant to the practice of occupational medicine that hazardous situations are recognized and information on the absorption and detoxification of chemicals is considered alongside a detailed knowledge of their potential toxic effects.

An additional factor is that within the general population there may be interindividual variation in specific

Table 6.1 *Toxicity rating of chemicals by probable lethal oral dose in adults*

Toxicity rating	Lethal oral dose	Typical volume
1. Practically non-toxic	>15 g/kg	More than 1 quart
2. Slightly toxic	5–15 g/kg	Between pint and quart
3. Moderately toxic	0.5–5 g/kg	Between ounce and pint
4. Very toxic	50–500 mg/kg	Between teaspoonful and ounce
5. Extremely toxic	5–50 mg/kg	Between 7 drops and teaspoonful
6. Supertoxic	<5 mg/kg	A taste (less than 7 drops)

enzyme activities which may be markedly different (greater or lesser) than expected. These variations constitute subgroups or genetic polymorphisms in a population; some are small in size (poor metabolizers of debrisoquine constitute about 10% of the general population) or large (the general population are more or less equally divided into either fast or slow acetylators). Subgroups with greater activity may produce toxic metabolites more rapidly (fast acetylators are more likely to develop isoniazid hepatotoxicity), whereas poor metabolizers may be at risk because they are unable to detoxify a chemical adequately (slow acetylators are more likely to develop an isoniazid neuropathy and poor debrisoquine metabolizers a perhexiline neuropathy). The role of interindividual variation in susceptibility to toxicity requires more general consideration, since, in certain combinations of circumstances, it may contribute to the 'dirty worker' phenomenon. At present most work on genetic polymorphisms relates to drug metabolism and toxicity but it is anticipated that relevance to non-drug chemicals will become increasingly obvious.

Within species differences in susceptibility are usually of a lesser magnitude than the variation between species. Most toxicity data are derived from animal toxicity tests and the models generated applied to man. Apart from the ethical considerations related to this use of animals, serious scientific problems may arise in extrapolating from animal models to human health risks. Ideally, data generated from animals should be supplemented with information derived from human studies.

ABSORPTION AND DISTRIBUTION OF CHEMICALS

Foreign or exogenous chemicals (xenobiotics) must be absorbed from the surrounding environment and transported to their target site in the body for a toxic effect to occur. The chemical has to cross the many cell membranes which form a lipoprotein barrier to the outside as well as maintaining the integrity of the cell. The specific transport mechanisms that have evolved are to facilitate the absorption and distribution of nutrients rather than toxic chemicals. Consequently, most xenobiotics are transported by simple methods and not complex carrier-associated processes (exceptions do occur such as paraquat transport into lung cells[3]). A carrier is usually specific for an endogenous substance and unless the xenobiotic compound has a very similar structure it will not usually be able to bind to the carrier (cf paraquat and the carrier for endogenous diamines such as putrescine[4]).

Lipid solubility is one of the major factors determining the extent and rate of simple diffusion through a lipoprotein membrane. Lipophilic molecules diffuse more readily than those that are hydrophilic, the rate of transport being dependent on the partition coefficient (i.e. the ratio of solubility in octanol/water). Non-ionized molecules are often more lipophilic and ions generally more hydrophilic, so that the movement of electrolytes, such as organic acids and bases, is related to the degree of ionic dissociation and the lipid solubility of the non-ionized form of the compound.

The extent of dissociation is expressed by the Henderson–Hasselbach equation:

for an acid: $\qquad pK_a - pH = \log \dfrac{Cu}{Ci}$

for a base: $\qquad pK_a - pH = \log \dfrac{Ci}{Cu}$

where Cu is the concentration of the non-ionized form,
Ci is the concentration of the ionized form
pK_a is the negative log of the dissociation constant.

The cell membrane controls the movement of chemicals in or out of the cytoplasm and several methods have been identified by which xenobiotics are transported across membranes:

- *Simple diffusion* down a concentration gradient is the most common and simple method, does not require expenditure of energy and is the principal mechanism for the transport of most lipid soluble, non-ionized compounds.
- *Filtration* allows water, ionic and hydrophilic molecules of appropriate size to pass through small pores (about 0.4nm in diameter) in the cell membrane.
- *Facilitated diffusion* is carrier-mediated, transports chemicals with specific common structures across the cell membrane and at high concentrations may become saturated.
- *Active transport* allows the absorption of substances against a concentration gradient but requires the expenditure of energy and so is linked to the metabolic activity of the cell.
- *Phagocytosis and pinocytosis* enable particulates and solutions to be taken into a cell by the extrusion or invagination of an area of the membrane and engulfing of part of the extracellular environment.

These absorption processes, although at a cellular level, influence the degree and nature of absorption through the lungs, skin and gastrointestinal tract and are, therefore, relevant at the macro level of hazard assessment.

TOXICOKINETICS

The investigation and management of a patient exposed to toxic chemicals requires at least a basic knowledge of the concepts of toxicokinetics alongside an understanding of the mechanisms by which chemicals gain entry to the body and are biotransformed into non-toxic or, occasionally, toxic metabolites. Toxicokinetics is the study of the dynamic (kinetic) relationships between the concentration of a chemical (toxicon) in body fluids and tissues and its biological effects. Toxicokinetic analysis produces a mathematical description of the dynamics of absorption, distribution and elimination of a chemical. Although involving the descriptive use of mathematical expressions and models it has a practical value in that the understanding can be used to evaluate the significance of blood concentrations in biological monitoring and to determine the nature of exposure control (i.e. risk management). (*Pharmacokinetic* analysis quantifies the dynamic changes in the concentration of a drug (*pharmacon*) and has been incorporated into toxicokinetics since there are no fundamental differences between a drug and a toxin – the major toxic effect of a drug is often the main reason for its therapeutic use.)

The kinetic profile of a chemical can be used to estimate the *body burden* after workplace exposure and to predict the time required for near total elimination of a chemical from the body. Similarly, the rate at which a compound is absorbed or eliminated from the body can be quantified and applied to occupational health practice.[5,6]

Toxicokinetic concepts

The body is composed of a multitude of real 'compartments' in the form of cells, tissues and organs. However, the analysis of kinetic data necessarily models a limited number of theoretical compartments. These models are one solution to the analysis of data but it must always be remembered that models are fitted to data rather than data to models. It is sometimes difficult to be sure that a specific model accurately describes the processes involved; one method of checking is to perturb the model and see if the outcome follows the effects of a similar change in the real world (e.g. decreased ventilation, hepatic metabolism, renal blood flow etc.). Toxicokinetic concepts have led to the development of complex multi-compartment models for the absorption, distribution and elimination of chemicals by the body. The simplest of these is a single compartment model which considers the body as a homogeneous unit. More sophisticated analysis uses two, three or occasionally more, compartmental models (see Fig. 6.1).

The rate of absorption (k_{abs}) is dependent on several parameters that are often difficult to measure individually so that in the initial analysis of blood concentration data the rate of elimination (k_{el}) is determined since this often appears to be a simpler process (e.g. via the kidney). The majority of chemical substances are eliminated from blood by an *apparent* first-order process which is seen as an *exponential decay* (see Fig. 6.2) and described by the mathematical equation:

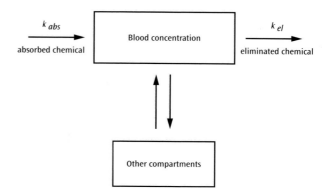

Figure 6.1 *Compartmental model.*

$$Ct = C_0.e^{-\beta t}$$

where C_t = plasma concentration at time t

C_0 = plasma concentration at $t = 0$
e = natural number (2.7182)
β = elimination rate constant (K_{el})

The elimination of some chemicals (e.g. phenytoin, ethanol) is non-linear and demonstrates zero order (saturation) kinetics. In *first-order* kinetics a constant fraction of the chemical is eliminated in unit time. In *zero-order* kinetics a constant mass of the chemical is eliminated in unit time and consequently the process can be saturated and toxic effects occur following a very small increase in dose.

The *half life* ($t_{1/2}$) of a chemical is the time period during which the blood concentration decreases by one-half and is inversely related to the elimination rate constant (β):

$$t_{1/2} = 0.693/\beta$$

(where 0.693 is $\log_e$ (ln) 2)

The half-life can be determined from the slope (elimination rate) of the log plasma concentration/time graph following a single dose of a compound (Fig. 6.2).

The concept of a half-life is useful for studying the uptake and elimination of compounds since it can be shown that after 3.3 half-lives the plasma concentration reaches 90% of the equilibrium concentration, and 95% after 5 half-lives. Hence $5 \times t_{1/2}$ is the time taken for 95% of a dose of chemical to be eliminated from the body after absorption, or to reach 95% of its steady-state value. The half-life is also the minimum time interval between chemical exposure (or drug administration) that avoids progressive accumulation. Data about the elimination half-life of a compound can be used to assess the importance of the duration of exposure and increase the value of either blood or breath monitoring of exposed workers.

The *volume of distribution* (V_D) is a theoretical estimate of the extent of the distribution of a chemical in the

Exponential decay curve for chemical elimination

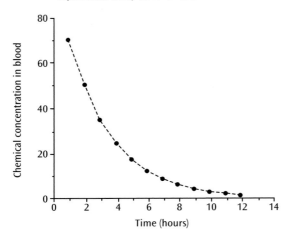

Exponential decay curve linearized by using log scale

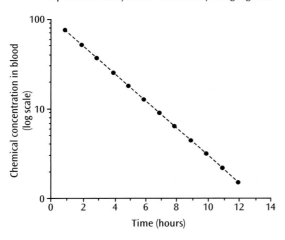

Figure 6.2 *Elimination of a chemical from blood by a first-order process. The rate of elimination is linearized when log values for Ct are used.*

body and provides a measure of the relative magnitude of differential tissue uptake.

V_D is expressed in units of litres or litres/kg:

$$V_D = \chi/C$$

where

χ = total amount of chemical = body burden (if bioavailability is 100%)
C = plasma concentration at t_0

Compounds with a large volume of distribution are widely and extensively distributed throughout the tissues

of the body and the plasma concentration constitutes a small fraction of the total body burden. A small volume of distribution implies limited tissue distribution and indicates that the plasma concentration is a good indicator of the total amount in the body (chemicals with a V_D approximating to blood volume (3–5 litre) are almost totally restricted to systemic circulation); V_D is apparent and not real so that a chemical which is concentrated in a tissue (such as fat) and has a low blood concentration, will have a high V_D that may markedly exceed the total volume of the body (e.g. >200 litre for some organic solvents).

Clearance (*Cl*) is the volume of the V_D that is completely cleared of a chemical per unit time (i.e. ml/min, litre/hour). Clearance is a more independent measure of elimination than half-life since it is a physiologically meaningful measure of the efficiency of elimination from the body. It provides the most reliable measurement of the elimination of a compound since clearance by a particular organ can be estimated (similar to renal clearance of insulin etc.).

In simple terms:

$$Cl = V_D \times k_{el}$$

Changes in the V_D may alter the $t_{1/2}$ but leave clearance unaltered. Chemicals with a large V_D may have a high clearance yet persist in the body and have a long $t_{1/2}$ of elimination.

The total systemic clearance is dependent on the specific clearances of each organ:

$$Cl_{systemic} = Cl_{renal} + Cl_{hepatic} + Cl_{other\ routes}$$

The clearance of a chemical by an organ (Cl_{organ}) can be measured and is principally dependent on blood flow and the degree of extraction (ER) of the chemical from blood:

$$Cl_{organ} = Q \times ER$$

where
Q = organ blood flow
ER = extraction ratio

The extraction ratio (*ER*) is determined from the arterial and venous concentration difference across an organ:

$$ER = \frac{CA - CV}{CA}$$

where
CA = concentration in blood flowing into organ (arterial)
CV = concentration in blood flowing out of organ (venous)

For those organs with a high *ER* (e.g. liver, kidney), clearance will be high and directly dependent on organ blood flow. Chemicals with a high liver clearance undergo extensive first-pass metabolism (e.g. nitrites). Organs with a low *ER* (e.g. muscle, bone) have a clearance that is not dependent on blood flow.

KINETICS OF EXPOSURE

The principal routes of exposure in the workplace are by inhalation or skin absorption.

Inhalation kinetics

The lungs enable the efficient transfer of gases between the body and the environment. The tissue barrier separating air and blood is only 0.5–1.0µ thick and the 300–400 million alveoli provide a large surface area for diffusion. In addition, the media on either side of this barrier are being continuously renewed; the air is changed 12–15 times per minute and the pulmonary blood flows at a rate of 3.5–5 litre per minute at rest. It is not surprising, therefore, that volatile chemicals can be efficiently both absorbed from and eliminated in the breath.[7]

Analysis of expired air has been used to diagnose diabetes and uraemia and more recently to detect ethanol in the blood of motorists (although only about 1% of the total body burden of ethanol is eliminated via this route). Real-time monitoring of the breath of workers exposed to volatile compounds in industry is a potentially useful non-invasive technique for determining the degree of absorption, but does require that the factors affecting the absorption, distribution, metabolism and elimination (i.e. the toxicokinetics) of compounds have been previously determined for this route in man.[8]

A number of volatile organic compounds can be identified in the breath of the normal general population[9,10] at concentrations of parts per billion; in industrial workers the concentrations are generally in parts per million; in hospital practice the inhalation kinetics of volatile compounds are of importance to the anaesthetist. Breath analysis has been used in experimental toxicology to study lipid peroxidation and in the investigation of defective intestinal absorption, but monitoring of marker metabolites in the expired breath remains a relatively unexploited technique (see Chapter 2). However, there is recent renewed interest in the diagnostic potential of breath monitoring in certain disease states.

In routine monitoring of the workplace the level of contamination of air with a compound is measured and assumed to be an indicator of exposure and, by implication, absorption. However, this is not a direct relationship; the environmental concentration merely indicates the potential for absorption. Under continuous exposure any change in the inhaled air concentration will have a corresponding effect on the alveolar air concentration. Increasing the duration of exposure produces a progressive increase in blood concentration towards a plateau value (equilibrium). A progressive saturation of blood and tissues with the compound involves a reduction in the difference between arterial and venous blood with less of the inhaled compound moving from the alveoli to capillary blood. For volatile compounds that are highly lipophilic and selectively taken up by fatty tissues, tissue saturation is never reached in the normal period of exposure in the workplace. In contrast, the elimination of such compounds from the body is extremely slow and the potential exists for progressive accumulation following frequent modest exposures.[11]

Other factors influencing the inhalation kinetics of a volatile compound include the environmental air concentration, duration of exposure, rate of alveolar ventilation, cardiac output, blood and tissue solubility and the degree of metabolism of the chemical. Volatile compounds are usually inhaled as a gas mixture with air and most are completely miscible in all proportions. The concentration of gases and volatile compounds in a mixture is expressed in terms of partial pressures, which often have been wrongly considered equivalent to concentrations; the relative concentrations of dissolved materials can be expressed in terms of partial pressures which add up to a total pressure of 100%. However, a limit is set on the concentration (wt/unit vol) which this represents by the solubility of the volatile materials. Solubility is inversely related to temperature and proportional to the pressure of the chemical in the surrounding gas. The partial pressures of constituent volatile compounds vary with the absolute pressure but, at a fixed pressure, the concentration of each gas or vapour varies directly with its partial pressure and indirectly with the total pressure of the gas/vapour mixture. A gas or vapour present at a partial pressures of 100% can still have its concentration (wt/unit vol) varied over a range that is determined by the absolute pressure.

The rate of delivery of an inhaled mixture of air and a volatile compound depends upon alveolar ventilation. A doubling of alveolar ventilation from 4 litre/min to 8 litre/min produces a minimal increase in the blood concentration of a poorly water soluble substance but an appreciable increase for highly water soluble substances. Cardiac output has an opposing effect on alveolar concentration and this is most noticeable for highly water soluble or extensively metabolized substances rather than poorly soluble compounds. An increase in cardiac output results in a larger amount of the inhaled substance passing from the lungs to the blood. A decrease has the opposite result and causes a rise in alveolar concentration.[12]

An insoluble substance that does not pass into the blood stream will increase in alveolar concentration until it is equal to the environmental air concentration, the time taken being equivalent to the lung wash-in time. A substance with an infinite solubility could in theory never increase the alveolar concentration and, although such substances do not exist, there is a broad range of solubilites. The concentration in alveolar or expired air, expressed relative to the environmental air concentration is inversely proportional to the blood solubility of a compound. Relative concentrations of >0.5 are poorly soluble and those <0.5 are highly soluble. The effect of solubility on alveolar concentration is seen in Fig. 6.3.

The aerodynamic particle sizes of aerosols, mists and sprays also affect their accessibility to alveoli and often large particles are deposited in the larger airways or in the pharynx and swallowed.

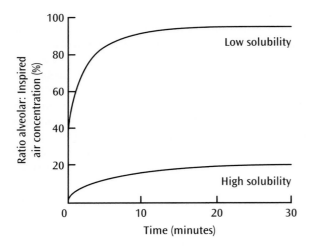

Figure 6.3 *Effect of solubility on the alveolar concentration of a chemical.*

The arterial concentration of an inhaled compound can be estimated from the alveolar concentration using the blood-air partition coefficient of the chemical (if partial pressure equilibrium is attained rapidly). This is not attained immediately but requires a finite time that depends on the half-life of the compound:

$$t_{1/2} = 0.693 \, V . \frac{Pc}{F}$$

Where
V is the tissue volume
Pc is the tissue-blood partition coefficient
F the rate of blood flow to the tissue

A high relative alveolar concentration is found for compounds that undergo little metabolism. As the degree of biotransformation increases so does the level of metabolites in pulmonary blood. The combined effects of metabolism and solubility affect the blood kinetics of a chemical. Extensive metabolism can significantly undermine the usefulness of biological monitoring of exhaled breath, unless a volatile marker metabolite predominates and there is no phenotypic variation in biotransformation within the population.

Routine measurement of the breath concentrations of industrial or therapeutic chemicals is poorly utilized for monitoring exposure or assessing body burden. Rigorous kinetic analysis is essential to establish its value and reliability as a non-invasive method of assessment. The necessary technology is widely available and simply requires more consideration.

Dermal absorption

The skin is an effective barrier to many environmental chemicals because the stratum corneum, acting to control the loss of water from the body, also functions as the principal barrier to dermal penetration by chemicals.[13] Direct absorption through the skin is a major route of exposure to pesticides and other workplace chemicals and accidental skin contamination by spillage or deposition on the skin surface may be followed by rapid systemic absorption. The lipid solubility of a chemical determines how easily it can cross the stratum corneum, the epidermis and upper dermis and enter the systemic circulation. Direct absorption through skin is utilized for those pharmaceutical compounds which are rapidly metabolized by first-pass metabolism in the gut wall or liver following oral administration. The drug, in a suitable formulation, is applied to the skin, enters the systemic circulation directly bypassing initial first-pass metabolism in the liver.

Dermal absorption has been considered a passive process limited only by the physical barrier function of the stratum corneum. The skin, however, is capable of metabolizing a range of xenobiotics and studies with whole skin homogenates and subcellular fractions have demonstrated significant metabolic activity, albeit less than that found in liver (about 10%). Mono-oxygenases, conjugation pathways and esterase activity have been identified. Consequently many compounds that penetrate the stratum corneum may undergo biotransformation to active metabolites before entering the systemic circulation. Some limited *in vivo* studies have indicated that metabolism takes place in the skin *in vivo* during absorption (e.g. aldrin, glycerol trinitrate and synthetic prostaglandins). However, reliable *in vitro* methods for modelling *in vivo* absorption processes are still required. Such models would predict the significance of dermal exposure in man. *In vitro* systems using animal tissue have been designed to simulate *in vivo* absorption profiles but involve the skin being in contact with a receptor fluid such as an ethanol/water mixture into which the penetrating chemical dissolves.[14] More recently this static cell model has been adapted into a flow through cell system that more closely simulates intact skin. These *in vitro* systems produce data for a number of compounds that are comparable with observed *in vivo* absorption both in animals and man.[15,16]

DETOXIFICATION AND ELIMINATION

Most toxic xenobiotics have no nutritional value and are metabolized primarily to reduce potential toxicity and facilitate their elimination from the body. The majority of compounds that gain entry most easily to the body are lipophilic and likely, therefore, to be retained and before they can be excreted must be converted into a form that is more easily eliminated. The liver is the major organ for the metabolism (biotransformation) of such compounds. There is, however, increasing evidence that other organs such as the skin, lungs, kidney and skeletal muscle may have a significant capability for biotransformation, albeit at a lower level of activity than the liver (Table 6.2). Detoxification does not always occur and, for some chemicals, toxicity may be enhanced as a result of biotransformation.

The metabolism of xenobiotics is carried out by a group of relatively non-specific enzymes. The key enzyme in this system is cytochrome P450, the active site of which contains an iron atom that can change between divalent and trivalent oxidation states. This enzyme combines with the substrate and molecular oxygen as part of the process through which the substrate is oxidized. The group of enzymes are classified as mixed function oxidases, the specific oxidizing enzyme, cytochrome P450, having a characteristic peak in the reduced form at 450nm in a carbon monoxide adduct difference spectrum. The enzyme requires an electron transport chain for its reduction which consists of a flavoprotein enzyme, cytochrome c reductase (cytochrome P450 reductase) that transfers e^- from the flavine to cytochrome P450. Cytochrome c reductase requires NADPH as a coenzyme; microsomal oxidation requires both NADPH and O_2. Cytochrome P450 exists as a family of isoenzymes with differing and overlapping specificities and more than eight gene families have been identified.[17,18]

Cytochrome P450 is abundant in the liver, which is the primary site of defence against systemic poisons, but may occur in other parts of the body such as the kidney, ovaries, testes and olfactory mucosa. The presence of the enzyme in the lungs, skin and gastrointestinal tract may reflect a defensive role in these organs against toxic xenobiotics. Oxidase enzyme activity is mainly associated with the smooth endoplasmic reticulum (ER). When tissues, such as liver, are homogenized the ER is broken down to form small vesicles known as microsomes. Microsomes are the fraction collected from centrifugation of tissue homogenate at about 100 000 g and essentially contain the rough and smooth endoplasmic reticulum and Golgi apparatus. There is evidence that the microsomal enzymes are associated with a lipid membrane and are lipid-dependent. Sonic vibration or the use of hypotonic solutions fail to solubilize them, whilst the treatment of microsomes with deoxycholic acid, which solubilizes lipid membranes, destroys the activity of oxidative enzymes.

Biotransformation of xenobiotics usually consists of two phases; phase 1, which involves oxidation (via the cytochrome P450-dependent mixed function oxygenases), reduction or hydrolysis of the parent compound and phase 2, in which the metabolite is conjugated to glucuronic acid, glutathione, glycine, sulphate or some other endogenous compound

In phase 1 a polar reactive group is introduced into the molecule to increase water solubility and make the compound suitable for phase 2 where the altered molecule is combined with an endogenous substrate to produce a water soluble conjugate that is more readily excreted in the urine. Consequently, the principal function of biotransformation is to facilitate the elimination of a foreign agent by its conversion to a more polar (water soluble) metabolite and is, therefore, a detoxification mechanism. In some cases the intermediate metabolites or final products may be more toxic than the parent compound (i.e. an entoxification). Such metabolites may be systemically toxic or, because they are produced locally by an organ, have toxic effects in the tissue of biotransformation. Most cells, particularly in the liver, have protective biochemical systems to prevent damage to vital cell processes from locally produced toxic metabolites.

Phase 1 reactions

Phase 1 metabolic transformations may result in the formation of compounds with a variety of properties

Table 6.2 *Comparative capability for biotransformation*

Organ	Approximate comparative capability for biotransformation of foreign agents (% relative to activity of liver)
Liver	100
Adrenal cortex	75
Lungs	30
Kidney	30
Testes	20
Skin	10
Gastrointestinal tract	10
Spleen	5
Heart muscle	3
Skeletal muscle	1

depending on whether toxicity has been increased or decreased.

INCREASED TOXICITY

Parathion, an organophosphate pesticide, is relatively non-toxic to man and in insects is rapidly metabolized (activated) by desulphuration to paraoxon, a potent cholinesterase inhibitor. There is some evidence for variability in man of parathion activation by P450 and of the activity of the enzyme, paraoxonase, which further metabolizes the paraoxon.[19]

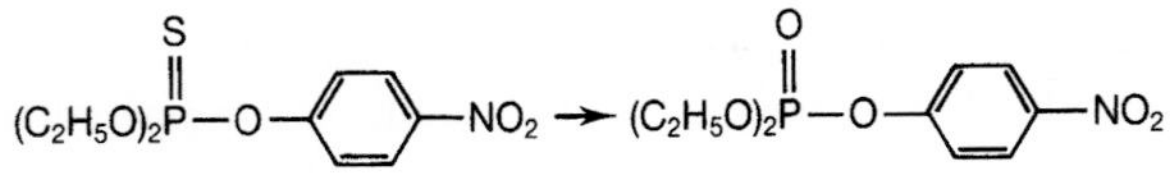

Parathion   Paraoxon

Although biochemical activation may present some human hazard, it can have a useful application in the development of new pesticides or pro-drugs that are converted into active products by metabolic transformation.

DECREASED TOXICITY

Phenobarbitone is detoxified by hydroxylation of the aromatic ring to form parahydroxyphenobarbitone. Amphetamines are similarly detoxified by aromatic hydroxylation to parahydroxyamphetamines and by deamination to a benzyl methyl ketone. Both of these metabolites are less active than the parent compound.

Specific chemical reactions can occur in phase 1 metabolism:

Epoxidation

Epoxidation is the insertion of an oxygen atom between two carbon atoms. It is an important mechanism for the initial metabolism of aromatic compounds and cytochrome P450 is involved. This reaction may increase the toxicity of the parent compound but many epoxides are unstable and undergo further reactions such as hydroxylation. Unstable epoxides are often toxic because they bind to proteins and other macromolecules. For example, vinyl chloride is converted to an intermediate, chlorethylene oxide, which spontaneously transforms to chloracetaldehyde. The two metabolites are mutagens and considered to act as proximate carcinogens.

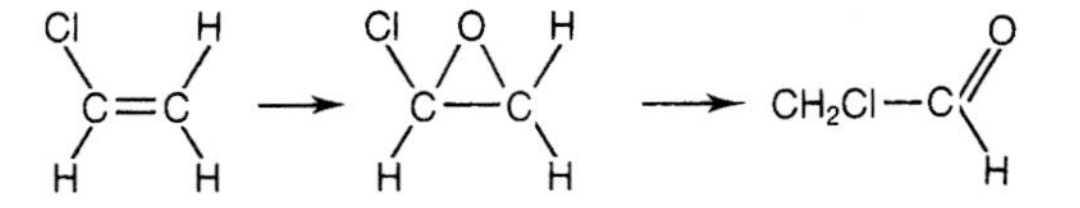

Vinyl chloride   Chlorethylene oxide   Chloracetaldehyde

Since both of these intermediates can bind directly with cellular macromolecules, such as DNA and proteins, it might be anticipated that local hepatic biotransformation of vinyl chloride would be associated with liver damage. Many epidemiological studies have confirmed the association of chronic vinyl chloride exposure with the development of a hepatic angiosarcoma, an otherwise rare primary liver cancer. Carcinogenicity appeared to follow chronic exposure to relatively low levels of vinyl chloride (50–100 ppm or less). Chronic exposure to higher levels of exposure (500–1000 ppm) was more commonly associated with serious hepatotoxicity, the hepatocytes dying before malignant transformation could occur. Vinyl chloride-induced angiosarcoma of the liver appears to have a latency of between 15 and 40 years. As a result of stringent workplace controls limiting exposure to below 1 ppm, vinyl chloride-associated diseases are now rarely seen (see Chapters 8, 43).

Another example of epoxide formation is the conversion of the pesticide aldrin to dieldrin, a stable epoxide.

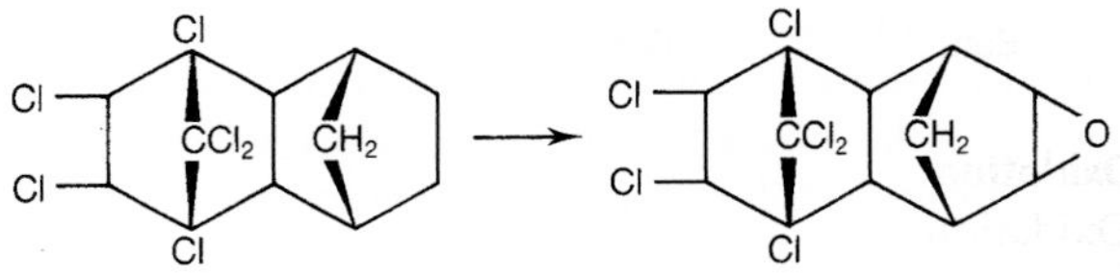

Aldrin   Dieldrin

Hydroxylation

Hydroxylation is the attachment of a hydroxyl group to hydrocarbon chains or rings and may follow epoxidation. One example is the metabolism of benzene epoxide, an intermediate in the biotransformation of benzene, to phenol.

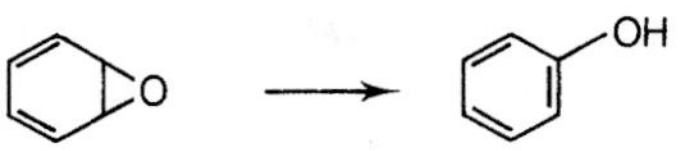

Benzene epoxide   Phenol

Benzene is initially metabolized by oxidation, primarily in the liver, with phenol as the major metabolite. Other metabolites that can be formed by hydroxylation of the aromatic ring include hydroquinone, catechol and 1,2,4-trihydroxybenzene. These hydroxylated metabolites can be further oxidized to quinones and semiquinones. Urinary excretion of muconic acid, a short chain dicarboxylic acid, suggests that the benzene ring may be opened by biotransformation.

The principal target organ for benzene toxicity is bone marrow. Marrow cells contain peroxidases and mixed function oxidases capable of metabolizing benzene. The metabolites produced may bind covalently to cell macromolecules causing disruption of cell growth and replication. The specific target of benzene is probably the DNA in the pluripotential stem cells and lymphocytic cells. Cytogenetic abnormalities of bone marrow cells and circulating lymphocytes have been observed in workers exposed to benzene. Myelodysplasia may be seen in the bone marrow of individuals with chronic exposure to benzene. Benzene-induced leukaemia has a latency period of 5–15 years and in many cases is preceded by an aplastic anaemia (see Chapter 44).

Hydroxylation may involve the addition of one or more epoxide groups and both reactions are responsible for making several xenobiotic compounds more toxic such as the production of the carcinogenic 7,8-diol-9,10-epoxide of benzo[a]pyrene. Benzo[a]pyrene is classified, therefore, as a procarcinogen since metabolic activation is required to convert it to a carcinogenic species.

Benzo[a]pyrene   Benzo[a]pyrene-7,8-diol-9,10-epoxide

Oxidation

Oxidation of nitrogen, sulphur or phosphorus is another important metabolic reaction in biotransformation that may increase toxicity. The oxidation of nitrogen in 2-acetylaminofluorene produces the carcinogen *N*-hydroxy-2-acetylaminofluorene.

2-Acetylaminofluorene (AAF)   *N*-Hydroxy-2-acetylaminofluorene

In parathion the oxidative desulphuration of phosphorus produces paraoxon which is more effective than the parent compound as an inhibitor of acetyl-cholinesterase (see above).

Dealkylation

Dealkylation is the removal of an alkyl group (such as a methyl group) and its replacement by a hydrogen atom. The reactions are carried out by mixed function oxidases. Examples include O-dealkylation of methoxychlor insecticides, N-dealkylation of the insecticide carbaryl, and S-dealkylation of dimethyl mercaptan.

Reduction

Reduction of some of the major functional groups in xenobiotics is carried out by reductases. Examples include the reduction of nitro groups by nitroreductases which are found mainly in the liver but to a lesser extent in other organs such as the lung and kidney. They may occur also in intestinal bacteria and reduction of xenobiotics may take place locally in the intestinal tract (e.g. dinitrotoluene).

Hydrolysis

Hydrolysis is the addition of water to a molecule preceding its division into two chemical species. Two types of compounds that undergo hydrolysis are esters (such as organophosphates) and amines many of which are pesticides. Hydrolases occur predominantly in the liver, but also in the gastrointestinal tract, nervous tissue, blood, kidney and muscle. Aromatic esters are hydrolysed by the action of aryl esterases and alkyl esters by carboxy-lesterases (an example being the metabolism of synthetic pyrethroids). Esterases were originally subdivided into A, B, or C esterases on the basis of their interaction with organophosphates.[20]

Depending on their degree of water solubility the products of metabolic transformation are either excreted directly or undergo further metabolism by conjugation (phase 2 reaction).

Phase 2 reactions

In phase 2 reactions the functional groups on a molecule (e.g. carboxyl, amino, hydroxyl and sulphydryl groups) are conjugated with endogenous compounds such as glutathione, glucuronic acid, amino acids (e.g. glycine) or sugars to form water soluble, polar derivatives that can be more readily excreted and are less toxic. A reduction in lipid solubility decreases the ability to diffuse back across membranes.

Conjugation with glucuronic acid is the most important and most common mechanism. The enzyme UDP-glucuronyltransferase catalyses the transfer of glucuronic acid from uridine diphosphate glucuronic acid. Glucuronide conjugation products are classified by the site of bindings; a hydroxyl functional group forms an ether glucuronide, a carboxyl acid group an ester glucuronide. Glucuronides may be attached directly to nitrogen as the linking atom (e.g. aniline glucuronide) or through an intermediate oxygen atom such as occurs in the conjugation product in *N*-hydroxyacetylaminoglucuronide. In contrast to the usual decrease in toxicity that results from glucuronide conjugation, this is a more potent carcinogen than the parent compound, *N*-hydroxyacetylaminofluorene.

Glutathione, a tripeptide of glutamic acid, cysteine and glycine, is another endogenous compound used in phase 2 reactions. The thiol groups (SH) groups in glutathione form covalent bonds with xenobiotic compounds and glutathione conjugates may be excreted directly or after further metabolism to mercapturic acids (compounds with *N*-acetylcysteine attached). The enzyme glutathione transferase is generally required for the conjugation process and is found throughout the body.

Sulphate conjugates are completely ionized, and therefore highly efficient in eliminating xenobiotics in the urine. The major species that form sulphate conjugates are alcohols, phenols and arylamines. Phenols are conjugated with either glucuronic acid or sulphate to form phenol glucuronide and phenol sulphate. Sulphation is a saturable pathway and so may have limited capacity for detoxification.

Other reactions can occur; acetyltransferase involves acetylation such as in the final step in the production of a mercapturic acid conjugates, amino acids, such as glycine, form peptide conjugates. Some compounds, such as salicylic acid, can be metabolized by several different mechanisms as well as glucuronide conjugation. Cyanide is detoxified by conjugation with sulphur to form thiocyanate (which can be monitored in blood or urine).

Most compounds undergo both metabolic transformation and conjugation but occasionally only one of these reactions. Biotransformation may produce a metabolite that is sufficiently water soluble to be easily excreted so that conjugation may not be necessary. If the compound already possesses groups which will easily conjugate then phase 1 metabolism may not be required.

OTHER MECHANISMS

Some xenobiotics are detoxified by linkage to a large molecule, such as a protein. This produces a complex that is less toxic and which can be stored in the body. Metallothionein, a low molecular weight cysteine rich protein, binds to heavy metals such as cadmium, zinc and copper and is found in high concentrations in the liver and kidneys.

Other sites of xenobiotic biotransformation

The liver is not always the most important site of metabolism. Reactions can occur in extrahepatic sites as a result of the activity of both microsomal and non-microsomal enzymes. For example, microsomal UDP-glucuronyltransferase is found in skin and the gastrointestinal tract. Many non-microsomal enzymes occur in plasma, the gastrointestinal tract, lungs and kidneys. Alcohol dehydrogenase in the liver, kidney and lungs oxidizes an alcohol to its aldehyde and a number of amino-oxidases and esterases are found in plasma. Bacterial flora in the gut may also have a role in xenobiotic metabolism (see **Reduction**, section on p. 75) and their first-pass metabolism by this route of exposure.

If these metabolic reactions did not occur then xenobiotics of high lipid solubility would remain and accumulate in the body with the resultant risk of toxicity. A more detailed review of the principles of biochemical toxicology can be found in standard texts.[21]

Pulmonary biotransformation

Over 40 histologically different cell types have been identified in the lungs but the susceptibility of a lung cell to toxic compounds or metabolites depends partly upon the specific biochemical activity of that cell.[22] The lungs may be the target organ for toxicity and, in some cases, there is a selective toxicity to a particular type of lung cell.[23] The level of metabolic activity of a cell depends upon its degree of specialization and the nature of the enzymes and substrates.

The lung is capable of metabolizing many xenobiotics by both phase 1 and phase 2 reactions.[24] The non-ciliated bronchiolar or Clara cell is the most metabolically active lung cell and has a high activity of mixed-function oxidases.[25] The mycotoxin 4-ipomeanol has been widely studied in animals as a model substrate for investigating organ-specific toxicity since it undergoes selective metabolism and activation in the lung. It appears that the Clara cell metabolizes ipomeanol to a reactive metabolite.[26,27] Significant amounts of the cytochromes P450 2B1 and P450 4B1 are found in the Clara cell of the rabbit lung. *In vitro* these isoenzymes are effective at converting ipomeanol to its reactive metabolite. A specific Clara cell lesion is seen also following the administration of the hepatotoxin, 1-nitronaphthalene.

Carbon tetrachloride (CCl_4) is a recognized hepatotoxin producing fatty degeneration and centrilobular necrosis of the liver (see Chapter 43). Biotransformation of carbon tetrachloride takes place in the liver and toxicity is believed to be linked to the production of a $CCl_3^{\cdot}$ radical that causes lipid peroxidation and irreversible damage to membrane systems. Bioactivation of CCl_4 is a classical model for free radical-induced toxicity. The first metabolic step is the formation of the trichloromethyl free radical ($CCl_3^{\cdot}$) by a cytochrome P450 enzyme. This free radical binds directly to microsomal lipids and other cellular macromolecules causing the breakdown of membrane structure, energy production and protein synthesis. The trichloromethyl free radical may also undergo both anaerobic and aerobic reactions leading to the further production of toxic metabolites.

Although the liver is the target organ of toxicity for this chemical, damage to the metabolically active Clara cells as well as types 1 and 2 alveolar epithelial and pulmonary endothelial cells has been reported. Gould and Smuckler[28] found focal atelectasis and haemorrhages with ultrastructural changes in type 2 cells, which suggested damage to the pulmonary surfactant system. Carbon tetrachloride probably has toxic effects on lung phospholipids since the main route of elimination of unchanged carbon tetrachloride is via the breath.

The profile of the isoenzymes of cytochrome P450-dependent monooxygenases in the lung cells is important for understanding of the toxicity of substances that undergo metabolic activation. The heterogeneity of cellular distribution and the high levels of enzyme activity in certain cells can explain specific cell toxicity for some compounds (such as ipomeanol for the Clara cell) but it is not so clear why other toxins (butylated hydroxytoluene and trialkylphosphorothioates) appear to be specifically toxic to the type 1 alveolar epithelial cells. Butylated hydroxytoluene appears to be species-specific in causing murine lung damage but despite extensive human safety evaluation, the potential for butylated hydroxytoluene in food to cause toxic lung damage in man has not been determined. Similarly, the trialkylphosphorothioates, as impurities in many organophosphorus thionates manufactured for use as pesticides (e.g. malathion), may be environmental causes of cell-specific lung damage in man. The type 1 alveolar epithelial cells do not demonstrate significant cytochrome P450 activity and their potential for xenobiotic biotransformation is unknown. It is possible that there is metabolic activation in another cell type or even organ and transport of the toxic metabolite to the type 1 cell. There is some evidence to suggest that certain conjugates may dissociate at a remote site after conjugation and release the toxic compound. Type 1 cells are derived from type 2 which have demonstrable metabolic capability but in vitro the total enzyme activities of a lung preparation cannot be accounted for by the sum of just the Clara and type 2 cells. The other enzyme systems that may be involved in the activation of toxins in the lung include pulmonary flavin-monooxygenases (Clara and alveolar type 2 cells) and pulmonary prostaglandin synthetase which is capable of activating chemicals by co-oxidation with prostaglandin precursors. This pathway, in particular, could be relevant to the pulmonary toxicity of α-naphthylthiourea (ANTU) and N-methylthiobenzamide. The latter compound has a similar toxicity profile to ANTU and has been shown to be metabolized by a pulmonary flavin adenine dinucleorotide (FAD)-dependent monooxygenase. ANTU produces severe, non-haemorrhagic pulmonary oedema with fibrin-rich pleural effusions in animals and has been used as a model for the study of the pathophysiology of pulmonary oedema. Pulmonary prostaglandin H-synthase mediated co-oxygenation has been shown to activate procarcinogens such as benzo[a]pyrene and aflatoxin B1.

The role of glutathione (GSH) in pulmonary detoxification has been investigated for ipomeanol and naphthalene, both of which selectively damage Clara cells in mice. GSH and GSH-S transferase concentrations are lower in the lungs than in liver and the cellular distribution is unclear although there appears to be more activity in the Clara cells than the type 2 cells. Consequently the protective detoxification mechanisms of the lungs are less effective than those of the liver. Low glutathione transferase activity in the lung compared with aryl hydroxylase activity has been associated with the increased risk of lung cancer in tobacco smokers.

The lung is a target organ for toxicity of many other compounds.[29] Some of the mechanisms involved in systemic lung toxicity have been identified in animal toxicity models. Administration of paraquat to animals causes lung fibrosis, the herbicide entering types 1 and 2 lung cells by a selective active uptake process.[30,31] Hydrazine given intraperitoneally in mice can produce lung tumours, and chlorphentermine, after chronic oral dosing, accumulates in the fatty tissue of the lung (and the adrenals) and causes a phospholipidosis. Polycyclic aromatic hydrocarbons may be activated in the lungs or metabolized elsewhere and transported to the lungs. There are significant species differences between animals and humans in susceptibility to the toxic effects of butylated hydroxytoluene (BHT), the trialkylphosphorothioates, ANTU, ipomeanol and paraquat.[32]

Dermal biotransformation

The importance of dermal metabolism during absorption through the skin in vivo is being increasingly recognized. Dermal absorption and metabolism can be assessed with either tissue samples or in vitro flow through diffusion systems using split-thickness skin. The viability of skin in these systems and the maintenance of metabolic capacity are important but still require complete verification. Studies of percutaneous absorption and cutaneous metabolism of some pesticides (aldrin, carbaryl and the herbicide fluazifop butyl) have been carried out to determine the relationship between physicochemical properties and the capacity of skin to absorb and metabolize the compounds in in vitro systems.[33]

Several studies have shown that metabolism occurs during percutaneous absorption for many compounds both in vivo and in vitro. The degree of skin metabolism depends on the physicochemical characteristics of the compound, the rate of absorption as well as the capacity of any metabolizing enzymes. A suitable choice of model systems is important to reflect not only absorption characteristics in vivo, but also metabolic capacity.[34] Metabolism may be relatively unimportant quantitatively in vivo compared with metabolism by the liver but may be highly significant when conversion to toxic metabolites causes local toxicity or where rapid detoxification follows absorption and enables the skin to act as a protective metabolic barrier against a toxic xenobiotic entering the system circulation. The lower metabolic capacity of human skin compared with animals must be considered when extrapolating from animals to man in quantitative risk assessment.

SUMMARY

It has been assumed to date that measurement of air concentrations of hazardous chemicals in the workplace is sufficient to adequately assess the health risks to individual workers. For most of these chemicals there are very few data on the factors affecting absorption, distribution, metabolism and elimination or the mechanism of toxicity in humans to justify this assumption. Toxicokinetic data suggest that for some compounds the degree of workplace exposure is not directly related to individual risk. Similarly, greater understanding of the mechanisms involved in the development of toxic effects in humans and the frequent discrepancies from the results of animal toxicity studies, indicate a need for more information from human studies. In addition, as with the effects on drug toxicity of genetic differences in drug metabolism, so the role of genetic polymorphisms in susceptibility to the toxic effects of hazardous chemicals must be defined. The application of more extensive human data in toxicology to the assessment of health risks in the workplace should not necessarily increase the complexity of controls but will increase their direct relevance. Experience in the workplace can then be applied to the more contentious issues of general environmental exposure.

REFERENCES

1 Klaassen CD, Amdur MO, Doull J (eds). *Casarett and Doull's Toxicology: The Basic Science of Poisons*. New York: McGraw-Hill, 1996.

2 Deichmann WB, Henschler D, Holmstedt B, Keil G. What is there that is not poison? A study of the Third Defense by Paracelsus. *Arch Toxicol* 1986; **58**: 207–13.

3 Rose MS, Smith LL, Wyatt I. Evidence for energy-dependent accumulation of paraquat into rat lung. *Nature* 1974; **252**: 314–5.

4 Smith LL. The identification of an accumulation system for diamines and polyamines into the lung and its relevance to paraquat toxicity. *Arch Toxicol* 1982; **5**(Suppl): 1–14.

5 Woollen BH, Guest EA, Howe W, Marsh JR, Wilson HK *et al.* Human inhalation pharmacokinetics of 1,1,2-trichoro-1,2,2- trifluorethane (FC113). *Int Arch Occup Environ Hlth* 1990; **62**: 73–8.

6 Woollen BH, Marsh JR, Mahler JD, Auton TR, Makepeace D *et al.* Human inhalation pharmacokinetics of chlorodifluoromethane (HCFC22). *Int Arch Occup Environ Hlth* 1992; **64**: 383–7.

7 Blain PG. Inhalation kinetics. In: Brewis RAL, Gibson GJ, Geddes DM eds. *Textbook of Respiratory Medicine*. London: Baillière Tindall, 1990; 158–62.

8 Pietrowskie J. *The Application of Metabolic and Excretion Kinetics to Problems of Industrial Toxicology*. Washington DC: US Government Printing Office, 1971.

9 Conkle JP, Camp BJ, Welch BE. Trace composition of human respiratory gas. *Arch Environ Hlth* 1975; **30**: 290–5.

10 Krotoszynski B, Gabriel G, O'Neil H. Characterisation of human expired air; a promising investigation and diagnostic technique. *J Chromatogr Sci* 1977; **15**: 239–44.

11 Fiserova Bergerova V, Vlach J, Cassady JC. Predictable 'individual differences' in uptake and excretion of gases and lipid soluble vapours. Simulation study. *Br J Ind Med* 1980; **37**: 42–9.

12 Kelman GR. Theoretical basis of alveolar sampling. *Br J Ind Med* 1982; **39**: 259–64.

13 Scott RC, Dugard PH. The properties of skin as a diffusion barrier and route of absorption. In: Greaves MW, Shusters eds. *Pharmacology of the Skin II*. Heidelberg: Springer Verlag, 1989: 93–114.

14 Scott RC. Percutaneous absorption. *In vitro* technique as an alternative to *in vivo* assessment. In: Wang RGM, Franklin CA, Honeycutt RC, Reinert JC eds. *Biological Monitoring for Pesticide Exposure*. Washington DC: American Chemical Society, 158–68.

15 Scott RC, Walker M, Dugard PH. A comparison of the *in vitro* permeability of human and some laboratory animal skins. *Int J Cosmet Sci* 1986; **8**: 189–92.

16 Dick IP, Blain PG, Williams FM. The influence of vehicle on the distribution of lindane in stratum corneum using *in vivo* and *in vitro* systems and its significance in skin absorption. In: Brain KR, James VJ, Walters KA eds. *Prediction of Percutaneous Penetration* Vol. 4b. Cardiff: STS Publishing, 1966: 146–9.

17 Nebert DW, Nelson DR, Adesnik M, Coon MJ, Estabrook RW *et al.* The P450 superfamily: updated listing of all genes and recommended nomenclature for the chromosomal loci. *DNA* 1989; **8**: 1–13.

18 Nelson DR, Koymans L, Kamataki T, Stegeman JJ, Feyereisen R *et al.* P450 superfamily: Update on new sequences, gene mapping accession numbers and nomenclature. *Pharmacogenetics* 1996; **6**: 1–42.

19 Williams FM, Mutch E, Blain PG. Paraoxonase distribution in Caucasian males. *Chem Biol Interact* 1993; **87**: 155–60.

20 Aldridge WN. Two types of esterase (A and B) hydrolysing p-nitrophenylacetate, propionate and butyrate, and a method of their determination. *Biochem J* 1900; **53**: 110–17.

21 Hodgson E, Guthrie FE (eds). *Introduction to Biochemical Toxicology*. New York: Elsevier North Holland Inc, 1984.

22 Sorokin SP. The cells of the lungs. In: Nettesheim P, Hanna MG, Deatherage JW eds. *Conference on Morphology of Experimental Carcinogenesis*. Washington DC: Atomic Energy Commision, 1970; 3–43.

23 Kehrer JP, Kacew S. Systematically applied chemicals that damage lung tissue. *Toxicology* 1985; **35**: 251–93.

24 Blain PG. Toxic lung injury: Ingested agents. In: Brewis RAL, Gibson GJ, Geddes DM eds. *Textbook of Respiratory Medicine*. London: Baillière Tindall, 1990: 1488–97.

25 Boyd MR. Biochemical mechanisms in chemical-induced lung injury: roles of metabolic activation. *CRC Crit Rev Toxicol* 1980; **7**: 103–76.

26 Boyd MR, Burka LT, Wilson BJ, Sasame HA. *In vitro* studies on the metabolic activation of the pulmonary toxin 4-

ipomeanol by rat lung and liver microsomes. *J Pharmacol Expl Ther* 1978; **207**: 677–86.

27 Boyd MR, Burka LT. *In vivo* studies in the relationship between target organ alkylation and the pulmonary toxicity of a chemically reactive metabolite of 4-ipomeanol. *J Pharmacol Expl Ther* 1978; **207**: 687–97.

28 Gould VE, Smuckler EA. Alveolar injury in acute carbon tetrachloride intoxication. *Arch Intern Med* 1971; **128**: 109–17.

29 Brewis RAL, Keaney NP. Respiratory disorders. In: Davies DM ed. *Textbook of Adverse Drug Reactions*. Oxford: Oxford University Press, 1986: 172–204.

30 Rose MS, Lock EA, Smith LL, Wyatt I. Paraquat accumulation: tissue and species specificity. *Biochem Pharmacol* 1976; **25**: 419–23.

31 Blain PG. Aspects of pesticide toxicology. Adverse drug reactions. *Acute Poisoning Rev* 1990; **9**: 37–68.

32 Marino AA, Mitchell JT. Lung damage in mice following intraperitoneal injection of butylated hydroxytoluene. *Proc Soc Expl Biol Med* 1972; **140**: 122–5.

33 Macpherson SE, Scott RC, Williams FM. Metabolism of pesticides during percutaneous absorption. In: Scott RC, Guy RH, Hadgraft J eds. *Prediction of Percutaneous Penetration*. Vol. 1. London: IBC Technical Services Ltd. 1990: 135–9.

34 Williams FM. Metabolism of xenobiotics during percutaneous absorption *in vivo* and in *in vitro* systems. In: Scott RC, Guy RH, Hadgraft J eds. *Prediction of Percutaneous Penetration*. Vol. 2 Southampton: IBC Technical Services Ltd, 1990: 270–8.

7

Metals

LINDSAY MORGAN, ALAN SCOTT

Toxic versus essential	81	Nickel	109
Lead	82	Osmium	110
Mercury	89	Platinum	110
Cadmium	93	Selenium	111
Arsenic	95	Silver	112
Phosphorus	97	Tellurium	112
Aluminium	99	Thallium	113
Antimony	100	Tin	113
Barium	101	Tungsten	115
Beryllium	101	Uranium	115
Chromium	104	Vanadium	116
Cobalt	105	Zinc	116
Copper	107	Zirconium	117
Manganese	107	References	117
Molybdenum	109		

'Metal' is a general term referring to elements (e.g. silver, gold, copper and mercury) with a typical lustrous appearance, which are good conductors of heat and electricity and which take part in chemical reactions as positive ions (cations). Some elements (e.g. tellurium) have the physical properties of a metal and the chemical properties of a non-metal. Metalloids (e.g. arsenic) have properties intermediate between metals and non-metals. In this chapter the term 'metals' is used to cover comprehensively true metals and metalloids.

Metals have been poisoning man almost since the day he first learned to use them. Seven metals were known in antiquity – gold, silver, copper, iron, tin, lead and mercury – and, of these, lead and mercury were well-recognized for their toxic effects. In succeeding years many more metals have been discovered. Some of these have bestowed benefits because of their physical and chemical purposes. Others have exacted a severe toll.

Monitoring of exposure and the application of correct controls to maintain exposure within stipulated guidelines will facilitate the safe use of metals and their compounds. This will minimize the risk of occupational disease while enabling the beneficial uses of these substances to be maximized.

TOXIC VERSUS ESSENTIAL

A number of the metals considered to be toxic in an occupational setting, for example, manganese, chromium, cobalt and selenium are essential for some metabolic processes and there is even evidence, at least in some laboratory animals, that lead and perhaps cadmium may be essential trace elements.

The division of metals into 'toxic' and 'essential' is somewhat abitrary as even the essential metals may be toxic if they are present in excess. Moreover, if their concentration in the body is too low, symptoms of deficiency will eventually be produced. For this reason the concentration of essential metals in the blood is kept within narrow limits which are sometimes referred to as 'concentration windows', and elaborate mechanisms have evolved to maintain these concentration windows under normal circumstances.

Factors affecting toxicity

The toxicity of any metal depends upon a number of factors, including its mode of entry to the body, its particle size (only particles that are of respirable size penetrate to the alveoli and thus become available for absorption from the lung), the chemical species, and its interactions with other metals. These mechanisms and also the activities of the metals in the biological matrix are subject to the laws of physics and chemistry, and consequently many of the biological features of metals can be deduced from the metal's place in the periodic table.[34,205]

As a general rule, absorption from the lung is more effective than from the gut, about 40% of an inhaled dose of a metallic aerosol may be retained in the lung, whereas usually only 10% or less of an ingested dose will be absorbed. Relatively few factors affect uptake from the lung apart from particle size and solubility but several must be taken into account when considering uptake from the gut. Age is an important criterion and, again as a general rule, the uptake of metals from the gut varies inversely with age. This may not be thought of as relevant to occupation, but child labour is by no means uncommon in some parts of the world and in the developed world environmental issues are bringing non-occupational childhood poisoning to the fore. There are also some interactions with other constituents of the diet which may affect the rate of uptake from the gut. For example, the absorption of lead varies inversely from the amount of calcium and iron in the diet and it may also be influenced by the presence of fat, protein and vitamin D in the gut. The uptake of cadmium is affected by the zinc content of the diet and that of manganese by the iron content.

Recognition of 'speciation' is fundamental to the understanding of metal toxicology. This concept of speciation includes the organic and inorganic compounds as well as the elemental metal, and is important because the toxicological properties are dependent upon the physicochemical ones including, very importantly, solubility and valency. As a general rule the water-soluble forms are associated with acute toxicity while the insoluble ones are more generally inert in the body. However, those forms that are slightly soluble in the biological matrix, if they allow a slow release of toxic ions, are frequently associated with chronic disease such as fibrosis or malignancy. Therefore it is important, when studying metal-related occupational disease, to know the metal species concerned and its solubility.

Diagnosis

It is important for the clinician to remember that the diagnosis of occupational metal poisoning is not always easy, for few cases present as clear clinical entities and, usually, an occupational cause will be part of a list of different possibilities. Exposure to a metal (or, indeed, any other substance) at work does not prove that it is the cause of the patient's illness. Epidemiological studies may give us a feel for the range of exposure that may be toxic but when one patient is being considered there may be considerable individual variation in susceptibility. It is therefore necessary to obtain reliable information as explained in Chapters 1 and 2 about the circumstances of exposure and their relationship to the course of the patient's illness. Also, the important difference between hazard (the inherent property of a substance to cause harm) and risk (the likelihood of harm being caused because of the way in which the substance is handled at work) should be emphasized. The clinician will also need to know what laboratory tests may be available to aid diagnosis and where such tests are best carried out. Further, it may be necessary to seek specialist advice, perhaps from a university department of occupational medicine, a poisons centre or from organizations with statutory responsibility for health and safety at work or other government agencies (in the UK, the Health and Safety Executive and, in the United States of America, the National Institute of Occupational Safety and Health, and the Occupational Health and Safety Administration).

LEAD

Lead has been used for at least 6000 years and is a most attractive metal for cultures that employ simple technology. It is easy to extract from its principal ores, has a low melting point so that it can be cast and moulded with ease, is malleable and so can be worked without undue effort. It can easily be joined together with moderate heat and it resists corrosion by the elements. Moreover, galena (lead sulphide), which was the ore from which lead was derived in antiquity, contains variable amounts of silver; indeed, it was for its silver and not its lead that galena was first mined and the so-called silver mines of the ancient world were, in fact, lead mines.

During the mediaeval period in Europe the practice developed of adulterating wines of modest vintage with lead and this must have caused much harm. The pernicious habit persisted well into the eighteenth century and there were also a number of epidemics of lead poisoning attributable to the drinking of wines that were (accidentally or deliberately) contaminated with lead. The Devonshire colic was extensively investigated in 1767 by Sir George Baker who showed, by a mixture of observation and experimentation, that it was caused by lead being incorporated into the Devonshire cider during the course of its production, from the cider pounds and presses which had lead in their structure.

In Europe, the eighteenth and nineteenth centuries were the heyday for lead poisoning and there are dozens of remarkable accounts of the conditions to which lead workers were subjected. Most workers in the lead trades could expect to develop symptoms of some sort and, in the potteries, women who dipped the wares into lead glazes had a stillbirth rate which might approach 60%.

Lead poisoning also afflicted great numbers of the general population who were exposed to contaminated water supplies and to adulterated food.

Because of its widespread occurrence, physicians in the nineteenth century became expert on lead poisoning, perhaps none more so than Tanquerel des Planches whose *Traite des maladies de plomb ou saturnines* in 1839 was a synthesis of his experience with more than 120 patients with lead poisoning whom he had treated in Paris. One of the features of lead poisoning that Tanquerel described was the blue line on the gums which was described in the *Lancet* the following year by Burton and which has since been known (in English-speaking countries at least) as the burtonian line; clearly Burton had not read the *Traite*!

Concern about occupational lead poisoning in the second half of the nineteenth century contributed to the establishment of the Medical Inspectorate of Factories; Thomas Legge devoted much energy to reducing the toll from this disease, which he accomplished with considerable success.

In more recent years much has been written about lead poisoning but perhaps the most influential work has been that of Robert Kehoe who first put forward the notion that, if the blood lead concentration was kept below 80 µg/dl, the probability of a worker contracting lead poisoning was remote. Although this concept has been challenged in recent years, with the possibility that 'subclinical' forms of lead poisoning might occur, experience has tended to support Kehoe's point of view and it is only in recent years that the maximum blood lead concentration considered safe for male lead workers has been lowered from 80 µg/dl.

Present day exposures

In developed countries, lead poisoning no longer occupies the predominant position it once did and few physicians will see a case during their working lifetime. By contrast, in developing countries, lead poisoning is still commonplace, and on a worldwide scale it remains the most common of the occupational poisonings.

Worldwide, about 2.5 million tonnes of lead are produced each year, almost half of which is consumed in the USA. Workers engaged in primary or secondary lead smelting may have heavy exposures and they may also be exposed at the same time to other metals such as arsenic or cadmium. Primary lead smelting is the process by which lead is extracted from its ore, usually lead sulphide (galena). High temperatures are used and, although large amounts of respirable lead oxide fume are evolved, the processes are usually well enclosed and ventilated. Secondary smelting involves the melting of scrap lead to reclaim the metal. This is usually carried out at temperatures below 500°C, with little evolution of lead oxide fume provided that temperature control is effective. The 'dross'

(oxidized lead) that is skimmed off the surface of the molten metal may, however, give rise to considerable quantities of lead-bearing dust which may be inhaled or ingested by workers. Lead in any of its forms may be processed by secondary smelting but lead storage batteries are the main source. There is a considerable demand for this type of lead in the UK for the building industry, and significant quantities of lead are still used in some countries in the manufacture of motor vehicles.

Airborne lead dust, sufficient to cause poisoning, may be produced during the manufacture of lead batteries, paints and colours, lead compounds, rubber products and glass, and during the dry disking, grinding and cutting by power tools of lead. Exposure may also arise from 'sanding down' (rubbing down) and from the application of lead paints and glazes, unless they are low solubility lead compounds or conform to BS 4310/68 or a similar standard. Poisoning from the inhalation of lead oxide fume may occur in the demolition industry where lead-painted metalwork is cut up with gas-powered burning torches.

Firearms instructors and members of rifle clubs have also been found to have increased lead absorption resulting from exposure to lead dust from bullets and lead azide fume from the explosive charge. Some enthusiasts have been known to make their own bullets on the kitchen stove.

Lead compounds such as dibasic lead phthalate, lead chlorosilicate and basic lead carbonates are frequently incorporated into polyvinyl chloride (PVC) plastics when thermal stability and high tensile strength are needed. Some exposure to lead may occur during the manufacture of these plastics, although there is no risk from the finished materials.

Organic lead compounds have been added to petrol as anti-knock agents for over half a century. The most important additives are tetraethyl and tetramethyl lead; the former is extremely toxic but the latter is not. Exposure may result from the handling of these compounds in refineries or during the cleaning out of tanks that have contained leaded petrol. Because of the strict control measures in industrialized countries, lead poisoning among workers who put the additives into petrol is exceptionally rare. Poisoning has also been reported when leaded petrol has been inadvertently used as a solvent in the manufacture of cheap shoes or as a degreasing agent. A few cases of organic lead poisoning have also occurred in those who habitually sniff petrol.

The uptake of lead

The rate of absorption from both gut and lungs depends upon the solubility of the lead compound in body fluids; lead chromate is highly insoluble whereas lead oxide is highly soluble and for this reason the toxicity of the chromate is considerably less than the oxide.

At one time, it was customary to give lead workers a pint of milk a day in order to protect them against the toxic effects of the metal. This well meant gesture would have had little protective effect, however, for the presence of calcium in the gut cannot influence the uptake of lead from the lung and, moreover, the large amounts of lactose in the milk might have had the effect of actually increasing the uptake from the gut. Nevertheless, it was commonly observed that the general health of lead workers improved when they were given milk to drink – almost certainly a comment on their poor diet.

Inhalation is still the major route of entry for those with occupational lead exposure but the risk from ingestion tends sometimes to be overlooked. Ingestion is often the principal route of entry, particularly where good standards of personal hygiene are not insisted upon. Lead workers who are allowed to eat or drink in their workplace without first carefully washing their hands are unnecessarily increasing the risk they run, as are those who smoke at work. Inorganic lead compounds are not significantly absorbed through the skin but organic ones may be.

Distribution of lead in the body

Lead circulates in the blood bound to haemoglobin molecules, and substantially less than 5% of the total blood lead is in the plasma; clinicians should not therefore request serum lead analyses in a suspected case of lead poisoning. Lead has a long biological half-life and the total body burden increases with time. For the sake of simplicity the total body burden can be considered to consist of three pools: a rapidly exchangeable pool in the blood and soft tissues; an intermediate pool in the soft tissues; and the skeletal pool. The skeletal pool may be further subdivided into an intermediate exchangeable pool in the marrow and the trabecular bone, and a very slowly exchangeable pool in the compact bone and dentine. By far the greatest part of the total body burden is in the skeletal tissues.

The rapidly exchangeable pool in the blood is toxicologically the most important although it represents only about 2% of the total body burden and has a biological half-life of about 30 days. The blood lead concentration is the most commonly used index of lead exposure but it

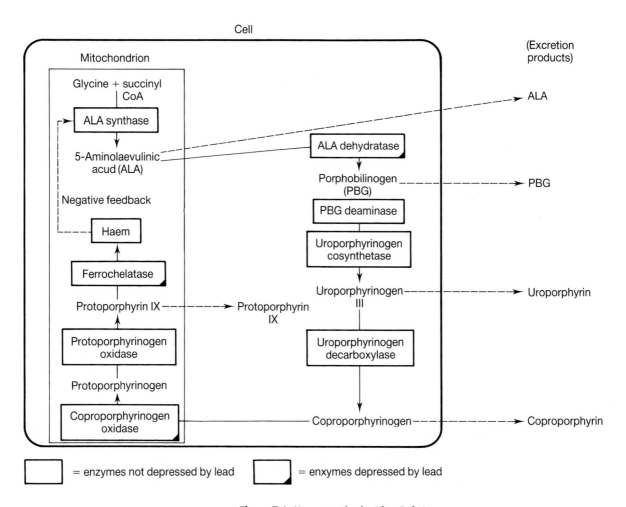

Figure 7.1 *Haem synthesis. After Ref. 1.*

should be remembered that it reflects only recent exposure and is not necessarily related in any way to the total body burden.

Lead is excreted through the kidney, and the urinary lead concentration was used, for many years, to estimate exposure until reliable methods of blood lead analysis became available. Furthermore, there is a considerable circadian variation in excretion but, although urinary lead analyses no longer have a role in the monitoring of inorganic lead exposure, they are the most useful form of monitoring exposure to organic lead. A small amount of lead is excreted into the bile to appear in the faeces but most of the lead in faeces is that which was ingested but not absorbed.

Small amounts of lead are also eliminated in other body fluids e.g. sweat, saliva and breast milk but they are not important routes of excretion compared with urine.

Tetraethyl lead is dealkylated in the liver to the triethyl form which then spontaneously dealkylates to the diethyl form. Diethyl lead is excreted into the bile and is further dealkylated in the gut to ionic lead. Diethyl lead is the only metabolite of the tetraethyl form that appears in the urine.

Biochemical effects of lead

Lead has three important biochemical properties that largely determine its toxic manifestations. First, it has a very high affinity for sulphydryl (-SH) groups and thus is able to inhibit the activity of enzymes which depend upon -SH groups for their proper functioning. Two enzymes that are inhibited by lead are of particular interest. They are 5-aminolaevulinic acid dehydratase (ALAD) and ferrochelatase, and are both concerned with haem synthesis (Fig. 7.1).

Second, the metabolism of lead mimics that of calcium in many respects and it is able competitively to inhibit the action of calcium at some important sites such as the synapse, and during mitochondrial respiration. It is this feature of its metabolism that determines its bone-seeking properties.

Finally, lead may affect both DNA and RNA *in vitro* but the biological implications of this – if indeed there are any – are not at all clear. Certainly there is no convincing evidence that lead is a human carcinogen although it has been found to induce renal and some other tumours in animals.[2]

Inorganic lead poisoning

Lead gradually accumulates until critical body burdens are reached, when symptoms may appear suddenly and progress rapidly, although subclinical manifestations (e.g. depression of ALAD activity, reduced motor nerve conduction velocity) will have been demonstrable earlier. The outline of haem synthesis is shown in Fig. 7.1,

beginning with the reaction of glycine and succinyl coenzyme A to form 5-aminolaevulinic acid (ALA). Two molecules of ALA move from the mitochondrium into the cell where they condense to form porphobilinogen (PBG) through the action of ALA dehydratase (ALAD); from PBG are formed a series of porphyrinogens and porphyrins. The molecule then moves back into the mitochondrium where final rearrangement of the side chains produces protoporphyrin IX. The incorporation of ferrous iron into protoporphyrin IX, through the action of ferrochelatase, leads to the formation of haem. Normal functioning of this synthetic pathway is essential for the production of both haemoglobin and the oxidative enzymes in all body tissues.

Depression of ALAD and of ferrochelatase, results in increased amounts of ALA in the urine and increased amounts of protoporphyrin in the circulating red cells. Because of the ferrochelatase suppression, protoporphyrin forms a metal chelate with zinc instead of with iron, giving increased amounts of zinc protoporphyrin (ZPP). Other stages of the synthetic pathway are also affected and large amounts of coproporphyrin III are excreted in the urine.

The rate-limiting enzyme in this series is ALA synthase, so decreased formation of haem has the effect of increasing the amount of ALA formed. This process produces what is essentially a lead-induced porphyria. Depression of haem synthesis in many tissues (not only the erythropoietic) leads to progressive impairment of their ability to synthesize oxidative enzymes. There may also be competitive inhibition by ALA of transmission by gamma-aminobutyric acid (GABA), a putative brain neurotransmitter. The similarity in their chemical structures is shown in Fig. 7.2.

$NH_2CH_2COCH_2CH_2COOH$
5-aminolaevulinic acid (ALA)

$NH_2CH_2CH_2CH_2COOH$
gamma-aminobutyric acid (GABA)

Figure 7.2

This pattern of effects is unique to lead poisoning and may be a useful adjunct in arriving at the diagnosis. The effects on ALAD occur at very low blood lead levels (less than 20 µg/dl; 1 µmol/litre), and somewhere around 85% of the activity of this enzyme may be suppressed before an increase in ALA in the blood is observed. Frank anaemia is usually a late phenomenon in lead poisoning. The mild anaemia of lead poisoning is mainly due to the impairment of haem synthesis but there is also some evidence that red cell life span is somewhat shortened.[3] This may be due to an increase in the mechanical or osmotic fragility of the red cells which, in turn, may be related to a loss of potassium caused by the inhibition of Na-K-ATPase.[4]

SYMPTOMS AND SIGNS

Classically, the patient with lead poisoning presents with a history of abdominal pain, colic and constipation. However, in developed countries not many patients now reach that stage. More likely they will complain of the premonitory symptoms of undue fatigue, lassitude, generalized aches and pains in the muscles and joints with, perhaps, some abdominal discomfort. A few patients have diarrhoea; some may have a bad taste in the mouth. Because these symptoms are non-specific the diagnosis of lead poisoning is not immediately considered but a careful occupational history will be an important pointer. The diagnosis is a clinical one and the term 'lead poisoning' should not be used for asymptomatic workers who simply have abnormal biological tests.

The later stage of peripheral neuropathy which is almost always motor and tends to produce weakness in the muscles that are most frequently used (particularly the long extensors of the limbs), is rarely encountered in the developed countries at the present day (Fig. 7.3).

Mild changes in the central nervous system are characterized by progressive fatigue and lethargy (see Chapter 42). This is often first noted by family members and may become so severe as to disturb the patient's work and social life. It is not unusual to hear the spouse complain that the patient has 'changed'; he or she may lose interest in domestic and social activities and may come home from work, sit down and immediately fall asleep.

Severe encephalopathy with impaired consciousness, confusion and bizarre neurological signs is rare in adults in the developed countries but is a common mode of presentation of lead poisoning in children. Occasionally, patients with inorganic lead poisoning may have psychiatric symptoms and the condition resembles a mixed affective organic state. It would be very unusual if these were presenting symptoms following occupational exposure but the possibility that exposure to lead may exacerbate preexisting psychiatric symptoms should be borne in mind.

Arthralgia has been recognized as a manifestation of acute lead poisoning for well over 100 years, but is usually a non-specific symptom. Lead also interferes with normal urate metabolism and may precipate attacks of gout sometimes associated with nephropathy.[5] The condition affects those who consume large quantities of home-distilled spirits, which may contain significant quantities of lead derived from solder within the still – hence 'saturnine gout'.

When occupational exposures were considerably greater, renal damage was common (see Chapter 41). The early effects of lead poisoning on the kidneys are directed against the cells of the proximal tubule, but with continued exposure severe and progressive renal insufficiency may develop with interstitial fibrosis and secondary hypertension. Lead workers formerly had an increased mortality from cerebrovascular disease but recent studies suggest that this is no longer the case.[6] In adults with lead poisoning, renal effects are not likely to loom large in the clinical picture, but in children, renal tubular dysfunction, leading to a Fanconi-like syndrome, with aminoaciduria, glycosuria and hyperphosphaturia is much more common.

It has been a concern in the past that occupational and general population exposure to lead was associated with raised blood pressure and possible cardiovascular disease, but the evidence for such effects is today considered inadequate.

There are few clinical signs to aid the diagnosis of lead poisoning. The patient may be pale and there may be some muscle weakness if there is a peripheral neuropathy; wrist drop is one of the classic signs of lead poisoning but is now rare (Fig. 7.3). A burtonian or blue line may be present on the dental margin of the gums. It is caused by bacterial deposition of lead sulphide, is associated with poor dental hygiene and is absent from the edentulous. It indicates lead exposure, not lead poisoning. There may be general tenderness of muscles and joints and on palpation of the abdomen. The pallor of lead poisoning is not caused by anaemia, but by cutaneous vasoconstriction.

Laboratory investigations are important in the diagnosis of lead poisoning. About a century ago the appearance of basophilic granules in the red blood cells was recognized as a concomitant, almost as a sign, of lead poisoning. By the 1920s, before the advent of microchemistry, the stippled cell count was used to monitor the exposure of lead workers. That has now been replaced by the biochemical measures described below. Stippled cells are not unique, as was at one time thought, but may be found, for example, in severe secondary anaemia, malignant disease and malaria. The importance of stippled cells today is that the haematologist may spot them in the blood film of a patient 'under investigation' and alert the clinician to con-

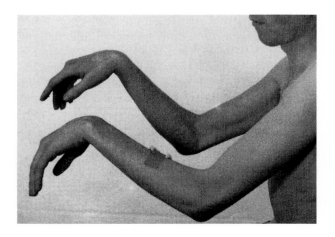

Figure 7.3 *Lead palsy in a ship-breaker. He had bilateral wrist drop which took several months to recover. Courtesy of Professor RI McCallum.*

sider the possibility of lead poisoning. In lead poisoning, iron entering the erythrocyte precursors is not fully utilized and accumulates. This non-haem iron, together with ferrigenous micelles, fragments of damaged mitochondria, and some RNA is believed to comprise the basophilic granules (see Chapter 44).

The blood lead concentration in the normal UK population is less than 10 µg/dl (0.5 µmol/litre). Occupationally exposed workers may have levels much higher than this but poisoning seldom occurs if the blood lead level is below 80 µg/dl (4 µmol/litre). In the UK, lead workers may continue such work until the level reaches 60 µg/dl (3.0 µmol/litre), although a restriction of 30 µg/dl (1.5 µmol/litre) is imposed on women of reproductive capacity to protect the fetus. A high blood lead is not synonymous with lead poisoning so further tests are required. The ZPP level in the normal population is usually less than 2.0 µg/g Hb. It begins to rise when blood lead concentrations reach the range 35–45 µg/dl (1.75–2.25 µmol/litre) in males or 25–35 µg/dl (1.25–1.75 µmol/litre) in females. Levels rise rapidly at blood lead concentrations higher than 50 µg/dl (2.5 µmol/litre). In lead poisoning, the ZPP level will be above 20 µg/g Hb, often at least one order of magnitude greater. The only other common condition that causes a rise in ZPP is iron deficiency anaemia. It is important, however, to remember that the ZPP does not immediately increase following lead exposure as it depends upon the formation of new red cells, and lag periods of up to 2 months have been reported. For recent exposures, it is better to measure urinary ALA concentrations. Normal values for subjects not exposed to lead are less than 5 mg ALA/g creatinine (4 µg/mmol creatinine) and the increase consequent upon lead exposure reflects that of ZPP. The lag period is only 2 weeks and levels in persons suffering from lead poisoning will be above 20 mg ALA/g creatinine (16 µg/mmol creatinine). If the exposure period is less than 2 weeks, it may be possible to have the blood ALAD activity measured: the normal level is greater than 6 European units.

Data on the clinical effects of lead have been summarized in publications such as the Environmental Health Criteria on inorganic lead (IPCS 1995).[7] Abdominal colic and renal effects are unlikely to arise if blood leads are below 100 µg/dl. This risk of developing significant anaemia is small – below 50 µg/dl. As far as neurological effects are concerned, life-threatening encephalopathy is unlikely to occur at blood levels below 100–120 µg/dl in adults and 80–100 in children. There are no firm quantitative data for the development of the classical sign of peripheral neuropathy. There is limited evidence for an effect on sperm quality above 40 µg/dl, but inadequate information on infertility.

Above a blood level of 10 µg/dl, epidemiological studies of children and environmental exposure to lead have shown subtle changes in brain development from the time of birth to the age of 5 years when the brain is most vulnerable to its effects: a loss of two IQ points on average for a rise in blood levels from 10 to 20 µg/dl[8] (See Chapter 2).

A band of increased density may be seen on radiographs at the growing ends of the long bones and the phalanges in children with lead poisoning, but not in adults. This increased density is caused by an alteration in the architecture of the bone and not by deposition of lead. This may be comparable to 'growth arrest lines'. In severe cases there may be changes in the shape of the bone, which revert gradually to normal once the child is removed from exposure and recovers.

At blood lead concentrations lower than those which cause frank neuropathy, motor nerve conduction velocity, especially of the slower fibres, is reduced.[9] There is no evidence of a dose–effect relationship. Changes in performance in psychometric tests have been reported in lead workers with blood lead levels below 70 µg/dl (3.5 µmol/litre). There is almost no consistency in the pattern of changes observed and, although some improvement in test scores is reported following a reduction in exposure,[10] the changes are of little long-term significance and the subjects are not themselves aware of any deterioration in their performance. These changes in the peripheral and central nervous systems are, however, of little value in the diagnosis of acute lead poisoning.

TREATMENT

The basis of the treatment of lead intoxication is immediate removal from occupational exposure to lead. In the UK, there is a statutory requirement for doing this for young persons (under 18 years) with blood lead levels above 50 µg/dl (2.5 µml/litre), in asymptomatic men with blood lead levels greater than 60 µg/dl (3 µml/litre) and women of reproductive capacity with blood lead levels above 30 µg/dl (1.5 µml/litre). All such cases are reportable by the employer to the Health and Safety Executive and poisoning by lead or compound of lead is also a prescribed disease (see Chapter 4).

If symptoms are mild, further treatment is unnecessary and blood lead level will gradually fall towards normal and should be monitored periodically. The process may take up to several months, so blood testing every few days is unnecessary and the clinician should not be anxious provided the patient's condition is improving. If the condition is more severe, treatment with chelating agents should be considered but should be based on symptoms and not on biochemical or haematological measurements. In some countries chelation is carried out simply because the blood lead level is high: there is no evidence that this confers any long-term benefit and there is always the risk of an adverse reaction to the drug.

The agents most commonly used for chelation are penicillamine and sodium calcium edetate. Penicillamine is given orally, 1 g per day for adults in divided doses for 5 days. If after a few days the blood lead rises again and the symptoms recur, the course of treatment might have to be repeated. Sodium calcium edetate is used at 50–75 mg/kg per day in two divided doses as a slow intravenous infusion for 5 days.[11] This will relieve colic within a few hours. With both drugs, the full blood count should be tested at the beginning and end of each treatment period. Because of their nephrotoxicity the urine should be tested for proteinuria and haematuria although renal disturbance is unlikely with the doses and the relatively short duration of therapy in acute lead poisoning. During the course of treatment, 24-hour specimens of urine should be taken to monitor the rate of lead excretion; this should be continued for 5–7 days after the end of treatment. Blood lead concentrations should be estimated at 48 hours and at 5 days by which time symptoms will usually have subsided.

After treatment it is important that no further exposure occurs until symptoms have completely remitted and the patient's blood lead concentration has returned to an acceptable level, preferably below 40 µg/dl (2.0 µmol/litre). It follows that once workers have developed symptoms they must be carefully supervised thereafter. If they require further treatment it is prudent that they should not have any further exposure to lead.

If symptoms persist or recur it may be necessary to repeat the chelation, or perhaps use one of the newer chelating agents such as 3-dimercaptopropane sulphonate (DMPS) or dimercaptosuccinic acid (DMSA), both of which are derivatives of dimercaprol (BAL). Occasionally, workers who have been removed from exposure, or treated for lead poisoning, will have blood lead concentrations that persist above the levels that are generally considered safe. They may be asymptomatic, with normal levels of ZPP. Usually these are workers who have been exposed to lead for many years and may have accumulated such large skeletal burdens that their blood levels will never return to normal. It seems likely that the lead distribution between red cells and plasma is much more in favour of the red cells than is normal, probably because they are able to produce lead-binding proteins within the red cell in greater quantities than is usual. These workers appear to be unaffected by their high blood leads and may represent an unusually resistant 'survivor population'. No further treatment is necessary and they may continue working with lead provided that blood tests are repeated at least every 3 months and the ZPP levels remain normal.

Organic lead poisoning

Poisoning with tetraethyl lead causes a toxic organic psychosis and so the picture is dominated by psychiatric

---

Mr A.T.

Petrol refinery work at . . . . since 1969. Aged 47 years.

Occupational history

– 1975	Worked on plant extracting sulphur compounds.
1975 – present	On TEL plant, adding TEL into large covered tanks.
	Work is carried out in covered workplace.
	TEL arrives in drums and is pumped under pressure into opening of tank.
	Spills occur 'many times' on to head, face and arms.
	Wears gloves, boots and long-sleeved cotton overalls, which are often splashed.
	Provided with a 'filter mask'.

Medical history

Symptoms began with numbness in head and hands
Developed: dizziness, headaches and vertigo
Later: blurred vision, especially in dim twilight
Heard strange sounds
Insomnia: could not sleep well because felt disturbed and agitated

Investigations

Date	Blood lead (µg/dl)	Urine lead (µg/dl)
1986	40	173
13.02.89	41	131
18.02.89	11	259
22.02.89	7	655
05.07.89	3	475
12.02.90	33	141
03.10.90	27	130
08.01.91	–	414

Figure 7.4 *A case report of a man with tetraethyl lead (TEL) poisoning. Courtesy of Professor WR Lee.*

symptoms which may appear suddenly. There is nothing in the clinical picture that is pathognomonic of organic lead poisoning and the diagnosis is made by establishing exposure. Occupational cases are uncommon and, as noted previously, usually occur in those who have been cleaning out tanks in which leaded petrol has been stored or who have been using leaded petrol inappropriately as a solvent or degreasing agent – tetraethyl lead is well absorbed through the skin. Occasionally, cases are seen arising from the abuse of solvents containing organic lead compounds.

Tetraethyl lead decomposes slowly in air, rapidly in bright sunlight, to yield needle-like crystals of tri-, di- and monoethyl lead compounds with a garlic-like odour. In their dry state they may be dispersed mechanically in air to be inhaled or deposited on the skin. Their inhalation induces vigorous, often paroxysmal sneezing, irritation of the upper respiratory tract and, in sufficient dosage, mild organolead poisoning. In contact with warm, moist skin, or unprotected ocular membranes, they induce itching, burning and transient redness.

The symptoms found in inorganic lead poisoning do not occur in organic poisoning although patients may have some abdominal discomfort and anorexia. It is, however, important to remember that both forms of lead poisoning may occur together, particularly in workers involved in the demolition or refurbishment of leaded-fuel storage tanks, which may be lead painted. The blood lead is usually not raised above 50 µg/dl (2.5 µmol/litre) and sometimes not at all, and ZPP and porphyrin levels are usually within normal limits. A raised urinary lead is the most important confirmatory laboratory test.

Poisoning is not seen at concentrations below 150 µg/dl (0.7 µmol/litre) but may occur at concentrations above 350 µg/dl (1.8 µmol/litre). The use of chelating agents in the treatment of organic lead poisoning is of little value and symptomatic therapy such as with diazepam is required. Adequate sedation (which may need to be prolonged) and nutritional support are important and, because sedation is symptomatic, it should be used only so long as is necessary to control symptoms. Complete recovery is usual but the illness may be prolonged and characterized by periodic and sudden psychotic relapses. The main features of a clinical case are shown in Fig. 7.4.

MERCURY

Mercury, like lead, was one of the metals of antiquity and it also has a long history of inflicting harm upon those who use it or work with it. The quicksilver mines in Spain, which the Romans exploited, had an even more terrible reputation than the lead mines, and all the uses to which mercury was put until recent times involved great risks to health. Mercury gilding and the silvering of mirrors were two especially dangerous occupations.

Gold or silver were amalgamated with mercury and applied to a manuscript or to glass and the mercury was allowed to vaporize with or without the application of heat; exposures of artist or artisan were consequently considerable. Ramazzini, in his *De morbus artificum diatriba*, had something to say about both gilders and mirror makers. Of the former he states:

> We all know what terrible maladies are contracted from mercury by goldsmiths, especially those employed in gilding silver and copper objects . . . craftsmen of this sort very soon become subject to vertigo, asthma and paralysis. Very few of them reach old age, and even when they do not die young their health is so terribly undermined that they pray for death.

Of the mirror makers, he wrote:

> They learn by experience just like gilders how malignant is mercury when, as is the custom, they coat with quicksilver huge sheets of glass so that the other side may give a clearer reflection. Those who make mirrors become palsied and asthmatic from handling mercury.

Kussmaul's classic work of 1861 on mercury poisoning was based on his experience among the silverers of mirrors in Fürth and Nuremberg. Mirrors were backed with an amalgam of tin and mercury. The working conditions were so bad that he was hardly able to find an adult male in the trade with a single tooth in his head. In addition to salivation and stomatitis, he described reddening of the pharynx (Kussmaul's sign) and ulceration of the buccal mucosa and palate. He described how the condition advanced in three clinical stages: erethism (abnormal irritability), tremor and cachexia. Publication of his findings led to stringent regulations which resulted in the mercurial silvering of mirrors being abandoned altogether.

During the nineteenth century, mercurial poisoning was so common among hat makers, who used mercuric nitrate in the carotting of felt – a process in which the hairs obtained from rabbit pelts were flattened and meshed together to form felt, that phrases such as 'hatter's shakes' and 'mad as a hatter' passed into common use. As an aside, the Mad Hatter in Alice in Wonderland almost certainly did *not* have mercurial poisoning despite the many assertions that he did.

The toxicity of mercury became clearer during the eighteenth century, when the use of mercurial ointments to treat syphilis became popular. When the patient complained of excessive salivation or his teeth began to blacken and fall out his physician could be sure that he was complying with the therapeutic regimen and that large amounts of mercury were being absorbed. Ramazzini noted that the surgeons who themselves rubbed ointment into their patients were by no means immune from its harmful effects.

Mercury is unique among all the toxic metals in that it has accounted for several epidemics of environmental poisoning. The best known of these, but by no means the most serious, was Minamata disease which was first noted at the end of 1953 when an unusual neurological disorder began to affect the villagers living on Minamata Bay on the southwest coast of the most southerly of the main islands of Japan. It was commonly referred to as *kibyo*, that is, the mystery illness. Both sexes and all ages were affected and the signs and symptoms were those of a polyneuropathy with cerebellar ataxia, dysarthria, deafness and disturbance of vision. The prognosis for the condition was poor; many patients became disabled and bed-ridden and the case fatality rate was about 40%.

The source of the mercury was traced to effluent released into the bay from a factory manufacturing vinyl chloride and using mercuric chloride as a catalyst. It is claimed that inorganic mercury was released by the factory. Some bacteria in the sediment of the bay are capable of detoxifying the metal by methylating mercury, but the rate of conversion is extremely slow, much too slow to have accounted for the large amounts of methyl mercury that are calculated to have accumulated in the waters of the bay. It is therefore more likely that the mercury was actually released in an organic form; at the time there were no regulations forbidding this in Japan.

Large-scale outbreaks of organic mercury poisoning have also occurred from eating bread made from seed grain that had been treated with mercurial fungicides. Outbreaks have been reported in Pakistan and Guatemala but the most severe have been in Iraq. The largest epidemic occurred in 1971–72 when over 6000 patients were admitted to hospital, of whom more than 500 died.[12] Many of those afflicted lived in remote country districts and the true scale of this episode has never fully been determined.

Uses of mercury

The annual production of mercury is approximately 7000 tonnes and it has many uses. Its largest single use is as a liquid electrode in the electrolytic production of chlorine from sodium chloride, by the so-called chloroalkali process. Mercury is also used in the production of fungicides, biocides (slimicides) and special antifouling paints, in switchgear, laboratory apparatus, thermometers and batteries, for the manufacture of some detonators and in dental amalgam.

The metabolism of mercury

Mercury is encountered in many different forms, as the metal, and as mercurous, mercuric or organic compounds, the last of which are grouped into alkyl, aryl and alkoxyl categories. The different forms have very different properties which help to determine their uptake, distribution and toxicity; the elemental, inorganic and alkyl forms are much the most toxic.

UPTAKE OF MERCURY

Mercury and its compounds generally cross biological membranes with ease and they may be absorbed by any of the three common routes: inhalation, ingestion and the skin.

Inhalation

Mercury vapour and compounds are well absorbed from the lung, and inhalation of vapour, aerosol or dust poses a high risk. This applies particularly to the metal itself which has a relatively high vapour pressure at room temperature: saturated air contains 20 mg/m^3 of mercury (2.37 ppm) at 25°C, i.e. 800 times the UK exposure standard. Few of those who regularly come into contact with elemental mercury, such as laboratory workers and dental nurses, realize that the metal vaporizes at room temperature and is readily absorbed through the lungs. Compounds of mercury are also rapidly absorbed through the lungs.

Ingestion

The organic compounds of mercury are more readily absorbed from the gut than are the inorganic. Mercury may be swallowed safely because only 0.01% of an ingested dose is absorbed. Ingested methyl and phenyl mercury are taken up quickly and virtually completely. About 10% of an ingested dose of mercuric salt is absorbed but uptake of mercurous salts is about 80% less. Many inorganic and aryl compounds including bichloride, nitrate, phenyl, butyl are corrosive when swallowed.

The skin

Mercury vapour is not absorbed through the skin but soluble and insoluble compounds, both inorganic and organic, appear to be absorbed at similar rates. Absorption is, however, too slow to cause acute poisoning but may lead to chronic intoxication.

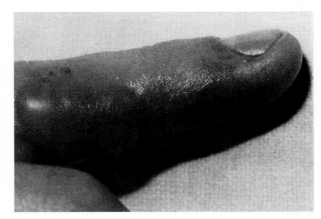

Figure 7.5 *Blister on the finger of a chemist who worked with butyl mercury nitrate. Courtesy of Professor RI McCallum.*

Some organic mercury compounds such as phenyl or butyl salts can cause chemical burns and blistering (Fig. 7.5).

DISTRIBUTION IN THE BODY

Mercury has a great affinity for thiol groups and is distributed bound to sulphur-containing ligands. Its affinity for thiol groups explains a number of its toxic effects for, like lead, it is able to combine with, and inhibit the action of, enzymes containing -SH groups. Following the absorption of elemental mercury it is transformed intracellularly into the divalent ionic form; the aryl, alkoxy and alkyl compounds also tend to release divalent mercuric ions in the tissues.

In the blood, inorganic mercury is distributed almost equally between the red cells and the plasma whereas the alkyl compounds (such as methyl mercury) are concentrated 10- or 20-fold in the red cells. The principal target organs for mercury are the central nervous system and the kidney. Within the kidney, mercury binds to metallothionein and the resultant metal protein complex may protect against the toxic effects of the free metal, and only when the metallothionein receptors are saturated does renal damage occur. The blood–brain barrier is crossed rapidly and readily by elemental mercury and by alkyl mercury compounds but not so well by inorganic compounds.

The post mortem findings in a man, who developed classical signs of mercurialism after working for 18 months filling mercury thermometers, and who died 16 years later after a slow but incomplete recovery, are interesting. Whilst there was no histological evidence of mercury toxicity, mercury was detected in lysosomal dense bodies in many nerve cells. It is not clear, however, how the presence of neuronal mercury was related to the mental and psychological state of the patient.[13]

By contrast, inorganic mercury accumulates rapidly in the cortex of the kidney but more slowly in the brain. These differences in distribution obviously contribute to the different toxic effects exerted by the various mercury compounds but it is not merely a matter of tissue concentration. Methyl mercury concentrations in the kidney, for example, are considerably higher than those in the central nervous system but, whereas the brain may be severely affected in methyl mercury poisoning, renal damage occurs only rarely.[14]

EXCRETION

Mercury is excreted in the urine and faeces and may also be found in the sweat, saliva and breast milk. The concentration of mercury in breast milk may be as much as 5% of the concentration in the blood and so be a risk to breast-fed infants of mothers who are exposed to mercury. Organomercury compounds are excreted in bile and reabsorbed from the gut.

The half-life of mercury compounds in the body is about 70 days; thus the excretion of absorbed material is slow and there is a tendency for the metal to accumulate with time. The urinary excretion of mercury shows considerable circadian variation and urinary concentrations are not always a good indicator of exposure but are used for the monitoring of exposed workers over a period of time. Blood mercury concentrations, on the other hand, reflect absorption well, once equilibrium has been achieved.[15] In the UK, the urine and blood concentrations for unexposed persons are less than 2.0 nmol/mmol creatinine (4.0 µg/litre) and 16 nmol/litre (3.2 µg/litre) respectively.

MERCURY POISONING

Acute poisoning

Acute poisoning usually results from the accidental or deliberate ingestion of mercury compounds and seldom from occupational exposure although acute industrial poisoning has been reported from the inhalation of mercury vapour at a concentration as low as 1 ppm. The toxicity of inorganic compounds is proportional to their solubility in gastric juice and, for example, the ingestion of less than 100 mg of mercuric chloride may cause severe symptoms.

Many compounds are corrosive and that may dominate the clinical picture. Acute effects include pain, inflammation, oedema and necrosis of the oropharyngeal mucosa. There may be nausea, vomiting and severe abdominal pain. Renal damage with both proximal tubular and glomerular lesions can develop rapidly and there may be albuminuria, haematuria, oliguria and excretion of casts.

In severe cases, acute papillary necrosis will occur. A chemical colitis may develop after 24–72 hours with the passage of bloody diarrhoea containing mucosal slough. There may be shock, oedema, tremor and ataxia. Specific diagnostic tests are of limited value but will demonstrate raised blood mercury levels and increased urinary and faecal excretion.

Poisoning from the inhalation of large amounts of mercury may cause an acute chemical pneumonitis with cough, dyspnoea, retrosternal pain, basal, late-inspiratory crackles, abnormal blood gases and patchy shadowing on chest radiograph. In severe cases, there will be expectoration of blood-stained sputum and pulmonary oedema.

Chronic poisoning

The classic symptoms of chronic mercury poisoning (noted by Kussmaul) are tremor, gingivitis and erethism (Gk *erethismos* = irritate). In addition, there may be evidence of renal damage and organic damage to the central nervous system.

The earliest findings are usually gingivitis, hypersalivation (mercurial ptyalism) and an unpleasant, bitter, metallic taste in the mouth. A bluish line on the dental margin of the gums, similar to that seen in lead workers, and a slate-grey or reddish, punctate pigmentation of the buccal mucosa are sometimes described but rarely seen. Gingivitis is most marked in those with poor oral hygiene and may be severe enough to cause loosening or loss of teeth.

Tremor, generally considered to be the first neurological indication of poisoning by elemental mercury or its inorganic compounds, is usually present at rest especially in the hands. It may be slight and accompanied by mild motor retardation (mercurial micro-parkinsonism). There is often an intentional component to the tremor, resembling that seen in cerebellar disease, which may seriously impair the ability to carry out fine and complex movements such as handwriting. The tremor in mercury poisoning may fluctuate in severity and be accompanied by ataxia resulting in difficulties in walking and in speaking. In poisoning with methyl mercury, cerebellar ataxia and dysarthria predominate, sometimes with constriction of the visual fields as the result of damage to the visual cortex. The clinical picture may resemble parkinsonism, multiple sclerosis or cerebellar disease but nystagmus is not a feature. Inability to release an object gripped in the hand has also been reported but, unlike the situation found in myotonia, it persists after repeated movements.

When the term 'erethism' was first coined, towards the end of the eighteenth century, it was used to describe the whole range of symptoms of mercury poisoning, but it is now reserved for the psychogenic manifestations. It is a form of toxic organic psychosis characterized by excessive timidity, morbid irritability, mental hyperactivity and outbursts of temper. There may be other features such as impairment of memory, difficulty in concentration, depression and somnolence. Short-term memory may also be slightly impaired in workers exposed to mercury who are otherwise normal.[16]

Mercury poisoning may present as a peripheral neuropathy which is predominantly sensory and is most common in those with organic mercury poisoning. Prolonged distal latencies in nerve conduction have been reported in some asymptomatic mercury workers and the neurophysiological changes correlate with time-integrated urinary mercury concentrations.[17] In advanced cases there are paraesthesiae of the extremities and around the mouth. In fatal cases, the dorsal and ventral roots of the spinal cord have been found to have undergone axonal degeneration and to have suffered a loss of myelin (see Chapter 42).[18]

The usual effect on the kidneys is tubular damage. Necrosis is more common in inorganic than organic poisoning. The glomerulus may also be damaged, leading to albuminuria in workers who have been exposed to mercury for many years. Rarely, a nephrotic syndrome may present as a manifestation of inorganic mercury poisoning.[19] Poisoning by mercury or a compound of mercury is a prescribed disease in the UK (see Chapter 4).

LABORATORY DIAGNOSIS

There are no laboratory tests that are particularly helpful in the diagnosis of chronic mercury poisoning but the finding of mercury in the urine or blood of those exposed to elemental mercury or to its inorganic or organic compounds confirms that absorption has occurred. Blood mercury concentrations in those exposed to methyl mercury are a good index of exposure as the alkylated compounds are mainly eliminated. If poisoning has occurred the blood mercury concentration may be well above 95 mmol/litre and the urinary level above 120 nmol/mmol creatinine for inorganic compounds and 15 nmol/nmol creatinine for organic compounds.

TREATMENT OF MERCURY POISONING

Acute mercury poisoning is a medical emergency and is dealt with in texts on poisoning, the purpose of treatment being to encourage the excretion of mercury and to limit gastrointestinal and renal damage. First-aid treatment involves the administration of four glasses of milk as an emulsient. If there is corrosive damage to the oropharynx, attention must be paid to the patency of the airway, and emergency tracheostomy performed if necessary. A stomach tube should be passed and gentle (bearing in mind the corrosive action of some mercury compounds) gastric lavage carried out using, preferably, warm, 10% sodium bicarbonate solution. If organomercury is involved, 3–6 sachets of the basic anion-exchange resin cholestyramine should be administered before the tube is withdrawn, as sequestration of bile salts increases faecal excretion of these compounds. Chelation therapy should be started, using either intravenous infusion of sodium calcium edetate or oral penicillamine (1–4 g daily, in four divided doses). It has been suggested[20] that in chronic mercury poisoning, though penicillamine may hasten the excretion of an easily mobilized extracellular fraction, it does not increase the excretion of mercury over a long period of time.

Care must be exercised as the chelation of mercury may enhance its passage across the blood–brain barrier and for this reason the use of dimercaprol (BAL) is contraindicated in poisoning with organic mercury compounds.[21] It is, however, extremely effective in the treatment of acute poisoning with inorganic mercurials when given by intramuscular injection. The recommended dose is 2.5 mg/kg body weight, repeated at 4-hour intervals for 2 days; after this the injections are given twice daily for 10 days or until recovery is complete. In the absence of these drugs intravenous administration of 100 ml of 5% sodium sulphate or

500–1000 ml of Ringer–Locke solution may be helpful. There is some evidence that alkaline diuresis, as described for salicylate poisoning in standard medical textbooks, with physiological saline, 5% dextrose and 1.26% bicarbonate solution affords the kidney some protection against mercury damage and might prevent the onset of anuria. This technique, however, is not without serious risk and ought to be carried out under continuous observation of fluid replacement and of electrolyte and acid-base status, as in an intensive care or high dependency unit.

Inhalation of large quantities of mercury vapour may lead to the onset of chemical pneumonitis 24–48 hours after exposure, with the onset of retrosternal discomfort and dyspnoea. Physical signs include tachypnoea, coarse basal crackles and, frequently, fever that may be treated symptomatically with oxygen and bronchodilators. Intercurrent infection will necessitate the use of appropriate antibiotics. If the condition is severe and respiratory failure threatens, mechanical ventilation may be required. If risk of permanent damage is high, it would be prudent to give steroids prophylactically but these have no proven value once the condition has developed.

There is no effective treatment for chronic mercury poisoning. Penicillamine and BAL may be tried, but are unlikely to alter the course of the illness, and the neurological effects of intoxication may never completely reverse. Mercaptopropionyl glycine has been used for the treatment of organic mercury poisoning in Japan. This drug produces a sustained increase in urinary excretion but has little effect on the clinical picture.[22]

SUPERVISION OF MERCURY WORKERS

The monitoring of mercury workers is generally based upon the periodical measurement of mercury in the urine. Because of the considerable circadian variation in the rate of urinary excretion it is important to ensure that samples are taken at the same time of day and not after several days away from exposure. It is usual to take samples at the end of the last working shift of the week.

For the UK, the upper 95% limits for urinary mercury are <2 µmol/mol creatinine (<3.5 µg/litre) for unexposed persons; the equivalent unexposed blood range is 0.6–19 nmol/litre. The occupational exposure standard is 0.025 mg/m^3 and the corresponding urine value is 20 µmol/mol creatinine (35 mg/g creatinine) and the blood threshold is 45 nmol/litre mercury.

It may be useful to test the urine for albumin at the same time using a simple dipstick method.

CADMIUM

Cadmium is one of the 'newer' metals, having been isolated by Strohmeyer in 1817. It occurs in nature with zinc and it is recovered as a by-product during the smelting of zinc ores and also from the smelting of some lead ores. It is used in electroplating, to make pigments, as a stabilizer in plastics and as one of the components in cadmium nickel batteries.

Cases of poisoning with the metal were first recorded in 1858 in Belgium, in domestic servants who had been polishing silver with a powder containing cadmium. In the UK, Legge reported three cases of cadmium poisoning with one fatality in 1924 in men in a paint factory where ingots of cadmium were melted down in a poorly ventilated room. Sporadic cases were subsequently reported from the UK until 1944 when Ross described mass poisoning in which 23 workers were affected by cadmium oxide fume. Finely divided cadmium dust from a cadmium recovery chamber ignited when a cigarette end was dropped by one of the workers. In a few minutes the cadmium dust became incandescent and emitted large clouds of cadmium oxide fume. The men affected complained of irritation of the eyes, headache, vertigo, dryness of the throat, cough, constriction of the chest and weakness of the legs. Three hours later they noticed further symptoms of shivering, nausea, epigastric pain and shortness of breath; none of them died.

Metabolism

Cadmium is poorly absorbed from the gut and only about 6% of an ingested dose is taken up whereas up to 40% may be retained in the lungs, depending on the particle size and solubility. In the blood, about 70% is bound to the red cells and it tends to accumulate in the liver and kidney, these two organs containing about 50% of the total body burden. The half-life of cadmium in the body is about 10 years and so, with continued exposure, it accumulates with age. The body burden in smokers is higher than in non-smokers although the increase is small compared with occupational causes.[23]

In the tissues, cadmium is largely bound to metallothionein which is a zinc storage protein with an unusual component of amino acids and containing between 30 and 35% of cysteine, 12% serine and 13% lysine or arginine. It has no aromatic amino acids in its structure and no histidine. The high proportion of sulphur-containing amino acids enables it to bind heavy metals and each molecule is able to bind seven divalent cations, usually zinc or copper but also cadmium, mercury and a number of other metals. Its synthesis is induced by the presence of zinc, cadmium, copper and mercury.

Cadmium is excreted in the urine, largely as a cadmium–metallothionein complex, but the rate of excretion is low (hence the long biological half-life) unless there is concomitant kidney damage. Small amounts of cadmium may also appear in the bile, saliva, hair and nails.

Cadmium poisoning

Acute effects may be noted after the inhalation of cadmium oxide fumes which are yellow and may be copious and are generated from welding or brazing on cadmium or its alloys. There is generally a lag period of up to 10 hours after the inhalation of the fumes before any untoward effects become apparent. The patient then notices retrosternal pain, dyspnoea and cough. With heavy exposure, pulmonary oedema may develop after 1–2 days; in some cases, symptoms similar to those seen in metal fume fever may develop (see Chapter 9). In all but the most severe cases, total resolution of the symptoms is usually complete within a week.

In chronic cadmium poisoning the kidney is the principal target organ. The earliest sign of cadmium poisoning is tubular proteinuria; the appearance of low molecular weight proteins (such as retinol binding protein, β2-microglobulins or a urinary enzyme such as N-acetyl-β-D-glucosaminidase (NAG)[24]) is particularly characteristic. The proteinuria may be accompanied by other evidence of tubular damage such as aminoaciduria, glycosuria and phosphaturia. There may be an increase in urinary calcium excretion, and renal stone formation has been reported in the UK and Sweden though not in other countries.

Renal damage is unlikely to occur until the concentration of cadmium in the renal cortex reaches about 200 ppm. When it reaches 215 ppm, renal dysfunction is likely to develop in about 10% of male workers occupationally exposed to the metal.[25] However, although the concept of a critical concentration refers to the total amount of cadmium in the renal cortex, it is only the small amount of the metal *not* bound to metallothionein that is capable of causing nephrotoxicity. It has been suggested that the concentration of free cadmium which will produce β_2-microglobulinuria is 2 ppm or 1% of the critical concentration of the total cadmium concentration in the kidney. There is some evidence that factors such as the capacity to synthesize metallothionein and ageing may decrease the critical concentration of cadmium which is associated with the development of tubular damage.

Some studies have shown that cadmium workers may also have an increased urinary excretion of albumin[26] which may occur with or without the excretion of tubular proteins, suggesting that, in some workers at least, cadmium also induces glomerular damage, but the mechanism by which this is brought about is obscure.

Although the concentrations of cadmium in the liver are high, liver damage is not a prominent feature of chronic cadmium poisoning.

The other important sequel of long-term exposure to cadmium is the development of emphysema, which was a common feature in a number of studies of cadmium workers, although some authorities dispute the extent to which cadmium may damage the lungs.[27] Lung function tests, which have sometimes been reported to be abnormal in cadmium workers, do not seem to show any dose–response relationship and are certainly not such sensitive indicators of cadmium damage as the excretion of tubular proteins.[28] Anosmia was also reported in early studies, as was anaemia, thought to be due to an interference with copper metabolism. Yellowing of the teeth also sometimes occurs.

There is some evidence that cadmium workers have a higher than expected incidence of prostatic cancer and also of lung cancer.[29] None of this evidence is overwhelming, however, and the risk, if it exists at all, is probably small. Poisoning by cadmium is a prescribed disease in the UK (see Chapter 4).

Itai-itai disease

Itai-itai disease was the name given to an outbreak of osteomalacia found in multiparous women in Japan. The women in whom the condition was first noted lived in an area where the crops had become contaminated with cadmium from water that had drained through an old zinc mine and had been used for irrigation. The women had pains in the back and legs (*itai-itai* literally means 'ouch-ouch') and a number developed pathological fractures. The occurrence of osteomalacia in cadmium workers has been considered by Stanbury and Mawer.[30] The cause of the osteomalacia is still not clear. Because cadmium may induce a Fanconi-like syndrome, a hypophosphataemic osteomalacia may occur (and not be recognized unless sought). In addition, cadmium, as noted above, accumulates in the cells of the renal tubules and there is evidence from radioisotopic studies of some failure of calcitrol formation in these cells. More recent findings in a study of smelter workers with continuous long-term exposure to cadmium suggest that perturbation of the vitamin D metabolic pathway arises through an interaction of cadmium with renal mitochondrial hydroxylases of the vitamin D_3 endocrine complex.[31]

Hypertension

It has been suggested that cadmium in the environment may be concerned in the aetiology of hypertension.[32] In experimental animals, exposure to cadmium modifies a number of mechanisms that regulate cardiovascular function but there are some important differences between species.[33] In epidemiological studies, cadmium workers have not had an increased prevalence of hypertension, and, if cadmium has a role in the aetiology of hypertension in those who are exposed to it only in the general environment, it is certainly not a simple one.

Diagnosis and treatment

Only a careful occupational history of exposure in a patient with renal or respiratory disease, in the absence of a more likely explanation, will lead to a diagnosis of cadmium poisoning. An elevated urinary cadmium concentration will be a guide to increased exposure, especially when renal damage is well established, but that cannot be used alone as the basis of a diagnosis.

Chelating agents such as BAL and EDTA increase the urinary excretion of cadmium but their effectiveness diminishes with time,[11] primarily because they remove only that cadmium not bound to metallothionein. They are not recommended as there have been reports that this treatment may cause kidney damage. There is little to be done in the case of chronic poisoning except to ensure that the patient is removed from further exposure, monitored for renal function and subclinical osteomalacia, and given whatever general treatment seems appropriate.

Supervision of cadmium workers

The interrelationships between cadmium exposure and cadmium concentration in blood and urine are complex and reflect the accumulation of cadmium in liver and kidney over considerable periods of time. It is generally accepted that the concentration of cadmium in blood reflects to some extent the level of exposure over the preceding 3–6 months. The concentration of cadmium in urine rises with liver and kidney accumulation following either environmental or occupational exposure. When the 'critical level' in the kidney is recorded there may well be a considerable rise in the urinary excretion of cadmium, related to the onset of renal tubular dysfunction.

Biological monitoring of cadmium workers is necessary to prevent excessive uptake leading to renal damage.[35] The urinary cadmium concentration that corresponds to the 'critical level' in the kidney is reported to be between 10 and 15 nmol/mmol creatinine (11.2 and 16.8 µg/litre). Because of the varying relationships between blood and urine concentrations during cadmium accumulation, both blood and urine concentrations should be measured. Ideas about appropriate cut-off levels vary between 90–180 nmol/litre blood (10–20 µg/litre) and 10–20 nmol/mmol creatinine (11.2–22.4 µg/litre) in urine. There is little epidemiological evidence to distinguish between them. The UK Health and Safety Executive recommends that blood levels below 90 nmol/litre (10 µg/litre) and urine levels below 10 nmol/litre mmol creatinine (11.2 µg/litre) indicate adequate control of exposure. Urinary levels greater than 15 nmol/mmol creatinine (16.8 µg/litre) indicate excessive cadmium accumulation in the renal cortex and the need for measurement of urinary proteins and an investigation into work practices and exposure.

The routine measurement of low molecular weight proteins in the urine is frequently used to assess the integrity of the proximal tubules in cadmium workers. Traditionally, β_2-microglobulins were measured, but because they are unstable in acid urine and because they may increase simply as a result of increased production (pregnancy, infection, malignancy), it is essential to measure blood levels as well. Alternatively, the measurement of NAG or of urinary retinol-binding protein is often used instead.

It is now possible to measure cadmium concentrations in liver and kidney in vivo using neutron activation analysis.[36] This technique is non-invasive, produces negligible amounts of radiation and uses transportable equipment but it is presently a research tool.

The assessment of renal function depends on the measurement of the excretion of both low and high molecular weight proteins. Increased excretion of low molecular weight proteins indicates tubular damage and failure of reabsorption, while the excretion of high molecular weight proteins, such as albumen, reflects glomerular damage. Metals may injure glomeruli and tubules, resulting in combined excretion of both high and low molecular weight proteins.

Measurement of urinary β_2-microglobulin has been widely used as an indicator of tubular function. This protein is, however, degraded rapidly in the bladder when urinary pH is less than 5.5. Because the rate of excretion depends upon endogenous production within the body, serum levels must also be measured. Retinol-binding protein (RBP) is stable at all urinary pH values and is therefore a more suitable indicator for tubular function (see Chapter 2).

More recent developments in this field have included measurement of NAG, a renal tubule enzyme, in urine. It is also possible to measure urinary concentrations of laminin, a glycoprotein component of glomerular basement membrane, and serum antibodies to this and other components of renal tissue. These have all been found in increased quantities following hydrocarbon[37–39] and chlorocarbon[40]-induced renal damage. These newer tests have not been widely applied to metal nephropathies.[41] Whether or not they will add diagnostic or prognostic value to the problem is debatable (see Chapter 2).

ARSENIC

Arsenic was known in antiquity through its sulphides but it was not extracted and used in its elemental form as were the other metals of antiquity. It occurs as an impurity in the ores of copper, lead and zinc and has been found in considerable quantities in some bronzes from archaeological sites. There have been suggestions that arsenical bronzes may have caused toxic symptoms in persons who worked with them and that many of the mythological smith gods were lame because polyneuropathy was an occupational disease among their mortal counterparts. Equally it has been argued that the lame from birth were turned out to become smiths. *Post hoc or propter hoc*? A pitfall well known to present day epidemiologists.

Arsenic is found in industry in its inorganic or organic forms and is also a constituent of the gas arsine which is used in the electronics industry. Most arsenic is used nowadays in pesticides and herbicides but exposure may occur in smelting, in the chemical, pesticide and pharmaceutical industries. Most workers are exposed to the inorganic compounds and, of these, the trivalent compounds are generally more toxic than the pentavalent.

Arsenical pigments were commonly used, especially during the nineteenth century, the most popular being Paris green (cupric acetoarsenite) and Scheele's green (cupric arsenite). Paris green was prepared by mixing together a copper salt, arsenious oxide and acetic acid but the exact method was kept a secret until it was published in 1822 by Liebig. In the middle of the nineteenth century the use of these pigments was so common that chronic arsenical poisoning from their dusts was widespread. The symptoms noted included coryza, vomiting, conjunctivitis, laryngitis and dermatitis.

Another hazard from the use of green arsenical pigments in wallpaper arose from the mould *Scopulariopsis brevicaulis* which was often a contaminant of wallpaper to form the gas dimethylarsine which escaped into the room. A variety of symptoms were sometimes considered to be associated with the use of these wallpapers and it has even been suggested that the death of Napoleon was due to arsenic given off from the wallpaper in the house in which he was confined on Elba. As late as 1931, a child died in the Forest of Dean from dimethylarsine poisoning; the arsenic was in a constituent of the plaster on the mouldy walls of the damp house in which he lived.

Metabolism

Arsenic has a half-life in blood of about 60 hours and, whatever the compound, is rapidly eliminated through the kidney either unchanged or after biotransformation. Cacodylic acid is excreted unchanged whereas monomethyl arsonic acid is partially methylated (to the extent of about 10%) to cacodylic acid (Fig. 7.6). About 75% of a dose of inorganic arsenic is excreted in the methylated form as either monomethyl arsonic acid or cacodylic acid. The methylated forms are much less toxic than inorganic arsenic and so this *in vivo* methylation represents a true detoxification process. With normal renal function, the biological half-life of arsenic in the urine after exposure to inorganic arsenic is between 1 and 2 days. During the first hours after exposure the arsenic is excreted mainly in the inorganic form but after about 8 hours the organic forms predominate as the methylation process starts. Some,

Figure 7.6 *Excretion products of arsenic.*

however, is retained in the dermal tissues of skin, hair and nails.

Acute poisoning

Acute arsenic poisoning may follow the ingestion of deliberately or accidentally contaminated food or drink. The presenting symptoms are abdominal pain, profound vomiting, rice water stools, dehydration and shock. These may be followed by stupor, coma, convulsions and death. The underlying lesion appears to be dilatation and increased permeability of the small blood vessels in the gut and elsewhere.

Chronic poisoning

This is the more common form of arsenical poisoning and can affect many systems of the body, including the skin, peripheral nerves, liver, cardiovascular system, blood and the respiratory system.

Chronic exposure to arsenic may induce a variety of changes in the skin, including eczematous or follicular dermatitis, ulceration, hyperkeratosis of the palms and the soles and hyperpigmentation (raindrop pigmentation). The most serious effects on the skin, however, are the production of skin cancer, and three types have been associated with exposure to arsenic: basal cell carcinoma, squamous cell carcinoma and Bowen's disease.

Priority for drawing attention to the carcinogenic properties of arsenic is generally given to Jonathan Hutchinson who, in 1888, described some cases of skin cancer in patients treated with arsenical mixtures for psoriasis and other skin conditions. Cases were later described in sheep dippers but the numbers were always small.

The peripheral neuropathy of arsenic poisoning is a form of dying back neuropathy of mixed sensorimotor type (see Chapter 42) and is caused by interference with glycolysis within the neuron. Arsenic inhibits the conversion of pyruvate diphosphoglycerate from glyceraldehyde-3-phosphate. The earliest symptoms are paraesthesiae with a glove and stocking distribution. Loss of vibration sense may be the earliest sign of the neuropathy. Electrophysiological studies show a decrease in the amplitude and a moderate reduction in the conduction velocity in the sensory nerves.[42] There may be pains in the limbs, especially in the calf muscles, and these may be followed by muscular weakness, especially in the legs. There is some evidence that the neuropathy is at least partially reversible once exposure is discontinued. Treatment of the condition with BAL has been tried with variable success and a therapeutic trial may be worth while.

Acute encephalopathy, which may resolve completely, is a rare sequel of exposure to arsenic. In one case, treatment with BAL was given but did not appear to affect the outcome materially.[43]

Exposure to arsenic is also associated with liver enlargement and with hepatic cirrhosis (see Chapter 43). This hepatocellular toxicity may be the result of the inhibition of enzymes concerned with intracellular respiration. Trivalent arsenic has a particular avidity for -SH groups and is thus able to interfere with the enzymes that rely on this group for their normal function.[44]

A megaloblastic anaemia has been associated with chronic arsenic exposure, and in experimental animals arsenic is found to interfere with -SH group enzymes concerned with haem synthesis in a manner analogous to lead. There is no good evidence of this occurring in persons with occupational exposure.

The characteristic lesion in the respiratory tract is a perforation of the nasal cartilaginous septum due to inflammatory and erosive lesions in the mucosa. It is generally painless and may occur within a short time of starting work entailing exposure to arsenic. Poisoning by arsenic is a prescribed disease in the UK (see Chapter 4).

Arsenic and cancer

In addition to skin cancer, exposure to arsenic has also been linked with angiosarcoma of the liver (in persons treated in the past with Fowler's solution or other arsenical medications) and lung cancer. An excess of lung cancer was noted among sheep dippers in the first half of this century but the numbers were small and it was unclear whether the effect was real. Since then an increased mortality from lung cancer has been reported in several studies of workers exposed to arsenic in different occupations and in different countries. In one study at least, a positive dose–response effect was noted with a rise in standardized mortality ratio (SMR) associated with an increasing degree of exposure (see Chapter 39).[45]

Study of the carcinogenicity of arsenic has been hampered because man is the only species in whom arsenic is known to induce tumours, and in this respect it appears to be unique.

Arsine

Arsine (AsH_3) is a colourless gas which is odourless at low concentrations but smells of garlic at high concentrations. It is formed whenever arsenic comes into contact with nascent hydrogen.

Arsine is a potent intravascular haemolysin and the symptoms that occur in arsine poisoning follow upon this central event (see Chapters 8, 44).

ORGANIC DERIVATIVES OF ARSINE

The organic derivatives of arsine have no commercial applications but were widely developed during the world wars as potential chemical weapons. They are highly vesicant and irritant to the lungs and mucous membranes. Their study led to the development of BAL (British anti-lewisite) as an antidote for chlorovinyldichloroarsine (lewisite). BAL is a dithiol compound which was found to be particularly effective both at preventing the toxic effects of some of the war gases and at reversing them once they had occurred. It was later used to treat some forms of poisoning with heavy metals which are known to have a special affinity for thiol groups.

Supervision of workers exposed to arsenic

The determination of arsenic in the urine provides a reliable index of recent exposure. In persons exposed to inorganic arsenic the determination of inorganic arsenic, monomethyl arsonic acid and cacodylic acid is required and the sum of these three arsenical compounds does not usually exceed 200 µg/g creatinine when the time-weighted average airborne concentrations are about 50 µg/m³. Because arsenic is a human carcinogen the aim must be to keep exposure as close to background levels as possible, in which case the urinary arsenic concentrations would be unlikely to exceed 50 µg/litre.

Total arsenic concentration in the urine may be misleading in workers who eat a lot of fish or shellfish, as some marine organisms may contain relatively high concentrations of organoarsenicals that are not toxic but are rapidly excreted unchanged in the urine.[46]

For workers exposed to monomethyl arsenic or cacodylic acids, the direct estimation of their concentration in the urine is an adequate measure of absorption.

Arsenic in hair and in nails has long been used by forensic scientists to determine exposure to arsenic in cases of suspected poisoning. Hair concentrations give a reliable indication of exposure to inorganic arsenic during the growth of the hair but they have little application for monitoring occupational exposure.

PHOSPHORUS

Phosphorus does not occur free in nature because it oxidizes extremely rapidly in contact with air. It is, however, widely distributed in the form of phosphate rock which is impure calcium phosphate, and as chlorapatite and fluorapatite. There are three allotropes of phosphorus: white (or yellow), red and black, of which the white variety is by far the most toxic.

The metal was discovered in 1674 by Hennig Brandt, a German alchemist and physician working in Hamburg. He hoped to make gold from human urine or at least convert silver into gold. Instead he produced a soft, white, waxy substance which glowed in the dark even when cold. No doubt Brandt was disappointed by his failure to prepare gold from urine but he was nevertheless able to make a living by demonstrating his glowing phosphorus in darkened rooms and by advertising it as a therapeutic agent.

In modern industry, phosphorus and its compounds have many uses including the manufacture of munitions, fireworks, explosive and incendiary devices, the production of chemicals, fertilizers, sugar, detergents, animal foods, pharmaceuticals, chlorinated organic compounds, insecticides and rodenticides. They are also used in electropolishing, engraving, photography, metal cleaning and water treatment and in the manufacture of semi-conductors and electroluminescent coatings.

The history of the use of phosphorus in match making is one of the most important and interesting in occupational medicine. The first friction match contained no phosphorus and was not very ignitable. This was the lucifer match sold in 1829 by Samuel Jones. The first match to contain white phosphorus was manufactured in 1832 in Austria by J Siegel and in Germany by C Kammerer. These matches, known as congreves after Sir William Congreve, were ignited by rubbing the head against any hard surface. In fact they were *too* ignitable and houses were set on fire by boxes of matches which had been left in the sun, or on shelves, or shaken. Despite this, the congreve match became extremely popular and remained in use in the UK until about 1870.

The use of white phosphorus in match-making ushered in what Donald Hunter referred to as 'the greatest tragedy in the whole story of occupational disease'. This was phosphorus-induced necrosis of the jaw – phossy jaw. The first cases were reported in 1844, 12 years after phosphorus matches were first manufactured, and within a few years they had been reported in almost every country in the world. The onset of the disease was generally quite slow, an average of about 5 years being required for the symptoms to develop from first exposure, although in susceptible cases the effects might become apparent within a few months.

In its full blown form, phossy jaw was an extremely painful and disfiguring condition; the mandible became necrotic with the formation of osteoporotic sequestra and abscesses which discharged foul-smelling pus. The mortality rate was about 20%, death being brought about most frequently by septicaemia. The only prospect of a cure lay in surgical removal of half or all the mandible; the fact that any patients at all submitted to this terrible operation gives some indication of their horror of the disease.

Although there could be no disputing the extremely harmful effects that white phosphorus could produce, it took many years for its use in match-making to be abolished altogether. The first country to abolish the use of white phosphorus was Finland, in 1872. Denmark followed suit 2 years later, Switzerland in 1898 and the Netherlands in 1901. By the Berne Convention of 1906 all the important countries of Europe agreed to forbid the manufacture and import of white phosphorus matches, and the use of white phosphorus was made illegal in England in 1910. In the USA, white phosphorus continued to be used in the mistaken belief that cases of phossy jaw did not occur there. Within a few years of the Berne Convention, however, 150 cases and four deaths had been recorded, and in 1931 the US government placed a prohibitive tax on white phosphorus matches and forbade their import and export. This almost immediately brought their use to an end.

In cases of chronic exposure, white phosphorus appears to act on the periosteum, leading to the formation of very compact tissue with thickening of the periosteum.[47] Necrosis, however, does not supervene until the occurrence of bacterial infection. Tooth extraction (necessitated sometimes because of the action of phosphorus on the tooth) allows bacterial access through the socket and the onset of 'phosphorus necrosis'.

Phossy jaw in modern times

White phosphorus is now used for the manufacture of munitions and explosives, and it is one of the constituents of napalm. Phossy jaw may still occur in those who manufacture these items or produce the white phosphorus itself, but improved dental hygiene and the use of antibiotics has ensured that the clinical picture is very different from that of earlier days. Nevertheless, some modern cases have developed sequestra requiring surgical removal.[48]

Other toxic effects of phosphorus

In addition to causing bony necrosis, white phosphorus causes serious burns on contact with the skin and these must be treated as rapidly as possible with a solution of cellulose and 3% copper sulphate with a small amount of lauryl sulphate added to enhance surface contact with the particles of phosphorus that adhere to the skin.[49]

Phosphoric acid and phosphoric sulphides are irritant to the eyes, the mucous membranes and the respiratory tract. The trichloride, pentachloride and oxychlorides of phosphorus are also extremely irritant, forming phosphoric and hydrochloric acids on contact with water;

this may occur in the tissue fluids in the upper respiratory tract or the eyes. Chronic exposure to the trichloride and pentachloride may be associated with the development of chronic bronchitis. Poisoning by phosphorus compounds is a prescribed disease in the UK (see Chapter 4).

Phosphine

Phosphine (PH_3) is a gas formed in a number of different circumstances, including the manufacture of acetylene, in the quenching of some metal alloys with water, when either zinc phosphide or aluminium phosphide is wetted, in the cleaning out of sulphuric acid tanks, during the rust proofing or handling of ferrosilicon and during the handling of yellow phosphorus explosives (see Chapter 8).

Supervision of workers exposed to phosphorus

Workers exposed to white phosphorus should have a rigorous pre-employment dental examination, and those with poor dental hygiene and untreated carious teeth should be advised to seek treatment before they can be considered for employment. Periodic dental examinations should be undertaken on those at work.

ALUMINIUM

Aluminium is a light, white metal which is used more widely throughout industry than any other non-ferrous metal, for the manufacture of alloys, engine and aircraft components, electric wires and cables, window frames, roofs and cladding, and beverage or food containers.

There has been great debate over the years about whether exposure to aluminium can cause disease. Traditionally it was considered that aluminium was poorly absorbed from the lung and gut, but subsequent evidence suggests that this may not always be so. It has been suggested that increased absorption of aluminium may be associated with increased risk of developing pulmonary fibrosis and Alzheimer's disease.

Occupational studies have included workers involved in the manufacture of alumina (aluminium oxide) abrasives, gold and uranium miners, aluminium smelter workers and those involved in the manufacture of aluminium powder.

In 1947 Shaver and Riddell reported cases of pulmonary fibrosis in workers who had been engaged in the manufacture of alumina abrasives and who commonly developed dyspnoea and pneumothorax. As they had also been exposed to silica and iron oxide fume, the precise cause of the disease was not clear.

Aluminium was given prophylactically to some Canadian gold and uranium miners between 1944 and 1979, in the mistaken belief that it prevented silicosis. Men were exposed to 20 000–34 000 ppm. 'McIntyre powder', consisting of 85% aluminium oxide and 15% aluminium for 10 minutes before each shift. Follow-up over 22 years has not revealed any cases of pulmonary fibrosis and the pattern and the prevalence of respiratory disease were similar to that in gold miners who had not been exposed to aluminium.[50] A more recent study failed to show any excess of neurological disease, but demonstrated a dose-related impairment on cognitive function testing.[51] Other recent studies have not confirmed these findings. There is still no firm conclusion as to whether occupational aluminium exposure can result in neuropsychological disorder.[52,53,54]

A number of studies have demonstrated an association between aluminium smelting and the development of an asthma-like syndrome.[55,56] There is also an increased prevalence of chronic airway disease (but not fibrosis), but it is difficult to say whether these effects are due to aluminium or to other substances such as sulphur dioxide and tar pitch volatiles, to which smelter workers are also exposed (see Chapter 8). A number of cases of pulmonary fibrosis associated with occupational exposure to aluminium powder have, however, been reported.[57–59] A study of workers at one of the factories, engaged in 'stamping' aluminium for use in pyrotechnics, found that six out of 30 had evidence of pulmonary fibrosis.[60] Subsequently, a series of pathological studies revealed that 'stamped' rather than granular aluminium powders were more likely to produce fibrosis.[61] Some authors have speculated that these cases may result from inhalation of aluminium particles of submicron size or, perhaps, aluminium fibres.[62]

Occupational absorption of aluminium has also been studied,[63] and it appears that exposed workers can absorb through their lungs, and excrete in urine, considerable quantities of aluminium. Unfortunately, that study did not document airborne levels, so it is not possible to put the results into the context of other industrial exposures.

Outside the occupational setting, aluminium has been implicated in the aetiology of Alzheimer's disease[64–66] and encephalopathy in patients undergoing renal dialysis.[67] Raised aluminium levels have been found in the brains of patients dying with Alzheimer's disease and also in the blood of renal patients, with or without encephalopathy, undergoing dialysis or taking oral aluminium hydroxide as a phosphate binder.

Under normal circumstances, aluminium is poorly absorbed from the gut. Once absorbed, more than 95% is transported in high molecular weight complexes, mainly bound to the glycoprotein, transferrin, which avidly binds metals. The remainder is associated with low molecular weight complexes, probably citrates. The spare binding capacity of transferrin is so great that it is very difficult to overwhelm it with aluminium by the oral route. Intravenous administration in dialysis fluid may, however, favour the formation of low molecular weight complexes of aluminium which cross the blood-brain barrier with relative ease, whereas high molecular weight complexes do not. Aluminium can only be released from transferrin into cells with surface transferrin receptors, and brain tissue has very few of these. Intravenous absorption of aluminium might possibly explain the development of encephalopathy and renal disease might enhance gut absorption of aluminium, but patients with renal failure do not appear to develop Alzheimer's disease more frequently than the general population. This question is discussed in Chapter 42. Recent research, using radioactive gallium as an analogue of aluminium, has suggested that patients suffering from Alzheimer's disease or Down's syndrome, which predisposes to the disease, may have a genetically determined defect of transferrin which impairs its ability to bind aluminium.[68] The study of [26]Al tracer absorption, using high energy accelerator mass spectrometry (AMS) may throw more light on this aspect.[69]

Accidental contamination of the water supply to the Camelford area of England with 8% aluminium sulphate solution, resulted in a number of consumers developing acute gastrointestinal symptoms and nasopharyngeal ulcers. No cases of encephalopathy were reported. Water aluminium concentrations at the time ranged from 30 to 620 mg/litre, well above the maximum of 0.2 mg/litre in the European Community Drinking Water Directive. Two sufferers were subsequently investigated.[70] Plasma aluminium levels were within normal limits (less than 10 μg/litre); 24-hour urine aluminium was slightly raised above UK normal range of up to 15 μg. Aluminium concentrations in bone biopsy specimens were normal (range 1.5–13.3 μg/g) but the pattern of deposition suggested a short period of enhanced aluminium absorption. A 3-year follow-up study of 55 affected individuals found evidence of damage to cerebral function which was not related to anxiety.[206]

There is no evidence that aluminium metal or any of its compounds are carcinogenic. However, an excess of pulmonary cancer has been observed in aluminium smelter workers. This is now attributed to the benzo pyrenes liberated from the carbon arc during smelting.[71] The process has been recognized by the International Agency for Research on Cancer (IARC)[72] as causing human cancer.

Contact dermatitis to aluminium has been recognized and can be confirmed with patch tests[73] but is relatively rare.

Determination of aluminium in body tissues has more of a place as a research tool than as a routine form of biological monitoring, and is infrequently used in the workplace.[63] The upper reference limit for urinary aluminium in those not occupationally involved is 0.6 μmol/litre.

ANTIMONY

A brittle, silver-white metalloid, antimony is usually obtained from the sulphide ore stibnite, found in commercially usable deposits in China, South America, Canada and several European countries. Its main use is as a flame retardant for plastics, paint, textiles, paper, rubber and adhesives, in the form of the trioxide. Its use in storage batteries as an alloy with lead in the grids has greatly decreased in the UK. Pentavalent organic compounds of antimony are used in the treatment of leishmaniasis where they act by inhibiting the enzyme phosphofructokinase, but in the treatment of schistosomiasis antimony has been superseded by other drugs.

Antimony is frequently found together with arsenic, and some of the toxic effects that have been ascribed to antimony may well have been due to arsenic. In the past, irritation of mucous membranes and dermatitis (antimony spots) have been common in antimony process workers but working conditions have improved considerably in recent years, so they are now uncommon. Nosebleeds, laryngitis and bronchitis were also described. A simple pneumoconiosis used to be common in antimony process workers and in antimony miners in whom it was combined with silicosis. In the process workers, the pneumoconiosis appeared as fine nodular opacities in the radiograph, the opacities often being close to the hilum.[74] Lung function is not greatly impaired and pathological studies in animals have not demonstrated fibrosis of the lung. With heavy and prolonged exposure to the processing of antimony a variety of gastrointestinal symptoms, including pain, nausea and vomiting, diarrhoea and a metallic taste in the mouth, have been reported,[75] together with perforation of the nasal septum. The actual cause of these symptoms, however, may in part be related to materials other than antimony involved in the processing, including arsenic.

Abnormalities in the electrocardiograph in workers exposed to antimony trisulphide have been reported,[76] including widening of the QRS complex, prolongation of the ST interval and flattening of T waves. Whilst it is known that ECG changes can occur in patients who have been treated for schistosomiasis with antimony compounds, and that organic antimony compounds have been shown to cause ECG changes in patients under long-term treatment, controlled observations on industrially exposed workers are lacking and there is no confirmatory evidence of toxic action on the cardiovascular system.[77]

One epidemiological study of antimony workers has shown an excess of lung cancer deaths in process and maintenance workers. It cannot be assumed, however, that the cause of this was antimony or its compounds; arsenic, which was used at one time to make an antimony arsenic alloy, could have been implicated.[78] Animal work has suggested that antimony may be carcinogenic but there are serious reservations about the limited available experiments and further work is required to clarify the problem.

Stibine, antimony hydride (SbH_3), is formed by the reaction between acids and metals containing antimony. It has also been evolved from batteries, whose lead plates contained some antimony, during charging. In its toxicity, it strongly resembles arsine with which it is sometimes associated, and it can cause a profound haemolytic anaemia followed by acute tubular necrosis and death (see Chapter 8). No specific treatment is described; exchange transfusions and dialysis have been suggested.

BARIUM

Barium, discovered by Sir Humphry Davey in 1808, is a soft alkaline earth metal that is so reactive that it does not occur in the natural state. The principal ores are barytes (barium sulphate) and witherite (barium carbonate). Commercial preparation of the metal is by heating the oxidic form in a vacuum with aluminium or by electrolysis. Barium is used as an alloy with nickel and other metals in the automative industry and in electronics. Barium sulphate is used as a contrast medium in clinical radiology and also in the manufacture of rubber, paint, soap and ceramics. Barium nitrite is used in fireworks, and barium carbonate has been utilized as a rat poison.

Baritosis is a benign, generally symptomless, pneumoconiosis resulting from the inhalation of finely divided barium sulphate dust. The radiological appearance is of circumscribed nodules, evenly distributed throughout the lung fields, which resolve on cessation of exposure.[79] No long function abnormalities occur in spite of the bizarre x-ray picture.

A study of welders[80] using barium-containing stick electrodes in an experimental situation indicated that exposure to soluble forms of barium exceeded the limit value for total welding fume of 5 mg/m³ and soluble welding fume of 0.5 mg/m³. The urinary barium reached 102 µg/litre, five times that of unexposed persons, but no adverse health effects were noted.

BERYLLIUM

Beryllium is a rare and extremely light metal with an atomic weight of 9. It occurs in nature as beryllium aluminium silicate, or beryl. There are three forms of beryl: emerald, the green colour of which is derived from chromium oxide; the gemstone aquamarine; and the yellow chrysoberyl. Beryllium is a hard shiny metal which resembles steel in appearance and lustre but its chemical properties are similar to those of aluminium and magnesium. The principal use of beryllium is in the manufacture of alloys, of which beryllium copper is the chief,

although beryllium nickel and beryllium aluminium are also in use. When 2–3% of beryllium is added to copper, the resultant alloy is hard, non-rusting, non-sparking and non-magnetic, and it has great tensile strength. The alloys can be temper hardened, when they behave like spring steel, and their electrical conductivity is similar to that of copper. They are also used for high performance, high reliability electrical connectors, in computers, telecommunications, automobiles and domestic appliances; undersea applications, oil drilling equipment, aircraft landing gear bearings, plastic moulding tools and non-sparking tools. Beryllium is highly transparent to x-rays and is used as a 'window' material in x-ray generators and detectors. It also has attractive thermal properties (high melting point, specific heat and conductivity) and is a very efficient neutron moderator, used in nuclear reactors.

Beryllia, the oxide of beryllium also has important commercial applications as an electrical insulator and is a very good thermal conductor. In ceramic form it is used as a heatsink insulator in electrical circuitry, microwave transmitters and lasers. It was formerly used in preparing the powdered phosphors zinc beryllium manganese silicate, zinc beryllium silicate and beryllium oxide for fluorescent strip lights. The fluorescent tubes were coated on the inside by pumping in a liquid suspension of the phosphor, the excess of which was drained away. Dry mixing of the powders, spillage and brushing clean the ends of the tubes produced considerable amounts of dust, and many cases of chronic beryllium disease were noted in workers engaged in this work. Beryllium phosphor has not been used in fluorescent tubes for 40 or more years.

The first cases of beryllium poisoning were seen in Germany in 1933 in people employed in extracting the metal from beryl. Cases were also described in the 1930s in Russia among workers preparing beryllium steel. Harriet Hardy in the USA contributed greatly to the understanding of this disease and described it in employees of a firm manufacturing fluorescent lights in Salem, Massachusetts. She noted the resemblance between beryllium disease and sarcoidosis and thus it came to be called Salem sarcoid. In 1952 she established the Beryllium Case Register to collect information about patients with the disease.

Acute poisoning

Beryllium may act as a direct irritant to the respiratory tract, leading to nasopharyngitis, tracheobronchitis or chemical pneumonitis. The severity of the symptoms is proportional to the inhaled dose, and the signs and symptoms are non-specific but may include dyspnoea, chest pain, cough with blood-stained sputum, tachycardia and cyanosis. Radiographs of the chest show diffuse or localized infiltrations. Heavy exposure can cause a fatal chemical pneumonitis but the clinical picture is variable. With less intense exposures, complete resolution of the symptoms can be expected following removal from exposure and treatment with bed rest, and oxygen if there is evidence of hypoxaemia. Corticosteroids are indicated in the most severe cases. Acute berylliosis is nowadays rare (see Chapter 35).

An insidious form of acute beryllium disease was reported by early workers in this field. It was observed as early as 3 weeks after commencing exposure.[81,82]

Skin disease

The implantation of beryllium compounds beneath the skin leads to the formation of a non-caseating granuloma. Granulomata have also been reported in patients in whom the only exposure has been through the inhalation of the dust of the metal or its compounds. These lesions were relatively common in those who cut themselves on broken fluorescent tubes coated with beryllium phosphor, and there was often a prolonged delay before the granulomata appeared.

Beryllium may also act as a sensitizer, producing a contact dermatitis which may be accompanied by periorbital oedema, conjunctivitis and upper respiratory tract involvement.

Chronic beryllium disease

Chronic beryllium disease is a condition associated with pulmonary granulomata formed as the result of inhaling beryllium dust. There is a latent period lasting from several months to several years between first exposure and the appearance of symptoms, but this generally lies between 10 and 15 years.

The first symptom is shortness of breath on exertion, followed by fatigue and weight loss, chest and joint pains and cough. On examination, skin rashes, lymphadenopathy, hepatosplenomegaly, crackles at both bases and finger clubbing may all be found.

The clinical course is extremely variable; some patients have a stable course in which they experience no worsening of symptoms for years whereas others show a progressive deterioration. This condition is also discussed further in Chapter 35.

RADIOGRAPHIC CHANGES

Standard chest radiography reveals a diffuse pulmonary infiltration and hilar lymphadenopathy. The opacities may be granular, nodular, linear or a mixture of all three. Hilar lymphadenopathy occurs in up to 50% of patients and is usually bilateral and not very marked. In beryllium disease it is very rare in the absence of parenchymal disease. That contrasts with the appearance in sarcoido-

sis. In addition there may be evidence of collapse of (usually the upper) lobes with overinflation of the adjacent lung tissue, calcification in the parenchymal opacities and hilar lymph nodes, pleural thickening, cysts and pneumothorax.

PULMONARY FUNCTION

Although abnormalities of pulmonary function are not uniform, three factors have been associated with chronic beryllium disease.[83] There may be a restrictive defect with a reduction in the FVC and a normal FEV_1/FVC ratio; there may be an interstitial defect, with normal lung volumes and air flows but a reduced TLCO, or there may be an obstructive defect which is associated with granulomata in the peribronchial regions.

The prognosis depends to some extent upon the pattern of alterations found in pulmonary function. Thus patients with interstitial defects tend to do best whereas the pulmonary function of those with obstructive or restrictive deficits often deteriorates despite treatment with steroids.

DIAGNOSIS

Beryllium disease has many of the features of sarcoidosis and the distinction between the two conditions may not be easy even after lung biopsy. In both, non-caseating granulomata are present in the lungs and in other organs. The pathological changes have been divided into two groups, I and II.[84] In group I there is a moderate or marked cellular infiltration comprising histiocytes, lymphocytes, plasma cells and giant cells. This group is further subdivided into types A and B depending upon the presence (B) or absence (A) of well formed granulomata. Group II, which comprises about 20% of cases, is characterized by slight or absent infiltration but there are numerous well formed granulomata. The appearances in group II are virtually indistinguishable from sarcoidosis and this group generally has a better response to treatment with steroids and a better overall prognosis.

Demonstration of beryllium sensitivity is by the beryllium lymphocyte proliferation test performed with lymphocytes retrieved by bronchoalveolar lavage.[99] Newman and others[82] considered that the following criteria were required for a diagnosis of beryllium disease.

1 Establishment of significant exposure to beryllium based upon the occupational history and, preferably, the results of environmental monitoring.
2 Objective evidence of pulmonary disease and a clinical course consistent with berylliosis.
3 Radiographic evidence of interstitial fibronodular disease.
4 Evidence of impairment in pulmonary function.
5 Histopathological changes of non-caseating granulomata and/or mononuclear infiltrates in biopsy specimens from the lung and/or thoracic lymph nodes.

6   The presence of beryllium in tissue specimens or in the urine.

7   Positive bronchoalveolar lavage lymphocyte transformation test.

Laboratory tests may show an elevation in serum gamma globulins (particularly IgA and IgG), a raised ESR, and sometimes hyperuricaemia, hypercalcaemia and hypercalciuria. Renal calculi have been reported in patients with beryllium disease and they may occasionally be the presenting feature. A beryllium patch test[85] using a 1% aqueous solution of $BeSO_4$ and also estimation of serum neopterin may clarify the sensitization status and assist in distinguishing between beryllium sensitivity and chronic beryllium disease.[86]

DIFFERENTIATION FROM SARCOIDOSIS

Chronic beryllium disease should be considered in any beryllium worker with lung disease.

Some features of sarcoidosis, including uveitis, neurological involvement and bone lesions, have never been reported in beryllium disease. In addition, the Kveim test is negative and spontaneous remission of radiographic changes is rare, while this commonly happens in sarcoidosis. In general, tissue levels will be elevated in beryllium-exposed workers but estimation of tissue levels in a beryllium worker probably adds no information specific to the diagnosis.

PATHOGENESIS

An immunological or hypersensitivity reaction has been postulated to underlie the pathological changes found in chronic beryllium disease. Blast transformation of lymphocytes occurs in a substantial proportion of patients and there is a good correlation between the amount of transformation and the severity of the disease.[87] The lymphocytes of patients with the disease and workers exposed to beryllium produce a macrophage migration inhibition factor and it was suggested that the workers with positive results had become sensitized to beryllium.[88] It is likely that the pathogenesis involves a combination of immunological and hypersensitivity reactions.

NEIGHBOURHOOD CASES

There is good evidence for cases of beryllium poisoning occurring in persons with no occupational exposure to the metal. In 1949, ten cases were described in individuals who had lived within three-quarters of a mile of a plant producing beryllium oxide, beryllium metal and beryllium copper. Atmospheric beryllium concentrations in the vicinity ranged from 0.01 to 0.1 $\mu g/m^3$.[89] Further cases have since been reported to the Beryllium Case Register, most of whom had been exposed to beryllium dust brought home on working clothes. Several others had lived near to such factories and been exposed to dust brought home by their relatives. In a small number of cases, the source of the beryllium was not clear. The number of neighbourhood cases has fallen considerably as more rigorous control measures have been introduced so that, for example, in the USA where, before 1949, 11% of cases were due to non-occupational exposures, the figure was only 3% for cases registered between 1949 and 1973; between 1973 and 1977 only one neighbourhood case was reported.[90,91] As more vigorous control measures in the workplace have been introduced, the occurrence of neighbourhood cases has become virtually non-existent. Poisoning by beryllium is a prescribed disease in the UK (see Chapter 4).

Carcinogenicity of beryllium

Beryllium is able to cause sarcomas in the soft tissues and bones of rabbits following intravenous injections or inhalation. Lung cancer also has been induced in rats and monkeys by intratracheal injections or inhalation of airborne particles.[92] In 1970, Mancuso reported that lung cancer was a frequent sequel of respiratory disease in workers extracting beryllium[93] and this has since been confirmed by others.[94–96] On the basis of this evidence IARC has determined that beryllium is carcinogenic. A retrospective study[97] of 9000 men employed at seven beryllium processing plants demonstrated an overall standardized mortality ratio of 1.26 (CI 1.12–1.42). The high cancer incidence was located at one plant where there was considerable exposure to acid mist but where there were also the greatest number of cases of chronic beryllium disease indicating high exposure. There remains controversy as to whether beryllium dusts are carcinogenic to man.[97,98]

Treatment of beryllium disease

The most important therapeutic measure in beryllium disease is to recognize it early. Affected workers have been advised to avoid further exposure although there are few hard data to support such a course of action. Corticosteroids generally produce symptomatic and radiograph improvement in early cases but do not reverse the pathological changes in later stages. Steroid treatment is generally given for life. Steroid-resistant cases may be given other immunosuppresive agents as adjuncts, e.g. cyclophosphamide. Standard treatments for hypoxaemia or right heart failure are given as necessary, and any chest infection must be dealt with promptly and effectively.

Prognosis

Spontaneous remission of symptoms and x-ray appearances has been observed but this is extremely rare.[99] The prognosis is variable. Patients with interstitial defects tend to do better than those with obstructive or restrictive deficits who often deteriorate despite treatment with steroids. All workers exposed to beryllium, salts or alloys are at risk of developing chronic beryllium disease. Workplace and worker monitoring are therefore essential.[100] Medical surveillance involves periodic review of chest symptomatology, chest x-rays and pulmonary function testing. The beryllium blood lymphocyte proliferation test has become the principal means of specifically diagnosing and screening for chronic beryllium disease in the beryllium-using industries in the USA. The test is identical to the procedure for bronchoalveolar lavage lymphocytes except that the growth period for lymphocytes is extended to 5–7 days.[101] To establish the diagnosis, persons with positive tests are referred for fibreoptic bronchoscopy with lavage and biopsy.

Occupational hygiene

The current US standard is 2 μgBe/m³ but exposure should be kept as low as is reasonably achievable.[102] Clinical surveillance performed in conjunction with job history and exposure information identifies jobs or work areas associated with beryllium disease, which should be targeted for priority industrial hygiene improvement.

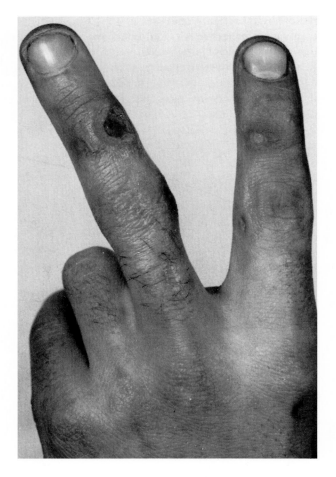

Biological monitoring to assess exposure, e.g. urinary beryllium, is not generally performed.

Supervision of beryllium workers

There are no reliable methods of biological screening for monitoring exposure although beryllium can be found in the urine of beryllium workers. Exposure must be reduced to the minimum by standard hygiene procedures and by providing efficient respiratory protection. Periodic chest radiographs and pulmonary function tests are important in detecting beryllium disease at an early stage and the beryllium-specific lymphocyte proliferation test may also have a role in health surveillance (see Chapter 35).

CHROMIUM

Chromium is a hard, silver white metal which is used for chrome plating and in the manufacture of special steels, such as stainless steel and ferrochrome. A number of its compounds are important as mordants in dyeing silk, wool and other textiles, as tanning agents and as pigments. Those chromium compounds which are commercially important occur in two valency states: trivalent (including chromic oxide and chromic sulphate) and hexavalent (including chromium trioxide, chromic acid and the dichromates of a number of metals). The trivalent compounds are generally considered to be virtually non-toxic, whereas the hexavalent salts are irritant, corrosive and, in some instances, carcinogenic.

Metabolism and action

Chromium is an essential element; it is required for normal carbohydrate metabolism and it potentiates the action of insulin. Its hexavalent salts can be absorbed from the lungs, the gut and, to a certain extent, through the intact skin. Trivalent chromium, however, is very poorly absorbed. Chromium is rapidly excreted in the urine with a half-life of between 15 and 41 hours.

All chrome compounds are sensitizers and may cause contact dermatitis; some may be a cause of occupational asthma. Chrome ulcers (chrome holes) are circular, well demarcated lesions which look as if they have been punched out of the skin (Fig. 7.7). They are only slightly painful and tend to heal spontaneously but may be troublesome if secondarily infected. They can, however, be treated adequately with a 10% solution of calcium EDTA. Long-term exposure to chromium compounds

Figure 7.7 *Chrome ulcers in various stages of activity on the hand of a fitter who worked in a chromium plating shop maintaining the plating tanks. Courtesy of Professor Rl McCallum.*

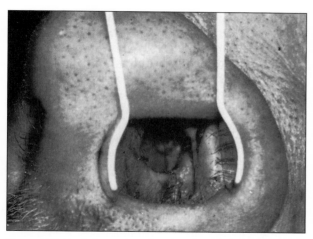

Figure 7.8 *Healed nasal perforation from inhalation of the vapour from a chrome-plating tank. Courtesy of Professor RI McCallum.*

may cause perforation of the cartilaginous nasal septum (Fig. 7.8) and occasionally lead to chronic rhinitis and chronic bronchitis. It may also induce conjunctivitis, keratitis and ulcerations on the eyelids.

The inhalation of large concentrations of hexavalent chromium compounds may cause coughing, wheezing, inspiratory pain, fever and loss of weight. Prolonged skin contact may lead to local irritation and, if skin damage is extensive, sufficient of the compound may be absorbed to cause renal damage and death.

The carcinogenicity of chrome salts

The most serious consequence of exposure to chromium compounds is the risk of developing lung cancer (see Chapter 39). It is generally considered that only the hexavalent compounds are carcinogenic and that the carcinogenicity is confined to those compounds of limited solubility. An increased risk of lung cancer has been demonstrated in workers engaged in primary chromate production and in the chrome pigment industry. The evidence relating to workers in the plating and ferrochromium industries is inconclusive. Stainless steel welders have also been studied because about 70% of the chromium in the aerosol is in the hexavalent form as soluble potassium or sodium monochromates; here, too, the results are inconclusive.

In short-term tests, hexavalent chromium produces mutations in bacterial systems without prior activation and, *in vitro*, the mutagenic potential of soluble and slightly soluble compounds does not differ. Trivalent chromium has a limited mutagenic effect although it has been shown to be 20 times more potent in decreasing the fidelity of DNA synthesis *in vitro* than the hexavalent form.

It may be that, in fact, the trivalent form of the metal is the proximate carcinogen having been produced by intracellular reduction of the hexavalent form. The apparent inactivity *in vivo* is thought to result from poor absorption. Bound to certain ligands, trivalent chromium is able to cross cell membranes. The carcinogenic effect may not be due to the trivalent form at all, however, but to some reactive intermediate formed during the reduction of hexavalent chromium, perhaps a pentavalent compound.[103]

Lung cancer was prescribed in 1986 under the Social Security Act for occupations involving the use or handling of or exposure to the dust of zinc chromate, calcium chromate or strontium chromate (see Chapter 4).

Monitoring of workers exposed to chromium

Special attention should be given to the skin and nose of chrome workers. It may also be prudent to conduct periodic tests of lung function if cases of asthma are suspected.

The chromium concentration in the urine at the end of a work shift is an index of recent exposure to soluble hexavalent chromium compound. Levels in unexposed persons are below 12 nmol/litre in blood and 0.2–3 μmol/mol creatinine in urine.[104]

COBALT

Cobalt is a silvery grey, magnetic metal which owes its name to the miners of Saxony who, in the fifteenth century, were so perplexed at not obtaining silver by smelting smaltite (CoAs2) despite its colour, that they thought there must be a kobold, or goblin, in the ore to account for this unreasonable behaviour. Nowadays cobalt is mainly recovered as a byproduct from copper and silver mining. The main production centres are in Central Africa, Canada, Russia, Australia and Central America. The metal form of cobalt is primarily used in the manufacture of high temperature thermally resistant alloys, called super alloys, principally used in jet engines. Hard metal, used for cutting and machining steel and rock consists of a thermally bonded mixture of cobalt and tungsten carbide. The metal has wide application in the chemical, electronic and metallurgical industries. It is used in magnets and as a catalyst in the petroleum industry. Cobalt salts are used as dryers in the paint industry and as pigments and coating agents in paint and pottery. Recently, cobalt has been used in the active ingredient of lithium ion rechargeable batteries. In nickel-cadmium and nickel metalhydride batteries several cobalt compounds are used as additives, for either the positive or negative electrode. Radioactive cobalt (Co^{60}) is used as a source of high energy gamma radiation in radiotherapy and industrial radiography.

Cobalt is an essential element and central to the action

of vitamin B$_{12}$. The absorption from the gut varies considerably from 5 to 45%, and about 30% of an inhaled dose of cobalt oxide is absorbed. It is stored in liver, spleen, kidney, muscle and fat, and is mainly (80%) excreted in the urine, the remainder in the faeces.

The inhalation of cobalt powder has been associated with the development of an interstitial lung fibrosis, termed 'hard metal disease'[105] (see Chapter 35). This disease can range in severity from a giant cell pneumonitis to an end-stage pulmonary fibrosis. Typical symptoms are wheezing, shortness of breath and chest tightness, and lung function tests show restrictive effects (reduced FVC) with a reduction of the diffusion capacity.

With progression, the pulmonary effects become irreversible and may lead to cor pulmonale and death.[106] Individual susceptibility probably plays an important role as the prevalence is estimated to be very low (less than 1%). The disease has only been diagnosed in workers in the hard metal and diamond polishing industries, where exposure is mixed, being not only to cobalt but also to different carbides and diamond particles.[107,108] Experimental findings, both *in vitro* and *in vivo*, indicate that the biological reactivity of the mixture of cobalt powder with different carbides is much higher than that of pure cobalt powder.[109] This is supported by an epidemiological study in a large cobalt refining plant which showed the absence of impaired lung function among workers exposed to pure cobalt.[110] The study suggests that simultaneous exposure to cobalt and other substances may be necessary in the causation of this disease.

There is ample evidence that cobalt may cause bronchial asthma. A specific IgE against cobalt has been detected and a Type 1 allergic reaction is therefore suspected.[111] Typical symptoms are wheezing, dyspnoea and cough, which disappear after removal from exposure. Lung function tests show obstructive lung disease. Occupational asthma has been recorded in all industry sectors with exposure to cobalt, either alone or in association with other constituents.[112,113]

In 1990 the IARC concluded that there was sufficient evidence to classify cobalt metal powder and cobalt (ii) oxide as being carcinogenic in experimental animals. Further evidence in respect of carcinogenicity of cobalt compounds came in 1996 when the National Toxicology Program in the USA reported that a 2-year inhalation bioassay with cobalt sulphate had shown an increased cancer incidence.[114] Consequently in 1998 the European Union classified cobalt metal and all metal compounds as Category 2 carcinogens i.e. 'May cause cancer in experimental animals'. With one exception, epidemiological surveys among workers in the cobalt producing industry, where exposure is only to cobalt, have not indicated an excess of lung malignancy.[115] In Denmark a cohort of porcelain workers showed a slight increase in lung cancer. Although this was attributed to cobalt the numbers were small and the results were not conclusive. However, studies in the hard metal industry have shown an increase in lung cancer risk. These findings add further weight to the hypothesis that concomitant exposure to cobalt and other substances such as occur in the hard metal industry might increase the risk of pulmonary cancer.[116] An interaction between hard metal exposure and tobacco smoking is a possible mechanism.[117]

At one time cobalt salts were added to beer as a foam stabilizer and a number of outbreaks of congestive cardiomyopathy were linked to that use. Those affected suffered from an abrupt onset of left ventricular failure with pericardial effusion and polycythaemia. It was generally considered that the aetiology was multifactorial since the amount of cobalt consumed, even by the most heavy drinkers, was far less than that given therapeutically for anaemia. The fact that the condition was seen almost exclusively in heavy drinkers suggested that there was a synergistic action between the cobalt in the beer, the direct effects of alcohol on the myocardium and an inadequate intake of proteins and vitamins.[118]

Cobalt also has an effect on thyroid function. It inhibits tyrosine iodinase which prevents the synthesis of thyroxine. This in turn leads to an oversecretion of thyroid-stimulating hormone and to thyroid hyperplasia.

The polycythaemia induced by cobalt is probably due to an increased release of erythropoietin from the kidney as the result of tissue hypoxia. This may be caused by the inactivation of 2,3-diphosphoglycerate (2,3-DPG), by the impaired release of oxygen from red cells depleted of 2,3-DPG, or by the formation of cobaltohaemoglobin with a consequent shift of the oxygen dissociation curve to the left.

Medical surveillance of cobalt workers

Workers exposed to pure cobalt powder or to cobalt-containing dusts should be submitted to periodic health checks, including clinical examination with special attention to the lungs and skin. Pulmonary function testing and periodic chest radiographs should be included in the surveillance programme. The retention time of cobalt in the human body is short. Excretion is biphasic, a rapid phase of elimination lasts approximately 2 days after which a second phase of prolonged and low-level elimination follows. Where exposure is to soluble cobalt compounds (e.g. salts), to the metal or to hard metal dust, measurement of cobalt in the urine at the end of the working week will give an indication of the extent of recent exposure. However, when exposure is to cobalt oxides, the urinary concentration of cobalt does not correlate well with recent exposure.[119,120] Whether routine estimation of urinary cobalt should be carried out and if so how frequently will depend upon the purpose but if undertaken it is best done at the end of the last shift of the working week. In some plants this is made to coincide with the clinical review already mentioned.

For unexposed persons, the level of urinary cobalt is < 3 μmol/mol creatinine. In Germany the Biological Exposure Index Value[121] (MAK) is 100 μmol/mol creatinine which is considered to equate with an atmospheric exposure of 0.1 mg/m³.

COPPER

Copper, particularly when alloyed with tin, has been used since prehistoric times, and copper-containing artefacts including coins and cooking vessels have been found associated with most early civilizations.

Copper is a very important industrial metal, principally because of its excellent electrical conductivity, corrosion resistance, malleability and ductility. Metallic copper is used, amongst other purposes, for electric wiring, plumbing, roofing and electroplating. Many important alloys are formed with copper: brass when alloyed with zinc; bronze with tin and monel with nickel. Copper beryllium alloys are also of increasing use. Copper-containing chemicals are used to dissolve cellulose in the manufacture of rayon, as pigments, fungicides (Bordeaux mixture) and algaecides. They are also used as food supplements and as fertilizers in agriculture.

The ores are frequently sulphidic, although oxides or carbonates also occur and the copper has been found in the metallic state. The ores, after preliminary separation by grinding and flotation, are smelted and then further refined to a high state of purity by electrolysis.

Copper is an essential element for many biological processes and is found in a variety of organisms across all phyla. It influences specific gene expression and serves as a cofactor for several oxidative enzymes including superoxide dismutase, cytochrome C oxidase and lysyl oxidase. It is also required as a cofactor for amino laevulinic acid dehydratase and is a constituent of dopamine-b-hydroxylase. Although an essential element, it is toxic at high concentrations and metabolic balance is achieved by an efficient homeostatic mechanism. Thus a gene on the X chromosome controls absorption and another, Xq13.3, is associated with the accumulation of copper in the body.[122] These genes involve the intestine as a barrier and organ of excretion and the liver for storage.[123] It is absorbed from the intestine by peptides or amino acids and either transported to the liver or bound within the mucosal cells by a metallothionein-like protein which is induced when plasma copper concentrations are high. Copper stored in the mucosal cells is lost when they are desquamated. Some copper is also directly incorporated into superoxide dismutase in the gut mucosa. Copper transported to the liver is bound to caeruloplasmin which contains 95% of the total copper in the plasma.

Excess copper is excreted in the bile where it is firmly bound to amino acids preventing reabsorption. Copper is able to bind to sulphydryl groups and its toxic effects are due to the inhibition of -SH group enzymes such as glucose-6-phosphate dehydrogenase and glutathione reductase which are important in protecting the cell from free oxygen radicals.[124]

Apart from metal fume fever (see Chapter 9), adverse effects resulting from exposure to copper in industry are rare although some workers develop dermatitis in response to contact with copper dust. Very high exposures may produce a symptomless, greenish discolouration of the tongue and hair, and superficial green staining of the teeth.[125]

Copper salts may be ingested accidentally or deliberately – taking copper sulphate is a favoured method of committing suicide in India – and produce nausea, vomiting, a haemorrhagic gastritis and diarrhoea. These symptoms are followed several hours later by the development of a haemolytic anaemia and acute tubular necrosis.[126] Some cases of acute copper poisoning were reported in patients undergoing renal dialysis when copper tubing was used in a heating coil.[127]

A granulomatous disease of the lung has been described in workers spraying grape vines with copper sulphate solutions to prevent mildew. The chest radiographs in vine sprayer's lung may show diffuse bilateral linear and nodular opacities and the disease may progress with the development of interstitial fibrosis. Granulomata are also found in the liver.[128] There is an increased risk of lung cancer among vine sprayers and, although this has been attributed to solutions containing arsenic, the excess has been noted even among sprayers who use only copper solutions.[129]

Copper miners in China have been shown to have increased lung cancer mortality. While copper is a possible aetiological agent, the author suggests that silica exposure and smoking are the more probable causes.[130]

Copper poisoning from occupational causes is very rare, and could be treated by penicillamine in the same way as in Wilson's disease. However, a report of an 86-year-old woman who ingested a zinc copper sulphate solution suggested that chelation therapy had been of little value in aiding her recovery.[131,132]

MANGANESE

Pure manganese is a silvery white metal but, as usually prepared, it is reddish grey, brittle and extremely hard. It was discovered by Scheele in 1774 in Sweden, the oxide has been known since ancient times and was used in the manufacture of glass by the Greeks.[133]

Manganese is found in recoverable quantities in the ore pyrolusite (manganese dioxide) in the Ukraine, South Africa, Chile, Canada, Australia, China and the USA. The pure metal is prepared by igniting an ore concentrate with aluminium powder (Thermit process) or electric arc furnacing.

The most important use is in the preparation of hardened steels, including ferromanganese, silicomanganese and manganin. Manganese dioxide is used in dry cell batteries and other compounds are found in pigments in paints, varnishes and inks, in matches, fireworks, fertilizers and drugs. Permanganate compounds are used in the ceramics and glass industries as decolourizing agents and pigments, and also used as oxidizing agents (e.g. potassium permanganate). Another possible source of exposure is the fumes from welding alloys containing manganese.[134]

Manganese is an essential element required for enzymes critical for the normal functioning of the central nervous, skeletal and reproductive systems e.g. glutamine synthetase and manganese superoxide dismutase.

It is extremely poorly absorbed from the gut and crosses biological membranes with difficulty. In the blood it is bound predominantly to red cells; it is excreted mainly through the bile and only small amounts appear in the urine. The uptake of manganese from the gut is enhanced by iron deficiency and the supposed susceptibility of some miners to the effects of manganese was probably because of a concomitant dietary iron deficiency causing an increased uptake of manganese.

Manganese poisoning

Many manganese compounds are mildly irritant to the eyes, skin and mucous membranes. Potassium permanganate, which is a powerful oxidizing agent, can cause considerable damage to the skin and the eyes.

In 1921, Brezina reported a high incidence of pneumonia in workers handling manganese ores and this observation has been confirmed by others. The inhalation of manganese probably produces an inflammatory reaction in the lungs which, because of its effect on the clearance of particles from the lungs by the pulmonary macrophages, increases susceptibility to bacterial infections.

The most serious consequence of manganese poisoning is the production of a condition that resembles Parkinson's disease. It was described first in 1837 by Couper in five men who were employed in the grinding of manganese dioxide in the manufacture of chlorine for bleaching powder in France. Couper's observations were apparently forgotten, unlike Parkinson's. The disease was rediscovered more than half a century later in workers employed in drying manganese dioxide in Austria in 1901, and further cases were reported in Boston in 1919. The first cases in the UK were reported by Charles in 1922 in men who had been exposed to the dust from manganese ores for between 9 months and 3 years.

The development of manganese poisoning is insidious and said to pass through three stages.[135] In the first, there are no specific signs or symptoms but workers may complain of anorexia, lassitude, apathy, excessive tiredness, headaches, weakness in the legs, muscular cramps, joint pains and irritability. The second stage is characterized by the development of such signs as dysarthria, disturbances of gait and excessive salivation. These signs may be accompanied, or preceded, by an organic psychosis (so-called manganic madness) which frequently disappears when the true parkinsonian symptoms supervene. The third and final stage of the disease is characterized by akinesia and rigidity, most pronounced in the lower limbs, and by debility, muscle pains, paraesthesiae and disturbances of speech. The tremor present in manganese poisoning is frequently an intention tremor and not a resting tremor as in idiopathic parkinsonism, and another difference between the two conditions is that there is often some degree of dystonia present in manganese poisoning. The disease is generally reversible if detected in the early stages but the development of parkinsonian features denotes permanent damage to the central nervous system. Poisoning by manganese is a prescribed disease in the UK (see Chapter 4).

In true parkinsonism, the area of the brain most commonly affected is the substantia nigra; the striatum and pallidum are generally little affected although their dopamine concentration is much reduced. In patients with manganese poisoning, it is the striatum and the pallidum that bear the brunt of the toxic effects and the substantia is altered very little. There is, however, a reduced concentration of dopamine in the substantia nigra as well as in the striatum (see Chapter 42).[136]

In workers exposed to low levels of manganese (less than 1 mg/m³) an effect on the performance of psychometric tests and neuropsychiatric symptoms has been observed.[137,138]

Treatment with L-dopa has been successful when hypokinetic and dystonic features predominate. Some authors have reported an improvement in symptoms following removal from exposure and treatment with EDTA. More recently, sodium para-aminosalicylic acid has been used successfully as the chelating agent in the treatment of manganese poisoning.[139]

Two cases of clinical parkinsonism after chronic exposure to the fungicide Maneb (manganese ethylene-bis-dithiocarbamate) have been reported.[140] The CT and MRI scans showed asymmetry of the ventricular system. In another series of four cases of manganese-induced parkinsonism the MRI was abnormal in only one case.[141]

Individual susceptibility to manganese

An individual susceptibility to the effects of manganese is well recognized and is due to an interaction with iron metabolism. Thus, individuals who take up an increased amount of iron from the gut also take up increased amounts of manganese; anaemic subjects may take up twice as much manganese as those who are not.[142] Moreover, the binding capacity of the plasma of anaemic animals is more than twice that of healthy animals and the increase in transport capacity to the blood-brain barrier is one explanation for the very much higher levels of manganese in the brains of anaemic rats.[143]

Supervision of manganese workers

Manganese workers should all receive periodic medical examinations, with particular attention given to the detection of behavioural changes and neurological changes such as hypertonia or tremor. It is important to detect any alterations at the earliest possible stage in order to prevent permanent damage.

There is no useful biological measure of exposure although the mean urinary manganese concentration in a group of workers may be useful for grading exposure.

Workers exposed to fumes from welding alloys containing manganese should be included in a monitoring programme.[144] Behavioural studies may have a place in the detection of early neurotoxic effects in asymptomatic exposed workers.[138] Estimation of plasma malondialdehyde can be used as an index of lipid peroxidation induced by manganese exposure.[145]

MOLYBDENUM

Molybdenum is a silver white metal used as a hardener in steels, in the production of some special alloys, ceramics and pigments, and in electrical wire. It is also added to fertilizers as some plants require it in order to fix nitrogen. It is an essential element for humans and is required for the enzyme xanthine oxidase. It has complex metabolic interactions with other metals and exists in animal tissues in inverse relationship to copper concentrations. In animals the ingestion of plants with a high molybdenum content causes a variety of effects, including anaemia, stunted growth and deformities of the bones and joints and, in sheep, degeneration of the central nervous system. All these effects are thought to be due to interference with normal copper metabolism.[146] Molybdenum also interacts with iron and it may increase the haematopoietic response to iron in iron deficiency anaemias.[147]

In humans, adverse effects are likely to follow exposure to molybdenum trioxide, which may occur during the production of molybdenum compounds at high temperatures. It is irritant to the mucous membranes.

NICKEL

Nickel is a hard silvery metal. It was first isolated by Cronstedt in 1751 and takes its name from 'Old Nick'

because of the 'devilish' difficulties it caused during the refining of Saxony copper ores.

It is a transition metal and is thus capable of having a number of oxidation states with markedly different properties. Some of the water insoluble or slightly soluble salts are soluble in biological matrices. Nickel forms important alloys, a number of oxides and also organometallic compounds. Nickel tetracarbonyl is remarkable in being a gaseous metallic compound at ambient temperatures. Although nickel tetracarbonyl was known to be acutely toxic little was known of any other hazards associated with the refining or use of nickel until in 1923 when a case of nasal cancer at a refinery in Wales, saw the beginning of modern nickel toxicology. The cancer problem was subsequently noted in other refineries processing sulphuride ores at high temperatures.

Nickel is widely distributed in the earth's crust. Mining, crushing and grinding and flotation followed by pyrometallurgy and then electrodeposition, or the carbonyl process are used to recover the metal.[148]

Ninety percent of nickel is used in alloys, mostly stainless steel, but the high nickel alloys (containing around 30–50% nickel) are important in the aero engine industry, desalination plants and where corrosion resistance is needed. Other uses include plating, foundry work and catalysts. Electroplated nickel silver (EPNS) is used on cutlery. Nickel powders find application in rechargeable batteries and other uses include the coating of fibres and foam for use in electronics. In combination with other metal oxides nickel oxide forms commercially important alloys, called spinels.

A high incidence of pulmonary and nasal sinus cancer has been observed at certain nickel refining operations. The problem was thought to be associated with arsenic exposure or nickel carbonyl gas but more recently has been attributed to the very high levels of dust and fume pertaining in these early workplaces.[149] An epidemiological study[150] to try to determine which form(s) of nickel had been the cause identified nickel sulphides (especially the subsulphide) and oxides involved in the processes as being the principal culprits. The influence of soluble nickel, however, could not be excluded, possibly as a promoter. The subject was reviewed by the IARC in 1990.[149] Subsequently the National Toxicology Program in the USA undertook an animal inhalation study. They exposed both rats and mice to three different nickel compounds.[151] The investigators found that nickel subsulphide was the most potent metal species, nickel oxide less so and nickel sulphate, which is a soluble salt, did not cause cancer under the conditions of the study. Modern processes technology has essentially eliminated the exposure of workers to the hazards. There is no firm evidence of any excess cancer risk in user industries, including welding of stainless steel.

Primary sensitization may result from 'close and prolonged contact' which may be occupational or domestic, especially skin piercing with the subsequent use of nickel in 'sleepers' to maintain the patency of the skin. The skin reaction may be local or remote.[152] Sensitized persons may subsequently react to contact with nickel at work or in clothing or jewellery. Since the introduction of automation and improved hygiene in the workplace, as well as new legislation limiting nickel in jewellery, 'nickel itch' is now less common but occupational nickel contact dermatitis has been observed in persons handling nickel plated instruments or tools. Clinical diagnosis is by patch tests and the lymphocyte proliferation test.

Asthma may be associated with the inhalation of droplets of soluble nickel and also possibly the fine nickel oxide fume resulting from welding of nickel containing alloys. As with dermatitis if a casual relationship is clearly established then affected workers should be removed from further exposure.[153]

Ingestion of soluble nickel is toxic and has occurred in the workplace, due to accidental contamination of the drinking water supply.[154]

Biological monitoring cannot differentiate between inhalation or ingestion. It is not therefore recommended as a routine procedure in the absence of skilled interpretation except in nickel carbonyl poisoning where it has a health guidance value and in exposure to soluble nickel, such as in nickel platers.[155]

Nickel carbonyl

Nickel tetracarbonyl gas was discovered by Ludwig Mond and co-workers in 1888. It is formed when carbon monoxide is passed over finely divided nickel at ambient temperatures and it decomposes at 180°C to deposit nickel metal of extremely high purity. This is the basis of the Mond process. The gas is acutely dangerous and similar in toxicology to phosgene. Its use is limited to a few refineries and to coating applications.

It has an immediate acute effect including giddiness, nausea and headache followed after an interval of 12–18 hours, by a severe chemical pneumonitis. Treatment is discussed in Chapter 8.

Poisoning by nickel carbonyl is a prescribed disease in the UK (see Chapter 4).

OSMIUM

Osmium is one of the platinum group of metals. An extremely dense, bluish white metal, it is three times as heavy as iron. An alloy with iridium (osmiridium) is very hard and used to tip fountain pen nibs and for making engraving tools and watch bearings. Osmic acid (osmium tetroxide) is used as a histological stain and, because it turns black on contact with oil and fat, aqueous solutions were once used for taking fingerprints. This practice was stopped when it was realized that it caused dermatitis.

Osmium itself is non-toxic but when heated in air or when left in a finely divided form it rapidly oxidizes to osmic acid, the vapour of which is exceedingly irritant to mucous membranes. Exposure may produce conjunctivitis and the appearance of haloes around bright lights. It may also cause headaches and difficulties in breathing and it may produce transient haematuria, proteinuria and pyuria. In experimental animals degeneration of the renal tubules has been observed. With chronic exposure, corneal ulceration and opacification have been noted[156] and contact dermatitis may also result. Because of these effects, osmic acid should always be handled with great care and, in the laboratory, kept and used within an efficient fume cupboard.

PLATINUM

Platinum is a beautiful silvery white metal, exceptionally corrosion resistant, malleable, ductile and electroconductive. It is found as the native metal in alluvial deposits in Russia. It is also found in mineral ores in Canada, South Africa, Australia and South America. In view of the considerable value of the material much of the platinum coming to refineries is reclaimed from scrap.

The metal and its alloys have uses in electronics, glass production, laboratory ware, jewellery and dental alloys and as industrial and motor exhaust catalysts. Cisplatin and carboplatin are used as cytotoxic drugs for treating testicular cancers and other solid tumours.

After pyrometallurgical preparation of a precious metal concentrate platinum salts are produced by solvent refining and then precipitation. The complex salts are converted to the pure metal by thermal decomposition. Donald Hunter,[157] who was the principal author of one of the earliest papers looking into the epidemiology and causation of platinum related asthma, recognized that the problem was related to the soluble complex chloroplatinate salts. They cause type 1 allergy. The highest risk of sensitization is in the first 3 years of employment. Smoking carries a relative risk of five- to eightfold for sensitization whereas atopy, once considered to be a risk factor is not relevant when smoking has been taken into account.[158,159] The soluble platinum compound tetramine platinum dichloride, used in the manufacture of autocatalysts has recently been shown not to be allergenic under normal conditions of industrial exposure.[160]

The results of skin prick tests using sodium and ammonium chloroplatinate correlate well with the clinical syndrome of allergic rhinitis and asthma.[161] This is useful for medical surveillance as the results are repeatable and specific.[162] Improvements in process engineering, with restriction of the use of allergenic chloroplatinates and increased use of non-allergenic platinum compounds has significantly reduced the incidence of adverse health effects. Nevertheless, as with other occupational asthmagens, in order to prevent induction of persistent bronchial hyperresponsiveness correct management of cases requires removal from exposure, as soon as sensitization is so detected.[163]

Earlier studies have indicated that the skin may demonstrate primary irritant or allergic contact dermatitis to complex platinum salts. In the conditions prevailing in modern refineries, skin problems are now uncommon.

Urinary platinum can be estimated by the highly sensitive technique of absorptive voltametry. Nurses caring for patients treated with the anti-cancer drug, cisplatin, have been observed to have increased blood platinum levels, most probably from patient contact.[164]

SELENIUM

Selenium was discovered in 1817 by Berzelius and named by him after the Greek word for the moon, owing to its resemblance to tellurium which had been discovered a few years before and named after the earth. It is a metalloid, i.e. a non-metal which nevertheless has some of the properties of a metal. Elemental selenium is recovered as a byproduct in the sludges and sediments of electrolytic refining of copper and also from the flue dusts produced in the manufacture of sulphuric acid.

Selenium and its compounds have a number of uses in industry. In its elemental form it is used in the production of photographic chemicals, rectifiers and photoelectric cells. It is also made into an alloy with copper and steel, and used as a vulcanizing agent for rubber and to decolorize green glass. Selenite salts are used as red pigments in the production of glass and enamels. Selenium diethyldithiocarbamate is a fungicide and the hexafluoride is used in transformers as a gaseous electrical insulator. Two additional selenium compounds may be encountered as byproducts of other processes. Selenium dioxide may be produced during copper or nickel smelting, during silver refining or when selenium alloys are welded or heated. Hydrogen selenide is produced when water or acids react with metal selenides (as may occur during the manufacture of sulphuric acid by the lead chamber process) or when hydrogen reacts with soluble selenium compounds.

Selenium is one of the essential trace elements, its function being related to the detoxification of free radicals. It is also antagonistic to the toxic effects of mercury. Soluble selenium compounds are readily absorbed through the lungs and from the gut and are methylated in the liver to the trimethylselenium ion and excreted in the urine. Urinary excretion is rapid and is the major route of elimination. Under conditions of very high exposure the volatile metabolite dimethylselenide is formed and this is also eliminated through the lungs.

Dimethylselenide has a garlicky smell which appears on the breath of those who are heavily exposed. It was this characteristic of selenium exposure that led Berzelius to discover the element after his housekeeper complained that he had eaten too much garlic for lunch when in fact he had been examining a selenium-bearing deposit formed from pyrites in a sulphuric acid chamber.

Selenium dioxide dusts are irritant to the eyes, nose and upper respiratory tract, and inhalation of high concentrations may induce pulmonary oedema. In liquid form, selenium dioxide is highly vesicant and causes serious skin burns. A particularly painful burn may follow if selenium dioxide gets under the finger nail. Burns caused by selenium dioxide are treated by copious washing with a 10% solution of sodium thiosulphate followed by the local application of 10% thiosulphate cream. Continued skin contact with selenium dioxide may result in a local or generalized dermatitis. Some workers exposed to selenium dioxide develop a form of conjunctivitis associated with pink, oedematous eyelids which is generally referred to as 'rose eye'.

Chronic selenium poisoning is characterized by respiratory irritation, gastrointestinal disturbances, hair loss and a strong garlic odour to the breath. Aggressive or depressive mood changes have been observed and anosmia reported. In a study of coal miners the blood selenium levels were found to be negatively related to coal exposure and tobacco consumption.[165] It is postulated that this may be an interaction between the irritant effects of the coal dust or smoking and the selenium, again connected with the anti-oxidant properties of the selenium ion.

Hydrogen selenide is an extremely toxic gas but is rapidly converted to elemental selenium on contact with water, such as may occur on the surfaces of mucous membranes. Exposure may cause acute irritation of the eyes and upper respiratory tract and coughs, sneezes and tightness in the chest. In some cases, pulmonary oedema follows some 6–8 hours after exposure. No chronic effects have been reported to follow exposure.

Dimethylselenide is a powerful irritant which may cause upper respiratory tract symptoms; it has also been reported to cause a granulomatous disorder with prolonged exposure.[166]

There is some debate about the carcinogenicity of selenium. In areas where there are high levels of selenium in the environment, there may be a low incidence of colonic cancer and some patients with gastrointestinal cancers have lower selenium levels in their blood than controls. On the basis of these observations, it has been suggested that the antioxidant properties of selenium may be protective against some gut carcinogens.[167] Experiments with animals, however, have shown that, although selenium may protect against the development of tumours in some instances, under other conditions it may actually be carcinogenic.[168] There is no good evidence that it is carcinogenic in man.

Supervision of workers exposed to selenium

Selenium concentrations in the blood and urine reflect recent exposure.[170] The Quebec Toxicology Center[171] recommends the following biological exposure indices: a) unexposed: 1.0 μmol/litre; b) level below which chances of exhibiting toxicity are almost zero: 2.5 μmol/litre; c) level above which toxicity is likely: 6.0 μmol/litre.

SILVER

Silver is a beautiful white metal, extremely ductile and malleable and with very good electrical conductivity. Its major use is in the preparation of photographic film but it is still widely used in jewellery. It is also used in the electronics industry, in special solders, in silver plating and small amounts are used to make inks and dyes. Some silver salts, of which the most familiar is silver nitrate, are corrosive and will cause serious burns to the eyes, skin and mucous membranes. Anyone swallowing silver nitrate will suffer the corrosive effect that this compound can have on the gut epithelium. Areas of the skin that are splashed with silver nitrate may become pigmented due to the local deposition of silver protein complexes. Pigmentation may also occur if metallic silver penetrates beneath the skin, as may happen to silversmiths. These pigmented areas look rather like tattoos and are somewhat similar in appearance to the tattooing that affects coal miners.

Repeated exposure to soluble compounds of silver leads to an accumulation of silver within the body, since very little of the metal is excreted. After many years' exposure, a slate grey pigment forms in the conjunctiva, the skin, the nail beds and the buccal mucosa. This condition, argyria, is permanent, somewhat unsightly but benign. The internal organs may also be pigmented but this is only found *post mortem*. Silver may deposit in the posterior lamina (Descemet's membrane) which if severe may impair night vision. Argyria does not occur with exposure to the elemental metal.[172,173]

'Silver polishers' lung' is a benign pneumonoconiosis from the inhalation of jewellers' rouge (iron oxide) and minute particles of silver. Interestingly, in this condition, as a histologist might expect, the elastic tissue is stained black.

Supervision of workers exposed to silver

Workers exposed to the soluble salts should be examined at regular intervals for early signs of argyria. Absorbed silver, either from the gastrointestinal tract or the lungs, is mainly excreted in the faeces, the retained fraction being deposited in tissue. Blood measurements are preferred to estimate occupational exposure and levels below 25 μg/litre are not thought to lead to argyria.[174]

TELLURIUM

Tellurium was discovered in 1782 by Muller von Reichenstein and named in 1798 by Klaproth from the Latin *tellus*, the earth. It behaves in a manner very similar to selenium.

Tellurium is a byproduct of copper, lead and bismuth smelting. It greatly hardens lead and increases its resistance to acids. A tellurium lead alloy has about twice the tensile strength of ordinary lead, enabling sheet lead to be worked without fracturing. Tellurium is also added to iron, steels and copper, and is used as a vulcanizing agent for rubber, and in the production of glass, solder, coins and ceramics. Metal tellurides and some organic compounds of tellurium are used as bactericides, in plating and etching solutions and in some photographic and water treatment reagents. Tellurium dioxide is formed when metals containing tellurium are heated or welded, and hydrogen telluride is produced by the action of acids on metal tellurides.

Not much is known about the metabolism of tellurium in man but it is converted to dimethyl-telluride and excreted through the lungs, kidney and faeces; the relative importance of these routes of elimination is not well established. Organic compounds of tellurium may be absorbed through the skin.

Exposure to tellurium gives a garlic smell to the breath and in much smaller quantities than are required to produce this effect with selenium. The administration of ascorbic acid seems to be effective in abolishing the smell on the breath by interfering with the metabolism of dimethyltelluride.

The toxicity of tellurium and its compounds is greater than that of selenium. Exposure to hydrogen telluride and tellurium dioxide causes irritation of the eyes, nose and upper respiratory tract. Tellurium hexafluoride is a respiratory irritant which causes delayed pulmonary oedema.

Long-term exposure to tellurium and its inorganic compounds may cause an illness which is characterized by a reduction in the ability to sweat, and a metallic taste in the mouth, nausea, anorexia and somnolence, with possibly blue-black discolouration of the finger webs.[175,176]

In experimental animals it has been found that exposure to tellurium is teratogenic and may cause testicular damage[177] but no such effects have been reported in humans.

Supervision of workers exposed to tellurium

The concentration of tellurium in the urine is probably a reflection of recent exposure and it has been suggested that, to avoid the smell of garlic, urinary tellurium concentrations should be less than 1 μg/litre.[178] In view of the reported teratogenic properties, exposure of women of child-bearing age should be avoided or minimized.

THALLIUM

Thallium is a soft, heavy metal which is a by-product from the smelting of copper, lead or zinc. It was discovered by Crookes in 1861 and named by him after the brilliant green line that distinguishes its spectrum. In its pure state thallium is silvery white in colour but when molten it becomes black owing to the formation of its oxide. It is used in the optical industry in the manufacture of lenses because its salts are characterized by their unusually high refracting power. It is also used in the manufacture of semi-conductors and electronics, imitation jewellery, in dyes and pigments, and thallium sulphate is used as a rodenticide. Thallium-201 is used for radionuclide imaging in the investigation of cardiac ischaemia. In the environment, water draining old lead or zinc mines may contain high concentrations of thallium and it has also been found in concentrations up to 420 parts per billion in table salt consisting of potassium rather than sodium chloride.[179]

Thallium is an extremely toxic metal, more toxic than lead and about as toxic as arsenic. It is well absorbed by any route, including the skin. In the blood, about 70% is bound to the red cells. It is mainly excreted slowly by the kidney, the half-life in urine being 15–30 days. Thallium crosses the placenta and may cause fetal toxicity.

In the body, thallium behaves as though it were potassium, which it will displace competitively. It is able to inhibit oxidative phosphorylation by virtue of its ability to bind to sulphydryl groups.

There are many reports of thallium poisoning, often with rat poison, some accidental and some with homicidal intent. In a 1995 review of these Wax[180] recalled that 31 deaths were caused in a single episode in California in 1932 when grain treated with thallium sulphate, to be used as a rodenticide to kill squirrels, was accidentally added to flour used to make tortillas for human consumption. Recently reported cases of occupational exposure include a man handling raw materials for glass manufacture which contained thallium[181] and a Chinese laboratory worker exposed to thallium.[182]

Acute intoxication, such as may follow the deliberate ingestion of a thallium-containing rat killer, frequently results first in hypotension and bradycardia as a direct result of its action on the sinus node and on the contractility of the cardiac muscle. These initial effects are then followed by hypertension and tachycardia which is thought to be due to degeneration of the vagus.[183]

The signs of chronic thallium poisoning consist of a dying back peripheral neuropathy, gastroenteritis and loss of hair. So characteristic is this combination that, in many cases, the diagnosis can safely be made over the telephone. The progression of the neuropathy may sometimes mimic a Guillain–Barré syndrome except that the deep tendon reflexes are lost relatively late in the course of thallium poisoning. The neuropathy resembles that induced by riboflavine deficiency and the mechanism is the same, a disruption in the transport of electrons during intracellular respiration.[184] In many cases the presenting symptoms are those of abdominal pain and bloody diarrhoea. Centrilobular hepatic necrosis and necrosis of the renal tubules may develop, together with focal necrosis in the skeletal and cardiac muscles. The loss of hair comes on relatively late in the disease although a dark line can be seen at the base of the hair shaft within a few days of the ingestion of a large dose of the metal.

Thallium poisoning has been treated with oral Prussian blue (potassium ferrihexacyanoferrate) in a dose ranging from 88 to 416 mg/kg per day[185] Thallium displaces potassium from the Prussian blue molecule and, after oral administration, thallium ions are sequestered in the gut and their absorption is hindered. The plasma levels of thallium fall rapidly following the administration of Prussian blue, and the progress of treatment can be followed by monitoring the urinary concentration. Thallium can be detected in the faeces when the urinary concentration is extremely low, and administration of Prussian blue should continue until there is no longer any thallium in the faeces. If the patient is constipated, a purgative such as magnesium sulphate or mannitol should also be given. The concurrent administration of intravenous potassium in doses of 4.0–4.5 mmol/litre in physiological saline and/or 5 per cent glucose will enhance the excretion of thallium into the gut and speed up its elimination. Continuous ECG monitoring and repeated measurements of plasma potassium are necessary to prevent the development of hyperkalaemia. Potassium supplements should not be given by mouth because they will interfere with the exchange between potassium and thallium in the Prussian blue molecule.

There are no specific means by which those exposed can be monitored. In our present state of knowledge, the most that can be said is that the concentration of thallium in the urine is probably a better indicator of recent exposure than its concentration in blood.[186]

TIN

Tin is a soft, silver-white metal with many industrial uses in both its inorganic and its organic forms. Tin metal is used for plating steel, in the manufacture of solder and alloys, of which the most common are bronze, brass, gunmetal, type metal and pewter. It exists in two valency forms: divalent (II) with stannous compounds, and tin (IV) with a valency of 4 and stannic compounds. Inorganic compounds such as stannous chloride are used as stabilizers in soaps and perfumes, in dyes and inks, in the textile industry as a mordant, in some processes for the strengthening of glass and in toothpastes to combat caries. Organotin compounds are also widely used. Thus dibutyl- and tributyltin oxides are used as catalysts and stabilizers in the production of rubber and other polymers, and dioctyltin is used as a stabilizer in PVC film. Triphenyltin is used in antifouling paints, in bactericides, fungicides and wood preservatives.

Metabolism

Inorganic tin compounds are poorly absorbed from the gut but tin (II) is more readily absorbed than tin (IV). Absorbed tin rapidly leaves the blood stream and is deposited preferentially in lung, kidney, liver and bone. Tin concentrations in the lung increase with age but this is not so in other organs. The main route of excretion is through the kidney, probably less than 15% being excreted into the bile.

Organotin compounds are, in general, better absorbed from the gut, and trialkyltin is well absorbed through the intact skin. The highest concentrations of organotin compounds are generally found in the liver. Most organotin compounds undergo biotransformation, mostly in the liver although dealkylation of diethyltin compounds seems to take place also in the gut and in some other organs. One important reaction from the toxicological point of view is the conversion of tetraalkyltin compounds to their more toxic tri forms. The route of excretion depends upon the chemical form; ethyltin seems to be excreted mainly in the urine whereas diethyltin is excreted in both the urine and the bile. The route of excretion for many of the organotin compounds, however, is not known. In many cases, they have long biological half-lives and are slow to clear from the body.

Toxicity of tin and its compounds

INORGANIC TIN

Inhalation of elemental tin does not produce any untoward effects in man although prolonged inhalation of tin (IV) oxide dust and fumes produces a benign pneumoconiosis, stannosis. The radiograph may show an alarming preponderance of small, extremely radiodense opacities but there is no impairment in lung function, no fibrosis and the individual is symptom free. The ingestion of foods with a high tin content may cause nausea, vomiting and diarrhoea but there are no sequelae.

ORGANIC TIN

In general the monoorgano- and diorganotin compounds are less toxic than the triorganotin compounds and the toxicity of the trialkyltins decreases as the number of carbon atoms in the alkyl chain increases. A number of the organotin compounds are potent irritants but the alkyl and aromatic tin compounds are also neurotoxic.

Burns have been reported in workers handling dibutyl- and tributyltin. These burns itch but they heal without scarring if there is no secondary infection. Splashes of tributyltin in the eye may cause permanent damage, and inhalation may result in intense respiratory irritation, apparently with no permanent damage.

Intoxication with triethyltin produces widespread interstitial oedema throughout the white matter of the brain, with splitting and vacuolation of the myelin sheaths and degeneration of nerve fibres.[187] Symptoms such as headache, vertigo, nausea and vomiting and visual disturbances have been reported in patients suffering from organotin poisoning, and there is sometimes evidence of raised intracranial pressure and diffuse and focal EEG changes which are generally reversible.[188,189]

In experimental animals dibutyltin compounds cause inflammatory changes in the bile duct, and some other compounds may produce fatty degeneration in the renal cortex and a mild haemolytic anaemia. These effects are rare in cases of human intoxication.

A serious outbreak of organotin poisoning occurred in France in 1954, caused by a proprietary preparation used for the treatment of staphyloccocal infections. It was dispensed in capsules containing 15 mg of diiododiethyltin and 100 mg of isolinoleic acid esters (and called 'vitamin F'). The capsules were on the market for about 6–7 months before any adverse effects were noted. In all, about 210 people suffered from organotin poisoning and 102 died; many of the survivors were nevertheless left with permanent CNS sequelae. The first symptom to appear was headache, usually starting on about the fourth day after taking the capsules. It was extremely severe and accompanied by repeated vomiting, disequilibrium and retention of urine. Diplopia occurred in some cases and in severe cases there was clouding of consciousness proceeding to coma and death. In those patients who came to autopsy or to surgery, there was evidence of cerebral oedema.[190]

Of those who survived the episode, only 10 recovered completely. The remainder were left with symptoms such as headache and weakness which persisted for at least 4 years.[191]

An increased incidence of lung cancer among tin

miners in the UK has led the Industrial Injuries Advisory Council to recommend its prescription under the Social Security Act (see Chapter 4). There is, however, no direct evidence of a causal link with any specific substance but it is possible that radon or radon daughters are involved.

Treatment of organotin poisoning

There is no satisfactory treatment for organotin poisoning although BAL has been suggested as an effective agent against poisoning with the dialkyltin compounds. It is not effective in cases of poisoning with trialkyltin because these compounds do not react readily with sulphydryl groups.[192] Steroids and/or surgical decompression may be required in cases where there is severe cerebral oedema.

Supervision of workers exposed to organotin compounds

There are no established methods of biological monitoring to assess exposure to organotin compounds. Exposed workers should receive regular medical supervision, particular attention being given to the eyes, skin and central nervous system.

TUNGSTEN

Tungsten is an extremely hard metal which is highly resistant to heat. It is used in the filaments of incandescent light bulbs and in the steels used to produce tools. Most of the tungsten used in industry, is in the manufacture of sintered tungsten carbide. In this process a mixture of metals, including tungsten carbide powder cobalt, nickel and chromium, are shaped into the form of cutting tools and then fired at high temperatures to produce machine tools that are almost as hard as diamond. Some of the soluble compounds of tungsten, such as tungsten molybdenate, are used in the textile industry as mordants or fireproofing agents, and some of the highly coloured tungsten salts are used as pigments in paints, inks, ceramics and textiles.

The principal hazard associated with the use of tungsten carbide is hard metal disease (see Cobalt and Chapter 35). The putative toxic agent is cobalt since animal experiments have shown that pure tungsten carbide crystals are inert.[193] The chest radiographs of affected workers may show either diffuse, patchy, linear shadows or nodulations of various patterns. There is usually a significant decline in vital capacity before any radiographic changes become evident but there is also a wide range of individual variation in response to exposure to hard metal.

Because hard metal contains nickel and chromium, those who handle it may develop contact dermatitis.

URANIUM

Uranium oxide was extracted from pitchblende by Klaproth in 1789 and named by him in honour of Herschel's discovery of the planet Uranus in 1781. The metal itself was not obtained from the oxide until 1851. The radioactive properties of uranium were discovered by Henri Becquerel in 1896 when he found that salts of the metal emitted radiations that were able to blacken a photographic plate. The major use for uranium has been in the production of atomic weapons and as a fuel in nuclear power stations.

Uranium ores contain, in addition to the metal itself, all its decay products – which include radium and its immediate daughter product, radon. This gas diffuses out of the rocks into the atmosphere of the mine, where it decays to give isotopes of polonium, bismuth and lead. All these daughter products, with the exception of ^{210}Pb, have short half-lives and if inhaled, decay on the bronchial epithelium before being exhaled. Radon and polonium emit alpha particles which may produce a significant dose to the cells in the respiratory tract. It was the presence of the alpha emitters that caused the high death rates from bronchial carcinoma in the miners of Joachimstal and Schneeberg, commented upon by Agricola in *De Re Metallica*. It has been estimated that between 30 and 70% of the deaths in these miners were caused by lung cancer.[194]

The risk of bronchial carcinoma is still present for those who mine uranium, and several epidemiological studies have shown a relationship between exposure to radiation and the prevalence of lung cancer. In a study of Czechoslovakian miners, the lowest excess seems to occur with an exposure of about 50 working level months.[195] An excess rate of lung cancer in Canadian miners has, however, been found to be associated with doses that are lower than this.[196] Uranium mill miners do not appear to share this risk.[197]

In the early studies of uranium miners in the USA it was found that almost every miner was a smoker and it was considered that smoking was the major contributing factor in the development of the lung cancer seen in these workers. That was later conclusively shown not to be the case[198] although there is undoubtedly an additive or multiplicative relationship between smoking and exposure to radon daughters.

All types of bronchogenic carcinoma have been found in uranium miners but the undifferentiated type appears to predominate. Some attempts have been made to detect those miners who are most at risk, using sputum cytology, without success. It has been shown that a latent period of about 10–20 years is required for the development of the tumour.[199]

An increase in lung cancer has been reported in several other groups of miners, including those engaged in the extraction of iron ore, fluorspar, zinc and lead. In each case, the proximate cause is the presence of radon and its daughter products in the air in the mines (see Chapter 19).

In addition to the radiation hazards described above, uranium also exhibits chemical toxicity. When absorbed as a soluble salt it is toxic to the proximal tubules, leading to albuminuria, aminoaciduria and the release of catalase and phosphatase. This has been employed in a test using catalase in urine as an index of the renal damage. It has been suggested that to prevent renal damage, the post-shift urinary concentration should not exceed 250 mg/litre.[200] The hexafluoride seems to be particularly toxic but the dioxide, oxide and tetrafluoride are very harmful too.

After absorption, uranium rapidly leaves the blood and is deposited in the tissue; hexavalent compounds seem to have a predilection for kidney and bone[201] and tetravalent forms are particularly absorbed by the liver. In poisoning, the critical organs seem to be the kidneys and bone and, by inhalation, the lungs. Experimentally, uranium compounds have been recovered from placenta, fetus and milk. Soluble compounds have a short biological half life and about 50% is excreted in the first day. Conversely, insoluble compounds are only poorly eliminated.

Uranium poisoning is usually caused by soluble compounds and is characterized by tubular necrosis and, perhaps, renal failure.[202,203] Inhalation of uranium hexafluoride may cause acute respiratory tract damage and pulmonary oedema.

Chronic poisoning has been associated with a range of injury including pulmonary fibrosis, anaemia and suppression of white cells. These changes appear to be independent of the radioactive properties of these compounds.

Details of radiation protection are to be found in Chapter 19.

VANADIUM

Vanadium was discovered in iron ore in Sweden in 1830 and romantically named after the Swedish goddess Freya Vanadin. The metal has many uses in industry; the alloy ferrovanadium contains only 0.5% vanadium but its tensile strength is twice that of normal steel. It is also widely employed in non-ferrous alloys, mainly with titanium, for use in the manufacture of jet engines and airframes. Vanadium salts are widely used as catalysts in, for example, the oxidation of sulphur dioxide to sulphur trioxides and in the production of synthetic rubber. Vanadium pentoxide is used as a catalyst in dye mordants, in paint and varnish drying and in the manufacture of glass, ink, pesticides and photographic chemicals. It occurs in oils from a number of regions including Venezuela, Iran and parts of the USA. The ash from these oils may be rich in vanadium and is a hazard to those who clean out oil-fired furnaces or who handle the fly ash.

Vanadium is an essential element concerned with normal lipid metabolism. It is poorly absorbed from the gut. In the blood it is almost entirely bound to transferrin and is rapidly excreted in the urine; very little appears in the faeces.

The principal hazard is to those who clean out oil-fired furnaces and who handle the fly ash or clean the heat exchanger tubes of gas turbines. The metal and its compounds are irritant to the eye and the respiratory tract. Exposure may result in conjunctivitis, dyspnoea, wheezing and a cough. Those affected may complain of a metallic taste in the mouth and, following particularly heavy exposure, there may be a greenish black discoloration of the tongue. The symptoms usually remit quickly after removal from exposure but cough may persist for several weeks.

The rate of excretion in the urine is chemical species dependent, with the half-life of the metal ion being 15–40 hours. Urinary monitoring of workers (end of shift samples) is feasible.

ZINC

Zinc is another of the silver white metals and is widely used in a number of common alloys such as brass and bronze and for galvanizing.

It is an essential element and a vital constituent of more than 200 metalloenzymes, including carbonic anhydrase and DNA polymerase. Its absorption from the gut is enhanced by the secretion of a pancreatic scavenger, probably prostaglandin E_2. It is bound to transferrin for transport to the liver and transferred within the liver to albumin and α_2-macroglobulin. Its uptake from the gut also depends upon a mucosal metallothionein, the formation of which is induced by plasma zinc levels and which sequesters zinc within the mucosal cells. The hepatocytes also contain metallothionein and they are able to sequester zinc intracellularly. The levels of zinc within the body are regulated by metallothionein uptake and zinc is lost from the body to a substantial degree by the desquamation of intestinal mucosal cells.

Two of the salts of zinc, zinc oxide and zinc chloride, produce adverse effects in humans. Zinc oxide is highly volatile at relatively low temperatures and so is evolved during any operations in which the molten metal is used. Welding on galvanized metal can also produce dense clouds of white zinc oxide fumes, inhalation of which produces a condition known as metal fume fever (see Chapter 9). Zinc is not alone in producing this condition, which may also follow the inhalation of fumes from copper, magnesium, aluminum, antimony, cadmium, iron, manganese, nickel, selenium, silver and tin. Most cases, however, are caused by zinc, copper or magnesium fumes.

ZIRCONIUM

Zirconium is a silvery white hard brittle metal which in powder form is very reactive and flammable. The metal may be alloyed with other metals to increase wear- and corrosion-resistance. Other uses of zirconium compounds include in foundry sands, ceramics and refactories. The principal modern use is in nuclear reactors as a cladding material because of its high temperature-resistance and corrosion-resistance properties. It is also used in vacuum tubes to remove traces of oxygen. A study of men exposed to zirconium compounds did not find any evidence of respiratory symptoms, or any adverse effect on pulmonary function or abnormal radiological findings.[204]

REFERENCES

1 Lee W R. What happens in lead poisoning? *J R Coll Phys* 1981;**15**:48–54.

2 International Agency for Research on Cancer. *Evaluation of Carcinogenic Risk of Chemicals to Man* Vol I. Lyon: IARC, 1972.

3 Leiken S, Eng G. Erythrokinetic studies of the anemia of lead poisoning. *Pediatrics* 1963;**31**:996–1002.

4 Secci GC, Alessio L, Cambiogghi G. Na/K-ATPase activity of erythrocyte membrane. *Arch Environ Hlth* 1973;**27**:399–400.

5 Batumen V, Maesaka JK, Haddad B *et al*. The role of lead in gout nephropathy. *N Engl J Med* 1981;**304**:520–3.

6 Gerhardsson I, Lundstrom NG, Nordberg G, Wall S. Mortality and lead exposure: a retrospective study of Swedish smelter workers. *Br J Ind Med* 1986;**43**:707–12.

7 International Programme on Chemical Safety (IPCS). *Inorganic Lead. Environmental Health Criteria 165.* Geneva:World Health Organization, 1995.

8 Pocock SJ, Smith M, Baghurst P. Environmental lead and children's intelligence:a systematic review of the epidemiological evidence. *Br Med J* 1994;**309**:1189–97.

9 Seppalainen AM, Hernberg S, Kock B. Relationship between blood levels and nerve-conduction velocity. *Neurotoxicology* 1979;**1**:313–32.

10 Baker EL, White RF, Pothier LJ *et al*. Occupational lead neurotoxicity: improvement in behavioural effects after reduction of exposure. *Br J Ind Med* 1985;**42**:507–16.

11 Hardman JG, Limbird LE, Molinoff PB, Ruddon RW (eds). *Goodman and Gilman's Pharmacological Basis of Therapeutics* 9th edn. New York: McGraw-Hill, 1996.

12 Bakir F, Damluji SF, Amin-Zaki I *et al*. Methyl mercury poisoning in Iraq. *Science* 1973;**181**:230–41.

13 Hargreaves RJ, Evans JG, Janota I, Magos L, Cavanagh JB. Persistent mercury in nerve cells 16 years after metallic mercury poisoning. *Neuropathol Appl Neurobiol* 1988;**14**:443–52.

14 Clarkson TW. The pharmacology of mercury compounds. *Ann Rev Pharmacol* 1972;**12**:375–406.

15 Buchet JP, Roels A, Bernard A, Lauwerys R. Assessment of renal function of workers exposed to inorganic lead, cadmium or mercury vapor. *J Occup Med* 1980;**22**:741–50.

16 Smith PJ, Langold GD, Goldberg J. Effects of occupational exposure to elemental mercury on short term memory. *Br J Ind Med* 1983;**40**:413–19.

17 Levine SP, Cavender GD, Langold GD, Albers JW. Elementary mercury exposure: peripheral neurotoxicity. *Br J Ind Med* 1982;**39**:136–9.

18 Takeuchi T, Morikawa N, Matsumoto H *et al*. A pathologic study of Minamata disease in Japan. *Acta Neuropathol* 1962;**2**:40–57.

19 Kazantzis G, Schiller KFR, Asscher AW *et al*. Albuminuria and the nephrotic syndrome following exposure to mercury and its compounds. *Q J Med* 1962;**31**:403–18.

20 Gledhill RF, Hopkins AP. Chronic inorganic mercury poisoning treated with *N*-acetyl-D-penicillamine. *Br Med J* 1972;**29**:225–8.

21 Magos L. Effect of 2,3-dimercaptopropanol (BAL) on urinary excretion and brain content of mercury. *Br J Ind Med* 1968;**25**:152–4.

22 Tsubaki T, Trukayama K. *Minamata Disease*. Amsterdam: Elsevier, 1977.

23 Friberg L, Elinder C, Kyellstrom T. *Cadmium and Health: Toxological and Epidemiological Appraisal* Vol. I. Boca Raton: CRC Press, 1986.

24 Kawada T, Koyama H, Suzuki S, Cadmium, NAG activity, and β_2-microglobulin in the urine of cadmium pigment workers. *Br J Ind Med* 1989;**46**:52–5.

25 Lauwerys R, Bernard AM. Cadmium and the kidney. *Br J Ind Med* 1986;**43**:433–5.

26 Elinder CG, Edling C, Lindberg E, Kagedal B, Vesterberg A. Assessment of renal function in workers previously exposed to cadmium. *Br J Ind Med* 1986;**42**:754–60.

27 Parkes WR. *Occupational Lung Disease* 3rd edn. London: Heinemann, 1994.

28 Edling C, Elinder CG, Randma E. Lung function in workers using cadmium containing solders. *Br J Ind Med* 1986;**43**:657–68.

29 Elinder CG, Kjellstrom TK, Hogstedt C, Andersson K, Span G. Cancer mortality of cadmium workers. *Br J Ind Med* 1985;**42**:651–5.

30 Stanbury SW, Mawer EB. Metabolic disturbances in acquired osteomalacia. In: Cohen RD, Lewis B, Albert KCMM, Denman AM eds. *The Metabolism and Molecular Basis of Acquired Disease* Vol 2. London: Baillière Tindall, 1990: 1717–82.

31 Chalkley SR, Richmond J, Barltrop D. Measurement of vitamin D_3 metabolites in smelter workers exposed to lead and cadmium. *Occup Environ Med* 1998; **55**: 446–52.

32 Staessen J, Bulpitt CJ, Roels H *et al*. Urinary cadmium and lead concentrations and their relation to blood pressure in a population with low exposure. *Br J Ind Med* 1984;**41**:241–8.

33 Boscolo P, Carmignani M. Mechanisms of cardiovascular regulation in male rabbits chronically exposed to cadmium. *Br J Ind Med* 1986;**43**:605–10.

34 Frausto da Silva JRR, Williams RJP. *The Biological Chemistry of the Elements*. Oxford: Oxford University Press.

35 Lauwerys R, Roels H, Regniers M *et al*. Significance of cadmium concentrations in blood and in urine in workers exposed to cadmium. *Environ Res* 1979;**20**:375–91.

36 Al-Haddad IK, Chettle DR, Fletcher JR, Fremlin JH. A transportable system for measurement of kidney cadmium *in vivo*. *Int J Appl Rad Isotopes* 1981;**32**:109–12.

37 Yaqoob M, Bell GM, Percy DF, Finn R. Primary glomerulonephritis and hydrocarbon exposure: a case-control study and literature review. *Q J Med (New Ser)* 1992;**82**:409–18.

38 Vian C, Bernard A, Lauwerys R. A cross-sectional survey of kidney function in oil refinery employees. *Am J Ind Med* 1987;**11**:177–87.

39 Yaqoob M, Bell GM, Stevenson A *et al*. Renal impairment with chronic hydrocarbon exposure. *Q J Med* 1993;**86**:165–74.

40 Mutti A, Alinvoi R, Bergamaschi E *et al*. Nephropathies and exposure to perchloroethylene in dry-cleaners. *Lancet* 1992;**340**:189–93.

41 Gerhardsson I, Chettle DR, Englyst V *et al*. Kidney effects in long term exposed lead smelter workers. *Br J Ind Med* 1992;**49**:186–92.

42 LeQuesne PM, McLeod JG. Peripheral neuropathy following a single exposure to arsenic. *J Neurol Sci* 1977;**32**:437–51.

43 Beckett WS, Moore JL, Keogh JP, Bleecker ML. Acute encephalopathy due to occupational exposure to arsenic. *Br J Ind Med* 1986;**43**:66–7.

44 Schiller CM, Fowler BA, Woods JS. Effects of arsenic on pyruvate dehydrogenase activity. *Environ Hlth Perspect* 1977;**19**:205–7.

45 Mabuchi K, Lilienfels AM, Snell LM. Lung cancer among pesticide workers exposed to inorganic arsenicals. *Arch Environ Hlth* 1979;**34**:312–20.

46 Buchet JP, Lauwerys R, Roels H. Comparison of several methods for the determination of arsenic compounds in water and in urine. *Int Arch Occup Environ Hlth* 1980;**46**:11–29.

47 Finkel AJ. *Hamilton and Hardy's Industrial Toxicology*. London:John Wright, 1983 : 117.

48 Hughes JPN, Baron R, Buckland DH *et al*. Phosphorus necrosis of the jaw:a present-day study. *Br J Ind Med* 1962;**19**:83–99.

49 Ben-Hur N, Gilardi A, Appelbaum J *et al*. Phosphorus burns:the antidote:a new approach. *Br J Plast Surg* 1972;**25**:245–9.

50 Muller J, Kusiak RA, Suranyi G *et al*. *Study of Mortality of Ontario Miners 1955–77*, part ii. Toronto:Ontario Ministry of Labour Special Studies Branch, 1986.

51 Rifat SL, Eastwood MR, Crapper McLachlan DR *et al*. Effect of exposure of miners to aluminium powder. *Lancet* 1990;**336**:1162–5.

52 Bast-Pettersen R, Drables PA, Goffeng LO *et al*. Neuropsychological deficit among elderly workers in aluminum production. *Am J Ind Med* 1994;**25**:649–52.

53 Sim M, Dick R, Jusso J *et al*. Are aluminium potroom workers at increased risk of neurological disorders? *Occup Environ Med* 1997;**54**:229–35.

54 Graves AB, Rosner D, Echererria D *et al*. Occupational exposure to solvents and aluminium and estimated risks of Alzheimer's disease. *Occup Environ Med* 1998; **55**:627–33.

55 Field GB. Pulmonary function in aluminium smelters. *Thorax* 1984;**39**:743–51.

56 Saric M, Marelja J. Bronchial hyperreactivity in potroom workers and prognosis after stopping exposure. *Br J Ind Med* 1991;**48**:653–5.

57 Mitchell J. Pulmonary fibrosis in an aluminium worker. *Br J Ind Med* 1959;**16**:123–5.

58 Jordan JW. Pulmonary fibrosis in a worker using an aluminium powder. *Br J Ind Med* 1961;**18**:21–3.

59 McLaughlin AIG, Kazantzis G, King E *et al*. Pulmonary fibrosis and encephalopathy associated with the inhalation of aluminium dust. *Br J Ind Med* 1962;**19**:253–63.

60 Mitchell J, Manning GE, Molyneux M *et al*. Pulmonary fibrosis in workers exposed to finely powdered aluminium. *Br J Ind Med* 1961;**18**:10–20.

61 Corrin B. Aluminium pneumoconiosis. *In vitro* comparison of stamped aluminium powders and a granular aluminium powder. *Br J Ind Med* 1963;**20**:264–7.

62 Abramson MJ, Wlodarczyk JH, Saunders NA *et al*. Does aluminium smelting cause lung disease? *Am Rev Respir Dis* 1989;**139**:1042–57.

63 Ljunggren KG, Lidums V, Bengt S. Blood and urine concentrations of aluminium among workers exposed to aluminium flake powders. *Br J Ind Med* 1991;**48**:106–9.

64 Martyn CN, Barker DJP, Osmond C *et al*. Geographical relation between Alzheimer disease and aluminium in drinking water. *Lancet* 1989;**i**:59–62.

65 Perl DP. Relationship of aluminium to Alzheimer disease. *Environ Hlth Perspect* 1985;**63**:149–53.

66 Crapper McLachlan DR, Lukiw WJ, Kruck TPA. New evidence for an active role of aluminium in Alzheimer disease. *Can J Neurol Sci* 1989;**16**:490–7.

67 Alfrey AC, LeGendre GR, Kaehny WD. The dialysis encephalopathy syndrome. Possible aluminium intoxication. *N Engl J Med* 1976;**294**:184–8.

68 Farrar G, Altmann P, Welch S *et al*. Defective gallium-transferrin binding in Alzheimer disease and Down syndrome:possible mechanism for accumulation of aluminium in brain. *Lancet* 1990;**335**:747–50.

69 Day JP, Barker J, Evans LJA *et al*. Aluminium absorption studied by [26]aluminium tracer. *Lancet* 1991;**337**:1345.

70 Eastwood JD, Levin GE, Pazianas M *et al*. Aluminium deposition in bone after contamination of drinking water supply. *Lancet* 1990;**336**:462–4.

71 Romundstad P, Haldorsen T, Rennberg A. Exposure to PA11 and fluoride in aluminium reduction plants in Norway. Historical estimation of exposure using process parameters and industrial hygiene measures. *Am J Ind Med* 1999; **35**: 164–74.

72 International Agency for Research on Cancer. Monographs on the evaluation of the carcinogenic risks of chemicals to humans: 34. *Polyaromatic Compounds*, Part 3 *Industrial exposures in aluminium production, coal gasification, coke production and iron and steel founding*. Lyon: IARC, 1984.

73 Veiren NK. Routine patch testing with aluminium trichloride. *Contact Derm* 1996; **35**: 126–33.

74 Cooper DA, Pendergrass EP, Vorwald AJ *et al*. Pneumoconiosis in workers in an antimony industry. *Am J Roentgen* 1968;**103**:496–508.

75 Renes LE. Antimony poisoning in industry. *Arch Ind Hyg Occup Med* 1953;**7**:99–108.

76 Brieger H, Semisch CW, Stasneg J *et al*. Industrial antimony poisoning. *Ind Med Surg* 1954;**23**: 521–3.

77 Ball E, Smith A, Northage C *et al*. *Antimony and Antimony Compounds. Criteria Document for An Occupational Exposure Limit*. London:Health and Safety Executive, 1997.

78 Jones RD. Survey of antimony workers:mortality 1961–92. *Occup Environ Med* 1994;**51**:772–6.

79 Gombos B. Pulmonary nodulation from inhalation of barium dust. *Pracov Lek* 1957; **9**: 399.

80 Zschiesche W, Schaller KH, Weltie D. Exposure to barium compounds: an interventional study in arc welders. *Int Arch Occup Environ Hlth* 1992; **64**: 12–23.

81 Hardy, Trabshaw IR. Delayed chemical pneumionitis in workers exposed to beryllium compounds. *J Ind Hyg Toxicol* 1946; **28**: 197.

82 Newman LS, Kriess K, King TE *et al*. Pathologic and immunologic alteration in early stages of beryllium disease. Re-examination of disease definition and natural history. *Am Rev Respir Dis* 1989; **139**: 1479–86.

83 Andrews JL, Hazemi H, Hardy HL. Patterns of lung disease in chronic beryllium disease. *Am Rev Respir Dis* 1969;**100**:791–800.

84 Freiman DG, Hardy HL. Beryllium disease *Hum Pathol* 1970;**1**:25–44.

85 Bobka CA, Stewart LA, Engleker PC. Comparison of *in vivo* and *in vitro* measures of beryllium sensitivity. *J Occup Environ Med* 1997; **39**: 540–1.

86 Harris J, Bartelson BB, Baker E *et al*. Serum neopterin in chronic beryllium disease. *Am J Ind Med* 1997; **32**: 21–8.

87 Deodhar SD, Barna B, van Ostrand HS. A study of immunologic aspects of chronic berylliosis. *Chest* 1973;**63**:309–13.

88 Price CD, Pugh A, Pioli EM *et al*. Beryllium macrophage inhibition test. *Ann NY Acad Sci* 1976;**278**:204–11.

89 Eisenbud M, Warita RC, Dunstan C *et al*. Non-occupational berylliosis. *J Ind Hyg Toxicol* 1949;**31**:282–94.

90 Hasan FM, Kazemi H. Chronic beryllium disease. *Chest* 1974;**65**:289–93.

91 Sprince NL, Kazemi H, Fanburg BL. *Serum Angi-otensin-1-converting Enzyme in Chronic Beryllium Disease*. Cardiff:Proceedings of 8th International Conference on Sarcoidosis, 1980.

92 Groth DH. Carcinogenicity of beryllium: review of the literature. *Environ Res* 1980;**21**:56–62.

93 Mancuso TF. Relation of length of employment and prior respiratory illness to respiratory cancer among beryllium workers. *Environ Res* 1970;**3**:251–75.

94 Waggoner JK, Infante PF, Bayliss DL. Beryllium: an etiologic agent in the induction of lung cancer, neoplastic respiratory disease, and heart disease among industrially exposed workers. *Environ Res* 1980;**21**:15–34.

95 Infante PF, Waggoner JK, Sprince NL. Mortality patterns from lung cancer and non-neoplastic respiratory disease among white males in the beryllium case register. *Environ Res* 1980;**21**:35–43.

96 Ward E, Okun A, Ruder A *et al*. A mortality study of workers at seven beryllium processing plants. *Am J Ind Med* 1992;**22**:885–904.

97 Beryllium Industry Scientific Advisory Committee. Is beryllium carcinogenic in humans? *J Occup Environ Med* 1997; **39**: 205–8.

98 Vanio H, Rice JM. Beryllium revisited [Editorial]. *J Occup Environ Med* 1997; **39**: 203–4.

99 Kriess K, Mroz MM, Zhen B *et al*. Risks of beryllium disease related to work processes at a metal alloy, and oxide production plant. *Occup Environ Med* 1997; **54**: 605–12.

100 Balkinssoon RC, Newman LS. Beryllium copper alloy (2%) causes chronic beryllium disease. *J Occup Environ Med* 1999; **41**: 304–8.

101 Kriess K, Wasserman SL, Mroz MM *et al*. Beryllium disease screening in the ceramics industry: Blood lymphocyte test performance and exposure disease relations. *J Occup Med* 1993; **35**: 267–72.

102 Kriess K, Mroz M, Newman LS *et al*. Marking risk of beryllium disease and sensitization with median exposure below 2 μg/m³. *Am J Ind Med* 1996; **30**: 16–25.

103 Norseth R. The carcinogenicity of chromium and its salts. *Br J Ind Med* 1986;**43**:649–51.

104 McAughey JJ, Samuel AM, Baxter PJ, Smith NJ. Biological monitoring of occupational exposure in the chromate production industry. *Sci Total Environ* 1988;**71**:317–22.

105 Cullen A. Respiratory diseases from hard metal or cobalt exposure. A continuing enigma. *Chest* 1984;**86**:513–4.

106 Fishbein EA. Clinical findings amongst hard metal workers. *Br J Ind Med* 1992;**49**:17–24.

107 Meyer-Bisch C, Pham QT, Mur JM. Respiratory hazards in hard metal workers:a cross sectional study. *Br J Ind Med* 1989;**46**:302–9.

108 Nemery B, Casier P, Rousels D *et al*. Survey of cobalt exposure and respiratory health in diamond polishers. *Am Rev Respir Dis* 1992;**145**:610–6.

109 Lison D, Lauwerys R, Demedts M *et al*. Experimental research into the pathogenesis of cobalt/hard metal lung disease. *Eur Respir J* 1996;**9**:1024–8.

110 Sivennen B, Buchet JP, Stanescue D *et al*. Epidemiological survey on workers exposed to cobalt oxides, cobalt salts and cobalt metal. *Br J Ind Med* 1993;**50**:835–42.

111 Shirakawa T, Kusaka T, Fujimura N *et al*. The existence of specific antibodies to cobalt in hard metal asthma. *Clin All* 1988;**18**:451–60.

112 Leysens B, Aurerx J, Van Den Eeckhout A *et al*. Cobalt-induced bronchial asthma in diamond polishers. *Chest* 1989;**88**:740–4.

113 Kusaka Y, Iki M, Kumagai S. Epidemiological study of hard metal asthma. *Occup Environ Med* 1996;**53**:188–99.

114 NTP Technical Report on the Toxicology and carcinogenesis studies of cobalt sulfate heptahydrate in rats and mice (inhalation studies). *NIH publication No 96-3951* 1996.

115 Moulin JJ, Wild P, Mur JM *et al*. A mortality study of cobalt production workers: an extension of the follow-up. *Am J Ind Med* 1993;**23**:281–8.

116 Lasfargues G, Wild P, Moullin JJ *et al*. Lung cancer mortality in a French cohort of hard metal workers. *Am J Ind Med* 1994;**26**:585–95.

117 Leonard S, Lauwerys R. Mutagenicity, carcinogenicity and teratogenicity of cobalt metal and cobalt compounds. *Mutat Res* 1990; **239**: 17–27.

118 Alexander CS. Cobalt-beer myopathy. *Am J Med* 1972;**53**:395–417.

119 Lauwerys R, Hoet P. *Industrial Chemical Exposure Guidelines for Biological Monitoring* 2nd edn. London: Lewis Publishers, 1993.

120 Lison D, Buchet J-P, Swennen B *et al*. Biological monitoring of workers exposed to cobalt metal, salts, oxides and hard metal dust. *Occup Environ Med* 1994; **5**: 447–50.

121 *Maximum Concentration at the Workplace and Biological Tolerance Values*. Report no.31. Deutsche Forschungsgemeinschaft, VCH, 1999.

122 Walsh JM. Copper: not too little, not too much but just right. *J Roy Coll Phys Lond* 1995; **29**: 280–8.

123 Schroeder HA, Nason AP, Fifton IH *et al*. Essential trace metals in mass:copper. *J Chronic Dis* 1966;**19**: 1007–34.

124 Deiss A, Lee GR, Cartwright GE. Hemolytic anemia in Wilson's disease. *Ann Intern Med* 1970;**73**:413–18.

125 O'Donogue AM, Ferguson MM. Superficial staining of the teeth in a brass foundry worker. *Occup Med* 1996;**46**:3 : 233–4.

126 Metz EN. Mechanism of hemolysis by excess copper. *Clin Res* 1969;**17**:32 [abstract].

127 Klein WJ, Metz EN, Price AN. Acute copper intoxication: a hazard of hemodialysis. *Arch Intern Med* 1972;**129**:570–82.

128 Pimental JC, Manzes AP. Vineyard sprayers' lung. *Am Rev Respir Dis* 1975;**111**:189–95.

129 Villar TG. Vineyard sprayers' disease. *Am Rev Respir Dis* 1974;**110**:545–55.

130 Chen R. An analysis program for occupational cohort mortality and update of cancer risk in copper mines. *Int J Occup Environ Hlth* 1996;**9**:301–8.

131 O'Donohue JW, Reid MA, Varghese BP *et al*. Micronodular cirrhosis and acute liver failure due to chronic copper self-intoxication. *Eur J Gastroent Hepat* 1993; **5**: 651–2.

132 Hanston P, Lievens M, Mahieu P. Accidental ingestion of a zinc and copper sulphate preparation. *J Toxicol Clin Toxicol* 1996; **34**: 725–30.

133 Browning E. *Toxicity of Industrial Metals*. Oxford: Butterworth, 1969.

134 Sjogren B, Iregren A *et al*. Effects on the nervous system among welders exposed to aluminium and manganese. *Occup Environ Med* 1996; **53**: 32–40.

135 Saric M, Markicevic A, Hrustic O. Occupational exposure to manganese. *Br J Ind Med* 1977;**34**:114–18.

136 Jacobs JM, LeQuesne PM. Toxic disorders. In: Adams JH, Duchen LW eds. *Greenfield's Neuropathology* 5th edn. London:Edward Arnold, 1992 : 894–7.

137 Wennberg A. Neurotoxic effect of metals. *Scand J Work Environ Hlth* 1994;**20**:65–71,

138 Iregren A. Using psychological tests in the early detection of neurotoxic effects of low levels of manganese exposure. *Neurotoxicology* 1994;**15**:671–7.

139 Ky SQ, Deng HS, Xie PY, Hu N. A report of two cases of chronic serious manganese poisoning treated with sodium para-aminosalicylic acid. *Br J Ind Med* 1992;**49**:66–9.

140 Meco G, Bonifati V, Vanacore N, Fabrizo E. Parkinsonism after chronic exposure to the fungicide MANEB (manganese ethylene-bis-dithiocarbamate). *Scand J Work Environ Hlth* 1994;**20**:301–5.

141 Wolters EC, Huang CC, Clark C *et al*. Positron emission tomography in manganese intoxication. *Ann Neurol* 1989;**26**:647–51.

142 Mena I, Horiuchi K, Burke K, Cotzias GC. Chronic manganese poisoning:individual susceptibility and absence of iron. *Neurology* 1969;**19**:1000–6.

143 Mena I, Horiuchi K, Lopez G. Factors enhancing entrance of manganese to the brain. *J Nucl Med* 1974;**15**: 516.

144 Sjogren B, Iregren A *et al*. Effects on the nervous system among welders exposed to aluminium and manganese. *Occup Environ Med* 1996;**53**:32–40.

145 Yin S-J, Lin FH, Shih T-S. Lipid peroxidation in workers exposed to manganese. *Scand J Work Environ Hlth* 1996; **22**: 381–6.

146 Bremner I. The toxicity of cadmium, zinc and molybdenum and their effects on copper metabolism. *Proc Nutr Soc* 1979;**38**:235–42.

147 Seelig M. Copper-molybdonum in iron deficiency and storage diseases. *Am J Clin Nutr* 1973;**26**:657–72.

148 Habashi F (ed). Nickel. In: *Handbook of Extractive Metallurgy*. Weinheim, Germany: Wiley-VCH, **19**: 716–90.

149 International Agency for Research on Cancer. Monographs on the evaluation of carcinogenic risks to humans: 49. *Chromium, Nickel and Welding*. Lyon: IARC, 1990.

150 Doll R. Report of the International Committee on nickel carcinogenesis in man. *Scand J Work Environ Hlth* 1990;**16**.

151 Dunnick JK, Elwell MR *et al*. Comparitive effects of nickel subsulfide, nickel oxide or nickel sulphate hexahydrate chronic exposures in the lung. *Cancer Res* 1995;**55**:5251–156.

152 Maibach HI, Menne T (eds). Nickel and the skin. In: *Immunology and Toxicology*. Boca Raton, Florida: CRC Press, 1989.

153 Bright P, Burge PS, O'Hickey SP *et al*. Occupational asthma due to chrome and nickel electroplating. *Thorax* 1997;**52**:28–32.

154 Sunderman FW Jr, Dingle B, Hopfer SM *et al*. Acute nickel toxicity in electroplating workers who accidentally ingested a solution of nickel sulphate and chloride. *Am J Ind Med* 1988; **14**: 257–66.

155 Kiilunen M, Utela J, Rantanen T *et al*. Exposure to soluble nickel in electrolytic nickel refining. *Ann Occup Hyg* 1997; **41**: 167–88.

156 Smith IC, Carson BL, Ferguson TL. Osmium. An appraisal of environmental exposure. *Environ Hlth Perspect* 1974;**8**:201–13.

157 Hunter D, Milton R, Perry KM. Asthma caused by complex salts of platinum. *Brit J Ind Med* 1945;**2**:92.

158 Venables KM, Dally MB, Nunn AJ *et al*. Smoking and occupational allergy in workers in a platinum refinery. *Br Med J* 1989; **299**: 939–2.

159 Calverley AE, Rees D, Dodswell RJ *et al*. Platinum salt sensitivity in refinery workers: incidence and effect of smoking and exposure. *Occup Environ Med* 1995; **52**: 661–6.

160 Linnett PJ, Glyn Hughes FG. 20 Years of medical surveillance on exposure to allergenic and non-allergenic platinum compounds: the importance of chemical speciation. *Occup Environ Med* 1999; **56**: 191–6.

161 Pepys J, Pickering CAC, Hughes EG. Asthma due to inhaled chemical agents – complex salts of platinum. *Clin All* 1972; **2**: 391–6.

162 Niczborala M, Garnier R. Allergy to platinum salts: a historical prospective cohort study. *Occup Environ Med* 1996; **53**: 252–7.

163 Cleare MJ, Hughes EG, Jacoby B *et al*. Immediate (type 1) allergic response to platinum compounds. *Clin All* 1976; **6**: 183–95,

164 Nygren O, Lundgren C. Determination of platinum in workroom air and in blood and urine from nursing staff attending patients receiving cisplatin chemotherapy. *Int Arch Occup Environ Hlth* 1997; **70**: 209–14.

165 Oryszezyn MP, Godin J, Frette C *et al*. Decrease in sele-

166 Diskin DJ, Tomasso CL, Alper JC *et al*. Long term selenium exposure. *Ann Intern Med* 1979;**139**:824–6.

167 Shamberger RJ, Rukovena E, Longeld AR *et al*. Antioxidants and cancer:selenium in the blood of normal and cancer patients. *J Natl Cancer Inst* 1973;**50**: 863–70.

168 Griffin AC. Role of selenium in the chemoprevention of cancer. *Adv Cancer Res* 1979;**29**:419–42.

169 Spallholz JE. On the nature of selenium toxicity and carcinostatic activity (a review). *Free Radical Biol Med* 1994; **17**: 45–64.

170 Robberecht H, Deeistra H. Selenium in human urine. Determination, speciation and concentration levels. *Tantala* 1984; **31**: 497–508.

171 Vaillancourt C, Robin JP. Medical surveillance of workers exposed to selenium. Proceedings of the Selenium Tellurium Development Association fifth international symposium. Brussels. 1994: 29–32.1

172 Weir FW. Health hazard from occupational exposure to metallic copper and silver salts. *Am Ind Hyg Assoc J* 1979;**40**:245–7.

173 Williams N, Gardner J. Absence of symptoms in silver refiners with raised blood silver levels. *Occup Med* 1995;**45**:205–8.

174 Armitage SA, White M, Wilson KH. The determination of silver in whole blood and its application to biological monitoring of occupationally exposed groups. *Ann Occup Hyg* 1996;**40**:331–8.

175 Shi MP, Deeds FE. *The Importance of Tellurium as a Health Hazard in Industry*. US Publ Hlth Serv Publ Hlth Rep 1920; **35**: 939.

176 Blackadder ES, Manderson WG. Occupational absorption of tellurium: a report of two cases. *Br J Ind Med* 1975; **32**: 59–61.

177 Geary DL, Myers RC, Nachreiner DJ *et al*. Tellurium and tellurium dioxide:single endotracheal injections in rats. *Am Ind Hyg Assoc J* 1978;**39**:100–9.

178 Amdur ML. Tellurium. *Occup Med* 1947;**3**:386–91.

179 Toots H, Parker RB. Thallium in salt substitutes. *Environ Res* 1977;**14**:327–8.

180 Wax PM. Tortilla thallotoxicosis. *Clin Toxicol* 1995; **33**: 265.

181 Hirata M, Taoda K, Ono-Ogaswara M *et al*. *Ind Hlth* 1998; **36**: 300–3.

182 Lee RV. In: Harbison R ed. *Hamilton and Hardy's Industrial Toxicology* 5th edn. Chicago: Mosby Year Book Inc, 1998: 124–6.

183 Lameijer W, van Zweiter PA. Acute cardiovascular toxicity of thallium. *Arch Toxicol* 1976;**35**:49–61.

184 Cavanagh JB, Gregson M. Some effects of a thallium salt on the proliferation of hair follicle cells. *J Pathol* 1978;**125**:179–91.

185 Barbier F. Treatment of thallium poisoning. *Lancet* 1974;**2**:965.

186 Schaller KH, Manke G, Raithel HJ *et al*. Investigation of

thallium-exposed workers in cement factories. *Int Arch Occup Environ Hlth* 1980;**47**:223–31.

187 Piver WT. Organotin compounds. *Environ Hlth Perspect* 1973;**4**:61–79.

188 Prull G, Rompell K. EEC changes in acute poisoning with organotin compounds. *Electroencephalogr Clin Neurophysiol* 1970;**29**:215.

189 Prull G. Neurological and cerebro-electrical disturbances in acute poisoning due to organotin compounds. *Nervenarzt* 1976;**41**:516–20.

190 'Stalinon':a therapeutic disaster. *Br Med J* 1958;**1**:515.

191 Barnes JM, Stoner HB. The toxicity of tin compounds. *Pharmacol Rev* 1959;**11**:211–31.

192 Barnes JM, Magos L. The toxicology of organometallic compounds. *Organometal Chem Rev* 1968;**3**:137–50.

193 Coates EO, Watson JHL. Diffuse interstitial lung disease in tungsten carbide workers. *Ann Intern Med* 1971;**75**:705–16.

194 Kunz E, Seve J. Lung cancer in man in relation to different time distribution of radiation exposure. *Hlth Phys* 1979;**36**:699–706.

195 Seve J, Kunz E, Placek V. Lung cancer in uranium miners and long-term exposure to radon daughter products. *Hlth Phys* 1976;**30**:433–7.

196 Hewitt D. In:*Report of the Royal Commission on the Health and Safety of Workers in Mines*. Toronto: 1976.

197 Archer VE, Waggoner JK, Lundin FE. Pulmonary function of uranium miners. *J Occup Med* 1973;**15**:11–14.

198 Whitmore AS, McMillan A. Lung cancer mortality among US uranium miners:a reappraisal. *J Natl Cancer Inst* 1983;**71**:489–99.

199 Saccomanno G, Archer VE, Auerback O *et al*. Development of carcinoma of the lung as reflected in exfoliated cells. *Cancer* 1974;**33**:256–70.

200 Heid KR, Walsh WP, Houston JR. In:*Conference on Occupational Health Experience with Uranium*. Washington DC:US Energy Research and Development Administration, 1975.

201 Chen PS, Terepka R, Hodge HC. The pharmacology and toxicology of bone thickness. *Ann Rev Pharmacol* 1969; **1**: 369–393.

202 Thun MJ, Baker DB, Steenland K. Renal toxicity in uranium mill workers. *Scand J Work Environ Hlth* 1985; **11**: 83–90.

203 Ghadially FN, Lalonde JA, Young-Steppuha S. Uraniosomes produced in cultured rabbit cells by uranyl acetate. *Virchows Arch (Cell Pathol)* 1982; **39**: 21–30.

204 Marcus RL, Turner S, Cherry NM. A study of lung function and chest radiography in men exposed to zirconium compounds. *Occup Med* 1996;**46**:109–13.

205 Duffus JH (ed.) *Carcinogenicity of Inorganic Substances: Risks from Occupational Exposure*. London: The Royal Chemistry Society, 1997.

206 Altmann P, Cunningham J, Dhanesha U, Ballard M, Thompson J, Marsh F. Disturbance of cerebral function in people exposed to drinking water contaminated with aluminium sulphate: retrospective study of the Camelford water incident. *Br Med J* 1999; **319**: 807–11.

8

Gases

PETER J BAXTER

Definitions	124	Investigation of gassing accidents	134
Classification of gases according to their health effects	124	Gases in the ambient air	135
Characteristics of hazardous gases	125	Properties and effects of gases	137
Occupational exposure to gases in industry	125	Primary irritant gases	147
Exposure to gases in the outdoor and indoor air	125	Irritant gases with systemic toxic effects	162
Exposure to gases in industrial accidents and fires	126	Gases with anaesthetic action: General anaesthetics	167
Principles of first aid and treatment in gassing accidents	131	Mixed exposure to gases	171
		References	173

Inhalation accidents have been a threat to workers since early times from encounters with gases in fires, mines and fermentation processes. Volcanic and geothermal gases formed the earliest atmosphere of the earth. Scientists laid the foundations of the chemical industry with the isolation and identification of individual gases. The foremost of these, Joseph Priestley (1733–1804) is credited with the discovery of 'alkaline air' (ammonia), vitriolic acid air (sulphur dioxide), nitrous oxide, nitrogen dioxide and methane, as well as isolating what he called 'dephlogisticated air', or oxygen, in 1774 whilst working as a schoolmaster in England. Early experience with gases in manufacturing industries inevitably included accidental deaths amongst workers from leaks or faulty working practices; today, however, deaths from occupational exposure to gases are rare, even though inhalation incidents are not uncommon. In the United Kingdom during a 5-year period 1989–1994, a total of 1180 cases was reported to SWORD, a national scheme for the surveillance of work-related and occupational respiratory diseases involving occupational and chest physicians. Gases and combustion products comprised by far the largest group of agents (45%), with chlorine and oxides of nitrogen the most commonly reported gases.[1]

Flammable and toxic gases stored in large quantities under pressure are an important cause of disaster. In 1974 an explosion at a chemical plant in Flixborough, England, caused by a leak of cyclohexane vapour, had an explosive force equivalent to 32 tonnes of TNT, killing 28 workers on site and causing extensive damage to houses and shops as far as 10 kilometers away.

In 1984 over 500 people died in Mexico City when a liquid petroleum gas plant exploded. Even greater hazards are posed by the release of a cloud of toxic irritant gas, which may cause death or pulmonary injury in populations for many kilometres downwind, as irritant gases are often extremely dangerous in even very dilute concentrations. The disaster at Bhopal, India, in 1984 involving the release of methyl isocyanate was the world's worst industrial incident of this kind, resulting in 4000 deaths and 100 000 survivors with respiratory injury. These incidents have led to a concerted and successful worldwide effort by national and international agencies to reduce the hazard of accidental toxic releases during chemical manufacture, storage and transport.[2]

Chemical and other industrial installations may also become military or terrorist targets. The first recorded mass civilian casualty incident due to a toxic release in warfare was during the London Blitz, when 47 people were overcome by ammonia gas. They were sheltering in a brewery cellar which received a direct hit in a heavy air raid and a fragment of flying metal pierced a pipe of an ammonia condenser.[3] The use of gases as military weapons has a long history, but in modern combat dates from the First World War.

In recent years renewed attention has been given to air pollution and respiratory health with the belated recognition of the effects that exhaust emissions from the growing number of motor vehicles are having on air quality. Carbon dioxide, carbon monoxide, sulphur dioxide, and nitrogen oxides are produced in the combustion of fossil fuels, whether as coal or petroleum products, and so are common pollutants of the outdoor and indoor air. The worst episodes of air pollution occurred during the era when coal burning was the prime source of energy. The most dramatic of these was the London Smog of December 1952 when there were an estimated 4000 excess deaths over a 5-day period provoked by a dense blanket of pollutants which included smoke and sulphur dioxide.

DEFINITIONS

A gas is any gaseous substance that is above its critical temperature and therefore is not capable of being liquefied by pressure alone. A vapour is the gaseous form of a substance which may condense at high concentrations, or is capable of being liquefied by pressure alone; aerosol (particulate) forms may coexist with the vapour. A vapour diluted with air behaves like a gas, so long as none of the substance is available in the liquid form. The same sampling devices can be used for the collection of gases and vapours.

Not all industrial 'gases', however, are true gases according to this definition. Examples are chlorine, ammonia, propane and butane which when handled in bulk are liquefied under pressure. Examples of 'true' or 'permanent' gases that require cooling as well as pressure to turn them into liquids are oxygen, nitrogen and methane.

Aerosols are solid or liquid particles dispersed in the atmosphere as dust, fumes, smoke, mists and fogs: stability is an essential characteristic.

A fume, strictly, is the solid particles generated by condensation from the gaseous state, generally after volatilization from melted substances and often accompanied by a chemical reaction such as oxidation. A cloud, or mist, of acid droplets (e.g. formed by the contact of hydrogen chloride gas with moist air) is often, but technically incorrectly, referred to as a fume.

The concentration of gases and vapours in the air can be expressed in at least four ways:

1   parts by volume (e.g. parts per million or ppm);
2   weight per volume (mg/m^3) of air;
3   partial pressure (mmHg);
4   percentage by volume.

Parts by volume (ppm) is most commonly used, but some comparisons of toxicity are on a weight per volume (mg/m^3) basis. The two expressions are interchangeable using the following conversion formula:

$$\text{Concentration in ppm} = \frac{\text{molecular volume}}{\text{molecular weight}} \times \frac{\text{concentration (as mg/m}^3}{\text{or } \mu\text{g/litre)}}$$

where molecular volume = $22.41 \times T/273 \times 1013/P$ litres

(T is the ambient temperature (K) and P is the atmospheric pressure (in millibars)).

CLASSIFICATION OF GASES ACCORDING TO THEIR HEALTH EFFECTS

Most of the common gases described in this chapter may be categorized according to the original classification of Henderson and Haggard.[4]

Irritant gases

The irritant gases are as a rule substances which chemically are regarded as corrosive. They injure surface tissues and induce inflammation of the air passages and the parenchymal region. *Primary irritants* are those which have little or no systemic toxic effect in the concentrations that cause death. *Secondary irritants* produce systemic toxic effects in addition to the surface irritation.

Workers may sometimes be exposed to a mixture of irritant gases, for example in welding. In these circumstances there is little information on how different gases interact, but additive or synergistic effects should be allowed for when assigning exposure limits to workers. Thus if the effects of the different gases are believed to be additive the mixed exposure should be assessed using the formula:

$$C_1/L_1 + C_2/L_2 + C_3/L_3$$

where C_1, C_2, etc. are the concentration of contaminants in the air and L_1, L_2, etc. are the corresponding exposure limits. The sum of the C/L fractions should not exceed unity.

Asphyxiant gases

This group of gases interferes with the supply and utilization of oxygen in the body. *Simple asphyxiants*, for example methane and hydrogen, exclude oxygen from the lungs. *Chemical asphyxiants* cause death by preventing the transportation of oxygen by the blood (e.g. carbon monoxide) or inhibit cellular respiration (e.g. hydrogen cyanide). Many simple asphyxiants are odourless and are not readily detectable. They are not given occupational exposure standards and the best means of ensuring safety is by monitoring the oxygen content of the air. Under normal atmospheric pressures the oxygen content of the air should not be allowed to fall below a minimum of 18% by volume. Simple asphyxiants do not come under the UK Control of Substances Hazardous to Health (COSHH) Regulations.

Drug-like gases and vapours

This group includes anaesthetic gases, hydrocarbons and solvents. They have a drug-like action after they have been absorbed through the lungs into the blood.

Thus in this chapter gases have been classified as follows:

1 asphyxiant gases: simple asphyxiants; chemical asphyxiants;
2 irritant gases: primary irritants with little or no systemic toxic effects; secondary irritants which produce systemic effects;
3 drug-like gases.

CHARACTERISTICS OF HAZARDOUS GASES

Flammable gases have lower and upper flammable (explosive) limits within which the resultant mixture with air may ignite. When ignited in a confined space an explosion may result but in an unconfined space, such as the open air, the consequence may be a flash fire. Most flammable gas clouds cease to be dangerous when diluted to about 2% by volume. Alarm levels for flammable gases are set at 20% of the lower explosive/flammable level so as to avoid the risk. Liquefied petroleum gases are stored or transported by road, rail and sea in large amounts and are major fire and explosion hazards. The flammability limits of flammable gases are usually much higher than the toxic levels, except for gases which spontaneously ignite on contact with air (pyrophoric gases), such as silane. Other exceptions are the flammable, simple asphyxiant gases such as hydrogen and methane whose lower flammable limits are exceeded before they can cause asphyxia by displacing air.

The general characteristics of gases which most relate to their hazard are density, water solubility and flammability. The air has a relative molecular mass of about 29 and the relative density of a gas compared with air is important in determining its tendency to disperse or accumulate at normal temperature and atmospheric pressure. The localization of the effects of irritant gases in the respiratory tract depends upon the water solubility and concentration of the gas. At low-to-moderate concentrations of highly soluble gases, such as ammonia, hydrogen chloride, hydrogen fluoride and hydrogen bromide, injury is greatest from the nasopharynx to the bronchi. Nose breathing of these gases may confine injury to the nasal passages. For less water-soluble gases, for example, nitrogen dioxide, the main localization is from the proximal to the distal acinus. At high concentrations of soluble gases, or if the gases are dissolved in fine aerosols, damage may extend throughout the respiratory tract. Solubility will also determine whether the gas will be rapidly taken up by suspended droplets in the workplace atmosphere, for example hydrogen chloride and hydrogen fluoride will readily combine with water to form hydrochloric and hydrofluoric acids, respectively. Inhalation kinetics are dealt with further in Chapter 6.

OCCUPATIONAL EXPOSURE TO GASES IN INDUSTRY

In practice, zero exposure to gases and other agents is an unattainable goal in industry and instead exposure limits are set to protect the worker. Under UK legislation the Health and Safety Executive defines a maximum exposure limit (MEL) as the maximum concentration of an airborne substance, averaged over a reference period, to which employees may be exposed by inhalation under any circumstances. Many gases have been given occupational exposure standards (OES) – the concentration that is not likely to be injurious, averaged over a reference period. These limits for many gases are long-term time-weighted average (TWA) (8 hours) and short-term exposure limit (STEL) (15 minutes) for peak exposures.[5] The worker's sense of smell is not a reliable guide to the presence of a gas, let alone a safe level. Apart from individual variability some gases, for example hydrogen sulphide and hydrogen cyanide, actually induce olfactory fatigue at higher and more dangerous concentrations. Nevertheless information on olfactory levels may be useful for a clinician when taking a patient's history. Objective measures of exposure require the use of chemical sensors or infrared detectors, colorimetric detection tubes and other special sampling devices.

EXPOSURE TO GASES IN THE OUTDOOR AND INDOOR AIR

The main sources of outdoor air pollution in the developed world today are motor vehicle emissions. Primary pollutants are those released directly into the air, and include carbon monoxide and nitric oxide, as well as benzene and particulate material. Diesel engines burn an excess of air and so produce little carbon monoxide, but they do give out more nitrogen dioxide and fine particles. The main single sources of sulphur dioxide are coal-fuelled electric power stations. Secondary pollutants are those formed by chemical changes to the primary pollutants. Thus nitrogen dioxide is produced by rapid atmospheric oxidation of nitric oxide emitted by motor vehicles, and subsequently may undergo photochemical oxidation to form ozone. Important combustion sources of gases in the home are gas cookers, which produce much higher concentrations of nitrogen dioxide inside houses compared with the ambient air, and faulty gas or paraffin heaters emitting carbon monoxide. Ambient air quality standards for pollutants set on health criteria alone are invariably lower than occupational exposure standards, including for gases. No standards have yet been established for indoor air. Carbon dioxide levels are sometimes used in office buildings as a surrogate measure of the rate of air exchange.

EXPOSURE TO GASES IN INDUSTRIAL ACCIDENTS AND FIRES

Industrial accidents

In modern industry with control measures in place the worker is only likely to receive heavy exposure to an industrial gas through a failure in the plant or other accidental event.

Information on the effects of single exposure to toxic gases and vapours in humans is sparse and consists mainly of reports of accidental exposures to one or a few individuals without the recording of exposure level or duration. Yet it is following just such accidental exposures that the physician will be consulted for advice. Toxicity data relating to routes of exposure other than inhalation should be treated with caution unless it is known that the toxicokinetics and sites of action for different routes are comparable. Knowledge of the long-term effects of single exposures, such as carcinogenicity, teratogenicity and other target organ damage, is very inadequate. Extrapolation from single exposure studies in animals to humans is also fraught with problems, but in practice most reliance is placed upon such studies.

The ultimate harm caused by an acute high exposure to a toxic gas will depend primarily upon the concentration of gas and the period of exposure.[6] Experimental studies suggest the following general relationship may hold for acute lethality for many gases and vapours.

$$\text{toxic load} = \text{concentration}^n \times \text{time}$$

where n is any number other than zero. Thus a given health effect of an irritant gas is not necessarily the product of the concentration in the inhaled air and duration of exposure (Haber's rule). For accidents involving exposure to chlorine lasting between 5 and 20 minutes the concentration is more important than the duration in determining the effects on health. In practice most releases will last a short time until emergency measures at the plant bring the release under control.

Any assessment of the toxic impact of a release into the general population must take into account the presence of young, old, pregnant and diseased individuals, particularly those who may be already suffering from acute or chronic respiratory illness at the time of the release. Little information is available about the susceptibility of these vulnerable groups.

Occupational exposure limits are set for workers who receive repeated daily exposures to hazardous substances on the basis of 8-hour work days over a working lifetime and are set to protect as far as is reasonably practicable against acute and chronic effects. For many substances the Health and Safety Executive lays down STELs for brief exposure which, for measurement purposes have a 15-minute reference period; this is typically used to protect against effects which may occur rapidly such as irritation of the eyes or nose/throat.[5] This is a different concept from the single exposure in an emergency, when a worker may have to be able to perform an urgent repair or close a valve, to rescue a victim or to be able to escape in a sudden accidental release of a large quantity of a gas or in a fire. The usual occupational exposure limits do not incorporate risks of unconsciousness, incapacitation or intolerable irritation which would greatly reduce the chances of escape in an emergency. Various agencies[7,8] have attempted to set guideline exposure levels for workers and the general population for emergency purposes (Table 8.1). A different concept again is the exposure to gases such as nitrogen dioxide and carbon monoxide as pollutants of indoor air in offices and homes. In such cases, where workers are being inadvertently exposed to gases in indoor or outdoor ambient air, then separate air quality criteria (and lower guideline values) should be applied, not occupational exposure limits.[9]

Major toxic releases

Major chemical disasters can be caused by large vapour or flammable gas explosions, fires and toxic releases. The accidental release of gases and chemicals during their distribution by pipeline, water, rail or road can also have severe consequences.[10] The gases that most often feature in toxic releases from plants are chlorine, ammonia, sulphuric acid, hydrogen chloride, phosgene, hydrogen sulphide and nitrous fumes.

In accordance with the EC Seveso directive, the UK introduced the Control of Industrial Major Accident Hazards (CIMAH) Regulations 1984 which included a requirement for emergency planning to be undertaken for on-site and off-site air releases at plants storing or using dangerous substances in larger than the threshold quantities laid down in the Regulations; these chemicals include commonly used toxic or flammable gases.[11] Chlorine is the must common gas for which emergency planning has been undertaken and is an example of a denser than air, highly corrosive gas that can cause injury to the respiratory tract ranging from irritation to incapacity or death from bronchospasm, laryngeal oedema or toxic pulmonary oedema.[12] Computer models of the dispersion of chlorine and other dense gases can be applied to determine risk contours around hazardous installations, so that the impact of a gas release on a nearby populated area can be predicted for different likely wind and weather conditions. The probability and size of accidental releases can be estimated to determine the serious but reasonably foreseeable event, such as a fracture of a liquid gas pipe or failure of a road tanker delivery coupling to a storage tank (Fig. 8.1). Plotting the concentration contours for a predicted plume on to maps of the area around a plant is a useful planning guide for police, fire brigade and ambulance services, and the method can also be applied to estimate broadly the numbers of deaths and acute casualties that may be

Table 8.1 *Health effect levels for certain irritant gases*

	Occupational exposure limit (ppm)		Air quality standard	Detection level (odour) (ppm)	Severe sensory irritation (humans) (ppm)	30 min lethal concentration (mammals) (ppm)	ERPG – 1 (ppm)	ERPG – 2 (ppm)	ERPG – 3 (ppm)
	15 min	8 h							
Ammonia	35	25	–	–	700–1700	1400–8000	25	200	1000
Carbon dioxide	5000	15 000	–	50,000 (dyspnoea)	–	15%	–	–	–
Chlorine	1	0.5	–	0.02–0.2	9–20	100	1	3	20
Hydrogen chloride	5	–	–	0.8	100	1600–6000	3	10	30
Hydrogen cyanide	10	–	–	2–5		100	NA	10	25
Hydrogen fluoride	3	–	–		120	900–3,600	3	20	100
Hydrogen sulphide	10	15	7 µg/m³ (30 min)	0.02	100	1000	0.1	30	100
Nitrogen dioxide	5	3	150 ppb (1 hour)	0.5	80	60–250	–	–	–
Sulphur dioxide	5	2	100 ppb (15 min)	1	120	300–500	0.3	3	15

American Industrial Hygiene Association: Emergency Response Planning Guidelines (1 hour exposures without protection)[7,8]

ERPG – 1   Capable of causing mild, transient and reversible effects
ERPG – 2   Concentrations may cause irreversible effects
ERPG – 3   Concentrations are considered life-threatening

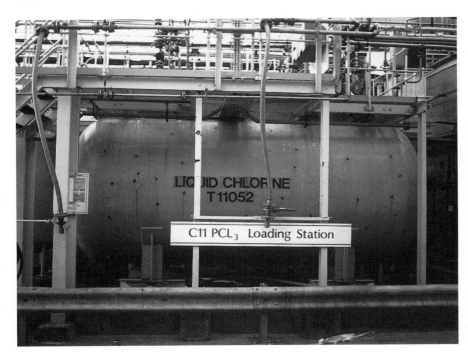

Figure 8.1 *Chlorine storage tank in a chemical factory.*

caused – important information for hospital disaster plans. An example of such a calculation for a factory in a populated area is shown in Table 8.2: the number of severely ill casualties in this (real) example would overwhelm the emergency capability of several large hospitals in the event of a reasonably foreseeable release of chlorine gas. Fortunately, no large-scale releases of chlorine gas have occurred in recent times, the last being in Romania in 1936 when 40 people were killed. Whilst engineering measures directed towards successful con-

tainment of stored gases such as chlorine are clearly proving to be successful, small-scale releases of gases and other chemicals do inevitably occur from fixed sites or during their transportation. Thus, in the USA, one of the few countries with comprehensive reporting, chlorine remains the most common substance involved in hazardous chemical releases resulting in personal injury.

Regulatory authorities will advise the local planning authority on developments of land near major hazard sites. An example is shown in Fig. 8.2. Estimated risk lev-

Table 8.2 *Calculation of the number of casualties to be expected in a release of 2.8 kg/s of chlorine for 20 min in an urban setting (population density 2000/km²)*

	Hazard zone for people located outdoors			Hazard zone for people located indoors		
	Fatal	**Danger**	**Distress**	**Fatal**	**Danger**	**Distress**
			Daytime release			
1 Hazard range (m) in $D_{4.4}$ conditions	400	1200	3700	250	850	2500
2 Hazard area (km²) (sector angle = 40)	0.056	0.51	4.8	0.022	0.25	2.2
3 No. of people affected = $(2000 \times (2) \times$ % present)	22	204	1920	35	400	3520
			Night-time release			
4 Hazard range (km) in F_2 conditions				750	1800	6000
5 Hazard area (km²)	All indoors			0.2	1.13	12.5
6 No. of people affected = $(2000 \times (5))$				400	2260	25 000

From ref. 9 with permission.
For daytime releases the total number of people affected in each hazard zone will be the sum of those outdoors and indoors at the time; it is assumed that 80% will be indoors during the day compared with 100% at night.
$D_{4.4}$, typical day conditions (neutral stability, wind speed 4.4 m/s); F_2, typical night conditions (very stable, wind speed 2 m/s).
Codes used by meteorologists to describe weather conditions.

els are computed from risk models and plotted on a map of the location to determine whether the proposed development falls inside or outside the contours of risk. Where do the risk values come from? They are derived by the Health and Safety Executive using historic data on the average failure rate of containment in the chemical industry. New regulations in the form of the Control of Major Accident Hazards Regulations 1999 (COMAH) place additional emphasis on the risk of chemical releases to the natural environment.

Fires

The main threats to life in fires are toxic gases, heat and oxygen deficiency.[13] The temperature in a room in a house fire can easily reach 500–1000°C, and as many as 400 toxic compounds can be demonstrated in the smoke. The principal toxic constituents of smoke are soot, carbon monoxide, carbon dioxide, nitrogen oxides, hydrogen cyanide, hydrogen chloride, sulphur dioxide, hydrogen fluoride, hydrogen sulphide, isocyanates, acrolein, benzene, phenol, formaldehyde and a range of chlorinated hydrocarbons. Carbon monoxide is an important factor in 50–80% of all fire fatalities. The role of hydrogen cyanide is less clear though it is formed in many fires especially those involving wool, silk, nylon and polyurethane products.[13,14]

Smoke comprises a mixture of gases, liquid and solid particles which arise as pyrolysis and combustion products. Predicting the products of combustion (oxidative degeneration) and pyrolysis (thermal decomposition) of burning materials is not easy, and so determining in retrospect the effects of exposure of firemen or other victims to the constituents of a smoke plume is not straightforward. Some general principles can be considered.[14] Materials consumed by fires contain carbon, hydrogen and oxygen as their main elements, and hence the bulk of all combustion products will consist of compounds formed from these, for example carbon monoxide and carbon dioxide. The next important elements are halogens (mostly chlorine) and nitrogen, with smaller amounts of elements such as sulphur and phosphorus. Almost all the inorganic anions are released as the irritant acid gases, hydrogen chloride and hydrogen fluoride, if fluorine is present. For the nitrogen present the products depend upon the availability of oxygen: in well ventilated fires oxides of nitrogen are released, but in large fires in buildings, where the ventilation is poorer, a larger proportion of the nitrogen is released as hydrogen cyanide. Organic compounds may form a number of partially decomposed products, for example formaldehyde, acrolein, crotonaldehyde and possibly free radicals that add to the irritancy of the smoke. Other compounds, such as decomposition products from isocyanates, styrene and phenol, may also be important.[14] Fires in warehouses storing chemicals will potentially

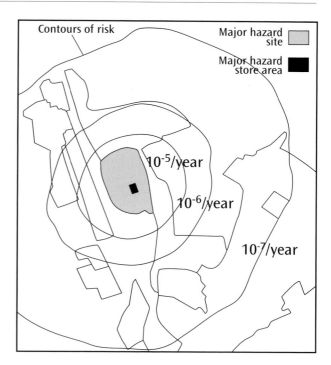

Figure 8.2 *Contours of individual risk around a major hazard site. Source: HSE Risk Criteria for Land-use Planning in the Vicinity of Major Industrial Hazards. London: HMSO, 1989.*

release a cocktail of irritants and toxic substances which may greatly add to the hazard of the fire plume.

Polyvinyl chloride (PVC) is the most widely used plastic and fires involving large amounts of this material at storage sites and recycling installations are not uncommon and attract notoriety because they are difficult for the fire services to put out whilst they generate toxic plumes.[15] At over 300°C, PVC decomposes to form hydrogen chloride and carbon monoxide together with small amounts of about 50 various hydrocarbons. About 50% of the polymer's weight comes off as hydrogen chloride, and the irritancy of the plume is added to by the presence of acrolein, ammonia, sulphur dioxide, nitrogen dioxide, aldehydes and particles. Phosgene is produced only in rare circumstances. There is now no doubt that dioxins are formed whenever chlorinated plastics are burned: in a large-scale plastics fire typically involving 500–1000 tonnes of PVC as much as 1–2 kg of dioxins could be produced.[15]

In the Gulf War in February 1991 about 600 naturally pressurized oil wells were set alight in Kuwait.[16] Close to the fires the smoke rained oil drops which coated large areas of desert. The plume contained carbon dioxide, carbon monoxide, sulphur dioxide and particles including soot. The major health concern revolved around the particle fallout that contained elemental carbon, rock/soil particles, metal oxides, silicates, vanadium, nickel and polycyclic aromatic hydrocarbons. Exposure studies and air monitoring started too late to ascertain the health risk to ground troops or the general population. Aplastic anaemia has been reported in a Gulf War veteran and a Kuwait child exposed to the fumes.[17] Fortunately, the fires were extinguished by November 1991.

Even if not directly fatal themselves, carbon monoxide and hydrogen cyanide singly or in combination may lead to the rapid incapacitation of the individual who is then unable to escape.[14] The other toxic gases can cause acute airways and lung injury or may obscure vision through causing eye irritation. An elevated carbon dioxide level will induce hyperventilation and hyperpnoea, and increase exposure to the combustion gases. In most fires these toxic factors are usually more important to survival than heat. However, intense fires can lead to severe burning from hot convected air or thermal radiation and in some fires direct burning from the heat of the flame can be the cause of death. Thermal injury to the airways and lungs is not as common as toxic damage, since the upper respiratory tract rapidly conducts away heat from the inspired air. Nevertheless air containing hot respirable particles or steam can cause injury as deep as the bronchioles. Less important is oxygen depletion except in major conflagrations or in intense building fires.

In the past, many firefighters did not always use respiratory protection equipment but nowadays as the equipment and training have improved breathing apparatus is routinely worn in the event of likely smoke exposure (Fig. 8.3). As a result firefighters are much less likely now to be exposed to the injurious

effects of smoke than in the past. However, accidental inhalation exposure may occur if the firefighters make a faulty judgement on their assessment of the fire conditions, or if the smoke plume unexpectedly blows towards unprotected firefighters, or if an immediate rescue of a victim has to be made. Skin contamination by noxious combustion products may also occur when the protective clothing is removed unless decontamination procedures are adequate.

The effects of single and repeated inhalation exposures to smoke therefore need to be considered. A fire victim will have a history of smoke exposure and the skin and clothing may be stained by smoke. The possibility of inhalational injury must be considered if there is production of carbonaceous sputum, reactive conjunctivitis and a hoarse voice. If the skin on the face and in the inside of the mouth or pharynx has been badly burned then thermal injury to the airways and lungs should be suspected; oedema of the glottis and larynx may develop rapidly and upper airways intubation with continuous positive airways ventilation should be urgently considered. Smoke can cause a chemical tracheobronchitis, the inflammation of the airways being associated with denudation of airway epithelium, ulceration and oedema with cellular infiltration. The inflammatory changes may give rise to an increase in airways reactivity even in patients without a previous history of asthma, and despite an apparently full clinical recovery the patient may go on to develop mild airways obstruction which can persist for months.[18] Firefighters who have received acute exposure to smoke should therefore be considered for early referral for an assessment of lung function as it may be advisable to begin early treatment with inhaled anti-inflammatory drugs.

Reports of unusual symptoms following smoke exposure are uncommon. Neurological symptoms were reported in a group of firemen heavily exposed to the fumes of toluene diisocyanate for several hours. The majority of the men developed persistent poor memory, personality change, emotional instability or depression.[19] Medical attendants should therefore be alert to the possibility of injury to other organs as well as the lungs in fire victims, particularly as it may be impossible to confirm the identity of materials and other combustion products in fires, for example in warehouses or chemical plants.

In the 1970s the concerns of firefighters that they were at high risk of premature death became a subject of epidemiological investigation.[20] No consistent trend of ill-health in firefighters has been demonstrated despite suggestions of a more rapid loss of lung function than expected and an increase in non-specific respiratory symptoms. An increased risk of heart disease was a concern but it seems unlikely that carbon monoxide is an occupational risk factor for ischaemic heart disease except where an elevated carboxyhaemoglobin precipitates ischaemia in a person with pre-existing coronary

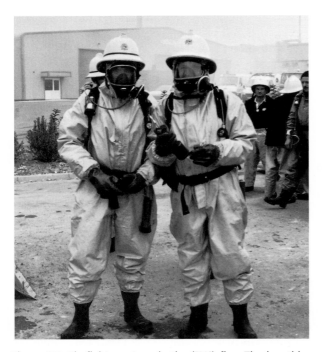

Figure 8.3 *Firefighters at a plastics (PVC) fire. The breathing apparatus and chemical suits protect the firemen from smoke which contains hydrogen chloride and carbon monoxide together with other combustion and pyrolysis products.*

atheroma. The risk of cancer of the respiratory tract may be increased by respiratory irritants impairing ciliary clearance mechanisms, thereby enhancing exposure to carcinogens adsorbed on particles, or from direct exposure to inhaled carcinogenic chemicals or polycyclic aromatic hydrocarbons in smoke. Despite the limited evidence for occupationally induced pulmonary impairment in firefighters the extensive and routine use of respiratory equipment to protect against smoke exposure is now widely advocated.

Nuclear reactor incidents

The processing of uranium involves a variety of hazardous substances. Hydrazine, chlorine and ammonia are used in nuclear power facilities and may be released into the atmosphere in an incident and threaten local populations. In 1985 a uranium processing plant in Gore, Oklahoma, released a cloud of hydrogen fluoride. A plume from a nuclear reactor incident may contain radioactive inert gases which are fission products of uranium. At Three Mile Island in 1979 very slight amounts of krypton-85 and xenon-133, together with iodine-131, were emitted following core damage to this commercial reactor. In the fire in the graphite reactor at Chernobyl in 1986 which lasted for several days several million curies of these gases, together with radioactive iodine, caesium, strontium and plutonium, were released in radioactive clouds that blew across Europe, making this event the worst nuclear accident in the world.[21] Since 1992, several tens of cases of thyroid cancer in children have appeared in the region around Chernobyl, and these are being attributed to exposure to iodine-131.[22]

PRINCIPLES OF FIRST AID AND TREATMENT IN GASSING ACCIDENTS

Regardless of the kind of gas involved the victim should be moved immediately to fresh air. If breathing has stopped or cardiac arrest has supervened then cardiopulmonary resuscitation should be begun. If hydrogen cyanide poisoning is suspected then a manual resuscitator should be used to maintain respiration so that mouth-to-mouth resuscitation is avoided.

Simple asphyxiant gases or lack of oxygen will cause loss of consciousness without irritation of the eyes or mucous membranes of the respiratory tract, but complications may include patchy consolidation of the lungs. Unless the hypoxia is severe the victim will recover consciousness in fresh air. If the patient is breathing and if oxygen is available, 100% oxygen should be given by oronasal mask until more specific treatment can be instituted. The treatment of overexposure to anaesthetically active gases is similar.

Inhalation of irritant gases and smoke gives rise to similar effects on the respiratory tract ranging from mild irritation and cough with bronchospasm to severe non-cardiogenic pulmonary oedema and respiratory failure. Irritant gases in high concentrations may kill the victim outright after a few deep breaths and before pulmonary oedema has had time to develop, an effect probably due to oxygen having been displaced from the air: there may be no sign of a death struggle. Exposure of the eyes or skin to corrosive gases should be treated by thorough irrigation or washing with water or sterile physiological (0.9%) saline, and all contaminated clothing must be removed.

Victims of gassing accidents should be assumed to be hypoxic. Central cyanosis (a blue colouration of the tongue and mucous membranes) is a variable clinical finding and when present is a sign of central hypoxia, though hypoxia may occur in the absence of cyanosis. Methaemoglobinaemia is another cause of cyanosis and hypoxia. In carbon monoxide and cyanide poisoning the skin retains its pink colour even in the presence of tissue hypoxia.

Even in the absence of signs of hypoxia or respiratory distress the patient can nevertheless be severely hypoxic and may collapse on slight exertion. This was first emphasized in First World War casualties in the management of phosgene gassing on the battlefield, and which is attributed in phosgene poisoning to the increased efflux of pulmonary oedema fluid during exercise.[23] In hospital, arterial blood gases should be tested at the earliest opportunity to assess the degree of hypoxaemia (PaO_2), partial pressure of carbon dioxide ($PaCO_2$), and acid-base state. Hypoxaemia is treated with oxygen therapy, but in advanced respiratory failure the patient may require endotracheal intubation and mechanical ventilation. The possibility of laryngeal oedema causing respiratory obstruction should not be forgotten, for example after ammonia exposure, but also in fire victims if burns are present on the face and around the mouth and lips, or soot is found in the anterior nares and larynx.

High concentration oxygen treatment (100% given by a tight fitting oronasal mask or IPPV and hyperbaric oxygen in severe cases) is essential in carbon monoxide poisoning despite a normal PaO_2, as the oxygen will compete with carbon monoxide for haemoglobin binding sites and reduces the half-life of carboxyhaemoglobin from about 320 to 80 minutes. Pulse oximetry can be misleading in carbon monoxide poisoning as it detects carboxyhaemoglobin as oxyhaemoglobin, and thus may overestimate the actual concentration of oxyhaemoglobin; erroneous readings may also arise in methaemoglobin states.[24] The use of hyperbaric oxygen should be urgently considered in cases of poisoning by the chemical asphyxiant gases (carbon monoxide, hydrogen sulphide and hydrogen cyanide). Most experience of this treatment has been gained with carbon monoxide.

Skin burns from corrosive gases and vapours should

be treated as for chemical burns. Contaminated clothes, jewellery, boots, etc., should be removed, and all affected areas should be washed or showered with water for at least 10 minutes. It is widely assumed that burns caused by corrosive gases and vapours will cause damage similar to thermal burns, for example irritation, erythema and bullae formation, but there is a dearth of hard fact on this in the literature. Certain agents, such as methyl bromide and vesicant warfare agents, are recognized as causing bullae formation, and erythematous lesions which may progress to intraepidermal or subepidermal vesicles or bullae with sweat gland necrosis can occur in some cases of coma caused by carbon monoxide poisoning. The mechanism of bullae formation in human skin is not understood. Bullae can occur in prolonged coma from various causes, for example in barbiturate poisoning, and could be caused by pressure, hypoxia or direct toxic effects.

Cold injury from the accidental contact of the unprotected skin with the liquid, vapour or gas of very cold liquefied gases resembles the local effects of severe cold which are described in Chapter 15, together with their treatment. The damage to the skin can be similar to heat burns, or to frostbite if exposure of unprotected parts is prolonged or severe.

The hospital management of victims of poisoning by irritant gases such as chlorine is outlined in Table 8.3. It should be noted that the treatment of the high permeability pulmonary oedema caused by irritant gases has not been well studied. In response to damage to the capillary endothelium, water accumulates in the interstitial space and then in the alveoli. The value of diuretics has not been confirmed and these should be used cautiously, if at all. Glucocorticosteroids may not be of value. Chest infection is common after severe gassing because of the denuded bronchial epithelium; vigorous antibiotic therapy is often required. Unlike cardiogenic oedema, the oedema fluid has a high protein content which may coagulate and the residual coagulum may become the skeleton on which lung fibrosis develops.[25]

Convulsions caused by certain gases, e.g. methyl bromide, should be treated with anticonvulsant drugs as appropriate, though more intensive therapy may be needed if they prove resistant.

Even mild gassing incidents can induce severe anxiety if individuals suddenly experience respiratory symptoms such as acute tightening of the chest and difficulty breathing, especially if they are asthma sufferers. Further alarm can be generated if their or other lives are perceived to be at imminent risk. Health professionals called to such incidents need to be aware that affected individuals may subsequently suffer post-traumatic distress syndrome or other emotional disturbances requiring psychological support. Several of the physical conditions arising from inhalation of toxicants are described below.

Lung injury

With many inhaled toxicants the principal location of deep lung injury is in the bronchioalveolar region. Ozone has been the most extensively studied gas, and its inflammatory mechanisms may apply to irritant gases in general.[26] The cells most susceptible to damage are Type I cells which line the alveoli and form part of the barrier for gaseous exchange between the air and the blood. With their loss and exposure of the basement membrane, stimulation of inflammatory cascades and increased fluid leak from the capillaries occurs, together with an increase in macrophages, neutrophils and alveolar surface protein in the interstitial and alveolar spaces. This is accompanied by the release of surfactant and other secretions by the epithelial Type 2 cells, which like the Clara cells, normally produce surfactant which prevents alveolar collapse and helps to keep the alveoli 'dry'. Biochemical changes induced in the lung by inhaled oxidants of free radical nature, such as ozone and nitrogen oxides are complex and not understood, but include lipid peroxidation. Both the upper and lower respiratory tract have a considerable range of protective antioxidants, with intracellular reduced glutathione (GSH) being one of the major ones of the lower respiratory tract. Clara cells have a major role in chemical detoxification by being a major site for the metabolism of inhaled and systemically administered chemicals by means of GSH, NADPH and P-450 monooxygenases; they also provide the bulk of the antioxidant molecules of the liquid lining of the airways.[26]

Adult (acute) respiratory distress syndrome

The inhalation of irritant agents may produce a common reaction in the lungs of rapid onset referred to as high permeability pulmonary oedema, or pulmonary oedema of non-cardiogenic origin, otherwise known as chemical pneumonitis. Pathologically, there is diffuse alveolar damage.[27] Mild cases recover rapidly and most without residual effects, but many authorities would nowadays regard chemical pneumonitis as belonging to the less severe end of a clinical spectrum that extends to adult (acute) respiratory distress syndrome (ARDS). This syndrome is diagnosed in a severe, acute lung injury after inhaling a toxic fume or gas if there is high-permeability pulmonary oedema present with widespread pulmonary infiltrates visible on chest radiographs, accompanied by a severe oxygenation defect in the presence of a normal pulmonary artery pressure.[28]

ARDS is a diagnosis in critical care settings for severe respiratory failure with an expected high mortality and which, in those patients surviving more than 3 days, is mainly caused by sepsis and multiple organ failure following intensive treatment.[29]

Table 8.3 *Chlorine poisoning: hospital management*

Immediate decontamination on arrival at hospital
(ideally decontamination should occur at the scene of the incident)
- *Remove all contaminated clothing* and thoroughly wash skin and eyes as necessary

Assessment of patient
- Examine *mucous membrane, eyes,* and *skin* for signs of corrosive injury
- Check *lung sounds, peak flow,* and *vital signs*: if patient is known to have been heavily exposed or has a cough or difficulty in breathing at rest perform baseline chest x-ray examination
- Take brief *medical history,* with particular attention to any history of respiratory or cardiovascular disease

Initial treatment
- *Oxygen*: all patients identified as being at risk (see Assessment of patient, above) should initially receive 100% oxygen, humidified if possible (unless this is contraindicated by their medical history). Oxygen concentration may subsequently be adjusted to the comfort of the patient
- *Bronchodilators*: salbutamol or terbutaline, used by nebulizer, may help relieve respiratory difficulties
- *Dose*:
  Salbutamol
     adults 2.5–5 mg as required
     children 2.5–5 mg as required
  Terbutaline
     adults 2.5–10 mg as required
     children up to 200 µg/kg
- *Corticosteroids* have not been proved to produce improvement in chlorine poisoning but have caused pronounced improvement after smoke inhalation. If patient exposed less than 4 hours previously and at risk of pulmonary injury (as defined above) steroids should be given
- *Dose*:
  Methylprednisolone
     adults 2 g iv stat (or equivalent)
     children 400 mg iv stat (or equivalent)
- *Laryngeal oedema*: give corticosteroids (dosage as above) if patient develops laryngeal oedema. Obtain early and expert help from anaesthetist as intubation may be needed
- *Skin burns* should be treated as thermal burns
- *Eye damage* requires ophthalmic referral

Monitoring
- Monitor respiratory function, particularly respiratory rate, and arterial blood gases regularly:
- Pulmonary oedema may occur up to 24 hours after exposure
- Patients who are well 24 hours after exposure may be discharged

Pulmonary oedema
- If pulmonary oedema occurs give humidified oxygen by facemask
- If PO_2 still cannot be maintained above 60 mmHg, or the respiratory rate >40 bpm, intubate the trachea and start mechanical ventilation
- Intravenous fluids should be given with great caution as fluid overload is extremely dangerous in such patients: if this occurs diuretics such as frusemide are indicated

Bronchiolitis obliterans

This uncommon condition is due to damage to the epithelium of the small airways and usually manifests itself pathologically as a proliferation of tufts or plugs of granulation tissue in the lumen of bronchioles. Diffuse alveolar damage (see above) and epithelial injury may occur together after inhalation exposure to a single noxious agent. Bronchiolitis obliterans with organizing pneumonia (BOOP) arises when the bronchiolitis obliterans is part of a more widespread inflammatory process affecting the alveoli and interstitium, leading to a restrictive ventilatory defect; it has been recorded with organizing respiratory tract infections, as well as inhalation agents, and in ARDS. Constrictive bronchiolitis obliterans is a pathologically distinct entity with narrowing of the bronchioles and fibrotic thickening of their walls, and it is associated with a progressive obstructive ventilatory defect.[27]

Bronchiolitis obliterans is a recognized complication in gassing accidents involving nitrogen dioxide, and sporadic cases have been reported after incidents with ammonia, fire smoke, sulphur dioxide, chlorine, hydrogen selenide, and hydrogen bromide.[27] The treatment of this condition is referred to under NITROGEN DIOXIDE (see p. 158).

Reactive airways dysfunction syndrome

Incidents involving high level exposure to irritant gases may cause this inflammatory response of the airways which results in an increase of airways reactivity lasting for months or even years.[30] Asthma-like symptoms arise abruptly within minutes or hours of exposure to excessive concentrations of an irritating gas, vapour, fume or dust. On investigation, bronchial reactivity is present on methacholine challenge testing. Treatment is the same as for mild obstructive airways disease. Once acquired, the patient with reactive airways dysfunction syndrome may respond with asthma-like symptoms when exposed to noxious agents in the general environment, such as cigarette smoke, perfumes and household chemicals. Many medical practitioners remain unaware of this condition since its description by Brooks and others[30] in their paper published in 1985, despite its occurrence being reported since in association with a long list of irritant gases, fumes and vapours.[31] In consequence, the association with the workplace exposure may be too easily ignored. The criteria for the diagnosis of the condition in individual patients remains controversial, however (see Chapter 33). For example, it is usually impossible to objectively confirm that there was normal bronchial responsiveness prior to the exposure, which is one of the main diagnostic tenets and, instead, reliance is placed on the individual reporting an absence of previous related symptoms. Nevertheless, the risk of acquiring reactive airways dysfunction syndrome (RADS) is one of the main reasons why workers should assiduously avoid inhaling excessive concentrations of irritant gases and vapours. Gases reported to induce reactive airways dysfunction syndrome in accidental exposures form a long list which includes hydrogen sulphide, nitrogen dioxide, sulphur dioxide (and sulphuric acid), ammonia, chlorine, ethylene oxide, phosgene, welding fumes and smoke.[27]

Hypoxic brain injury

Simple asphyxiant gases will reduce the inspired oxygen concentration and cause hypoxic hypoxia, or low blood levels of oxygen. Acute, severe hypoxic hypoxia does not usually lead to brain damage or long-term neurological signs and symptoms unless accompanied by cardiac arrest, when the neurological picture resembles global ischaemia as seen after cardiac arrest from any cause.

Hydrogen cyanide and hydrogen sulphide inhibit cellular respiration and induce histotoxic hypoxia. As before, poisoning by these agents does not usually cause brain damage unless hypotension supervenes, when injury to the cerebral cortex and hippocampus may arise in a distribution resembling that seen in global ischaemia after cardiac arrest. Both gases are potent and immediate depressors of blood pressure, however, and the 'knock down' which occurs in sudden apnoea with hydrogen sulphide poisoning may possibly be the result of cardiac hypotension or cardiac standstill.

The action of carbon monoxide is undoubtedly more complex than either of these agents, but the mechanism is poorly understood. Focal damage to the globus pallidus and substantia nigra is more often seen in severe carbon monoxide poisoning, as is delayed neurological deterioration associated with the late destruction of white matter and demyelination. However, much the same pattern of injury may arise occasionally in patients who have suffered global ischaemia from other causes, including cyanide poisoning.[32]

The electroencephalogram, magnetic resonance imaging and computed tomography scans may all be normal in some patients with permanent hypoxic injury.

INVESTIGATION OF GASSING ACCIDENTS

In all gassing accidents investigations should be undertaken to determine or confirm the agent involved together with the degree of exposure whenever possible. Where biological tests for specific gases are available for verifying exposure, these are mentioned in the subsequent text. It is important that this task is done as part of the overall management of the patient and not as an afterthought. Thus blood (5 ml EDTA [ethylenediaminetetraacetic acid]) and urine (50 ml universal container) samples should always be stored and collected at the earliest opportunity in case investigative tests are required later.

The post-mortem appearances are often non-specific. Corrosive gases will cause macroscopic injury to the airways. Pulmonary oedema, however, may be found in rapid hypoxic and anoxic deaths from any cause as well as from gassing by corrosive gases, and is due to increased capillary permeability. In asphyxiated victims the viscera may show little change apart from congestion, oedema and petechial haemorrhages; conjunctival petechiae may also be present.

Survivors of gassing accidents should always be followed up for the development of short- and long-term psychological and physical sequelae. Accidental exposures to gases in industry may be life-threatening and there are few follow-up studies of incidents in the literature. Pulmonary function testing should be undertaken after exposure-incidents involving irritant gases, and referral for neurological and neuropsychological investigations should be considered in all patients who have experienced a severe exposure to a simple or chemical asphyxiant gas, with or without a period of unconsciousness.

GASES IN THE AMBIENT AIR

Air is a mixture of gases, the average composition of which stays remarkably constant (Table 8.4) and sustains life on earth. Lovelock has proposed that the biosphere maintains and regulates the atmosphere in a way analogous to homoeostasis.[33] Fears over global warming led to the Kyoto Protocol agreement in 1997, which requires industrialized nations to cut total anthropogenic emissions of six greenhouse gases, namely carbon dioxide, methane, nitrous oxide, hydrofluorocarbons, perfluorocarbons and sulphur hexafluoride.

Table 8.4 *Composition of the earth's atmosphere*

Gas	Vol (%)
Nitrogen (N$_2$)	78.094
Oxygen (O$_2$)	20.946
Argon (Ar)	0.934
Carbon dioxide (CO$_2$)	0.035
Neon (Ne)	1.82×10^{-3}
Helium (He)	5.24×10^{-4}
Methane (CH$_4$)	1.72×10^{-4}
Krypton (Kr)	1.14×10^{-4}
Hydrogen (H$_2$)	5×10^{-5}
Nitrous oxide (N$_2$O)	3.1×10^{-5}
Xenon (Xe)	0.86×10^{-5}
Ozone (O$_3$)	up to 10^{-5}
Carbon monoxide (CO)	up to 10^{-5}
Radon (Rn)	6×10^{-18}
Water (average)	0.1–4

Oxygen lack

Oxygen-deficient atmospheres can be encountered in mines and other underground or confined spaces. The main danger of suddenly entering an atmosphere devoid of oxygen is that it will lead to an almost immediate loss of consciousness without warning; even very quiet breathing will produce sudden loss of consciousness within 50 seconds when all the remaining oxygen in the lungs has gone.[34]

It is the partial pressure of oxygen, not its percentage, which is of physiological importance. A drop of 3–4% of oxygen by volume is of little physiological significance in humans, but it will extinguish a candle flame. (A candle flame will continue to burn at levels of atmospheric pressure well below those at which humans will be asphyxiated: it will not go out until 10% of normal pressure.) The level of oxygen has to fall to 13% volume (equivalent to a 33% asphyxiant gas in air mixture) before symptoms become very noticeable.

The effects of low oxygen concentration are as follows:

Oxygen (% in air)

- 16–13% Dizziness and shortness of breath on exertion; pulse rate accelerated and volume of breathing increased. Ability to maintain attention is diminished but it can be restored with conscious mental effort.
- 13–10% Judgement faulty. Rapid fatigue and fainting on exertion. Severe injuries cause no pain. Emotional lability.
- 10–6% Nausea and vomiting. Loss of ability to perform any vigorous muscular movements or even to move at all.
- <6% Loss of consciousness with fainting or coma. Rapidly fatal.

Oxygen excess

Industrial and medical oxygen supplies can enrich atmospheres in a room to dangerous levels. At 25% oxygen in air even damp vegetation will continue to burn once a fire has started, and substances which do not normally burn easily in air may burn vigorously. Lubricants must never be used on oxygen equipment as they may react explosively with pressurized oxygen. Even in the open air oxygen may remain trapped in clothing which can then be readily ignited and cause severe burns. Oxygen and other compressed gases should only be used in well-ventilated areas.

Anaerobic fermentation

Natural biological processes produce toxic gases in the absence of oxygen. In anaerobic fermentation bacteria that are methanogens or sulphate reducers remove hydrogen ions in the form of methane or hydrogen sulphide, respectively. The digestive function of the colon in healthy people may produce predominantly one or other of these gases in the breakdown of carbohydrates and the concentration of methane in the bowel can occasionally be high enough to be an explosion hazard during surgical operations. Excessive or abnormal colonic gas production may be an important factor in the pathogenesis of irritable bowel syndrome[35] and inflammatory bowel disease.[36] Human flatus may typically contain nitrogen (68%), oxygen (less than 1%), carbon dioxide (9%), hydrogen (16%) and methane (6%). In contrast, the rumen of animal species such as the cow, sheep, goat and deer contain mostly methanogenic bacteria.

Fermentation of human or animal excrement releases toxic gases which can be a threat to sewer workers or workers in confined spaces on farms and in swine confinement buildings, amongst others (Fig. 8.4). Farm animal-house air can be contaminated by ammonia,

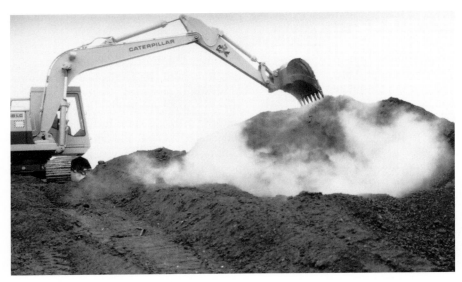

Figure 8.4 *Gas clouds released from untreated sewage sludge being added to topsoil on a toxic waste reclamation site. A machine driver collapsed from the gas which turned out to be ammonia.*

hydrogen sulphide and carbon dioxide. The mixing or pumping of slurry, for example in cow sheds, can release lethal amounts of hydrogen sulphide into enclosed spaces.

Anaerobic fermentation of sheep intestines and their contents can cause hydrogen sulphide keratoconjunctivitis in sausage makers, the same condition that Ramazzini recorded in workers who emptied jakes (privy vaults). Sewer gas is methane with small amounts of hydrogen sulphide and it also occurs in septic tanks and cesspits. Gases from decaying fish can be a hazard to workers unloading catch from poorly refrigerated and unventilated holds.

Decay of organic matter generally provides hydrogen sulphide, ammonia, methane and carbon dioxide; levels of carbon monoxide in air can sometimes also be dangerously elevated in manure storage areas. Bacterial action on nitrogenous compounds may form nitrogen dioxide, and fermentation of silage can produce high concentrations of this gas within 2 days of silo filling. Carbon dioxide and methane concentrations, if elevated, depress oxygen levels, or oxygen may be depleted anyway. Following gassing accidents in confined spaces it is important to measure as soon as possible for oxygen depletion and elevated levels of carbon dioxide, as well as the full range of gases mentioned above, to determine what was responsible for the incident.

A condition occasionally, but not exclusively, reported in hog farmers is organic dust toxic syndrome, which may present as an acute systemic illness characterized by fever, malaise, aches and pains in the limbs, vomiting and a dry cough. The onset is within a few hours of heavy exposure to endotoxin-producing Gram-negative bacteria, as may occur in swine confinement buildings. The condition, which resolves completely within 72 hours, should not be confused with the toxic effects of gases produced by fermentation. Pig farming exposes workers to a mixture of ammonia, organic dusts and high levels of endotoxins, and the types of disinfectants in regular use can contain respiratory sensitizers.[37]

Confined spaces

Confined spaces include trenches, pits, tanks, sewers, tunnels and also submarines and spacecraft. Working in enclosed spaces with inadequate natural ventilation is a well known cause of death from asphyxia due to oxygen deficiency or from a build-up of toxic gases and vapours, such as carbon dioxide, carbon monoxide, methane, ammonia, hydrogen sulphide, petroleum vapour and liquid petroleum gas. In addition, the presence of flammable gases such as butane, propane and petrol, all of which are normally heavier than air, can be responsible for explosions in tanks. The risk of fire and explosion may be increased by enrichment of the air by oxygen in the event of a leak from an oxygen cylinder forming part of welding equipment. Toxic substances can accumulate where workers are welding or flame-cutting.

Oxygen deficiency in pits can arise from an ingress of methane or absorption of oxygen by certain constituents of soils. The rotting of vegetation and the rusting of metalwork inside tanks also consume oxygen. Manholes, tunnels and trenches in limestone soils can partly fill with carbon dioxide formed by the action of acid groundwater. Apparently safe atmospheres can become suddenly dangerous if the residues and sludges in tanks or in sewers are disturbed by the worker walking in them, or by water surges following sudden heavy rainfall. Underground spaces may be in ground which is contaminated or near old refuse tips, or they may be connected to sewers. In the construction industry, pipe-freezing work is carried out using liquid nitrogen to solidify soil to enable drilling to be performed in wet conditions and fatalities have occurred from the cold gas pushing out the available air.

In order to avoid gassing accidents, safe systems of work must be adhered to and these often require the use of electronic monitors or detector tubes to test for toxic, flammable and asphyxiating gases before initial entry to a confined space and whilst the work continues. The space should be well ventilated before entry, otherwise appropriate breathing apparatus has to be worn. In the UK safe working practices are followed under the Confined Spaces Regulations, 1997.[38]

There is no formal medical examination laid down for workers in confined spaces in the UK, but the competent person who carries out the risk assessment under the Regulations[38] will need to consider the physical suitability of the individuals involved and to check that they are of suitable build. Medical advice on an individual's suitability may be needed. A history of claustrophobia, fits, blackouts and fainting attacks would be reasons for exclusion, as are chronic respiratory problems such as asthma, bronchitis or exertional dyspnoea, and other evidence of lack of fitness to wear breathing apparatus. The presence of heart disease or severe hypertension might also be a contraindication. Physical limitations such as deafness, lack of a sense of smell, visual defects, and problems with balance (e.g. Ménière's disease) should also be considered. Prospective workers with limited mobility from back or joint trouble, certain physical handicaps or psychiatric problems may also be unsuitable.

Routine sewer work is normally safe so long as standard measures to detect toxic and flammable gases and oxygen deficient atmospheres are performed. However, the possibility of unusually toxic substances entering sewage systems must always be borne in mind.

In an unusual incident in Aberdeen, Scotland, a group of 26 workers went down a sewer to investigate an unusual smell, and 14 became unwell. The symptoms, which included cough, chest discomfort, breathlessness and fatigue, developed over several days. The more severely affected also complained of thirst, sweating, irritability and loss of libido. Five workers with persistent symptoms were investigated and in one a desmopressin test was abnormal and he was diagnosed as suffering from cranial diabetes insipidus; other endocrine organ tests included thyroid function, follicular stimulating hormone, luteinizing hormone, prolactin and testosterone which were all normal. The causal agent and its possible source were not identified, but the coincidence of autonomic symptoms and diabetes insipidus suggested that the gas exposure was responsible. Organic sulphur compounds with intense odours, such as dimethyldisulphide, were also considered.
                                        Watt *et al.* 1997[39]

This episode shows the importance of all workers donning full positive pressure breathing apparatus when investigating unusual problems in sewers.

Mines

Black damp was the name given to the residual gas encountered in mines where the oxygen has been removed by chemical oxidative processes such as oxidation of coal, timber and iron sulphide.[40] It typically contains 12–15% carbon dioxide but can be higher, with the rest of the gas as nitrogen. *Fire damp* is methane which is present under pressure in coal seams and may be given off with carbon dioxide and nitrogen with audible hissing noises during mining. The main hazard is explosion. After an explosion of methane and coal dust the mixture of gases produced in the mine is called *afterdamp*: it contains toxic levels of carbon monoxide, and it has been responsible for the deaths of miners and rescuers in numerous mining disasters. The introduction of a form of safety lamp by Sir Humphrey Davy in 1812 helped to reduce the risk of explosion in mines. The flame is surrounded by a fine metal gauze, which offers little resistance to gases, but which leads heat away from them so effectively that the flame cannot cross it. The oil flame gave warning of the presence of fire damp (1–4% methane makes the flame burn brighter) and is also extinguished before the oxygen levels fall to dangerous levels.

PROPERTIES AND EFFECTS OF GASES

Simple asphyxiant gases

METHANE (CH₄)

[CAS no. 74–82–8]
Relative density: 0.56
Flammability in air: 5.0–15.4% (vol.)

Methane is a colourless flammable gas with a nondetectable or a sickly sweet oily odour which is normally too faint to provide warning of its presence. The main global sources of methane are rice paddies and wetlands from the anaerobic fermentation of organic material, but it is released from coal mining, biomass burning, the leakage of natural gas from the earth as well as pipelines and well-heads, landfills and enteric fermentation in mammals (mainly ruminants). Total global emissions of methane are about 500 million tonnes a year, two-thirds of which come from anthropogenic sources. It is second only to carbon dioxide as a cause of global warming. Natural gas contains methane as a major constituent combined with significant amounts of ethane, propane and butane, together with diethyl sulphide as a deodorant. Some natural gas sources contain substantial amounts of mercury, which can be an occupational hazard.[41] Coal gas, which it replaced as a fuel, contains methane together with hydrogen and a little carbon

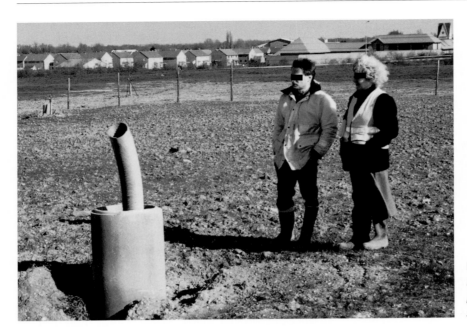

Figure 8.5 *Methane outlet on a municipal waste landfill site. Note the proximity of local housing (hazard of soil seepage of gas).*

monoxide and ethylene plus small amounts of carbon dioxide, nitrogen, oxygen, ammonia and hydrogen sulphide. Marsh gas is mostly methane with a little hydrogen, carbon dioxide and nitrogen. It has been widely believed that marsh gas can undergo a spontaneous combustion, producing a pale, ghostly light (Will o' the Wisp or Jack o' Lantern), but another fermentation product is likely to be responsible.

> One minute it darted like a kingfisher, and the next it entirely disappeared. At times it grew as big as an ox's head, and then straightaway shrank to a cat's eye . . . finally . . . it returned to frisk in the reeds.
>
> George Sand 1848[42]

Mixtures of methane and air do not ignite spontaneously, otherwise flames would be seen around the tails of cows. Methane burns with a hot, yellowish flame and not cold, bluish white. Fermentation may also produce traces of phosphine, PH_3, but this does not ignite spontaneously in air either, although it commonly contains an impurity, P_2H_4, which does.

As methane is much lighter than air it can accumulate as an upper layer in the air of poorly ventilated spaces where it may cause asphyxia, or there is a risk of explosion at much lower concentrations if ignited by a flame or spark. A major incident involving methane took place at Abbeystead, England, in 1984 when 34 local residents and eight employees were visiting the valve house at the local water pumping station. The pipe system had been drained down and, unknown to the engineers, methane gas from the surrounding methane-rich soils had permeated the pipes. When the pumping began, the methane entered the atmosphere of the valve house and exploded, killing 16 people. Carboniferous geological strata are methane rich and soil emissions may increase

with rapid falls in atmospheric pressure. The air near the ground in oil-rich regions may contain as much as 1% methane.

Another important methane mixture is landfill gas produced by putrefaction of municipal and other wastes buried in an excavation and covered with clay and topsoil. Huge amounts of landfill gas may be generated containing typically a methane/carbon dioxide mixture in the ratio 60:40. Volatile organic compounds may also enter and add to the toxicity of the gas. The gas can migrate long distances through the ground and cause a hazard to workers by flooding into trenches. Nearby residential areas may be at risk from soil gas. To help avoid these hazards special vents are incorporated into landfill sites to provide adequate escape for the copious amounts of gas produced (Fig. 8.5)

CARBON DIOXIDE (CO_2)

[CAS no. 124–38–9]
Exposure limits
LTEL (8 h TWA) 5000 ppm or 0.5% (9000 mg/m³)
STEL (10 min) 15000 ppm or 1.5% (27 000 mg/m³)
Relative density: 1.53

Joseph Priestley was the first to establish the biological properties of this gas and in 1772 came upon the art of manufacturing carbonated water, which was made popular by Joseph Schweppes who started a business in Bristol in 1794. The dangers of carbon dioxide were, however, known to wine producers in Roman times, if not earlier. Today carbon dioxide is encountered in numerous ways, for example as a refrigerant, in fire extinguishers, arc welding, breweries and wineries, flue gases, fermentation processes which deplete oxygen (including in unventilated mines, wells, tunnels) and in the manufacture and use of dry ice. It is often regarded as a simple asphyxiant, yet it has been known since the turn of this century that it has a toxic action which is independent of oxygen deficiency. The toxic properties of carbon dioxide were demonstrated on a large scale in the disaster at Lake Nyos, Cameroon, in 1986, where over 1700 people were killed when as much as a quarter of a million tonnes of carbon dioxide held in the depths of the lake under hydrostatic pressure were suddenly released and flowed down into the nearby valleys (Fig. 8.6). The sparse medical findings and the accounts of survivors[43] strongly suggested that the carbon dioxide had mixed with air to give rise to prolonged states of coma due to carbon dioxide narcosis in many of the victims. Skin bullae were another unusual finding. This unprecedented massive release contrasts with accidents in industry when isolated deaths from carbon dioxide are normally attributed to oxygen lack or simple asphyxia, and there are no characteristic findings on autopsy.

Carbon dioxide is dangerous because it is colourless and odourless, but when breathed from an anaesthetic machine it has a faintly acid smell. The effects of breathing the gas are very characteristic.[44] A 2–3% carbon dioxide level in air will pass unnoticed at rest but tidal volume is increased by 30% and the minute volume by 5%; on exertion there may be marked shortness of breath. At 3% carbon dioxide in air, breathing becomes noticeably deeper and more frequent at rest, with the effect becoming more marked until at 5% carbon dioxide in air there is severe dyspnoea, which limits exposure for most people. Subjects complain of headache and are sweaty and have a bounding pulse. At 10% carbon dioxide in air, respiratory distress develops rapidly with loss of consciousness in 10–15 minutes, even though the

oxygen concentration is reduced to 19% only. Exposures to carbon dioxide levels above 15% are intolerable, and rapid loss of consciousness ensues after a few breaths of a mixture of 30% carbon dioxide in air. Even at this level the oxygen concentration is 15%, not enough to cause loss of consciousness from hypoxia, but death will occur if the carbon dioxide level is maintained. Thus it is important to note that monitoring oxygen in air is an inadequate guide to the carbon dioxide hazard; carbon dioxide should be directly measured. A working or living area should be immediately evacuated when concentrations exceed 1.5% by volume (the occupational short-term exposure limit value). Experimental studies show that carbon dioxide exerts a narcotic action at the higher concentrations through a disturbance of acid-base balance resulting in a fall in pH of arterial blood and the cerebrospinal fluid.[44]

Industrial carbon dioxide poisoning is a rare occurrence. Survival after severe intoxication by carbon dioxide has been described (in a patient in Bristol in 1972).[45]

A 34-year-old male worker was overcome by an accidental release of the gas from a fire extinguishing system, filling the room 'like a cold, thick fog.' There were two others present, one died and the other managed to rescue the patient and save himself. The patient was given artificial respiration, but breathed by himself within a very short time whilst remaining deeply unconscious. On admission to hospital within 15–20 min of the accident he was still deeply unconscious, but was maintaining a free airway. He had a respiratory rate of 24 per minute, but was grossly hypernoeic, flushed and markedly vasodilated. He was normotensive, with a heart rate of 120 per minute, and his chest was clear. He became rousable after 35

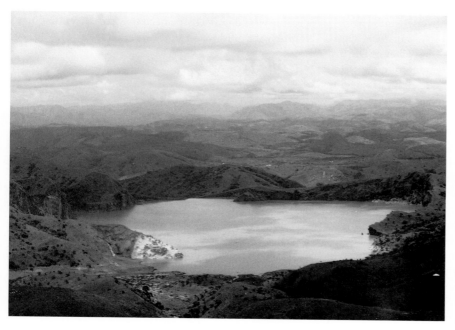

Figure 8.6 *Lake Nyos, Cameroon. On 21 August 1986 carbon dioxide was suddenly degassed from the lake and flowed down into the adjacent valleys in this remote region. The lake, 200 m deep, is replenished from a bottom spring rich in carbon dioxide. This event was the first recorded exposure of a population to a wide scale release of carbon dioxide.*

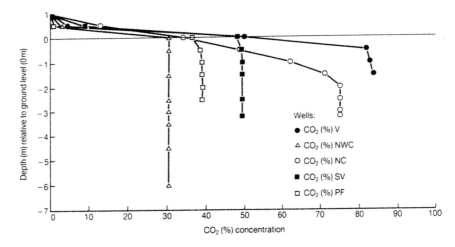

Figure 8.7 *Carbon dioxide concentrations measured with an infrared analyser in five domestic water wells in Vulcano, Sicily. Carbon dioxide measured from the top of the well above ground level to the water surface. The carbon dioxide concentration is lethal (> 30%) in all the wells within 1 m of the top and a worker would lose consciousness almost immediately on entry using a ladder. On this volcanic island carbon dioxide diffuses into wells from the soil. Courtesy of Jean Claude Baubron.*

minutes in the hospital whilst being treated with oxygen through an MC mask. Soon he was rational, and complained of headache and feeling stiff all over. He developed pre-renal uraemia, which spontaneously resolved over several days, and he was eventually discharged well.

Brighten 1976[45]

Soil gas emissions in volcanic and geothermal areas can be a silent hazard to workers. In Mammoth Mountain, California, a popular ski resort, park rangers have been overcome due to an unsuspected increase in gas flow associated with volcanic unrest.[46] In the largest island of the Azores, San Miguel, the town of Furnas is built in an active caldera where soil gas emissions have overwhelmed workers digging roads. The phenomenon is not new, with Loudon reporting in 1832 on the famous 'Valley of Death' in Java which contained the skeletal remains of many wild animals and birds that had strayed into the layer of carbon dioxide floating above the ground.[44]

The danger of entering an enclosed space containing carbon dioxide is illustrated by the concentration gradient of the gas in wells on Vulcano, Sicily, a volcanic island with areas which have strong ground emissions of carbon dioxide (Fig. 8.7). The breathing zone of a worker entering such a well by ladder will be at a narcotic level of carbon dioxide without warning and within a very short descent (less than 2 m) below the top. The worker would lose consciousness after a few breaths and fall to the bottom of the well. The carbon dioxide gradient is so steep that there would be no opportunity for the worker to become aware himself that he was hyperventilating before consciousness was lost. Spaces where carbon dioxide may build up can therefore be much more dangerous than is commonly supposed because of diffusion of the gas. It has been known from ancient times (in wine production) that the flame of a candle can be used to give adequate warning of the presence of lethal levels of carbon dioxide. A vertically held lit candle or oil lamp is normally extinguished when the oxygen level falls to 17.6% in the presence of nitrogen, but carbon dioxide has a stronger effect, causing the flame to be extinguished at 18.8–18.9% (or 8–10% carbon dioxide).

Carbon dioxide levels can be used to measure the quality of indoor air. At a ventilation rate of 4.6 m^3/min per person the carbon dioxide level in an office would be expected to be approximately 800–1000 ppm in the absence of unvented combustion sources. Higher levels of carbon dioxide would indicate the need to increase ventilation to improve the outdoor air supply (see Chapter 36).[47]

ARGON A (A or Ar)

[CAS no. 7440–37–1]
Relative density: 1.4

Argon is the most abundant 'rare' gas in the atmosphere and, together with helium and neon, makes up nearly 1% of air: all three gases are of inorganic origin. Argon is inactive, colourless and odourless. It is used in the control of high technology refining and semiconductor processes. It is also used in lamps, as a shielding gas in welding, and in many gas-filled devices.

HELIUM (He)

[CAS no. 7440–59–7]
Relative density: 0.14

Helium is colourless, inert, non-flammable and very

light. It is found with natural gas deposits in the USA and Poland. Extraction from air is not commercially viable. It is used as a shielding gas in welding, in electric lighting tubes, as a substitute for nitrogen in diving gas mixtures and as a balloon gas.

HYDROGEN (H₂)

[CAS no. 1333–74–0]
Deuterium D_2 or $^2H_2$
Relative density: (H_2) 0.07

Hydrogen is very light, colourless and flammable. It is used for hydrogenation of fats and in chemical synthesis. Deuterium is a heavier stable isotope of hydrogen and is used as a tracer. Hydrogen burns with a bluish, non-luminous flame.

KRYPTON (Kr)

[CAS no. 7439–90–9]
Relative density: 2.9

Krypton is a rare gas present in the atmosphere at about 1 ppm. It is colourless, non-flammable and has applications in electrical equipment. Its radioactive isotope ^{85}Kr is used in respiratory and cardiac studies.

NEON (Ne)

[CAS no. 7440–01–9]
Relative density: 0.7

Neon is a rare gas present in the atmosphere at about 18 ppm. It is colourless and non-flammable, used in fluorescent tubes, and as a cryogenic refrigerant.

XENON (Xe)

[CAS no. 7440–63–3]
Relative density: 4.5

Xenon is a rare gas present in the atmosphere at about 0.086 ppm. It is colourless, non-flammable and is used for specialized lighting.

NITROGEN (N₂)

[CAS no. 7727–37–9]
Relative density: 0.97

Nitrogen is the major constituent of air, comprising about 78% by volume. It is very widely used as an inerting agent and in freezing processes of many varieties including food, earth freezing in civil engineering projects and metal shrinkage in machinery manufacture. Because the uses are ubiquitous, nitrogen is not infrequently implicated in anoxic deaths or incidents. Under increased pressure it induces narcosis.

Liquid nitrogen and argon are commonly stored in cylinders in laboratory areas, and may have to be transported in the confined space of a lift. The worst scenario can be calculated if the full contents of the vessel are released to atmosphere over a short period of time.

Calculate the worst scenario on the basis that the full contents of the vessel are released to atmosphere over a short period of time:

Resulting oxygen concentration %

$$\% O_2 = \frac{100 \times V_o}{V_r}$$

where for argon and nitrogen

$$V_o = 0.2095\ (V_r - V_g)$$

and for oxygen

$$V_o = 0.2095\ (V_r - V_g) + V_g$$

V_g = maximum gas release which is the liquid volume capacity of the vessel $V \times$ gas expansion

V_r = room volume

Gas expansion being for

nitrogen 682.7

oxygen 842.1

argon 823.8

An example of such a calculation is:

LC 200 containing 200 liquid litres of nitrogen in a room 20 m × 20 m × 3 m

$V_r = 20 \times 20 \times 3 = 1200$ cubic metres

$V_g = 200$ litres × 682.7 = 136540 litres = 136.5 cubic metres

$V_o = 0.2095\ (1200-136.5) = 222.80$

$\% O_2 = 100 \times 222.8/1200 = 18.6\%$

If the calculation suggests an oxygen content in the atmosphere lower than 18% then either

- site the vessel outside the building and pipe gas to the point of use; or
- pipe the pressure release valve and bursting disc to vent gas outside the building; and/or
- fit a permanent oxygen monitor;
- ensure personnel use/wear personal monitors;
- fit a forced ventilation system triggered by the permanent oxygen monitor.

Source: BOC Guidance Note: *Siting of liquid cylinders or vessels in buildings*

Chemical asphyxiant gases

CARBON MONOXIDE (CO)

[CAS no. 630–08–0]
Exposure limits
  LTEL (8 h TWA) 50 ppm (58 mg/m³)
  STEL (15 min) 300 ppm (349 mg/m³)

Relative density: 0.97
Flammability range: 12.5–74.2% (vol.)
Ambient air quality standard (UK): 10 ppm (running 8-hour average).

Carbon monoxide is a colourless, odourless, non-irritating gas which is slightly soluble in water and burns in air with a bright blue flame. It is the most widely encountered toxic gas in industry and the general environment, commonly as the result of incomplete combustion of fossil fuels. Although Ramazzini (1633–1714) remarked on the danger of gases from burning coal and Harmant in France gave the first clinical description of coal gas poisoning in 1775, it was Leblanc in 1842 who identified carbon monoxide as the toxic agent. The potential for dangerous exposures to carbon monoxide arises in metal production in iron foundries, steel works and electrical arc furnaces; in the chemical industry, in the manufacture of methanol, the catalytic cracking of hydrocarbons, around gas generating and purification plant, and in the synthesis of carbon black. Vehicle exhausts may pose hazards from carbon monoxide to workers in roll-on/roll-off vehicle ferries as well as in multi-story car parks and enclosed garages.

Typical carbon monoxide concentrations in gas mixtures are: blast furnace gas 20–25%; coal and coke oven gas 7–16%; petrol or LPG (liquid petroleum gas) engine exhaust gas 1–10%; and diesel engine exhaust gas 0.1–0.5%. Water gas is formed by passing steam through a bed of white-hot coke and consists of carbon monoxide and hydrogen. A mixture of carbon monoxide and nitrogen, known as producer gas, is used to fire metal-making furnaces and is produced by passing air over hot coke.

Potentially dangerous sources of carbon monoxide in homes and workplaces are faulty heaters that produce excessive fumes or burn in a restricted air supply, whether using natural gas, propane, butane, coal, coke or wood. Reducing ventilation in buildings in the winter to conserve heat may unwittingly elevate carbon monoxide levels in the indoor air to hazardous levels. Carbon monoxide from faulty gas appliances kills nearly 30 people in the UK every year, and at least 100 are known to suffer ill-health from this cause. The elderly and the very young are most at risk. In the USA, approximately 600 accidental deaths due to carbon monoxide poisoning are reported each year, whilst the number of intentional carbon monoxide-related deaths is 5–10 times higher. The use of catalytic converters in car exhausts has reduced carbon monoxide emissions, making suicide more difficult by inhaling exhaust gases in an enclosed space; death may in certain circumstances be more likely due to carbon dioxide instead.

Propane-fuelled equipment is commonly believed to be safe, but hazardous emissions of carbon monoxide have been reported in indoor environments with the use of ice resurfacing machines[48] and in forklift trucks with maladjusted carburettors.[49]

Carbon monoxide is a chemical asphyxiant because it combines with haemoglobin with an affinity some 250 times that of oxygen to form carboxyhaemoglobin (COHb). Carbon monoxide also increases the oxygen affinity of haemoglobin and causes the oxygen dissociation curve to shift to the left by impeding the release of oxygen to the tissues. With 50% saturation of the blood with COHb the oxygen pressure must fall to less than half the usual value in order to dissociate half the oxygen present.[50] The clinical manifestations of poisoning and tissue hypoxia are known to be greater than can be accounted for by loss of the oxygen-carrying capacity of the blood alone. Experimental studies suggest that carbon monoxide exerts a direct action by combining with other haem-containing proteins in cells such as cytochrome oxidase, myoglobin, and cytochrome P450. The interaction with cytochrome oxidase may result in mitochondrial dysfunction and a prolonged impairment of oxidative metabolism. An alternative hypothesis is that carbon monoxide damages mitochondria by provoking the release of free nitric oxide. Central nervous system injury may also be due to reoxygenation injury as a result of the production of partially reduced oxygen species, which in turn can oxidize essential proteins and nucleic acids, and induce brain lipid peroxygenation.

Normal metabolism produces some endogenous carbon monoxide and the normal COHb concentration is less than 1%. Tobacco smoke contains carbon monoxide and it is the commonest cause of an elevated blood COHb. Cigarette smokers on average have a COHb level of 5–6% and heavy smokers can have levels in excess of 10%. Typically urban non-smokers will have levels of 1–2% COHb. A level greater than 5% in non-smokers and 10% in most smokers suggests a source of carbon monoxide in the inhaled air. Levels in excess of 10% can sometimes be found in groups such as drivers, firefighters, garage employees and dock workers, especially if they are smokers.[50]

The proportions of COHb and oxyhaemoglobin in blood depend upon the partial pressure of carbon monoxide and oxygen. Several empirical equations have been proposed for estimating per cent COHb at different levels of exposure to carbon monoxide in combination with sedentary, light or heavy work and which take into account the duration of exposure, pulmonary ventilation and the COHb present before inhalation of contaminated air. The relation is not necessarily a simple one and therefore exposure should be assessed measuring both COHb and the levels of carbon monoxide in the air, but the following formula first proposed by Forbes and others[51] may be used:

$$\% \text{ COHb} = k \times \% \text{ CO in air} \times \text{minutes of exposure}$$

The constant k is 3 for an individual at rest, 5 for light activity, 8 for light work, and 11 for heavy work. More refined formulae, such as Coburn–Forster–Kane equations,[52] are also available. Figure 8.8 can be used to predict COHb in an individual with a continuing exposure to a specified concentration of carbon monoxide at different levels of exertion.

Performance of light-to-moderate work (up to 70% of maximum aerobic capacity) is not affected at low levels of carbon monoxide, that is COHb levels of 4–6%, but short-term maximal exercise duration is reduced in young healthy men. The effect is small and is only likely to be of concern for competing athletes. Subtle impairment of mental functioning has been reported in volunteers when COHb levels exceed about 5%. These changes include impairment of memory, learning ability, attention span, coordination, and abstract thinking.[50]

A less well-known hazard arises from the use of methylene chloride (dichloromethane), a widely used solvent and a main ingredient of commonly used removers of paint and varnish from wood. Dichloromethane is readily absorbed through skin contact and in the lungs as a vapour and is metabolized in the liver. Carbon monoxide is an important metabolite of dichloromethane and forms COHb: peak levels can occur within 3 hours of exposure associated with elevated alveolar carbon monoxide levels, and there is a return to pre-exposure levels in 24–48 hours after the exposure has ceased.[53] Approximately 5% COHb saturation is obtained following exposure of non-smokers to 200 ppm dichloromethane for 4–8 hours. High exposure to this solvent by inhalation as a result of stripping paint in an inadequately ventilated working area for 2–3 hours may result in levels of COHb high enough to precipitate angina or myocardial infarction in workers with pre-existing cardiovascular disease.[54]

Clinical features of carbon monoxide poisoning

Acute poisoning Exposure to carbon monoxide resulting in levels of 10–30% COHb may produce throbbing headaches and mild exertional dypnoea. At 30–50% additional symptoms include dizziness, nausea, weakness and collapse. Acute heavy exposures may result in loss of consciousness without warning, followed by coma, convulsions and death. Fatal levels of COHb in healthy persons are usually in excess of 50%; anaemia predisposes to carbon monoxide poisoning (see Chapter 2). The classic cherry pink colour of the skin is a rare sign, and if present suggests a carboxyhaemoglobin level over 30%, but venous blood frequently looks arterial. Carboxyhaemoglobin levels in heparinized blood samples are measured by dedicated co-oximeters or by spectrophotometry by second derivative.[55] In post-mortem blood, gas chromatographic analysis is the preferred method because of the breakdown of haemoglobin.

There is no diagnostic symptom complex for carbon monoxide poisoning and the diagnosis can be easily missed. The clinical presentation can vary widely, with vomiting, headaches, malaise, weakness, fatigue, chest pain, palpitations and dyspnoea. It is as well to know that the signs and symptoms of non-lethal exposure may mimic those of a non-specific viral illness.[56] Whilst blood carboxyhaemoglobin concentrations are diagnostic, the levels are not a good guide to prognosis and the clinical condition is more important, especially if the patient is or has been unconscious. Without adequate treatment, 10–30% of severely poisoned patients may develop late neuropsychiatric manifestations 3–240 days after exposure.[56] The prevention of this adverse outcome is the main reason for advocating aggressive early treatment.

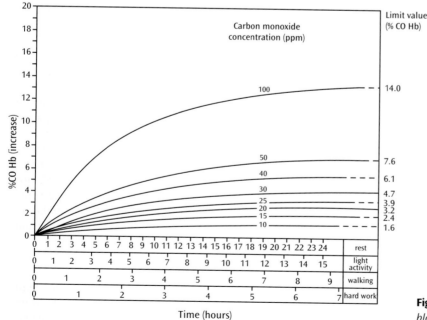

Figure 8.8 *Uptake of carbon monoxide by blood. Adapted from Ref. 64, with permission.*

The half-life of COHb is normally about 4 hours (longer if induced by methylene chloride exposure) but without treatment coma can last for 24 hours or longer. The relatively short half-life of COHb means that by the time the patient is seen, measurement of COHb may not be a good guide to the initial exposure. Therapy is directed towards reducing the half-life of COHb which falls to 80 minutes when the patient is given 100% oxygen at sea level. Most authorities now advocate giving hyperbaric oxygen where there is access to a hyperbaric chamber.[57] Hyperbaric oxygen at 2.5 atmospheres (252 kPa) reduces the half-life to 20 minutes and increases the amount of oxygen dissolved in the blood to a concentration sufficient to meet the needs of the body even without functioning haemoglobin.

Hyperbaric oxygen should be considered for pregnant women and for patients who have evidence of:

- A period of unconsciousness
- Neurological or psychiatric symptoms
- Cardiac complications
- Carboxyhaemoglobin levels above 40%

Neuropsychiatric damage can be immediate or a clear period of several days may be followed by the development of neuropsychiatric symptoms within the next 2–3 weeks or longer (see Chapter 42). Neurological manifestations such as vegetative state, akinetic mutism, parkinsonism, agnosia, visual impairment, and amnestic-confabulatory states have all been described.[56,58,59] The patient can develop changes in personality typified by increased irritability, verbal aggressiveness, violence, impulsiveness and moodiness. Up to 40% of patients develop memory impairment, and 33% can suffer late deterioration of personality. Depression and suicidal tendencies are also reported. Although many patients improve after some months, a proportion will be found not to have improved 3 years later.[60] The syndrome of delayed neurological sequelae is more characteristic of carbon monoxide poisoning than other types of anoxia, and the cause remains speculative, but it seems likely that carbon monoxide has a specific cytotoxic action. Bilateral necrosis of the globus pallidus is common, and lesions may also be found in the basal ganglia, hippocampus and white matter on computerized axial tomography or MRI scanning,[61,62] but delayed neurological sequelae may also occur in the absence of such findings. Positron emission tomography scanning can detect regions of the brain affected by ischaemia in the acute poisoning stage, and which may be at risk of late complications, but the technique is no better at predicting the eventual outcome.[63] Neuropsychometric assessment will show impairment in acute poisoning and may reveal cognitive deficiency consistent with organic brain damage in the delayed syndrome. The diagnosis of delayed neurological sequelae may be missed, and the patient assumed to have even made a good recovery, until a return to work reveals a failure to perform to the expected level (see Chapter 42).

Ambient air By far the principal source of carbon monoxide in the general outdoor atmosphere is general pollution by vehicle exhausts. Uptake of carbon monoxide from multiple sources, such as smoking and traffic, is not additive. Smokers who already have a carboxyhaemoglobin level above the equilibrium value that would be reached by breathing air in their surroundings are liable to act as 'source', breathing out carbon monoxide rather than absorbing more. Air quality standards therefore in effect protect non-smokers from peak concentrations close to heavy traffic. The most important adverse health impact from environmental exposure to carbon monoxide is the effect on people with angina and disease from the coronary arteries. In the UK the air quality standard has been set at a level at which the carboxyhaemoglobin should not exceed 2.5% in people breathing the air over a prolonged period, that is, 10 ppm measured as a running 8-hour average.[64] This level equates to 25 ppm for 1 hour, 50 ppm for 30 minutes, and 87 ppm for 15 minutes when breathing at maximum levels of activity. The reader should note that this standard is substantially below the OES for an 8-hour period, and its rationale highlights the need to ensure the adequate protection of people who suffer from ischaemic heart disease if they are likely to come into contact with the gas.

Recent studies indicate that even a circulating blood concentration of COHb of 2–3.9% is associated with impairment of cardiovascular function in patients with angina pectoris, who may show detectable changes in the cardiac ischaemic threshold on light-to-moderate exercise (as assessed on the electrocardiogram (ECG) by a reduction in time to the ST end point) and an earlier development of angina pectoris.[65] In healthy workers there is no clear evidence that these levels of COHb (or indeed levels as high as 10% COHb) impair the functioning of the central nervous system. Nevertheless, deterioration in maximum work capacity or maximum aerobic capacity can be demonstrated with increasing levels of COHb. It is possible that healthy individuals are able to adapt to the mild hypoxia of chronic exposure to carbon monoxide. Experimental studies have shown that carbon monoxide has an atherogenic effect in rabbits and rats but it is not generally accepted that low-level occupational exposures contribute to atherosclerosis in man; more information is needed on the effects of carbon monoxide on vascular endothelium and lipid metabolism. An epidemiological study of a cohort of bridge and tunnel workers regularly exposed to traffic fumes concluded that carbon monoxide may be a contributory factor in increasing cardiovascular mortality, but the mechanism was not clear.[66]

There is no available evidence to suppose that carbon monoxide is mutagenic or carcinogenic, but exposure is suspected to be a contributory factor for low birthweight in the babies of pregnant women who smoke. The teratogenic effects of carbon monoxide have been attributed to the transfer of carbon monoxide across the placenta and a consequently reduced oxygen supply to the fetus. Studies have predicted significant changes in fetal oxygenation as a result of maternal carboxyhaemoglobin levels of about 5%. Severe acute exposures have caused fetal death; and developmental and other neurological abnormalities have been recorded in live births.[67]

The pregnant worker should avoid occupational exposure to carbon monoxide or methylene chloride and undue exposure to carbon monoxide should be prevented in workers with symptomatic ischaemic heart disease. It is also important to appreciate that the effects of carbon monoxide in people living or working at high altitude (or at a reduced partial pressure of oxygen) are greater than at sea level.

HYDROGEN CYANIDE (HCN)

[CAS no. 74–90–8]
Maximum exposure limit (STEL) 15 ppm (11 mg/m³)
Relative density: 0.95
Flammability limits: 6–41% (vol.)

As well as hydrogen cyanide the gaseous cyanides include cyanogen $(CN)_2$, once used as a fumigant, and cyanogen chloride (CICN), a fumigant and industrial intermediate. Exposure to cyanide in industry may also be the result of the accidental or intentional ingestion of cyanide salts (e.g. sodium, potassium, calcium and copper cyanide) and from exposure to the vapour of nitrites such as acrylonitrile (vinyl cyanide, see p.), and acetonitrile (methyl cyanide). Cyanide salts are used widely for metal cleaning or hardening, in metal refining, gold extraction and film recovery and electroplating. Historically hydrogen cyanide used to be widely used as a fumigant, but today its main industrial usage is in the production of acrylonitrile and methyl methacrylate. The gas is also evolved when acids come into contact with cyanide salts. Firemen may be exposed to the gas in fires involving the combustion of nitrogen-containing synthetic materials. The main route of poisoning by hydrogen cyanide is inhalation though in solution it can also readily penetrate the skin.

At room temperature hydrogen cyanide is a clear, highly volatile liquid (boiling point 26°C). The gas has a characteristic odour of bitter almonds which is recognizable at 2–5 ppm but its detection by odour is unreliable; at higher concentrations it causes olfactory fatigue. At 18–36 ppm warning symptoms of poisoning may occur, such as irritation of the eyes, nose and throat, dizziness, nausea, general weakness and headaches, flushed or occasionally pale skin, and palpitations. Rapid and sudden loss of consciousness and cessation of breathing may occur on exposure to levels over 100 ppm. Levels of hydrogen cyanide above cyanide plating baths normally vary around 1–5 ppm and workers do not complain of symptoms; headache and vertigo may be reported at slightly higher concentrations.

Cyanide paralyses mitochondrial respiration by binding reversibly with enzymes containing ferric ions, in particular cytochrome aa3, thereby blocking intracellular respiration. Its direct action on the respiratory centre may also induce respiratory failure.

Victims of acute poisoning present with headache, dizziness and vertigo. There may be marked agitation and confusion, with nausea and vomiting. Dyspnoea is accompanied by hyperpnoea due to lactic acidosis. Acute cyanide poisoning induces sustained seizures, endogenous catecholamine release and cardiovascular shock. On examination the external findings may be normal with a pink appearance even when the blood pressure is immeasurable. The diagnosis can be confirmed by measuring cyanide in a sample of heparinized whole blood. Cyanide is concentrated in the red blood cells and plasma cyanide measurements are not recommended. Concentrations greater than 50 mmol/litre are associated with altered consciousness, and the lethal level is above 100 mmol/litre. Blood thiocyanate is a metabolite which can be measured after the acute event. Other useful tests include plasma lactate and arterial blood gases. In fatal cases there are no specific pathological changes and in particular the blood remains well oxygenated

The treatment of cyanide poisoning remains controversial because the effectiveness of the recommended antidotes, and so the treatment of choice, is not proven. Immediate first aid measures include removing the patient to fresh air, keeping the patient warm and at rest, and removing contaminated clothing. Contaminated skin should be washed thoroughly. Oxygen should be administered if available. First aiders should wear suitable protective clothing, including impervious gloves, to avoid skin absorption of cyanide. Where there is the potential for a large release of hydrogen cyanide, first aiders should be trained in the use of self-contained or airline breathing apparatus for the rescue of victims. However, in most biological laboratories the amount of cyanide in routine use does not normally warrant this precaution.

The UK Health and Safety Executive issued new advice on the first aid treatment of cyanide poisoning at work in 1997. The Executive no longer recommends the use of any antidote in the first aid treatment of cyanide poisoning and does not require employers to keep supplies. Instead, the administration of oxygen is regarded as the most useful initial treatment using a bag and mask device connected to an oxygen supply. The new advice is summarized in Table 8.5. There is growing animal and human evidence that oxygen is itself an antidote to cyanide or improves the response to treatment with specific antidotes.

The main antidotes recommended in the UK are amyl nitrite and dicobalt edetate. A conservative approach to

Table 8.5 *Overall outline of first aid treatment for cyanide poisoning*

- **Speed is essential. Obtain immediate medical attention**
- Protect yourself and the casualty from further exposure during decontamination and treatment

Inhalation

Remove patient from exposure. Keep warm and at rest. Oxygen should be administered. If breathing has ceased apply artificial respiration using oxygen and a suitable mechanical device such as a bag and mask. Do not use mouth-to-mouth resuscitation

Skin contact

Remove all contaminated clothing immediately. Wash the skin with plenty of water. Treat patient as for inhalation

Eye contact

Immediately irrigate with water for at least 10 minutes. Treat patient as for inhalation

Ingestion

Do not give anything by mouth. Treat patient as for inhalation

Source: Health and Safety Executive

their use is recommended. Any patient exposed to hydrogen cyanide who reaches hospital fully conscious will probably not need treatment with antidotes, their use being reserved for the patient who is unconscious or who has a clear history of exposure to cyanide and has deteriorating physical signs.[68] To be effective the antidotes should be administered immediately the diagnosis of cyanide poisoning is made, but the problem is that the uninitiated could readily mistake an ordinary collapse for poisoning. Accidental cyanide poisoning is rare in British industry today, but the risk of suicide bids from swallowing cyanide in solid form or in liquids such as acetonitrile is also a possibility which occupational physicians need to be aware of.

The rationale of treatment is the rapid fixation of cyanide ion either by direct fixation with dicobalt edetate or by methaemoglobin formation. Experience with gassing incidents suggests that after the unconscious casualty has been removed from further exposure he should be observed for any deterioration of vital signs before administering cyanide antidotes as patients often recover spontaneously and quickly from apparently severe poisoning. A rapid method of diagnosing cyanide poisoning is to test the patient's breath for hydrogen cyanide with a gas detector tube. Amyl nitrite by inhalation and oxygen delivered by face mask are relatively safe and may be administered if the patient is conscious. A capsule of amyl nitrite is broken into a handkerchief and the patient inhales the vapour for 15–30 seconds. This process must be repeated every 2–3 minutes until the

capsule is exhausted. If the patient is comatose, or starts to become drowsy and has the features of cyanide poisoning, then dicobalt edetate (300 mg in 20 ml glucose solution) should be administered by slow intravenous injection over 3–4 minutes. The second-line treatment, if there is no return to consciousness, is to give sodium thiosulphate (12.5 g – i.e. 25 ml of 50% solution) intravenously over 5–6 minutes. Dicobalt edetate is a chelating agent that combines with cyanide to form an inert complex, cobalticyanide. This agent is not innocuous and if administered in the absence of cyanide will cause cobalt poisoning, hence the need to be cautious about its use. Amyl nitrite produces methaemoglobin which promotes the binding of cyanide. Thiosulphate is a sulphur donor and accelerates the detoxification of cyanide by assisting in its conversion to the non-toxic thiocyanate.

If the patient is not breathing then artificial respiration should be commenced using a manual resuscitator. Mouth-to-mouth artificial respiration may put the first aider at risk of absorbing cyanide from the patient's mouth or breath. The manual methods of artificial ventilation, such as Holger Nielsen, are no longer recommended because they have poor efficiency and cause problems in maintaining an adequate airway.

Hydrogen cyanide may be formed when cyanides come into contact with acids. The cyanogen halides cyanogen chloride (CNCl) and cyanogen bromide (CNBr) also have local irritant effects on the eyes and respiratory tract and can cause inflammation of the bronchioles and pulmonary oedema, as well as having a similar toxic action as hydrogen cyanide. The cyanonitriles have a slower rate of intoxication than cyanide gas or cyanide salts as the cyanide is released when they are metabolized by the body over several hours; they also have their own toxic properties. Cyanide is not produced in the metabolism of isocyanates or diisocyanates.

Despite evidence that hydrogen cyanide can be inhaled in fires the use of dicobalt edetate is not recommended. The relatively safe antidotes amyl nitrite and sodium thiosulphate, as well as hyperbaric oxygen, have been used to treat fire casualties in hospital. Hydroxocobalamin (Vitamin B12), which reacts with cyanide to form cyanocobalamin, is advocated by some experts as an alternative in such patients.[69]

The evidence for chronic health effects arising from long-term exposure to cyanides at work is limited. Workers may experience recurrent mild acute, or subacute, symptoms if exposures are not being adequately controlled.[70] In the clinical setting, a neurotoxicological role for cyanide has been suggested in tobacco amblyopia, and tropical ataxic neuropathy associated with the ingestion of certain types of cassava which have not been adequately prepared before cooking. Cyanides are mostly metabolized to thiocyanates in the body, and a toxic side-effect of thiocyanate administration was found to be goitre when it was advocated in the past for the treatment of hypertension. Evidence for goitre, but not for neurological complications, has been reported in association with chronic cyanide exposure in a group of electroplating workers.[71]

PRIMARY IRRITANT GASES

CHLORINE (Cl₂)

[CAS no. 7782–50–5]
Exposure limits
   LTEL (8 h TWA) 0.5 ppm (1.5 mg/m³)
   STEL (15 min) 1 ppm (2.9 mg/m³)
Relative density: 2.47

Chlorine is a greenish, highly irritant gas with a pungent odour; it is moderately soluble in water. It is widely used in the manufacture of chemicals, the bleaching of pulp and paper, for disinfecting water and in waste treatment. Workers may also be exposed in the production of chlorine by diaphragm cell or mercury electrolytic cell processes. Chlorine is used in the manufacture of polyvinyl chloride and thousands of organochlorine compounds, most of which do not occur in nature and persist in the environment, the most toxicologically potent being the 'dioxins'.

Chlorine was discovered by the Swedish pharmacist, CW Scheele, in 1774, who was the first to observe its bleaching properties. Chlorine-based bleaching agents have been used in the pulp industry for more than a century. Chlorine dioxide was first synthesized in 1811 by Humphrey Davy, but was not introduced in the pulp and paper industry until 1946. This gas is at least as toxic as chlorine.[72] Exposure to workers and occasionally the public is by the accidental release of chlorine from closed systems under pressure. In the UK it is the most common hazardous chemical stored in large quantities at industrial installations.

Despite its widespread commercial exploitation since before the First World War, human data on dose-effect relations are sparse and instead the results of animal experiments extrapolated to man are used to estimate lethal or dangerous concentrations of chlorine gas. Its odour can be detected by most people at 0.2 ppm and by some at 0.02 ppm and irritant effects on the eyes and mucous membranes are felt at 3–15 ppm. In susceptible individuals significant changes in lung function occur at 1 ppm after 4 hours. Exposures in the ranges 15–150 ppm may be dangerous after 5–10 minutes, particularly at the higher end of this range or in susceptible individuals, for example with chronic respiratory disease. At 400–500 ppm the gas is estimated to be fatal in 50% of active healthy people exposed for 30 minutes, and exposure to 1000 ppm will be fatal after a few breaths. Chlorine is a strong oxidizing agent and when dissolved in tissue water will produce hypochlorite and hydrogen chloride as well as damaging oxygen free radicals.

The effects of chlorine are mainly confined to the respiratory system.[73] Because of its solubility it will act in the upper and lower respiratory tract. Acute exposure causes irritation of the mucous membranes of the eyes, nose and throat, producing cough, choking, substernal pain and tightness. Abdominal pain, nausea and vomiting have also been reported in accidents. Upper respiratory tract obstruction from laryngeal oedema should always be considered but the most frequently encountered effect is interstitial oedema which leads to impairment of gas diffusion and hypoxaemia; a restrictive and obstructive defect in lung function may be due to bronchospasm or interstitial oedema. Death may occur from respiratory failure or cardiac arrest due to non-cardiogenic pulmonary oedema. Irritation and necrosis of the skin can be caused by contact with a jet of gas, but mild erythema resembling first-degree burns may follow lesser exposure. Most mildly affected patients will settle quickly with rest, but symptomatic treatment for cough and soreness of eyes and throat may need to be given. Symptomless casualties should rest for 12 hours and be told to report any change in their health to a doctor. The treatment of severe chlorine poisoning is as for irritant gases in general (see PRINCIPLES OF FIRST AID AND TREATMENT IN GASSING ACCIDENTS (p. 131)).

After acute gassing incidents with chlorine RADS may occur, and associated respiratory symptoms, bronchial obstruction or bronchial hyper-responsiveness may persist for at least 18–24 months later.[74] There is little doubt that pre-existing bronchial hyperresponsiveness may also be aggravated in some individuals for weeks or months afterwards. In most persons, however, the evidence of a deterioration in airway function is transient. More studies are needed to determine whether chronic low-level exposures to chlorine can lead to long-term respiratory effects.[75,76] The recent follow-up studies of acute chlorine gassing among pulpmill and other groups of workers do indicate that the health effects of major incidents involving the accidental release of the gas may be much more extensive and persistent than was previously supposed for irritant exposures.[77]

Chlorination of public swimming pools results in free chlorine reacting with nitrogenous compounds (sweat and urine) introduced by bathers to form chloramines, especially nitrogen trichloride with dichloramine (NHCl₂) and monochloramine (NH₂Cl). These can be in the atmosphere in the form of droplets or gas and are irritant in their own right, but they may also decompose to form hydrochloric acid and ammonia. Nitrogen trichloride is an upper airway irritant as powerful as chlorine and may build up in the air of indoor pools and trigger acute eye and nasal irritation, as well as wheeze in susceptible bathers and swimming pool attendants.[78] Free chlorine and hypochlorite are unlikely to be present in the swimming pool atmosphere. A similar problem can arise in the processing of green salads in water containing hypochlorite.[79]

Cleaners have suffered near fatal pulmonary oedema from chlorine liberated by the mishandling of standard household bleaches (5.25% sodium hypochlorite solution – NaOCl), for example by mixing bleach with a cleaning agent containing acids, such as phosphoric acid, when chlorine gas and water are released.[80] Another hazard may arise in the chlorination of swimming pools using hydrochloric acid and sodium hypochlorite if the two chemicals are accidentally mixed in a way to cause a release of a cloud of chlorine gas.[81] Mixing bleach with a solution of ammonia produces monochloramine and dichloramine, and an accident, involving cleaning agents has led to a mass casualty event involving inhalation of chlorine gas.[82]

There is no evidence that chlorine is carcinogenic or that typical industrial exposures affect reproductive outcome. The use of chlorine to disinfect drinking water has been one of the greatest public health advances of the twentieth century, saving countless lives, but chlorine reacts with organic matter in untreated water to form trihalomethanes – of which chloroform is the most common – and these might cause cancer.[83]

PHOSGENE (COCl$_2$)

[CAS no. 75-44-5]
Exposure limit
    LTEL (8 h TWA) 0.02 ppm (0.08 mg/m^3)
    STEL (15 min) 0.06 ppm (0.25 mg/m^3)
Relative density: 3.48

Phosgene is a colourless, relatively insoluble gas.[84] At low concentrations (1 ppm) it smells like new-mown hay, but is pungent and irritating at higher levels. The gas dissolves in water and moist air to form carbon dioxide and hydrogen chloride but only a small amount will hydrolyse in the upper and lower airways when inhaled, most of the reaction taking place in the alveoli. It is not reported to affect the skin. The danger of phosgene is that it may cause only mild transient irritation of the mucous membranes of the eyes and respiratory tract at concentrations which can nevertheless cause delayed and fatal damage to lung tissue, the symptoms of which may not begin until 30 minutes to 48 hours later. In having a latent asymptomatic period following exposure the gas resembles nitrogen dioxide, but the mechanism of its toxicity is unknown.

Exposure is usually confined to the chemical industry where it is used in many organic syntheses requiring chlorination, such as in the manufacture of isocyanates, polyurethane, and polycarbonate resins. Gassing may occur from accidental releases from plant. It may also arise whenever a volatile chlorine compound or its vapour comes into contact with a flame or very hot metal and this could give rise to dangerous exposures in confined spaces; for example welders in the hold of a ship in Sweden welding steel plates which had been degreased by trichloroethylene all suffered pulmonary oedema. In fires, polystyrene may burn to form phosgene as well as chlorine.

The odour of phosgene is recognizable at concentrations exceeding 0.5 ppm, above which level it is probably dangerous to inhale the gas for prolonged periods. At exposures above 10–20 ppm for 1–2 minutes severe lung injury can follow, and inhalation of 90 ppm is said to be rapidly fatal. The main feature of phosgene poisoning is massive pulmonary oedema.[23] In most fatal cases pulmonary oedema reaches a maximum in 12 hours followed by death in 24–48 hours. The trachea and bronchi are usually normal in appearance, which contrasts with chlorine poisoning in which there is typically damage to the epithelial lining with desquamation. Exposure to high concentrations may also cause severe conjunctivitis and subsequent turbidity of the cornea. Chronic bronchitis and emphysema have been reported as a consequence of acute exposure.

No animal studies are available on the carcinogenicity of phosgene. No information is available on its reproductive toxicity or carcinogenicity in humans.[84] Because it is a highly reactive electrophilic compound it would be expected to bind in biological systems at the point of contact and so systemic absorption of unchanged phosgene by the inhalation or dermal route of exposure is not likely to be significant.

A notable escape of phosgene gas from storage tanks occurred in Hamburg in 1928, leaving at least 11 people dead and 250 casualties.

HYDROGEN CHLORIDE (HCl)

[CAS no. 7647-01-0]
Exposure limit
    STEL (15 min) 5 ppm (7.6 mg/m^3)
Relative density: 1.27

Hydrogen chloride gas is colourless and has a sharp, suffocating odour perceptible at 0.8 ppm. It is highly soluble in water and will produce a mist containing hydrochloric acid in moist air. Occupational exposure will therefore usually be to a mixture of gas and aerosol. It has a wide range of uses in the chemical industry. In parallel with chlorine consumption anhydrous HCl is used in the synthesis of vinyl chloride and other chlorinated hydrocarbons, and in steel pickling. Hydrogen chloride is also formed in the exhaust gases of many types of missile. The maximum levels of exposure that can be sustained over several hours are 10–50 ppm, though partial tolerance does occur. Throat irritation is caused by brief exposures to 35 ppm. A lethal level in air is often quoted as 500–1000 ppm for short exposures, but this is probably an overestimate of toxicity. The gas is highly irritant to the eye, causing conjunctival irritation and superficial corneal damage; on contact with the skin it will dissolve in the perspiration and produce epidermal inflammation. Repeated elevated exposures to the mist may cause ulceration of the nasal septum. Inhalation can cause choking, coughing, laryngeal oedema and non-cardiogenic pulmonary oedema depending upon the severity of exposure. Chronic, elevated exposures to the mist can give rise to erosion of teeth, particularly the incisors. It is some 30 times less irritant to the respiratory tract than chlorine and major incidents involving the public have not been recorded.[73]

Hydrogen chloride was one of the first gases to have its factory emissions controlled by legislation with the passing of the Alkali Acts in 1863. The alkali industry of the nineteenth century manufactured sodium sulphate which was used in glass making and to produce alkalis such as sodium carbonate and sodium hydroxide. The Leblanc process was based upon the reaction of common salt with sulphuric acid, and the unwanted byproduct hydrogen chloride was discharged into the air around the factories where it blighted vegetation over wide areas.[85] Hydrogen chloride is one of the most common gases emitted by volcanoes and it readily dissolves in rainwater to form acid rain. The gas is also formed in voluminous white clouds when liquid lava flows into sea water.

Hydrogen chloride is emitted from a variety of industrial sources including incinerators and coal-burning power plants. It is not one of the major ambient air pollutants. It undergoes rapid dry deposition from the air and low ambient air levels do not seem to pose a direct health risk. Asthmatic subjects do not appear to respond with adverse respiratory effects on exercising whilst breathing air containing less than 2 ppm hydrogen chloride.[86] Limited experimental and epidemiological studies do not provide any evidence that the gas is a human carcinogen.[87]

Compounds which hydrolyse to hydrochloric acid

The following gases are highly soluble in water and hydrolyse to hydrochloric acid; the treatment of overexposure is the same as hydrogen chloride and for irritant gases in general (p. 131).

BORON TRICHLORIDE (BCl₃)

[CAS no. 10294-34-5]
Exposure limit not established
Relative density: 4.1

Boron dichloride is a colourless gas which will form a mist in moist air to give hydrochloric acid and boric acid. It has a sharp odour and is non-flammable. It is used in metal refining and as a catalyst.

DICHLOROSILANE (SiH₂Cl₂)

[CAS no. 4109-96-0]
Exposure limit not established
Relative density: 3.5

Dichlorosilane is colourless and produces a mist in moist air. It is used in the semiconductor industry for the deposition of silicon.

NITROSYL CHLORIDE (NOCl)

[CAS no. 2696-92-6]
Exposure limit not established]
Relative density: 2.3

Nitrosyl chloride is a reddish brown, non-flammable, highly irritant gas. It is used in diazo reactions and other organic preparations. It reacts rapidly with water to form HCl and nitrogen oxides which makes it a highly dangerous irritant gas with both immediate and delayed effects on mucous membranes and lungs.

Other hydrogen halides

Both of these gases are more corrosive than HCl.

HYDROGEN BROMIDE (HBr)

[CAS no. 10035-10-6]
Exposure limit
    STEL (15 min) 3 ppm (10 mg/m³)
Relative density: 2.8

Hydrogen bromide is a colourless, fuming, corrosive and non-flammable gas with a strong acidic odour, usually found in solution in water up to a strength of 48% HBr. Exposure to 2–6 ppm for several minutes causes nasal and throat irritation, but no eye irritation. It is used as a chemical reagent in the manufacture of inorganic bromides, in organic synthesis, in the processing of ores and as an alkylation catalyst.

HYDROGEN IODIDE (HI)

[CAS no. 10034-85-2]
Exposure limit not established]
Relative density: 4.5

Hydrogen iodide is a colourless, corrosive, very heavy, fuming gas and the most unstable of the hydrogen halides. It is used as a reducing agent and in the preparation of iodides.

Fluorine and hydrogen fluoride

FLUORINE (F₂)

[CAS no. 7782-41-4]
Exposure limit
    STEL (15 min) 1 ppm (1.6 mg/m³)
Relative density: 1.31

Flourine is a pale yellow acrid gas which is highly reactive and rarely exists in the elemental state in nature. It is more toxic than hydrogen fluoride. Its effects on the eyes and respiratory tract resemble hydrogen fluoride, but gaseous fluoride is capable of reacting with the skin to induce severe thermal or chemical burns depending upon the duration of exposure.

The element fluorine is widely distributed in the environment, being present in virtually all rocks, normal soils, surface waters, sea water and air. Low concentrations of fluoride in drinking water (about 1 ppm) are beneficial in preventing dental caries, but excessive ingestion or inhalation of fluoride over prolonged periods causes fluorosis in humans and livestock. Since 1974 chlorofluorocarbons (CFCs or 'freons') have been implicated in stratospheric ozone depletion. Hydrofluorocarbons (HFCs) are less destructive of ozone, but they and CFCs are 'greenhouse' gases.

HYDROGEN FLUORIDE (HF)

[CAS no. 7664-39-3]
Exposure limit]
    STEL (15 min) 3 ppm (2.5 mg/m³)
Relative density: 1.86

Hydrogen fluoride, or anhydrous hydrofluoric acid, is a colourless, corrosive liquid which boils at 19.4°C and reacts in moist air to form a mist. Its main uses are in the manufacture of fluorocarbons, the etching and polishing of glass and as a fluoridating agent in organic and inorganic reactions; it is handled in the form of gaseous hydrogen fluoride or as an aqueous solution of hydrofluoric acid which on contact with the skin can cause severe burns.

Industrial exposure to fluoride may also arise in mining and use of fluoride-containing materials. Fluorspar (CaF₂) is mined in many countries (in Derbyshire, England, local deposits are known as 'Blue John') and is used throughout the world as a flux in high temperature smelting and refining processes for the production of metals and alloys. It is reacted with concentrated sulphuric acid to produce hydrogen fluoride. Cryolite (₃NaF AlF₃) used to be mined in Greenland until deposits became exhausted and is now produced by chemical synthesis instead: it is used in the manufacture of aluminium. Fluorapatite (CaF₂₋₃Ca₃(PO₄)₃) is present in rock phosphate which is mined in vast quantities in the production of phosphate fertilizers, phosphoric acid and phosphorus.

Exposure to hydrogen fluoride and silicon tetrafluoride, as well as fluoride particulates, may occur in a wide range of processes. Silicon tetrafluoride is also produced when hydrofluoric acid is used to etch glass and in water this toxic gas hydrolyses to form fluosilicic acid (H_2SiF_6) which is the agent most commonly used to fluoridate water. Processes with the potential to create large fluoride emissions include: phosphate fertilizer production, which involves the crushing and drying of phosphate rock; the manufacture of bricks, tiles, pottery and cement products when fluoride is released during the firing of clays containing fluoride; glass enamel and glass fibre production; metal casting; steel and petroleum refining; coal combustion; and aluminium production. Calcium fluoride and other inorganic fluorides are used as fluxing agents in arc welding. In uranium processing plants, isotopes of uranium are separated using the extremely corrosive solid uranium hexafluoride: emissions of fluoride compounds are usually negligible but a cloud of hydrogen fluoride was released from a uranium plant in Gore, Oklahoma, in 1985, killing one worker and affecting numerous others.

In 1989, an accidental release of about 24 tonnes of hydrogen fluoride occurred over a 48-hour period at a petroleum plant in Texas; 94 local residents were hospitalized and many others suffered from the irritant effects of the gas 'fog'.[88]

Acute health effects of hydrogen fluoride and fluorides[89]

In industrial exposures to gaseous and particulate fluoride, absorption of fluoride is mainly through the respiratory tract. Of fluoride in the body 99% is found in the skeleton since fluoride is not retained in soft tissue and is not metabolized. There is rapid renal excretion of an acutely absorbed dose so that about half is lost in the urine in a few hours. Only a very small amount is excreted in sweat or in the faeces. Occupational fluoride exposure has not been shown to cause liver or kidney injury and evidence is inadequate to implicate hydrogen fluoride and fluoride-derived gases as carcinogens or teratogens.

The maximum concentration of hydrogen fluoride in air tolerated by humans for 1 minute is about 120 ppm when it causes smarting of the skin, conjunctivitis and irritation of the respiratory tract.[90] The gas has a sour taste. At 60 ppm there are no skin symptoms but irritation of the eyes and nose with discomfort in the pharynx and trachea is present. A level of 30 ppm can be tolerated for several minutes.[91] In magnitude of acute toxicity, studies of human volunteers and experimental animals suggest that the halide gases hydrogen fluoride, hydrogen chloride and hydrogen bromide are of the same order;[92] their high water solubility ensures a rapid absorption in the nose and upper respiratory tract.

Accidental inhalation of high levels of hydrogen fluoride can cause rapid death from intense inflammation of the respiratory tract and gross haemorrhagic pulmonary oedema.[93] Inhalation of hydrogen fluoride and fluorine and most fluorine-derived gases may cause coughing, choking and chills lasting 12 hours after exposure.[94] After an asymptomatic period of 1 or 2 days pulmonary oedema may develop followed by regression over a period of 10–30 days. Advice to patients who have been in gassing accidents involving fluorine gases should therefore be cautious and should include the need for admission to hospital for 24–48 hours' observation.

Healthy volunteers who underwent bronchiolar lavage had a detectable inflammatory cell response after 1 hour of exposure to concentrations below 6 ppm. Pronounced eye and upper (burning throat) and lower (cough with expectoration) respiratory symptoms are reported above 3 ppm. Occupational exposures should therefore be kept well below the current exposure limit.[94]

Chronic fluoride toxicity – osteofluorosis

Osteofluorosis was first recognized as an occupational disease in Danish cryolite workers in 1932, since when cases have been reported in aluminium production, magnesium foundries, fluorspar processing and superphosphate manufacture. The accumulation of fluoride in the skeletal tissues is associated with pathological bone formation. The condition appears to be identical to endemic skeletal fluorosis found in parts of the world where drinking water contains fluoride in excess of 10 ppm and which was first described several years after a report of the first case of occupational fluorosis was published.[95]

The disease is detected by the radiological changes in spongy and other bones. There may be no symptoms even in the presence of radiological changes but back stiffness and vague joint pains are common. Initially there may be increased density of vertebral and pelvic bones but as the disease advances the bone contours and trabeculae become uneven and blurred. The bones of the extremities show irregular periosteal thickening with calcification of ligaments and muscular attachments. The cortex of the long bones is thick and dense and the medullary cavity is diminished. Radiological thickening of the bone may cause confusion with Paget's disease or osteoblastic metastases. In severe cases exostoses and osteophytes develop and calcification of ligaments, tendons and muscle insertions may lead to fusion of the spine and the development of a 'poker back' which clinically resembles ankylosing spondylitis.

Diagnosis is based upon the radiological findings and a history of prolonged fluoride exposure, together with raised urinary fluoride levels. Urinary excretion may remain high for several years after long-term heavy industrial exposure. There is evidence that the condition at least partially regresses if occupational exposure ceases, unless exposure has been prolonged in a patient suffering from poor nutrition.

The daily limit that may be ingested without risk of developing the disease is 4–5 mg of fluoride. The normal daily dietary fluoride intake does not exceed 1 mg, but in areas of endemic fluorosis the level of ingestion often exceeds 8 mg daily and in industrial situations absorption of 15–20 mg daily may unusually occur due to the inhalation of fluoride dust and gases. The current occupational exposure standard for gaseous and particulate fluorides (as fluorine) is 2.5 mg/m³. Inorganic fluoride exposure at 3.4 mg/m³ has resulted in an increase in bone density. Persistent urinary concentrations of fluorides above 5–7 ppm are quoted in the literature as unsafe, whilst the urinary biological exposure limits published by the American Conference of Governmental Industrial Hygienists (ACGIH) are 18 mol/mmol creatinine pre-shift and 60 mol/mmol creatinine post-shift.

Plasma fluoride levels correlate with concentrations of inhaled hydrogen fluoride, but they are not used for routine monitoring.[94]

Workers exposed to fluorides are not at risk of developing dental fluorosis as the mottling occurs when enamel is being laid; beyond 12–14 years of age a person's teeth can no longer be mottled, whatever the fluoride intake. Roholm, however, described three different family cases of dental fluorosis arising in the children of female cryolite workers in which the exposure to fluoride was believed to have been through the mother's breast milk.[95] The manifestations of dental fluorosis range from chalky white flecks on the teeth in mild forms to brown discolouration and pitting in the severe cases (Fig. 8.9). There are many parts of the world dependent on

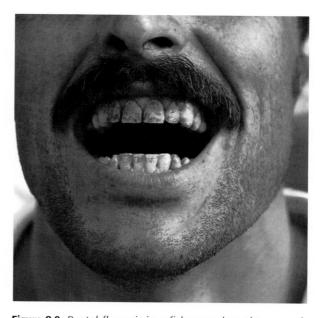

Figure 8.9 *Dental fluorosis in a fisherman brought up on the volcanic islands of the Azores. Until recently, his village water supply came from a spring fed by groundwater contaminated with fluoride (> 5 ppm).*

groundwater supplies for drinking which are contaminated by fluorides in geological strata. Developing, particularly permanent, teeth are extremely sensitive to fluorides during their formation.

Pot room asthma in aluminium production

Aluminium is produced by the reduction of alumina (Al_2O_3) which is obtained from bauxite, an ore produced mainly in South America and Australia. Since 1936 reports of asthmatic symptoms in pot room workers engaged in the manufacture of aluminium have suggested that respiratory irritants in the working atmosphere (hydrogen fluoride, sulphur dioxide and fluoride particles) may cause asthma or chronic obstructive pulmonary disease. Despite numerous studies the relation between exposure agents and disease is not resolved, but exposure to irritant gases such as hydrogen fluoride can cause a bronchial inflammatory reaction and a reactive airway dysfunction syndrome.[96]

The traditional Hall–Heroult process for producing aluminium was invented over a century ago and involved the extraction of alumina ore from bauxite and then placing the ore in a reduction cell, or 'pot'. Bauxite, the chief ore of aluminium, contains aluminium oxides and hydroxides with fluorides present as impurities. The prebake method uses carbon anodes prepared from calcine, petroleum pitch and coal pitch. In the prebake process the carbon anodes burn out releasing carbon dust, sulphur dioxide, carbon dioxide and carbon monoxide. In the Soderberg process, on the other hand, carbon paste is dropped into a steel casing hanging over the pot and the ore is baked *in situ* using separate, vertically placed, anodes.

The manufacture of carbon anodes in the carbon plant is associated with the release of polycyclic aromatic hydrocarbons from coal tar pitch volatiles and substantial exposure to these in the past has been found to be associated with an excess risk of lung cancer in several epidemiological studies.[97] Gaseous and particulate fluoride are given off in the two reduction processes.[98]

Exposure of susceptible individuals to the pot room atmosphere may provoke bronchial hyperreactivity or precipitate symptoms in those with subclinical asthma, but the mechanism is probably irritant rather than allergic. The syndrome tends to persist in some individuals even after stopping exposure. A study of Norwegian potroom workers over 6 years of follow-up found an increased decline in FEV_1 (see Chapter 35).[99]

Occupational systemic poisoning by fluorides

Acute systemic toxicity may arise from the ingestion of fluoride salts, e.g. sodium fluoride, or from absorption of fluoride in hydrofluoric acid burns.[100] There is no single cause of death in fluoride poisoning. Fluoride causes enzyme inhibition involving vital functions, such as the origin and transmission of nerve impulses. Calcium complex formation, with a rapid fall in plasma calcium, may interfere with blood clotting and cell membrane permeability. Deaths associated with profound hypocal-

caemia, hypermagnesaemia and hyperkalaemia have all been reported. In addition there may be specific organ injury involving cell damage and necrosis. Terminally there is a shock-like syndrome in which tetany is a prominent characteristic. There is no specific treatment except for the slow infusion of intravenous calcium gluconate which may be life-saving.[101]

Accidental exposure of the skin to hydrofluoric acid solutions can cause severe deep tissue injury. The treatment is beyond the scope of this chapter but it relies on immediate removal of contaminated clothing, thorough washing of the skin with water and rigorous topical application of 2.5% calcium gluconate gel which should always be available for use at locations where workers may be exposed. In hospital, subcutaneous injections of 5% calcium gluconate solutions may be necessary. Systemic effects from skin burns may be fatal; in one patient as little as 2.5% of the body surface area was affected.[101]

Other gases which hydrolyse to hydrofluoric acid

The following gases hydrolyse to hydrofluoric acid. Their effects and treatment of overexposure are as for hydrogen fluoride.

BORON TRIFLUORIDE (BF₃)

[CAS no. 7637–07–2]
Exposure limit
   STEL (15 min) 1 ppm (2.8 mg/m³)
Relative density: 2.4

Boron trifluoride is colourless and forms a mist in moist air to give hydrogen fluoride and boric acid. It is highly corrosive and has severe irritant effects on body tissues. It has a sharp odour and is non-flammable. It is used mainly as a catalyst in many chemical processes.

CHLORINE TRIFLUORIDE (ClF₃)

[CAS no. 7790–91–2]
Exposure limit
   STEL (15 min) 0.1 ppm (0.38 mg/m³)
Relative density: 3.2

Chlorine trifluoride is extremely reactive. The utmost care must be taken in ensuring that no contact with living tissue is possible. It is used for specialized purposes, such as rocket propellants and fluorinating agents.

CARBONYL FLUORIDE (COF)

[CAS no. 353–50–4]
Exposure limit not established
Relative density: 2.29

Carbonyl fluoride is a colourless, pungent gas used mainly for the preparation of organic fluorine compounds. It is also produced during the thermal decomposition of polytetrafluoroethylene (PTFE).

PERCHLORYL FLUORIDE (ClO₃F)

[CAS no. 7616–94–6]
Exposure limits
   LTEL (8 h TWA) 3 ppm (13 mg/m³)
   STEL (15 min) 6 ppm (26 mg/m³)
Relative density: 3.6

Perchloryl fluoride is a colourless, stable, non-flammable, sweet smelling gas. It is a strong oxidizing agent used in fluorination processes and for rocket fuels.

PHOSPHORUS PENTAFLUORIDE (PF₅)

[CAS no. 7647–19–0]
Exposure limit not established
Relative density: 4.5

Phosphorus pentafluoride is a colourless gas with a sharp odour. It produces a mist in contact with moist air. With large quantities of water it will ultimately yield phosphoric acid. It is used in laboratory and experimental work.

PHOSPHORUS TRIFLUORIDE (PF₃)

[CAS no. 7783–55–3]
Exposure limit not established
Relative density: 3.0

Phosphorus trifluoride is a colourless gas. It is odourless at concentrations which can cause toxic effects. It is used in specialized small chemical processes for the fluorination of some metals. The gas is highly toxic but only slowly hydrolyses to hydrogen fluoride.

SILICON TETRAFLUORIDE (SiF₄)

[CAS no. 7783–61–1]
Exposure limit not established
Relative density: 3.6

Silicon tetrafluoride is a colourless non-flammable gas with an overwhelming odour, and produces a dense white mist in air. It is used to manufacture fluosilicic acid (H₂SiF₆) and thence cryolite and aluminium fluoride. Fluosilicic acid has the same general effect as hydrogen fluoride and the treatment is the same.

SULPHUR TETRAFLUORIDE (SF₄)

[CAS no. 7783–60–0]
Exposure limits
   LTEL (8 h TWA) 0.1 ppm (0.45 mg/m³)
   STEL (15 min) 0.3 ppm 1.3 mg/m³)
Relative density: 3.8

Sulphur tetrafluoride is a very reactive, colourless and corrosive gas with a sharp odour. It is rapidly hydrolysed to hydrogen fluoride and thionyl fluoride, which in turn is slowly hydrolysed further into hydrogen fluoride and sulphur dioxide. It is used to batch produce fluorinated compounds by replacing oxygen with fluorine.

TETRAFLUOROHYDRAZINE (N₂F₄)

[CAS no. 10036–47–2]
Exposure limit not established
Relative density: 3.7

Tetrafluorohydrazine is a colourless gas with a musty odour and which slowly hydrolyses to hydrazine and hydrogen fluoride. Hydrazine is suspected of being a potential carcinogen in man. Tetrafluorohydrazine is used for the preparation of specialized fluorides.

OXYGEN DIFLUORIDE (OF₂)

[CAS no. 7783–41–7]
Exposure limit not established
Relative density: 1.9

Oxygen difluoride is a highly toxic, colourless gas with a foul smell. It is a very strong oxidizing agent used in the preparation of complex fluorides.

SULPHUR HEXAFLUORIDE (SF₆)

[CAS no. 2551-62-4]
   LTEL (8 hour TWA) 100 ppm (6070 mg/m³)
   STEL (15 min) 1250 ppm (7590 mg/m³)
Relative density: 5.1

This is an inert, heavy, colourless and odourless gas used by the electrical supply industry to insulate high voltage circuit breakers and cables. It is also frequently added to emissions to track the spread of pollution. The gas may also be used in loudspeakers and gas-filled cushions in the soles of training shoes. It is harmless except in a confined space where it displaces air, but electric sparking in the presence of oxygen will produce the irritant breakdown products sulphur oxyfluoride, sulphur dioxide and sulphuryl fluoride. A group of repair workers were inadvertently exposed to these gases by inhalation and suffered severe irritant effects.[102] It is one of the most potent greenhouse gases known.

NITROGEN TRIFLUORIDE (NF₃)

[CAS no. 7783–54–2]
Exposure limits
   LTEL (8 h TWA) 10 ppm (30 mg/m³)
   STEL (15 min) 15 ppm (44 mg/m³)
Relative density: 2.46

This gas is used as an oxidizing agent in rocket fuel and in fluorination reactions. Its principal hazard on inhalation is that it readily oxidizes haemoglobin to form methaemoglobin.

SULPHURYL DIFLUORIDE (SO_2F_2)

[CAS no. 2699–79–8]
Exposure limits
    LTEL (8 h TWA) 5 ppm (21 mg/m³)
    STEL (15 min) 10 ppm (42 mg/m³)
Relative density: 3.7

Sulphuryl difluoride is a colourless, odourless non-flammable gas with minimal smell. Its main use is as a fumigant. Overexposure has been reported to cause respiratory tract irritation, nausea and vomiting with crampy abdominal pain.

The following gases contain fluorine and are usually relatively inert, but they can undergo pyrolysis to produce respiratory irritants.

Fluorinated hydrocarbons

These gases are more widely known by their trade names. They are heavy, colourless, usually non-flammable and are used as refrigerants, specialized solvents and aerosol propellants. The usage of CFCs grew rapidly in the 1950s and 1960s as aerosol spray can propellants and blowing agents for foam insulation and foam packaging containers. CFCs are not biologically reactive and, being insoluble in water, are not removed from the air by rain. In the stratosphere they undergo photodissociation, the chlorine atom reacting with ozone to form chlorine monoxide (CIO) and oxygen. The destruction of the ozone layer by CFCs has been recognized since 1974, but the dramatic discovery by investigators from the British Antarctic Survey of an ozone hole above Antarctica in 1985 led scientists to confirm that the depletion was due to the increase of CFCs and related halocarbons (especially methyl chloroform-1,1,1,-trichloroethane and halons). This development gave greater weight to the Montreal Treaty which was then under negotiation. The most important CFCs responsible are CFC-11 (or Freon-11) and CFC-12. The 1980 global concentrations of these two gases were 0.18 and 0.28 ppb vol respectively, with lesser amounts of CFC-13, 113 and 114. The troposphere residence times of these compounds ranges from 65 to 400 years. There are now plans to phase out the world-wide usage of the fully hydrogenated CFCs. As the CFCs are also greenhouse gases, limiting their production will also substantially help efforts to counter global warming. The hydrogenated partially halogenated chlorofluorocarbons are being introduced as substitutes for the unacceptable fully hydrogenated chlorofluorocarbons; these are designated as HCFCs.

Although CFCs mainly pose an occupational hazard by displacing oxygen in confined spaces, they are not all as innocuous as has been supposed. Most cause narcosis at high concentrations and skin contact with the compounds with low boiling points can cause skin irritation or frostbite. In animal studies mixtures of over 1% (vol) cause respiratory depression, bronchoconstriction and reduced pulmonary compliance. The pyrolysis products of CFCs include chlorine, hydrogen chloride, hydrogen fluoride and phosgene, and these may be a hazard to firefighters. CFC-22 (chlorodifluoromethane) has been reported to cause cardiac arrhythmias (palpitations) in hospital workers who sprayed tissue with an aerosol preparation in order to 'speed up' the work of a cryostat machine,[103] but these adverse effects have not been found in studies of refrigerator repairmen. CFC-113 (Freon-113 or Genetron-113) has been implicated in fatalities from cardiac arrhythmia, asphyxiation or both in those working in confined spaces or in poorly ventilated areas.

The following gases are representative of the group and include some related compounds.

DICHLORODIFLUOROMETHANE (FREON-12, GENETRON-12) (CCl_2F_2)

Exposure limit
    LTEL (8 h TWA) 1000 ppm (5030 mg/m³)
    STEL (15 min) 1250 ppm (6280 mg/m³)

CHLOROTRIFLUOROMETHANE (FREON-13, GENETRON-13) ($CClF_3$)

TETRAFLUOROMETHANE (FREON-14) (CF_4)

This substance occurs naturally in significant traces in natural gas and is a potent greenhouse gas, being inert like silicon hexafluoride.

DICHLOROFLUOROMETHANE (FREON-21) ($CHCl_2F$)

CHLORODIFLUOROMETHANE (CFC-22; FREON-22) ($CHClF_2$)

Exposure limit
    LTEL (8 h TWA) 1000 ppm (3590 mg/m³)
    STEL – none

FLUOROFORM (FREON-23) (CHF_3)

1,1,2-TRICHLORO-1,2,2-TRIFLUOROETHANE (FREON-113) (CCl_2FCClF_2)

1, 2-DICHLOROTETRAFLUOROETHANE (FREON-114, GENETRON-114) ($C_2Cl_2F_4$)

HEXAFLUOROETHANE (FREON-116) (C_2F_6)

CHLOROPENTAFLUOROETHANE (GENETRON-115) (C_2ClF_5)

1,1-DIFLUOROETHYLENE (GENETRON-1132A) (H₂C: CF₂)

1,1-DIFLUORO-1-CHLOROETHANE (GENETRON-142B) (H₃ CCClF₂)

1,2-DIBROMOTETRAFLUOROETHANE (FLUOROCARBON-114 B2) (C₂BR₂F₄)

1,1,1,2-TETRAFLUOROETHANE (HCFC-134a)

LTEL 1000 ppm (proposed)

This is used as a new ozone sparing propellant, and is being used in asthma inhalers, for example. No human data on its health effects are available. At high concentrations in animal studies, delayed fetal development has been found. For a review of the health effects of the fully halogenated chlorofluorocarbons, see reference.[104]

Substitutes for the phased out chlorofluorocarbons are the partially halogenated hydrochlorofluorocarbons (HCFCs), the most important being 1,1-dichloro-2,2,2-trifluoroethane (HCFC 123) and 1-chloro-1,2,2,2-tetrafluoroethane (HCFC 124). These have only recently become available for commercial and industrial use.[105,106] An outbreak of liver disease has recently been reported in workers who received repeated accidental exposure to a mixture of these two compounds.[107] They were drivers of an overhead gantry in a secondary smelting depot and were exposed to a leaking air-cooling system in their cabin. Three out of nine workers presented with acute hepatitis, the remainder progressively developed varying degrees of liver abnormalities. Liver biopsy showed hepatocellular necrosis which was prominent in perivenular zone three and focally extending from portal tracts to portal tracts and centrilobular areas. Autoantibodies against human liver cytochrome P450 2E1 and P58 protein disulphide isomerase isoform (P58) were found in the serum of five of the workers.[107]

BROMOTRIFLUOROMETHANE (HALON 1301) (CF₃Br)

[CAS No 75–63–8]
   LTEL (8 h TWA) 1000 ppm (6190 mg/m³)
   STEL (15 min) 1200 ppm (7430 mg/m³)

This gas is commonly used as a fire extinguishant in computer and high technology facilities. A group of workers exposed in an accidental discharge of a halon fire-extinguishing system reported irritation symptoms of the eyes, nose and throat, and light headedness, but there may also have been exposure to irritant breakdown products of halon 1301 and Freon-22.[108]

SULPHUR DIOXIDE (SO₂)

[CAS no. 7446–09–5]
  Exposure limits
  LTEL (8 h TWA) 2 ppm (5.3 mg/m³)
  STEL (15 min) 5 ppm (13 mg/m³)
  Relative density: 2.26
  Ambient air quality standard: 100 ppb (15 min)

Sulphur dioxide is a colourless, highly irritating, non-flammable toxic gas. It is a common pollutant of urban air wherever fossil fuels are burnt. Being moderately soluble in water, it will dissolve easily in the layer of fluid on the surface of the epithelium of the nasal passages and upper airways. The upper respiratory tract and the large bronchi are the major site of absorption and toxicity of sulphur dioxide, but at high concentrations it behaves like other soluble irritant gases in causing airways injury, pulmonary oedema and corneal burns.[109] Survivors of gassing accidents may develop reactive airways dysfunction syndrome.

Sulphur dioxide from anthropogenic sources, such as coal- or oil-fired power stations, is oxidized in the atmosphere to sulphate at a rate of about 1–5% per hour,[110] but it can be faster in the presence of catalysts such as metals or their particulate compounds in a plume. Sulphate is much more soluble than the gas and readily forms fine sulphuric acid aerosols or combines with rainwater and cloud droplets to produce acid rain, often at long distances from the source of the pollution. Acid rain has no direct health impact, but it blights vegetation, acidifies surface waters and corrodes buildings. The major natural sources of sulphur dioxide are volcanic activity, and the oxidation of dimethyl sulphide released from marine organisms.

Occupational exposures to the gas may arise in petroleum processing, wood pulping, food preservation, sulphuric acid production, and in paper mills. The uses of sulphur dioxide include bleaching and refrigeration. Quite high exposures to sulphur dioxide are common in many smelting operations since most ores contain sulphide; it is also a contaminant of the air of non-ferrous metal foundries. Explosions of sulphide dust may occur when blasting in massive sulphide ores, and workers may become exposed to dangerously elevated concentrations of sulphur dioxide in such accidents.[111,112] Particulate matter will arise during many industrial processes as well as in the combustion of fossil fuels and the respiratory effects of the accompanying particle concentrations may also need to be considered.

Sulphur dioxide concentrations of 3–5 ppm in the air are easily noticeable and at these levels a few sensitive individuals will show a fall in pulmonary function at rest. Healthy individuals do not respond to sulphur dioxide below 1 ppm but may respond on exercise or deep breathing at levels of 1–5 ppm; most healthy individuals will show an effect with an increase in air flow resistance when exposed to concentrations of 5 ppm or higher. Asthmatic individuals, on the other hand, are especially sensitive to sulphur dioxide and can respond at rest to concentrations below 0.5 ppm and on exercise as low as 0.2 ppm, though no discernible threshold exists. The odour threshold is in excess of 1 ppm and so this criterion does not provide warning of potentially harmful lower levels. In the past, regular exposures in industry to over 30 ppm have been recorded, but marked irritation of the eyes, throat and upper respiratory tract usually occur at concentrations around 10 ppm. The maximum concentration that healthy individusals can endure for a few minutes is 150 ppm,[113] a level which can be fatal in the elderly asthma sufferer.[114]

'Dark-room disease' is a term coined in some quarters for radiographers reporting eye and upper respiratory irritation during the course of working in x-ray film processing under poorly ventilated conditions. Although the precise cause has not been ascertained, a study showed that the main airborne contaminants were sulphur dioxide and acetic acid at concentrations of about 0.1 ppm, as well as detectable glutaraldehyde.[115]

Much attention has been paid to sulphur dioxide as one of the main pollutants in smogs that occurred in cities in the nineteenth century and the first half of the present century as a result of the widespread burning of coal in homes and factories. With changing patterns of energy production the emissions of the gas have been much reduced and in the UK peak levels may be mainly found 30–40 km downwind of fossil-fuel power stations where the plume reaches ground level.[116] At low concentrations sulphur dioxide is thought to act on contact with the nose, throat and bronchi by stimulating neural reflexes which cause the smooth muscle of the airways to contract. This causes a reflex cough, irritation, and a feeling of chest tightness. Other mechanisms contributing to airway narrowing include the development of mucosal oedema, vascular congestion of the mucosa and increased airways excretions. Although exposure studies have focused on people suffering from asthma, it is likely that similar effects may be observed in patients with other chronic lung diseases. The UK air quality standard is 100 ppb measured over an average 15 minute period and is directed towards protecting these susceptible groups in the population.[116] The evidence for longer term effects and whether exposure to sulphur dioxide actually causes lung disease rather than simply provoking attacks of asthma, remains conflicting. It is noteworthy that the ambient air quality standard, which is based solely on health criteria, is much lower than the current UK occupational exposure standard.

Accordingly, pre-employment health screening in workplaces where exposure to sulphur dioxide is high enough to affect susceptible individuals should aim to advise patients with asthma or other chronic lung dis-ease to seek other employment, though the occupational physician should carefully evaluate individual cases.

A proportion of the population are, when exposed to inhaled irritants over time, prone to develop mucous gland hyperplasia and chronic obstructive pulmonary disease. Epidemiological studies of smelter and pulp mill workers exposed to sulphur dioxide at regular concentrations of 1–5 ppm or over have shown inconclusive results on measures of respiratory symptoms or chronic reduction in pulmonary function. Because of its irritant properties, sulphur dioxide has been thought possibly to act as a co-carcinogen in the causation of lung cancer. Studies of workers in copper smelters have shown an increased risk in relation to exposure to arsenic, but no independent effect of sulphur dioxide was seen.[117] There is little information available on teratogenic effects, but the gas is not considered to be a human carcinogen.[87]

'Smelter Disease' has been recognized in workers replacing pipes in sulphuric acid manufacturing plants. Characterized by dyspnoea, diarrhoea, colicky pain, muscle pain and dermatitis, it was attributed to sulphur dioxide in the past, but a recent study has shown it is due to mercury fume exposure when burning through the pipes containing sludge.[118]

SULPHUR TRIOXIDE (ANHYDRIDE OF SULPHURIC ACID) (SO_3)

[CAS no. 7446–11–9]

Oleum ('fuming sulphuric acid') is a complex mixture of sulphuric acid and sulphur trioxide. Sulphur trioxide can exist as a gas, liquid or solid, and is used primarily as a sulphating or sulphonating agent, for example in the manufacture of detergents, dyestuffs, drugs and insecticides. Dense clouds of sulphuric acid mist are formed when sulphur trioxide comes into contact with moisture in the air.

Sulphuric and other inorganic acid mists

Erosion of the enamel of the teeth has been reported with occupational exposure to sulphuric and other strong inorganic acid mists (nitric, hydrochloric and phosphoric acids).[119] They are irritating to mucous epithelia and provoke respiratory symptoms and changes in pulmonary function and, at high concentrations, death.[73,114,120] Acid mists may also cause pulmonary irritation by adhering to fine particles. There is sufficient evidence that occupational exposure to strong inorganic mists containing sulphuric acid is carcinogenic; laryngeal and lung cancer have been implicated in certain strong acid processes.[87,120]

An interesting incident demonstrating the impact of factory emissions containing concentrated sulphuric acid aerosols occurred in Japan between 1960 and 1969 when asthmatic symptoms were reported in about 600 individuals living within 5 km of a titanium dioxide plant during this period.[121]

AMMONIA (NH₃)

[CAS no. 7664–41–7]
Exposure limits
LTEL (8 h TWA) 25 ppm (18 mg/m³)
STEL (15 min) 35 ppm (25 mg/m³)
Flammability limits in air: 15–28 per cent (vol.)
Relative density: 0.59

Anhydrous ammonia is a colourless gas with a distinctive pungent odour. It is extremely soluble in water, forming a caustic alkaline solution of ammonium hydroxide. Ammonia is one of the most widely used industrial gases, as a catalyst and reagent, and has been used for many years as a refrigerant and in the manufacture of fertilizers. Although the gas is lighter than air it can behave paradoxically in an accidental release from storage in liquid form under pressure by undergoing rapid cooling to form a dense cloud that hugs the ground.

Most people will recognize the odour of ammonia at 30–50 ppm. At or above 50 ppm the gas is irritant to the eyes and mucous membranes of the respiratory tract though partial tolerance does develop. Being readily hydroscopic it is absorbed by the mucous coating of the upper respiratory tract. Human data are sparse but the only clearly established effect arising from exposure to low concentrations (<200 ppm) in humans is irritation of the skin, eyes and upper respiratory tract. There is no evidence that ammonia is genotoxic, carcinogenic or reprotoxic. Exposure to concentrations up to 500 ppm for a few minutes can be tolerated by healthy adults but at this level there is cough, hoarseness and tightness of the throat as well as marked eye irritation and conjunctivitis. At estimated levels of between 5000 and 10000 ppm ammonia is likely to damage the lower respiratory tract and be life-threatening, and concentrations in excess of 10000 ppm may be rapidly fatal.[122,123] At life-threatening levels the gas causes chemical burns of the nose, mouth and throat which become red and raw, and corneal burns. The tracheal epithelium and bronchi may become denuded of epithelium. Pulmonary oedema by itself or with subsequent bronchopneumonia is the main cause of death, but fatalities can also be caused by the very rapid onset of acute laryngeal oedema which initially can manifest itself by hoarseness and dyspnoea.[124,125]

The strongly irritant nature of ammonia has led to the oft-repeated view that laryngeal spasm is a frequent cause of death in gassing accidents, but it is more likely to be due to rapid onset of laryngeal oedema.[122] Although spasm of the glottis could persist long enough to induce asphyxia the spasm would normally relax during unconsciousness and then breathing would recommence.

Apart from respiratory tract irritation, injury to the eyes at these high concentrations can be severe. Irrigation of the eyes should be instituted immediately after exposure to prevent rapid absorption of ammonia by the eye. Ophthalmic sequelae include corneal opacities, cataract and glaucoma. A jet of anhydrous ammonia on to the moist skin can cause second-degree burns, as will splashes of liquid ammonia. The literature reports a case of severe gastritis continuing for months after a gassing accident.[124]

There is good evidence that some individuals who have survived an acute gassing incident may go on to develop permanent respiratory disability with complications such as progressive airway obstruction, diminishing diffusion capacity (low transfer factor), bronchiolitis obliterans, bronchiectasis, and continuing cough and sputum.

In contrast, exposure to ammonia in pig farmers is around a few ppm. Respiratory symptoms are common in these workers. But exposure to dust, disinfectants and endotoxins may contribute to the respiratory irritants in the air of livestock confinement buildings.[37,126]

Alkyl amine gases
The following aliphatic amine gases are used widely in industrial processes and pharmaceutical manufacturing:

MONOMETHYLAMINE (CH₃NH₂)

DIMETHYLAMINE (CH₃)₂NH

[Cas no. 124–40–3]
Exposure limits
LTEL 10 ppm (19 mg/m³)

TRIMETHYLAMINE (CH₃)₂N

[Cas no. 75–50–3]
Exposure limits
LTEL 10 ppm (25mg/m³)
STEL 15 ppm (37mg/m³)

They are flammable, highly soluble, alkaline, colourless gases which have a fishy odour at low concentrations and an ammoniacal odour at higher concentrations. They are all denser than air and act as irritants to the eyes, nose, throat, respiratory tract and skin. Trimethylamine (TMA) is a major component of the odour produced by decaying fish. In Fish Odour Syndrome, an uncommon inherited autosomal recessive condition, the oxidation of trimethylamine in the body is impaired. Unoxidized trimethylamine is increased in urine, breath, sweat and other secretions, causing the fish smell.[127]

OZONE (O₃)

[CAS no. 10028–15–6]
Exposure limits
STEL (15 min) 0.2 ppm (0.40 mg/m³)
Relative density: 1.66

Ambient air quality standard: 50 ppm (running 8-hour average)

Ozone is a faintly bluish gas with a characteristic pungent odour. Because it is irritant to mucous membranes and only moderately soluble in water, it readily penetrates to the small airways and alveoli, even with brief exposure, and at elevated concentrations causes pulmonary oedema. Exposure to moderately elevated levels of ozone causes a measurable fall in FEV_1 and FVC (forced vital capacity) associated with symptoms in susceptible adults, and children. These changes are compatible with an inflammatory bronchiolitis causing reflex inhibition of respiration. They are related to the duration of exposure and to exercise and have been recorded at concentrations as low as 0.08 ppm over periods of 6.6 hours.[26,128] There is no evidence that asthmatics or subjects with chronic obstructive pulmonary disease are more sensitive to ozone than others. Distinct irritation to the eyes and respiratory tract occurs at 0.5 ppm and prolonged exposure to this concentration is reported to cause pulmonary oedema or could increase susceptibility to respiratory infections (bacterial and viral). Even brief exposure to 1 ppm is inadvisable as it may cause severe cough and malaise. The lethal level is not known precisely but inhalation of 50 ppm for 30 minutes is regarded as a potentially fatal exposure.

Ozone is used in industry as an oxidizing agent in chemical reactions, for water fumigation and for the bleaching of synthetic and natural fibres, oils, paper and flour. It is also generated by electrical storms and by discharges in electrical equipment, for example during processes involving arc welding or emission of ultraviolet radiation. In offices with poor ventilation electrostatic photocopiers which utilize the action of high intensity discharge lamps, and laser printers, particularly older models, may produce sufficient ozone to cause symptoms such as headache and eye and throat irritation in some workers. Laser printers have ozone filters and it is important that the machines are regularly serviced according to the manufacturer's instructions.

Much attention has been focused on ozone as the major oxidant in photochemical smog. In terms of producing inflammation of the respiratory tract, ozone is the most toxic of the common air pollutants. Ozone may also increase bronchial responsiveness to allergens in atopic asthmatic subjects.[128] and the response to other bronchoconstrictor pollutants such as sulphuric acid or sulphur dioxide. The UK Department of Health has advised that those healthy or asthmatic individuals who are particularly sensitive to ozone should limit heavy exercise out of doors in the afternoon, the time of day when ozone levels reach a peak during periods of poor air quality, if peak hourly levels are likely to exceed 0.1 ppm.[26] The UK ambient air quality standard is 50 ppb as a running 8-hour average.[128]

There is no information in humans on whether long-term exposure to levels of ozone at the current occupational exposure standard (0.2 ppm) can cause chronic pulmonary health effects or adverse reproductive effects. In practice, most industrial exposures tend to be brief and related to attending specific processes. Monitoring methods should be in place to detect leaks so that ozonators can be shut down if abnormal operating conditions prevail. Leak detection by nose is not satisfactory because even slight leaks cause the sensation of smell to be numbed.

Nitrogen oxides

NITRIC OXIDE (NO)

[CAS no. 10102–43–9]
Exposure limits
    LTEL (8 h TWA) 25 ppm (31 mg/m³)
    STEL (15 min) 35 ppm (44 mg/m³)
Relative density: 1.04

Certain conditions, e.g. septic shock, result in enhanced endogenous synthesis of nitric oxide via induction of a nitric oxide synthase in endothelial and vascular smooth muscle cells, leading to vasodilatation and hypotension. A 40 ppm NO/air inspired mixture acts as a highly selective pulmonary vasodilator and reduces pulmonary hypertension. Its therapeutic properties are under study in patients requiring assisted ventilation, as in adult respiratory distress syndrome. Endogenous nitric oxide production probably accounts for most of the methaemoglobin in the blood of normal subjects. At 40 ppm nitric oxide the increase in methaemoglobin is small and clinically insignificant, but at over 100 ppm methaemoglobinaemia and pulmonary oedema are the principal hazards of the gas. Much of the toxicity is accounted for by the formation of nitrogen dioxide, which is not a vasodilator.

NITROGEN DIOXIDE (NO₂)

[CAS NO. 10102 44–0]
Exposure limits
    LTEL (8 h TWA) 3 ppm (5.7 mg/m³)
    STEL (15 min) 5 ppm (9.6 mg/m³)
Relative density: 2.62

Ambient air quality standard: 150 ppb (hourly average)

Nitric oxide is a colourless and odourless gas which rapidly oxidizes in air to nitrogen dioxide, a reddish-brown gas with a pungent odour apparent to most people at about 0.5 ppm. Both are found in nitrous fumes produced by fuming nitric acid, but nitric oxide is non-irritant whilst nitrogen dioxide is the more hazardous. Nitrogen dioxide is non-flammable and hydrolyses in water to form nitrous and nitric acid. Nitric oxide and nitrogen dioxide are formed in the combustion of fossil fuels or from biomass burning, the amount depending upon the nitrogen content of the fuel and the combustion temperature. Some fuels, such as natural gas, contain negligible amounts of nitrogen, but nitrogen oxides are also formed during the combustion of all fuels in the regions of peak flame temperature. In the UK, some 50% of the atmospheric nitrogen dioxide is produced by motor vehicles and some 25% by power stations. The most significant indoor source of nitrogen dioxide is cooking with gas. Like ozone, nitrogen dioxide is an oxidant gas with free radical properties and these may be responsible for its injurious effects on the pulmonary parenchyma by damaging cell membranes and proteins, though the gas is considerably less irritant than ozone. The formation of nitrous and nitric acid in dissolved nitrogen dioxide may also injure the airways. Mild asthmatics are more sensitive than normal subjects to exposure to nitrogen dioxide. At relatively high concentrations the gas causes acute inflammation of the airways. Nitrogen dioxide reduces mucociliary clearance and in animal studies has been shown to affect the immune cells of the airways and increase susceptibility to bacterial and viral respiratory infections.[129,130]

In the indoor environment the burning of natural gas as a cooking fuel in homes is an important source of nitrogen dioxide as are paraffin space heaters: indoor air concentrations may readily exceed those outside the home. An unvented gas cooker may typically provide peak levels of 200–400 ppb in a kitchen.

In industry nitrogen dioxide is released as a byproduct whenever nitric acid acts on metals or on organic materials, such as in the nitration of cotton or other cellulose, and in the manufacture of many chemicals. Certain welding operations also produce nitrogen dioxide. Fermentation of silage will produce high concentrations of gas within 2 days of silo filling and exposure to farmers entering the confined silo space may give rise to acute fatalities or the respiratory effects of exposure to nitrogen dioxide known as 'silo fillers' disease'. The hazard from oxides of nitrogen in silos was first reported from the USA where farmers commonly silage maize stalks.[131,132] Under certain growth conditions, for example drought or in soils with elevated nitrates, the content of nitrate in the grass or maize stalks used for silage may be increased enough to release an abundance of nitrous acid during fermentation which then breaks down into oxides of nitrogen. Warning signs to farmers are dead birds or rodents and a yellow-brown haze around the silage surface. Elevated carbon dioxide and reduced oxygen concentrations may also occur at the same time. Similar reactions can arise if silage grass is treated with ammonium salts. To prevent the build-up of gases silos should have adequate mechanical ventilation. Nitro-explosive fumes contain oxides of nitrogen, and when dynamite or gun cotton burn quietly instead of detonating, nearly the whole of the nitrogen is given off as nitric oxide instead of free nitrogen. Thus numerous inhalation accidents have occurred in mining and tunnelling

from the imperfect detonation of nitro-explosives, or from dynamite catching fire in poorly ventilated spaces. Armed services personnel may also be exposed to the fumes in gun-pits, armoured vehicles, ships' magazines and turrets.

Increased airways resistance has been measured in healthy human volunteers exposed to 2-hour concentrations as low as 2.5 ppm of nitrogen dioxide. Asthma sufferers may respond at concentrations as low as 0.3 ppm when exercising and exposure may enhance their response to common allergens.[133] The main danger of nitrogen dioxide is that it is only a mild upper respiratory tract irritant so that exposure to up to 50 ppm may produce no immediate symptoms to warn of its potential hazard. However, exposure to 4–25 ppm may result in severe cough, haemoptysis, chest pain. Exposure for less than an hour to 100–150 ppm can result in fatal pulmonary oedema arising between 3 and 72 hours later, with the initial irritant effects comprising throat irritation, cough, headaches, tightness in the chest, and sweating, all of which may pass off within 30 minutes. Thus persons who are believed to have received significant exposure should be admitted to hospital and placed under observation for 48 hours. At more elevated concentrations a few breaths can produce severe and immediate hypoxaemia which may be fatal. In less severe cases the delayed symptoms will be dyspnoea, chest pain with haemoptysis, and headache followed by an uneventful recovery in most patients, though the cough may last several weeks.

Apollo astronauts were accidentally exposed in an incident to an average of 250 ppm of nitrogen dioxide for 4 minutes before splashdown. They developed chest symptoms and evidence of pneumonia over the next day.[134]

Poisoning by oxides of nitrogen is a prescribed disease (see Chapter 4).

The initial treatment of nitrogen dioxide poisoning is as for non-cardiac pulmonary oedema induced by irritant gases. However, with this gas a second episode of pulmonary oedema may occur, and following apparent recovery bronchiolitis obliterans may develop after an asymptomatic period that can last up to 6 weeks. This complication, which appears as a fine, widely scattered nodular infiltration on the chest radiograph, may be fatal. Treatment with glucocorticosteroids should be continued for at least 2 months.

Nitrogen dioxide exposure should always be considered in workers who have suffered an acute onset of pulmonary symptoms with haemoptysis associated with minimal evidence of preceding respiratory irritation. Such incidents have also involved ice hockey players and spectators due to nitrogen dioxide emitted by malfunctioning combustion engines in ice surfacing machines that use propane.[135] Methaemoglobin determinations should be routinely performed: in an accident involving deaths of three men entering a silo that had been filled with corn the previous day postmortem blood samples showed a methaemoglobinaemia in the range of 38–44% in the three men.[136]

Information on the effects of chronic low-level occupational exposures is currently inadequate. A meta-analysis of epidemiological studies of the effects of exposure to nitrogen dioxide in the indoor air from domestic gas cookers on respiratory disease in children was inconclusive.[129] Nitrogen dioxide is not considered to be carcinogenic or teratogenic.[129] on present evidence.

HYDROGEN SULPHIDE (H₂S)

[CAS no. 7783 06–4]
Exposure limits
   LTEL (8 h TWA) 10 ppm (14 mg/m³)
   STEL (15 min) 15 ppm (21 mg/m³)
Relative density: 1.19
Flammability limits: 4.3–46% (vol)

Hydrogen sulphide is a colourless gas which burns in air with a pale blue flame and is moderately soluble in water. It is rapidly converted to sulphur dioxide in the atmosphere by a reaction with hydroxyl groups and carbonyl sulphide. In the body the sulphide ion is oxidized to thiosulphate and sulphate in the liver and kidneys and is mostly eliminated in the urine. The toxic effects of the gas are caused through the inhibition of cytochrome oxidase and through a direct depressant effect on the respiratory centre of the brain.[137]

Hydrogen sulphide poisoning is a frequently met hazard in the oil, gas and petrochemical industries where the risks of exposure are well known. Less well recognized are the dangers from the release of hydrogen sulphide as a result of the fermentation of proteinous material, e.g. the decay of 'trash' fish in boat holds and on farms which store slurry and liquid manure. It may also be found in dangerous concentrations in the vicinity of fumaroles and the craters of volcanoes, as well as in geothermal and hot spring areas (Fig. 8.10). Occupations associated with hydrogen sulphide exposure include carbon disulphide production, viscous rayon production, sewer and tunnel work and mining, petroleum production or processing, rubber vulcanizing, pulp industry, sulphuric acid production, tanning and glue manufacture. Its characteristic smell of rotten eggs is normally readily detectable below 1 ppm: the threshold of detection of the gas is 0.02 ppm and the rotten egg smell is detectable at levels several times higher. However, the sense of smell to hydrogen sulphide is soon lost at over 20 ppm and so the worker may have little, if any, warning of the presence of the gas at dangerous concentrations. Inhalation of concentrations of 10 ppm hydrogen sulphide has no effect on pulmonary function in exercising healthy subjects,[138] and levels of 20 ppm can be tolerated for some hours without harm (Fig. 8.10), and there is no cumulative action. Asthmatic subjects do not appear to so readily respond to low levels of hydrogen sulphide as they may do to sulphur dioxide.[139] On volcanoes, scientists can be totally unaware of hydrogen sulphide because its smell may be undetectable, even at low levels, in mixtures of fumarolic gases for reasons which are not clear. As with other toxic gases a safe system of work that includes air monitoring is essential. Whilst the toxic hazard of hydrogen sulphide depends upon the duration of exposure as well as its concentration, levels above 500 ppm should be regarded as very dangerous and immediate evacuation from a contaminated atmosphere should begin well below this level.

The symptoms of acute intoxication (> 1000 ppm) are rapid breathing and distress, with nausea and vomiting, and these may be rapidly followed by loss of conscious-

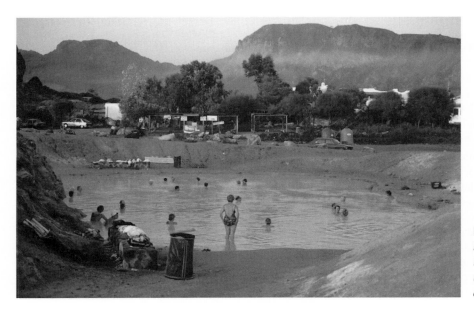

Figure 8.10 *Bathers in a volcanic mudpool on Vulcano Island, Italy. Hydrogen sulphide concentrations up to 20 ppm can be measured above the surface of the water.*

ness usually in association with cessation of breathing. Loss of consciousness without warning can occur on sudden exposure to a high concentration of hydrogen sulphide (>2000 ppm) after only one or two breaths ('knockdown') and there is a high probability of death unless emergency resuscitation is commenced. Hydrogen sulphide is also a pulmonary irritant and brief exposures above 500 ppm may cause acute non-cardiogenic pulmonary oedema; this potentially fatal complication can occasionally occur with prolonged exposures at concentrations exceeding 250 ppm. Hydrogen sulphide keratoconjunctivitis is usually a feature of subacute intoxication by the gas that may arise after prolonged exposure above 50–60 ppm, the symptoms being related to blepharitis and irritant conjunctivitis with lacrimation and photophobia. Sensations of grittiness or pain in the eye are associated with superficial punctate corneal erosions. Usually the eyes recover within 24 hours following removal from exposure, or after treatment with chloramphenicol eye ointment, but corneal ulceration and acute keratitis have been recorded. Upper respiratory tract irritation and conjunctivitis may also accompany acute inhalation poisoning.[137]

With prompt first aid and hospital treatment the overall fatality rate from hydrogen sulphide poisoning with loss of consciousness is low and recovery is normally complete.[140] However, in a small minority of patients neurological sequelae may be found after an episode of unconsciousness. There is no specific treatment for hydrogen sulphide poisoning and the use of nitrite therapy is controversial. There is no specific finding at autopsy. Blood sulphide concentrations can be measured in fatal and non-fatal poisonings using an ion-selective electrode method,[141] but blood and urine thiosulphate are believed to be more reliable by most laboratories,[142,143] though experience remains limited. As sulphaemoglobin is not formed in vivo by hydrogen sulphide, sulphaemoglobinaemia is not evidence of exposure to the gas.[144]

Evaluating the effects of hydrogen sulphide poisoning is complicated when case-reports often lack good information on exposure levels, in particular, the presence or absence of other gases, such as ammonia and carbon monoxide, which may be present due to fermentation processes. There is also dearth of good follow-up studies. Reports of interstitial fibrosis and chronic disability following pulmonary oedema (pneumonitis) are uncommon.[145] Clinical experience and animal experiments suggest that neurological damage due to hydrogen sulphide poisoning is similar to hypoxic brain damage from any other cause, and case-reports of delayed sequelae as in carbon monoxide poisoning are rare.[146] However, there is a group of patients occupationally exposed to hydrogen sulphide who present with non-specific symptoms such as hypersusceptibility to gas smells and other strong odours, fatigue, lack of energy, poor memory, irritability, decreased libido, and disturbances of equilibrium. There may even be signs of vestibular dysfunctioning on clinical investigation. Ahlborg concluded that the majority of these patients have suffered repeated episodes of intoxication without loss of consciousness.[147] There is insufficient evidence in the literature to justify the entity of chronic hydrogen sulphide intoxication at prolonged exposures at 50–100 ppm, and such levels above the occupational exposure standard should not be regularly encountered anyway in modern industry.

Chronic exposures to low levels in the environment, such as in geothermal areas, as well as at workplaces, have not been shown to be harmful though its unpleasant smell can be a considerable nuisance. The New Zealand city of Rotorua sits on a geothermal field, and the air is polluted by low levels of hydrogen sulphide, but there is an absence of scientific data on which to base opinions on the carcinogenicity, teratogenicity or reproductive effects of the gas in this or other locations.[148,149] The World Health Organization has issued a guideline concentration limit in ambient air of 7 $\mu g/m^3$ (30-minute averaging period), based on odour annoyance.[9] Natural gas may contain as much as 50% hydrogen sulphide that must be removed through refining. An escape of hydrogen sulphide from a refining plant into the local neighbourhood occurred in Poza Rica, Mexico, in 1950, resulting in 320 hospitalized persons and 22 deaths.[150]

Malodorous sulphur compounds

Hydrogen sulphide and methyl mercaptan are present in the breath of individuals with halitosis as a result of proteolytic activity by microorganisms residing on the tongue and teeth. Both substances, together with dimethyl sulphide and dimethyl disulphide are the principal air pollutants emitted by pulp mills. For safety reasons, odourants are added to natural domestic gas, namely diethyl sulphide, tertiary butyl mercaptan, ethyl mercaptan and methyl ethyl sulphide. Evidence for health effects of low level exposure to reduced sulphur compounds in the ambient air rests in studies of communities in the vicinity of sulphate paper mills in Finland, where concentrations of total reduced sulphur compounds in excess of 40 $\mu g/m^3$ (1-h or daily means) have been associated with daily reported symptoms of headache, depression, tiredness and nausea.[151] Dimethyl sulphide is allegedly the principal component of foetor hepaticus.[152]

CARBONYL SULPHIDE (COS)

[CAS no. 463–58–1]
Exposure limit not established
Relative density: 2.1
Flammability range: 12–29% (vol.)

The most abundant sulphur species in the atmosphere is carbonyl sulphide, being naturally produced from soil decomposition, wetlands and marshes, etc. The gas is often encountered with hydrogen sulphide in processes involving the destructive distillation of coal and the purification of petroleum. It is a colourless gas with an odour of rotten eggs that decomposes in moist air to carbon dioxide and hydrogen sulphide. The gas is less irritant to the lungs than hydrogen sulphide and probably acts in the same way on the central nervous system to cause respiratory paralysis.

SILANE (SiH$_4$)

[CAS no. 7803–62–5]
Exposure limits
   LTEL (8 h TWA) 0.5 ppm (0.67 mg/m^3)
   STEL (15 min) 1 ppm (1.3 mg/m^3)
Relative density: 1.1

Silane is a colourless gas with a repulsive odour and even at low concentrations is spontaneously flammable in air at room temperature. When silane burns in pipelines carrying the gas, silicon oxide dust is formed. The main use of silane is in the semiconductor industry as a source of high purity silicon where, because of its fire hazard, it has to be used under special control technology with the result that human exposure has tended to be minimal. There is little information on the effects of human exposure, but as it will form silicic acid in the presence of moisture it is assumed that silane will have an irritant effect on the eyes, mucous membranes and respiratory tract.

METHYL MERCAPTAN (METHANETHIOL) (CH$_3$SH)

[CAS no. 74–93–1]
Exposure limit
   LTEL (8-h TWA) 0.5 ppm (1 mg/m^3)
Relative density: 1.7
Flammability limits: 3.9–21.8%

Methyl mercaptan (methanethiol) is colourless and flammable with a very foul odour detectable at very low concentrations. It is reported to have similar toxic properties to hydrogen sulphide, being capable of causing central respiratory paralysis and pulmonary oedema. In a rare case of death by overexposure acute severe haemolytic anaemia and methaemoglobinaemia were found in the comatose victim, though this effect was probably unique to the patient who, in addition, suffered from glucose-6-phosphate dehydrogenase deficiency.[153]

HYDROGEN SELENIDE (H$_2$Se)

[CAS no. 7783–07–5]
Exposure limit
   LTEL (8 h TWA) 0.05 ppm (0.17 mg/m^3)
Relative density: 2.8

Hydrogen selenide is an irritant gas capable of causing pulmonary oedema. In one reported case of acute poisoning the effects were acute severe cough and wheeze which were followed by a lasting obstructive lung disorder.[154] Effects of chronic selenium exposure include extreme lassitude and fatiguability, garlic odour on the breath, tremor, excess perspiration, abdominal pain and vomiting and a metallic taste in the mouth. The gas is used in the preparation of selenides and is important as a doping gas in the semiconductor industry, but routine biological monitoring for selenium is not undertaken.

IRRITANT GASES WITH SYSTEMIC TOXIC EFFECTS

ARSINE (AsH$_3$)

[CAS no. 7784 42–1]
Exposure limit
   LTEL (8 h TWA) 0.05 ppm (0.16 mg/m^3)
Relative density: 2.69

Arsine is a colourless, non-irritating gas with a garlicky odour and is moderately soluble in water. Apart from its use in the manufacture of semiconductors in the microelectronics industry, its evolution is almost always accidental.[155] It can be produced by the action of water on a metallic arsenide, and an ore contaminated with arsenic will liberate arsine when treated with acid. Poisoning may arise in metal smelting and extraction, but exposure may also occur in galvanizing, soldering, etching and lead plating as well as in the disposal of toxic waste containing arsenic or arsenides (see Chapter 7).

The gas may lead to incidents in the most unexpected ways. In a classical incident off the British coast involving the *Asiafreighter*, a cylinder of arsine stored in the ship's hold leaked through a cylinder valve: four crew members who inspected the hold were inadvertently exposed to the gas. They suffered severe poisoning but exchange transfusion was lifesaving, the diagnosis having been made by a physician-toxicologist over the telephone.[156] The occupational and general physician should be alert to arsine poisoning and its characteristic features. The gas is a powerful haemolytic agent and its effects are usually fatal if exposure is severe enough to cause anuria, unless the diagnosis is made quickly and exchange transfusion is employed as a mainstay of treatment (see Chapter 44).

The presenting symptoms are nausea, vomiting and headache which can arise 2–24 hours after a casual exposure to arsine which may have lasted only 1–2 minutes. There may be no olfactory or other warning of the presence of the gas. Exposure to only 3–10 ppm of arsine in air can produce symptoms after several hours of exposure and 25–50 ppm for 30 minutes is potentially lethal in humans. The victim may early on pass dark red urine, and the combination of haemoglobinuria (without intact red blood cells in the urine), jaundice and abdominal pain should alert one to the diagnosis. The abdominal pain and jaundice typically arise in 24–48 hours and anuric or oliguric renal failure sets in by 72 hours.

Other causes of haemoglobinuria to be considered in the differential diagnosis are leptospirosis, malaria and paroxysmal nocturnal haemoglobinuria. Other chemical agents capable of causing haemoglobinuria include potassium chlorate, pyrogallic acid and stibine gas.

Diagnosis is made on the history of exposure and the finding of elevated urinary arsenic.

Because acute poisoning produces rapid and fulminant haemolysis, many body organs, particularly the kidney, are at risk from the sludging of red cell debris within the microcirculation, hypoxia and the direct effect of arsine, but the mechanisms involved are not fully understood. There is reticulocytosis and leucocytosis with an elevated plasma haemoglobin, and methaemoglobin may form in the plasma and urine. Renal failure from severe tubular necrosis is the main clinical complication and requires treatment with exchange transfusion to remove the arsine adequately.[157] In mild cases of haemoglobinuria forced diuresis is recommended. Recovery from the acute tubular necrosis may be followed by the development of chronic renal failure with glomerular sclerosis, atrophic tubules and interstitial fibrosis. A wide spectrum of clinical manifestations may arise including damage to the liver, myocardium, nervous system and bone marrow.

A chronic form of poisoning from low-level exposure to arsine has been described in workers engaged in the cyanide extraction of gold and in zinc smelting. This gave rise to severe anaemia, mildly elevated serum bilirubin and raised urinary arsenic.[155]

STIBINE (SbH₃)

[CAS no. 7803–52–3]
Exposure limits
LTEL (8 h TWA) 0.1 ppm (0.5 mg/m³)
STEL (15 min) 0.3 ppm (1.5 mg/m³)

Stibine is a highly toxic, colourless gas which is formed when an acid reacts with a metal containing antimony as an impurity, or when nascent hydrogen comes into contact with metallic antimony or a soluble antimony compound. The gas is not used in industry and its evolution is accidental. Exposure may occur in metallurgy or chemical laboratories but, unlike arsine, it has an extremely unpleasant odour. Stibine poisoning is rare in industry. The manifestations of poisoning and the physiological action of the gas resemble arsine, but are less fulminant. Haemolysis, myoglobinuria, haematuria, renal failure, nausea, vomiting, and headache have been reported after inhalation (see Chapter 44). Antimony trioxide is used as a fire retardant in plastics manufacture, and the release of stibine from PVC cot mattresses was considered, and later discounted, as a cause of sudden infant death syndrome. Urine antimony measurements may be used as a guide to overexposure to the gas in workers.

GERMANE (GeH₄)

[CAS no. 7782–65–2]
Exposure limits
LTEL (8 h TWA) 0.2 ppm (0.64 mg/m³)
STEL (15 min) 0.6 ppm (1.9 mg/m³)
Relative density: 2.6

Germane is flammable and colourless and has a pungent odour. Unlike its cousin arsine it is not encountered as an incidental product in ore or scrap processing. It is used to deposit pure germanium in semiconductor manufacturing.

The toxicity of the family appears to be in the order Ge, As, Sb. Although germane produces haemolysis, no industrial poisonings have been reported. By analogy with arsine, any victim of significant exposure should be removed to an intensive care facility and assessment of blood, kidney and cerebral function continued for some days.

PHOSPHINE (PH₃)

[CAS no. 7803–51–2]
Exposure limit
STEL (15 min 0.3 ppm (0.42 mg/m³)
Relative density: 1.18

Phosphine or hydrogen phosphide is a colourless, flammable gas which can auto-ignite at ambient temperatures if it contains other phosphorus anhydrides as impurities. Pure phosphine will auto-ignite above 38°C and forms an explosive mixture in air at concentrations greater than 1.8% by volume. The pure gas is considered odourless, but impurities will give it a characteristic smell of dead fish or garlic which may be imperceptible at low but hazardous concentrations.[158]

Phosphine is used as an intermediate in the synthesis of organophosphines and organic phosphonium derivatives. It is widely used in its pure form as a dopant in the manufacture of semiconductors, but it has chiefly gained notoriety through its use as a fumigant against insects and rodents in grain stores, in grain elevators and on board ships. It is an unwanted byproduct in various metallurgical reactions and in the manufacture of acetylene using impure calcium carbide. It may also be generated when water or acids come into contact with metals containing phosphide as a contaminant, such as ferrosilicon and spheroidal graphite iron.

Aluminium phosphide is a common poison used in suicide in India where it is widely used to fumigate stored grains. When consumed it reacts with hydrochloric acid in the stomach to liberate phosphine which then becomes a hazard to pathologists performing autopsies because the gas will escape when the stomach is opened. Phosphine may arise transiently in the anaerobic degradation of phosphorus-containing matter, as in marsh gas, but is otherwise rare in nature.

Aluminium or magnesium phosphide pellets are

inserted into the cargo of wheat on board ships for fumigation purposes. The moisture causes a chemical reaction which releases phosphine and leaves a harmless residue of aluminium hydroxide. Peak concentrations will arise in a sealed hold during a voyage and it is necessary that the gas is dissipated by opening the hatches to the air for at least 24 hours before the cargo is discharged. Accidental poisoning incidents continue to be reported with grain cargoes when gas escapes into living or working areas of the ship.[159] If the cargo is too dry, the gas is liberated after the hold is opened when the phosphide pellets come into contact with moist air: workers in the mill processing of the discharged cargo can then be affected.

Initial symptoms of exposure to low concentrations include headache, weakness, fainting, pain in the chest, cough, chest tightness and difficulty in breathing. With prolonged exposure, nausea, vomiting and diarrhoea may occur. The main hazard is pulmonary oedema which usually occurs within 24 hours, but may be delayed for up to 2 days. Central nervous system signs and symptoms, progressing to convulsions, coma and death, have been reported as have gastrointestinal symptoms such as nausea, vomiting, diarrhoea and severe epigastric pain.[158] Unlike arsine, phosphine does not cause haemolysis but one case of purpura ascribed to phosphine poisoning is known.[158] However, some sources of exposure to phosphine may also lead to exposure to arsine whose haemolytic effects should therefore be looked for. Chronic poisoning does not appear to have been recorded.

The reported maximum concentration that can be tolerated for several hours is 7 ppm. A level of 2000 ppm is regarded as rapidly fatal and the maximum exposure that can be tolerated for 30–60 minutes without serious effects is 100–200 ppm. Recovery from phosphine poisoning is usually complete.[158]

The evidence for genotoxic effects of phosphine in humans is inconclusive.[160]

METHYL BROMIDE (BROMOMETHANE) (CH₃Br)

[CAS no. 74–83–9]
Exposure limits
   LTEL (8 h TWA) 5 ppm (20 mg/m³)
   STEL (15 min) 15 ppm (59 mg/m³)
Relative density: 3.36
Flammability limits: 10–16% (but practically non-flammable)

Methyl bromide (bromomethane) is a colourless, odourless and relatively insoluble gas, but it is said to have a faintly detectable sweet odour at high concentrations. The gas is widely used as a fumigant, being toxic against mammals, insects, mites and pathogenic organisms in soil and compost.[161] Thus, it is used to fumigate soil in compost under gasproof sheets; fruit in ships' holds or freight containers; and in aircraft and special fumigation chambers. Fire extinguishers containing methyl bromide are no longer manufactured.

Methyl bromide is the most abundant gaseous bromine species in the atmosphere, being emitted from a wide range of natural as well as industrial sources. Atom for atom, bromine is about 50 times more effective than chlorine in destroying stratospheric ozone, and hence some countries are already moving to cease production and importation of methyl bromide. The gas is scheduled to be phased out in industrialized countries by the year 2005.

Sporadic cases of acute poisoning may still occur but, because of its severe toxicity and low warning properties, only qualified operators are normally permitted to work with this gas and they are well versed in the dangers and protective measures.

Occupational exposure is by inhalation or skin absorption. Although the hazards are well known, serious exposure incidents continue to occur due to lapses in the standard protective measures laid down for working with this gas. At low but dangerous concentrations, it has no irritating effects, thus dangerous exposure may occur without adequate warning, with onset of symptoms usually delayed from 30 minutes up to 48 hours later. Symptoms of mild exposure can come on within a few hours and include headache, eye and nose irritation, cough, nausea and malaise. At high exposures, the gas typically causes injury to the central nervous system as well as the lungs, producing headache, nausea, vomiting, pulmonary oedema (up to 30 h after exposure), tremors and convulsions followed by coma; the convulsions may not respond to standard anticonvulsant therapy. Health effects may also arise from chronic exposure to lesser concentrations, resulting in nervous system involvement with manifestations such as numbness (especially of the feet), visual disturbance (including optic atrophy), mental confusion, psychiatric disturbances and tremor (see Chapter 42).[161]

Exposure above 25 ppm is dangerous and acute central nervous system symptoms with possible permanent effects on the vision, hearing and balance are reported to occur above 120 ppm. Concentrations greater than 250 ppm are associated with pulmonary oedema, coma and convulsions. Exposure of the skin to high concentrations of vapour or liquid produces erythema and blister formation and severe burns, particularly if the gas or liquid is trapped under clothing. Blisters are usually large and surrounded by areas of redness and swelling; they may take a long time to heal. Severe inflammation of the eyes induced by the vapour may lead to conjunctivitis and temporary blindness.

First-aiders must not use mouth-to-mouth resuscitation. Treatment of acute poisoning should concentrate on controlling the convulsions and, if there is no response to drug therapy, muscular paralysis and positive pressure ventilation should be considered early on. The toxic mechanism is unknown and no specific antidotes are recognized, but the administration of dimercaprol and glutathione have been suggested.[162,163]

Regular users of methyl bromide should notify the

local hospital of the hazard and appropriate treatment measures. Biological monitoring should be undertaken by measuring serum bromide levels. According to the UK Health and Safety Executive a level of serum bromide of 0.18 mmol/litre (1.45 mg/dl) or more suggests occupational exposure, and above 0.35 mmol/litre (2.8 mg/dl, equivalent to a concentration of 28 ppm methyl bromide in air) symptoms may arise, but dietary intake should also be excluded as a cause of increased levels.[164] The toxic symptoms of methyl bromide are not directly related to the levels of circulating bromide and so the results must be interpreted with caution.

Methyl bromide is a methylating agent and is mutagenic in short-term tests, but is not carcinogenic in rodents.[165]

Poisoning by methyl bromide is a prescribed disease (see Chapter 4).

METHYL CHLORIDE (CHLOROMETHANE) (CH_3Cl)

[CAS no. 74–87–3]
Exposure limits
   LTEL (8 h TWA) 50 ppm (105 mg/m³)
   STEL (15 min) 100 ppm (210 mg/m³)
Relative density: 1.78
Flammability limits: 10.7–17.4 per cent

Methyl chloride is a colourless, flammable and sweet smelling gas which is widely used in the chemical industry, for example to produce methyl silicone polymers and resins, as a methylating agent in the production of butyl rubber and tetramethyl lead and as a blowing agent for polystyrene foams. The gas is a natural source of chlorine in the atmosphere, being released from the oceans and biomass burning.

The effects of methyl chloride and methyl iodide are similar to methyl bromide in that their primary target organs are the brain, liver, kidneys and lungs. All three are mutagens and potential carcinogens, and methyl chloride is a suspect occupational teratogen. However, the evidence for carcinogenicity or teratogenicity in humans is inadequate.

Because methyl chloride is almost odourless, hazardous levels of exposure may occur with little warning. In mild poisoning there is a staggering gait, dizziness, headaches, nausea and vomiting resembling acute alcoholism, followed by recovery. In more severe cases, symptoms and signs include vertigo, confusion, drowsiness, seizures, ataxia and diplopia; these effects may last for weeks and even months or lead on to coma and death.

METHYL ISOCYANATE (NCOCH₃)

[CAS no. 624–83–9]
Maximum exposure limits (as NCO)
   LTEL (8 h TWA) 0.02 mg/m³
   STEL (15 min) 0.07 mg/m³:
Relative density: 2

Methyl isocyanate is not a widely used chemical, but it gained worldwide notoriety after its disastrous release from the Union Carbide pesticide plant in Bhopal in India in 1984.[166] There it had been used in the chemical synthesis of carbaryl pesticides, and had been stored in liquid form in two steel tanks. The cause of the incident is still not known, but at 00:30 on 3 December 1984 an exothermic reaction took place in one of the storage tanks, resulting in the escape over a few hours of 40 tonnes of methyl isocyanate. A dense cloud of methyl isocyanate flowed over an area of the city about 40 square kilometres at a time when there was a temperature inversion and a light wind. At least 4000 people were killed and up to 100 000 injured. It is noteworthy that at the time of the accident there was scarcely any toxicological information available on the effects of methyl isocyanate in man.

Respiratory involvement was the most common serious health problem, with many victims suffering breathlessness, cough, throat irritation or choking, chest pain and haemoptysis. Death was mostly from bronchial necrosis or pulmonary oedema. An unknown proportion of survivors was reported to have developed bronchiolitis obliterans or interstitial fibrosis. Eye reactions were also prominent, and included severe watering, photophobia, lid oedema and corneal ulceration.

A follow-up study of survivors after 3 years reported an increased risk of eye infections and hyper-responsive phenomena, possibly related to immune disturbance.[167]. Unfortunately, follow-up studies of the survivors have been inadequate to document long-term pulmonary changes, as well as damage to other organs or teratogenic effects, and many questions on the chronic effects of this momentous event remain unanswered. A cross-sectional survey conducted 10 years after the gas leak suggested that many survivors had symptoms commensurate with persistent small airways obstruction and with obliterative bronchiolitis.[168] This incident showed the potential for disastrous releases into populated areas of chemicals of unknown but severe toxicity, and the need for the rapid setting up of investigative studies to evaluate the acute and long-term medical effects in order to assist the medical management of the exposed population.

ETHYLENE OXIDE (CH_2CH_2O)

[CAS no. 75–21–8]
Maximum exposure limit:
   LTEL (8 h TWA) 5 ppm (9.2 mg/m³)
Relative density: 1.49
Flammability limits in air: 3.0–80% (vol)

The main use of ethylene oxide is as a chemical intermediate in the production of ethylene glycol, polyester fibres and detergents, but it has been used on a much smaller scale since the 1950s as a sterilizing agent for medical supplies and foodstuffs. Most hospital gas sterilizers are automatic general purpose sterilizers and many of these use ethylene oxide, the gas being mixed with dichlorodifluoromethane to reduce the flammability and explosion risk. Exposures are controlled using exhaust systems, and air levels should be routinely monitored using sensor and alarm systems. The odour detection level is at least 500 ppm and is therefore of no value in warning the worker of significant exposure.[169]

Ethylene oxide is a narcotic and depresses the central nervous system as well as being a primary irritant of the respiratory tract. Acute exposure to high concentrations leads to nausea, vomiting and headache; also reported are excitement, muscular weakness, sleeplessness and diarrhoea. Four men were exposed to an intermittently leaking sterilizer (around 500 ppm) for 2–8 weeks and three developed a reversible peripheral neuropathy, and one reversible acute encephalopathy. Irreversible neuropathy and encephalopathy have been described in other operators of leaking sterilizers at similar levels of intermittent exposure[169] (see Chapter 42).

The gas condenses to a liquid at 10°C and is infinitely soluble in water. Excessive exposure to the vapour causes irritation of the eyes, whilst contact of the skin with even dilute solutions may cause erythema, oedema, blistering and necrosis. Allergic contact dermatitis has also been reported.

Ethylene oxide is considered to have potential for causing cancer and adverse reproductive effects in humans. It is a highly reactive epoxide and a direct alkylating agent, as well as being a recognized animal carcinogen associated with leukaemia and brain cancer in rodents. Chromosome aberrations and sister chromatid exchange have been found in studies of exposed workers. Epidemiological studies have not unequivocally demonstrated an association with human cancer, in particular of the haemopoietic system, but it is viewed as a probable human carcinogen by the International Agency for Research on Cancer (IARC).[170,171]

Medical surveillance of exposed workers using complete blood count and differential was recommended in the USA (lymphocytosis had been reported in symptomatically exposed workers), but no longer. Ethylene oxide is a potent sensitizing agent: occupational asthma associated with measurable IgE antibodies to ethylene oxide used to sterilize latex gloves and adsorbed on to the glove powder has been reported in a health care-worker.[172]

HEXAFLUOROACETONE (F_3CCOCF_3)

[CAS no. 684–16–2]
Exposure limit
   LTEL (8 h TWA) 0.1 ppm (ACGIH)
Relative density: 5.7

Hexafluoroacetone is colourless, non-flammable, fumes in moist air, and has a stale smell. It is very reactive and is used to prepare a variety of chemicals.

It is irritating to mucous membranes and especially

to the lung. Chronic exposure has been shown to lead to cumulative effects in the testes, kidney and bone marrow of experimental animals. It is teratogenic in rats.

DIBORANE (B_2H_6)

[CAS no. 19287–45–7]
Exposure limit
LTEL (8 h TWA) 0.1 ppm (0.12 mg/m³)
Relative density: 0.96
Flammability limits in air: 0.9–98.0%

As well as a doping agent for semiconductor manufacture diborane has uses in organic syntheses and in rocket fuel. It is a colourless gas with a sickly sweet odour. The ability to detect the odour is rapidly lost with exposure. It is spontaneously flammable in air, but because its ignition temperature (40–50°C) is above room temperature it may remain for several days in air at room temperature without igniting. Diborane is used as a dopant gas, a catalyst in polymer manufacture, and as a rubber vulcanizer. It is hydrolysed to boric acid in the moisture of the respiratory tract and exposure can cause dizziness, headache, drowsiness, chest tightness, cough and nausea. Severe poisoning with boranes is marked by convulsions and pulmonary oedema. The gas is also irritant to the eyes and skin and should be treated with the same respect as phosgene or chlorine.

The other boron hydrides are pentaborane and decaborane. These are more toxic than diborane and they can be readily absorbed through the skin and conjunctivae as well as by inhalation. Boranes are neurotoxic.

NICKEL CARBONYL (TETRACARBONYLNICKEL) ($Ni(CO)_4$)

[CAS no. 13463–39–3]
Exposure limit: (as nickel)
STEL (10 min) 0.1 ppm (0.24 mg/m³)
Relative density: at 50°C: 5.95
Lower flammability limit in air: 2% (vol.)

Nickel carbonyl is actually a liquid with a boiling point at 43°C but its vapour is highly toxic. It has a 'brick dust' odour detectable at 1–3 ppm. Nickel carbonyl is prepared by passing carbon monoxide over finely divided nickel. In the Mond process the gas is used to isolate nickel from its ore. The effects of occupational exposure have only been documented in workers engaged in the Mond process where occupational exposure has also been associated with an elevated incidence of carcinoma of the nasal cavities, lung and pharynx.

Exposure to raised levels of the vapour will cause the rapid onset of headache, dizziness, nausea, vomiting and dyspnoea, which rapidly disappear on removal from exposure. The worker should be kept under observation or admitted to hospital because potentially lethal sequelae may arise for up to 36 hours later with a risk of interstitial pneumonitis, pulmonary oedema, cerebral oedema and cerebral haemorrhage. The patient becomes febrile and cyanosed with a rapid pulse and develops a leucocytosis. Delirium may precede other central nervous system changes. Death may follow in 4–11 days after exposure. Exposure to 30 ppm, for 30 minutes is said to be potentially lethal in humans.

Nickel carbonyl is rapidly absorbed by the lungs and nickel levels rise in the blood and urine soon after exposure. Measurement of nickel in the blood and urine is an important guide for diagnosis and management. In severe cases, therapy with chelating agents to remove nickel from the body is recommended as well as treatment with oxygen and corticosteroids. Concomitant poisoning by carbon monoxide from the Mond process should be excluded by measuring carboxyhaemoglobin.

Mild cases present with giddiness, headache, nausea and weakness of the limbs and an affected worker can return to work if these symptoms pass off quickly. Close supervision is, however, necessary in more severe cases. The delayed stage generally starts 12–18 hours after the first symptoms, and is marked by retrosternal or epigastric tightness or pain that is aggravated by deep breathing or exertion. Conventional therapy is to start disulfiram (Antabuse®) in standard dosage as soon as possible, a drug normally used for the treatment of alcoholism but which also has chelating properties. A short course of oral prednisolone should also be given (starting with prednisolone 5 mg four times a day initially and tailed off over 5 days). The patient should be warned not to consume alcohol whilst receiving disulfiram.[173]

The degree of poisoning can be assessed by monitoring urinary nickel levels. The unexposed level is <50 µg/litre.

Poisoning by nickel carbonyl is a prescribed disease (see Chapter 4).

GASES WITH ANAESTHETIC ACTION: GENERAL ANAESTHETICS

The first deliberate use of an inhaled gas to produce anaesthesia for the performance of surgical operations was in animals, being carried out by Henry Hill Hickman in 1823 using carbon dioxide, but his work went unrecognized by medical opinion at the time (Later in the century, carbon dioxide was tried out on humans, but was unsuitable as it induced convulsions at anaesthetic concentrations). The first general anaesthetic to be used in surgery was diethyl ether in 1846 by William Morton in the Massachusetts General Hospital and later that year in a leg amputation performed by Robert Liston at University College Hospital, London. This agent was subsequently replaced by chloroform as the most widely used inhalational agent following its introduction by Sir James Simpson and James Snow in 1847.

Snow was later to achieve fame in public health when he ordered the removal of the Broad Street pump handle in the cholera epidemic of 1854. Joseph Priestley discovered nitrous oxide in 1772 and in 1800 Humphrey Davy had proposed the use of the gas as an anaesthetic.

Trichloroethylene later became popular in obstetrics, but it has now been discontinued in the USA and UK. Cyclopropane was popular for induction anaesthesia in children until the 1980s. Since 1956 the CFC halothane (CF3CHClBr) has been one of the most popular agents. Isoflurane has been used since 1971 and, because about 2% of the gas inhaled is biotransformed compared with 18% of halothane, it is considered safer for patients. Other agents in use are methoxyflurane and enflurane. Methoxyflurane, isoflurane and its isomer flurane undergo significant metabolic breakdown to fluoride compounds which can be nephrotoxic if given to a patient for 2–3 days, but this is not a consideration for the occupational exposure of anaesthetists.

Most concern over the health effects of anaesthetic gases has centred on the hazard to the reproductive system in anaesthetists and operating theatre staff. This was first highlighted in 1968 in a report describing a marked increase in spontaneous abortions amongst a group of female anaesthetists in the USSR. The combined results of subsequent epidemiological studies in Denmark, USA and the UK seemed at first to confirm this finding and in addition raised the possible risk of congenital abnormalities in pregnant women and in the offspring of male anaesthetists. In 1976 the UK Department of Health released a circular advising the use of scavenging systems in operating theatres. By 1980 the considered opinion was that spontaneous abortions in operating room staff were likely to be linked with exposure to inhalational agents. However, in the mid-1980s detailed evaluation of the evidence available then did not show support for any of the risks raised.[174,175] The current prudent view is that exposure to anaesthetic gases should be kept to a minimum and active or passive scavenging should be incorporated into operating theatre design (Fig. 8.11). A recent meta-analysis of the epidemiological studies based on data in the prescavenging era indicated an increased risk of spontaneous abortion.[176] Some of the earlier reports of adverse reproductive outcome may have been related to much higher exposures than occur today. Even now high levels of nitrous oxide can be achieved in poorly ventilated delivery rooms where a mixture of half nitrous oxide and half oxygen (Entonox, BOC Gases Ltd) is used for analgesia. These high levels could impair mood and cognitive functions in staff but in a study of more typical average time weighted exposure levels (nitrous oxide 58 ppm and halothane 1.4 ppm average) no changes were found.[177] However, high levels of nitrous oxide may impair fertility in female staff.[178]

Suspicion that the health of anaesthetists is poorer than other medical specialists keeps recurring and studies have suggested a higher risk of suicide, lymphomas

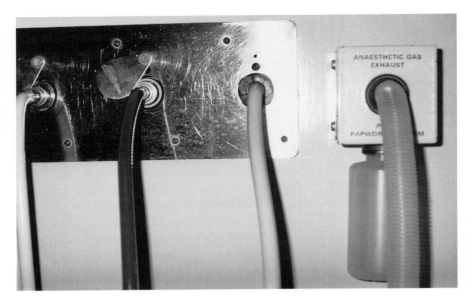

Figure 8.11 *Modern wall gas connections for operating threatre anaesthetic gas machine showing scavenging outlet.*

and reticuloendothelial tumours as well as an increased rate of early retirement on grounds of ill-health.[179] A mortality study of British anaesthetists found a doubling of deaths from suicide compared with other men in social class 1 but the rate was not significantly different from that amongst doctors as a whole.[179] It may be speculated that adverse health effects could be related to job factors such as sustained mental stress, long hours or inadequate time to rest and eat.

Occupational hygiene studies in the UK have shown that the geometric mean time weighted average exposure to nitrous oxide amongst anaesthetists is 94 ppm in unscavenged theatres compared with 32 ppm in scavenged theatres, the corresponding means for halothane being 1.7 ppm and 0.7 ppm. Active scavenging systems are much more effective than passive ones.[180] A further study by the Health and Safety Executive in 14 veterinary practices showed similar results though the duration of exposure of veterinarians and nurses was shorter than in hospital operating room staff; halothane is the most common inhalational agent used in veterinary practice.[181] Dental practices may also operate with inhalational agents for only a few hours a week. A high level of efficient forced general ventilation is important for reducing exposure levels by removing contaminants not handled by scavenging. Leakages readily occur from mask use, and intubation is to be preferred whenever it is clinically feasible.

Occupational exposure standards for anaesthetic gases were introduced in the UK in 1996, and these are equally applicable to manufacturing facilities as well as hospitals.[182] These are (8 h TWA): halothane 10 ppm (82 mg/m^3), enflurane 50 ppm (383 mg/m^3) and isoflurane 50 ppm (383 mg/m^3). As anaesthetic gases are toxic agents they all call for consideration under the Control of Substances Hazardous to Health Regulations (1988). In hospitals, compliance with the occupational exposure standards is achievable through balanced supply and extract ventilation with high rates of air change in, e.g. delivery rooms and recovery areas, as well as by the use of gas scavenging equipment in operating theatres.[175]

NITROUS OXIDE (N$_2$O)

[CAS no. 10024−97−2]
Exposure limit
  LTEL (8 h TWA) 100 ppm (183 mg/m^3)
Relative density: 1.5

Nitrous oxide is a stable, toxic gas which has been shown experimentally to interfere with DNA synthesis by inactivating vitamin B12, a coenzyme for methionine synthase activity. It is not normally used for prolonged periods, as in intensive care, because it may cause megaloblastic changes in the bone marrow if exposure goes on for longer than 24 hours. Excessive occupational exposure to the gas in dentists has been reported to cause measurable bone marrow changes from depression of vitamin B12 activity.[183] Agranulocytosis and subacute combined degeneration of the spinal cord have also occurred after repeated exposure in patients. Experimental studies of nitrous oxide in animals indicate that at subanaesthetic levels it may reduce fetal weight and growth, but there is no evidence of teratogenicity or mutagenicity. However, a study of female dental assistants suggested that exposure to high levels of unscavenged nitrous oxide may impair fertility as measured by an increased time before conception.[178] Nitrous oxide neuropathy has been reported in abusers of the gas. Abusers may develop addictive behaviour, tolerance and psychological dependence, and anaesthetists are an at-risk group because of their access to the gas. Deaths have occurred in health care workers who have tried to obtain a 'high' without using supplementary oxygen. (Nitrous oxide abuse has also been reported in the restaurant trade where it is used in power whipped cream dispensers and as a non-tainting foaming agent for dairy products.) Overall, there is no convincing evidence that exposure to nitrous oxide in the workplace has caused developmental defects in the fetus or any other reproductive health effects, but this lack of evidence should not foster complacency in its usage.

Other common anaesthetically active gases

ACETYLENE (ETHYNE) (C₂H₂)

[CAS no. 74–86–2]
Exposure limit not established
Relative density: 0.9

Acetylene is a colourless, highly flammable gas. It is regarded as a simple asphyxiant, but marked intoxication will occur at 20% mixture in air. Very pure acetylene has a pleasant sweet smell but commercial acetylene smells of garlic. It burns at a very high temperature with oxygen, up to approximately 3500 °C.

Acetylene is used in the manufacture of many organic chemicals and polymers. Its fierce flame is used for oxy-acetylene cutting and welding and wherever there is an application for great heat.

CYCLOPROPANE (C₃H₆)

[CAS no. 79–19–4]
Exposure limit: 400 ppm (ACGIH)
Relative density 1.4

Cyclopropane is colourless, flammable and smells like ether. It is used for chemical synthesis and was popular as a general anaesthetic, mainly in children.

DIMETHYL ETHER (CH₃OCH₃)

[CAS no. 115–10–6]
Exposure limits
LTEL 400 ppm (766 mg/m³)
STEL 500 ppm (958 mg/m³)
Relative density: 1.6

Dimethyl ether is colourless, flammable and is used as a refrigerant and as a fuel gas in welding. It has a lesser anaesthetic action than diethyl ether.

METHYL VINYL ETHER (CH₃OCH:CH₂)

[CAS no. 109–92–2]
Exposure limit not established
Relative density: 2.0

The principal physiological effect of this gas is its anaesthetic action, but it is much less than that produced by dimethyl ether.

2,2-DIMETHYL PROPANE C(CH₃)₄

[CAS no. 463–82–1]
Exposure limit not established
Relative density: 2.5

2,2-Dimethyl propane is a colourless, flammable gas. It is used in the manufacture of synthetic rubber.

ETHANE (CH₃CH₃)

[CAS no. 74–84–0]
Exposure limit not established
Relative density: 1.0

Ethane is colourless, odourless and flammable. It is regarded as a simple asphyxiant, and is used as a low temperature refrigerant and an antiknock agent.

ETHYL CHLORIDE (CHLOROETHANE) (C₂H₅Cl)

[CAS no. 75–00–3]
Exposure limits
LTEL (8 h TWA) 1000 ppm (2700 mg/m³)
STEL (10 min) 1250 ppm (3280 mg/m³)
Relative density: (gas) 2.2

Ethyl chloride is colourless and flammable, with an ethereal odour. It is used as a refrigerant, a local spray anaesthetic and as a specialized solvent. At 40 000 ppm (4%) it produces stupor and eye irritation almost at once.

ETHYLENE (CH₂CH₂)

[CAS no. 74–85–1]
Exposure limit not established
Relative density: 0.98

Ethylene is a colourless, flammable and sweet smelling gas which is regarded as a simple asphyxiant. It is used in horticulture for ripening fruit and increasing plant growth rates, and in specialized welding. It is an important feedstock in the production of ethylene oxide and many polymers.

ISOBUTANE ((CH(CH₃)₃)

[CAS no. 75–28–7]
Exposure limit not established
Relative density: 2.1

Isobutane is the simplest isoalkane. It is a colourless, flammable gas which is mainly used as an intermediate in the production of aviation fuel and various organic chemicals.

ISOBUTYLENE ((CH₃)₂CCH₂)

[CAS no. 75–28–5]
Exposure limit not established
Relative density: 1.9

Isobutylene is a colourless, flammable gas used in the manufacture of butyl rubber.

Liquefied petroleum gases

N-BUTANE (CH₃CH₂CH₂CH₃)

[CAS no. 106–97–8]
Exposure limits
 LTEL (8 h TWA) 600 ppm (1450 mg/m³)
 STEL (15 min) 750 ppm (1810 mg/m³)
 Relative density: 2.1
 Flammability limits: 1.8–8.4% (vol.)

Butane is a colourless, flammable gas with a mild aromatic odour, widely used in the petrochemical industry and as a fuel.

PROPANE (CH₃CH₂CH₃)

[CAS no. 744–98–6]
Exposure limit not established
Relative density: 1.5
Flammability limits: 2.2–9.5% (vol.)

Propane is colourless and flammable. It is widely used as a fuel gas, in welding, as a solvent and as a refrigerant.

PROPYLENE (CH₃CHCH₂)

[CAS no. 115–07–1]
Exposure limit not established
Relative density: 1.5
Flammability limits: 2.0–11.1% (vol.)

Propylene is a colourless, flammable gas. It is a widely used chemical feedstock.

VINYL BROMIDE (CH₂CHBR)

[CAS no. 693–60–2]
Exposure limit
 LTEL (8 h TWA) 5 ppm (20 mg/m³)
Relative density: 3.79
Flammability limits: 9–14% (vol.)

Vinyl bromide is a colourless, flammable gas with a pleasant smell. It is a chemical intermediate, a flame retardant and is used to manufacture acrylic fibres. Easily polymerized, it is used as a fire retardant in plastics. It behaves like an anaesthetic gas, inhalation of very high concentrations leading to coma and death. Liquid splashes are irritant to the eyes and skin. The gas is mutagenic and induces liver angiosarcoma and hepatocellular carcinoma in laboratory animals exposed through inhalation; it is therefore a suspect human carcinogen.

VINYL CHLORIDE (CH₂CHCl)

[CAS no. 75–01–4]
Maximum exposure limits
 Day: LTEL (8 h TWA) 7 ppm *Year*: mean not to exceed 3 ppm

Relative density: 2.21
Flammability limits: 4–22% (vol.)

The main use of vinyl chloride monomer (VCM) is to manufacture PVC, the most widely used plastic polymer. Production took off after the Second World War. Polymerization is a batch process undertaken in autoclaves. In the past workers entered the autoclaves after each batch to clean them from inside; unfortunately VCM was regarded as very safe and many workers failed to use adequate respiratory protection. As a result, very high levels of exposure to VCM occurred until 1974. when the first human cases of angiosarcoma of the liver were reported in workers (see Chapters 39, 43).

Health problems associated with these high exposures had begun to be recognized in the mid-1960s. Acro-osteolysis typically affected the terminal phalanges of the hands, giving rise to 'pseudo-clubbing', with clinical and radiological appearances which resemble those seen in some patients with hyperparathyroidism. Other bones could also be affected. Scleroderma and Raynaud's phenomenon were also reported.

Animal studies were undertaken to reproduce acro-osteolysis experimentally and these unexpectedly led to the discovery that VCM caused angiosarcoma of the liver, with the first report of the tumour in VCM workers emerging from the USA in 1974. Since then over 150 cases associated with the industry have been reported worldwide. Angiosarcoma of the liver is an extremely rare tumour in the general population,[184] but sporadic cases without obvious causal factors arise in all age groups. Almost all of the occupational tumours have been reported in highly exposed VCM autoclave workers, though many other chemical workers had some contact with VCM before its dangers were known and its usage came under strict control (in 1974 in the UK and USA). Hepatic injury from this chemical also produces non-cirrhotic periportal fibrosis and portal hypertension. Workers exposed in the PVC manufacturing industry before 1974 are at potential risk of manifesting these problems.

The adverse effects of VCM are unlikely to be seen arising from present-day working conditions in the UK and USA, but chemical firms should ensure that general practitioners have a history of exposure to vinyl chloride in the individual's medical record. There are, however, no screening tests of use in the early detection of angiosarcoma of the liver or periportal fibrosis, including special imaging. There is presently insufficient evidence to implicate VCM exposure in humans as a causal factor in primary cancers at other sites such as lung and brain (see Chapter 4).

Heating plastic packaging film will form thermal degradation products which may be associated with symptoms known as 'meat wrappers' asthma'. All heated plastics will generate carbon monoxide but PVC also gives off hydrogen chloride and plasticizers such as dioctyl phthalate and di-octyl adipate. The polyolefin plastics (polyethylene and polypropylene) can produce formaldehyde and acrolein. The degradation products are normally quickly dispersed and diluted, but attention needs to be paid to the correct operation of manual heating sealing machines to ensure temperature regulation, and the cleanliness and maintenance of the sealing head. Inhalation incidents have been reported in PVC film manufacture if the film is accidentally overheated.

VINYL FLUORIDE (CH$_2$CHF)

[CAS no. 75–02–5)
Vinyl fluoride, a chemical intermediate, is a relatively non-toxic gas.

MIXED EXPOSURE TO GASES

Irritant and nerve gases

The earliest efforts to use gases as weapons were in classical times with the lighting of bonfires and the hurling of pitch and sulphur.[23] Chlorine was the first chemical warfare agent used in modern times when it was exploited by the German army against the Allies at Ypres in 1915. Subsequently the Germans mixed chlorine with phosgene, or phosgene was deployed alone. Blister agents, mustard gas and arsenicals were also introduced in the First World War, and altogether chemical agents were responsible for approximately 1.3 million casualties, of which at least 90 000 were fatal. Mustard gas was the most widely used agent by the end of the First World War, but phosgene was responsible for most of the deaths.[23]

Much more poisonous than these irritant gases are the nerve 'gases' or organophosphorus compounds that inhibit tissue cholinesterase in man at small dosages. The first to be discovered was tabun in 1936 which was in production by the Second World War; sarin and soman were developed subsequently. The nerve gases and blister agents are not really gases, but are encountered as vapours or liquids.

The nerve agents are closely related to organophosphorous pesticides which have similar clinical manifestations and the treatment of poisoning is the same (see Chapter 10). However, it is unlikely that these agents would be used in warfare in their pure form and quite unexpected clinical features could arise in exposed combatants or civilians. The terrorist attack with sarin on the Tokyo subway on 20 March, 1995, caused 12 deaths and more than 5000 people attended hospital.[185] The same agent was used in an incident in a residential area in the city of Matsumoto in 1994, when seven people died and about 600 residents and rescue staff were poisoned.[186,187] Hydrogen cyanide is a potential chemical warfare agent because it is used in a wide range of chemical industries

and its production for sinister purposes could go undetected, but it would have to be released in high concentrations to be effective against populations.

In the Gulf War in 1990–1991 the Iraqi forces had stocks of shells of mustard gas and tabun which in the event were not used. The threat against civilian as well as military targets led to extensive defensive preparations by the Allies and the Israeli Civil Defence. This war showed that the deployment of chemical weapons remains a likely option for aggressors in future hostilities around the world. Studies of British and US Gulf War veterans are continuing in response to a wide array of medical complaints reported by veterans and their families, but evidence for a specific Gulf War Syndrome is lacking[188] (see Chapter 42). The UK ceased manufacture of chemical weapons in 1957. The disposal of stockpiles of chemical weapons presents considerable problems for worker safety and environmental protection.

Vesicant agents

The blister or vesicant agents include sulphur mustard (mustard gas), nitrogen mustard and the arsenical agents such as lewisite. Mustard gas is a liquid which gives off a dangerous vapour which has a delayed onset, with a vesicant action on the skin and injury to the eyes and respiratory tract. Typically there are no effects immediately on exposure but acute conjunctivitis develops between 30 minutes and 3 hours later. This is followed by an irritant bronchitis with sore throat and coughing. Within a few hours the symptoms become more pronounced and the voice is husky. Gastric pain, nausea and vomiting may develop and the exposed skin starts to itch and become erythematous. Death almost never occurs during the first day. On the second day the inflammation of the respiratory tract becomes severe and expectoration may contain large sloughs of tracheal mucosa. Potentially fatal complications are bronchopneumonia and depression of the bone marrow about 2 weeks after exposure.[23,189]

The vesicant agents attack mainly moist areas of the skin, causing blister formation in the groins, genitalia, buttocks, axillae and inner thighs. Lewisite is more volatile and more acutely irritant than mustard gas, and arsenic can be detected in the tissues and urine following exposure sufficient to cause symptoms. Mustard gas was deployed in combat in the Iraq/Iran war. Civilian medical and nursing attendants were at risk of being contaminated themselves when handling casualties. Victims of mustard gas poisoning should therefore be well decontaminated before being treated, but the blister fluid does not contain the toxin.

CS GAS (C$_{10}$H$_5$ClN$_2$)

[CAS no. 2698-41-1]
The riot control agent most widely used by police and military forces is CS gas (O-chlorobenzylidene malanonitrile). It is fired in cartridges from tear gas guns or in

grenades into crowds when it produces irritating and disabling effects if it comes in contact with the eyes, or if it is inhaled.[23] It is a powder, not a gas, or it can be dispersed as a smoke. Release of CS into the confined spaces of houses can cause fatalities.

The toxic basis of this agent is uncertain, but the pronounced irritation is due to the local formation of hydrochloric acid. The victim suffers a burning sensation in the eyes with lacrimation, rhinorrhoea, sneezing, irritation of the skin, coughing and difficulty in breathing. Higher concentrations produce nausea and vomiting with conjunctivitis, tracheitis and bronchitis. Asthma sufferers may develop bronchospasm. Treatment is symptomatic and recovery is usually rapid on exposure to fresh air.

Because CS solidifies on the skin and clothes, the use of CS batons can become an occupational health issue for police officers, police doctors, ambulance and hospital personnel. As used by UK police forces, it is dissolved at 5% weight per volume (w/v) methyl iso-butyl ketone (MiBK) with nitrogen as a propellant. Accident and emergency staff receiving contaminated persons should wear impermeable gloves and close fitting goggles. Clothing should be removed and placed in sealed plastic bags, but irrigating the face and eyes with water is not advised.[190] Instead, dry air should be blown directly on the eyes with an electric fan. If the skin effects persist for 30 minutes, showering in water for at least 15 minutes is recommended. Severe dermatitis and ocular injuries, including keratitis, have been reported. Further investigations of the safety of CS are warranted.[191]

Semiconductor industry

The production of semiconductor chips is at the centre of computer manufacture and the modern electronic industry, and toxic and flammable gases are among the most hazardous materials employed. These include ammonia, hydrogen chloride, silane, phosphine, arsine, diborane, hydrogen, chlorine, trichlorosilane, germane, boron trifluoride, boron bichloride, and silicon tetrafluoride. The processes are complex and multistaged. Silicon chips are wafers of silicon or, as in special applications such as laser and optical fibres, of gallium arsenide. Electronic circuits are imprinted by a photolithograph process that requires the use of solvents such as isopropanol, methanol, methyl ethyl ketone, methyl n-butyl ketone, glycol ethers and chlorobenzene. The circuits are etched on to the silicon wafer using hydrofluoric or hydrochloric acids. The electrical properties of the wafer are then altered by exposing it to dopant gases such as arsine, phosphine or diborane. Toxic gases are also employed in plasma deposition and plasma etching processes.

To ensure a high degree of purity of the gases, closed and automated gas handling systems are required which will incidentally reduce the potential for human exposure. In addition, the gases silane, diborane and phosphine are pyrophoric, and silane in particular has been responsible for fires and explosions in the industry in the past. These gases are piped into furnaces and chambers with carrier gases such as nitrogen which is also used to purge the lines. Automatic monitoring for toxic gases may be undertaken, particularly for arsine which can be difficult for a worker to detect at low concentrations in the working atmosphere.

The worker is usually at most risk of a hazardous exposure when connecting up the gas cylinders: a safe system of work is essential. The cylinders supplying gas to the closed lines are kept in gas cabinets which are exhaust ventilated to the outside to prevent a build-up of gases from leaks.

Despite these precautions concerns have arisen for the health of workers with potential exposure to the numerous solvents, acids, gases and metals used. In particular, epidemiological studies of adverse reproductive outcomes in female workers in US semiconductor manufacturing facilities have suggested that an elevated risk of spontaneous abortion and low birthweight is associated with solvent or other chemical exposures.[192,193] Regular urinary arsenic estimations in workers exposed to arsine are undertaken in some firms but these are unlikely to be abnormal where continuous air monitoring for arsine is routinely undertaken.

Geothermal power

The possibility of using hydrothermal energy to produce heat and electricity arises in parts of the world where there is active volcanism or where magma (liquid rock) lying close to the earth's surface forms shallow bodies of hot rocks and fluids (Fig. 8.12). The world's first geothermal steam field was built at Larderello, Italy, in 1904 and today the world's largest, The Geysers, California, produces nearly 2000 megawatts of electricity. In Reykjavik, Iceland, all the hot water needs of the city are provided by geothermal sources.

The occupational and environmental problems of utilizing geothermal power must be assessed separately in different parts of the world as the technology needed to generate electricity from steam turbines using geothermal energy and the toxic compounds arising in geothermal fluids may vary widely.[192,193] In the steam fields in Utah and California hydrogen sulphide, ammonia, carbon dioxide, methane and radon-222 are the chief gases emitted. Of these, hydrogen sulphide is the most important, but in fields elsewhere in the world it may be only a minor component. Leaks from geothermal steam wells may expose workers to gases and toxic compound such as mercury, arsenic, boron, selenium, lead, cadmium and fluoride. Steam leaving turbines is passed through a condenser and it

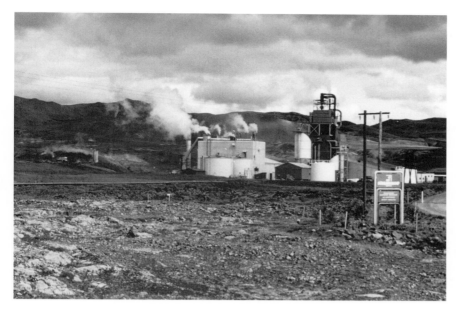

Figure 8.12 *The Icelandic Diatomite Plant at Lake Myvatn uses geothermal steam to dry algal deposits dredged from the lake bottom, and power is fed directly from the nearby Krafla geothermal power plant. Elsewhere in the world diatomaceous earth (kieselguhr) is obtained by open-cast mining.*

gases and entrained substances from leaks inside the plant or by working on or near drilling rigs. Carbon dioxide may pose a risk of asphyxiation in confined spaces, and accidental blow-outs of wells can occur.

REFERENCES

1 Sallie B, McDonald C. Inhalation accidents reported to the SWORD Surveillance Project 1990–1993. *Ann Occup Hyg* 1996; **40**: 211–21.
2 Organization for Economic Co-operation and Development. OECD Monograph No. 81. *Health Aspects of Chemical Accidents*. Paris: OECD, 1994.
3 Caplin M. Ammonia-gas poisoning. Forty-seven cases in a London shelter. *Lancet* 1941; **ii**: 95–6.
4 Henderson Y, Haggard HW. *Noxious Gases* 2nd edn. New York: Reinhold, 1943.
5 Health and Safety Executive. *EH40/99. Occupational Exposure Limits 1999*. Norwich:HMSO, 1999.
6 Illing HPA. Assessment of toxicity for major hazards: some concepts and problems. *Hum Toxicol* 1989; **8**: 369–74.
7 Rusch GM. The history and development of emergency response guidelines. *J Hazardous Materials* 1993; **33**: 193–202.
8 McCunney RJ. Emergency response to environmental toxic incidents: the role of the occupational physician. *Occup Med* 1996; **46**: 397–401.
9 World Health Organization. *Air Quality Guidelines for Europe*. Copenhagen: WHO, 1987.
10 Health and Safety Commission. Advisory Committee on Dangerous Substances. *Major Hazard Aspects of the Transport of Dangerous Substances*. London: HMSO, 1991.
11 Health and Safety Executive. *The Control of Industrial Major Accident Hazards Regulations (CIMAH): Further Guidance on Emergency Plans*. London: HMSO, 1985.

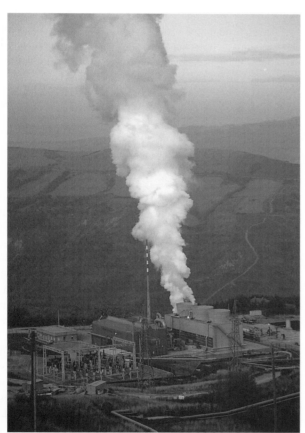

Figure 8.13 *Steam venting from a geothermal power plant in Tuscany, Italy. Mount Amiata is an extinct volcano where mercury ore was mined until 1980.*

is the 'non-condensable' gases and toxic compounds that will enter cooling towers and a portion of these will escape into the air (Fig. 8.13). The drift from the cooling tower may waft around and be deposited in the vicinity. Workers may also be exposed to hazardous

12 Baxter PJ, Davies PC, Murray V. Medical planning for toxic releases into the community: the example of chlorine gas. *Br J Ind Med* 1989; **46**: 277–85.

13 National Research Council. *Fire and Smoke: Understanding the Hazards.* Washington: National Academy Press, 1986.

14 Purser DA. Toxicity assessment of combustion products. In: *SFPE Handbook of Fire Protection Engineering* 2nd edn. Boston: National Fire Protection Association, 1995: 2.85–2.146.

15 Baxter PJ, Heap BJ, Rowland MGM, Murray VSG. Thetford Plastics fire, October 1991: the role of a preventive medical team in chemical incidents. *Occup Environ Med* 1995; **52**: 694–8.

16 Hobbs PV, Radke LF. Airborne studies of the smoke from the Kuwait oil fires. *Science* 1992; **256**: 987–90.

17 Stern SCM, Kumar R, Roberts IAG. Aplastic anaemia after exposure to burning oil. *Lancet* 1995; **346**: 183.

18 Kinsella J, Carter R, Reid WH, Campbell D, Clark CJ. Increased airways reactivity after smoke inhalation. *Lancet* 1991; **337**: 595–7.

19 Axford AT, McKerrow CB, Jones AP, Le Quesne PM. Accidental exposure to isocyanate fumes of a group of firemen. *Br J Ind Med* 1976; **33**: 65–71.

20 Guidotti TL, Clough VM. Occupational health concerns of firefighting. *Ann Rev Publ Hlth* 1992; **13**: 151–71.

21 Medvedev ZA. *The Legacy of Chernobyl.* London: Blackwell, 1990.

22 Smith R. Chernobyl and public health. *Lancet* 1998; **316**: 952–3.

23 Marrs TC, Maynard RL, Sidell FR. Chemical warfare agents. *Toxicology and Treatment.* Chichester: Wiley, 1996.

24 Williams AJ. Assessing and interpreting arterial blood gases and acid-base balance. *Br Med J* 1998; **317**: 1213–6.

25 Pritchard JS. Pulmonary oedema. In: Weatherall DJ, Ledingham JGG, Warrell DA eds. *Oxford Textbook of Medicine* 3rd edn. Oxford: Oxford University Press, 1996: 2495–505.

26 Department of Health. *Advisory Group on the Medical Aspects of Air Pollution Episodes: Ozone.* London: HMSO, 1991.

27 Wright JL, Churg A. Diseases caused by gases and fumes. In: Churg A, Green FHY eds. *Pathology of Occupational Lung Disease* 2nd edn. Baltimore: Williams and Wilkins, 1998: 57–75.

28 Beale R, Grover ER, Smithies M, Bihari D. Acute respiratory distress syndrome (ARDS): no more than a severe acute lung injury? *Lancet* 1993; **307**: 1335–39.

29 Zapol WM, Lemaire F. *Adult Respiratory Distress Syndrome.* New York: Marcel Dekker, 1991.

30 Brooks SM. Occupational asthma. *Chest* 1985; **87** (Suppl): 218–22.

31 Alberts AM, Do Pico GA. Reactive airways dysfunction syndrome. *Chest* 1996; **109**: 1618–26.

32 Aver RA, Benveniste H. Hypoxia and related conditions. In: Graham DI, Lantos PL eds. *Greenfield's Neuropathology* 6th edn. London: Arnold: 1997: 263–314.

33 Lovelock J. *The Ages of Gaia.* Oxford: Oxford University Press, 1989.

34 Haldane JS, Priestley JG. *Respiration.* Oxford: Clarendon Press, 1935.

35 King TS, Elia M, Hunter JO. Abnormal colonic fermentation in irritable bowel syndrome. *Lancet* 1998; **352**: 1187–9.

36 Cummings J, Pitcher M. Hydrogen sulphide: a bacterial toxin in ulcerative colitis? *Gut* 1996; **39**: 1–4.

37 Preller L, Heederik D, Boleij JSM, Vogelzang PFJ, Tielen MJM. Lung function and chronic respiratory symptoms of pig farmers: focus on exposure to endotoxins and ammonia and use of disinfectants. *Occup Environ Med* 1995; **52**: 654–60.

38 Health and Safety Executive. Safe work in confined spaces. *Confined Spaces Regulations 1997. Approved Code of Practice Regulations and Guidance.* Norwich: HMSO, 1997.

39 Watt MK, Watt SJ, Seaton A. Episode of toxic gas exposure in sewer workers. *Occup Environ Med* 1997; **54**: 277–80.

40 Haldane J. The air of mines. In: Oliver T ed. *Dangerous Trades.* London: John Murray, 1902: 540–56.

41 Boogaard PJ, Houtsma A-T AJ, Journée HL, Van Sittert NJ. Effects of exposure to elemental mercury on the nervous system and the kidneys of workers producing natural gas. *Arch Environ Hlth* 1996; **51**: 108–14.

42 Sand G. *La Petite Fadette.* Paris: Garnier Flammarion, 1967.

43 Baxter PJ, Kapila M, Mfonfu D. Lake Nyos disaster, Cameroon, 1986: the medical effects of large scale emission of carbon dioxide? *Br Med J* 1989; **298**: 1437–41.

44 Stupfel M, Le Guern F. Are there biomedical criteria to assess an acute carbon dioxide intoxication by a volcanic emission? *J Volcanol Geothermal Res* 1989; **39**: 247–64.

45 Brighten P. A case of industrial carbon dioxide poisoning. *Anaesthesia* 1976; **31**: 406–9.

46 Farrar CD, Sorey ML, Evans WC. Forest-killing diffuse CO_2 emissions at Mammoth Mountain as a sign of magmatic unrest. *Nature* 1995; **376**: 675–7.

47 Norbäck D, Björnsson E, Janson C, Widström J, Boman G. Asthmatic symptoms and volatile organic compounds, formaldehyde, and carbon dioxide in dwellings. *Occup Environ Med* 1995; **52**: 388–95.

48 Centers for Disease Control. Carbon monoxide poisoning at an indoor ice arena and bingo hall. *Morbid Mortal Weekly Rep* 1996; **45**: 265–7.

49 Fawcett TA, Moon RE, Fracica PJ, Mebane GY, Theil DR, Piantadosi CA. Warehouse workers' headache. Carbon monoxide poisoning from propane-fueled forklifts. *J Occup Med* 1992; **34**: 12–15.

50 World Health Organization. *Carbon Monoxide: Environmental Health Criteria 13.* Geneva: WHO, 1979.

51 Forbes WH, Sargent F, Roughton FJW. The rate of carbon monoxide uptake by normal men. *Am J Physiol* 1945; **143**: 594–608.

52 Coburn RF, Forster RE, Kane PB. Considerations of the

physiological variables that determine the blood carboxyhaemoglobin concentration in man. *J Clin Invest* 1965: **44**: 1899–1910.

53 Illing HPA, Shillaker RO. Dichloromethane (methylene chloride). *Toxicity Review 12*. Health and Safety Executive. London: HMSO, 1985.

54 Stewart RD, Hake CL. Paint-remover hazard. *JAMA* 1976; **235**: 398–401.

55 Barnett K, Wilson JF. quantification of carboxyhaemoglobin in blood: external quality assessment of techniques. *Br J Biomed Sci* 1998; **55**: 123–6.

56 Ernst A, Zibrak JD. Carbon monoxide poisoning. *N Engl J Med* 1998; **339**: 1603–8.

57 Thom SR, Taber RL, Mendiguren II, Clark JM, Hardy KR, Fisher AB. Delayed neuropsychologic sequelae after carbon monoxide poisoning: prevention by treatment with hyperbaric oxygen. *Toxicology* 1995; **25**: 474–80.

58 Hardy KR, Thom SR. Pathophysiology and treatment of carbon monoxide poisoning. *Clin Toxicol* 1994; **32**: 613–29.

59 Choi IS. Delayed neurologic sequelae in carbon monoxide poisoning. *Arch Neurol* 1983; **40**: 433–5.

60 Sidney Smith J, Brandon S. Morbidity from acute carbon monoxide poisoning at three-year follow-up. *Br Med J* 1973; **1**: 318–32.

61 Sawada Y, Takahasi M, Ohashi N. Computerised tomography as an indication of long-term outcome after acute carbon monoxide poisoning. *Lancet* 1980; **i**: 783–84.

62 Vieregge P, Klostermann W, Blüm RG, Borgis KJ. Carbon monoxide poisoning: clinical, neurophysiological, and brain imaging observations in acute disease and follow-up. *J Neurol* 1989; **236**: 478–81.

63 De Reuck J, Decoo D, Lemahieu I, Strijckmans K, Boon P *et al*. A positron emission tomography study of patients with acute carbon monoxide poisoning treated by hyperbaric oxygen. *J Neurol* 1993; **240**: 430–4.

64 Department of the Environment. *Expert Panel on Air Quality Standards: Carbon Monoxide*. London: HMSO, 1994.

65 Allred EN, Bleecker ER, Chaitman BR *et al*. Short-term effects of carbon monoxide exposure on the exercise performance of subjects with coronary heart disease. *N Engl J Med* 1989; **321**: 1426–32.

66 Stern FB, Halperin WE, Hornung RW, Ringenburg VL, McCammon CS. Heart disease mortality among bridge and tunnel officers exposed to carbon monoxide. *Am J Epidemiol* 1988; **128**: 1276–88.

67 Norman CA, Halton DM. Is carbon monoxide a workplace teratogen? A review and evaluation of the literature. *Ann Occup Hyg* 1990; **34**: 335–47.

68 Peden NR, Taha A, McSorley PD, Bryden GT, Murdock IB, Anderson JM. Industrial exposure to hydrogen cyanide. *Br Med J* 1986; **293**: 538.

69 Houeto P, Hoffman JR, Imbert M, Levillain P, Baud FJ. Relation of blood cyanide to plasma cyanocobalamin concentration after a fixed dose of hydroxocobalamin in cyanide poisoning. *Lancet* 1995; **346**: 605–8.

70 Blanc P, Hogan M, Mallin K, Hryhorczuk D, Hessl S, Bernard B. Cyanide intoxication among silver reclaiming workers. *JAMA* 1985; **253**: 367–71.

71 El Ghawabi SH, Gaafar MA, El-Saharti AA, Ahmed SH, Malash KK, Fares F. Chronic cyanide exposure: a clinical, radio isotope and laboratory study. *Br J Ind Med* 1975; **32**: 215–9.

72 Toren K, Blanc PD. The history of pulp and paper bleaching: respiratory health effects. *Lancet* 1997; **349**: 1316–8.

73 World Health Organization. *Chlorine and Hydrogen Chloride. Environmental Health Criteria 21*. Geneva: WHO, 1982.

74 Bherer L, Cushman R, Courteau J-P, Quevillon M, Cote G *et al*. Survey of construction workers repeatedly exposed to chlorine over a 3–6 month period in a pulpmill: II. Follow-up of affected workers by questionnaire, spirometry, and asessment of bronchial responsiveness 18–24 months after exposure ended. *Occup Environ Med* 1994; **51**: 225–8

75 Wegman D, Eisen EA. Acute irritants, more than a nuisance. *Chest* 1990; **97**: 773–5.

76 Schwartz DA, Smity DD, Lakshminarayan S. The pulmonary sequelae associated with accidental inhalation of chlorine gas. *Chest* 1990; **97**: 820–5.

77 Kennedy SM, Enardson DA, Janssen RG, Chan-Yeung M. Lung health consequences of reported accidental chlorine gas exposures among pulpmill workers. *Am Rev Respir Dis* 1991; **143**: 74–9.

78 Massin N, Bohadana AB, Wild P, Hery M, Toamain JP, Hubert G. Respiratory symptoms and bronchial responsiveness in lifeguards exposed to nitrogen trichloride in indoor swimming pools. *Occup Environ Med* 1998; **55**: 258–63.

79 Hery M, Gerber JM, Hecht G, Subra I, Possoz C *et al*. Exposure to chloramines in a green salad processing plant. *Ann Occup Hyg* 1998; **42**: 437–51.

80 Centers for Disease Control. Chlorine gas toxicity from mixture of bleach with other cleaning products – California. *Morbid Mortal Weekly Rep* 1991; **40**: 619–29.

81 Deschamps D, Soler P, Rosenberg N, Baud F, Gervais P. Persistent asthma after inhalation of a mixture of sodium hypochlorite and hydrochloric acid. *Chest* 1994; **105**: 1895–96.

82 Pascuzzi TA. Mass casualties from acute inhalation of chloramine gas. *Milit Med* 1998; **163**: 102–104.

83 Sim M, Fairley C, McIver J. Drinking water quality: new challenges for an old problem. *Occup Environ Med* 1994; **53**: 649–51.

84 International Programme on Chemical Safety (IPCS). *Phosgene. Environmental Health Criteria 193*. Geneva: WHO, 1997.

85 Brimblecombe P. *The Big Smoke*. London: Routledge, 1987.

86 Stevens B, Koenig JQ, Rebolledo V, Hanley QS, Covert DS. Respiratory effects from the inhalation of hydrogen chloride in young adult asthmatics. *J Occup Med* 1992; **34**: 923–9.

87 International Agency for Research on Cancer. Monographs on the Evaluation of Carcinogenic Risks to Humans: 54. *Occupational Exposures to Mists and Vapours from Strong Inorganic Acids, and Other Industrial Chemicals.* Lyon: IARC, 1992.

88 Wing JS, Sanderson LM, Brender JD, Perrotta DM, Beachamp RA. Acute health effects in a community after a release of hydrofluoric acid. *Arch Environ Hlth* 1991; **46**: 155–60.

89 World Health Organization. *Fluorine and Fluorides. Environmental Health Criteria 36.* Geneva: WHO, 1984.

90 Turner RM, Fairhurst S. *Toxicology of Substances in Relation to Major Hazards: Hydrogen Fluoride.* London: HMSO/Health and Safety Executive, 1990.

91 Machle W, Thamann F, Kitzmiller K, Cholak J. The effects of the inhalation of hydrogen fluoride. I. The response following exposure to high concentrations. *J Ind Hyg* 1933; **16**: 129–145.

92 Stavert DM, Archuleta DC, Behr MJ, Lehnert BE. Relative toxicities of hydrogen fluoride, hydrogen chloride and hydrogen bromide in nose- and pseudo-mouth-breathing rats. *Fundament Appl Toxicol* 1991; **16**: 636–55.

93 Chela A, Reig R, Sanz P, Huguet E, Corbella J. Death due to hydrofluoric acid. *Am J Forensic Med Pathol* 1989; **10**: 47–8.

94 Lund K, Ekstrand J, Boe J, Sostrand P, Kongerud J. Exposure to hydrogen fluoride: an experimental study in humans of concentrations of fluoride in plasma, symptoms, and lung function. *Occup Environ Med* 1997; **54**: 32–7

95 Grandjean P. Occupational fluorosis through 50 years: clinical and epidemiological experiences. *Am J Ind Med* 1982; **3**: 227–36.

96 Abramson MJ, Wlodarczyk JH, Saunders NA, Hensley MJ. Does aluminium smelting cause lung disease? *Am Rev Dis* 1989; **139**: 1042–57.

97 Armstrong B, Tremblay C, Baris D, Therault G. Lung cancer mortality and polynuclear aromatic hydrocarbons: a case-cohort study of aluminium production workers in Arvida, Quebec, Canada. *Am J Epidemiol* 1994; **139**: 250–62.

98 Burgess WA. *Recognition of Health Hazards in Industry: A Review of Materials and Processes* 2nd edn. New York: Wiley, 1995.

99 Søyseth, Boe J, Kongerud J. Relation between decline in FEV$_1$ and exposure to dust and tobacco smoke in aluminium pot room workers. *Occup Environ Med* 1997; **54**: 27–31.

100 Upfal M, Doyle C. Medical management of hydrofluoric acid exposure. *J Occup Med* 1990; **32**: 726–31.

101 Tepperman PB. Fatality due to acute systemic fluoride poisoning following a hydrofluoric acid skin burn. *J Occup Med* 1980; **22**: 691–2.

102 Kraut A, Lilis R. Pulmonary effects of acute exposure to degradation product of sulphur hexafluoride during electrical cable repair work. *Br J Ind Med* 1990; **47**: 829–32.

103 Speizer FE, Wegman DH, Ramirez A. Palpitation rates associated with fluorocarbon exposure in a hospital setting. *N Engl J Med* 1975; **292**: 624–6.

104 International Programme on Chemical Safety (IPCS). *Fully Halogenated Chlorofluorocarbons. Environmental Health Criteria 113.* Geneva: WHO, 1990.

105 International Programme on Chemical Safety (IPCS). *Partially Halogenated Chlorofluorocarbons (Methane Derivatives). Environmental Health Criteria 126.* Geneva: WHO, 1991.

106 International Programme on Chemical Safety (IPCS). *Partially Halogenated Chlorofluorocarbons (Ethane Derivatives): Environmental Health Criteria 139.* Geneva: WHO, 1992.

107 Hoet P, Graf M-LM, Bourd M, Pohl LR, Duray PH *et al.* Epidemic of liver disease caused by hydrochlorofluorocarbons used as ozone-sparing substitutes of chlorofluorocarbons. *Lancet* 1997; **350**: 556–9.

108 Holness DL, House RA. Health effects of halon 1301 exposure *J Occup Med* 1992; **34**: 722–5.

109 Charan NB, Myers CG, Lakshminarayan S, Spencer TM. Pulmonary injuries associated with acute sulfur dioxide inhalation. *Am Rev Respir Dis* 1979; 119>: 555–60.

110 Eatough DJ, Caka FM, Farber RJ. The conversion of SO$_2$ to sulfate in the atmosphere. *Israel J Chem* 1994; **34**: 301–14.

111 Harkonen H, Nordmann H, Korhonen O, Winblad I. Long-term effects of exposure to sulfur dioxide. Lung function four years after a pyrite dust explosion. *Am Rev Respir Dis* 1983; **128**: 890–3.

112 Piirila PL, Nordmann H, Korrhonen OS, Winblad I. A thirteen-year follow-up of respiratory effects of acute exposure to sulfur dioxide. *Scand J Work Environ Hlth* 1996; **22**: 191–6.

113 World Health Organization. *Sulfur Oxides and Suspended Particulate Matter. Environmental Health Criteria 8.* Geneva: WHO, 1979.

114 Huber AL, Loving TJ. Fatal asthma attack after inhaling sulfur fumes. *JAMA* 1991; **266**: 2225.

115 Scobie E, Dabill DW, Groves JA. Chemical pollutants in x-ray film processing departments. *Ann Occup Hyg* 1996; **40**: 423–35.

116 Department of the Environment. *Expert Panel on Air Quality Standards: Sulphur Dioxide.* London: HMSO, 1995.

117 Enterline PE, Marsh GM, Esmen NA, Henderson VL, Callaghan CM, Paik M. Some effects of cigarette smoking, arsenic, and SO$_2$ on mortality among US copper smelter workers. *J Occup Med* 1987; **29**: 831–8.

118 Koizumi A, Aoki T, Tsukada M, Naruse M, Saitoh N. Mercury, not sulphur dioxide, poisoning as cause of smelter disease in industrial plants producing sulphuric acid. *Lancet* 1994; **343**: 1411–12.

119 Turner RM, Fairhurst S. *Toxicology of Substances in Relation to Major Hazards. Sulphuric Acid Mist.* London: HMSO, 1992.

120 Coggan D, Pannett B, Wield G. Upper aerodigestive cancer in battery manufacturers and steel workers exposed to mineral acid mists. *Occup Environ Med* 1996; **53**: 445–9.

121 Kitagawa T. Cause analysis of the Yokkaichi asthma episode in Japan. *J Air Pollution Control Assoc* 1984; **34**: 743–6.

122 Payne MP, Delic J, Turner RM. *Toxicology of Substances in Relation to Major Hazards: Ammonia.* London: HMSO, 1990.

123 World Health Organization. *Ammonia. Environmental Health Criteria 54.* Geneva: WHO, 1986.

124 Leung CM, Foo CL. Mass ammonia inhalational burns – experience in the management of 12 patients. *Ann Acad Med* 1992; **21**: 624–9.

125 De la Hoz R, Schlueter DP, Rom WN. Chronic lung disease secondary to ammonia inhalation injury: a report on three cases. *Am J Ind Med* 1996; **29**: 209–14.

126 Dongham KJ, Reynolds SJ, Whitten P, Merchant JA, Burmeister L, Poppendorf WJ. Respiratory dysfunction in swine production facility workers: dose-response relationships of environmental exposures and pulmonary function. *Am J Ind Med* 1995; **27**: 405–418.

127 Ayesh R, Mitchell SC, Zhang A, Smith RL. The fish odour syndrome: biochemical, familial and clinical aspects. *Br Med J* 1993; **307**: 655–7.

128 Department of the Environment: Expert Panel on Air Quality Standards. *Ozone.* London: HMSO, 1994.

129 International Programme on Chemical Safety. *Nitrogen Oxides. Environmental Health Criteria 188.* 2nd edn: Geneva: WHO, 1997.

130 World Health Organization. *Oxides of Nitrogen. Environmental Health Criteria 4.* Geneva: WHO, 1977.

131 Grayson RR. Silage gas poisoning: nitrogen dioxide pneumonia, a new disease in agricultural workers. *Ann Intern Med* 1956; **45**: 393–408.

132 Ramirez RJ, Dowell AR. Silo-filler's disease: nitrogen dioxide induced lung injury. *Ann Intern Med* 1971; **74**: 569–76.

133 Department of the Environment: Expert Panel on Air Quality Standards. *Nitrogen Dioxide.* London: HMSO, 1996.

134 Hatton DV, Leach CS, Nicogossian AE, Di Ferrante N. Collagen breakdown and nitrogen dioxide inhalation. *Arch Environ Hlth* 1977; **32**: 33–6.

135 Brauer M, Spengler JD. Nitrogen dioxide exposures inside ice skating rinks. *Am J Publ Hlth* 1994; **84**: 429–33.

136 Fleetham JA, Tunnicliffe BW, Munt PW. Methemoglobinemia and the oxides of nitrogen. *N Engl J Med* 1978; **298**: 1150.

137 World Health Organization. *Hydrogen Sulfide.* Geneva: WHO, 1981.

138 Bhambani Y, Burnham R, Snydmiller G, MacLean I, Lovlin R. Effects of 10 ppm hydrogen sulfide inhalation on pulmonary function in healthy men and women. *J Occup Environ Med* 1996; **38**: 1012–7.

139 Jäppinen P, Vilkka V, Marttila O, Haahtela T. Exposure to hydrogen sulphide and respiratory function. *Br J Ind Med* 1990; **47**: 824–8.

140 Arnold IMF, Dufresne RM, Alleyne BC, Stuart PJW. Health implication of occupational exposure to hydrogen sulfide. *J Occup Med* 1985; **27**: 373–6.

141 Jappinen P, Tenhunen R. Hydrogen sulphide poisoning: blood sulphide concentration and changes in haem metabolism. *Br J Ind Med* 1990; **47**: 283–5.

142 Kage S, Takekawa K, Kurosaki K, Imamura T, Kudo K. The usefulness of thiosulfate as an indicator of hydrogen sulfide poisoning: three cases. *Int J Legal Med* 1997; **110**: 220–2.

143 Kangas J, Savolainen H. Urinary thiosulphate as an indicator of exposure to hydrogen sulphide vapour. *Clin Chim Acta* 1987; **164**: 7–10.

144 Finch CA. Methemoglobinemia and sulfhemoglobinemia. *N Engl J Med* 1948; **239**: 470–8.

145 Parra O, Monso E, Gallego M, Morera J. Inhalation of hydrogen sulphide: a case of subacute manifestations and long term sequelae. *Br J Ind Med* 1991; **48**: 286–7.

146 Tvedt B, Skyberg K, Aaserud O, Hobbesland A, Mathiesen T. Brain damage caused by hydrogen sulfide: a follow-up study of six patients. *Am J Ind Med* 1991; **20**: 91–101.

147 Ahlborg G. Hydrogen sulfide poisoning in shale oil industry. *Ind Hyg Occup Med* 1951; **3**: 247–66.

148 Bates MN, Garrett N, Graham B, Read D. Air pollution and mortality in the Rotorua geothermal area. *Aust NZ J Publ Hl* 1997; **21**: 581–6.

149 Bates MN, Garret N, Graham B, Read D. Cancer incidence, morbidity and geothermal air pollution in Rotorua, New Zealand. *Int J Epidemiol* 1998; **27**: 10–14.

150 McCabe LC, Clayton GD. Air pollution by hydrogen sulfide in Poza Rica, Mexico. *AMA Arch Ind Hyg Occup Med* 1952; **6**: 199–213.

151 Partti-Pellinen K, Marttila O, Vilkka V, Jaakkola JJK, Jäppinen P, Haahtela T. The South Karelia air pollution study: effects of low-level exposure to malodorous sulphur compounds on symptoms. *Arch Environ Hlth* 1996; **51**: 315–20.

152 Tangerman A, Meuwese-Arends MT, Jansen JBMJ. Foetor hepaticus. *Lancet* 1994; **343**: 1569.

153 Schults WT, Fountain EN, Lynch EC. Methanethiol poisoning. *JAMA* 1970; **211**: 2153–4.

154 Schecter A, Shanske W, Stenzler A, Quintilian H, Steinberg H. Acute hydrogen selenide inhalation. *Chest* 1980; **77**: 554–5.

155 Fowler BA, Weissberg JB. Arsine poisoning. *N Engl J Med* 1974; **291**: 1171–4.

156 Wilkinson SP, McHugh P, Horsley S *et al.* Arsine toxicity aboard the Asiafreighter. *Br Med J* 1975; **3**: 559–63.

157 Hesdorffer CS, Milne FJ, Terblanche J, Meyers AM. Arsine gas poisoning; the importance of exchange transfusions in severe cases. *Br J Ind Med* 1986; **43**: 353–5.

158 World Health Organization. *Phosphine and Selected Metal*

Phosphides. *Environmental Health Criteria 73*. Geneva: WHO, 1988.

159 Wilson R, Lovejoy FH, Jaeger RJ, Landrigan P. Acute phosphine poisoning aboard a grain freighter. *JAMA* 1980; **244**: 148–50.

160 Barbosa A, Bonin AM. Evaluation of phosphine genotoxicity at occupational levels of exposure in New South Wales, Australia. *Occup Environ Med* 1994; **51**: 700–5.

161 International Programme for Chemical Safety (IPCS). *Methyl bromide. Environmental Health Criteria 166*. Geneva: WHO, 1995.

162 Yang RS, Witt KL, Alden CJ, Corkerham LG. Toxicology of methyl bromide. *Rev Environ Contam Toxicol* 1995; **142**: 65–85.

163 Behrens RH, Dukes DCD. Fatal methyl bromide poisoning. *Br J Ind Med* 1986; **43**: 561–2.

164 Health and Safety Executive. *Fumigation Using Methyl Bromide. Guidance Note CS12*. London: HMSO, 1991.

165 Garnier R, Rambourg-Schepens M-O, Müller A, Hallier E. Glutathione transferase activity and formation of macromolecular adducts in two cases of acute methyl bromide poisoning. *Occup Environ Med* 1996; **53**: 211–5.

166 Mehta PS, Mehta AS, Mehta SJ, Makhijani AB. Bhopal tragedy's health effects: a review of methyl isocyanate toxicity. *JAMA* 1990; **264**: 2781–7.

167 Andersson N, Ajurani MK, Mahashabde S, Tiwari MK *et al.* Delayed eye and other consequences from exposure to methyl isocyanate: 93% follow-up of exposed and unexposed cohorts in Bhopal. *Br J Ind Med* 1990: **47**: 553–8.

168 Cullinan P, Acquilla S, Ramana Dhara V. Respiratory morbidity 10 years after the Union Carbide gas leak at Bhopal: a cross-sectional survey. *Br Med J* 1997; **314**: 338–42.

169 World Health Organization. *Ethylene Oxide. Environmental Health Criteria 55*. Geneva: WHO, 1985.

170 Steenland K, Stayner L, Grief A *et al.* Mortality among workers exposed to ethylene oxide. *N Engl J Med* 1991; **324**: 1402–7.

171 Shore RE, Gardner MJ, Pannett B. Ethylene oxide: an assessment of the epidemiological evidence on carcinogenicity. *Br J Ind Med* 1993; **50**: 971–97.

172 Verraes S, McChel O. Occupational asthma induced by ethylene oxide. *Lancet* 1995; **346**: 1434.

173 Kurta DL, Dean BS, Krenzelok EP. Acute nickel carbonyl poisoning. *Am J Emerg Med* 1993; **11**: 64–6.

174 Tannenbaum TN, Goldberg RJ. Exposure to anesthetic gases and reproductive outcome. *J Occup Med* 1985; **27**: 659–68.

175 Spence AA. Environmental pollution by inhalation anaesthetics. *Br J Anaesth* 1987; **59**: 96–103.

176 Boivin J-F. Risk of spontaneous abortion in women occupationally exposed to anaesthetic gases: a meta-analysis. *Occup Environ Med* 1997; **54**: 541–8.

177 Stollery BT, Broadbent DE, Lee WR, Keen I, Healy TEJ, Beatty P. Mood and cognitive functions in anaesthetists working in actively scavenged operating theatres. *Br J Anaesth* 1988; **61**: 446–55.

178 Rowland AS, Baird DD, Weinberg CR, Shore DL, Shy CM, Wilcox AF. Reduced fertility among women employed as dental assistants exposed to high levels of nitrous oxide. *N Engl J Med* 1992; **327**: 993–7.

179 Neil HAW, Fairer JG, Coleman MP, Thurston A, Vessey MP. Mortality among male anaesthetists in the United Kingdom, 1957–83. *Br Med J* 1987; **295**: 360–1.

180 Gardner RJ. Inhalation anesthetics – exposure and control: a statistical comparison of personal exposures in operating theatres with and without anaesthetic gas scavenging. *Ann Occup Hyg* 1989; **33**: 159–73.

181 Gardner RJ, Hampton J, Causton JS. Inhalation anaesthetics – exposure and control during veterinary surgery. *Ann Occup Hyg* 1991; **35**: 377–88.

182 Health and Safety Commission: Health Service Advisory Committee. *Anaesthetic Agents: Controlling Exposure Under COSHH*. London: HMSO, 1995.

183 Sweeney B, Bingham RM, Amos RJ, Petty AC, Cole PV. Toxicity of bone marrow in dentists exposed to nitrous oxide. *Br Med J* 1985; **291**: 567–9.

184 Elliott P, Kleinschmidt I. Angiosarcoma of the liver in Great Britain in proximity to vinyl chloride sites. *Occup Environ Med* 1997; **54**: 14–18.

185 Okumura T, Takasu N, Ishimatsu S, Miyanoki S, Mistuhashi A *et al.* Report on 640 victims of the Tokyo subway sarin attack. *Ann Emerg Med* 1996; **28**: 129–35.

186 Morita H, Yanagisawa N, Nakajima T, Shimuzu M, Hirabayashi H *et al.* Sarin poisoning in Matsumoto, Japan. *Lancet* 1995; **346**: 290–3.

187 Nakajima T, Sato S, Morito H, Yanagisawa N. Sarin poisoning of a rescue team in the Matsumoto sarin incident in Japan. *Occup Environ Med* 1997; **54**: 697–701.

188 Unwin C, Blatchley N, Coker W, Ferry S, Hotopf M *et al.* Health of UK servicemen who served in Persian Gulf war. *Lancet* 1999; **353**: 169–78.

189 Ministry of Defence. *Medical Manual of Defence against Chemical Agents*. London: HMSO, 1987.

190 Yih J-P. CS gas injury to the eye. *Lancet* 1995; **311**: 276.

191 Jones GRN. Are CS sprays safe? *Lancet* 1997; **350**: 605.

192 Pastides H, Calabrese EJ, Hosmer DW, Harris DR. Spontaneous abortion and general illness symptoms among semi-conductor manufacturers. *J Occup Med* 1988; **30**: 543–51.

193 Lipscomb JA, Fenster L, Wrensch M, Shusterman D, Swan S. Pregnancy outcomes in women potentially exposed to occupational solvents and women working in the electronics industry. *J Occup Med* 1991; **33**: 597–604.

194 Nicholson K. *Geothermal Fluids: Chemistry and Exploration Techniques*. Berlin: Springer, 1993.

9

Welding, fumes and inhalational fevers

GRANT HG McMILLAN

Introduction	179	Health effects of exposure to welding fumes	182
Principal manual electric arc welding processes	179	Inhalation fevers	185
Source, nature and variation of emissions	180	References	187

Studies in recent years have largely re-focussed concerns over the health risks associated with electric arc metal welding from chronic bronchitis and siderosis to the apparent excess risk of lung cancer among welders compared with the general population, occupational asthma, the toll of wear and tear on the musculoskeletal system and, most recently, the possibility that metals inhaled as part of welding fumes may facilitate pneumonic infections. There is a continuing need for proactive measures to recognize, evaluate and control exposure to welding fumes and to increase the involvement of welders in protecting their own health.

INTRODUCTION

Metal welding is a generic term for any of the processes, ubiquitous in industry, of joining metals at areas or points softened or liquefied by the application of heat, sometimes with associated local pressure. The heat required may be derived in a variety of ways including friction, electron beams, ultrasound or the combustion of fuel gases but the most common source is an electric arc struck between two electrical conductors. Further consideration of the health hazards of welding here will be limited largely to these electric arc processes.

The emissions from these processes comprise ultraviolet and infrared radiation, visible light, and an airborne, dynamic and often biologically active mixture of particles and gases, termed 'welding fume'. This is derived from evaporation, condensation, oxidation, decomposition, pyrolysis and combustion of materials involved in the process. Though much welding is now automated, manual electric arc welding is still very common, estimates suggesting that perhaps as many as a million workers[1] use it to some extent in their work while many others work in their vicinity and may be exposed to emissions. With such numbers involved, should the emissions be sources of significant hazards due to their composition and concentration and if exposure to them is inadequately controlled then there is the potential risk for many workers to be harmed.

While interest in health effects of welding commonly is concentrated on those attributed to gaseous, particulate, ultraviolet and infrared emissions, it should not be forgotten that inadequately controlled risks of fire, burns or electric shock, high levels of noise, musculoskeletal damage due to poor ergonomics (including difficult access or egress, contorted or otherwise stressing body postures and heavy lifting) may play an important part in the causation of injury and illness among welders.

PRINCIPAL MANUAL ELECTRIC ARC WELDING PROCESSES

A basic understanding of the principal electric arc welding processes helps one to appreciate the source and nature of the emissions and the potential which exists to control them; more information and technical details are widely available elsewhere.[2-4] The Welding Institute has much useful information in the Job Knowledge section of its internet site [http://www.twi.co.uk/bestprac/].

In general terms, the great heat generated by an electric arc struck, usually between an electrode held by the welder in a handpiece and the workpiece, melts the abutting edges of the pieces of metal to be joined sufficiently for these to contribute molten metal to a common weld pool which, when cool, forms a solid joint. When the workpiece cannot contribute sufficient metal to the pool, metal may be added from a filler wire held in the arc or weld pool. Alternatively the filler wire may also conduct electric current and act as the electrode which is the source of the arc. It is then called a 'consumable' electrode. The wire may have a core or coating with specific properties to improve the quality of the weld. It is usual for a gas shield to be formed round the arc and weld pool, creating a bubble-like, stable and reproducible microenvironment restricting access of oxygen and ozone and thus minimizing oxidation and other inclusions which could weaken the weld. This shield may be produced indirectly by combustion of components of the coating or core of the consumable or be provided directly as a flow of inert or active gas, such as argon or carbon dioxide respectively.

There are three main categories of electric arc welding processes, described below in increasing order of the relative amount and complexity of emissions.

Tungsten inert gas welding

The arc in tungsten inert gas (Fig. 9.1) arises from a non-consumable electrode formed by a conical spike of tungsten, often alloyed with 1–4% thorium, which must be kept correctly contoured by periodic grinding at intervals up to several weeks. The arc and weld pool are shielded by a shroud of inert shielding gas such as argon and/or helium. Metal may be added from a filler wire fed into the weld pool.

Metal inert gas and metal active gas welding

In metal inert gas and metal active gas welding the electrode is a continuous consumable small diameter wire fed through the welding handpiece or 'gun'. This is melted in its own arc to contribute directly to the weld pool. The pool, the tip of the electrode and the arc are shrouded by a shield of piped gas; in metal inert gas this is inert while in metal active gas the gas shield contains an active gas such as carbon dioxide.

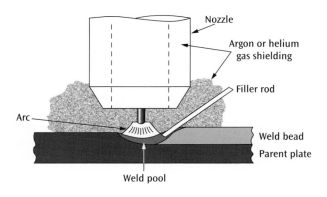

Figure 9.1 *Schematic diagram of tungsten inert gas welding.*

Manual metal arc welding

In manual metal arc welding (Fig. 9.2) the most commonly used electric arc welding process, the arc is struck between a short, consumable electrode, in a hand-piece, and the work piece. The wire of the electrode is usually coated with a mixture of chemicals and alloying metals. In addition to forming a shield of combustion gases this coating may contribute much to the properties of the weld. It forms a temporary residue 'slag' over the weld bead to reduce oxidation and slow cooling before being chipped off.

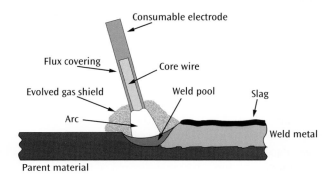

Figure 9.2 *Schematic diagram of manual metal arc welding.*

SOURCE, NATURE AND VARIATION OF EMISSIONS

The fume composition is very largely determined by the composition of the filler metal and the flux, the composition of the parent metal having only a relatively minor effect unless it bears low melting point contaminants which may make a significant contribution (see below). The formation and emission rates and composition of welding fumes vary both between and within welding processes.[5-7] This may be used to advantage to select and perhaps modify processes to reduce the risk of harm from their emissions.[8]

Variations within a process are influenced by many factors including the materials to be welded, those in the filler wire or consumable, electrical parameters and shield gas[8-13] and the skill and self-protection measures of the individual welder,[14] the latter being a powerful influence which can be reinforced by good training and education. The dynamism of the fume can present challenges to meaningful sampling. When assessing exposure the fume should be sampled behind the welder's face shield.[15,16] It may be imprudent to extrapolate results obtained in one situation to another[14] or to seek to assess exposure by means of one universal exposure indicator such as the maximum additive hygiene limit value. The content of the fume measured in the welder's breathing zone may include significant contributions from neighbourhood activities such as grinding, welding or degreasing with chlorinated hydrocarbons.

Particulate emissions

Two main groups of particles may be emitted from electric arc welding processes.[18,19] Fractionated mixed metal oxide particles are formed from metal which is vapourized in the high temperature of the arc then condensed, often reacting with oxygen in the air, to form chains and aggregates reflecting the composition of the electrode but with the more volatile constituents predominating. Most of these particles are in the respirable range with many small enough to penetrate to the periphery of the lung.[7,20–22] It has been estimated that 50% of inhaled fume reaches the lower respiratory tract[23] and 35% reaches to alveolar level[24] with most then being exhaled.[25] The second group of particles is termed 'spatter'. These are coarser, discreet, unfractionated particles of electrode, usually larger than the respirable range but providing a secondary source for the formation of smaller, respirable oxide particles as the hot metal reacts with oxygen in the air, often explosively.

A wide range of metallic oxides may be present in the fume, usually with iron oxide predominating. In the current climate of concern over occupational asthma and cancer, nickel and chromium compounds merit special mention as they are known sensitizers and, with regard to welding, possible carcinogens, as discussed below.

Nickel is found in welding fumes almost exclusively as nickel oxide and only when welding with pure nickel or nickel alloy filler material.[26] The choice of welding process has a strong influence on the emission rate.[27–28] Nickel carbonyl has not been identified in welding fume.[29,30]

Trivalent, and hexavalent chromium compounds are found in fume from welding on or with materials that contain chromium or chromates. These include high chromium nickel alloys and low alloy steels, high alloy flux covered wires, chromate paints and coatings, and chromium plating. While trivalent compounds are considered to be harmless in themselves, they provide a source of hexavalent chromium through oxidation. Between the processes the highest emissions of hexavalent chromium compounds are associated with manual metal arc welding with lower levels in metal inert gas welding and the lowest with tungsten inert gas welding. Water soluble hexavalent chromium compounds may cause irritation of the respiratory tract but do not enter the cell efficiently and are thought not to be carcinogenic. On the other hand, the water insoluble chromium compounds such as zinc chromate, calcium chromate, lead chromate and barium chromate enter cells by phagocytosis and have been found to have a carcinogenic effect on the human organism in some industries – but there is no proof of this regarding welding fume. That

said, the International Agency for Research on Cancer (IARC) has classified welding fume as possibly carcinogenic.[31]

Gaseous emissions

The principal gases formed are ozone, oxides of nitrogen and carbon monoxide. The arc plays a key role in their formation. As manual welding, and thus arcing, is not a continuous process, gas formation and emission peaks during and diminishes or is absent between arcing, so welders may be exposed for repeated short periods to concentrations higher than those indicated by an averaging sampling and measuring technique.

The generation of ozone by welding processes is due to photolysis of molecular oxygen in the ambient air by direct or reflected ultraviolet radiation emitted from the arc. The gas forms in two distinct regions relative to the arc; approximately half within a 10–15 cm radius of the arc by the action of ultraviolet in the 130–175 nm range and the remainder in relatively low concentrations up to a metre from the arc by ultraviolet radiation of wavelengths between 175 and 240 nm.

Ozone concentration is affected by anything which influences the magnitude of ultraviolet radiation in the critical ranges and by the ozone decomposition rate. The presence of other gases, fumes or dust slows the production and accelerates the decomposition of ozone to oxygen and so ozone concentrations are higher in processes with lower fume emission. The most significant factors are the composition of the workpiece and filler wire, the welding process and, most complex and variable, the composition of the shield gas. Levels are likely to be very low in manual metallic arc welding, low to moderate in tungsten inert gas and metal active gas welding and highest in metal inert gas welding, especially the latter on aluminum. The addition of helium or carbon dioxide to argon-based shielding gas mixtures may result in a significant reduction in the welder's exposure to ozone. The sampling site for ozone is of paramount importance in assessing the risk of harm to the welder as the concentration within the face shield may be an order of magnitude less than that close to the arc due to decomposition on contact with the shield.

Nitrogen oxides are generated in welding processes by the oxidation of atmospheric nitrogen first to nitrogen monoxide, a gas of very low toxicity, in contact with the very hot gas emanating from the arc and weld pool. This then oxidizes at room temperature to the highly active, and thus potentially biologically active gases, nitrogen dioxide and peroxide. Nitrogen oxide levels peak during arcing then drop dramatically at other times. Harmful concentrations may develop in poorly ventilated enclosed spaces but are unlikely in an open workshop. The rate of formation of nitric oxide is initially slower than the rate of ozone production since it is partly dependent on the workpiece achieving a high temperature whereas the ozone production reaches a peak within a fraction of a second of the arc being struck and ultra-violet radiation being emitted.[15]

Carbon monoxide is generated during metal active gas welding with carbon dioxide or mixed shield gases by thermal decomposition of the carbon dioxide and in all processes through combustion of materials. Coated or contaminated surfaces and substances in the ambient air may also be sources of harmful gases.

Influence of coatings and contaminants

The composition and amount of particulate fume and gases produced may be significantly influenced when the metal to be welded has a surface coating or is contaminated by materials.[32,33] Surface coatings may be paints, plastics or metals applied by spraying, galvanizing or electroplating to prevent corrosion, reduce friction, improve insulation or enhance appearance. Contaminants may be oil or grease, degreasers or, in the case of plant repair welding, process residues such as lead, manganese and vanadium. Welding on these materials can produce a wide range of substances of varying complexity and potential for causing harm[32,34,35] as may the action of ultraviolet radiation from the arc on aliphatic hydrocarbon degreaser vapour in the ambient atmosphere. Surface coatings and contaminants should be removed whenever possible.

HEALTH EFFECTS OF EXPOSURE TO WELDING FUMES

Harm to several body systems has been attributed to the emissions from welding processes. Each will be considered in turn. From within a few years of welding becoming a relatively commonly used process in the first quarter of the twentieth century, greatest attention has been paid to the respiratory system and so it will be discussed first.

Respiratory system

While the fact of a cause–effect relationship is seldom a matter of contention for acute effects of inhalation of welding fumes on the respiratory system, the possibility and nature of chronic effects of exposure have long been the subjects of research studies and, as the results have not been at all consistent, these remain a matter of debate. Probable reasons for the variations in conclusions include a requirement for more subjects than there have been welders available to give sufficient power to test the hypothesis of individual studies satisfactorily; the variety in the nature of welding work and thus of fume exposure between welders; failure to appreciate

this variety when seeking to consolidate small, possibly disparate, groups of welders into a large and supposedly homogeneously exposed study group; the absence of contemporaneous records of work or exposure from which some estimate of dose might be made; and failure to take account of confounding factors such as cigarette smoking and asbestos exposure in a group with a generally higher rate of smoking and greater chance of occupational exposure to asbestos than most. Moreover, many of the effects of metal fumes and gases on the respiratory system remain poorly understood.

ASPHYXIA

A fortunately rare, and sometimes fatal, acute condition suffered by welders is asphyxia through working in inadequately ventilated confined spaces where oxygen has been displaced by inert shielding gases or depleted by combustion or rusting of ferrous structures. Foolish measures taken to counter the risk of asphyxia by 'freshening the air' in such workplaces with oxygen provided as a fuel gas have led to fires in the 'oxygen enriched' workplace – some with fatal consequences. There is merit in reducing the risk of such unauthorized practices by odourizing the oxygen supplied as a fuel gas in workplaces.

METAL FUME FEVER

One of the most common acute harmful effects of electric arc welding, metal fume fever is considered with other inhalational fevers[36] at the end of this chapter.

CHRONIC PULMONARY DISEASES

Chronic bronchitis

Over the years the studies reporting no excess prevalence of chronic bronchitis in welders[37–46] have almost been matched by those which have found an excess of the symptom complex[47–57] or of individual symptoms,[56–82] especially if the welders were tobacco smokers.[41,43,47,49,53,55–57,60] There is some evidence suggesting a dose–response relationship.[54,56,62–64] (For a more detailed account see Chapter 31.)

Occupational asthma

Occupational asthma (see Chapter 32) may be caused by inhalation of irritants or sensitizing agents; welding fume can be rich in both. One comes almost to expect inconsistency of results between studies of welders and this is borne out to some extent regarding asthma. Overall, reports of occupational asthma in relation to welding are few in comparison with the other health effects. This suggests an infrequent occurrence of the disease in association with welding. National reporting schemes may contribute to the confusion by categorizing as 'welders' craftsmen such as braziers and solderers who are likely to be exposed to well recognized causes of asthma to which welders are not exposed. That said, welders were among the highest occupational groups self-reporting asthma in Sweden (647 per million),[65] small to moderate excesses over other occupations have been demonstrated,[66,67] there have been case reports of welders developing asthma attributable to fume exposure,[58,68] and it has been implied that fume from welding mild steel in a modern shipyard may have been critical in causing asthma in about 1% of workers.[69] In contrast, other studies have shown no excess prevalence of the disease in welders.[64,70,71]

Welding stainless steel implies potential exposure to hexavalent chromium, a recognized but uncommon cause of asthma,[72] but while there are reports of asthma in stainless steel welders,[73] probably due to inhaled chromium or nickel in the fume, the disease has also been found in individuals undertaking only mild steel welding[68,69] and epidemiological studies have demonstrated that the prevalence of the disease may be similar in stainless steel and mild steel welders.[66,67]

Several aspects of **pulmonary function** have been studied. The majority of short-term or cross-shift studies of pulmonary function of welders has shown no significant changes[38,46,59,66–78] while others have shown slight, but statistically significant reversible reductions in pulmonary function tests[62,79,80] and even an increase in forced expiratory volume in 1 second (FEV_1) and peak expiratory flow (PEF).[67] Many studies seeking a chronic decline in pulmonary function in groups of welders have been completed over the years. Almost all have been cross-sectional. Despite the apparent excess of chronic bronchitis symptoms described above, even when account can be taken of smoking habits, most have failed to find significant effects on pulmonary function of having been employed as a welder.[39,41–43,46,55,57,62,80–88] A small number of studies has shown predominance of changes attributable to obstructive airways disease,[57,58,89,90] but an excess number of welders with restrictive disease has also been found.[91] Yet another study demonstrated an excess of welders with a mixture of patterns of diminished lung function, more with obstructive patterns than restrictive. This was said to indicate that 'the lungs of the welders were physiologically 10–15 years older than those of the control group'.[92] Some recent studies have used the methacholine challenge test of airways hyperreactivity and, true to form, while some have found no evidence of enhanced reactivity,[62,67] others have found evidence of a permanent effect[69,93,94] with the suggestion of a dose relationship in one.[69]

Only three longitudinal studies designed to identify accelerated and chronic decline in lung function have been reported. The first confirmed the small bronchi obstruction which had been identified in excess in the study welders 5 years previously but found that the disorder had not evolved more than in the control group in the intervening period.[45] The second,[95] an exceptionally well designed and executed study, has shown there to be a work-related irreversible decline in lung function. The third study,[62] also well designed, has yet to run long enough for there to be opportunities for optimal detection of such a change.

Iron oxide is deposited from welding fume in the lungs of welders of ferrous materials. There is considerable variability between individuals in the amount of lung dust in a group with apparently homogenous exposure.[96] **Siderosis** is a radiologically apparent pulmonary nodulation exhibited by varying proportions of electric arc welders as a result of inhaling this iron oxide in welding fume.[39,41,42,46,48,49,58,60,82,83,89,94,97–107] It is unusual to find siderosis before 5 years' welding experience and more often after 15 years with prevalence then increasing steadily with time.[83,99,100,106] Iron clears from the lungs progressively after exposure to ferrous fume has ceased.[108] Radiological regression of opacities has been reported after exposure to welding fume has ceased,[78,109–111] a phenomenon unlikely to be seen if the opacities were due to fibrosis. The majority of experimental, clinical, respiratory function and histological studies of welders with siderosis have revealed no significant abnormalities indicating fibrosis, supporting the hypothesis that siderosis is a benign condition without related fibrosis or pulmonary dysfunction.[39,58,83,89,99,104,109–111,115–127]

There is, however, no doubt that siderosis and parenchymal fibrosis may co-exist in the lungs of welders. With one exception,[128] evidence that siderosis is a fibrogenic condition comes from individual cases or small series, some with gross overexposure.[106,107,129–132] Other workers have found siderosis and fibrosis to co-exist in welders but have not attributed this solely to iron, alternatives suggested including a mixed exposure during occupation as a welder; perhaps to oxides of nitrogen,[133,134] zinc,[135] silica,[91,131,136–138] hexavalent chromium,[140,141] nickel compounds,[140] asbestos,[142] aluminium,[143–145] or an as yet unidentified fibrogenic agent in the fume.[107,129,134,141,147–148] Alternatively the fibrogenic exposure may have been in another occupation.

The risk of welders who have been exposed to fumes in the past developing **lung cancer** is about 30% greater than for that of the general population.[148–154] Compounds of nickel and chromium, proven carcinogens in other industrial circumstances, were initially thought to be the cause.[152,155,156] The excess, however, is not confined to stainless steel welders who are most likely to be exposed to fume containing these compounds, but it is also found in those who weld only mild steel and thus have no such occupational exposure.[151–154]

The excess may be explained in part by tobacco smoking, welders having been found to smoke more than many other groups,[157] and/or with previously inhaled asbestos,[157] a risk factor found especially in shipyard welders. It has been suggested that radioactive thorium dust inhaled following grinding of tungsten inert gas electrodes might cause some lung cancer[158] but there appears to be neither a concentration of cases, nor indeed excess morbidity,[159] among tungsten inert gas welders. The IARC, whilst acknowledging the confounding variables of smoking and asbestos exposure, has classified all welding fumes as possibly carcinogenic (Category 2B).[31]

The electromagnetic fields created by welding apparatus also came under suspicion as carcinogenic but the evidence weighs against this being the case.[160]

Welders are also at significant risk of developing mesothelioma[142,153] and the other asbestos-related diseases consequent upon occupational exposure to asbestos dust (see Chapter 35). Such exposure could explain the excess incidence of lung cancers (other than pleural mesothelioma).[161]

So what is the summary position for diseases of the respiratory system? First, it must be emphasized that the results of published studies relate mainly to exposures some time in the past and are not necessarily relevant for present day conditions in modernized industries. That said, given the evidence of the potentially irritant nature of the fume and the positive results of many studies, one might feel justified in concluding that prolonged occupational exposure to high concentrations of welding fumes, such as those which may be found in poorly ventilated work areas, is likely to be associated with at least aggravation of signs and symptoms of chronic bronchitis, however caused, and probably with a progressive decline in lung function. It may also be concluded that, while asthma may be caused by inhalation of specific constituents of welding fume, such as compounds of chromium, nickel or an irritating gas, there is to date insufficient justification for classifying welding fume in general as a cause of occupational asthma.

Welders commonly develop siderosis, usually a benign condition, which may be found in association with parenchymal fibrosis. Many welders are at risk of developing the whole range of asbestos-related diseases including mesothelioma. While tobacco smoking and asbestos exposure are likely to be important contributory factors to the excess of lung cancer seen in welders internationally, there is good justification in the classification of welding fume as 'possibly carcinogenic to humans' there being limited evidence of carcinogenicity in humans and inadequate evidence in animals for a more definite conclusion to be drawn.

Central and peripheral nervous system

Workers welding aluminium may progressively develop raised serum and urine levels and internal loads of the metal, retaining a significant proportion of it in the tissues, especially the skeleton. This metal is excreted very slowly.[162,163] The brain is a recognized target for aluminium toxicity; long-term exposure to aluminium-containing welding fumes may be related to an excess of neuropsychiatric symptoms[164] and, on testing, deficiencies in short-term memory, attention and motor function, with some evidence of a dose–effect relationship suggesting cumulative toxicity due to aluminium exposure[163,165–167] (see Chapter 7). Welders may be sufficiently exposed to manganese fume during welding operations to suffer toxic consequences exhibited as encephalopathy and disturbed motor dysfunction[167–170] but the evidence to date is less than convincing of a significant hazard in a typical well run welding workplace. Absorption of manganese-containing welding fume is likely to be much less than if the manganese compunds were simple and pure.

Reproductive system

Welders of mild or stainless steel may run a small risk of occupationally induced reduced fertility[171–177] but the evidence is by no means constant.[178–180] Observed effects on semen quality appear to be irreversible in the short term[180] but increasingly reversible as the years pass after exposure to welding has ceased.[174] Suggested causes include exposure to radiant heat or to metals such as chromium, nickel, manganese and cadmium in welding fume (see Chapter 40).

Physical injuries

MUSCULOSKELETAL SYSTEM

Injuries and wear and tear conditions of the musculoskeletal system are a main cause of short- and long-term absence from work, restricted employability and chronic invalidity in welders in several countries.[37,62,181–185] There is a particular risk of shoulder pain due to inflammatory changes in the rotator cuff notably in those who weld at or above shoulder level.[186–189] Much of the damage to the musculoskeletal system could be prevented by better training, better equipment and better design of the workplace.[190,191]

SKIN

Ultraviolet and infrared from electric arc processes commonly cause 'ray burn' (erythema) and, ultimately, persistent pigmentation in unprotected areas of skin;[192] notably the neck and chest exposed at the V opening of an unbuttoned shirt or overall, wrists, forehead and, the front of the ankles in welders who squat to work and allow their trouser legs to ride up.[193] The back of the ears may be affected by reflected radiation as when welding within an aluminium container. Many welders have been burned by sparks, spatter and droplets of metal or slag and bear the scars of these repeated injuries, with feet and forearms most commonly affected. The occupational stigmata of 'ray burn' and multiple small burn scars found on many welders can cause difficulties in 'blinding' controlled studies. Welding may affect the exposed skin in other ways including siderosis,[194] and contact[195] and photodermatitis.[196,197] No skin cancers attributed to welding have been reported in the literature.

High velocity metal fragment projectiles causing deep penetrating injuries with residual foreign material may be emitted during spot or resistance welding, probably due to poor cleaning and maintenance of the equipment.[198,199]

EARS AND HEARING

Burns inside the ear are relatively uncommon but particularly painful. These may have serious complications including perforation of the tympanic membrane with deafness and facial paralysis and unusually high rates of residual and recurring perforations.[200–203] The high sound pressure levels which can be found as background in welding shops and are emitted by some welding and cutting processes may cause noise-induced hearing loss[204] (see Chapter 13).

EYES

Welders have a high incidence of eye injuries,[193,205] especially due to foreign bodies when chipping slag from manual metal arc welds and from the arc's ultraviolet radiation, the latter causing arc-eye and, reportedly, an excess of pterygium.[206] Arc-eye is an acute high flux ultraviolet injury to the corneal epithelium causing a punctate superficial keratitis in the welder (and/or others in the area) whose eyes have not been adequately protected when he or a neighbour has struck the electric arc to begin welding. Some injuries are caused by reflected radiation. The incidence is said to decline with increasing age; perhaps because more older welders wear prescription spectacle lenses at work,[207] as even clear lenses can afford significant protection from a brief overexposure.[208] Care must be taken to ensure that such lenses are not used as a substitute for the correct tinted protective welding lens. Typically, presentation occurs 4–6 hours after exposure when the damaged epithelial cells have sequestered into the tear film. The patient complains of pain, photophobia, excessive lachrymation and a feeling of grittiness. The injury stains diffusely with fluoroscein. As most of the pain appears to be caused by spasm of the iris and ciliary muscle it has been reported that the most effective treatment is temporary cycloplegia with cyclopentolate 1%, rather than prescribing local anaesthetic drops, a single drop being usually all that is necessary.[209] Patients should be discouraged from driving until the effect of this agent has worn off, usually after about 8–12 hours.

Accounts of contact lenses adhering to the comea following exposure to ultraviolet radiation from welding circulate periodically; none have been substantiated.

There is no evidence to support the contention that welders should not wear contact lenses provided they take normal precautions and adhere to recommended wear times, and cleaning procedures are observed. While the cornea and lens can absorb ultraviolet radiation and prevent it reaching the retina, the radiation in the visible spectrum is not absorbed and may cause retinal damage. Fortunately this appears to be a very rare consequence of welding[210–212] and is limited to unprotected exposure.

Other systems

There is no evidence to link welding with diseases of the urinary, gastrointestinal or blood forming systems.

Two concerns have been voiced in regard to the cardiovascular system. The first was a fear, now discounted, that the toxic effects of soluble barium in fumes from certain filler wires and consumable electrodes,[213–215] shown to be toxic in animals,[216] might have cardiotoxic effects in man. The second was the possibility of electromagnetic fields created by welding apparatus disrupting the normal activity of cardiac pacemakers and implanted defibrillators. This appears to cause no significant problems with modern models of these appliances.[217–221]

That said, although the balance of evidence shows that electric and magnetic fields created have no other adverse effects on health,[160] it would be prudent to reduce the risk of any harm as much as possible by reducing welders' exposure by ensuring that welders do not work between current carrying cables or unnecessarily close to power sources (see Chapter 21).

INHALATION FEVERS

The term inhalational fever[36] collectively describes a group of acute, non-allergic, usually benign and self-limiting flu-like illnesses caused by heavy exposure to certain inhalable environmental pollutants. The most common of these is metal fume fever, with polymer fume fever some considerable way behind in incidence, followed by a raft of disorders including humidifier fever (bioaerosols from air conditioning and humidifier systems), organic dust syndrome[222] (dust from organic matter such as mouldy hay, compost, wood chips), grain fever (grain dust), mill fever (dusts of flax, cotton, hemp or kapok) and Pontiac fever (bioaerosols containing the bacterium *Legionella pneumophila*). Each usually resolves with 2–3 days. Treatment of the uncomplicated case is supportive only (see Chapter 36).

Metal fume fever

Metal fume fever is one of the few ancient occupational diseases[223] still encountered in modern industrial practice, is quite common among welders, the percentage reporting an attack when asked specifically has been variously reported as 10% and 31%.[224–225]

It is an unpleasant but, in its uncomplicated form, self-limiting acute flu-like illness caused by a single exposure to freshly formed metal oxide fumes. The concentration need not be high; inhalation of zinc oxide for 2 hours at 5 mg/m³, the 8-hour weighted threshold limit value, produced fever, symptoms and elevation in plasma of the pyrogen interleukin 6 in healthy and normal individuals.[226,227] Symptoms usually begin within a few hours of exposure with bouts of intense shivering, muscle and joint pains, undulating low grade fever, but sometimes high fever, difficulty in keeping warm and, in more severe cases, chest pain, abdominal pain and vomiting.[228–234]

Physical examination may reveal rales and rhonchi.[235,236] Pulmonary function is commonly unaffected[237] or there may be transient acute impairment[238] with reduced lung volume and transfer factor, usually followed by complete recovery.[239] Rarely, there is an asthma-like response.[240] A subclinical cross-shift reduction in lung function has been attributed to occupational exposure to small quantities of zinc oxide.[241] The chest radiograph is typically normal and there is a peripheral leucocytosis.

If asked, the affected welder will usually admit to welding on zinc-containing material, galvanized metal being most commonly involved, but the oxides of several other metals have been implicated.[238,242–245]

Usually the affected worker recovers completely within 24 hours, apparently without long-term sequelae.[237,240,246] While it is difficult to accept that there should be no long-term health penalty to pay for repeated or severe attacks, long-term sequelae are reported but rarely. The rapid and full recovery from metal fume fever leads to the illness often passing unreported and thus it is underestimated in studies based on recorded sickness absence.

Some welders believe that an attack early in the week confers temporary immunity or resistance,[245] but it may be simply that the welder is more cautious of his exposure in the days following such an unpleasant illness.[247] Rarely the welder may develop pneumonitis and pulmonary oedema when the concentration of fumes has been particularly high or when the illness is complicated by specific acute metal toxic damage as in cadmium pneumonitis.

The pathogenesis of metal fume fever has not been established. Particles of freshly formed metal oxide can reach the alveoli. Histological and bronchoalveolar lavage results from animal and human exposure studies indicate that zinc oxide fume inhalation results in marked pulmonary inflammation, especially at the periphery, with cytokine release in the lungs and raised levels of the pyrogen interleukin 6 having been measured in subjects exposed to zinc fume who developed symp-

toms. In some evaluations data shows a dose – response relationship. Taken together, the findings of various studies indicate that the lung itself plays a principal role in initiating metal fume fever rather than only acting as the point of absorption.[226,233,236,237,239,248–257] This view is supported by observations that neither ingestion nor intravenous injection of toxic levels of zinc oxide in humans is associated with symptoms resembling those of metal fume fever.[257–259] The hypotheses for the initiating process which gains most favour currently is production of an endogenous pyrogen, possibly one or several cytokines released from pulmonary and blood cells.[226,237,250,255,257,260–263] Tumour necrosis factor is reported to play an important role in mediating metal fume fever.[260,264] *In vitro* studies indicate that the mechanism for formation of these substances is zinc oxide stimulation of mononuclear cells.[264]

Many components of emissions from or related to welding processes have been associated with cases of chemical (or toxic) and hypersensitivity pneumonia/pneumonitis including cadmium, beryllium, manganese, oxides of nitrogen, ozone and phosgene. Toxic pneumonitis may occur on the first exposure to such fumes while, in contrast, hypersensitivity pneumonitis, which also develops some 4–6 hours after exposure, requires at least one or more previous sensitizing exposures to the offending substance and characteristically occurs in the context of repeated episodes of increasing severity prior to diagnosis (whereas repeated episodes of metal fume fever appear to vary in severity with exposure). A mild episode of hypersensitivity pneumonia may be self-limiting without chronic residual effect but a single severe episode or repeated episodes may lead to chronic destruction of functional lung. A case of recurrent bronchoalveolitis thought to be due to hypersensitivity pneumonitis has been described in a zinc smelter.[265] Typically, a sensitized person will develop symptoms and pulmonary infiltrates with levels of exposure that do not affect others similarly exposed in the same work place.[266]

Welding on cadmium metal or its alloys, often unsuspectingly when it is present as a surface coating, is probably the most common cause of toxic pneumonitis in welders, sometimes with a fatal outcome. Measuring the urinary cadmium concentration can be useful in differentiating between metal fume fever and chemical pneumonitis early in the course of the illness,[267] and may be lifesaving.

Four successive national surveys of occupational diseases in England and Wales, covering several decades, have shown there to be an excess risk of death from pneumonia in men of working age in the occupational group which contains welders. Toxic pneumonitis was suspected as the explanation but this has not proved to be the case.[268] The diversity of trades other than electric welders which may include the analysis group, and which is to be found on certificates of cause of death in the first three surveys (including gas, spot and blacksmith welders), suggested that the cause was not specific to arc welding[269] and the observation of a similar pattern in coremakers and furnacemen has prompted the hypotheses that inhaled metal fume is the common factor and may have an immunotoxic effect or that accumulated iron in the lung might facilitate infection.[270] A controlled study to determine if lobar pneumonia is an occupational disease of welders is being undertaken.[270]

Polymer fume fever

First described in 1951, this inhalational fever may follow within 8 hours or so the inhalation of pyrolytic products of fluorocarbon polymers or copolymers, the most commonly reported of which is polytetrafluoroethylene (PTFE) or Teflon®. Under normal usage Teflon® is among the most inert non-toxic and non-flammable substances, but if heated above 250°C it will begin to decompose to form hydrogen fluoride, tetrafluoroethylene, hexafluoropropylene and octofluoroisobutylene. Other common pyrolysis products include organic fluorides, carbonyl fluoride and perfluoropropane, depending upon the fluorocarbon polymer and the temperature and humidity at which it is burnt. Cigarettes rolled or smoked in the work place contaminated with particles of polymer may be a source of the fever, pyrolysis products being inhaled with the cigarette smoke. A no-smoking rule should be strictly enforced and employees should be instructed to wash their hands before eating or rolling or smoking cigarettes.

Outbreaks of polymer inhalation fever have been described in workers using electronic instrument boards and mould release sprays containing polymers,[271] in people using shoes sprays containing fluoropolymers,[272] the manufacture of synthetic fabric,[273] and in the manufacture of plastics or chemicals, and in rubber stamps, paint and an aircraft repair shop.[274]

In common with other inhalation fevers, the symptoms of polymer fever begin a few hours after exposure and can usually be expected to resolve completely within 24–36 hours. It is usually a relatively benign self-limiting flu-like illness with dyspnoea, chest tightness and a mild dry cough. There may be nausea, vomiting, weakness and myalgia. Some patients have a leucocytosis with a left shift and raised erthrocyte sedimentation rate. Occasionally following severe exposure, pulmonary function tests (FEV_1 and FVC) may become transiently abnormal. Mild pulmonary oedema or pneumonitis that resolves over a few days has been reported. Though permanent lung damage is rare, polymer fever has been associated with the development of chronic obstructive pulmonary disease when workers have suffered multiple exposures/episodes and/or have an underlying pulmonary disease.[273] There has been a single report of a fatal outcome, due to respiratory complications.[275]

As with metal fume fever, repeated exposures to the causative agent(s) are said to lead to the attacks subsiding, only to recur on re-exposure after a period of absence from such work. The causal mechanism for these inhalation fevers is unknown though, as mentioned in regard to metal fume fever, there are several theories. Recent work on the toxicity of ultrafine particles of relatively inert materials, in particular PTFE, has demonstrated that lung inflammation may be caused in rats when inhaled or instilled in nanometer-sized particulate form.[276] The role of ultrafine particles in fume fevers may become a fruitful area of research.

REFERENCES

1 Stern RM, Berlin A, Fletcher AC, Tarvisaio T (eds). *Health Hazards and Biological Effects of Welding Fumes and Gases*. Amsterdam:Elsevier, 1986.

2 American Welding Society. Classification of the welding processes. *Weld J* 1976;**55**:270–2.

3 Akelsson KR. Arc characteristics and their significance in welding. *Br Weld J* 1979;**7**:73–8.

4 McMillan G. Meet the welding processes. *Occup Hlth* 1985; October: 447–53.

5 American Welding Society. *Characterisation of Arc Welding Fume*. Miami: AWS, 1983.

6 Hewett P. The particle size distribution, density and specific surface area of welding fumes from SMAW and GMAW mild and stainless steel consumables. *Am Ind Hyg Assoc J* 1995;**56**:128–35.

7 Hewett P. Estimates of the regional pulmonary deposition and exposure for fumes from SMAW and GMAW mild and stainless steel consumables. *Am Ind Hyg Assoc J* 1995;**56**:136–41.

8 Hewitt PJ, Hirst AD. A systems approach to the control of welding fumes at source. *Ann Occup Hyg* 1993;**37**:297–306.

9 Stenback N. *Ozone Reduction with Mison Gases – Basic Facts*. Lidingo, Sweden: Research and Development Department, AGA AB, 1989.

10 Hewitt PJ. Reducing fume emission through process parameter selections. *Occup Hyg* 1994;**1**:35–45.

11 Dennis JH, Mortazavi SB, French MJ, Hewitt PJ, Redding CR. The effects of welding parameters on ultraviolet light emissions, ozone and Cr^{vi} formation in MIG welding. *Ann Occup Hyg* 1997;**4**:95–104.

12 Dennis JH, French MJ, Hewitt PJ, Mortazavi SB, Redding CR. Reduction of hexavalent chromium concentration in fumes from metal cored arc welding by addition of reactive metals. *Ann Occup Hyg* 1996;**40**:339–44.

13 Paskevich IR, Rykov OA. Vaporisation and oxidation of electrode metal during gas shielded arc welding. *Automat Weld* 1971;**24**:15–8.

14 Evans MJ, Ingle J, Molyneux MK, Sharp GT, Swain J. An occupational hygiene study of a controlled welding task

using a general purpose rutile electrode. *Ann Occup Hyg* 1979;**22**:1–17.

15 Anderson P, Wiktorowicz R. Ozone and the breathing zone- health and safety using gas shielded processes. *Weld Inst Bull* 1995;**1**:4–7.

16 Liu D, Wong H, Quinlan P, Blanc PD. Welding helmet airborne fume concentrations compared to personal breathing zone sampling. *Am Ind Hyg Assoc J* 1995;**565**:280–3.

17 Matczak W, Chmielnicka J. Relation between various chromium compounds and some other elements in fumes from manual metal arc stainless steel welding. *Br J Ind Med* 1993;**50**:244–51.

18 Stern RM. *A Chemical, Physical and Biological Assay of Welding Fumes*. Part 1. Publication 77.08. Copenhagen: The Danish Welding Institute, 1977.

19 Hewitt PJ, Hicks R. Neutron activation analysis of blood and body tissues from rats exposed to welding fume. In: *Nuclear Activation Techniques in the Life Sciences*. Vienna: International Atomic Energy Authority, 1972 : 129.

20 Ulfvarson U. Survey of air contaminants from welding. *Scand J Work Environ Hlth* 1981;**1**(Suppl 2):28pp.

21 Hewitt PJ, Hicks R, Lam HF. The generation and characterisation of welding fumes for toxicological investigations. *Ann Occup Hyg* 1978;**2**:159–67.

22 Stettler LE, Groth DH, McKay GR. Identification of stainless steel welding fume particulates in human lung and environmental sampling using electron probe microanalysis. *J Am Ind Hyg Assoc* 1977;**38**:76.

23 Piscator M. Health hazards from inhalation of metal fumes. *Environ Res* 1976;**11**:268–70.

24 Ross DS, Hewitt PJ. Welding fumes and welders' health. *Occup Hlth* 1976;**28**:520–7.

25 Hewitt PJ, Hicks R. An investigation of the effects of inhaling welding fume in the rat. *Ann Occup Hyg* 1973;**16**:213–21.

26 Naheme G. *Literature Review Update on Nickel Containing Welding Fumes (1988-mid-1994)*. Report RC512. Welding Institute of Canada, 1995.

27 Akesson B, Skerfving S. Exposure in welding of high nickel alloy. *Int Arch Occup Environ Hlth* 1985;**56**: 111–7.

28 Angerer J, Lehnert G. Occupational chronic exposure to metals: II Nickel exposure of stainless steel welders – biological monitoring. *Int Arch Occup Environ Hlth* 1990;**62**:7–10.

29 Hallne U, Hallberg BO. *Problems of the Work Environment Due to Welding*, Undersokning rapport 1982. 11. Arbetarskyddastyresen, Publikations-service 17184 Solna, Sweden.

30 Wiseman LG. No nickel carbonyl detected when welding stainless steel or nickel alloys. *Weld Res Suppl* 1989;May:192s–7s.

31 International Agency for Research on Cancer. Monographs on the evaluation of carcinogenic risk to humans: 49. *Chromium, Nickel and Welding*. Lyon: IARC, 1990.

32 McMillan G. Cleaner metal – cleaner air. *Occup Hlth* 1985; December: 552–60.

33 Peterson JE. Toxic pyrolysis products of solvents, paints and polymer films. *Occup Med* 1993;**8**:533–47.

34 Rinzema LC, Silverstein LG. Hazards from chlorinated hydrocarbon decomposition during welding. *J Am Ind Hyg Assoc* 1972; **33**:35–40.

35 Dahlberg JA, Myrin LM. The formation of dichloroacetyl chloride and phosgene from trichloroethylene in the atmosphere of welding shops. *Ann Occup Hyg* 1971;**14**:269–74.

36 Rask-Andersen A, Pratt DS. Inhalation fever: a proposed unifying term for febrile reactions to inhalation of toxic substances. *Br J Ind Med* 1992;**49**:40.

37 McMillan GHG, Molyneux M. The health of welders in Naval Dockyards:the work situation and sickness absence patterns. *J Soc Occup Med* 1981;**31**:43–60.

38 McMillan GHG, Heath J. The health of welders in Naval Dockyards:acute changes in respiratory function during standardised welding. *Ann Occup Hyg* 1972;**22**:19–32.

39 McMillan GHG, Pethybridge RJ. A clinical, radiological and pulmonary function case-control study of 135 dockyard welders aged 45 years and over. *J Soc Occup Med* 1984;**34**:3–23.

40 McMillan GHG. The health of welders in Naval Dockyards: welding, tobacco smoking and absence attributed to respiratory disease. *J Soc Occup Med* 1981;**31**:112–8.

41 Fogh A, Frost J, Georg J. Respiratory symptoms and pulmonary function in welders. *Ann Occup Hyg* 1969;**12**:213–78.

42 Peters JM, Murphy RLH, Ferris BG. Pulmonary function in shipyard welders. *Arch Environ Hlth* 1973;**26**:28–31.

43 Hayden SP, Pincock AC, Hayden J, Tyler LE, Cross KW, Bishop JM. Respiratory symptoms and pulmonary function of welders in the engineering industry. *Thorax* 1984;**39**:442–7.

44 Mur JM, Teculescu D, Pham QT, Gaertner M, Massin N *et al*. Lung function and clinical findings in a cross-sectional study of arc welders. *Int Arch Occup Environ Hlth* 1985;**57**:1–17.

45 Mur JM, Teculescu D, Massin N, Meyer-Bisch C, Moulin J *et al*. Arc welders, respiratory health evolution over 5 years. *Int Arch Occup Environ Hlth* 1989;**61**:321–7.

46 Swaminathan V, Sivaramakrishman M. *Respiratory Symptoms and Pulmonary-Functions in Different Groups of Welders*. International Institute of Welding Document VIII-1516-90; Abington, Cambridge, UK: The Welding Institute.

47 Sevcik M, Chalupa B, Klhufkova E, Hrazdira CL. Gesund heit schaden bei Elektrascheitrern. *Z Arbeitsmed* 1960;**10**:77.

48 Donoso H, Segura E, Vallejos ME, Lorono R. Arc welders' siderosis. *Rev Med Child* 1974;**102**:202–7.

49 Barhad B, Teculescu D, Cracium O. Respiratory symptoms, chronic bronchitis and ventilatory function in shipyard welders. *Int Arch Occup Environ Hlth* 1975;**36**:137–50.

50 Slepicka J, Tesar Z, Skoda V, Mirejovsky P. The effect of

electric arc welding pneumoconiosis upon the respiratory tract of welders. *Pracov Lek* 1974;**26**:295–302.

51 Dobrzynski W. Chronic non-specific disease of the respiratory systems among electric welders. *Roczn Pom Akad Med Swierczewskiego* 1974;(Suppl.10): 277–94.

52 Bergert KD, Krause M, Mahrlein W. Possibility of the effect of a long-term activity as a welder on the development of chronic obstructive airways disease. *Z Ges Inn Med* 1978;**33**:779–80.

53 Fawer RF, Gardner AW, Oakes D. Absences attributed to respiratory diseases in welders. *Br J Ind Med* 1982;**39**:149–52.

54 Groth M, Lyngenbo O. Respiratory symptoms in Danish welders. *Scand J Soc Med* 1989;**17**:271–6.

55 Sjogren B, Ulfvarsson U. Respiratory symptoms and pulmonary function among welders working with aluminium, stainless steel and railway tracks. *Scand J Work Environ Hlth* 1985;**11**:27–32.

56 Cotes JE, Feinmann EL, Male VJ, Rennie FS, Wickham CAC Respiratory symptoms and impairment in shipyard welders and caulker/burners. *Br J Ind Med* 1989;**46**:292–301.

57 Ozdemir O, Numanoglu N, Gonullu U, Savas I, Alper D, Gurses H. Chronic effects of welding exposure on pulmonary function tests and respiratory symptoms. *Occup Environ Med* 1995;**52**:800–3.

58 Hunnicutt TN, Cracovaner DJ, Myles JT. Spirometric measurement in welders. *Arch Environ Hlth* 1964;**8**:661–9.

59 Keimig DG, Pomrehn PR, Burmeister LF. Respiratory symptoms and pulmonary function in welders of mild steel: a cross-sectional study. *Am J Ind Med* 1983;**4**:489–99.

60 Zober A, Welte D. Cross-sectional study of respiratory effects of arc welding. *J Soc Occup Med* 1985;**35**:79–84.

61 Chandrasekaran NK. *A Comparative Study of Pulmonary Function and Respiratory Morbidity among Ex-welders and Non-welding Controls. International Institute of Welding Document* VIII-1517-90; Abington, Cambridge, UK: The Welding Institute.

62 Beckett WS, Pace PE, Sferlazza SJ, Periman GD, Chen AH, Xu XP. Airway reactivity in welders; a controlled prospective cohort study. *J Occup Environ Med* 1996;**38**:1229–38.

63 Naslund P-E, Hogstedt P. Welding and bronchitis. *Eur J Respir Dis* 1982;**S118**:69–72.

64 Sferlazza SJ, Beckett WS. The respiratory health of welders. *Am Rev Respir Dis* 1991;**143**:1134–48.

65 Toren K. Self reported rate of occupational asthma in Sweden 1990–92. *Occup Environ Med* 1996;**53**:757–61.

66 Antti-Poka M, Nordman H, Koskenvuo M, Kaprio J, Jalava M. Role of occupational exposure to airway irritants in the development of asthma. *Int Arch Occup Environ Hlth* 1992;**64**:195–200.

67 Wang ZP, Larsson K, Malmberg P, Sjogren B, Hallberg B-O, Wranngskong K. Asthma, lung function, and bronchial

responsiveness in welders. *Am J Ind Med* 1994;**26**:741–54.

68 Vandenplas O, Dargent F. Auverdin JJ. Boulanger J, Bossiroy JM *et al.* Occupational asthma due to gas metal arc welding on mild steel. Late and dual asthmatic reactions in one welder. *Thorax* 1995;**50**:587–8.

69 Beach JR, Dennis JH, Avery AJ, Bromly CL, Ward RJ *et al.* An epidemiological investigation of asthma in welders. *Am J Respir Crit Care Med* 1996;**154**:1394–400.

70 Ross DJ, McDonald JC. Asthma following inhalation accidents reported to the SWORD Project. *Ann Occup Hyg* 1996;**40**:645–50.

71 Siruttanapruk S, Burge PS. The impact of COSHH regulations on workers with occupational asthma. *Occup Med* 1997;**47**:101–4.

72 Williams CD Jr. Asthma related to chromium compounds. Report of two cases and review of the literature on chromatic diseases. *N Carolina Med J* 1969;**30**:482.

73 Keskinen H, Kalliomaki PL, Alanko K. Occupational asthma due to stainless steel welding fumes. *Clin All* 1980;**10**:151–9.

74 Ouw KM, Jones R, Young I, Reece R, Shandar A, Hayes M. *Welding Fumes, their Effect on Man.* International Institute of Welding Document 1977 VIII-713–77; Abington, Cambridge, UK: The Welding Institute.

75 Oxhoj H, Bake B. Wedel H. Wilhelmsen L. Effects of electric arc welding on ventilatory function. *Arch Environ Hlth* 1979;**24**:211–7.

76 Akesson B, Skerfving S. Exposure in welding of high nickel alloy. *Int Arch Occup Environ Hlth* 1985;**56**:111–7.

77 Kilburn KH, Warshaw RH, Boyken CT, Thronton JC. Respiratory symptoms and functional impairment from acute (cross-shift) exposure to welding gases and fumes. *Am J Med Sci* 1989;**298**:341–9.

78 Marquart H, Smid T, Heederik D, Visschers M. Lung function of welders of zinc-coated mild steel:cross-sectional analysis and changes over five consecutive work shifts. *Am J Ind Med* 1989;**16**:289–96.

79 Akbar-Khanzadeh F. Short-term respiratory function changes in relation to workshift welding fume exposures. *Int Arch Occup Environ Hlth* 1993;**64**:393–7.

80 Donoghue AM, Glass WI, Herbison GP. Transient changes in the pulmonary function of welders: a cross sectional study of Monday peak expiratory flow. *Occup Environ Med* 1994;**51**:553–6.

81 Francis TJR. A study of the immediate effects of welding fume on pulmonary function. *J Roy Nav Med Serv* 1982;**68**:136–44.

82 Ahlmark A, Lonneberg B. A clinical examination of workers with more than 5 years continuous welding experience. *Nord Hyg Tidskr* 1953;**34**:238–49.

83 Haglind O. Lung changes in electric welders. *Proc XII International Congress on Occupational Hlth* 1957;**III**:169.

84 Kleinfeld M, Messite J, Kooyman O, Shapiro J. Welders' siderosis. *Arch Environ Hlth* 1969;**19**:70–3.

85 Antti-Poika M, Hassi J, Pyk L. Respiratory diseases in arc welders. *Int Arch Occup Environ Hlth* 1977;**40**:225–30.

86 Ross DS. Welders' health; the respiratory system and welding. *Metal Construct* 1978;**10**:119–21 : 204.

87 Schneider WD, Rebohle E. Early diagnosis by means of flow volume curves in workers with respiratory exposure. *Z Erkr Atmungsorgane* 1981;**157**:291–6.

88 Kalliomaki P-L, Kalliomaki K, Korhonen O, Rahkonen E, Vaaranen V. Respiratory study of stainless steel and mild steel welders. *Scand J Work Environ Hlth* 1982;**8**:117–21.

89 Sander OA. Further observations on lung changes in electric welders. *J Ind Hyg* 1944;**26**:79–85.

90 Panjwani RC. A study of lung function tests among welders. *Am J Ind Med* 1984;**30**:107–15.

91 Kierst W, Uselis J, Graczyk M, Krynick A. Pulmonary changes in shipyard welders. *Bull Mar Med Inst Ddansk* 1964;**15**:149–56.

92 Lyngenbo O, Groth S, Groth M, Olsen O, Rossing N. Occupational lung function impairment in never-smoking Dabish welders. *Scand J Soc Med* **17**:157–64.

93 Hjortsberg U, Orbaeck P, Arborelius M. Small airways dysfunction among non-smoking shipyard arc welders. *Br J Ind Med* 1992;**49**:441–4.

94 Nielsen J, Dahlqvist M, Welinder H, Thomassen Y, Alexandersson R, Skerfving S. Small airways function in aluminium and stainless steel welders. *Int Arch Occup Environ Hlth* 1993;**65**:101–5.

95 Chinn DJ, Cotes JE, El Gamal FM, Wollaston JF. Respiratory health of young shipyard welders and other tradesmen studied cross sectionally and longitudinally. *Occup Environ Med* 1995;**55**:33–42.

96 Kalliomaki P-L, Korhonen O, Vaaranen V, Kalliomai K, Koponen M. Lung retention and clearance of shipyard arc welders. *Int Arch Occup Environ Hlth* 1978;**42**:83–90.

97 Britton JF, Walsh EL. Health hazards of electric welding *J Ind Hyg Toxicol* 1940;**22**:125–151.

98 Grohr JA. Benign pulmonary changes in arc welders. *Ind Med* 1944;**13**:598–601.

99 Schuler P, Maturana V, Cruz E, Guijon C, Vasquez A *et al.* Arc welders' pulmonary siderosis. *J Occup Med* 1962;**4**:353–8.

100 Lucionni R, Charpin T, Mosinger M. Pulmonary siderosis in arc welders. *Arch Mal Prof* 1966;**27**:803–7.

101 Stanescu DC, Pilat L, Gavrilescu N, Teculescu PB, Cristescu I. Aspects of pulmonary mechanics in arc welders, sierosis. *Br J Ind Med* 1967;**24**:143–7.

102 Kleinfeld M, Messite J, Kooyman O, Shapiro J. Welders' siderosis. *Arch Environ Hlth* 1969;**19**:70–73.

103 Pikulskaya AF, Gulko SN. External respiration and drainage function of the bronchi in electric welders. *Vrach Delo (USSR)* 1975;**1**:127–30 (English summary).

104 Spacilova M, Koval Z. Pulmonary x-ray and function findings in electric arc welders. *Int Arch Arbeitsmed* 1975;**34**:231–36.

105 Attfield M, Ross DS. Radiological abnormalities in electric arc welders. *Br J Ind Med* 1978;**35**:117–22.

106 Charpin J, Chemin-Roche T, Bonneau H, Coste P. Lung siderosis in arc welders. *J France Med Chir Thor* 1965;**19**:197–205.

107 Einbrodt Hi, Maas W, Josten HG, Stecher W. Examination of lung changes in arc welders. *Off Geundh-Wes* 1971;**33**:286.

108 Kalliomaki P-L, Alanko K, Korhonen O, Mattsson T, Vaaranen V, Koponen M. Amount and distribution of welding fume lung contaminants among arc welders. *Scand J Work Environ Hlth* 1978;**4**:122–30.

109 Doig AT, McLaughlin AIG. Clearing of x-ray shadows in welders, siderosis. *Lancet* 1948;**i**:789–91.

110 Gamuszewski Z, Dobrzynski W. Regression of pulmonary radiological changes in dockyard welders after cessation of exposure to welding fumes. *Polish Med J* 1967;**6**:610.

111 Kujawska A, Marek K, Domagalik L, Kalemba K. Evolution of radiological changes and functional disturbances in arc welders, pneumoconiosis. *Med Pracy* 1975;**26**:307–14. (English abstract)

112 Enzer N, Sander OA. Chronic lung changes in electric arc welders. *J Ind Hyg Toxicol* 1938;**20**:333–50.

113 Harding HE. Radiographic and histological appearances of the rat lung after intratracheal injection of rouge (Fe_2O_3). *Br J Ind Med* 1945;**2**:32–35.

114 Harding HE, Grout JLA, Lloyd Davies AT. The experimental production of x-ray shadows in the lungs by inhalation of industrial dusts – iron oxide. *Br J Ind Med* 1947;**4**:223–224;232.

115 Harding HE, McLaughlin AIG, Doig AT. Clinical, radiological and pathological studies of the lungs of electric arc and oxyacetylene welders. *Lancet* 1958;**ii**:294–400.

116 Enzer N, Simonson E, Evans AM. Clinical, physiological observations on welders with pulmonary siderosis and foundry men with nodular uncomplicated silicosis. *J Ind Hyg Toxicol* 1945;**27**:147.

117 Schiotz EH. Welding regarded from the medical point of view. *Acta Med Scand* 1945;**121**:537.

118 Morgan WCC, Kerr HD. Pathologic and physiologic studies of welders' siderosis. *Ann Int Med* 1963;**58**:293–304.

119 Malik E, Ulrich L. Roentgenologic changes in the lungs of electrowelders after several years exposure. *Pracov Lek* 1975;**27**:314–17.

120 Mouton N. Study of three cases of pulmonary siderosis in arc welders. *Arch Mal Prof* 1976;**37**:413–8.

121 Barrie H, Harding HE. Argyro-siderosis of the lung in silver finishers. *Br J Ind Med* 1947;**4**:225.

122 Mann BT, Lecutier ER. Arc welders' lung. *Br Med J* 1957;**2**:921–2.

123 McLaughlin AIG, Grout JLA, Barrie Hi Harding HE. Iron oxide dust and the lungs of silver finishers. *Lancet* 1945;**i**:337–41.

124 Hamlin L, Webber Hi. Siderosis: clinical, roentgenological and industrial hygiene study of foundry cleaning employees. *Ind Med* 1950;**19**:4.

125 Vorward AJ, Pratt PC, Durkan TM, Delahan AB, Bailey DA. An experimental study of the pulmonary reaction following inhalation of dust generated by cleaning room operations. *Ind Med* 1950;**19**:22.

126 Vorwald, AJ, Pratt PC, Durkin TM, Delahant AB, Bailey DA.

Siderosis; a benign pneumoconioisis due to the inhalation of iron dust. *Ind Med Surg* 1950;**19**:170–80.

127 Hamlin LE. Siderosis; additional observations over a period of 8 years on 69 foundry cleaning room employees. *J Occup Med* 1959;**1**:79.

128 Schneider WD, Maintz G, Reimer W, Schmidt G, Tittelbach U. Functional significance of lung siderosis in electrode welders. *Z Gesamte In Med* 1987;**42**:126–30.

129 Charr R. Pulmonary changes in welders – a report of three cases. *Ann Int Med* 1956;**44**:806–812.

130 Friede E, Rachow DO. Symptomatic pulmonary disease in arc welders. *Ann Int Med* 1961;**54**:121–7.

131 Irmscher G, Beck B, Ahlendorf W, Anspach M, Konetzke G *et al*. Experience in expert assessment of dubious lung fibrosis from effect of welding fumes. *Z Ges Hyg* 1975;**21**:562–66.

132 Wagner U, Meerbach W, Fischer W, Otto J, Jahn R, Schneider WD. A case report of welder's lung. *Z Erkr Atmungsorgane* 1990;**174**:1149–154.

133 Lewis TR, Campbell KL, Vaughan TR. Effects on canine pulmonary function via induced nitrogen dioxide impairment. *Arch Environ Hlth* 1969;**18**:596.

134 Stem RM, Pigott GH, Abraham JL. Fibrogenic potential of welding fume. *J Appl Toxicol* 1983;**3**:18–30.

135 Glass WI, Taylor DR, Donoghue AM. Chronic interstitial disease in a welder of galvanised steel. *Occup Med* 1994;**44**:158–60.

136 Meyer E, Kratzinger SF, Miller WH. Pulmonary fibrosis in arc welder. *Arch Environ Hlth* 1967;**15**:462–8.

137 Patel KC, Sheth SM, Kamat SR. Arc welders' lung. *J Postgrad Med* 1977;**23**:35–38.

138 Stettler LE, Groth DH, Mackay GR. Identification of stainless steel welding fume particulates in human lung and environmental samples using electron probe microanalysis. *Am Ind Hyg Assoc J* 1977;**39**:76–82.

139 Guidotti TL. The higher oxides of nitrogen:inhalation toxicity. *Environ Res* 1978;**15**:443.

140 Hicks R, Klam HF, Al-Shamma KJ, Hewitt PJ. Pneumoconiotic effects of welding fume particles from mild and stainless steel deposited in the lungs of the rat. *Arch Toxicol* 1984;**55**:1–10.

141 Stem RM, Pigott GH. *In vitro* RPM fibrogenic potential assay of welding fumes. *Environ Hlth Perspect* 1983;**51**:231–6.

142 McMillan GHG. The health of welders in Naval dockyards: the risk of asbestos-related diseases occurring in welders. *J Occup Med* 1983;**25**:27–730.

143 Vallyathan V, Bergeron WN, Robichaux PA, Craighead JE. Pulmonary fibrosis in an aluminium arc welder. *Chest* 1982;**81**:372–4.

144 Herbert A, Sterling G, Abraham J, Corrin B. Desquamative interstitial pneumonia in an aluminium welder. *Hum Path* 1982;**13**:694–99.

145 Cole BM, Benton RE, Skalsyk HL. Pulmonary fibrosis in an aluminium arc welder. A complex issue. *Chest* 1983;**83**:291–292.

146 Funahashi A, Schlueter DP, Pintar K, Bemis EL,

Siegesmund KA. Welders, pneumoconioisis:tissue elemental microanalysis by energy dispersive x-ray analysis. *Br J Ind Med* 1988;**45**:14–18.

147 Billings CG, Howard P. Occupational siderosis and welders' lung: a review. *Monaldi Arch Chest Dis* 1993;**48**:304–14.

148 Meokild A, Langard S, Anderseon A, Stray-Tionnesen JN. Incidence of cancer among welders and other workers in a Norwegian shipyard. *Scand J Work Environ Hlth* 1989;**15**:387–94.

149 Moulin JJ, Portefaix P, Wild P, Mur JM, Smagghe G, Mantout B. Mortality study amongst workers producing ferroalloys and stainless steel in France. *Br J Ind Med* 1990;**47**:537–43.

150 Danielsen TE, Langard S, Andersen A, Knudsen O. The incidence of cancer among welders of mild steel and other shipyard workers. *Br J Ind Med* 1993;**50**:1097–103.

151 Moulin JJ, Wild P, Haguenoer JM, Faucon D, de Gaudemaris R *et al*. A mortality study among mild steel and stainless steel welders. *Br J Ind Med* 1993;**50**:234–43.

152 Langard S. Nickel related cancer in welders. *Sci Tox Environ* 1994;**148**:303–9.

153 Danielson TE, Langard S, Andersen A. Incidence of cancer among Norwegian boiler welders. *Occup Environ Med* 1996;**53**:231–4.

154 Lauritsen JM, Hansen KS. Lung cancer mortality in stainless steel and mild steel welders; a nested case-referent study. *Am J Ind Med* 1996;**30**:383–91.

155 Stern RM. 1983 Assessment of risk of lung cancer for welders. *Arch Environ Hlth* 1983;**38**:148–55.

156 Langard S, Stem RM. Nickel in the human environment. *IARC Scient Public* 1984;**53**:95–103.

157 Jockel KH, Ahrens W, Bolm-Audorff U. Lung cancer risk and welding – preliminary results from an ongoing case control study. *Am J Ind Med* 1994;**25**:805–12.

158 Vinzents P, Poulsen OM, Ligaard R, Simonsen H, Hansen EB *et al*. Cancer risk and thoriated welding electrodes. *Occup Hyg* 1994;**1**:27–33.

159 McElearney N, Irvine D. A study of thorium exposure during tungsten inert gas welding in an airline engineering population. *J Occup Med* 1993;**35**:707–11.

160 Heath C. Electromagnetic field exposure and cancer; a review of the epidemiologic evidence. *CA Cancer J Clin* 1996;**46**:29–44.

161 Becker N. Cancer mortality among arc welders exposed to fumes containing chromium and nickel. *J Occup Environ Med* 1999;**41**:294–303.

162 Elinder C-G, Ahrengart L, Lidums V, Pettersson E, Sjogren B. Evidence of aluminium accumulation in aluminium welders. *Br J Ind Med* 1991;**48**:735–8.

163 Hanninen H, Matikainen E, Kovala T, Valkonen S, Riihimaki V. Internal load of aluminium and the central nervous system function of aluminium welders. *Scand J Work Environ Hlth* 1994;**20**:279–85.

164 Sjogren B, Gustavsson P, Hogstedt C. Neuropsychiatric symptoms among welders exposed to neurotoxic metals. *Br J Ind Med* 1990;**47**:704–7.

165 Altman P, Dhanesha U, Hamon C, Cunningham J, Blair J, Marsh F. Disturbance of cerebral functions by aluminium in haemodialysis patients without overt aluminium toxicity. *Lancet* 1989;**ii**:7–11.

166 Sjogren B, Elinder CG. Proposal of a dose response relationship between aluminium welding fume exposure and effect on the central nervous system. *Med Lavora* 1992;**83**:484–8.

167 Sjogren B, Iregen A, Frech W, Hagman M, Johansson L *et al*. Effects on the nervous system among welders exposed to aluminium and manganese. *Occ Environ Med* 1996;**53**:32–40.

168 Kolmodin-Hedman B, Wenngren B-I, Rudell B, Carstensen U, Hammarstrom U, Jonsoon E. Suspected functional disorder of the brain in welders from two industries. *Arbete Halsa* 1991;**33**:1–14.

169 Wechsler LS, Checkoway H, Franklin GM, Costa LG. A pilot study of occupational and environmental risk factors for Parkinson's disease. *Neurotoxicity* 1991;**12**:387–92.

170 Fairfax RE. Manganese exposure during welding operations. *App Occup Environ Hyg* 1994;**9**:537–8.

171 Rachootin P, Olsen J. The risk of infertility and delayed conception associated with exposures in the Danish workplace. *J Occup Med* 1983;**25**:394–402.

172 Mortensen JT. Risk from reduced sperm quality among metal workers, with special reference to welders. *Scand J Work Environ Hlth* 1988;**4**:7–30.

173 Bonde JP. Subfertility in relation to welding. A case reference study among male welders. *Dan Med Bull* 1990;**1**:105–8.

174 Bonde JP, Hansen KS, Levine RL. Fertility among Danish male welders. *Scand J Work Environ Hlth* 1990;**16**:315–22.

175 Bonde JP. Semen quality and sex hormones among mild steel and stainless steel welders: a cross sectional study. *Br J Ind Med* 1990;**47**:508–14.

176 Bonde JP. Semen quality in welders exposed to radiant heat. *Br J Ind Med* 1992;**49**:5–10.

177 Moskova P, Popov I. Occupational damage to fertility in welders (Bulgarian). *Akush Ginekol* 1994;**33**:29–31.

178 Jelnes JE, Knudsene L. Stainless steel welding and semen quality. *Reproduct Toxicol* 1988;**2**:209–12.

179 Kandracova E. Fertility disorders in welders. *Ceskoslov Dermatolog* 1981;**56**:342–5.

180 Bonde JP. Semen quality among welders at follow up after three weeks of non-exposure. *Br J Ind Med* 1990;**47**:515–8.

181 Torell G, Sanden A, Jarvholm B. Musculosketal disorders in shipyard workers. *J Soc Occup Med* 1988;**38**:109–12.

182 Health Risks Study Group to the Swedish Commission on Working Conditions. *Report of a Survey of Jobs Posing Special Risks to Health*. Stockholm:Ministry of Labour, 1990.

183 Naheme GJ. Welding injuries. *Occup Hlth Safety Canada* 1993; May/June:74–5.

184 E Torner M, Zetterberg C, Anden U, Hansson T, Lindell V. Workload and musculoskeletal problems;a comparison

185 Wanders SP, Zielhuis GA, Vreuls HJH, Sielhuis RL. Medical wastage in shipyard welders; a forty year historical cohort study. *Int Arch Occup Environ Hlth* 1992;**64**:281–90.

186 Herberts P, Kadefors R. A study of painful shoulder in welders. *Acta Orthop Scand* 1976;**44**:4381–7.

187 Kadefors R, Petersen I, Herberts P. Muscular reaction to welding work;an electromyographic investigation. *Ergonomics* 1976;**19**,543–58.

188 Herberts P, Kadefors R, Hogfors C, Sigholm G. Shoulder pain and heavy manual labour. *Clin Orthop* 1984;**191**:166–78.

189 Hagberg M, Wegman DH. Prevalence rates and odds ratios of shoulder neck diseases in different occupational groups. *Br J Ind Med* 1987;**44**:602–10.

190 Jarvholm U, Palmerud G, Kadefors R, Herbert P. The effect of arm support on supraspinatus muscle load during simulated assembly work and welding. *Ergonomics* 1991;**34**:57–66.

191 Kadefors R. A model for assessment and design of workplaces for manual welding. In: Marras WS, Karwowski W, Smith J, Pacholski L eds. *The Ergonomics of Manual Work* London, Washington DC:Tayor and Francis, 1993 : 601–4.

192 Tenkate TD, Collins MJ. Personal ultraviolet radiation exposure of welders in a welding environment. *Am Ind Hyg Assoc J* 1997;**58**:33–48.

193 McMillan GHG. Protection of dockyard welders. *Safety Practitioner* 1983;May:8–16.

194 Jirasek L. Occupational exogenous siderosis of the skin. *Contact Derm* 1979;**5**:334.

195 Weiler KJ. Nickel contact eczema caused by electric welding. *Derm Berud Umweldt* 1979;**27**:142.

196 Shehade SA, Roberts PI, Diffey, Foulds IS. *Br J Dermatol* 1987;**1**: 117–19.

197 Elsner P, Hassam S. Occupational UVC-induced exacerbation of atopic dermatitis in a welder. *Contact Derm* 1996;**335**:180–1.

198 Giddins GE, Wilson-Macdonald J. Spot weld injuries of the hand. *J Hand Surg* 1994;**19**:165–7.

199 Shanahan EM, Hanley SD. Soft tissue injury in resistance welding. *Occup Med* 1995; **45**:137–40.

200 Stage J, Vinding T. Metal spark perforation of the tympanic membrane with deafness and facial paralysis. *J Laryng Otol* 1986;**100**:699–700.

201 Fisher EW, Gardiner Q. Tympanic membrane injury in welders. *J Soc Occup Med* 1991;**41**:86–8.

202 Mertens J, Bubmann M, Reker U. Welding spark injuries of the ear. *Laryngorhinootologie* 1991;**70**:405–8.

203 Panosian MS, Dutcher PO. Transtympanic facial nerve injury in welders. *Occup Med* 1994;**44**:99–101.

204 Rodgers L. Hearing conservation in fabrication shops. *Welding Metal Fabric* 1993;May/June:417–22.

205 Rees MR, Dufresne RM, Suggett D, Alleyue BC. Welder eye injuries. *J Occup Med* 1989;**31**:1003–6.

206 Karai I, Horigichi S. Pterygium in welders. *Br J Ophthalmol* 1984;**68**:347–9.

207 Ross DS. Welding injury accidents. *Metal Construct Br Weld J* 1973;July:261.

208 Horstman S, Ingram JW. A critical evaluation of the protection provided by common safety glasses from ultraviolet radiation in welding operations. *Am Ind Hyg Assoc J* 1979;**40**:770.

209 Vernon S. External eye problems. *Pulse* 1996;Sep:86.

210 Naidoff MA, Sliney DH. Retinal injury from a weldering arc. *Am J Ophthalmol* 1979;**77**:663.

211 Brittan GPH. Retinal burns caused by exposure to MIG welding: report of two cases. *Br J Ophthalmol* 1988;**72**:570–5.

212 Fich M, Dahl H, Fledelius H, Tinning S. Maculopathy caused by welding arcs. A report of 3 cases. *Acta Opthalmol* 1993;**71**:402–4.

213 Dare PRM, Hewitt PJ, Hicks R. Barium in welding fume. *Ann Occup Hyg* 1984;**28**:445–8.

214 Moreton J, Jenkins N. Barium in welding fume. *Ann Occup Hyg* 1985;**29**:443–5.

215 Yeo RBG. Barium in welding fume. *Ann Occup Hyg* 1986;**30**:515–7.

216 Hicks R, Caldas LQ, Dare PR, Hewitt PJ. Cardiotoxic and bronchoconstrictor effects of industrial metal fumes containing barium. *Arch Toxicol Suppl* 1986;**9**:416–20.

217 Embil JM, Geddes JS, Foster D, Sandeman J. Return to arc welding following defibrillator implantation. *Pacing Clin Electrophysiol* 1993;**16**:2313–8.

218 Balbi M, Bertero G, Bellotti S. The effects of electromagnetic interference on pace makers of the new generation. *Cuore* 1992;**9**:523–8.

219 Bourton MA. *A Review of Arc Welding and Electromagenetic Compatibility*. Technology Briefing 490. Cambridge: The Welding Institute. 1994.

220 Weman K. Health hazards caused by electro-magnetic fields during welding. *Svetsaren* 1994;**48**:14–6.

221 Fetter JG, Benditt DG, Stanton MS. Electromagnetic interference from welding and motors on implantable cardioverter-defibrillators as tested in the electrically hostile work site. *J Am Coll Cardiol* 1996;**28**:423–7.

222 Rask-Andersen A. The organic dust toxic syndrome – a review. *Agricultural Health and Safety: Workplace, Environment, Sustainability*. McDuffle HH, Dosman JA, Semchuk KM, Olenchock SA, Senthilselvan A eds. Boca Raton, FL: Lewis Publishers, 1995 : 101–103.

223 Thackrah CT. *The Effects of Arts, Trades and the Professions and of Civic States and Habits of Living on Health and Longevity*. London: Longman, 1832 : 101.

224 Dressen WC, Brinton HP, Keenan RG, Thomas TR, Place EH, Fuller JE. *Health of Arc Welders in Steel Ship Construction*. Public Health Bulletin No 298. Federal Security Agency, US Public Health Service. Washington: United States Government Printing Office, 1947.

225 Ross DS. The short term effects on health of manual arc welding. *Trans Soc Occup Med* 1973;**23**:92–5.

226 Fine JM, Gordon T, Chen LC, Kinney G, Becket WS. Metal fume fever: characterisation of clinical and plasma IL-6 responses in controlled human exposures to zinc oxide at or below the threshold limit value. *J Occup Environ Med* 1997;**39**:722–26.

227 Beckett WS, Chen LC, Cosma G, Fine J, Garte S *et al. Metal Fume Fever. Occupational Medicine Program*. New Haven, Connecticutt: Yale University, 1996.

228 Hamilton A. *Industrial Poisons in the United States*. New York: McMillan, 1925 : 276–90.

229 Sturgis CC, Drinker P, Thompson RM. Metal fume fever. I. Clinical observations of the effect of the experimental inhalation of zinc oxide by two apparently normal persons. *J Ind Hyg* 1927;**9**:88–97.

230 Petit DW. Some respiratory hazards of welding. *Stanford Med Bull* 1943;**1**:136–42.

231 Drinker P, Nelson KW. Welding fumes in steel fabrication. *Texas J Med* 1944;**40**:275–8.

232 Papp JP. Metal fume fever case report. *Postgrad Med* 1968;**43**:160–3.

233 Fishburn CW, Zenz C. Metal fume fever; a report of a case. *J Occup Med* 1969;**11**:142–4.

234 Department of Employment and Productivity. *Fumes from Welding and Flame Cutting. Report on the Shipbuilding and Ship Repair Industry*. London: HMSO, 1970.

235 Dula DJ. Metal fume fever. *J Am Coll Emerg Physicians* 1978;**7**:448–50.

236 Armstrong CW, Moore LW, Hackler RL, Miller GB, Stroube RB. An outbreak of metal fume fever. *J Occup Med* 1983;**25**:886–8.

237 Blanc P, Wong H, Bernstein MS, Boushey HA. An experimental human model of metal fume fever. *Ann Intern Med* 1991;**114**:930–6.

238 Anthony JS, Zamel N, Alberman A. Abnormalities in pulmonary function after brief exposure to toxic metal fumes. *J Can Med Assoc* 1978;**119**:586–8.

239 Vogelmeier C, Konig G, Bencze K, Fruhmann G. Pulmonary involvement in zinc fume fever. *Chest* 1987;**92**:946–8.

240 Gordon T, Fine JM. Metal fume fever. *Occup Med State Art Rev* 1993;**8**:504–17.

241 Pasker HG, Peeters M, Genet P, Clement J, Nemery B, Van de Woestijne KP. *Eur Resp J* 1997;**10**:1523–9.

242 Brodie J. Welding fumes and gases – their effects on the health of the worker. *Calif West Med* 1943;**59**:13–18.

243 Rohrs CL. Metal fume fever from inhaling iron oxide. *Arch Int Med* 1957;**100**:44.

244 Glass WI. Mercury fume fever. *NZ Med J* 1970;**71**:297–8.

245 Ross DS. Welders' metal fume fever. *J Soc Occup Med* 1974;**24**:125–9.

246 Blanc P, Boushey HA. The lung in metal fume fever. *Semin Respir Med* 1993;**14**:212–25.

247 McMillan G. Metal fume fever. *Occup Hlth* 1986;May:148–9.

248 Drinker KR, Drinker P. Metal fume fever. Results of the inhalation by animals of zinc and magnesium oxide fumes. *J Ind Hyg* 1928;**10**:56–70.

249 Mori T, Akashi S, Nukada A. Effects of the inhalation of

catalytically active metallic oxide fumes on rabbits. *Int Arch Occup Environ Hlth* 1975;**36**:29–39.

250   Migally N, Murthy RC, Daye A, Zambernard F. Changes in pulmonary alveolar macrophages in rats exposed to oxide of zinc and nickel. *J Submicrosc Cytol* 1982;**14**:621–6.

251   Lam HF, Conner MW, Rogers AE, Fitzgerald S, Amdur MO. Functional and morphologic changes in the lungs of guinea pigs exposed to freshly generated ultrafine zinc oxide. *Toxicol Appl Pharmacol* 1985;**78**:29–38.

252   Conner MW, Flood WH, Rogers AE, Amdur MO. Lung injury in guinea pigs caused by multiple exposures to untrafimne zinc oxide:changes in pulmonary lavage fluid. *J Toxicol Environ Hlth* 1988;**25**:57–69.

253   Blanc PD, Bigby B, Bernstein MS, Wong H, Boushey HA. The role of lung inflammation in metal fume fever. *Am Rev Respir Dis* 1990;**141**:A594.

254   Gordon T, Chen LC, Fine JM, Schleinger RB, Su WY *et al*. Pulmonary effects of inhaled zinc oxide in human subjects, guinea pigs, rats and rabbits. *Am Ind Hyg Assoc J* 1992;**53**:503–9.

255   Blanc PD, Boushey HA, Wong H, Wintermeyer SF, Bernstein MS. Cytokines in metal fume fever. *Am Rev Respir Dis* 1993;**147**:134–8.

256   Kuschner WG, D'Alessandro A, Wintermeyer SF, Wong H, Boushey HA, Blanc PD. Pulmonary responses to purified zinc oxide fume. *J Occup Med* 1995;**43**:371–8.

257   Callender GR. Acute poisoning by the zinc and antimony content of limeade prepared in a galvanised iron pan. *Mil Surg* 1937;**80**:67–71.

258   Murphy J. Intoxication following ingestion of elemental zinc. *JAMA* 1970;**212**:2119–20.

259   Brocks A, Reid H, Glazer G. Acute intravenous zinc poisoning. *Br Med J* 1977;**1**:1390–1.

260   Pemis B, Vigliani EC, Cavagna G, Finulli M. Endogenous pyrogen in the pathogenesis of zinc fume fever. *Med Lav* 1960;**51**:579–86.

261   McCord CP. Metal fume fever as an immunological disease. *Ind Med Surg* 1960;**12**:101–07.

262   Farrell FJ. Angioedema and urticaria as acute and late phase reactions to zinc fume exposure with associated metal fume fever-like symptoms. *Am J Ind Med* 1987;**12**:331–7.

263   Kuschner WG, D'Alessandro A, Wong H, Blanc PD. Early pulmonary cytokine responses to zinc oxide inhalation. *Environ Res* 1997;**75**:7–11.

264   Kuschner WG, D'Alessandro A, Wong H, Blanc PD. Tumour necrosis factor-alpha and interleukin-release from U937 human mononuclear cells exposed to zinc oxide *in vitro*. Mechanistic implications for metal fume fever. *J Occup Environ Med* 1998;**40**:454–59.

265   Ameille J, Brechot JM, Brochard P, Capron F, Dore MF. Occupational hypersensitivity pneumonia in a smelter exposed to zinc fumes. *Chest* 1992;**101**:862–63.

266   Sferlazza SJ, Beckett WS. The respiratory health of welders. *Am Rev Respir Dis* 1991;**143**:1134–48.

267   Ando Y, Shibata E, Tsuchiyama F, Sakai S. Elevated urinary cadmium concentrations in a patient with acute cadmium pneumonitis. *Scand J Work Environ Hlth* 1996;**22**:150–53.

268   Coggon D, Inskip H, Winter P, Pannett B. Lobar pneumonia: an occupational disease in welders. *Lancet* 1994;**344**:41–3.

269   McMillan GHG, Pethybridge RJ. The health of welders in naval dockyards; proportional mortality study of welders and two control groups. *J Soc Occup Med* 1983;**33**:75–84.

270   Coggon D. New occupational diseases. *J Roy Coll Phys* 1997;**31**:202–5.

271   Goldstein M, Weiss H, Wade K, Penek J, Andrews L, Brandt-Rauf P. An outbreak of fume fever in an electronics instrument testing laboratory. *J Occup Med* 1987;**29**:746–49.

272   Centers for Disease Control. Severe acute respiratory illness linked to use of shoe sprays. Colorado, November 1993. *Morbid Mortal Weekly Rep* 1993;**42**:885–87.

273   Kales SN, Christiani DC. Progression of chronic obstructive pulmonary disease after multiple episodes of an occupational inhalation fever. *J Occup Med* 1994;**36**:No 1, 75–8.

274   Shusterman DJ. Polymer fume fever and other fluorcarbon pyrolysis-related syndromes. *Occup Med State Art Rev* 1993;**8**:519–531.

275   Lee CH, Guo YL, Tsai PJ, Chang HY, Chen CR *et al*. Fatal acute pulmonary odema after inhalation of fumes from polytetrafluoroethylene (PTF). *Europ Resp J* 1997;**10**:1408–11.

276   Johnston CJ, Finkelstein JN, Gelein R, Baggs R, Oberdorster G. Characterisation of the early pulmonary response associated with PTFE fume exposure. *Toxicol Appl Pharmacol* 1996;**140**:154–163.

10

Pesticides and other agrochemicals

ALISON L JONES, ALEX T PROUDFOOT

Definitions	195	Poisoning with insecticides	204
Classification of pesticide poisoning	196	Exposure to rodenticides	212
Epidemiology of pesticide poisoning	197	Exposure to fungicides	212
Prevention of health impairment by pesticides	197	Exposure to molluscicides	213
Principles of management of pesticide exposures	199	Accidental self-injection with veterinary products	213
Poisoning with herbicides	200	References	214

A pesticide is any physical, chemical or biological agent that will kill an undesirable plant or animal pest. Pesticides are therefore almost as diverse as their targets. Over the centuries many have been developed. Sulphur was used as a fumigant by the Chinese before 1000 BC and in the nineteenth century in Europe against powdery mildew in fruit. Arsenic-containing compounds were also used as insecticides in the sixteenth century and as weed killer in the late nineteenth century. By the 1920s the extensive use of arsenicals caused public concern because some fruit and vegetables were found to contain toxic residues. The 1930s saw the development of a variety of synthetic pesticides such as alkyl thiocyanate insecticides, dithiocarbamates and ethylene dibromide some of which have been superseded by numerous new compounds developed in the post-war era.

All pesticides are inherently toxic to some living organism, otherwise they would be of no value. There is therefore no such thing as a completely safe pesticide. Despite modern day agents being second- and third-generation derivatives of earlier chemicals, the target species specificity of pesticides is not as well developed as might be hoped and non-target species are often affected because they possess physiological or biochemical systems that are similar to those of the target organisms. However, many present a very low risk to human health when applied in accordance with product recommendations.

In recent years there has been a backlash against pesticide use in general, largely because of the misuse and abuse of some by a few individuals in a relatively small number of well publicized incidents.[1] In developed countries the public are becoming increasingly aware and suspicious of pesticide residues and other chemicals in the environment and the possibility that they may be responsible for currently unexplained ill health.[2] As a result, ingestion of residues on fruits or vegetables has been alleged to be the cause of numerous chronic non-specific symptoms, allergies, reduced sperm counts,[3] neurological disorders and a variety of malignant tumours. Despite the controversy surrounding these claims and the presence of low levels of residues in food, groundwater and air, pesticides and other agrochemicals are important components of integrated approaches to efficient crop production. They have helped provide society with an abundance and variety of inexpensive fruits and vegetables that was unthinkable only 50 years ago. Between the extremes of unrestricted use and prohibition must be a position of effective use compatible with safety for operators, consumers and the environment. However, as long as pesticides continue to be used, accidental and/or deliberate poisoning of some wildlife, domestic animals and even humans can be anticipated and will require management.

DEFINITIONS

Pesticides include a variety of agents that are more specifically classified on the basis of their target organisms:

- herbicides e.g. paraquat,
- insecticides e.g. organophosphorus compounds,
- molluscicides e.g. metaldehyde,
- fungicides e.g. carbamates,
- rodenticides e.g. superwarfarins.

CLASSIFICATION OF PESTICIDE POISONING

Pesticide poisoning can be classified according to the circumstances of exposure. The main varieties are occupational, accidental and deliberate (Table 10.1).

Table 10.1 *Classification of pesticide poisoning*

Occupational
Major chemical disasters
During manufacture
During preparation for dilution and application
Harvesting and packing

Accidental
Consumption of residues
Bystander exposure
Ingestion and other exposures in children
Major chemical disasters

Deliberate
Use for parasuicide, suicide or homicide

Exposures during manufacture

Major chemical disasters apart, occupational exposure to pesticides is theoretically possible during the manufacture of pesticides but is rare because of the elaborate engineering controls and other safety measures built into manufacturing processes.

Exposure during dilution and application

Occupational exposure is potentially a problem during the dilution and application of pesticides such as within the lawn, tree, or care service industries and apple orchard workers.[4,5] The biggest risk is during handling of concentrates, particularly while mixing or loading[6] and during application itself. During these activities the most important route of exposure is through the skin with inhalation a secondary route. Clearly, when the pesticide is a fumigant being used in a closed environment, e.g. in greenhouses, the respiratory route is the dominant one.

Failure to read and comply with the recommendations on the product label, ignoring advice on the wearing of appropriate personal protective equipment, poorly designed pesticide containers with necks that make 'glugging' and splashing during pouring unavoidable and badly maintained application machinery are important contributors to dermal contamination with pesticides. The care with which pesticides are diluted, mixed and applied by farmers and small independent contractors is likely to vary but failure to comply with operator safety recommendations is probably common and is dif-

ficult, if not impossible, to eradicate. Reduction of exposures depends on education but the extent to which workers are trained in the safe use of pesticides varies enormously.

An analysis of occupationally related pesticide exposures, by category, in 1988 in California revealed that ground applicators were at greatest risk whereas aerial applicators and workers involved in mosquito abatement programmes had the least pesticide-related illness.[7] However, such data may not be representative of the rest of the world.

Exposure during harvesting and packing

Dislodgable residues may well be present on some crops and ornamental plants at the time of harvesting or packaging making possible further dermal absorption. This type of exposure can be minimized by observing recommended intervals between the last application of the pesticide and harvesting. Washing the crop may only be practicable when it reaches the consumer.

Consumption of foods containing pesticide residues

Regulatory authorities throughout the world take great care to ensure that the proper use of any pesticide should result in residues on crops that are so small that the risk to the public from consuming them is infinitesimally low. However, good agricultural practice is not universal. Monitoring reveals that undesirably high, but not necessarily toxic, residues on food can occur for a variety of reasons including incorrect application rates and harvesting too soon after pesticide application.[8] Many incidents of contamination of potable water, fish stock or wildlife by pesticides have been reported. Occasionally, the reason for high residue levels is the illegal use of an agent. Amongst the best known examples are several incidents where the carbamate insecticide, aldicarb, was used on hydroponically grown melons and cucumbers.

Bystander exposure

Bystanders and passers by can be exposed to off-target drift from spraying resulting in subsequent claims of ill health such as hypersensitivity.[9]

Accidental ingestion or skin contamination

Children are at particular risk from ingestion of pesticides around their homes.[10] Careless storage or decanting them into unlabelled bottles or soft drinks containers are contributory factors.

Major disasters

Major disasters at manufacturing plants are potentially the events most likely to result in severe and life-threatening, accidental pesticide poisoning. Fortunately these events are rare.

Deliberate ingestion

Not surprisingly, the most serious and potentially lethal effects of pesticides result from their deliberate consumption. They are rarely injected. Paraquat and organophosphate insecticides are well recognized examples of pesticides that are ingested. The agents used, vary from one culture to another and some have attracted notoriety because of this form of abuse.

EPIDEMIOLOGY OF PESTICIDE POISONING

It has been estimated that there are approximately 3 million pesticide poisonings annually world-wide, with some 220 000 deaths though there is probably considerable under-reporting.[11] The sad reality is that approximately two of every three pesticide poisonings is deliberate and self-inflicted.[12] The apparent increase in the number of cases in recent years may not simply be the result of increased use of pesticides by a larger population; the availability of better statistics from some countries may have contributed.[13] Pesticides are estimated to be responsible for less than 4% of deaths from all types of accidental poisoning but pesticide poisoning is 13 times more common in developing countries than in the highly industrialized societies that consume 85% of the crops produced using pesticides.[14–16] For example, in the United Kingdom in 1992 there were fewer than 20 occupational poisonings with organophosphates[17] whereas 8268 were reported in Thailand in a population of 100 000 agricultural workers.[12] This is partly because the registration and sale of pesticides is less well regulated in developing countries[14] and because the steady increase in their use has not been matched by the development of systems to educate users in the safe handling of these toxic substances. It is perhaps surprising that despite the number of new active ingredients that have become available in recent years, poisoning with pesticides remains largely dominated by older compounds.[11]

PREVENTION OF HEALTH IMPAIRMENT BY PESTICIDES

The risk of pesticides causing adverse effects on health can be minimized by a number of mechanisms. These probably have a higher profile in developed countries.[18]

They include:

- manufacturing regulations,
- pesticide regulations,
- personal protective equipment,
- biological monitoring of operators,
- monitoring pesticide residues in food and water,
- education,
- measures to deter or reduce the consequences of deliberate ingestion.

Manufacturing regulations

Work practices and levels of exposure are defined in such a way that they do not present an unacceptable health risk although they do not necessarily eliminate risk completely. Interindividual variability in susceptibility to the adverse effects of chemicals may be important at low level exposure e.g. bronchospasm being more likely induced in those with pre-existing asthma.

Regulation of pesticides

To ensure as far as possible the health and safety of those who apply pesticides and those who consume produce treated with them, many developed countries have established regulatory bodies that advise on the pesticides that can be marketed for professional use in agriculture, horticulture and public premises and also those for amateur use in homes and gardens. They also specify the approved target organisms for each pesticide, the rate at which it may be applied (dose per application and number of applications), the crop(s) to which it may be applied, minimum application/harvest intervals (where appropriate), obligatory hazard warnings to be carried on product labels and other conditions of use including the level of protective equipment for operators. The impact of use on the environment is also an important component of the evaluation of each pesticide. Both the active ingredient and the formulated product must be assessed. The range and volume of data required to make informed decisions on such disparate matters is enormous. Much animal toxicity testing may be necessary to enable assessment of the human health risks. Provision of data on safety and efficacy is the statutory responsibility of the manufacturer who meets the costs of generation of the required data and assessment by the regulatory authorities.

In the UK, assessment of pesticides is the responsibility of the statutory and independent Advisory Committee on Pesticides. This committee makes recommendations to relevant government departments whose ministers make the final decision and the departments then issue the formal approval for use. Investigation of non-compliance with the conditions of storage, use and disposal of pesticides rests with the Health and Safety

Executive inspectorate. To avoid unnecessary duplication of animal studies and effort, and to achieve harmonization, the UK government now collaborates with those of other European Union states in evaluating pesticides. For pesticide operators, evaluation allows permissible exposure levels and levels of personal protective equipment to be set in addition to determining the potential of the active ingredient and the formulated product to irritate or sensitize the skin. Unfortunately, legislation cannot prevent the accidental or deliberate misuse of pesticides.

Animal studies can provide only a best guess of the toxicity of a chemical for humans. For example dioxin is less toxic on acute exposure on a weight-for-weight basis to humans than other mammalian species because of the lower affinity with which it binds to its receptor.[19] Some chemicals may be more carcinogenic to rodents than humans because of interspecies differences. In contrast, skin and gastrointestinal carcinomas after excessive ingestion of arsenic in humans have not been reproduced in carcinogenicity studies in animals.[20] Similarly respiratory sensitizers may be missed in animal studies and so far no predictive tests have been validated for respiratory sensitization in humans.[21]

Personal protective equipment

In addition to observing good practice, exposure to pesticides can be reduced by wearing gloves, goggles, suitable protective clothing and respiratory protection depending on what is appropriate to the product being applied. The level of protection is advised by the regulatory authorities. However, personal protective equipment may make performance of some tasks more difficult and together with blatant disregard, climatic conditions and operators' perceptions of their image may result in precautions being ignored e.g. in sheep dipping.

Biological monitoring and health surveillance

The difficulty of extrapolating the results of animal testing to workers involved in the manufacture and application of pesticides makes careful clinical surveillance of them important. Their exposure may be assessed qualitatively (e.g. by job classification or questionnaire) or quantitatively by ambient (such as factory air monitoring) or personal monitoring or by measurement of serum concentrations of pesticides.[22,23] Some pesticides (e.g. DDT [dichlorodiphenyltrichloroethane]) have long biological half-lives and the timing of sampling is not critical.[24] For those with a short elimination time, timing may be critical and the sample is usually collected during exposure, at the end of the exposure period or before resuming work after the weekend.[25]

Biological monitoring evaluates the health risk of either the amount of chemical absorbed recently or the total amount stored in various body compartments i.e. the body burden. The ideal biological monitor measures the amount of active chemical bound to critical sites of action and is a better measure of risk than ambient air monitoring as it takes account of variable absorption, inter-individual variation in response and personal hygiene habits.[26] Because of its ability to evaluate the overall exposure, biological monitoring can also be used to test the efficacy of various protective measures such as gloves, masks or barrier creams.[22,26]

Biological monitoring is of no value for assessing exposure to substances that exhibit their toxic effects at the tissues of first contact (e.g. lung irritants) or are poorly absorbed. In these cases measurement of exposure or of the direct toxic effect is more appropriate. Biological monitoring may provide different information, dependent on our current knowledge of relationships between external exposure, internal exposure and the risks of adverse health effects. If only the relationship between external exposure and the internal dose is known, this parameter can be used as an index of exposure, but if a quantitative relationship between internal dose and health effects is established, then biological-effects monitoring allows for direct health risk assessment.[25,26] Unfortunately, too few published data have defined the relationship between internal dose and exposure, most merely concentrating on the external dose applied. Thus in relatively few cases can biological-effects monitoring allow for direct health risk assessment.

Various factors influence the fate of pesticides *in vivo*. Sex, weight, fat mass, pregnancy and diseases, particularly those of the liver and kidneys may alter the metabolism of pesticides as do competition for metabolic pathways, enzyme induction and interactions with alcohol, food additives, drugs or even tobacco. All of these factors must be considered when interpreting results of biological exposure tests. Interpretation of the values for a given individual level is possible only if the individual's response varies little and the specificity of the effect is high.

Health surveillance is not merely the diagnosis of occupational disease. It should be carried out even when exposure is below permitted levels. The main objectives are:

- to detect hypersensitivity reactions as early as possible,
- to detect other adverse biological effects as early as possible,
- to test the safety of the permissible operator exposure level.

Health surveillance is particularly important when a new pesticide is being used and should include measurement of both exposure and possible health effects.[27] The latter is based on knowledge of the mechanism of action and target organs obtained from animal studies. However, detection of early health impairment is difficult as the features are often subtle and there may be considerable inter-individual variations. Similarly, the diagnostic tools of clinical medicine are frequently less sensitive than is desirable and may not detect adverse effects sufficiently early for corrective action to reverse them. For example, the glomerular filtration rate must be reduced by more than 60% before serum creatinine concentrations rise significantly and standard liver function tests tell us more about cell death and leakage of enzymes into serum than they do about function. The results must therefore be compared statistically with those for unexposed workers matched for variables such as age, sex, socioeconomic status and smoking habits; comparison with the general population is less valid.

Reports of the consequences of accidental or deliberate acute intoxication with a pesticide can also be of value since they establish beyond doubt the features that occur in humans and identify measures that may be of value in the management of poisoning. However, they do not help to determine the no-effect level.

Monitoring residues

Monitoring of pesticide residues in staple items of the national diet is an important way of ensuring that food is being produced in accordance with good agricultural practice. The continuous monitoring programme that operates in the UK occasionally identifies residues that exceed limits (e.g. organophosphate insecticides in carrots in the UK in 1997) and though they probably do not pose any risk to the health of consumers, the causes can be investigated and corrective action taken if the crop is home grown. Dealing with excessive pesticide residues in imported produce is more difficult.

Education

Education of professional pesticide operators is vital for the protection of their own health and that of the wider public. The Health and Safety Executive, the National Farmers Union and other concerned organizations arrange a variety of courses and provide educational material to encourage safe handling and application of pesticides.

Preventing deliberate ingestion of pesticides

Legislation can never prevent the deliberate misuse of pesticides. As indicated earlier, most deaths from pesticide poisoning are the result of suicide attempts and the use of pesticides rather than other agents in these cases reflects local custom, the toxins that are most readily

available and perceptions about which might be most lethal. Thus suicide by means of paraquat poisoning is unusually high in Japan, aluminium and other metal phosphides in India and organophosphate insecticides in a number of countries including Sri Lanka. The relatively low concentrations of active ingredients in products on sale to the public reduce the likelihood of massive poisoning but more concentrated formulations sporadically find their way into unauthorized hands with fatal consequences. The addition of emetics or stenching agents to some products may also minimize the quantity deliberately ingested or retained.

PRINCIPLES OF MANAGEMENT OF PESTICIDE EXPOSURES[28]

Be prepared

In all places where pesticides are handled, or manufactured, notices should be posted giving the name and telephone number of the:

- first aider,
- nearest doctor,
- nearest hospital emergency department.

Immediate responses

The basic steps in the event of acute pesticide exposures include:[29]

- ensure that you do not become a victim yourself;
- remove the victim from further exposure;
- establish a clear airway and commence artificial respiration if necessary;
- if practicable, get the victims to remove soiled clothing and wash contaminated skin thoroughly with soap and water; helpers who have to perform this task should wear appropriate personal protective equipment;
- if the pesticide has been ingested consider the need for gut decontamination (see below);
- advice on the management of pesticide-poisoned patients is available 24 hours a day from the centres of the National Poisons Information Service in the UK (Table 10.2);
- if there are multiple victims, the contaminated area, the area of containment and a safe area in which no further exposure can take place should be defined; fire-officers are well trained in setting up such areas as are physicians working for larger agrochemical companies – the concern is for smaller companies with no experience or preparedness for chemical incidents.

Table 10.2 *NPIS telephone numbers*

Belfast	028 20 240503
Birmingham	0121 507 5588/9
Cardiff	024 76 709901
Dublin	00353 1 8379964
Edinburgh	0131 536 2300
London	0207 635 9191
Newcastle	0191 232 5131

Reassurance

Individuals who have ingested excessive amounts of pesticides should be observed. In general, if symptoms do not develop within about 4–6 hours, it is unlikely that they will do so at all and the patient can be reassured. It then remains to determine the reasons for the incident and prevent repetition. The onset of toxic features can be expected to be slower after excessive dermal exposures and the period of observation may need to be extended.

Exposure to unknown pesticides

Exposure to an unknown pesticide with symptoms or features of toxicity developing should be treated with supportive and symptomatic care. Care must be taken to maintain the airway, breathing and circulation. High flow oxygen should be given, convulsions should be controlled with diazepam (10 mg intravenously for an adult), fluid losses should be replaced and acid-base abnormalities corrected. Clusters of symptoms and signs may give clues to the type of pesticide to which the patient has been exposed (Table 10.3).

Table 10.3 *Distinctive symptoms or signs giving clues to the type of pesticide to which patients have been exposed*

Distinctive symptoms or signs	Type of pesticide
Muscle fasciculation Weakness Respiratory failure Bronchorrhoea Arrhythmias	Organophosphates and carbamates
Bleeding gums Gastrointestinal bleeding	Warfarins and superwarfarins
Buccal ulceration Pulmonary infiltrates Renal failure	Paraquat/diquat
Transient burning of skin and conjunctivae	Permethrins
Nausea Vomiting Abdominal pain Methaemoglobinaemia	Chlorates

POISONING WITH HERBICIDES

Herbicides kill or severely injure plants. In the past two decades herbicides have represented the most rapidly growing section of the agrochemical industry. Amongst the most important from a toxicological point of view are the bipyridyl herbicides (paraquat and diquat), phenoxyacetate compounds and glyphosate-containing products.

Paraquat

Paraquat is tightly adsorbed to clay and by virtue of this is inactivated almost instantly on contact with soil. If used according to the label recommendations, it is safe[30] because little, if any, is absorbed across intact skin or by inhalation of spray. However, occupational poisoning has occurred by transdermal absorption when concentrated sprays solutions have leaked from back packs (see below). In terms of human poisoning, paraquat is the herbicide that has been used most commonly as a means of suicide by deliberate ingestion and has a high case fatality rate. Paraquat poisoning is common in countries such as Japan, the West Indies, Samoa and Taiwan.[31] In Japan, it is estimated that at least 1000 adults die each year as a result of deliberate ingestion of paraquat. Stenching agents, dyes and emetics have been added to some formulations to deter ingestion and reduce its consequences.

TOXICOKINETICS AND MECHANISM OF TOXICITY

Paraquat is poorly absorbed through intact skin or the respiratory tract.[31] When ingested, only about 5–10% of the dose is absorbed although the percentage may be enhanced by the presence of emulsifiers or solvents. Liquid formulations enter the small intestine rapidly and plasma concentrations reach a peak at 1–2 hours.[32] Absorbed paraquat is sequestered in the lungs, the main target organ, by an active adenosine triphosphate (ATP)-dependent, diamine/polyamine transport system.[33,34] It then undergoes a complex sequence of changes that result in the production of hydrogen peroxide and superoxide anions which attack polyunsaturated lipids present in cell membranes and cause cell death. An acute alveolitis develops causing haemorrhagic pulmonary oedema or adult respiratory distress syndrome.

Subsequently, collagen is deposited in and between alveolar spaces leading to fibrosis.[35] Paraquat is not extensively metabolized; most is excreted unchanged in the urine within the first 24 hours after ingestion.[36] Urinary elimination may continue for days or weeks after exposure as paraquat stored in lung and muscle is slowly released back into the blood.

CONSEQUENCES OF OCCUPATIONAL EXPOSURE

Occupational exposure to paraquat results in irritative and corrosive effects on mucous membranes, the cornea and skin – the magnitude of which is mainly determined by the concentration of paraquat in the contaminating fluid and to a lesser extent by the duration of contact. If splashes on skin are promptly removed and the skin washed they seldom cause further problems. However, prolonged contact, even with paraquat concentrations as low as 5 g/litre, can result in burns which, if they involve a large surface area, may allow enough paraquat to be absorbed to cause systemic poisoning and death.[32,37,38] Spraying higher concentrations (28 and 40 g/litre) from a leaking knapsack or shoulder-carried applicator has also caused death.[37,39] Reversible changes in finger nails such as guttate lesions and corrosive changes also occur.

Splashes in the eye cause lacrimation and blepharospasm. Corneal ulceration may result from concentrated solutions.[35] Features may not develop until 12–24 hours after the exposure. Inhaled droplets may produce a sore throat and nose bleeds.[40]

Swan[41] found no detectable lung changes in workers exposed to sprays 6 days per week for 12 weeks. Senanayake et al.[42] demonstrated no changes in pulmonary function tests in Sri Lankan tea workers with chronic exposure to paraquat aerosols. Others have however developed pulmonary damage due to absorption through the skin.[43]

FEATURES OF DELIBERATE INGESTION

Serious and fatal paraquat poisoning is most commonly due to deliberate ingestion of concentrates intended only for professional use. The lethal dose for an adult is estimated to be of the order of 3–5 g.[32] Therefore, as little as 10–15 ml of a 20% solution can be fatal. The features of upper gastrointestinal and respiratory tract damage reflect the concentration of the solution swallowed while the systemic features are more due to the amount ingested (Table 10.4).[40] Death is usually due to critically

impaired gas exchange secondary to the pulmonary toxicity of paraquat and occurs about a week after ingestion but there is considerable variation. Very large doses are commonly fatal within 24 hours while death may be delayed for 3–4 weeks after smaller doses. Rarely, death can occur before the results of laboratory investigations become grossly abnormal.[35] The development of renal failure compromises the only efficient method of eliminating absorbed paraquat and for that reason it frequently heralds the demise of many patients. In one series, 19 of 20 who developed this subsequently died.[44]

DIAGNOSIS OF PARAQUAT POISONING

The diagnosis of poisoning is usually made on the basis of a history of ingestion. Rarely, undisclosed poisoning presents to ear, nose and throat departments, respiratory physicians and to renal units. Absorption of paraquat is confirmed if a blue-green colour develops when a knife-point each of sodium bicarbonate and sodium dithionite is added to about 5 ml of urine voided within 4 hours of alleged exposure.[31,45] A negative test at this time indicates that not enough has been absorbed to cause problems and is of great reassurance value in cases of accidental inhalation or alleged ingestion.

MANAGEMENT OF ACUTE PARAQUAT POISONING

The prognosis for an individual who has ingested paraquat can be predicted from a nomogram which relates plasma paraquat concentrations at given times after ingestion to the probability of survival.[31] Patients whose plasma paraquat concentrations exceed the line have very poor prognosis, regardless of treatment and therefore should be kept as comfortable as possible and their families given appropriate emotional support and counselling.

Table 10.4 *Time course, features and outcome of paraquat poisoning is dependent on the amount ingested*

Amount ingested	> 6 g for an adult or > 40 mg paraquat/kg	>3–6 g for an adult or >20–40 mg paraquat/kg	>1.5–3 g for an adult or >10–20 mg paraquat/kg
Time course and outcome	Fatal in 24–48 hours	More protracted course but still fatal	
Features	Nausea and vomiting Abdominal pain Diarrhoea Ulceration Cardiovascular shock Metabolic acidosis Impaired consciousness Convulsions Breathlessness and cyanosis due to acute pneumonitis	Painful buccal ulceration Dysphagia Coughing and breathlessness Crepitations and central cyanosis may be present by 5–7 days and progress relentlessly until death Renal failure Rarely, perforation of oesophagus with mediastinitis Rarely, jaundice due to hepatocellular damage	Nausea and vomiting Diarrhoea Mild renal tubular damage Throat pain Respiratory damage starts between 10–21 days after ingestion and includes breathlessness, basal crepitations and bilateral opacities on chest radiograph. Death due to respiratory failure may occur as late as 5–6 weeks

After Ref. 40.

A range of treatment options are available for those whose plasma paraquat concentrations lie below the line but the efficacy of each is unproven.[31,35] Despite the corrosive actions of paraquat on the upper alimentary tract, it is usual to carry out gastric lavage if the patient presents within 1–2 h of ingestion of a potentially serious amount. Further gut decontamination including the administration of absorbents such as fuller's earth, bentonite and activated charcoal is traditional; activated charcoal is probably as effective as any absorbent and has the advantage of being more readily available. Symptomatic measures including anti-emetics, mouth washes and analgesics help and rigorous rehydration may be needed to replace gastrointestinal fluid losses. Experimentally, oxygen administration has been shown to enhance paraquat toxicity[46] and supplemental oxygen therapy is therefore best avoided.

Such is the distress caused by paraquat poisoning to patients and their carers that physicians have resorted to all manner of ingenious and often heroic treatments; usually to no avail. The occasional apparent success usually raises more questions than it answers. It is doubtful if elimination techniques such as forced diuresis, dialysis or haemoperfusion have any role. Paraquat has a very high volume of distribution which militates against them being successful and experience shows that they clear only very small amounts of the herbicide.[31] Similarly, corticosteroids, free-radical scavengers, immunosupressives and lung irradiation[47] and transplantation have all had their days but there is no evidence that they reduce mortality.

Diquat

Few acute diquat intoxications have been reported to date.[48] Unlike paraquat, diquat does not accumulate in the lungs or cause pulmonary injury.[33] Ulceration of mucous membranes, skin burns,[49] gastrointestinal symptoms, acute renal failure, hepatic damage and central nervous system effects appeared to be more severe. No fibrosis was evident in the lungs at autopsy of one poisoned individual who died as a result of cardiac arrest.[33]

Chlorates

Sodium chlorate and potassium chlorate are powerful oxidizing agents and highly toxic if ingested.[50] The fatal dose for an adult may be as little as 20 g.[50] Serious chlorate poisoning is rare and results from deliberate ingestion but accidental cases have been reported. Significant absorption through intact skin is unlikely. Even though the manufacturers emphasize care in handling sodium chlorate its toxic nature is often underestimated, perhaps because of its resemblance to castor sugar.

FEATURES OF ACUTE POISONING

Features of acute chlorate toxicity include nausea, vomiting, diarrhoea and abdominal pain.[50] Red blood cells and haemoglobin are damaged and Heinz bodies can be seen in peripheral blood films and intravascular haemolysis results in hyperkalaemia, haemoglobinaemia, haemoglobinuria, jaundice and acute renal failure.[51] The presence of cyanosis indicates that methaemoglobinaemia has developed. Methaemoglobin catalysis[52] also contributes to the development of renal failure.

MANAGEMENT OF ACUTE POISONING

Gastric lavage should be carried out if the patient presents within 1–2 hours of ingestion and administration of activated charcoal is recommended. The haemoglobin, haematocrit and plasma potassium concentrations will need to be monitored and hyperkalaemia treated as necessary. Methylene blue (1–2 mg/kg body weight by slow intravenous injection) is usually advised for methaemoglobinaemia exceeding 30% but its efficacy in chlorate-induced methaemoglobinaemia has been questioned[52] and there is concern that its use could lead to production of chlorite and further methaemoglobin production.[51] Transfusion may be required to replace the oxygen-carrying capacity of the blood lost by haemolysis but it is not an effective treatment for methaemoglobinaemia. Haemodialysis removes chlorate and may be required for treatment of renal failure.[50,53] Plasmapheresis may also have a role.[50]

Chlorophenoxyacetate herbicides

The chlorophenoxyacetate herbicides (Table 10.5) are widely used in agriculture and by the public. These herbicides are popularly known as 'hormone' weedkillers and in plants mimic the action of auxins, though no hormonal activity is seen in mammals. Despite their widespread availability for the past 50 years, reports of poisoning with chlorophenoxyacetates have been remarkably rare[54,55] and some of their apparent toxicity may be attributable to the dicamba, ioxynil and bromoxynil with which they are often co-formulated. While dicamba is of low toxicity, ioxynil and bromoxynil are powerful uncouplers of oxidative phosphorylation.[54]

The oral dose of 2,4-dichlorophenoxyacetic acid (2,4-D) required to elicit symptoms is 50–60 mg/kg. A 75 kg male died after intentionally ingesting 6 g (80 mg/kg)[56] and a further patient survived a substantial ingestion.[57] Pulmonary and gut oedema and necrosis, degeneration of the renal tubules and necrosis and fatty infiltration of the liver are found at autopsy.[58] In contrast, the daily ingestion of 500 mg over 3 weeks elicited no symptoms in another case.[59]

A simple high-performance liquid chromatographic assay is possible to confirm ingestion or aid diagnosis of

Table 10.5 *Chlorophenoxyacetate herbicides*

Chemical name	Other names
2,4-dichlorophenoxyacetic acid	2,4-D
4-(2,4-dichlorophenoxy)butyric acid	2,4-DB
2-(2,4-dichlorophenoxy)propionic acid	2,4-DP
	DCPP, dichloroprop
2,4,5-trichlorophenoxyacetic acid	2,4,5-T
2-(2,4,5-trichlorophenoxy) propionic acid	2,4,5-TP, fenoprop
4-chloro-2-methylphenoxyacetic acid	MCPA
4-(4-chloro-2-methylphenoxy)butyric acid	MCPB
2-(4-chloro-2-methylphenoxy)propionic acid	MCPP, mecoprop

acute poisoning with eight chlorophenoxy and two benzonitrile herbicides (bromoxynil and ioxynil).[60]

OCCUPATIONAL EXPOSURE TO CHLOROPHENOXYACETATE HERBICIDES

Early studies in Sweden suggested that exposure to chlorophenoxy herbicides and chlorophenols produced a sixfold increase in soft tissue sarcomas, Hodgkin's lymphoma (HL) and non-Hodgkin's lymphoma (NHL), whether or not the chemicals were contaminated by polychlorinated dibenzodioxins and dibenzofurans.[61] A review by Morrison *et al.*[62] concluded that there was reasonable evidence that occupational exposure to phenoxy herbicides resulted in an increased risk of developing NHL. However, an analysis of cancer mortality in workers exposed to chlorophenoxy herbicide using an international database[63] showed no excess of NHL or HL but sixfold and ninefold excesses of soft tissue sarcomas in workers and sprayers respectively. More recent investigations conclude that the impact of chlorophenoxyacetates on the incidence of human cancer has been negligible.[64] 2,4,5-Trichlorophenoxyacetic acid (2,4,5-T) and 2,4-D have not been shown to be teratogenic in primates or man.[65]

FEATURES OF DELIBERATE INGESTION

Ingestion of large amounts of chlorophenoxyacetates causes burning of the mouth and throat with nausea, vomiting, diarrhoea and abdominal pain. The face of the victim may be flushed and there is often profuse sweating and hyperventilation. Headache, dizziness, hyperthermia and hypotension may be features. More serious poisoning is associated with pulmonary oedema and depression of the central nervous system with prolonged, deep coma.[66] Transient albuminuria and oliguria has been observed in some cases. Reported laboratory abnormalities include hypoglycaemia, hypocalcaemia severe enough to cause carpopedal spasm and metabolic acidosis.[67]

Rarely, a proximal myopathy with aching and tender muscles occurs. Electrophysiologically proven peripheral neuropathies beginning several hours to one month after exposure and progressing to severe pain, paraesthesiae and paralysis have been reported.[68] Recovery may be incomplete even after several years. In one fatal case, extensive plaques of acute demyelination similar to those observed in multiple sclerosis were found in all parts of the brain.[69] However, neuropathies have not been observed in recent years, either with occupational or accidental exposure to high concentrations of these agents and it has been suggested that they were related to a contaminant, 2,3,7,8-tetrachlorodibenzo-*p*-dioxin (TCDD)[70] (see Chapter 12).

MANAGEMENT OF ACUTE POISONING

Gastric lavage should be carried out if ingestion has occurred within the previous 1–2 hours. Supportive measures for the airway, ventilation and blood pressure should be implemented if indicated. Renal function, acid-base status, and blood glucose and serum calcium concentrations should be measured in severe cases; repeat measurements may be necessary. Fortunately, although there is no antidote, the elimination of 2,4-D,[66] dichloroprop and mecoprop can be considerably enhanced, shortening the duration of poisoning and reducing morbidity and possibly mortality. Alkalinization of the urine is the treatment of choice, even when poisoning is severe since it is as effective as haemodialysis, is relatively non-invasive, requires little expertise or equipment and can be instituted almost anywhere.[55] Intravenous infusion of 1.26% sodium bicarbonate at a rate sufficient to achieve and maintain a urine pH of 7–8 is indicated. Attempting to force a diuresis is of no value and is potentially dangerous.

Urinary alkalinization is ineffective with other phenoxyacetates or ioxynil[71] but these compounds can be removed by haemodialysis which should therefore be considered for seriously poisoned patients.

Glyphosate-containing herbicides

Glyphosate-containing herbicides have been introduced relatively recently. They contain the isopropylamine salt together with a surfactant (polyoxyethylene amine) which was almost certainly the cause of much of the toxicity of the products initially marketed.[72] The surfactant has now been changed to a less toxic alternative.

OCCUPATIONAL EXPOSURE

Accidental exposure to skin, and eating vegetables sprayed with glyphosates does not produce symptoms.[73] Inhalation of mist may cause oral and nasal discomfort.

FEATURES OF DELIBERATE INGESTION

Ingestion commonly leads to buccal irritation, nausea, vomiting, dysphagia and diarrhoea.[74] The features of severe poisoning include systemic hypotension, tachy-cardia, bradycardia, pneumonitis, oliguria, haematuria and metabolic acidosis.[74] Gastrointestinal haemorrhage secondary to erosions has been reported[73] but deaths are usually due to a combination of irreversible systemic hypotension and adult respiratory distress syndrome.[73]

MANAGEMENT

Management is predominantly supportive.[75] The toxico-kinetics in man are not known and the role of elimination measures is uncertain.

Triazine herbicides

Triazine herbicides are so widely used that concentrations of atrazine and simazine in UK drinking water occasionally exceed statutory European limits. Amitrole (aminotriazole) is readily absorbed after ingestion and excreted in the urine, usually within 24 hours.[76]

OCCUPATIONAL EXPOSURE

There is no evidence that exposure by any route to even large amounts of atrazine and simazine causes serious effects in man.[77] Amitraz exposure has similarly been reported.[78,79]

The toxicity of herbicides containing amitrole (aminotriazine) was once thought to be confined to irritation of the skin or eyes[76] but the possibility of severe pulmonary damage after inhalation has been raised by one case of occupational exposure. Features developed within 6 hours and included crepitations, extensive bilateral radiographic lung infiltrates and effusions and a restrictive defect on pulmonary function tests. Fortunately, the effects were reversed by high-dose corticosteroids.[80]

In two studies, 2683 workers (especially long-term employees) with definite or probable exposure to triazines had a lower mortality than the general population – possibly a healthy worker effect.[81] Adjustment for the use of other pesticides reduced most of the calculated associations between atrazine and NHL.[77]

While amitrole is goitrogenic in animals,[82] data held by manufacturers and that on field workers chronically exposed to triazines have never reported health effects.[77] A possible link of chronic use with a two- to threefold increased risk of epithelial ovarian cancer was reported by Donna *et al.*[83] However, this and subsequent studies have been challenged because they contained various sources of possible bias.[84]

DELIBERATE INGESTION

One death has been reported after deliberate ingestion of ammonium thiocyanate and amitrole.[85] Cyanosis, sweating, vomiting and diarrhoea, systemic hypotension, heart block, convulsions, coma and oliguric renal failure developed. Bilateral alveolar opacities were present on the chest radiograph and oesophagitis and gastritis was found at endoscopy. The role of amitrole in this case is uncertain as the thiocyanate concentration alone was compatible with a fatal outcome.

MANAGEMENT OF DELIBERATE INGESTION

Gastric lavage is recommended in patients who present within 1–2 hours. Activated charcoal may be given though there is no good evidence for its efficacy. Haemodialysis would be expected to remove thiocyanate to some extent.[85] The hypothesis that thiocyanate toxicity is due to generation of cyanide has led to suggestions that treatment with antidotes to cyanide could be tried.[86]

POISONING WITH INSECTICIDES

The chemical insecticides in use today act by poisoning the nervous systems of the target organisms. It is perhaps not surprising therefore that they evoke similar effects in higher forms of life and that the dose dictates the intensity of effect. Organochlorine compounds and pyrethroids affect axonal membranes and the transport of sodium, potassium, calcium and chloride ions while organophosphorus and carbamate esters act on enzymes, particularly cholinesterases, affecting transmission at synapses and neuromuscular junctions.

Organophosphorus insecticides

Organophosphorus compounds (OPs) were initially developed as chemical warfare agents. They now comprise the most commonly used pesticides in the world with more than 200 different OPs formulated into thousands of products. Their toxicity varies widely.

MECHANISMS OF TOXICITY

Although OPs have numerous complex actions their principal effect is to attach to serine sites on the surface of cholinesterases, particularly acetylcholinesterase (AChE), thus inhibiting their activity.[87] AChE is responsible for the hydrolysis of acetylcholine (ACh) liberated at nerve endings. It therefore limits the duration of action of the transmitter at junctions between neurons and between neurons and muscles. Inhibition of the enzyme causes accumulation of ACh and continuing electrical activity. The organophosphate–AChE complex may either be hydrolysed to yield functional AChE again or, depending on time, the organophosphate component may undergo chemical change that prevents hydrolysis and reactivation of AChE, a process commonly referred to as ageing. Ageing is more common with some OPs than others. The onset of symptoms and severity of acute organophosphorus (OP) insecticide poisoning is thus dependent on:

- the rate at which AChE is inactivated,
- the rate of dissociation of inactivated AChE to release active enzyme,
- the rate at which ageing occurs,
- synthesis of new AChE by the liver (this takes weeks).

The activity of AChE in blood is reduced in a number of conditions but is mainly determined genetically. About 4% of UK, French and American individuals have reduced AChE activities that render them more susceptible to organophosphate toxicity than others.[88] Some OPs must undergo biotransformation before becoming active.

PATTERNS OF POISONING AND MANAGEMENT

Acute poisoning with OPs is rare in the UK but much more common in developing countries.[89,90] Most acute organophosphate poisonings admitted to hospital in India, were the result of suicide attempts; fewer were the result of accidents in manufacture.[91] Deliberate ingestion and occupational dermal exposure are most common and mortality of organophosphate exposure depends on dose and route of exposure.[92] Chronic poisoning is also a common problem in modern society.

Chronic organophosphate poisoning

A variety of chronic symptoms have been reported after acute OP insecticide poisoning. They include tiredness, insomnia, inability to concentrate, depression and irritability and whether they can be attributed to acute poisoning with OPs or can develop without previous acute intoxication is hotly debated.[93] The latter is a matter of concern for some sheep farmers who experience considerable dermal contamination in the process of dipping sheep to protect them against scab.[94] Proving a causal relationship is virtually impossible. The chronic symptoms attributed to organophosphate poisoning are extremely common in the general population and overlap considerably with those of the chronic fatigue syndrome, Gulf War illness, myalgic encephalomyelitis, multiple chemical sensitivity and agoraphobia.[93,95] In addition, farmers who have used OPs have almost certainly used other pesticides and chemicals. Similarly, solvents[96,97] and chemicals used in hobbies are potential confounding factors.

Only subtle abnormalities can be detected on neurological examination.[98] Behavioural and psychological effects which have been attributed to organophosphate poisoning have taken several months to regress.[99,100] However, few controlled studies in man have been reported. Levin and Rodnitzy[101] found that when organophosphate exposure had been sufficient to depress plasma or red blood cell cholinesterases, some or all of the following variables might subsequently be impaired:

- cognition: vigilance, information processing, psychomotor speed and memory,
- speech: both performance and perception,
- psychiatric state: increased depression, anxiety and irritability,
- electroencephalogram (EEG) records: faster frequencies and higher voltages.

Subsequent investigations have confirmed these findings. Savage et al.[102] compared 100 matched pairs of individuals with previous organophosphate poisoning and non-poisoned controls and found differences in neuropsychological tests. They believe there are chronic neurological sequelae after acute organophosphate poisoning but that they are so subtle that 'clinical neurological examination, EEG, and ancillary laboratory testing cannot discriminate poisoned from non-poisoned subjects'. Stephens et al.[100] also found subtle abnormalities on neurobehavioural testing but their relevance to what are often major symptoms is unclear. Acetylcholinesterase activity is considerably greater in some areas of the brain than in others and it has been postulated that inhibition in specific areas could explain some of the symptoms of alleged chronic OP poisoning as shown in Table 10.6.[103]

Principles of management of chronic organophosphate poisoning

Dealing with alleged chronic organophosphate poisoning is difficult and the relationship between the doctor and the patient is likely to be even more fragile than usual.[93] The physician who, out of hand, dismisses the patient's perception of the cause of his symptoms has little prospect of

Table 10.6 *Possible clinical correlates of region-specific brain AChE inhibition*

Brain area	Symptoms
Cerebellar cortex (molecular layer)	Impairment of co-ordination, ataxia, slurred speech
Frontal cortex	Impaired cognition, psychomotor slowing, impaired reading, comprehension, expressive language defect
Temporal cortex	Amnestic word-finding disturbance
General	Impaired arousal, memory and mood

establishing the trust and confidence required to help the patient and psychological or psychiatric diagnoses are likely to be met with incredulity and indignation. The features attributed to organophosphate exposure are commonly disabling and not infrequently devastate people's lives. Whether or not the doctor believes that they are caused by OPs is largely irrelevant, he can neither prove nor disprove it. His duty to advise and help the patient is best served by showing interest, adopting a sympathetic approach and taking time to discuss options (see Chapter 2).

Clinical features such as lethargy, irritability and poor concentration are vague and do not lend themselves to easy measurement. Each complainant must be examined and investigated, more to exclude other possible causes than to confirm that the symptoms are the result of pesticide exposure. Renal and liver dysfunction, hypothyroidism, diabetes mellitus and vitamin B_{12} deficiency are readily eliminated. Measurement of plasma or red cell cholinesterase activity is unlikely to be of value in alleged chronic organophosphate poisoning unless there has been exposure within the past day or two. A chest radiograph should be taken to exclude bronchial carcinoma and the brain scanned to rule out a space-occupying lesion. Nerve conduction studies and neurobehavioural tests help measure effects in individuals but require considerable expertise, careful interpretation and are only available in specialist centres. Early suggestion of psychiatric evaluation is often counterproductive.

Conventional medicine has no specific treatment to offer. Physical and psychiatric illness, particularly depression, should be managed appropriately but symptomatic treatment and sympathy are usually all that can be offered. Depending on the state of the doctor–patient relationship, some patients will accept consultation with a clinical psychologist or psychiatrist. Most therapeutic approaches are ineffective and patients commonly turn to alternative medicine and self-help groups.

Subclinical organophosphate poisoning

Minor exposure to OPs may cause subclinical poisoning in which there is reduction of cholinesterase activity but no symptoms or signs. It most commonly results from local absorption of the compounds from the conjunctiva, upper respiratory tract and skin during agricultural work.[89] Management of subclinical poisoning includes observation for 24 hours to ensure that delayed toxicity does not develop. During this observation time the respiratory peak flow rate and degree of tiredness is monitored. Depression of AChE activity of 20–25% is indicative of exposure but not necessarily toxicity. Depression of 30–50% is an indication for removal from further contact with pesticides until AChE levels return to normal.

Acute organophosphate poisoning

Features Ingestion of organophosphate causes typical signs and symptoms within an hour or two. They include nausea, vomiting, abdominal pain, diarrhoea with tenesmus, sweating, hypersalivation and chest tightness due to bronchoconstriction.[93] Anxiety, restlessness, insomnia, nightmares, tiredness, dizziness, headache and loss of memory have also been reported. Miosis may be present and although bradycardia would be predicted from the mechanism of action of the insecticides, tachycardia occurs in about 30% of cases. Later, fasciculation and flaccid paralysis of limb muscles, respiratory muscles and occasionally extraocular muscle palsies occur.

Respiratory muscle paralysis and bronchial narrowing secondary to bronchoconstriction and the presence of copious respiratory secretions contribute to respiratory failure but animal experiments suggest that depression of respiratory drive is the single most important factor. Respiratory complications are the major cause of death in severely poisoned patients.[104] Coma is present in severe poisoning and convulsions may also occur. Rarely, hyperglycaemia, complete heart block and arrhythmias may occur.[105] In general, clinical features are more helpful than cholinesterase measurements in determining severity of intoxication and prognosis but there is a rough correlation between the two, e.g. 50% cholinesterase activity in subclinical poisoning, 20–50% activity in mild poisoning, 10–20% activity in moderate poisoning and <10% of normal cholinesterase activity in severe poisoning.[93]

The intermediate syndrome A small minority of patients develop what has been termed the intermediate syndrome. It is characterized by cranial nerve and brainstem lesions and a proximal neuropathy commencing 1–4 days after acute poisoning[106] and lasting for approximately 3 weeks. Respiratory depression is a complication and urgent ventilatory support is usually required as it is unresponsive to atropine and oximes. The syndrome has been said to be due to inadequate oxime therapy but the aetiology is probably much more complicated (see Chapter 42).

Organophosphate-induced delayed neuropathy This starts 2 weeks or more after exposure and is the result of degeneration of large myelinated motor and sensory fibres secondary to phosphorylation of neuropathy target esterase. The initial flaccidity and muscle weakness in the arms and legs gives rise to a clumsy shuffling gait and is followed later by spasticity, hypertonicity, hyperreflexia and clonus. In many patients, recovery is limited to the arms and hands and damage to the lower extremities such as foot drop and spasticity is permanent.[107] The problem was first identified during the prohibition years in the USA after consumption of an extract of Jamaican ginger contaminated with mixed tolyl phosphate esters.[108] Not all OPs cause delayed neuropathy and those that do have been phased out of use in most developed countries.

Management Emergency measures such as clearing the airway, ensuring adequate ventilation and giving high flow oxygen are implemented as necessary.[93] If exposure has been dermal, remove soiled clothing and wash the skin thoroughly with soap and water. Allowing the victim to do this, if practicable, avoids the rescuer becoming contaminated. If the compound has been ingested do not induce emesis. Give activated charcoal (50–100 g for an adult) if it is readily available. The patient should be hospitalized as quickly as possible. Gastric lavage may then be undertaken if the organophosphate was ingested within the preceding 1–2 hours. It is wise to confirm the diagnosis by measuring AChE activity, preferably in both red blood cells and plasma.

Patients who are severely poisoned with OPs should be managed in an intensive care area. Appropriate supportive measures are implemented as necessary and convulsions controlled with 10–20 mg diazepam intravenously. Definitive treatment involves administration of atropine to counteract some of the cholinergic features and oximes to reactivate inhibited AChE.

Atropine (2 mg intravenously for an adult) reduces bronchorrhoea, bronchospasm, salivation, abdominal colic and bradycardia and should be repeated every 10 minutes until signs of atropinization (flushed dry skin, tachycardia, dilated pupils and dry mouth) develop. Up to 30 mg atropine or more may be required in the first 24 hours and the drug may have to be continued for prolonged periods.[109] If titrated correctly, atropine has few serious side-effects but particular care must be taken with its use in warm climates because of inhibition of sweating. It may also precipitate ventricular arrhythmias in hypoxic patients.

Cholinesterase reactivators such as the oximes pralidoxime mesylate (P2S), pralidoxime chloride (2-PAM chloride, 2-PAMCl) and obidoxime (toxogonin)[109] are helpful if given before the organophosphate–cholinesterase enzyme complex ages.[110] However, concern that ageing may have occurred should not deter the use of oximes. Pralidoxime is preferred because it is less likely to cause hepatocellular damage and information on the location of supplies in the UK is available from the National Poisons Information Service Centres (Table 10.2). It should be given in addition to atropine to every symptomatic patient. The dose is 30 mg/kg body weight by slow intravenous injection. Clinical improvement (cessation of convulsions and fasciculation, improved muscle power and recovery of consciousness) usually occurs within 20–30 minutes. The use of oximes in the early stages of intoxication reduces the amount of atropine needed to ensure survival. The need for further therapy is guided by clinical improvement together with monitoring of cholinesterase activity. If necessary, further doses of pralidoxime can be given 4-hourly or by continuous infusion (7.5 mg/kg body weight/hour). Side-effects are seen at high doses or rates of administration (> 500 mg/min). They include tachycardia, muscle rigidity, neuromuscular

blockade, hypertension and laryngospasm. Repeated doses chelate calcium causing hypocalcaemic tetany. Intravenous calcium gluconate may be required. Toxogonin (obidoxime chloride) and more recently the H-series compounds (such as HI-6) have also been used as antidotes for organophosphate poisoning but differences between them and other oximes in pesticide poisoning are less clear than with nerve agents.[111] Haemoperfusion and haemodialysis have been used to remove OPs from the circulation but they are of doubtful benefit.

Detecting exposure to organophosphates and carbamates

Detection is easier if there is a history of exposure.

Measurement of cholinesterase activity Exposure can easily be confirmed by measurement of cholinesterase activity in plasma or red blood cells.[88,93] Depression of plasma ChE reflects recent and moderate exposure to OPs and carbamates and is the most sensitive measure of exposure.[112] Red cell cholinesterase activity may better reflect AChE activity in the central and peripheral nervous system though it does not correlate well with the clinical severity of acute poisoning.[93]

There do not appear to be differences in the activity of either AChE or plasma cholinesterase between racial groups but there are significant inter- and intra-person variations which make interpretation of isolated values difficult. These are less within individuals than between individuals and also less for AChE than ChE.[93] AChE but not plasma ChE activity decreases with age in adults. Laboratory factors are also important and may account for as much as 40% of the variability in AChE activity and 24% in plasma ChE activity.[113] Apparent reduction in cholinesterase activity may also result from contamination and poor sample handling (see below).

Organophosphate metabolites Recent exposure to some OPs can also be confirmed by demonstrating the presence of their metabolites in urine, particularly alkyl phosphates and p-nitrophenol. Peak excretion occurs approximately 8–9 hours after exposure and metabolites may be found when exposure has been insufficient to lower cholinesterase activity. Urinary free and conjugated 1-naphthol metabolites, the main urinary metabolites of carbaryl, may be a practical means of assessing the severity of exposure to this carbamate. Concentrations above 4 mg/litre are considered to represent significant exposure[114] but insufficient human data exist for meaningful biological monitoring of the majority of carbamate insecticides.

Electrophysiology Electromyography may be used to detect the effects of exposure to OPs. Unfortunately, while it is a simple, non-invasive technique it requires specialized equipment and skills and may not be sufficiently sensitive to detect early changes. Reproducibility varies with many factors and the changes reported tend not to be dose-related.[99]

Monitoring Screening for excessive exposure to anti-cholinesterases protects workers from harm and helps to identify unsatisfactory work practices. The exposure level which should trigger monitoring has not yet been adequately defined. Whole blood cholinesterase activity is the most widely used measurement for monitoring occupational exposure to OPs and carbamates but is probably only practical in large companies employing stable work forces. It is not practicable for small farms. The samples are best taken immediately after exposure but sampling towards the end of the day avoids the 'diurnal variation' effect.[115] It is clearly important that the blood should not be contaminated by exposure to anti-cholinesterases in the air or on the skin of the donor or sampler. Cholinesterases are unstable when kept at room temperature for long periods and samples should therefore by stored on ice or frozen prior to analysis. If activity is reduced to 30% or more of the pre-exposure level, the test should be repeated.[93] Other results are managed as detailed under the heading **Subclinical organophosphate poisoning** (p. 206).

Pre-employment assessment Pre-placement medical examination assesses the suitability of applicants to work with anticholinesterases. The crucial elements of this process involve:

- an initial occupational history;
- a comprehensive medical history especially asking about frequency of headaches, dizziness, chest tightness, dimness of vision and or difficulty of focus;
- evaluation of alcohol consumption to identify problem drinkers in whom neurobehavioural impairment may later be erroneously attributed to organophosphate exposure;
- physical examination including cardiovascular system, central nervous system, visual acuity and abdomen, especially kidneys;
- urinalysis;
- baseline cholinesterase determination (two tests performed at least 3 days apart but not more than 14 days apart);
- assessment of the ability to tolerate protective clothing and respirators.

Carbamate insecticides

The majority of carbamate insecticides in use are *N*-monomethylcarbamic acids, more simply referred to as methylcarbamates.

MECHANISM OF TOXICITY

Carbamate insecticides inhibit a number of tissue esterases the most important of which are the nervous tissue, erythrocyte and plasma cholinesterases.[93] There is,

therefore, accumulation of acetylcholine at nerve endings in the brain, ganglia and neuromuscular junctions. The inhibition of function is of much shorter duration than that of OPs as the carbamate–cholinesterase complex tends to dissociate spontaneously with a half-life of the order of 30–40 minutes depending upon the carbamate. Indeed dissociation is sufficiently rapid that carbamates are frequently considered to be poor inhibitors of cholinesterases that turn over slowly.

ROUTES OF EXPOSURE

Poisoning with carbamates is usually the consequence of ingestion and attempted suicide and less commonly accidental dermal exposure. In man the more potent carbamates such as propoxur, methomyl or aldicarb are most often involved. Poisoning with illegal rodenticides containing mainly aldicarb is common in Brazil.[116] Gupta[117] has reviewed carbofuran toxicity. Foodborne outbreaks of carbamate poisoning have also been reported. Three individuals died when methomyl instead of salt was used accidentally in the preparation of bread.[118] More recently several incidents have resulted from consumption of water melons[119] and hydroponically grown cucumbers, crops on which the use of this insecticide is not approved because of its high degree of water solubility.

CHRONIC TOXICITY

The chronic toxicity of carbaryl has been extensively reviewed.[120] Volunteers who took carbaryl (0.06 or 0.13 mg/kg bodyweight/day orally) for a period of 6 weeks did not develop haematological or biochemical effects other than small reversible decreases in the ability of the proximal renal tubule to reabsorb amino acids.[120] There is little evidence of prolonged neurological effects following the exposure of humans to carbamates other than the few instances described below (see also Chapter 42). Studies of orchard and forest spraymen, mixers and handlers of carbamate esters have revealed that exposures did occur and that there was a direct relationship between the length of time in the occupation and the severity of neurological defects. However, it was impossible to identify individual causative agents from the variety of chemical pesticides and solvents which many of the workers handled during a short time.[93]

FEATURES OF ACUTE TOXICITY

Since carbamate insecticides act in the same way as OPs, the features of poisoning are similar but not usually so severe. However, deaths have been reported.[121] Despite prompt gastric lavage and antidote administration, a 39-year-old man died after ingesting 0.5 litre of an 80% concentrate of carbaryl.[120] Acute pancreatitis, occurring within 2 days of deliberate ingestion of aldicarb has also been reported.[122] Propoxur has a shorter duration of action than carbaryl and thus recovery may occur within 1 hour.

COMPLICATIONS OF ACUTE POISONING

Delayed neurotoxicity has been reported following acute exposure to carbamate insecticides (see Chapter 42). A patient who ingested 27 g of carbaryl developed sensory loss and weakness in the arms and legs accompanied by electrophysiological alterations consistent with a peripheral axonal neuropathy. Loss of vibration sensation and proprioception in the toes and reduced tactile perception below mid-calf persisted.[123] In another case involving metolcarb (metoyl methyl carbamate) electron microscopy revealed denervated Schwann cell clusters, collagen pockets and myelinated nerve fibres with degenerate axons.[124] By 3 months following exposure, numbness was reduced and the motor symptoms had improved although deep tendon reflexes remained absent. By 6 months no further neurological signs were observed.

In 1989, 318 sheep became poisoned with aldicarb after contamination of grazing areas. All but 30 of them died within a few hours. Of six previously healthy men present in the field that day, three required hospital admission and two were seen as outpatients the next day with features of cholinesterase poisoning. Two developed a chronic fatigue syndrome, with dyspnoea on exposure to hairsprays or perfumes while a third continued to complain of night sweats, abdominal pain, blurred vision, alcohol intolerance and dyspnoea 3 years later. He was found to have hereditary coproporphyria. No long-term information was available on the remaining three.[125]

MANAGEMENT OF ACUTE POISONING

The management of acute carbamate insecticide poisoning requires that patients receive the same intensive supportive care as that given to those poisoned with OPs but in other respects there are two important differences. The first is that only symptomatic cases require an antidote; rapid recovery tends to occur with supportive therapy alone.[126] The second is that the use of oximes is contraindicated partly because they are of limited efficacy and partly because carbamyolated oximes are themselves potent inhibitors of AChE.[127] Despite this, oxime use in severe poisoning by unidentified cholinesterase inhibitors can be justified.[128] In severe carbamate poisoning atropine may be given intravenously in frequent small doses (0.5 mg–1.0 mg) until signs of atropinization develop. Several milligrams may be required.[129] Diazepam (10 mg given orally or intravenously) may be used to relieve anxiety.

Organochlorine insecticides

The organochlorine insecticides include DDT, aldrin, dieldrin, chlordane and lindane (gamma benzene hexachloride or hexachlorocyclohexane). Until recent years they were used extensively in all aspects of agriculture and forestry but concerns about the slow rates at which they underwent biotransformation and their persistence in the food chain led to them being withdrawn from use in many developed countries. However, they continue to be used in developing nations because they are cheap and effective. Organochlorine insecticides are highly lipid-soluble and as a result are sequestered in the liver, kidneys, nervous system, adipose tissue and milk.[130] They also have potent oestrogenic and enzyme-inducing properties.

MECHANISMS OF TOXICITY

Nerves poisoned by DDT show a characteristic prolongation of polarization of the action potential as a result of reduced permeability to potassium ions and slow closure of sodium channels. In addition, DDT inhibits neuronal ATPases which play vital roles in neuronal repolarization. The nerve membrane remains partially depolarized and partially repolarized and is extremely sensitive to minor stimuli.[131] Thus following exposure to DDT, repetitive stimulation of the peripheral sensory nerves by touch or sound is magnified causing generalized tremors throughout the body (see Chapter 42).

The actions of cyclodiene, benzene and cyclohexane insecticides are more central than those of DDT. They mimic the action of picrotoxin, a nerve excitant and gamma-aminobutyric acid (GABA) antagonist resulting in excitation. Cyclodiene insecticides also inhibit Ca/Mg ATPase at synaptic membranes causing release of further neurotransmitter from storage vesicles. Kepone® is thought to interfere with metabolic processes in Schwann cells.[121]

ROUTES OF EXPOSURE

Poisoning with organochlorines may occur by deliberate ingestion or by occupational exposure. There has also been controversy over the use of lindane in head-lice shampoos as significant dermal absorption has been demonstrated.[132] Chlorinated cyclodienes are therefore a significant hazard to those working with them unless appropriate protective equipment is worn. In contrast, DDT is poorly absorbed through the skin.

Occupational and chronic exposure

Forestry workers planting seedlings treated with lindane developed non-specific 'flu-like' symptoms.[133] In two workers plasma concentrations of lindane exceeded 70 nmol/litre. Even low doses of chlorinated cyclodiene insecticides cause convulsions. They usually follow headaches, nausea, vertigo, clonic jerks, motor hyperexcitability and hyper-reflexia. Chronic exposure to low or moderate concentrations leads to muscle twitching, headaches, psychological disorders including insomnia, convulsions, chest pains, arthralgia, ataxia, inability to focus and fixate, depression, muscle weakness and impairment of spermatogenesis. Two unprotected workers with confirmed chronic exposure to aldrin, lindane and heptachlor developed clinical and electromyogram (EMG) evidence of motor neuron disease.[134]

Carelessness during manufacture of an organochlorine called Kepone® caused a severe syndrome of tremors, ataxia, behavioural changes, arthralgia, headaches, chest pains, hepatomegaly, splenomegaly and impotence 30 days after exposure. The symptoms persisted for several months[131] (see Chapter 42).

There has been enormous controversy about a potential role for environmental organochlorines, particularly lindane, in the development of breast cancer. However, the data provide reassurance rather than concern.[135] Similarly, the allegation that lindane is a cause of aplastic anaemia rests on a series of anecdotal reports of bone marrow injury temporally associated with environmental exposure.[136] Regional variations in diagnostic criteria do not aid assessment but aplastic anaemia is such a rare disease that the data are unlikely ever to be sufficient to establish a causal relationship.

CLINICAL FEATURES OF ACUTE POISONING

Exposure to high oral doses of DDT results in paraesthesiae of mouth and face, apprehension, irritability, light sensitivity, dizziness, vertigo, tremor and convulsions. Fine tremors associated with voluntary movements progress to coarse tremors in moderate to severe poisoning. Symptoms tend to appear within 6–24 hours of exposure to large doses. It has been estimated that a dose of 10 mg/kg body weight will cause signs of poisoning in humans. Little toxicity is thought to result from dermal exposure to DDT.

Dicofol has been associated with nausea, dizziness, double vision, ataxia, confusion and disorientation in a 12-year-old whose clothes were saturated in an accident.[137] Headaches, blurred vision, nystagmus, paraesthesiae, pain in legs, memory loss and impulsive behaviour with reduced academic performance continued over the next 8 months.

A 30-year-old woman was exposed to chlordane over several weeks through careless domestic use.[138] Her early symptoms included numbness around the mouth, anorexia, nausea and fatigue. Myoclonic jerks started after a delay of 1 month. She still had malaise 6 months after the exposure.

Hexachlorocyclohexane (lindane or gamma-benzene hexachloride) is widely used for the treatment of scabies and pediculosis. It is absorbed through the skin[132,139] resulting in features identical to those that follow ingestion.[140,141] They include rapid loss of consciousness, myoclonus, tremors, ataxia, hypertonia, hyperreflexia,

convulsions and rhabdomyolysis.[142] Metabolic acidosis, disseminated intravascular coagulation (DIC), renal tubular and hepatocellular necrosis also occur in severe cases.[143] Pancreatitis and proximal myopathy have been reported.[142]

MANAGEMENT OF ACUTE POISONING WITH ORGANOCHLORINES

Management of poisoning with organochlorine insecticides is supportive and symptomatic. Gastric lavage should be undertaken if lindane has been ingested within 1–2 hours. Activated charcoal or cholestyramine should be given. Both adsorb lindane and in a murine model, cholestyramine is more effective.[144] Experience with chlordecone (Kepone®) intoxication has shown that administration of cholestyramine resulted in a 3- to 18-fold enhancement of excretion by interrupting enterohepatic circulation of the pesticide, accompanied by enhanced rate of recovery.[145] Whether this approach would be of value in poisoning with other organochlorines in unknown but would depend on the extent of enterohepatic circulation. Seizures should be controlled and ventilation ensured. Skin decontamination should be performed if appropriate.

Aluminium phosphide

Tablets and pellets of aluminium and magnesium phosphides are used extensively against rodents which infest grains in stores and during transportation. They react with moisture in the air liberating phosphine which is said to smell like newly mown hay or garlic. Phosphine, being heavier than air, sinks slowly through the grain.

ROUTES OF EXPOSURE

Inhalation is the usual route of occupational and accidental poisoning. Suicidal ingestion appears to be common in India.

MECHANISM OF TOXICITY

Metal phosphides have direct effects on the gastrointestinal tract. Phosphine generated on contact with fluid and acid in the stomach is thought to be absorbed and inhibit cytochrome C oxidase, thus impairing the ability of cells to utilize oxygen.[146]

OCCUPATIONAL AND ACCIDENTAL EXPOSURE

Sixty-seven workers involved in loading and unloading grain to which aluminium phosphide had been admixed developed nausea, epigastric pain, diarrhoea, headache, chest tightness and breathlessness. They were considered to have been exposed to phosphine in concentrations of up to 35 parts per million (ppm) and though they were aware of the smell of the gas most of the time they only developed symptoms when it was stronger than usual.[147] Similar features were reported in further cases.[148,149] Haemolysis is not a feature and clinical jaundice was not confirmed by laboratory tests. Reduced cholinesterase activity has been found in some occupational exposures[150] but not in others.[149] Deaths due to suspected phosphine poisoning have been reported after exposure to treated grain[151,152] and other pesticidal uses of metal phosphides[153] (see Chapter 8).

DELIBERATE INGESTION

Intentional ingestion of aluminium phosphide causes retrosternal discomfort, vomiting, epigastric discomfort, watery diarrhoea, gastrointestinal bleeding, haemodynamic shock, metabolic acidosis and renal failure due to acute tubular necrosis in addition to the features above.[154] The vomitus may smell of rotten fish, suggesting the diagnosis. Jaundice with liver function tests reflecting centrilobular necrosis may also occur. Myocardial injury manifested by a variety of electrocardiogram (ECG) abnormalities (ST depression, ST elevation, T wave changes, QRS widening), elevated cardiac isoenzymes, arrhythmias (atrial fibrillation, ventricular tachycardia), heart block and sinus arrest is common.[155] Pericardial effusion has been reported in as many as 30% of cases.[156] Patients with moderate to severe poisoning developed tachypnoea, cyanosis and bilateral rales and adult respiratory distress syndrome has also been reported. Although altered sensation is common during shock, central nervous system symptoms are not a major feature of aluminium phosphide poisoning though headache, diplopia, paraesthesiae, dizziness and tremors have rarely been reported.[157] Mortality is invariably high – as high as 100% in some series.[154]

MANAGEMENT OF POISONING

Management is symptomatic and supportive. Most occupational and accidental exposures to phosphine will not require specific measures. When phosphide pesticides have been ingested the stomach should be emptied if the patient presents within 2 hours. The use of a lavage solution containing 1:5000 potassium permanganate has been recommended to oxidize the remaining aluminium phosphide in the stomach[155] but evidence for its efficacy is lacking. Intravascular fluid volume replacement and positive inotropic agents should be given if required. Intravenous hydrocortisone may be of value since adrenal function is compromised in severe poisoning.[155] The use of vegetable oils and liquid paraffin to inhibit the release of phosphine from phosphides may be of use therapeutically in future.[158]

Pyrethrum and pyrethroids

The synthetic pyrethroids, the newest major class of insecticides, entered the market in the 1980s. They are synthetic analogues of dried pyrethrum extracts from chrysanthemums and are considered amongst the safest insecticides available.[159] Their rapid 'knock-down' effect on insects is particularly prized and they are used extensively, not only in agriculture but also in anti-flea products for pets and plant sprays for home and greenhouse use.

MECHANISMS OF TOXICITY

The pyrethroids are thought to block sodium ion channels in neuronal membranes thus causing repetitive sensory and motor discharges similar to DDT.[159] Certain pyrethroids cause a persistent depolarization and a frequency-dependent conduction block in sensory and motor axons[131] which alone could account for the cutaneous symptoms of exposure (see Chapter 42). Permethrin, cypermethrin and deltamethrin inhibit Ca/Mg ATPase leading to neurotransmitter release and post-synaptic depolarization in the squid axon.

ACCIDENTAL AND OCCUPATIONAL EXPOSURE

Use indoors and in enclosed spaces has produced toxicity in humans. The characteristic feature of exposure to synthetic pyrethroids is cutaneous paraesthesiae or a stinging or burning sensation on the skin. These effects are most likely to occur after occupational exposure to products containing the alpha-cyano substituent deltamethrin, cypermethrin or fenvalerate. They are noticed several hours following exposure and may last from 12 to 18 hours.[160] The largest incident, involving over 500 cases, occurred in China.[161] Contact dermatitis may also occur. Spillage on the head, face and eyes results in pain, lacrimation, photophobia and oedema of the eyelids.[161] Systemic toxicity has been reported in a farmer who dipped sheep with a product containing flumethrine.[162]

Inhalation caused dyspnoea, nausea, headaches and irritability when cypermethrin was inadvertently introduced into air-conditioning ducts in an office.[163] Upper respiratory tract irritation, dyspnoea with productive cough, repeated vomiting and diarrhoea have been reported after exposure to commercial strength flea and tick spray containing 0.15% pyrethrins.[164] Allergic reactions to pyrethrins are well documented[165] and one fatality due to bronchospasm has been reported after inhalation of a pyrethrin shampoo.[166]

CHRONIC POISONING

The potential for chronic poisoning from pyrethroids has been evaluated by a Altenkirch et al.[167] Of 64 patients evaluated, a number had other neurological diseases to account for their symptoms, some had multiple chemical sensitivity and in no case was there evidence of irreversible peripheral or central nervous system lesions.

INGESTION

Ingestion of pyrethroids causes epigastric pain, nausea and vomiting, headache, dizziness, anorexia, fatigue, chest tightness, blurred vision, paraesthesiae, palpitations and coarse muscular fasciculations. Coma, convulsions and pulmonary oedema are the most serious consequences of ingestion but only occur in the most severe cases.[161]

MANAGEMENT OF POISONING

The features of occupational and accidental exposure to pyrethroids appear to be reversible. Patients should be reassured that long-term consequences do not occur. Symptomatic and supportive care is all that can be offered for the treatment of serious poisoning.[161]

EXPOSURE TO RODENTICIDES

Warfarin and other anticoagulants

Anticoagulant-containing rodenticides are widely used. Warfarin remains the most common agent but resistance of rodents to it has led to the introduction of brodifacoum, bromodiolone, coumatetralyl, diphacinone, difenacoum, chlorophacinone and floumafen, the so-called 'superwarfarins' which have durations of action lasting weeks and months.[168]

Ingestion is the only important route of exposure to anticoagulant rodenticides and occupational poisoning should not occur. However life-threatening haemorrhage has been reported after dermal exposure.[169] Children commonly ingest prepared baits available to the public but seldom develop toxicity. Deliberate ingestion by adults occurs infrequently but the potential for serious consequences is higher. Rarely, ingestion is surreptitious[170] and presents as a bleeding diathesis, the cause of which may be difficult to determine unless the clinician has a high index of suspicion.

The features of intoxication are entirely the result of the anticoagulant action of the rodenticides. Spontaneous bleeding may occur from the nose, gums and gastrointestinal or urinary tracts. Less commonly cerebral haemorrhage may occur. The diagnosis is confirmed by finding an increased prothrombin time.

Life-threatening haemorrhage may require administration of fresh frozen plasma or clotting factor concentrates, but fortunately few cases are so serious. If only a small amount has been ingested, monitoring of the prothrombin time over the next 48 hours is all that is required. Vitamin K_1 intravenously, or phytomenadione by mouth, may be given as a prophylactic measure. Repeated doses may be necessary particularly if one of the superwarfarins is involved. In such cases months of treatment may be required. Oral cholestyramine reduces absorption of recently ingested anticoagulant and also shortens the half-life of that already absorbed.

Alpha-chloralose

Alpha-chloralose is used in cereal baits for rodents (4%) and in technical form (about 90%) against moles. It is sometimes used for self-poisoning.

Toxic amounts (approximately 1 g for an adult and 20 mg/kg body weight for a child) cause central nervous system excitation with hypertonia, hyperreflexia, opisthotonus and convulsions. Rhabdomyolysis, coma and respiratory depression may follow.

Supportive measures are necessary if very large amounts of bait have been ingested. Gastric lavage may provoke seizures and is not recommended. Repeated oral doses of activated charcoal may be of value.

EXPOSURE TO FUNGICIDES

These include a wide variety of substances from simple inorganic chemicals such as sulphur to derivatives of thiocarbamic acid. Foliar fungicides provide a physical and chemical barrier to fungi while soil fungicides act either by vapours released or by systemic properties. Dressing fungicides are used on crops which have been harvested. With few exceptions, they are of low toxicity to mammals.

Organomercurials

Methyl or methoxyethyl-mercuric chloride, phenylmercuric acetate, tolylmercuric acetate and similar compounds were used as seed dressing fungicides until the 1980s. They were neurotoxic and also toxic to the gastrointestinal tract and kidney.[171]

Pentachlorophenol

This has largely been phased out of use because of the finding that many commercial products were contaminated by polychlorinated dibenzodioxins and dibenzofurans. Whilst such congeners are less toxic than TCDD, animal data point to contaminants as being responsible for the toxicity of pentachlorophenol.

Poisoning has occurred with occupational use of pentachlorophenol (PCP), particularly as a result of poor hygiene.[172] It is readily absorbed through skin and may be detected in the urine. High dose exposure has resulted in death caused by hyperthermia, profuse sweating and dehydration, possibly secondary to uncoupling of oxidative phosphorylation. Chest tightness, exertional dyspnoea, weakness, ataxia and coma have also been reported.[171] Survivors frequently display dermal irritation, cough and autonomic dysfunction (see Chapter 12).

EXPOSURE TO MOLLUSCICIDES

Metaldehyde is one of the most popular molluscicides and is available for amateur use in the form of pellets for killing slugs. The route of exposure is ingestion. Nausea, vomiting, abdominal pain and diarrhoea often occur 1–3 hours after ingestion of any amount while more than 100 mg/kg may cause hypertonia, convulsions, impaired consciousness and metabolic acidosis. Hepatocellular damage and renal tubular necrosis may occur after 2–3 days.

Management is supportive and symptomatic. Gastric lavage should be considered if more than 50 mg/kg has been ingested within 2 hours.

ACCIDENTAL SELF-INJECTION WITH VETERINARY PRODUCTS

Every year millions of animals including sheep, cattle, birds and fish are routinely vaccinated or given antibiotics, trace elements or other agents to protect them against disease. It has been estimated in Norway that 60 million salmon alone were vaccinated against furunculosis in 1991.[173,174] In spite of this intense activity and a survey of veterinary workers suggesting that accidental self-injection with veterinary products is 'common'[175] remarkably little has been written about the problem.

Epidemiology of self-injection incidents

Vaccination is carried out manually using multiple-dose syringes or guns and inevitably the need to treat large numbers of uncooperative subjects in a short period of time results in accidents. Needlestick injuries were reported in 19/199 veterinarians (9.4%) inoculating cattle.[176] In contrast, only 12 self-injections occurred in a prospective survey of 12 operators who vaccinated almost 2.5 million salmon.[177] The difference between fish vaccinators and others is presumably explained by the difficulties of adequately restraining large animals. Incidents known to us were spread throughout the year and involved six different groups of veterinary pharmaceuticals: vaccines, antihelminthics, copper supplements, synthetic prostaglandins, antibacterial agents and neuroleptic sedatives (Table 10.7), with vaccines comprising the largest group. Most vaccines are formulated in a mineral oil emulsion which causes a local reaction and enhances the immune response.[178] Some contain preservatives and adjuvants which can irritate.

Table 10.7 *Self-injection of veterinary products*

Age/sex	Injection	Injection site	Clinical features	Treatment	Progress
55, M	Heptavac	Finger	Pain, swelling	Intravenous and oral antibiotics	Treatment for 11 days, hospitalized
30, M	Heptavac P	Leg	Cellulitis	Antibiotics	Uneventful recovery
43, M	Heptavac P	Knee	Effusion	Intravenous antibiotics	Hospitalized 1 night
37, M	Heptavac P	Knee	Pain, redness	Antibiotic, antihistamine, magnesium sulphate dressings	Full recovery in 3 days
20, M	Ovivac P	Hand	Swelling, reduced function	Analgesic, antibiotics	Full recovery in 3 days
45, M	Quarivexin	Leg	Cellulitis	Rest, elevation, oral antibiotics	Gradual improvement
32, M	Trivexin T	Finger	Pain, swelling	Antibiotics	Resolved 8–9 days
23, M	Biojec	Thumb	Cellulitis	Incised, irrigated, antibiotics	Hospitalized 3 days
23, M	Biojec	Hand	Swelling, inflammation	Incised, irrigated	Hospitalized several days
20, M	Biojec	Thumb	Cellulitis followed by necrosis	Incised, irrigated, antibiotics. Day 6 debridement	Unknown
27, F	Estrumate	Arm	Severe pelvic cramps	Ice pack, analgesia	Settled over 1 hour
19, M	Stresnil	Wrist	Drowsy, constricted pupils, slurred speech	Unknown	Unknown

Clinical sequelae of accidental vaccination with veterinary products

There is very limited information about the outcome of veterinary inoculation accidents. The near fatal and fatal consequences of accidental injection with etorphine, a veterinary neuroleptanalgesic with opioid properties, have, however, received wide publicity. Needle guards have been developed to help avoid such accidents.

If experience with grease guns and high pressure guns is relevant, injection of veterinary vaccines into soft tissues may have potential for serious sequelae.[179] Those that contain an oil base are poorly absorbed and pressure effects and an overwhelming inflammatory reaction to the chemicals can cause constriction of the surrounding blood vessels.[179,180] The features in cases known to us are shown in Table 10.7. Serious systemic features, other than those secondary to intense local reactions are unlikely as the organisms contained in vaccines are either killed or attenuated. However, the possibility has been raised that one case of acute brucellosis may have been the result of accidental injection with a vaccine.[181] Occasionally, a flu-like illness has occurred after injection of fish vaccines[174] and repeated accidents may induce hypersensitivity which increases the local inflammatory response to further incidents. Serious anaphylactic reactions were reported in three fish vaccinators who had repeated accidents; all needed hospitalization but survived.[173]

Systemic toxicity may also result from the pharmacological properties of the agent injected. Thus accidents involving cloprostenol and azaperone resulted in predictable effects in our series. Tilmicosin may be cardiotoxic.[182] Antihelminthics and copper solutions do not appear to cause problems.

MANAGEMENT

The key to managing injection injuries with veterinary products is swift diagnosis and decompression of the injected area but delays remain common. Because of the small volume injected, some injuries sometimes resolve satisfactorily without exploration and are simply treated with corticosteroids.[178,183] If this option is favoured, the patient requires observation in hospital so that decompression of the injury site can be urgently implemented should swelling and inflammation extend.

Alternately, immediate local decompression may be preferred, with removal of necrotic fat and some of the oil. The wound should be loosely sutured to allow discharge of serum and oil into dressings and the hand elevated on a volar slab in the position of function (metacarpophalangeal joint flexion and interphalangeal joint extension). Physiotherapy should be started early.

Amputation, however, may be necessary in some severe cases. Burke and Brady[178] described a farmer who injected 2 ml of oil-based parvovirus vaccine into his thumb. Over ensuing months he suffered repeated episodes of inflammation that were not controlled by further debridement. This was thought to be due to the mineral oil component of the vaccine and amputation at the carpometacarpal joint was required to control pain and inflammation.

Systemic symptoms should be treated conventionally but the possibility of zoonoses should be considered by any physician treating agricultural or veterinary workers.

REFERENCES

1 Pesticide concerns. *JAMA* 1997; **278**: 536.
2 Berry C. Can chemicals be loved? – a problem for 2000. *Toxicol Lett* 1995; **82/83**: 725–9.
3 de Kretser DM. Declining sperm counts. Environmental chemicals may be to blame. *Br Med J* 1996; **312**: 457–8.
4 Gadon M. Pesticide poisonings in the lawn care and tree service industries. A review of cases in the New York State Pesticide Poisoning Registry. *J Occup Environ Med* 1996; **38**: 794–9.
5 Occupational pesticide poisoning in apple orchards – Washington 1993. *Morbid Mortal Weekly Rep* 1994; **42**: 993–5.
6 Albertson TE, Cross CE. Pesticides in the workplace: a world-wide issue. *Arch Environ Hlth* 1993; **48**: 364–5.
7 Kilgore W. Human exposure to pesticides. In: Newberne PM, Shank RC, Ruchirawat M eds. *International Toxicology Seminar: Environmental Toxicology*. Bangkok: Chulalongkorn Research Institute and Mahidol University, 1988.
8 Ferrer A, Cabral R. Recent epidemics of poisoning by pesticides. *Toxicol Lett* 1995; **82/83**: 55–63.
9 Bartle H. Quiet sufferers of the silent spring. *New Scientist* 1991; **130**: 30–5.
10 Zweiner RJ, Ginsburg CM. Organophosphate and carbamate poisoning in infants and children. *Pediatrics* 1988; **81**: 121–6.
11 World Health Organization. *Public Health Impact of Pesticides Used in Agriculture*. Geneva: WHO, 1990.
12 Jeyaratnam J. Acute pesticide poisoning: a major global health problem. *World Hlth Stat Quarterly* 1990; **43**: 139–44.
13 Pelfrene AF. Acute poisonings by carbamate insecticides and oxime therapy. *J Toxicologie Clinique Exp* 1986; **5**: 313–18.
14 Forget G, Goodman T, deVilliers A (eds). *Impact of Pesticide Use on Health in Developing Countries*. Ottawa, Canada: International Development Research Centre, 1993.
15 Chan TYK, Critchley JAJH, Chan AYW. An estimate of the incidence of pesticide poisoning in Hong Kong. *Vet Hum Toxicol* 1996; **38**: 362–4.
16 Yamashita M, Matsuo H, Ando Y, Tanaka J. Analysis of

1,000 consecutive cases of acute poisoning in the suburb of Tokyo leading to hospitalization. *Vet Hum Toxicol* 1996; **38**: 34–5.

17 Weir S, Minton N, Murray V. Organophosphate poisoning; the UK National Poisons Unit experience during 1984–1987. In: Ballantyne B, Barrs TC eds. *Clinical and Experimental Toxicology of Organophosphates and Carbamates*. Oxford: Butterworth-Heinemann, 1992: 463–70.

18 Lyznicki JM, Kennedy WR, Young DC *et al.* Educational and informational strategies to reduce pesticide risks. *Prev Med* 1997; **26**: 191–200.

19 Kimbrough RD. Uncertainties in risk assessment. *Appl Occup Environ Hyg* 1991; **6**: 759–63.

20 ATSDR (Agency for Toxic Substances and Disease Registry): *Toxicological Profile for Arsenic* Atlanta: US Department of Health and Human Services, 1993.

21 Briatico-Vangosa G, Braun CLJ, Cookman G *et al.* Respiratory allergy: hazard identification and risk assessment. *Fund Appl Toxicol* 1994; **23**: 145–58.

22 Lauwerys R. Basic concepts of monitoring human exposure. *IARC Sci Publ* 1984; **59**: 31–6.

23 Mikheev MI, Lowry LK. WHO global project on biological monitoring of chemical exposure at the workplace. *Int Arch Occup Environ Hlth* 1996; **68**: 387–8.

24 Maizlish N, Rudolph L, Dervin K. The surveillance of work-related pesticide illness: an application of the Sentinal Event Notification System for Occupational Risks (SENSOR). *Am J Publ Hlth* 1995; **85**: 806–11.

25 Angerer J, Gundel J. Biomonitoring and occupational medicine. Possibilities and limitations. *Ann Ist Super Sanita* 1996; **32**: 199–206.

26 Anwar WA. Biomarkers of human exposure to pesticides. *Environ Hlth Perspect* 1997; **105** (Suppl 4): 801–6.

27 Ordin DL, Fine LJ. Surveillance for pesticide-related illness – lessons from California. *Am J Publ Hlth* 1995; **85**: 762–3.

28 O'Malley M. Clinical evaluation of pesticide exposure and poisonings. *Lancet* 1997; **349**: 1161–6.

29 Hillman JV. Emergency care of insecticide poisonings. *J Fla Med Assoc* 1994; **81**: 750–2.

30 Hart TB. Paraquat – a review of safety in agricultural and horticultural use. *Hum Toxicol* 1987; **6**: 13–18.

31 Bismuth C, Hall AH (eds). *Paraquat Poisoning – Mechanisms, Prevention, Treatment*. New York: Marcel Dekker, 1995.

32 Smith JG. Paraquat poisoning by skin absorption: a review. *Hum Toxicol* 1988; **7**: 15–19.

33 Gordonsmith RH, Brooke-Taylor S, Smith LL, Cohen GM. Structural requirements of compounds to inhibit pulmonary diamine accumulation. *Biochem Pharmacol* 1983; **32**: 3701–9.

34 Smith LL. Mechanism of paraquat toxicity in the lung and its relevance to treatment. *Hum Toxicol* 1987; **6**: 31–6.

35 Pond SM. Manifestations and management of paraquat poisoning. *Med J Aust* 1990; **152**: 256–9.

36 Smith LL. The toxicity of paraquat. *Adv Drug React Acute Poison Rev* 1988; **7**: 1–17.

37 Levin PJ, Klaff LJ, Rose AG, Ferguson AD. Pulmonary effects of contact exposure to paraquat: a clinical and experimental study. *Thorax* 1979; **34**: 150–60.

38 Garnier R, Chataigner D, Efthymiou M-L, Moraillon I, Bramary F. Paraquat poisoning by skin absorption: report of two cases. *Vet Hum Toxicol* 1994; **36**: 313–15.

39 Jaros F. Acute percutaneous paraquat poisoning. *Lancet* 1978; **i**: 275.

40 Vale JA, Meredith TJ, Buckley BM. Paraquat poisoning: clinical features and immediate general management. *Hum Toxicol* 1987; **6**: 41–7.

41 Swan AAB. Exposure of spray operators to paraquat. *Br J Ind Med* 1969; **26**: 322–9.

42 Senanayake N, Gurunathan G, Hart TB *et al.* An epidemiological study of the health of Sri Lankan tea plantation workers associated with long-term exposure to paraquat. *Br J Ind Med* 1993; **50**: 257–63.

43 Papiris SA, Maniati MA, Kyriakidis V, Constantopoulos SH. Pulmonary damage due to paraquat poisoning through skin absorption. *Respiration* 1995; **62**: 101–3.

44 Bismuth C, Schermann JM, Garnier R, Baud FJ, Pontal PG. Elimination of paraquat. *Hum Toxicol* 1987; **6**: 63–7.

45 Braithwaite RA. Emergency analysis of paraquat in biological fluids. *Hum Toxicol* 1987; **6**: 83–6.

46 Rhodes ML, Zavala DC, Brown D. Hypoxic protection in paraquat poisoning. *Lab Invest* 1976; **35**: 496–500.

47 Franzen D, Baer F, Heitz W *et al.* Failure of radiotherapy to resolve fatal lung damage due to paraquat poisoning. *Chest* 1991; **100**: 1164–5.

48 Williams PF, Jarvie DR, Whitehead AP. Diquat intoxication: treatment by charcoal haemoperfusion and description of a new method of diquat measurement in plasma. *Clin Toxicol* 1986; **24**: 11–20.

49 Manoguerra AS. Full thickness skin burns secondary to an unusual exposure to diquat dibromide. *Clin Toxicol* 1990; **28**: 107–10.

50 Helliwell M, Nunn J. Mortality in sodium chlorate poisoning. *Br Med J* 1979; **2**: 119.

51 O'Grady J, Jarescsni E. Sodium chlorate poisoning. *Br J Clin Prac* 1971; **25**: 38–9.

52 Steffen C, Wetzel E. Chlorate poisoning: mechanism of toxicity. *Toxicology* 1993; **84**: 217–31.

53 Bloxham CA, Wright N, Hoult JG. Self-poisoning by sodium chlorate – some unusual features. *Clin Toxicol* 1979; **15**: 185–8.

54 Friesen EG, Jones GR, Vaughan D. Clinical presentation and management of acute 2,4-D oral ingestion. *Drug Safety* 1990; **5**: 155–9.

55 Schmoldt A, Iwersen S, Schlüter W. Massive ingestion of the herbicide 2-methyl-4-chlorophenoxyacetic acid (MCPA). *Clin Toxicol* 1997; **35**: 405–8.

56 Nielsen K, Kaempe B, Jensen-Holm J. Fatal poisoning in man by 2,4-dichlorophenoxyacetic acid (2,4-D). Determination of the agent in forensic materials. *Acta Pharmacol Toxicol* 1965; **22**: 224–34.

57 Durakovic Z, Durakovic A, Durakovic S, Ivanovic D.

Poisoning with 2,4-dichlorophenoxyacetic acid treated by hemodialysis. *Arch Toxicol* 1992; **66**: 518–21.

58 Hayes WJ Jr. *Pesticides Studied in Man*. Baltimore: Williams and Wilkins, 1982.

59 Berwick P. 2,4-Dichlorophenoxyacetic acid poisoning in man. Some interesting clinical and laboratory findings. *JAMA* 1970; **214**: 1114–17.

60 Flanagan RJ, Ruprah M. HPLC measurement of chlorophenoxy herbicides, bromoxynil, and ioxynil, in biological specimens to aid diagnosis of acute poisoning. *Clin Chem* 1989; **35**: 1342–7.

61 Hardell L, Sandstrom A. Case-control study: soft-tissue sarcomas and exposure to phenoxyacetic acids or chlorophenols. *Br J Cancer* 1979; **39**: 711–17.

62 Morrison HI, Wilkins K, Semenciw R, Mao Y, Wigle D. Herbicides and cancer. *J Natl Canc Instit* 1992; **84**: 1866–74.

63 Saracci R, Kogvinas M, Bertazzi PA *et al.* Cancer mortality in workers exposed to chlorophenoxy herbicides and chlorophenols. *Lancet* 1991; **338**: 1027–32.

64 Bond GG, Rossbacher R. A review of potential human carcinogenicity of the chlorophenoxy herbicides MCPA, MCPP and 2,4-DP. *Br J Ind Med* 1993; **50**: 340–8.

65 Pearn JH. Herbicides and congenital malformations: a review for the paediatrician. *Aust Paediatr J* 1985; **21**: 237–42.

66 Prescott LF, Park J, Darrien I. Treatment of severe 2,4-D and mecoprop intoxication with alkaline diuresis. *Br J Clin Pharmacol* 1979; **7**: 111–16.

67 Kancir CB, Andersen C, Olesen AS. Marked hypocalcaemia in a fatal poisoning with chlorinated phenoxy acid derivatives. *Clin Toxicol* 1988; **26**: 257–64.

68 O'Reilly JF. Prolonged coma and delayed peripheral neuropathy after ingestion of phenoxyacetate weedkillers. *Postgrad Med J* 1984; **60**: 76–7.

69 Dudley AW Jr, Thapar NT. Fatal human ingestion of 2,4-D, a common herbicide. *Arch Pathol* 1972; **94**: 270–5.

70 Courtney KD, Moore JA. Teratology studies with 2,4,5-trichlorophenoxyacetic acid and 2,3,7,8-tetra-chlorodibenzo-dioxin. *Toxicol Appl Pharmacol* 1971; **20**: 396–403.

71 Flanagan RJ, Meredith TJ, Ruprah M, Onyon LJ, Liddle A. Alkaline diuresis for acute poisoning with chlorophenoxy herbicides and ioxynil. *Lancet* 1990; **335**: 454–8.

72 Menkes DB, Temple WA, Edwards IR. Intentional self-poisoning with glyphosate-containing herbicides. *Hum Exp Toxicol* 1991; **10**: 103–7.

73 Talbot AR, Shiaw M-H, Huang J-S *et al.* Acute poisoning with a glyphosate-surfactant herbicide ('Round-up'): a review of 93 cases. *Hum Exp Toxicol* 1991; **10**: 1–8.

74 Chang S, Hung CS, Chow W, Wu T. Endoscopy survey of glyphosate-surfactant intoxication. *Clin Toxicol* 1995; **33**: 553.

75 Tominack RL, Yang G, Tsai W-J, Chung H, Deng J. Taiwan National Poison Center survey of glyphosate-surfactant herbicide ingestions. *Clin Toxicol* 1991; **29**: 91–109.

76 International Programme on Chemical Safety (IPCS).

Amitrole. Environmental Health Criteria 158. Geneva: WHO, 1994.

77 Loosli R. Epidemiology of atrazine. *Rev Env Contamin Toxicol* 1995; **143**: 47–57.

78 Jorens PG, Zandijk E, Belmans L, Schepens PJC, Bossaert LL. An unusual poisoning with the unusual pesticide amitraz. *Hum Exp Toxicol* 1997; **16**: 600–1.

79 Kennel O, Prince C, Garnier R. Four cases of amitraz poisoning in humans. *Vet Hum Toxicol* 1996; **38**: 28–30.

80 Balkisson R, Murray D, Hoffstein V. Alveolar damage due to inhalation of amitrole-containing herbicide. *Chest* 1992; **101**: 1174–6.

81 Sathiakumar N, Delzell E, Austin H, Cole P. A follow-up study of agricultural chemical production workers. *Am J Ind Med* 1992; **21**: 321–30.

82 Alexander NM. Antithyroid action of 3-amino-1,2,4-triazole. *J Biol Chem* 1959; **234**: 148–50.

83 Donna A, Crosignani P, Robutti F *et al.* Triazine herbicides and ovarian epithelial neoplasms. *Scand J Work Environ Hlth* 1989; **15**: 47–53.

84 Minder CE. Re Triazine herbicides and ovarian epithelial neoplasms. (letter) *Scand J Work Environ Hlth* 1990; **16**: 445–7.

85 Legras A, Skrobala D, Furet Y *et al.* Herbicide: fatal ammonium thiocyanate and aminotriazole poisoning. *Clin Toxicol* 1996; **34**: 441–6.

86 Domazalski CA, Kolb LC, Hines EA. Delirious reactions secondary to thiocyanate therapy of hypertension. *Proc Mayo Clin* 1953; **28**: 272–80.

87 Fukuto TR. Mechanism of action of organophosphorus and carbamate insecticides. *Environ Hlth Perspect* 1990; **87**: 245–54.

88 Jokanovic M, Maksimovic M. Abnormal cholinesterase activity: understanding and interpretation. *Eur J Clin Chem Clin Biochem* 1997; **35**: 11–16.

89 Ganendran A. Organophosphate insecticide poisoning and its management. *Anaesth Intens Care* 1974; **4**: 361–63.

90 Saadeh AM, Al-Ali M, Farsakh NA, Ghani MA. Clinical and sociodemographic features of acute carbamate and organophosphate poisoning: a study of 70 adult patients on North Jordan. *Clin Toxicol* 1996; **34**: 45–51.

91 Agarwal SB. A clinical, biochemical, neurobehavioural, and sociopsychological study of 190 patients admitted to hospital as a result of acute organophosphorus poisoning. *Environ Res* 1993; **62**: 63–70.

92 Yamashita M, Yamashita M, Tanaka J, Ando Y. Human mortality of organophosphate poisonings. *Vet Hum Toxicol* 1997; **39**: 84–5.

93 Ballantyne B, Marrs TC. *Organophosphates and Carbamates*. Oxford: Butterworth-Heinemann, 1992.

94 Rees H. Exposure to sheep dip and the incidence of acute symptoms in a group of Welsh farmers. *Occup Environ Med* 1996; **53**: 258–63.

95 Spyker DA. Multiple chemical sensitivities – syndrome

and solution. *Clin Toxicol* 1995; **33**: 95–9.

96 White RF, Feldman RG, Travers PH. Neurobehavioural effects of toxicity due to metals, solvents and insecticides. *Clin Neuropharmacol* 1990; **13**: 392–412.

97 Ames RG, Steenland K, Jenkins B, Chrislip D, Russo J. Chronic neurologic sequelae to cholinesterase inhibition among agricultural pesticide applicators. *Arch Environ Hlth* 1995; **50**: 440–4.

98 Beach JR, Spurgeon A, Stephens R *et al.* Abnormalities on neurological examination among sheep farmers exposed to organophosphorus pesticides. *Occup Environ Med* 1996; **53**: 520–5.

99 World Health Organization. *Planning Strategy for the Prevention of Pesticide Poisoning.* Geneva: WHO, 1986.

100 Stephens R, Spurgeon A, Calvert IA *et al.* Neuropsychological effects of long-term exposure to organophosphates in sheep dip. *Lancet* 1995; **345**: 1135–9.

101 Levin HS, Rodnitzy RL. Behavioural effects of organophosphate pesticides in man. *Clin Toxicol* 1976; **9**: 391–405.

102 Savage EP, Keefe TJ, Mounce LM, Heaton RK, Lewis JA, Burcar PJ. Chronic neurological sequelae of acute organophosphate pesticide poisoning. *Arch Environ Hlth* 1988; **43**: 38–45.

103 Finkelstein Y, Taitelman U, Biegon A. CNS involvement in acute organophosphate poisoning: specific pattern of toxicity, clinical correlates and antidotal treatment. *Ital J Neurol Sci* 1988; **9**: 437–46.

104 Tsao TC-Y, Juang Y-C, Lan R-S, Shieh WB, Lee C-H. Respiratory failure of acute organophosphate and carbamate poisoning. *Chest* 1990; **98**: 631–6.

105 Saadeh AM, Farsakh NA, Al-Ali MK. Cardiac manifestations of acute carbamate and organophosphate poisoning. *Heart* 1997; **77**: 461–4.

106 Senananyake N, Karalliede L. Neurotoxic effects of organophosphorus insecticides. *N Engl J Med* 1987; **316**: 761–3.

107 Morgan JP, Penovich P. Jamaica ginger paralysis. Forty-seven year follow up. *Arch Neurol* 1978; **35**: 530–2.

108 Woolf AD. Ginger Jake and the blues: a tragic song of poisoning. *Vet Hum Toxicol* 1995; **37**: 252–4.

109 LeBlanc FN, Benson BE, Gilg AD. A severe organophosphate poisoning requiring the use of an atropine drip. *Clin Toxicol* 1986; **24**: 69–74.

110 Worek F, Bäcker M, Thiermann H *et al.* Reappraisal of indications and limitations of oxime therapy in organophosphate poisoning. *Hum Exp Toxicol* 1997; **16**: 466–72.

111 Besser R, Weilemann LS, Gutmann L. Efficacy of obidoxime in human organophosphorus poisoning: determination by neuromuscular transmission studies. *Muscle Nerve* 1995; **18**: 15–22.

112 Rider JA, Moeller HC, Puletti EJ, Swader JI. Toxicity of parathion, systox, octamethyl-pyrophosphoramide and methyl parathion in man. *Toxicol Appl Pharmacol* 1969; **14**: 603–11.

113 Yager J, McLean H, Hudes M, Spear RC. Components of variability in blood cholinesterase assay results. *J Occup Med* 1976; **18**: 242–4.

114 Baselt RC. *Biological Monitoring Methods for Industrial Chemicals.* Foster City, CA: Chemical Toxicology Institute, Biomedical Publications, 1980.

115 Kahn E. Outline guide for performance of field studies to establish safe re-entry intervals for organophosphate pesticides. *Residue Rev* 1979; **70**: 27–43.

116 Lima JS, Alberto C, Reis G. Poisoning due to illegal use of carbamates as a rodenticide in Rio de Janeiro. *Clin Toxicol* 1995; **33**: 687–90.

117 Gupta RC. Carbofuran toxicity. *J Toxicol Environ Hlth* 1994; **43**: 383–418.

118 Liddle JA, Kimbrough RD, Needham LL *et al.* A fatal episode of accidental methomyl poisoning. *Clin Toxicol* 1979; **15**: 159–67.

119 Goldman LR, Smith DF, Neutra RR *et al.* Pesticide food poisoning from contaminated watermelons in California, 1985. *Arch Environ Hlth* 1990; **45**: 229–36.

120 Cranmer MF. Carbaryl. A toxicological review and risk analysis. *Neurotoxicol* 1986; **7**: 247–328.

121 Ecobichon DJ, Joy RM. *Pesticides and Neurological Diseases* 2nd edn. Boca Raton, Fl: CRC Press, 1994.

122 Moritz F, Droy JM, Dutheil G, Melki J, Bonmarchand G, Leroy J. Acute pancreatitis after carbamate insecticide intoxication. *Intens Care Med* 1994; **20**: 49–50.

123 Dickoff DJ, Gerber O, Turovsky Z. Delayed neurotoxicity after ingestion of carbamate pesticide. *Neurology* 1987; **37**: 1229–31.

124 Umehara F, Izumo S, Arimura K, Osame M. Polyneuropathy induced by m-tolyl methyl carbamate intoxication. *J Neurol* 1991; **238**: 47–8.

125 Grendon J, Frost F, Baum L. Chronic health effects among sheep and humans surviving an aldicarb poisoning incident. *Vet Hum Toxicol* 1994; **36**: 218–23.

126 Sterri SH, Rognerud B, Fiskum SE, Lyngaas S. Effect of toxogonin and P2S in the toxicity of carbamates and organophosphorus compounds. *Acta Pharmacol Toxicol* 1979; **45**: 9–15.

127 Kurtz PH. Pralidoxime in the treatment of carbamate intoxication. *Am J Emerg Med* 1990; **8**: 68–70.

128 Morgan DP. *Recognition and Management of Pesticide Poisonings* 3rd edn. Washington DC: US Government Printing Office, 1982: 11.

129 Mortensen ME. Pharmacological and toxicological considerations in the treatment of carbamate intoxications. *Am J Emerg Med* 1990; **8**: 83–84.

130 Abbott DC, Goulding R, Holmes DC, Hoodless RA. Organochlorine pesticide residues in human fat in the United Kingdom 1982–1983. *Hum Toxicol* 1985; **4**: 435–45.

131 Joy RM. Chlorinated hydrocarbon insecticides. In: Ecobichon DJ, Joy RM. *Pesticides and Neurological Diseases* 2nd edn. Boca Raton, FL: CRC Press, 1994.

132 Lange M, Nitzsche K, Zesch A. Percutaneous absorption of lindane in healthy volunteers and scabies patients.

Dependency of penetration kinetics in serum upon frequency of application, time and mode of washing. *Arch Dermatol Res* 1981; **271**: 387–99.

133 Drummond L, Gillanders EM, Wilson HK. Plasma gamma-hexachlorocyclohexane concentrations in forestry workers exposed to indane. *Br J Ind Med* 1988; **45**: 493–7.

134 Fonseca RG, Resende LA, Silva MD, Camargo A. Chronic motor neurone disease possibly related to intoxication with organochlorine insecticides. *Acta Neurol Scand* 1993; **88**: 56–8.

135 Key T, Reeves G. Organochlorines in the environment and breast cancer. *Br Med J* 1994; **308**: 1520–1.

136 Morgan DP, Stockdale EM, Roberts RJ, Halter AW. Anemia associated with exposure to lindane. *Arch Environ Hlth* 1980; **35**: 307–10.

137 Lessenger JE, Riley N. Neurotoxicities and behavioural changes in a 12 year-old male exposed to dicofol, an organochlorine pesticide. *J Toxicol Environ Hlth* 1991; **33**: 255–61.

138 Garrettson LK, Guzelian PS, Blanke RV. Subacute chlordane poisoning. *Clin Toxicol* 1984–5; **22**: 565–71.

139 Ginsburg CM, Lowry W, Reisch JS. Absorption of lindane (gamma benzene hexachloride) in infants and children. *J Pediatrics* 1977; **91**: 998–1000.

140 Davies JE, Dedhia HV, Morgade C, Barquet A, Maibach HI. Lindane poisonings. *Arch Dermatol* 1983; **119**: 142–4.

141 Etherington JD. Major epileptic seizures and topical gammabenzene hexachloride. *Br Med J* 1984; **289**: 228.

142 Munk ZM, Nantel A. Acute lindane poisoning with development of muscle necrosis. *Can Med Assoc J* 1977; **117**: 1050–4.

143 Sunder Ram Rao CV, Shreenivas R, Singh V, Perez-Atayde A, Woolf A. Disseminated intravascular coagulation in a case of fatal lindane poisoning. *Vet Hum Toxicol* 1988; **30**: 132–4.

144 Kassner JT, Maher TJ, Hull KM, Woolf AD. Cholestyramine as an adsorbent in acute lindane poisoning: a murine model. *Ann Emerg Med* 1993; **22**: 31–5.

145 Cohn WJ, Boylan JJ, Blanke RV, Fariss MW, Howell JR, Guzelian PS. Treatment of chlordecone (Kepone) toxicity with cholestyramine. Results of a controlled clinical trial. *N Engl Med J* 1978; **298**: 243–8.

146 Nakakita H. The mode of action of phosphine. *J Pesticide Sci* 1987; **12**: 299–309.

147 Jones AT, Jones RC, Longley EO. Environmental and clinical aspects of bulk wheat fumigation with aluminium phosphide. *Am Ind Hyg Assoc J* 1964; **25**: 376–9.

148 Misra UK, Tripathi AK, Pandey R, Bhargwa B. Acute phosphine poisoning following ingestion of aluminium phosphide. *Hum Toxicol* 1988; **7**: 343–5.

149 Wilson R. Acute phosphine poisoning aboard a grain freighter. *JAMA* 1980; **244**: 148–50.

150 Potter WT, Garry VF, Kelly JT, Tarone R, Griffith J, Nelson RL. Radiometric assay of red cell and plasma cholinesterase in pesticide appliers from Minnesota. *Toxicol Appl Pharmacol* 1993; **119**: 150–5.

151 Garry VF, Good PF, Manivel JC, Perl DP. Investigation of a

fatality from nonoccupational aluminium phosphide exposure: measurement of aluminium in tissue and body fluids as a marker of exposure. *J Lab Clin Med* 1993; **122**: 739–47.

152 CDC. Deaths associated with exposure to fumigants in railroad cars-United States. *Morbid Mortal Weekly Rep* 1994; **43**: 489–91.

153 Schoonbroodt D, Guffens P, Jousten P, Ingels J, Grodos J. Acute phosphine poisoning? A case report and review. *Acta Clin Belg* 1992; **47**: 280–4.

154 Gupta S, Ahlawat SK. Aluminium phosphide poisoning – a review. *Clin Toxicol* 1995; **33**: 19–24.

155 Khosla SN, Nand N, Khosla P. Aluminium phosphide poisoning. *J Trop Med Hyg* 1988; **91**: 196–8.

156 Bhasin P, Mittal HS, Mitra A. An echocardiographic study in aluminium phosphide poisoning. *J Assoc Physicians India* 1991; **39**: 851.

157 Bajaj R, Wasir HS, Agarwal R. Aluminium phosphide poisoning. Clinical toxicity and outcome in 11 intensively monitored patients. *Natl Med J India* 1988; **1**: 270–4.

158 Goswami M, Bindal M, Sen P, Gupta SK, Avasthi R, Ram BK. Fat and oil inhibit phosphine release from aluminium phosphide – its clinical implication. *Ind J Exp Biol* 1994; **32**: 647–9.

159 Dorman DC, Beasley VR. Neurotoxicology of pyrethrin and the pyrethroid insecticides. *Vet Hum Toxicol* 1991; **33**: 238–42.

160 Miyamoto J, Kaneko H, Tsuji R, Okuno Y. Pyrethroids, nerve poisons: how their risks to human health should be assessed. *Toxicol Lett* 1995; **82/83**: 933–40.

161 He F, Wang S, Liu L, Chen S, Zhang Z, Sun J. Clinical manifestations and diagnosis of acute pyrethroid poisoning. *Arch Toxicol* 1989; **63**: 54–8.

162 Box SA, Lee MR. A systemic reaction following exposure to a pyrethroid insecticide. *Hum Exp Toxicol* 1996; **15**: 389–90.

163 Lessenger JE. Five office workers inadvertently exposed to cypermethrin. *J Toxicol Environ Hlth* 1992; **35**: 261–7.

164 Paton DL, Walker JS. Pyrethrin poisoning from commericial-strength flea and tick spray. *Am J Emerg Med* 1988; **6**: 232–5.

165 Feinberg SM. Pyrethrum sensitisation: its importance and relation to pollen allergy. *JAMA* 1994; **102**: 1557–8.

166 Wax PM, Hoffman RS. Fatality associated with inhalation of a pyrethrin shampoo. *Clin Toxicol* 1994; **32**: 457–60.

167 Altenkirch H, Hopmann D, Brockmeier B, Walter G. Neurological investigations in 23 cases of pyrethroid intoxication reported to the German Federal Health Office. *Neurotoxicol* 1996; **17**: 645–52.

168 Rauch AE, Weininger R, Pasquale D *et al.* Superwarfarin poisoning: a significant public health problem. *J Commun Hlth* 1994; **19**: 55–65.

169 Abell TL, Merigian KS, Lee JM, Holbert JM, McCall JW. Cutaneous exposure to warfarin-like anticoagulant causing an intracerebral hemorrhage: a case report. *Clin Toxicol* 1994; **32**: 69–73.

170 McCarthy PT, Cox AD, Harrington DJ *et al*. Covert poisoning with difenacoum: clinical and toxicological observations. *Hum Exp Toxicol* 1997; **16**: 166–70.

171 Edwards R, Ferry DG, Temple WA. Fungicides and related compounds. In: Hayes WJ Jr, Laws ER Jr eds. *Handbook of Pesticide Toxicology. Classes of Pesticides.* New York: Academic Press, 1991: 1409–70.

172 Jorens PG, Schepens PJC. Human pentachlorophenol poisoning. *Hum Exp Toxicol* 1993; **12**: 479–95.

173 Leira HL, Baalsrud KJ. Self-injection of fish vaccine can cause anaphylaxis. *Scand J Work Environ Hlth* 1992; **18**: 410.

174 Leira HL, Berg RE, Baalsrud KJ, Eggen BM, Olafsson K. Health risks of vaccination of farmed fish. *Tidsskr Nor Laegeforen* 1993; **113**: 1563–5.

175 Constable PJ, Harrington JM. Risks of zoonoses in a veterinary service. *Br Med J* 1982; **284**: 246–8.

176 Patterson CJ, LaVenture M, Hurely SS, Davis JP. Accidental self-inoculation with *Mycobacterium paratuberculosis* bacterin (Johne's bacterin) by veterinarians in Wisconsin. *J Am Vet Med Assoc* 1988; **192**: 1197–9.

177 Dyrkorn S, Saegrov BH, Saegrov S. Frequency and clinical consequences of self-injection among salmon vaccinators. *Tidsskr Nor Laegeforen* 1993; **113**: 1566–8.

178 Burke F, Brady O. Veterinary and industrial high pressure injuries. *Br Med J* 1996; **312**: 1436.

179 Proust AF. Special injuries of the hand. *Emerg Med Clin N Am* 1993; **11**: 767–79.

180 Duncan K. Accidental self-inoculation with veterinary vaccine. *Br Med J* 1980; **280**: 795.

181 Squarcione S, Maggi P, Lo Caputo S, De Gennaro M, Carbonara S. A case of human brucellosis caused by accidental injection of animal vaccine. *G Ital Med Lav* 1990; **12**: 25–6.

182 McGuigan MA. Human exposures to Tilmicosin (MICOTIL). *Vet Hum Toxicol* 1994; **36**: 306–8.

183 Couzens G, Burke FD. Veterinary high pressure injection injuries with inoculations for larger animals. *J Hand Surg (Br)* 1995; **20**: 497–9.

11

Aliphatic chemicals

LEONARD S LEVY

Alkanes	224	Carboxylic acids	249
Alkenes	232	Esters	249
Dienes	237	Amides	250
Alkynes	239	Ethers	251
Alcohols	239	Epoxides	252
Diols	243	Nitriles	253
Carbonyl compounds	244	Sulphur-containing compounds	253
Aldehydes	244	Aliphatic mixtures: petroleum solvents	255
Ketones	246	References	256

The main reason for a clinician to know about the actions of industrial chemicals is to help with the recognition, diagnosis and rational management of cases of poisoning (whether acute or long-term), or suspected poisoning, occurring at the patient's workplace. This introductory section reviews some general principles related to those objectives.

The recognition and diagnosis of any occupational disease depend principally on thinking about the possibility of industrial poisoning and taking adequate occupational and medical histories. In the case of chemically induced occupational disease, the effects of the suspect material are uppermost in the mind of the clinician but a flexible approach should always allow the possibility that another industrial chemical or indeed a non-occupational cause might be responsible.

Because the components of an adequate occupational history are considered more fully in Chapter 1, it will be sufficient here to mention the main points. Care should be taken to determine, as exactly as possible, all the chemical substances to which the patient has been exposed. Nearly all industrial chemicals enter the body through the respiratory tract and a lesser but important number by dermal absorption. Ingestion of chemicals at the workplace is extremely uncommon in the United Kingdom.

Useful estimates of the degree of exposure and uptake may very often be obtained from careful questioning about the duration of exposure, including overtime, and whether the patient knows (and he/she frequently does) if the material was present in unusual amounts, or if an accident or excessive exposure occurred. Absorption, if through the respiratory tract, might have been diminished by 'protective' measures such as masks, airline hoods, or if through the skin, by gloves, impermeable aprons, etc. (Figs 11.1, 11.2). Occasionally, gloves increase skin, absorption by accidentally retaining liquids in contact with the skin, and this possibility should not be overlooked.

Throughout this chapter mention is made of metabolites of industrial chemicals which can be measured in the urine or the blood, and also occasionally of the suspected chemical being found in expired air. Many hospital laboratories will not be equipped to undertake such analysis immediately. It is worth considering, therefore, if help might be available from elsewhere. Two useful sources in the UK are first a doctor from the Employment Medical Advisory Service (EMAS), which for the present purpose might be thought of as the medical branch of the Health and Safety Executive – and so be found under that heading in the telephone directory, and second the medical department (if there is one) of the factory where the suspected poisoning occurred. However, in recent years many people tend not to be employed in large enterprises with their own medical department, but in smaller to medium-sized enterprises where such medical expertise will not be available.

The term 'solvent', frequently encountered in the literature of occupational medicine (and in this chapter), is sometimes confusing. 'Solvents' may be regarded as almost a marketing term describing a group of liquids, many of which are organic chemicals. Whilst they differ

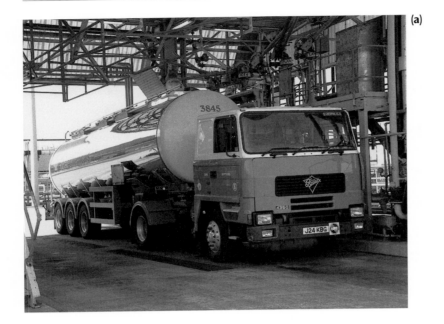

(a)

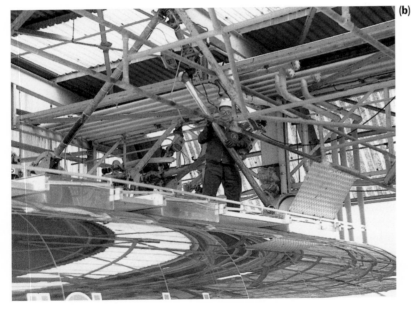

(b)

Figure 11.1 *(a) Top loading of roadcar with solvent at refinery. (b) Close-up of operative on top of roadcar. Note personal protective equipment. Photograph courtesy of Shell UK Limited.*

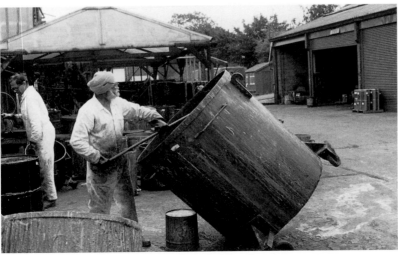

Figure 11.2 *Solvent exposure in a paint factory: a worker using solvents to clean a vessel for mixing paints. Exposure to vapour is reduced by carrying out the operation outdoors and skin absorption is prevented by protective gloves. The effectiveness of these measures may be assessed by occupational physicians using biological monitoring.*

widely in chemical structure (and therefore in metabolism and biochemical action), they nevertheless share important physical characteristics. They are nearly all volatile liquids at room temperature. They are strongly lipophilic and thus may depress the central nervous system if absorbed in quantity (inhalation anaesthetics are solvents).

Diagnosis and rational management depend, particularly in acute poisonings, on an understanding of both the actions and the mechanisms of action of the suspect chemical. Because the descriptions of the aliphatic chemicals considered in this chapter bear this in mind, an outline of the general principles of management may be useful here.

Prevention of further absorption, in industrial toxicology, is confined to first aid measures such as removal from exposure for respiratory hazards or skin cleansing in the case of possible dermal absorption. Because absorption from the gastrointestinal tract is virtually unknown in industry, measures to prevent further absorption by that route, such as gastric lavage, emesis or the administration of activated charcoal, are hardly ever called for.

Active measures, such as haemodialysis, to increase the *elimination* of absorbed substances are rarely needed in cases of poisoning by industrial chemicals. If, however, the chemical has been swallowed, and therefore a much larger dose has entered the body, as in methanol or ethylene glycol poisoning, such active measures may well be appropriate.

Attention in this chapter is, therefore, directed to the metabolic effects so that treatment can help control the adverse effects and accelerate the metabolism of the substance, where this may be done safely. Besides considering the effects on target organs such as the central nervous system, liver or kidney, it may be important, particularly in acute cases, to pay particular attention to the intensive monitoring of both the acid-base balance and the electrolyte balance.

Acute poisoning from industrial chemicals is uncommon today in developed countries. The principal measures in such cases are not different from poisoning by drugs. Thus for acute overexposure to solvent vapour all that is generally necessary is removal from exposure, followed by supportive measures. Heroic treatments such as haemoperfusion to remove trichloroethanol derivatives, for example, are practically never necessary.

In the very rare instances of severe acute poisoning, general measures of intensive therapy may be considered. Metabolic acidosis might occur and hyperkalaemia must be guarded against to prevent the development of cardiac arrhythmias. Forced alkaline diuresis is a metabolically invasive procedure to be undertaken only where frequent biochemical monitoring is available with experienced medical and nursing staff.

Carcinogenic and reproductive effects, and alleged carcinogenic and reproductive effects, are dealt with in detail in Chapters 39 and 40 and will not be exhaustively covered here.

Sources of information

Several million chemicals have been identified, some of them with recognized toxicological properties, but very many more where the toxicological properties are completely unknown. Most of these are organic chemicals, often with complex structures and nomenclature which might seem to make occupational toxicology too huge a subject to grasp. But many organic chemicals contain the same functional groups, which have similar biochemical actions, and this often provides some assistance to the understanding of this apparently overwhelming problem.

Furthermore:

1   The number of chemicals which are in common use in the workplace and may represent a health hazard to exposed workers has been variously estimated to range from 40 000 to 100 000.

2   Information and practical advice on assessment and clinical management of those industrial chemicals which are commonly used is becoming increasingly accessible on computerized databases – not only as raw data but sometimes, and more usefully, as evaluated summaries. Often this information may be available from a local poisons centre unit and, in the UK, from the Health and Safety Executive; in the USA from The National Institute of Occupational Safety and Health (NIOSH). Additionally, university departments of occupational health are frequently able to assist.

Organic chemical compounds

In the same way that organic compounds were originally named to indicate those compounds formed by living matter but are now better described as those compounds containing carbon, so the two main groupings of organic chemicals, aliphatic and aromatic compounds, are better described by their present rather than by their earlier etymological meanings (aliphatic = oily; aromatic = fragrant). Aliphatic now describes open-chain compounds together with those cyclic compounds which chemically resemble open-chain compounds. Aromatic now describes ring compounds such as benzene together with other compounds which resemble benzene in chemical properties. They are discussed in Chapter 12.

Table 11.1 lists some of the main families of aliphatic organic chemicals of interest to industrial toxicology along with specific substances which are described in this chapter. The table also indicates their structural formulae which to some extent determines their toxic effects. As mentioned earlier, the description of each chemical will mention:

1   those characteristics of its chemistry and use in industry which may be useful to the clinician;

2   briefly, its metabolism and biochemical effects;

3   the clinical manifestations (immediate and where relevant long-term) of poisoning by the chemical;

4   suggestions for management.

Table 11.1 *Some of the major aliphatic families and examples*

Chemical family	Formula	Examples
Alkanes and their halogenated compounds (chloroalkanes)	C_nH_{2n+2} (with halogen substitution for H where appropriate)	n-Hexane Dichloromethane Carbon tetrachloride Chloroform 1,2-Dichloroethane 1,1,1-Trichloroethane 1,2-Dibromoethane
Alkenes and their chlorinated compounds (chloroalkenes)	C_nH_{2n} (with halogen substitution for H where (appropriate)	Trichloroethylene Tetrachloroethylene Vinylidene chloride
Dienes	-HC=C=CH- (allene) -HC=C(H)-(H)C=CH- (diene)	1,3-Butadiene
Alkynes	C_nH_{2n-2}, e.g. acetylene HC≡CH	Dichloroacetylene
Alcohols	R-OH	Methanol 2-Propanol 1-Butanol 2-Butanol tert-Butanol iso-Butanol
Diols	-C=C- | | HO OH	1,2-Propylene glycol
Aldehydes	RCOH	Formaldehyde Acetaldehyde Glutaraldehyde
Ketones	R-C-R₁ (‖ O)	Methyl n-butyl ketone Methyl iso-butyl ketone Methyl ethyl ketone
Carboxylic acids and their chlorinated compounds	RCOOH	Trichloroacetic acid
Esters	RC=OOR'	Methyl methacrylate
Amides	$RCONH_2$	Acrylamide Dimethylformamide
Ethers	R-O-R'	Bis(chloromethyl) ether
Epoxides	O (=C—C=)	Epichlorohydrin
Acid nitriles (cyanides)	R-C≡N	Acrylonitrile
Sulphur-containing compounds	Aliphatic compounds containing sulphur	Carbon disulphide
Aliphatic mixtures	—	White spirits

ALKANES

The general formula for alkanes is C_nH_{2n+2} and the first member of the series is methane (CH_4) where n = 1. This is followed by ethane, propane and butane, etc. (n = 2, 3, 4 etc.). These compounds are gases and the last two are commonly used as fuels (liquid petroleum gas-LPG).

As the number of carbon atoms in the chain increases, so do the boiling and melting points as well as the number of possible isomers. Straight-chain alkanes containing 18 or more carbon atoms are low-melting point waxy

Table 11.2 *Linear and branched alkanes*

n	Name
1	Methane
2	Ethane
3	Propane
4	Butane
5	Pentane
6	Hexane
7	Heptane
8	Octane
9	Nonane
10	Decane
11	Undecane
12	Dodecane

solids and mixtures of some of these are used to produce paraffin waxes. Table 11.2 gives examples of the alkane family. For values of n greater than 3, there are branched isomers. The linear isomer may be indicated by the prefix *n*-and branched isomers by the prefixes such as *iso-*, *sec-*, *tert-*, *neo-*; but in modern nomenclature promulgated by the International Union of Pure and Applied Chemistry (IUPAC), the alkanes are named as substituents of the longest chain, thus:

$$CH_3—CH_2—CH_2—CH_2—CH_2—CH_3 \qquad \text{Hexane}$$

2-Methylpentane

3-Methylpentane

2,2'-Dimethylbutane

2,3-Dimethylbutane

The alkanes exist as open-chain compounds, such as *n*-hexane which is described in detail below, and some also in cyclic forms such as cyclohexane. In the cyclic forms, the carbon atoms loop round so that the hydrogen atoms are removed from the two end atoms and the carbon atoms are joined together (the formula of cyclohexane is, thus, C_6H_{12} whereas that of *n*-hexane is C_6H_{14}).

In general, alkanes have a central nervous system depressant action at increasing concentrations and at higher concentrations may act as simple asphyxiants by the displacement of oxygen in the air. Perhaps more important, the handling of these compounds carries an explosion hazard. In 1974 an accident with cyclohexane at Flixborough, England killed 28 and injured 36 persons, causing extensive structural damage. That tragedy was caused by an *explosion* and *not* by *toxicity*.

n-HEXANE (C₆H₁₄)

[CAS no. 110-54-3]

Characteristics and use

n-Hexane, the straight unbranched isomer, is a colourless liquid, insoluble in water but miscible with many other organic solvents. It is stated to have a mildly disagreeable odour with an odour threshold of around 80–150 parts per million (ppm). Whilst pure *n*-hexane will only be encountered as a laboratory reagent, most *n*-hexane occurs as a component of commercial hexane mixtures or petroleum hydrocarbon products (Fig. 11.3). Special boiling point mixtures (SBPs), often used as solvents for adhesives, contain up to 25% *n*-hexane and even petrol may contain up to 5%. *n*-Hexane is mainly used as a solvent in the chemical industry, a seed-oil solvent and a diluting solvent for adhesives, paints and inks.

The main route for occupational absorption is by inhalation. Skin absorption appears to be limited. There is a wide potential for exposure in industry but when it is used as a solvent, exposure will often be mixed because, as noted above, *n*-hexane is generally used with other organic solvents. Because of its potential for

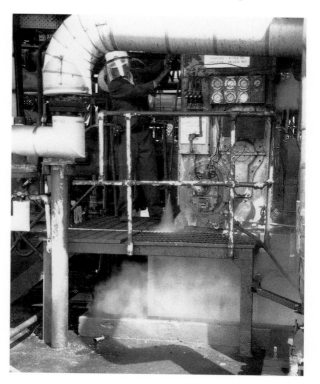

Figure 11.3 *Industrial alkane plant at refinery showing protected operative steaming out compressor before maintenance. Photograph courtesy of Shell UK Limited.*

causing peripheral neuropathy, occupational exposures should be controlled to below 20 ppm (UK occupational exposure limit in 1999).

Metabolism/biochemical effects

The most serious toxic effect of repeated overexposure, first observed in the 1960s and 1970s in outworkers and small enterprises in the shoe-manufacturing industry in Japan and Italy, is a sensorimotor peripheral neuropathy. Subsequent studies on its metabolism demonstrated that the neurotoxic effects are due to the toxic metabolite 2,5-hexanedione which, possibly by cross-linking with neurofilaments as a primary action on the neuroskeleton, leads to paranodal neurofilament accumulations. An alternative explanation is that the γ-diketone moiety (of 2,5-hexanedione) inhibits glycolysis in the neurons. That is followed by secondary thinning and retraction of the myelin sheath.

n-Hexane has a low acute toxicity in experimental animals, although repeated exposure by inhalation over 6 months at 500 ppm has led to peripheral neuropathy. No clinical or pathological effects have been seen following repeated exposure to 125 ppm or less. The neurotoxic effects of n-hexane can be enhanced, so that they appear more quickly and possibly from a lower exposure, by concomitant exposure to methyl ethyl ketone (MEK)[1] (p. 248) or methyl iso-butyl ketone (MiBK) (p. 247) which, by themselves, are not neurotoxic.

Clinical manifestations

n-Hexane is a mild irritant to skin. The sparse human data on acute toxicity suggest that it is of low acute toxicity. As with many organic solvents, narcotic effects on the central nervous system such as drowsiness, vertigo and giddiness have been reported from exposure to commercial hexane at concentrations between 1000 and 5000 ppm over 10–60 minutes.[2]

After exposures lasting for several months the subject may develop paraesthesiae in the extremities and possibly signs of peripheral motor, and less commonly, sensory neuropathy, with decreased nerve conduction velocity. The clinical features and electrophysiological features are indistinguishable from other causes of sensorimotor neuropathy. Recovery is generally slow after removal from exposure,[3] taking months or years, and in some cases may be incomplete.

There is some difficulty in deciding at what concentrations neuropathy occurs. Symptomless workers, in an Italian shoe factory, exposed to n-hexane, with MEK and cyclohexane, showed both decreased motor nerve conduction velocities in upper and lower limbs and an increased prevalence of symptoms of early narcosis compared with controls. Clinically overt neuropathy will probably develop if the air concentration of n-hexane exceeds 100 ppm but workers exposed to levels less than 100 ppm showed significantly decreased motor nerve conduction velocities.[4]

Management

The first step is obviously removal from further exposure. In case of acute overexposure, clinical management will be as for any 'solvent' overexposure. For chronic sensiorimotor neuropathy, besides continued exclusion from further exposure, additional supportive measures as for peripheral neuropathy will be required.

Halogenated alkanes

Another particularly important group of alkanes used in industry is the halogenated alkanes. These are alkanes in which one or more of the hydrogen atoms have been substituted by halogens, usually chlorine, bromine or fluorine. These compounds generally share toxic effects including depression of the central nervous system and toxic effects on the liver and kidney.

The hepatotoxicity may be demonstrated by increased levels of enzymes of injury, e.g. alanine aminotransferase (ALT), serum glutamic-pyruvic transaminase (SGPT), and aspartate aminotransferase (AST), or serum glutamic-oxaloacetic transaminase (SGOT), in the serum. This is discussed in greater detail below under CARBON TETRACHLORIDE (p. 228). The halogenated alkanes may be ranked in the following order of decreasing hepatotoxicity:

- tetrachloroethane
- carbon tetrachloride
- 1,1,2-trichloroethane
- chloroform
- perchloroethylene
- trichloroethylene
- methylene dichloride
- 1,1,1-trichloroethane

Only some of the better known of these are described here. Methylene chloride (dichloromethane) is also mentioned as it has an unusual further toxic action.

Hitherto, disturbances of renal function resulting from exposure to these chemicals were explored employing commonly used tests for renal disease. In recent years symptomless groups of workers exposed to these materials have been studied using a wide range of tests which give very early indication of alteration to renal structure/function (see Chapter 41). One such study is discussed under perchloroethylene (tetrachloroethylene). Most of these studies are cross-sectional and, as occurs in similar situations elsewhere in occupational toxicology, the significance of such abnormalities may be debatable. Do they indicate more than just a shift of physiological adaptation/response to the various xenobiotics? The longitatudinal (follow-up studies) which might help to elucidate those problems are, at present, few and far between.

Another, again epidemiological, approach has been to compare past exposure to hydrocarbons in groups of patients with glomerulonephritis and control groups.[5,6]

A study of past hydrocarbon exposure together with a thorough review of the literature[7] concluded that occupational exposure to hydrocarbons is likely to play a role in the pathogenesis of primary glomerulonephritis and, further, that the risk of developing glomerulonephritis is greatest in those subjects exposed to petroleum products. Harrington's study,[8] with negative findings, was criticized on the grounds that over 50% of the patients therein had those types of glomerulonephritis which are usually secondary to an underlying systemic disorder and so are less likely to be associated with hydrocarbon exposure.

Three further points are worthy of note. First, whilst the evidence for an association between primary glomerulonephritis and hydrocarbon exposure continues to strengthen, it must be remembered that primary glomerulonephropathy is a relatively rare condition and such studies do not relate the risk of such renal disease to the total population of persons exposed to hydrocarbons. That total population must be very large.

Second, is it possible to form a hypothesis relating these findings to those of the group of studies mentioned above wherein very early changes to the nephron are associated with hydrocarbon exposure? In this connection it has been suggested that constant low-grade tubular damage from chronic hydrocarbon exposure might, in susceptible individuals, release sequestered or altered tubular antigens which then provoke local autoimmunity.

Third, and of some importance to both general and occupational physicians, patients with glomerulonephritis who continue heavy hydrocarbon exposure appear to have an accelerated progression of renal failure.

METHYLENE CHLORIDE (DICHLOROMETHANE) (CH_2Cl_2)

[CAS no. 75-09-2]

Characteristics and use
Methylene chloride (dichloromethane) boils at 40°C and has a vapour pressure of 400 mmHg at room temperature 24°C. It is, therefore, very volatile and is used as a solvent and extracting agent where a high degree of volatility is desired. It has been a common ingredient of paint strippers. Unless stringent precautions are instituted, toxic concentrations will readily occur. If it is allowed to come in contact with a naked flame or hot metal, as in welding, phosgene may be produced.

Metabolism/biochemical effects
Methylene chloride is readily absorbed through the lungs and then oxidized to carbon monoxide (CO), producing up to 40% carboxyhaemoglobin (COHb), measured the morning after a 6-hour exposure to paint remover in an unventilated room. Furthermore, the half-life, in the body, of COHb resulting from methylene chloride exposure is about 13 hours, i.e. some two-and-a-half times longer than the half-life of COHb resulting

from CO inhalation (see Chapter 8). This has been explained by the slow release, and oxidation to COHb, of methylene chloride stored in the body fat. Thus, it is possible for raised levels of CO to persist long after the immediate narcotic symptoms have passed and, perhaps, to cumulate with successive daily exposures.

One area of potential concern has been the possibility of carcinogenicity of methylene chloride. This stems from a standard carcinogenicity bioassay carried out in the USA under the National Toxicology Program (NTP). In this study, no tumours were induced in rats but there was an increase in liver and lung tumours in mice. This raised the concern regarding the possibility of carcinogenicity in humans although available epidemiology did not show such a risk. Metabolic and toxicokinetic studies were able to show that there were two principal metabolic pathways for the elimination of methylene chloride and that the one favoured by mice was essentially a minor pathway for rats, hamsters and humans, hence the mouse-specific tumour response. Thus, although research work is still being carried out on methylene chloride, it is not generally regarded as presenting a cancer risk to humans.

Clinical manifestations
Prolonged skin contact with the liquid may produce chemical burns[9] The principal action is on the central nervous system as a narcotic causing headache, giddiness, irritability and numbness and tingling of the limbs. Higher concentrations may cause light-headedness, drowsiness, unconsciousness and, eventually but rarely, death. As noted earlier, it has a relatively low hepatotoxicity compared with other chlorinated hydrocarbons.

In a middle-aged man, who developed serious cerebral impairment after 3 years' exposure to concentrations estimated as somewhere between 500 and 1000 ppm, the accompanying dementia was attributed to the endogenous production of carbon monoxide.[10] Similarly, a 66-year-old man with no previous history of heart disease suffered three attacks of myocardial infarction within a period of less than a year, each of them following within a very few hours of working with methylene chloride for about 3 hours, in a basement workshop.[11] It is important to recognize, however, that used carefully under controlled conditions (atmospheric concentration less than 100 ppm) methylene chloride does not produce any evidence of long-term brain damage, detectable by careful psychological and neurophysiological testing (although there was an excess of self-reported neurological symptoms found in the exposed men).[12]

Management
Removal from further exposure and supportive measures are obvious immediate measures. It is important to be aware of the possibility of carbon monoxide poisoning, particularly in the middle aged where the heart or brain, which are vulnerable to anoxaemia because of atherosclerosis, can be at risk.

CARBON TETRACHLORIDE (CCl₄)

[CAS no. 56-23-5]

Characteristics and use

Carbon tetrachloride has the structural formula:

$$\begin{array}{c} Cl \\ | \\ Cl - C - Cl \\ | \\ Cl \end{array}$$

It is a colourless, volatile and non-flammable liquid with a sweet odour. The odour threshold is in the range 20–100 ppm. Thousands of tonnes of carbon tetrachloride are manufactured in the UK annually by the chlorination of short-chain hydrocarbons. It is, however, no longer used for dry-cleaning or as a fire extinguishant, having been replaced by other, less toxic, chlorinated alkanes and it is now used mostly in the production of some CFCs (chlorofluorocarbons), although even this use is likely to decline in the next few years. It is also used in the production of chlorinated rubber, as a solvent in the production of pharmaceuticals and pesticides and the production of anti-knock agents for petrol.

Metabolism/biochemical effects

Carbon tetrachloride, because it is a fat solvent, may be absorbed through the skin. In addition its relatively high vapour pressure (113 mmHg at 25°C) means that absorption by inhalation is a serious risk. It is stored in the adipose tissue, liver, bone marrow, brain and kidneys. It is slowly eliminated, over 50% being exhaled unchanged.[15] In a case of poisoning by ingestion, carbon tetrachloride was detected unchanged in the breath 3 weeks later.[16] The suggested metabolic pathway involves microsomal cleavage by the P450 system to Cl- and the trichloromethyl free radical, CCl₃, followed by oxidation to the unstable intermediate CCl3COH. That breaks into hydrogen chloride (HCl) and carbonyl chloride, COCl₂ (which is found also during the metabolism of chloroform). Carbonyl chloride, whilst being the major source of the ultimate product, carbon dioxide (CO₂), is not believed to be the intermediate which binds onto lipid and protein.[15]

The mechanisms of liver damage have been clearly summarized by Finkel[16] (see also Chapter 41). The two principal histopathological changes, fatty degeneration and necrosis, may be related to lipid peroxidation and to the formation of free radicals as described above. Lipid accumulation is related to injury of the endoplasmic reticulum and disruption of the transport of lipid out of the liver cells by impairment of the coupling of triglycerides to the lipoprotein carrier. Cellular necrosis may be related to release of lysosomal enzymes mediated by the free radical CCl₃.

Cells which do not actively metabolize carbon tetrachloride appear to be relatively resistant to its effects whereas stimulation of endoreticular activity and enzyme induction enhance its effects. Thus the increased vulnerability of alcoholics to the hepatotoxicity of carbon tetrachloride (and to other hepatotoxic chlorinated aliphatic hydrocarbons) might be associated with enzyme induction by ethanol leading to overload of free radicals, beyond the capacity of normal cellular antioxidants.

Carbon tetrachloride is a nephrotoxin causing widespread damage and death of proximal tubular cells. Like other nephrotoxins, high concentrations may also cause intense vasoconstriction, leading to ischaemic damage which is randomly distributed and may affect any part of the nephron (Fig. 11.4). The glomeruli remain unaffected although glomerular filtration may be severly reduced.

Liver cancer has been reported in workers exposed to carbon tetrachloride[17] but then only where cirrhosis was already present. Based on these findings, the International Agency for Research on Cancer (IARC) classified carbon tetrachloride as a Group 2B carcinogen in 1992, 'the agent is possibly carcinogenic to humans'[18] (see Chapter 39). Generally, carbon tetrachloride has not been demonstrated to be mutagenic; thus any carcinogenicity is probably based on a nongenotoxic mechanism and only in compromised or damaged tissue.

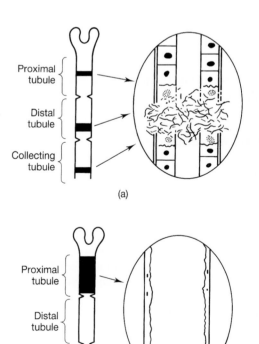

Figure 11.4 (a) Ischaemic lesion of tubular necrosis. (b) Nephrotoxic lesion of tubular necrosis. Adapted from Ref. 151.

Clinical manifestations

Quantitative analysis of expired air or blood for carbon tetrachloride (on occasion for up to 2 weeks after the incident, see above) will establish unequivocally that exposure has occurred and provide strong evidence in diagnosis. Nausea and vomiting have been reported in workers exposed to concentrations about 45–97 ppm and albuminuria at about 170 ppm. These disappeared when concentrations were brought down to around 10 ppm. Constriction of the visual colour fields, toxic amblyopia and optic atrophy have been reported. Exposure to higher concentrations of carbon tetrachloride will lead to narcosis and sometimes coma. There has been an isolated report of Parkinsonism in a chemist following exposure for 3 months due to a leaking faulty evaporator.[19]

Acute toxic hepatitis can ensue within a few days of overexposure and, although milder cases may run an anicteric course, jaundice and an enlarged tender liver can develop with increase of serum bilirubin and raised transaminase levels. The course of the disease varies, generally lasting a few weeks, although in more severe cases acute necrosis may ensue. The increased vulnerability of alcoholics possibly results, as observed above, from induction of the metabolizing enzymes on the endoplasmic reticulum.

Renal damage may occur in the absence of toxic hepatitis. The clinical picture follows the usual phases of oliguria, diuresis and postdiuresis. Oliguria may at first be unrecognized (particularly if attention is directed toward concurrent liver damage). The development of azotaemia or hyperkalaemia might call for dialysis to be considered. The start of recovery is accompanied by the onset of diuresis which should be managed in the usual way with attention to urinary loss of sodium and potassium. The post-diuretic phase develops imperceptibly with subsequent gradual improvement in renal function over several months.

Management

The management of acute toxic hepatitis and of threatened, or actual, renal failure will be along the usual lines. However, because of the free radical action of the toxic metabolite CCl_3, anti-oxidant therapy might be considered. It can be directed at several points.[20]

1 Removing/inhibiting the source of excessive free radicals.
2 Mopping up the primary metabolites of oxygen.
3 Intercepting the free radical attack by a mixture of preventive and chain-breaking anti-oxidants.
4 Repleting key cellular ingredients, e.g. adenosine triphosphate (ATP), S-adenosylmethionine (SAM), glutathione (GSH).
5 Damage limitation by removing toxic metabolites (e.g. by exchange transfusion) and/or providing agents to inhibit secondary effectors of cellular injury.

CHLOROFORM (TRICHLOROMETHANE) (CHCl$_3$)

[CAS no. 67-66-3]

Characteristics and uses

Chloroform (trichloromethane) has the structural formula:

It is a colourless, volatile liquid having a characteristically sweet smell with an odour threshold around 200 ppm. It is manufactured on a substantial scale in the UK, much going into the production of chlorodifluoromethane. It is also used in laboratory work and as an industrial solvent, for example in the production of laminated windscreens. It is no longer used as an anaesthetic and nowadays probably no more than 2000 UK workers are regularly exposed to chloroform. However, laboratory use will no doubt continue but here exposure is intermittent and highly variable.

Metabolism/biochemical effects

Chloroform is readily absorbed through the lungs, skin or from ingestion and is believed to be transformed, first, by oxidation to trichloromethanol and then to the trichloromethyl free radical (CCl_3, see CARBON TETRACHLORIDE (p. 228)) and possibly via carbonyl chloride (phosgene) and a chlorinated compound of formaldehyde before hydrolysis to carbon dioxide.

Clinical manifestations

Liquid chloroform is highly irritating to the eyes and skin, although the vapour is less so. It is of low-to-moderate acute toxicity in animals via the oral, dermal, or inhalation route. Delayed deaths from hepatotoxic effects have been reported following anaesthesia. Anaesthetic concentrations, however, were in the range of 10 000–20 000 ppm. In occupational situations chloroform at concentrations of about 21–77 ppm has led to a variety of minor symptoms such as headache, tiredness, depression and digestive disturbances.

An increased incidence of hepatomegaly has been reported at concentrations of 205 ppm. and greater,[21] whilst toxic jaundice is associated with exposure to concentrations of more than 400 ppm.[22] Toxic effects on the liver are generally seen only after heavy exposure and may be accompanied by centrizonal necrosis and fatty degeneration (see Carbon tetrachloride)

By a mechanism which is not clearly understood and hence often called 'sensitization of the myocardium' sudden death from heart failure can occasionally occur at high exposures. This has also been reported for trichloroethylene and other halogenated solvents,[23] and has happened in anaesthetic use and with 'sniffers' who may expose themselves to concentrations of several thousand parts per million, albeit for short periods. As it has followed the administration of catecholamines, the administration of drugs of this category in cases of chloroform intoxication is contraindicated.

Although a number of animal studies have indicated that chloroform can induce some liver and kidney tumours, the results of most tests for genotoxicity have been negative so it is likely that if chloroform is carcinogenic, it is probably related to a non-genotoxic mechanism and follows general liver damage. There is no human evidence either to refute or support these suspicions.

Management

Management of acute poisoning would be along the lines indicated under CARBON TETRACHLORIDE, remembering the warning above regarding catecholamines.

1,2-DICHLOROETHANE (ETHYLENE DICHLORIDE) ($ClCH_2CH_2Cl$)

[CAS no. 107-06-2]

Characteristics and use

1,2-Dichloroethane has the following structural formula:

$$H-\underset{\underset{H}{|}}{\overset{\overset{Cl}{|}}{C}}-\underset{\underset{H}{|}}{\overset{\overset{Cl}{|}}{C}}-H$$

and is also called ethylene dichloride or, sometimes in industry, simply ethylene chloride. (Its isomer, 1,1-dichloroethane is sometimes referred to as ethylidene dichloride or simply ethylidene chloride).

It is a colourless volatile oily liquid (the vapour pressure at 29°C is 100 mmHg) with a chloroform-like odour and sweet taste. In the USA 80% of the 1,2-dichloroethane produced is used as a starting material for vinyl chloride and other structurally related chlorinated chemicals, as a constituent of anti-knock compounds, as a grain and seed fumigant and as a commonly used solvent. Because most 1,2-dichloroethane is used in enclosed systems, poisoning is uncommon, occurring mostly from leaks.

Metabolism/biochemical effects

Inhalation of the vapour is generally the main route of exposure in industry although skin absorption from the liquid is also possible.

Studies of its metabolism show progressive oxidation:

$ClCH_2\text{-}CH_2Cl \rightarrow ClCH_2\text{-}CH_2OH \rightarrow ClCH_2\text{-}COOH$
1,2-dichloro-   2-chloro-   monochloro-
ethane   ethanol   acetic acid

Animal studies show that up to 40% is exhaled unchanged, up to 15% is exhaled as carbon dioxide. As much as 50% may be recovered from the urine as 1,2-dichloroethane or quite probably its metabolites. There are few case reports of human poisoning and these confirm, albeit indirectly, that it is metabolized. In an early study Bryzhin[24] analysed the remainder of liquid drunk by some deceased subjects as well as the chemicals found in the internal organs. The liquid contained ethylene chloride but the internal organs contained 'an organic chloride – ethylene chloride was not found'. In another report[25] the amount of ethylene dichloride in exhaled breath samples of workers was highest just after exposure and then decreased, whilst milk samples taken from exposed working and nursing mothers showed that the concentrations of ethylene dichloride in milk increased after leaving work, reached a maximum after 1 hour and then diminished. This suggests rapid elimination, either by excretion or metabolism.

Post-mortem and other reports of victims of poisoning indicate renal and hepatic effects, similar to those seen from exposure to a number of other chlorinated alkanes. In the kidney, there is tubular degeneration with casts in the lumen of the nephron, and in the liver, necrosis and fatty degeneration are reported.

Animal studies indicate that the occurrence of hepatic and renal effects is both dose and species related. Dogs were unaffected by exposure to 800 ppm, even after 8 months. Higher doses resulted in fatty degeneration of the liver and renal tubular degeneration.[26] Monkeys, on the other hand, showed marked degeneration and vacuolation of liver cells and moderate degeneration of the epithelium of the renal tubules after eight 7-hour exposures at 400 ppm, whereas 148 exposures for 7 hours at 200 ppm produced no histopathological changes.[27]

Clinical manifestations

1,2-Dichloroethane is irritant to the respiratory tract and to the conjunctivae, although earlier reports that it might cause corneal opacities appear to have been discounted.[28] It is absorbed through the respiratory tract and through the skin. Eye splashes cause pain and irritation. Short-term exposures to high concentrations of the vapour will produce eye, nose and throat irritation. Prolonged skin contact may cause roughening, cracking and chapping, leading to dermatitis. Nausea and vomiting are frequently mentioned in case reports, although whether this is a central effect or an effect on the lining of the upper part of the gastrointestinal tract is not clear.

Exposure by any route can lead to increasing dose-related depression of the central nervous system with headaches, weakness, drunkenness, incoordination, drowsiness, coma and ultimately death. Evidence of renal and hepatic damage (renal tubular necrosis and acute toxic hepatitis), similar to those seen from exposure to a number of other chlorinated alkanes, appears from clinical reports of poisonings.

In a rat study, both sexes showed an increase in hepatomas. Based on this information, and the data which showed that 1,2-dichloroethane is mutagenic in a number of test systems, the IARC gave it the classification of Group 2B, 'The agent is possibly carcinogenic to humans'[17,18] (see Chapter 39). There are no human carcinogenicity data on which to confirm or refute these findings on animals.

Management
No case reports have been found indicating the success of any measures other than those mentioned under carbon tetrachloride.

1,1,1-TRICHLOROETHANE (METHYL CHLOROFORM) (CH_3CCl_3)

[CAS no. 71-55-6]

Characteristics and uses
1,1,1-Trichloroethane (methyl chloroform) is commonly

marketed, in the UK, as Genklene and has the following structural formula:
It is a colourless volatile liquid with a heavy chloroform-like sweetish smell and an odour threshold around 100 ppm. It is non-flammable but decomposes on heating beyond 360°C to hydrochloric acid and phosgene. In the UK about 35 000 workers in the engineering and electronics industry are regularly exposed to it during degreasing and cleaning. A further 20 000 workers in furniture and upholstery industries are also estimated to be exposed. It is also used as a solvent and thinner for adhesives, paints, varnishes, inks and as a propellant for aerosol cans.

Metabolism/biochemical effects
It is readily absorbed by inhalation but is poorly absorbed through the skin. Clearance from the body is slow, most of the compound being eliminated unchanged through the lungs (see Fig. 11.5). Only a small fraction is metabolized. Two metabolites which have been identified in the urine, 2,2,2-trichloroethanol and trichloroacetic acid, have been suggested for use in occupational medicine for the biological monitoring of exposed workers (see Chapter 2).

1,1,1-Trichloroethane has been extensively tested for mutagenicity and the force of evidence suggests that it

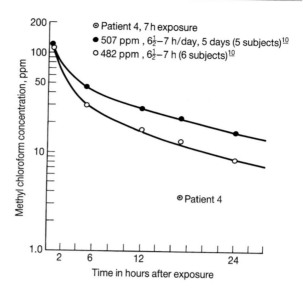

Figure 11.5 *Excretion of 1,1,1-trichloroethane is slow and exponential. Adapted from Ref. 30.*

does not have a mutagenic potential. It has been tested for carcinogenicity in mice and rats with no evidence of carcinogenicity.

Clinical manifestations
Quantitative analysis of expired air or blood for 1,1,1-trichloroethane will confirm uptake.

Acute inhalation at high concentrations has a depressant action on the central nervous system and may produce narcosis. Early effects are dizziness, lassitude and headaches but very high concentrations may produce loss of consciousness and death. Fatalities have occurred in confined spaces at concentrations estimated to be between 5000 and 50 000 ppm (the saturated vapour pressure at 25°C is 160 000 ppm) but accurate reconstruction of exposures in such circumstances is always difficult. The fact that the six cases of fatal poisoning due to 1,1,1-trichloroethane, reported to the Health and Safety Executive in the UK over a 5-year period, were all males of 20 years of age or younger has led to the suggestion that the possibility of deliberate sniffing should always be considered.[29]

Inhalation studies with human volunteers showed no central nervous system effects following 3-hour exposures to between 400 and 500 ppm although some eye irritation was noted. At 900–1000 ppm for 20 minutes there was some light-headedness. There is no evidence of the severe hepatic and renal effects which are associated with carbon tetrachloride, although in one worker rendered unconscious by over-exposure, urinary urobilinogen was increased on the 4th day and remained elevated for 4 days.[30] There was an increase in urobilinogen, after 7 days, in one experimental subject following 20 minutes of exposure to 900 ppm, but there was no note of how long this effect persisted.[31]

Management

The absence of reports of serious systemic effects, apart from narcosis after gross overexposure, indicates that treatment for hepatic or renal effects is extremely unlikely to be required, nevertheless it would be prudent, after an acute over exposure, to check hepatic and renal function.

1,2-DIBROMOETHANE (ETHYLENE DIBROMIDE) (CH₂BrCH₂Br)

[CAS no. 106-93-4]

Characteristics and uses

1,2-Dibromoethane, sometimes known as ethylene dibromide, has the following structural formula:

It is a colourless, dense liquid with a sweetish odour. With a boiling point of 130°C, its vapour pressure at 20°C is only 11 mmHg which fortunately reduces the chances of inhalation. It is used as a scavenger for lead in anti-knock agents in petrol, as a fumigant and as a constituent of some pesticides. It will readily penetrate protective clothing, including natural rubber and neoprene.

Metabolism/biochemical effects

It is converted to bromoacetic acid which is then excreted in the urine.

Clinical manifestations

Ethylene dibromide is a severe irritant and prolonged contact with the skin leads to redness, oedema and blistering. The vapour, too, is irritant, affecting both the upper respiratory tract and the lungs, causing pulmonary oedema. Although it is a central nervous system depressant, such systemic effects from inhalation are uncommon in industry. Toxic effects to the liver and kidneys have been reported from animal studies.

Ethylene dibromide is, structurally, somewhat similar to dibromochloropropane (DBCP):

CH₂Br-CH₂Br   CH₂Br-CHBr-CH₂Cl

Ethylene dibromide; EDB

Dibromochloropropane; DBCP

(1,2-Dibromoethane)

(1,2-Dibromo-3-chloropropane)

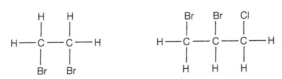

which is known to impair testicular function and to reduce fertility in male workers (see Chapter 40). Ethylene dibro-

mide also had been shown to be gametotoxic in rodents, probably in the premeiotic spermatogonial rather than postmeiotic stage.[32] Therefore, the reproductive history of 297 male employees engaged in ethylene dibromide manufacture in four plants in the US was studied.[33] For the four plants as a whole the standardized birth ratio (compared with the expected number derived from national fertility tables) was close to unity. The problems besetting this sort of investigation may be illustrated by the facts that in one of the plants the observed/expected births ratio was consistently and significantly low, although in that plant the average exposure level was below 5 ppm and the prevalence of vasectomy at that plant was the highest among the four and somewhat higher than that in that country as a whole. Caution has been advocated, however, before ethylene dibromide is accepted as completely harmless in this respect.[34]

It is mutagenic in a range of test systems and an animal carcinogen both in rats and mice but the reported studies, in humans, do not permit a clear evaluation. The available evidence is, however, sufficient for 1,2-dibromoethane to be labelled R45, 'may cause cancer', within the European Community.

ALKENES

Alkenes, sometimes referred to as olefins, comprise a group of open-chain hydrocarbons which contain a carbon–carbon double bond (C=C). The physical properties of alkene compounds are essentially the same as alkanes–insoluble in water, soluble in several organic solvents and weakly polar. Corresponding alkenes and alkanes have similar boiling points. The carbon–carbon double bond (C=C) is the functional group of the alkenes and it determines their chemical properties. The presence of the double bond means that alkenes are chemically reactive compounds. The simplest compound in the alkene group is ethylene (C₂H₄), followed by propylene (C₃H₆) and then the isomers of butene (1-butene, 2-butene and isobutylene).

The most commonly encountered are the chlorocompounds which include ethylene derivatives such as trichloroethylene, tetrachloroethylene and vinylidene chloride. Vinyl chloride is considered in Chapters 8 and 43.

Chloroalkenes

TRICHLOROETHYLENE (Cl₂C=CHCl)

[CAS no. 79-01-61]

Characteristics and uses

Trichloroethylene ('trike') has the following structural formula:

Trichloroethylene is a colourless liquid with a pleasant, sweet odour. Commercial grade material contains approximately 1% stabilizers such as epoxides (e.g. epichlorohydrin), amines or esters. Its main use is as a metal degreasant. Other uses include textile treatment, dry-cleaning industry, the production of inks, coating and adhesives, polyvinyl chloride production and fire retardants. It is also used as a rubber solvent. Large numbers of workers may be exposed to trichloroethylene – an estimated 10 000 degreasing units are currently considered to exist in the UK (Fig. 11.6). Its use as a general anaesthetic was abandoned because of the availability of better anaesthetic agents and because of the possibility of the generation of dichloroacetylene by reaction of the trichloroethylene with soda lime in carbon dioxide absorbers in closed circuit anaesthetic apparatus.

Metabolism/biochemical effects

The principal route of absorption in industry is through inhalation of vapour although it must be remembered that trichloroethylene liquid is also readily absorbed both through the skin and from the gastrointestinal tract. Following absorption a large proportion is exhaled unchanged. The absorbed trichloroethylene is oxidized in the liver to chloral hydrate which is then either reduced to trichloroethanol or oxidized to trichloroacetic acid. The trichloroethanol is either oxidized to trichloroacetic acid or excreted as the glucuronide after conjugation with glucuronic acid:

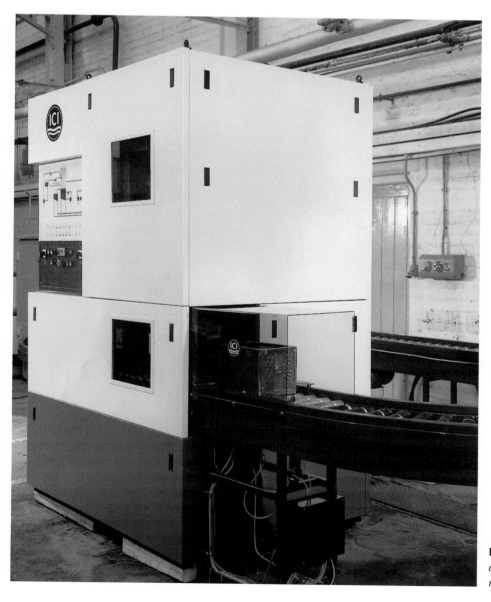

Figure 11.6 *Modern, totally enclosed degreasing equipment. Courtesy of ICI.*

$$CCl_2 = CHCl \rightarrow CCl_3CHO.H_2O \rightarrow CCl_3CH_2OH \rightarrow + GluAc \rightarrow Glucuronide$$

Trichloroethylene   Chloral hydrate   Trichloroethanol

$$CCl_3COOH$$
Trichloroacetic acid

(GlucAc = Glucuronic acid)

In occupational medicine the urinary concentrations of the conjugated trichloroethanol and trichloroacetic acid in samples collected towards the end of the working week provide a useful method of biological monitoring for estimating trichloroethylene absorption (see Chapter 2).

Clinical manifestations

High concentrations of vapour cause eye irritation (200 ppm) and nasal irritation (1000 ppm). The liquid is slightly irritating to the skin and splashes to the eyes may cause reversible damage to the corneal epithelium. Short-term exposure to vapour at concentrations of 300 ppm and above causes dizziness, fatigue, headache, nausea, visual disturbance, mental confusion, loss of co-ordination and narcosis. Coma and death may occur in extreme cases and several fatalities have been reported amongst workers exposed to high concentrations.

The sudden deaths of four men had some features in common: they had all been fairly heavily exposed whilst working on degreasing tanks; the levels of trichloroethylene had been sufficiently high to cause symptoms of the central nervous system disturbance; all had continued at work despite repeated complaints of drowsiness, dizziness, nausea and vomiting. Three had died suddenly within hours of leaving work (the fourth was a night watchman who did degreasing and was found dead in the morning); post-mortem examinations did not show macroscopic evidence of coronary heart disease or any other apparent cause of death. It was suggested that the cause of death was ventricular fibrillation.[35] The accounts of sudden death, which are very uncommon and seem to follow high exposures, are generally attributed to catecholamines causing ventricular arrhythmias. The effect can occur with other chlorinated aliphatics.[36] There is animal experimental evidence to support this view and one particular study has demonstrated that the induction of trichloroethylene-induced arrhythmias, in this case specifically premature ventricular contractions, can be potentiated by caffeine.[37]

In most instances and even after heavy exposure the symptoms clear within a few hours of removal from exposure (as was the experience when trichloroethylene was used as a general anaesthetic). Residual headache and psychological symptoms, such as fatigue or loss of memory, have occasionally been reported.[38–40] In a patient recovering from overexposure to the warm vapours from a degreasing machine, nerve conduction velocity in the ulnar nerve was slowed, returning to normal in about 9 weeks, whereas conduction velocity of the facial nerve took about 18 months to recover.[41]

The evidence for hepatotoxicity and nephrotoxicity is not strong.[16]

Trichloroethylene has been evaluated in recent years by the IARC (see Chapter 39). It came to the conclusion that trichloroethylene *is probably carcinogenic to humans* (Group 2A).[42] This evaluation was based on a number of epidemiological studies which had demonstrated an elevated risk for cancer of the liver and biliary tract and non-Hogkins lymphoma. These observations were supported by animal carcinogenicity data in rats and mice and, although a rodent-specific mechanism involving peroxisome proliferation has been postulated for liver tumours induced in mice, it cannot hold for tumours induced at other sites.

Consumption of alcohol after working with trichloroethylene may lead to transient reddening of the face and neck, know as 'degreaser's flush'. This condition is sometimes more severe than a simple blushing as it may be accompanied by a sensation of fullness in the chest and difficulty in breathing. It passes off after a few hours but will recur the next time alcohol (even one half pint of beer) is consumed. Although the clinical features may resemble the flushing and breathlessness associated with carcinoid syndrome (which can also be induced by alcohol), the symptoms invariably remit within 5–7 days once exposure to trichloroethylene has stopped. The mechanism of this striking phenomenon, which occurs in only a small minority of exposed workers, is little understood. Suggestions concerning some interference with the aldehyde dehydrogenase pathways leave much unexplained.

Management

Whilst treatment for hepatotoxicity or renal complications following trichloroethylene exposure is extremely rarely needed, it would be prudent to consider checking hepatic and renal function after overexposure.

TETRACHLOROETHYLENE (PERCHLOROETHYLENE) ($Cl_2C{=}CCl_2$)

[CAS no. 127-18-4]

Characteristics and uses

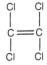

Commonly known as perchloroethylene or 'perk', tetra-chloroethylene ($Cl_2C=CCl_2$) is a colourless liquid with a pleasant, ethereal odour and a boiling point of 121.2 °C. The commercial product contains small quantities of stabilizers, such as epoxides, amines or esters which may be associated with some adverse effects.

Tetrachloroethylene is used predominantly in the dry-cleaning industry. It is also used as a chemical interme-diate in the production of fluorocarbons and hexachloroethane, in the textile industry, as a metal degreasant, and in the production of adhesives, cleaning agents and thinners. In 1987 an estimated 15 000 work-ers were reported to be exposed to tetrachloroethylene in the UK, mainly in dry-cleaning premises.

Metabolic/biochemical effects

Although tetrachloroethylene may be absorbed through the skin, that is only to a limited extent.[43] The main route of absorption is by inhalation. During an experimental exposure to 194 ppm for 3 hours, the concentration of tetrachloroethylene in blood was reaching a plateau by the end of the 3 hours. After exposure it disappeared from the blood in about 30 minutes.[44] More useful to the clinician is its persistence in expired air – for 2 weeks in one subject (Fig. 11.7), estimated to have been exposed to about 275 ppm for 3 hours and then to around 1400 ppm for 30 minutes before he was discovered unconscious. His urinary bilinogen and total serum bilirubin increased on the 9th post-exposure day and remained so for only a few days.[45]

Its toxicological properties are similar to those of trichloroethylene.[16] The metabolism of tetrachloroethyl-ene has been extensively studied in experimental systems and in humans with the result that a number of urinary metabolites have been identified.[46] There are two princi-pal metabolic pathways, one involving cytochrome P450 and the other glutathione s-transferase.

Clinical manifestations

Tetrachloroethylene liquid is a skin irritant and the vapour, at concentrations of 100 ppm and above, causes eye irritation.

The principal effect of tetrachloroethylene is its depressant action on the central nervous system. Minimal central nervous system effects have been reported with exposure as low as 100 ppm. Cases of fatal central nervous system and respiratory depression have resulted from the use of sleeping bags which had not been thoroughly cleared of the solvent before use.

The hepatotoxicity of tetrachloroethylene is ranked below that of carbon tetrachloride and chloroform but greater than that of 1,1,1-trichloroethane. Serum AST (SGOT) and ALT (SGPT) reach their peak values about 3 days after exposure (although with workers under well controlled conditions these enzyme levels are not gener-ally raised). Raised urinary urobilinogen may be found in asymptomatic persons for up to 10 days after expo-sure.

A promising development in the medical surveillance of exposed workers is the use of isoenzyme separation of serum γ-glutamyltransferase (γGT)[47] (Fig. 11.8). In a comparison of workers and control subjects (matched for: evidence of current liver disease, low alcohol intake, no drugs affecting enzyme activity, and other possible confounding factors) the total γGT was higher in the exposed group, this mean increase being mainly due to increase in the isoenzyme γGT2. Furthermore, the isoen-zyme γGT4, which is considered to reflect hepatobiliary impairment (Fig. 11.8), appeared only in exposed work-ers when the total γGT activity was about 17 U/litre.[48]

A study of nephropathies in 50 drycleaners, exposed to low levels of perchloroethylene (median 15 ppm) dis-closed early diffuse structural and functional changes along the length of the nephron including the

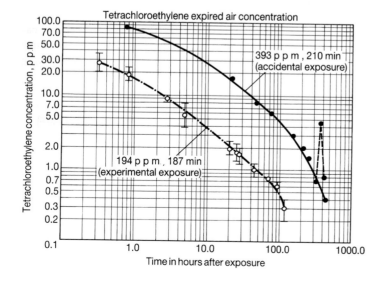

Figure 11.7 *Tetrachloroethylene expired air concentra-tions, following vapour exposure. Note that time scale is logarithmic. Adapted from Ref. 45.*

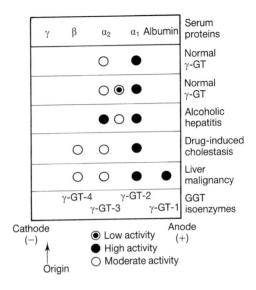

Anode (+)

◉ Low activity
● High activity
○ Moderate activity

Figure 11.8 *Separation of γGT isoenzymes in health and selected diseases. Adapted from Refs 47 and 48.*

glomerulus.[49] The latter changes, however, were attributed to loss of charge rather than size-selectivity of the glomerular barrier. The authors speculated on generalized membrane disturbance produced by the solvent itself or by reactive metabolites. The possibility of a very early widespread lesion (Fig. 11.4)) was not apparently considered.

Two further points require emphasis. First, there was a lack of association between renal damage/dysfunction and the intensity or duration of exposure. Second, the significance of the subtle changes which were found need more consideration. As the authors concluded: 'The significance of such abnormalities cannot be easily assessed, since they could be accounted for by a shift of physiological adaption/response to various stimuli. Alternatively these subtle abnormalities may represent an early stage of clinically silent but potentially progressive renal disease'.

Acute renal failure is rarely observed in cases of overexposure.[16]

Long-term occupational exposure may result in symptoms such as headache, fatigue, nausea and lightheadedness, although there is no firm evidence of central nervous system effects resulting from chronic exposure.[50]

A number of studies have suggested that there is a positive association between exposure to tetrachloroethylene and the risks for oesophageal, and cervical cancer and non-Hodgkin's lymphoma. However, it should also be noted that information on smoking, alcohol consumption and socioeconomic status, all important confounders, was not adequately addressed in the studies. Based on these results, and other evidence the IARC concluded in 1995 that tetrachloroethylene is *probably carcinogenic to humans* (Group 2A).[51]

Management

Apart from removal from exposure and supportive measures, active treatment is rarely required. It would, nevertheless, be prudent to consider checking hepatic and renal function after overexposure.

VINYLIDENE CHLORIDE (1,1-DICHLOROETHYLENE) ($CH_2=CCl_2$)

[CAS no. 75-35-4]

Characteristics and uses

Vinylidene chloride, also known as 1,1-dichloroethylene (or 1,1-dichloroethene), is a colourless liquid with a sweet odour and is insoluble in water. Technical grade material contains small quantities of methyl ether of hydroquinone (MEHQ) stabilizer. It is used mainly with other vinyl monomers, particularly vinyl chloride, in the production of polymers. Vinylidene chloride polymers have a variety of applications including food packaging, extrusion resins, barrier coatings and reinforcement materials. Exposure occurs both in factories producing the monomer and in polymerization plants.

Metabolism/biochemical effects

The main route of absorption of vinylidene chloride is by inhalation. The extent of dermal absorption is uncertain. It can be absorbed from the gastrointestinal tract although, as pointed out at the start of this chapter, that would be most unlikely in industry. Some animal studies show 1,1-dichloroethylene to be more hepatotoxic than carbon tetrachloride and some other chloroethylenes such as vinyl chloride and trichloroethylene. Whereas the latter group primarily involves the mixed function oxidase system on the smooth endoplasmic reticulum, 1,1-dichloroethylene preferentially affects the mitochondria, although it is not clear why it does. It is metabolized, presumably on the smooth endoplasmic reticulum, via epoxide to acid chloride. Why these acid chlorides then apparently move to cause mitochondrial damage and do not damage the endoplasmic reticulum, where they are formed, is not at present explained.[52,53,54]

In view of the above it is interesting that there are no clinical reports of acute poisoning by 1,1-dichloroethylene. An epidemiological mortality study of 138 vinylidene chloride workers, who were not concomitantly exposed to vinyl chloride, showed no increase of deaths from malignant disease. (One who had died from cirrhosis was stated to have a history of heavy drinking.) Comparison of some liver function studies on 23 workers with matched control subjects revealed that three of the exposed had increased values (one had increased SGOT, but normal SGPT and γGT, the other two had increased alkaline phosphatase values).[55]

Clinical effects

Concentrations of vapour at about 25 ppm cause upper respiratory tract irritation and the liquid is irritating to the skin and eyes (although these irritant effects may be in part due to the presence of the MEHQ stabilizer). Short-term exposure to high concentrations of vinylidene chloride (4000 ppm has been quoted) produces depression of the central nervous system in humans, with symptoms of inebriation leading to unconsciousness. Complete recovery generally follows cessation of exposure.

As noted above, although there is some experimental evidence to suggest that it may cause hepatic effects and possibly renal damage, clinical evidence to support this is sparse. The long-term effects of vinylidene chloride in humans are largely undetermined.

With regard to its potential to cause cancer, inadequate data currently prevent any conclusions being drawn. Furthermore, workers in polymerization plants are often concurrently exposed to vinyl chloride. The reproductive effects of vinylidene chloride in humans similarly remain undetermined.

Management

Generally, all that is required in case of poisoning is removal from further exposure and, if necessary, supportive measures. After exposure it would be prudent to check hepatic and renal function. More severe effects might require treatment as recommended under CARBON TETRACHLORIDE (p. 228).

DIENES

Dienes contain two carbon–carbon double bonds. both of which are chemically reactive. The chemical properties of such compounds depend on the relative positions of the double bonds and on the length of the carbon chain. Rubber is a naturally occurring diene and is a polymer of isoprene (CH_2=C(CH_3)-CH=CH_2 namely 2-methyl-1,3-butadiene with a structural formula:

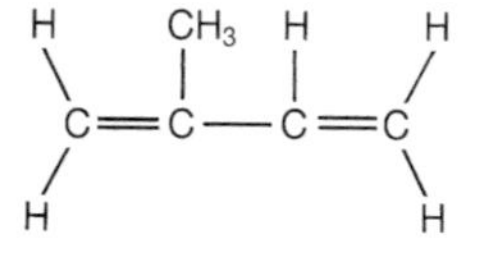

Synthetic rubbers mostly resemble natural rubber in having a series of double bonds in their polymer chain. Butadiene, therefore, usually comprises one of the monomers used in their manufacture, e.g. styrene butadiene rubber and is the only diene of much consequence encountered in occupational medicine.

1,3-BUTADIENE (CH$_2$=CH-CH=CH$_2$)

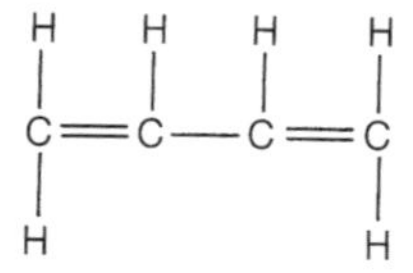

[CAS no. 106-99-0]

Characteristics and uses

1,3-Butadiene is a colourless gas with a slightly aromatic odour which is easily liquefied (boiling point −4.4°C). Exposure occurs in butadiene manufacture and in styrene butadiene rubber production plants, in some areas of rubber manufacturing plants and it is widely used in the manufacture of synthetic rubber for tyres. It is also used as a plastics copolymer with styrene and acrylonitrile (e.g. ABS plastics). These latter situations will, however, always involve mixed exposures (making the determination of toxicity difficult). In 1983, in Western Europe, 1.5 million tonnes of 1,3-butadiene were produced and, in the USA, in 1983 it was ranked 36th among all chemicals produced. In 1984 it was estimated that 65 000 workers in the USA were exposed to 1,3-butadiene.

The principal route of exposure in humans is probably by inhalation.

Metabolism/biochemical effects

The metabolism of 1,3-butadiene differs in different species, which makes interpretation of animal data rather difficult. Whereas mice achieve higher blood concentrations of reactive metabolites than do rats, blood levels of toxic metabolites in monkeys are lower than in rodents.[56] Dahl and his colleagues suggest possible pathways for metabolism (Fig. 11.9). In small mammals (after exposure to a wide range of concentrations) the route of elimination of 1,3-butadiene metabolites was largely via the urine, whilst for monkeys (after exposure to 10 ppm) elimination was mostly by carbon dioxide exhalation. Because the initial metabolism of 1,3-butadiene by either route probably involves the formation of a mutagenic epoxide, the toxicological importance of this difference in routes of metabolism is not clear. Another interesting observation has been the demonstration of butadiene metabolite adducts with globin. Such adducts may, in the future, serve occupational physicians as dosimeters of exposure.[57]

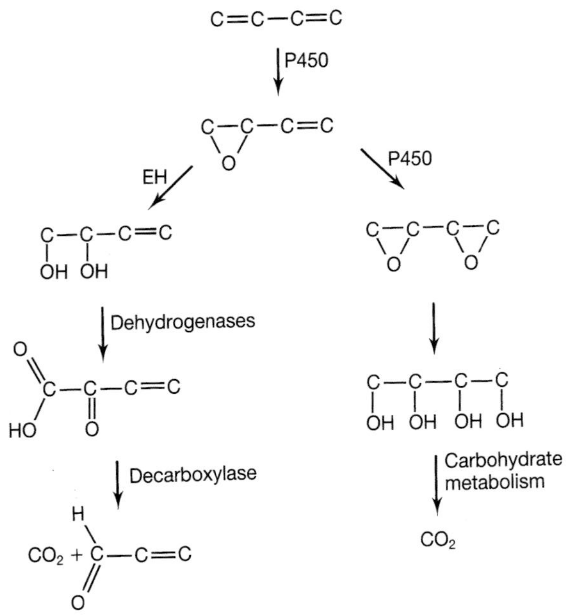

Figure 11.9 *Some possible pathways for metabolism of 1,3-butadiene to carbon dioxide. Adapted from Ref. 56.*

Clinical manifestations

Acute exposure to high concentrations of gas can cause irritation of the respiratory tract and anaesthetic effects. Humans have tolerated concentrations up to 8000 ppm for up to 8 hours with no ill-effects other than slight irritation of the eyes, nose and throat.[58] These irritant properties may be attributable to the presence of impurities or stabilizers in the chemical tested. Inhalation of excessive levels of the gas, as from accidental large spills or leaks, might result in respiratory paralysis and death.[59]

In a National Toxicology Program (NTP) carcinogenicity study,[60] long-term exposure to 1,3-butadiene (625 or 1250 ppm) resulted in an increased incidence of several different tumour types in mice – malignant lymphomas, alveolar/bronchiolar carcinomas and adenomas, granulosa-cell tumours of the ovary and haemangiosarcoma of the heart. This latter tumour is extremely rare. An earlier carcinogenicity study in rats used up to 8000 ppm 1,3-butadiene over 2 years and provided no clear evidence of its carcinogenicity in that species.[61] The IARC concluded nevertheless, that there is *sufficient evidence for its carcinogenicity in animals* and has recently concluded that 1,3-butadiene is *probably carcinogenic to humans*.[18] In the USA the NIOSH estimated that there could be 597 excess cancers per 10 000 workers having 45 years of exposure to 2 ppm, based upon the use of a linear-risk model.

However, the alleged carcinogenic properties of 1,3-butadiene came under critical scrutiny in an editorial in *Science*.[62] By contrast with these NIOSH extrapolations, a cohort of 2582 butadiene monomer workers has been followed from first employment, in 1943–1945, through to the end of 1985. Their SMR from all causes was 84 and from cancer was 80.[63] The explanation for this wide discrepancy might lie (as noted earlier) in the differences in metabolic rates between different species.

- After exposure to 10 ppm, blood levels of the metabolite, butadiene epoxide, were 590-fold greater in mice than in monkeys.
- Mice differ from rats, monkeys and humans in a propensity to oxidize the monoepoxide to a diepoxide, which has been shown to participate in the formation of DNA-DNA and DNA-protein cross-links in the mouse. In particular, the mouse strain used (B6C3F1) is postulated to possess an endogenous retrovirus, not present in the NIH Swiss strain which does not share these results with 1,3-butadiene, the reactive mono- and diepoxides interacting, it is suggested, with molecules involved in virus expression.[64]
- *In vitro* studies with liver and lung microsomes have shown that metabolism of the butadiene monoepoxide in humans also proceeds to the non-DNA-reactive product.

The critical scrutiny in the *Science* editorial noted above, was challenged,[65,66] although it is probably fair to state that the challenge is based less on new evidence regarding humans than on a reiteration of the claims regarding the validity of extrapolating animal results to humans, together with the subsequent cautionary action by the United States Occupational Health and Safety Administration which appears to be based on the results of those animal experiments. This latter proposal is to reduce the occupational exposure standard from 1000 ppm to 2 ppm In spite of these uncertainties and different extrapolations and modelling, there seems to be reasonably consistent scientific opinion that 1,3-butadiene should be regarded as a human carcinogen and, rather like benzene, capable of causing an increase in lymphatic and haemopoietic cancers. Because 1,3-butadiene, like benzene, is ubiquitous in the environment (from engine exhaust emissions) as well as in some working environments, both stringent occupational and environmental air quality standards have been set in many countries.[67] The UK air quality standard is 1ppm ($2.25\mu/m^3$) as a running annual mean.[67]

Fetotoxic effects have been reported in animal studies, with delayed fetal development occurring in rats exposed to 200 ppm 1,3-butadiene during days 6–15 of pregnancy. However, there appears to be no evidence of teratogenicity. The fetotoxic effects which have been observed in animal studies suggest that exposure to 1,3-butadiene may present a specific risk to pregnant women.

Management

Persons who have been exposed to very high concentrations must obviously be removed immediately and may require emergency supportive therapy.

Although dermatitis from skin exposure is reported in the literature, it seems possible that a chemical with a boiling point of $-4.4°C$ might well cause frostbite on the affected areas.

ALKYNES

Alkynes have the general formula C_nH_{2n-2}. They are characterized by a carbon–carbon triplebond ($C \equiv C$) which determines the chemical properties of the family. The simplest member of the alkyne family is ethyne (acetylene). The next homologue is propyne, and then 1-butyne and 2-butyne. All of these alkynes are gases at room temperature; the higher homologues are liquids. Acetylene itself has a low toxicity with a simple asphyxiant action.

Chloroalkynes

DICHLOROACETYLENE (CCl≡CCl)

[CAS no. 7572-29-4]

Characteristics and uses

Dichloroacetylene is a volatile liquid with the chemical formula $ClC \equiv CCl$. It is not produced commercially and has no industrial uses. It is of interest as a thermal degradation product, for example, when trichloroethylene was passed through carbon dioxide absorbing canisters during closed circuit anaesthesia. It has been detected in environmental life support systems, e.g. in the US space programme and in the atmosphere of a nuclear submarine. It may also be formed when trichloroethylene is used to remove wax coatings from floors.

Metabolism/biochemical effects

Dichloroacetylene is absorbed through the lungs. It affects the sensory trigeminal nucleus, causing chromatolysis, disintegration of Nissl bodies and cell shrinkage. Other acute effects reported include fatty degeneration of the liver and tubular necrosis in the kidney, occurring after repeated short-term exposure. The reported respiratory effects were possibly due to phosgene.

Clinical manifestations

After a period of 1–3 days, extreme nausea and vomiting may develop and has been reported after prolonged exposure to only 0.5–1 ppm of dichloroacetylene.[68] That may be followed by violent headache, pain in the jaw and by paresis and neuralgia in cranial and cervical nerves which may persist for several days up to several years. A curious feature is the development of facial and oral herpes. Oedema of the brain has been reported in fatal cases.

Animal studies provide limited evidence for the carcinogenicity of dichloroacetylene.

Management

No specific treatment is known for the effects of dichloroacetylene.

ALCOHOLS

Alcohols are chemicals with the general formula R-OH. The functional group is the hydroxyl (OH) which determines their chemical properties. The R-group in the general formula represents different alkyl groups attached to the hydroxyl group. Thus, when R is the methyl group (CH_3), the alcohol is methanol (CH_3OH).

Alcohols are classified as primary, secondary or tertiary according to the number of carbons attached to the

Table 11.3 *Examples of members of the alcohol family*

Name	Formula	Physical form at room temperature
Methanol	CH_3OH	Liquid
Ethanol	CH_3CH_2OH	Liquid
n-Propanol	$CH_3CH_2CH_2OH$	Liquid
Isopropanol	$CH_3CHOHCH_3$	Liquid
n-Butanol	$CH_3(CH_2)_3OH$	Liquid
iso-Butanol	$(CH_3)_2CHCH_2OH$	Liquid
sec-Butanol	$CH_3CH_2CHOHCH_3$	Liquid
tert-Butanol	$(CH_3)_3COH$	Solid/Liquid (mp = 25 °C)
n-Hexanol	$CH_3(CH_2)_5OH$	Liquid
n-Lauryl alcohol	$CH_3(CH_2)_{11}OH$	Solid/Liquid (mp = 24 °C)
Ethylene glycol	$HOCH_2CH_2OH$	Liquid
Glycerin	$HOCH_2CHOHCH_2OH$	Solid/Liquid (mp = 18 °C)

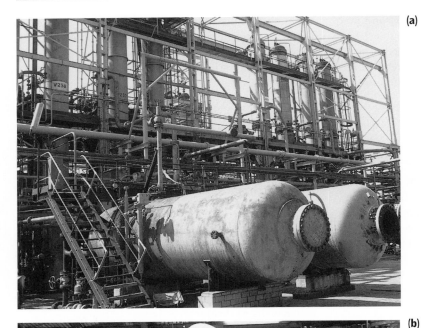

(a)

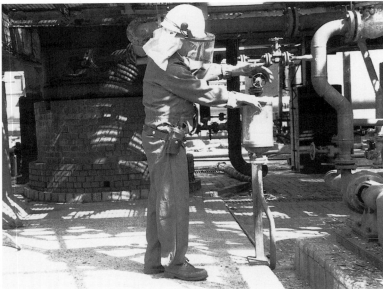

(b)

Figure 11.10 *(a) Industrial alcohol plant at refinery showing reactors (vertical columns) and settling/separating vessels (horizontal). (Photograph courtesy of Shell UK Limited.) (b) Industrial alcohol plant at refinery showing protected operator taking sample using bottle in sample cabinet. Photograph courtesy of Shell UK Limited.*

carbon bearing the hydroxyl group, e.g. *n*-butanol and *iso*-butanol are primary alcohols; *sec*-butanol is a secondary alcohol; *tert*-butanol is a tertiary alcohol (Fig. 11.10).

Table 11.3 lists some of the common alcohols.

METHANOL (CH₃OH)

[CAS no. 67-56-1]

Characteristics and uses

Methanol is the simplest alcohol and has the following structural formula:

$$H - \overset{\displaystyle H}{\underset{\displaystyle H}{\overset{|}{\underset{|}{C}}}} - OH$$

It is a clear, colourless, volatile and flammable liquid with a mild odour at a threshold of around 8–10 ppm, which is well below its current occupational exposure limit in the UK. Most methanol production is based on the synthesis from mixtures of hydrogen, carbon monoxide and carbon dioxide gases in the presence of metallic catalysts. Much of its toxicology is known from its *ingestion* (in place of ethanol), whether accidental, deliberate or misguided.

Methanol is now a common ingredient of antifreeze solutions. It is also widely used as an industrial intermediate, as a solvent and also as a fuel. Much is used to produce formaldehyde, acetic acid and a range of methyl esters. In industry most uptake will be from *inhalation* although the liquid is well absorbed following ingestion or skin contact.

Metabolism/biochemical effects

Although non-occupational methanol poisoning is well described, occupational poisoning is still reported, either by the inadvertent consumption, at work, of methanol in place of industrial methylated spirits, which is about 95% ethanol and 5% methanol,[69] or by percutaneous absorption in a hot climate.[70]

The metabolism of methanol is slow compared with ethanol. It is successively oxidized to formaldehyde and then to formic acid and carbon dioxide:

$$CH_3OH \rightarrow HCOH$$
Methanol   Formaldehyde
$$\downarrow$$
$$CO_2 \leftarrow HCOOH$$
Carbon dioxide   Formic acid

Formaldehyde, although forming part of this pathway, is not detected in body fluids or tissues in animal experiments, although formates are found. This metabolic process can, of course, lead to metabolic acidosis.

The dynamics of this process have received some attention in recent years. In primates, including humans, the rate of formate metabolism to carbon dioxide proceeds at only about half the rate as in the rat, explaining why formate accumulates in methanol poisoned monkeys (and humans) but not rats. Furthermore, the rate of elimination of formate is markedly reduced in folate-deficient monkeys and it is postulated that a folate-dependent pathway is a major route for formate metabolism.[71] For this reason, folinic acid has been successfully used in the treatment of experimental methanol poisoning in monkeys and its use advocated in human cases[72,73] (see below). Because of the slow metabolism repeated exposures will have cumulative effects.

Clinical manifestations

Liquid methanol can cause defatting of the skin and dermatitis. Uptake through the skin can be sufficient to cause optic neuritis (see below) and metabolic acidosis. In humans, eye irritation has occurred at 950–1100 ppm over 25 minutes and headaches with exposure to 800–1000 ppm over 4 hours. Acute poisoning by inhalation can occur but is rare, although a fatality has occurred at exposure to 4000–13 000 ppm.[74]

The exposure levels which cause systemic poisoning have been poorly characterized. Repeated exposure for 200–375 ppm[75] has been related to reports of headaches in duplicating machine workers whilst levels of 760–7600 ppm over 10 years have led to reduced visual acuity in another group of workers.[76]

Clinical knowledge of the more serious effects is mainly derived from patients poisoned by *ingestion* and may be divided into three stages:

1 narcotic stage, similar to ethanol;
2 a latent period of up to 24 hours;
3 development of more serious central nervous system symptoms, visual disturbances, concomitant with onset of metabolic acidosis.

In the first stage the patient is confused and ataxic and there is often epigastric pain and vomiting. After several hours, together with the appearance of metabolic acidosis, the serious visual complications may start. They include blurred vision, flashing lights and perhaps a grey mist sensation. This may be accompanied by pain or tenderness of the eyes and photophobia. On examination hyperaemia of the disc with blurred margins is seen.

Computerized tomography has shown symmetrical areas of low attenuation in the putamen.[77] This might be related to the development of a Parkinson-like syndrome which sometimes appears after successful treatment of methanol poisoning.[78]

Formate, one of the metabolites, has been suggested as responsible for the retinal changes which comprise optic disc oedema with a normal vascular bed and intracellular oedema with intra-axonal swelling. The vulnerability of the retina, which has a high oxygen consumption, is attributed to the impairment of retinal cytochrome oxidase activity by formate.[79]

Management

Treatment should be instituted without delay and its aims are:

1 correction of metabolic acidosis;
2 inhibition of methanol oxidation;
3 removal, if necessary, of circulating methanol and its metabolites.

Because substantial amounts of bicarbonate may be necessary to correct the metabolic acidosis, careful attention should be given to the possibility of hypernatraemia and hypervolaemia.

Ethanol, by competitive inhibition of alcohol dehydrogenase, inhibits methanol oxidation if administered early on in poisoning. On the other hand, if most of the methanol has already been metabolized (methanol blood level well below 50 mg/100 ml) the administration of further alcohol might exacerbate the acidosis. A loading dose of about 50 g orally is followed by intravenous infusion at about 10–12 g ethanol/h. Slightly higher rates may be required if ethanol removal is being increased, for example, by preexisting enzyme induction (history of alcohol or drug abuse) or by concurrent haemodialysis (see below). The aim is to achieve an ethanol blood concentration of about 1 g/litre. 4-Methylpyrazole, which inhibits alcohol dehydrogenase activity, has been used successfully in the treatment of methanol poisoning in monkeys and it is possible that it may eventually be used in the treatment of severe methanol poisoning in man.[80]

Severe poisoning, for example, blood methanol greater than 500 mg/litre; severe metabolic acidosis; developing visual or fundiscopic abnormalities would be indications to consider haemodialysis. The electroretinogram (ERG), it has recently been suggested, might have to be used as an early non-invasive diagnostic test with which to assess the degree of retinal toxicity.[81]

Intravenous folinic acid (30 mg) has been recommended as a protection against ocular toxicity by accelerating formate metabolism (see above), although there has been no formal controlled trial.

Propanol

There are two isomers of propanol (propyl alcohol): *n*-propanol and 2-propanol. *n*-Propanol has toxic properties similar to ethyl alcohol and will not be discussed further.

2-PROPANOL (ISOPROPYL ALCOHOL) (CH₃CHOHCH₃)

[CAS no. 67-63-0]

Characteristics and uses
2-Propanol (isopropyl alcohol) is a highly flammable liquid with an odour, said to resemble that of a mixture of acetone and ethanol. The odour threshold is variously given as between 3 and 50 ppm.

It is widely used as a solvent in industry, for household and personal products and as a process solvent for many natural products, including foodstuffs. It is used in polymers, varnishes, paints and inks as well as a cleaning and drying agent for metal and glass components.

Metabolism/biochemical effects
It is very rapidly absorbed following inhalation or ingestion and either excreted unchanged or metabolized to acetone.[82]

Clinical manifestations
No case of industrial poisoning has been reported. Some reports, however, in the 1950s and 1960s raised the question of its possible carcinogenicity to the nasal sinuses, mostly in manufacturing plants. It was subsequently shown that the causative agent was most likely to be the alkyl sulphates, produced during the strong acid process and not 2-propanol itself[83] (see below).

Butanols

The butanols are an example of the existence of more than one industrially important isomer of a chemical substance. They all have some toxicological similarities

(although none severe) because of their general structure but there are also some differences. There are four isomers; 1-butanol, 2-butanol, *tert*-butanol and *iso*-butanol and all have the empiral formula C₄H₁₀O. Their individual structural formulae are:

- 1-Butanol (*n*-butyl alcohol) CH₃-CH₂-CH₂-CH₂-OH
- 2-Butanol (*sec*-butyl alcohol) CH₃-CH₂-CH(OH)-CH₃
- *tert*-Butanol (2-methylpropan-2-ol)

$$CH_3 - \underset{\underset{CH_3}{|}}{\overset{\overset{CH_3}{|}}{C}} - OH$$

- *iso*-Butanol (2-methylpropan-1-ol)

$$CH_3 - \underset{\underset{H}{|}}{\overset{\overset{CH_3}{|}}{C}} - CH_2OH$$

All are synthesized from petrochemicals and used widely as solvents and intermediates in chemical and allied industries.

1-BUTANOL (*n*-BUTYL ALCOHOL)

[CAS no. 71-36-3]

Characteristics and uses
1-Butanol is manufactured by the petrochemical industry and is a flammable colourless liquid having a slightly rancid/sweet odour. It also occurs naturally in some alcoholic beverages, as a product of carbohydrate fermentation. It is widely used as an organic solvent for waxes, natural resins, paints and lacquers and in silk screen printing. It is also used as a flavouring agent in butter cream, rum and whisky; and in cosmetics.

Metabolism/biochemical effects
It is readily absorbed by lungs, skin and gastrointestinal tract and metabolized by alcohol dehydrogenase to the corresponding acid via the aldehyde (hence the intoxicant effects) and to carbon dioxide.

Clinical manifestations
Because of its low volatility, the practical hazards associated with its production and use are low. It may cause headache, drowsiness, alcoholic intoxication and narcosis. A slightly reduced erythrocyte count has been reported (but not explained). The effect may be analogous to that seen with ethanol.[84]

Management
As for ethyl alcohol intoxication.

2-BUTANOL (*SEC*-BUTYL ALCOHOL)

[CAS no. 78-92-2]

Characteristics and uses

2-Butanol is a flammable, colourless liquid with a sweet-ish odour. It occurs naturally in food at low levels. In industry it is used as a solvent and chemical intermediate as well as in hydraulic brake fluids and as an industrial cleaning compound.

Metabolism/biochemical effects

It is metabolized in a similar way to 1-butanol. Animal studies indicate that at high concentrations it is more narcotic and lethal than *n*-butyl alcohol.

Clinical manifestations

2-Butanol is irritating to the eyes but not the skin. The main harmful effect is likely to be alcoholic intoxication. No other adverse systemic effects have been reported.

Management

As before, no specific measures exist.

TERT-BUTANOL (2-METHYLPROPAN-2-OL)

[CAS no. 75-65-0]

Characteristics and uses

tert-Butanol is a colourless liquid or white crystalline solid (melting point 25°C) with a camphor-like smell. Again, it is used as an industrial solvent, as a dehydrating agent and in the manufacture of perfumes.

Metabolism/biochemical effects

Unlike its isomers, which are rapidly metabolized by alcohol dehydrogenase, *tert*-butanol is metabolized more slowly, probably involving direct conjugation of the hydroxyl (OH) group with glucuronic acid followed by oxidation of one or more of the alkyl (CH$_3$) substituents.

Clinical manifestations

No industrial ill-effects have been reported other than mild irritation of the skin.[85]

Management

As before, no specific treatment is indicated.

ISO-BUTANOL (2-METHYLPROPAN-1-OL)

[CAS no. 78-83-1]

Characteristics and uses

iso-Butanol is a flammable, colourless liquid with a sweet odour (similar to amyl alcohol). Like other butanols, it occurs in trace amounts in alcoholic beverages as a fermentation product of carbohydrates. It is synthesized in the petrochemical industry and is used as an organic solvent, a plasticizer, an intermediate, in the production of perfumes and as a flavouring agent.

Metabolism/biochemical effects

It is well absorbed by all exposure routes and metabolized by alcohol dehydrogenase to *iso*-butyric acid via the aldehyde.

Clinical manifestations

The liquid is a mild skin irritant. Vapour concentrations above 100 ppm will cause eye irritation and blurred vision together with nausea, vomiting and headache. Industrial poisoning has not been reported.

Management

No specific treatment is called for.

DIOLS

Diols are dihydroxy alcohols which contain two OH groups on adjacent carbon atoms. They are commonly known as glycols.

1,2-PROPYLENE GLYCOL (PROPANE-1,2-DIOL) (CH$_3$CHOHCH$_3$OH)

[CAS no. 57-55-6]

Characteristics and uses

Propylene glycol (propane-1,2-diol) is a clear, colourless, slightly viscous liquid with a very slight odour and a bitter sweet taste. It has a wide range of uses; in antifreeze mixtures, in heat exchange and hydraulic fluids (due to its stability), as a solvent in the plastics and chemical industry, and in pharmaceutical formulations (because of its low toxicity). It is also used as a plasticizer for resins, as a humectant in textiles and tobacco and sometimes in smoke generation in discotheques and the theatre. Although many people are exposed to the liquid because the vapour pressure at 20°C is only 0.08 mmHg, workplace exposures are not normally likely to be other than very low.

Metabolism/biochemical effects

Propylene glycol can be absorbed from the respiratory tract (when vaporized or in aerosol form), the gastrointestinal tract and through the skin. Metabolism by oxidation to lactic acid and pyruvic acid (normal constituents of carbohydrate metabolism) is fairly rapid and unchanged propylene glycol is excreted by the kidneys.

Clinical manifestations

Propylene glycol is not particularly toxic in animal investigations. The very low vapour pressure makes inhalation unlikely and in industry it has no toxicological importance.[86] Clinical experience suggests that a small proportion of individuals may develop skin sensitization.[87] Based on industrial experience, there is no evidence of respiratory sensitization. Its use in theatrical fogging machines has the potential for high exposures to both vapour and aerosol, albeit for short periods, but has not led to any reports of ill-effects, to date.

CARBONYL COMPOUNDS

Several families of chemicals are collectively referred to as carbonyl compounds. These are compounds which contain the bivalent carbonyl (C=O) group and as a result possess characteristic chemical properties. Examples of carbonyl compound families include aldehydes, ketones, carboxylic acids, esters, acid anhydrides and amides.

ALDEHYDES

Aldehydes have the following general formula (where one of the available valencies, of the carbonyl group, is occupied by a hydrogen atom):

$$R—C{=}O$$
$$|$$
$$H$$

Aldehydes are polar compounds, generally liquids, which are soluble in most organic solvents. The lower aldehydes are also soluble in water.

FORMALDEHYDE (CH$_2$O)

[CAS no. 50-00-0]

Characteristics and uses
Formaldehyde is the simplest carbonyl compound and, unlike most other aldehydes, is a gas. It has the structural formula:

$$H—C{=}O$$
$$|$$
$$H$$

The gas is colourless with a pungent odour which is detectable at low concentrations (odour threshold of about 0.8 ppm). Formaldehyde is generally available as a 37% aqueous solution, formalin, commercial grades of which might contain up to about 10% of methyl alcohol, or in solid form as paraformaldehyde (CH$_2$O)$_n$, or trioxane, (CH$_2$O)$_3$.

Its major use is in the production of resins such as urea–formaldehyde, phenolic (bakelite), melamine and polyacetyl resins. These resins are widely used in the wood industry for the production of particle-board and plywood, furniture manufacture and paper finishing. They are also used in insulation materials, textile finishing, moulded plastic products and foundry moulds. Formaldehyde is also used as a preservative in foodstuffs, cosmetics, detergents and embalming fluid and as a sterilant in several medical applications.

Metabolism/biochemical effects
Systemic toxic effects are not described, probably because it is so irritant, producing a severe burning sensation of the upper respiratory tract with coughing, conjunctivitis and lacrimation, thus preventing exposure to much more than 5 ppm. The metabolism of formaldehyde has been extensively studied in experimental animals and to a lesser amount in humans. Formaldehyde is an essential metabolic intermediate in all cells and is produced endogenously. There is some evidence that, as well as being absorbed by inhalation, it can also penetrate skin. This may account for the allergic contact dermatitis reported. Following absorption, formaldehyde can be oxidized to formate and carbon dioxide, or can be incorporated into biological macromolecules via tetrahydrofolate-dependent one-carbon biosynthesis pathway (see Fig. 11.11).

Clinical manifestations
The strong irritant action of formaldehyde, particularly on the upper respiratory tract, has been noted above. Lower concentrations allow it to penetrate deeper into the respiratory tract and it has been described as a cause of occupational asthma, although that seems to be quite rare.[88]

There has been a continuing debate over whether or not formaldehyde is able to cause cancer in exposed workers. Experimental studies in the mid 1980s demonstrated that rats inhaling 14.3 ppm formaldehyde for up to 2 years developed squamous-cell carcinomas of the nasal cavities. This was confirmed in other studies at similar levels. There have been a wide range of epidemiological studies looking at cancer in a range of formaldehyde-exposed workers. Most recently, the **IARC** evaluated in 1995 all the available studies and concluded that there is a causal relationship between exposure to formaldehyde and nasopharyngeal cancer although the strength of evidence is weak.[89]

However, the epidemiological studies do no more than suggest a causal role between occupational exposure to formaldehyde and squamous-cell carcinoma of the nasal cavities and paranasal sinuses. The overall evaluation of Group 2A (*probably carcinogenic to humans*) was based on an individual evaluation of *limited evidence in humans* for the carcinogenicity of formaldehyde and *sufficient evidence in experimental animals for the carcinogenicity* of formaldehyde. Other bodies have classified formaldehyde in other ways based on the same evidence. In the USA it has been classified as a suspected human carcinogen by the ACGIH[90] and in the European Union a Category 3 carcinogen requiring the label *R40 Risk of irreversible effects.*

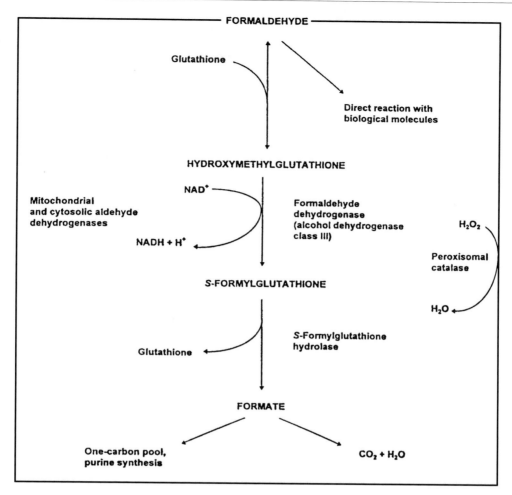

Figure 11.11 *Metabolism and fate of formaldehyde. Adapted from Ref. 89.*

ACETALDEHYDE (CH₃CHO)

[CAS NO. 75-07-0]

Characteristics and uses

Acetaldehyde has the structural formula

$$CH_3 - \overset{\displaystyle H}{\underset{}{C}} = O$$

and is a colourless liquid with a pungent, suffocating odour. Its main use is as a chemical intermediate mostly in the production of acetic acid but also in the production of vinyl acetate and acetic esters. Other minor applications include its use as a food additive and as an alcohol denaturant. Occupational exposure to acetaldehyde occurs mainly in the industrial organic chemical industry. Acetaldehyde may also occur as a decomposition product of some polymers. The trimer, paraldehyde, may still be used in some places for the treatment of status epilepticus.

Metabolism/biochemical effects

Acetaldehyde can be absorbed by inhalation or through the skin. Its metabolism to carbon dioxide and water is well recognized.

Clinical manifestations

It is an irritant to the eyes, skin and to the upper respiratory tract if inhaled. Industrial poisoning is not described.

In animal carcinogenicity studies inhalation of acetaldehyde vapour induced carcinomas of the nasal mucosa in rats and laryngeal carcinomas in hamsters. Genotoxic activity has been demonstrated in several *in vitro* assays using bacterial and mammalian cells, and in some *in vivo* experiments. With regard to its carcinogenic potential in humans, there is at present insufficient formal data to make any reliable evaluation.

The IARC currently classify acetaldehyde as a Group 2B carcinogen, that is *sufficient evidence* for carcinogenicity in animals but *inadequate evidence* for carcinogenicity in humans.[91]

Management
Treatment would be for its irritant effects on the portal of entry although it must be said that acetaldehyde is not commonly regarded as a poison in industry.

GLUTARALDEHYDE (1,5-PENTANEDIAL) (CHO(CH₂)₃CHO)

[CAS no. 111-30-8]

Characteristics and uses
Glutaraldehyde (1,5-pentanedial) has two carbonyl groups and has the following structural formula:

It is a liquid with an acidic, extremely irritating odour which is perceptible at 0.04 ppm. Generally it is supplied as a 50% or 25% aqueous solution. Glutaraldehyde readily reacts with proteins and may polymerize unless kept at a cool temperature. Because of its antimicrobial properties it is widely used, for example in endoscopy units where it is used in a 2 buffered alkaline solution (pH 7.5–8.5) as a cold-sterilizing agent. It is also used as a biological fixative in laboratories, in tanning and chemical synthesis, and as an embalming fluid.

Metabolism/biochemical effects
Glutaraldehyde is rapidly absorbed through mucous membranes of the respiratory tract, and via the skin and eyes. Systemic effects from glutaraldehyde are not described in industry although it does have a narcotic action. It may irritate at the portal of entry, generally the skin or respiratory tract, and may cause sensitization there (see below).

Clinical manifestations
Skin contact with glutaraldehyde can result in irritation and repeated contact may lead to allergic dermatitis. During its use as a sterilizing agent glutaraldehyde is generally 'activated' by sodium bicarbonate or bisulphite, a process which exacerbates its irritant properties.

Although the vapour pressure over a 2% solution at 20°C is reported to be only 0.0012 mgHg, glutaraldehyde vaporizes sufficiently at room temperature to cause irritation of the respiratory tract and eyes. It has caused some concern as a cause of occupational asthma.[92] Asthma due to exposure to glutaraldehyde is a prescribed disease (see Chapter 4). In one survey, hospital staff, who were intermittently exposed to low levels of glutaraldehyde (the highest, in a ward with poor ventilation was only 0.13 mg/m³ compared with the Swedish 15-min occupational exposure limit of 0.8 mg/m), reported increased prevalence of airway symptoms such as nasal and throat irritation, skin disorders which included eczema and rash, and general symptoms such as headache and nausea.[93]

Recent years have seen an increasing number of reported cases of occupational asthma, particularly among health-care workers handling or exposed to glutaraldehyde-containing sterilizing solutions. A precise mechanism for such an effect has yet to be identified. Within the European Union, the classification criteria for substances causing occupational asthma has been widened in recent years and this has permitted glutaraldehyde to attract the risk phrase: R42 *May cause sensitization by inhalation.*

One report concerns a radiographer who developed occupational asthma and who responded, on challenge to the stirring of developer and fixer solutions, by an immediate fall-off in the FEV₁ (forced expiratory volume in one second), lasting 2–3 hours. Acetic acid, glutaraldehyde, formaldehyde and sulphur dioxide are released from the combined developer and fixer solutions. The patient was not, however, challenged by these constituents separately.[94]

The limited data currently available provide neither indication about its reproductive effects in humans nor its carcinogenic potential.

Management
This will be for the presenting conditions, occupational dermatitis or occupational asthma.

KETONES

The general formula of a ketone is:

Like aldehydes, ketones contain the carbonyl (C=O) group and therefore aldehydes and ketones have many similar chemical and toxicological properties. The simplest aliphatic ketone is acetone where R and R′ are methyl groups. The other ketones are named according to the groups (R and R′) attached to the carbon, e.g. methyl ethyl ketone has a methyl (CH₃) and an ethyl group (C₂H₅) attached (see Table 11.4).

METHYL n-BUTYL KETONE (2-HEXANONE, MnBK) (CH₃CO(CH₂)₃CH₃)

[CAS no. 591-78-6]

Characteristics and use
Methyl *n*-butyl ketone (2-hexanone, M*n*BK), like *n*-hexane, has been used as an industrial solvent and a varnish remover.

Table 11.4 *Some common members of the ketones family*

Name	Formula	Physical form (at room temperature)
Acetone	CH_3COCH_3	Liquid
Methyl ethyl ketone	$CH_3COCH_2CH_3$	Liquid
Methyl *iso*-butyl ketone	$(CH_3)_2CHCH_2COCH_3$	Liquid
Diethyl ketone	$CH_3CH_2COCH_2CH_3$	Liquid
3-Hexanone	$CH_3CH_2COCH_2CH_2CH_3$	Liquid
t-Butyl methyl ketone	$(CH_3)_3CCOCH_3$	Liquid
Cyclopentanone	$(CH_2)_4CO$	Liquid
Cyclohexanone	$(CH_2)_5CO$	Liquid
Methyl vinyl ketone	$CH_3COCH=CH_2$	Liquid
Mesityl oxide	$CH_3COCH=C(CH_3)_2$	Liquid
Acetylacetone	$CH_3COCH_2COCH_3$	Liquid

Metabolism/biochemical effects

It can be absorbed through the skin as well as by inhalation.

MnBK is an intermediate metabolite, possibly via 5-hydroxy-2-hexanone, in the conversion, *in vivo*, of *n*-hexane to the toxic metabolite 2,5-hexanedione[95] (see *n*-Hexane) and subsequently to CO_2:

n-Hexane

$CH_3(CH_2)_4CH_3$

MnBK

$CH_3CO(CH_2)_3CH_3$

2,5-Hexanedione

$CH_3CO(CH_2)_2COCH_3$

The biotransformation is increased by the simultaneous administration of phenobarbitone or the inhalation of methyl ethyl ketone, presumably by enzyme induction. In experimental animals, MnBK itself induces hepatic microsomal cytochrome P450 and may, therefore, enhance the toxicity of other chemicals (including chloroform and carbon tetrachloride). As these effects necessitated fairly high doses of MnBK their importance in human industrial exposure requires careful consideration.

Because it acts by their common metabolite (2,5-hexanedione), MnBK produces the same neurohistological changes as those produced by *n*-hexane.

Clinical manifestations

Peripheral neuropathic symptoms, typically of numbness and tingling, generally come on within 1 year of first exposure. In the more severe cases affected subjects are unable to work within a few weeks of the onset and, eventually, may be unable to walk. See *n*-Hexane. Following removal from further exposure recovery takes place, but, in the more severely affected, may not be complete. Thankfully, the more restricted use of MnBK and better adherence to control measures means that reports of such effects are quite rare.

Management

See *n*-Hexane.

METHYL *ISO*-BUTYL KETONE (M*i*BK) (($CH_3)_2$ CHCH$_2$COCH$_3$)

[CAS no. 108-10-1]

Characteristics and uses

Methyl *iso*-butyl ketone (M*i*BK) has the structure:

It is a colourless liquid with a sweet odour and a reported odour threshold of 0.4 ppm. It is produced commercially by acetone condensation followed by catalytic hydrogenation. M*i*BK is used in lacquers such as cellulose and polyurethane lacquers. It is also used as a solvent in paint and as an extraction solvent in pharmaceutical and other products.

Metabolism/biochemical effects

The metabolism of M*i*BK has been studied in animals and it would appear that the two principal metabolites are 4-hydroxy-4-methyl-2-pentanone and 4-methyl-2-pentanol. The importance of this biochemical route of metabolism is that it is different from that of the straightchain ketone considered above. It does not necessarily suggest a method of monitoring exposure or confirming a case of suspected poisoning, because when volunteers were exposed for 2 hours to 200 ppm, the concentrations in urine of those two metabolites were below the level of detection, 5 nmol/litre.[96]

The molecular structure of M*i*BK and its metabolites precludes the metabolic production of γ-diketone, such as 2,5-hexanedione, the neurotoxic agent which is formed from both *n*-hexane and methyl *n*-butyl ketone (see *n*-Hexane).

Clinical manifestations

Short-term exposures to levels up to 100 ppm causes irritation of the eyes and throat and up to 200 ppm leads to headache, nausea and vertigo. Workers repeatedly exposed to around 500 ppm for up to 30 minutes a day and around 80 ppm for the rest of the day exhibit a range of symptoms, including weakness, loss of appetite, headache, eye irritation, nausea and vomiting, and sore throats.[97]

Because its metabolic pathway is different from that of methyl *n*-butyl ketone, methyl isobutyl ketone is frequently regarded as a less (or non-)toxic substitute for the former. There is, however, one report of a demyelinating sensorimotor distal polyneuropathy starting 1 week after its use for a few hours in spray painting, using a mixture of toluene and several aliphatic hydrocarbons. Sural nerve biopsy showed a spongiform myelin sheath giving rise to axonal compression and no neurofilament accumulations[98] (i.e. different from *n*-hexane and M*n*BK neuropathy which appears to be primarily axonal with paranodal neurofilament accumulations and secondary thinning and retraction of the myelin sheath). Attempts to reproduce this in a number of animal models have not been successful.[99]

Whilst the contention that M*i*BK is neurotoxic must remain unproven, there is, nevertheless, experimental evidence that M*i*BK induces certain hepatic microsomal P450 enzymes (which *n*-hexane itself does not) thereby accelerating the oxidation of *n*-hexane to its more toxic metabolites.

METHYL ETHYL KETONE (MEK) (CH₃COCH₂CH₃)

[CAS no. 78-93-3]

$$CH_3 - \overset{\displaystyle \underset{\|}{C}}{\underset{O}{}} - CH_2 - CH_3$$

Characteristics and uses

Methyl ethyl ketone (MEK) is a volatile, water-soluble, colourless liquid with an acetone-like smell. It is highly flammable and has a wide range of industrial applications as a solvent. It is used in vegetable-oil extraction and separation in the petrochemical industry. Other applications involve production of antioxidants, flavours and perfumes. The major solvent uses include vinyl coatings, nitrocellulose coatings, adhesives and acrylic coatings.

Metabolism/biochemical effects

MEK is rapidly absorbed through the skin, respiratory tract and gastrointestinal tract. It is well distributed in body tissues and studies in exposed workers suggest that it is metabolized to, and partly excreted as, 3-hydroxy-2-butanone and 2,3-butanediol. Part is said to be metabolized to methanol which accounts, perhaps, for occasional reports of optic nerve injury such as to an aircraft fitter who developed retrobulbar neuritis after less than 2 hours of using MEK. Methanol and formaldehyde were detected in the urine. His ocular condition resolved after some 6 days.[100]

The previous ingestion of ethanol seems to interfere with the metabolism of 2,3-butanediol leading to increase in the serum levels and in the urinary excretion.

Clinical manifestations

Its irritant properties are similar to those of acetone but are more severe. Reports of toxic effects are uncommon. There are reports of peripheral neurotoxicity associated with exposure to methyl ethyl ketone. These refer mainly to an acceleration or a potentiation of the effects of *n*-hexane or of methyl *n*-butyl ketone from the induction, by MEK, of one or more of the P450 enzyme group. There is, however, an isolated report of MEK alone as a cause of polyneuropathy.[101]

Management

Normally, the only treatment required is for the narcotic effect and removal from further exposure is generally all that is needed. As explained above, a diagnosis of peripheral neuropathy due to exposure to MEK alone should only be entertained after most careful occupational investigation has been undertaken.

Comment

The effects of these ketones, and of *n*-hexane, whose catabolic pathway includes M*n*BK, on the peripheral nervous system merit some comment. Whilst *n*-hexane and M*n*BK are accepted as being able to cause peripheral neuropathy, the evidence for a similar action by MEK and by M*i*BK is very weak, if not altogether absent. The last two are not, however, without any reported effect in this regard. On present knowledge it seems that both MEK and M*i*BK may enhance the effects of n-hexane and M*n*BK by enzyme induction.

It behoves the physician, therefore, to enquire not simply into 'solvent' use by his patient or even whether the patient has been working with, or exposed to, *n*-hexane and/or M*i*BK, but also to enquire carefully whether or not there was exposure to MEK and/or M*i*BK as well. The physician should remember that solvents, when used in industry, are rarely single chemicals but, frequently, several are used together – and the possibilities exist that a neurotoxin may be used with an enzyme inducer which enhances its effects. That is, peripheral neuropathy occurs sooner and after less exposure than might otherwise have been expected (see also Chapter 42).

CARBOXYLIC ACIDS

The general formula for carboxylic acids is RCOOH. Aliphatic carboxylic acids contain the carboxyl group:

$$-\underset{\underset{O}{\|}}{C}-OH$$

This functional group contains a carbonyl group with a hydroxyl group attached to the carbon atom. The behaviour of chemicals in this family is determined by this functional grouping. Compounds with one carboxyl group are called monocarboxylic acids, dicarboxylic acids contain two carboxyl groups, and so on. The simplest member of this group is formic acid, but the most common compound is acetic acid (vinegar). Formic and acetic acids are soluble in water, forming weak acids as they dissociate to a small extent (about 1–2%). The lower molecular weight monocarboxylic acids are liquids with pungent odours, such as acetic acid. Butyric acid and higher acids are responsible for the smell of rancid butter resulting from the hydrolysis of some of their esters. Long-chain monocarboxylic acids are used in the manufacture of soaps and detergents.

TRICHLOROACETIC ACID (TCA) (CCl_3COOH)

[CAS no. 76-03-9]

Characteristics and uses
Trichloroacetic acid (TCA) forms colourless, deliquescent crystals with a sharp pungent odour. The structural formula is:

$$Cl-\underset{\underset{Cl}{|}}{\overset{\overset{Cl}{|}}{C}}-\underset{\underset{O}{\|}}{C}-OH$$

TCA and its sodium salt are used as a herbicide, marketed under names such as Amchem® grass killer, Konesta® and Varitox®. Medically it has been used as an astringent; and a cauterizing agent, and in dentistry to remove excess gingival tissue.

Metabolism/biochemical effects
TCA, and other chloroacetic acids, are highly reactive chemically. Because of its great irritancy, protective reflexes limit absorption, through the respiratory tract, to any but extremely low concentrations. TCA is formed in drinking water during chlorination and it has been estimated that a 60 kg person will have a daily intake of 0.25–6.67 g/kg from drinking water.[102]

Animal studies suggest that, with systemic poisoning, the liver and kidney are the target organs. It has been shown to cause hepatomegaly and hepatocarcinoma but preceded by peroxisome proliferation.[103,104]

Clinical manifestations
Precipitation of proteins at the site of application results in the destruction of the epidermis and dermis. A 20% solution on the skin provokes mild erythema and a burning sensation and a 35% solution causes necrosis. Workers in the tropics, spraying sodium trichloroacetate mists daily for 5.5 months outside for weed control, experienced cough, sore throats, chest pains and eye irritation.[105]

Functional derivatives of carboxylic acids

Esters, anhydrides and amides are chemical families known as functional derivatives of carboxylic acids. In these compounds the hydroxyl (OH) part of the carboxyl group has been replaced with another functional group: OR′ in esters; RCO_2 in acid anhydrides; and NH_2 in amides.

The presence of the carbonyl (C=O) group in these carboxylic acid derivatives makes them polar compounds. In the case of amides, the strong intermolecular bonding causes them to have fairly high boiling points.

ESTERS

An ester is a product of the reaction between a carboxylic acid and an alcohol. Ethyl acetate, for instance, is derived from the condensation of ethanol and acetic acid. They are neutral liquids with pleasant fruity smells.

METHYL METHACRYLATE ($CH_2C(CH_3)CO_2CH_3$)

[CAS no. 80-62-6]

$$CH_2=\underset{\underset{O}{\|}}{\overset{\overset{CH_3}{|}}{C}}-C-O-CH_3$$

Methyl methacrylate, $CH_2C(CH_3)CO_2CH_3$, is one of the monomers used in the manufacture (by polymerization) of acrylic resins; tough, weather resistant and translucent

(Perspex). The monomer, dissolved in an organic solvent such as styrene, may be used as an adhesive – forming a strong bond when the solvent evaporates. Because the polymers are not irritating to tissues they have been widely used in medicine and dentistry.

Metabolism/biochemical effects

With a boiling point of 100°C and a vapour pressure, at room temperature, of only 40 mmHg, methyl methacrylate is unlikely to enter the body unless it is used in an exothermic reaction which it frequently is. The monomer is a mild irritant to the skin and in large amounts the vapour is narcotic.

Clinical manifestations

There is clinical evidence that methyl methacrylate can act as an irritant, a skin sensitizer[106] and in addition dental technicians and others, handling the monomer with bare hands, may sometimes complain of numbness, paraesthesiae and coldness. Those complaints are more pronounced in the hand which has handled the monomer more (e.g. the right hand in right-handed persons) and are more common in persons with a longer history of exposure. Reduced sensory conduction velocities in the region of the affected areas have been described but these findings did not correlate with current dermatitis.[107,108]

There is an isolated, carefully presented account of generalized peripheral neuropathy occurring in a dental technician after working with methyl methacrylate monomer for nearly 40 years. The histological picture after sural nerve biopsy was described as being similar to that found in acrylamide poisoning.[109]

Methyl methacrylate has received the occasional report as a causative agent in occupational asthma,[110] although it is not generally accepted that it is a proven asthma-inducing substance.

A condition referred to as 'cement hepatitis', with raised liver enzymes and, less often, serum bilirubin, accompanied by anorexia, nausea and/or vomiting, is described in patients after hip and knee replacement, the rise in serum γ-glutamyl transpeptidase being related to the weight of cement inserted.[111,112] There is no record of this effect as a problem in occupational medicine.

Management

Management is of the presenting condition, occupational dermatitis or suspect occupational asthma.

AMIDES

Amides have the following general structural formula:

$$R - \underset{\underset{O}{\|}}{C} - NH_2$$

Examples of aliphatic amides include acrylamide and dimethylformamide.

ACRYLAMIDE ($CH_2=CHCONH_2$)

[CAS no. 79-06-1]

Characteristics and uses

$$CH_2 = CH - \underset{\underset{}{\overset{O}{\|}}}{C} - NH_2$$

Acrylamide is a white, crystalline solid with no odour. It is used mainly as an intermediate in the production of water-soluble polymers, such as polyacrylamide and copolymers, used in chemical processing, water treatment, mineral separations, surface coatings and adhesives. It is used also in the production of electrophoresis gels. Acrylamides are employed as flocculants in water and sewage treatment. Occupational exposure may occur during its manufacture, and in the polymer-production and surface-coatings industries.

Metabolism/biochemical effects

Poisoning results from acrylamide *monomer* and not from the *polymers*. The principal route of occupational exposure to acrylamide is by skin absorption. To a lesser extent absorption through the lungs may occur, following inhalation of acrylamide dust or vapour, or aerosols of acrylamide in solution, and this will contribute to the total body burden. Absorption from the gastrointestinal tract following ingestion is also possible.

Acrylamide is metabolized to the epoxide glycidamide. Both acrylamide and glycidamide are able to react directly with haemoglobin *in vivo*, but DNA adducts results only from the formation of glycidamide. It has been suggested that the toxic action leading to peripheral neuropathy is mediated via effects on the axons and myelin sheaths resulting in a 'dying back' neuropathy (see Chapter 42).

There is evidence for its carcinogenic activity in animals, inducing testicular tumours in male rats and several other tumour types in females. Genotoxicity tests which have been conducted using *in vitro* systems and whole animals indicate that acrylamide possesses mutagenic activity which may cause heritable genetic disorders. Although the available epidemiological evidence did not produce any evidence of a cancer risk, the small size of these studies coupled with the positive finding in experimental animals, its mutagenicity and its ability, together with that of its epoxide metabolite, to form DNA adducts and haemoglobin adducts led the IARC to conclude in 1994 that is is *probably carcinogenic to humans* (group 2A).[113]

Clinical manifestations

Short-term exposure results in irritation to the eyes, skin, nose and throat. Blistering of the skin, particularly the hands, may result from prolonged contact.

Acrylamide is readily absorbed through the skin and signs of toxicity may be delayed for days or weeks after exposure. Repeated exposure induces axonal neuropathy with numbness, paraesthesiae, muscle weakness and sometimes muscle atrophy. Central effects, such as ataxia, tremor and dysarthria, are consistent with mid-brain lesions. Recovery from these neurotoxic effects generally ensues after exposure has stopped but may take several months. In severe poisoning the neurological sequelae may be permanent. Drinking water contaminated with acrylamide has resulted in central nervous system effects such as drowsiness, disturbance of balance, confusion, memory loss and hallucination.

There is no information at present available regarding the carcinogenic potential of acrylamide in humans. However, on the basis of non-human data, noted above, the IARC have classified acrylamide as *possibly carcinogenic to humans*.[91] Similarly there are no human data which indicate any reproductive effects, although it should be noted that acrylamide has the potential to damage germ cells and can also cross the placenta from the pregnant mother to the fetus.

Management

This will be along usual lines for the neurological effects. There is no specific treatment.

DIMETHYLFORMAMIDE (DMF) (HCON(CH₃)₂)

[CAS no. 68-12-2]

Characteristics and uses

Dimethylformamide (DMF) is a colourless or slightly yellow liquid with a slight amine odour and is an excellent solvent, being miscible in water and several organic liquids (alcohols, ketones and both unsubstituted and halogenated hydrocarbons). It is used as a solvent for polymers and resins. In vinyl-based polymers it is used in the production of fibres, coatings, films, adhesives and inks. It is also widely used in the production of poly-acrylonitrile fibres and films and in polyurethane lacquers where it is used in synthetic leather manufacture. It is also used in leather tanneries and is commonly encountered in chemical laboratories.

Metabolism/biochemical effects

DMF is readily absorbed through the skin and by inhalation of the vapour. It may also be absorbed after oral ingestion.

It is successively demethylated, via monomethylfor-mamide, also called *N*-methylformamide (NMF) (a fact used in occupational medicine for the 'biological monitoring' of exposed workers) to formamide and then to carbon dioxide. In humans, NMF appears to be the main identifiable metabolite although the amount recovered from urine represents only 2–6% of the amount of DMF inhaled. It is rapidly eliminated, within about 24 hours of exposure.

Clinical manifestations

Skin contact results in mild irritation with drying and cracking of the skin. Eye irritation may be induced by vapours or splashes of liquid.

The symptoms of poisoning noted below may be related to the central nervous system, the gastrointestinal system and to 'degreasers' flush' (alcohol intolerance) described under TRICHLOROETHYLENE (p. 232).

The central nervous system symptoms are those of solvent intoxication and include dizziness, unsteadiness, lassitude, and headache.

The gastrointestinal symptoms result from liver damage which has been reported in several studies of exposed workers but because they are associated both with acute exposure to high concentrations and with long-term exposure, such manifestations, at the clinical level, are unusual amongst DMF workers. Symptoms include anorexia, nausea, dyspepsia, vomiting and upper abdominal pain. Clinical examination may reveal a large and tender liver, while laboratory tests may show increase of alkaline phosphatase and bilirubin together with an increase in the serum transaminases with the ratio of aspartate aminotransferase (AST) to alanine aminotransferase (ALT) as less than 1– the reverse of that generally found in alcohol poisoning. Liver biopsy specimens show hepatic cellular necrosis and steatosis as seen with some of the chlorinated aliphatic compounds.[114]

The potential carcinogenicity of DMF has received some attention in recent years following reports of a small number of cases of testicular germ-cell tumours (which has an incidence, in the USA, of about 5 in 100 000 white men aged from 20 to 64 years) among DMF-exposed workers.[115,116] Genotoxicity assays have not provided supportive evidence for the mutagenicity of DMF. The IARC concluded in 1989 on the basis of human data that DMF is *possibly carcinogenic in humans* and therefore should be classified as a Group 2B carcinogen.[117]

ETHERS

Ethers have the general formula R-O-R'. When R and R' are the same the compound is termed a simple ether and, when different, mixed ethers, The simplest ether is dimethyl ether CH₃OCH₃ the next is methyl ethyl ether CH₃OC₂H₅, and so on. The most commonly encountered member of this family is diethyl ether or simply ether.

BIS (CHLOROMETHYL) ETHER (BCME) (ClCH₂OCH₂Cl)

[CAS no. 542-88-1]

Characteristics and uses

Bis(chloromethyl) ether, BCME, is a chlorinated ether with the structural formula:

$$CH_2-Cl$$
$$|$$
$$O$$
$$|$$
$$CH_2-Cl$$

It is a colourless liquid, with a boiling point of 104°C and a vapour pressure, at 25°C, of 41 mmHg. It decomposes rapidly in water to hydrochloric acid and formaldehyde, although it is relatively stable in humid air. It is used in polymer production and in textile manufacture. It may be a contaminant (1–8%) of chloromethyl ether (CME).

Metabolism/biochemical effects

Evidence from animal studies indicate that BCME is highly irritant and corrosive to the skin, eyes and respiratory tract. Similarly, inhalation experiments have produced congestion, oedema and haemorrhages in the lungs.[118]

It is a biologically active alkylating agent.

Clinical manifestations

Acute effects are uncommon in industry. Following an accidental soaking in BCME in a chemical plant, a worker experienced irritation to the conjunctivae, turbidity of the cornea, and mild irritation to the facial skin. Over the subsequent hours, second- and third-degree burns developed on the skin directly in contact with the liquid. He developed atrophy of the optic nerves and then bilateral pneumonia which led to pulmonary fibrosis and death. Further details on the time course were not reported. A brief exposure of five men to BCME in a chemical plant resulted in nausea and 'cramp-like' pains in the eyes. Three of the exposed developed keratitis punctata with secondary iritis.

The long-term effects of BCME have been reported on a number of occasions. In one German chemical company, eight deaths due to lung cancer were reported during an 8-year period. Six had been preparing and/or processing BCME, comprising one-third of the total workers in that department.[119] In a Japanese chemical company producing dyestuffs, five of 32 workers who had worked with BCME died from lung cancer, against an expected value of 0.024. Smoking histories were not known. One tumour was histologically identified as an oat-cell carcinoma.[120] McCallum and colleagues[121] have stressed the interesting point that the most important factor affecting the number of deaths from lung cancer in their study was the degree of exposure to the process, rather than the duration of exposure.

Lung cancer due to exposure to bis(chloromethyl) ether is a prescribed disease (see Chapter 4).

Management

For acute effects management is primarily symptomatic. For long-term effects preventive measures are called for.

EPOXIDES

Epoxides are compounds containing the three-membered ring:

$$\begin{array}{c} \diagdown \quad / \\ C-C \\ / \diagup O \diagdown \diagdown \end{array}$$

They are cyclic ethers but are highly reactive due to the ease of opening of their highly strained three-membered ring. Perhaps, equally interesting, is that many double-bonded organic chemicals (e.g. vinyl chloride, benzene, styrene) are thought to form epoxides as intermediates as the double bonds are broken during metabolic detoxification.

EPICHLOROHYDRIN (1-CHOLORO-2,3-EPOXYPROPANE) (CH₂OCHCH₂Cl)

[CAS no. 106-89-8]

$$CH_2-CH-CH_2Cl$$
$$\diagdown_O\diagup$$

Characteristics and uses

Epichlorohydrin is a colourless liquid, widely used in the manufacture of epoxy resins, surface-active agents, pharmaceuticals, solvents and many other products.

Metabolism/biochemical effects

The presence of the chlorine atom enhances the reactivity of the epichlorohydrin molecule which is much more reactive than ethylene oxide or propylene oxide.

Clinical manifestations

In contact with the skin, epichlorohydrin may cause erythema, papules, oedema and even blisters. In animal experiments it has caused pulmonary oedema and damage to renal tubules.

Whilst mutation experiments indicate that epichlorohydrin is a mutagen and animal studies indicate that it is a carcinogen, analysis of data on exposed workers indicates a non-significant excess of lung cancer.[122] The IARC evaluates epichlorohydrin as *probably carcinogenic to humans* (Group 2A).

Similarly, although a rapidly reversible effect on sperm motility and fertility has been observed in male rats, limited data on male employees, working with epichlorohydrin, revealed normal sperm counts.[123]

Management

Apart from local measures for acute local effects, no management for acute cases is called for.

NITRILES

Nitriles are organic cyanides containing a cyano group, i.e. a carbon with a triple bond to a nitrogen atom. The general formula is $RC \equiv N$. Nitriles are extremely reactive and are therefore used as intermediates in chemical syntheses.

ACRYLONITRILE (VINYL CYANIDE) ($CH_2 = CHC \equiv N$)

[CAS no. 107-13-1]

Characteristics and uses

Acrylonitrile, vinyl cyanide, $CH_2=CHC \equiv N$, is a colourless liquid with a pungent garlic-like odour.

About 1000–2000 workers in the UK are estimated to be exposed. Commercial acrylonitrile may contain hydroquinone monomethyl ether as an inhibitor. Acrylonitrile is used in the plastics and resin industry and, in the materials and clothes industry, it is used in the manufacture of acrylonitrile fibre, a polymer sold under the trade name Orlon® and a copolymer with vinyl acetate called Acrilan®; ABS rubber is made from 30% acrylonitrile with butadiene (20%) and styrene (50%).

Metabolism/biochemical effects

Acrylonitrile is readily absorbed both by inhalation and through the skin. Leather gloves and footwear readily absorb acrylonitrile, which may lead to skin absorption and systemic effects as well as local effects such as blistering. It is an acute irritant to the skin and eyes. It is slowly broken down, releasing cyanide ions which block the ferric ion of cytochrome oxidase, producing tissue anoxia. In an earlier edition of this book Jackson wrote, 'The level of cyanide is an indication of absorption but not necessarily a measure of lethality'.[124]

Clinical manifestations

As would be expected from the somewhat slower release of cyanide ions noted above, symptoms of poisoning may develop more slowly than in exposure to hydrogen cyanide but when they appear the victim can have significant levels of cyanide in his blood. 'The symptoms derive from tissue anoxia and are in order of onset: limb weakness, dyspnoea, burning sensation in the throat, dizziness and impaired judgement, cyanosis[sic], nausea, collapse, irregular breathing, convulsions and death'. Some persons appear hysterical or may even be violent.

Any deviation of this sort from normal is deeply suspect'.[125] It is important that, in an acrylonitrile worker, such departures from normal are regarded very seriously.

Acrylonitrile caused tumours in rodents of the forestomach, brain and Zymbal gland following long-term feeding or inhalation studies, and was positive with microsomal enhancement in bacterial mutagenicity tests.[126,127] Although carcinogenic in animals, there are no conclusive epidemiological studies of exposed workers which show an increased risk of lung cancer.[128] A statistically significant increase in prostatic cancer noted in one study was treated with some reserve by the authors.[129]

Embryotoxicity was seen after administration of acrylonitrile to pregnant mice. Exposure to acrylonitrile orally or by inhalation caused birth defects in offspring of rats but only at doses which caused some toxicity to the mothers.[130]

Management

The management of acute acrylonitrile poisoning is the same as for cyanide poisoning. The slower release of the cyanide ion from acrylonitrile, with the consequent slower onset of symptoms, described above, means that very careful attention must be paid to the onset of the premonitory symptoms, however vague they may appear.

SULPHUR-CONTAINING COMPOUNDS

The most common organic chemical containing the C=S grouping is carbon disulphide.

CARBON DISULPHIDE (CS_2)

[CAS no. 75-15-0]

Characteristics and uses

Pure carbon disulphide (CS_2) is a clear, colourless, highly combustible, volatile liquid. Industrial forms, however, contain impurities which give it an unpleasant acrid sulphurous odour and a faint yellow colour. Most carbon disulphide is manufactured from the catalysed reaction of sulphur vapour with methane. It has been used in the past as a good solvent for oils, fats, rubber and other materials. Now, in the European Union, its use is decreasing. Some is used in the production of carbon tetrachloride (as an intermediate for CFC propellants and refrigerants) but it is employed also in the manufacture of rayon and cellulose fibres.

Carbon disulphide is used as a solvent for fats, lipids, resins and in laboratory analysis.

Metabolism/biochemical effects

Carbon disulphide is well absorbed by the respiratory tract, skin and gastrointestinal tract but inhalation is the principal route for occupational exposure. Not all the inhaled carbon disulphide is retained and absorbed.

About 90% of absorbed carbon disulphide is metabolized. The metabolism has been extensively studied,[131] the metabolic pathway leading, at first, to the formation of dithiocarbamates, which are claimed to be involved in some of the neurotoxic effects. Conjugation reactions with glutathione (see below) and microsomal oxidation yielding reactive sulphur are other established pathways, although the relative activities of the various metabolic pathways are not known.

The iodine-azide reaction, which is catalysed by organic – SH and C=S compounds, used to be employed for the 'biological monitoring' of workers and is believed to depend on the presence of thiazolidine in the urine. It is, however, relatively insensitive and non-specific and has been replaced by measurement of urinary 2-thiothiazolidine-4-carboxylic acid (TTCA), a conjugation product of CS_2 and glutathione.

The measurement of urinary TTCA seems to be a reliable and sensitive technique for the 'biological monitoring' of exposed workers for the uptake of carbon disulphide even though it appears to comprise only about 0.7–2.3% of absorbed CS_2. The excretion kinetics of TTCA exhibit two phases, a fast one with a half-life of about 6 hours and a slower phase with a half-life of about 60–70 hours. The slow phase may be related to mobilization of CS_2 from body fats in which it is readily soluble.[132]

Clinical manifestations

The toxic effects of carbon disulphide have been recognized for about 150 years. Up to about the end of the First World War workers who were exposed to extremely high concentrations, particularly in the cold vulcanization of rubber, developed acute and subacute psychoses. At the beginning of the twentieth century, Thomas Oliver wrote that the maniacal condition of some of the workers, both male and female, led them to precipitate themselves from the top rooms of the factory to the ground (his book was truly titled *Dangerous Trades*).[133] The next sentence of his account was not perhaps intended to sound ominous: 'In consequence of bisulpide of carbon being extremely explosive, vulcanization by means of it has generally to be carried on in rooms, one side of which is perfectly open. This open front is usually protected by iron bars.' Somewhat lower concentrations encountered from then up to about the end of the Second World War led, predominantly, to peripheral neuropathy.

Following gassing accidents in which loss of consciousness has occurred, psychiatric disturbances as well as permanent peripheral and central nervous system damage have ensued. Chronic poisoning is said to result in headaches, muscle weakness, anorexia, anaemia, disturbance of cardiac rhythm, visual disturbances and paraesthesiae.

The World Health Organization[134] attempted to classify the wide range of syndromes related to overexposure to carbon disulphide (sometimes using International 'English' which sounds strange to UK clinicians):

- psychoses (mainly manic and depressive symptomatology and disorientation);
- polyneuropathy of lower extremities, sensory disturbances and decrease of motor and sensory conduction velocity in peripheral nerves;
- gastrointestinal tract disturbances such as chronic hyper- and hypoacidic gastritis and duodenal ulceration;
- myopathy of calf muscles;
- neurasthenic syndrome in automatic nervous system;
- optic neuritis;
- atherosclerotic vasculoencephalopathy.

The different clinical pictures have also been well summarized by Finkel.[135]

With modern control systems such effects no longer occur. Nevertheless, recent studies continue to demonstrate disturbances, albeit more subtle, of the peripheral and central nervous system, including diminished peripheral nerve conduction velocity, impaired performance on the Wechsler Adult Intelligence Scale, electroencephalographic abnormalities and electromyographic evidence of neuropathy.[136,137] These are reported to have persisted for 10 years following the last recorded exposure. Impaired colour discrimination has been demonstrated amongst workers currently exposed to concentrations below 20 ppm. but who might have been exposed transiently to higher concentrations for short periods in the past. As the observed defects did not relate to specific pattern defects in colour discrimination, it was suggested that the abnormal findings indicated an impairment in the receptiveness of the ganglion cells or demyelination of the optic nerve fibres.[138]

A relationship between exposure to carbon disulphide and coronary heart disease has been demonstrated in a number of countries. Recent findings suggest that this may be controlled by reduction of exposure,[139] and interestingly, by removal from further exposure either by leaving or retirement. That has led to the suggestion that carbon disulphide has some sort of reversible, direct cardiotoxic or thrombotic effect.[140]

There have been reports of effects on male and female reproductive functions. For women, it is conflicting in relation to effects on menstrual cycle and a slight increase in miscarriages and further complicated by concomitant exposure to hydrogen sulphide. In males, hypospermia and abnormal sperm morphology were reported concomitant with presentation of chronic poisoning. Here levels were reported at average concentrations of 13–26 ppm but with peaks of up to 250 ppm.[141,142]

Overall, it seems that the most serious effects from repeated exposure to carbon disulphide are cardiotoxic and neurological effects. The most recent reports in the literature seem to suggest that the threshold for the earliest subclinical manifestations for both these effects is around 20 ppm.[137,143-144]

Management

Acute poisoning by carbon disulphide is nowadays very rare.

With current exposure levels it seems that, for early effects on the nervous system, the prognosis is good if they have been detected early and the patient removed from further exposure. Otherwise prognosis should be guarded until the patient has been observed over several months.

As to the enhanced risk of coronary heart disease, it is reassuring that modern control measures appear to be able to reduce the excess number of deaths and that the increased risk of death diminishes after removal from further exposure.

ALIPHATIC MIXTURES: PETROLEUM SOLVENTS

Petroleum solvents are complex mixtures of aliphatic and aromatic hydrocarbons which are generally grouped into three classes based on their volatility and aromatic content: (1) special boiling-range solvents; (2) high-boiling aromatic solvents; and (3) white spirits. For the purposes of this chapter white spirits have been selected as a useful example due to their widespread use in the paint and coatings industry.

WHITE SPIRITS

Characteristics and uses

White spirits is a petroleum distillate, produced in the petroleum refining industry which contains a complex mixture, of variable composition, containing open-chain aliphatic alicyclic and aromatic hydrocarbons (Fig. 11.12). 'White spirits' is the term generally encountered in Europe although elsewhere other names exist: mineral spirits, Stoddard solvent (in USA), solvent naphtha, turpentine substitute. Other authorities would also include in this group (which, after all, is a petroleum distillate defined by its boiling *temperature range* – rather than a precise boiling *point*) petroleum ether, petrol (gasoline) and benzine (not benzene, see Chapter 12).

From the foregoing it will be seen that the chemical composition of 'white spirits' may vary and is largely determined by the production process used, either hydrogenation or hydrosulphurization. A typical example has the following chemical composition: aromatics 15% (predominantly C_9 and C_{10} alkylbenzenes); 48% open-chain aliphatics (mainly C_9, C_{10} and C_{11} compounds); and 37% alicyclics (26% monocyclo-compounds, 11% dicyclo-compounds). The boiling point

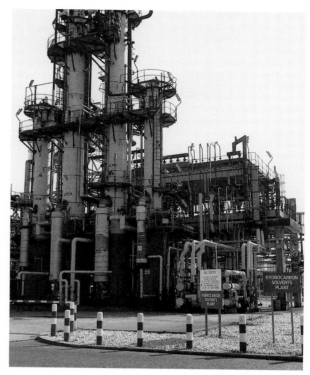

Figure 11.12 *General view of special boiling point processing plant in a refinery. Photograph courtesy of Shell UK Limited.*

range generally falls between 150° and 205°C. White spirits with both lower and higher aromatic content are commercially available, although recent years have seen a move towards hydrogenated types which have a lower aromatic content. The composition in Table 11.5 has been given by Carpenter.[145]

White spirit is a clear, colourless liquid with a kerosene-like odour and is principally encountered in paints, varnishes and lacquers. To a lesser degree it is used as an industrial degreasant and cleaner, in wood treatment and in some chemical processes.

Metabolism/biochemical effects

The main route of absorption for white spirits is through the lungs. Beyond that it is impossible to attempt to cite metabolic pathways for such a mixture of straight, branched and cyclic carbon compounds, the composition of which varies according to the origin of the crude oil and the subsequent molecular modifications and additions made at the refinery.

Clinical manifestations

Prolonged moderate exposure (hours) to vapours of these materials will give rise to symptoms like those of the longer chain aliphatic hydrocarbons: giddiness, vertigo, nausea and vomiting and generally with a headache. Irritation of the respiratory tract may be only moderate and not sufficient to discourage further exposure. Gross

Table 11.5 *Composition of white spirit*

	API mass spectrographic data	API gas-liquid chromatography
Light hydrocarbon to C_8	1.4	3.0
C_9 hydrocarbons	18.5	12.6
C_{10} and higher molecular weight hydrocarbons	65.0	69.0
Aromatics	15.1	15.4

From Ref. 145.

overexposure, as might occur from entering a tank containing, or recently containing, these materials will rapidly lead to stupor and unconsciousness.

Over the least 15 years, some authors, particularly in Scandinavian countries, have described an increased incidence of non-specific psychiatric symptoms in workers exposed, over longer periods of time, to only moderate amounts. Thus, 30 workers exposed to an average concentration of some 300 mg/m³ 'jet fuel' (distillation range, 50–250°C and comprising: aromatic hydrocarbons 12 vol%, olefin hydrocarbons 0.5 vol%, saturated hydrocarbons (paraffins, cycloparaffins, etc.) 87.5 vol% – see above) showed an increased prevalence of 'psychiatric' symptoms (37 different symptoms from the Comprehensive Psychopathological Rating Scale) and decreased performance on some psychological tests when compared with a matched group of non-exposed control subjects.[146] Overall, there is certainly a body of evidence that long-term exposure to a range of organic solvents, including white spirit, can give rise to a range of increased subclinical neurobehavioural and neurophysiological effects although no mechanism has been elucidated.[147–149]

Although some cases of cancer have been reported in epidemiological studies of workers exposed to white spirits, any causal association with white spirits currently remains undetermined. At the present time the overall conclusion of the IARC is that petroleum solvents are not classifiable with regard to their carcinogenicity in humans.[150] For the same reasons reports of adverse pregnancy outcomes amongst women exposed to white spirits and other solvents are difficult to evaluate.

Management

The management of acute overexposure is generally a matter for first aid. Because of the indefinite composition of these materials it would be prudent to consider whether any of the components might have the hepatic or renal toxicity of other aliphatic compounds and, therefore, to check hepatic and renal function.

It is not yet clearly established whether recovery from the non-specific psychiatric symptoms described above is complete after removal from exposure.

REFERENCES

1 Altenkirch H, Mager J, Stoltenburg G *et al*. Toxic polyneuropathies after sniffing glue thinner. *J Neurol* 1977;**214**:137–52.

2 Yamada S. Intoxication polyneuritis in workers exposed to *n*-hexane. *Jap J Ind Hlth* 1967;**9**:651–9.

3 Paulson GW, Waylonis GW. Polyneuropathy due to *n*-hexane. *Arch Intern Med* 1976;**136**:880–2.

4 Wang JD, Chang YC, Kao KP, Huang CC, Lin CC, Yeh WY. An outbreak of *n*-hexane induced polyneuropathy among press proofing workers in Taipei. *Am J Ind Med* 1986;**10**:111–18.

5 Bell GM, Gordon ACH, Lee P *et al*. Proliferative glomerulonephritis and exposure to organic solvents. *Nephron* 1985;**40**:161–5.

6 Hotz P, Pilliod J, Soderstrom JD, Rey F, Boillet MA, Savolainen H. Relation between renal function tests and a retrospective organic solvent exposure score. *Br J Ind Med* 1989;**49**:815–19.

7 Yaqoob M, Bell GM, Percy DF, Finn R. Primary glomerulonephritis and hydrocarbon exposure: a case-control study and literature review. *Q J Med* 1992;**83**:409–18.

8 Harrington JM, Whitby H, Gray CN, Reid FJ, Aw TC, Waterhouse JA. Renal disease and occupational exposure to organic solvents: a case referent approach. *Br J Ind Med* 1989;**49**:643–50.

9 Wells GG, Waldron HA. Methylene chloride burns (letter). *Br J Ind Med* 1984;**41**:420.

10 Barrowcliff DF, Knell AJ. Cerebral damage due to endogenous chronic carbon monoxide poisoning caused by exposure to methylene chloride. *J Soc Occup Med* 1979;**29**:12–14.

11 Stewart RD Hake CL. Paint-remover hazard. *JAMA* 1976;**235**:398–401.

12 Cherry N, Venables H, Waldron HA *et al*. Some observations on workers exposed to methylene chloride. *Br J Ind Med* 1981;**38**:351–5.

13 McCollister DD, Beamer WH, Atchison GJ, Spencer HC. Absorption, distribution and elimination of radioactive carbon tetrachloride by monkeys upon exposure to low vapor concentrations. *J Pharmacol Exp Ther* 1951;**102**:112–24.

14 Stewart RD, Boettner EA, Southworth RR, Cerny JC. Acute carbon tetrachloride intoxication. *JAMA* 1963;**183**:994–7.

15 Shah H, Hartman SP, Weinhouse S. Formation of carbonyl chloride in carbon tetrachloride metabolism by rat liver in vitro. *Cancer Res* 1979;**39**:3942–7.

16 Finkel AJ. *Hamilton and Hardy's Industrial Toxicology* 4th edn. London: John Wright, 1983 : 230–37.

17 International Agency for Research on Cancer. Monographs on the evaluation of carcinogenic risks to humans: 20. *Some Halogenated Hydrocarbons.* Lyon: IRAC, 1979: 371–99.

18 International Agency for Research on Cancer. Monographs on the evaluation of carcinogenic risks to humans: 54. *Strong Acid Mists and Other Industrial Exposures.* Lyon IRAC, 1992: 272–4.

19 Melamed E, Lavy S. Parkinsonism associated with chronic inhalation of carbon tetrachloride. (letter) *Lancet* 1977;**i**:1015.

20 Braganza JM. Towards antioxidant therapy for gastrointestinal disease. *Curr Med Lit Gastroenterol* 1989;**8**:99–106.

21 Bomski H, Sobelewska A, Strakowski A. Toxic damage of the liver by chloroform in chemical industry workers. *Arch Gewerbepath Gewerbehyg* 1967;**24**:127–34.

22 Phoon WH, Goh KT, Lee LT et al. Toxic jaundice from occupational exposure to chloroform. *Med J Malaysia* 1983;**38**:31–4.

23 McCarthy TB, Jones RD. Industrial gassing poisonings due to trichloroethylene, perchlorethylene and 1-1-1 trichloroethane, 1961–1980. *Br J Ind Med* 1983;**40**:450–5.

24 Bryzhin FF. [Pathomorphological changes of internal organs in connection with poisoning by ethylene dichloride through the digestive tract.] *Farmakol Toksikol* 1945;**8**:43–9. (Russian)

25 Urusova TP. [About a possibility of dichloroethane absorption into milk of nursing women when contracted under industrial conditions]. *Gig Sanit* 1953;**18**:36–7. (Russian)

26 Torkelson TR, Rowe VK. In: Clayton GD, Clayton FE eds. *Patty's Industrial Hygiene and Toxicology* 3rd edn. New York: John Wiley, 1981;3491–7.

27 Spencer FIC, Rowe VK, Adams EM, McCollister DD, Irish DD. Vapour toxicity of ethylene dichloride determined by experimentation etc. *Arch Ind Hyg Occup Med* 1951;**4**:482–93.

28 National Institute of Occupational Safety and Health *Criteria for a Recommended Standard . . . Occupational Exposure to Ethylene Dichloride (1,2dichloroethane).* Washington, DC: NIOSH 1976;76–139 : 19.

29 Jones RD, Winter DP. Two case reports of deaths on industrial premises attributed to 1,1, 1-trichloroethane. *Arch Environ Hlth* 1983;**38**:59–61.

30 Stewart RD. Methyl chloroform intoxication; diagnosis and treatment. *JAMA* 1971;**215**:1789–92.

31 Stewart RD, Gay HH, Erley DS, Hake CL, Schaffer AW. Human exposure to 1,1,1-trichloroethane vapour: relationship of expired air and blood concentrations to exposure and toxicity. *Am Ind Hyg Assoc* 1961;**22**:252–62.

32 Lowery MC, Au WW, Adams PM, Whorton EB Jr, Legator MS. Male mediated behavioural abnormalities. *Mutat Res* 1990;**229**:213–29.

33 Wong O, Utidjian HMD, Karten VS. Retrospective evaluation of reproductive performance of workers exposed to ethylene dibromide (EDB). *J Occup Med* 1979;**21**:98–102.

34 Dobbins JG. Regulation and the use of 'negative' results from human reproductive studies: the case of ethylene dibromide. *Am J Ind Med* 1987;**12**:33–45.

35 Kleinfeld M, Tabershaw IR. Trichloroethylene toxicity – report of five fatal cases. *AMA Arch Ind Hyg Occup Med* 1954;**10**:134–41.

36 Reinhardt CF, Mullin LS, Maxfield ME. Cardiac sensitization potential of some common industrial solvents. *Ind Hyg News Rep* 1972;**15**:3–4.

37 White JF, Carlson CP. Epinephrine-induced cardiac arrhythmias in rabbits exposed to trichloroethylene: potentiation by caffeine. *Fundam Appl Toxicol* 1982;**2**:125–9.

38 Smith GF. Trichloroethylene: a review. *Br J Ind Med* 1966;**23**:249–62.

39 Grandjean E, Munchinger R, Turian V, Haas PA, Knoeffel H-K, Rosenmund H. Investigations into the effects of exposure to trichloroethylene in mechanical engineering. *Br J Ind Med* 1955;**12**:131–42.

40 Fielder FJ, Lowng RK, Shilaker RO et al. *HSE Toxicity Review* 6: Trichloroethylene: London: HMSO, 1982.

41 Feldman RG, Mayer RF. Studies of trichloroethylene intoxication in man. *Neurology* 1968;**18**:309.

42 International Agency for Research on Cancer. Monographs on the evaluation of carcinogenic risks to humans: 63. *Trichlorethylene.* Lyon: IRAC, 1995: **63**:75

43 Stewart RD, Dodd HC. Absorption of carbon tetrachloride, trichloroethylene, tetrachloroethylene, methyl chloride, and 1,1,1-trichloroethane through the human skin. *Am Ind Hyg Assoc* 1964;**25**:439–46.

44 Stewart RD, Gay HH, Erley DS, Hake CL; Schaffer AW. Human exposure to tetrachloroethylene vapor. *Arch Environ Hlth* 1961;**2**:516–22.

45 Stewart RD, Erley DS, Schaffer AW, Gay H. Accidental vapor exposure to anesthetic concentrations of a solvent containing tetrachloroethylene. *Ind Med Surg* 1961;**30**:327–30.

46 Dekant et al. Absorption, elimination and metabolism of trichloroethylene: a quantitative comparison between rats and mice. *Xenobiotica* 1986;**16**:143–52.

47 Nemesanszky E, Lott JA. Gamma-glutamyltransferase and its isoenzymes: progress and problems. *Clin Chem* 1985;**31**:797–803.

48 Gennari P, Naldi M, Motta R et al. Gammaglutamyltransferase isoenzyme pattern in workers exposed to tetrachloroethylene. *Am J Ind Med* 1992;**21**:661–71.

49 Mutti A, Alinovi R, Bergamaschi E et al. Nephropathies

and exposure to perchloroethylene in dry-cleaners. *Lancet* 1992;**340**:189–93.

50 Illing HPA, Mariscotti SP, Smith AM. *HSE Toxicity Review 17: Tetrachloroethylene*. London: HMSO, 1987.

51 International Agency for Research on Cancer. . Monographs on the evaluation of carcinogenic risks to humans: 63. *Tetrachloroethylene* Lyon: IRAC, 1995: 159–221.

52 Jenkins LJ, Trabulus MJ, Murphy SI). Biochemical effects of 1,1-dichloroethylene in rats: comparison with carbon tetrachloride and 1,2-dichloroethylene. *Toxicol Appl Pharmacol* 1972;**23**:501–10.

53 Reynolds ES, Moslen MT, Szabo S, Jaeger RJ, Murphy SI. Hepatotoxicity of vinyl chloride and 1,1-dichloroethylene. *Am J Pathol* 1975;**81**:219–36.

54 Reynolds ES, Moslen MT, Boor PJ, Jaeger RJ. 1,1-Dichloroethylene hepatotoxicity. *Am J Pathol* 1980;**101**:331–44.

55 Ott MC, Fishbeck WA, Townsend JC, Schneider Ej. A health study of employees exposed to vinylidene chloride. *J Occup Med* 1976;**18**:735–8.

56 Dahl AR, Bechtold WE, Bond JA *et al*. Species differences in the metabolism and disposition of inhaled 1,3-butadiene and isoprene. *Environ Hlth Perspect* 1990;**86**:65–9.

57 Lee WR. What should we do about work related cancer? *Br Med J* 1986;**292**:1155–6.

58 Weaver NK. Butadiene. In: *ILO Encyclopaedia of Occupational Health and Safety*. Geneva: International Labour Organization, 1983 : 347–8.

59 Illing HPA, Shillaker RO. *HSE Toxicity Review 11. 1,3-Butadiene and Related Compounds*. London: HMSO, 1985.

60 National Toxicology Program. *Toxicology and Carcinogenesis Studies of 1,3-butadiene in B6C3F1 Mice (inhalation studies)>*. NTP Technical Report Series No. 28 NIFI Publication 84–2544, 1984.

61 Owen PE. *The Toxicity and Carcinogenicity of Butadiene Gas Administered to Rats by Inhalation for Approximately 24 months*. Report No. 2653–522/2. Harrogate Hazleton Laboratories Europe Ltd 1981 (Confidential report prepared for the International Institute of Synthetic Rubber Producers Inc. New York).

62 Abelson PH. Editorial. Exaggerated carcinogenicity of chemicals. *Science* 1992;**256**:1609.

63 Divine BJ. An update on mortality among workers at a 1,3-butadiene facility – preliminary results. *Environ Hlth Perspect* 1990;**86**:119–28.

64 Irons RD, Stillman WS, Cloyd MW. Selective activation of endogenous ecotropic retrovirus in hematopoietic tissues of B6C3F1 mice during the preleukemic phase of 1,3-butadiene exposure. *Virology* 1987;**161**:457–62.

65 Melnick RL, Huff J, Matanoski CM. Carcinogenicity of 1,3-butadiene. *Lancet* 1992;**340**:724–5.

66 Infante PF, Book SA. Chemicals and human cancer. *Lancet* 1992;**340**:1408–9.

67 Department of the Environment. Expert Panel on Air Quality Standards: *1,3 Butadiene*. London: DOE, 1994.

68 Saunders RA. A new hazard in closed environmental atmospheres. *Arch Environ Hlth* 1967;**14**:380–4.

69 Braddick MR. Are hazard warnings sufficient? *Br J Ind Med* 1986;**43**:431.

70 Downie A, Khattab TM, Malik MIA, Samara IW. A case of percutaneous industrial methanol toxicity. *Occup Med* 1992;**42**:47–9.

71 McMartin KE, Martin-Amat G, Makar AB, Tephly TR. Methanol poisoning. V. Role of formate metabolism in the monkey. *J Pharmacol Exp Ther* 1977;**201**:564–72.

72 Noker PE, Tephly TR. The role of folates in methanol toxicity. In: Thurman RG ed. *Alcohol and Aldehyde Metabolizing Systems* Vol. 4. New York: Plenum Press, 1980 : 305–15.

73 Noker PE, Eells JT, Tephly TR. Methanol toxicity: treatment with folic acid and 5-formyltetrahydrofolic acid. *Alcohol Clin Exp Res* 1980;**4**:378–83.

74 American Conference of Governmental and Industrial Hygienists. *Documentation of the Threshold Limit Values for Chemical Substances in the Workroom Environment. Methanol*. Cincinnatti: ACGIH, 1986.

75 Klaassen CD, Admar MO, Doull J (eds). *Casarett & Doulls' Toxicology. The Basic Sciences of Poisons*. 4th edn. Oxford: Pergamon, 1991 : 702.

76 Swedish Criteria Group for Occupational Standards. *Arbete och Halsa* 1985;32 (ed. P. Lundberg). Scientific basis for Swedish Occupational Standards VI. Quoted. In: *Solvents in Common Use: Health Risks to Workers*. Royal Society for Chemistry Publ.no. EUR 11553 CEC Luxembourg, 1988 : 179.

77 Aquilonius S-M, Askmark H, Enoksson P, Lundberg PO, Mostrom V. Computerized tomography in severe methanol intoxication. *Br Med J* 1978;**2**:929–30.

78 McLean DR, Jacobs H, Mielke BW. Methanol poisoning: a clinical and pathological study. *Ann Neurol* 1980;**8**:161–7.

79 Martin~Amat G, McMartin KE, Hayreh SS, Hayreh MS, Tephly TR. Methanol poisoning: ocular toxicity produced by formate. *Toxicol Appl Pharmacol* 1978;**45**:201–8.

80 Meredith RJ, Vale JA. Poisoning from alcohols and glycols. In: Wetherall DJ, Ledingham JGG, Warrell DA eds. *Oxford Textbook of Medicine*. Oxford: Oxford University Press, 1983.

81 Eelis JT. Methanol-induced visual toxicity in the rat. *J Pharmacol Exp Ther* 1991;**257**:56–63.

82 International Program on Chemical Safety (IPCS). *Environmental Health Criteria 103. 2-Propanol*. Geneva: WHO, 1990.

83 Alderson M. *Occupational Cancer*. London: Butterworth, 1986 : 93.

84 Herbert V, Tisman G. Hematologic effect of alcohol in medical consequences of alcohol. *Ann NY Acad Sci* 1941; **42**:307–15.

85 International Program on Chemical Safety (IPCS). *Butanols – four isomers: 1-butanol, 2-butanol tert-butanol and isobutanol. Environmental Health Criteria 65*. Geneva: WHO, 1987.

86 American Industrial Hygiene Association (AIHA). Workplace environmental exposure level guide: polyethylene glycols. *Am Ind Hyg Assoc* 1980;**41**: A55–7.

87 Fisher AA. Immediate and delayed allergic contact reactions to polyethylene glycol. *Contact Dermatitis* 1978;**4**:135–8.

88 Smith AE. Formaldehyde. *Occup Med* 1992;**42**:83–8.

89 International Agency for Research on Cancer. Monographs on the evaluation of carcinogenic risks to humans: 62. *Wood dust and formaldehyde.* Lyon: IARC, 1995;**62**:217–362.

90 American Conference of Governmental Industrial Hygienists. 1991–1992 *Threshold Limit Values for Chemical Substances and Physical Agents and Biological Exposure indices.* Cincinnati: ACGIH, 1991 : 22.

91 International Agency for Research on Cancer. Monographs on the evaluation of carcinogenic risks to humans: 7. *Overall Evaluation of Carcinogenicity – An Updating of Volumes 1 to 42.* Lyon: IRAC, 1987, 77–8.

92 Benson WG. Case report exposure to glutaraldehyde. *J Soc Occup Med* 1984;**34**:63–4.

93 Norback D. Skin and respiratory symptoms from exposure to alkaline glutaraldehyde in medical services. *Scand J Work Environ Hlth* 1988;**14**:366–71.

94 Trigg Q, Heap DC, Herdman MJ, Davies RJ. A radiographer's asthma. *Respir Med* 1992;**86**:167–9.

95 Bos PMJ, de Mik G, Bragt: PC. Critical review of the toxicity of methyl *n*-butyl ketone: risk from occupational exposure. *Am J Ind Med* 1991;**20**:175–94.

96 Hjelm EW, Hagberg M, Iregren A, Lof A. Exposure to methyl isobutyl ketone: toxicokinetics and occurrence of irritative and CNS symptoms in man. *Int Arch Occup Environ Hlth* 1990;**62**:19–26.

97 Armeli G, Linari F, Martorano G. Clinical and haematological examinations in workers exposed to the action of the higher ketone (MiBK) repeated after five years. *Lav Um* 1968;**20**:418–24.

98 Aubuchon J, Robins HI, Viseskul C. Peripheral neuropathy after exposure to methyl-isobutyl ketone in spray paint. *Lancet* 1979;**ii**:363–4.

99 Lapadula 13M, Habig C, Cupta RP, Abu-Urnia MB. Induction of cytochrome P450 isoenzymes by simultaneous inhalation exposure of hens to *n*~hexane and methyl *iso*-butyl ketone (MiBK). *Biochem Pharmacol* 1991;**41**:877–83.

100 Berg EF. Retrobulbar neuritis. A case report of presumed solvent toxicity. *Ann Ophthalmol* 1971;**3**:1351–3.

101 Dyro FM. Methyl ethyl ketone polyneuropathy in shoe factory workers. *Clin Toxicol* 1978;**13**:371–6.

102 Uden PC, Miller JWC. Chlorinated acids and chloral in drinking water. *J Am Waterworks Assoc* 1983;**75**:524–7.

103 De Angelo AB, Daniel PB, McMillan L, Wernsurg P, Savage RE. Species and strain sensitivity to the induction of peroxisome proliferation by chloracetic acids. *Toxicol Appl Pharmacol* 1989;**101**:285–98.

104 Herren-Freund SL, Pereira MA, Khoury MD, Olsen G. The carcinogenicity of trichlorethylene and its metabolites, trichloroacetic acid and dichloroacetic in mouse liver. *Toxicol Appl Pharmacol* 1987;**90**:183–9.

105 Hayes WJ (ed). Trichloroacetic acid. In: *Pesticides Studied in Man.* Baltimore: Williams and Wilkins, 1982 : 537.

106 Fisher AA. Acrylic bone cement sensitization and dermatitis. *Cutis* 1973;**12**:333–7.

107 Seppalainen AM, Rajaniemi R. Local neurotoxicity of methyl methacrylate among dental technicians. *Am J Ind Med* 1984;**5**:471–7.

108 Rajaniemi R. Clinical evaluation of occupational toxicity of methyimethacrylate monomer to dental technicians. *J Soc Occup Med* 1986;**36**:56–9.

109 Donaghy M, Rushworth G, Jacobs JM. Generalized peripheral neuropathy in a dental technician exposed to methyl methacrylate monomer. *Neurology* 1991;**41**:1112–16.

110 Pickering CAC, Bainbridge D, Birtwistle IH *et al.* Occupational asthma due to methylmethacrylate in an orthopaedic theatre sister. *Br Med J* 1986;**292**:1362–3.

111 Ritter MA, Gioe Tj, Sieber JM. Systemic effects of polymethylmethacrylate. *Acta Orthop Scand* 1984;**55**:411–13.

112 Pope IK, Philips H. Bone cement and the liver: a dose related effect? *J Bone Jt Surg* 1988;**70B**:364–6.

113 International Agency for Research on Cancer. Monographs on the evaluation of carcinogenic risks to humans: 60. *Acrylamide.* Lyon: IARC, 1994: 389–433.

114 Redlich CA, Beckett WS, Sparer J *et al.* Liver disease associated with occupational exposure to the solvent dimethylformamide. *Ann Intern Med* 1988;**108**: 680–6.

115 Ducatman AM, Conwill DE, Crawl J. Germ cell tumours of the testicle among aircraft repairmen. *J Urol* 1986;**136**:834–6.

116 Levin SM, Baker DB, Landrigan PJ *et al.* Testicular cancer in leather tanners exposed to dimethylformamide. *Lancet* 1987;**ii**:1153.

117 International Agency for Research on Cancer. Monographs on the evaluation of carcinogenic risks to humans: 47. *Dimethylformamide.* Lyon: IARC, 1989: 171–97.

118 *HSE Toxicity Review 22: Bis(chloromethyl) ether.* London: HMSO, 1990.

119 Norpoth K. Fatal cases of lung carcinoma due to BCME in the federal republic of Germany. In: Travenius SZM ed. *Symposium on Bis(chloromethy)ether (BCME) 1981.* Sweden: Perstorp AB, 1981.

120 Sakabe H. Lung cancer due to exposure to bis (chloromethyl) ether. *Ind Hlth* 1973;**11**:145–8.

121 McCallum RI, Woolley V, Petrie A. Lung cancer associated with chloromethyl methyl ether manufacture: an investigation at two factories in the United Kingdom. *Br J Ind Med* 1983;**40**:384–9.

122 Enterline PE. Importance of sequential exposure in the production of epichlorohydrin and isopropanol. *Ann NY Acad Sci* 1982;**381**:344–9.

123 Hine C, Rowe VK, White ER, Darmer KI Jr, Youngblood GT. Epoxy compounds. In: Clayton CD, Clayton FE eds. *Patty's Industrial Hygiene and Toxicology* 3rd edn. New York: John Wiley, 1981 : 2245.

124 Jackson JR. Aliphatic and aromatic compounds. In: Raffle PAB, Lee WR, McCallum RI, Murray R eds. *Hunter's Diseases of Occupations*. London: Edward Arnold, 1987 : 396.

125 Bryson DD. Acrylonitrile. In: *ILO Encyclopaedia of Occupational Health and Safety*. Geneva: International Labour Organization, 1983 : 55.

126 Maltoni C, Ciliberti A, Di Maio V. Carcinogenic bioassays on rats of acrylonitrile administered by inhalation and by ingestion. *Med Lav* 1977;**68**:41011.

127 de Meester C, Poncelet F, Roberfroid M Mercier M. Mutagenic activity of acrylonitrile. *Toxicology* 1978;**11**:19–27.

128 Werner JB, Carter JT. Mortality of United Kingdom acrylonitrile polymerisation workers. *Br J Ind Med* 1981;**38**:247–53.

129 O'Berg MT, Chen JL, Burke CA, Wallrath J, Pell S. Epidemiologic study of workers exposed to acrylonitrile: an update. *J Occup Med* 1985;**27**:83540.

130 Joharmsen FR, Levinskas Gj, Berteua PE, Rodwell DE. Evaluation of the teratogenic potential of three aliphatic nitriles in the rat. *Fundam Appl Toxicol* 1986;**7**:33–40.

131 Brieger H, Teisinger J (eds). *Toxicology of Carbon Disulphide*. Amsterdam: Excerpta Medica, 1967.

132 Riihimake V, Kivisto H, Peltonen K, Helpio E, Aitio A. Assessment of exposure to carbon disulfide in viscose production workers from urinary 2-thiothiazolidine-4-carboxylic acid determinations. *Am J Ind Med* 1992;**22**:85–97.

133 Oliver T. *Dangerous Trades*. London: John Murray, 1902 : 472–73.

134 World Health Organization. *Environmental Health Criteria 10: Carbon Disulphide*. Geneva: UNEP/WHO, 1979.

135 Finkel AJ. *Hamilton and Hardy's Industrial Toxicology* 4th edn. London: John Wright, 1983 : 264–5.

136 Grasso P, Sharatt M, Davies DM, Irvine D. Neurophysiological and psychological disorders and exposure to organic solvents. *Food Chem Toxicol* 1984;**22**:819–52.

137 Ruijten MWMM, Salle HJA, Verberk MM, Muisser H. Special nerve functions and colour discrimination in workers with long term low level exposure to carbon disulphide. *Br J Ind Med* 1990;**47**:589–95.

138 Raitta C, Teir H, Tolonen M, Nurminen M, Helpid E, Malstróm S. Impaired color discrimination among viscose

rayon workers exposed to carbon disulfide. *J Occup Med* 1981;**23**:189–92.

139 Nurminen M, Hernberg S. Effects of intervention on the cardiovascular mortality of workers exposed to carbon disulphide: a 15 year follow up. *Br J Ind Med* 1985;**42**:32–5.

140 Sweetnam PM, Taylor SWC, Elwood PC. Exposure to carbon disulphide and ischaemic heart disease in a viscose rayon factory. *Br J Ind Med* 1987;**44**:220–7.

141 Beauchamp RO, Irons RD, Richett DE, Couch DB, Hamms TE Jr. A critical review of the literature on carbon disulphide toxicity. *Crit Rev Toxicol* 1983;**11**:33–84.

142 Lancranjan J, Popescu HI. Changes of the gonadic function in chronic carbon disulphide poisoning. *Med Lav* 1969;**60**:566–71.

143 Drexler H, Ulm K, Hardt R, Hubmann M, Göen T et al. Carbon disulphide IV. Cardiovascular function in workers in the viscose industry. *Int Arch Occup Environ Hlth* 1996;**69**:27–32.

144 Price B, Bergman TS, Rodriguez M, Henrich RT, Moran EJ. A review of carbon disulfide exposure data and the association between carbon disulfide exposure and ischaemic heart disease mortality. *Reg Tox Pharm* 1997;**26**:119–28.

145 Carpenter CP. White spirits. In: *ILO Encyclopedia of Occupational Health and Safety* Geneva: International Labour Organization, 1983;2300–1.

146 Knave B, Olson BA, Elofsson S et al. Long-term exposure to jet fuel. II: A cross-sectional epidemiologic investigation on occupationally exposed industrial workers with special reference to the nervous system. *Scand J Work Environ Hlth* 1978;**4**:19–45.

147 Spurgeon A, Grey CN, Sims J et al. Neurobehavioral effects of long-term occupational exposure to organic solvents: two comparable studies. *Am J Ind Med* 1992;**22**:325–35.

148 Baker EL. A review of recent research on health effects of human occupational solvents: a critical review. *J Occup Med* 1994;**36**:1079–1092.

149 Seaton A. Organic solvents and the nervous system: time for a reappraisal? *Q J Med* 1992;**84**:637–9.

150 International Agency for Research on Cancer. Monographs on the evaluation of carcinogenic risks to humans: 49. *Some Petroleum Solvents*. Lyon: IARC, 1989:43–77.

151 De Wardner. *The Kidney*. Edinburgh: Churchill Livingstone, 1985:144.

12

Aromatic chemicals

TAR-CHING AW

Benzene and common benzene derivatives	261	Other aromatic compounds	273
Aromatic amines	267	Acknowledgements	275
Phenol and phenol derivatives	271	References	275
Fused ring aromatic compounds	272		

Aromatic organic compounds constitute more than 50% of the different chemicals in common use in occupational settings worldwide. This group of chemicals consists of unsaturated cyclic compounds based on the benzene ring – benzene being the simplest homologue within the group. The term 'aromatic' originally stemmed from the pleasant odour characteristic of the earlier recognized compounds in the group (e.g. some esters used in perfumes and flavourings). However, many of the aromatic hydrocarbons today are odourless.

Benzene was first demonstrated in coal tar in 1845, and most aromatic compounds were previously isolated from the coal tar fraction of coal distillation. Destructive distillation of coal at 1000–1300°C yields coke, coal gas, coal tar and water-soluble volatile compounds, with the coal tar fraction containing over 200 different organic chemicals. The main source of aromatic organic compounds nowadays is petroleum.

While there are considerable animal data on the health effects of these compounds, acute and/or chronic effects in humans have only been documented for a few. Reports of ill-health in humans tend to be based on clinical cases of occupational or intentional (suicide or homicide) overexposure, or on epidemiological studies of exposed workers. Occupational epidemiological data related to exposure to only one compound are uncommon. Workplace exposures tend to be to a mixture of related or unrelated compounds or within a particular process; in a specified job category, or in a common industry. The aromatic compounds discussed in this chapter are primarily those with recognized human health effects related to occupational exposure. Some compounds with sparse data on human effects but with animal and laboratory toxicological data are included where there are relevant exposures to them in the workplace.

BENZENE AND COMMON BENZENE DERIVATIVES

BENZENE (BENZOL) (C_6H_6)

[CAS no. 71-43-2]

Benzene is a volatile, colourless, clear flammable liquid, and a natural constituent of crude oil. It has been used as a solvent in adhesives and paint removers, in the rubber and shoe industry,[1] and as a starter material for synthesis in the production of plastics and explosives. Exposures from these uses in the past have been responsible for chronic benzene poisoning. Currently, large-scale commercial and industrial use of benzene is strictly controlled. In the UK, up to 5% benzene is allowed in unleaded petrol, although there is a European Union Directive requiring the amount to be reduced to 1%. This takes effect in January 2000. Benzene is sometimes confused with the less toxic benzine, which is a mixture of hydrocarbons (generally straight chained) obtained from petroleum distillation and used as a motor fuel and a solvent.

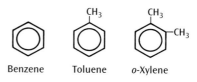

Benzene   Toluene   o-Xylene

Figure 12.1 *Benzene and some methylated derivates.*

Clinical effects

Benzene is absorbed systemically by inhalation and skin absorption. Acute effects on the nervous system include headache, tiredness, nausea, dizziness, narcosis and loss of consciousness. These acute symptoms occur at high exposures e.g. air concentrations of 7500 parts per million (ppm) for more than 30 minutes causes narcosis leading to death, but there is considerable individual variability in responses to benzene.

Chronic effects include depression of the bone marrow and an increased risk of aplastic anaemia and leukaemia (see Chapter 4). It is also suspected of causing multiple myeloma. The most common type of leukaemia reported is acute non-lymphocytic myeloblastic myeloid leukaemia, but chronic myelocytic leukaemia, chronic lymphatic leukaemia and erythroleukaemia have also been reported.[2,3] The latent period for the development of leukaemia at high exposure levels is around 10 years (see Chapter 4).[3]

Haemopoietic effects of exposure to benzene are leucocytopenia, thrombocytopenia, or pancytopenia, and in severe cases fatal aplastic anaemia. Splenomegaly with haemolysis, hyperbilirubinaemia, punctate basophilia of erythrocytes, and marrow hyperplasia may occur. Reduction of granulocytes with a relative increase in monocyte and lymphocyte count, and therefore a reversal of granulocyte/monocyte ratio have also been reported. In some workers exposed to high benzene levels, as have occurred in the past, the haematological changes persisted for months after exposure had ceased. An evaluation of routine data collected for workers with low-level benzene exposure showed that no lymphopenia nor other haematologic changes were noted at average benzene exposure levels of 0.55 ppm (see Chapter 4).[4]

Chronic benzene poisoning affecting the nervous system may present as behavioural and psychomotor changes, and labyrinthine, vestibular, or acoustic impairment. Effects on the myocardium and arrhythmias have occurred following high levels of exposure.

In inhalation studies benzene produced lymphomas in mice. Benzene is non-mutagenic in the Ames test, but there is experimental evidence showing it to be a genotoxic carcinogen (see Chapters 38, 39).

Chromosome aberrations in white blood cells are associated with chronic benzene poisoning. These abnormalities persist for many years after exposure but their role in the development of leukaemia is uncertain. Chromosome aberrations have frequently been noted in patients both with benzene-induced and with spontaneous leukaemia. It is possible that such aberrations in bone marrow cells may give rise to leukaemic clones. The International Agency for Research on Cancer (IARC) has evaluated benzene and determined that there is limited evidence that it is carcinogenic in experimental animals, and sufficient evidence that it is carcinogenic in humans (see Chapter 39).[5] The American Conference of Governmental Industrial Hygienists (ACGIH) has designated benzene a confirmed human carcinogen.[6,7]

Metabolism and monitoring

About 50% of absorbed benzene is excreted unchanged in exhaled breath. The half-life is triphasic, with metabolism occurring via the cytochrome P450 system in the liver (see Chapter 6). Among the metabolites that appear in the urine are phenol, catechol and quinol. Benzene toxicity is linked to the dihydroxy metabolites. Urinary phenol has been used for biological monitoring of benzene-exposed workers,[8] but for exposures around 1 ppm or less, this is of little value. The ACGIH has suggested S-phenylmercapturic acid in urine for biological monitoring, with a biological exposure index (1999) of 25 µg/g creatinine for an end-of-shift urine sample.[7] In addition, an end-of-shift urine sample for another metabolite – t,t-muconic acid, has recently been proposed.[7] Benzene in exhaled breath[9] and blood benzene[10] have also been tried for biological monitoring, although these presently remain as experimental procedures. Cigarette smoke and burning polyvinyl chloride (PVC) are sources of benzene and exposure to these increase benzene in exhaled breath.[11]

Exposure limits for benzene in air vary according to different agencies. The US Occupational Health and Safety Administration (OSHA) has a permissible exposure level (PEL) of 1 ppm; the National Institute of Occupational Safety and Health (NIOSH) has a threshold limit value (time-weighted average; TWA) of 0.5 ppm (designated an A1 carcinogen); and the Health and Safety Executive in the UK set the 1999 occupational exposure limit for benzene at 5 ppm as a maximum exposure limit (MEL).[12] Various risk assessments have estimated from 15 to 25 lifetime excess leukaemia deaths per 1000 workers exposed to 10 ppm of benzene for 30 years.[13,14] These assessments may have overestimated the risk, and a re-evaluation resulted in the proposal that for a lifetime exposure to benzene of 1 ppm, the excess leukaemia deaths would be between 0.5 and 1 per thousand.[15]

Aplastic anaemia from occupational exposures

Benzene and ionizing radiation, are well recognized causes of aplastic anaemia although benzene derivatives, such as toluene and xylene, have not been implicated. Case reports have linked exposure to organic arsenicals and some organochlorine compounds, e.g. pentachlorophenol and lindane, with aplastic anaemia, but epidemiological evidence for this is lacking. The diagnosis of aplastic anaemia should include an enquiry into occupational and environmental exposures.

Occupational exposure to benzene should now be a rare cause of aplastic anaemia in the UK as exposures are generally controlled to levels well below the occupational exposure limits. In the management of a patient with aplastic anaemia, removal of the individual away from further exposure to the suspected agents and to other chemicals that can affect the haemopoietic system should be considered.

Periodic haematological screening has been advocated as a means of health surveillance for benzene-exposed workers. The rationale is that early haematological changes may indicate an adverse effect from benzene exposure, and early detection of these abnormalities and removal of the worker from exposure allows reversal of adverse effects. The usefulness of screening at current low levels of occupational exposure to benzene in the UK is debatable. There is no good evidence for the effectiveness of early treatment for benzene-induced leukaemia. Furthermore, at low levels of benzene exposure (0.01–1.4 ppm), no haematological abnormalities appear to be detectable.[16,17] Periodic health surveys of workers exposed to 1–30 ppm of benzene have not shown significant haematological abnormalities, with transient reduction in red cell count being the only abnormality mentioned. Hence, routine periodic haematological screening for benzene-exposed workers is of limited value.

Preventive measures have therefore focused on elimination or substitution of benzene, or on reduction of exposure. Cases of poisoning by benzene, or its nitro-, chloro-, amino-derivatives or by homologues of benzene are prescribed diseases (see Chapter 4) and are reportable by employers in the UK under the Reporting of Injuries, Diseases, and Dangerous Occurrences Regulations, 1985 (RIDDOR).

TOLUENE (METHYL BENZENE, TOLUOL) ($C_6H_5CH_3$)

[CAS no. 108-88-3]

Toluene is a monomethyl derivative of benzene. It is used extensively as an industrial solvent for paints and coatings, resins, oils and rubber. Following inhalation, most of the toluene is oxidized by microsomal mixed function oxidases to benzoic acid and in turn conjugated with glycine to form hippuric acid; 10–20% is conjugated with glucuronic acid to yield benzoyl glucuronide.

Clinical effects

Acute exposure to concentrations of toluene above 200 ppm results in headache, dizziness, irritation of the eyes, nose and throat, paraesthesia, incoordination, confusion and narcosis. Chronic exposure may give rise to muscle weakness, abdominal pain, cerebellar abnormalities, optic neuropathy, peripheral neuropathy, and an altered mental state (see Chapter 42). Hepatomegaly and neurobehavioural effects have also been documented.[18]

Effects on the haemopoietic system similar to benzene

have been attributed to benzene being present as a contaminant in some commercial batches of toluene. Toluene is regarded as a relatively safe organic solvent in its use in modern industry. The health effects described are rarely encountered in situations with strict control of occupational exposures.

Monitoring

Biological monitoring can be performed using urinary hippuric acid and/or urinary *ortho*-cresol.[19,20] Hippuric acid also appears in the urine from dietary sources, e.g. foods preserved with benzoates (benzoic acid is metabolized to hippuric acid) such as fruits, preserved meats and some beverages. Urinary hippuric acid is unreliable for biological monitoring for low levels of exposure to toluene. The 1999 UK occupational exposure limit for toluene is 50 ppm (8-hour TWA reference period) with a short-term exposure limit of 150 ppm.[12] The rate of hippuric acid excretion over the last 4 hours of a workshift correlates with toluene uptake. The ACGIH recommended biological exposure indices (BEI) for toluene exposure are:

- 1.6 g/g creatinine for hippuric acid in urine samples collected at the end of shift,
- 0.5 mg/litre for *ortho*-cresol in urine samples collected at the end of shift, or
- toluene in venous blood level of 0.05 mg/litre for a blood sample taken prior to the last shift of a working week.[7]

Urinary hippuric acid from non-occupational exposure is in the range of 0.5–1.5 g/g creatinine.[10]

XYLENE (XYLOL; DIMETHYLBENZENE) ($C_6H_4(CH_3)_2$)

[CAS no. 1330-20-7]

Xylene exists in three isomeric forms: *ortho*-, *meta*- and *para*-isomers (or 1,2-, 1,3-, and 1,4-isomers respectively). It is a volatile, flammable, colourless liquid derived from coal tar distillation. Xylenes are among the highest-volume chemicals in production.[21]

Commercial xylenes contain a mixture of all three isomers, and ethyl benzene can also be present as an impurity.[22] Xylene is a constituent of aviation grade fuel and cleaning fluids. It is also used as a petrol additive, as a solvent in paints, inks, lacquers, adhesives, protective coatings, dyes and cosmetics, in the production of plasticizers, fibres and resins, and in histopathology laboratories for the processing of microscopic slide preparations of tissue specimens.[23] Benzoic acid (a food preservative), benzaldehyde, and phthalic acid are produced using xylene as a starter material.

Clinical effects

Acute exposure to xylene produces irritant effects on the skin, mucous membranes, and respiratory tract.[21] Significant systemic absorption follows skin contact, and it has been shown that immersion of both hands in xylene for 15 minutes is equivalent to being exposed to 100 ppm of xylene (the current UK occupational exposure limit) for the same duration.[24,25] Systemic absorption also follows inhalation of xylene vapour. Acute effects are similar to those described for other organic solvents acting on the central nervous system. These are headaches, nausea, vomiting, dizziness, drowsiness, confusion, and coma. Xylene-exposed individuals have also reported vague symptoms as 'a floating sensation', a 'heavy feeling in the head' and experiencing 'an unusual taste'.[26] Central nervous system symptoms have been reported at inhalation exposure levels around 700 ppm.[27] Exposure to high levels (over 10 000 ppm) of xylene in paint in a poorly ventilated, confined space has resulted in death from acute pulmonary oedema with centrilobular liver congestion, and petechial haemorrhages in the brain. Survivors suffered a prolonged period of loss of consciousness, with transient hepatic and renal effects. These included elevated serum transaminase and urea levels and reduced creatinine clearance.[28] Glue sniffing as a form of solvent abuse can involve exposure to xylene. This has been shown to cause renal tubular acidosis.[29]

Splashes of xylene into the eyes result in photophobia, reduced visual acuity, ocular discomfort and pain. Ocular damage includes corneal erosion, conjunctival hyperaemia, and conjunctival epithelial loss. These effects are similar to alkali-induced burns.[30]

Low-level chronic exposure to organic solvents, such as xylene and white spirit have been thought to cause non-reversible central nervous system damage (see Chapter 4). This condition has been referred to as the 'psycho-organic syndrome',[31,32] the 'Danish painters' syndrome' (from the early descriptions of the syndrome in Denmark), or the 'neurasthenic syndrome'. The disorder is characterized by headache, irritability, fatigue, dizziness and personality changes, with impaired concentration and memory. Studies in Scandinavia and the Netherlands have shown that chronic exposure to paints containing mixed solvents, of which xylene is the main component, have resulted in mood changes, effects on balance, fatigue, decreased nerve conduction and other neurophysiological and behavioural effects.[33] Studies of dockyard painters with heavy and prolonged exposure to paint solvents including xylene and methylethyl ketone, showed an excess of psychological and neurological symptoms.[34,35] However, these neurotoxic findings have not been replicated in other studies of painters or paint manufacturers.[36]

In rodent experiments, delayed fetal development has been found with inhalational exposure to xylene, and increased malformations after oral administration of high doses to mice. In a study of university laboratory employees exposed in the first trimester of pregnancy to a variety of solvents including xylene, miscarriage rates were slightly increased but not significantly different from pregnancies where no solvent exposure occurred.[37] There are no adequate epidemiological data confirming xylene to be a reproductive hazard in humans.[27]

Metabolism and monitoring

The main routes of systemic absorption from occupational exposures are by inhalation and through skin contact. The metabolic pathway for xylene involves primarily microsomal oxidation followed by glycine conjugation to produce methylhippuric acid in the urine.[38] Around 50% of absorbed xylene is rapidly cleared in 0.5–1 hour. There is some storage in body fat, and this component is metabolized at a slower rate.[39] Unlike hippuric acid which can appear in urine from sources other than toluene exposure, urinary methylhippuric acid is specific for exposure to xylene; hence its usefulness for biological monitoring. If a worker exposed to xylene has taken aspirin the methylhippuric acid concentration could be artefactually reduced as aspirin is also eliminated by glycine conjugation.[40] Alcohol consumption may also decrease the metabolic clearance of xylene leading to reduced excretion of urinary methylhippuric acid, although this may only occur with substantial alcohol consumption.[41] Both aspirin and alcohol consumption should be excluded when using urinary methylhippuric acid for biological monitoring of xylene exposure.

High performance liquid chromatography can separate the different isomeric forms of methylhippuric acid, which indicate the extent of exposure to the isomers of xylene.[42,43] When expressed as total methylhippuric acids in urine for an end-of-shift urine sample, a biological exposure index of 1.5 g/g creatinine has been suggested by the ACGIH for exposure to xylenes.[7] This correlates well with exposure to 100 ppm (the current ACGIH and HSE occupational exposure limit for xylene)[7,12] and moderate work activity.

STYRENE (VINYL BENZENE, PHENYLETHYLENE) ($CH_2CHC_6H_5$)

[CAS no. 100-42-5]

Styrene is a colourless to yellow fat-soluble and sparingly water-soluble liquid. It is used in the production of polymers (e.g. polystyrene), copolymers, and reinforced plastic products (e.g. fibre glass boats),[44] car parts, bathtubs (Fig. 12.3) and shower bases. In the production of glass reinforced plastics, styrene is used as a solvent. Resin is applied between layers of fibrous glass, and as the resin cures, the styrene vaporizes and can lead to exposures to styrene vapour of 100 ppm or more. Styrene is also an ingredient for producing plastics based on acrylonitrile-butadiene-styrene (ABS), and in styrene-butadiene rubber (SBR).[45]

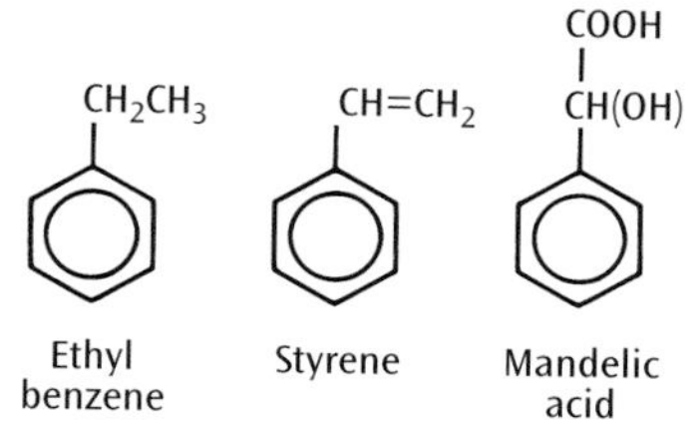

CH₂CH₃   CH=CH₂   COOH | CH(OH)

CH_2CH_3 $CH=CH_2$ $\begin{array}{c}COOH\\ |\\ CH(OH)\end{array}$

Ethyl benzene   Styrene   Mandelic acid

Figure 12.2 *Mandelic acid and its precursors.*

Clinical effects

Acute effects from exposure to styrene above 100 ppm are mucosal irritation, drowsiness, nausea and incoordination. Styrene has been reported to cause central nervous system depression and peripheral nerve damage, manifesting as electroencephalographic abnormalities and sensory nerve conduction deficit[46] (see Chapter 42). The acute behavioural effects of styrene may be related to the rate at which mandelic acid is cleared from the body.[47] Contradictory findings have been obtained in studies on possible neurobehavioural effects at low levels of exposure. Some studies indicate no acute effects that can impair vigilance at levels below 50 ppm,[48] (half the 1999 UK occupational exposure limit for styrene),[12] although minor impairment of performance in psychometric tests were noted. The clinical significance of such test findings is uncertain.

Styrene exposure has also been associated with chromosomal aberrations in peripheral lymphocytes, and is mutagenic following metabolic activation in laboratory studies. Although the IARC has classified styrene as a group-2B possible human carcinogen,[49] the epidemiological evidence for this is weak. There is also no good evidence for a teratogenic risk in man, nor of an increase in spontaneous abortions in exposed female workers.

Metabolism and monitoring

Styrene is absorbed mainly by inhalation; percutaneous absorption is not significant. A small amount (3%) of absorbed styrene is excreted unchanged in exhaled breath. Most of the styrene absorbed is metabolized in the liver via the cytochrome-P450 monooxygenase system to styrene-7,8 oxide. Further detoxification involves several biochemical mechanisms: hydrolysis, conversion by microsomal epoxide hydrolase to styrene glycol, and conjugation with glutathione.[50] The final metabolites are mandelic acid (up to 90%) and phenylglyoxylic acid (10%) which are both excreted in the urine. The amounts of the two urinary metabolites have been used in the biological monitoring of styrene-exposed individuals.[51,52]

For 1999, the ACGIH biological exposure indices (BEIs) for exposure to styrene are 800 mg of urinary mandelic acid/g creatinine for an end-of-shift urine sample; and 300 mg of urinary mandelic acid/g creatinine for a urine sample taken prior to the next shift. Using urinary phenylglyoxylic acid as an index for styrene exposure, the ACGIH BEIs are 240 mg/g creatinine at the end of shift; and 100 mg/g creatinine prior to the next shift. Styrene in blood has a BEI of 0.55 mg/litre at the end of shift, and 0.02 mg/litre prior to the next shift.[7]

Consumption of alcohol during the working day delays the excretion of mandelic acid, and so end-of-shift urine samples may be spuriously low in mandelic acid in such workers.[53]

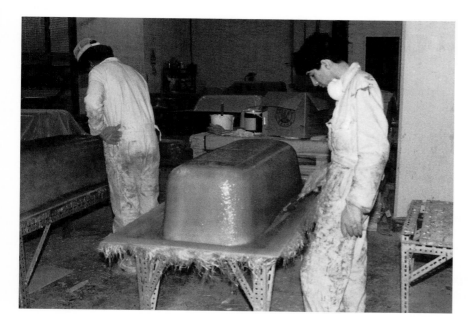

Figure 12.3 *Manufacture of bath tubs using glass fibre and resin containing styrene.*

ETHYL BENZENE (PHENYLETHANE) (CH₃CH₂C₆H₅)

[CAS no. 100-41-4]

Ethyl benzene is a colourless liquid with a sweet odour, and is produced from benzene and ethylene. Its odour threshold in air is about 2 mg/m³.[54] It is used mainly to manufacture styrene, and is also present in paint thinners, degreasing agents and some typewriting correction fluids.[55] The main source for ethyl benzene emission into the environment is from the use of fuel and solvents.

Clinical effects

The number of reports on the health effects from ethyl benzene exposure are limited. The agent is known to cause skin and mucosal irritation. While it is a solvent to which painters are exposed, its role in the development of the psycho-organic syndrome is uncertain (see p. 264). Like styrene, it is metabolized to mandelic acid and phenylglyoxylic acid,[56] and urinary levels of mandelic acid have been used for biological monitoring. Care must be exercised in the interpretation of urinary mandelic acid results where there is concomitant exposure to both styrene and ethyl benzene.

CUMENE (CUMOL 2-PHENYLPROPANE, ISOPROPYLBENZENE, 1-METHYLETHYL BENZENE) ((CH₃)₂CHC₆H₅)

[CAS no. 98-82-8]

Cumene is a colourless flammable liquid. It is used as a paint thinner, as acomponent in aviation fuel, in the perfume industry, and for styrene production. Animal studies and reports on adverse effects in man have shown it to cause respiratory tract irritation and central nervous system depression. Exposure to high concentrations cause headaches, dizziness, loss of coordination, and loss of consciousness.[57] However, there are no well documented toxic effects in occupationally exposed workers.[58]

Nitro-, amino- and chloro-derivatives of benzene or its homologues

Nitro- and amino-derivatives are easily absorbed via the skin and lungs and can cause methaemoglobinaemia and haemolytic anaemia.[59] Poisoning by nitro-, amino-, and chloro-derivatives of benzene or a homologue of benzene is a prescribed industrial disease in the UK (see Chapter 4).

Nitrobenzene [CAS no. 98-95-3] is used as a solvent, for refining, in lubricating oils, and as an ingredient in polishes, perfumes, and soaps. Most of the nitrobenzene used commercially is converted to aniline which is a starter chemical for production of other industrial products. In common with other organic solvents, it can cause mucosal irritation, dermatitis, and central nervous system depression.

p-Diaminobenzene (para-Phenylenediamine; [CAS no. 106-50-3]) is an ingredient in some hair dyes, and is used in dye manufacture and as a developer in photography. It is a well-recognized skin sensitizer and is a common cause of dermatitis in the dye trades. (see Chapter 37) Acute poisoning can result in hepatosplenomegaly, renal and respiratory effects, and death.[57]

Monochlorobenzene (benzene chloride) [CAS no. 108-90-7] exposure has been reported to cause headache, dizziness, stupor and difficulty with micturition. Isomers of dichlorobenzene, in particular 1,2-dichlorobenzene (o-dichlorobenzene) [CAS no. 95-50-1] cause mucosal and skin irritation, narcosis and central nervous system depression. The 1,3-isomer (m-dichlorobenzene) [CAS no. 541-73-1] has been detected as an environmental pollutant, and the 1,4- isomer (p-dichlorobenzene) reported to cause haematological effects following occupational exposure (see section below).

p-DICHLOROBENZENE (1,4-DICHLOROBENZENE) (C₆H₄Cl₂)

[CAS no. 106-46-7]

p-Dichlorobenzene is used as an insecticide and disinfectant. Workers exposed to p-dichlorobenzene at levels in air of 50–80 ppm may suffer eye and nasal irritation, but tolerance develops with repeated exposures. Case reports have referred to purpura and various haematological effects in heavily exposed workers. These effects include methaemoglobinaemia, lymphocytopenia and thrombocytopenia. Haemolytic anaemia has occurred following ingestion of p-dichlorobenzene. Other less common effects are jaundice and cirrhosis following acute liver injury, and cerebellar ataxia.[60]

HEXACHLOROBENZENE (PERCHLOROBENZENE) (C₆Cl₆)

[CAS no. 118-74-1]

Hexachlorobenzene and other polyhalogenated aromatic compounds induce porphyria in man and animals by inhibiting uroporphyrinogen decarboxylase. Hexachlorobenzene gained notoriety in Turkey in the 1950s when its use as a fungicidal seed dressing led to contamination of a supply of wheat for bread, causing an outbreak of acquired porphyria.

Affected individuals suffered dermal photosensitivity with hyperpigmentation, skin bullae and hypertrichosis as well as hepatomegaly and porphyrinuria. In all, 10% of these patients succumbed to the poisoning, and there was also a high mortality rate among infants of poisoned mothers. Other clinical effects were neuropsychiatric symptoms, extrapyramidal signs, and sensory neuropathy with reduced muscle tone and weakness.[61] There are no reports of occupational exposures causing similar health effects. The main current concerns centre around the possible long-term effects of this compound which like the polychlorinated biphenyls persist in the environment.[62] Hexachlorobenzene has been shown to be carcinogenic in rodents, but there is no evidence of increased malignancy in those affected by the contaminated bread incident in Turkey.

Acquired hepatic porphyria

The porphyrias are a group of disorders with congenital or acquired abnormalities in porphyrin metabolism. Porphyrins are pigments with a structure based on four pyrrole rings linked by methylene bridges, and are normally present in haemoglobin, myoglobin and cytochromes.

Porphyrias have been classified into hepatic and erythropoietic porphyrias based on the major site of abnormal porphyrin production, and into acute and non-acute porphyrias based on the clinical presentation. The form of porphyria due to hexachlorobenzene poisoning was a non-acute hepatic porphyria with cutaneous manifestations (porphyria cutanea tarda). The main clinical features were liver function abnormalities and other indicators of liver damage, photosensitivity, and abnormal porphyrin biochemistry.

In addition to hexachlorobenzene, forms of hepatic porphyria have also been described following exposure to vinyl chloride, some halogenated biphenyls, chlorinated naphthalenes, and organophosphorus and organochlorine pesticides[63] (see Chapter 43).

AROMATIC AMINES

Aromatic amines or arylamines are aromatic hydrocarbons where one or more hydrogen atoms are replaced by amino (-NH_2) groups. They include anilines and phenylenediamines, benzidines, naphthylamines, and aminoazobenzenes.[64]

ANILINE (BENZENAMINE, PHENYLAMINE, AMINOBENZENE) ($C_6H_5NH_2$)

[CAS no. 62-53-3]

Aniline is an oily, colourless liquid used as a starter material for the synthesis of dyes, rubber accelerators and antioxidants, drugs, photographic chemicals, herbicides and fungicides. It is a recognized cause of methaemoglobinaemia.

o-TOLUIDINE (2-METHYLBENZENAMINE, 2-AMINOTOLUENE, 2-METHYLANILINE) ($CH_3C_6H_4NH_2$)

[CAS no. 95-53-4]

o-Toluidine is a light yellow liquid which rapidly darkens on exposure to light and air. It is used mainly as an inter-mediate in the manufacture of dyes, rubber chemicals, pharmaceuticals and pesticides. o-Toluidine is also a known cause of methaemoglobinaemia. It can cause microscopic haematuria, probably from renal damage rather than from bladder abnormalities. Neoplasms have been produced at various sites in rodent studies and there are case reports of bladder tumours in workers primarily exposed to o-toluidine and excess bladder tumours in groups of workers exposed to a number of dyestuffs which included o-toluidine. The IARC designated it as a group 2B (*possibly carcinogenic to humans*) carcinogen in 1987. ACGIH has categorized it as a group A3 carcinogen (*confirmed animal carcinogen with unknown relevance to humans*).[7] The UK Health and Safety Executive has designated o-toluidine as a carcinogen and assigned it a maximum exposure limit of 0.2 ppm (0.89 mg/m³).[12]

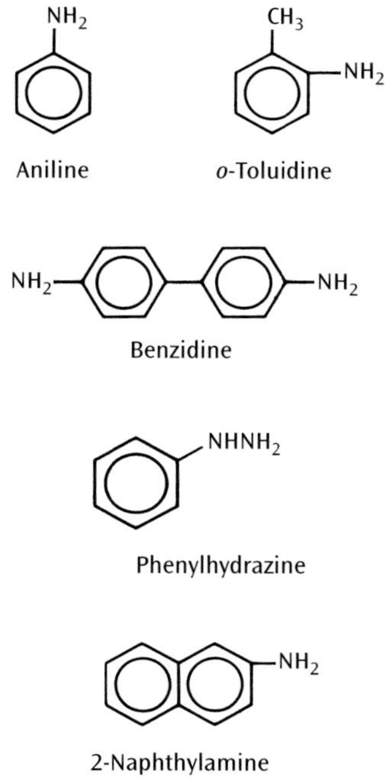

Figure 12.4 *Aniline; o-toluidine; benzidine; phenylhydrazine; 2-naphthylamine.*

BENZIDINE ($NH_2C_6H_4C_6H_4NH_2$)

[CAS no. 92-87-5]

Benzidine is a white or slightly reddish crystalline material which darkens on exposure to light and air. It can be absorbed by inhalation, ingestion, and through the skin. The main use of benzidine was in the production of dyestuffs, and as a laboratory reagent. Benzidine is a recognized human bladder carcinogen (see Chapter 39), and regulated in most countries as one (see Chapter 4).

PHENYLHYDRAZINE ($C_6H_8N_2$)

[CAS no. 100-63-0]

Phenylhydrazine is produced commercially from aniline through an azo intermediate compound. It is used to produce pharmaceuticals, agrochemicals, and photographic chemicals. Case reports of incidents involving splashes onto the skin of workers indicated a potential for causing haemolysis. Affected workers had reduced haemoglobin and erythrocyte counts, and in one case there was methaemoglobinaemia and haemolytic jaundice. Skin effects from contact with the hydrochloride include acute irritation, papules and bullae, and skin sensitization.[65]

2-NAPHTHYLAMINE (β-NAPHTHYLAMINE) ($C_{10}H_7NH_2$)

[CAS no. 91-59-8]

2-Naphthylamine (β-naphthylamine) is a white-to-reddish crystalline compound that has little commercial usage today, mainly because of it being associated with bladder cancer in humans (see Chapter 39). It was previously present in dyestuffs, as a contaminant in the manufacture of rubber tyres, and used as a reagent in research laboratories.

Methaemoglobinaemia

Over 600 episodes of occupationally induced methaemoglobinaemia have been published in the scientific literature.[66] Aromatic compounds were responsible for 88% of these episodes, with 3% being due to aliphatic compounds, 7% due to inorganic chemicals, and 2% from unidentified chemicals. The main biochemical change in methaemoglobinaemia is the oxidation of the iron in haem from the ferrous state to the ferric. In ferric form, the oxygen-carrying capacity of haem is diminished. Under normal circumstances about 1% of haemoglobin is present as methaemoglobin. Reduced nicotinamide adenine dinucleotide ($NADH_2$) and its phosphate ($NADPH_2$) and reduced glutathione help to maintain most of the haemoglobin in reduced form.

Methaemoglobinaemia can arise from an inherited deficiency of methaemoglobin reductase (autosomal recessive) or as an inherited abnormal haemoglobin M (autosomal dominant). These inherited disorders are uncommon, and it would be reasonable to advise affected individuals and their employers regarding placement in jobs with occupational exposure to chemical agents capable of causing methaemoglobinaemia. Exposure to these chemical agents could aggravate the pre-existing haemoglobinopathy.

Chemicals that can cause methaemoglobinaemia include aniline, nitrobenzene, naphthalene, nitroglycerin, p-dichlorobenzene, nitrites, chlorates, quinones, and other nitro- and amino-organic compounds. Among the more potent inducers of methaemoglobin are phenylhydroxylamine, p-dinitrobenzene, m-dinitrobenzene, o-aminophenol, and nitrosobenzene. Exposure to nitric oxide and nitrogen dioxide can lead to methaemoglobin formation. Drugs known to cause methaemoglobinaemia following ingestion include amyl nitrite, phenacetin, primaquine, dapsone, and sulphanilamide.

The main clinical manifestation is cyanosis – most noticeable in the face and fingernails, with symptoms of respiratory distress, throbbing headaches, dizziness and muscle weakness. Symptoms are related to the degree of methaemoglobinaemia and its speed of onset. In more serious cases, there is marked cyanosis with nausea, vomiting, colic and collapse. Symptoms usually occur at methaemoglobin levels of more than 15%. Heinz bodies in erythrocytes, diffuse or punctate polychromasia, and other features of anaemia are seen in peripheral blood films of patients with methaemoglobinaemia.

Treatment involves the slow intravenous administration of methylene blue (1% solution) using a dose of 75–100 mg administered over 5 minutes. A further dose can be given if cyanosis persists after an hour of the initial dose. The basis for using methylene blue is to introduce a reducing agent to convert the oxidized iron in haem back to its ferrous state. Ascorbic acid has also been used as an antidote, either administered alone or in conjunction with methylene blue. The reducing agent is given in addition to general supportive measures such as oxygen therapy, removal of contaminated clothes, and cleaning of contaminated areas of skin. Caution must be exercised in the administration of methylene blue because excessive amounts may aggravate methaemoglobinaemia, and it can cause haemolysis especially in those with glucose-6-phosphate dehydrogenase (G6PD) deficiency.[67] The total dose of methylene blue given should not exceed 7 mg/kg body weight. Features of excessive methylene blue include dyspnoea, restlessness, chest pain, and reduced R waves and flattened or inverted T waves in the electrocardiogram.

Sulphaemoglobinaemia

Sulphaemoglobin is a blood pigment that has some similarities to methaemoglobin – the presence of either leads to cyanosis. Both can be formed following exposure to chemicals such as naphthalene and oxidant drugs such as phenacetin and acetanilide. Sulphaemoglobin is also associated with abnormal haemoglobin, e.g. haemoglobin M, and G6PD deficiency. Unlike methaemoglobin, sulphaemoglobin is not reversed in the presence of cyanide or by the administration of reducing agents. It is only reversible by the progressive replacement of the affected red cells at the normal rate. Thus sulphaemoglobin disappears steadily over a period of weeks and months rather than days. It can also be produced *in vitro* from reacting hydrogen sulphide and oxyhaemoglobin. However, it is not formed *in vivo* in hydrogen sulphide poisoning. The pigment is often formed in the absence of any exposure to exogenous sources of sulphur, hence it has been suggested that it might be better termed 'pseudosulphaemoglobin'.

Occupational bladder tumours from aromatic amines

Rehn in 1895 described the first cases of occupational bladder cancers in workers making aniline-based synthetic dyes (see Chapter 39). These workers were exposed to compounds such as benzidine and 2-naphthylamine. Hueper in 1938 induced bladder tumours in dogs by prolonged oral administration of 2-naphthylamine. This chemical was also present as a contaminant in antioxidants employed as compounding ingredients in the rubber tyre industry. The relevant antioxidants were Nonox 'S' and Agerite resin, and both were withdrawn from use in Great Britain in 1949. The 'at-risk' areas for exposure to these agents included stores, compounding, mixing and milling, calendering, and inner-tube manufacture.[68] Following its description as a cause of bladder tumours, 2-naphthylamine was prohibited in many countries. In the UK it was designated a prohibited carcinogenic substance under the Carcinogenic Substances Regulations 1967 which were superseded by the Control of Substances Hazardous to Health regulations, 1988 (COSHH). Its accompanying Carcinogens Approved Code of Practice prohibits the 'manufacture and use, including any process resulting in the formation of 2-naphthylamine, benzidine, 4-aminodiphenyl, 4-nitrodiphenyl and their salts and any substance containing any of these compounds in a total concentration greater than 0.1%'. The importation of these four compounds is also prohibited. However, their presence as a contaminant in amounts less than 0.1% concentration is still technically permitted if that occurs as a chemical reaction byproduct.[69]

Medical surveillance is required under the UK COSHH regulations for exposure to aromatic amines which were listed in the 'controlled substances' part of the Carcinogenic Substances Regulations 1967. These substances are 1-naphthylamine, *o*-toluidine, dianisidine, dichlorobenzidine and their salts in processes involving manufacture, formation, or use of these substances. Two other dyes which meet the requirement for medical surveillance are auramine and magenta in processes that involve their manufacture only.

Urothelial tumours of occupational origin are prescribed for benefits in the UK and there is available guidance to urologists and other physicians on the detection and reporting of such cases.[70] For compensation for a primary neoplasm (including papilloma, carcinoma *in situ* and invasive carcinoma) of the epithelial lining of the urinary tract (renal pelvis, ureter, bladder, and urethra) under the Prescribed Diseases regulations, there must have been occupational exposure to substances including 1-naphthylamine, 2-naphthylamine, or methylene-bis-orthochloroaniline, benzidine or a diphenyl substituted by at least one nitro or primary amino group, auramine or magenta (see Chapter 4). For auramine and magenta, prescription is limited to the manufacture but not the use of these compounds. The maintenance or cleaning of plant or machinery or cleaning of contaminated clothing may constitute relevant exposure. There is evidence suggesting that pure 1-naphthylamine is not a carcinogen. Previous descriptions of bladder cancer cases in those exposed to commercial 1-naphthylamine could be due to the presence of 2-naphthylamine as an impurity.[71]

The term 'aniline tumours' was first used because of the initial suspicion of aniline as the carcinogen, though this view was later not substantiated. Aniline itself was not thought to be carcinogenic.[72] However, a 1991 retrospective cohort study of bladder cancer at a chemical plant producing an antioxidant for tyre manufacture showed an excess of bladder cancer in workers exposed to both *o*-toluidine and aniline. It was suggested that as *o*-toluidine was the more potent animal carcinogen, it was more likely to be the implicated carcinogen.[73] This view was reinforced by a further study involving monitoring of aromatic amine exposure by personal air sampling and by measurement of aromatic amine-haemoglobin adducts in workers from the same plant.[74] Post-shift urinary *o*-toluidine levels were also higher in exposed workers compared to controls. Though structurally similar to 2-naphthylamine, there is no evidence suggesting that other isomers of toluidine (*m*- and *p*-toluidine) are human bladder carcinogens.

Cigarette smoking is a risk factor for bladder tumours. Other occupational groups where associations with bladder tumours have been described, and where there have been previous documented exposures to carcinogenic aromatic amines are rubber workers[75] those in gas, coke, printing, and textile industries, chemical manufacture, aluminium refining, machinists, and hair dressers.[76] Exposure to traces of 2-naphthylamine occurred in the 1950s in rodent operators using a rat poison containing 1-naphthylthiourea (trade name ANTU).

The latent period between initial exposure to occupational bladder carcinogens and the subsequent development of malignancy is on average 25 years.[70] Systems for health surveillance of workers exposed to bladder carcinogens have included periodic urine examination for microscopic haematuria and cytology. Staining of cells with a Papanicolaou stain and looking for features of malignancy have formed the basis of early detection of bladder tumours. Periodic cystoscopy, once widely used, has been largely discontinued due to the practical difficulty of continuing such a programme and the discomfort of the procedure. It is uncertain whether these screening procedures lead to any improvement in survival time for those cases of bladder cancer detected early. The value of screening programmes for bladder cancer has not been adequately evaluated.[77,78] Continuing health surveillance for workers who have left a plant could present some practical difficulties, particularly if they move to an area distant from the worksite. In the UK difficulties with continuing surveillance have been overcome by coordination between the plant occupational health departments, the workers' general practitioners, the British Rubber Manufacturers Association, and the Employment Medical Advisory Service of the Health and Safety Executive.

Occupational dermatitis from aromatic amines

Many of the primary amines cause irritant contact dermatitis because of their alkaline properties. Allergic dermatitis also follows contact with aromatic amines, one of the best examples being dyes, rubber products and other formulations containing p-phenylenediamine. This causes a delayed hypersensitivity reaction (type IV allergy) which can be detected by skin patch testing (see Chapter 37). There is cross-reaction between p-phenylenediamine and other anilines and benzidines. m-Phenylenediamine used as a curing agent for epoxy resins also causes both irritant and allergic contact dermatitis. Rubber gloves made using phenylenediamine derivatives as antioxidants may cause or worsen dermatitis instead of offering skin protection (see Chapter 37).

4,4′-METHYLENEDIANILINE (DIAMINODIPHENYLMETHANE) ($NH_2C_6H_4CH_2C_6H_4NH_2$)

[CAS no. 2644-71-9]

The Epping jaundice incident occurred in Epping, Essex, in 1965 and was due to mass exposure to bread contaminated with 4,4′methylenedianiline (MDA).[79] This aromatic amine had contaminated a bag of baking flour when it was being transported to the bakery in a van. Eighty-four individuals who ate bread made from the contaminated flour developed cholestatic jaundice. Liver biopsy revealed a characteristic histological picture with portal inflammation, eosinophilic infiltration, cholangitis, and cholestasis.[80] The jaundice was reversible on recovery. An attempt to trace the individuals affected resulted in documentation of 18 deaths among 68 individuals successfully traced.[81] There was a single death from cancer of the biliary tract, and no other hepatobiliary causes of death. Four of the individuals traced had experienced further episodes of jaundice, although there

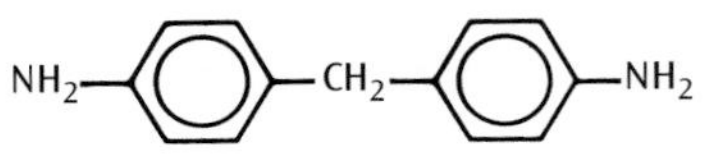

Figure 12.5 *4,4′Methylenedianiline.*

was a suggestion that this may not be related to the earlier exposure to MDA.

Occupational exposure to MDA resulting in acute toxic hepatitis has been reported following its use as an epoxy resin hardener in the manufacture of insulating material.[82] Skin absorption was thought to be the major route of entry. The affected workers had severe right upper abdominal pain, high fever, chills and jaundice. There was no evidence of chronic liver disease as a sequel. Complete recovery with normal liver function tests was documented within 7 weeks.

4,4′-METHYLENE *bis*(2-CHLOROANILINE) (MbOCA) ($CH_2(C_6H_3ClNH_2)_2$)

[CAS no. 27342-75-2]

MbOCA is an aromatic amino compound used as a curing agent for epoxy-resin bonding systems, in the manufacture of rigid plastic car mouldings, and for the manufacture of polyurethane foam. It is used in the form of a pure powder or a liquid, and can be absorbed systemically through the skin and the respiratory tract. Oral administration in rodent experiments has resulted in liver and lung tumours, and dogs fed MbOCA developed transitional cell carcinomas of the bladder. Mutagenicity tests showed MbOCA or its metabolites to cause genetic damage in a variety of organisms. There have been clinical case reports of bladder cancer in MbOCA exposed young male non-smokers,[83] This is a prescribed disease in the UK (see Chapter 4). Exposure to MbOCA results in detectable urinary levels of free MbOCA and its N-acetyl metabolites.[84] Detection of these compounds in the urine is a method for biological monitoring.[85] However, no biological exposure index has yet been set by the ACGIH, as they considered the current available data insufficient.[7] The Health and Safety Executive in the UK has produced a benchmark guidance value for biological monitoring of MbOCA-exposed workers, and this is set at 15 μmol total MbOCA/mol creatinine in post-shift urine.[12] Benchmark guidance values are not health-based but represent practicable, achievable values based on monitoring at workplaces with good occupational hygiene practices.[12]

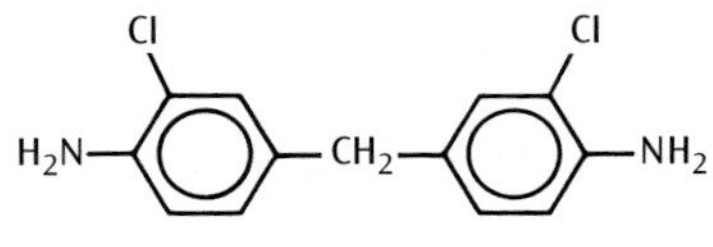

Figure 12.6 *MbOCA.*

PHENOL AND PHENOL DERIVATIVES

PHENOL (CARBOLIC ACID) (C₆H₅OH)

[CAS no. 108-95-2]

Phenol is used in disinfectants, glues and resins, paints and paint removers, as an ingredient of antiseptic medicines, in wood preservation, in laboratories, and in rubber, plastics, and explosives. Its germicidal properties were first shown by Lister in 1867. It denatures protein and is an irritant to the skin and mucous membranes. Solutions of more than 5% concentration are corrosive to the skin. Phenol produces effects on the central nervous system, liver and kidneys when absorbed through the skin, lungs and gastrointestinal tract. Phenol vapours and aerosols are readily absorbed through the lungs.

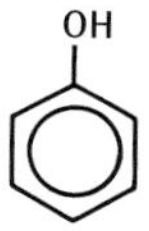

Figure 12.7 *Phenol.*

Splashes on the skin lead to deep skin burns and gangrene without vesiculation, but these may go unnoticed because of a local anaesthetic effect of phenol. The affected area of skin becomes white and opaque. There may be a grey white slough and, after prolonged contact, necrosis of subcutaneous tissue. Management of phenol splashes consists of removal of contaminated clothing, and swabbing the skin with cotton wool soaked in glycerol, polyethylene glycol, or isopropyl alcohol.[86] Application of a polyethylene glycol/methylated spirit mixture for at least 10 minutes is also effective.[87] Immediate and repeated application of polyethylene glycol and silver sulphadiazine has been used successfully for phenol burns.[88] Prompt removal of contaminated clothing is important because sufficient amounts of phenol may be retained in clothing to cause systemic absorption, leading to death. First-aiders should use gloves and avoid any direct contact with phenol.

Acute systemic poisoning leads to cardiorespiratory collapse presenting as cyanosis, dyspnoea, loss of consciousness and death. Other effects are muscle weakness, reduced reflexes, convulsions, altered body temperature and pulse rate. Chronic phenol poisoning is unlikely from current usage, though it was a problem in healthcare workers in the days of antiseptic surgery when phenol was sprayed in the air during surgical procedures. Phenol is excreted in the urine unchanged or as conjugated phenol metabolites (sulphates and glucuronides). These metabolites can result from exposure to both phenol and benzene.

Following incidents involving environmental contamination of drinking water by phenol, symptoms reported by those who consumed the contaminated water were mainly gastrointestinal.[89] These included diarrhoea, mouth sores, dark urine, and burning of the mouth.[90] Follow-up of some of the affected individuals indicated no residual health effects 6 months later.

Other phenol derivatives

Phenol-based compounds include a wide range of chemicals including catechols, hydroquinone, butyl and amyl phenols – all of which can cause leucoderma (vitiligo; see p. 272). In addition, derivatives of some of the substituted phenols such as *p*-tert-butylphenol used in shoe adhesives, and *p*-tert-butylcatechol used in some paints, rubber, and plastics products can also cause occupational irritant and allergic dermatitis.[91,92]

Nitroderivatives of phenol include dinitrophenol (DNP) and dinitro-*o*-cresol (DNOC), both of which exists as several isomers. DNP is used in explosives, dyestuffs, photograph developers and wood preservatives and DNOC is a herbicide, and was used as a weight loss agent until this was discontinued because of the side-effects experienced. These compounds can all affect mitochondrial oxidative phosphorylation (see p. 272). Thymol, menthol and hexachlorophene are used in medicinal preparations. Creosote is a timber preservative and is a mixture of phenolic compounds.

Chlorophenols are used as fungicides, in wood preservatives and in the production of phenoxyherbicides.

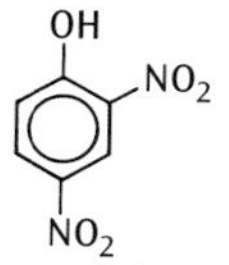

Figure 12.8 *2,4-Dinitrophenol; 4,6-dinitro-o-cresol; pentachlorophenol.*

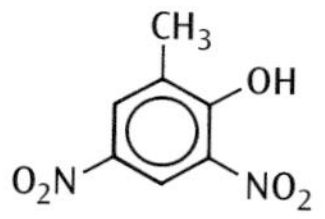

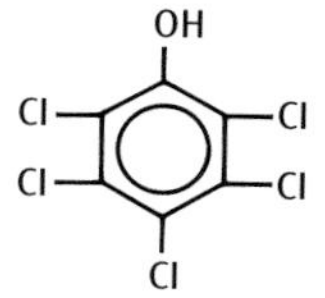

There is a suspected link between chlorophenol exposure and non-Hodgkins lymphoma and Hodgkin's disease, although the evidence is inconsistent[93,94] (see Chapter 4). For Hodgkin's disease, the evidence is better for a causative link with Epstein–Barr virus infection than following occupational exposure to chemicals.[95] Pentachlorophenol is a chlorinated phenolic compound used as a pesticide. It is rapidly absorbed through the skin and acts similarly to DNP and DNOC in affecting oxidative phosphorylation.

Occupational leucoderma

Occupational leucoderma (see Chapter 37) (occupational vitiligo) refers to depigmentation of the skin following contact with chemicals in the work environment. These chemicals include catechols such as methyl catechol, pyrocatechol, 4-isopropyl catechol, and *p*-tert-butyl catechol. Phenol derivatives causing similar depigmentation are *p*-tert-butylphenol, *p*-amyl phenol, *o*-phenylphenol, and chloro-2 amino-4 phenol. Another depigmenting agent hydroquinone is used as a photographic developer and as an antioxidant in paints and fuels, and in the manufacture of dyes.

Occupational leucoderma usually presents as hypopigmented and depigmented patches on the exposed areas of the forearms and hands. The occurrence of these lesions is related to the duration and intensity of exposure to the compounds mentioned, causing damage to melanocytes. The affected areas can be mottled, patchy, confluent or symmetrical. Exposure to bright sunlight may occasionally cause redness, irritation and pain. Removal from exposure can lead to a slow repigmentation.

Clinically, occupational leucoderma is indistinguishable from non-occupational vitiligo. Non-occupational causes of skin depigmentation should be considered in the differential diagnosis. The relevant conditions include use of steroid preparations on the skin, autoimmune disorders, and idiopathic cases which are more commonly seen in females of dark skin complexion. Occupational vitiligo is a prescribed occupational disease in the UK[59] (see Chapter 4).

Uncoupling oxidative phosphorylation

Oxidative phosphorylation is a mitochondrial process by which cells produce adenosine triphosphate (ATP) from adenosine diphosphate (ADP). This is part of cellular energy transfer which involves a chain of intracellular electron carriers and enzymes. DNP, DNOC and pentachlorophenol act by uncoupling the chain of oxidative phosphorylation. This results in blocking the phosphorylation of ADP. The energy generated is dissipated by an increase in metabolic rate. Hence, in systemic poisoning by these compounds, hyperthermia, tachycardia, tachyp-

noea, prolific sweating and rapid dehydration are common.[96] Hepatic and renal damage may follow, leading to coma and death.

FUSED RING AROMATIC COMPOUNDS

These consist of two or more fused benzene rings. Examples are naphthalene (two fused benzene rings), anthracene and phenanthrene (both with three fused rings), naphthacene and 1,2-benzanthracene (with four fused rings), and 1,2-benzpyrene or benzo[a]pyrene (with five fused benzene rings). Those with several fused rings are also referred to as polycyclic aromatic hydrocarbons (PAHs). Benzo[a]pyrene is a PAH present in polluted urban atmospheres, in cigarette smoke, and from combustion of coal. It has been identified as an experimental carcinogen.

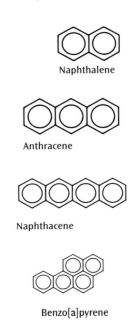

Naphthalene

Anthracene

Naphthacene

Benzo[a]pyrene

Figure 12.9 *Naphthalene; anthracene; naphthacene; benzo[a]-pyrene.*

NAPHTHALENE ($C_{10}H_8$)

[CAS no. 91-20-3]

Naphthalene is a white solid at ambient temperature. As it has a moderately high vapour pressure, it volatilises easily to produce a characteristic pungent odour. It is a starter material for the manufacture of phthalic anhydride – a component of epoxy-resins, and in the production of azo dyes. It is also used in the synthesis of biocides in the wood industry, and as a moth repellent in 'mothballs'. Naphthalene is a major constituent of creosote – which has applications in timber treatment.

Alkyl naphthalenes are present in carbon paper. Chlorinated naphthalene is used as a synthetic insulating wax.

Naphthalene can precipitate haemolysis in individuals with glucose-6-phosphate dehydrogenase (G6PD) deficiency. This may follow contact with naphthalene-impregnated clothing or via inhalation of the vapour. Apart from exposure to naphthalene, ingestion of broad beans and antimalarial drugs such as primaquine, chloroquine and quinine can also cause haemolysis in such individuals. G6PD deficiency is a common red cell enzyme defect which is genetically determined and is prevalent in Oriental, Afro-Caribbean, and Mediterranean populations. Workers with this enzyme defect should be counselled regarding occupational exposure to naphthalene and other oxidizing agents capable of precipitating acute haemolysis. It has been suggested that workers with the A-variant of G6PD deficiency should not be excluded from work involving exposure to oxidant gases such as ozone and nitrogen dioxide, as the levels of these gases need to be considerable before haematological effects occur.[97]

Chlorinated naphthalene when heated volatilizes and produces fumes or particles which may be inhaled or which can come into contact with exposed skin. Clinical effects include chloracne and focal liver damage resulting in acute necrosis and jaundice. Acute yellow atrophy of the liver and death may occur. Simultaneous exposure to carbon tetrachloride fumes increases the likelihood of liver damage[59] (see Chapter 43). Poisoning by chlorinated naphthalene is a prescribed disease (Chapter 41) in the UK, although the occurrence of this condition is now rare.

Polycyclic aromatic hydrocarbons (PAHs)

These compounds often referred to as PAHs or PNAs (polynuclear aromatics) cause cancer in experimental animals. Dibenz[a,h]anthracene was the earliest PAH to be shown to be an animal carcinogen. Benzo[a]pyrene was the first pure carcinogen to be isolated from coal tar by Cook in 1933.[98,99] PAHs are formed from the incomplete combustion of organic material, as an ingredient in cigarette smoke, in exhaust fumes, and forest fires.

Because of their low vapour pressures, some PAHs are present at ambient temperatures both as a gas and associated with particles. The lighter PAHs, such as phenanthrene, are found almost exclusively in the gas phase: the heavier PAHs, such as benzo[a]pyrene, are almost totally adsorbed onto particles. Whether as gases or adsorbed onto particles they are inhaled into the lungs. Exposure of humans to single PAHs does not occur because these chemicals are always encountered as complex mixtures containing many different PAH constituents. The best monitoring approach is still to regard benz[a]pyrene as a marker for the carcinogenic potential of the total PAH

mixture. The designation of any single chemical as a human carcinogen is difficult, but the three potent animal carcinogens benzo[a]pyrene, benz[a]anthracene and dibenz[a,h]anthracene are classified as 'probably carcinogenic to humans' by the IARC (see Chapter 39).

Occupational exposure to PAHs occurs in gas production, coke oven work, use of coal tar in roofing, from bitumen and asphalt in road paving, and in the production of graphite from pitch. Epidemiological studies of coke oven workers have shown an increased risk of lung and urothelial cancers. Unrefined mineral oils have a high aromatic hydrocarbon content, and chronic direct skin contact with such oils has caused scrotal cancer. Solvent refining, oleum treatment and hydrotreatment of these oils in metalworking fluids have reduced their aromatic hydrocarbon content which, together with increased awareness of the hazards and improved personal and work hygiene, has led to the reduction of the risk.[100]

Detection of metabolites of PAHs in the urine have indicated a possibility for biological monitoring. The main metabolite is 1-hydroxypyrene. Excretion of this metabolite is increased in workers exposed to PAHs in bitumen fumes. While levels of the metabolite in urine can indicate the extent of exposure to PAHs, the relationship to genotoxic effects in those exposed is unclear. Findings from various studies have been inconsistent.[101–103]

OTHER AROMATIC COMPOUNDS

POLYCHLORINATED BIPHENYLS

[CAS no. 1336-36-3]

Polychlorinated biphenyls (PCBs), chlorinated dioxins (PCDDs), chlorinated dibenzofurans (PCDFs), and polychlorinated quarterphenyls (PCQs) are related compounds based on the biphenyl moeity.

Different isomers of PCBs are produced by the chlorination of biphenyl; there are over 200 possible isomers. The extent of chlorination affects the resistance to temperature, high chemical stability, and electrical resistance – hence the use of PCBs as a heat insulator medium in heavy-duty electric transformers and capacitors. In the UK they are only allowed in some hydraulic mining machinery, and some electrical and heating equipment. PCBs are difficult to destroy; natural degradation is slow and they therefore persist in the environment for many years. Together with sufficient evidence for liver tumours in rodents, and limited evidence for carcinogenicity of

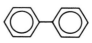

Figure 12.10 Unsubstituted biphenyl.

PCBs in humans[49] this is part of the reason for concerns regarding the fate of such chemicals in the environment.

Occupational exposure to PCBs have been documented in transformer fires when firefighters were at risk, and from leaks from capacitors and transformers whilst being stored, repaired, maintained or transported. Following exposure and absorption, PCBs accumulate in body fat and will persist in the body for long periods. Clinical effects include chloracne and liver function abnormalities. Chloracne is a refractory follicular dermatosis caused by a range of halogenated aromatic compounds including polyhalogenated naphthalenes, biphenyls and dibenzofurans, dioxins, and contaminants of 3,4-dichloroaniline (see also Chapter 37). There is a suggestion of an increased risk of hepatobiliary cancers in humans from PCB exposure.[49]

Workers who have had inadvertent exposure to PCBs can have PCB levels measured in serum and, if necessary, in adipose tissue. This will only confirm that exposure to PCBs has occurred. There are continuing difficulties with the current laboratory methods used, and part of this is related to the attempt at detecting small amounts of the chemical in the biological sample (measured in parts per million or parts per billion). Although laboratory analytical methods for these compounds are available to quantify levels as low as several parts per trillion, the risk to health related to the detection of such low levels in biological samples is unknown. Caution should be exercised before proceeding with determination of PCB levels in blood or adipose tissue as a routine occupational health procedure, or even in the investigation of an incident involving exposure to PCBs.

PCBs are no longer manufactured for commercial purposes. The oil used in electrical equipment has also been replaced by less toxic insulating fluids.

Yusho incident

An accident in the production of rice oil in a factory in southern Japan in 1968 led to the contamination of the oil with Kanechlor 400. This compound contains PCB and it was used as a medium for heat transfer in the production process. About 10 000 people were affected after consuming the oil. The clinical manifestations included chloracne, meibomian gland hypersecretion, skin pigmentation and liver damage with hypercholesterolaemia.

In 1979 a similar incident involving contaminated rice bran oil in central Taiwan led to a further outbreak of what is now known as Yusho, or 'rice oil' disease.[104] Analysis of the contaminated oil in both incidents showed the presence of PCDFs and PCQs. The health effects were almost certainly the result of exposure to these more toxic contaminants of the PCBs rather than the PCBs themselves. Studies of the infants born to mothers exposed to PCBs indicated that the effects on offspring included transient hyperpigmentation, and subsequent abnormalities of growth and development. These two incidents have shown that PCBs and their toxic contaminants are teratogenic.

TCDD (2,3,7,8-tetrachlorodibenzo-p-dioxin) ($C_{12}H_4Cl_4$)

[CAS no. 1746-01-6]

TCDD is often referred to as dioxin. It is an animal carcinogen and teratogen and may be produced as a toxic byproduct in the manufacture of certain defoliant herbicides produced from 2,4,5-trichlorophenol. One of the most widely used of these phenoxyacetic acid herbicides in the last 40 years has been 2,4,5-T (2,4,5-trichlorophenoxyacetic acid). The herbicide mixture called Agent Orange, which was used as a defoliant by the US Military in the Vietnam war, contained 2,4,5-T and 2,4-D (2,4-dichlorophenoxyacetic acid). Claims by US veterans that health problems and birth defects in their offspring had been caused by exposure to dioxin in Agent Orange have not been fully substantiated by epidemiological studies.

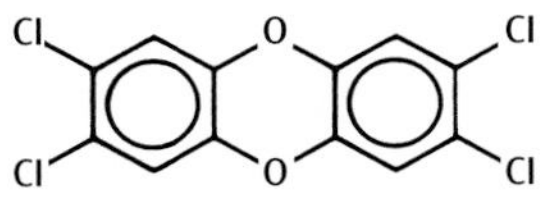

Figure 12.11 *2,3,7,8-Tetrachlorodibenzo-p-dioxin (TCDD).*

Dioxin gained further notoriety in the Seveso incident in Italy in 1976 when the exothermic reaction in the synthesis of 2,4,5 trichlorophenol at the Icmesa factory went out of control. There was a release of 1.3 kg of TCDD in a chemical cloud over a wide geographical area near the town of Seveso. Several similar industrial accidents have exposed workers to dioxin in other 2,4,5-trichlorophenol plants around the world.

The clinical effects observed in exposed workers include chloracne, peripheral neuropathy, hepatic damage, hypercholesterolaemia and hepatic porphyria (see Chapter 43). Despite the enormous publicity surrounding the Seveso incident, the death of many birds and animals, and the fears of long-term health effects, the only substantiated acute human health effect in the community was chloracne in a group of 178 children. Concerns that dioxin may be a human carcinogen[105–107] were confirmed by the IRAC in 1997, based largely on an excess of all cancers combined in four highly exposed industrial cohorts.[108,109] In an epidemiological study involving a large international cohort of workers exposed to phenoxy herbicides, including some contaminated with dioxin, there was a small excess of soft-tissue sarcomas and non-Hodgkins lymphoma. The excesses were however not statistically significant.[110] Follow-up of a group of individuals with chloracne from the Seveso incident showed reversal of the acne and no significant persistence of hepatic or neurological function deficit several years after the incident.[111]

A 10-year mortality study[112] revealed an increased occurrence of cardiovascular diseases that might be related to stressors caused by the disaster. Increased risks of leukaemia in men and hepatobiliary cancer were found. The incidence of multiple myeloma and soft tissue sarcomas was also raised.

In early 1999, an incident in Belgium involving contamination of animal feed with dioxin led to the withdrawal of poultry, pork, beef, eggs and egg products from farm animals fed with the contaminated material. This caused several countries to impose restrictions on the supply of such products from Belgium. It also culminated in the resignation of two Belgian government ministers from office.

POLYBROMINATED BIPHENYLS

[CAS no. 59536-65-1]

Polybrominated biphenyls (PBBs) were associated with an outbreak of poisoning in farm animals in Michigan in 1973 when a fire retardant ('Firemaster' BP-6) was inadvertently substituted for an animal feed ('Nutrimaster'). As a result PBBs contaminated dairy products from affected cattle. A follow-up study of Michigan residents showed levels of PBB in body fat above 10 ppb with some individuals showing immunological abnormalities. Investigation of the workers employed in the plant manufacturing the PBBs showed that some had chloracne, abnormal sweating, altered fingernail growth, and hair loss. Despite studies in rodents showing liver malignancy,[49] there was no evidence of an excess cancer risk in these workers.

Other aromatic compounds

There is increasing concern about the public and environmental health effects of a wide range of chlorinated organic compounds. These include aromatic compounds such as the pesticides DDT (dichlorodiphenyltrichloroethane), pentachlorophenol and dieldrin, and plasticizers. Regional differences exist for plasma levels of DDT metabolites and urinary chlorophenols.[113] Levels tend to be higher in Asia and Africa where such pesticides continue to be widely used. (see Chapter 10 on pesticides) There are also current concerns regarding the possible endocrine-disrupting potential and immunological effects of these chemicals. This follows reports of

a decline in sperm quality in Western populations,[114] and alterations of male/female ratio in aquatic and marine life thought to be related to an oestrogenic effect from environmental contamination with such chemicals.

ACKNOWLEDGEMENTS

Thanks are due to Dr A Vale and staff of the National Poisons Information Service (Birmingham Centre), City Hospital NHS Trust for their assistance and advice.

REFERENCES

1 Karacic V, Skender L, Prpic-Majic D. Occupational exposure to benzene in the shoe industry. *Am J Ind Med* 1990; 18: 68–70.
2 Aksoy M. Benzene as a leukemogenic and carcinogenic agent. *Am J Ind Med* 1985; 8: 9–20.
3 Aksoy M. Malignancies due to occupational exposure to benzene. *Am J Ind Med* 1985; **7**: 395–402.
4 Collins JJ, Ireland BK, Easterday PA, Nair RS, Braun J. Evaluation of lymphopenia among workers with low-level benzene exposure and the utility of routine data collection. *J Occup Environ Med* 1997; **39**: 232–237.
5 International Agency for Research on Cancer. Monographs on the evaluation of carcinogenic risks to humans: 29: *Some Industrial Chemicals and Dyestuffs.* Lyon: IRAC, 1982.
6 American Conference of Governmental Industrial Hygienists. Notice of intended changes – benzene. *Appl Occup Environ Hyg* 1990; **5**: 453–63.
7 American Conference of Governmental Industrial Hygienists. *1999 Threshold Limit Values for Chemical Substances and Physical Agents and Biological Exposure Indices.* Cincinnati: ACGIH, 1999.
8 Inoue O, Seiji K, Kasahara M *et al.* Quantitative relation of urinary phenol levels to breathzone benzene concentrations: a factory survey. *Br J Ind Med* 1986; **43**: 692–7.
9 Money CD, Gray CN. Exhaled breath analysis as a measure of workplace exposure to benzene. *Ann Occup Hyg* 1989; **33**: 257–62.
10 American Conference of Governmental Industrial Hygienists. *Documentation of the Biological Exposure Indices.* Cincinnati: ACGIH, 1989.
11 Wallace LA, Pellizzari E, Hartwell T, Perritt R, Ziegenfus R. Exposures to benzene and other volatile compounds from active and passive smoking. *Arch Environ Hlth* 1987; **22**: 272–9.
12 Health and Safety Executive. EH40/99 *Occupational Exposure Limits.* Sudbury: HSE Books, 1999.
13 Austin H, Delzell E, Cole P. Benzene and leukaemia: a review of the literature and a risk assessment. *Am J Epidemiol* 1988; **127**: 419–39.
14 Rinsky RA, Smith AB, Hornung R *et al.* Benzene and

leukemia: an epidemiologic risk assessment. *N Engl J Med* 1987; **316**: 1044–9.

15 Yardley-Jones A, Anderson D, Parke DV. The toxicity of benzene and its metabolism and molecular pathology in human risk assessment. *Br J Ind Med* 1991; **48**: 437–44.

16 Yardley-Jones A, Anderson D, Jenkinson PC, Lovell DP, Blowers SD, Davies MI. Genotoxic effects in peripheral blood and urine of workers exposed to low level benzene. *Br J Ind Med* 1988; **45**: 694–700.

17 Collins JJ, Conner P, Friedlander BR, Easterday PA Nair RS, Braun J. A study of the hematologic effects of chronic low-level exposure to benzene. *J Occup Med* 1991; **33**: 619–26.

18 Meulenbelt J, de Groot G, Savelkoul TJF. Two cases of acute toluene intoxication. *Br J Ind Med* 1989; **47**: 417–20.

19 Hasegawa K, Shiojima S, Koizumi A, Ikeda M. Hippuric acid and *o*-cresol in the urine of workers exposed to toluene. *Int Arch Occup Environ Hlth* 1983; **52**: 197–208.

20 de Rosa E, Bartolucci GB, Sigon M, Callegano R, Perbellini L, Brugnone F. Hippuric acid and ortho-cresol as biological indicators of occupational exposure to toluene. *Am J Ind Med* 1987; **11**: 529–37.

21 Fay M, Eisenmann C, Diwan S, De Rosa C. ASTDR evaluation of health effects of chemicals. V. Xylenes: health effects, toxicokinetics, human exposure, and environmental fate. *Tox Ind Hlth* 1998; **14**: 571–97.

22 European Chemical Industry Ecology and Toxicology Centre. *Xylenes. Joint Assessment of Commodity Chemicals* No. 6. Brussels: ECETOC, 1989.

23 Lowry LK, Thorburn TW, Phipps FC, Gunter BJ, Sollenberg J. Xylene exposure in a histology laboratory investigated by environmental and biological monitoring. In: Ho MH, Dillon MK eds. *Biological Monitoring of Exposure to Chemicals: Organic Compounds*. New York: John Wiley, 1987: 143–53.

24 Engstrom K, Husman K, Riihimaki V. Percutaneous absorption of m-xylene in man. *Int Arch Occup Environ Hlth* 1977; **39**: 181–9.

25 Grandjean P. *Skin Penetration: Hazardous Chemicals at Work*. London: Taylor & Francis, 1990.

26 Uchida Y, Nakatsuka H, Ukai H, Watanabe T, Liu Y-T, Huang M-Y *et al*. Symptoms and signs in workers exposed predominantly to xylenes. *Int Arch Occup Environ Hlth* 1993; **64**: 597–605.

27 Bell GM, Shillaker RO, Padgham MDJ, Standring P. Health and Safety Executive. Toxicity Review 26: *Xylenes*. London: HMSO, 1992.

28 Morley R, Eccleston DW, Douglas CP, Greville WEJ, Scott DJ, Anderson J. Xylene poisoning: a report on one fatal case and two cases of recovery after prolonged unconsciousness. *Br Med J* 1970; **3**: 442–3.

29 Elzinga LW. Renal toxicity of xylene. *JAMA* 1989; **261**: 2258.

30 Ansari EA. Ocular injury with xylene – a report of two cases. *Human Exp Toxicol* 1997; **16**: 273–5.

31 Errebo-Knudsen EO, Olsen F. Organic solvents and presenile dementia (the painters' syndrome): a critical review of the Danish literature. *Sci Total Environ* 1986; **48**: 45–67.

32 Grasso P, Sharratt M, Davies DM, Irvine D. Neurophysiological and psychological disorders and occupational exposure to organic solvents. *Food Chem Toxicol* 1984; **22**: 819–52.

33 Ruijten MWMM, Hooisma J, Brons JT, Habets CEP, Emmen HH, Muijser H. *Neurotox* 1994; **15**: 613–20.

34 Chen R, Dick F, Seaton A. Health effects of solvent exposure among dockyard painters: mortality and neuropsychological symptoms. *Occup Environ Med* 1999; **56**: 383–387.

35 Chen R, Wei L, Seaton A. Neuropsychological symptoms in Chinese male and female painters: an epidemiological study in dockyard workers. *Occup Environ Med* 1999; **56**: 388–90.

36 Bleeker ML, Bolla KI, Agnew J, Schwartz BS, Ford DP. Dose-related subclinical neurobehavioral effects of chronic exposure to low levels of organic solvents. *Am J Ind Med* 1991; **19**: 715–28.

37 Axelsson G, Lutz C, Rylander R. Exposure to solvents and outcome of pregnancy in university laboratory employees. *Br J Ind Med* 1984; **41**: 305–312.

38 Ogata M, Taguchi T. Quantitative analysis of urinary glycine conjugates by high performance liquid chromatography: excretion of hippuric acid and methylhippuric acids in the urine of subjects exposed to vapours of toluene and xylenes. *Int Arch Occup Environ Hlth* 1986; **58**: 121–9.

39 Laine A, Savolainen K, Riihimaki V, Matikainen E, Salmi T, Juntunen J. Acute effects of m-xylene inhalation on body sway, reaction times, and sleep in man. *Int Arch Occup Environ Hlth* 1993; **65**: 179–88.

40 Campbell L, Marsh DM, Wilson HK. Towards a biological monitoring strategy for toluene. *Ann Occup Hyg* 1987; **31**: 121–33.

41 Kaneko T, Wang P-Y, Sato A. Enzyme induction by ethanol consumption affects the pharmacokinetics of inhaled m-xylene only at high levels of exposure. *Arch Toxicol* 1993; **67**: 473–7.

42 Huang M-Y, Jin C, Liu Y-T, Li B-H, Qu Q-S *et al*. Exposure of workers to a mixture of toluene and xylenes: I. Metabolism. *Occup Environ Med* 1994; **51**: 42–6.

43 Inoue O, Seiji K, Kawai T, Watanabe T, Jin C *et al*. Excretion of methylhippuric acids in urine of workers exposed to a xylene mixture: comparison among three xylene isomers and toluene. *Int Arch Occup Environ Hlth* 1993; **64**: 533–9.

44 Ikeda M, Koizumi A, Miyasake M, Watanabe T. Styrene exposure and biological monitoring FRP boat production plants. *Int Arch Occup Environ Hlth* 1982; **49**: 325–39.

45 Lemasters G, Carson A, Samuels SS. Occupational styrene exposure for twelve product categories in the reinforced-plastics industry. *Am J Hyg Assoc* 1985; **46**: 434–41.

46 Cherry N, Gautrin D. Neurotoxic effects of styrene: further evidence. *Br J Ind Med* 1990; **47**: 29–37.

47 Cherry N, Rodgers B, Venables H, Waldron HA, Wells GG.

Acute behavioural effects of styrene exposure: a further analysis. *Br J Ind Med* 1981; **38**: 346–50.

48 Jegaden D, Amann D, Simon JF, Habault M, Legoux B, Galopin P. Study of the neurobehavioural toxicity of styrene at low levels of exposure. *Int Arch Occup Environ Hlth* 1993; **64**: 527–31.

49 International Agency for Research on Cancer. IARC monographs on the evaluation of the carcinogenic risk of chemicals to humans. *An updating of IARC Monographs Vols 1 to 42*, Suppl 7, Lyon: WHO, 1987.

50 Gadberry MG, DeNicola DB, Carlson GP. Pneumotoxicity and hepatotoxicity of styrene and styrene oxide. *J Toxicol Env Hlth* 1996; **48**: 273–94.

51 Sollenberg J, Bjurstrom R, Wrangskog K, Vestberg O. Biological exposure limits estimated from relations between occupational styrene exposure during a workweek and excretion of mandelic and phenylglyoxylic acids in urine. *Int Arch Occup Environ Hlth* 1988; **60**: 365–70.

52 Gullemin MP, Berode M. Biological monitoring of styrene: a review. *Am Ind Hyg Assoc J* 1988; **49**: 497–505.

53 Wilson HK, Robertson SM, Waldron HA, Gopertz D. Effect of alcohol on the kinetics of mandelic acid excretion in volunteers exposed styrene vapour. *Br J Ind Med* 1983; **40**: 75–8.

54 International Programme on Chemical Safety (IPCS). Environmental Health Criteria: 186. *Ethylbenzene*. Geneva: WHO, 1996.

55 Ong CN, Koh D, Foo SC, Kok PW, Ong HY, Aw TC. Volatile organic solvents in correction fluids: identification and potential hazards. *Bull Environ Contam Toxicol* 1993; **50**: 787–93.

56 Korn M, Gfrorer W, Herz R, Wodarz I, Wodarz R. Stereometabolism of ethylbenzene in man: gas chromatographic determination of urinary excreted mandelic acid enantiomers and phenylglyoxylic acid and their relation to the height of occupational exposure. *Int Arch Occup Environ Hlth* 1992; **64**: 75–8.

57 Richardson ML, Gangolli S (eds). *The Dictionary of Substances and their Effects*. Cambridge: Royal Society of Chemistry, 1993.

58 Standring P. Health and Safety Executive. Toxicity Review 25: Part 2: *Cumene*. London: HMSO, 1991.

59 Department of Health and Social Security. *Notes on the Diagnosis of Occupational Diseases*. London, HMSO, 1983.

60 Fairhurst S. Health and Safety Executive. Toxicity Review 25: Part 3: *Paradichlorobenzene (p-DCB)* London: HMSO, 1991.

61 Peters HA, Cripps DJ, Gocmen A, Erturk Bryan GT, Morris CR. Neurotoxicity of hexa-chlorobenzene-induced porphyria turcica. In: Morris CR, Cabral JRP eds. *Hexachlorobenz. Proceedings of an International Symposium, Lyon, France, 1985*. Lyon: IARC Scientific Publications No. 77, 1986: 575–9.

62 To-Figueras J, Barrot C, Rodamilans M, Gomez-Catalan J, Torra M *et al*. Accumulation of hexachlorobenzene in humans: a long standing risk. *Hum Exp Toxicol* 1995; **14**: 20–3.

63 Strik JJTWA. Porphyrins in urine as an indication of exposure to chlorinated hydrocarbons. *NY Acad Sci* 1987; **514**: 219–21.

64 Shuker LK, Batt S, Rystedt I, Berlin M. *The Health Effects of Aromatic Amines – A Review*. MARC Report Number 35. London: Monitoring and Assessment Research Centre, 1986.

65 Brooke IM, Cain JR, Cocker J, Groves JA. *Phenylhydrazine: Risk Assessment Document* EH72/1 Sudbury: HSE Books, 1997.

66 Beer ST, Bradberry SM, Vale JA. The use of methylene blue in occupational methaemoglobinaemia. Abstract: European Association of Poisons Centres and Clinical Toxicologists (EAPCCT) Scientific Meeting, July 1997. Oslo, Norway.

67 Blanc P. Methemoglobinemia. In: Olson KR ed. *Poisoning and Drug Overdose*. Connecticut: Appleton & Lange, 1990: 204–6.

68 Veys CA. Bladder cancer as an occupational disease in the British rubber industry: an in-depth factory study to show the past extent of the problem and confirmation of its subsequent disappearance. *Progress Rubber Plastics Technol* 1992; **8**: 1–14.

69 Wallace DMA. Occupational urothelial cancer. *Br J Urol* 1988; **61**: 175–82.

70 The BAUS Subcommittee on industrial bladder cancer. Occupational bladder cancer. *Br J Urol* 1988; **61**: 183–91.

71 Searle CE (ed). *Chemical Carcinogens* 2nd edn. American Cancer Society Monograph 182. Washington DC: ACS, 1984.

72 Case RAM, Pearson JT. Tumours of the urinary bladder in workmen engaged in the manufacture and use of certain dyestuff intermediates in the British chemical industry. Part II. Further consideration of the role of aniline, and of the manufacture of auramine and magenta (fuchsin) as possible causative agents. *Br J Ind Med* 1954; **11**: 213–16.

73 Ward E, Carpenter A, Markowitz S, Roberts D, Halperin W. Excess number of bladder cancers in workers exposed to orthotoluidine and aniline. *J Natl Cancer Inst* 1991; **83**: 501–6.

74 Ward EM, Sabbioni G, DeBord DG, Teass AW, Brown KK *et al*. Monitoring of aromatic amine exposures in workers at a chemical plantwith a known bladder cancer excess. *J Natl Cancer Inst* 1996; **88**: 1046–52.

75 Veys CA. *A study of the Incidence of Bladder Tumours in Rubber Workers*. Liverpool: University of Liverpool, 1973. MD Thesis.

76 Steineck G, Plato N, Norell SE, Hogstedt C. Urothelial cancer and some industry-related chemicals: an evaluation of the epidemiologic literature. *Am J Ind Med* 1990; **17**: 371–91.

77 Schulte PA. Screening for bladder cancer in high risk groups: delineation of the problem. *J Occup Med* 1990; **32**: 789–92.

78 Cartwright RA. Bladder cancer screening in the United Kingdom. *J Occup Med* 1990; **32**: 878–80.

79 Kopelman H, Robertson MH, Saunders PG, Ash I. The Epping jaundice. *Br Med J* 1966; **1**: 514–6.

80 Kopelman H, Scheuer PJ, Williams R. The liver lesion of the Epping jaundice. *Q J Med* 1966; **35**: 553–64.

81 Hall AJ, Harrington JM, Waterhouse JAH. The Epping jaundice outbreak: a 24-year follow-up. *J Epidemiol Commun Hlth* 1992; **46**: 327–8.

82 McGill DB, Motto JD. An industrial outbreak of toxic hepatitis due to methylenedianiline. *N Engl J Med* 1974; **291**: 278–82.

83 Ward E, Halperin W, Thun M *et al*. Bladder tumours in two young males occupationally exposed to MBOCA. *Am J Ind Med* 1988; **14**: 267–72.

84 Cocker J, Wilson HK. Determination of 4,4′-methylene-bis-(2-chloroaniline) in urine. *Clin Chem* 1989; **35**: 506.

85 Osorio AM, Clapp D, Ward E, Wilson HK, Cocker J. Biological monitoring of a worker exposed to MBOCA. *Am J Ind Med* 1990; **18**: 577–89.

86 Hunter DM, Timerding BL, Leonard RB, McCalmont TH, Schwartz E. Effects of isopropyl alcohol, ethanol, and polyethylene glycol/industrial methylated spirits in the treatment of acute phenol burns. *Ann Emerg Med* 1992; **21**: 1303–7.

87 Conning DM, Hayes MJ. The dermal toxicity of phenol: an investigation of the most effective first-aid measures. *Br J Ind Med* 1970; **27**: 155–9.

88 Horch R, Spilker G, Stark GB. Phenol burns and intoxications. *Burns* 1994; **20**: 45–50.

89 Jarvis SN, Straube RC, Williams ALJ, Bartlett CLR. Illness associated with contamination of drinking water supplies with phenol. *Br Med J* 1985; **290**: 1800–2.

90 Baker EL, Landrigan PJ, Bertozzi PE, Field PH, Basteyns BJ, Skinner HG. Phenol poisoning due to contaminated drinking water. *Arch Environ Hlth* 1978; **33**: 89–94.

91 Zimersson E, Bruze M, Goossens A. Simultaneous *p*-tert-butylphenol formaldehyde resin and *p*-tert-butylcatechol contact allergies in man and sensitizing capacities of *p*-tert-butylphenol and *p*-tert-butylcatechol in guinea pigs. *J Occup Environ Med* 1999; **41**: 23–8.

92 Tarvainen K, Kanerva L. Occupational dermatoses from plastic composites. *J Environ Med* 1999; **1**: 3–17.

93 Rothman N, Cantor K, Blair A *et al*. A nested case-control study of non-Hodgkins lymphoma and serum organochlorine residues. *Lancet* 1997; **350**: 240–4.

94 Garabedian MJ, Hoppin JA, Tolbert PE, Herrick RF, Brann EA. Occupational chlorophenol exposure and non-Hodgkins lymphoma. *J Occup Environ Med* 1999; **41**: 267–8.

95 McCunney RJ. Hodgkin's disease, work, and the environment: a review. *J Occup Environ Med* 1999; **41**: 36–46.

96 Bidstrup PL, Payne DJH. Poisoning by dinitro ortho-cresol: report of eight fatal cases occurring in Great Britain. *Br Med J* 1951; **2**: 16–19.

97 Amoruso MA, Ryer J, Easton D, Witz G, Goldstein BG. Estimation of risk of glucose 6-phosphate dehydrogenase-deficient red cells to ozone and nitrogen dioxide. *J Occup Med* 1986; **28**: 473–8.

98 Cook JW, Hewett CL, Hieger I. The isolation of a cancer-producing hydrocarbon from coal tar. *J Chem Soc* 1933; **1**: 395–405.

99 Lindstedt G, Sollenberg J. Polycyclic aromatic hydrocarbons in the occupational environment. *Scand J Work Environ Hlth* 1982; **8**: 1–19.

100 Health and Safety Executive. Guidance note EH62. *Metalworking Fluids – Health Precautions*. London: HMSO, 1991.

101 Jarvholm B, Nordstrom G, Hogstedt B, Levin J-O, Wahlstrom J *et al*. Exposure to polycyclic aromatic hydrocarbons and genotoxic effects on nonsmoking Swedish road pavement workers. *Scand J Work Environ Hlth* 1999; **25**: 131–6.

102 Bentsen-Farmen RK, Botnen IV, Note H, Jacob J, Ovrebo S. Detection of polycyclic aromatic hydrocarbon metabolites by high-pressure liquid chromatography after purification on immunoaffinity columns in urine from occupationally-exposed workers. *Int Arch Occup Environ Hlth* 1999; **72**: 161–8.

103 Kuljukka T, Savela K, Vaaranrinta R, Mutanen P, Veidebaum T *et al*. Low response in white blood cell DNA adducts among workers in a highly polluted cokery environment. *J Occup Environ Med* 1998; **40**: 529–37.

104 Hsu ST, Ma CI, Hsu KH, Wu SS, Hsu NHM, Yeh CC. Discovery and epidemiology of PCB poisoning in Taiwan. *Am J Ind Med* 1984; **5**: 71–9.

105 Eriksson M, Hardell L, Adami HO. Exposure to dioxins as a risk factor for soft tissue sarcoma: a population-based case-control study. *J Natl Cancer Inst* 1990; **82**: 486–90.

106 Fingerhut MA, Halperin WE, Marlow DA *et al*. Cancer mortality in workers exposed to 2,3,7,8-tetrachlorodibenzo-p-dioxin. *N Engl J Med* 1991; **199**: 212–8.

107 Manz A, Berger J, Dwyer JH, Flesch-Janys D, Nagel S, Waltsgott H. Cancer mortality among workers in chemical plant contaminated with dioxin. *Lancet* 1991; **338**: 959–64.

108 International Agency for Research on Cancer. Monographs on the evaluation of carcinogenic risks to humans: 69. *Polychlorinated dibenzo-para-dioxins and polychlorinated dibenzofurans*. Lyon: IARC, 1997: 1–631.

109 Steenland K, Piacitelli L, Deddens J, Fingerhut M, Chang LI. Cancer, heart disease and diabetes in workers exposed to 2,3,7,8-tetrachorodibenzo-p-dioxin. *J Natl Cancer Inst* 1999; **91**: 779–86.

110 Saracci R, Kogevinas M, Bertazzi P-A, Bueno de Mesquita BH, Coggon D *et al*. Cancer mortality in workers exposed to chlorophenoxy herbicides and chlorophenols. *Lancet* 1991; **328**: 1027–32.

111 Assennato G, Cervino D, Emmett EA, Longo G, Merlo F. Follow-up of subjects who developed chloracne

following TCDD exposure at Seveso. *Am J Ind Med* 1989; **16**: 119–25.

112 Bertazzi P A *et al*. Cancer incidence in a population accidentally exposed to 2,3,7,8-tetra chloro-dibenzo-para-dioxin. *Epidemiology* 1993; **4**: 398–406.

113 Schmid K, Lederer P, Goen T, Schaller KH, Strebl H *et al*. Internal exposure to hazardous substances of persons from various continents: investigation on exposure to different organochlorine compounds. *Int Arch Occup Environ Hlth* 1997; **69**: 399–406.

114 Kolstad HA, Bonde JP, Spano M, Giwercman A, Zschiesche W *et al*. Change in semen quality and sperm chromatin structure following occupational styrene exposure. *Int Arch Occup Environ Hlth* 1999; **72**: 135–41.

Diseases associated with physical agents

Sound, noise and the ear	283
Vibration (hand–arm and whole body)	307
Heat and cold	325
Raised barometric pressure	343
Flying	361
Working at high altitude	383
Ionizing radiations	397
Non-ionizing radiation and the eye	419
Extremely low frequency electric and magnetic fields	439

Diseases associated with physical agents

13

Sound, noise and the ear

RICHARD T RAMSDEN, SHAKEEL R SAEED

The physics of sound	283	Non-organic (or exaggerated, or functional)	
Anatomy and physiology of the ear	285	hearing loss	300
Occupational noise-induced hearing loss	289	Electric response audiometry (evoked response	
Acoustic trauma and blast trauma	294	audiometry)	300
Assessment of hearing disability	294	Occupational noise-induced tinnitus	303
Age-associated hearing loss	295	Occupational noise-induced vertigo	303
Hearing conservation programmes	295	Infrasound and ultrasound	304
Management	299	References	304

There has been an awareness for several centuries that exposure to high levels of sound may be detrimental to an individual's hearing. The objectives of this chapter are to review the response of the ear to normal and hazardous sound levels, examine the issues of assessment and management of patients presenting with possible noise-induced afflictions of the ear, and discuss the legal provisions available for such individuals.

THE PHYSICS OF SOUND

The application of a mechanical force to an elastic medium such as air results in the displacement of the particles or molecules that constitute that medium. The energy in the displacing force effectively overcomes the mass or inertia of the molecules. This displacement is resisted by a force that tends to return the molecule or particle to its resting position, that is the elasticity. In effect, the displacing force sets up an oscillation or vibration in that medium, which is essentially sound. This oscillation would continue indefinitely if it were not for the frictional resistance that is also inherent to any vibrating system. As a result of this frictional resistance, the energy in the initial displacing force is dissipated as heat and the vibration ceases. The transfer of kinetic energy between vibrating molecules, however, leads to a propagation of the sound through the medium. This

generates alternating areas of condensation (with a rise in ambient pressure) and rarefaction (with a fall in ambient pressure) within the medium (Fig. 13.1). There is no net movement of the medium as such but rather the movement of changes in pressure in the medium, which is a sound wave and takes the form of a sine wave when the pressure changes are plotted against time. A sound wave thus has two fundamental properties: its intensity (amplitude of the peak of the wave form), correlating subjectively with loudness, and its frequency, which has the subjective correlate of pitch.[1]

Sound wave intensity

By definition, the intensity of a sound wave is its power per unit area (expressed in Watts per metre squared) and depends on the peak pressure of the sound wave and the peak velocity of the air molecules. The peak pressure and peak velocity are proportional to each other, the constant of proportionality being the impedance of the medium through which the wave is being propagated. The ambient pressure of a sound wave depends on the point on the sinusoid wave form at which it is measured and therefore the relationship between the intensity and the peak pressure will also vary in this manner. In order to overcome this during quantification, the average or root mean square value (RMS) of the pressure is calculated from pressure measurements at points along the wave-form. This allows the intensity of the sound to be calcu-

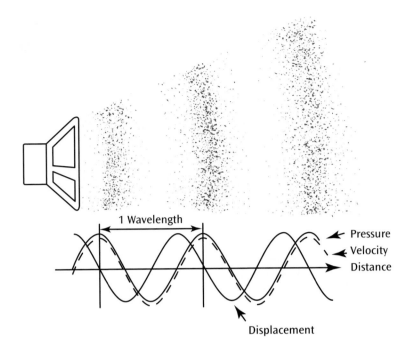

1 Wavelength

Pressure
Velocity
Distance

Displacement

Figure 13.1 *A sound wave generated by alternating areas of condensation and rarefaction of the medium through which it travels. Reproduced with permission from Ref. 1.*

lated from the RMS pressure for a medium with a known impedance. Unlike intensity, sound pressure can be readily measured with a microphone and is expressed in newtons per square metre (N/m^2) (pascals (Pa)). The auditory system, however, is sensitive to a vast range of sound pressures: 2×10^{-5} N/m^2 for the threshold of hearing to around 1×10^{8} N/m^2 next to a jet aircraft at take-off. With such a wide numerical range the impracticalities of quantification and calculation are obvious. Second, the ear does not respond in a linear manner to linear changes in sound pressure. In fact the ear perceives changes in intensity more closely to logarithmic changes in power or sound pressure. The use of the logarithm of the ratio of the measured pressure to a reference pressure or ratios of intensity or indeed power overcomes the two difficulties cited.

Logarithms to the base 10 of these ratios are termed 'bels' after Alexander Graham Bell as the scale was first used in telephony. In practical terms, one tenth of a bel or decibel (dB) is more convenient for the sizes of the numbers involved. Thus:

Sound pressure
level in bels (SPL) = $\log_{10}$ $\dfrac{\text{RMS measured sound pressure}}{\text{reference sound pressure}}$

Sound pressure
level in dB (SPL) = $10 \log_{10}$ $\dfrac{\text{RMS measured sound pressure}}{\text{reference sound pressure}}$

To express the sound intensity which varies as the *square* of the pressure:

Intensity (dB SPL) = $20 \log_{10}$ $\dfrac{\text{RMS measured sound pressure}}{\text{reference sound pressure}}$

Using this decibel scale for measuring sound pressure levels (SPL), the reference sound pressure is $2 \times 10^{-5} N/m^2$ (20 µPa), 0 dB SPL corresponds to the threshold of hearing and 130 dB SPL the threshold of pain. Audiometrically, however, the reference pressure is frequency dependent as the threshold sensitivity of the human ear is frequency dependent (see below). These reference pressures have been defined by the International Standards Organization (ISO 389:1991)[2] and are the same as those of the British Standards Institution (BS 2497:1992).[3] Using these reference pressures, an audiometric sound level of say 30 dB is written as 30 dB HL (hearing level) and if this corresponds to the threshold of hearing of an individual's ear then the threshold is said to be 30 dB HTL (hearing threshold level) for that ear.[4] Conveniently, the minimum detectable change in intensity is 1 dB SPL and an increase of 10 dB SPL gives a subjective sensation of doubling the loudness of a sound though the intensity of the sound has increased tenfold.

Table 13.1 shows the internationally agreed reference levels for the calculation of decibels of sound with respect to power, sound pressure and intensity. One other relevant consideration relating to sound intensity

Table 13.1 *The internationally agreed reference levels for the calculation of decibels of sound*

Scale	Abbreviation	Reference quantity
Power level	PWL	1.0 pW (10^{-12} W)
Intensity level	IL	10^{-12} W/m^2
Pressure level	SPL	20 µPa (20×10^{-6} N/m^2)

is the effect of distance from the sound source. For a theoretical point sound source in an homogenous medium, the intensity of the sound is a function of the power per unit area. Since the area increases as the square of the distance from the source, the intensity is inversely proportional to the square of the distance from the source of the sound. In reality, the presence of physical obstructions with the resultant reflection, diffraction and absorption effects tend to confound this relationship.

Sound wave frequency

The number of complete cycles of a sound wave per second is its frequency, expressed in Hertz (Hz). At sea level with an ambient temperature of 15°C, the velocity of sound waves is 330 metres per second in free air. Therefore, a sound wave with a frequency of 330 Hz has a wavelength of 1 metre and as the frequency increases, the wavelength decreases. The human ear in a child or young adult has a frequency perception range of around 20 Hz–20 kHz. The high frequency sensitivity diminishes with age such that few adults over the age of 30 years can detect sound with a frequency greater than 16 kHz.

The frequency of a sound broadly correlates with the subjective sensation of pitch. The threshold of human hearing, however, varies with frequency with maximum sensitivity between 2 and 3 kHz which encompasses the important speech sounds. This necessitates the use of a correction factor or weighting when measuring sound pressure levels or hearing thresholds and several such weighting curves exist. Of these, the 'A' weighting scale (low and extremely high frequencies weighted less heavily) is commonly utilized as it best correlates measured and perceived sound. A statement of a sound pressure level should also, therefore, indicate the weighting utilized by means of a suffix e.g. 30 dB (A) SPL.

As with sound intensities, the ear subjectively responds to incremental changes in frequency ratios rather than in a linear manner. Hence doubling the frequency of a tone produces a perceived change in pitch of one octave. Conventionally therefore, tuning fork tests and audiometric testing is undertaken in multiples of 256 Hz (middle C) though amongst musicians, middle C corresponds to a frequency of 261 Hz. Everyday sounds, of course, are more complex than those of a simple sinusoid (sine wave). Analysis of a complex waveform by breaking it down into its component sinusoids (Fourier analysis) allows the relative contribution of the components to be determined by frequency and relative amplitude. Periodic sounds (waveforms in the same time interval) are shown to have components that are multiples of the fundamental frequency or harmonics. These in part give a musical note, for example, its particular timbre. For non-periodic sounds such as the spoken voice, analysis shows that rather than discrete component frequencies there is a continuous range of frequencies or spectrum.

Noise

The preceding discussion examines sound in terms of its physical properties. Physically, noise is a complex sound whose characteristics are not easily amenable to analysis and has little or no measurable periodicity. Physiologically, noise is an uninformative signal with variable intensity. Psychologically, any sound that is unpleasant, noxious or unwanted is noise irrespective of its waveform.[5] Noise may be classified as continuous (steady-state or fluctuant) or intermittent (impulse or impact). Impulse noise, such as the noise generated from a gun blast, is characterized by its short duration and shock-front pressure waveform. Impact noise, such as in pile driving is characterized by little or no shock-front but considerable reverberant sound. The characteristics of intermittent noise merge into those of continuous noise if the former is repeated very rapidly.

ANATOMY AND PHYSIOLOGY OF THE EAR

Structurally and functionally the human ear is divided into three parts, namely the outer ear, middle ear and inner ear (Fig. 13.2). Together with the central connections of the ear in the brain, each part plays a role in the process of hearing and therefore merits further consideration.

The outer ear

The outer or external ear comprises the auricle (pinna) and the external auditory canal. Collectively these serve to modify incoming sound in two specific ways. First, the combination of the auricle behaving as an ear trumpet, concentrating sound from a large area to the smaller area of the external canal and the natural resonances of the external canal itself serves to increase the sound pressure level at the tympanic membrane by about 10 dB over a frequency range of 2–7 kHz.[1] Second, based on the above phenomenon and the fact that a proportion of incident sound is reflected off the head in a manner dependent on the direction of the sound, the outer ear provides some information about sound localization.

The middle ear

Embryologically derived from the outer and middle ear, the tympanic membrane (drumhead) constitutes the

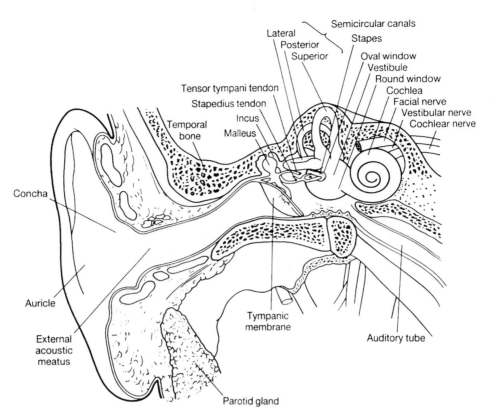

Figure 13.2 *The external, middle and inner ears. Reproduced with permission from Ref. 86.*

major component of the lateral or outer wall of the tympanic cavity. Within this cavity are the three ossicles, the malleus, incus and stapes, linking the drumhead to the inner ear. The middle ear cavity communicates with the pharynx at the back of the nose by the Eustachian tube and with the mastoid air cells by the *aditus ad antrum*. The fundamental function of the middle ear is mechanically to couple acoustic energy to the cochlea. To do this effectively, the middle ear has to match the impedance of air to the considerably higher impedance of the inner ear fluids, that is, function as an acoustic sound pressure transformer. The effect of this, in combination with the effects of the outer ear already described means that up to 50% of the incident sound energy is transmitted to the inner ear as opposed to the expected 1% in the absence of the transformer.[6] This is achieved by two mechanisms. The leverage of the malleus and incus about their axis of rotation gives a ×1.3 mechanical gain. The difference in the functional surface area between the drumhead and the stapes footplate which sits in the oval window gives rise to a 14-fold hydraulic effect.[7] Combining the two provides an increase in pressure at the oval window by a factor of around 18.

The second consideration is that the cochlear fluids, like any fluid are incompressible. The ossicular chain preferentially directs acoustic energy to the stapedial end of the cochlear compartment. The other end of this compartment is closed by the round window membrane which is able to deform in response to the pressure change in the cochlear fluids. Relative to the oval window, the incident acoustic energy at the round window is very small due to the effect of the ossicular chain and the presence of air (via the Eustachian tube) in the middle ear cavity (Fig. 13.3).

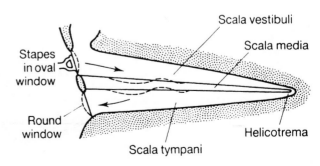

Figure 13.3 *Schematic diagram of an unrolled cochlea showing the transmission of vibrations from the oval window to the round window. Reproduced with permission from Ref. 87.*

The inner ear

The inner ear consists of two parts: the osseous labyrinth and the corresponding membranous labyrinth which lies within it. Descriptively, the labyrinth comprises the semicircular canals and vestibule which house the sensory end organs of balance and the cochlea within which is the hearing organ (Fig. 13.4). Lying in the medial wall of the middle ear, the cochlea is shaped like a snail's shell with two and three-quarter turns, 5 mm in height and 9 mm across the base.[8] The central bony axis of the cochlea (modiolus) has a spiral bony lamina projecting from it along its length which is completed by the basilar membrane. On this lies the cochlear duct (membraneous labyrinth) effectively dividing the cochlear lumen into three compartments, the scala vestibuli (in continuity with the vestibule, containing perilymph), the scala tympani, (in continuity at the apex of the cochlea with the scala vestibuli and closed by the round window membrane) and the scala media (containing endolymph), within which is the organ of Corti (Fig. 13.5). The organ of Corti is a specialized area of the lining of the cochlear duct that runs the whole length of the cochlear spiral and is around 35 mm long.[9] The sensory cells of the organ of Corti are arranged in one inner row and three to five outer rows. Microfilaments (stereocilia) from the sensory cell surface have given rise to the descriptive term sensory hair cells (Fig. 13.6). This rep-

resents the interface where mechanical energy is converted to electrical energy: the organ of Corti is thus a specialized transducer. From the sensory cells, afferent nerve fibres pass together as the cochlear nerve to the brainstem and ultimately to the auditory cortex of the brain.

The incident mechanical energy at the oval window sets up a series of waves in the perilymph of the scala vestibuli which in turn distort the membranes of the cochlear duct. In the 1940s Békésy introduced the concept of the travelling wave (Fig. 13.7) following a series of experiments in which he observed the movements of cadaveric basilar membranes in response to high intensity sounds at different frequencies.[7,10] The travelling waves for higher frequencies peaked at the basal end of the cochlear whilst the lower frequencies produced a peaked wave towards the apex. He correctly concluded that the basilar membrane had the property of frequency selectivity. More recent work has shown that the mechanical response of the basilar membrane (by way of tuning or frequency-threshold curves) and indeed the tuning curves for hair cells and the auditory neurons is very narrow.[11,12] There is thus a sharp band pass frequency for a given point on the basilar membrane, the hair cells in the organ of Corti at that point and the auditory neurons from those sensory cells.[13] The auditory system thus exhibits sensitivity and frequency selectivity probably as an active as well

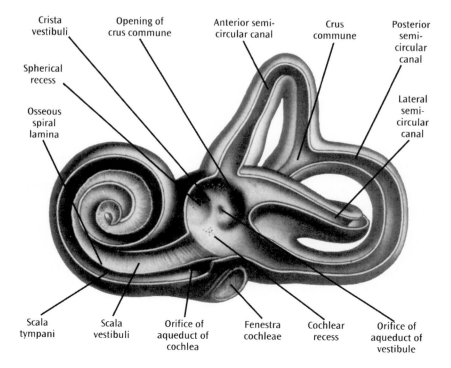

Crista vestibuli
Opening of crus commune
Anterior semi-circular canal
Crus commune
Posterior semi-circular canal
Spherical recess
Lateral semi-circular canal
Osseous spiral lamina
Scala tympani
Scala vestibuli
Orifice of aqueduct of cochlea
Fenestra cochleae
Cochlear recess
Orifice of aqueduct of vestibule

Figure 13.4 *The interior of the osseous labyrinth showing the cochlea, vestibule and the semicircular canals. Reproduced with permission from Ref. 8.*

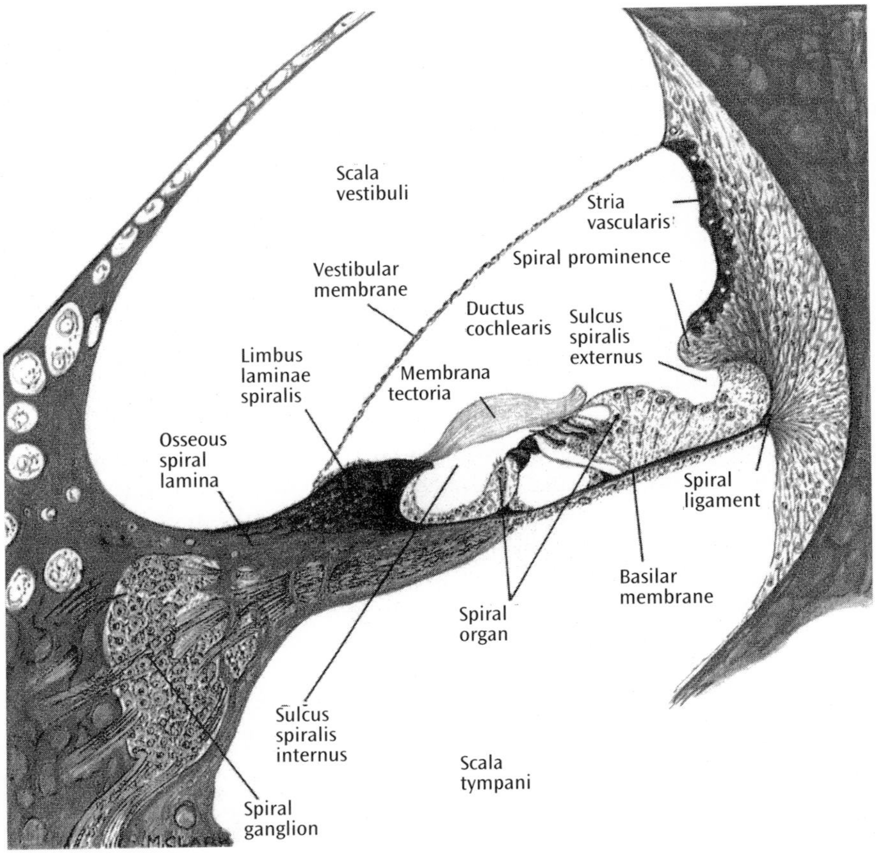

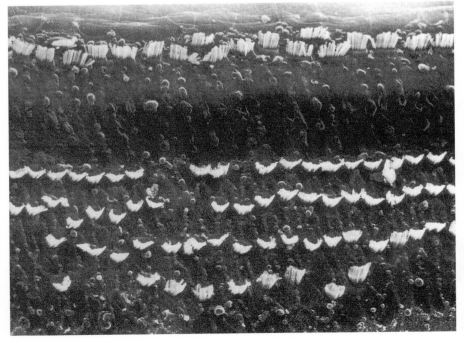

Scala
vestibuli

Stria
vascularis

Spiral prominence

Vestibular
membrane

Ductus
cochlearis

Sulcus
spiralis
externus

Limbus
laminae
spiralis

Membrana
tectoria

Osseous
spiral
lamina

Spiral
ligament

Spiral
organ

Basilar
membrane

Sulcus
spiralis
internus

Scala
tympani

Spiral
ganglion

Figure 13.5 *Section through the cochlea showing the organ of Corti. Mallory's stain. Reproduced with permission from Ref. 8. See colour plate section.*

Figure 13.6 *Scanning electron micrograph of part of the human organ of Corti. There is a single row of inner hair cells and several rows of outer hair cells. Reproduced with permission from Ref. 88.*

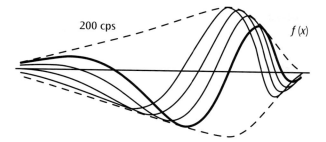

200 cps   f (x)

Figure 13.7 *The cochlear travelling wave according to Békésy. The solid lines depict displacement at four successive instants and the dotted lines show the static envelope. Reproduced with permission from Ref. 1.*

as passive mechanical process in the basilar membrane.[1] The deflection of the basilar membrane results in deflection of the stereocilia of the sensory cells in the organ of Corti. Depending on the relative movements of the stereocilia, ion channels in the sensory cell membrane are either opened or closed.[14] The resultant movement of potassium and calcium ions from the endolymph into the hair cells and change in their relative electrical potentials leads to the release of neurotransmitters in the synapses at the base of the hair cells giving rise to action potentials in the auditory nerve fibres. This then completes the process of transduction as the inner hair cells are in contact with 95% of the afferent fibres of the auditory nerve.

OCCUPATIONAL NOISE-INDUCED HEARING LOSS

Historical aspects

One of the earliest descriptions of the adverse effects of noise on hearing was by Francis Lord Bacon in 1627.[15] He wrote: 'A very great sound, near hand, hath strucken many deaf.' He relates his own experience of what was a temporary threshold shift: '. . . myself, standing near one that lured (whistled loudly to call back a falcon) loud and shrill, had suddenly an offence, as if somewhat had broken or been dislocated in my ear; and immediately after a loud ringing (not an ordinary singing or hissing, but far louder and differing) so I feared some deafness But after some half quarter of an hour it vanished'.

Nearly a century later, a report by Ramazzini recognized the relationship between copper hammering and hearing impairment[16] and in 1782, Admiral Lord Rodney

was deafened for 2 weeks following the firing of 80 broadsides from his ship *HMS Formidable*.[17] Fosbroke in 1831 accurately described noise-induced hearing loss in blacksmiths and coined the phrase 'blacksmith's deafness'.[18] It was the arrival of the Industrial Age, however, that led to a more widespread recognition of the deleterious effects of intense or prolonged noise on hearing: Roosa and Holt in the United States of America, Bezold in Germany and Barr in Great Britain.[5]

The work of Thomas Barr merits further consideration. He undertook field studies comparing the hearing in 100 boilermakers, 100 iron moulders and 100 postmen.[19] He wrote: 'It is familiarly known that boilermakers and others who work in very noisy surroundings are extremely liable to dullness of hearing. In Glasgow, we would have little difficulty in finding hundreds whose sense of hearing has thus been damaged, by the noisy character of their work. We have therefore in our city ample materials at hand for investigation on this subject'. Barr found that 75% of the boilermakers had difficulty in hearing at church or at a public meeting compared with 12% of the ironmoulders and 8% of the postmen. Four years later, in 1980, the pathology of noise-induced hearing loss was described by Habermann. Partial loss of the organ of Corti with destruction of the hair cells, particularly in the basal turn was noted.[20]

Following the introduction of audiometry, Fowler in 1929 observed the characteristic 4kHz dips and the first systematic audiometric studies were reported in 1939 by Bunch and by Larsen.[21-23] The technological advancements seen after the Second World War were paralleled by ever increasing noise levels in the workplace. Whilst loss of earnings due to hearing loss caused by acute trauma at work was compensatable from the early part of this century, it is only in the last 25 years that the legislative bodies of developed countries have recognized occupational noise-induced hearing loss, put into place mechanisms to confer responsibility on the manufacturing industries and compensate those individuals deemed to suffer this disorder.

Epidemiology

Occupational noise-induced hearing loss is considered one of the most common occupational disorders in industrial countries. Apparently between 1 and 4% of the population are exposed to harmful or potentially harmful noise levels and the presence or effectiveness of hearing conservation programmes will dictate the proportion of these individuals who do not have a noise-induced hearing deficit.[4] The paucity of hard data on hearing impairment in the adult population prompted the Medical Research Council to fund a multicentre epidemiological study which was carried out in the 1980s. This rigorous study, (UK National Study of Hearing) found that 12% of adults in Britain had a sensorineural hearing defect. Around one-third of these was accounted for by age and 5% by noise.[24] This would imply that around 1 in 200 of the adult population has noise-related sensorineural hearing impairment. Putting aside principal factors such as the level and nature of noise exposure, its duration and hearing conservation programmes, adjunctive factors are also recognized. Variations in individual susceptibility are now considered to be multifactorial but nonetheless a real entity.[25] The evidence for differences in susceptibility between men and women or between dark and fair skinned individuals is conflicting.[25,26] Indeed, a recent pilot study showed that in view of their ambivalence to their disorder, women with noise-induced hearing loss are less likely to be reported than men in studies examining noise-induced hearing loss.[27] With regard to children, a study that screened over 14000 Swedish schoolchildren found a greater than 20 dB 4 kHz dip in 2.3% with nearly two-thirds having an identifiable noise exposure factor such as firearms and crackers.[28] Perhaps the greatest area of concern, however, is that whilst developed countries are slowly bringing noise under control, the developing nations are witnessing an ever increasing level of urban and industrial noise.

Effects of sound stimulation and hazardous noise

ADAPTATION (PRE-STIMULATORY FATIGUE)

This is an immediate physiological phenomenon that occurs when a sound is presented to the ear. For sound pressure levels up to 80 dB the greatest elevation in threshold occurs at the same frequency of the stimulating tone. There follows an exponential recovery which occurs within 1 second. Electrophysiological animal studies have shown that adaptation correlates with a reduction in auditory nerve action potentials.[29] For higher stimulating sound intensities, true temporary threshold shift sets in though the intensity of stimulation required varies from individual to individual and depends on the frequency of the stimulating tone.

TEMPORARY THRESHOLD SHIFT (POST-STIMULATORY FATIGUE)

The magnitude of a temporary threshold shift is proportional to the intensity and duration of the stimulus and the recovery, unlike adaptation is slow. Recovery usually occurs within 16 hours but may take several days with higher intensities. The risk of developing permanent threshold shift has been studied by Mills and is complex.[30] Interactions between the level, nature and number of noise exposures, their duration and frequency and the susceptibility of the individual are all factors (Fig. 13.8). Classically, there is a high frequency rise in threshold with a characteristic notch at 4 kHz (Fig. 13.9) though the notch may centre at 3 or 6 kHz. This is often accompanied by tinnitus and after a short rest period, the rise in threshold recovers. With repeated exposure there is a tendency to acquire resistance to the auditory effects in that the degree of temporary threshold shift lessens[31] though at some arbitrary point, continued exposure leads to a permanent threshold shift.

PERMANENT THRESHOLD SHIFT

This is characterized by irreversible audiometric effects and pathological changes in the cochlea. The 4 kHz notch tends to deepen but also insidiously widen, encompassing adjacent high frequencies (Fig. 13.10). Once the audiometric changes encroach upon the speech frequencies (2 and 3 kHz in particular) the affected individual becomes aware of the diminished acuity in his or her hearing. Speech discrimination with background noise becomes difficult and the associated tinnitus (which is highly variable in character) may become intrusive. The rate of progression again depends on the noise parameters cited previously and on individual susceptibility. Generally, progression at 4 kHz is initially rapid but slows down after 10–12 years. Progression to involve the lower frequencies

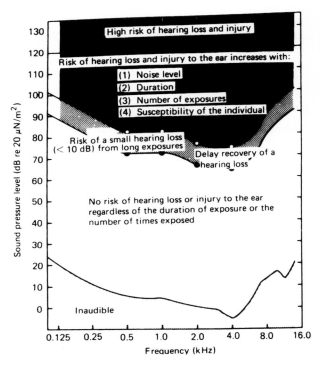

Figure 13.8 *Most of the range of human audibility categorized with respect to the risk of hearing loss and injury. Reproduced with permission from Ref 5.*

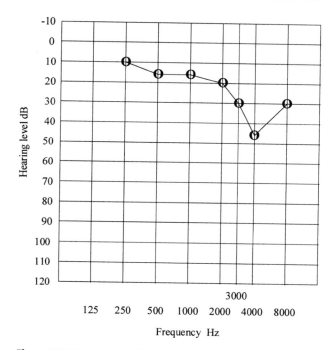

Figure 13.9 *Pure tone audiogram, right ear, showing the typical 4 kHz notch after excessive noise exposure.*

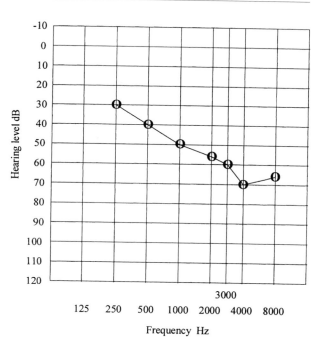

Figure 13.11 *Pure tone audiogram, right ear, showing a rise in the thresholds across the mid and high frequencies after protracted exposure to noise.*

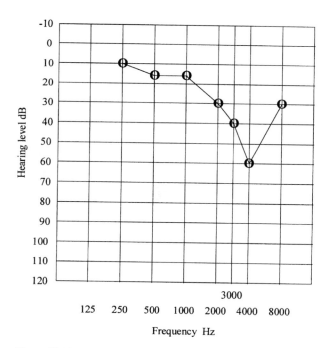

Figure 13.10 *Pure tone audiogram, right ear, showing a deepening of the 4 kHz notch and involvement of adjacent frequencies.*

is associated with a flattening of the audiogram in the highest frequencies (Fig. 13.11) such that the characteristic notched audiogram is not prerequisite for a diagnosis of occupational noise-induced hearing loss. At this stage,

the impaired speech discrimination in noise is accompanied by the complaint of sound generally being too quiet.[5]

With the progression of time, the increasing effects of ageing on auditory function come into play and this aspect assumes importance in the evaluation process of those being assessed with possible occupational noise-induced hearing loss (see below).

Pathology

As mentioned previously, the correlation of occupational noise-induced hearing loss with cochlear pathology was first described by Habermann in 1890. He reported that it was the organ of Corti, particularly the sensory hair cells and occasionally the spiral ganglion cells of the auditory nerve fibres that were affected.[20] Studies by Igarashi and colleagues[32] and Bredberg[33] showed that the site of predilection in the organ of Corti was 11 mm and 10.5–14 mm respectively from the beginning of the basal turn of the cochlea. This corresponds to an area that is responsive to sound frequencies around 4 kHz.

The work of Békésy in the 1940s not surprisingly led to attempts to tie in his mechanical travelling wave theories with pathological changes in the cochlea. If the maximal excursion of the basilar membrane in response to a travelling wave is in its central relatively unsupported part, then the shearing stress is exerted maximally at this point and would explain why the supporting cells of the inner hair cells and the first row of the outer hair cells are the structures that sustain most injury.[34] As the limitations of the Békésy model were realized and technological advances such as electron microscopy became available, the ultrastructure and function of the hair cells themselves has become the focus of attention.

Progressive degrees of stereocilial damage and hair cell death correlate with temporary and permanent threshold shifts (Fig. 13.12).[35,36] The sensitivity of the afferent inner hair cells depend in part on the function of the efferent outer hair cells[37] and it is postulated that dysfunction of the latter has an adverse effect on the function of the former. The time honoured belief that the pathological site correlated with the threshold shift has also been challenged as there is a variation in the distribution of the hair cell loss and loss of cochlear sensitivity, related perhaps to the response of the middle ear muscles to different types of hazardous sound stimulation.[38] In addition to these mechanical factors, metabolic and vascular factors have been postulated.[39] Disruption of mitochondrial ion concentrations and enzyme systems of the hair cells would certainly be detrimental to function, particularly if the hair cells play an active role in fine frequency – sensitivity tuning. The precise sequence of events leading from injurious noise exposure to permanent threshold shift thus remains obscure though ultrastructural and biochemical investigation continues to clarify the picture.

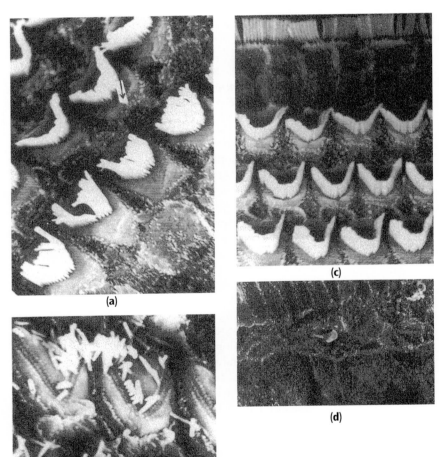

(a)

(b)

(c)

(d)

Figure 13.12 *Change in the stereocilia of guinea pigs. (a) Exposure to 110 dB for 30 min; half an hour after exposure there is swelling of the cuticular plate (arrow) × 2800. (b) Exposure to 110 dB for 30 min; 80 days after exposure, 9.5 mm from the round window. The inner and outer hair cells appear normal as was the hearing threshold, ×1900). (c) Exposure to 120 dB for 150 min; half an hour after exposure there is total loss of the stereocilia on the outer hair cells (×4300). (d) Exposure to 120 dB for 150 min; 80 days after exposure, 9 mm from the round window. The surface is devoid of both sterocilia and hair cells, correlating with a 30–35 dB permanent threshold shift at 2 and 4 kHz. Reproduced with permission from Ref 5.*

The effects of middle ear disease

The widely held belief that a conductive hearing loss due to middle ear disease serves to protect the inner ear from hazardous noise is open to debate as the literature is somewhat conflicting. Alberti and colleagues studied a group of individuals with otosclerosis and presumed occupational noise-induced hearing loss and found that there was no difference in the bone conduction threshold curves between the operated and non-operated ear even though the individuals concerned had continued to work in a noisy environment after their surgery.[40] Similarly, Simpson and O'Reilly could not demonstrate a protective effect on the inner ear in a worker with chronic middle ear disease.[41] In contrast, a study by McShane and colleagues examined the hearing in workers with unilateral unoperated otosclerosis and demonstrated a small protective effect (around 4 dB) in the affected ear at 4 kHz.[42]

Hinchcliffe has discussed the reasons for such disparate findings and reduces them to two main factors.[4] Firstly, the two most common causes of adult conductive hearing loss, otosclerosis and chronic inflammatory middle ear disease, may be associated with sensorineural hearing loss – the former as cochlear otosclerosis and the latter as a complication of the disease. The pathological status of the middle ear in terms of extent, nature and activity also has a bearing on inner ear function. Ossicular fixation (whether due to otosclerosis or otherwise) alters the middle ear resonance and may give rise to the 2 kHz Carhart notch in the bone conduction threshold. Second, the temporal relationship between the onset of the conductive hearing loss and noise exposure is also relevant. Clearly the interaction between middle ear disease and inner ear function is complex and one cannot draw the intuitive conclusion that a conductive hearing loss acts as some form of hearing protective device.

The diagnosis of occupational noise-induced hearing loss

The process of establishing a diagnosis of occupational noise-induced hearing loss should be no different from the process of reaching a diagnosis when faced with any other clinical problem. The fundamental principles of taking a comprehensive and pertinent history, conducting a thorough examination and undertaking appropriate investigations are just as applicable. However, certain factors cloud this process and as a result the diagnosis is usually circumstantial.[5] When faced with an individual with hearing loss and a history of occupational noise exposure, the clinician has to make a decision as to whether the former is a result of the latter. This gives rise to the first problem. Of the 12% of adults found to have

a sensorineural hearing loss in the Medical Research Council study cited previously, only 40% of these could be accounted for by the effects of age or noise exposure.[24] Some of the remaining 60% were no doubt due to the myriad of less common or rare disorders (in population terms) that cause a sensorineural hearing loss but a significant proportion were idiopathic (cause unknown). If the diagnostic process is one of exclusion of known causes, Williams has put forward the argument that attempting to exclude that which cannot be identified defies logic.[43] However, appraisal by an appropriately trained clinician remains paramount as there is no reason why the prevalence of other otological disorders should be any different in the individual with noise-induced deafness than in the general population. The Department of Health and Social Security publication *Occupational Deafness* (1973) states that apart from the characteristic audiometric changes, there are no signs or symptoms specific to noise-induced deafness.[44] This implies that the diagnosis of occupational noise-induced hearing loss is an audiometric one. However, the characteristic audiogram with its 4 kHz notch is not a pathognomonic feature of noise-induced deafness. The notch may be lie between 3 and 6 kHz (a notch centred at 6 kHz is considered to be an artefact), and with progression over time the notch may widen and be lost as the thresholds at the higher frequencies rise. Additionally, noise exposure is not the only cause of a 4 kHz notch and the hearing loss may not necessarily be symmetrical.[45]

The history must include not only audiovestibular symptoms but also details of previous and intercurrent focal and systemic disorders that may affect the ear. This includes the administration of potentially ototoxic drugs. The history of noise exposure, whether occupational, military or otherwise can be difficult to construct in temporal terms as individuals may have difficulty in recalling past events and employment accurately. Increasing recognition of non-syndromic familial sensorineural deafness and the familial nature of otosclerosis and some cases of Ménière's disease underlines the importance of obtaining a good family history. Autoimmune deafness may be associated with systemic symptoms and these should be enquired about. The examination of the ear, nose and throat must be complete. Much information regarding the health of the external and middle ear can be gleaned from pneumatic otoscopy and if the clinician is in any doubt, microscopic examination of the ear should be readily available, if nothing else, to clear the external meatus of wax that precludes a view of the drumhead. Aside from the audiometric evaluation additional investigations are dictated by the clinical assessment and include haematological, serological and relevant immunological laboratory tests in addition to radiology if indicated. Evaluation of the historical, clinical and investigative evidence usually allows, if present, the causal relationship between hearing loss and noise exposure to be established but as there is currently no single clinical or investigative feature unique to noise-induced hearing loss the diagnosis remains one of clinical probability and audiometric compatibility.

ACOUSTIC TRAUMA AND BLAST TRAUMA

The preceding discussion has primarily focused on the auditory effects of *prolonged* exposure to hazardous noise. The term acoustic trauma describes permanent hearing loss following *brief* exposure to a single very loud noise. This encompasses, for example, the effects of gunfire but also includes the effects of industrial impulse noise associated with drop forging and riveting. Gunfire noise in particular has the potential to be extremely hazardous. Peak sound pressure levels of 160 dB for hand-held weapons to 190 dB for field weapons have been recorded and therefore permanent injury to the inner ear may arise from the first exposure.[5] It is worth bearing in mind that with rifle fire, the forward ear (left ear in a right-handed individual) is closer to the muzzle thereby bearing the greater brunt of the acoustic trauma than the opposite ear and this is often discernible audiometrically. Second, in view of the historical events of this century, occupational noise-induced hearing loss and acoustic trauma may co-exist in the same individual.

Blast trauma (otic blast injury) is due to the effects of an explosion such as a bomb blast but may also be a component of the acoustic trauma from large calibre weapons. It is characterized by a greater severity and may be associated with damage to the tympanic membrane and the middle ear structures.[46] The shock wave from an explosion is longer than that of hazardous sound and consists of a short (5 milliseconds) positive pressure followed by a longer (30 ms) negative pressure. Clinically there may be a history of bleeding from the ear following the injury and examination shows a spectrum of tympanic membrane changes ranging from hyperaemia to frank perforation of the *pars tensa* which may be 'clean' or ragged. It is the initial positive pressure that perforates the drumhead and the subsequent negative pressure that leads to the characteristic everted edges of the perforation. The resultant deafness and tinnitus is immediate and severe but recovery, though incomplete for the higher pitches is not uncommon and over three-quarters of drumhead perforations heal spontaneously.[46]

ASSESSMENT OF HEARING DISABILITY

Impairment, disability and handicap

These consequences of disease are differentiated by the World Health Organization.[47]

Impairment relates to a loss or impairment of the structure or function of an organ or system. Within the auditory system there are a number of impairments of function which could be measured. The one which has most relevance for the assessment of hearing disability is the alteration in the pure tone threshold.

Disability is an index of the loss of an individual's functional performance as a consequence of impairment to the diseased organ or system. It thus represents a disturbance at the level of the individual. Hearing disability has been described as the restriction or lack of ability to perceive everyday sounds in the manner that is considered normal for healthy young people.[48]

Handicap encompasses the disadvantages experienced by an individual as a consequence of impairments and disabilities. It thus reflects interactions between the individual and his social and working environment. Hearing handicap is the disadvantage to an individual resulting from a hearing impairment or disability, that limits or prevents the fulfilment of a role that is normal for that individual. Disability and handicap are thus seen to be multifaceted. A given degree of hearing impairment could represent a much greater handicap for a professional musician than for a sculptor for example. The complex picture of disability and handicap that may result from occupational noise-induced hearing loss has been painted by Hetu *et al.*[49]

In 1981 a working party of members of the British Association of Otolaryngologists (BAOL) and the British Society of Audiologists (BSA) was set up to address the problem of assessment of hearing disability for the purpose of compensation. Up to then there was a plethora of conflicting recommendations, from a number of different sources. The results of the working party's deliberations were published in the so-called 'Blue Book' of 1983.[50] Because of some misgivings about its conclusions a new group called the Inter-Society Working Group was established in 1986 with a wider membership including representatives of the British Association of Audiological Physicians (BAAP), and the British Association of Audiological Scientists (BAAS).

The results of this group's efforts are published in *Guidelines for Medicolegal Practice.*[48] They considered every aspect of hearing disability and its assessment. They stated that 'hearing disability assessment should provide an accurate quantitative assessment of the actual disability suffered by the individual, appropriately weighted according to the way he uses his auditory facilities and the extent to which difficulties in hearing interfere with those activities'. The authors recognize, however, that the ideal is impossible to attain in an easily measurable, scientific and quantitative way because of the subjective nature of disability and handicap and the great variability between individuals. They identify instead a typical (median or average) individual and relate disability to that notional individual, and they recognize that such a concept may underestimate disability in some persons and overestimate it in others. They also recognize the need to identify an audiometric surrogate (i.e. a measure of impairment) as a means of quantifying disability.

Several studies have been carried out to identify the audiometric descriptors which best relate with disability including those by Atherley and Noble,[51] Lutman et al.[52] and the Medical Research Council's National Study of Hearing from the early 1980s. These studies by and large looked at the different patterns on pure tone audiometry which were the best predictors of disability. It was concluded that the three-frequency average of 1,2 and 3 kHz was the best predictor. Errors were introduced by the inclusion of 0.5 Hz and 6 kHz.[53] It may seem strange that 4 kHz is excluded from this formula, when one considers that this is the frequency most likely to be affected by occupational noise; however the notches at 4 kHz may be narrow but quite deep, so that there is a danger of obtaining an inflated average hearing threshold measurement which does not truly reflect the degree of disability. Furthermore it is convenient not to include 4 kHz in the estimate because of the difficulty in obtaining accurate bone conduction thresholds above 3 kHz. Finally the three-frequency average coincides with the UK statutory hearing loss criteria, even though the fence values of the latter may be subject to some criticism.

Fence values

The low fence is that notional point on the continuum of elevation of the hearing threshold level at which disability is deemed to commence. It has never been satisfactorily identified, and indeed cannot be seen as anything other than an artifice erected for administrative convenience, with little relevance to the individual case. Robinson et al. identified a 30 dB hearing threshold level averaged over 1, 2 and 3 kHz as the threshold of disability,[54] and this coincides with British Standard BS 5330 (1976).[55] A low fence as high as 50 dB HL (1, 2, 3 kHz average) is employed in the UK statutory compensation scheme. Even the much lower value of 26 dB (0.5, 1, 2 kHz) that prevailed under the American Academy of Otolaryngology and Ophthalmology (AAOO) scheme underestimated the disability of those individuals who began life with hearing that was 'normal'. The high fence is that point in the continuum of elevation of hearing threshold level at which disability is deemed to be total. High fence values have been judged to be any level from 70 dB upwards, and are just as arbitrary as low fence values.

AGE-ASSOCIATED HEARING LOSS

Ageing is associated with a progressive loss of auditory function, a condition which has been described in the past as presbyacusis. It is recognized that most of the impairment arises as a result of progressive cochlear dysfunction with loss of hair cells from the organ of Corti, affecting the higher frequencies first, but advancing through the cochlea to affect eventually the whole frequency range to some extent. Other structures may also undergo degenerative change, for example the auditory nerve and the central auditory pathways. There may also be a central loss of cognitive function. It is clearly important to be able to make some allowance for the effects of 'natural' ageing on the hearing of those middle-aged and elderly individuals who have also been exposed to the harmful effects of noise during their working lives.

Data on this subject are available from many sources. International Standard ISO 7029 (1984)[56] gives values of age-associated hearing loss as deviations relative to the median thresholds of young otologically normal subjects. The data are available for sex, for the age range 20–70 years, for frequencies ranging from 125 Hz to 8 kHz, and for percentiles of the population from the 5th to the 95th. They are available in table form for ease of reference so that allowance can be made in the individual case for the effects of ageing.[57]

The International Standard ISO 1999 (1990)[58] *Determination of Occupational Noise Exposure and Estimation of Noise-induced Hearing Impairment* assumes a direct additive effect between noise and age effects, although that is not true at profound levels of deafness. A word of caution is necessary, however. Burns and Robinson[59] and Robinson[60] have drawn attention to the complicated interrelationship of occupational noise-induced hearing loss and ageing. The former tends to produce an elevation in threshold which is initially rapid but slows down with subsequent exposure. Age-related hearing loss takes a progressively accelerating course with time. Thus the contribution of occupational noise-induced hearing loss to the total sensorineural hearing loss decreases with age, and by the age of 80 it would make virtually no difference what the noise had been.[43]

HEARING CONSERVATION PROGRAMMES

There are several areas in which employers may help to minimize the risks to the hearing of employees from the harmful effects of industrial noise:

- noise measurement and reduction,
- provision of personal ear protection,
- audiometric testing,
- education.

Noise measurement: the relationship of hearing loss to noise exposure

With the development of more precise methods of measuring both the noise stimulus and the hearing level, more precise determinations of the relationship of hearing loss and noise exposure have become possible. Burns and Robinson[59] reduced the number of significant parameters to two: the noise level and the duration of exposure. Daily personal exposure to noise (LEPd) can be established from the measured values of A-weighted sound pressure levels and the duration of exposure at work, and reference made to a nomogram (Fig. 13.13). Calculation is easiest when there is only one significant level of noise during the day, but is more complex when there are different periods of exposure to more than one significant noise level, or when one wants to know the LEPd caused by repeated 'single event' noise such as impact or cartridge-operated tools. Peak pressure meters provide rapid information and are easy to use. If the reading exceeds 125 dBA more accurate measures should be made. An integrating sound level meter (BS 6698: IEC 804) is the most convenient instrument for general use. It computes the equivalent continuous sound pressure level according to the equal energy principle. Personal sound dosemeters may be worn by an individual to determine a personal dose of noise over a given period. A daily personal noise exposure of 85 dBA is defined as

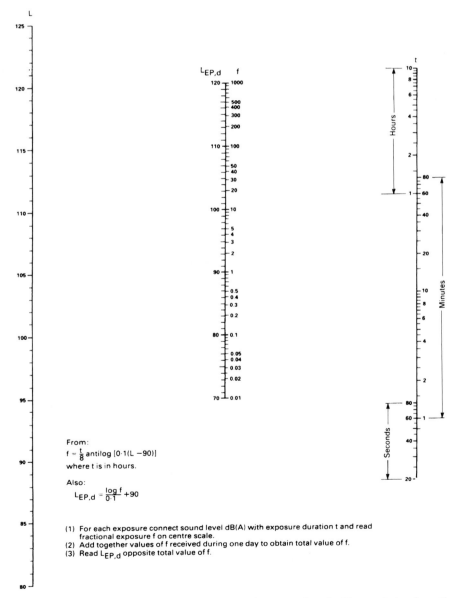

From:

$$f = \frac{t}{8} \text{ antilog } [0{\cdot}1(L - 90)]$$

where t is in hours.

Also:

$$L_{EP,d} = \frac{\log f}{0{\cdot}1} + 90$$

(1) For each exposure connect sound level dB(A) with exposure duration t and read fractional exposure f on centre scale.
(2) Add together values of f received during one day to obtain total value of f.
(3) Read $L_{EP,d}$ opposite total value of f.

Figure 13.13 *Reference nomogram for calculation of exposure to noise. Reproduced with permission from the Health and Safety Executive, UK. (Crown copyright.)*

the 'first action level'. This is the level at which ear protectors should be available on demand. A daily personal noise exposure of 90 dBA is defined as the 'second action level'. At this level the use of protectors is mandatory. A peak sound pressure of 200 Pascals is defined as the 'peak action level'. At this level the use of protectors is mandatory. It is clearly essential that the measurement equipment is accurate and regularly calibrated.[61]

Noise reduction

This can be helped, inter alia, by the enclosure of noisy machines, the use of mufflers, damping, silencers and antivibration mountings, the treatment of reflective surfaces with absorbing materials, the limitation of the use of noisy equipment to times when it is actually required, and the distancing of workers from the areas of maximum noise, There are many more suggestions for the reduction of noise in the workplace in the Consultative Document *Prevention of Damage to Hearing from Noise at Work* published by the Health and Safety Commission in 1987.[62] The publication *Sound Solutions* published by the Health and Safety Executive (1995) provides employers with many examples of techniques to reduce noise in the workplace.[63]

ACTIVE NOISE CONTROL

The principles of active noise control (or active cancellation) have been known for 50 years but the techniques remain rather experimental. One sound is cancelled by the introduction of a second sound of equal amplitude but reversed phase, derived electronically from the first sound. There are considerable difficulties in designing and commissioning these systems, but the technique does show considerable promise in the reduction of low frequency noise where control by passive measures can be difficult. Commercial interest in the technique is increasing.

EAR PROTECTION

Ear protection provides a system of attenuation of the incoming sound and thus minimizes the sound arriving at the tympanic membrane. Various types of protector are available.[64,65]

Ear muffs

Ear muffs (Fig. 13.14) fit over the ears and are sealed to the side of the head by soft cushion seals filled with soft plastic foam or a viscous fluid. They are usually held in position by means of a headband, but may alternatively be attached to a safely helmet. Attenuation may be 'frequency selective', protecting some frequencies more than others, particularly the higher frequencies rather than the speech frequencies. 'Amplitude selective' devices are designed to provide attenuation that increases with sound level. Such a device usually has a small hole which

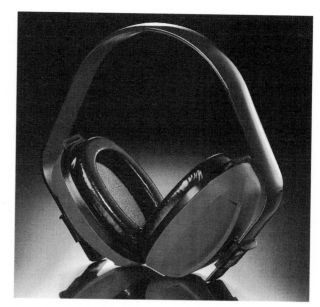

Figure 13.14 *Sound-excluding ear muffs. Reproduced with permission from Bilsom International Ltd., Fountain House, Odiham, Hook, Hampshire RG29 1LP, UK.*

acts as a mechanical filter, allowing low sound pressures to pass but offering more resistance at high pressures. 'Active devices' incorporate electronic circuitry which limits the transmission of sound at high intensity, and are of value when workers are exposed to short bursts of high intensity sound or impulsive sounds. 'Antinoise' devices incorporate circuitry which cancels out incident noise especially at low frequency. These devices are still largely experimental. Many of the newer muffs incorporate an inbuilt communication system.

Whilst ear muffs usually provide an effective level of attenuation, their value may be limited by any effect which decreases the efficiency of the seal, for example spectacle frames, goggles, beards and long hair, or scarves worn under the muffs. Furthermore, wear and tear may decrease the efficiency of the seal. It should also be emphasized that if protection is removed in noisy areas, even for a short period, the amount of protection will be severely limited. For example if a protector with an 'assumed protection' of 20 dB(A) is removed for 30 minutes per day the actual reduction in noise dose received by the wearer will be only 12 dB(A).

Ear plugs

Ear plugs are generally thought to be less efficient attenuators of sound than muffs but have the advantage that they are easy to use. They may be disposable or permanent. Disposable plugs are made of a compressible or conformable material and fit most people without individual fitting. They are readily available commercially, but have a finite 'life expectancy' after which their effectiveness decreases. Permanent and custom moulded plugs have a longer survival, and are usually comfortable if made by an experienced technician. One of the main disadvantages of plugs is the increased propensity to otitis externa, although this too can occur with muffs.

Dual protection with the use of both muffs and ear plugs may be indicated when the noise levels are extremely high (e.g. when LEPd exceeds about 115 dBA)

Noise-excluding helmets

At extremely high levels of sound (e.g. in tunnelling) the protection offered by muffs and plugs either alone or in combination may be insufficient. Sound may still reach the ears through the nose, mouth, eye sockets and the skull itself. Experimental studies with helmets to protect the whole skull are at present under evaluation.

The attenuation provided by a protector should comply with British Standard BS 5108[66] (ISO 4869),[67] and the basic design features should comply with BS 6344.[68] The 'assumed protection' of a device will vary with frequency and most will attenuate higher frequency sound better than low frequency sound. The 'assumed protected level' of noise exposure is obtained by subtracting the assumed protection of the device at each octave band frequency from the sound pressure level at each frequency.

Conversion should then be made to A-weighted sound levels (dBA). All this sounds complicated. Attempts to simplify the rating of devices by using a 'single number' rating which does involve frequency analysis, tends to sacrifice accuracy in the cause of simplicity. It is important that ear protection zones be identified within which use of ear protectors are advisable or mandatory.

Measurement of hearing: audiometry in the workplace

Measurement of hearing using electroacoustic devices is generally referred to as audiometry. Pure tone audiometry records the threshold for each ear separately, at a series of test frequencies at octave intervals covering the frequencies most commonly encountered in everyday life and in particular in everyday speech. The frequencies usually tested in the clinical setting are 125 Hz, 250 Hz, 500 Hz, 1 kHz, 2 kHz, 4 kHz, and 8 kHz. In the medicolegal and compensation fields 3 kHz is always tested, and 6 kHz may be. Air and bone conduction thresholds are measured to establish the presence or absence of a conductive component of the overall hearing loss. Bone conduction thresholds are inaccurate above 3 kHz. Audiometry may be carried out by an audiometrician (manual audiometry) or using a self-recording audiometer.

Hinchcliffe has pointed out the possible shortcomings of manual audiometry.[4] Two different audiometricians might obtain significantly different thresholds at 3 kHz and 4 kHz on the same patient on the same day. Test–retest reliability on the same patient by the same audiometrician may yield differences of up to 25 dB. Self-recording audiometry eliminates the variability due

to the audiometrician. By utilizing a combination of continuous and pulsed test tones there is a greater likelihood of picking up a spurious (non-organic) hearing loss. A permanent record is obtained without the need for transcription with the risk of errors. Sweep frequencies are used because this technique may pick up notches at intervals not tested on fixed frequency audiometry. Thus the preferred technique is sweep frequency self-recording audiometry using both continuous and pulsed tones. An audiometry programme ideally should consist of a pre-employment test followed by tests at regular intervals. Important side issues include the calibration of equipment, the acoustic requirements of the test area, instructions to the subject and the format and storing of records. These are all covered in detail in the Discussion Document *Audiometry in Industry* published by the Health and Safety Executive.[69] Electric Response Audiometry is an objective method of assessing hearing thresholds which has no place in the routine evaluation of hearing loss, but has a role in the medicolegal arena. It will be described later in this chapter.

Information and education

Workers at risk of occupational noise-induced hearing loss need to be educated about the harmful effects of noise and the importance of hearing conservation measures. They need to understand the importance of wearing properly fitting and appropriate ear protectors. The attitude that it is somehow 'macho' not to wear ear protectors must be changed. Workers should recognize and report the first symptoms of deafness such as temporary threshold shift and tinnitus. Warning signs should be attached to machines or displayed in all areas likely to cause workers to receive a daily personal noise exposure of 90 dBA or a peak pressure of 200 Pa (the levels at which the use of ear protectors becomes mandatory). Oral explanations, individual counselling and lectures, as well as leaflets, posters, films and videos may all be employed. Education must be extended to management so that their responsibilities are clearly defined, and managers exposed to potentially damaging sound levels must themselves be seen to be conscientious in their observation of safety measures.

LEGAL DUTIES OF EMPLOYERS

The general obligations of employers in the UK to safeguard the health of their employees (including hearing) were laid out under the Health and Safety at Work Act of 1974. Specific requirements with regard to hearing are covered by the Noise at Work Regulations 1989, which came into force on 1 January 1990. The reader is referred to *Noise at Work: Guidance on Regulations* published by the Health and Safety Executive for full details,[61] but certain salient points can be highlighted here.

The Regulations require the employer to take certain

basic steps where an employee is likely to be exposed to noise at or above the first action level. These together with additional action, must also be taken where an employee is likely to be exposed at or above the second or the peak action level (Regulation 2).

Every employer shall, when any of his employees are likely to be exposed to the first action level or above or to the peak action level or above, ensure that a competent person makes a noise assessment that is adequate for the purpose of a) identifying which of his employees are so exposed, and b) providing him with such information with regard to the noise to which those employees may be exposed as will facilitate compliance with his duties (Regulation (4.1).

Following any noise assessment the employer shall ensure that an adequate record of that assessment is kept until a further noise assessment is made (Regulation 5).

Where employees are exposed at or above the second or peak action levels the employer will have to reduce exposure as far as reasonably practicable by means other than provision of personal ear protectors (Regulation 7). (This entails the use of measures to reduce the actual sound levels themselves as outlined earlier in this chapter.)

Where employees are exposed between the first and second action levels, Regulation 8(1) requires the employer to provide protectors for those who ask for them. Regulation 8(2) requires the employer to provide protectors for all workers likely to be exposed above the second or peak action levels. (This regulation also deals with the need to ensure that the protectors comply with the recommended standards and are suitable for the job in question, and that there are adequate arrangements for the distribution of protectors.)

In addition, the Regulations define the responsibilities of the employer in the provision of ear protection zones, in the maintenance and use of equipment and the provision of information, instruction and training to employees. The employees' obligations under the Regulations are also emphasized. The document also deals with the legal obligations of designers, manufacturers, importers and suppliers of plant and machinery for use at work to provide noise information and control the noise emission of machinery.

MANAGEMENT

With the exception of the transient phenomenon of temporary threshold shift, the hearing loss caused by noise exposure is permanent and is due to the loss of or damage to the organ of Corti and neuronal structures in the inner ear. There is as yet no medical or surgical treatment that can reverse the damage to these structures. Management of occupational noise-induced hearing loss is therefore based on prevention of further damage, suit-

able amplification with hearing aids, and the provision where indicated of other assistive devices. It is generally felt that the process of injury to the inner ear ceases when the subject is removed from, or protected from, his noisy working environment, but subjects should be warned of further possible damage from other sources such as recreational noise exposure.

These effects on the inner ear are, as has been previously stated, most marked in the high frequencies commencing at 4 kHz but spreading downwards across the frequency range. The early effects therefore are most marked for the high frequency components of speech, the consonants, the sibilants and fricatives. It is these elements which convey most of the meaning in speech. Neuronal damage causes a further loss of speech discrimination which may not be correctable by simple amplification. In addition there are other psychoacoustic deficits which may come into play and for which hearing aids cannot compensate, such as impaired frequency discrimination, frequency selectivity or temporal acuity. Furthermore the phenomenon of recruitment, a feature of cochlear deafness, may limit the usefulness of amplification. This is characterized by a disproportionately great increase in the perceived loudness for a small increase in the actual sound pressure level. This is a major factor in causing distortion with hearing aids, and may limit their use. The ability to discriminate speech in the presence of background noise is lost early in the evolution of sensorineural deafness, and involves factors other than a simple elevation of the hearing threshold. It is not restored by fitting a hearing aid and it remains one of the main grievances of hearing aid users who find it impossible to converse with one individual in a noisy environment such as a bar, cocktail party, or if the television or a stereo system is on.

Despite these shortcomings it is, however, clear that individuals with noise-induced hearing impairment can derive appreciable benefit from hearing aids provided that careful attention is given to the type of aid and the design and engineering of the ear mould.

Different hearing aids have different frequency responses. Some preferentially amplify the higher frequencies and this would intuitively seem a sensible type of device for a subject with a high frequency hearing loss. The prescription of an aid with a customized frequency response for an individual hearing loss is beguiling and has commanded much attention in recent years. It is nevertheless a much more challenging problem than the prescription of spectacles for a simple refractive error, for reasons mentioned earlier in this section. Different hearing aids have different gain or amplification (i.e. some are stronger than others), and again it is clearly important to have the appropriate aid for the severity of the deafness. Hearing aids like car engines have a point or a range at which they function best. If one attempts to get more performance from an underpowered aid there is a marked falloff in the efficiency of the device. It is better to get a stronger aid and have it working at its most efficient level. Compression aids incorporating automatic gain control, attempt to overcome the problem of the loud sound which exceeds the discomfort level of the listener.

Systems which address the problems of understanding speech in the presence of background noise have been developed and in the UK are at present only available in the private health sector, where they cost considerably over £1000.

The other factor of considerable importance is the design and fitting of the hearing aid mould. The aid must fit comfortably in the ear, but must be secure enough to prevent acoustic feedback problems – the whistling that one often associates with hearing aids is usually the result of a poorly fitting mould or an underpowered aid with the volume setting too high. The effect of occlusion of the ear canal may be to cause otitis externa in susceptible individuals. Some wearers develop an allergic reaction in the skin of the meatus to the mould material. Hypoallergenic alternatives are available to overcome such problems.

The physical properties of the mould have an effect on the acoustic output of the aid and modifications to the mould may influence the performance of the device. Venting entails the creation of a second hole next to the existing sound tube. This has a considerable effect in increasing the low frequency responses of the aid. It also incidentally may decrease the tendency to otitis externa by decreasing the greenhouse effect within the ear canal. Funnelling of the outlet tube where the sound leaves the mould may increase the high frequency response. Acoustic filters can be introduced into the tube. These may alter the shape of the frequency response curve. All of these facilities are available in the UK on the standard ear level hearing aids. The National Health Service does not, at present, provide small in-the-ear aids.

In addition to hearing aids there are other assistive devices or environmental aids that can be used with or independent of conventional hearing aids[70] including amplifying devices, alerting and alarm systems, telephone modifications and speech to text transcription. They are not necessarily expensive and may provide significant personal benefit. They include induction loop systems, television listening aids, tactile and visual devices activated by sound stimuli (door bells, fire alarms, alarm clocks, telephone). Inductive coupling between coils in the handpiece and the hearing aid greatly helps telephone conversation. Text telephones using a computer link, or a relay service via an operator may help the very deaf. Speech to text transcription such as Palantype is a major help at public meetings, but is expensive and the system operators are relatively few. A simple overview of the devices available is given by Martin.[70]

Cochlear implantation

The cochlear implant is an electric device inserted into the inner ear of certain profoundly deaf individuals to take the place of a severely damaged organ of Corti and convey to the brain a processed sequence of electric stimuli which the brain perceives as sound. Cochlear implants have now reached such a level of sophistication that the best implantees can converse almost effortlessly even over the telephone. To 'qualify' for an implant, a subject must have a degree of deafness that cannot be aided with any conventional hearing aid. Pure occupational-induced hearing loss very rarely if ever produces deafness of that degree of severity, and with the present selection criteria for implantation, cochlear implantation is not a treatment option for such individuals. There are indications, however, that selection criteria may become less strict in the future.

NON-ORGANIC (OR EXAGGERATED, OR FUNCTIONAL) HEARING LOSS

In the medicolegal context, with the attendant lure of financial gain from compensation, the doctor assessing an industrial deafness case has to be constantly aware of the possibility of exaggeration of a hearing loss. Experienced clinicians and audiometricians may develop a finely honed sixth sense, based on the inappropriate or pantomimic behaviour of an individual subject. There may be a clear discrepancy between the perceived hearing of the subject in interview, and the volunteered thresholds on pure tone audiometry. Further discrepancies may exist between the pure tone thresholds and the score on speech audiometry. There may be test-retest unreliability on audiometry, and there may be a lack of agreement between pure tone thresholds obtained with ascending and descending stimulus intensity. Sweep frequency audiometry may reveal a pattern suggestive of non-organic hearing loss. Suspicion may be heightened if the threshold for the stapedial reflex (acoustic reflex) is found to be close to, or better than, the volunteered pure tone threshold. Sometimes these contradictions can be ironed out, and the true threshold established, by the employment of low cunning on the part of the tester. Not infrequently, however, one may have to turn to electric response audiometry for verification.

ELECTRIC RESPONSE AUDIOMETRY (EVOKED RESPONSE AUDIOMETRY)

Electric response audiometry (ERA) provides a method of objectively estimating the auditory thresholds, by the recording of the electrical events which occur in the auditory pathways following the exposure of the ear to an acoustic stimulus. The stimuli used are either broad band clicks containing a wide spectrum of frequencies, or more frequency specific stimuli such as filtered clicks or tone bursts. A single such stimulus will give rise to electrical potential changes in a series of neural structures from the cochlea to the auditory cortex. These events have a characteristic form and latency depending upon which part of the auditory pathway is being studied.

The cochlea and eighth nerve give rise to near field potentials of very short (or no) latency such as the cochlear microphonic (CM), the summating potential (SP) and the eighth nerve action potential (AP). The components of the auditory brainstem response (ABR or BSER) have a latency of up to 7–8 ms, and arise from structures in the lower to mid brainstem. The middle latency response (MLR) takes origin higher in the brainstem and at higher subcortical levels. The slow vertex response (SVR), recorded on cortical ERA (CERA) is thought to take origin from the highest levels in the auditory pathways and naturally has the longest latency (50–300 ms).

Most of these responses are recorded through simple disc electrodes located on the skin of the scalp and are thus non-invasive. The exception is the recording of cochlear potentials by the process of electrocochleography (ECochG, ECoG) which entails the siting of a recording electrode deep in the ear canal on the surface of the ear drum, or sometimes from the medial wall of the middle ear by means of a transtympanic needle electrode. The potentials recorded are of very low voltage, and are difficult to differentiate from random background electrical activity. They have to be extracted by the process of 'time domain averaging' of the responses to a series of stimuli, then amplified for display on a visual display/computer unit where they can be studied, manipulated and stored for future recall. The better the signal-to-noise ratio of the response the fewer stimulus repetitions will be required to produce a reliable recording. Near field responses such as ECochG, therefore, require fewer stimuli that far field responses such as the ABR. A greater number of stimuli are needed to produce a response as the threshold is approached.

Electric response audiometry is employed in the neuro-otological diagnosis of certain disease states. For example, ECochG, yields typical patterns in Ménière's disease. The ABR frequently demonstrates latency abnormalities in tumours of the cerebellopontine angle or brain stem of which vestibular schwannoma is the most common example. The other main use for ERA is to help establish the true hearing threshold when it is difficult to obtain reliable thresholds using conventional techniques. In addition to its role in the case of suspected non-organic hearing loss it is used to test very young children, or children or adults with multiple handicaps who are unable to co-operate in the performance of standard hearing tests. The great advantage of the tech-

nique is that the patient cannot influence the generation of the potentials.

There are, however, certain disadvantages with ERA, some of which are common to all techniques, and some of which are specific to the individual test. Subjectivity on the part of the tester remains, in that it is not always easy, when tracing an ever-decreasing response to a stimulus of decreasing intensity, to determine at exactly what point the response disappears (the end point). Thus the threshold estimation is not always as precise as one might wish. All ERA techniques tend to give more accurate information about high frequency thresholds than about thresholds at frequencies below 1 kHz. In the industrial deafness case this is not always such a problem as in pure clinical work, because most of the desired information is in the higher frequencies anyway. One misconception about ERA needs to be corrected. It is not a better test of hearing than conventional hearing tests. The best estimate of hearing is a standard pure tone audiogram carried out on a willing and co-operative subject; ERA is used when that ability or willingness are absent. The preferred technique in the evaluation of a subject suspected of exaggerated hearing loss is CERA, but two other techniques (ABR and ECochG) are occasionally employed and will also be described.

The auditory brainstem response

The ABR comprises a series of five potentials (N1-N5) which occur in the first 7–8 ms after acoustic stimulation. The generators of these potentials are still the subject of debate, but have been suggested to be:

N1 cochlear nerve/nucleus,
N2 cochlear nucleus,
N3 superior olivary complex,
N4 lateral lemniscus,
N5 inferior colliculus.

Of these, the largest component and the one most usually employed in the estimation of hearing threshold is N5 (Fig. 13.15). Stimuli are presented initially at a moderately high intensity, say 70 dB, and if an N5 response is observed the stimulus intensity is decreased stepwise. As threshold is approached the latency of the N5 response increases and the amplitude decreases, until it is no longer recordable. In a subject with normal hearing, the N5 response can usually be recorded down to stimulus intensities of 25–30 dB. The reason it cannot be recorded at lower intensities is largely due to the small voltage of the response and distance of the recording scalp electrodes from the generators in the brain stem. Most workers in this field would state that if responses are recordable down to 25–30 dB, the hearing is likely to be close to normal.

The advantages of ABR are that in the hands of an experienced audiologist it produces clear and

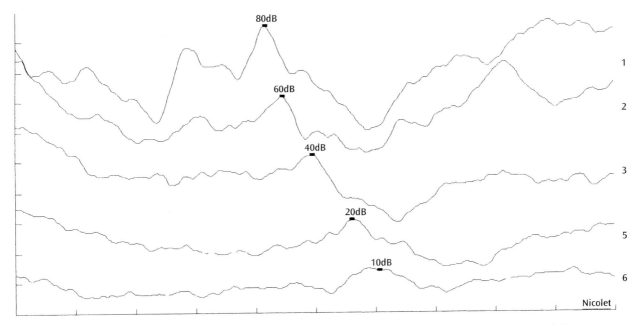

Figure 13.15 *Auditory brainstem response. The stimulus intensity is marked on wave N5. Note that the latency of the N5 response increases and the amplitude decreases as the hearing threshold is approached.*

reproducible waveforms, is non-invasive and carries no risk to the subject. It is also unaffected by general anaesthesia, which is of value in the assessment of the young and uncooperative. There are certain disadvantages. It is quite time-consuming because as the threshold is approached many hundred stimuli may be required to produce a good response, and in order to demonstrate reproducibility the test may have to be repeated several times. The information it yields is greatest in the high frequencies, though as stated above this may be less of a problem in the industrial deafness case.

Electrocochleography

The most important component of the ECochG is the eighth nerve action potential. The signal noise ratio is much more favourable than with ABR, so large and reliable responses can be obtained after very few stimuli, even at quite low stimulus intensities, at which the response again decreases in amplitude and increases in latency. Threshold estimation is usually more accurate than with ABR (probably to within 10–15 dB) but as with ABR the higher frequency responses are more reliable than the low. The main disadvantage is the fact that the recording electrode has to be sited in the ear. An ear canal electrode may be satisfactory but the best responses are obtained from a transtympanic electrode which has to be passed through the tympanic membrane to lie on the cochlea. This is done under topical anaesthesia using Emla® (eutectic mixture of local anaesthetics) cream, and the tiny perforation created nearly always

heals rapidly. Nevertheless the invasiveness of the technique means that it is not the technique of first choice, although there are occasions when its reliability might be desirable.

Cortical evoked response audiometry

CERA records a response, the slow vertex response (SVR) which occurs between 50 and 250 ms after the delivery of sound to the ear (Fig. 13.16). This long latency suggests that it is not a primary response. It is best recorded from scalp electrodes placed at the vertex.[71] The precise generators of the response are unclear, but it is known to arise from cortical structures. It thus has the theoretical advantage over ABR and ECochG of getting closer to recording 'hearing' than the other techniques which record events lower in the auditory pathway. The components of the waveform are two vertex positive waves and one vertex negative wave (the P1, N1, P2 complex).

Although frontal lesions do not affect the waveform, extensive temporoparietal lesions may eliminate the N1 component, but not P1. The SVR is influenced by general anaesthesia and to a lesser extent by sedation so it is of little value in children. It is also influenced by EEG alpha activity so is best tested with the subject's eyes open. In about 5% of subjects high levels of alpha activity make it very difficult to obtain an accurate SVR threshold.[70] In such a situation ABR or ECochG might be preferred. The test is carried out with the subject reclining, perhaps reading. The scalp electrodes are non-

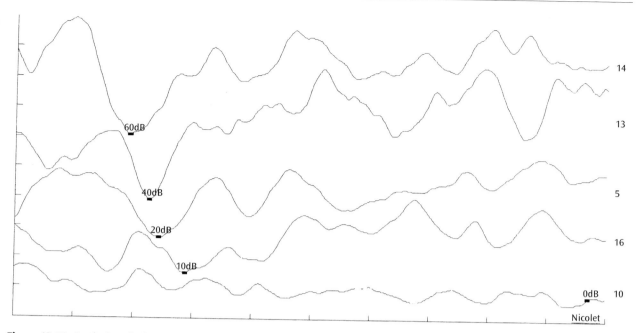

Figure 13.16 *Cortical evoked response audiometry showing the slow vertex response. The vertex negative N1 wave is marked with the stimulus intensity.*

invasive. In most cases an audiogram at 500 Hz, 1 kHz, 2 kHz and 3 kHz can be obtained in an hour. In adults it is usually accurate to about 10 dB of the true threshold[73] and furthermore its frequency specificity is better than that of ABR and ECochG. It is the technique of choice for verification of the pure tone audiogram in cases of suspected NOHL. If the pure tone threshold and the SVR threshold agree to within 10 dB the behaviour threshold is confirmed. If the pure tone threshold exceeds the SVR threshold by 15 dB or more, exaggerated hearing loss should be strongly suspected.[78]

OCCUPATIONAL NOISE-INDUCED TINNITUS

Many individuals have experience of the tinnitus that occurs after exposure to loud music such as that of a rock concert or discotheque. This temporary tinnitus may be short-lived or last for days, depending on the duration and intensity of the exposure and may be associated with a measurable temporary threshold shift.[74] Similarly, tinnitus is reported often to accompany industrial noise exposure and whilst initially it is temporary, over a period of years it may become permanent in as many as 60%, particularly in those exposed to impact noise.[75,76] There is some debate, however, regarding the importance of tinnitus in the assessment of occupational noise-induced hearing loss: Hinchcliffe and King suggest that tinnitus is often a symptom of those seeking compensation.[77] In contrast, a study of 647 individuals with occupational noise-induced hearing loss, showed a prevalence of tinnitus in 23.3%, nearly one-third of

whom felt that the tinnitus was intrusive to the point of having an effect on daily activities.[78] The issue is complicated further by the observation that solicitors advertising their services to potential claimants may do so with provocative statements linking noise exposure at work with tinnitus.[4] The debate then is not so much as to whether tinnitus and occupational noise-induced hearing loss go hand in hand but the weight that should be attributed to the tinnitus component during the evaluation of a claimant.

OCCUPATIONAL NOISE-INDUCED VERTIGO

Temporary vestibular disturbance in response to loud noises is referred to as the Tullio phenomenon. In a state of health, high sound intensities are required to evoke this response. In various otological disorders however, lesser sound levels may have a similar effect in certain individuals. Firm evidence that occupational noise-induced vertigo is a real entity is lacking. However, three more recent studies merit consideration. Shupak and colleagues demonstrated a reduced vestibulo-ocular reflex and reduced caloric response of the inner ear in 22 individuals with occupational noise-induced hearing loss compared with 21 controls though all those evaluated were sub-clinical in terms of vestibular complaints[79] Manabe and colleagues evaluated 36 patients with occupational noise-induced hearing loss cases, half of whom complained of vertigo. In the symptomatic group, a reduced caloric response was also shown as were electrophysiological changes suggestive of endolymphatic hydrops.[80] Histopathological evidence of endolymphatic hydrops in two patients with late onset vertigo and noise-induced hearing loss was provided by Kemink and Graham.[81] Thus there is some evidence to substantiate a link between acoustic trauma and delayed endolymphatic hydrops but further investigation into this aspect of hazardous noise exposure is required.

INFRASOUND AND ULTRASOUND

Evidence that excessive sound above or below the normal human auditory range may have an adverse effect on inner ear function remains scant.

Infrasound (conventionally sound below 20 Hz), is commonly felt as vibration rather than heard and is a component of natural phenomena such as earthquakes and thunder.[82] Heavy industrial machinery, high speed car travel with open windows and ship's engine rooms are potential sources of infrasound. More specifically, Pyykkö and colleagues examined 203 lumberjacks over a 6-year period, compared the hearing in those with and without vibration-induced white finger syndrome and found a statistically significant difference in thresholds at 4 kHz in those with the syndrome than those without.[83] They postulated that the higher thresholds in the lumberjacks with vibration-induced white finger was due to reflex sympathetic vasoconstriction in cochlear blood vessels in response to vasospasm of the hands rather than a direct mechanical effect on the cochlea (see Chapter 14).

The auditory effects of ultrasound (sound above 20 kHz) have been reviewed by Acton. These include a full feeling in the ear, tinnitus and headaches.[84] Utilizing low frequency ultrasound (10 kHz to 28 kHz) in guinea pigs, Ishida and colleagues noted auditory electrophysiological effects including alteration in the cochlear microphonic and increased thresholds.[85] Currently, the adverse auditory effects of hazardous levels of both infrasound and ultrasound in humans remain to be defined.

REFERENCES

1   Pickles JO. Physiology of hearing. In: Kerr AG ed. *Scott-Brown's Otolaryngology* Vol 1. Oxford: Butterworth-Heinemann, 1997: 2/1–34.

2   International Standards Organization. ISO 389. *Acoustics – Standard Reference Zero for the Calibration of Pure-tone Air Conduction Audiometers* (3rd edn). Geneva: ISO, 1991.

3   British Standards Institution BS 2497. *Specification for Standard Reference Zero for the Calibration of Pure-tone Air Conduction Audiometers*. London: BSI, 1992.

4   Hinchcliffe R. Sound, infrasound and ultrasound. In: Raffle PAB, Adams PH, Baxter PJ, Lee WR eds. *Hunter's Diseases of Occupations*. 8th edn. London: Arnold, 1994: 271–94.

5   Alberti PW. Noise and the ear. In: Kerr AG ed. *Scott-Brown's Otolaryngology* Vol 2. Oxford: Butterworth-Heinemann, 1997: 11/1–34.

6   Rosowski JJ, Carney LH, Peake WT. The radiation impedance of the external ear of the cat: measurements and applications. *J Acoust Soc Am* 1990; **84**: 1697–1708.

7   Ludman H. Physiology of hearing and balance In: Ludman H ed. *Mawson's Diseases of the Ear*. London: Edward Arnold, 1988: 74–101.

8   Williams PL, Warwick R (eds). Auditory and vestibular apparatus. In: *Gray's Anatomy*. Edinburgh: Churchill Livingstone, 1996: 1367–97.

9   Ulehlova L, Voldrich L, Janisch R. Correlative of sensory cell density and cochlear length in humans. *Hearing Res* 1987; **28**: 147–51.

10 Békésy G von. The variation of phase along the basilar membrane with sinusoidal variations. *J Acoust Soc Am* 1947; **19**: 452.

11 Sellick PM, Patuzzi R, Johnstone BM. Measurement of basilar membrane motion in the guinea pig using the Mossbauer technique. *J Acoust Soc Am* 1982; **72**: 131–141.

12 Robles L, Ruggero MA, Rich NC. Basilar membrane mechanics at the base of the chinchilla cochlea. I. Input-output functions, tuning curves and response phases. *J Acoust Soc Am* 1986; **80**: 1364–74.

13 Cody AR, Russell IJ. Acoustically induced hearing loss: intracellular studies in the guinea pig cochlea. *Hearing Res* 1988; **35**: 59–70.

14 Pickles JO, Corey DP. Mechanoelectrical transduction by hair cells. *Trends Neurosci* 1992; **15**: 254–9.

15 Bacon FL. *Sylva Sylvarum: or A Natural History*. London: W Rawley, 1627:

16 Ramazzini B. In: Wright WC. *Diseases of Workers*. Translated from the Latin *De Morbis Artificum*. New York: Hafner, 1964: 438–9.

17 Ludman H. Inner ear trauma. In: Ludman H ed. *Mawson's Diseases of the Ear*. London: Edward Arnold, 1988: 593–604.

18 Fosbroke J. Practical observations on the pathology and treatment of deafness II. *Lancet* 1831; 644–8.

19 Barr T. Enquiry into the effects of loud sound upon the hearing of boiler makers and others who work amid noisy surroundings. *Trans Phil Soc Glasgow* 1866; **17**: 223–9.

20 Habermann J. Über die Schwerhörigkeit des Kesselschmiede. *Arch Ohrenheilk* 1890; **30**: 1–25.

21 Fowler EP. Limited lesions of basilar membrane. *Trans Am Otolaryngol Soc* 1929; **19**: 182.

22 Bunch CC. Traumatic deafness. In: Fowler EP ed. *Nelson Loose Leaf Medicine of the Ear*. New York: Thos Nelson, 1939: 349–67.

23 Larsen B. Investigations of professional deafness in shipyard and machine factory labourers. *Acta Otolaryngologica Suppl* 1939; **36**: 3–255.

24 Browning GG, Davis AC. Clinical characterisation of the hearing of the adult British population. *Adv Oto-rhino-laryngol* 1983; **31**: 219–23.

25 Henderson D, Subramaniam M, Boettcher FA. Individual

susceptibility to noise induced hearing loss: an old topic revisited. *Ear and Hearing* 1993; **14**: 153–68.

26 Barrenås ML, Lindgren F. The influence of eye colour on susceptibility to TTS in humans. *Br J Audiol* 1991; **25**: 303–7.

27 Hallberg LR, Jansson G. Women with noise-induced hearing-loss: an invisible group? *Br J Audiol* 1996; **30**: 340–5.

28 Rytzner B, Rytzner C. School children and noise. The 4kHz dip-tone screening in 14391 school children. *Scand Audiol* 1981; **10**: 213–6.

29 Botte MC, Monikheim S. Psychoacoustic characterization of two types of auditory fatigue. In: Dancer AL, Henderson D, Salvi RJ, Hamerick RP eds. *Noise Induced Hearing Loss*. St Louis: Mosby Year Book, 1992: 259–68.

30 Mills JH. Effects of noise on auditory sensitivity, psychophysical tuning curves and suppression. In: Hamernik RP, Henderson D, Salvi R eds. *New Perspectives on Noise Induced Hearing Loss*. New York: Raven Press, 1982: 249–63.

31 Ryan AF, Bennett TM, Woolf NK, Axelsson A. Protection from noise induced hearing loss by prior exposure to a non-traumatic stimulus: role of the middle ear muscles. *Hearing Res* 1994; **72**: 23–8.

32 Igarashi M, Schuknecht HF, Myers EN. Cochlear pathology in humans with stimulation deafness. *J Laryngol Otol* 1964; **78**: 115–23.

33 Bredberg G. The human cochlea during development and ageing. *J Laryngol Otol* 1967; **81**: 739–58.

34 Beagley HA. Acoustic trauma in the guinea pig. II Electron microscopy including the morphology of cell functions in the organ of Corti. *Acta Otolaryngologica* 1965; **60**: 479–95.

35 Liberman MC. Chronic ultrastructural changes in acoustic trauma: serial section reconstruction of stereocilia and cuticular plates. *Hearing Res* 1987; **26**: 25–88.

36 Goa WY, Ding DL, Zheng XY, Ruan FM, Liu YJ. A comparison of changes in the stereocilia between temporary and permanent hearing losses in acoustic trauma. *Hearing Res* 1992; **62**: 27–41.

37 Reuter G, Gitter AH, Thurm U, Zenner HP. High frequency radial movements of the reticular lamina induced by outer hair cell mobility. *Hearing Res* 1992; **60**: 236–46.

38 Saunders JC, Cohen YE, Szymko YM. The structural and functional consequences of acoustic injury in the cochlea and peripheral auditory system: a five year update. *J Acoust Soc Am* 1991; **90**: 136–46.

39 Saunders JC, Dear SP, Schneider ME. The anatomical consequences of acoustic injury: a review and tutorial. *J Acoust Soc Am* 1985; **78**: 833–60.

40 Alberti PW, Hyde ML, Symons FM, Miller RB. The effect of prolonged exposure to industrial noise on otosclerosis. *Laryngoscope* 1980; **90**: 407–13.

41 Simpson DC, O'Reilly BF. The protective effect of a conductive hearing loss in workers exposed to industrial noise. *Clin Otolaryngol* 1991; **16**: 274–7.

42 McShane DP, Hyde ML, Finkelstein DM, Alberti PW. Unilateral otosclerosis in noise-induced hearing loss. *Clin Otolaryngol* 1991; **16**: 70–5.

43 Williams RG. The diagnosis of noise-induced hearing loss. *J Audiol Med* 1996; **6**: 45–58.

44 Department of Health and Social Security. *Occupational Deafness*. London: HMSO, 1973.

45 Alberti PW, Symons F, Hyde ML. The significances of asymmetrical hearing thresholds. *Arch Otolaryngol* 1979; **87**: 255–63.

46 Kerr AG, Byrne JET. Concussive effects of bomb blast on the ear. *J Laryngol Otol* 1975; **89**: 131–43.

47 World Health Organization. *International Classifications, Disabilities and Handicaps*. Geneva: WHO, 1980, 27, 73.

48 King PF, Coles RRA, Lutman ME, Robinson DW. Assessment of hearing disability. In: *Guidelines for Medicolegal Practice*. London: Whurr Publishers, 1992.

49 Hetu R, Riverin L, Getty Lalande N, St-Cyr C. Quantitative analysis of the handicap associated with occupational hearing loss. *Br J Audiol* 1988; **22**: 251–64.

50 British Association of Otolaryngologists and British Society of Audiology. *Method for assessment of hearing disability*. London: BA04 BSA, 1983.

51 Atherley GRC, Noble WG. Clinical picture of occupational hearing loss obtained with the hearing measurement scale. In: Robinson DW ed. *Occupational Hearing Loss*. London: Academic Press, 1971: 193–206.

52 Lutman ME, Brown EJ, Coles RRA. Self reported disability and handicap in the population in relation to pure tone threshold, age, sex and type of hearing loss. *Br J Audiol* 1987; **21**: 45–58.

53 Robinson DW. Relation between hearing threshold level and its component parts. *Br J Audiol* 1991; **25**: 93–103.

54 Robinson DW, Wilkins PA, Thyer NJ, Lawes JF. *Auditory Impairment and the Onset of Disability and Handicap in Noise-induced Hearing Loss*. ISVR Technical Report no. 126. Southampton: University of Southampton, 1984.

55 British Standards Institution BS 5330. *Method of Estimating the Risk of Hearing Handicap Due to Noise Exposure*. London: BSI, 1976.

56 International Standards Organization. ISO 7029. *Acoustics – Threshold of Hearing by Air Conduction as a Function of Age and Sex for Otologically Normal Persons*. Geneva: ISO, 1989.

57 Shipton MS. *Tables Relating Pure-tone Audiometry Threshold to Age*. National Physics Laboratory Report 94. Teddington: National Physics Laboratory, 1979.

58 International Standards Organization. ISO 1999. *Acoustics – Determination of Occupational Noise Exposure and Estimation of Noise-induced Hearing Impairments* (2nd edn). Geneva: ISO, 1990.

59 Burns W, Robinson DW. *Hearing and Noise in Industry*. London: HMSO, 1970.

60 Robinson DW. Impairment and disability in noise-induced hearing loss. In: *Advances in Audiology*. Basel: Karger, 1988: 5: 71–81.

61 Health and Safety Executive. *Noise at Work. The Noise at Work Regulations. Guidance on Regulations*. Sudbury, Suffolk, UK: HSE Books, 1989.

62 Health and Safety Commission. *Prevention of Damage to Hearing from Noise at Work. Draft Proposals for Regulations and Guidance. Consultative Document.* London: HMSO, 1987.

63 Health and Safety Executive. *Sound Solutions. Techniques to Reduce Noise at Work.* Sudbury, Suffolk, UK: HSE Books, 1995.

64 Health and Safety Executive. *Noise at Work. Noise Assessment, Information and Control. Noise Guides* 3–8. Sudbury: HSE Books, 1990.

65 Alberti PW (ed) *Personal Hearing Protection in Industry.* New York: Raven Press, 1982.

66 British Standards Institution BS 5108. *Sound Attenuation of Hearing Protectors.* London: BSI, 1991.

67 International Standards Organization. ISO 4869. *Acoustics – Hearing Protectors.* Geneva: ISO, 1989, 1990.

68 British Standards Institution BS 6344. *Industrial Hearing Protectors.* London: BSI, 1988, 1989.

69 Health and Safety Executive. *Audiometry in Industry. Discussion Document.* London: HMSO, 1978.

70 Martin M. In: Ballantyne J, Martin MC, Martin A eds. *Deafness.* London: Whurr Publishers, 1993: 270–9.

71 Davis H, Zerlin S. Acoustic relations of the human vertex potential. *J Acoust Soc Am* 1966; **39**: 109–16.

72 Hyde M, Alberti P, Matsumoto N, Yao-Li L. Auditory evoked potentials in the audiometric assessment of compensation and medicolegal patients. *Ann Otol Rhinol Laryngol* 1986; **95**: 514–19.

73 Lutman ME. Diagnostic audiometry. In: Kerr AG ed. *Scott-Brown's Otolaryngology* Vol 2. Oxford: Butterworth-Heinemann, 1997: 12/22–23.

74 Coles RRA. Tinnitus. In: Kerr AG ed. *Scott-Brown's Otolaryngology* Vol 2. Oxford: Butterworth-Heinemann, 1997: 18/1–34.

75 McShane DP, Hyde ML, Alberti PW. Tinnitus prevalence in industrial hearing loss compensation claimants. *Clin Otolaryngol* 1988; **13**: 323–30.

76 Axelsson A, Barrenäs ML. Tinnitus in noise-induced hearing loss. In: Dancer AL, Henderson D, Salvi RJ, Hamerick RP eds. *Noise Induced Hearing Loss.* St Louis: Mosby Year Book, 1992: 269–76.

77 Hinchcliffe R, King PF. Medicolegal aspects of tinnitus. I, II, III. *J Audiol Med* 1992; **1**: 38–58, 59–79, 127–47.

78 Phoon WH, Lee HS, Chia SE. Tinnitus in noise-exposed workers. *Occupat Med* 1993; **43**: 35–38.

79 Shupak A, Bar-El E, Podoshin L, Spitzer O, Gordon CR, Ben-David J. Vestibular findings associated with chronic noise induced hearing impairment. *Acta Otolaryngol* 1994; **114**: 579–85.

80 Manabe Y, Kurokawa T, Saito T, Saito H. Vestibular dysfunction in noise-induced hearing loss. *Acta Otolaryngologica Suppl* 1995; **519**: 262–4.

81 Kemink JL, Graham MD. Hearing loss with delayed onset of vertigo. *Am J Otol* 1985; **6**: 344–8.

82 Westin JB. Infrasound. A short review of effects on man. *Aviat Space Environ Med* 1975; **46**: 1135–43.

83 Pyykkö I, Starck J, Farkkila M, Hoikkala M, Korhonen O, Nurminen M. Handarm vibration in the aetiology of hearing loss in lumberjacks. *Br J Ind Med* 1981; **38**: 281–9.

84 Acton WI. Exposure to industrial ultrasound: hazards, appraisal and control. *J Soc Occup Med* 1983; **33**: 107–13.

85 Ishida A, Matsui T, Yamamura K. The effects of low-frequency ultrasound on the inner ear: an electrophysiological study using the guinea pig cochlea. *Eur Arch Oto-Rhino-Laryngol* 1993; **250**: 22–6.

86 Kessel RG, Kardon RH. *Tissues and Organs: A Text-Atlas of Scanning Electron Microscopy.* San Francisco: Freeman, 1979.

87 Pickles JO. *An Introduction to the Physiology of Hearing.* New York: Academic Press, 1982.

88 Wright A. Anatomy and ultrastructure of the human ear. In: Kerr AG ed. *Scott-Brown's Otolaryngology* Vol I. Oxford: Butterworth-Heinemann, 1997.

Colour plates

These illustrations also appear in the text in black and white

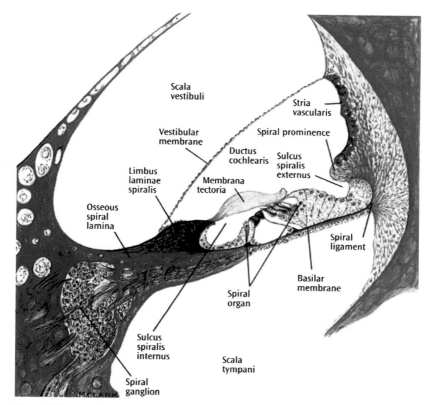

Plate 1 (Figure 13.5) *Section through the cochlea showing the organ of Corti. Mallory's stain.*

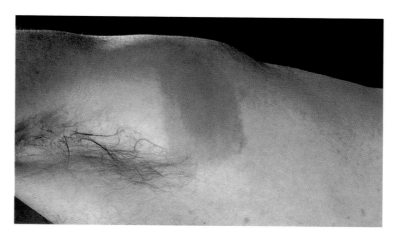

Plate 2 (Figure 24.1) *Erythema migrans: the patient had been picnicking in an area known to be infested with* Ixodes ricinus, *the tick responsible for transmission of* Borelia burgdorferi.

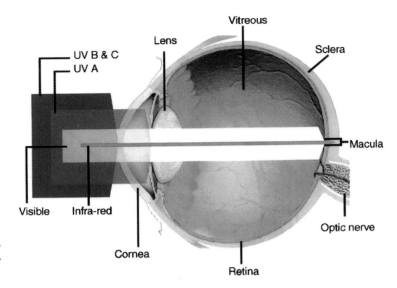

Plate 3 (Figure 20.3) *The penetration/absorption of ultraviolet, visible and infrared radiation by the different structures of the eye.*

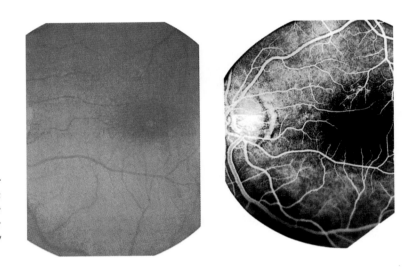

Plate 4 (Figure 20.5) *Photographs of solar retinopathy. The fundus photograph shows pigmentary disturbance at the fovea and the angiogram confirms a focal window defect in the pigment epithelium at the fovea. Provided by Professor D McLeod, Manchester.*

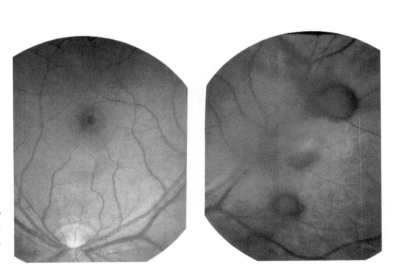

Plate 5 (Figure 20.6) *Photographs of an accidental laser lesion causing a macular hole, a cuff of surrounding subretinal haemorrhage and choroidal bleeding into the surrounding vitreous. Provided by Professor A Bird, Moorfields Eye Hospital, London.*

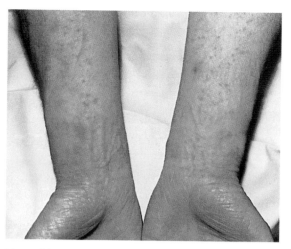

Plate 6 (Figure 37.1) *Scabies mimicking contact eczema.*

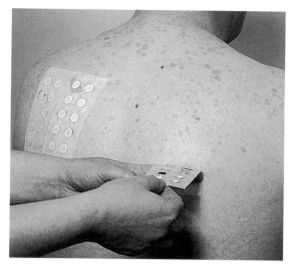

Plate 8 (Figure 37.3) *Patch tests being applied.*

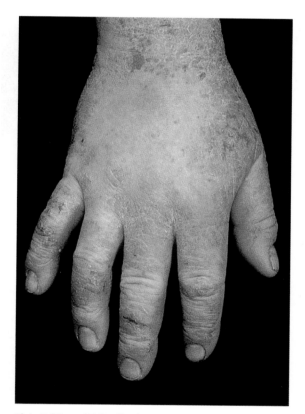

Plate 7 (Figure 37.2) *Allergic contact dermatitis from chromate in cement.*

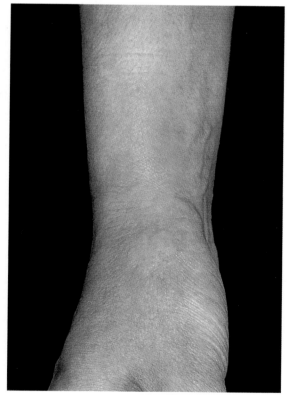

Plate 9 (Figure 37.4) *Immunological contact urticaria from natural rubber latex gloves.*

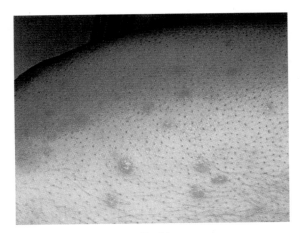

Plate 10 (Figure 37.5) *Oil folliculitis.*

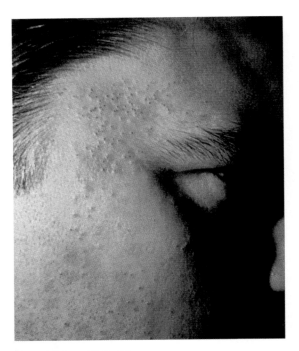

Plate 11 (Figure 37.6) *Chloracne.*

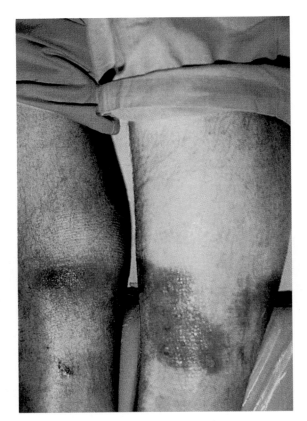

Plate 12 (Figure 37.7) *Burns from quick-setting cement.*

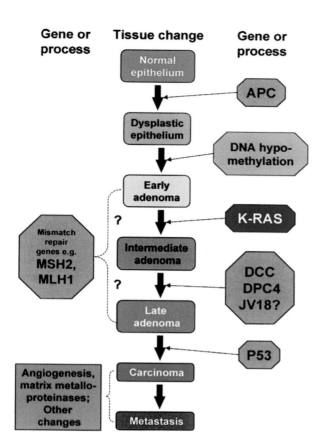

Gene or process | **Tissue change** | **Gene or process**

Normal epithelium

APC

Dysplastic epithelium

DNA hypo-methylation

Early adenoma

?

Mismatch repair genes e.g. MSH2, MLH1

K-RAS

Intermediate adenoma

?

Late adenoma

DCC DPC4 JV18?

P53

Angiogenesis, matrix metallo-proteinases; Other changes

Carcinoma

Metastasis

Plate 13 (Figure 38.1) *A genetic model for colorectal tumorigenesis, based on Ref. 20. 'Tissue changes' refers to the pathological changes that occur during the development of human colorectal cancer. 'Gene or process' refers to the genes or processes that are perturbed or changed during carcinogenesis. The genes depicted in pale blue are tumour-suppressor genes (see Table 38.2 for details). During carcinogenesis, tumour suppressor genes are inactivated by mutation and other genetic events that lead to the loss of both alleles. DCC, DPC4 and JV18 are candidate tumour-suppressor genes. K-RAS is an oncogene (Table 38.1) which requires point mutation in just one of its two alleles for its activation. DNA hypomethylation may allow inappropriate gene expression. Inactivation of mismatch repair genes increases the mutability of affected cells. The precise timing of mismatch-repair inactivation is unknown.*

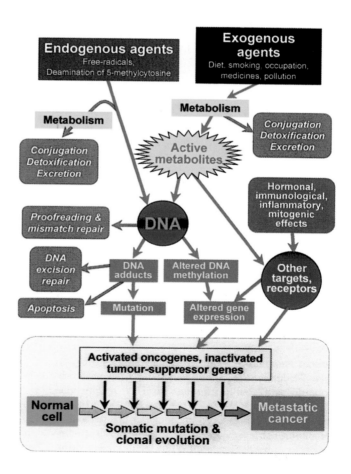

Plate 14 (Figure 38.2) *Pathways in carcinogenesis. The text in green boxes and the green arrows denote protective pathways and processes. The text in red boxes and the red arrows depict deleterious pathways and processes.*

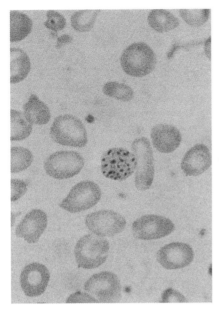

Plate 15 (Figure 44.3) *Basophilic stippling.*

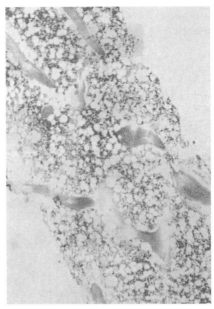

Plate 17 (Figure 44.5a) *Normal marrow.*

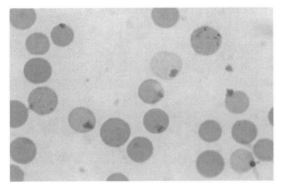

Plate 16 (Figure 44.4) *Heinz bodies.*

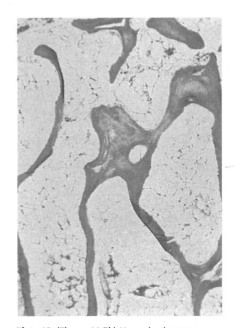

Plate 18 (Figure 44.5b) *Hypoplastic marrow.*

14

Vibration (hand–arm and whole body)

PETER L PELMEAR

Hand–arm vibration	308
Whole-body vibration	317
References	319

Vibration is a physical stressor to which many people are exposed either at work, in the home or in their social activities. The oscillatory motion from a source e.g. vehicle, work station or tool, may be a simple harmonic sine wave with displacement, velocity and acceleration; a multiple wave complex differing in frequency and acceleration; or a random non-repeating series of complex waves.

To analyse and quantify the characteristics of any vibratory wave form, one needs to take note of the following points.

1 *The displacement.* This is the distance travelled by the wave form or object (in millimeters or inches); the velocity which is the speed (m/s, ft/s) of the displacement; and the acceleration which is the rate of change of speed or velocity expressed as distance/time/time (m/s/s or ft/s/s).

2 *The frequency.* Another characteristic of motion is that it can repeat itself over and over again. One full cycle of motion completed in 1 second(s) is the frequency of vibration. This is measured in cycles/s or hertz (Hz).

3 *The peak value.* This is the maximum instantaneous acceleration measured during the time period.

4 *The root mean square (rms) value.* This refers to the instantaneous accelerations measured during the time period (Fig. 14.1). It is calculated as the square root of the mean of the sum of squares of all these measurements.

5 *The crest factor.* This is the ratio between the peak value and the rms value. The more impulsive a vibration, the higher the crest factor.

Vibration is also a vector quantity and the linear motion can move up-and-down, back-and-forth, or side-to-side in three mutually perpendicular directions or axes

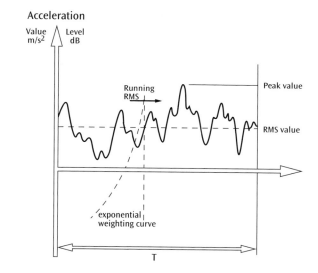

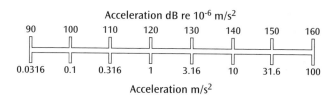

Figure 14.1 *Vibration measurement.*

(X,Y,Z). Around each of these axes, rotational motion can occur – i.e. pitch, yaw, and roll. For simplicity, usually only the linear motion is measured. Three vibration transducers (accelerometers) have to be used, one for each axis, and they need to be as light as possible. The minute electrical signals, which are recorded simultaneously, are amplified and computer analysed.

The latter, known as the Fourier spectrum analysis, will characterize the acceleration levels at the respective frequencies in each linear X, Y, and Z axis, and the data can then be compared with reference standards. It is important to appreciate that humans, like physical structures, respond characteristically to certain critical vibration frequencies at which there is maximum energy transfer from source to receiver. It may even be enhanced. At these specific resonant frequencies, which differ for the different organs in the body, the adverse effects from exposure will be exacerbated. In general, the larger the system mass the lower the resonant frequency. In humans, the principal resonance frequencies by body part when standing are whole body 4–7 Hz; head and shoulder 1–2 Hz; lower arm 15–30 Hz; hand 30–150 Hz; legs 2–20 Hz; and knees 1–3 Hz range. When sitting or reclining the principal resonances by body part are foot 16–31 Hz; knees, abdomen and chest 4–8 Hz; eye-balls 20–25 Hz; and skull 50–70 Hz range.[1]

It is common to distinguish two different types of vibration exposure in humans:

1 hand–arm vibration (HAV) (segmental) when contact with the source is through the fingers and hands;
2 whole-body vibration (WBV) when the body is supported on a vibrating surface (usually a seat or the floor).

HAND–ARM VIBRATION

Health effects

Adverse health effects from exposure to HAV have been recognized since 1911 when Loriga reported dead fingers amongst the Italian miners who used pneumatic tools. Such tools had been introduced into the French mines in 1839 and were being extensively used by 1890. In the United States of America pneumatic tools were first introduced into the limestone quarries of Bedford, Indiana about 1886. The health hazard from their use was subsequently investigated by Dr Alice Hamilton and her colleagues in 1918.

Since then there have many reports in the literature from all over the world.[2–5] First reports of the syndrome in specific tool users occurred as follows: compressed air tools (1911 and 1918); grinding wheels (1931); cutlery grinding (1940); pneumatic drills, fettlers, riveters, caulkers, and polishers (1945); jack-leg and stoper drills (1962); chain saws (1964); brush cutters (1979); speed-way motorcycles (1982); surgical instruments (1994);[6] power screwdrivers (1996);[7] and pneumatic knives (1999).[8]

It is now evident that adverse health effects can result from almost any vibrating source in contact with the hands (and the feet in some situations) if the vibration is sufficiently intense over the frequency range 4–5000 Hz for a critical period of time. The time exposure necessary may range from 1 month to 30 years.

The most important sources of HAV are pneumatic tools (air compressed and electrical) e.g. grinders, sanders, drills, fettling tools, impact wrenches, jack hammers, rivetting guns etc. Users of chainsaws, brush saws, hedge cutters and grass trimmers are also at risk (Table 14.1).

The predominant health effect is known as the Hand–Arm Vibration Syndrome (HAVS),[9] and some of the occupations associated with it and the types of tool used are shown in Table 14.2.

HAVS is a disease entity with the following separate peripheral components:

- *Circulatory disturbances* (vasospasm with local finger blanching 'white finger').
- *Sensory and motor disturbances* (numbness, loss of finger co-ordination and dexterity, clumsiness and inability to perform intricate tasks).
- *Musculoskeletal disturbances* (muscle, bone and joint disorders).

While arterial disruption or spasm is necessary to stop the blood flow, vasospasm in the skin venules is essential

Table 14.1 *Some tools associated with hand-arm vibration*

Drills	Sanders/Buffers
Jack-leg	Orbital sanders
Stoper	Oscillating (jitter-bug)
Plugger	Rotary burrs
Hammer	Floor polishers/buffers
Jack hammer	
Spade	**Saws**
Diamond	Chain
Dental	Brush
	Band
Guns	Concrete
Hilte	Block
Rivetting	
Chipping	**Other**
Fettling	High pressure hoses
Needle	Swaging
Kango	Vibrating pokers (concrete)
	Grass trimmers
Impact	
Wrenches	
Pneumatic screwdrivers	
Pneumatic knives	
Grinders	
Pedestal grinders	
Disc grinders	
Swing-beam grinders	
Angle grinders	
Straight grinders	
Orthodontic	

Table 14.2 *Some occupations associated with hand–arm vibration syndrome and type of tool*

Occupations	Type of tools
Assembly workers aircraft vehicle	Wrenches, screwdrivers, grinders, sanders, buffers
Autobody shop workers	Wrenches, screwdrivers, grinders, sanders, buffers, pneumatic knives
Bricklayers	Block saws
Drop forge workers	Handles, tongs
Carpenters	Saws, screwdrivers, wrenches, needle guns
Construction workers	Guns (various), jack hammers, vibrating pokers
Die shop workers	Drills (various)
Electricians	Hilte guns, screwdrivers
Foresters	Chainsaws, brush saws
Foundrymen	Grinders (various), fettling, chipping guns
Iron workers	Wrenches, grinders (various)
Labourers	Jack hammers, vibrating pokers, concrete saws
Mechanics	Wrenches, grinders
Millwrights	Grinders, impact wrenches
Miners	Drills (various)
Pipe fitters	Hilte guns
Press operators	Handles, tongs
Rivetters	Rivetting guns, wrenches
Welders	Grinders, fettling tools

to produce the blanching. All components may not be recognized in a patient at the same time, and although there is an association between the vascular and sensorineural components of HAVS the two components appear to occur and progress independently of each other. There may be a delay in onset of one or more components, and in the recovery phase the vascular disturbance usually clears before the sensory disturbance.

The most commonly observed component is vasospasm, also known as Raynaud's phenomenon, hence the occupational disease was called 'vibration white finger' initially. Raynaud's phenomenon, is precipitated by exposure to cold and/or damp conditions, and sometimes HAV exposure itself. The time period between first exposure to HAV and its onset is termed the 'latent interval.' There is considerable variation because of individual susceptibility, however, the shorter the mean latent interval period in a work situation, the greater the risk to workers of early onset and progression of severity. The blanching is accompanied by numbness, and as the circulation to the digits recovers, with return of colour from white to blue (cyanosis) to red (reactive hyperaemia), there is usually pain. Tingling and paraesthesia may precede the onset of blanching in many subjects.[10]

The blanching is initially restricted to the tips of one or more fingers but progresses as the vibration exposure time increases. The thumbs are usually the last to be affected. The existence of sensory and vascular components in HAVS led to the adoption of the Stockholm

Table 14.3 *The Stockholm Workshop Scale for classification of hand–arm vibration syndrome*

Stage	Grade	Description
Cold-induced Raynaud's phenomenon[a]		
0	–	No attacks
1	Mild	Occasional attacks affecting only the tips of one or more fingers
2	Moderate	Occasional attacks affecting distal and middle (rarely also proximal) phalanges of one or more fingers
3	Severe	Frequent attacks affecting all phalanges of most fingers
4	Very severe	As in stage 3, with trophic skin changes in the finger tips
Sensorineural effects[a]		
0_{SN}	–	Exposed to vibration but no symptoms
1_{SN}	–	Intermittent numbness, with or without tingling
2_{SN}	–	Intermittent or persistent numbness, reduced sensory perception
3_{SN}	–	Intermittent or persistent numbness, reduced tactile discrimination and/or manipulative dexterity

[a]The staging is made separately for each hand. In the evaluation of the subject, the grade of the disorder is indicated by the stages of both hands and the number of affected fingers on each hand e.g. 2L(2)/1R(1),-/3R (4).

grading,[11,12] based on the subjective history supported by the results of clinical tests, to stage the severity (Table 14.3). The vascular and sensorineural symptoms and signs are evaluated separately, and for both hands.

In advanced cases the peripheral circulation becomes sluggish, giving a cyanotic tinge to the skin of the digits, and in very severe cases trophic skin changes (gangrene) will appear at the finger tips. Smoking tends to accelerate the onset of finger blanching and has been shown to increase the risk in several studies. Recovery from HAVS is also delayed if the addiction continues.

In addition to tactile, vibrotactile, and thermal threshold impairment, which may differ in severity from subject to subject, impairment of grip strength is a common symptom in the longer exposed worker,[13] both with respect to power and the ability to sustain. Discomfort and pain in the upper limbs is also a common complaint.

The toes can be affected if directly subjected to vibration from a local source (such as a vibrating platform), or they may be affected by reflex sympathetic spasm in subjects with severe hand symptoms.[14–19] Reflex sympathetic vasoconstriction may also account for the increased severity of noise-induced hearing loss in HAVS subjects.[20,21]

Swelling of the fingers and hands is usual following exposure to HAV. Normally it is mild and may persist,[22] but sometimes it is more severe and episodic angioedema with secondary carpal tunnel syndrome (CTS) has been reported.[23]

Bone cysts and vacuoles, although often reported,[24,25] are more likely to be caused by forceful manual activity of the hands because of adverse biodynamic and ergonomic factors.

Recent studies indicate that the hearing of subjects with HAVS is particularly vulnerable to noise. Pyykkö et al.[26] studied 72 lumberjacks in 1972 and 203 in 1978, and grouped them according to their history, age, duration of chainsaw use, and use of hearing protectors. They were exposed to noise at 95–107 dBA Leq (the average noise exposure level over a defined time interval). The hearing level at 4000 Hz was used as a measure of noise-induced hearing loss. A statistically significant difference ($p < 0.001$) in hearing level was found between lumberjacks with and without HAVS. These findings were confirmed by Pelmear et al.[27] in a study of 227 hard-rock miners exposed in 1985 and 1987 to noise levels of 107–117 dBA Leq. It is unlikely that vibration from hand-held tools is transmitted to the inner ear in amounts sufficient to cause a direct mechanical effect on the cochlea structures, so the explanation is presumably reflex sympathetic vasoconstriction from vasospasm in the hands, with consequent ischaemia and hair cell destruction.[28]

The condition of HAVS caused by continuous HAV exposure is now well recognized,[29] but the association with impact vibration has been less well identified by researchers.

Khilberg[30] studied the acute effects and symptoms of workers with vibrating hand-held powered tools. He found that workers using non-impact tools (grinders) had a lower prevalence of elbow and shoulder symptoms than those using low-frequency impact tools (chipping hammers), but did not differ in this respect from workers using high-frequency impact tools. Work with impact tools in general was associated with a higher prevalence of pain in the wrist than work with non-impact tools. He suggests that an explanation for these findings may be that low-frequency impact vibration is transmitted to the upper arm, thus constituting a potential hazard to the elbow and shoulder as well as to the muscles in the arm and shoulder. Independent of frequency, impact vibration is transmitted to the wrist, which may therefore be affected.

In a recent analysis of 141 HAV-exposed workers examined for HAVS,[31] a strong association was found between the development of finger blanching and the use of high vibration level impact pneumatic tools (identified by a 20 dB or more difference between the weighted Leq component and the corresponding weighted peak acceleration in the dominant direction). The impulsive tools included jack hammers, electric hammers, stoper drills, and impact guns. Starck et al.[32] had drawn attention to this association of impulsiveness with pedestal grinders using zirconium corundum wheels as it had not been reported previously in the literature from other work situations. The importance of impulsiveness was emphasized again in subsequent papers.[33,34]

A more recent report[35] of HAVS being associated with impact vibration in ten spot-welding and punch press operators provides further evidence that impact vibration, in addition to continuous vibration, is a potential hazard to health. Hence, impact vibration (high impulsiveness) is a critical factor which needs to be addressed in the design of vibratory tools and in the hazard risk assessment of tools in use.

Diagnosis

The assessment of patients with HAVS seeking diagnostic evaluation is an on-going activity which is increasing, particularly in the area of compensation (see Chapter 2). Their grading according to the Stockholm Workshop scales[11,12] is a well established protocol now in clinical practice and in field studies. However, there may be a significant disparity in the level of agreement between ratings based on history alone, and ratings verified by clinical tests,[36] because with health education and the avoidance of cold, many workers are able to reduce the number of blanching attacks. Consequently the frequency factor in the scales can be misleading, so the provisional history grading for each hand needs to be verified with the results of clinical tests.

In general the diagnosis of HAVS is based on the symptoms, the history of HAV exposure, and the exclusion of other causes of Raynaud's phenomenon i.e. Primary Raynaud's phenomenon (Raynaud's disease or constitutional white finger), local trauma to the digital vessels, thoracic outlet syndrome, drugs (e.g. β-adrenoceptor blocking agents and cytotoxic drugs such as bleomycin or vinblastine medication), peripheral vascular disease, and the collagen diseases, including scleroderma.

The simple clinical tests for vascular assessment include Adson's test[37] – palpation of wrist pulse pressure reduction on rotation of the neck with inspiration, to detect thoracic outlet obstruction, and Allen's test[38] – radial and ulnar artery compression and release at the level of the wrist with observation of any delay in the return of colour to the hand and fingers, to evaluate arterial circulation at or distal to the wrist.

The laboratory vascular tests[39] for the upper limbs (the lower limb as well when indicated) may include Doppler studies (to check the patency of the limb blood vessels and the blood pressure ratios in the peripheral vessels), plethysmography (on the digits to evaluate the pulse waves before and after cold stress), finger systolic pressure measurement[40,41] (to compare the blood pressure of an affected digit pre- and post-cold stress), and cold air or water provocation tests[42] (immersion of the digits in water or air for 2–10 minutes at 5–15°C with recording of skin temperature) to note any reactive hyperaemia while immersed, and delay in recovery afterwards. The cold-stress tests are used to verify that vasospasm occurs on cold exposure, and the severity grade may be determined from the results.

The recommended pre-examination regimen prior to an assessment is that the patient should have avoided HAV exposure for 16 hours; should be conditioned for 30 minutes prior to the test in a room temperature at 20–24°C; should preferably have a minimum hand temperature of 30°C; and should not have smoked on the day of the test.

The sensorineural tests[39] may include subjective tests e.g. Tinel's[43] – median nerve percussion at the wrist, and Phalen's tests[44] – wrist hyperflexion; pin prick, cotton wool, or monofilament hairs (von Frey or Semmes–Weinstein); callipers for two-point discrimination; depth sense and two-point appreciation[45] (plastic blocks with split levels and widening groves); grip strength; finger tip vibration threshold[46] at 8–500 Hz with vibrometer instrumentation;[47] thermal hot/cold perception (using Minnesota thermal discs[48] or instrumentation[49–51]); and current perception threshold tests[52,53] (detection of a 0–10 milliamperes current at 5250 and 2000 Hz). The only objective test available is nerve conduction and although this is advantageous because it eliminates the reporting bias of patients it can only evaluate the large medullated fibres. When the results are abnormal the patient has to be graded in Stage 3 SN sensorineural.

Finally urine and blood analyses need to be conducted to identify any systemic diseases (e.g. diabetes, rheumatoid and collagen disease, blood dyscrasias).

The use of multiple tests[54,55] to identify and quantify the severity of the neuropathy in HAVS patients is also important information for the surgeon hoping to relieve a supposedly median nerve compression from CTS. By definition there cannot be an ulnar neuropathy in CTS and it is unusual for repetitive strain injuries to produce it. An ulnar neuropathy on the other hand is quite often present together with a median neuropathy in HAVS.[56] If previous HAV exposure is recognized needless CTS surgery and poor surgical results, will be avoided.

There is a need for the diagnostic tests used in the examination of HAVS patients to be standardized and the results statistically analysed to provide normative data. This will permit physicians to correctly establish the severity and impairment of HAVS in those subjects seeking compensation.

It is usual when evaluating the merits of clinical tests to consider sensitivity and specificity. The usual gold standard is the presence or absence of disease. With respect to HAVS the reference standard varies e.g. history alone or history plus laboratory tests. Furthermore, there are grades of severity which are identified by the different tests. Hence the sensitivity and specificity of a specific test will depend on the severity grade e.g. plethysmography is usually very sensitive and specific for early mild cases, while cold immersion is better for prolonged and sustained vasospasm. Similarly finger systolic pressure using the thumb as a reference digit, and nerve conduction are only highly sensitive and specific in the severe stages.[56] A superficial comparison of the test results published by researchers will lead to erroneous conclusions with respect to the value of a test, and the enlightened researcher will avoid this.

There is a need for an ongoing evaluation of the numerous administrative and treatment regimens used for patients suffering from vibration-induced disease. In follow-up studies of HAVS subjects, the health effects should be evaluated in response to medication and therapy, as well as a reduction in HAV exposure. Many HAVS patients receive no medication at all, and in those that do there is little if any statistical evaluation of the results of specific medication and therapy.

Pathophysiology

An understanding of the pathophysiology of HAVS is still evolving. It is now generally agreed that due to the mechanical stimulus, specific anatomical changes occur in the small arteries and arterioles of the digits i.e. vessel wall muscle hypertrophy which ultimately leads to narrowing of the lumen, and endothelial cell damage.[57–62] In addition, intimal fibrosis is seen sometimes, especially in severe cases.[58] In the initial stages there is extrusion of fluid into the tissues, and this oedema, together with the subsequent spasmodic ischaemia from the cold-induced vasospasm, damages the mechanoreceptor nerve endings and non-medullated fibres. Subsequently a demyelinating neuropathy of the peripheral nerve trunks develops. So, the principal pathological changes in the digits of the hand are arterial medial muscular hypertrophy, a demyelinating neuropathy, and an increase in connective tissue with collagen.[59,60] Medial muscular hypertophy and narrowing in small arteries have also been observed in toe biopsies.[61,62]

Angiographic studies of the upper limbs have demonstrated organic stenoses and occlusions of the digital arteries in workers exposed to vibration,[63,64] and arterial obstructions are occasionally also found in the palmer arches of the ulnar artery[65] (hypothenar hammer syndrome). No definite relationship between arteriographic changes and blanching sites has been established and no correlation was found in a finger biopsy study.[62]

The vascular response to cold with vasoconstriction and subsequent decrease in skin temperature and blood flow, often accompanied by palmar sweating, is mediated through the sympathetic system.[66–73] These responses can occur in the unexposed hand[63–68,70,71] and also feet.[70,72]

Microneurographic techniques have shown that vibration will evoke and increase sympathetic activity in the nerves supplying the hand and foot, a somatosympathetic reflex.[74–76] However, vibration may also inhibit smooth muscle contraction and cause vasodilation,[77–79] even with a nerve block. Hence, acute vibration exposure may induce both a direct vasodilation and a reflex vasoconstriction response on peripheral blood vessels. Studies have suggested that low amplitude (10–25 microns (μ)) and high frequency (150–250 Hz) induce vasodilation, while high amplitude (100–200 μ) at frequencies 30–500 Hz cause vasoconstriction.[76] The optimum frequencies for vasoconstriction have been reported to be 30–60 Hz, 125 Hz, or 125–500 Hz.[76–82] These responses may be mediated by the pacinian corpuscles which are easily excited by vibration at frequencies above 50 Hz, and most easily at 250 Hz; and Meissner's corpuscles which are activated at 5–50 Hz, and most sensitively at 30 Hz.[83]

It is probable that the cold-induced pathological closure of the digital arteries and end vessels is mainly mediated by α2-adrenoceptors in the wall of the arterioles and veins. It has been demonstrated that the α2-receptors are more receptive to the cold stimulus. In HAVS it is postulated that there is selective damage of α2-receptors, hence the cold stimulus is more effective.[84–86]

The endothelium also plays a vital role because cold, as well as vessel wall injury e.g. from vibration, causes platelet aggregation and skin vasconstriction as a net effect of the liberation of various vasoactive substances.[87] Vibration can produce arterial shear stress[88,89] to induce endothelial damage, and acute exposure to vibration also increases plasma norepinephrine, a neurotransmitter released from the peripheral sympathetic nerve ending and the adrenal medulla.[90] The release of serotonin (5-hydroxytryptamine, 5-HT) promotes further release of 5-HT from the platelets, and the increased concentration stimulates smooth muscle to contract. Besides promoting contraction, serotonin may also contribute to vasodilation by inducing the release of endothelium-derived relaxing factor and prostacyclin from the endothelial cells. Acetylcholine and its agonist metacholine, acting through the muscarine receptors on the endothelial cell stimulates endothelium-derived relaxing factor (probably nitric oxide), while nitric oxide and its agonists, nitroprusside and nitroglycerine, release prostacyclin. The prostacyclin and endothelium-derived relaxing factor besides inhibiting platelet aggregation, stimulate the production of cyclic adenosine monophosphate (cAMP) and cyclic guanosine monophosphate (cGMP) in the smooth muscle cell. The latter substances inhibit calcium utilization by the smooth muscle cells so they do not contract. A delicate balance between smooth muscle contraction and relaxation is produced by these mechanisms interacting simultaneously (Figs 14.2, 14.3, 14.4).

It has been demonstrated that prolonged exposure to vibration causes a peripheral neuropathy with damage to the mechanoreceptor nerve endings,[58,91] loss of myelin sheaths and axon deterioration. Lundborg et al.[92] demonstrated in rats that following exposure to vibration, oedema developed in the epineurium of the sciatic nerve. Such an effect may result in nerve function disturbance through interference with nerve fibre nutrition. Subsequently, Ho and Yu[93] exposed rabbits to vibration at 60 Hz and found that it induced disruption of the myelin sheath and constriction of the axon proportional to the vibration dose. Previously, Takeuchi et al.[59,60] in their finger biopsy reports on subjects with vibration syndrome had noted a demyelinating neuropathy and increased collagen in the connective tissue, intraneurally and extraneurally.

Recent studies of skin biopsies using immunohistological techniques have demonstrated in patients with primary Raynaud's phenomenon, and Raynaud's phenomenon secondary to HAVS and systematic sclerosis that there is a reduction of digital nerve fibres containing the powerful vasodilator and sensory neuropeptide–calcitonin gene-related peptide, as well as protein gene product 9.5 immunoreactive nerve fibres.[94,95] The loss of calcitonin gene-related peptide will influence the severity of vasospasm, while the reduced protein gene product immunostaining indicates generalized structural neuronal damage which could account for the pain and paraesthesia characteristic of HAVS. Thus the vibration-induced sensorineural symptoms may arise from vascular insufficiency of the nerve endings and distal digital branches of the ulnar and median nerves, and/or their nerve trunks. In the early stages HAVS patients often

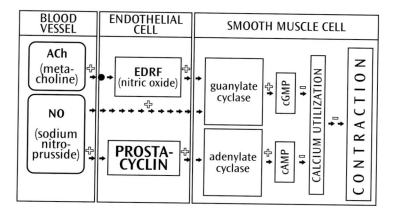

Figure 14.2 *Schematic representation of endothelial vasoactive mechanisms. Reproduced from Ref. 29 with permission.*

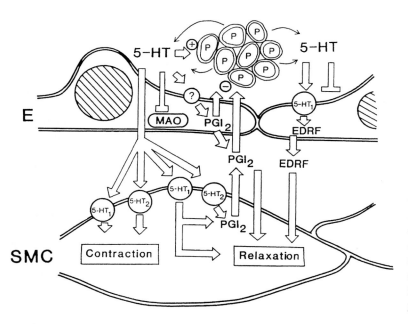

Figure 14.3 *Interactions between platelets (P), endothelium (E), and smooth muscle cells (SMC) involving serotonin (5-HT). ERDF = endothelium–derived relaxing factor; MAO = monoamine oxidase (metabolizing some of the serotonin); PGI2 = prostaglandin I2 (prostacyclin); 5-HT1 and 5-HT2 = different types of serotonin receptors. Reproduced from Ref. 29 with permission.*

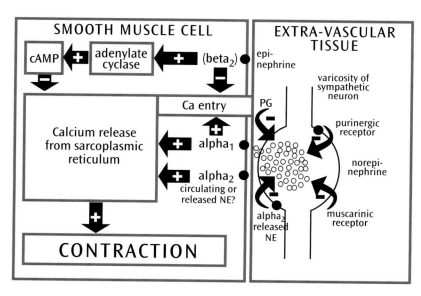

Figure 14.4 *Schematic representation of skin vasoregulation. Reproduced from Ref. 29 with permission.*

have a reactionary oedema of the fingers and hands, and a nocturnal increase whilst in the prone position is common. The median nerve axon and myelin sheath are thereby affected (as indicated by nerve conduction studies) and also the ulnar nerve in two-thirds of the cases.[36] Less frequently the ulnar nerve axon and myelin sheath alone is involved. When the median nerve myelinated fibres are involved at the wrist level, there can be confusion with CTS nerve entrapment because the symptoms and signs are similar (Table 14.4). Indeed CTS and HAVS may coexist[96] in some HAV exposed workers.

From the results of research reports it is very probable that HAVS subjects have an increased sympathetic outflow in response to cold,[97] and that this is the cause of the exaggerated vasospastic response when coupled with the peripheral vessel abnormalities i.e. medial muscular hypertrophy, chemical interactions, etc.

Treatment

To reduce the frequency of blanching attacks, the central body temperature must be kept high, and cold exposure must be avoided. Mitts rather than gloves should be worn, together with extra socks if feet are affected. Discontinuation of smoking is a further essential requirement, because of the adverse action of nicotine and carbon monoxide on the digital arterial system.

With effective health education the prevalence and severity of Raynaud's phenomenon have decreased remarkably in many occupations and HAVS has been shown to be reversible, except perhaps in the very advanced cases.[98]

To reverse the pathology and achieve recovery further exposure to HAV should be avoided. If this is not possible a modified work routine with reduction in HAV exposure time, and instruction to grip the tools as lightly as possible to reduce vibration transmission, is necessary to slow down progression.

Recent advances in drug therapy have focussed on three aspects;

- use of calcium channel antagonists to produce peripheral vasodilation;
- use of drugs to reduce platelet aggregation in combination with the above;
- drugs to reduce blood viscosity and emboli formation.

The necessity for medication increases with the severity of the Raynaud's phenomenon and the age of the subject. The results to date with calcium channel antagonist usage have been encouraging in all stages of HAVS and in all age groups when patients do not abandon medication because of drug intolerance, the predominant adverse symptoms being lassitude, light headedness, indigestion and impotence. While the majority of patients who are working discontinue the medication for this reason, its prescription is justified in workers still exposed to HAV to delay progression, and it may have to be taken for several years after discontinuing exposure to promote recovery. The response to medication is more favourable when smoking and HAV exposure have been discontinued, but it needs to be evaluated by vascular tests as subjective impressions are not reliable. When the response is poor a condition causing Raynaud's phenomenon in addition to HAVS has to be considered, in particular Raynaud's disease or scleroderma.

The use of additional drugs to reduce platelet aggregation and blood viscosity in HAVS patients is not justified unless the vasospasm is severe with trophic changes in the digital skin. Even in these circumstances their benefit is questionable. Cervical sympathectomy is never helpful, so surgical interference must be limited to digital resection as necessary.

The sensorineural component always takes longer to recover. Wrist splints at night with medication will provide some relief, but surgery to release a supposed carpal tunnel compression is rarely if ever justified. The failure rate is high due to a vibration-induced neuropathy rather than a simple median nerve compression, as mentioned earlier, and a further reduction in grip strength occurs invariably. The latter will be an additional handicap and further reduce the possibility of a worker returning to meaningful labouring work without HAV exposure. Retraining for alternative work, with academic upgrading, will then be necessary and this is difficult, if not impossible, for many.

In most jurisdictions the impairment rating for compensation purposes is determined using the Guides to the Evaluation of Permanent Impairment by the American Medical Association or their equivalent. The Guides provide that assessment of impairment of the upper extremity be made based on pain, discomfort, sensory deficit, loss of strength, and cold sensitivity.[99] In the UK, HAVS (vibration white finger, Raynaud's phenomenon) is a prescribed disease for the circulatory disturbance. The claimant has to satisfy the diagnostic and work criteria, and has to have a minimum impairment assessment of 14% to be entitled to benefit.[100]

Related conditions

CARPAL TUNNEL SYNDROME (see Chapter 22)

When the sensorineural symptoms predominate the diagnosis may be confused with CTS, although the two conditions may co-exist. In the diagnosis of work-related CTS (including repetitive strain injuries and cumulative trauma diseases) patients typically have sleep disturbance with nocturnal pain, paraesthesia, and numbness involving the median-enervated fingers which awaken them. The pain may radiate up the arm towards or even beyond the elbow. These symptoms may also occur during the day, particularly following unaccustomed or excessive movement of the hands. Thenar weakness and atrophy are late findings. It is known that CTS is associated with pregnancy and with various systemic disorders including hypothyroidism, rheumatoid arthritis, acromegaly and amyloid.[101] There is some evidence that patients with CTS have restricted carpal tunnels, as seen on computed tomography scanning[102,103] and many of the associated conditions increase the bulk of the contents of the carpal tunnel, narrowing the canal volume, with resulting increase in canal pressure. This increased pressure is postulated as producing intermittent intraneural ischaemia and compression.[104]

Often CTS occurs for no obvious reason. In those patients where occupational factors appear to be relevant there is usually a history of work involving one or more of the following activities before the development of symptoms:

- frequent repetitive use of the same movements of the hand;
- regular tasks requiring high force or grip;
- regular tasks requiring awkward hand positions;
- regular use of vibratory tools;
- frequent or prolonged pressure over the wrist or base of the palm.

The ergonomic design of tools and machines with work rotation or rest periods is essential to prevent the onset of CTS. Treatment in order of preference is:

- work modification;
- wrists splints (preferably at night);
- anti-inflammatory medication;
- cortisone (local injection or by iontophoresis);
- surgery.

The diagnosis of CTS rests upon the nature of the work, tools and posture, clinical history, signs and symptoms, and nerve conduction testing. Examination may reveal some sensory impairment in the median-enervated digits, and wasting and/or weakness of the abductor pollicis brevis muscle. The pathophysiology, aetiology, clinical picture, and treatment of CTS have been well reviewed by Carragee and Hentz.[105] Although the pathophysiology of the median nerve neuropathy is incompletely understood these authors conclude that median nerve entrapment is likely to involve both mechanical and ischaemic factors. The main distinctions between HAVS and CTS are given in Table 14.4.

It is apparent that the diagnosis and treatment of patients with HAVS and CTS varies considerably from country to country. Hadler[106] has drawn attention to this. There is clearly a need for more in-depth knowledge of the respective conditions – HAVS and CTS, their management at work, and the response to conservative treatment regimens. If the frequency of wrist surgery which escalated dramatically in the USA in the 1980s is to be reduced in HAVS patients, a comparison of surgical intervention with more conservative treatment regimens needs to be appraised. In addition to the surgical failures in HAV exposed workers, the post-surgical reduction in grip strength is a serious handicap for them.

Epidemiological studies have shown that in high risk occupation groups the incidence and prevalence of HAVS can be 80% or more.[2,107] While excessive vibration has been accepted as the causal agent for HAVS, in many work situations workers are exposed to other ergonomic stress factors at the same time.[108] In such situations where workers develop degenerative changes in the tissues it can be difficult to differentiate between the direct effects

Table 14.4 *HAVS vs CTS comparison*

History/symptoms	HAVS	HAVS and CTS	CTS
Exposure to vibration	Yes	Yes	No
Exposure to repetitive strain	No	Yes	Yes
Finger			
numbness tingling	Yes	Yes	Yes
median nerve	Yes	Yes	Yes
ulnar nerve	Yes	Yes	Rarely
Sleep disturbance	Unusual	Common	Common
Muscle cramps	Common	Common	Unusual
Aches and pains in arms and shoulders	Common	Common	Unusual Less common
Grip strength reduced	Common	Common	Unusual
Raynaud's phenomenon	Yes[a]	Yes[a]	No

Reproduced with permission from Ref. 96. [a]May not be apparent to the subject in the early stage.

of vibration and those of heavy manual work involving forceful and repetitive movements. Misdiagnosis occurs and this is confirmed by a study of US compensation claimants which showed that some workers who had CTS surgery were not diagnosed as having HAVS even though they met the diagnostic criteria.[109]

Silverstein et al.[110,111] in a study of 652 active workers in 39 jobs in seven different industrial sites investigated occupational risk factors of CTS. Four of the jobs which were classified as high-force involved nearly continuous exposure to vibration (buffing, grinding, cutting) while none of the control jobs involved vibration exposure. The data suggested that when accompanied with nearly continuous vibration exposure, the risk of CTS for low-repetitive, low-force work is increased by a factor of 6 and that the risk of CTS for high-force, high-repetitive work is elevated by a factor of 2. While hand and wrist tendinitis were highly associated with high-force, high-repetitive work, no association with vibration was found.

Studies by Radwin et al.[112] have demonstrated that hand–tool vibration can introduce disturbances in neuromuscular force control, through the tonic vibration reflex, resulting in excessive grip force when holding vibrating handles. Therefore upper extremity cumulative trauma diseases involving peripheral nerves, such as CTS, may occur directly through increased forcefulness, as an alternative to direct injury to the nerve tissue arising from the vibratory energy.[2] Cannon et al.[113] in a case-control study of workers in an aircraft engine manufacturing company found that the use of vibratory tools was strongly associated with CTS.

When the results of numerous studies are aggregated, where appropriate, they provide strong evidence of a causal relationship between repetitive, forceful work and the development of musculoskeletal disorders of the tendons and tendon sheaths in the hands and wrists, and nerve entrapment of the median nerve at the carpal tunnel.[114] Silverstein et al.[115] concluded that although it seems likely that vibration is an independent risk factor in CTS, no study so far has adequately disentangled the role of vibration as separate from the role of force, awkward postures, or repetitiveness. The more recent National Institute of Occupational Health and Safety (NIOSH) review of musculoskeletal disorders and workplace factors concluded that there is evidence for a positive association between jobs with exposure to vibration and CTS.[116]

DUPUYTREN'S CONTRACTURE

This contraction of the fascial components of the lateral aspect of the palm of the hand normally affects white males over 45 years, and is usually bilateral (see Chapter 22). Women may also be affected, the prevalence increasing with age, and sometimes it seems to be familial. There is an increased incidence in association with diabetes, alcoholism and epilepsy, in particular with

patients taking anti-convulsant medication (phenytoin). It is well known to follow a single injury to the palm.[117] The association with HAV exposure was thought to be less certain,[118] but there is some evidence of a dose–response relationship,[119] and Liss and Stock[120] from a literature review have concluded that there is good support now for an association between vibration exposure and Dupuytren's contracture.

SCLERODERMA

Systemic sclerosis or scleroderma is an uncommon multisystem disease with a reported incidence of two to 12 cases per million people per year (see Chapter 37). The clinical and pathological features can be grouped into three main categories, those relating to fibrosis, to vascular abnormalities, and to immunological abnormalities. Raynaud's phenomenon is an early symptom and trophic skin changes are likely to occur.

A possible association between scleroderma and workers exposed to HAV, silica or solvents has been suggested by reports in the literature since the early 1900s.[121] Pelmear et al.[122] recently reported a further four cases, one with HAV exposure alone and the others to mixed silica and HAV exposure.

It has been established that HAV exposed workers are prone to endothelial cell damage and collagen production, hence the pathophysiological evidence is very supportive of a causative association. However, the miners (exposed to both HAV from their drills and silica dust) who developed scleroderma, rarely had radiological diagnosable silicosis of their lungs so the intensity of silica exposure rather than the duration was suggested as being the important factor.[123] Since HAVS was not recognized by the researchers in the mines they postulated that silica dust stimulated an immunological reaction. It has also been suggested that other environmental factors such as exposure to polyvinyl chloride, immunological adjuvant (paraffin, silicone) epoxy resins, organic solvents, drugs (bleomycin), contaminated rapeseed oil, and trichloroethylene may be associated with scleroderma or scleroderma-like syndromes.[124]

Prevention

The measurement of vibration on hand-held tools or hand-guided machinery is necessary to determine the vibration dose by combining the measured vibration accelerations with the time history over which the tool is used during a typical working day, and also to compare the vibrations from different tools or machinery or different models of the same tool.[125]

The development of HAVS is dose-related so control measures should first be directed to reducing the intensity of vibration at the source, then the use of isolation and damping techniques to reduce transmission. Old tools should be properly serviced and maintained, and replaced as necessary with anti-vibration tools conforming to recommended safety limits for commercial use. Follow-up studies in Finland[126,127] on chainsaw users have confirmed that the use of anti-vibration chainsaws has reduced the prevalence of HAVS. Workers using anti-vibration chainsaws develop HAVS more slowly, but these chainsaws can elicit or maintain symptoms initiated by former exposure to more intense HAV.[128]

All hand-tools should also be ergonomically designed to place minimum strain on the user; have a high power-to-weight ratio; have low torque with a cut-off rather than slip-clutch mechanism; and the handles should have a non-slip surface to reduce the need to grip tightly.

The wearing of gloves at all times is recommended, if feasible. They will maintain hand temperature, reduce the risk from cuts and abrasions, and attenuate some of the high frequency vibration. So-called anti-vibration gloves provide some additional protection,[129] particularly if they can be used as inserts.

Administrative controls should be introduced in high-risk situations to reduce exposure time by means of job rotation or rest periods. Alternative vibration-free work should be made available to workers with HAVS if they request it.

All workers should be advised of the potential hazard and receive training on the need to service their tools regularly; to grip the tools as lightly as possible within the bounds of safety; to use the protective equipment provided; to attend for periodic medical surveillance; and to report all signs and symptoms of HAVS as soon as they develop. The potential harmful sources of vibration are summarized in Table 14.5.

Standards

There are numerous standards for the measurement of HAV together with reference levels to reduce the risk from human exposure. In addition to the UK standard-BSI DD ENV:25349:1993/ISO 5349[130] and the International standard (ISO 5349),[131] there are USA standards – ACGIH-TLV,[132] ANSI S3.34,[133] and the NIOSH criteria document,[134] while the EC has issued numerous directives.[125, 135–138]

WHOLE-BODY VIBRATION

Health effects

To suffer health effects from WBV exposure the frequency range 1–100 Hz is crucial. In the occupational situation several vibration frequencies are usually present simultaneously in the spectrum, and one or more are predominant. Depending on the magnitude, direction (axis), frequency, and duration of exposure to vibration, the health effects will range from sensations of pleasure, discomfort or pain; to interference with performance (reading and hand control); to acute or chronic illness with physiological and pathological changes.

The occupational groups most exposed to WBV are: drivers e.g. of tractors, trucks, heavy construction vehicles, and buses; workers on vibrating stationary or quasi stationary equipment e.g. cranes, excavators, and drilling platforms; and pilots of helicopters. Helicopters vibrate in all major axes at frequencies related to both rotor speeds and flight conditions, while further vibrations are produced by the engines, gearboxes, and rotors. The effect of these vibrations, usually at a frequency of 1–50 Hz and sometimes with considerable energy, is primarily on the musculoskeletal system.[139]

Studies on the subjective assessment of vibration levels[140,141] have permitted reliable comparison of the discomfort produced by most common vibration exposures, and this information is used by vehicle designers (see Table 14.6). The maximum subjective discomfort level occurs in the 4–8 Hz frequency band.

The effects of vibration on performance are known to be highly dependent on the activity, so any adverse effect

Table 14.5 *Potentially harmful sources of vibration*

Whole-body	Segmental (HAND–ARM)
Vehicles	**Tools**
Agricultural e.g. tractor, tree fellers, back-hoe, etc.	*Air compressed drills* e.g. jack hammer, jack-leg, stoper, concrete, etc
Construction e.g. bulldozer, grader, etc.	*Air compressed grinders* e.g. disc, rotatory, jitter-bug, etc.
Transport e.g. bus, train, helicopter, jeep, truck, motorcycle, motorboat, snowmobile, etc.	*Air compressed impact* e.g. impact wrench, hilte gun, rivetting gun, etc.
	Air compressed hose
	Electrical e.g. drills, saws, etc.
Mining e.g. jumbo drill, trucks, trains, etc.	*Combustion engine* e.g. chain saw, brush saw, etc.
Work platforms	**Vehicles**
e.g. drilling, crane, etc.	e.g. snowmobile, motorcycle, all terrain vehicle, etc.

Table 14.6 *Guidance for acceptable values of whole-body vibration for comfort*

<0.315 m/s²	Not uncomfortable
0.315–0.63 m/s²	A little uncomfortable
0.5–1.0 m/s²	Fairly uncomfortable
0.8–1.6 m/s²	Uncomfortable
1.25–2.5 m/s²	Very uncomfortable
<2.0 m/s²	Extremely uncomfortable

can usually be reduced by designing the task to be less demanding. It should be noted that manual tracking capability is most seriously affected at 5 Hz, and visual acuity is most severely impaired in the 20–25 Hz range.

Knowledge of the health effects of WBV is less certain than with HAV, and is incomplete.[142] Ship motion studies have shown that WBV exposure in the region of 0.1–0.5 Hz is generally associated with motion sickness (kinetosis) in susceptible people, if the motion is sustained with an ongoing periodicity. Heavy-equipment operators, do not suffer motion sickness at these levels because of the transient nature of the motion.

Epidemiology

Epidemiological studies have revealed that the most frequently associated long-term effects of WBV exposure are low back complaints with degenerative changes in the spine.[143–145] The response is most apparent at 4.5–6 Hz. It is a significant problem not only in terms of pain and lost productivity, but also in terms of societal cost.[146] The symptoms and signs may be aggravated or caused by adverse ergonomic factors related to machine design and seating, or bad driving posture. These factors and the operating movements of the worker in some situations enhance the likelihood that the spine will buckle and degenerate. Such degeneration occurs most frequently in the middle and lower thoracic spine, the upper lumbar, and to a lesser extent in the lower lumbar spine. Changes are usually localized in one part of the spine, a feature which is generally in favour of an external cause. Reported symptoms in the cervical spine are more likely to be caused by a forced posture rather than vibration. Different long-term effects dependent on WBV frequency cannot be derived from the literature. However, intense WBV with frequencies below, as well as above 20 Hz, have induced disorders in the spine; and WBV at 40–50 Hz applied to standing workers through the feet have been followed by osteoporosis and arthrosis of the feet.[147]

A higher incidence of inguinal hernia, muscular weakness and incoordination, and disorders of the digestive system including lower bowel and anal complaints have been reported.[1] Digestive disorders appear to be less if exposures are to frequencies above 20 Hz.

In women exposed to WBV, there seems to be a higher risk of menstrual disorders, proneness to abortion, and other complications of pregnancy including hyperemesis gravidarum and varicose veins. There is a distinct increase in blood volume during the phases of ovulation and menstruation.

Following long-term exposure in both sexes there is decreased vestibular excitability and a higher incidence of other vestibular disturbances, including subjective complaints of dizziness. The interaction with noise could be an important factor. The question of long-term exposure to WBV below 20 Hz on the central nervous system remains open.

With the circulatory system a variety of symptoms and diseases have been reported including varicose veins, haemorrhoids, varicoceles, ischaemic heart disease, and hypertension. To date there is little, if any, statistical evidence so there is a need for further studies to validate the findings before any of these common conditions can be presumed, in some cases, to be caused by WBV exposure.

Finally it is well recognized that after a prolonged period of WBV exposure, a general morbidity with malaise, lassitude and temporary disablement occurs. There is full recovery after a period of freedom from exposure. The potential harmful sources of vibration are summarized in Table 14.5.

Prevention

Back problems respond out of phase with a vibratory stimulus. The delay is based on a musculoskeletal response characteristic over which we have no conscious control. For these reasons it is important to isolate the spine from jolt/vibration conditions, especially in the mechanically extreme, seated position. Although work hardening is appropriate under conditions in which the muscles can control and optimize the loading of the hard and soft tissues, it is not appropriate for the complex, seated, jolt/vibration environment.[148] As a rule, it is only possible to protect people effectively from mechanical vibration by means of a combination of various measures – identification, elimination or reduction at source, isolation, and monitoring of the health of exposed persons.[142] Any preventive measure proposed by technologists, organizations, individuals or occupational physicians should be evaluated and supported if feasible.

Standards

Because of the difficulty recognizing and quantifying WBV-induced health effects, the majority of the data upon which to base a standard have been from laboratory and field studies. Such data have provided the basis for the development of guidelines and standards such as the American Conference of Government Industrial Hygienists (ACGIH) threshold limit value for Whole

Body Vibration,[132] the American National Standards Institute (ANSI) standard S3.18,[149] the International Standards Organization (ISO) standard 2631–1,[150] the British Standard 6841,[151] and the EC Directive for Whole Body Vibration.[135–138]

REFERENCES

1 Dupuis H, Zerlett G. *The Effects of Whole Body Vibration.* Berlin: Springer-Verlag, 1986: 162.

2 Pelmear PL. Epidemiology of hand-arm vibration syndrome. In: Pelmear PL, Wasserman DE eds. *Hand-Arm Vibration: A Comprehensive Guide for Occupational Health Professionals* 2nd edn. Beverly Farms, MA: OEM Press, 1998: 103–26.

3 Wilder DG, Wasserman DE, Pope MH, Pelmear PL, Taylor W. Vibration. In: Wald PH, Stave GM eds. *Physical and Biological Hazards in the Workplace.* New York: Van Nostrand Reinhold, 1994: 64–83.

4 Pelmear PL. Vibration-related occupational injuries. In: Herington TN, Morse LH eds. *Occupational Injuries: Evaluation, Management, and Prevention.* St Louis: CV Mosby, 1995: 411–21.

5 Pelmear PL. Noise and vibration. In: McDonald JC ed. *The Epidemiology of Work Related Diseases.* London: BMJ Publishing Group, 1995: 185–205.

6 Cherniack MG, Mohr S. Raynaud's phenomenon associated with the use of pneumatically powered surgical instruments. *J Hand Surg* 1994; **19**A: 1008–15.

7 Kåkosy T, Martin J, Diner J, Székely A. Hand-arm vibration syndrome caused by power screwdrivers. *Cen Eur J Occup Environ Med* 1996; **2**: 175–80.

8 Pelmear PL. Hand-arm vibration syndrome from exposure to pneumatic knives. *J Low Freq Noise Vib Active Control* 1999; **18**: 1–7.

9 Gemne G, Taylor W (eds) Foreword: Hand-arm vibration and the central nervous system. In: Gemme G, Taylor W eds. *Special Volume. J Low Freq Noise Vib* 1983; XI.

10 Pelmear PL. Clinical picture (vascular, neurological, and musculoskeletal). In: Pelmear PL, Wasserman DE eds. *Hand-Arm Vibration: A Comprehensive Guide for Occupational Health Professionals* 2nd edn. Beverly Farms, MA: OEM Press, 1998: 27–43.

11 Gemne G, Pyykkö I, Taylor W, Pelmear PL. The Stockholm Workshop scale for the classification of cold-induced Raynaud's phenomenon in the hand-arm syndrome (revision of the Taylor-Pelmear scale). *Scand J Work Environ Hlth* 1987; **13**: 275–8.

12 Brammer AJ, Taylor W, Lundborg G. Sensorineural stages of the hand-arm vibration syndrome. *Scand J Work Environ Hlth* 1987; **13**: 279–83.

13 Färkkilä M, Aatola S, Stark J, Korhonen O, Pyykkö I. Hand-grip force in lumberjacks: Two year follow-up. *Int Arch Occup Environ Hlth* 1986; **58**: 203–8.

14 Hedlund U. Raynaud's phenomenon of fingers and toes of miners exposed to local and whole-body vibration and cold. *Int Arch Occup Environ Hlth* 1989; **61**: 457–61.

15 Sakakibara H, Akamatsu Y, Miyao M, Kondo T, Furuta M *et al.* Correlation between vibration induced white finger and symptoms of upper and lower extremities in vibration syndrome. *Int Arch Occup Environ Hlth* 1988; **60**: 285–9.

16 Sakakibara H, Hashiguchi T, Furuta M, Kondo T, Miyao M, Yamada S. Circulatory disturbances of the foot in vibration syndrome. *Int Arch Occup Environ Hlth* 1991; **63**: 145–8.

17 Toibana N, Ishikawa N. Ten patients with Raynaud's phenomenon in fingers and toes caused by vibration. In: Okada A, Taylor W, Dupuis H eds. *Hand-Arm Vibration.* Kanazawa, Japan: Kyoei Press, 1990: 245–8.

18 Kindo T, Sakakibara H, Miyao M, Akamatsu Y, Yamada S. Effect of exposure to hand-transmitted vibration on digital skin temperature changes. *Ind Hlth* 1987; **25**: 41–53.

19 Egan CE, Espies BH, McGann S, McKenna KM, Allen JA. Acute effects of vibration on peripheral blood flow in healthy subjects. *Occup Environ Med* 1996; **53**: 663–9.

20 Pyykkö I, Starck J, Färkkilä M, Hoikkala M, Korhonen O, Nurminen M. Hand-arm vibration in the aetiology of hearing loss in lumberjacks. *Br J Ind Med* 1981; **38**: 281–9.

21 Iki M, Kurumantani N, Satoh M, Matsuura F, Arai T *et al.* Hearing of forest workers with vibration induced white finger: A five year follow up. *Int Arch Occup Environ Hlth* 1989; **61**: 437–42.

22 Pelmear PL, Taylor W, Pearson JCG. Clinical tests for vibration white finger. In: Taylor W, Pelmear PL eds, *Vibration White Finger in Industry.* London: Academic Press, 1975: 53–81.

23 Wener MH, Metzger WJ, Simon RA. Occupationally acquired angioedema with secondary carpal tunnel syndrome. *Ann Int Med* 1983; **98**: 44–6.

24 James PB, Yates JR, Pearson JCG. An investigation of the prevalence of bone cysts in hands exposed to vibration. In: Taylor W, Pelmear PL eds. *Vibration White Finger in Industry.* London: Academic Press, 1975: 43–51.

25 Gemne G, Saraste H. Bone and joint pathology in workers using hand-held vibratory tools – an overview. *Scand J Work Environ Hlth* 1987; **13**: 290–300.

26 Pyykkö I, Strack J, Färkkilä M, Hoikkala M, Korhonen O, Nuriminen M. Hand-arm vibration in the aetiology of hearing loss in lumberjacks. *Br J Ind Med* 1981; **38**: 281–9.

27 Pelmear PL, Leong D, Wong L, Roos J, Pike M. Hand-arm vibration syndrome and hearing loss in hard rock miners. *J Low Freq Noise Vib* 1987; **6**: 49–66.

28 Iki M, Kurumatani N, Moriyama T, Ogata A. Vibration-induced white finger and auditory susceptibility to noise exposure. *Kurume Med J* 1990; **37**: 33–4.

29 Pelmear PL, Taylor W, Wasserman DE eds. *Hand-Arm Vibration: A Comprehensive Guide for Occupational*

Health Professionals. New York: Van Nostrand Reinhold, 1992: 226.

30 Khilberg S. Acute effects and symptoms of work with vibrating hand-held powered tools exposing the operator to impact and reaction forces [Thesis]. *Arbete och Hälsa* 1995; **10**: 1–50.

31 Pelmear PL, Kusiak R, Leong D. Hand-arm vibration syndrome associated with impact vibration. *J Low Freq Noise Vib* 1995; **14**: 73–9.

32 Starck J, Färkkilä M, Aatola S, Pyykkö I, Korhonen O. Vibration syndrome and vibration in pedestal grinding. *Br J Ind Med* 1983; **40**: 426–433.

33 Starck J. High impulse acceleration levels in hand-held vibratory tools. An additional factor in the hazards associated with hand-arm vibration syndrome. *Scand J Work Environ Hlth* 1984; **10**: 171–8.

34 Starck J, Pekkarinen J, Pyykkö I. Physical characteristics of vibration in relation to vibration induced white finger. *Am Ind Hyg Assoc J* 1990; **51**: 179–84.

35 Pelmear PL, Wills M. Impact vibration and hand-arm vibration syndrome. *J Occup Environ Med* 1997; **39**: 1092–6

36 Pelmear PL, Wong L, Dembek B. Laboratory tests for the evaluation of hand-arm vibration syndrome. In: Dupuis H, Christ E, Sandover J, Taylor W, Okada A eds. *Proceedings of the 6th International Conference on Hand-Arm Vibration, Bonn*, 1992: 817–27.

37 Adson AW. Surgical treatment for symptoms produced by cervical ribs and the scalenus anticus muscle. *Surg Gynecol Obstet* 1947;**85**:687–700.

38 Ashbell TS, Kutz JE, Kleinert HE. The digital Allen test. *Plast Reconstr Surg* 1967; **39**: 311–12.

39 Pelmear PL. Clinical evaluation. In: Pelmear PL, Wasserman DE eds. *Hand-Arm Vibration: A Comprehensive Guide for Occupational Health Professionals* 2nd edn. Beverly Farms, MA: OEM Press, 1998: 73–94.

40 Nielsen SL, Lassen NA. Measurement of digital blood pressure after local cooling. *J Appl Physiol* 1997; **43**: 907–10.

41 Bovenzi M. Finger systolic pressure during local cooling in normal subjects aged 20 to 60 years: reference values for the assessment of digital vasospasm in Raynaud's phenomenon of occupational origin. *Int Arch Occup Environ Hlth* 1988; **61**: 179–81.

42 Pelmear PL, Roos J, Leong D, Wong L. Cold provocation test results from a 1985 survey of hard rock miners in Ontario. *Scand J Work Hlth* 1987; **13**: 343–347.

43 Mossman SS, Blau JN. Tinel's sign and carpal tunnel syndrome. *Br Med J* 1987; **294**: 680.

44 Heller L, Ring H, Costeff H, Solzi P. Evaluation of Tinel's and Phalen's signs in diagnosis of carpal tunnel syndrome. *Ear Neurol* 1986; **25**: 40–2.

45 Carlson WS, Samueloff S, Taylor W, Wasserman DE Instrumentation for measurement of sensory loss in the fingertips. *J Occup Med* 1979; **21**: 260–4.

46 Lundborg G, Sollerman C, Stromberg T, Pyykkö I, Rosen B. A new principle for assessing vibrotactile sense in

vibration-induced neuropathy. *Scand J Work Environ Hlth* 1987; **13**: 375–9.

47 Lundborg G, Lie-Stenström A, Sollerman C, Strömberg T, Pyykkö I. Digital vibrogram: A new diagnostic tool for sensory testing in compression neuropathy. *J Hand Surg* 1986; **11A**: 693–9.

48 Dyck PJ, Curtis DJ, Bushek W, Offord K. Description of Minnesota thermal dices and normal values of thermal discrimination in man. *Neurology* 1974; **24**: 325–30.

49 Ekenvall L, Nilsson BY, Gustavsson P. Temperature and vibration thresholds in vibration syndrome. *Br J Ind Med* 1986; **43**: 825–9.

50 Hirosawa I. Original construction of thermo-esthesiometer and its application to vibration disease. *Int Arch Environ Hlth* 1983; **52**: 209–14.

51 McGeogh KL, Taylor W, Gilmour WH. The use of objective tests as an aid to the assessment of hand-arm vibration syndrome by the Stockholm classification. In: Dupuis H, Christ E, Sandover J, Taylor W, Okada A eds. *Proceedings of the 6th International Conference on Hand-Arm Vibration, Bonn*, 1992: 783–792.

52 Katims JJ, Naviasky EH, Rendell MS, Ng LKY, Bleecker ML. Constant current sine wave transcutaneous nerve stimulation for the evaluation of peripheral neuropathy. *Arch Phys Med Rehab* 1987; **68**: 210–3.

53 Katims JJ, Rouvelas P, Sadler BT, Weseley SA. Current perception threshold. Reproducibility and comparison with nerve conduction in evaluation of carpal tunnel syndrome. *Trans Am Soc Art Int Org* 1989; **35**: 180–284.

54 Pelmear PL, Kusiak R, Dembek B. Cluster analysis of laboratory tests used for the evaluation of hand-arm vibration syndrome. *J Low Freq Noise Vib* 1993; **12**: 98–109.

55 Pelmear PL, Kusiak R. Clinical assessment of hand-arm vibration syndrome. *Nagoya J Med Sci* 1994; **57** (Suppl): 27–41.

56 Pelmear PL, Wong L, Dembek B. Laboratory tests for the evaluation of Hand-arm Vibration Syndrome. In: Dupuis H, Christ E, Sandover J, Taylor W, Okada A eds. *Proceedings 6th International Conference of Hand-arm Vibration, Bonn*, 1992: 817–27.

57 Ashe WF, Cook WT, Old JW. Raynaud's phenomenon of occupational origin. *Arch Environ Hlth* 1962; **5**: 333–43.

58 Walton KW. The pathology of Raynaud's phenomenon of occupational origin. In: Taylor W ed. The *Vibration Syndrome*. London: Academic Press, 1974: 109–21.

59 Takeuchi T, Imanishi H. Histopathological observations in finger biopsy from thirty patients with Raynaud's phenomenon of occupational origin. *J Kumanato Med Soc* 1984; **58**: 56–70.

60 Takeuchi T, Futatsuka M, Imanishi H, Yamada S. Pathological changes observed in the finger biopsy of patients with vibration-induced white finger. *Scand J Work Environ Hlth* 1986; **12**: 280–3.

61 Hashiguchi T, Yanagi H, Kinugawa Y, Sakakibara H, Yamada S. Pathological changes of finger and toe in

patients with vibration syndrome. *Nagoya J Med Sci* 1994; **57** (Suppl): 129–36.

62 Hashiguchi T, Yanagi H, Kinugawa Y, Sakakibara H, Yamada S. Pathological changes of the small arteries in finger and toe biopsies from patients with vibration syndrome. In: Dupuis H, Christ E, Sandover J, Taylor W, Okada A eds. *Proceedings 6th International Conference on Hand-Arm Vibration, Bonn*, 1992: 157–63.

63 Wegelius U. Angiography of the hand. Clinical and postmortem investigations. *Acta Radiologica* 1972; (Suppl)**315**: 1–115.

64 James PB, Galloway RW. Arteriography of the hand in men exposed to vibration. In: Taylor W, Pelmear PL eds. *Vibration White Finger in Industry*. London: Academic Press, 1975: 31–41.

65 Kaji H, Honma H, Usui M, Yasono Y. Saito K. Hypothenar hammer syndrome in workers occupationally exposed to vibrating tools. *J Hand Surg* 1993; **18**: 761–6.

66 Hyvärinen J, Pyykkö I, Sundberg S. Vibration frequencies and amplitudes in the aetiology of traumatic vasospastic disease. *Lancet* 1973; **i**: 791–4.

67 Nasu Y. Changes in skin temperature caused by local vibration stimulation in normals and patients with vibration syndrome. *Yonago Acta Med* 1977; **21**: 83–99.

68 Färkkilä MA, Pyykkö I. Blood flow in the contralateral hand during vibration and hand grip contraction of lumberjacks. *Scand Work Environ Hlth* 1979; **5**: 368–74.

69 Welsh CL. The effect of vibration on digital blood flow. *Br J Surg* 1980; **67**: 708–10.

70 Kindo T, Sakakibara H, Miyao M, Akamatsu Y, Yamada S. Effect of exposure to hand-transmitted vibration on digital skin temperature changes. *Ind Hlth* 1987; **25**: 41–53.

71 Egan CE, Espies BH, McGann S, McKenna KM, Allen JA. Acute effects of vibration on peripheral blood flow in healthy subjects. *Occup Environ Med* 1996; **53**: 663–9.

72 Hashiguchi T, Sakakibara H, Yamada S. Changes of skin blood flow in the finger and dorsum of the foot during chain saw operation. In: Okada A, Taylor W, Dupuis H eds. *Hand-Arm Vibration*. Kanazawa: Kyoei Press, 1990: 455–8.

73 Sakakibara H, Kondo T, Koike T, Miyao M, Furuta M *et al*. Combined effects of vibration and noise on palmar sweating. *Eur J Appl Physiol* 1989; **59**: 195–8.

74 Sakakibara H, Iwase S, Mano T, Watanabe T, Kobayashi F *et al*. Skin sympathetic activity in the tibial nerve triggered by vibration applied to the hand. *Int Arch Occup Environ Hlth* 1990; **62**: 455–8.

75 Okada A, Naito M, Ariizumi A, Inaba R. Experimental studies on the effects of vibration and noise on sympathetic nerve activity in skin *Eur J Appl Physiol* 1991; **62**: 324–31.

76 Sato A, Schmidt RF. Somato-sympathetic reflexes: afferent fibres, central pathways, discharge characteristics. *Physiol Rev* 1973; **53**: 916–47.

77 Lijung B, Sivertsson R. Vibration-induced inhibition of

smooth muscle contraction. *Blood Vessels* 1975; **12**: 38–52.

78 Azuma T, Ohhashi T, Sakaguchi M. An approach to the pathogenesis of white finger induced by vibratory stimulation: acute but sustained changes in vascular responsiveness of canine hind-limb to noradrenaline. *Cardiovasc Res* 1980; **12**: 725–30.

79 Lindblad LE, Lorenz RR, Shepherd JT, Vanhoutte PM. Effect of vibration on a canine cutaneous artery. *Am J Physiol* 1986; **250**: H519–23.

80 Greenstein D, Kester RC. Acute vibration – its effect on digital blood flow by central and local mechanisms. Proc *Inst Mech Engrs* 1992; **206**: 105–8.

81 Nohara S, Okamoto K, Okada A. Peripheral circulation and nervous response to various frequencies of local vibration exposure. *Scand J Work Environ Hlth* 1986; **12**: 382–4.

82 Furuta M, Sakakibara H, Miyao M, Kondo T, Yamada S. Effect of vibration frequency on finger blood flow. *Int Arch Occup Environ Health* 1991; **63**: 221–4.

83 Lundström R. Responses of mechanoreceptive afferent units in the glaborous skin of the human hand to vibration. *Scand J Work Environ Hlth* 1986; **12**: 413–6.

84 Ekenvall L, Lindblad LE. Is vibration white finger a primary sympathetic injury? *Br J Ind Med* 1986; **43**: 702–6.

85 Ekenvall L, Lindblad LE, Norbeck O, Etzell BM. Alpha-adrenoceptors and cold-induced vasoconstriction in human finger skin. *Am J Physiol* 1988; **255**: H1000–3.

86 Bodelsson M, Arneklo-Nobin B, Nobin A, Owman C, Sollerman C, Törnebrandt K. Cooling enhances alpha 2-adrenoceptor mediated vasoconstriction in human hand veins. *Acta Physiol Scand* 1990; **138**: 283–91.

87 Moulds RFW, Iwanov V, Medcalf RL. The effects of platelet-derived contractile agents on human digital arteries. *Clin Sci* 1984; **66**: 443–51.

88 Nerem RM. Vibration induced arterial shear stress. The relationship to Raynaud's phenomenon of occupational origin. *Arch Environ Hlth* 1973; **26**: 105–10.

89 McKenna KM, McGrann S, Blann AD, Allen JA. An investigation into the acute vascular effects of riveting. *Br J Ind Med* 1993; **50**: 160–6.

90 Harada N, Iwamoto M, Hirosawa I, Ishii F, Yoneda J, *et al*. Combined effect of noise, vibration and cold exposures on the autonomic nervous system. In: Dupuis H, Christ E, Sandover J, Taylor W eds. *Proceedings of the 6th International Conference on Hand-Arm Vibration, Bonn*, 1992: 465–73.

91 Ekenvall L, Nilsson BY, Gustavsson P. Temperature and vibration thresholds in vibration. *Br J Ind Med* 1986; **43**: 825–9.

92 Lundborg G, Dahlin LB, Hansson HA, Pyykkö I. Intramural oedema following exposure to vibration. *Scand J Work Environ Hlth* 1987; **13**: 326–9.

93 Ho ST, Yu HS. Ultrastructural changes of the peripheral nerve induced by vibration: an experimental study. *Br J Ind Med* 1989; **46**: 157–64.

94   Goldsmith PC, Molina FA, Bunker CB, Terenghi G, Leslie TA *et al*. Cutaneous nerve fibre depletion in vibration white finger. *J Roy Soc Med* 1994; **87**: 377–81

95   Dowd PM, Goldsmith PC, Bull HA, Runistock G, Foreman, JC, Marshall T. Raynaud's phenomenon. *Lancet* 1995; **346**: 283–90

96   Pelmear PL, Taylor W. Carpal tunnel syndrome and hand-arm vibration syndrome. A diagnostic enigma. *Arch Neurol* 1994; **51**: 416–20.

97   Sakakibara H. Pathophysiology and pathogenesis of circulatory, neurological, and musculoskeletal disturbances in hand-arm vibration syndrome. In: Pelmear PL, Wasserman DE eds. *Hand-Arm Vibration: A Comprehensive Guide of Occupational Health Professionals* 2nd edn. Beverly Farms, MA: OEM Press, 1998; 45–72.

98   Färkkilä M. Vibration induced injury. [Editorial] *Br J Ind Med* 1986; **43**: 361–2.

99   American Medical Association. *Guides to the Evaluation of Permanent Impairment* 3rd edn. Milwaukee WI: AMA, 1988: 262.

100   Neusner D, Arkell CL. Legal and compensation aspects of hand-arm vibration syndrome. In: Pelmear PL, Wasserman DE eds. *Hand-Arm Vibration: A Comprehensive Guide for Occupational Health Professionals* 2nd edn. Beverly Farms, MA: OEM Press, 1998: 201–19

101   Editorial. *Lancet* 1985; **ii**: 854–5.

102   Castelli WA, Evans G, Diaz-Perez R, Armstrong TJ. Intraneural connective tissue proliferation of the median nerve in the carpal tunnel. *Arch Phys Med Rehab* 1980; **61**: 418–22.

103   Phalen GS. Reflection on twenty-one years with the carpal tunnel syndrome. *JAMA* 1970; **212**: 1363–7.

104   Bleecker ML, Bohlman M, Moreland R, Tipton A. Carpal tunnel syndrome: role of carpal canal size. *J Neurol* 1985; **35**: 1599–604.

105   Carragee EJ, Hentz VR. Repetitive trauma and nerve compression. *Orthoped Clin North Am* 1988; **19**: 157–64.

106   Hadler NM. Arm pain in the workforce. A small area analysis. *J Occup Med* 1992; **34**: 113–9.

107   Pelmear PL. Noise and Vibration. In: McDonald JC ed. *Epidemiology of Work Related Diseases*. London: BMJ Publishing Group, 1995: 185–205

108   Radwin RG, Armstrong TJ, Van Bergeijk E. Hand-arm vibration and work related disorders of the upper limb. In: Pelmear PL, Wasserman DE eds. *Hand-Arm Vibration: A Comprehensive Guide for Occupational Health Professionals* 2nd edn. Beverly Farms, MA: OEM Press, 1998: 127–57.

109   Miller RF, Lohman WH, Maldonado G, Mandel JS. An epidemiologic study of carpal tunnel syndrome and hand-arm vibration syndrome in relation to vibration exposure. *J Hand Surg* 1994; **19A**: 99–105.

110   Silverstein BA, Armstrong TJ, Fine LJ. Hand wrist cumulative trauma disorders in industry. *Br J Ind Med* 1986; **43**: 779–84.

111   Silverstein BA, Fine LJ, Armstrong TJ. Occupational factors and carpal tunnel syndrome. *Am J Ind Med* 1987; **11**: 340–58.

112   Radwin RG, Armstrong TJ, Chaffin DB. Power hand tool vibration effects on grip exertions. *Ergonomics* 1987; **30**: 833–55.

113   Cannon LJ, Bernacki EJ, Walter SD. Personal and occupational factors associated with carpal tunnel syndrome. *J Occup Med* 1981; **23**: 255–8.

114   Stock SR. Workplace ergonomic factors and the development of musculoskeletal disorders of the neck and upper limbs: A meta-analysis. *Am J Ind Med* 1991; **19**: 87–107.

115   Silverstein BA, Fine JF, Armstrong TJ. Carpal tunnel syndrome: Causes and a preventive strategy. *Semin Occup Med* 1986; **1**(3): 213–21.

116   National Institute for Occupational Safety and Health. *Musculoskeletal Disorders and Workplace Factors. A Critical Review of Epidemiologic Evidence for Work-related Musculoskeletal Disorders of the Neck, Upper Extremity, and Low Back*. DHHS (NIOSH) publication No 97–141, 1997.

117   McFarlane RM. Dupuytren's contracture. In Green D ed. *Operative Hand Surgery*. New York: Churchill Livingston, 1988: 608–616.

118   McFarlane RM. Dupuytren's disease: Relation to work and injury. *J Hand Surg* 1991; **16A**: 775–8.

119   Bovenzi M. Hand-arm vibration syndrome and dose-response relation for vibration induced white finger among quarry drillers and stone carvers. *Occup Environ Med* 1994; **51**: 603–11.

120   Liss GM, Stock SR. Can Dupuytren's contracture be work related?: Review of the evidence. *Am J Ind Med* 1996; **29**: 521–32.

121   Bovenzi M, Barbone F, Betta A, Tommasini M, Versini W. Scleroderma and occupational exposure. *Scand J Work Environ Hlth* 1995; **21**: 289–92.

122   Pelmear PL, Roos JO, Maehle WM. Occupationally-induced scleroderma. *J Occup Med* 1992; **34**: 21–2.

123   Sluis-Cremer GK. Silica, silicosis and progressive systemic sclerosis. *Br J Ind Med* 1985; **42**: 838–43.

124   Masi AT. Clinical-epidemiological perspective of systemic sclerosis (scleroderma). In: Jayson MIV, Black CM eds. *Systemic Sclerosis Scleroderma*. New York: John Wiley, 1988: 7–31.

125   European Standard DD ENV 25349. *Mechanical Vibration – Guidelines for the Measurement and the Assessment of Human Exposure to Hand-Transmitted Vibration*. 1993: 1–16.

126   Pyykkö I, Korhonen OS, Färkkilä MA, Stark JP, Aatola SA. A longitudinal study of the vibration syndrome in Finnish forestry workers. In: Brammer AJ, Taylor W eds. *Vibration Effects on the Hand and Arm in Industry*. New York, John Wiley, 1982: 157–67.

127   Pyykkö I, Korhonen OS, Färkkilä MA, Stark JP, Aatola SA, Jäntti V. Vibration syndrome among Finnish forestry workers: a follow-up from 1972 to 1983. *Scand J Work Environ Hlth* 1986; **12**: 307–12.

128 Kivekäs J, Riihimäki H, Husman K, Hänninen K, Härkönen H et al. Seven year follow-up of white finger symptoms and radiographic wrist findings in lumberjacks and referents. *Scand J Work Environ Hlth* 1994; **20**: 101–6.

129 Reynolds D, Weaver D, Jetzer T. Application of a new technology to the design of effective anti-vibration gloves. *Cent Eur J Publ Health* 1996; **4**: 140–4.

130 British Standards Institute. BS DD ENV:25349: 1993/ISO 5349 : 1986 *Mechanical Vibration Guidelines for the Measurement and Evaluation of Human Exposure to Vibration Transmitted to the Hand*. London: BSI, 1993.

131 International Standards Organization. ISO 5349. *Guidelines for the Measurement and Assessment of Human Exposure to Hand-Transmitted Vibration*. Geneva: ISO, 1986.

132 American Conference of Government Industrial Hygienists. *Threshold Limit Values (TLVs) for Chemical Substances and Physical Agents and Biological Exposure Indices (BEIs)*. Cincinnati, OH, 1999.

133 American National Standards Institute. S3.34. *Guide for the Measurement and Evaluation of Human Exposure to Vibration Transmitted to the Hand*. New York, N Y: ANSI, 1986.

134 National Institute of Occupational Safety and Health. *Criteria for a Recommended Standard: Occupational Exposure to Hand-Arm Vibration*. DHHS (NIOSH) publication No 89–106, 1989.

135 Council of the European Communities Directive 89/392 EEC of 14 June 1989 on the approximation of the laws of the Member States relating to machinery. *Offic J Eur Communities* L 183: 9–32.

136 Council of the European Communities Directive 91/368 EEC of 20 June 1991 amending Directive 89/392 EEC on the approximation of the laws of the Member States relating to machinery. *Offic J Eur Communities* L 198; **34**: 16–32.

137 Commission of the European Communities. Proposal for a Council Directive on the minimum health and safety requirements regarding the exposure of workers to the risks arising from physical agents. COM (92) 560 final – SYN 449. *Offic J Eur Communities* 23 December 1992: 1–74.

138 Commission of the European Communities. Amended proposal for a Council Directive on the minimum health and safety requirements regarding the exposure of workers to the risks arising from physical agents. COM 230. *Offic J Eur Communities* 19 August 1994: 3–29.

139 Gerhart JR. Response of the skeletal system to helicopter-unique vibration. *Aviat Space Environ Med* 1978; **49**: 253–6.

140 Seidal H, Heide R. Long-term effects of whole-body vibration: a critical survey of the literature. *Int Arch Environ Hlth* 1986; **58**: 1–26.

141 Hulshof C, van Zanten BV. Whole-body vibration and low back pain: a review of epidemiological studies. *Int Arch Occup Environ Hlth* 1987; **50**: 205–20.

142 Griffin, M.J. *Handbook of Human Vibration* London: Academic Press, 1990: 988.

143 Frymoyer JW, Pope MH, Clements JH, Wilder DG, MacPherson B, Ashikaga T. Risk factors in low back pain: an epidemiological survey. *J Bone J Surg* 1983; **65**A: 213–6.

144 Kelsey JL, Githens PB, O'Conner T et al. Acute prolapsed lumbar intervertebral disc: an epidemiological study with special reference to driving automobiles and cigarette smoking. *Spine* 1984; **9**: 608–13.

145 Behrens V, Seligman P, Cameron L, Mathias T, Fine L. The prevalence of back pain, hand discomfort, and dermatitis in the US working population. *Am J Publ Hlth* 1994; **84**: 1780–5.

146 Cats-Baril W, Frymoyer J. The economics of spinal disorders. In: Frymoyer J, Ducker T, Hadler N, Kostuik J, Weinstein J, Whitecloud T eds. *The Adult Spine*. New York: Raven Press, 1991: 85–105.

147 Seidel H, Heide R. Long-term effects of whole-body vibration: a critical survey of the literature. *Int Arch Occup Environ Hlth* 1986; **58**: 1–26.

148 Wasserman DE, Wilder DG, Pope MH, Magnusson M, Aleksiev AR, Wasserman JF. Whole-body vibration and occupational work hardening. [Editorial] *J Occup Environ Med* 1997; **39**: 403–6.

149 American National Standards Institute. ANSI S3.18: *Guide for the Evaluation of Human Exposure to Whole-Body Vibration*. New York: ANSI; 1979.

150 International Standards Organization. ISO 2631/1-1985(E). *Evaluation of Human Exposure to Whole Body Vibration*. Geneva: ISO; 1985.

151 British Standards Institution. BS 6841 *Measurement and Evaluation of Human Exposure to Whole-Body Mechanical Vibration and Repeated Shock*. London: BSI, 1987.

15

Heat and cold

E HOWARD N OAKLEY

The principles of heat balance	325	The principles of the reduction of thermal strain	337
Cold stress	327	References	340
Heat stress	333		

In contrast to other animals, humans achieve much of their thermoregulation by conditioning their ambient environment. Even the Inuit bask in a tropical microclimate. It is a combination of application, engineering feasibility and economy which determines whether this is accomplished by clothing or shelter. Examples of environmental conditioning range from the use of highly insulative clothing by those working outdoors in polar climes, to the mass chilling of air to supply high-rise office blocks in the tropics. Compromises and shortcomings in such environments impose thermal stress, resulting first in physiological and then pathological changes.

Previously, environmental medicine has emphasized the occurrence and prevention of life-threatening disorders arising from heat and cold stress. Whilst these remain at the forefront in certain industries such as offshore oil exploration, on a global scale more subtle adverse effects, which endanger performance, are both more common and of greater importance. The numbers of deaths resulting directly from hypothermia and heat illness are relatively low, in comparison with the number of fatal incidents in which thermal stress is expected to have been a contributory factor.

Throughout this chapter, careful distinction will be made between the terms 'stress' and 'strain'. In accordance with their engineering origins, these will be used rigorously: 'stress' is the force applied to an object (in a thermal context, the thermal load to which the body is subjected), whilst 'strain' is the response within that object to the applied stress (thermally, the physiological and behavioural responses which result from thermal load). A surprisingly large proportion of gross domestic product, natural energy reserves, and each of our lives are devoted to the minimization of thermal strain, in the face of the stress applied by climate, weather, and industrial processes. The usefulness of this distinction should

not be underestimated: for example, the measurement of stress is useful in predicting the safe exposure for groups, whilst measurement of strain can assess how well a given individual is coping with a certain stress, and thus whether or not that person should be withdrawn or treated.

This chapter reviews the fundamental factors in human heat exchange, describes the reactions to thermal stress and their adverse consequences, and outlines approaches to the modification of both stress and strain. Although coverage includes discussion of local cold injury, thermal burns are omitted in deference to authoritative accounts elsewhere.

THE PRINCIPLES OF HEAT BALANCE

The foundation of all thermal physiology is the application of the law of conservation of energy to human heat balance. This is succinctly expressed in the equation:

$$M + (R + C + K - E) = S$$

where: M is the heat generated by metabolism (always positive); R is the radiant heat exchange with the environment (negative for net loss); C is the convective heat exchange with surrounding fluid (negative for net loss), K is the conductive heat exchange with any contacting solid (negative for net loss); E is the evaporative heat loss resulting from the evaporation of liquid from the body or its clothing (almost always positive, i.e. loss from the body, or zero); and S is the heat stored (positive) or lost (negative) by the body.

Metabolic heat generation consists of a basal component, which may be reduced by hypothermia and in some pathological conditions, and an augmentation resulting from physical activity. Such activity ranges from the slight, as when maintaining a seated position, to the severe, as might be achieved by a fit athlete exercising close to his or her maximum oxygen uptake. In addition to voluntary exercise, the involuntary exercise of shivering may increase metabolic heat generation in those exposed to the cold. Non-shivering thermogenesis within brown fat is only of significance in infant humans, but basal metabolism rises in all ages following a meal (the 'specific dynamic effect').

The four modes of heat exchange (R, C, K and E above) are each governed by physical laws which, in theory at least, allow their precise computation. In practice though, information is seldom sufficiently complete, and more empirical relationships have to be used. Most popular are lumped equations analogous to Ohm's law of electrical resistance:

$$q = t/h$$

where: q is the heat flux by that route, t is the thermal differential driving that mode of heat exchange, typically the difference between the surface and ambient temperatures, but notably the difference between fourth powers of temperatures in the case of radiant heat transfer (R), and h is the coefficient of resistance to that mode of heat exchange.

Although empirical, such equations are valuable in demonstrating the crucial importance of temperature gradients in determining the direction and size of heat flows. Heat cannot flow against a temperature gradient.

The magnitude of each mode of heat exchange is thus set by a combination of environmental conditions, including ambient radiation, air movement, temperature and water content, together with skin temperature and clothing worn. For example, some industrial environments impose a high radiant heat load (R) from hot machinery, molten metals and flame; this can be usefully attenuated by garments coated with an outer metallized reflective layer. However this may in turn render the garments impermeable to water vapour transfer, resulting in evaporative heat loss (E) falling to zero. Another major factor which affects thermal resistance is the difference in physical properties of fluids: convective exchange with water is much greater than that with air.

A common error in the application of physics to human thermoregulation is to assume that the body can be treated as a single inert and undifferentiated entity. Regulatory mechanisms respond to central (or 'core') temperatures quite differently from those in the periphery. When someone who is hyperthermic immerses the hands in cold water, peripheral vasodilatation is maintained and they can lose substantial amounts of heat into the water;[1] euthermic or hypothermic subjects will not only vasoconstrict on (cold) hand immersion, but may not be able to vasodilate even if the hands are immersed in warm water.

Should heat production not match heat loss, heat will either be gained or lost from the body, according to the sign of S above, and it is this which results in a change in body temperature. The oversimplistic single-element model of the body then fails to show the change which occurs in internal thermal gradients. If excessive heat is being lost from the skin, the peripheries will cool first and there will be little effect on the 'core' other than its shrinking in effective volume. Insufficient heat loss and a rising 'core' temperature tends to externalize the core by reducing thermal gradients with the peripheries, and increasing the volume of the body at core temperature.

Responses to cold

The primary physiological responses to cold exposure are peripheral vasoconstriction, piloerection, and the increase in metabolic heat production by shivering. Skin temperature falls first, a result of local cooling without a corresponding increase in the delivery of heat to the skin by the flow of blood. This fall in skin temperature stimulates peripheral cold receptors and leads to both locally mediated and centrally regulated vasoconstriction, which in turn allows a further fall in skin temperature.

If the rest of the body is sufficiently warm, cyclical cold vasodilatation ('cold induced vasodilatation', or the 'hunting reaction') may ensue, with skin temperatures falling below 12°C, rising with the vasodilatation, and then falling again. This phenomenon probably results from cold paralysis of blood vessels, but is very variable between and within individuals, and absent if the rest of the body is cold. Sustained peripheral vasoconstriction may be accompanied by fluid shifts resulting in a reduction in plasma volume.

Shivering first appears as short bursts in a few groups of muscles, becoming continuous and generalized as a rectal temperature of about 35°C is reached. Further cooling or exhaustion results in shivering gradually tailing off, until it is replaced by generalized rigidity and finally the flaccidity of imminent death.

Responses to heat

Under heat stress, changes in blood flow to the periphery are again the earliest response, followed by an increase in evaporative heat loss by sweating. The normally low nutrient skin capillary flow is augmented by the opening of arteriovenous anastomoses in the skin, which allow high rates of heat transfer from the deeper body to its surface without altering capillary exchange. This increases skin temperature, driving higher rates of heat loss so long as the ambient temperature is lower than that of skin. When this temperature difference becomes too small to support adequate heat loss, or is actually reversed, the only significant means by which the body can lose heat is by the evaporation of sweat, which also makes high demands on peripheral blood flow.

These responses conflict with the requirement to perfuse working muscle during exercise, which may of course be the cause of the thermal stress. Fluid loss in sweat also threatens plasma volume, which is in turn essential to the maintenance of peripheral vasodilatation and sweating. A further problem is that thermally effective sweating requires evaporation from the skin (or, less effectively, the outermost layers of clothing); sweat which drips from the body makes no contribution to the loss of heat, whilst remaining a drain on fluid reserves. Failure of evaporation in humid conditions, with little air movement, or impermeable clothing, explains many cases of heat illness in relatively moderate dry bulb temperatures.

COLD STRESS

Assessment of cold stress

The dominant components of cold stress are the temperature and nature (air or water) of the fluid surrounding the body. Wind speed, and to a lesser extent water movement, can also be important. A simple thermometer and a wind speed indicator are the main measuring instruments needed. Anemometers need not be complex: one of the cup type is best for outside use, whilst vane and hot wire systems are preferred in enclosed spaces. The measurement of radiant heat exchange is more difficult to measure accurately, although it is generally small except under a clear night sky.

Evaporative loss is even harder to assess, and is small in cold–dry systems. But if the clothing is wet, evaporative losses alone can exceed 700 W, more than the total of other modes of heat loss; simple techniques such as repeated weighing to estimate water loss can then only give a crude overestimate. Although convective losses in water are much greater than in air of the same temperature, partial immersion presents a particularly complex situation. Subtle differences in behaviour and conditions can result in large changes in heat loss, as the body switches from convective cooling in water, through evaporative cooling of wet surfaces in air, to dry convective cooling. The delayed evaporative cooling of sweat-soaked garments after exercise is also difficult to quantify but of potentially great significance in those working hard in cold conditions.

Siple and Passell[2] were the first to attempt to incorporate dry bulb air temperature and wind speed into a single figure, now referred to as 'wind chill equivalent temperature' (Table 15.1). Models for this vary and none is universally applicable; for example the effect of wind depends greatly on whether the individual is wearing windproof clothing. However, such models give a useful first approximation of cold stress.

Assessment of cold strain

Any fall in core temperature below 35°C, the accepted threshold for hypothermia, is the best guide to a serious degree of general cold strain. Rectal measurement, at least 10 cm and preferably 15 cm beyond the anal sphincter, is the most reliable in cold conditions, though tympanic, oesophageal, gastric, vaginal, deep arterial and deep venous sites can each be used in different circumstances; detailed discussion is given in ISO 9886.[3] All require careful calibration of probes, and measures to prevent the transmission of infections such as hepatitis B and human immunodeficiency virus (HIV). Oral temperature is never reliable in the cold, as it is depressed by cold saliva, and infra-red tympanic techniques may also be misleading.[4]

Skin temperatures can give warning of lesser degrees of general cold strain, and are necessary measures of local cold strain, particularly when there is a risk of cold

Table 15.1 *Wind chill equivalent temperatures °C*

Wind speed				Dry bulb air temperature (°C)							
Beaufort	**miles/h**	**kt**	**m/s**	**−1**	**−7**	**−12**	**−18**	**−23**	**−29**	**−34**	**−40**
0	0	0	0	−1	−7	−12	−18	−23	−29	−34	−40
2	4	3	2	−3	−9	−15	−21	−26	−32	−38	−44
3	9	8	4	−9	−16	−23	−30	−36	−43	−50	−57
4	13	12	6	−14	−21	−29	−36	−43	−50	−58	−65
4	17	15	8	−16	−24	−32	−40	−47	−55	−63	−71
5	22	19	10	−18	−26	−34	−42	−51	−59	−67	−76
6	26	23	12	−19	−28	−36	−44	−53	−61	−70	−79
6	35	31	16	−21	−30	−38	−46	−55	−64	−73	−82
									Wind chill equivalent temperature (°C)		

Derived from the work of Siple and Passell,[2] applicable to naked exposed fingers. The equivalent temperature indicated in the main body of the table for a given combination of wind speed (at the left) and dry bulb temperature (at the top) is claimed to be that at which there is an equal rate of heat loss, given a wind speed of 0 m/s. For example, at a wind speed of 15 kt and a dry bulb air temperature of −12°C, the wind chill equivalent temperature is indicated to be −32°C, i.e. the risk of cold injury is the same as that for a wind speed of 0 kt and a dry bulb temperature of −32°C.

injury. Techniques are based on thermistors or thermo-couples, or infra-red emission measurement systems for uncovered skin. Electromyography (EMG) and oxygen uptake can be used to assess shivering and total metabolic heat production, although these are of limited value outside the laboratory.

Adaptation and habituation

Repeated brief exposures to cold produce clear reductions in both the vasoconstrictor and metabolic responses to cold stress. A course of just eight repeated cold (15°C for 40 minutes) immersions has been shown to attenuate the initial hyperventilation and tachycardia found during the initial responses to cold immersion.[5] Adaptation of more sustained responses has been seen to be more variable and difficult to demonstrate, although they may play a part in the physiology peculiar to long-distance sea swimmers,[6] and in the reduced response to cold by aboriginal peoples in Australia, and Ama divers. It may be that this 'hypothermic' adaptation has an advantage in increasing comfort during cold exposure, in particular permitting sleep, though it could be hazardous in cold exposure of longer duration. Many other attempts to demonstrate central adaptation or acclimatization to prolonged cold have failed to provide clear or consistent effects. The signal exception to this is earlier and more marked cold vasodilatation, which may be a result of reduced vasoconstriction, described in occupational groups subjected to repeated peripheral cold exposure such as fish filleters.[7]

Freezing cold injury

Local freezing of tissues, the most rapid and dramatic form of cold injury, may occur when people are exposed to temperatures below 0°C without adequate protection or opportunities to return to warm environments when the extremities become chilled.

The areas most commonly affected include fingers and toes, followed by nose, cheeks and ears, and occasionally the male genitalia. The last can occur in association with alcoholic episodes, or as a result of running without windproof underwear.[8] Such injuries may be associated with hypothermia, in which case the potentially life-threatening condition must be treated first, or with local or general trauma.[9] Although most commonly seen in wartime and the military, freezing cold injury is also seen in those undertaking winter sports, and in outdoor workers in cold climes, sometimes when the air temperature is not particularly low.[10] Cases do occur in cold stores and other processing plants, but the widespread use of effective protection and safe working practices normally prevents these. The damage is mainly caused by high concentrations of electrolytes left in tissue fluids when most of the water turns to ice. While

frozen, the skin is white and hard; on thawing, there is first hyperaemia and then, in severe cases, pallor and a woody feel to the skin as local blood vessels become occluded by red cells.

FROSTNIP

'Frostnip' is popularly used to describe mild freezing cold injury in which the superficial tissues (which are the only layer affected) recover completely within 30 minutes of starting rewarming; such recovery must include the return of normal sensation. Classically it involves any combination of the loss of peripheral sensation and the slight freezing of superficial tissues. Typically one or more finger or toe tips are blanched, the skin is leathery to the touch but not of wooden feel (which usually indicates deeper freezing), and anaesthetic. The immediate and diagnostic treatment is to rewarm the affected periphery against the warm skin of an understanding colleague; hands and feet may conveniently be placed in an axilla or groin, whilst portions of the nose, cheeks or ears are best rewarmed by firm contact with a hand or fur patch on the back of a mitten. Rubbing, massage and direct heat should be avoided. Provided that recovery is complete within the 30 minute period, no further treatment is necessary. However those who have not returned to normal should then be treated for superficial frostbite.[11] Thereby hangs the dilemma, in that this diagnosis is dependent on the outcome of field treatment; an adverse outcome has serious consequences in terms of further management.

SUPERFICIAL FROSTBITE

More severe freezing injury which would not recover so rapidly is usually termed 'frostbite'. If confined to the skin and most peripheral layers of tissue, it can usefully be qualified as being 'superficial'. Initial appearances may be indistinguishable from frostnip, but in the hours and days following thawing, gross discoloration may occur, with haemorrhagic patches and blisters containing fluid varying from clear serous exudate to the frankly haemorrhagic. Later still, small and superficial areas of dry gangrene may develop, with skin peeling and nail loss.

The standard treatment for superficial frostbite remains conservative. Rapid rewarming in a stirred waterbath at 40–42°C should be prolonged and thorough, with analgesic cover (typically using a paracetamol compound preparation).[12] Care must be taken to ensure that patches do not remain partially defrosted on removal from the waterbath. For some, rewarming is an exquisitely painful process which may even merit intravenous morphine at a rate adjusted to give freedom from pain, but sublingual buprenorphine may both suffice and be more convenient. Although objective evidence of other beneficial effects is still wanting, moderate quantities of alcohol can reduce the requirement for analgesia and improve general well-being, and a twice daily 'tot' of spirits is recommended. Infection must be prevented with liberal use of topical antibacterials such as povi-done–iodine preparations, preferably in combination with twice daily 'whirlpool' baths at 40°C. Tetanus prophylaxis is also required in cases where there is likely to be any significant amount of necrotic tissue, but systemic antibiotics are normally only considered when there is active infection or deeper tissues are involved.

Blisters should not be burst or aspirated because of the risk of infection. Their resolution will be aided by the elevation of the injured part, which should be kept comfortably warm but not too hot. Early physiotherapy to restore functional movement is very important, particularly when hands are affected, as is the restraining of overenthusiastic surgeons; in the absence of any other threat to the injured tissues, surgery should be avoided for at least 4 and preferably 6 months. Careful conservative management will normally result in the loss of much less tissue than might originally be expected from appearances in the first few weeks after injury. One decisive factor is the avoidance of premature or incomplete rewarming. In spite of the diagnostic definition of frostnip, rewarming should never be attempted until it is certain that further freezing cannot occur, and that the affected part will not be used or further damaged. For this reason, rewarming is generally best avoided in remote areas, unless the casualty can be evacuated by stretcher and in guaranteed warmth.

An almost complete lack of good clinical trials of adjuvant drugs makes it impossible to recommend pharmacological intervention. Different groups have advocated colloidal infusions, various vasodilators, even derivatives of snake venoms. To date the only addition to the conservative regimen which might hold promise is the use of *Aloe vera* derived inhibitors of thromboxane, but few are licensed and evidence still scant.[12]

DEEP AND COMPLICATED FROSTBITE

Freezing of muscles and other deeper tissues, including their blood vessels, is much rarer and more serious. Almost unseen in ordinary working situations, it is mainly a product of wartime and occasionally in mountaineering accidents. Whole limbs may freeze solid, and victims are invariably hypothermic. Rapid rewarming should only be attempted in hospital under full biochemical control, as massive release of potassium from damaged cells can otherwise cause sudden death. Surgical decompression of tissue spaces may be needed before rewarming, to limit the rise of tissue pressures which results from the volume expansion accompanying the melting of ice crystals. The amount of tissue likely to be dead or dying demands the utmost care in preventing tetanus and gas gangrene.[13] Even so, proper conservative management may result in the salvage of much of the limb.[14]

Cyclical freezing, thawing and refreezing is even more destructive of cells, and can result in the very worst end result. Early and radical amputation, 2 to 3 months following injury, may be preferred in these cases, as it might in cases where infections are established.[12]

LONG-TERM SEQUELAE OF FREEZING COLD INJURY

Military campaigns and civil disaster may leave swathes of the population recovering from the acute effects of freezing cold injury. Although often not as severe as the long-term consequences of non-freezing cold injury, those resulting from freezing injuries may be just as frequent.[11,15] Reviews of veterans as long as 45 years after their original injuries reveal many suffering from chronic problems as a result. The proportion so affected is hard to determine, but likely to lie between 10% and 50%.

Commonest sequelae include cold sensitization (which is more usually associated with non-freezing cold injury, see below), chronic pain, residual neurological deficit, joint pain and stiffness, hyperhydrosis, and skin and nail abnormalities. Persistent neurological deficits most usually range from loss of fine touch to complete anaesthesia, with the densest deficit in the most distal of the affected parts.

Radiographic examination may reveal characteristic appearances of 'frostbite arthritis', which include small local subarticular punched-out lesions possibly representing subchondral cysts from vascular injury.[16] Long-term changes in gait from sensory ataxia and chronic foot disorders may be responsible for less specific joint pain. Whilst hyperhydrosis may lead to chronic fungal infection, the skin is often dry and scaly, and may crack painfully; topical application of lanolin cream, or preparations intended for the care of cows' udders, can alleviate this. Fungal infections of the nails may respond little to treatment and, together with disturbances of nail growth, can result in thickening and frank onychogryphosis, making a high standard of podiatary essential if mobility is to be maintained.

More unusual sequelae include recurrent ulceration and breakdown of old scars, which may in turn lead to an increased risk of local skin cancers. It is not clear whether this is specifically related to the frostbite, or is common to other causes of recurrent ulceration (Marjolin's ulcer). Although rarely the major finding, complete local loss of proprioception in someone with a history of cold injury is a characteristic neurological association. In the hands, this can make dressing very hard, whilst in the feet the resulting sensory ataxia may threaten mobility.

Non-freezing cold injury

Longer exposures to less severe temperatures, particularly when coupled with other conditions (such as limb dependency and constrictive clothing) liable to cause circulatory stasis, can result in injuries which appear generally mild in comparison with frostbite. A wide variety of terms have been applied to non-freezing cold injury (NFCI) since it was first described in the eighteenth century, including trench foot, immersion foot, shelter limb, and Flanders foot, depending on the circumstances in which the variant was described. It often co-exists with freezing injury, but in spite of its apparent innocence during the acute phase, NFCI frequently results in more severe long-term sequelae.

The great majority of cases of NFCI affect the feet alone, although it has been described in the hands as well. Apart from military personnel in cold wet climates, the main groups affected by classical NFCI are survivors in the water or in liferafts. Immersion of a hand for as little as 45 minutes in water at 0°C may produce mild NFCI, but 3 hours are needed to result in overt injury. Because seawater freezes at a temperature below 0°C (normally around −1.9°C), tissues immersed in very cold seawater may sustain freezing rather than non-freezing injury. Although circumstantial evidence points to dependence on a function of duration of exposure and low temperature, variation between individuals may obscure this. In the same person, the same injury might result from a short period at a low temperature, or a longer period exposed to a milder temperature. There also appear to be relationships with other similar conditions: long immersion in luke-warm water results in 'paddy foot', which is clinically indistinguishable from NFCI. The pathogenesis of these conditions remains obscure; factors which have been proposed include the direct effect of cooling on nerves, prolonged ischaemia during cold exposure, and the liberation of reactive oxygen compounds during reperfusion. Some or all of these may be important in the evolution of vibration injuries, reflex sympathetic dystrophy, and other similar syndromes.[12]

PRESENTATION AND MANAGEMENT

Clinical appearances have been divided into four stages:

1 injury: in which the foot is very cold, ischaemic, and numb;
2 rewarming: in which the foot becomes mottled blue-pink and exquisitely painful;
3 hyperaemia: in which the pulses are full and bounding, but there is slow capillary refill, marked swelling, some degree of anaesthesia and paraesthesia, and severe pain (primarily nocturnal);
4 recovery: in which the foot gradually returns towards normal, with residual sequelae including cold sensitization.

Stage 1 is seen throughout the period in which the injury is actually occurring, ranging from minutes to days in duration. It is therefore usually only witnessed by the patient, who may provide the diagnostic description of numbness or other sensory impairment. Stage 2 is seen fleetingly during rewarming, typically lasting just a few minutes. The majority of cases present in stage 3, which lasts for several days or weeks. Stage 4 may then supervene for months, years, and possibly last throughout the lifetime.

Although NFCI is best managed using similar conservative principles to those for freezing injury, it has been established that rapid rewarming in a waterbath exacerbates both damage and pain. Slow (or 'passive') rewarming is therefore preferred. The management of early pain can be fraught: bedclothes should be cradled over the feet at night, and conventional analgesics (simple, non-steroidal anti-inflammatory, or even narcotic) are invariably ineffective. Although some have claimed benefit from the nocturnal administration of quinine, the standard approach is to give a single daily dose of amitriptyline (50–200 mg) in the evening. Morphine does not affect the pain but the patient no longer cares about the discomfort, whilst regional analgesia is highly effective but short-lived.[12] Untreated, this pain usually lasts for several days or weeks, or may subside by about 3 months into less severe chronic pain.

Late consequences are common and may last for life, even after subclinical NFCI, which may only present years later as a result of chronic sequelae. It is likely that the majority of those suffering NFCI are still symptomatic 6 months after injury, but less than 10% suffer from significant symptoms at 5 years. Most prominent is a prolonged vasoconstrictive response to further cold exposure; when a patient complains of this as a symptom, it is termed 'cold sensitivity', but assumes the diagnosis of 'cold sensitization' when supported by physical findings. A cold stimulus as innocuous as a 2-minute immersion in water at 15°C may precipitate a cold, vasoconstricted foot for 4 or more hours afterwards. This predisposes to further injury, and is a prime reason for following up those who have sustained NFCI and investigating those claiming cold sensitivity. Such assessment should include infrared thermography to investigate rewarming following a mild cold stress, and measurement of warm and cool sensory thresholds in affected digits.

The cause of cold sensitization remains ill-understood. It was originally supposed that it resulted from a sympathetic denervation supersensitivity, but most recent assessment of vascular sympathetic nerve function in sensitized feet has shown this not to be the case.[17] The cause may lie in a vascular endothelial abnormality (and NFCI is known to result in endothelial injury), or the devascularization which is known to arise when local blood flow is chronically reduced. No effective treatment is known, although exposure to heat may be ameliorative. Severe cases may enjoy slow and slight benefit from sustained-release nifedipine, but thymoxamine has not so far been of use. Assessing the outcome to treatment is complicated by the variable natural course: whilst in some cases the complaint appears to resolve spontaneously after 1–15 years, the condition of other patients may worsen (particularly if they undergo further cold exposure), or remain unchanged. Patients should be advised to avoid further cold exposure, to adopt effective measures to minimize local cold stress which might include the wearing of gloves or mittens even in relatively warm conditions, and should be given an honest account of the prognosis. Other long-term sequelae are common and include all those mentioned for freezing cold injury above.[12]

Hypothermia on land

Taken across the working population as a whole, hypothermia is comparatively rare without immersion, and as a cause of death it is quite unusual. Even in social groups deemed to be at particular risk, notably the very young and very old in poorer circumstances, hypothermia is considerably less common than is usually portrayed. In those of working age, cases tend to occur in clusters when groups involved in military or leisure activities are exposed to particularly harsh conditions, frequently in association with inadequate planning and preparation.

On land, its onset is usually gradual, over a period of hours, when heat loss is greatly increased by evaporation from precipitation or accumulated sweat, but heat production is falling due to physical exhaustion. In many cases, victims have been maintaining thermal balance by hard physical exertion and then start to tire; as their fatigue causes them to reduce the rate of work, heat loss starts to exceed heat production, and core temperature falls. Inadequate replenishment of energy and fluid, insufficient physical fitness, and previous alcohol intake (which can produce sustained hypoglycaemia)[18] are all common predisposing factors.

Detailed clinical descriptions of hypothermia and its management are given elsewhere.[19] From early subtle changes in affect and behaviour, as body temperature falls further, so the signs become more gross. Shivering intensifies until it dominates attempts at any other activity, although it can be attenuated or even absent. Once the core temperature falls below the threshold of definition of hypothermia, 35°C, so a progressive decline in all body functions supervenes. At first, the victim may lapse into light sleep, then into an unrousable unconsciousness. Bradycardia and slow, shallow breathing may make vital signs almost undetectable by a core temperature of about 30°C. Electrocardiogram (ECG) recordings typically show prolonged QT intervals, and J deflections below 31°C. Muscle rigidity, the successor to shivering, eventually becomes flaccidity with absent reflexes, as potentially lethal temperatures are reached below about 28°C. However, the only reliable way to establish death is to demonstrate failure to revive following a determined attempt to rewarm.

In the field, actions should be directed at reducing further heat loss and evacuating the casualty. Although the risks of circum-rescue collapse and cardiac dysrhythmias associated with rough handling and postural change (sometimes inevitable during evacuation across harsh terrain) are thought to be lower on land than following immersion, evacuation should be careful and considered rather than rushed. Those providing assistance should not neglect the risk of others in the party succumbing to hypothermia: it may be necessary for them to be placed in shelter, or for their evacuation after that of the immediate casualties. Issues relating to rewarming are discussed below.

Successful rewarming from the most profound hypothermia can be curative, or complications may result in a more stormy course. Although hypothermia usually provides some measure of protection from hypoxia, organ failure will eventually occur, and a significant number of those revived from combined hypothermia and anoxia (such as those rescued after falling through ice-covered water) will have permanent neurological sequelae. This is not helped by the tendency to cardiac dysrhythmias, including ventricular fibrillation, and their resistance to treatment until the myocardium has been rewarmed. Metabolic acidosis should be corrected by intravenous sodium bicarbonate, but cardioversion delayed until the core temperature has reached about 30°C. More remarkable is the high frequency of pancreatitis, which has been reported post mortem in up to 80% of cases of hypothermic death. In survivors, it is responsible for raised serum amylase levels, but other evidence of pancreatic damage may be lacking. Haemorrhagic gastric erosions also appear common, possibly reflecting 'stress ulceration'.

Immersion hypothermia and 'cold shock'

Immersion poses more threats than hypothermia alone. Many of those who die in the water do so because of drowning, although even then this simple diagnosis obscures a complex causal sequence. Golden and Hervey[20] have divided up the hazards of cold immersion into four phases according to the time since entry into the water: the initial 2–3 minutes of 'cold shock', the next 10–15 minutes of 'swimming failure', from 30 minutes onwards from hypothermia and drowning, and the period during and after rescue.

Sudden immersion in cold water produces dramatic physiological responses, which have been reviewed by Tipton.[21] In the great majority of adults, any tendency to the potentially protective effects of the 'diving response' is usually overwhelmed by an inspiratory gasp followed by hyperventilation, tachycardia, and peripheral vasoconstriction: the cardinal responses of 'cold shock'. If trapped in a ditched helicopter or capsized vessel, useful breath-hold time diminishes almost to zero, making underwater escape almost impossible; underwater breathing apparatus (particularly if not based on pressurized gas, with its concomitant risk of arterial gas embolism) can be invaluable in enabling successful escape. Hyperventilation not only makes the inhalation of water, thus primary drowning, more likely, but its effects on blood chemistry can be disabling. Cardiovascular responses may be dramatic, such as the sudden onset of cardiac arrhythmias ranging from frequent extrasystoles to ventricular fibrillation. When just a tachycardia, they combine with peripheral vasoconstriction to produce a sharp rise in blood pressure, which may be sufficient to burst arterial aneurysms.

Those who survive the first 2 or 3 minutes of cold water immersion may drown in the ensuing 10–15 minutes, apparently failing to swim even though they may be close to safety. Such 'swimming failure' is largely independent of warm water swimming ability, and appears related to the direct cooling of peripheral nerves (making muscular control harder), failure to synchronize breathing with swim-stroke, and other subtle effects. It is only when the casualty has been immersed for more than about 20 minutes that immersion hypothermia becomes a serious threat, and even then it may lead to disablement and thus drowning long before core temperatures reach lethal levels below about 28°C.

Divers appear prone to two forms of hypothermia which may occur with minimal physiological responses. One affects saturation divers who are dependent on careful control of breathing gas temperature and their hot water suits to maintain thermal balance.[22] If their inspired gas is slightly too cool, large amounts of heat can be lost from the core, whilst skin temperatures are held high. In the absence of stimulus to the peripheral cold receptors, the body may make little or no physiological response to the falling core temperature. The other form of insidious hypothermia affects slightly underdressed free-swimming divers in water temperatures between about 20° and 25°C. Although cold enough to result in falling core temperature, such water may not elicit any sensation of cold, and once again peripheral vasoconstriction and shivering may not occur.

The hazards of immersion do not stop when rescue starts. As many as 20% of all those conscious but thought to be hypothermic at the time of rescue die during the following minutes. Golden et al.[23] have reviewed the causes, which are related to the mode of rescue and subsequent treatment. Because the ailing circulation receives substantial hydrostatic support during immersion, during which the margin for cardiac compensation is being eroded, vertical modes of recovery can result in sudden loss of venous return and complete circulatory collapse. The adoption of horizontal modes of rescue, such as double rescue strops, can reduce this risk, provided that they do not compromise the chances of successful recovery.

Another risk following rescue is that of rewarming collapse, which appears to be the result of peripheral vasodilatation during rewarming. For this reason, casualties should not be left unattended nor rewarmed in an upright position, for example in a shower. Hot baths are often the method of choice for those who are cold but not clinically hypothermic. Aggressive or active rewarming techniques should be avoided unless they are applied in sophisticated medical facilities such as intensive therapy units; they may hasten complex and life-threatening problems during rewarming, and good evidence that they improve outcome is still lacking. Another pitfall is the decision to start external cardiac massage (ECM) should it be thought that cardiac output is insufficient in the hypothermic. Because this is likely to ensure that the heart is in ventricular fibrillation (if still alive), and the cold heart cannot be defibrillated, starting ECM commits the first-aider to maintaining it – effectively – until the casualty is delivered to a place of definitive care. If this will only take 30 minutes, ECM may prove life-saving; if evacuation could take many hours or even days, it is probably wisest to avoid starting ECM for this reason.

Those who have inhaled insufficient water to cause primary drowning may exhibit signs of respiratory distress during the first 1–3 days after immersion; this is secondary drowning and requires immediate aggressive intensive therapy. Clinical manifestations are those of an adult respiratory distress syndrome, with dyspnoea, cough, copious frothy and blood-stained sputum, progressing to respiratory failure and death. All those who have become immersed and could have aspirated water, and thus could be at risk of secondary drowning, should be cautioned about the unlikely but possible chance of the condition, and the need to seek medical aid as a matter of urgency should they show signs of respiratory deterioration such as shortness of breath and cough.

The ideal protection from cold immersion is an integrated survival system, consisting of personal protective equipment to provide appropriate buoyancy and thermal protection, if necessary with underwater escape supported by a breathing system.[24] For longer term survival, as when abandoning a ship in the ocean, dry-shod entry into a seaworthy and thermally effective liferaft should be the goal. In spite of some earlier pessimistic predictions of human survival times, a recent large survey of immersion incidents in UK waters[25] has proposed that average survival times are better: provided that the casualty is rescued within a reasonably survivable period, half of the subjects would be expected to be alive at the time of rescue after 3 hours in water at 5°C, 6 hours at 10°C, and 12 hours at 15°C.

The effect of cold on performance

Although opinion and anecdote invariably assert the deleterious effects of cold on a wide range of aspects of human performance,[26] objective assessments such as tests of manual performance and visual–motor tasks are less frequent and not as clear-cut.[27] There are many methodological problems to be overcome before the body of scientific evidence can be considered to be substantial enough either to confirm opinion or to modify it. The presence of large variations between individuals, and differences between performances of the same individual on different occasions, have been of particular hindrance. Broadly speaking, cold has been described as impairing three different aspects of performance: sensory, motor, and higher brain function. The first two are commonly combined in measures of dexterity, which are reduced either by cooling, or by the protective clothing worn to prevent cooling. Where studies have been able to show significant effects on dexterity, they are usually related to both local and central cooling.[28] In actual occupational settings, impairment of performance is commonly a result of many factors. The combination of cold, physical exertion and protective clothing can be particularly dangerous, as rest periods may result in rapid and severe peripheral cooling,[29] whilst the metabolic cost of submaximal work increases, and maximal aerobic performance falls.

Observations that accident rates increase during cold periods of the year[26] are too crude to permit conclusions to be drawn about the influence of moderate cold on higher mental functions. However, a particularly disturbing study by Coleshaw *et al.*[30] demonstrated that even slight levels of body cooling (above those diagnosed as hypothermia) can have dramatic effects on simple measures of mental function such as memory registration and the speed of reasoning.

HEAT STRESS

Assessment of heat stress

At warmer temperatures, air has a greater capacity to contain water vapour. This is of importance to human thermoregulation, because of the increasing significance of the evaporation of sweat as a means of cooling the body as air temperatures increase. Accordingly, the simple dry measures made in cold environments are insufficient to assess warmer conditions quantitatively. The one exception to this is when personnel are clad almost entirely in impermeable clothing, as they might be when working in toxic or radioactive environments, for instance. In such clothing, sweating cannot be thermally effective, as no evaporation can occur, so that measures of heat stress can be simplified.

Most measures of heat stress therefore attempt to combine weighted values of dry bulb temperature with some estimate of humidity, together with radiant heat load and sometimes other variables. Although different indices come into vogue at different times and for different purposes, that with perhaps the best all-round record is the Wet Bulb Globe Temperature (WBGT) index, which also has the advantages of being simple to compute and easily measured with compact instruments. More detailed studies may require a psychrometric chart on which the relationship between air temperature, moisture content and relative humidity is shown. Body heat production is again an important consideration, and can be measured in the field by expired gas analysis using a portable respiratory system, or more crudely estimated from activity levels against standard scales. Methods for doing this are given in ISO 8996.[31]

WET BULB GLOBE TEMPERATURE

ISO 7243[32] prescribes a standard method for the estimation of heat stress using three temperature measurements: those of a standard dry bulb, a wet bulb, and one inside a blackened globe of 150 mm diameter. The three temperatures are combined using the following equation, into the WBGT index:

$$\text{WBGT} = 0.7T_{\text{wet bulb}} + 0.2T_{\text{globe}} + 0.1T_{\text{dry bulb}}$$

Under this ISO standard, it is permissible to ignore the dry bulb temperature if there is little difference between it and that of the globe (e.g. indoors with little radiant heat load), in which case the equation becomes:

$$\text{indoor WBGT} = 0.7T_{\text{wet bulb}} + 0.3T_{\text{globe}}$$

The standard provides a set of reference index values for five levels of metabolic rate for both acclimatized and unacclimatized persons, which may be of value in assessing the relative stress.

Related indices can be derived for environments in which formal measurement of the WBGT index is not possible. For example, Nunneley and Stribley developed a 'Fighter Index of Thermal Stress' (FITS)[33] for the cockpit of aircraft at low altitude but using measurements taken at ground level on clear days:

$$\text{FITS} = 0.83T_{\text{psychrometric wet bulb}} + 0.35T_{\text{dry bulb}} + 5.08$$

PSYCHROMETRIC CHARTS

In many situations, radiant heat loads are fairly small in comparison with the heat exchange by convection and evaporation. The psychrometric chart, reproduced in Fig. 15.1, is a clear graphical way of understanding the effect of changing humidity and temperatures alone. Use of the chart requires a measurement of the water content of the air (e.g. by some form of psychrometer capable of yielding relative or absolute humidity values) and the dry bulb temperature. Limits may be defined on the chart appropriate to a given group of individuals for specified activities and clothing, thus allowing the user to make recommendations as to how their physiological requirements may be met. The chart may also be used to under-

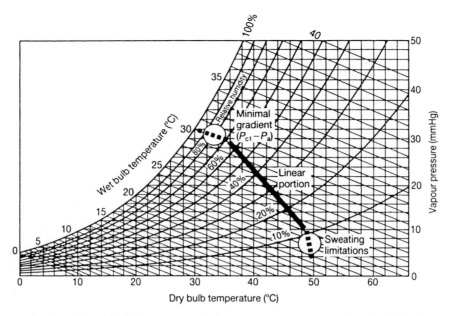

Figure 15.1 *A psychrometric chart. The grid is laid over a graph of water vapour pressure against dry bulb air temperature. On this, curves of equal percentage relative to humidity are superimposed, as are lines of equal wet bulb temperature. Thus, the graph may be entered using any pair of dry bulb air temperature, water vapour pressure, relative humidity or wet bulb temperature. For a given garment assembly and work rate, it is possible to plot a straight line which determines the upper limit of the exposure envelope, marked as the 'linear portion' in this figure. Those conditions to the left of and below this line are acceptable. However, there are two additional linear segments which are also shown: at higher relative humidifies, the small vapour pressure gradient from clothing to ambient limits tolerance, whilst at low relative humidities sweating endurance is limited and thus restricts the envelope.*

stand the relative effects of lowering air temperature and humidity when trying to control an environment.

OTHER INDICES

Although the WBGT index is simple to measure quite accurately, it is only indirectly linked with heat strain. In most circumstances operators prefer to employ measures which can give a more direct assessment of heat strain, and to this end many alternatives have been proposed. These have been compared by Parsons,[34] and more formally in ISO 11399.[35] A potentially very attractive approach to the assessment of heat stress is to attempt to relate it to the amount of evaporative heat loss required for thermal balance; this was originally incorporated into a 'predicted 4-hour sweat rate' (P4SR), but has more recently evolved into the 'required sweat rate', as defined in ISO 7933.[36] Measurement essentially consists of a semi-empirical solution of the equation of heat balance, to arrive at an estimate of the sweat rate required for the maintenance of thermal equilibrium. It is thus considerably more complex than the WBGT index, and more suited to experimental investigations rather than routine monitoring. The latest studies have confirmed its efficacy in predicting averages and limits to exposure,[37] although modifications may be required to the calculation of the evaporative efficiency of sweating.[38]

More moderate thermal stress may need to be assessed by more complex methods than the simple WBGT index, as the transfer of heat by each physical mode is usually more sensitive to subtle changes. Detailed accounts of the 'Predicted Mean Vote' (PMV) and 'Predicted Percentage of Dissatisfied' (PPD) indices are given in ISO 7730,[39] based on measurements of air temperature, mean radiant temperature, humidity, air velocity, metabolic rate, and clothing insulation. Indeed in any situation in which clothed individuals are being assessed, reference will need to be made to the estimation of the thermal insulation and resistance to evaporative heat loss imposed by clothing; ISO 9920[40] provides a sound practical basis for this.

Assessment of heat strain

The principal measurement of heat strain, like that of cold, is core body temperature. However, core temperature can rise rapidly in the heat and the fact that rectal temperature changes later and more slowly than other sites makes it less suitable for safety purposes. Accordingly, it is more common to estimate deep body temperature in the heat from a tympanic membrane or auditory canal reading; this has the added advantage that this site should usually be a good indicator of the temperature of the brain, which is not only the central temperature controller, but is also one of the more critical organs in heat illness.

Three other variables are commonly recorded in heat studies: heart rate is the simplest of all to measure, loss of body mass due to sweating is also very easily determined, whilst skin temperatures are sometimes of value if judiciously interpreted.

Heart rate is directly correlated with heat strain, provided that changes due to exercise are allowed for. It is often used, in conjunction with aural temperature, in establishing criteria for the withdrawal of persons exposed to heat loads. The simple estimate of body weight loss is a useful measure of fluid loss in laboratory conditions. Skin temperatures can prove misleading, as they fall if there is good evaporation from the skin, but climb close to core if evaporation is limited or absent. These methods are described in ISO 9886.[3]

Acclimatization

Temperate residents cannot perform as well under heat stress as those used to living in the tropics. Careful studies during the middle of the twentieth century demonstrated that unacclimatized temperate residents show significant acclimatization after only 2 weeks of exposure to heat.[41] This can be produced by prolonged exposure to an environmental heat load (e.g. by living in the tropics, or working in hot conditions), or by repeatedly raising the body temperature by undertaking sustained physical exercise, or by a combination of both. Pure fitness training produces similar changes to heat acclimatization and so improves tolerance to heat stress.

During the first week of acclimatization, the ability of the body to sweat is increased, so that thermal sweating occurs more rapidly under heat stress, and the amount of sweat produced is progressively increased. Simultaneous cardiovascular changes sustain peripheral vasodilatation and the blood flow required by active sweat glands. Towards the end of this period, salt is retained by the kidneys and salt content of the sweat starts to decline, so that increased sweating does not result in severe sodium deficiency. This is achieved by an early peak in renin, followed by an increase in aldosterone levels. Consequently some individuals need to increase dietary salt intake during the first week of acclimatization, but seldom after that. It should be noted that required water intake may actually be increased in those who are acclimatized: popular belief that those conditioned to living in the tropics are also able to do without water, or even worse to substitute alcohol, is completely erroneous.

The process of acclimatization continues more gradually over the remainder of the first 3 months or so spent in the tropics, at the end of which the temperate-born individual is almost physiologically indistinct from those who have spent their entire lives under a heat stress. However, behavioural adaptation, in which dress and habits are changed to those most appropriate in the heat, may never occur.

Immediate consequences of heat strain

The continuing popularity of prolonged physical exercise in temperate climates, such as marathons and triathlons in the populous countries of the northern hemisphere, reinforces the need to move away from the traditional classification of heat illness. The latter, evolved during British Imperial days, endeavoured to distinguish acute, subacute and chronic disorders involving overheating and water and electrolyte losses in a complex and probably misleading terminology. Setting aside a few discrete disorders such as prickly heat, salt and water deficiencies, true heat illness can be spread along a continuum from heat exhaustion to heat stroke.[42] At the one extreme, this consists of little change in body temperature and overt hyperventilation, and at the other, a core temperature in excess of 41°C, absence of sweating, and complete circulatory collapse. Patients can move rapidly from minor heat exhaustion to life-threatening heat stroke; so no matter how mild the symptoms may appear to be, anyone suffering from a heat illness should be considered to be in incipient heat stroke and thus in imminent danger of death.

HEAT EXHAUSTION

Heat exhaustion is typified by the moderately well trained athlete competing in a marathon during the warmer months in a temperate country. It may also be seen in military personnel during fitness training in similar conditions and in groups of manual workers with moderate environmental heat loads. The first sign of impending heat exhaustion is usually hyperventilation, in someone who appears ill at ease with the exercise which they are performing, and this appears to be the cause of most symptoms and signs.[42]

Classic signs and symptoms from the disturbance of the body's acid-base balance and the calcium–phosphate ratio in the blood follow, with dizziness, nausea, carpopedal spasm, paraesthesiae in the peripheries and around the mouth, progressing to confusion, collapse, vomiting and even fits. Core temperature at this stage is below 40°C, and usually between 37° and 39°C. Early cases respond rapidly to rest in a recumbent position, rebreathing from a paper bag to restore end-tidal CO_2 levels, and simple cooling. Fluids may also be beneficial and should always be given by appropriate means. If these patients are allowed or even encouraged to continue exercising, they may rapidly develop frank heat stroke.

HEAT STROKE

Those working in very hot surroundings, particularly when evaporative cooling is ineffective due to high humidity, may undergo a rapid rise in core temperature, to the point at which thermoregulation fails.[43] The classic victims of heat stroke have stopped sweating and are dry to the touch. They may still maintain peripheral circulation and thus be red, or may have undergone circulatory collapse, in which case their skin colour is not diagnostic. They are very hot, semi-conscious or comatose and prone to cardiac and respiratory arrest. The onset of this dramatic illness may have been very rapid, although many will have shown evidence of earlier heat exhaustion.

Cooling is best achieved in the field by stripping the patient in the shade, drenching with tepid water, and fanning if there is little natural wind. Cold water or ice is less useful because of the intense vasoconstriction which it can precipitate, which limits heat transfer from the core to the skin. Alternating litres of isotonic dextrose and saline intravenously are the best means of fluid administration. The precise quantity given may be based on an estimate of fluid loss, but in unconscious cases it is probably best to give the first litre over 15 minutes or less, thereafter reducing the rate of infusion according to clinical indications and the perceived risk of hypervolaemia leading to pulmonary oedema. Such fluids should not be warmed, but neither should they be cooled below 15°C. Elevation of the legs to assist venous return, administration of oxygen, and possibly sedatives, are of value. However, vasodilators and platelet inhibitors such as aspirin should be avoided. Rapid but careful evacuation to an intensive care unit is essential, where urinary output, blood biochemistry and direct measurement of the central venous pressure can be monitored closely. Cooling is normally discontinued when the rectal or aural temperature has reached 38°C, lest it overshoot.

Unfortunately, the outcome of true heat stroke is not good. If core temperature rises to around 45°C, irreversible heat denaturation of proteins causes multiple organ failure or disseminated intravascular coagulation. If this is not immediately fatal, renal dialysis may be necessary during recovery. Heat illness, associated with exercise, can produce subacute rhabdomyolysis (necrosis of muscle) which may in turn lead to late renal failure because of myoglobinuria.

OTHER CONDITIONS

Traditional salt depletion, due to salt loss in sweat while on a low salt diet, with adequate water intake, is now rarely seen. The classic accompaniment of cramp (e.g. miner's cramp) only occurs in association with hard exercise and is now very unusual. Plasma sodium only falls in more severe cases, with milder cases showing a fall in extracellular fluid volume with normal plasma sodium. In the worst cases, vigorous treatment with oral or intravenous saline may be required. Subacute and other variants of this condition, sometimes attributed to different combinations of water and electrolyte depletion and 'disacclimatization', are similarly uncommon. They are best treated by cooling, rest, rehydration and the restoration of a normal diet. Those whose appetite has been suppressed and who have overindulged in alcohol should recover quickly in this way. The blind oral administration of salt, even with the copious quantities of fluid which are required, is potentially dangerous and should be avoided.

One possible danger is that of hyperkalaemia; many young people often rehydrate following exercise in the heat using some form of orange juice, or a 'sports rehydration' fluid, which may be high in potassium. They should be advised to ensure that their rehydration fluid is well diluted with water.

Perhaps the most common of the 'mild' heat disorders is prickly heat, or miliaria rubra, which results from blocking of the orifices of sweat glands. Because of the blockage, the glands rupture their ducts, raising a weal within an erythematous area, which is extremely itchy. Removal from the heat both abolishes sweating and prevents the body overheating as a result of its impaired ability to sweat. Other less well understood conditions which may appear during heat stress include a transient ankle oedema (which may result from the thermal attenuation of the venoarteriolar reflex) and mild muscular cramps. Some individuals experience dizziness and fainting which may have a common aetiology.

The effect of heat on performance

Reconciling the subjective and objective is no easier for the possible effects of heat than was noted above for cold. Ramsey has reviewed[44] more than 150 studies which attempted to find differences in 'perceptual motor performance' in the heat, and commented on the remarkable lack of objective evidence of dominant effects. It appears that there is no significant detectable impairment in the performance of the great majority of tasks until the level of heat stress reaches a WBGT index of approximately 30°C. This is broadly in accordance with the criteria originally laid down by the US National Institute of Occupational Safety and Health (NIOSH) in their original recommended exposure limit (REL).[45] Paradoxically, when revised 14 years later, NIOSH omitted this REL because of lack of supporting evidence.[46]

A few studies cast interesting and potentially different light on the area. There is much stronger support for adverse effects in circumstances in which core temperature has risen; when core temperature is 38°C or greater, a prominent effect is an increase in irritability independent of the rise in subjective discomfort.[47] Critics of studies which have used more artificial and perhaps oversimplified measures of performance may find some comfort in the work of Wyon et al.,[48] who examined the effect of moderate heat stress on driving performance. Whilst they observed a heat-related increase in overt driving errors, it was found to occur only in women.

Perhaps the most useful tool (beyond tenuous attempts to relate accident statistics to heat stress or strain) in the practical examination of performance effects is the expression of subjective judgement scales. ISO 10551[49] lays down a standard approach to these, which allows inclusion of comfort, acceptability and tolerance in the assessment of thermal environments.

THE PRINCIPLES OF THE REDUCTION OF THERMAL STRAIN

Given that there are many industrial processes and situations which could lead to injury or illness resulting from cold or heat, and the potential consequences of such injuries or illnesses, the importance of prevention cannot be overemphasized. In addition to specific remarks in previous sections, the following provides general principles to form the basis of systematic plans for prevention. There are already a number of good examples of codes of practice which illustrate how preventive measures can be implemented.[50–53]

The worker

Working in particularly cold or hot environments makes many demands of the individual. The body and mind may be taken to the limits, something which is often viewed as an attraction for those who voluntarily expose themselves to thermal extremes in their leisuretime pursuits. Any condition which impairs the physiological mechanisms responsible for compensating for heat or cold stress risks the safety of the individual, and thus is contraindicated in workers exposed. Margins for such compensation generally decline with age, although experience in coping behaviourally increases with maturity, and the very young may be limited on both counts. The additional metabolic and cardiovascular demands of pregnancy make exposure to heat stress inadvisable for women during those times. Any form of concurrent illness, especially if febrile, increases risks whether the worker is exposed to heat or cold. The consumption of alcohol or drugs of abuse, even in small quantities, or of most medications, can compromise some or all of the physiological mechanisms; in the case of medication, it needs to be ascertained from recognized pharmacological authorities that the treatment in question is not likely to do this. On the other hand, general physical fitness of a cardiorespiratory or endurance nature is usually a great benefit.

If called upon to assess the fitness of an individual to undergo thermal stress, detailed knowledge of the environment, activities and clothing to be worn are essential. For those undertaking work in the cold, obesity is actually highly undesirable, as it impairs the mobility of someone required to wear already bulky protective clothing, and increases the likelihood of their being subject to heat stress when wearing that clothing. The level of physical fitness required is at least that of a person undertaking the same activity in more comfortable temperatures whilst carrying the whole protective clothing ensemble.

Sedentary work in the heat, particularly following acclimatization, is not normally too physically demanding. However, those who have to wear restrictive protective clothing or breathing apparatus and then have to perform arduous physical work need to be physically very fit. For example, in both laboratory and field studies of firemen,[54] it is more usual that their ability to carry out work is limited by physical exhaustion than by dangerous elevation of body temperature; factors of particular importance include the duration of work and the use of breathing apparatus. In the face of these demands, firemen should have good pulmonary and cardiovascular function, and significant pathology such as myocardial ischaemia or lung disease should contraindicate further exposure. Formal tests of physical fitness, such as step tests and even the measurement of maximal oxygen uptake, are only guides in the overall assessment of individuals. In all cases, the examining doctor should ask whether the person presenting for examination is capable of undertaking the specific tasks in the given environment in reasonable safety, and not whether they have achieved an arbitrary standard in an artificial test.

Good progressive training, coupled with conditioning or acclimatization, is very valuable in preparing the individual for work in stressful environs. In the case of heat, every effort should be made to allow personnel to acclimatize before they are required to carry out any exercise in the heat. Once they do start, the period for which they work should be carefully controlled according to the heat stress and strain, making due allowance for accidents and emergencies which might happen. For example, fire-fighting teams wearing breathing apparatus are limited in duration by the air supply which they carry with them; this supply should not encourage them to stay so long in the full heat of the fire that they suffer from heat illness, but at the same time it must allows for delays in withdrawing once their anticipated working time is over. The total number of teams should allow for a reasonable number of entries to be made, with adequate cooling and rest periods in between. In some cases, three teams will be needed to provide these breaks, but each team may then be limited in the number of entries that it can make. It should be borne in mind that, in these circumstances, cooling down takes longer than heating up.

In environments in which all other methods have failed, and personnel are required to work hard physically, the only solution may be to plan that they undertake only brief periods of work, interspersed with rest periods in which they may cool. Although many factors have to be taken into consideration, guideline WBGT indices above which this may be required are 29–33°C for the sedentary, 24–28°C for those working moderately hard, and 20–26°C for those performing heavy exercise. Those who have acclimatized to the heat can generally tolerate higher temperatures for longer periods (provided that they are both kept well hydrated and are able to sweat effectively), and at higher work rates increased air movement may also reduce heat stress at a given WBGT index. In extremely hot environments, such as coke ovens, it may be necessary to restrict exposure to a very short period, which must be strictly enforced.

Although there is little physiological advantage to progressive training in the cold, it is psychologically and behaviourally of great benefit. Circumstantial evidence suggests that the experienced individual develops many small but very effective techniques for minimizing their cold stress, such as an ability to don and doff clothing quickly and with minimum cooling. The naive person in a cold environment can quickly run into trouble, particularly when things start going wrong or there is an accident or emergency. On the other hand, those who have had adverse effects, such as previous cold injury or any other evidence of cold intolerance, should be prevented from further cold exposure. This includes a small number of people with conditions which predispose to local cold injury, including those with vibration white finger, any form of Raynaud's complex, impaired circulation, skin grafts, or other cold sensitivity. Similarly, those with a history of previous heat illness should only be re-exposed under careful supervision, as further episodes are likely, and anyone with a skin or neurological disorder which impairs thermally effective sweating should avoid heat stress. Such disorders include exfoliative dermatitis and anhydrotic regions following sympathectomy, with the 'rule of nines' (for assessing the percentage surface area of burns) a useful guide to the quantitative impact of local lesions.

Care also needs to be taken in considering the nature of work to be performed, with regard to the effects of its impairment. In spite of the equivocal results from experimental work discussed above, those operating plant and machinery, in particular vehicle drivers, should only ever be permitted to be exposed to very mild heat or cold stress. An extreme example of this is in aircrew, in whom even very subtle psychological impairment resulting from thermal stress may have disastrous consequences. Careful consideration should always be given to the potential role of thermal stress and its consequences in the investigation of all incidents and accidents.

Personal protective equipment

Hot or cold working environments are often those in which there are more serious thermal hazards (e.g. in the steel industry, or firefighting) or other serious threats (e.g. chemical or radioactive contamination), and personal protective equipment (PPE) is frequently required to counter the thermal and other hazards.

The use of PPE in the heat is a more serious problem, as almost all PPE adds to the heat stress. Garments which are worn necessarily increase the resistance to heat loss from the body, and may of course abolish all effective evaporative transfer; equipment which is carried increases the amount of work performed for a given task, and thus it increases the metabolic heat generated. In some cases, workers who are required to wear effective PPE to protect them from a high radiant heat load, flame and contact burns, such as firefighters, find that this PPE imposes a great heat stress on them (Fig. 15.2). Apart from the impaired performance which results, there is the real risk that workers will not use the PPE completely or correctly, in an effort to increase their comfort, and there is the constant danger that their discomfort will

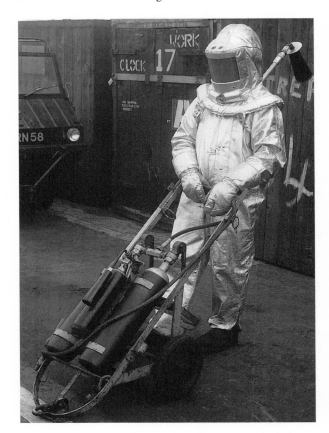

Figure 15.2 *Specialist clothing for firefighters may include metallized garments which reflect the high radiant heat load. Below the reflective surface is a thick insulative layer to minimize heat gain by the body, which forms an almost complete barrier to heat loss from the body, even when worn in cold conditions (Crown copyright).*

detract from performance in an emergency, resulting in an accident.

There are no easy solutions to these problems. Active cooling systems still require substantial chilling plants and power, and may not always work with the body; a liquid-conditioned garment, for example, may be cooled with water so cold that it induces vasoconstriction in the skin and thus slows cooling, or with tepid water which must have a very high flow rate to remove sufficient heat. Workers who need to be mobile can often only carry the cooling plant with them, which may make matters still worse. A promising approach just being introduced into some industries is the use of regional cooling, for example periodic immersion of the hands in cold water, which does not result in vasoconstriction but may lead to substantial heat loss.[55] Another useful advance is in the availability of vapour-permeable materials, such as Goretex® which can sometimes replace impermeable protective layers, yet allowing evaporative cooling to occur through them. Garments using vapour-permeable materials are becoming very popular in many circumstances, for example in affording firemen a water-impermeable and chemical-resistant layer. Consideration still needs to be given to the essential function of the garment, though, as failure to achieve that cannot be excused by the improvement of thermal comfort.

Selecting protective clothing for cold environments is also fraught with difficulty. The amount of thermal insulation provided by clothing is approximately proportional to its thickness (actually, it is more accurate to refer it to the thickness of air trapped within), so the greater the insulation, the more cumbersome the garments. As the body sweats, so water may condense within these layers, and reduce insulation. This is worst if the individual overdresses when working, leading to extensive wetting of their clothing, and then stops to rest; they may then become cold surprisingly rapidly. Workers who enter very cold environments only intermittently, such as those in cold stores, should always doff their protective clothing as soon as they return to warmer conditions, or they will quickly start to saturate the garments with sweat. Water may also mist or ice-up eye protection, causing the wearer to remove it (Fig. 15.3).

The most intractable problems in PPE for cold conditions are in protecting the hands and feet. Any form of glove reduces manual dexterity, whilst trying to work without in even cool conditions is just as deleterious to performance.[56] As temperatures fall below 0°C, gloves cannot provide sufficient insulation to keep the fingers warm, and mittens must be worn, very severely impairing work requiring tactile sensation and dexterity. Some of those working in cold conditions have additional protective requirements of their handwear, such as those preparing meat in cold rooms. Although metallic elements may be incorporated into their gloves, to reduce the risk of injury from knives and other cutting equipment, it must be remembered that metal is also an excel-

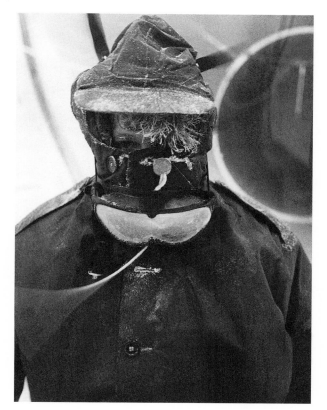

Figure 15.3 *This worker in an experimental refrigerated wind tunnel requires good facial protection, but he has had to remove his goggles because of icing (Crown copyright).*

lent conductor of heat, and will reduce the thermal protection of such clothing. The situation with regard to the protection of the feet has been reviewed by Oakley,[57] albeit in a military setting, but the same considerations are needed when choosing footwear for workers (see Fig. 15.4).

It is possible, using tables of thermal insulation and evaporative resistance for garments such as those in ISO 9920,[40] and the required values for the environment and physical activity (e.g. IREQ, the calculated clothing 'Insulation REQuired'),[58] to make provisional choices as to suitable clothing ensembles. However, careful trials and experience in use are required before firm decisions can be made, owing to the extreme complexity of the situation. For example, the efficacy of closures such as zips and cuffs may be critical in a cold environment. Although aided by national and international standards, the selection of PPE remains a difficult task, which requires detailed knowledge, possibly careful trials, and is often only a rough compromise.

Control of the environment

In an ideal world, of course, all working environments would be thermally neutral, and all the preceding material irrelevant. Whilst it is often impossible to achieve

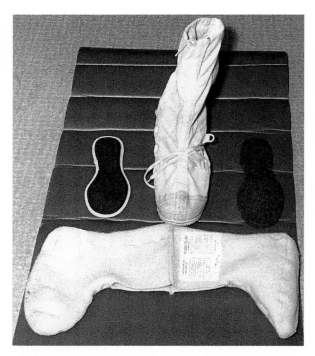

Figure 15.4 *A complete mukluk assembly, consisting of a canvas outer boot, insulative insoles, and a double felt inner boot, which has been used successfully in temperatures below −40°C (Crown copyright).*

this, most situations are capable of improvement to the extent that the untenable may become at least temporarily acceptable, or the uncomfortable become not unpleasant. A range of standards for different occupational settings has been offered by the leading national and international standards organizations.[46,58–61]

Careful application of the equation of heat balance given at the start of this chapter can be of great value. For example, if ambient air temperature and humidity cannot be controlled, then forced ventilation can increase cooling markedly; thus, in enclosed machinery spaces, a very effective way of providing 'cooling off stances' is to force-ventilate air into a number of places. Then workers can stand in a draught to cool down intermittently, and significantly extend their effective working time in the compartment. The provision of shade for those working exposed to the sun, and the wetting of surfaces and even clothing in dry heat, are other examples. However, such an approach in a cold storage facility is much more difficult to implement, as deliberately warming several areas would add greatly to the problem of refrigerating the rest. A parallel in cold environments might be to heat small shelters in a cold and windy outdoor setting, allowing workers as much time as possible within them, out of the high wind chill.

The involvement of a good heating and refrigeration engineer can also save much wasted effort. Simple physical facts, such as the rising of warmed air, can be harnessed and turned to advantage, rather than negating

what is being attempted; expert advice at the earliest stage can anticipate such problems. Indeed, the appalling environments often found in working places which have no real intrinsically severe thermal problems (modern electronic share dealing rooms, for example) usually arise because this has been neglected. For whilst heat and cold may be amongst man's oldest environmental enemies, there is a wealth of new and old technology available to control them.

REFERENCES

1 House JR, Davies N, Oakley EHN. The influence of local and deep body temperatures on skin blood flow in the human hand. *Proceedings of the Seventh International Conference on Environmental Ergonomics, Jerusalem, Israel, October 1996.*

2 Siple PA, Passell CP. Dry atmospheric cooling in sub-freezing temperatures. *Proc Am Phil Soc* 1945; **89**: 177–99.

3 International Standards Organization. ISO 9886. *Evaluation of Thermal Strain by Physiological Measurements.* Geneva: ISO, 1992.

4 Frim J, Ducharme MB. Physical properties of several infrared tympanic thermometers. *Proceedings of the Sixth International Conference on Environmental Ergonomics, Montebello, Canada, September 1994.*

5 Golden FStC, Tipton MJ. Human adaptation to repeated cold water immersions. *J Physiol (Lond)* 1988; **396**: 349–69.

6 Golden FStC, Hampton IFG, Smith DJ. Lean long distance swimmers. *J Roy Nav Med Serv* 1980; **66**: 26–30.

7 LeBlanc J. *Man in the Cold.* Springfield, Illinois: Charles C Thomas, 1975.

8 Hershkowitz M. Penile frostbite, an unforeseen hazard of jogging. *N Engl J Med* 1977; **296**: 178.

9 Andrews RP. Cold injury complicating trauma in the subfreezing environment. *Milit Med* 1987; **152**: 42–4.

10 Miller CW. Diseases of sprout pickers. *Occup Hlth Saf* 1983; **35**: 120–1.

11 Riddell DI. Is frostnip important? *J Roy Nav Med Serv* 1984; **70**: 140–2.

12 Francis TJR, Oakley EHN. Cold injury. In: Tooke JE, Lowe GDO eds. *A Textbook of Vascular Medicine.* London: Arnold, 1996; 353–70.

13 Killian H. *Cold and Frost Injuries.* Berlin: Springer-Verlag, 1981.

14 Mills WJ. Comment and recapitulation. *Alaska Med* 1993; **35**: 69–87.

15 Oakley EHN. *The Long-term Sequelae of Cold Injury Among 'The Chosin Few'.* INM Report no. 96043. Gosport, UK: Institute of Naval Medicine, 1996.

16 Blair JR, Schatzki R, Orr KD. Sequelae to cold injury in one hundred patients. Follow-up study four years after occurrence of cold injury. *JAMA* 1957; **163**: 1203–8.

17 Oakley EHN. Control of peripheral blood flow in subjects with non-freezing cold injury. In: Niimi H, Oda M, Sawada

T, R-J Xiu eds. *Progress in Microcirculation Research*. Oxford: Pergamon, 1994.

18 Haight JSJ, Keatinge WR. Failure of thermoregulation in the cold during hypoglycaemia induced by exercise and alcohol. *J Physiol (Lond)* 1973; **229**: 87–97.

19 Maclean D, Emslie-Smith D. *Accidental Hypothermia*. Oxford: Blackwell Scientific Publications, 1977.

20 Golden FStC, Hervey GR. The 'after-drop' and death after rescue from immersion in cold water. In: Adam JA ed. *Hypothermia Ashore and Afloat*. Aberdeen: Aberdeen University Press, 1981.

21 Tipton MJ. The initial response to cold-water immersion in man. *Clin Sci* 1989; **77**: 581–8.

22 Keatinge WR, Hayward MG, McIver NKI. Hypothermia during saturation diving in the North Sea. *Br Med J* 1980; **280**: 91.

23 Golden FStC, Hervey GR, Tipton MJ. Circum-rescue collapse: collapse, sometimes fatal, associated with rescue of immersion victims. *J Roy Nav Med Serv* 1991; **77**: 139–49.

24 Tipton MJ. The concept of an 'Integrated Survival System' for protection against the responses associated with immersion in cold water. *J Roy Nav Med Serv* 1993; **79**: 11–4.

25 Oakley EHN. *The Prediction of Survival During Cold Immersion: Results from the UK National Immersion Incident Survey*. INM Report no. 97011. Gosport, UK: Institute of Naval Medicine, 1997.

26 O'Neill R. Work in winter. *Occ Health Rev* 1995; Jan/Feb: 10–13.

27 Enander A. Performance and sensory aspects of work in cold environments: a review. *Ergonomics* 1984; **27**: 365–78.

28 Tanaka M, Tochihara Y, Yamazaki S, Ohnaka T, Yoshida K. Thermal reaction and manual performance during cold exposure while wearing cold-protective clothing. *Ergonomics* 1983; **26**: 141–9.

29 Rissanen S, Rintamäki H. Thermal responses and physiological strain in men wearing permeable and semipermeable protective clothing in the cold. *Ergonomics* 1997; **40**: 141–50.

30 Coleshaw SRK, van Someren RNM, Wolff AH, Davis HM, Keatinge WR. Impaired memory registration and speed of reasoning caused by low body temperature. *J Appl Physiol* 1983; **55**: 27–31.

31 International Standards Organization. ISO 8996. *Ergonomics – Determination of Metabolic Heat Production*. Geneva: ISO, 1990.

32 International Standards Organization. ISO 7243. *Hot Environments – Estimation of the Heat Stress on Working Man, Based on the WBGT-index (Wet Bulb Globe Temperature)*. Geneva: ISO, 1990.

33 Nunnely SA, Stribley RF. Fighter index of thermal stress (FITS): guidance for hot-weather aircraft operations. *Aviat Space Environ Med* 1979; **50**: 639–42.

34 Parsons KC. International heat stress standards: a review. *Ergonomics* 1995; **38**: 6–22.

35 International Standards Organization. ISO 11399. *Ergonomics of the Thermal Environment – Principles and Application of the Relevant International Standards*. Geneva: ISO, 1995.

36 International Standards Organization. ISO 7933. *Hot Environments – Analytical Determination and Interpretation of Thermal Stress Using Calculation of Required Sweat Rate*. Geneva: ISO, 1989.

37 Peters H. Testing climate indices in the field. *Ergonomics* 1995; **38**: 86–100.

38 Mairiaux P, Malchaire J. Comparison and validation of heat stress indices in experimental studies. *Ergonomics* 1995; **38**: 58–72.

39 International Standards Organization. ISO 7730. *Moderate Thermal Environments – Determination of the PMV and PPD Indices and Specification of the Conditions for Thermal Comfort*. Geneva: ISO, 1994.

40 International Standards Organization. ISO 9920. *Ergonomics of the Thermal Environment – Estimation of the Thermal Insulation and Evaporative Resistance of a Clothing Ensemble*. Geneva: ISO, 1995.

41 Clark RP, Edholm OG. *Man and his Thermal Environment*. London: Edward Arnold, 1985.

42 Oakley EHN. Heat exhaustion. *J Wld Accident Emerg Disast Med* 1987; **3**: 28–30.

43 Khogali M, Hales JRS (eds) *Heat Stroke and Temperature Regulation*. Sydney: Academic Press, 1983.

44 Ramsey JD. Task performance in heat: a review. *Ergonomics* 1995; **38**: 154–65.

45 National Institute of Occupational Safety and Health. *Criteria for a Recommended Standard – Occupational Exposure to Hot Environments*. HSM 72–10269. Washington DC: NIOSH, 1972.

46 National Institute of Occupational Safety and Health. *Criteria for a Recommended Standard – Occupational Exposure to Hot Environments. Revised Criteria 1986*. DDHS (NIOSH) 86–113. Washington DC: NIOSH, 1986.

47 Holland RL, Sayers JA, Keatinge WR, Davis HM, Peswani R. Effects of raised body temperature on reasoning, memory and mood. *J Appl Physiol* 1985; **59**: 1823–7.

48 Wyon DP, Wyon I, Norin F. Effects of moderate heat stress on driver vigilance in a moving vehicle. *Ergonomics* 1996; **39**: 61–75.

49 International Standards Organization. ISO 10551. *Ergonomics of the Thermal Environment – Assessment of the Influence of the Thermal Environment Using Subjective Judgement Scales*. Geneva: ISO, 1995.

50 Refrigerated Food Industry Confederation. *Guidance on Work in Cold Indoor Environments*. Bracknell, Berks: RFIC, undated.

51 British Standards Institution. *Draft British Standard: Ergonomics of the Thermal Environment – Code of Practice for the Design and Evaluation of Working Practices for Cold Indoor Environments*. London: BSI, 1996.

52 Griefahn B. *Arbeit in mässiger Kälte*. Report no. Fb 716. Dortmund, Germany: Bundesanstalt für Arbeitsschutz, 1995.

53 Malchaire J, Mairiaux P. Strategy of analysis and interpretation of thermal working conditions. *Ann Occup Hyg* 1991; **35**: 261–72.

54 Smith DL, Petruzzello SJ, Kramer JM, Misner JE. The effects of different thermal environments on the physiological and psychological responses of firefighters to a training drill. *Ergonomics* 1997; **40**: 500–10.

55 Allsopp AJ, Poole KA. The effect of hand immersion on body temperature when wearing impermeable clothing. *J Roy Nav Med Serv* 1991; **77**: 51–7.

56 Provins KA, Clarke RSJ. The effect of cold on manual performance. *J Occup Med* 1960; **2**: 169–76.

57 Oakley EHN. The design and function of military footwear: a review following experiences in the South Atlantic. *Ergonomics* 1984; **27**: 631–7.

58 International Standards Organization. ISO TR 11079.

Evaluation of Cold Environments – Determination of Required Clothing Insulation (IREQ). Geneva: ISO, 1993.

59 American Society of Heating, Refrigerating, and Air-Conditioning Engineers/American National Standards Institute. *ASHRAE/ANSI. Standard 55–81: Thermal Environmental Conditions for Human Occupancy*. Atlanta: ASHRAE/ANSI, 1981.

60 American Society of Heating, Refrigerating, and Air-Conditioning Engineers . *Standard 62–1989: Ventilation for Acceptable Indoor Air Quality*. Atlanta: ASHRAE, 1989.

61 COST. *Indoor Air Quality and its Impact on Man*. Brussels: Commission of European Community, Working Group 6: Ventilation Requirements, 1990.

16

Raised barometric pressure

DAVID H ELLIOTT

Diving procedures	343	Ear and skin infections in saturation diving	349
Basic physics and applied physiology	344	The decompression illnesses	350
Compression barotrauma	347	Long-term effects	356
Unconsciousness in the water	348	Fitness for diving	358
Medical emergencies in deep diving	349	References	358

Increased barometric pressure is a unique physiological parameter and one which affects all those who have to work in it. Barometric pressure is transmitted throughout the body just as it is through a fluid. Many of the effects of increased pressure are immediate but only transient, though a few of their consequences may be long-lasting. The immediate effects tend to include those that affect safety at work. The permanent effects of pressure exposure, which include the sequelae of pressure-related accidents, may affect the long-term health of the individual worker, but not necessarily his safety.

The increases of barometric pressure which have been experienced by man have been as great as 701 m (7000 kPa), some 70 times the normal barometric pressure present at the earth's surface.

The persons exposed to the effects of raised barometric pressure represent many different occupations. The first, historically, were the breath-hold divers who, through the centuries, have dived for sponges, shellfish and salvage. This type of diving is still a commercial activity in many parts of the world.

The simple diving bell is also centuries old and allowed a stay at depth of brief duration. This was extended in the seventeenth century by taking barrels of fresh air to the bell.[1] The invention of the force-pump by Smeaton in 1788[2] had the potential of extending this duration almost indefinitely. Since then the compressed-air worker (tunnel worker, caisson-worker or sand-hog), has been employed in building tunnels and bridges world wide where pressure is needed to keep out the water. The compressed-air worker usually has shifts of 4–8 hours at relatively shallow depths in a dry environment.[3] The occupational illnesses of this group of workers differ only little from those of divers. Another group

who work in a dry environment at raised barometric pressure are the medical and technical staff of hyperbaric units which are to be found in many hospitals for the treatment of problem wounds and other clinical conditions. Their exposure is to relatively low pressures and so, with the compressed-air workers, their occupational health hazards, though fewer, may be considered together with those of the divers.

DIVING PROCEDURES

Divers form the largest group of persons occupationally at risk from exposure to the hyperbaric environment. There are many types of diving and some understanding of this is needed in order to reach valid conclusions in the management of diving accidents. Although the diver's work is carried out in the water, they also spend time at raised pressure in a dry environment. A major difference between the 'wet' and the 'dry' exposures to pressure is the presence in water of a vertical hydrostatic pressure gradient over the height of the diver's body. Though this has a number of important consequences such as upon the physiology of breathing and the design of underwater breathing apparatus, there are no specific medical sequelae associated with this phenomenon.

The majority of divers use compressed air for breathing. This may be supplied to them by a hose from the surface or from bottles of compressed air which they carry (self-contained breathing apparatus: scuba). The gas must be made available on inspiration at the same pressure as that exerted by the depth of water around them. There are a number of devices which can achieve this, but some of them may provide additional hazards to the diver. Because of the narcotic consequences of raised partial pressures of nitrogen, the use of compressed air diving should be limited in depth. For professional divers in the North Sea this has been set at 50 m (600 kPa) though slightly deeper limits have been set in other parts of the world.

Beyond 50 m the divers breathe a mixed gas, usually oxy-helium which has no significant narcotic effect but which is expensive. Other gases may be substituted for helium or may be added to this mix. All diving at these depths is tethered, the diver being supplied by hose because he is unable to carry sufficient gas to meet his volumetric needs for a reasonable duration at these greater pressures. Some divers may use a semi-closed circuit or closed-circuit breathing apparatus at these depths but because this equipment is more complex, there is a greater risk of failure.

Other types of breathing equipment and dive procedures are needed for specific purposes. Examples include the use of closed-circuit oxygen apparatus in waters less than 8 m and of oxygen enriched oxy-nitrogen mixtures in semi-closed breathing apparatus to 50 m or so, for military purposes. With CO_2 being constantly scrubbed from the breathing circuit, such apparatus can present special hazards such as an insidious hypoxia if the flow rate becomes too low. Oxygen-rich oxy-nitrogen mixtures are also used when hose or scuba diving in shallow depths by some to reduce nitrogen uptake.

Most dives are made from the surface and, on completion of the task, the diver returns to the surface. In order to assist the safe elimination of respiratory gases which have become dissolved in his body during the dive, the diver may have to return to the surface by following a predetermined slow ascent. The selected decompression profile may require the diver to change respiratory gas mixtures during decompression. For compressed-air workers and divers, a technique known as 'surface decompression' or 'decanting' may be adopted, the individual returning rapidly to the surface in order to be repressurized and complete the process of dissolved gas elimination in the relative warmth and safety of a compression chamber. Whatever decompression procedure is used, the air divers and compressed-air workers can spend a significant portion of every working day in decompression.

Where much work is required on one location the technique of 'saturation diving' may be adopted. Though not the only method, this is the usual technique for diving to depths deeper than 50 m and is also used at shallower depths because more time can be spent at work and less in decompression. The diver and his colleagues live at raised environmental pressure in a compression chamber situated at the surface. Two (or, in some bells, three) men will begin a 'bell-run' by transferring into a diving bell which has been mated on to their living chamber at the same raised pressure. The connecting

doors are closed and the bell and its occupants are lowered to the working depth. The bell is small and crammed with controls and equipment. After equalization, the divers open the bell door in order to emerge and perform their in-water tasks. This may require them to make an excursion slightly deeper than their storage or living depth, to a depth known as the 'excursion depth'. A common routine is for one diver to work in the water for some 4 hours and then change places with the second diver who has remained in the bell as the 'standby diver' during this time. On completion of the work period, up to 8 hours normally, the lower door of the bell is closed and it is hoisted to the surface so that the divers can transfer under pressure back into their living chamber. Thus three shifts of saturation divers may be employed to work around the clock. On completion of their project, or after some 3 weeks, the entire team will commence their return to the surface at some 30 m per day, possibly having been replaced already by a new team of divers recently compressed to continue working from the same living depth.

Procedures are available for the many possible in-water emergencies such as impairment of consciousness, trauma and blow-up while other emergencies are associated with deep saturation diving. For each of these the diving team should have on call a diving medical specialist with a detailed knowledge of topics outlined below.

BASIC PHYSICS AND APPLIED PHYSIOLOGY

Some knowledge of the natural laws which relate to the hyperbaric environment is needed in order to understand the pathogenesis and management of the occupational illnesses of divers and compressed-air workers. A full account of the relevant aspects of environmental physiology is available elsewhere,[4,5] particularly for those who have a direct responsibility for the medical support of commercial diving or tunnelling activities but, for those who may be concerned with the sick diver or compressed-air worker only when after return to normal barometric pressure at the surface, a summary can suffice.

Gas pressure and volume

The ideal gas law is:

$$PV = nRT$$

where P is the absolute pressure, V is the volume of gas, n is the number of moles of gas, R is the universal gas constant and T is the absolute temperature. In other words, Boyle's law states that the volume of a given mass of gas is inversely proportional to the pressure. Thus 1 litre of gas at sea level (100 kPa) decreases to 0.25 litres at

30 m (400 kPa). Of equal importance to the pathogenesis of the dysbaric illnesses is the converse of this, that 1 litre of compressed gas at 30 m (400 kPa) will expand on ascent to 4 litres at the surface. An application of another gas law (Charles' law) explains the associated rise of temperature when a gas is being compressed and the 'misting' of chamber atmosphere in the coolness of decompression.

Partial pressures

The application of Dalton's law, that the partial pressure of a gas in a mixture is equal to the product of its fractional concentration and the absolute pressure, has a special importance in the hyperbaric environment. Thus at 50 m (600 kPa) the partial pressure of oxygen in compressed air is 126 kPa which is equivalent to breathing a hypothetical 126% oxygen at the surface.

Gas solubility and uptake

The amount of a gas which dissolves in a particular liquid with which it is in contact is, in accordance with Henry's law, proportional at constant temperature to the partial pressure of that gas. Some gases are more soluble than others and their solubilities in the watery and the fatty tissues of the body are not the same. Also, the uptake of the inert components of the respiratory gases into solution in the body depends upon the characteristics of the circulation during the transient dynamic phase until the steady state of tissue gas equilibrium ('saturation') has been achieved.

Oxygen effects

The well known toxic effects of oxygen on the lungs[6] and the central nervous system[7] are especially important in the hyperbaric environment where not only is partial pressure of oxygen in the air increased by descent, but also when pure oxygen and oxygen-enriched mixtures are used as a respiratory gas. The biochemical mechanisms of oxygen toxicity and its effects upon other organ systems are reviewed elsewhere.[8] For practical purposes the important aspects are those of recognition and prevention. Most compressed-air workers are exposed to such moderate pressures that oxygen toxicity does not usually occur.

Lack of oxygen is a particular hazard of some types of diving in which errors can be made in the content of the respiratory gas supplied to the diver or when there is a failure of complex breathing apparatus.

PULMONARY TOXICITY

The effects of oxygen upon the lung are relatively slow in onset. Though there is much individual variation it is generally considered that, below a partial pressure threshold of 50 kPa, oxygen effects will not occur. At greater partial pressures oxygen will progressively cause damage. A method of calculating a cumulative dose of oxygen to the lungs (Unit Pulmonary Toxic Dose: UPTD) is available as a guide to limiting the oxygen exposure occurring with changes of gas mixtures and changing depths,[9] but it is no substitute for clinical vigilance. The use of intermittent oxygen delivery in which, for example, 20 minutes of oxygen breathing is followed by a 5-minute interlude breathing compressed air before returning to oxygen, is known to delay the onset of pulmonary symptoms.

The onset of tracheal irritation and a dry cough are among the first manifestations of impending pulmonary oxygen poisoning, but similar symptoms can arise just from breathing a dry gas. Measurement of vital capacity will demonstrate a progressive impairment of pulmonary function with continued oxygen exposure. Though reversible at first, if lung impairment is severe, the effects can persist for months, or fatal pulmonary oedema may occur. In fact, awareness of the hazard has led to routine diving procedures which avoid this risk.

Pulmonary oxygen toxicity is likely to arise only when elevated partial pressures are used intentionally as in the treatment of divers and others for decompression sickness and other conditions. Treatment of pulmonary oxygen toxicity is to remove the cause by reducing the inspired gas partial pressure of oxygen to less than 50 kPa but, rarely, severe cases leading to pulmonary oedema may also require supportive treatment such as positive-pressure respiration.

NEUROTOXICITY

The partial pressure threshold for the neurological effects of oxygen is in excess of 150 kPa, but this form of oxygen toxicity is relatively quick in onset. Thus it is another diving hazard which usually can be avoided. Nitrogen narcosis, heavy exercise and carbon dioxide build-up are considered to be synergistic with oxygen in causing this toxicity. However, enriched oxygen mixtures make an important contribution in diving to improved decompression performance, provided that also they are used well within the threshold of pulmonary toxicity.

Though a number of prodromal symptoms have been reported,[10] the classic presentation is that of a sudden epileptiform convulsion. If this occurs in the water, the aqueous environment may contribute to a fatal outcome. It also occurs in the dry environment although, when at rest, most patients undergoing hyperbaric treatment can tolerate 280 kPa oxygen given intermittently for an hour or two. The treatment for an epileptiform attack is to remove the oxygen stimulus and provide conventional support to the fitting individual. Other than some amnesia, no permanent effects should occur.

HYPOXIA

With persons breathing compressed air, hypoxia should not be a hazard. A hazard arises when divers are required to breathe a gas mixture which is meant to be in the partial pressure range 20–150 kPa and either the wrong oxygen percentage is provided, or the oxygen make-up system of a closed-circuit or semi-closed-circuit breathing apparatus fails. With a scrubber in the circuit, as there is no concurrent accumulation of carbon dioxide then, unlike hypoxia from most other causes, its onset may not be noticed by the subject who gently passes through unconsciousness towards an anoxic death.

Carbon dioxide effects

Hyperventilation may be intentional, for the purposes of inducing hypocapnia to prolong breath-hold duration, or unintentional, in association with near panic. The latter is likely to be concurrent with other factors contributing towards a perceived in-water emergency and may contribute to an unfavourable outcome.

Hypercapnia may be due to extrinsic causes such as the failure of carbon dioxide scrubbing in closed-circuit breathing apparatus or intrinsic causes. Hypercapnia alone can account for dyspnoea and headaches, even fits and unconsciousness but it is perhaps more significant as just one of several synergistic factors in cases of unexpected loss of consciousness underwater. It has been established that, using the Read test, a proportion of experienced divers can be identified as 'carbon dioxide retainers'.[11] While this might be seen as an adaptive phenomenon, the failure of these divers to respond normally to raised carbon dioxide levels of intrinsic origin is considered to contribute towards the likelihood of an episode of underwater unconsciousness, particularly during hard physical exercise.[12] A raised partial pressure of oxygen and, if diving deeply on air, nitrogen narcosis are thought to be contributory. Because of individual variation and the lack of a recommended threshold response, it is unlikely that a test of CO_2 sensitivity would be a suitable routine screening examination for commercial divers.

Nitrogen narcosis

At increased partial pressures nitrogen behaves as a narcotic agent, the mechanism of its action being analogous to that of the volatile anaesthetics. Euphoric irresponsibility is not compatible with the safe use of complex procedures and equipment and for this reason commercial compressed-air diving is limited, in the North Sea, to 50 m. In other places slightly deeper limits may be in force but, in general, at deeper depths than this, nitrogen is replaced by helium as the necessary oxygen diluent. Compressed air in the past has been used successfully by experienced divers to 90 m but, much beyond that, there is the probability of narcosis leading to unconsciousness. Helium has no significant narcotic properties at depths down to around 700 m.

High-pressure neurological syndrome (HPNS)

A number of neurological manifestations become evident during compressions to depths beyond 200 m.[13] That similar effects develop in mice breathing oxygenated fluorocarbon oil, a non-absorbable fluid, suggests that these phenomena are not a form of helium narcosis but are a direct consequence of elevated hydrostatic pressure upon the cell, thus affecting neuromuscular transmission.

The most obvious manifestations are those of tremor, nausea and vomiting to the extent that these may impair the diver's ability to go to work safely for the next 12–24 hours. More subtle evidence of HPNS includes changes to the electroencephalogram (EEG) with increased theta and diminished alpha activity. Though epileptiform fits have occurred in animals at great depths it is considered that man at 700 m is still safely within the depth limits. The effects of HPNS are depth-related and improvement begins during the stay at depth and also on decompression.

The effects of HPNS can be ameliorated by the use of slow-staged compression rates, which have been developed in the light of experience, and by the addition of a narcotic agent, such as 5% nitrogen, to the breathing mixture[13] though this is not used for operational reasons.

Decompression theory

At the end of a period of time exposed to raised environmental pressure the diver or compressed-air worker must return to normal atmospheric pressure at the surface. To do so safely requires him to follow procedures designed to prevent the onset of a decompression illness.

While at pressure, his respiratory gases were being dissolved in the blood and tissues and would continue to do so until equilibrium were achieved (saturation). The body comprises a spectrum of fast and slow tissues and, for practical purposes, saturation occurs in them in just a few minutes or up to some 12 hours. Thus, in the majority of compressed-air divers, the process of tissue gas uptake is still in progress in many parts of the body at the time that decompression begins. When the diver or compressed air worker leaves maximum pressure, he may not have been there long enough to absorb sufficient gas to be at clinical risk of significant bubble formation, and thus he can make a direct ascent safely from what is termed a 'no-stop dive'. Beyond some threshold of depth and duration, a direct ascent is no longer safe. For instance, an indefinitely long dive could be made to just less than 10 m by many individuals, but only 20 minutes or so of exposure pressure is considered safe at 30 m depth. Beyond these 'no-stop' limits a slow ascent, usually by means of prescribed 'stops' at progressively shallower depths, is required. Many versions of these diving tables are available and most are derived from mathematical models based upon theoretical principles and modified by experience.[14,15] Some categories of working divers carry personal computers during the dive which, based upon input from a pressure transducer, use similar models to provide an on-line display of the specific calculated decompression profile.

The mathematical models are of many varieties and most can predict quite well provided that the prediction is made for a large population of divers. However, they are less accurate at predicting the decompression performance of an individual on any particular occasion. There are many factors that can contribute to what seems to be more than simple biological variation. Among the factors influencing the potential safety of a particular decompression will be whether or not there has been any degree of pulmonary barotrauma causing small bubbles of alveolar gas to enter the arterial circulation.

Venous gas emboli may form from dissolved gases during or after an ascent and are detectable by Doppler but without causing any symptoms. Normally these pass to the lungs where the gas is excreted but, if a right-to-left shunt exists, these bubbles may pass across to the arterial circulation and cause adverse effects.

Another factor is the degree of adaptation to regular decompressions which may develop in compressed-air workers[15] and divers, seemingly permitting them to take short cuts in their obligated decompression with impunity, but this 'acclimatization' is quickly lost during a break from work after which resumption of the same pattern of diving may no longer be associated with immunity from decompression problems. Laboratory studies suggest that a high level of C5a complement may be associated with a greater degree of susceptibility.[16] Other factors known to predispose an individual to decompression sickness include hangovers and dehydration, recent injury and, probably by influencing tissue gas uptake or elimination, heavy physical exercise at depth and cold exposure during decompression.

Thus the theoretical basis for calculating safe decompression procedures is subject to these and many other influences to the extent that, while a small number of decompression incidents may be regarded as unavoidable, the general success of the published diving tables can be considered a remarkable achievement.

However, one must remember that the apparent success of a particular table is based upon knowing the number of cases of decompression sickness that arise from it in relation to the total number of similar dives that are incident-free. Too often these data are not readily available and, when they are, they may not tell the whole story. There are often no objective criteria to confirm the diagnosis of decompression sickness and the individuals naturally vary in their threshold for reporting symptoms, just as their associates vary in their recording of such data. Because of the wide variety of dives undertaken by most divers it is not easy to assess the relative efficacy of different diving tables but, because of the greater consistency of pressure exposures in tunnelling, some useful information about the effectiveness of decompression procedures has been derived from studies of the bends and bone necrosis rates of compressed-air workers.[17]

COMPRESSION BAROTRAUMA

During descent, the reduction in volume of gas contained in the body needs to be compensated by the addition of an appropriate supplementary volume of compressed gas. Thus the respiratory gases must have easy access to compensate the gas-filled spaces of the sinuses and middle ear, otherwise the diminishing volumes of their gas may have to be replaced, for instance by a serosanguinous transudate.

'Reversed ear'

The external auditory meatus does not usually suffer barotrauma because, whether underwater or in the dry, it communicates directly with its surrounding environment. Rarely, due to wax, an ear-plug or the use of a tight-fitting hood during the dive, this equalization does not occur and the external meatus and tympanic membrane are subjected to a potential negative pressure relative to the middle ear. Sanguinous blisters occur in the skin of the canal and drum and, rarely, the drum may rupture outwards.

Middle ear barotrauma

The diver and compressed-air worker is fully aware of the need to 'clear his ears' right from the first moments of leaving surface if he is to 'stay ahead of the pressure'. He cannot always do so and the eustachian tube can lock in a closed position as shallow as 1 m, after which no Toynbee or Frenzel manoeuvre can be successful. The subject must then ascend to a shallower depth and, once he restores patency, try again to descend.

Persistence in making a descent without frequent equalization of the middle ear leads to middle ear barotrauma, characterized by pain in the affected ear, possibly radiating down the neck. Sudden relief of this pain may be due to tympanic rupture in which case there is a risk to a diver of immediate vertigo due to the entry of cold water into the middle ear.

Several categories of middle ear barotrauma are

described based upon otoscopic appearance, but the use of mild, moderate and severe is adequate. A mild barotrauma is no more than injection of the vessels of the drum perhaps with some apparent foreshortening of the handle of the malleus due to retraction of the drum. Moderate is a greater degree of injection with some evidence of serosanguinous transudate beyond the drum. Severe is rupture of the tympanic membrane.

Treatment is conservative with prophylactic antibiotics if there is fluid in the middle ear or if the drum is ruptured. Allowing some 6 weeks for healing of the drum, diving should not be resumed until there is full functional recovery.

The use of oral decongestants may seem to prevent the condition but after a day or two nasal sprays, because of a rebound phenomenon, may aggravate the difficulties of pressure equalization.

Alternobaric vertigo

A sudden sensation of disorientation or spinning during a dive, most often at the beginning of the ascent, is considered to be due to inequality of equalization of pressure between right and left middle ears. This phenomenon has been described also on blowing the nose after surfacing. It is transient. History and examination suggest middle ear barotrauma and no specific treatment is required.

Inner ear barotrauma

Forced Valsalva manoeuvres because of difficulty in clearing the ears during descent can lead to oval or round window rupture and fistula. The mechanism may be explosive, due to the transmission of raised cerebrospinal fluid pressure through the perilymph. The presentation may be a persistent vertigo and total or some degree of sensorineural hearing loss. If the leakage of fluid from the inner ear is slow, deafness may not be noticed until waking the morning after a dive. A high resolution computed tomography (CT) scan may reveal gas in the inner ear near the footplate.

An immediate operative repair is the treatment of choice though some patients respond to absolute bed rest, with the head kept up, for 3–5 days.

Sinuses, eyes, skin and teeth

Sinus pain during descent is usually sufficiently painful for the compression to be discontinued. No specific treatment is required other than to avoid compression until natural equalization is again possible.

Failure of a diver to add extra gas via his nose to his face mask during descent may cause a relatively negative pressure over his eyes resulting in conjunctival oedema and haemorrhage. A failure to add extra gas from a cylinder to a diver's dry suit will lead to a reduction of the contained volume of gas within the suit and severe pinching of the skin. No treatment is required.

A small gas-containing cavity in a tooth can also cause sharp pain on descent. The dive should be aborted and dental treatment sought. Teeth fillings have exploded during ascent.

Lungs

Compression barotrauma of the lungs is a hazard virtually confined to the use of the standard helmet diving dress which is no longer in use in the UK but still used commercially in other parts of the world.

The accident arises because it is necessary to pump down to the diver compressed air at the pressure of the depth at which he is working. Should the diver accidentally fall into deeper water, his attendants at the surface may fail to increase the supply pressure of the compressed air. Under these circumstances all the gas contained in his helmet and respiratory tract will be reduced in volume in accordance with Boyle's law. While some 'squeeze' can be compensated by an increase in pulmonary blood volume, in extreme cases divers have been killed by the crushing injury to the chest.

UNCONSCIOUSNESS IN THE WATER

A compressed-air worker may suffer a loss of consciousness while at raised pressure, but this is likely to be coincidental and the dry environment contributes little to the incident. A diver too may suffer a coincidental illness which leads to unconsciousness but, when underwater, there are other causes and consequences to be considered.

Unconsciousness occurring with the mouthpiece still in place may be due to the supply of a hypoxic breathing gas, nitrogen narcosis if at great depth, an oxygen fit, electric shock, cerebral gas embolism during ascent, 'shallow-water blackout', 'deep-water blackout' or a coincidental illness such as myocardial infarction.

Shallow-water blackout is a term that should be confined to otherwise unexplained unconsciousness associated with the use of closed circuit oxygen. Together with the effects of carbon dioxide build-up, whether associated with hard physical work or with the use of a soda-lime carbon dioxide scrubber, the cerebrovascular effects of increased oxygen tension are considered to lower the diver's syncope threshold. Similar effects may occur with semi-closed and other types of breathing apparatus but not with the use of open-circuit with oxy-helium or, in the customary ranges of depth, with compressed air.

In contrast, the term *deep-water blackout* is applied to otherwise unexplained unconsciousness occurring in compressed-air divers below some 60 m. Other than an additional contribution made by nitrogen narcosis, the precipitating causes may be the same as occur with pure oxygen at very shallow depths. The inspired oxygen tension on compressed air at 70 m is close to that of pure oxygen at the maximum depth usually permitted for military use (8 m, PO_2 180 kPa). While there is no question of CO_2 build-up due to scrubber inadequacies, the majority of these cases have been associated with hard physical work where the density of air is increased eightfold or more. Another contributory factor may be the fact that a small number of regular air divers can be identified as 'carbon dioxide retainers', showing a diminished ventilatory response to intrinsic or extrinsic carbon dioxide.

Rarely the use of closed-circuit breathing apparatus, at any depth, leads to a loss of consciousness due to hypoxia which, if not corrected quickly, will progress to death. This occurs if the oxygen supply becomes exhausted or fails, when the subsequent hypoxia will not be associated with a carbon dioxide build-up as it is in most dyspnoeic situations. This is because the carbon dioxide scrubber in the circuit removes any build-up of the CO_2 that might otherwise alert the diver. Without this warning the diver dies of a 'silent hypoxia'. In some apparatus the diver has the safeguard of checking the display from a PO_2 sensor.

A diver found unconscious but without a mouthpiece in place may have lost it due to panic as a result of entanglement or other perceived crisis, or it may be secondary to any one of the other causes above.

Cold exposure may be a contributory factor in any underwater accident but clinical hypothermia is not likely to be the sole cause of unconsciousness in a diver whose body should be thermally protected and whose duration of exposure to cold is usually quite brief.

Some other conditions may contribute to loss of consciousness underwater but may also cause injury without any loss of consciousness. One example is an underwater blast injury and while this may be thought of in a military context, the illegal use of dynamite for fishing has killed or injured diving marine scientists.

In certain parts of the world the possibility of a marine animal injury must also be considered. The sting of a box jellyfish is so painful that death by drowning can occur almost immediately. Quickly lethal but less obvious causes of unconsciousness are the toxins of sea snakes and cone shells. There is no experience of these in European waters and treatment is well described elsewhere.[18]

Treatment of the unconscious diver

Recovery of the unconscious diver from the water can be difficult. The treatment of near-drowning should follow standard clinical management procedures well described elsewhere. Consideration must also be given to the secondary onset of hypothermia, particularly after the uncon-

scious diver has been recovered from the water. Of greater urgency may be the need to treat the diver either prophylactically, because of omitted decompression stops, or for the onset of acute decompression illness. This may be of greater clinical significance than the original incident.

MEDICAL EMERGENCIES IN DEEP DIVING

Though the records from the North Sea show that deep diving is less hazardous than air diving, there are a number of occupational hazards specific to bell diving that require skilled technical rescue and may require medical intervention. Contingency planning is essential and occupational health service responsibilities include first aid training of divers and the provision of medical advice during the management of diving emergencies.

If a diver is unconscious in the water the standby diver has the task of recovering him into the diving bell, a cramped space where conventional resuscitation approaches the impossible. In the event of a seriously injured diver being transferred back to the deck chamber or if a serious coincidental illness occurs at depth, many conventional emergency and anaesthetic techniques are incompatible with the safety constraints of a closed compartment at raised pressure.

Should a diving bell become parted from the surface accidentally, it will be carrying only a limited supply of breathing gas and supplementary heat and there is a risk that the trapped divers may become hypoxic or, in spite of passive thermal protection and respiratory heat exchangers, hypothermic before rescue.

Medical advice may be sought during these and other unique diving emergencies. Practical action is to hold an immediate telephone conference with doctors experienced in the management at one or more of the diving treatment centres around the world. The immediate care of a sick or injured diver depends on his diving colleagues who are trained in first aid. This is because, even after a doctor arrives, compression time cannot be foreshortened without exacerbating the manifestations of HPNS which would diminish professional capabilities at the saturation depth. A surgeon and anaesthetist, if needed, should preferably be drawn from a pool of specialists with some previous experience of the effects of raised barometric pressure and the limitations that this imposes upon conventional techniques of treatment as well as upon communications.

EAR AND SKIN INFECTIONS IN SATURATION DIVING

The warm and humid living conditions of the chamber complex facilitate bacterial growth, particularly that of *Pseudomonas* species (usually *Ps. pyocynea*). Otitis externa is a debilitating condition but can largely be prevented by meticulous hygiene. Daily cleansing of the chamber interior is required, using antiseptics that are not toxic to the humans within its confined space. Each diver needs to be witnessed undertaking his aural toilet twice daily and again after each wet dive. The most common procedure is to fill each external ear canal in turn with a modified Burrow's solution for one full minute in order to restore and maintain the normal acid pH of the external ear canal. Swabs should be taken from the ears and other sites prior to and during the dive and thus the sensitivities of the bacteria will be known should treatment be necessary. The skin is also susceptible to infection, especially where it may have been damaged by chafing or perhaps due to minor scalds from the hot water supplied to the diver's suit for keeping him warm at depth. The lesions are usually mild but unresponsive to treatment.

THE DECOMPRESSION ILLNESSES

Any return from raised to normal atmospheric pressure may be associated with the development of clinical manifestations, some of which can be serious. There are two principal types of decompression illness. The first is from the expansion of gas in accordance with Boyle's law in the gas-containing spaces of the body and the second is due to the evolution of bubbles in the body from the gases which have become dissolved in the tissues during the stay at raised environmental pressure. Pulmonary barotrauma can come from any dive whereas decompression sickness requires a sufficient stay at depth for significant gas uptake. These two mechanisms can lead to clinical manifestations some of which are unique to one or the other of the two pathogenetic processes and to other manifestations, neurological in particular, that could be the end point of either pathological process. The pathogenesis of these illnesses is described fully elsewhere[19,20] and need be only outlined here. Because the immediate management of both conditions is so similar, the following description is based upon the clinical presentations rather than on the presumed underlying pathology. A previous classification, introduced by those concerned with decompression sickness among compressed-air workers, has been into type 1 decompression sickness ('mild') and type 2 decompression sickness ('serious').[21] A similar distinction was made in the treatment protocols published in the navy diving manuals. The attraction of such an approach is that the majority of cases must be treated immediately and without the presence of a medical officer, but even a simple algorithm is not foolproof. With the severe pain of a mild (type 1) manifestation the concurrent presence of a small neurological deficit may be overlooked, but this would make the case a serious type 2 illness. Indeed,

Rivera[22] reported that some 30% of persons with joint pain overlook a more serious manifestation. Unless this is spotted, the patient may then receive treatment for only the more minor condition, the limb pain, a circumstance which predisposes to neurological complications later.

The diagnosis and classification of the acute conditions which arise from decompression are often dependent upon a circumstantial guess concerning the underlying pathological mechanism, barotrauma or dissolved gas. A wrong diagnosis creates the potential for an inappropriate management and has led to a nomenclature which does not presume that the pathological pathways have been revealed at the time of presentation. The justification for this classification,[23] which is descriptive in nature, seems enhanced by a study which revealed the inability of some 50 doctors experienced in the decompression illnesses to make consistent diagnoses.[24] Adoption of a more logical classification in clinical practice might also provide a more accurate basis for therapeutic trials and for the epidemiological analysis of cases.

The traditional terminology (pulmonary barotrauma, gas embolism, decompression sickness) remains valid for discussion of the underlying pathology.

Pathogenesis

Pulmonary barotrauma occurs due to the expansion of gas retained in the lungs. This may be due to the failure of the diver to exhale adequately during the ascent, a potential problem that should be eliminated by appropriate training. Gas may be retained because of pulmonary disease. Thus divers with a 'chest cold' should stay out of the water. A good medical history, examination and chest x-ray can eliminate many causes of potential barotrauma. Pulmonary function tests are not sufficiently predictive and barotrauma can occur in those who exhale correctly and who are passed as medically fit. The condition is often associated with a rapid ascent to the surface and this suggests that dynamic airway collapse may occur[25] when the pressure differentials from alveolus to airway are large. The expansion of retained gas increases at an exponential rate during ascent and the greatest volume changes occur close to the surface. Thus the introduction of an arbitrary 'stop' at some 5 m for scuba divers is thought to have reduced the likelihood of barotrauma due to rapid ascent by making them improve buoyancy control during ascent in order to achieve this 'stop'. However, not much overpressure is needed and manifestations requiring treatment have followed as ascent from as shallow as 1 m.

The expanding alveolus can rupture its gas into the pleural cavity causing a pneumothorax which may be bilateral. The gas may track to the mediastinum and both pericardial and perirenal gas have been detected.

The gas may pass into the pulmonary veins and its subsequent embolic distribution usually includes the carotid and vertebrobasilar arteries.

The pathogenesis of 'classic' decompression sickness is quite different. The uptake at raised environmental pressure of the respiratory gases into the blood and tissues will continue until equilibrium (or saturation) is achieved. When decompression begins this dissolved gas needs to be eliminated and there will be a degree of supersaturation which may lead to bubble formation in the body. Much has been written about the extravascular and intravascular sites of origin of bubbles and their subsequent distribution. Some may cause their effects by simple expansion. However, the surface activity which occurs at the blood–gas interface of intravascular emboli can cause platelet aggregation and release, complement activation, Hageman factor activation, the release of vasoactive amines, and many other perturbations of both the cellular and non-cellular constituents of blood. A raised haematocrit is a common finding in severe decompression illness and hypovolaemia can complicate the treatment of difficult cases.

The cause of decompression sickness can be a failure to follow the published decompression procedures. The tables, designed to permit a safe elimination of dissolved gas by a succession of timed 'stops' at progressively shallow depths, may themselves be inadequate. Another cause of decompression sickness is personal idiosyncrasy which might be natural biological variation, an altered complement status,[16] recent injury or dehydration or, in compressed-air workers particularly, a loss of 'acclimatization' following time off work.[15] The use of individual decompression computers worn on the diver's wrist is not accepted for most military and commercial working dives where the divers are under the immediate control of a diving supervisor at the surface but these may be used by diving scientists or professional recreational instructors who have a greater degree of diving freedom and often make multilevel dives. Decompression sickness can arise even after a dive in which a safe decompression schedule or computer has been correctly followed.

Some clinical manifestations could be the end point of either arterial gas embolism or decompression sickness but in many cases the nature of the dive and its decompression may not provide evidence to distinguish between the possible causes. A few individuals may show some features characteristic of gas embolism and others characteristic of decompression sickness, sometimes when the dive has been within the safety of the 'no-stop' limits, i.e. in the absence of significant dissolved gas. A number of hypotheses, and some evidence, exist to account for such phenomena but, for the purposes of case management, treatment must be determined by the manifestations and not by the presumed aetiologies.

Cutaneous decompression illness

Itching of the skin may be reported in those parts that have been exposed to compressed air during the pressure exposure but not those parts that were immersed. Thus it may be due to the cutaneous absorption of nitrogen. This uncommon manifestation is not a serious condition but is associated with compressed-air dives of marginal safety. No specific treatment is required but the individual should remain under medical observation in case other manifestations follow.

A blotchy red or purple rash, usually over the upper trunk, may be due to superficial vasodilation and stasis. This rash, cutis marmorata, blanches under direct local pressure. Though mild in itself, this condition may be a warning of a possible onset of a more serious condition later and, if recompression facilities are readily available, treatment not only resolves the skin condition but may be prophylactic therapy for other manifestations later. Certainly a person with such a rash should be regarded as a candidate for recompression and, if no chamber is readily available, arrangements should be made to transfer the patient.

The lymphatic form of decompression illness is thought to be due to bubbles blocking the lymphatics and the lymphatic glands. Peau d'orange is usually seen in the limbs but the oedema can also appear on the face or trunk. Again the condition itself is not serious but, if the patient is recompressed for some other manifestation, the oedema also responds.

From the evidence of submarine-escape training casualties, in whom there is no significant gas load at the time of ascent, it can be concluded that cutis marmorata and peau d'orange are associated only with bubbles formed from dissolved gases.

Musculoskeletal pain

The 'bends' is the most widely known term among the manifestations of decompression sickness. In compressed-air workers and saturation divers musculoskeletal pain is more common in the knees whereas in compressed-air divers it is more common in the shoulders. It can, however, occur in almost any synovial joint, only the temporomandibular joint seems to be immune. Joint pain may be the presenting symptom in as many as 90% of compressed-air workers but it needs to be emphasized that it is not present in all cases. Also, in some 30%, limb pain may be associated with a less obvious but more serious neurological manifestation.

The pain can be discrete or diffuse, mild or intense, steady or fluctuating. It may be possible to distinguish between cases with sharp, localized and superficial pain and those with a more dull, diffuse and deeper pain. The pain may be in a single joint, flitting, or in multiple sites. There may be some associated redness, oedema or limitation of movement. If not treated by recompression the pain may rapidly regress (a 'niggle') or may slowly resolve over some days or even weeks. An association between limb pain and associated osteonecrosis is described later.

Constitutional manifestations

Malaise, anorexia and a degree of fatigue disproportionate to the amount of preceding activity, are common accompaniments to decompression illness and, if they occur alone, must be regarded as a warning that further manifestations may soon develop.

Cardiopulmonary decompression illness

Known to divers as the 'chokes' this condition is a severe form of decompression sickness thought to be due to the build-up of venous gas emboli and associated vasoactive products of surface activity in the pulmonary circulation.

It is not reported among submarine-escape training casualties and has been associated with ascents from deep dives of short duration rather than the slower decompressions of compressed air workers. It is relatively rare in professional diving.

The onset of a retrosternal pain which limits deep inspiration may be the first symptom of this form of decompression illness. A dry cough and shallow rapid respirations may presage the onset of circulatory collapse. Milder presentations occur, but all are serious.

Pulmonary barotrauma

Chest pain, particularly after a rapid ascent or occasionally when a diver is subjected to the buffeting of severe wave action, may be due to a pneumothorax. Decompression may expand the contained gas and the condition can be bilateral. The tracking of gas into the mediastinum is a less common cause of symptoms and, if present, crepitus over subcutaneous gas in the supraclavicular region is diagnostic.

These forms of pulmonary barotrauma are not necessarily associated with the neurological manifestations of arterial gas embolism. Rarely, pulmonary barotrauma and gas embolism may be present concurrently. Occasionally a pneumothorax remains undetected when a patient presents with gas embolism and is recompressed. During the subsequent decompression an expansion of gas in the pneumothorax may present as chest pain and dyspnoea which can be relieved by a few metres of further recompression. However, when it next recurs on decompression, it recurs at a deeper depth and requires a greater recompression to relieve it. Pleurocentesis at depth is essential. The early recognition of the possibility of a pneumothorax in an individual being treated for neurological decompression illness is an important feature of management.

Neurological decompression illness

Any neurological symptom or deficit arising within some 36 hours of completing a dive must be considered as a manifestation of decompression illness until shown otherwise and managed accordingly. Whereas the classic presentation of gas embolism due to pulmonary barotrauma is immediate loss of consciousness on surfacing, often leading rapidly to death, hemiplegia, monoplegia or vertigo, the classic presentation of decompression sickness due to bubbles from dissolved gas is an ascending paraplegia ('spinal bends'). This appears to be a phenomenon not found in general arterial embolic diseases but because it has a different pathogenesis, is unique to decompression sickness.[19]

Cerebral dysfunction can take the form of a feeling of 'spaciness', a detachment from reality, dysarthria, visual disturbances, behavioural changes or, occasionally, a psychosis. Any neurological manifestation may be met: a naturally bilingual diver remained able to converse in either Italian or English but became unable to interpret between the two. Sometimes there is a denial of illness even when the peripheral signs are self-evident.

The vertiginous form of decompression illness, 'the staggers', may be associated with nausea, vomiting and/or ipsilateral deafness and it is known that the underlying lesion can be anywhere in the end-organ or its central connections. Rarely, one or more of the other cranial nerves may be affected.

The onset of tingling or 'woolliness' in the feet ascending in minutes or maybe an hour or so into complete paraplegia or possibly quadriplegia is a classic presentation of spinal decompression sickness. The sudden onset of unilateral or bilateral girdle pain of the trunk is associated with an almost immediate paraplegia below that level. Pathology demonstrates that the lesions at this stage are usually small, discrete, multiple and multi-level. Thus almost any lesser peripheral neurological deficit can occur.

Reversed interpretation of hot and cold, and a diminished sense of vibration may be detected at the early stages. Impairment of the bulbocavernous reflex and of anal sphincter tone are early signs leading to retention of urine, rectal incontinence and impotence. The patient with only the phrenic nerves for respiration indicates one limit of survivable decompression illness but it must be understood that many minor cases do not progress very far and that a number recover spontaneously.

Many neurological presentations are compatible with either pathogenesis and only rarely does one meet the 'classical' decompression sickness or arterial gas embolism. Nevertheless there are a number of cases which demonstrate features of both classic presentations concurrently or sequentially.

CASE HISTORY

A 32-year old compressed air diver made an emergency rapid ascent from a 12-minute dive to a depth of 30 m sea water. This was followed immediately by an impairment of consciousness and hemiparesis which cleared spontaneously within minutes. Some 20 minutes later he noticed the onset of 'woolliness' in his feet which progressed into classic paraplegia. He was evacuated by air to a chamber where, some 24 hours later, he was recompressed but with little response. While in the chamber, a surgeon conducted a laparotomy 'because of paralytic ileus' and after decompression the wound dehisced. The patient emerged still paraplegic but, 6 months later, was able to walk with two sticks.

Diagnosis
Biphasic decompression illness.

Comment
It may be speculated that arterial emboli following this safe no-stop dive, besides causing his transient neurological manifestations of arterial gas embolism, passed through tissues loaded with nitrogen which otherwise would have been excreted symptom-free through the lungs after the dive. The nitrogen then diffused into these bubbles to a degree that spinal cord decompression sickness followed what would normally be considered to be a safe dive. The unnecessary laparotomy is relevant only in demonstrating a need for all doctors working in the vicinity of a recompression chamber to have some basic understanding of decompression sickness pathology and the potential effect of mild nitrogen narcosis on their own performance.

Latency

Loss of consciousness on arriving at the surface from a relatively rapid ascent is characteristic of the immediacy of conditions associated with arterial gas embolism. A delay of some minutes may occur before the onset of lesser neurological deficits such as weakness or disorientation but delays longer than this are not characteristic of presentations in submariners whose prior exposure was so brief that they did not acquire a significant gas load.

The onset of limb pain is not associated with such brief exposures but only with those dives in which there has been sufficient time to dissolve a significant mass of gas in the tissues. In both compressed-air workers and divers a latency of as long as 36 hours is possible though the onset is usually much quicker. Longer apparent latencies than this, though possible, may be due to the diver failing to recognize or report earlier symptoms.

In saturation divers particularly, the onset of limb pain and other manifestations characteristically associated with decompression sickness due to dissolved gas may arise during their multi-day decompression to the surface. Decompression illness can arise at any time after decompression has begun. This can be at the living depth of saturation divers if the causative dive was an excursion to a deeper working depth, or after arrival at the surface.

Diagnosis

Any symptom or sign arising within 36 hours of a decompression should first be considered to be a decompression illness. A reluctance to do so can lead to delay in treatment and a delay in treatment permits a progression of the underlying condition and also appears to render it less responsive to treatment.

CASE HISTORY

A 28-year old compressed-air diver working at a depth of 24.4 m sea water for less than 20 minutes on a hose returned to the surface apparently unconscious. As he had not been down long enough to incur an obligation for decompression stops, his colleagues decided that it could not possibly be decompression sickness, that therefore this must be the result of a venomous fish or jelly-fish, and rushed him to hospital. He heard these comments but was unable to speak as they carried him past the recompression chamber into the ambulance. He made a slow spontaneous recovery of speech over the next few days but was left with a residual lower monoparesis, a condition likely to have been reversed if he had been recompressed immediately.

Retrospective diagnosis
Arterial gas embolism.

CASE HISTORY

A 27-year old diving scientist made a dive to a depth of 30 m for 40 min in a calm sea with in-water decompression in accordance with a dive computer. He vomited several times during the decompression and felt nauseous at the surface. No medical advice or recompression chamber was available locally. For the next 24 hours he felt 'spaced out' and had frontal headaches with nausea and dizziness. He attended the outpatient department of a prestigious teaching hospital where it was concluded that he could not have decompression sickness because he did not have any 'limb-bends'. He was then taken by a fellow diver to a naval recompression chamber in which he made a rapid and complete recovery with no permanent residua.

Diagnosis
Cerebral decompression sickness.

Comment

The diagnosis can be made from the history alone. An examination may demonstrate physical signs, but these are not necessarily present. The need for immediate treatment may justify a foreshortening of the examination in urgent cases, but a full examination should be conducted as soon as time permits. If a compression chamber is on site, the examination of neurological or cardiopulmonary illness may be conducted at depth, after treatment has begun. This will establish a baseline of any residua against which subsequent progress can be judged. If there is no chamber on site, time for the full examination may be available while waiting for transport. In all cases the desire to complete the examination should be balanced against the probably greater need to minimize delay before definitive treatment can be started.

Those divers or compressed-air workers complaining only of limb pain, however, must be examined meticulously prior to recompression in order to discover any unsuspected neurological deficit.

Supplementary investigations are not often appropriate. This may be due to the urgency of treatment or because the diving site with its recompression chamber may be at an isolated location, perhaps at sea. Regulations do not require a recompression chamber to be at the site of all working dives and thus there may be a delay of some hours before the patient can be brought to a hyperbaric treatment centre. In these circumstances, if full medical facilities are available, but only if the patient's condition permits the delay, a chest radiograph and a blood sample for a haematocrit may be useful.

The use of ultrasound to detect bubbles has no place in the clinical management of persons who have symptoms.

Treatment

The earlier the onset of the presenting manifestation, the more rapid the progress of the illness and the more severe the condition may become. The earlier that recompression begins, the more responsive the illness is to treatment. There are exceptions to these general rules but the record of success justifies each case of decompression illness being considered as a medical emergency.

CASE HISTORY

A diving research assistant had just emerged from a complex deep air dive and, standing by the chamber, he suddenly complained of an encircling pain around his lower chest. As he clambered back into the chamber he became paraplegic and so he was lifted into the chamber by the doctor who had no time to make a formal examination. He was compressed within 2 minutes to 50 m and examined on arrival where he had no residual symptoms or signs.

Diagnosis

Decompression sickness of the spinal cord.

Comment

Such rapidity of onset is uncommon and implies a life-threatening prognosis. The complete and rapid response to an immediate recompression is characteristic also of the neurological manifestations of arterial gas embolism and demonstrates the urgency of recompression treatment where available.

The early return of the stricken diver or compressed-air worker to raised environmental pressure often provides an immediate and complete resolution of the illness and the subsequent therapeutic decompression is sufficiently slow to prevent a relapse. Residua are more likely if there has been a delay of some hours before recompression. The tables and algorithms to be followed during recompression are well established and each treatment centre will have its own recommended procedures to be followed according to the circumstances. Most chambers are run on site by personnel trained for the task and with the support of a nominated diving doctor experienced in such therapy. Most recompression algorithms are based on those of the US navy[26] but those that stem from the French navy are equally acceptable. Because a working diver with residua may be unfit to resume diving, maximum therapeutic gain must be derived from the initial recompression, if necessary extending it for many hours. Though some controversies exist concerning what the optimum treatment might be, especially of unresponsive or deteriorating cases, the details of such treatments are not needed by those doctors who are not on call to attend a recompression centre. Indeed, many divers have a better understanding of the natural history of these diseases than some attending doctors.

CASE HISTORY

A commercial diver noticed the onset of one-sided chest pain during decompression. This was relieved by recompression but recurred on resuming decompression.

Diagnosis

A diagnosis of pneumothorax was made by the diver himself as well as by his colleagues but they were overruled by the doctor called out to treat him with pleurocentesis.

Comment

The doctor perhaps did not appreciate the distortion of percussion and auscultation which occurs with increased gas density at depth and instead diagnosed and managed the diver as a case of pneumonia. The patient died of a tension pneumothorax during the subsequent decompression.

Where no chamber is readily available at the diving

site and the patient is awaiting transfer, there are a number of measures that should begin immediately at the surface. The first is giving 100% oxygen by close-fitting mask, preferably from a supply that can be maintained for more than 6 hours. If serious symptoms are present an intravenous infusion should be set up with isotonic saline or Ringer's solution. In milder cases oral fluids should be pushed until the urine is pale and copious. A fluid balance chart should be kept. Bladder catheterization or pleurocentesis may be required. Attention should be given to the pressure points of paralysed patients and the affected limbs regularly put through their full range of passive movement.

Controversy exists also over the efficacy of large doses of corticosteroids but it is generally accepted that they may reduce the neurological sequelae due to oedema or reperfusion injury. Controlled trials in acute decompression illness are not available. The use of diazepam is effective for the symptomatic relief of vertigo although the subsequent suppression of obvious symptoms may make the management of the underlying pathology more difficult. There are also a number of drugs which have been used in the past but about which there is now doubt. These include the use of very low doses of heparin, originally thought to be valuable for its anti-lipaemic activity, and of aspirin (acetylsalicylic acid) for its inhibition of platelet aggregation. In both cases the current concern is that their small anticoagulative side-effects may enhance haemorrhage, for example, in an inner ear already damaged by bubbles. In cases of severe limb pain the use during transport of nitrous oxide analgesia which is available in some ambulances should be discouraged because the nitrous oxide is known to enlarge bubble size by counter diffusion, albeit temporarily.

Decompression illness is a dynamic condition and an important feature of management is regular reassessment to detect any deterioration so that if any is found it can be treated as soon as possible. Patients should remain in the vicinity of the chamber for at least 24 hours after surfacing since a relapse is not uncommon.

For decompression illness arising at depth during a saturation dive, treatment follows the same principles. Recompression follows a prescribed emergency procedure and raised inspiratory tensions of oxygen are provided using oxy-helium mixtures by mask.

Although it can and has been done, there should be no place in professional diving for dressing the diver in his equipment again and sending him down for recompression in the water. The obvious difficulties of this are that the patient may not be capable of supporting himself, that he is inaccessible to medical intervention and that limitations of gas supply and supplementary heat will in turn limit the depth and duration of the recompression therapy. Because of this, many heroic attempts to alleviate decompression illness by returning the diver to depth in the water on compressed air have not succeeded; indeed some patients have been made worse. The only

exception has been where the procedure has been agreed before diving begins and the team have special equipment including oxygen and have had appropriate training to use it. A full facemask, a virtually unlimited oxygen supply, thermal protection and, in cold water, supplementary heat enable a modest recompression to 9 m (90 kPa) for 30–60 minutes with a slow decompression. As this is sufficient for only mild cases, a careful risk analysis is likely to favour the more expensive but more versatile alternative of a transportable recompression chamber on site.

Prognosis

The majority of patients, particularly those treated soon after the onset of manifestations, appear to make a full recovery, many immediately and most within 24 hours. Those with limb pain only may return to work some 24 hours after a full and uncomplicated recovery.

Some patients fail to respond in spite of the best of treatment and may suffer permanent neurological residua. Functional improvement of decompression paraplegia tends to occur over subsequent weeks and months, a person initially able to move only a toe may be able to resume some walking within some 3–6 months. This is perhaps a reflection of the multiple discrete lesions of spinal decompression sickness in contrast to the permanent nature of a cord transection. However, an individual should not return to diving if neurological residua can be detected. This guidance[27] was based on clinical signs but the use of special investigations enhances the sensitivity of the examination for fitness to return to diving. In compressed-air workers, who suffer predominantly limb pain decompression illness, it has long been considered by some that an episode of neurological decompression sickness, however mild, should debar the individual from working again at raised environmental pressure. (Dysbarism, including decompression sickness, barotrauma and osteonecrosis, is a prescribed disease in the UK; see Chapter 4).

The arguments here are complex. There is evidence[28] that, while functional recovery may be excellent, the scars of the original lesion in the spinal cord remain unchanged. On the other hand, a compressed-air worker who may have suffered transient paraesthesia is not likely to agree to give up his livelihood. The training of a diver is long, arduous and expensive and one must also consider the probable response of workers to the threat of medical disqualification: that of suppressing the symptoms and failing to report until the illness may be irreversible.

In summary, early treatment with complete resolution of all detectable neurological manifestations within 24 hours is compatible with continued work at pressure. Extreme views have ranged from no further pressure exposure ever for compressed-air workers (tunnellers) after any neurological manifestation even though rapidly and completely resolved and, in the USA, a return to diving if complete resolution is obtained within 8 weeks. Because these fitness assessments to resume diving are not straight-forward, each patient should be carefully examined, after a period of some 7 days (if sensory only) or 28 days (if other neurological manifestations were present), by a doctor experienced in diving. In the UK this means a Medical Examiner of Divers approved by the Health and Safety Executive.[27]

After neurological decompression illness, echocardiography should be considered to detect the presence of a right-to-left intracardiac shunt for possible transcatheter repair.[29] Incomplete resolution is considered as grounds for medical disqualification. In those whose full recovery takes longer than 24 hours there may be some loss of neuronal reserves and these individuals require counselling before they return to work at pressure should they wish to do so.

Equally difficult is any decision on the prognosis of an individual after pulmonary barotrauma. While a full clinical recovery is the general rule, the individual's lungs are considered to be at greater risk of damage during some future decompression. Pulmonary manifestations of barotrauma are considered by some to be a disqualification for future diving even after apparent recovery. Since the only manifestation of an underlying pulmonary pathology may have been transient neurological effects due to secondary arterial gas embolism, the retrospective diagnosis of the cause of a neurological illness, i.e. whether due to alveolar rupture or to the relatively less disruptive evolution of bubbles from dissolved gas, could be critical in the decision of whether or not to permit a return to work at raised environmental pressure. Indeed, the distinction may not be possible. At present the Diving Medical Advisory Committee (DMAC) recommends a minimum of 28 days after full recovery from known pulmonary barotrauma before an approved doctor considers a possible resumption of diving.

LONG-TERM EFFECTS

Some conditions exist which are considered to be occupational hazards of work at raised environmental pressure. These effects are not related specifically to known incidents of decompression sickness but some pose a threat to health.

Hearing loss

Audiometric examination of divers and compressed-air workers may demonstrate hearing loss greater than in age-matched controls. This may be due to one or more of many possible occupational causes,[30,31] including barotrauma to the inner ear, decompression sickness and excessive noise. The first two have been discussed already

and are important in groups of air divers not exposed to noise.[31] Noise-induced hearing loss should be preventable by using the principles of conventional hearing conservation programmes. However, noise dosimetry in chambers and diving helmets, though not easy, reveals some noise levels that should not be tolerated.

Pulmonary changes

There are a number of effects of diving upon respiratory function but the significance of some to the health of the individual are uncertain.[32] There is a diminished response in some divers to raised tensions of carbondioxide and these so-called 'carbon dioxide retainers' may be more susceptible than the normal population to otherwise unexplained loss of consciousness underwater.[12] An increase of vital capacity in divers is reported by some[33] though not all.[34] The maximum expiratory flow rate at 25% of forced vital capacity (FVC) is also reduced in divers,[35] suggesting an occupational narrowing of small airways. The diminution of transfer capacity (TLco) after some deep dives may persist for many months[36] but, while this may cause some functional impairment, there is no evidence yet that this will have a serious effect on health.

Neurological sequelae

The gross changes in the central nervous systems of compressed-air workers which were reported by Rozsahegyi[37] were in most cases associated with a past history of decompression sickness. The large cysts in the brain and other pathological changes described by him have not been confirmed by subsequent studies. Current concerns, however, are not about such gross lesions but about the possibility of subtle lesions in the central nervous system occurring even in the absence of any known history of decompression illness.[38]

There are some indications that such changes do occur[39–41] and, from fluorescein retinal angiography, that there may be associated cerebrovascular changes.[42] However, all these studies need the benefit of more data and, particularly, additional controls. As with magnetic resonance imaging[43] and electroencephalographic studies of divers,[44] there is also a need to define more precisely the investigative procedures to be followed and the diagnostic criteria used to evaluate the results. Without agreement between different centres on these fundamentals there can be no valid comparisons between them. Even when a boundary can be defined between the extremes of normality and the beginnings of pathology there is still one further unknown: what is the clinical significance of the changes found? As yet there is insufficient justification for the use of such special investigations as part of the periodic health screening of divers and compressed-air workers.

Dysbaric osteonecrosis

The first known cases of bone necrosis presented as joint pain in compressed-air workers. The crippling effects of articular collapse justified studies of prevalence and a search for preventive measures. Surveys began of the asymptomatic population of workers in order to detect lesions at an early stage. The radiological techniques to do so and the associated diagnostic criteria were defined by the Decompression Sickness Panel of the Medical Research Council (MRC),[17] that a bone lesion occurring in a person who is a compressed-air worker or diver is not likely to be due to natural causes. Indeed, most other causes of bone necrosis are incompatible with the guidelines of fitness for diving and this should be so also for compressed-air workers.

Clinical presentations of osteonecrosis are now rare because, with regular screening of those whose exposures to pressure are of the type that put them in an at-risk category, imaging techniques should detect a lesion before subchondral collapse becomes inevitable. Osteonecrosis of the subchondral portion of the head of the femur or the head of the humerus is regarded as sufficiently serious to recommend strongly to the individual

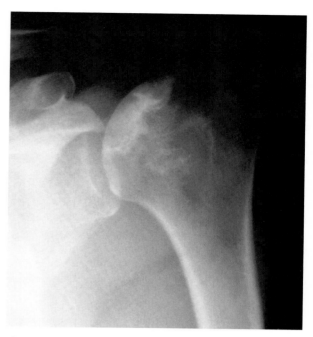

Figure 16.2 *An A3 lesion in the left humerus of a diving medical officer. This is a routine survey view and shows a developed lesion. Reproduced with permission from Ref. 4.*

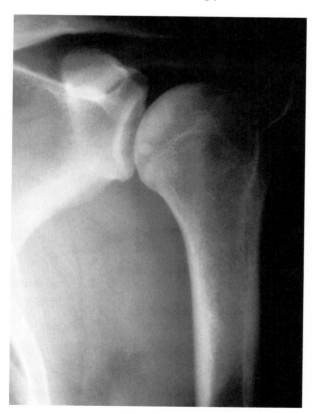

Figure 16.1 *A juxta-articular lesion (A2) in the head of the left humerus in a diver. The radiolucent line within the shoulder joint is a vacuum phenomenon known not to be related to decompression. Two bone islands are present and are not significant. The A2 lesion shows an increased density, is subcortical and is a typical 'snowcap' lesion. Reproduced with permission from Ref. 4.*

that he gives up further work at raised environmental pressure. There is no risk to safety for him and therefore this decision, which may involve significant loss of earnings, should be voluntary but it should be made.

The MRC radiological classification[45] of the subchondral or A lesions (Figs 16.1 and 16.2) has been used as the basis for a possible sequence of juxta-articular lesions which might be followed in an individual case.[46] The lesions in the heads of the long bones but distant from the subchondral area are, for the MRC classification, regarded as shaft or B lesions. These are relatively benign, do not lead to osteoarthritis but, extremely rarely, may be the site of malignant change.[47,48]

From those whose osteonecrosis has developed from a single exposure to raised environmental pressure, it is known that the radiological changes may not appear for at least 2 months and possibly not for up to 2 years after the causative incident. The use of technetium bone scans to detect lesions at a much earlier stage[49] has not been generally accepted because only a minority of 'hot spots' progress to a lesion which is confirmed by radiograph. Thus the number of doubtful and false-positive diagnoses does not provide sufficient guidance for case management. Magnetic resonance imaging of the bones also provides a very early indication of osteonecrotic changes which, though the technique has not been systematically evaluated, may prove to be reliable even though some apparent lesions appear to regress spontaneously.

The overall prevalence of osteonecrosis as determined radiologically is as high as 17% among compressed-air workers.[50] The prevalence in divers may be as high as

50% in some populations[51] but, among naval divers[52] and commercial divers in the North Sea,[53] it is as low as 4.2%. More important, however, is the prevalence of juxta-articular lesions.

No treatment is required for shaft lesions and affected individuals having been counselled may continue their occupation. The juxta-articular lesion justifies discontinuation of compressed-air work or diving and the reduction of stress and weight-bearing for the affected joint. Only a minority progress to articular collapse as defined radiologically and only a minority of this group progresses further to referable pain.

Prevention is not easy. It is known that there is a statistical association between those who have osteonecrosis and those who have been recompressed for decompression sickness.[53] However, this is not a one-to-one relationship. Many have been treated for 'bends' who do not subsequently develop bone necrosis and many have had no known decompression sickness but do develop bone necrosis. In those who have both bone necrosis and a history of limb bends, the sites rarely match. However, it is known that the more extreme pressure exposures or, more probably, their associated decompressions are associated with a greater likelihood of osteonecrosis. For instance, those who make dives of less than 4 hours' duration or to less than 30 m rarely develop bone necrosis whereas those who make deep saturation dives have a higher incidence of osteonecrosis than those who dive between these two exposure extremes.[53]

FITNESS FOR DIVING

Periodical medical examinations of working divers are required by many authorities. Their fundamental purpose is to detect any condition which might lead to an underwater accident. Correction of any detected problem or the medical disqualification of a diver is thus in the interests of the safety of the diver and those who might have to rescue him.

A secondary purpose is to protect the diver's health from the effects of diving. The surveillance for early osteonecrosis is an example of such medical screening.

The criteria for fitness for the professional divers[54] in the UK are given in detail by the Health and Safety Executive. Interpretation of the guidance for some conditions is not easy for the individual diver and each examination is required to be conducted by a doctor who should have the knowledge and experience to assess borderline cases and is formally approved by the Health and Safety Executive. With a candidate for diver training one can be very strict and aim for perfect health. As the diver gets older, assessment can become more difficult. Consultation between colleagues is accepted practice in order to achieve consistency among the uncertainties.

Following a medical disqualification the diver has the right to appeal after which the Health and Safety Executive will appoint a diving doctor and an appropriate specialist to review the case and advise them.

Assessment of fitness to return to diving after illness or injury, or after a diving accident, must be judged by the same guidance and principles, particularly in relation to the tasks that the diver will be expected to do.

The diver also needs to be physically fit. Beyond the minimum demands set by the Guidance Notes a more rigorous test may be considered for some divers. Most should be able to attain an oxygen uptake of 13 mets (metabolic equivalents), equivalent to 45 ml ($\dot{V}O_2$) per kg per minute. This is considered to be appropriate for the need by anybody underwater to cope with the sudden physical demands imposed by some unexpected in-water emergency.

REFERENCES

1 Halley E. The art of living underwater: Or, a discourse concerning the means of furnishing air at the bottom of the sea, in any ordinary depths. *Phil Trans Roy Soc* 1716; **29:** 492–9.

2 Bevan J. *The development of the diving helmet and dress in the UK during the 19th century.* PhD thesis, University of London, 1991.

3 McCallum RI. Increased barometric pressure. In: Raffle PAB, Lee WR, McCallum RI, Murray R eds. *Hunter's Diseases of Occupations* 7th edn. London: Hodder & Stoughton, 1986: 523–47.

4 Bennett PB, Elliott DH (eds). *The Physiology and Medicine of Diving* 4th edn. London: WB Saunders Co, 1993.

5 Elliott DH. Underwater physiology. In: Edholm OG, Weiner JS eds. *Principles and Practice of Human Physiology.* London: Academic Press, 1981: 30951.

6 Bert P. *La Pression Barometrique. Recherches de Physiologie Expérimentale.* Paris: Masson,

7 Smith JL. The pathological effects due to increase of oxygen tension in the air breathed. *J Physiol (Lond)* 1899, **24:** 19–35.

8 Clark JM. Oxygen toxicity. In: Bennett PB, Elliott DH eds. *The Physiology and Medicine of Diving* 4th edn. London: WB Saunders Co, 1993: 121–69.

9 Wright WB. *Use of the University of Pennsylvania Institute for Environmental Medicine Procedure for Calculation of Pulmonary Oxygen Toxicity.* US Navy: Experimental Diving Unit Report 2–72, 1972.

10 Donald KW. Oxygen poisoning in man. *Br Med J* 1947; **1:** 667–72.

11 Lanphier EH, Camporesi EM. Respiration and exertion. In: Bennett PB, Elliott DH eds. *The Physiology and Medicine of Diving* 4th edn. London: WB Saunders Co, 1993: 77–120.

12 Morrison JB, Florio JT, Butt WS. Loss of consciousness in divers. In: Smith G ed. *Proceedings of the Sixth International Congress on Hyperbaric Medicine*. Aberdeen: Aberdeen University Press, 1979: 377–81.

13 Bennett PB, Rostain J. The high pressure nervous syndrome in man. In: Bennett PB, Elliott DH eds. *The Physiology and Medicine of Diving* 4th edn. London: WB Saunders Co. 1993: 194–237.

14 Vann RD, Thalman RD. Decompression physiology and practice. In: Bennett PB, Elliott DH eds. *The Physiology and Medicine of Diving* 4th edn. London: WB Saunders Co, 1993: 376–432.

15 Paton WDM, Walder DN. *Compressed Air Illness. Special Report Series, Medical Research Council, No. 281*. London: HMSO, 1954.

16 Ward CA, Weathersby PK, McCullough D, Fraser WD. Identification of individuals susceptible to decompression sickness. In: Bove AA, Bachrach AJ, Greenbaum LJ eds. *9th International Symposium on Underwater and Hyperbaric Physiology*. Bethesda, MD: Undersea and Hyperbaric Medical Society Inc., 1987: 239–47.

17 McCallum RI, Walder DN. Bone lesions in compressed air workers with special reference to men who worked on the Clyde tunnels 1958 to 1963. Report of Decompression Sickness Panel, Medical Research Council. *J Bone Jt Surg [Br]* 1966; **48:** 207–35.

18 Edmonds C. Marine animal injuries. In: Bove AA, Davis J eds. *Diving Medicine* 2nd edn. Philadelphia: WB Saunders Co, 1990: 115–37.

19 Hallenbeck JM, Anderson J. Pathogenesis of the decompression disorders. In: Bennett PB, Elliott DH eds. *The Physiology and Medicine of Diving* 3rd edn. London: Baillière Tindall, 1982: 435–60.

20 Francis TJR. The pathophysiology of decompression sickness. In: Bennett PB, Moon RE eds. *Diving Accident Management*. Bethesda: Undersea and Hyperbaric Medical Society Inc., 1990:

21 Golding FC, Griffiths PD, Hempleman HV, Paton WDM, Walder DN. Decompression sickness during construction of the Dartford tunnel. *Br J Ind Med* 1960; **17:** 167–80.

22 Rivera J. Decompression sickness among divers: an analysis of 935 cases. *Milit Med* 1964; **129:** 314–34.

23 Francis TJR, Smith D (eds). *Describing Decompression Illness*. Bethesda, MD: Undersea and Hyperbaric Medical Society Inc., 1991.

24 Smith DJ, Francis TJR, Pethybridge RJ, Wright JM, Sykes JJW. Concordance: a problem with the current classification of diving disorders. *Undersea Biomed Res* 1992; **19** (suppl): 40.

25 Dayman H. Mechanics of air flow in health and in emphysema. *J Clin Invest* 1951; **30:** 1175–90.

26 US Navy. *Diving Manual. NAVSEA 0994–LP001–9010*. Washington DC: US Navy Department, 1985.

27 Diving Medical Advisory Committee. *Guidance on Assessing Fitness to Return to Diving. DMAC 013, Rev 1*. London: DMAC, 1994.

28 Palmer AC, Calder IM, McCallum RI, Mastaglia FL. Spinal cord degeneration in a case of 'recovered' spinal decompression sickness. *Br Med J* 1981; **283:** 888.

29 Wilmshurst P, Walsh K, Morrison L. Transcatheter occlusion of foramen ovale with a button device after neurological decompression illness in professional divers. *Lancet* 1996; **348:** 752–3.

30 Molvaer OI, Lehmann EH. Hearing acuity in professional divers. *Undersea Biomed Res* 1975; **12:** 311–12.

31 Edmonds C, Freeman P. Hearing loss in Australian divers. *Med J Aust* 1985; **143:** 446–8.

32 Longhair EH. Nitrogen-oxygen mixture physiology, phase 3. *US Navy Experimental Diving Unit Research Report 2–56*. Washington DC: US Navy Department, 1956.

33 Crosbie WA, Reed JW, Clarke MC. Functional characteristics of the large lungs found in commercial divers. *J Appl Physiol* 1979; **46:** 639–45.

34 Thorsen E, Hjelle J, Segedal K, Gulsvik A. Exercise tolerance and pulmonary gas exchange after deep saturation. *Undersea Biomed Res* 1988; **15** (Suppl): 34–5.

35 Davey IS, Cotes JE, Reed JW. Relationship of ventilatory capacity to hyperbaric exposure in divers. *J Appl Physiol: Respir Environ Exercise Physiol* 1984; **56:** 1655–8.

36 Thorsen E, Segedal K, Kambestad BK, Gulsvik A. Reduced pulmonary function in saturation divers correlates with diving exposure. *Undersea Biomed Res* 1990; **17** (Suppl): 70.

37 Rozsahegyi I. Late consequences of the neurological forms of decompression sickness. *Br J Ind Med* 1959; **16:** 311–17.

38 Todnem K, Nyland H, Kambestad BK, Aarli JA. Influence of occupational diving upon the nervous system: an epidemiological study. *Br J Ind Med* 1990; **47:** 708–14.

39 Palmer AC, Calder IM, Hughes JT. Spinal cord degeneration in divers. *Lancet* 1987; **ii:** 1365–6.

40 Palmer AC, Calder IM, Yates PO. Cerebral vasculopathy in divers. *Neuropathol Appl Neurobiol* 1992; **18:** 113–24.

41 Mork S. Selection of supplementary material. In: *MRC Open Meeting of Long Term Health Effects Working Group: Report*. London: Medical Research Council, 1988.

42 Polkinghorne PJ, Sehmi K, Cross MR, Manassian D, Bird AC. Ocular fundus lesions in divers. *Lancet* 1988; **ii:** 1381–3.

43 Brubakk AO, Rinck P, deFrancisco P, Svihus R. Central nervous system changes in professional divers as evaluated by MRI. *Undersea Biomed Res* 1990; **17** (Suppl): 88.

44 Todnem K, Nyland H, Dick APK, *et al*. Immediate neurological effects of diving to a depth of 360 metres. *Acta Neurol Scand* 1989; **80:** 333–40.

45 McCallum R, Harrison JAB. Dysbaric osteonecrosis: aseptic necrosis of bone. In: Bennett PB, Elliott DH eds. *The Physiology and Medicine of Diving*. London: Baillière Tindall, 1993: 563–84.

46 Kawashima M. Aseptic bone necrosis in Japanese divers. *Bull Tokyo Med Dent Univ* 1976; **23:** 71–92.

47 Dorfman HD, Norman A, Wolf H. Fibrosarcoma complicating bone infarction in a caisson worker. A case report. *J Bone Jt Surg [Am]* 1966; **48:** 528-32.

48 Kitano M, Iwaski H, Yoh SS, Kuroda K, Hayashi K. Malignant fibrous histiocytoma at site of bone infarction in association with DCS. *Undersea Biomed Res* 1984; **11:** 305–14.

49 Pearson RR, MacLeod MA, McEwan AJB, Houston AS. Bone

scintigraphy as an investigative aid for dysbaric osteonecrosis in divers. *J Roy Nav Med Serv* 1982; **68:** 61–8.

50 Trowbridge WP. Bone necrosis in British compressed air workers. In Evans A, Walder DN eds. *Aseptic Bone Necrosis: Proceedings of a Symposium of the European Undersea Biomedical Society*. London: CIRIA, 1977: 41–9.

51 Ohta Y, Matsunaga H. Bone lesions in divers. *J Bone Jt Surg [Br]* 1974; **56:** 3–16.

52 Elliott DH, Harrison JAB. Aseptic bone necrosis in Royal Navy divers. In: Lambertsen CJ ed. *Proceedings of the Fourth Symposium on Underwater Physiology*. New York: Academic Press, 1971: 251–67.

53 McCallum RI. Bone necrosis due to decompression. *Phil Trans Roy Soc Lond [Biol]* 1984; **304:** 185–91.

54 Health and Safety Executive. *Diving at Work Regulations 1997 (SI 1997 No 2776)*. Sudbury: HSE Books.

17

Flying

TM GIBSON

Pressure change	361	Food and drink	374
Gravitational stress	365	Exposure to chemicals	374
Extremes of temperature	366	Exposure to radiation	374
Noise and vibration	368	Aircraft accidents	374
Vision	369	Spaceflight	375
Spatial disorientation	371	Fitness for flight	377
Air sickness	372	References	379
Jet lag	373		

Flying is an exciting occupation, providing exposure to unfamiliar environmental stresses. Although over 200 years have passed since the first manned balloon flight by Pilatre de Rozier, François Laurent and the Marquis d'Arlandes, most of the understanding of the stresses of the aviation environment has come since 1900. In the last 100 years, when mankind has progressed from Kitty Hawk to the Moon, from bicycle goggles to night vision goggles, aeroplanes have flown ever higher, ever faster. Physiologically, man has evolved to live at ground level, at $+1$ G*, within strict temperature limits and with certain design limitations to his special senses and his psychology. Adaptation and acclimatization can increase the physiological range to an extent, while training can help to maximize performance. However, flying is usually an acute experience so the physiological processes have a limited role to play. Protection from the environment, by means of engineering solutions, can increase the operating range of the human but it also has limitations. The potential for failure of that protection necessitates the provision of back-up systems or a restriction in the operating envelope of the aircraft. Thus, human tolerances have increasingly set the limits to which aircraft can be engineered.

People work in the air in a variety of capacities. Astronauts and cosmonauts work in space, often for extended periods. Military aviators fly in aircraft ranging from helicopters to high speed, single seat jets. Crews of large transport aircraft will face different challenges when they are flying tactical missions than crews of military or civilian strategic transport aircraft. Civilian flight in small aircraft can range from instructional duties to recreational flight to crop spraying. Many people, of course, fly just as passengers but some also work while they are flying and many need to be fit for work on arrival at their destination. This chapter will outline the stresses and hazards of flight from low level to space, describe the ways of overcoming them, and consider fitness for flight, both for professional aviators and passengers.

PRESSURE CHANGE

As altitude increases, pressure decreases (see Fig. 17.1). For fliers, this gives rise to four potential problems: gas expansion, hypoxia, decompression sickness, and rapid decompression.

Gas expansion

As ambient pressure decreases, volume increases in accordance with Boyle's Law. When the gas in the human body is enclosed, this may cause problems. Gas is enclosed in the body after surgery. It is therefore unwise to fly within 10 days of laparotomy (unless a drainage tube remains), within 3 weeks of craniotomy or air contrast radiograph studies of the spinal canal, or within 2

---

*The ratio of the applied acceleration due to the gravity to the gravitational constant (g) is given the symbol G, further defined by a subscript (x, y, or z) describing the axis of acceleration.

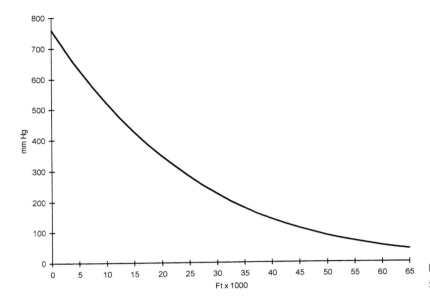

Figure 17.1 *Relationship of barometric pressure to altitude.*

weeks of thoracotomy or pneumothorax unless a Heimlich valve or similar device is in place. Similarly, penetrating injury of the eyeball can produce subluxation of the lens on ascent to altitude. Patients with these conditions may be flown but only if the cabin pressure of the aircraft is held at the ambient pressure of the departure airfield. Similarly, a small gas bubble beneath a badly filled tooth can cause excruciating pain on ascent (aerodontalgia) which usually improves on descent.

Where the gas is incompletely enclosed, there is less of a problem. The gut normally contains between 100 and 200 ml of gas at ground level. The rise in intra-abdominal pressure limits the volume increase. The usual symptom is of abdominal fullness or bloating and is reduced by eructation or passing flatus. The problem can be limited by avoiding dietary items that predispose to flatulence, such as fizzy drinks or pulses. Gas in the middle ear also has an outlet to ambient air. On ascent, the gas expands easily along the Eustachian tube and the ears 'pop' automatically. On descent, however, the increased pressure in the pharynx causes the Eustachian tube to act as a flap valve. The resulting pressure differential causes the eardrum to invert, causing pain (which is often severe) and deafness. In severe cases, vertigo and nausea may occur. The way to equalize pressures is to yawn, swallow or waggle the jaw if the pressure change is gradual, or to perform a Valsalva manoeuvre (holding the nose and straining against a closed glottis) or Frenzel (holding the nose and raising the pressure in the nasopharynx without increasing intrathoracic pressure) manoeuvre if the change is rapid. Topical decongestants before or during flight may be effective. Future developments may include the use of surfactants that play a role in maintaining patency of the Eustachian tube[1] or commercial insufflators.[2]

If descent is continued without the pressure equalizing, there is haemorrhage into the drum and it may actually perforate with subsequent relief from pain. Colds and upper respiratory tract infections predispose to this inability to 'clear the ears'. Since ear pain, deafness and vertigo are flight safety hazards, aircrew with these conditions should be discouraged from flying until they can clear their ears. Inability to clear the ears during flight can, if possible, be helped by a re-ascent to altitude and a more gradual descent. Otitic barotrauma usually clears spontaneously in 2–3 weeks.

The paranasal sinuses usually vent to ambient easily on ascent and equally easily repressurize on descent. Again, infection may interfere with this, causing pain. Nasal polyps or deviated nasal septum can also predispose to sinus barotrauma. Topical decongestants before or during flight may help. Symptomatic treatment may be required on the ground for a few days afterwards.

The respiratory passages can easily cope with the expansion of gas in the lung on ascent, except in explosive decompression when air embolus may occur. This is uncommon in flying and would be expected more when the pressure differential was high and the decompression itself likely to lead to loss of structural integrity of the aircraft.

Finally, at an altitude of 63 000 ft, the total ambient pressure is 47 mmHg. This is also the pressure exerted by water vapour at body temperature. At this altitude (known as the Armstrong line) body tissues begin to vaporize. Small pockets of gas appear beneath the skin within 2–3 seconds, there is gas evolution within the abdominal cavity in 10 seconds and in the heart in about 20 seconds. Although man can recover from brief exposures, it is better to protect the individual by means of a pressure cabin or pressure suit.

Hypoxia

At all altitudes, the fractional concentration of oxygen in the air remains at 21%. However, as pressure falls on ascent to altitude, the partial pressure exerted by that oxygen also falls, in accordance with Dalton's law of partial pressures. Up to an altitude of about 10 000 ft, the amount of oxygen available to the body remains almost the same because of the shape of the oxygen–haemoglobin dissociation curve. The oxygen saturation can fall below 90% even in commercial pressurized aircraft[3] and this may have detrimental effects on some patients.[4]

The most common causes of hypoxia in flight are ascent to altitude without supplementary oxygen, failure of personal breathing equipment to provide an adequate supply of oxygen and decompression of the cabin at high altitude. Human failure to turn on the supply, check hoses are connected or to ensure the mask seals to the face properly, accounts for 20% of hypoxia cases in military flying.[5]

The symptoms of hypoxia are insidious and include euphoria, loss of insight, impairment of cognitive functions, reduction of visual acuity, incoordination, cyanosis, hyperventilation and, eventually, loss of consciousness and death. It is widely quoted in the literature that mild hypoxia (8000 ft) impairs the learning of a novel task[6] but recent research has failed to confirm this.[7] Smokers may take longer to detect hypoxia than non-smokers.[8] Tolerance to hypoxia is reduced by exercise, exposure to cold, the presence of illness and after alcohol.

The following case history from a Halifax bomber in the Second World War is amusing but could have had a tragic outcome.

> The captain became very talkative and resented any suggestion that he was behaving abnormally . . . When we realised the aircraft was out of control the engineer trimmed the aircraft. The pilot resented this and assaulted the engineer. He then gave the order to bale out which we cancelled. He opened the window to look out, and was only prevented from falling out by the engineer who hauled him in. He said that he felt very happy, and had no feeling of fear, even when he tried to force land on a cloud, thinking he was near the ground . . . After being forced to take oxygen from the spare helmet and mask, he gradually recovered his senses . . .[9]

The insidious nature of the symptoms of hypoxia have led many military air forces to adopt a training regime in decompression chambers to allow aviators a greater chance of spotting hypoxia in themselves. The symptoms of hypoxia are very difficult to distinguish from those of hyperventilation.[10] Any symptoms in flight that could be either, must be treated as hypoxia until proved otherwise. On acute exposure to high altitude, either from failure of a pressure cabin or of the oxygen supply, the oxygen stored in the tissues allows a 'time of useful con-sciousness' before capability is lost. This time ranges from about 4 minutes at 25 000 ft to about 20 seconds at 40 000 ft and 10–15 seconds at 52 000 ft. Impairment of performance occurs sooner (45 seconds at 25 000 ft, 12–15 seconds at 40 000 ft).

Hypoxia can be prevented by ensuring that the aircraft does not fly above 10 000 ft, by providing supplemental oxygen to breathe or by pressurizing the aircraft to maintain a cabin pressure of less than 10 000 ft. The alveolar oxygen tension (P_AO_2) at sea level can be exceeded up to 33 000 ft by breathing 100% oxygen and the 10 000 ft equivalent can be exceeded up to 40 000 ft. However, there are two disadvantages to providing 100% oxygen. First, if the aircraft has an aerobatic capability, the gravitational forces may occlude small airways in the lung leading to absorption of all the oxygen distal to the occlusion. The localized pulmonary collapse is called acceleration atelectasis. Second, a similar problem may occur in the inner ear after landing, causing pain (oxygen ear). The usual solution is to provide an oxygen/air mix sufficient to allow a ground level P_AO_2 (103 mmHg) until 33 000 ft when 100% oxygen is supplied. The P_AO_2 then falls to a 10 000 ft equivalent at 40 000 ft.

Above this altitude, oxygen has to be provided under pressure to maintain adequate oxygenation (pressure breathing). In military aircraft, pressure breathing is usually applied through an oronasal mask. The barometric pressure at 40 000 ft is 141 mmHg. The aim of pressure breathing is to maintain that absolute pressure delivered to the lungs. Thus the breathing pressure will be (141-ambient pressure) mmHg. Breathing pressures up to 70 mmHg will protect against hypoxia at altitudes up to 56 000 ft. However, there are disadvantages.

Pressure breathing gives rise to physiological problems. The increased work of expiration, which is usually passive, produces discomfort, as does the distension of cheeks, mouth and respiratory passages. The nasolachrymal duct can be forced open causing severe blepharospasm and the Eustachian duct can also be forced open causing ear pain. Blood return to the heart is compromised. Peripheral pooling of the blood and the passage of fluid from the circulation into the tissues reduce effective blood volume, leading to reduced tolerance to gravitational stresses and syncope. The likelihood of syncope during pressure breathing is increased in the presence of hypoxia, hypocapnia, anxiety, infection or after alcohol.

The effects of pressure breathing can be minimized by providing counterpressure to bladders in a partial pressure jacket and to the anti-G trousers. An alternative in military aviation is to use a full pressure suit with either a full or a partial pressure helmet but these have the significant disadvantages of reduced mobility and increased heat load. In Concorde, protection is given by a combination of a rapid-don pressure mask and rapid descent to altitudes below 40 000 ft.

One significant flight safety hazard remains. It is very difficult to talk when pressure breathing. Sudden loss of cabin pressure in a large aircraft flying above 40 000 ft will lead to the requirement to read through check lists. Practice is vital.

Decompression sickness

Decompression sickness is dealt with fully in Chapter 16. It is commonly believed that altitude decompression sickness does not occur below 18 000 ft. However, bubbles have been recorded at altitudes down to 13 000 ft. Bubbles do not usually form at low altitude unless the individual has been diving in the preceding 24 hours. The occurrence of symptoms of decompression sickness is related to the final altitude and the time spent at altitude. Other predisposing factors are known susceptibility, exercise at altitude, female gender (two to four times more prone),[11] age,[12] body build, general health and previous exposure to altitude within the preceding 24 hours. Flying after diving is particularly dangerous. At least 12 hours should be spent at ground level after diving; this time should be doubled if the dive lasted more than 4 hours and redoubled if the subsequent flight is to be at a cabin altitude of 8000 ft.

The symptoms in one series of over 400 cases arising from decompression chamber experience ranged from joint pains (the 'bends' – 83% with the knee accounting for 70%), respiratory effects (the 'chokes' – 2.7%), skin symptoms (formication or the 'creeps' – 2.2%), paraesthesia (10.8%) to neurological manifestations (0.5%).[13] Visual symptoms include blurred vision, loss of vision, scintillation and scotoma. Neurological symptoms and collapse can occur after return to ground level (one study demonstrated a 45% incidence of symptoms at altitude, with 24% in the first hour after return to ground level and 21% between 1 and 6 hours).[14]

The incidence of decompression sickness in those individuals exposed to an altitude of 25 000 ft or less is low. The U-2 aircraft, however, flies at an altitude of more than 73 000 ft for more than 15 hours unrefuelled, at a cabin altitude of 29 500 ft. Despite precautions, more than 75% of U-2 pilots have experienced symptoms of decompression sickness, and 13% have had, at some stage, to alter the flight profile or abort the mission.[15]

Treatment[16] depends on the severity and resolution of the symptoms. If the symptoms clear on descent and neurological examination is normal, the patient should ideally breathe 100% oxygen for 2 hours and undergo aggressive oral rehydration. The patient should be observed for 24 hours. If symptoms (other than limb pain that clears with 100% oxygen) persist after descent, in addition to 100% oxygen and oral rehydration, the patient should be exposed to treatment in a hyperbaric chamber on US Navy Treatment Tables 5 or 6. Travel to the chamber should be by road. If air travel is absolutely necessary, then either a cabin altitude of sea level or an absolute aircraft altitude of 1000 ft should be maintained. The patient should be supine, intubated if necessary, or in the lateral decubitus position. Intravenous fluids should be either normal saline or Ringer's solution (i.e. isotonic), 1 litre in the first hour and then ~1.5 ml/kg/h. Avoid solutions (oral or intravenous) containing glucose. If there are spinal cord symptoms, there may be benefit in giving a bolus of 30 mg/kg of methylprednisolone and then 5.4 mg/kg/h for 23 hours. It is important to control the body temperature of the patient. On recovery from mild decompression sickness without central nervous system complications, the pilot can return to flying within 72 hours if there are no symptoms and examination is normal.

Prevention is based on three factors: selection of individuals who are not susceptible to decompression sickness by testing them in a decompression chamber limiting exposure to altitude by use of pressurized aircraft; and denitrogenation by breathing 100% oxygen before take-off. Pre-breathing schedules are a mixture of experience and pragmatism. Pre-oxygenation for 30 minutes will protect against short exposure to 48 000 ft as long as total time above 25 000 ft is less than 10 minutes. Exposure to 40 000 ft for 3 hours requires 3 hours of pre-oxygenation at ground level. U-2 pilots pre-breathe for 60 minutes. Recent evidence suggests that exercise while denitrogenating can reduce the time that pre-breathing is necessary whilst retaining the same level of protection.[17]

Rapid decompression

The effects of rapid decompression depend on the altitude at which the aircraft is flying, the pressure differential of the cabin, the volume of the aircraft and the size and location of the hole. Hypoxia, exposure to cold and, eventually, decompression sickness may all occur. The initial problem for aircrew in a rapid decompression is that the flow of air can raise dust and debris; visibility may also be restricted by the condensation of water vapour that occurs. Provided P_AO_2 remains above 30 mmHg, there will be no expected decrement in the aircrew's performance. The transient cabin altitude can be lower than outside because of the Venturi effect or it may be higher because of a ram air effect. The airblast can even suck passengers out of a window although the risk is only to those immediately next to the defect. The time of rapid decompression can be as little as 0.005 seconds for loss of a canopy in a military aircraft to 30 seconds if a window is lost in a large passenger aircraft. The incidence is low: $2–3/10^5$ flying hours for military aircraft and 30–40 a year worldwide for commercial aircraft.

Low differential pressure cabins, such as in military aircraft, require the aircrew to use oxygen equipment throughout. Provided it can give 100% oxygen at 33 000 ft and pressure breathing above 40 000 ft hypoxia is unlikely following rapid decompression. In civilian, high pressure differential aircraft, there is little risk of hypoxia in the crew provided they can don oxygen equipment delivering 100% oxygen within 5 seconds of cabin altitude exceeding 10 000 ft. The crew will then make an emergency descent to at least 10 000 ft. In Concorde, the protection is provided by designing the aircraft so that, even if a window were lost at 65 000 ft the cabin altitude would not exceed 36 000 ft provided emergency descent was started within 30 seconds.[18] Sufficient oxygen is carried on all commercial aircraft for passengers' P_AO_2 to be maintained above 50 mmHg in the event of a rapid decompression, although it is unlikely that they will all be able to use the drop-down masks successfully.

GRAVITATIONAL STRESS

The most common long duration accelerations experienced in flying are radial accelerations – those produced by change of direction of motion without change of speed. Acceleration is conventionally described by a three-axis system as shown in Fig. 17.2. The acceleration of most interest in military aviation is +/− G_z. Current agile aircraft can easily achieve +9.5G_z at onset rates of over 10 G/s. In these circumstances the limiting factor on the performance of the aircraft is the physiology of the aircrew. There is no evidence that relaxed +G_z tolerance and endurance on simulated air combat manoeuvring to levels up to +7G_z are any different in females than males.[19] In this respect, the shorter stature (and hence smaller heart-eye vertical distance) of females may compensate for lack of physical strength.

Effects of +G_z

The effects of acceleration are exacerbated by heat stress, hypoglycaemia, ingestion of alcohol, hyperventilation and intercurrent infection. Even at +2G_z, there is noticeable difficulty in moving the limbs and the face sags. At levels greater than +3G_z, it is impossible to escape unaided from an aircraft. Movement becomes more difficult as +G_z rises and raising the head once it is flexed becomes impossible at +8G_z even without a helmet. Head movement generally at high G_z is difficult, and will become more so with the new generation of helmets which carry helmet mounted sights and displays and, when required, night vision goggles. Exposure to high G flight causes a temporary diminution in height of up to almost 5 mm due to spinal compression[20] and musculoskeletal symptoms[21] and cervical disc bulges[22] have been reported.

Acceleration in the G_z axis has a hydrostatic effect on the circulation. The mean arterial pressure at the level of the heart is 100 mmHg at both +1 and +4G_z. At eye level, some 30 cm vertically above the heart, the respective pressures are 100 mmHg minus the hydrostatic pressure exerted by the column of blood (22 mmHg at +1G_z and 88 mmHg at +4G_z), i.e. 78 and 12 mmHg. Similarly, the corresponding pressures in the posterior tibial artery, some 80 cm below the heart in the sitting individual, can be calculated to be 157 and 324 mmHg. It is hardly surprising that there are many anecdotal accounts of increased incidents of haemorrhoids in aircrew exposed repeatedly to high +G_z levels.

The blood pressure effects at head level affect vision and the level of consciousness. Eyeball pressure is 20 mmHg. Thus, the blood pressure at head level has to be above that for retinal perfusion to occur. In the relaxed individual, peripheral vision starts to deteriorate

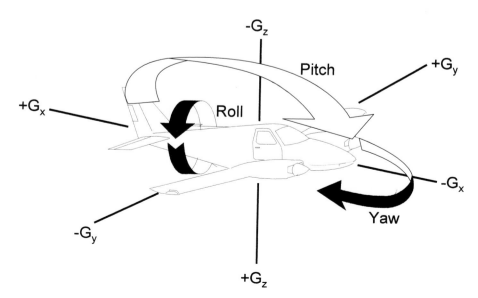

Figure 17.2 *G axes and vectors of motion in aviation.*

at about +3G$_z$ (grey-out) and totally disappears near +4G$_z$. The symptom takes a few seconds to develop because of retinal oxygen stores and at sustained, low rates of +G$_z$ will often recover in a few seconds because of adaptive changes in the circulation. At +5 to +6G$_z$, consciousness is lost (G-induced loss of consciousness, known as G-LOC) but at higher rates of +G$_z$, consciousness can be lost before visual symptoms arise. The incidence of G-LOC is lower than would be predicted because of various physiological mechanisms that tend to maintain regional cerebral perfusion. In one survey, 21% of aircrew reported that they had experienced blackout and 10% reported G-LOC.[23] Not all aircrew who experience G-LOC in centrifuge training remember the episode, so the incidence may be much higher than reported. The US Air Force reported seven fatal aircraft crashes attributed to G-LOC in one 22-year period.[24] Performance in a flight simulator 15 minutes after centrifuge G-LOC was satisfactory in 11 subjects but the 12th crashed.[25]

Below the heart, the effects of +G$_z$ produce pooling of blood in the periphery, transudation of fluid from the blood to the tissues and rupture of unsupported skin capillaries to produce petechiae. The pooling and loss of blood volume eventually produce intense peripheral vasodilation and bradycardia, leading to syncope.

Without an anti-G suit, increasing G$_z$ lowers the diaphragm, increasing the functional residual capacity. Inflation of the abdominal bladder of the anti-G suit reverses this. The closing volume of the lung increases linearly with +G$_z$, and use of an anti-G suit, by raising the diaphragm, increases the number of non-ventilated alveoli in the base of the lung. Thus there is a change to the ventilation/perfusion ratio from the apex to the base of the lung, with the apex tending to be ventilated but underperfused and the base tending to be perfused but underventilated. This is of particular importance when air enriched with oxygen is breathed for it assists in the development of acceleration atelectasis. The increased respiratory work of anti-G straining manoeuvres pro-

duces respiratory fatigue that may contribute to overall tolerance to prolonged +G$_z$.[26]

Negative acceleration (−G$_z$) is experienced during outside loops and spins and inverted flight. Tolerance is much lower than for positive G$_z$. The general effects include heaviness of the limbs, fullness and pressure in the head (which can produce severe headache), congestion of the air passages which can cause difficulty in breathing, bradycardia, epistaxis, eye discomfort, subconjunctival haemorrhages and petechiae in unsupported skin. The transition from −G$_z$ to +G$_z$ (a bunt, sometimes called 'push-pull') can reduce tolerance to +G$_z$[27] which is worsened by the duration of the preceding −G$_z$[28] and has even led to death.[29]

Protection against +G$_z$

The major ways of increasing tolerance to +G$_z$ are by use of an anti-G straining manoeuvre (AGSM), anti-G suits, posture, positive pressure breathing (PPB) and training, or by various combinations of these. The various benefits are summarized in Table 17.1. At high G, if the hands are 20 cm or more below the level of the heart, the rise in venous pressure causes arm pain, which is often worse with PPB.[30] The commonly used AGSMs, which all include isometric muscle tensing, are the M-1 manoeuvre (exhaling forcibly against a partially closed glottis with a rapid inspiration every 4–5 seconds), the L-1 manoeuvre (periods of raised intrathoracic pressure with a closed glottis separated by short inspiratory and expiratory gasps) and the Qigong manoeuvre (rapid panting with tensed muscles).[31]

EXTREMES OF TEMPERATURE

Details on heat and cold can be found in Chapter 15. This chapter will highlight those aspects relevant to flying.

Table 17.1 *Factors influencing grey-out threshold*

Factor	Increase in grey-out threshold (+G$_z$) over relaxed	Cumulative tolerance (+G$_z$)
Relaxed	–	3.0–4.0
Standard anti-G suit	1.0–1.5	4.0–5.5
Anti-G straining manoeuvre	2.0+	7.5+
Extended anti-G suit	2.0	8.0+
30° tilt to seat back	1.0	9.0+
Pressure breathing	2.0+	9.0+

Note that pressure breathing utilizes the same physiological mechanisms for protecting against absolute levels of +G$_z$ as the AGSM. Cumulative protection is not increased but tolerance to time at peak G is increased and fatigue is decreased.

Cold

Exposure to extreme cold may occur when operating at high altitude, in open cockpit aircraft or balloons, on the ground in very cold countries and following accidents in isolated locations. At very low cockpit temperatures, simple oxygen systems run the risk of the freezing open of the expiratory valve because of the accumulation of condensed and frozen water vapour from the expirate. This may lead to hypoxia because the inspiratory resistance of breathing in through a stuck open expiratory valve is less than that of cracking open an inspiratory valve. Most military oxygen systems overcome the problem by design of the expiratory valve, by the use of safety pressure in the mask above certain altitudes (which would lead to continuous flow being sensed and shown on the flow indicator if there was a leakage) and by the use of cockpit heating. Appropriate clothing is required for pilots of vintage, open cockpit aircraft and balloons.

Heat

There are several ways in which a flier may become hot in the aircraft. First, thermal radiation from the sun becomes trapped in the cockpit rather like a greenhouse. In small aircraft, the large relative size of the cockpit transparency exacerbates the problem. Surface temperatures of seats can exceed 60°C. Second, electrical components, of which there are many in military aircraft, consume power inefficiently, radiating heat to the aircrew. Third, aerodynamic heating of the aircraft exterior can conduct heat into the cockpit. Temperatures above 110°C have been recorded on the skin of aircraft flying at high speed and low level. Finally, the aircrew produce heat from their own metabolism. These sources of heat would not be an embarrassment to the aircrew if they were able to dissipate the heat load. Unfortunately, particularly in military aviation, the clothing worn interferes with heat loss by being bulky and insulating and also by incorporating materials impermeable to water vapour, thus preventing sweat evaporation. Moreover, the specialized flying ensemble of military aviators is multi-layered (see Fig. 17.3), increasing the work required to move whilst wearing it. Certainly, deep body temperatures of above 38°C have been measured in aircrew at cockpit temperatures below Wet Bulb Globe Temperature (WBGT) index of 30°C. Laboratory simulations of aircrew wearing ensembles including nuclear, biological chemical (NBC) protection, in cockpit temperatures previously measured in flight, suggest that

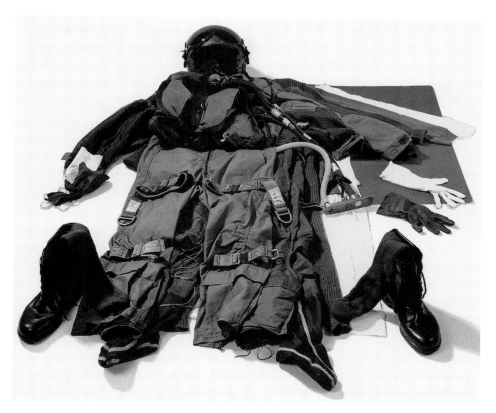

Figure 17.3 *Layers of clothing worn by a military fast-jet (Tornado) pilot in winter. Shown are long-limbed cotton underwear, cotton socks, knitted wool inner coverall, inner immersion coverall with integral immersion bootees, anti-G trousers, external coverall, long-sleeved life preserver with arm restraint system, upper and lower leg restraint garters, inner and outer gloves, boots, helmet and mask. Note that this does not include nuclear, biological, chemical clothing.*

sortie length may be limited in the heat[32] or performance affected.[33]

There are two main approaches to solving the problem of heat in the cockpit – cabin conditioning and personal conditioning systems. The former is frequently not as effective as it could be, occasionally even being de-rated to reduce cockpit noise. Furthermore, the aircrew are insulated from the cooling air by their flying clothing. Personal conditioning systems do have the advantage that the cooling fluid is circulated where it is most required – next to the skin. However, air systems cannot be used in potential NBC conditions and liquid systems, whilst physiologically effective, are not yet in widespread use. Both systems require the aircrew to wear yet another layer of clothing.

NOISE AND VIBRATION

Noise

Noise is covered in Chapter 13. The human tolerance to noise is exceeded in many aircraft with the risks of interference with and deterioration of performance of the flying task, degradations of communication, fatigue and hearing damage. Noise in flight arises from the aircraft power source, subsidiary noise from equipment, flow of air over aircraft surfaces and weapons firing. Sonic booms do not affect the occupants since the aircraft leaves the sonic boom behind. The noise profile will differ between aircraft types, seat positions and profiles flown. Cabin noise levels up to 120 dB have been measured when flying at 480 knots at 250 ft[34] with the highest peaks being in the 0.5–4.0 kHz range. Noise in helicopters is related to the rotors (at about 20 Hz) and the gearbox and transmission chains (from 400 to 600 Hz). In propeller-driven aircraft, the noise is primarily related to the number and the speed of rotation of the propeller blades. In jet passenger aircraft, the major noise contributors are aerodynamic noise and noise from the conditioning systems; the noise in a window seat may be as much as 6 dB higher than in the centre of the aircraft.

Protection is obtained by careful engineering of the aerodynamic properties of the aircraft and (less frequently) of the cabin conditioning system. In military aircraft, the aircrew helmet affords an important degree of protection. Attenuation is generally low at low frequencies but attenuation of 30 dB at 500 Hz to 50 dB at 4 kHz can be achieved. Careful attention to fitting can maximize the attenuation of perceived noise at the ear. In addition, active noise reduction (ANR – a mechanism of destructive interference by sampling the noise field, inverting the phase and then reintroducing it to the headset to cancel the original noise) can produce a further benefit of up to 10 dB. Passengers in noisy aircraft will benefit from the use of earplugs.

Vibration

Vibration is considered in detail in Chapter 14. This chapter will address only those aspects relevant to flying. Complex structures such as human bodies and aircraft can vibrate in one or more of the six geometric degrees of freedom (three rotational: yaw, pitch and roll; three translational: heave, surge and sway). In flying, the sources of vibration are the power source and the air through which the aircraft is travelling.

In helicopters, vibration is generally related to the rotor rate and to the number of rotor blades. The former is generally four revolutions per second, which gives rise to vibration within the helicopter of 4 Hz. The rotor rate multiplied by the number of blades gives the blade pass frequency which can give vibrations generally in the region of 8–20 Hz. Further vibration is generated at higher harmonics of the blade pass rate and also at levels related to the tail rotor. Vibration is usually similar in intensity in each of the x, y and z axes and is worse on transition to the hover. Vibration is one factor that affects helicopter crew comfort but poor seating is another.[35]

In fixed-wing aircraft, the vibration from the engines is usually at a higher frequency than in helicopters. A single-stage turbine usually produces vibration at about 130 Hz while a dual-stage turbine produces 230 Hz. In propeller-driven aircraft the blade-pass frequency is about 100 Hz although desynchronized propellers may give beating at lower frequencies. In fixed-wing aircraft, the atmosphere causes the most noticeable turbulence, for example, during cloud penetration, during low level flight or in 'clear air turbulence'. In military aircraft, the firing of weapons can also give rise to vibration.

The effects of vibration in the aviator can range from imperceptible to inconvenient to unpleasant. The body is least tolerant of vibration between 4 and 8 Hz. The main symptoms limiting tolerance in the laboratory are precordial and abdominal pain. In flying, the most important effect for the pilot is on vision. Outside the aircraft, the image is stable in space and at optical infinity. Other aircraft are unlikely to be moving across the image so fast that they exceed the angular velocity limitations of the pursuit reflex. However, the instrument panel and the pilot's eyes are usually vibrating out of phase. This results in degraded visual acuity. This is often exacerbated when helmet-mounted display systems are in use, particularly at frequencies of 4–6 Hz.[36] At normal levels of vibration in flight, there are no great effects on the cardiovascular system although there may be an increase in metabolic rate reflecting an increase in muscle activity required to maintain posture. It can cause hyperventilation.

A fall in arterial carbon dioxide pressure (P_aCO_2) to less than 25 mmHg has been recorded after 2 minutes of vibration at 9.5 Hz with an acceleration-amplitude of $1G_z$.[37] This is sufficient to reduce cerebral blood flow by 35%.[38] Vibration can also give rise to illusions of motion and to symptoms of motion sickness. It has also been implicated in orthopaedic problems in helicopter aircrew although seating, posture and ergonomic factors undoubtedly also play a part. Certainly, helicopter pilots have a greater incidence of prolapsed intervertebral disc[39] and backache than controls.[40] In addition, casualties from military operations tend to be evacuated by helicopter before definitive surgery. Vibration of unstabilized fractures can cause severe pain and may contribute to complications.

Protection can be afforded against vibration by careful engineering of the aircraft, the use of dynamic vibration absorbers and by vibration isolation of the aircrew seat or of stretcher mounts. Casualties evacuated by helicopter must be given adequate analgesia and their fractures adequately stabilized. Finally, if the source of vibration is turbulent air, the effects may be minimized by routing away from it, changing cruising altitude and by ensuring passengers remain in their seats with seat belts fastened.

VISION

The importance of vision in aviation was first recognized during the First World War.[41] Despite the increase in equipment to improve flight safety, vision is still important in collision avoidance and target identification. Intact colour vision is more than ever necessary in the 'glass cockpit' where displays and warnings are presented in more and more hues. Aircrew need to be protected from insults such as glare, lasers and chemicals with the addition of birdstrike, blast, explosive devices and nuclear flash in military aircraft. Visual illusions are covered later in this chapter.

When there are no visual clues, the eye tends to focus at a point 1–2 m away. This functional short sight, called empty field myopia, can reduce the chances of a pilot seeing another aircraft, since objects at infinity are blurred. This is an important cause of road accidents in fog. Pilots should be trained to look at their wing tips from time to time to relax their accommodation. If a pilot looks at his instruments and then outside again, his gaze can be distracted for 2.5 seconds or more and the requirement to refocus frequently from infinity to near vision can be fatiguing. It was for these reasons that the first Head-Up Display (HUD – where the instrument image is produced on a glass screen in front of the pilot, focused at infinity) was developed for the Beaufighter in the Second World War.[42] It can take up to 5 seconds from the time an image first falls on the pilot's retina for an aircraft to change course. During this time, it can cover almost a mile if travelling at 500 knots. However, if two aircraft are on a collision course, they will remain on a constant bearing from each other, thus denying the pilots the stimulus of a moving object in the visual field.

Objects are more easily seen in the peripheral visual fields, especially if they are moving. Tracking is optimal up to 30 degrees per second but visual acuity is halved at 40 degrees per second. Pilots must therefore be trained to maintain a good lookout at all times.

Spectacles and contact lenses

Approximately 27% of pilots, 51% of navigators and 40% of other aircrew in the US Air Force need to wear spectacles. Over 12% need bifocals.[43] Evidence suggests that there is no difference in civil accident rates or in US Naval carrier landing accidents in pilots who wear visual correction.[44]

Corrective flying spectacles need to provide as wide a visual field as possible and must be capable of integration with the rest of the aircrew equipment without impairment of hearing protection or interference with the seal of an oxygen mask. They must be comfortable, resistant to fogging, minimize internal reflections and not move under conditions of vibration or G. Tinted spectacles should not be worn with tinted visors (see below). Photochromatic lenses are not yet sufficiently reactive to respond quickly enough on entering a cloud layer from high sunlight. Many military aircrew have reported losing a lens from their spectacles in flight. It seems sensible to carry a spare pair. In the RAF, most spectacles and helmets are retained on the head during ejection. In the US Air Force, on the other hand, sorties were flown higher with clear visors up and up to 80% lost their eyewear.[45]

Both soft and hard contact lenses have been used in flight. High water content soft contact lenses are preferred in the low humidity of aircraft cockpits but hard contact lenses are still required in some conditions such as keratoconus. Rigid, gas-permeable lenses may offer advantages for this group in the future. The major difficulties quoted in flight are foreign body incursion and movement off-centre. In both of these, the incidence is greater for hard than soft contact lenses.[46] The greatest difficulty experienced in the Gulf War related to resupply problems with replacement lenses.[47] Some US Air Force aircrew have lost soft or hard lenses during ejection but the overall experience is small.[45] Radial keratotomy (RK) is incompatible with aircrew status because of the unpredictability of the outcome, daily fluctuations of visual acuity, glare and altitude induced changes. Excimer laser photorefractive keratotomy (PRK)[48] produces haze, glare and halos for 3–6 months and unstable refraction for 1 year (more in high myopes). There is a residual refractive error in 40% of cases. After 2 years, 10% still complain of glare at night. Therefore, PRK cannot therefore be recommended yet for the active aviator. There is not yet enough experience with laser in situ keratomileusis (LASIK) for its use to be recommended for professional aviators.

Night vision

During the Second World War, interceptors had to pick up their targets before they themselves were spotted, bomb-aimers needed to be able to place their bombs accurately despite the attentions of searchlights and tracer and pilots had to be capable of judging their landings correctly on darkened airfields. Thus, 'Night flying brings out in intensified form the difficulties of day flying'.[49] Much effort was given to dark adaptation of aircrew before take-off.

The relatively recent introduction of night vision goggles has changed things but has introduced new problems. Some accidents have been directly linked to their use. In effect, they present an isochromatic view of the world limited in contrast and detail. Visual acuity and visual fields are both degraded. For example, switching from forward-looking infra-red to night vision goggles gives a 4 second visual loss, a twofold reduction in visual acuity and a threefold reduction in contrast sensitivity.[50] The cockpit lighting needs to be compatible with the use of such devices. Careful fitting and training are required. In one study, training improved visual acuity from 6/15 to 6/12.[51]

Eye protection

In civil flight and military transport aircraft, sunglasses give protection from glare, while in high performance aircraft, visors attached to the helmet provide protection. Sunglasses and visors should have a transmittance of 10–15%. In addition to increasing visual acuity in bright sunlight, they also protect the eye from the effects of ultraviolet light.

Lasers, for example from sound and light shows, are more of a problem. The international aviation community is attempting to minimize the problem by legislation controlling the use of such devices near airfields. In military flying, lasers are used for target designation and thus may be deliberately aimed at aircraft. Protection is best provided by distance but visor coatings designed to protect against specific wavelengths may be necessary. These have the disadvantages that they only protect against specific threats, they produce a blending of surface colours and loss of terrain features, a reduction in depth perception and difficulties with warning lights and displays, maps and weapons displays.[52]

Military fast-jet aircrew usually wear helmets whose polycarbonate visors (one clear, one tinted) afford protection against glare, birdstrike and blast. Ideally the cockpit transparency should be tough enough to withstand birdstrike but this often conflicts with the need for rapid escape in an emergency. About 85% of birdstrikes occur below 500 ft[53] and the clear visor should be selected down for take-off, landings and high speed, low-level flight. Figure 17.4 shows the damage that may be caused by a small bird. The clear visor can also protect against lead spatter from canopy fragmentation devices used to clear the ejection path. Although lead spatter usually causes superficial damage only, cases of ocular penetration have occurred.

The fireball from a nuclear explosion can cause direct and indirect flash blindness and may even cause a retinal burn. The problem is worse at night when, theoretically, a pilot could be effectively blind for as long as a minute after exposure. Various protective devices have been proposed, ranging from an eyepatch which could be raised after exposure to complex electro-optical devices. For example, a sandwich of lead lanthanum zirconate titanate (PLZT) between two polarizers with their planes of polarization set at right angles to each other rotates the plane of polarization when a voltage is applied so that light is transmitted. When a flash stimulates a photodiode, the voltage is withdrawn so that light is no longer transmitted. Unfortunately PLZT is complex, expensive and has relatively low transmittance in the normal state.

Visors form an integral part of the overall protection against windblast during the ejection sequence. Design of the ensemble of helmet, visor and mask is important so that they remain on the head during ejection. Current RAF systems provide adequate protection up to 650 knots. Overall, sunglasses and visors should give as wide a field of vision as possible. The optical quality should be high and it may be necessary to incorporate anti-scratch and anti-reflection coatings.

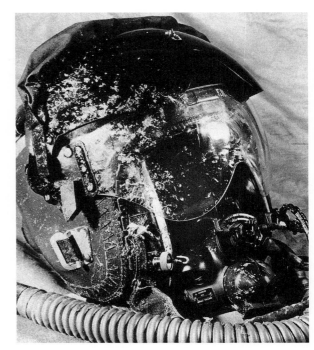

Figure 17.4 *Damage to a clear visor caused by bird strike penetrating the canopy of a Hawk aircraft flying at high speed and low level (Crown Copyright).*

SPATIAL DISORIENTATION

Spatial disorientation occurs when a pilot does not sense correctly the position relative to the ground, motion or attitude of himself or his aircraft. The broader term 'situational awareness' is taken to include a tactical appreciation of the position of other aircraft as well as a sense of geographical location. Spatial disorientation is caused by inadequate or erroneous cues to the brain and by central processing errors such as errors of perception or coning or attention.

Spatial disorientation is a significant cause of aircraft accidents. A major precipitating cause, particularly in private flying, is by continued flight into adverse weather. The majority of accidents occur in poor visibility, when the pilot may not be aware that his interpretation of aircraft attitude is incorrect, but some occur in good conditions when visual cues are misinterpreted. The type of incident where the pilot is aware that there is a mismatch between his aircraft instruments and what his brain is telling him is less likely, with appropriate training, to lead to an accident. Spatial disorientation is more likely in poor weather, at night, at high altitude and during flight over sea or featureless terrain. Certain flight manoeuvres contribute, such as prolonged linear acceleration or deceleration and prolonged angular motion particularly when combined with head movement. Transfer to Instrument Meteorological Conditions (IMC) when landing in helicopters, when the downwash from the rotor kicks up dust or snow, is also a potent cause of spatial disorientation. Sub-threshold changes in attitude are unlikely to be detected and thus can also lead to spatial disorientation. At times when the pilot has a high workload, or when he is undergoing treatment with certain drugs or when he has an upper respiratory tract infection, spatial disorientation is more likely to occur.

Types of illusion

Illusions may be caused by false information from the otoliths and kinaesthetic receptors during sustained acceleration (somatogravic illusions), on moving the head in an atypical force environment (G excess illusions), from the semicircular canals on recovery from prolonged rotation (somatogyral illusions) and on moving the head during rotation (cross-coupled or Coriolis illusions).

Man is habituated to expecting any sustained acceleration to be due to gravity. When a sustained acceleration is applied, the resultant combined acceleration is interpreted as the vertical. For example, when an aircraft accelerates on take-off, the resultant acceleration from the rearward inertial force and downwards gravity is between the two; the pilot senses this resultant force and mentally orientates it so that it is vertical. He thus senses that the aircraft nose is high and tends to want to push the stick forwards. A brief G_x acceleration of 5 G for 2–3 seconds, such as occurs in a catapult launch from an aircraft carrier, gives an apparent nose-up attitude of 5 degrees for a minute or more.[54] There is little time to overcome this particular illusion on take-off. If the pilot pushes the stick forward, he introduces a radial acceleration that will make matters worse. When performed at high altitude, pilots approaching the vertical in this bunt manoeuvre have reported feeling as if the aircraft was flipped on its back. Similarly, a pilot in a flat turn will feel as if he has rolled out of the turn and a pilot in a banked turn may feel himself to be level. Head movement during these manoeuvres can induce further illusions.

When external visual cues are inadequate, for example at night, the apparent movement of light sources in the external environment may be interpreted as a change in attitude of the aircraft. For example, during linear acceleration, the backward rotation of the resultant force vector may make a bright star appear to move upwards. This may be interpreted as a nose-down change in the aircraft attitude.

One of the most common illusions is 'the leans'. If a pilot is in a gentle turn to the right, at a rate below that which would stimulate the otoliths, he could feel that the wings are level. If he then rolls wings level abruptly, he can feel that he is banking to the left. Even though this can be recognized as level flight on the instruments, there is a distinct temptation to lean to align the body with the perceived vertical.

In the same way that the otoliths can misinterpret linear accelerations, so can the semicircular canals misinterpret angular accelerations in yaw, pitch and roll. At constant angular speed the body's sensors will only give the correct information during the first few seconds of the manoeuvre. During recovery from a prolonged spin, not only is there a somatogyral illusion that the aircraft is turning in the opposite direction but vision may also be degraded by the nystagmus induced by the spin; this will make reading of instruments difficult at a critical time. In reduced light conditions, oculogyric illusions may occur with an illusory perception of movement of an isolated light.

Movement of the head during angular accelerations can produce quite compelling sensations of movement by cross-coupled or Coriolis forces. For example, a head movement in roll from 45° left to 45° right whilst rotating at a steady speed about the z body axis will produce a strong sense of pitching forward. In new, highly manoeuvrable aircraft, there is a potential for cross-coupling illusions independent of pilot head motion.[55]

Imbalance between middle ear pressure on ascent or descent can also cause vertigo which, although usually lasting only seconds, can last minutes. It is more common when there is a respiratory tract infection. The flicker of propellers or rotor blades has also caused vertigo and nausea but the more usual presentation is irritation.

Occasionally, pilots in single seat aircraft at high altitude report a feeling of detachment, isolation or remoteness from the aircraft. Some even describe it as an 'out-of-body' experience, watching themselves controlling the aircraft. A similar 'break-off phenomenon' has been described in helicopters flying at lower altitudes but in conditions of limited visual cues.

Another form of misinterpretation is caused by the error of expectancy. When flying in cloud, the cloud is brighter in the direction of the sun. The brain interprets this direction as 'up' and stimulates the pilot to 'lean on the sun'. Another example of expectancy is when lights on fishing boats at night are interpreted as stars, which are expected to be above the aircraft; the pilot then inverts the aeroplane. Other errors can occur when interpreting heights of mountains or trees, in misinterpreting a short runway as a longer one seen from a greater height or in assuming a sloping cloudbank to be the horizontal.

Incidence

Spatial disorientation is surprisingly common. In one survey of Royal Navy helicopter pilots, only 2% stated that they had never been disorientated in flight and 68% had experienced more than ten incidents in their flying career.[56] Almost 70% of fixed-wing, military pilots reported experiencing 'the leans', 33% recorded break-off and 12% reported target fixation resulting in flying too close to the ground.[57] Similar estimates are not available for general aviation pilots although confidential reporting for commercial flights gives a much lower incidence.

Protection

There are some aircraft factors that can help to reduce spatial disorientation. The instruments should be reliable and able to be read clearly and unambiguously by day and night. The instruments should be able to cope with the manoeuvres flown by the aircraft and the conditions in which it will operate. A head-up display will also help. The instruments should be laid out so that they can be read without undue head movement.

Aircrew factors include rejection for licensing of those likely to be affected by spatial disorientation, for example those with Ménière's disease. Aircrew should not fly whilst suffering from upper respiratory tract infections or acute labyrinthitis, nor should they fly whilst taking medications whose potential side-effects include nausea, vertigo or sensory disturbance. Alcohol has been shown to compromise a pilot's ability to detect angular acceleration and this may continue even after blood alcohol level reaches zero.[58]

Training, in the air as well as on the ground, plays a major part in preventing spatial disorientation. Instrument flying must be continually practised. In military aviation, spatial disorientation familiarization devices used on the ground can give valuable experience in the various illusions that occur during flight.

AIR SICKNESS

Air sickness is a normal response to flying in the unadapted individual. The incidence is related to the intensity of the motion stimulus, the frequency spectrum of the motion and the time of exposure. The condition may have significant effects on flight safety. It is most commonly experienced during flying training, when the instructor may misinterpret the quietness and withdrawal it produces as disinterest or inaptitude. Severe airsickness in a trained aviator is uncommon unless the stimulus is unduly provocative, for example during flights to study hurricanes. Commercial flying as a passenger does not induce much airsickness but paratroopers or special forces, who may be flown tactically in more adverse weather may be particularly affected. Their performance on the ground immediately after landing may suffer adverse consequences.

Some people may not be affected at all, some may experience minor inconvenience whilst others will be prostrated. In addition to individual susceptibility, there is a gradual decrease in susceptibility with increasing age from 12 years onwards. Females are more susceptible than males. There is an indication that foods high in protein predispose males to airsickness, while a similar effect is seen in females for foods high in sodium such as preserved meat.[59]

Symptoms

The condition does not differ essentially from any of the other forms of motion sickness and presents commonly as nausea, vomiting, pallor and cold sweating. The first symptom is usually epigastric awareness, which progresses to nausea. Cold sweating with facial pallor then occurs. There is then a crescendo of symptoms (the avalanche phenomenon) with increased salivation, lightheadedness, yawning and often depression and apathy. Vomiting then follows, which often temporarily improves the symptoms. Feelings of lethargy and drowsiness can last for some hours after landing.

Prevention and treatment

The best treatment is adaptation, particularly for aircrew who should not fly whilst taking drugs for airsickness. Flying training should introduce exposure to the more adventurous flight manoeuvres gradually. Return to flying after a period away should follow the same principle. The distraction of flying the aircraft or other demanding mental activity rather than being a passenger often keeps the symptoms at bay. However, reading does not help because of the risk of introducing anomalous visual cues. Passengers generally can reduce their incidence by closing the eyes and limiting movement of the head.

About 5% of aircrew do not manage to adapt by normal means. In the RAF, about 85% of these have been salvaged by a programme of increasing exposure to cross-coupled stimuli on the ground before a similarly progressive exposure to aerobatic flight in a dual controlled aircraft.[60] More recent work has suggested that it is the number of challenges rather than the severity of malaise achieved that is the important factor determining habituation.[61]

The number of remedies available is large but none can completely prevent all persons from experiencing airsickness in all conditions. One of the most effective drugs is L-hyoscine hydrobromide (L-scopolamine hydrobromide in the USA; Kwells®). In conditions where 10% of the population would be airsick, 0.4 mg of the drug can increase protection so that only 2% suffer symptoms. In more severe conditions, when 50% would be sick untreated, 1.0 mg of the drug can provide protection for all but 8%.[62] Unfortunately, most of the drugs used have side-effects unacceptable for use by aircrew. Hyoscine can cause blurred vision, dry mouth, sedation, dizziness and significant performance decrements. Promethazine (Phenergan,® Avomine®) 25 mg can also impair psychomotor performance. Dimenhydrinate (Dramamine®, Gravol®) is a central depressant. For short-term protection in passengers, oral L-hyoscine hydrobromide (0.3–0.6 mg) is the drug of choice. For longer benefit, transdermal administration of hyoscine by patch may be useful if placed at least 6 h before protection is needed. Antihistaminic drugs like cinnarizine (Stugeron®) give protection for 6 h while related drugs, for example, promethazine can give protection for 12 h. Recent developments, such as wristbands claimed to work by pressure on the acupoints, have not proved effective.

JET LAG

Rapid and large time zone changes, coupled with sleep disturbance related to overnight flights, are particularly important in flying. Chapter 29 addresses the subject of shift work and extended hours of work. For the short-haul pilot, who has frequent early departures, late arrivals and night flights, sleep deficit generally accumulates until the night work ceases.[63] The long-haul pilot is affected by irregular hours of work as well as by time zone changes. On a 2-day layover after west transatlantic flight, aircrew experienced extended awake spans, increased sleepiness and a slow recovery on return home.[64] Older people tend to be more affected than younger individuals.

Time zone changes may lead to lethargy, loss of appetite, a general feeling of malaise and disruption to the normal pattern and quality of sleep. Until rhythms are resynchronized, the nadir of psychomotor perfor-

mance no longer coincides with sleep. After flight westward, when the normal sleep onset is delayed, individuals tend to fall asleep quickly and sleep more deeply. Sleep later in the night is more disturbed. By the third night, the sleep pattern is more adapted to the new time zone and this is reflected in daytime alertness and general wellbeing. Eastward flights impose an advanced sleep onset time. If sleep during the flight and during daytime at the destination is avoided, the first night's sleep may be good. However, once the immediate effects of sleep loss are overcome, the sleep pattern does not adapt to local time for several days. Sleep quality is reduced and there are more night-time awakenings. In one pilot operating an eastward schedule for one month, almost half of his sleep periods were 5 h or less.[63]

Protection

Airline scheduling is largely governed by commercial factors. In an ideal world, an overnight, eastward flight after a period of desynchronization caused by the flight west, would be timed to arrive when alertness and performance would be expected to be high. However, this is not always possible and flight safety is maintained by imposing statutory flight time limitations. Figure 17.5 shows one method of estimating acceptable and unacceptable duty times.[65] For aircrew required to work overnight, an anticipatory sleep of about 4 h in the afternoon or evening will improve overnight performance.

For the statesman or businessman, there are two ways of limiting the effects of time zone changes. One is to time the trip so that adaptation to the local time zone is complete by the time important business is transacted and to allow adequate time for recovery on return. Another is to travel by supersonic aircraft, conduct the business and then return by supersonic aircraft; adaptation to a new time zone is therefore unnecessary. For those who have neither the time nor the money to adopt these techniques, napping when necessary and the use of hypnotics may be the only answer.

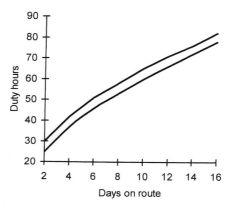

Figure 17.5 *Duty time compatible with effective sleep (lower line); upper line is limit above which effective sleep is unlikely. After Ref 65.*

Hypnotics have been used for some years in the RAF to impose sleep at unusual times or in unusual conditions. A rapidly absorbed drug with a short half-life, such as temazepam 10–20 mg has been found to have an acceptable margin of safety when used sparingly. It was used successfully in the Falklands campaign[66] and in the Gulf War. Psychostimulants have not been used by the RAF since the Second World War but dextroamphetamine (5 mg every 2–4 h) has been used extensively and effectively by the US Air Force.[67,68] More recently, attention has been focused on the use of melatonin, which has been reported to prevent jet lag symptoms in east and west transmeridian flight.[69] A dose of 10 mg can advance bed and rise times by 2–3 hours and maintain sleep duration between 7–8 hours compared with placebo and produces fewer performance errors on awakening than placebo.[70] Another stimulant that shows potential is pemoline (20 mg).[71]

FOOD AND DRINK

Food

Food has been recognized as an important factor in flight safety from the earliest days of flying.[72] First, gastrointestinal upsets are the commonest cause of in-flight incapacitation.[73] For this reason, flightdeck crew must select different menu items for meals both in-flight and when down the route. In addition, it is sensible, for obvious reasons, for the flightdeck crew to stagger their times of eating when in flight. Second, hypoglycaemia can reduce tolerance to $+G_z$ and has been cited as a significant finding in more than 50% of incidents of unconsciousness in the air.[74] This has led to a requirement to eat sensibly before flying and to provide in-flight rations during long flights.

Drink

The cabin air of all aircraft, and the breathing mixture provided by military aircraft oxygen systems, are dry. This, combined with fluid shifts in the body caused by sitting for long periods, produces dehydration.[75] In turn, dehydration can affect tolerance to $+G_z$ and to heat load and may contribute to an increased risk of deep venous thrombosis.[76] An adequate fluid intake on long flights is therefore important.

Professional pilots often have a drinking culture.[77] However, alcohol in large quantities is not sensible. Not only does alcohol itself contribute to dehydration, but it also affects performance, tolerance to $+G_z$, incidence of decompression sickness and can potentiate spatial disorientation. Most airlines and military air forces impose a 'bottle to throttle' time. The usual time allowance, of 8–12 h, could be considered insufficiently stringent bearing in mind its continuing contribution to accident rates.[78,79]

EXPOSURE TO CHEMICALS

Ordinarily, the aviator should not be exposed to noxious chemicals. However, there are four main circumstances in which exposure may occur: toxic fumes in the cockpit, fire, aircraft crash and deliberate release, for example crop spraying or when attacked by chemical warfare agents. The chemicals involved at a crash site include aviation fuels, hydraulic fluid, metals such as cadmium, beryllium, chromium, mercury and their salts, plastic resins and surface coatings and products of combustion. Unexploded ordnance like ejection seat cartridges when ejection was not initiated, may also be present.

Protection against toxic fumes in the cockpit is given by use of an oxygen system with 100% oxygen selected. Gas chromatography of blood samples taken as soon as possible after landing may identify the chemicals concerned. Exposure of crop sprayers to chemicals may require skin decontamination and systemic treatment.[80] Protection of aircrew against chemical warfare agents is provided by a spectrum of training, deployment of detection devices, a reporting system, protective clothing including respirators which maintain a positive internal pressure to prevent inward leaks, decontamination schedules, filtered accommodation for briefing and rest and, finally, medical treatment if required. Pyridostigmine 30 mg every 8 h may be given as pre-exposure treatment against some nerve agents.

EXPOSURE TO RADIATION

Radiation generally is covered in Chapter 19.

The atmosphere provides much of the protection against galactic radiation. Thus, it is hardly surprising that Concord crews have been shown to be exposed to twice the dose experienced by aircrew flying ordinary passenger aircraft. However, even this dose of 6 mSv is still less than one-third of the maximum allowable dose for radiation workers[81] although draft European Community Directive 96/27 identifies aircrew as 'exposed workers' who should have an annual exposure of less than 6.0 mSv.[82] The annual average for long-haul cabin crews flying the MD-11 has been reported to be 2.27 mSv.[82] Whilst there are reports that some cabin attendants have an increased risk of breast cancer[83], other factors than radiation could have contributed, such as heavy use of high-oestrogen oral contraceptives in the 1970s, delay in first pregnancy and delayed breast feeding. Current employment practice should lessen the impact of these factors in the present cohort of female attendants although, if pregnant, their fetuses may be exposed to more than the recommended total of 2.0 mSv.[84]

AIRCRAFT ACCIDENTS

Aircraft crashes are, fortunately, relatively rare events. Commercial flying is the safest form of mass transport.

Military flying, when conducted at high speed and low level, is inherently more dangerous but the risks are reduced by meticulous planning and training. Crashes can occur following engineering or design failure but most are caused by human factors that may include physiological or psychological causes. Spatial disorientation was a major contributing factor in 20% of one series of military aircraft crashes.[85] Aircraft are also used as a method of committing suicide.[86,87] The majority of crashes occur in the vicinity of an airfield, being related to take-off or landing. Many crashes occur during training; in one series of civilian crashes, an instructor was present for 50% of crashes following stalls and 32% of those resulting from fuel mismanagement.[88]

Most accidents involve ground impact. Injury can result from sudden deceleration, crushing loads on the fuselage, break-up of the floor structure or by fire. Protection from mechanical forces is given by restraint harnesses and, in military aircraft, energy-attenuating seating. The more efficient the restraint in the seat, the higher is the likelihood of survival. In one study of fire in 134 fatal civil aircraft accidents, 360 individuals had insignificant antemortem injury but carboxyhaemoglobin levels of more than 20%, enough to impair chances of escape.[89] Almost 60% of fires start during the impact sequence with another 17% occurring after the aircraft has come to rest. Terrain, bad weather and the dark then hamper rescue.[90] Smoke hoods for passengers have been developed but are still not in use by airlines.[91] Fire and crash sites are controlled by incident commanders who restrict access depending on risk.

Many military aircraft have ejection seats that can allow the aviator to be on a fully deployed parachute within 3 seconds of initiating ejection. The risks are of not initiating ejection soon enough, of back injury as a result of the forces of ejection, of collision with canopy or canopy fragments, windblast and flail injuries and landing injury. The design of the seat, the use of miniature detonating cord to fragment the canopy to clear the escape path and use of leg and arm restraint can minimize the risks. The miniature detonating cord can cause lead spatter to the face and eyes but this is not usually serious. Injury can occur during ejection, with anterior wedge fractures of the thoracolumbar region being most common. The risk is greater with taller and heavier aircrew,[92] although the risks to smaller, lighter (i.e. female) aircrew are not fully understood. After ejection, a full spinal radiographic screen from C1 to the sacrum should be carried out. Even with a negative screen, MRI or isotope bone scan will often demonstrate 'hot spots' indicative of fresh bony injury. Treatment is by total bed rest for 3 weeks in hospital, then gradual mobilization. Resumption of flying on ejection seats is possible after 3 months.

Escape from helicopters offers different challenges. Up to half of military helicopter accidents involve ditching in water.[93] The problems of escape include physical restriction from equipment or trapped air, limited air supply, poor underwater visibility, exit design and fear. The solutions include comprehensive training in a crash simulator, better design of exits and hatches, more streamlined personal equipment, underwater lighting and breathing aids.[94] The success rate of helicopter crashes over land depends on height and whether or not autorotation was possible. The death rate is increased by not using the shoulder restraint harness.[95]

SPACEFLIGHT

Spaceflight is an extreme form of flight at high altitude, experienced so far by a tiny minority of the population. Since Yuri Gagarin's first flight in 1961, over 500 men and women of more than 20 nations have spent a total of more than 12 000 days in space. Cosmonaut Valeriy Polyakov holds the record of 439 days spent continuously in space; the equivalent female record is 174 days by Yelena Kondova. The Apollo series of 11 missions had 29 astronauts spending over 600 man-hours on the moon's surface. In the period 1999–2001, there will be an increase in extra-vehicular activity to 240 hours a year (from an average of 50 hours in 1997 and 20 hours in 1995 and 1996) during the building of the Space Station. Longer periods in space should follow with the eventual expectation of manned trips to the nearer planets. The major irritating aspects of living in cramped environments are a relative lack of water, the inability to move freely, boredom and psychosocial factors.

Risks

So far, 13 astronauts and cosmonauts have died in spacecraft (seven in the Challenger accident, three in a flash fire during ground training, two in a rapid decompression and one on ground impact when the parachute did not deploy properly). In addition, several more have been killed in aircraft crashes during training. The clinical hazards of being in space are hypoxia, oxygen toxicity, decompression sickness, radiation and space motion sickness. As a consequence of working in spacecraft, personnel are exposed also to risks of collision with other orbiting objects or micrometeoroids, electric shock, trauma, thermal injury, burns and toxic contamination. Moreover, astronauts are expected to stay fit. In the US astronaut corps, averaging 90 individuals, there were 26 fractures and 36 serious ligamentous injuries in an 8-year period; the remedy is less running and competitive sport and more swimming.[96]

Outside barometric pressure is less than 1 mmHg and the temperature can range from +1500°C to −130°C. Re-entry can give rise to temperatures in the heat shield of more than 3000°C. G forces during launch are up to +4G_x (with the astronauts lying on their backs). During re-entry, the G exposure is -1.2 G_x for 17 minutes in the Space Shuttle and 3.0–4.0 G for Soyuz.[97] In orbit G forces range from 1×10^{-4} to 1×10^{-5} G with a rise to 1×10^{-3} G during some in-flight manoeuvres. Exposure to radiation comes from galactic radiation (protons, alpha particles and some heavy metal nuclei), solar radiation (mainly X-rays and high energy electrons and protons) and trapped radiation in the van Allen belts (energetic neutrons). Data suggest that space station personnel will receive 0.3 Sv (sieverts) in the worst case on a 180-day mission,[98] while measurements from Mir showed equivalent dose rates varying from 0.416 to 0.604 mSv per day.[99] Results from Skylab suggest that an astronaut could fly an 84-day mission annually for 25 years before reaching the career limit for radiation to the testis. Damage to the spacecraft, and thus risk to the crew, may be expected from micrometeoroids. A test area of 1200 cm^2 on Skylab was hit twice a day. Although the largest was estimated to be over 10 cm diameter, the wall was not breached.

There have been several toxic contamination incidents during the space programme. Nitrogen tetroxide was released in an Apollo capsule after decoupling from the Soyuz in a link-up in 1975; the three crewmembers suffered a pneumonitis and one even lost consciousness for a short while, despite donning oxygen masks quickly. Contaminants arise from hardware off-gassing, crew and microbial metabolism, leakage from fluid systems and payload experiments and from overheating. The major contaminants are non-toxic alcohols, ketones, alkanes, halocarbons and siloxanes. Occasional contaminants included methanol, acetaldehyde, tetrachloroethane and benzene.[100] Generally, the aggregate toxicity showed that air quality met acceptable limits. The risk of minor toxicological incidents was put at about 30% with a 3% risk of moderate incidents.

Space motion sickness is identical in presentation to ordinary motion sickness. However, about 30% of participants are affected rising to 50% in larger spacecraft. Adaptation takes 3–4 days. Microgravity causes a redistribution of body fluids in the first few days; one indication is a rise in eyeball pressure in the first few minutes.[101] This produces a 30% reduction in limb circumference and a feeling of nasal stuffiness and facial fullness. The increased fluid in the chest is interpreted by atrial stretch receptors as an increased circulating blood volume and this stimulates a diuresis. There is a fall in left ventricular mass and stroke volume that stabilizes after 2–3 months. These contribute to reduced orthostatic tolerance on return to Earth. Muscle atrophy (a reduction in size ranging from 4–11% in postural muscles after an 8-day mission[102]) and bone demineralization (about 8% in the calcaneum) occur and are linked to time in microgravity. Urinary nitrogen excretion rises by 25% and urinary calcium loss doubles. This last, together with dehydration, may dispose to renal stone; one such case has occurred in the Russian space programme.[103] There is

evidence of a decline in testicular androgens with a corresponding diminution in libido.[104] Muscular efficiency declines and there is a tendency to fatigue. All changes are reversible in days to months on return to Earth.

Medical problems have proved to be reassuringly few. Missions have been terminated thrice on medical grounds, once with a cardiac dysrhythmia, once with chronic prostatitis and once with intractable headaches. Problems are likely to have been minimized by careful selection. However, astronauts and cosmonauts have experienced adjustment and psychosomatic reactions, mood and thought disorders, post-mission personality change and martial problems. Folliculitis has developed where pressure, friction and moisture have combined to macerate the skin. Halitosis and gingivitis occurred until facilities for oral hygiene were introduced. Cardiac arrhythmia was noted during Apollo 15, which was thought to be a combination of dietary potassium deficiency before take-off and an exhausting extravehicular activity.

Protection

Protection against many of the potential stresses is given by the spacecraft and by the spacesuit. The spacecraft provides passive shielding against radiation and micrometeorites and its atmospheric control and waste management systems provide a habitable environment. The spacesuit controls breathing gases, temperature and humidity, provides waste management, protection against radiation and micrometeorites, communications, a propulsion system and the vital manoeuvrability to allow work to be performed. It has been calculated that a man should be able to carry up to 170% of his body mass for 8 hours without undue fatigue on the Moon and 50% on Mars.[106] This may limit the size and weight of the protective equipment provided. The Apollo Portable Life Support System weighed up to 86 kg. To minimize the time spent pre-breathing oxygen to protect against decompression sickness before extravehicular activity, the Space Shuttle decompresses to 10 000 ft cabin altitude and increases the PO_2 to a 3000 ft equivalent for 12 hours before extra-vehicular activity, following which the astronaut pre-breathes 100% oxygen before final depressurization to 222 mmHg for extravehicular activity.

Problems have been minimized by careful selection and training of astronauts, meticulous health care in the final few days before launch and by the provision of a medical kit on board. The Space Shuttle carried anti-dysrhythmic drugs and the crew take potassium supplements. The most commonly used medicaments have been painkillers, sedatives, nasal decongestants and anti-diarrhoeal preparations.[97] After the moon landings, the crews, their equipment and the module were quarantined for 21 days and the samples were isolated for up to 80 days. No microorganisms were ever isolated. The muscular changes are limited by providing exercise facil-

Table 17.2 *Types of Civil Aviation Authority medical certificate with period of validity*

Class	Applicability	Age at examination (years)	Validity (months)
1	Airline transport/ commercial pilot	40+	6
		<40	12
	Basic commercial pilot with public transport privileges		12
	Flight navigator		12
	Flight engineer		12
	Commercial airship pilot		12
		<40	24
	Air traffic control officer	40+	12
2	Flying instructors, Commercial balloon licence (public transport), ATCO (aerodrome control) licence	<40	24
		40–59	12
		60+	6
3	Student and private pilot licence, Commercial balloon licence (aerial work privileges), Self-launching motor glider pilot licence	<40	60
		40–49	24
		50–69	12
		70+	6

Adapted from the Civil Aviation Authority Guidance Notes for Aeromedical Examiners – June 1996.
Note that Class I licences are also valid for flying under Classes 2 and 3. Similarly, Class 2 licences are also valid for Class 3 flying.

ities on board. In-flight cardiac deconditioning and orthostatic intolerance on return is also helped by exposure in flight to lower body negative pressure. Tolerance to the gravitational stress of re-entry may also be aided by fluid loading beforehand.[107]

FITNESS FOR FLIGHT

It is a generally accepted principle that not only should aircrew be protected against the rigours of the aviation environment but also that the general public should be protected from accidents caused by aircrew illness. This is achieved by agreeing to medical standards that are the minimum compatible with professional flying. Aircrew who meet those standards are then selected for training. They are required to be not abnormally susceptible to the stresses of flying, either by disease or by unusual physiological response. Once the aircrew are trained, they are regularly examined to ensure that they continue to meet medical standards. Military aircrew are subject to the standards imposed by their parent armed force. Civilian aircrew in the UK are subject to licensing by the Civil Aviation Authority. Details are shown in Table 17.2.

The formation of the Special Royal Flying Corps Medical Board in 1916 significantly improved the proportion of candidates who passed flying training.[108] Nowadays it can cost over £1 million to train a military fast-jet pilot. The aircraft he flies can cost up to 100 times that figure. Moreover, medical factors frequently feature in accident reports. One study cited medical factors as causing or contributing to 4.7% of fatal accidents.[78] Aviation medicine policy must therefore balance the risks to individual health, flying safety and mission completion against conservation of resources, flying experience and training costs. Civilian aviation authorities have set a goal of one fatal accident in multicrew aircraft in each 10^7 flying hours.[109] If the medical contribution to this is an arbitrary 10%, then incapacitation in flight should cause an accident no more than once in every 10^8 flying hours. This is attainable if the risk to an individual pilot of incapacitation is less than 1% a year.[110] The actual figure for the US Air Force over a 10-year period was 1.9 in 10^7 flying hours.[111]

To allow any aircrew to fly with particular medical conditions, the following criteria must be satisfied:

- There must be minimal risk of sudden incapacitation.
- There must be minimal risk of subtle performance decrement.
- The condition must have resolved or be stable and be expected to remain so under the stresses of the aviation environment.
- If there is a risk of progression or recurrence, the symptoms and signs must be easily detectable and must not pose a risk to the safety of the individual or others.

In addition, for professional aircrew, the condition must not need exotic tests, regular invasive procedures or frequent absences to monitor for stability or progression. Finally, for military aircrew, the condition must be compatible with performance of sustained flying operations in austere environments worldwide.[112] The role of the doctor dealing with aircrew must be clearly understood. Most aviators regard doctors as only marginally better than the angel of death because of the risk of being grounded. The medical officer must work to obtain and hold the trust of the aircrew and make it clear that his main aim is to maintain their flying status – but that he also has a responsibility to the employer and the general public as one of the guardians of flight safety. The three most common conditions seen by the US Navy requiring a decision on fitness for flying are allergic rhinitis, obesity and decreased visual acuity.[113] In the final analysis, the decision on whether or not to return an aviator to flying rests with the appropriate national authorities, civil or military.

Use of therapeutic drugs

The use of therapeutic agents, whether by self-medica-

tion or prescribed, may be particularly dangerous in aviation. Most have side-effects, some of which may be hazardous in aviation. For example, a British Airways co-pilot took two tablets of a paracetamol-like painkiller which also contained codeine. Later in the flight he felt nauseated and lightheaded and collapsed in the lavatory. He was unable to contribute to the rest of the transatlantic flight.[114] It is more likely that the cause of the collapse was the condition for which he took the tablets but the packaging did warn about possible drowsiness and gave the advice not to operate machinery if affected. Figure 17.6 shows possible approaches to the considered use of medications when flying.[115] The key questions that have to be asked are:

- Does the condition for which the drug is being taken necessitate grounding in its own right?
- What monitoring of the condition is required?
- What are the potential side-effects relevant to aviation?
- Does the patient have any untoward reaction to the drug on the ground?

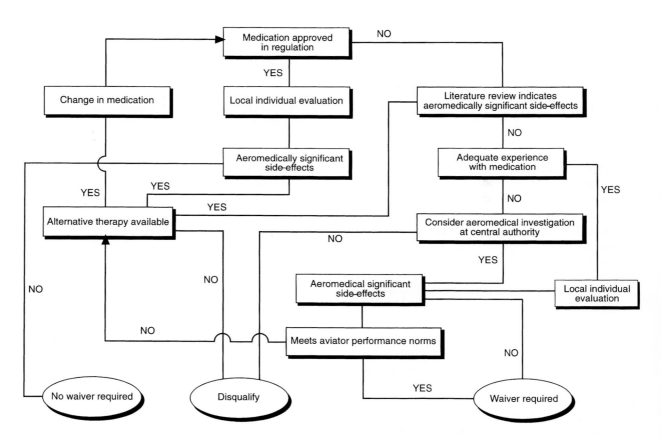

Figure 17.6 *Algorithm for medication approval in aircrew. The original version of this material was first published by the Advisory Group for Aerospace Research and Development, North Atlantic Treaty Organization (AGARD (NATO) in Conference Proceedings CP-553.*[115]

Fitness for flight as a passenger

Passengers fly with all sorts of medical conditions every day and survive. A survey by the Air Transport Association found that in-flight medical problems occurred in only 1 in 58 000 airline passengers. However, with some conditions there is a degree of risk. The doctor asked to advise a patient must bear in mind the inactivity of a long flight, the relative hypoxia, the low humidity, the excitement, the ready availability of alcohol and the time zone changes. Susceptible passengers may be at increased risk of deep vein thrombosis.[76,116] The swelling of legs may cause circulatory embarrassment to patients in plaster of Paris leg casts. Airlines expect that passengers with known medical conditions will need to be medically cleared before flight, either by their own or an airline doctor. When such patients are accepted as passengers, on-board oxygen, special diets or individual embarking, debarking or transfer arrangements may be made available. Kerbside check-in of baggage may be recommended. The airlines reserve the right not to accept infectious patients, patients who would be expected to deteriorate in flight or those whose conditions would be offensive to fellow travellers. Carriage of unstable patients is a skilled business, which should only be undertaken by specially trained operators.

Transmission of disease

Hundreds of millions of people fly commercially every year. Worldwide flight exposes aircrew and passengers, as well as ground personnel, to a variety of disease vectors. For example, transmission of *Mycobacterium tuberculosis* from one crew member to another on a single flight has been reported.[117] Communicable disease can enter the country by an infected person, infected vector or by infected material. International Health Regulations exist to detect, reduce and eliminate sources of infection, improve sanitation around airports and prevent the dissemination of vectors. Despite disinfection, cases of malaria have occurred in non-travellers living in the vicinity of airports in non-malarious countries. The regulations provide for notification of disease, health organization at airports, procedures at and between airports, documentation and disinfection. In the UK, the Public Health (Aircraft) Regulations 1979 cover cholera, plague, yellow fever, the viral haemorrhagic fevers and rabies.

Immunization and, for those potentially exposed, anti-malarial prophylaxis, are required. The number of mandatory immunizations is small but there are additional ones that may be recommended. Aircrew should not fly immediately after immunization because of the risk of side-effects. Aircrew for the same reason should not take some malaria prophylaxis, for example mefloquine. Chloroquine (300 mg weekly – despite an occasional, temporary effect on visual accommodation) and proguanil (200 mg daily) are the mainstay of malaria prophylaxis for aircrew with other drugs such as doxycycline being given in areas of chloroquine resistance. The main actions to be taken are avoidance – use of mosquito nets, sprays, long-sleeved and long-legged clothing.

REFERENCES

1 Jiang B. Studies on surfactant of Eustachian tube. Paper presented to Sino-American Symposium on Aerospace Medicine Xi'an, China, 1993.

2 Stangerup S-E, Tjernström Ö, Klokker M, Harcourt J, Stokholm J. Point prevalence of barotitis in children and adults after flight, and effect of autoinflation. *Aviat Space Environ Med* 1998; **69:** 45–9.

3 Cottrell JJ, Lebovitz BL, Fennell RG, Kohn GM. Inflight arterial saturation: continuous monitoring by pulse oximetry. *Aviat Space Environ Med* 1995; **66:** 126–30.

4 Bendrick GA, Nicolas DK, Krause BA, Castillo CY. Inflight oxygen saturation decrements in aeromedical evacuation patients. *Aviat Space Environ Med* 1995; **66:** 40–4.

5 Harding RM (revised by Gradwell D). Hypoxia and hyperventilation. In: Ernsting J, Nicholson AN, Rainford DJ eds. *Aviation Medicine* 3rd edn. Oxford: Butterworth-Heinemann, 1999: 45.

6 Denison DM, Ledwith F, Poulton EC. Complex reaction times at simulated cabin altitudes of 5000 feet and 8000 feet. *Aerosp Med* 1966; **37:** 1010–3.

7 Paul MA, Fraser WD. Performance during mild acute hypoxia. *Aviat Space Environ Med* 1994; **65:** 891–9.

8 Tomoda M, Yoneda I. Effect of smoking habit on the symptoms of hypoxia. *Aviat Space Environ Med* 1996; **67:** 711 (Abstr).

9 Ernsting J, Stewart WK. Introduction to oxygen deprivation at reduced barometric pressure. In Gillies JA ed. *A Textbook of Aviation Physiology*. Oxford: Pergamon Press, 1965: 212.

10 Gibson TM. Hyperventilation in flight. *Aviat Space Environ Med* 1984; **55:** 411–3.

11 Webb JT, Pilmanis AA. The gender aspect of altitude-induced decompression sickness susceptibility. *Aviat Space Environ Med* 1996; **67:** 682 (Abstr).

12 Sulaiman ZM, Pilmanis AA, O'Conner RB. Relationship between age and susceptibility to altitude decompression sickness. *Aviat Space Environ Med* 1997; **68:** 695–8.

13 Ryles MT, Pilmanis AA. The initial signs and symptoms of altitude decompression sickness. *Aviat Space Environ Med* 1996; **67:** 983–9.

14 Fitzpatrick DT. Visual manifestations of neurologic decompression sickness. *Aviat Space Environ Med* 1994; **65:** 736–8.

15 Bendrick GA, Ainsclough MJ, Pilmanis AA, Bisson RU. Prevalence of decompression sickness among U-2 pilots. *Aviat Space Environ Med* 1996; **67:** 199–206.

16 Moon RE, Sheffield PJ. Guidelines for treatment of

decompression illness. *Aviat Space Environ Med* 1997; **68:** 234–43.

17 Loftin KC, Conkin J, Powell MR. Modeling the effects of exercise during 100% oxygen prebreathe on the risk of hypobaric decompression sickness. *Aviat Space Environ Med* 1997; **68:** 199–204.

18 Preston FS. Medical aspects of supersonic travel. *Aerospace Med* 1975; **46:** 1074–8.

19 Dooley JW, Werchan PM. The USAF female acceleration tolerance enhancement (FATE) project. *Aviat Space Environ Med* 1996; **67:** 682 (Abstr).

20 Håmålåinen O, Vanharanta H, Hupli M, Karhu M, Kuronen P, Kinnunen H. Spinal shrinkage due to +Gz forces. *Aviat Space Environ Med* 1996; **67:** 659–61.

21 Kikukawa A, Tachibana S, Yagura S. G-related musculoskeletal spine symptoms in Japan Air Self Defense Force F-15 pilots. *Aviat Space Environ Med* 1995; **66:** 269–72.

22 Håmålåinen O, Visuri T, Kuronen P, Vanharanta H. Cervical disk bulges in fighter pilots. *Aviat Space Environ Med* 1994; **65:** 144–6.

23 Alvim KM. Greyout, blackout and G-loss of consciousness in the Brazilian Air Force: a 1991–92 survey. *Aviat Space Environ Med* 1995; **66:** 675–7.

24 Glaister DH, Prior ARJ. The effects of long duration acceleration. In: Ernsting J, Nicholson AN, Rainford DJ eds. *Aviation Medicine* 3rd edn. Oxford: Butterworth-Heinemann, 1999: 135.

25 Paul MA. Instrument flying performance after G-induced loss of consciousness. *Aviat Space Environ Med* 1996; **67:** 1028–33.

26 Bain B, Jacobs I, Buick F. Respiratory fatigue during simulated air combat maneuvering (SACM). *Aviat Space Environ Med* 1997; **68:** 118–25.

27 Prior ARJ, Adcock TR, McCarthy GW. In-flight arterial blood pressure changes during −Gz to +Gz manoeuvring. *Aviat Space Environ Med* 1993; **64:** 428 (Abstr).

28 Banks RD, Grissett JD, Saunders PL, Mateczun AJ. The effect of varying time at −Gz on subsequent +Gz physiological tolerance (Push-Pull effect). *Aviat Space Environ Med* 1995; **66:** 723–7.

29 Banks RD, Paul MA. Death due to push-pull effect. *Aviat Space Environ Med* 1996; **67:** 669 (Abstr).

30 Green NDC. Arm arterial occlusion cuffs as a means of alleviating high +Gz-associated arm pain. *Aviat Space Environ Med* 1997; **68:** 715–21.

31 Guo H-Z, Zhang S-X, Jing B-S. The characteristics and theoretical basis of the Qigong maneuver. *Aviat Space Environ Med* 1991; **62:** 1059–62.

32 Belyavin AJ, Gibson TM, Anton DJ, Truswell P. Prediction of body temperatures during exercise in flying clothing. *Aviat Space Environ Med* 1979; **50:** 911–6.

33 Gibson TM, Allan JR, Lawson CJ, Green RG. Effect of induced changes of deep body temperature on performance in a flight simulator. *Aviat Space Environ Med* 1980; **51:** 356–60.

34 Rood GM. Noise and communication. In Ernsting J, King P

eds. *Aviation Medicine* 2nd edn. London: Butterworth, 1988: 362.

35 Thomae MK, Porteous JE, Brock JR, Allen GD, Heller RF. Back pain in Australian military helicopter pilots: a preliminary study. *Aviat Space Environ Med* 1998; **69:** 468–73.

36 Wells MJ, Griffin MJ. Benefits of helmet-mounted display image stabilisation under whole-body vibration. *Aviat Space Environ Med* 1984; **55:** 13–18.

37 Ernsting J. Respiratory effects of whole body vibration. *Flying Personnel Research Committee Report* No 1164, 1961.

38 Gibson TM. Hyperventilation in aircrew: a review. *Aviat Space Environ Med* 1979; **50:** 725–33.

39 Mason KT, Harper JP, Shannon SG. Herniated nucleus pulposis: rates and outcomes among US Army aviators. *Aviat Space Environ Med* 1996; **67:** 338–40.

40 Sheard SC, Pethybridge RJ, Wright JM, McMillan GHG. Back pain in aircrew – an initial survey. *Aviat Space Environ Med* 1996; **67:** 474–7.

41 Wells HV. Some aeroplane injuries and diseases, with notes on the aviation service. *J Roy Nav Med Serv* 1916; **ii:** 65–71.

42 Gibson TM, Harrison MH. *Into Thin Air: A History of Aviation Medicine in the RAF* London: Hale, 1984: 201.

43 Miller RE, Kent JF, Green RP. Prescribing spectacles for aviators: USAF experience. *Aviat Space Environ Med* 1992; **63:** 80–5.

44 Still DL, Temme LA. Eyeglass use by US Navy jet pilots: effects on night carrier landing performance. *Aviat Space Environ Med* 1992; **63:** 273–5.

45 O'Connell SR, Markovits AS. The fate of eyewear in aircraft ejections. *Aviat Space Environ Med* 1995; **66:** 104–7.

46 Dennis RJ, Tredici TJ, Ivan DJ, Jackson WG Jr. The USAF aircrew medical contact lens study group: operational problems. *Aviat Space Environ Med* 1996; **67:** 303–7.

47 Moore RJ, Green RP. A survey of US Air Force flyers regarding their use of extended wear contact lenses. *Aviat Space Environ Med* 1994; **65:** 1025–31.

48 Ivan DJ, Tredici TJ, Perez-Becerra J, Dennis R, Burroughs JR, Taboada J. Photorefractive keratotomy (PRK) in the military aviator: an aeromedical perspective. *Aviat Space Environ Med* 1996; **67:** 770–6.

49 Corner H. *Flying Personnel Research Committee Report* No 75, 1939.

50 Rabin J, Wiley R. Switching from forward-looking infrared to night vision goggles: transitory effects on visual resolution. *Aviat Space Environ Med* 1994; **65:** 327–9.

51 DeVilbiss CA, Antonio JC, Fiedler GM. Night vision goggle (NVG) visual acuity under ideal conditions with various adjustment procedures. *Aviat Space Environ Med* 1994; **65:** 705–9.

52 Thomas SR. Aircrew laser eye protection: visual consequences and mission performance. *Aviat Space Environ Med* 1994; **65:** A108–15.

53 Smith PA. Vision in aviation. In: Ernsting J, Nicholson AN,

Rainford DJ eds. *Aviation Medicine* 3rd edn. Oxford: Butterworth-Heineman, 1999: 485.

54 Cohen MM, Crosbie RJ, Blackburn LH. Disorientating effects of aircraft catapult launchings. *Aerospace Med* 1973; **44:** 37–9.

55 Pancratz DJ, Bomar JB, Raddin JH. A new source for vestibular illusions in high agility aircraft. *Aviat Space Environ Med* 1994; **65:** 1130–3.

56 Benson AJ. Spatial disorientation – general aspects. In Ernsting J, King P eds. *Aviation Medicine* 2nd edn. London: Butterworth, 1988: 278.

57 Clark B. Disorientation incidents reported by military pilots across fourteen years of flight. In: *The Disorientation Incident*. Conference Report CP 95, Neuilly sur Seine: AGARD/NATO, 1971 A1: 1–6.

58 Ross LE, Maghni WN. Effect of alcohol on the threshold for detecting angular acceleration. *Aviat Space Environ Med* 1995; **66:** 635–40.

59 Lindseth G, Lindseth PD. The relationship of diet to airsickness. *Aviat Space Environ Med* 1995; **66:** 537–41.

60 Bagshaw M, Stott JRR. The desensitisation of chronically motion sick aircrew in the Royal Air Force. *Aviat Space Environ Med* 1985; **56:** 1144–51.

61 Golding JF, Stott JRR. Effect of sickness severity on habituation to repeated motion challenges in aircrew referred for airsickness treatment. *Aviat Space Environ Med* 1995; **66:** 625–30.

62 Brand JJ, Perry WLM. Drugs used in motion sickness. *Pharm Rev* 1966; **18:** 895–924.

63 Nicholson AN, Spencer MB. Aircrew: their work and rest. In: Ernsting J, Nicholson AN, Rainford DJ eds. *Aviation Medicine* 3rd edn. Oxford: Butterworth-Heinemann, 1999: 643–6.

64 Lowden A, Åkerstedt T. Sleep and wake patterns in aircrew on a 2-day layover on westward long distance flights. *Aviat Space Environ Med* 1998; **69:** 596–602.

65 Nicholson AN. Duty hours and sleep patterns in aircrew operating world-wide routes. *Aerospace Med* 1972; **43:** 138–41.

66 Baird JA, Coles PKL, Nicholson AN. Human factors and air operations in the South Atlantic campaign. *J Roy Soc Med* 1983; **76:** 933–7.

67 Emonson D, Vanderbeek R. The use of amphetamine in US Air Force tactical operations during Desert Shield and Storm. *Aviat Space Environ Med* 1995; **66:** 260–3.

68 Caldwell JA, Caldwell JL. An in-flight investigation of the efficacy of dextroamphetamine for sustaining helicopter pilot performance. *Aviat Space Environ Med* 1997; **68:** 1073–80.

69 Petrie K, Conaglen JV, Thompson L, Chamberlain K. Effect of melatonin on jet lag after long haul flights. *Br Med J* 1989; **298:** 705–7.

70 Comperatore CA, Lieberman HR, Kirby AW, Adams B, Crowley JS. Melatonin efficacy in aviation missions requiring rapid deployment and night operations. *Aviat Space Environ Med* 1996; **67:** 520–4.

71 Nicholson AN, Turner C. Intensive and sustained air operations: potential use of the stimulant, Pemoline. *Aviat Space Environ Med* 1998; **69:** 647–55.

72 Anderson HG. *The Medical and Surgical Aspects of Aviation*. London: Henry Froude and Hodder & Stoughton, 1919: 147.

73 Buley LE. Incidence, causes and results of airline pilot incapacitation while on duty. *Aerospace Med* 1969; **40:** 64–70.

74 Powell TJ, Carey TM, Brent HP, Taylor WGR. Episodes of unconsciousness in pilots during flight in 1956. *J Aviat Med* 1957; **28:** 374–86.

75 Carruthers M, Arguelles AE, Mosovich A. Man in transit: biochemical and physiological changes during intercontinental flights. *Lancet* 1976; **i:** 977–81.

76 Sahiar F, Mohler SR. Economy class syndrome. *Aviat Space Environ Med* 1994; **65:** 957–60.

77 Maxwell E, Harris D. Drinking and flying: a structual model. *Aviat Space Environ Med* 1999; **70:** 117–23.

78 Cullen SA, Drysdale HC, Mayes RW. Role of medical factors in 1000 fatal aviation accidents: case note study. *Br Med J* 1997; **314:** 1592.

79 Li G, Hooten EG, Baker SP, Butts JD. Alcohol in aviation-related fatalities: North Carolina, 1985–1994. *Aviat Space Environ Med* 1998; **69:** 755–60.

80 Cable GG, Doherty S. Acute carbamate and organochlorine toxicity causing convulsions in an agricultural pilot: a case report. *Aviat Space Environ Med* 1999; **70:** 68–72.

81 Harding RM (revised by Gradwell DP). The Earth's atmosphere. In: Ernsting J, Nicholson AN, Rainford DJ eds. *Aviation Medicine* 3rd edn. Oxford: Heinemann, 1999: 7.

82 Oksanen PJ. Estimted individual annual cosmic radiation doses for flight crews. *Aviat Space Environ Med* 1998; **69:** 621–5.

83 Lynge E. Risk of breast cancer is also increased among Danish female cabin attendants. *Br Med J* 1996; **312:** 253.

84 Geeze DS. Pregnancy and in-flight cosmic radiation. *Aviat Space Environ Med* 1998; **69:** 696–8.

85 Cheung B, Money K, Wright H, Bateman W. Spatial disorientation-implicated accidents in Canadian Forces 1982–92. *Aviat Space Environ Med* 1995; **66:** 579–85.

86 Ungs TJ. Suicide by use of aircraft in the United States. *Aviat Space Environ Med* 1994; **65:** 953–6.

87 Cullen SA. Aviation suicide: a review of general aviation accidents in the UK, 1970–96. *Aviat Space Environ Med* 1998; **69:** 696–8.

88 Baker SP, Lamb MW, Li G, Dodd RS. Crashes of instructional flights. *Aviat Space Environ Med* 1996; **67:** 105–10.

89 Chaturvedi AK, Sanders DC. Aircraft fires, smoke toxicity and survival. *Aviat Space Environ Med* 1996; **67:** 275–8.

90 Li G, Baker SP, Dodd RS. The epidemiology of aircraft fire in commuter and air taxi crashes. *Aviat Space Environ Med* 1996; **67:** 434–7.

91 Reader DC. Smoke hoods revisited. *Aviat Space Environ Med* 1997; **68:** 617 (Abstr).

92 Edwards M. Anthropometric measurements and ejection injuries. *Aviat Space Environ Med* 1996; **67:** 673 (Abstr).

93 Higenbottam C, Redman P. Underwater escape from helicopters. *J Defence Sci* 1997; **2:** 161–6.

94 Baker CO, Bellenkes AH. US Naval helicopter mishaps: cockpit egress problems. *Aviat Space Environ Med* 1996; **67:** 480–5.

95 Krebs MB, Li G, Baker SP. Factors related to pilot survival in helicopter commuter and air taxi crashes. *Aviat Space Environ Med* 1995; **66:** 99–103.

96 Jennings RT, Bagian JP. Musculoskeletal injury review in the US Space Program. *Aviat Space Environ Med* 1996; **67:** 672–6.

97 Harding RM. *Survival in Space*. London: Routledge, 1989.

98 Stanford M. Radiation concerns for exploratory manned spaceflight. *Aviat Space Environ Med* 1996; **67:** 704 (Abstr).

99 Vana N, Schöner W, Fugger M, Akatov Y, Shurshakov V. Determination of equivalent dose on board of space station Mir during Russian long term flight (RLF). *Aviat Space Environ Med* 1996; **67:** 706 (Abstr).

100 James LT, Limero TF, Leano HJ, Boyd JF, Covington PA. Volatile organic contaminants found in the habitable environment of the Space Shuttle: STS-26 to STS-55. *Aviat Space Environ Med* 1994; **65:** 851–7.

101 Draeger J, Schwartz R, Groenhoff S, Stern C. Self-tonometry under microgravity conditions. *Aviat Space Environ Med* 1995; **66:** 568–70.

102 LeBlanc A, Rowe R, Schneider V, Evans H, Hedrick T. Regional blood loss after short duration space flight. *Aviat Space Environ Med* 1995; **66:** 1151–4.

103 Billica RD, Simmons SC, Mathes KL, McKinlay BA, Chuang CC, Wear ML, Hamm PB. Perception of the medical risk of spaceflight. *Aviat Space Environ Med* 1996; **67:** 467–73.

104 Strollo F, Riondino G, Harris B, Strollo G, Casarosa E et al. The effect of microgravity on testicular androgen secretion. *Aviat Space Environ Med* 1998; **69:** 133–6.

105 Kanas N. Psychiatric issues affecting long duration space missions. *Aviat Space Environ Med* 1998; **69:** 1211–6.

106 Wickman LA, Luna B. Locomotion while load carrying in reduced gravities. *Aviat Space Environ Med* 1996; **67:** 940–6.

107 Schvartz E. Endurance fitness and orthostatic tolerance. *Aviat Space Environ Med* 1996; **67:** 935–9.

108 Gibson TM, Harrison MH. British aviation medicine to 1939. *Royal Air Force Institute of Aviation Med Rep* R593, 1981.

109 Chaplin JC. In perspective – the safety of aircraft, pilots and their hearts. *Eur Heart J* 1988; **9:** (Suppl G): 17–20.

110 Tunstall-Pedoe H. Risk of a coronary heart attack in the normal population and how it might be modified in fliers. *Eur Heart J* 1988; **9:** (Suppl G): 13–15.

111 McCormick TJ, Lyons TJ. Medical causes of in-flight incapacitation: USAF experience 1978–1987. *Aviat Space Environ Med* 1991; **62:** 884–7.

112 Gibson TM. Medical Waivers for Aircrew. *US Air Force Pamphlet* 1993; **48–132:** 1–162.

113 Bailey DA, Gilleran LG, Merchant PG. Waivers for disqualifying medical conditions in US naval aviation personnel. *Aviat Space Environ Med* 1995; **66:** 401–7.

114 *Daily Mail*, 6 June 1997.

115 Gibson TM, Giovanetti PM. Aeromedical risk management for aircrew. In: *The Clinical Basis for Aeromedical Decision Making*. AGARD-CP-553; Neuilly-sur-Seine: AGARD/NATO, 1994; 1.1–1.8.

116 Mercer A, Brown JD. Venous thromboembolism associated with air travel: a report of 33 patients. *Aviat Space Environ Med* 1998; **69:** 154–7.

117 Driver CR, Valway SE, Morgan WM, Onorato IM, Castro KG. Transmission of mycobacterium tuberculosis associated with air travel. *JAMA* 1994; **212:** 1031–5.

FURTHER READING

1 *Aviation, Space and Environmental Medicine*. Journal of the Aerospace Medical Association, 320 South Henry St, Alexandria, VA22314. e-mail: pday@asma.org

2 Davis JR. Medical issues for a mission to Mars. *Aviat Space Environ Med* 1999; **70:** 162–8.

3 Ernsting J, Nicholson AN, Rainford DJ (eds). *Aviation Medicine* 3rd edn. Oxford: Butterworth-Heinemann, 1999.

4 Gibson TM, Harrison MH. *Into Thin Air: A History of Aviation Medicine in the RAF*. London: Hale, 1984.

5 Gillies JA (ed). *A Textbook of Aviation Physiology*. Oxford: Permagon Press, 1965.

6 Harding RM, *Survival in Space*. London: Routledge, 1989.

7 Harding RM, Mills FJ. *Aviation Medicine* 2nd edn. London: BMA Publications, 1992.

8 Nicogossian AE, Huntoon CL, Pool SL (eds). *Space Physiology and Medicine* 3rd edn. Philadelphia: Lea & Febiger, 1993.

9 Rayman RB. *Clinical Aviation Medicine* 2nd edn. Philadelphia: Lea & Febiger, 1990.

18

Working at high altitude

PETER J G FORSTER

Illness at high altitude	383	Altitude sickness	390
At-risk groups	388	References	394
Sleep problems at high altitude	389		

ILLNESS AT HIGH ALTITUDE

The journals of intrepid mountaineers give clear testimony to the perils and discomfort of life at high altitude. In 1879, on Chimborazo in Ecuador, Edward Whymper, conqueror of the Matterhorn and the foremost mountaineer of his day, suffered intense headache and an 'indescribable feeling of illness which pervaded the whole body.'[1] Whymper succeeded in reaching the summit of Chimborazo (6290 m); however, Edward Fitzgerald failed to achieve his personal ambition of the first ascent of Aconcagua (6980 m), the highest mountain in the Western Hemisphere. Fitzgerald records: 'I got up, and tried once more to go but I was only able to advance from two to three steps at a time and then to stop, panting for breath, my struggles alternating with violent fits of nausea.'[2]

The discomfort experienced by mountaineers on ascent to high altitude is compounded by the additional hardships of exertion, fatigue, exposure, low temperature, gastrointestinal upsets and alteration in diet. Fitzgerald's discomfort was intensified by a diet which on Christmas morning 1896, camping cold and hungry at 4900 m, consisted of 'some tins of Irish Stew . . . melting the great white frozen lumps of grease slowly in our mouths, and then swallowing them'. In 1913, T H Ravenhill, medical officer to a mining district in the Chilean Andes, described the features of altitude sickness affecting miners transported by rail from Antofagasta, a seaport on the Pacific Ocean, to mines situated above 4600 m. The miners in Ravenhill's study were subject to the effects of altitude without other complicating influences. Ravenhill described three forms of altitude sickness – 'normal puna' (acute mountain sickness), 'cardiac puna' (high altitude pulmonary oedema), and 'nervous puna' (high altitude cerebral oedema).[3]

Acute mountain sickness is a self-limiting condition characterized by headache, insomnia, breathlessness on exertion, nausea, anorexia and cerebral symptoms such as profound lassitude, irritability, lack of concentration, and confusion. Physical signs include periorbital and peripheral oedema and manifestations of the physiological response to high altitude exposure such as periodic breathing (Cheyne–Stokes respiration), tachycardia and oliguria. Acute mountain sickness (AMS) affects unacclimatized visitors at elevations above 3000 m: symptoms become manifest after a period of approximately 6 hours at high altitude and reach their maximum severity at 24–48 hours. Symptoms subside gradually over 2–5 days providing ascent to greater altitude is not attempted.

The incidence of AMS in sea-level residents ascending to altitudes greater than 3000 m has been estimated from large population studies of trekkers and soldiers on single ascents. Hackett and Rennie reported an incidence of 43% in 200 hikers reaching Pheriche (4243 m) on the trail to Mount Everest.[4] One-third of the hikers were symptom free. Of the thousands of climbers making the rapid ascent to the summit of Mount Rainier (4392 m) every year, 50–75% suffer from AMS.[5] Singh *et al.* reported an 8.3% incidence of severe AMS in thousands of soldiers transported from sea level to above 3500 m.[6] These published studies have involved young, physically fit and predominantly male subjects; in a general population of visitors (age range 16–87 years, one-third female) to modest elevations (1900–3000 m) in the Rocky Mountains of Colorado, 25% suffered AMS within the first 12 hours of arrival.[7]

A study of sea-level residents transported rapidly to high altitude, similar to the experience of the Andean miners in Ravenhill's paper, was conducted on personnel manning astronomical observatories at the summit of

Mauna Kea (4200 m), on the island of Hawaii.[8,9] Seven major telescopes are situated at the summit which, because of the dry atmosphere, absence of pollution and ready access, is the pre-eminent site for terrestrial infrared and submillimetre astronomy (Figs 18.1, 18.2 and 18.3). Mauna Kea telescope personnel make frequent journeys by four-wheel drive vehicle from sea level to the summit with minimal provision for acclimatization above 3000 m. At the summit elevation, the barometric pressure is 625 mbars (475 mmHg) and the ambient partial pressure of oxygen is 60% of the sea-level value. The partial pressure of oxygen in inspired air is 12.6 kPa (95 mmHg) compared with 20 kPa (150 mmHg) at sea level and 7.6 kPa (57 mmHg) in alveolar air compared with 14 kPa (105 mmHg) at sea level. On Mauna Kea, 80% of the shift workers were affected by altitude sickness symptoms on the first day. Headache and breathlessness were the commonest and most troublesome complaints. Other common symptoms were insomnia, lethargy, poor concentration and impairment of memory.

After 5 days on the mountain, 60% of workers were free of symptoms, whilst the remainder continued to experience minimal symptoms of exertional dyspnoea, headache and insomnia. There was no difference in the incidence of AMS in shift workers who worked at the summit following a 4-day sojourn at sea level compared with a 30-day rest period at sea level; acclimatization to altitude achieved during 5 days above 3000 m was reversed within days of return to sea level. Telescope personnel who commuted to the summit for a single day did not suffer from severe AMS symptoms. However, commuters were only at an advantage if their exposure to high altitude was limited to less than 6 hours, the period of time that elapsed between arrival at 4200 m elevation and the development of AMS. The disadvantage of the commuter's work schedule was that commuters did not acclimatize.

If the symptoms of AMS are ignored and ascent to higher altitude is attempted the 'malignant' forms of altitude sickness, high altitude pulmonary oedema (HAPO) and high altitude cerebral oedema (HACO), may develop. Onset of HAPO occurs usually 1–3 days after ascent to altitudes above 3000 m. The signs of HAPO are

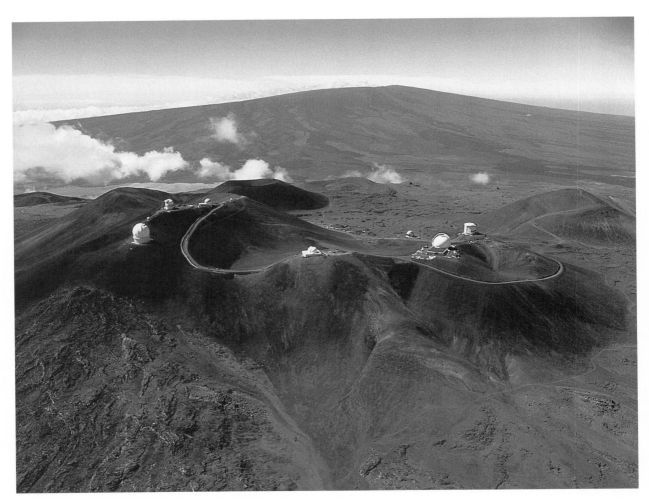

Figure 18.1 *Telescope domes on the summit of Mauna Kea, Hawaii. Copyright: Royal Observatory, Edinburgh.*

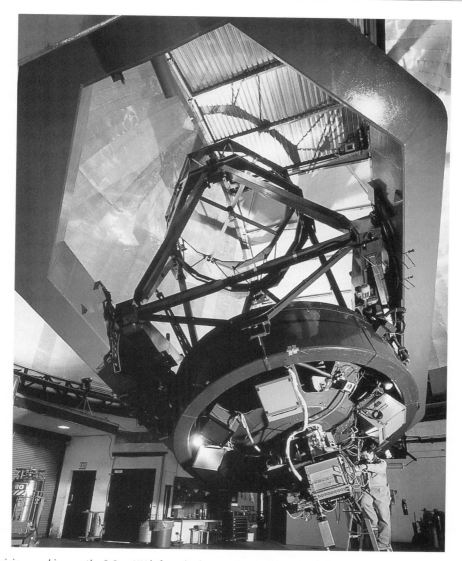

Figure 18.2 *Technician working on the 3.8 m UK infrared telescope (UKIRT) on Mauna Kea. Copyright: Royal Observatory, Edinburgh.*

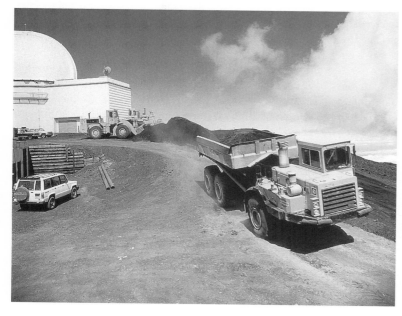

Figure 18.3 *Construction work at the summit of Mauna Kea. Copyright: Royal Observatory, Edinburgh.*

marked breathlessness at rest, a rapid respiratory rate (>30 breaths/min), and a cough which may be productive of white, frothy, or blood-streaked sputum. The victim appears deeply cyanotic and may complain of chest discomfort. Extensive bilateral crepitations are heard on auscultation. In extreme cases 'gurgling' sounds from the lungs may be audible to the victim and his companions without the use of a stethoscope. Signs of cardiac failure are not evident although tachycardia (pulse rate >120 beats/min) and a low systemic blood pressure are commonly present. Cardiac murmurs are not a feature of HAPO; however, the second heart sound is accentuated, and sometimes palpable, reflecting elevation of pulmonary artery pressure. An erroneous diagnosis of bronchopneumonia may be suggested by the presence of low grade pyrexia and moderate leucocytosis.

Arterial blood gas measurements confirm severe hypoxaemia and decreased arterial carbon dioxide tension ($PaCO_2$). Patchy infiltrates with prominence of pulmonary arteries seen in chest radiographs in early disease progress to homogeneous bilateral infiltration in severe cases. Right ventricular overload pattern is present on electrocardiogram tracings: echocardiography may demonstrate incompetence of the tricuspid valve. Cardiac catheterization studies performed on HAPO victims before treatment or descent confirm a high pulmonary arterial pressure and low or normal pulmonary artery wedge pressure.[10] Descent to low altitude and administration of oxygen lowers pulmonary artery pressure, clears radiographic pulmonary infiltrates within 1–2 days and relieves symptoms.

The development of HAPO is related to the speed of ascent, the altitude reached and the exertion involved. An incidence of HAPO has been reported as high as 15.5% in thousands of lowland troops flown up to the Himalayas.[11] Seven cases of HAPO were encountered amongst 278 unacclimatized hikers at 4243 m in Nepal, an incidence of 2.5%.[12] At the Regina Margherita hut (4559 m) in the Alps Valais, 4% of climbers were diagnosed as suffering from HAPO as indicated by pronounced pulmonary crepitations on auscultation.[13] On Mauna Kea, one case of HAPO was diagnosed in 41 shift workers during a 2-year study (Table 18.1). Calculated in terms of the 2000 ascents per annum to a single telescope, this low incidence of HAPO may reflect the lack of physical exertion involved in ascent to 4200 m.

Failure to descend or to treat HAPO effectively may result in a fatal outcome within a few hours of onset; the mortality rate is quoted in the range 4–11%. In a review of 166 reported cases of HAPO, untreated victims had a mortality rate of 44% compared with a 3% mortality in subjects who were treated by descent and oxygen administration.[14]

Cerebral oedema presents with intense headache, ataxia, impaired coordination, confusion and hallucinations. Cerebral oedema occurs usually in people exhibiting 'benign' AMS; the diagnosis may depend on a deterioration in existing AMS or the appearance of additional neurological signs such as ataxia on walking (inability to perform heel to toe walking) or sitting (truncal ataxia), extensor plantar responses, cranial nerve palsies and visual field loss.[15] Features of HAPO may be present and complicate the diagnosis and management. Papilloedema develops in over 50% of HACO victims although optic disc swelling may not be present in cases of moderate severity.[9] Retinal vein engorgement and retinal haemorrhage are of minor prognostic significance in HACO as these fundoscopic abnormalities are not uncommon in asymptomatic subjects at high altitude.[8] Rapid deterioration in conscious level leading to death has been widely reported.[16] Postmortem examination reveals extensive cerebral oedema, intracerebral haemorrhages and thrombosis in cerebral veins and dural venous sinuses.[17,18] In a study of 278 trekkers in the Himalayas, five cases were diagnosed at 4243 m, an incidence of 1.8% (compared with 2.5% for HAPO).[12] Singh et al. described 24 cases of 'severe' neurological abnormality amongst 1925 AMS victims at altitudes of 3350–5486 m.[6] A single episode of HACO occurred during the Mauna Kea study (Table 18.1).

Physical fitness offers no protection against altitude sickness. Ravenhill records in his 1913 paper: 'There is, in my experience, no type of man whom one may say that he will, or will not, suffer from puna (altitude sickness). Most of the cases I have instanced were men to all appearances perfectly sound. Young, strong and healthy men may be completely overcome: stout, plethoric individuals of the chronic bronchitic type may not even have a headache.'[3] A recent writer describes, pithily, that acute mountain sickness affects 'the young, the fit, the enthusiastic, the audacious and the physically hard working.'[19]

Anecdotal reports that males are more susceptible than females may reflect the gender bias of climbing expeditions and trekking groups. Ravenhill believed that women suffered less than men, a view supported by later studies suggesting a protective effect by the respiratory stimulant hormone progesterone.[19] Other studies do not support an advantage for females either at a high or moderate altitude.[4,7,12] The increasing number of women enjoying leisure pursuits at high altitude will permit definitive studies. Children are prone to the adverse effects of high altitude, and are more susceptible to HAPO than adults.[20]

Susceptibility to altitude sickness varies greatly between individuals; however, in general, individuals respond consistently on each ascent. On Mauna Kea mean arterial oxygen tension (PaO_2) recorded in the study group ranged from 4.4 kPa (33 mmHg) to 7.6 kPa (57 mmHg) at the summit. The worker with the highest PaO_2 during the first ascent (7.0 kPa, 52.5 mmHg) recorded the highest PaO_2 on a subsequent ascent (7.6 kPa, 57 mmHg): similarly one subject recorded the lowest PaO_2 (4.4 kPa, 33 mmHg: 5.1 kPa, 38 mmHg) on both ascents.[21] The reproducibility of individual

Table 18.1 *Medical emergencies at United Kingdom Infrared Telescope (UKIRT) on Mauna Kea*

Assuming a complement of three day staff and three night observers, approximately 2000 'man days' are worked each year at the UKIRT facility. An average working day constitutes 9 hours at the summit. During a 2-year period of study, the following medical emergencies occurred:

Case 1   High altitude pulmonary oedema

Male age 29

Progressive dyspnoea, tachypnoea, cyanosis; occurred at rest camp (3000 m elevation) following third night shift at summit

Treatment

- immediate descent and oxygen administration (6 litres/min)

Outcome

- clinical examination at sea level-symptoms and signs of HAPO resolved; chest radiograph normal; subsequent work at summit without recurrence of HAPO

Case 2   High altitude cerebral oedema

Male age 30

Slurred speech, frontal headache with neck stiffness, temporary loss of peripheral vision, impaired coordination, ataxic gait; Symptoms presented on first day at summit

Treatment

- descent and oxygen

Outcome

- complete resolution of signs and symptoms at sea level; no subsequent work at telescope

Case 3   Acute mountain sickness

Male age 30

Headache, nausea, lethargy, poor concentration, impaired memory, cyanosis, periodic respiration: no focal central nervous system signs

Symptoms present on first day of work at summit of every shift, necessitating descent; subject attempted, unsuccessfully, to ameliorate symptoms by gradual staging of ascent

Treatment

- acetazolamide prescription prior to ascent (dose 500 mg to 1.5 g/day); minimal reduction in AMS symptoms: occurrence of carbonic anhydrase inhibitor adverse effects – paraesthesia, diuresis

Outcome

- exemption from work at high altitude

Case 4   Migraine headache

Male age 29

History of classical migraine

Eighth day on mountain – symptoms of expressive dysphasia, loss of right peripheral visual field, numbness right arm; nausea: no headache

Treatment

- descent
- anti-emetic for nausea

Outcome

- neurological symptoms resolved at sea level
- EEG, isotope brain scan – normal

Case 5   Bronchopneumonia

Male age 34

Cough productive of purulent sputum, dyspnoea at rest, fever, anorexia, ataxic gait – following flu-like illness

Treatment

- descent under supervision by colleague (patient exhibited marked loss of insight)
- antibiotics
- bed rest

Outcome

- return to observatory after 4 days

Continued

Table 18.1 *Medical emergencies at United Kingdom Infrared Telescope (UKIRT) on Mauna Kea* – (cont.)

Case 6   Bronchopneumonia

Male age 30
Two episodes on consecutive visits to Mauna Kea
Cough productive of purulent sputum, severe dyspnoea, central cyanosis

Treatment
- descent to sea level
- antibiotics
- bronchodilators
- bed rest

Outcome
- completed work schedule at observatory after 3 days sojourn at sea level
- following second episode, persistent dyspnoea; astronomical research aborted, returned home
- subsequent examination by respiratory physician – no underlying chest disease

Case 7   Perforation of eardrum

Male age 55
Contracted coryza at sea level, developed right otitis media on Mauna Kea
Impaired hearing, 'pressure in right ear', discharge from ear

Treatment
- remained on mountain
- antibiotics
- decongestant

Outcome
- healing of perforation

---

response to high altitude exposure implies that the surest means of predicting an individual's performance at high altitude is their response on previous ascents. Inevitably, anomalies do occur: the healthy 29-year-old male astronomer who suffered from HAPO on Mauna Kea worked for 2 years before the episode of HAPO, and 3 years subsequently, without incident.

Predisposition to AMS may be related to individual sensitivity of hypoxic drive.[22] Subjects with a low ventilatory response to hypoxia are liable to develop AMS.[23] The magnitude of the increase in pulmonary arterial pressure in response to hypoxia is a further risk factor and has been implicated in the increased susceptibility of children to HAPO.[24]

AT-RISK GROUPS

Ischaemic heart disease

On the first day of work on the summit of Mauna Kea, mean PaO_2 was 5.6 kPa (42 mmHg) measured in 27 subjects on 40 ascents. Hypoxaemia induces increased sympathetic stimulation. As pulse rate increases, so does cardiac work. The increase in cardiac work can be expressed in terms of the 'double product' i.e., the product of heart rate and systolic blood pressure. In the

Hawaiian telescope workers, the mean sea-level 'double product' was 8925 units (mean resting pulse rate 75 × mean systolic blood pressure 119 mmHg). At 4200 m, the 'double product' rose to 10285 units, an increase in cardiac work of approximately 15%. By 5 days, with the development of acclimatization, sympathetic activity had fallen with a reduction in pulse rate and the 'double product' stood at 9840 units.

Modest increases in cardiac output at high altitude will have little deleterious effect on subjects with controlled ischaemic heart disease symptoms and these people can work safely at high altitude. However, subjects experiencing angina or exertional dyspnoea at sea level risk a worsening of symptoms shortly after arrival at high altitude when cardiac output is highest. The threat to coronary patients is greatest during the first 3 days at altitude and diminishes by 5–7 days. General advice should include gradual ascent, limitation of physical activity to less than the level that precipitates ischaemic symptoms at sea level and attention to control of blood pressure.[25] People whose level of activity is severely curtailed by ischaemic symptoms at sea level are likely to suffer a marked deterioration at high altitude and must be cautioned against ascent. For such people, facilities for rapid retreat down the mountain are mandatory, taking precedence over other precautions, for example provision of oxygen or medical supervision.

A single cardiac death occurred at the telescopes on Mauna Kea in the decade 1975–1985. At this site the population at risk number approximately 60 personnel each working day. The fatal event involved a 37-year-old astronomer, a cigarette smoker, who suffered a myocardial infarction at the summit; postmortem examination revealed severe coronary artery disease. Population studies indicate that adverse coronary events occur infrequently at high altitude. Shlim and Houston surveyed reports of illness in 148 000 trekkers in Nepal during a 3-year period. In the 23 fatalities, the causes of death were trauma (11), 'illness' (8) and AMS (3); no cardiac deaths were reported.[26] Hultgren reports that in the 25 years of his experience, the Chief Medical Officer at La Oroya (altitude 3750 m) never witnessed a myocardial infarction in a known sufferer from ischaemic heart disease amongst the hundreds of visitors who ascend each year from Lima, near sea level, to La Oroya.[27]

Respiratory disorders

Sea-level dwellers rendered hypoxic by chronic lung disease will experience a further reduction in PaO_2 at high altitude. At modest elevations, and if exertion is not excessive, subjects with moderate chronic obstructive pulmonary disease (COPD) may suffer no adverse consequences despite the presence of profound hypoxia.

Graham and Houston accompanied eight COPD patients, with average resting PaO_2 of 8.8 kPa (66 mmHg) at sea level, to an altitude of 1920 m.[28] Within 3 hours of ascent, resting PaO_2 fell to 6.9 kPa (52 mmHg). Six minutes on a treadmill produced severe arterial hypoxaemia [mean PaO_2 6.2 kPa (46.5 mmHg) compared with 8.4 kPa (63 mmHg) at sea level]. Despite levels of PaO_2 which would qualify as respiratory failure in COPD patients at sea level, none of the study patients came to harm and altitude sickness symptoms were trivial. In this study, tolerance of modest high altitude was facilitated by the exclusion criteria of coexistent disease (cor pulmonale, hypertension, angina) or elevated $PaCO_2$.

Many COPD patients will be afflicted by these complications and the results of this study must be interpreted with caution. Other factors may compromise high altitude tolerance in chronic lung patients. Smokers experience more profound arterial hypoxia than non-smokers at high altitude.[29] Obese individuals are more prone to sleep apnoea at high altitude,[30] during periods of apnoea, PaO_2 falls precipitously. (Marked nocturnal arterial desaturation contributes to the exaggeration of altitude sickness symptoms, in particular headache, present on morning waking in all AMS sufferers.)

Bronchial airway narrowing in asthmatics can be provoked by stimuli such as exercise and inhalation of cold air. Nevertheless, exposure to mountain air relatively free of air pollutants (tobacco smoke, petrol fumes) and exogenous allergens (house dust mites) is of benefit to asthmatics and treatment clinics have flourished in alpine regions at altitudes as high as 3200 m in the Northern Tien-Shan mountains in Kyrgyzstan. Asthmatics with well-controlled disease may be encouraged to go to high altitude: pre-treatment with carbonic anhydrase inhibitor drugs (acetazolamide) protects against AMS symptoms and lessens arterial desaturation during sleep.[31] In the Mauna Kea study, a 32-year-old asthmatic was unaffected by work at 4200 m. Bronchodilator therapy was used as symptoms dictated. The astronomer's worst attack of asthma was precipitated by participation in a cardiac stress test (Table 18.2 Case A).

Haemoglobinopathies

Sickle cell anaemia, the homozygous form of the disease with HbS accounting for more than 90% of haemoglobin, carries a high childhood mortality and considerable morbidity for adult survivors. However, people with the heterozygote sickle cell trait (HbA 60%; HbS 40%) are usually symptom free at sea level and, with normal respiratory function, are unlikely to be at risk at altitudes up to 3000 m. Above this altitude, there is a risk of splenic and renal infarction and hence workers should be screened for the sickle cell trait before they are employed to work at high altitude.

Avoidance of dehydration, caution in the event of infection and awareness of the significance of unexplained abdominal pain or haematuria will afford some protection to individuals with haemoglobinopathies who wish to venture to high places.[32]

SLEEP PROBLEMS AT HIGH ALTITUDE

Insomnia is a common complaint at high altitude. Periodic breathing (Cheyne–Stokes respiration) occurs during sleep and periods of apnoea interspersed with rapid respiration disturb the night. At relatively modest altitudes, below 1400 m, sleep duration is reduced and the sleep efficiency index (ratio of total sleep time to the time in bed) falls. Above 4000 m, sleep duration and efficiency deteriorate further; sleep onset latency is increased and rapid eye movement (REM) sleep is decreased.[33] Disruption of the normal respiratory rhythm produces marked hypoxaemia during sleep at high altitude. Sleep quality can be improved and sleep hypoxaemia alleviated by acetazolamide.[34] The use of hypnotic drugs by climbers at extreme altitude is not recommended because of the accompanying depression of ventilation which exacerbates nocturnal hypoxia. Nevertheless, the prescription of a benzodiazepine at low doses (e.g. 10 mg temazepam) in conjunction with acetazolamide reduces sleep-onset latency and increases sleep efficiency at 4000 m to values comparable with those at sea level.[33]

Table 18.2 *Effect of repeated exposure to high altitude (4200 m) on subjects with pre-existing medical conditions*

Case A   Bronchial asthma

Male age 32

Exercise-induced asthma since childhood; modest severity – no regular medication, bronchodilator by inhalation as required

No asthmatic attacks on mountain during 2½ year work programme; single attack of bronchospasm at 3000 m precipitated by cardiac exercise test – self-limiting, no medication required

Case B   Mitral valve prolapse and paroxysmal supraventricular tachycardia

Male age 34

Single episode of tachycardia during 3 years work on Mauna Kea; episode curtailed by carotid massage performed by subject

Case C   Paroxysmal atrial tachycardia

Male age 40

Self treatment with β-blocker drug (oxyprenolol 80 mg)

No episodes of tachycardia on mountain; cardiac stress test (3000 m) normal

Case D   Wolff–Parkinson–White syndrome (Pre-excitation syndrome)

Male age 26

No episodes on Mauna Kea

Normal cardiac stress test (3000 m)

Case E   Essential hypertension

Male age 45

Moderate increase in blood pressure on each ascent to 4200 m; no deterioration in blood pressure control during 3 years of supervision

Treatment
- salt restricted diet
- diuretic (hydrochlorthiazide)
- β-blocker (propranolol 80 mg three times daily)

Case F   Crohn's disease

Male age 29

No deterioration in bowel condition during 2 years at Mauna Kea telescopes

Treatment
- diet
- sulphasalazine
- corticosteroids (oral and rectal administration)

ALTITUDE SICKNESS

Prevention

Wise mountaineers who wish to lessen the debilitating effects of high altitude respect the maxims 'Climb high, sleep low' and 'Hasten slowly'. These precepts are of particular relevance for people with a previous history of altitude sickness. A slow ascent above 3000 m altitude of only 300 m per day for 2 days followed by a rest day thereafter is recommended.[23,35,36] Staging the climb, so that a rest day and 2 consecutive nights are spent at the same altitude every 2nd and 3rd day, facilitates acclimatization. By following these cautious guidelines, the majority of sea-level residents ascend safely; however, some susceptible individuals will develop altitude sickness above 3000 m. Common sense must prevail: an attempt to climb higher whilst in the throes of an attack of altitude sickness is foolhardy. Victims of altitude sickness must descend or, at least, remain at a safe moderate altitude until their condition improves.

General measures to ease discomfort include avoidance of strenuous exercise on arrival at high altitude, maintenance of an adequate fluid intake and abstinence from alcohol and tobacco. Cold exposure and lack of sleep aggravate the discomforts of a hypoxic environment. Concomitant infection, gastrointestinal or respiratory, is associated with a higher incidence of AMS and greatly increases the misery of altitude sickness; climbers with infections should ascend at a slower rate or, preferably, remain at an intermediate altitude.[37]

People whose work or leisure schedules do not allow gradual ascent can be offered prophylactic treatment with acetazolamide and this is a wise precaution if they have a previous history of altitude sickness. Acetazolamide, and methazolamide, inhibit the enzyme carbonic anhydrase which regulates CO_2 transport out of cells. Inhibition of the enzyme in the renal tubule promotes renal excretion of bicarbonate (HCO_3^-) and conserves hydrogen ion (H^+). The increased arterial H^+ concentration counteracts the respiratory alkalosis caused by hyperventilation in the low oxygen environment of high altitude. Respiratory alkalosis produces a negative feedback on central respiratory drive; carbonic anhydrase inhibition removes this negative feedback, thus enhancing respiratory activity and increasing oxygen uptake (Fig. 18.4).

Prophylactic treatment with acetazolamide raises arterial H^+ concentration and PaO_2 and ameliorates AMS symptoms.[38–41] Prescriptions of acetazolamide (250 mg 80 hourly or 500 mg/day, sustained-release tablet) or methazolamide (150 mg/day) should be given for 2 days before ascent and continued for 7 days at high altitude. Limited data are available on the consequences of discontinuing drug therapy at high altitude. Personal experience indicates that therapy does not impede the process of natural acclimatization and therefore medication can be stopped once sufficient time has elapsed for acclimatization to develop and AMS symptoms to abate. The period of time needed for acclimatization will depend upon the speed of ascent, the altitude achieved and the individual's

unique physiology. Adverse effects of carbonic anhydrase inhibitors include limb and perioral paraesthesia, which diminish with time, and an alteration of the taste of carbonated drinks.

Mountaineers recognize that individuals resistant to altitude sickness urinate profusely on reaching altitude – the 'Hohendiuresis' of the alpine climber. Although acetazolamide is a diuretic, the diuretic effect is short-lived and its efficacy in altitude sickness is not due to this property. Frusemide, a potent loop diuretic, has been advocated for the prevention of AMS; however, there is a danger of aggravating fluid depletion in climbers dehydrated by hyperventilation, intense physical activity and the twin scourges of vomiting and diarrhoea. Hypercoagulability of the blood and sequestration of platelets provoke pulmonary thrombosis at high altitude. The dehydrating effect of a powerful diuretic may aggravate this thrombotic tendency. The milder potassium-sparing diuretic and aldosterone antagonist spironolactone (75 mg/day commencing before ascent) has been recommended for prophylactic treatment on the basis of an uncontrolled trial and case report.[42] Other reports dispute the efficacy of spironolactone[43] and there is insufficient evidence to recommend spironolactone in preference to acetazolamide.

Dexamethasone, a potent synthetic glucocorticoid, has been demonstrated to reduce AMS symptoms when given prior to simulated ascent to high altitude (4570 m)[44] and during rapid ascent of Mount Rainier.[45] In the latter study, dexamethasone was administered at a 4 mg dose every 8 hours for 24 hours before ascent. The potentially serious adverse effects of this drug, such as adrenocortical insufficiency following withdrawal of the drug, limit the duration of prophylactic treatment. The mechanisms whereby dexamethasone exerts its beneficial effect are not known; dexamethasone has no effect upon oxygen consumption or carbon dioxide transport. However, on the assumption that hypoxia-induced cerebral oedema is present even in 'benign' AMS and responsible for the cerebral features (e.g. headache, lack of concentration) seen in this condition, dexamethasone may operate by reducing the extent of cerebral oedema. This action may be exerted by reduction of cerebral blood flow which is increased at high altitude or by decreasing cerebrospinal fluid formation.

Treatment with nifedipine, has no effect on AMS symptoms or gas exchange although pulmonary artery pressure is reduced.[47] The use of nifedipine in altitude-induced illness is confined to the prevention and treatment of HAPO: nifedipine cannot be recommended for AMS prophylaxis.

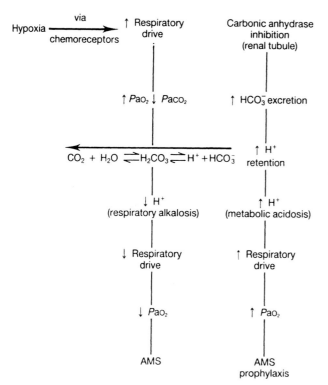

Figure 18.4 *Mode of action of carbonic anhydrase inhibitors in prophylaxis of acute mountain sickness (AMS)*

Treatment

Acute mountain sickness of moderate severity – without respiratory distress or neurological dysfunction such as ataxia – may be managed at intermediate altitudes between 3000 and 4000 m. Descent by only 300–500 m may produce a definite clinical improvement especially if the victim is enabled to sleep at a lower altitude.

Exercise induces sodium and water retention, decreases oxygen saturation and increases pulmonary artery pressure thus enhancing the pathophysiological processes leading to altitude sickness: rest is an important component of therapy for all grades of severity of AMS.[48] Abstinence from alcohol, adequate fluid intake and frequent, small, carbohydrate content meals are recommended.

Paracetamol has been the headache remedy traditionally favoured by AMS sufferers, although ibuprofen, a readily available non-steroidal anti-inflammatory drug, has been demonstrated to be effective in relieving high altitude headache in a placebo-controlled, double-blind trial.[49] The association of nausea, vomiting, and visual disturbance with headache led to the supposition that AMS headache could share a similar pathophysiological mechanism to classical migraine.[50] However, selective stimulation of 5-hydroxytryptamine receptors by sumatriptan (100 mg dose), although a rapid and comprehensive treatment for migraine, was not found to be efficacious in high altitude headache.[51] As the cost is £8 sterling for each 100 mg tablet, this finding will be a relief to financially hard-pressed members of the mountaineering community. To ease other altitude-associated discomforts anti-emetics may be administered, although sedatives should be avoided other than short-acting hypnotics (e.g. temazepam) prescribed at low doses.

The utility of carbonic anhydrase inhibitor treatment for established AMS has been investigated in two published studies. In a double-blind, placebo-controlled trial on Mt McKinley (4200 m) low dose acetazolamide (250 mg) was prescribed at diagnosis and 8 hours subsequently. Symptoms of AMS were relieved, arterial oxygenation improved and pulmonary gas exchange was stabilized.[52] High-dose acetazolamide (1.0–1.5 g) or methazolamide (400–500 mg) were studied on three separate expeditions at altitudes between 3200 and 5486 m; as in the low dose study, AMS symptoms and arterial oxygenation improved significantly.[53] High-dose acetazolamide was associated with more adverse effects, a quarter of subjects suffering from headache. This is sufficient reason to advocate the use of the lower dose treatment regime.

The treatment for severe AMS, HAPO and HACO is immediate descent to the lowest altitude feasible. All other therapeutic measures are of secondary importance. The consequences of delayed descent may be fatal pulmonary and cerebral disease. Once HAPO or HACO are established, oxygen therapy is not unequivocally beneficial even at the recommended flow rate of 6–8 litre/min,[36] the failure of supplementary oxygen to be invariably effective suggests that hypoxia, the initiating insult, precipitates a sequence of pathological events which can only be reversed by retreat from a hypoxic and hypobaric environment. In circumstances where descent is not possible, dexamethasone may be of benefit in AMS and HACO at a dose of 8 mg initially followed by 4 mg every 6 hours by mouth or by intramuscular injection.[54]

Subjects with a history of HAPO have a brisk pulmonary vasoconstriction response to hypoxia and an exaggerated elevation in pulmonary artery pressure at high altitude. Nifedipine, a calcium channel blocker, reverses hypoxic pulmonary hypertension and lowers pulmonary artery pressure; oxygenation improves and the clinical manifestations of HAPO are relieved.[55] As treatment for established HAPO, nifedipine (10 mg sublingually and 20 mg slow-release capsule immediately, 20 mg slow-release capsule every 6 hours until descent) is prescribed. It is known that HAPO is not caused by cardiac failure and the use of frusemide may worsen the condition of a hypotensive, shocked HAPO victim.

Nifedipine has been shown to be effective chemoprophylactic therapy for susceptible mountaineers with previous experience of HAPO.[56] Prescription of nifedipine (20 mg slow-release capsule) for 3 days prior to ascent and during 4 days sojourn at 4559 m reduced significantly the incidence of HAPO. Symptom scores fell, pulmonary artery hypertension was attenuated and oxygenation improved.

The practical problems of transporting oxygen cylinders to high altitude limits the availability of oxygen in an emergency. The alternative of a fabric hyperbaric chamber is now available. The Gamow Bag (weight 6.6 kg including foot pump) can be inflated to an inside pressure of 103 mmHg above ambient atmospheric pressure. At this inflation pressure, an altitude sickness patient inside the chamber experiences a simulated descent;[57] for example, at 4500 m altitude (ambient atmospheric pressure of 433 mmHg) a treated subject experiences a pressure of 536 mmHg equivalent to an altitude of 2780 m, a 'descent' of 1720 m[58] (Fig. 5).

Initial studies of the hyperbaric chamber's contribution to the treatment of altitude sickness reported that altitude symptoms were alleviated[59,60] and PaO_2 rose; however, PaO_2 falls within minutes of return to the outside atmospheric pressure. Later controlled randomized trials confirmed that 1 hour of hyperbaric treatment led to a short-lived improvement in AMS symptoms but there were no beneficial long-term effects.[61] Symptom relief was greater and quicker with pressurization treatment than with oral dexamethasone (8 mg initially, 4 mg after 6 hours) but the benefits of corticosteroid were of greater duration prompting the suggestion that the two forms of therapy should be jointly administered to AMS patients.[62] Other novel attempts to improve gas exchange and hence oxygenation at high altitude include the use of expiratory positive airway pressure in HAPO[48] and the addition of 3% carbon dioxide to inhaled air in AMS.[63] However, the value of these therapeutic interventions remains unproven (Table 18.3).

The experience derived from the operation of the telescopes on Mauna Kea has shown that moderate high alti-

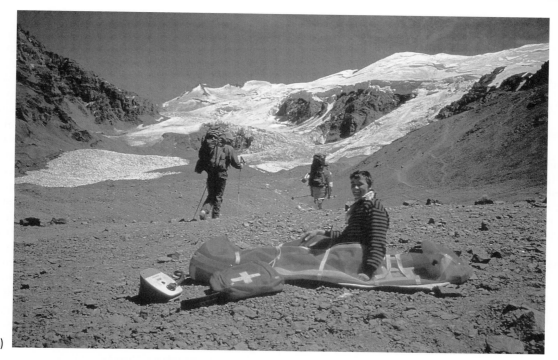

(a)

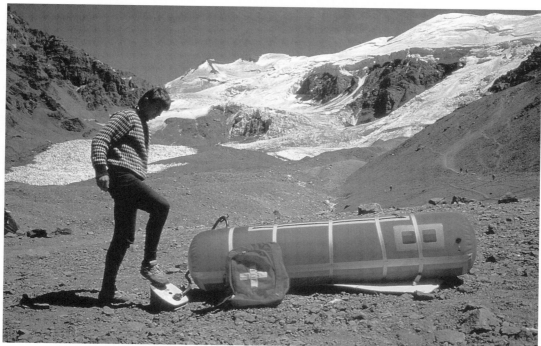

(b)

Figure 18.5 *The Gamow Bag modelled by Dr Ginette Harrison MD MRCGP on Aconcagua. (In 1995, Dr Harrison completed ascents of the seven summits – the highest peaks on each continent.)*

tude can be a safe working environment. Education is essential for safety at high altitude. Recognition of symptoms by a lay group of workers on Mauna Kea was encouraged by the display of a 'Red Alert' notice in the telescope dome (Table 18.4).

Over several decades of scientific endeavour on Mauna Kea, the calibre of astronomical research has

demonstrated that high altitude is not detrimental to high performance. Men endure high altitude for reasons more prosaic than gazing at the stars. At the Aucanquilcha sulphur mines in the Chilean Andes, native miners live and sleep at 5330 m and each day ascend to the mines at 5950 m. Miners refuse to inhabit the camp erected at the mine because of difficulty with

Table 18.3 *Management of altitude sickness*

Prophylaxis: 'Climb high, sleep low'

Slow ascent: above 3000 m, ascend only 300 m per day

Staging: 2 days sojourn at intermediate altitude (i.e. 3000 m)

Drugs for poor acclimatizers: Acetazolamide (250 mg three times a day or 500 mg sustained-release tablet) for 2 days before ascent and 7 days at high altitude; dexamethasone (4 mg three times a day) for 24 h prior to ascent

Treatment for Mild/moderate cases: 'If in doubt, go down'[35]

Rest

Abstinence from alcohol

Adequate fluid intake

Frequent small meals

Paracetamol or ibuprofen

Anti-emetics

Acetazolamide (500 mg sustained-release or 250 mg twice daily)

Severe cases: AMS, HAPO, HACO

Descent

Rest

Oxygen 6–8 litre/min

Hyperbaric pressurization (Gamow bag)

AMS: dexamethasone (8 mg initially, 4 mg every 6 h intramuscular route)

acetazolamide (250 mg 12-hourly or 500 mg slow release)

HAPO: nifedipine (10 mg sublingual and 20 mg slow release immediately, 20 mg slow release 6-hourly)

HACO: dexamethasone (as above)

Table 18.4 *'Red Alert' list*

Cerebral symptoms

Slurred speech

Loss of co-ordination

Loss of balance (when walking)

Impairment of vision (e.g. double or blurred vision)

Weakness of limbs

Disturbance of conscious level (e.g. confusion, disorientation)

Incapacitating headache

Hallucinations

Respiratory symptoms

Severe shortness of breath at rest

Shortness of breath when talking (at rest)

Cough productive of frothy or blood-stained spit

Marked increase in breathing rate at rest (e.g. > 30 min)

- If in doubt, descend from summit – *one* of the above symptoms is sufficient.
- Use common sense

Action to be taken

Inform fellow workers

Descend to sea level

Administer oxygen (6 litres/min)

Seek medical attention at sea level

sleep at the higher elevation nevertheless a gang of caretakers live at the mine in a galvanised iron hut. Each Sunday the caretakers descend to the comfort of 4220 m to play football.[64] Whether people ascend mountains for reasons of economics, curiosity, leisure or physical challenge, high altitude morbidity and mortality are, in part, predictable and preventable. High altitude is an environment which offers unique opportunities to explore and extend the knowledge of ourselves and our world.

REFERENCES

1 Whymper E. *Travels Amongst the Great Andes of the Equator*. London: John Murray, 1892.
2 Fitzgerald E A. *The Highest Andes. A record of the first ascent of Aconcagua and Tupungatoin Argentina and the exploration of the surrounding valleys*. London: Methuen & Co 1899.
3 Ravenhill T H. Some experiences of mountain sickness in the Andes. *J Trop Med Hyg* 1913; **16**: 313–20.
4 Hackett PH, Rennie D. Rales, peripheral edema, retinal haemorrhage and acute mountain sickness. *Am J Med* 1979; **67**: 214–18.

5 Roach RC, Larson EB, Hornbein TF, Houston R, Bartlett S *et al*. Acute mountain sickness, antacids and ventilation during rapid, active ascent of Mount Rainier. *Aviat Space Environ Med* 1983; **54**: 397–401.

6 Singh I, Khanna PK, Srivastava MC, Lal M, Roy SB, Subramanyam CSV. Acute mountain sickness. *N Engl J Med* 1969; **280**: 175–84.

7 Honigman B, Theis MK, Koziol-McLain J, Roach R, Yip R *et al*. Acute mountain sickness in a general tourist population at moderate altitudes. *Ann Int Med* 1993; **118**: 587–92.

8 Forster PJG. *Work at High Altitude: a clinical and physiological study at the United Kingdom Infrared Telescope, Mauna Kea, Hawaii*. Edinburgh: Royal Observatory, 1983.

9 Heath D, Williams DR. *High Altitude Medicine and Pathology*. Oxford: Oxford University Press, 1995.

10 Hultgren HN. High altitude pulmonary edema: Current concepts. *Ann Rev Med* 1996; **47**: 267–84.

11 Singh I, Kapila CC, Khanna PK, Nanda RB, Rao BDP. High altitude pulmonary oedema. *Lancet* 1965; **i**: 229–34.

12 Hackett PH, Rennie D, Levine HD. The incidence, importance and prophylaxis of acute mountain sickness. *Lancet* 1976; **ii**: 1149–54.

13 Maggiorini M, Buhler M, Waiter M, Oelz O. Prevalence of acute mountain sickness in the Swiss Alps. *Br Med J* 1990; **301**: 853–55.

14 Richalet JP. High altitude pulmonary oedema: still a place for controversy. *Thorax* 1995; **50**: 923–29.

15 Milledge JS. High altitude. In: Harries M, Williams C, Stanish WD, Micheli L eds. *Oxford Textbook of Sports Medicine*. Oxford: Oxford University Press, 1996: 217–30.

16 Houston CS, Dickinson J. Cerebral form of high altitude illness. *Lancet* 1975; **ii**: 758–61.

17 Dickinson J, Heath D, Gosney J, Williams D. Altitude related deaths in seven trekkers in the Himalayas. *Thorax* 1983; **38**: 646–56.

18 Rennie D. High altitude oedema – cerebral and pulmonary. In: Clarke C, Ward M, Williams E eds. *Mountain Medicine and Physiology*. London: Alpine Club, 1975: 85–98.

19 Harris CW, Shields JL, Hannon JP. Acute altitude sickness in females. *Aerosp Med* 1966; **37**: 1163–67.

20 Hultgren HN. High altitude medical problems. *Western J Med* 1979; **131**: 8–23.

21 Forster PJG. Reproducibility of individual response to high altitude exposure. *Br Med J* 1984; **2**: 1269.

22 Lakshminarayan S, Pierson DJ. Recurrent high altitude pulmonary oedema with blunted chemosensitivity. *Am Rev Respir Dis* 1975; **111**: 869–72.

23 Milledge JS. Acute mountain sickness. *Thorax* 1983; **38**: 641–45.

24 Fasules JW, Wiggins JW, Wolfe RR. Increased lung vasoreactivity in children from Leadville, Colorado, after recovery from high altitude pulmonary oedema. *Circulation* 1985; **72**: 957–62.

25 Alexander JK. Coronary problems associated with altitude and air travel. *Cardiol Clin* 1995; **13**: 271–78.

26 Shlim D, Houston R. Helicopter rescues and deaths among trekkers in Nepal. *JAMA* 1989; **261**: 1017–19.

27 Hultgren HN. Coronary heart disease and trekking. *J Wilderness Med* 1990; **1**: 154–61.

28 Graham WGB, Houston CS. Short term adaptation to moderate altitude. Patients with chronic obstructive pulmonary disease. *JAMA* 1978; **240**: 1491–94.

29 Brewer GJ, Eaton JW, Grover RF, Weil JV. Cigarette smoking as a cause of hypoxaemia in man at altitude. *Chest* 1971; **59**: 30S–31S.

30 Rennie D, Wilson R. Who should not go high. In: Sutton JR, Jones NL, Houston CS eds. *Hypoxia: Man at Altitude*. New York: Thieme–Stratton Inc, 1982: 186–90.

31 Mirrakhlmov M, Brimkulov N, Cieslicki J, Tobiasz M, Kudaiberdiev Z *et al*. Effects of acetazolamide on overnight oxygenation and acute mountain sickness in patients with asthma. *Eur Resp J* 1993; **6**: 536–40.

32 Winslow RM. Notes on sickle cell disease. In: Sutton JR, Jones NL, Houston CS eds. *Hypoxia: Man at Altitude*. New York: Thieme–Stratton Inc, 1982: 179–81.

33 Nicholson AN, Smith PA, Stone BM, Bradwell AR, Coote JH. Altitude insomnia: Studies during an expedition to the Himalayas. *Sleep* 1988, **11**: 354–61.

34 Sutton R, Houston CS, Mansell AL, McFadden MD, Hackett PH *et al*. Effect of acetazolamide on hypoxemia during sleep at high altitude. *N Engl J Med* 1979; **310**: 1329–31.

35 Pollard AJ. Altitude induced illness. *Br Med J* 1992; **304**: 1324–25.

36 Johnson TS, Rock PB. Acute mountain sickness. *N Engl J Med* 1988; **319**: 841–45.

37 Murdoch DR. Symptoms of infection and altitude illness among hikers in the Mount Everest region of Nepal. *Aviat Space Environ Med* 1995; **66**: 148–51.

38 Wright AD, Bradwell AR, Fletcher RF. Methazolamide and acetazolamide in acute mountain sickness. *Aviat Space Environ Med* 1983; **54**: 619–21.

39 Birmingham Medical Research Expeditionary Society Mountain Sickness Study Group. Acetazolamide in control of acute mountain sickness. *Lancet* 1981; **i**: 180–3.

40 Forward SA, Landowne M, Follansbee JN, Hansen JE. Effect of acetazolamide on acute mountain sickness. *N Engl J Med* 1968; **279**: 839–45.

41 Larson EB, Roach RC, Schoene RB, Hornbein TF. Acute mountain sickness and acetazolamide: clinical efficacy and effect on ventilation. *JAMA* 1982; **248**: 328–32.

42 Turnbull G. Spironolactone prophylaxis in mountain sickness. *Br Med J* 1980; **281**: 1453.

43 Meyers DH. Spironolactone prophylaxis of mountain sickness. *Br Med J* 1980; **281**: 1569.

44 Johnson ST, Rock PB, Fulco CS, Trad LA, Spark RF, Maher JT. Prevention of acute mountain sickness by dexamethasone. *N Engl J Med* 1984; **310**: 683–6.

45 Ellsworth AJ, Larson EB, Strickland D. A randomised trial of dexamethasone and acetazolamide for acute mountain sickness prophylaxis. *Am J Med* 1987; **83**: 1024–30.

46 Zell SC, Goodman PH. Acetazolamide and dexamethasone

in the prevention of acute mountain sickness. *Western J Med* 1988; **148**: 541–45.

47 Hohenhaus E, Niroomand F, Goerre S, Vock P, Oelz O, Bartsch P. Nifedipine does not prevent acute mountain sickness. *Am J Respir Crit Care Med* 1994; **150**: 857–60.

48 Bartsch P. Treatment of high altitude diseases without drugs. *Int J Sports Med* 1992; **1**: 71–74.

49 Broome JR, Stoneham MD, Beeley JM, Milledge JS, Hughes AS. High altitude headache: treatment with ibuprofen. *Aviat Space Environ Med* 1994; **65**: 19–20.

50 Bartsch P, Maggi S, Kleger GR, Ballmer PE, Baumgartner RW. Sumatriptan for high altitude headache. *Lancet* 1994; **344**: 1445.

51 Burtscher M, Likar R, Nachbauer W, Schaffert W, Philadelphy M. Ibuprofen versus sumatriptan for high altitude headache. *Lancet* 1995; **346**: 255–56.

52 Grissom CK, Roach RC, Sarnquist FH, Hackett PH. Acetazolamide in the treatment of acute mountain sickness: clinical efficacy and effect on gas exchange. *Ann Int Med* 1992; **116**: 461–65.

53 Wright AD, Winterborn MH, Forster PJG, Delamere JP, Harrison GL, Bradwell AR. Carbonic anhydrase inhibition in the immediate therapy of acute mountain sickness. *J Wilderness Med* 1994; **5**: 49–55.

54 Ferrazzini G, Maggiorini M, Kriemler S, Bartsch P, Oelz O. Successful treatment of acute mountain sickness with dexamethasone. *Br Med J* 1987; **294**: 1380–82.

55 Oelz O, Maggiorini M, Ritter M, Waber U, Jenni R *et al.* Nifedipine for high altitude pulmonary oedema. *Lancet* 1989; **ii**: 1241–44.

56 Bartsch P, Maggiorini M, Ritter M, Noti C, Vock P, Oelz O. Prevention of high altitude edema by nifedipine. *N Engl J Med* 1991; **325**: 1284–89.

57 Gamow RI, Geer GD, Kasic JF, Smith HM. Methods of gas balance control to be used with a portable hyperbaric chamber in the treatment of high altitude illness. *J Wilderness Med* 1990; **1**: 165–80.

58 Forster PJG, Bradwell AR, Winterborn MJ, Delamere JP, Harrison G and Birmingham Medical Research Expeditionary Society. Alleviation of hypoxia at high altitude: a comparison between oxygen, oxygen and carbon dioxide inhalation and hyperbaric compression. *Clin Sci* 1990; **79**: 1P.

59 King SJ, Greenlee R, Goldings HJ. Acute mountain sickness. *N Engl J Med* 1989; **320**, 1492.

60 Robertson JA, Shlim DR. Treatment of moderate acute mountain sickness with pressurization in a portable hyperbaric (Gamow) bag. *J Wilderness Med* 1991; **2**: 268–73.

61 Bartsch P, Merki B, Hofstetter D, Maggiorini M, Kayser B, Oelz O. Treatment of acute mountain sickness by simulated descent: a randomised controlled trial. *Br Med J* 1993; **306**: 1098–1101.

62 Keller HR, Maggiorini M, Bartsch P, Oelz O. Simulated descent versus dexamethasone in treatment of acute mountain sickness. *Br Med J* 1995; **310**: 1232–35.

63 Harvey TC, Raichle ME, Winterborn MH, Jensen J, Lassen NA *et al.* Effect of carbon dioxide in acute mountain sickness: a rediscovery. *Lancet* 1988; **ii**: 639–41.

64 West JB. *High Life: A History of High-altitude Physiology and Medicine.* New York: Oxford University Press, 1998.

19

Ionizing radiations

JOHN R HARRISON, CHRIS SHARP

Ionizing radiations	397	Basic plan for the handling of casualties following a nuclear reactor accident	413
Dose quantities	398		
Natural background radiation	399	Accidents and radiation risk	415
Detection of radiation	399	Summary	416
Health effects of ionizing radiation	399	References	416
Medical aspects	409	Additional reading on medical treatment of casualties	418
Health surveillance	409		

On 8 November 1895 Wilhelm Roentgen was examining the effects of passing an electric current through a glass tube from which air had been evacuated, when he found that a sheet of photosensitive paper glowed when the current was switched on. He had discovered x-rays and by the turn of the last century radiographs were being used in many fields, in particular for diagnostic purposes. In 1896 Henri Becquerel discovered that certain types of substances, in particular radium, darkened photographic plates. He called this phenomenon 'radiation' and, with a student who worked with him, Madame Marie Curie, continued to investigate and experiment in this field. Due to a lack of knowledge of the harmful biological effects that radiation could produce, they adopted no precautions or gave no thought to the hazards. As a result, Madame Curie received very high doses of radiation and died of leukaemia, possibly due to her radiation exposure. Similarly, many radiologists received high doses of radiation to their hands resulting in erythema and subsequently many died of radiation-induced cancers.[1] Throughout the twentieth century the use of radiation has increased so that now radiation sources and radioactive elements are found in wide and diverse environments, embracing, *inter alia*, nuclear medicine and therapy, non-destructive testing, nuclear power and smoke detectors.

Accident and emergency personnel, hospital specialists, occupational health and public health physicians are likely to become involved with radiation issues if the stringent statutory controls for radiation sources or equipments are bypassed or ignored. For example, the theft of a caesium-137 source in Goiânia, Brazil led to 50 people receiving significant exposure and four deaths.[2]

Large areas of land and property were affected. There have been many accidents with irradiator sources using non-destructive testing or irradiation of foods and materials where individuals have received very high doses, often leading to death. In the Chernobyl nuclear power plant accident 28 members of the workforce died of radiation-related injuries and the release of radioactivity led to widespread contamination of houses, land and foodstuffs.[3,4] These low probability events can lead to significant radiation exposures to both the workforce and the public and their clinical management would clearly involve hospital physicians, occupational and public health physicians, and general practitioners. Experience suggests that in all these scenarios both the individual employee's health outcome and the public's health concerns dominate the agenda and place a burden on health professionals. Coherent plans to deal with these events are essential.

IONIZING RADIATIONS

Atoms, radioactivity and radiation

All matter is made up of atoms. Each atom contains a nucleus around which electrons orbit. In the nucleus there are protons and neutrons. All atoms of the same chemical element have an identical number of positively charged protons in the nucleus and negatively charged electrons on the orbits. So an undisturbed atom is electrically neutral. The number of protons defines the atomic number of the element. The mass of the atom is determined by the number of protons and neutrons and

Table 19.1 *Properties of ionizing radiations*

Type	Range in air	Range in tissue	Hazard	Examples
Alpha (α)	Few cm	10s of μ	Internal	Plutonium
Beta (β)	Up to several metres	Few mm	External and internal	Caesium
Gamma (γ)	Many metres	Many cm	External and internal	Cobalt source
x-Rays	Many metres	Many cm	External	Hospitals
Neutrons	Many metres	Many cm	External	Reactors

Tables 19.1–19.10 created by, and reproduced with permission from National Radiological Protection Board, Chilton, Oxfordshire, UK.

the total number is called the mass number. The same element can have different numbers of neutrons and consequently different mass numbers. These variants of the elements are known as isotopes. Some of these isotopes are unstable and eventually transform into atoms of another element with the simultaneous emission of alpha(α)- or beta(β)-particles and accompanied usually by gamma (γ)-rays. This property of the unstable atom is called radioactivity; the change itself is called radioactive decay and the unstable atom is said to be a radionuclide. The time necessary to reach a stable form depends on the particular isotope and may take a few fractions of a second to several thousand years. The time for the activity to decay by one-half is termed the half-life ($t_{1/2}$). For example sodium-23 (^{23}Na) is the stable form of sodium and ^{24}Na is a radioactive isotope with a $t_{1/2}$ of 15 hours. The latter decays emitting a β-particle to become ^{24}Mg a stable isotope of magnesium. This activity is measured by the numbers of disintegrations per unit time. The unit by which radioactivity is measured is the becquerel (Bq) and one Bq equals one atomic disintegration per second; 60 Bq is the average amount of natural potassium-40 (^{40}K) in every kilogram of the average person. This means that about 15 million ^{40}K atoms disintegrate inside a person each hour.

What are ionizing radiations?

Ionizing radiation may be higher energy electromagnetic radiations (x-rays and γ-rays) or energetic subatomic particles such as α- and β-particles and neutrons. According to their energy, x-rays and γ-rays interact with matter and tissue and although the mechanisms may be different, they all produce positively and/or negatively charged ions, which then interact with the absorbing matter to produce physicochemical changes by adding or subtracting electrons. The energy of these electromagnetic radiations will also determine their penetration, higher energy photons penetrating further than low energy ones. When they do interact with tissues and cells, energy is deposited within the tissue.

The different radiations penetrate matter in different ways, the properties being determined by the size, charge and energy of each type; α-particles are stopped by a thin piece of paper or the dead layer of the skin, while β-particles can penetrate the hand and but will be stopped by a thin sheet of aluminium; x- and γ-rays penetrate the body and an aluminium sheet but are stopped by lead. Neutrons penetrate most materials but may be stopped by thick polythene or concrete (hydrogenous materials); high energy neutrons have a high penetrance in tissue but low energy neutrons can be absorbed in the body because of the body's high water content. (See Table 19.1.) These overall properties of radiation affect the degree of cellular damage following exposure and the methods needed for protection.

In general α-particles do not constitute a significant hazard as an external source, but are hazardous when taken into the body. When incorporated they can irradiate adjacent cells in, for example, the liver. Neutrons, because of their absence of electrical charge, produce ionization indirectly and tend to be more penetrating. Ionizing radiations have sufficient energy to break chemical bonds and ionize atoms and molecules, producing an ion pair. These ions are charged and capable of causing further ionization and energy deposition leading to physicochemical changes in cellular constituents.

DOSE QUANTITIES

Some of these changes may be of no biological consequence and others may be repaired, but there is a finite probability that damage may cause cell death or irreparable damage to vital cell constituents. The *absorbed dose* is a measure of the mean energy absorbed by unit mass of tissue, and the absorbed dose in gray (Gy) is equal to the deposition of one joule (J) of energy in 1 kilogram (kg) of tissue. Overall, the greater the dose, the greater the likelihood of a biological effect being seen. Energy is deposited along the path of ionizing radiation as it traverses tissues in the form of ionizations. The average deposition of energy per unit length is called the linear energy transfer (LET).

Charged particles tend to have higher LET values than x- or γ-rays. The International Commission on Radiological Protection (ICRP) has introduced a weighting factor related to LET to take into account these differences.[5] These radiation weighting factors (w_R) may range from 1 to 20 for different radiations. Thus photons, such as x- or γ-rays, are assigned a w_R of 1 (low LET) and α-particles 20 (high LET). Tissues are also assigned weighting factors (w_T) to differentiate the wide variation in tissue sensitivity to radiation, the lymphopoeitic stem cells and gonadal germ cell cells being the most sensitive and bone being relatively insensitive. These radiation and tissue weighting factors are used to convert the absorbed dose in grays to an effective dose in sieverts (Sv). This system allows external and internal exposures to be combined into one dose – on the basis of equality of risk. Once a radionuclide is incorporated it will continue to expose surrounding tissues until final decay or it is excreted. It is usual to calculate this committed effective dose following the ingestion or inhalation so that extra care can be taken to reduce future external exposures.

Submultiples of the sievert are commonly used, such as the millisievert (mSv), which is one-thousandth of a sievert; for example, the world average individual dose received due to exposure to natural background radiation is about 2.4 mSv per year compared with the occupational dose limit of 20 mSv per year.[6] It is sometimes useful to have a measure of the total dose to groups of people or a population. The quantity used to express this total is the collective effective dose: it is obtained by summing the product of all the doses in a group and the number of people in the group and is usually expressed in person sieverts. Throughout this chapter these various dose quantities will be referred to as dose, except where further clarification is required.

NATURAL BACKGROUND RADIATION

Radiation of natural origin pervades the whole environment. Cosmic rays reach the earth from outer space, the earth itself is radioactive, and natural activity is present in our diet and in the air. Everybody is exposed to natural radiation to a greater or lesser extent, and for most people it is the major source of exposure.

DETECTION OF RADIATION

Physical

Ionizing radiations cannot be directly detected by the human senses, but they can be detected and measured by a variety of means, such as photographic films, Geiger tubes and scintillation counters. There are also relatively new techniques using thermoluminescent materials and silicon diodes. Some of these techniques are used to measure individual doses on dosemeters (generally called film badges). Measurements made with such

dosemeters can be interpreted to represent the energy deposited in the body or in a particular part of the body by the radiation concerned.

Biological

When a radionuclide is deposited in an internal organ, for instance via ingestion or inhalation, doses are generally calculated because the activities are too small to be measured. The dose (or activity) can be assessed or measured by taking urine or blood samples and applying biokinetic models or be measured directly by special detection systems, e.g. whole body monitors. These systems are only available at special sites in the UK, such as British Nuclear Fuels, the Atomic Weapons Establishment, the National Radiological Protection Board (NRPB) or the United Kingdom Atomic Energy Authority.

In an accident situation, estimating the whole body dose by changes in circulating absolute lymphocyte counts in the first 48 hours is possible and by cytogenetic assays for chromosome aberrations in cultured lymphocytes. These techniques use either dicentric counting or more recently fluorescence *in situ* hybridization (FISH) painting of chromosomes and measuring the translocation of genetic material. The threshold for whole body dose validated chromosomal changes is around 1–200 mSv. More recently electron spin resonance techniques have been developed using teeth or, in the case of cadavers, bone, which permits a retrospective assessment of the dose. The accurate range for this technique is from around 100 mGy to lethal doses. Another technique using post-subcapsular lens opacities also offers a possible way to assess historic doses; however, its accuracy is not yet proven.

HEALTH EFFECTS OF IONIZING RADIATION

Any organ or tissue may be affected, the degree varying with the dose and the radiosensitivity of the given organ or tissue. Distinguishing two types of effects is possible, somatic and hereditary. The somatic effects relate to the individual who is exposed, and may be early or late, and in the embryo or fetus may be teratogenic. The hereditary effects would occur in the offspring, through genetic damage to germ cells of the exposed individual.

Somatic effects

Somatic effects are classified as *deterministic* and *stochastic*. Deterministic effects are those for which the severity increases with the dose and for which a threshold exists. Stochastic effects are those whose probability of occurrence increases with the dose and whose severity is independent of the dose and without a threshold. With deterministic effects, cause and effect can be seen. However, due to the random nature of the interaction of radiation with matter, for stochastic effects the inference of cause can only be based on an increase in the probability of that effect. Where the dose is low (as is likely in occupational exposures), only stochastic effects might be seen. The severity of stochastic effects is not dose dependent as it is with deterministic effects. So an increase in a dose produces an increase in the probability of a stochastic effect.

DETERMINISTIC EFFECTS

Generally, dose-response relationships are sigmoid in shape and exhibit a threshold. For each deterministic effect, the two main parameters to consider are the threshold dose (ED_0), at which the given effect may appear, and its relative severity. These effects are characterized by the median dose, ED_{50}, at which 50% of exposed individuals will exhibit the effect, and by the slope of the curve at the median. The dose-response relationships are generally quoted for acute exposure; protraction of exposure increases the median dose for the effect.[6-8]

Doses below which selected deterministic effects should not occur in a normally distributed population (ED_0) are given in Table 19.2. These levels take into account the individual variation and sensitivity rather than the average value. They are not complete and are for guidance only. The values should not be used in conditions of known radiosensitivity, e.g. ataxia telangiectasia.

Haematopoietic system

The bone marrow is the main organ of concern since exposure to penetrating radiation at high dose rate can

lead to death within a few weeks. This early mortality results from stem cell depletion in the marrow. The lymphocytes are the most sensitive indicators of injury to the bone marrow. Acute doses of 1–2 Gy reduce their concentration in blood to about 50% of their normal level within about 48 hours. Neutrophils and platelets also show a dose-related decrease in concentrations and the levels can be used to predict the likelihood of survival and the necessity for treatment. People with bone marrow aplasia show an increased susceptibility to infection and frequently spontaneous bleeding (from thrombocytopenia) as a direct result of damage to the immune and haematopoietic systems. In severe cases of radiation injury, marrow aplasia is the likely cause of death.[6,9]

Because of the lack of quantitative human data there has been considerable uncertainty about the dose-effect relationship for death due to irradiation of the bone marrow following acute or chronic radiation exposure. Extensive data have been published on the effects of whole-body irradiation in animals.[10] However, they cannot be used directly to predict dose-response relationships for man due to marked variation between species but they do provide information on the likely shape of the dose-response relationship.

The median lethal dose for humans is not precisely known. Several estimates have been published ranging from 2.4 to 5.1 Gy bone marrow dose. The higher values of the estimates of the LD_{50} involved cases where significant supportive and therapeutic medical treatment was provided. With minimal medical treatment involving no more than basic first aid, a value for LD_{50} of 3 Gy has been adopted by United Nations Scientific Committee on the Effects of Atomic Radiations (UNSCEAR)[6] the National Radiological Protection Board, UK (NRPB)[7]

Table 19.2 Approximate threshold levels of dose (ED_0) for deterministic effects (adult exposure)

Organ	Effect	ED_0 (threshold dose) (Gy)
Whole body	Early death	1.5
	Prodromal syndrome (e.g. vomiting)	0.5
Bone marrow	Early death	1.5
	Depression of haematopoiesis	0.5
Lung	Early death	6
	Pneumonitis	3–5
Skin	Prompt erythema, dry desquamation	>8
	Moist desquamation and necrosis	>15
Thyroid	Hypothyroidism	3
Lens of the eye	Detectable opacity	0.5–2
	Cataract with loss of vision	5
Testes	Temporary sterility	0.15
	Permanent sterility	3.5–6
Ovaries	Permanent sterility	2.5–6
Embryo or fetus	Teratogenesis	0.10

and the Nuclear Regulatory Commission, USA (NUREG).[11] For supportive medical treatment which includes procedures such as reverse isolation procedures, the use of antibiotics, white cell and platelet transfusions and intravenous feeding, NRPB[7] and NUREG[11] recommend a value for LD_{50} of 4.5 Gy. This is based partly on human and partly on animal data. Recent advances in rescuing depleted marrow with stem cell stimulating growth factors[12,13] would now be included in treatment. These offer hope that the LD_{50} will be raised, possibly to the point where death no longer depends on haematopoietic damage.

The lymphocyte count decreases within a few hours of irradiation and the platelet and granulocyte counts within a few days or weeks, while the erythrocyte count begins to decrease rather slowly only after a number of weeks. The exposed individual may die from infection or from haemorrhage. The consensus value for the median lethal dose within 60 days ($LD_{50/60}$) is estimated to range from 2.5 to 5 Gy, after homogeneous exposure. The slope of the dose-response curve is relatively steep, expressing a rapidly increasing probability of death for small increments of dose without medical treatment.

Gastrointestinal tract

There is considerable variation in response as the different parts of the gastrointestinal tract have markedly different radiosensitivity. The oesophagus and rectum are relatively radio-resistant, while the stomach and small intestine are much more sensitive.[14] The small intestine is the most sensitive because of the rapidly proliferating mucosal cells of the mucosal epithelium in the crypts of Lieberkühn.[15] Single acute doses to the abdomen of around 6–16 Gy produces early onset of nausea, vomiting and diarrhoea, the symptoms occurring earlier and being prolonged broadly in proportion to the dose. These symptoms are thought to be caused by the release of 5-hydroxytryptamine (5-HT) into the bloodstream which stimulates the nausea/vomiting centres in the brain and other 5-HT receptors.[16] There is a concomitant increase in bowel motility which may be caused by bile salts and other substances acting on the damaged mucosa. Very few human data are available on this gastrointestinal syndrome. It is known, however, that cancer patients given whole body doses of 10 Gy or more (generally as a single dose delivered in about 4 hours, in conjunction with bone marrow transplantation) have survived the gastrointestinal syndrome.[17] Data obtained from studies in which x-rays were used to irradiate acutely the gastrointestinal tract of rats indicate an LD_{50} of about 15 Gy, an LD_{10} of 10 Gy and an LD_{90} of 20 Gy.

For gastrointestinal symptoms the following figures are given as guidelines for adults; anorexia may be seen in 5% of those at 0.4 Gy and 95% at 3 Gy, nausea in 5% at 0.5 Gy and 95% at 4.5 Gy, vomiting in 5% at 0.6 Gy and 100% at 7 Gy, and diarrhoea in 5% at 1 Gy and over 20% at 8 Gy. If the time from exposure to onset of any of the above symptoms is less than 1 hour the whole body dose is likely to be >3 Gy, if more than 3 hours <1 Gy and if they last for more than 24 hours the dose is likely to be >6 Gy. The onset of symptoms within 30 minutes indicates an abdominal dose >3Gy. These signs and symptoms are sometimes referred to as the acute radiation syndrome.

Lung

The lung can be exposed to external radiation from a beam or internal radiation after inhalation of radioactive materials. Radiation pneumonitis appears some weeks or months after exposure. It is a complex phenomenon, including oedema, cell death, cell desquamation, fibrin exudate in the alveoli, fibrous thickening of alveolar septa and proliferative changes in the blood vessels. The main effect is interstitial pneumonitis, followed by pulmonary fibrosis, resulting principally from the damage and response of the fine vasculature and the connective tissues. Development of the lesions is highly influenced by the volume of the organ irradiated and the dose. An acute exposure of both lungs shows a threshold at about 6–7 Gy, with an ED_{50} at about 9 Gy.[18]

Thyroid

The adult thyroid is not especially sensitive to radiation; however, it should always be considered if iodine isotopes are inhaled or ingested by some employees as it accumulates rapidly in the gland. The radiation-induced diseases include acute radiation thyroiditis and hypothyroidism. Total ablation of the thyroid requires high doses, about 1000 Gy delivered within a short period (2 weeks).[18,19] Hypothyroidism is produced by much lower doses, with 50% incidence at about 60 Gy for acute external exposure and 300 Gy for prolonged internal exposure. The childhood thyroid is more sensitive to radiation (see below).

Skin

The skin is a relatively radio-resistant organ but is likely to be exposed in any type of accident. Skin responses depend upon various factors, such as size of the irradiated area, depth distribution of dose, duration of exposure and dose rate.[18] Radiation damage to the skin may be observed as erythema, moist desquamation and necrosis, with thresholds of 2 Gy, 12–20 Gy and >18 Gy respectively. Moist desquamation often results in chronic changes, with hyperkeratosis and telangiectasia of the capillaries and of superficial and deep blood vessels. The chronic phase may lead to ulceration, atrophy and necrosis.

Protraction of exposures for 1–14 days will increase the threshold and ED_{50} values by a factor of about 2 compared with acute exposure.[18] Recent experience[2,20] has demonstrated that some accidents may cause extensive damage to the skin. As radiation burns involving large areas can precipitate the same systemic effects as thermal injury, overall management may be complicated especially where other body systems have been affected, e.g. bone marrow.

Eye

Experience has shown that radiation doses received by the lens may result in cataracts. The eye may be exposed either after local irradiation – acute or protracted – or after whole body irradiation. The threshold level for detectable opacity is estimated at about 1 Gy.[5,6] Protraction does not increase the threshold so much as for some other organs. Unlike the previously discussed deterministic effects, the cataract does not appear early after exposure; the latent period varies from 6 months to 35 years, with an average of 3 years.

Gonads

The germ cells of the reproductive system are highly radiosensitive. The threshold dose for transient sterility lasting for several weeks averages 0.15 Gy for men and about 5–10 times higher for women.[5,6] Recovery time in men is dose dependent and may take many years. Doses of 2.5–6 Gy or more are required for permanent sterility in both men and women.

Embryo and fetus

The embryo and fetus should also be considered, as women in the workforce may become pregnant. The developmental effects of radiation in the embryo and fetus are strongly related to the gestational age at which the exposure occurs, i.e. whether it occurs during organogenesis.[21] The most serious health consequences of prenatal exposure are embryonic death, gross congenital malformation, growth retardation or severe mental retardation. For exposures at high dose rates, severe mental retardation has been shown for exposure occurring during the 8th–15th week and to a lesser degree during the 16th–25th week after conception. The threshold dose is estimated to be around 0.4 Gy between the 8th and 15th week and 0.1–0.2 Gy between the 16th and 25th respectively.[22]

Central nervous system

The acute central nervous system effects are generally reached only when the whole body radiation dose exceeds about 50 Gy. The survival time is usually less than 48 hours.[8,23] Death is believed to be a function of several causes including vascular damage, meningitis, myelitis and encephalitis. Fluid also infiltrates the brain causing marked oedema. However, any person who exhibits even mild symptoms of central nervous system syndrome would inevitably die from gastrointestinal or haematopoietic damage.

Effects of acute whole body radiation exposure

The effects which are likely to be seen following a homogenous whole body irradiation over a short period (minutes or hours) are shown in Table 19.3 below. Experience from several accidents has shown that most casualties have only part of their bodies exposed to the radiation. The non-uniform and heterogeneous nature of the exposure leads to variable signs and symptoms and the outcomes are different. Some high localized

doses do not present with the classical prodromal signs of nausea and vomiting. This complicates the initial triage and subsequent therapy. For example, in patients with severe but partial bone marrow irradiation residual stem cells in unaffected bone marrow can reject bone marrow grafts causing host-versus-graft disease. This was one of the prime reasons why most of the transplantations at Chernobyl were unsuccessful.[4]

Effects of whole body chronic radiation exposure

In a chronic exposure (measured in days, weeks, months) the symptoms are usually more subtle. The usual feature is of general malaise, with influenza type symptoms, fever and or diarrhoea and vomiting. Several cases have arisen where people have been exposed chronically to an industrial or a medical therapy radiation source, sometimes discarded or procured illegally. In a recent case (unpublished), where a radiation source had been taken into a house, it was only after an elderly member of the household died and others started to suffer from general malaise that radiation exposure was suspected. It has been reported that chronic radiation exposures have been implicated in life shortening, accelerated ageing and premature atherosclerosis, but the evidence is inconclusive; when the data were critically reviewed by UNSCEAR in 1982 most claims were not

Table 19.3 *Expected signs and symptoms following whole body irradiation*

Dose	Signs/Symptoms
0–100 mSv	No signs or symptoms Dose clinically undetectable
100–500 mSv	No signs or symptoms Expected laboratory findings: • Small decrease in lymphocyte count in blood (1–4 days) • Increase in accuracy of chromosome dosimetry from limit of sensitivity
500 mSv–2 Sv	Nausea and vomiting probable Onset usually >2 h Laboratory findings: • Diagnostic changes in blood within days • Accurate chromosome dosimetry
2–6 Sv	Nausea, vomiting and headache onset within 30 min to 2 h Laboratory findings: • Early diagnostic changes in blood • Accurate chromosome dosimetry *Note*: Lethal dose 50% without treatment ~3 Sv
>6 Sv	Rapid onset nausea, vomiting headache and pyrexia (within 30 min)
>8 Sv	Chromosome dosimetry becoming saturated Gastrointestinal syndrome – diarrhoea
10s of Sv	Rapid onset of apathy, prostration, convulsions and death

substantiated.[24] Chronic fatigue has also been reported in other accidents and is a characteristic seen in patients who have undergone radiotherapy.[25] Some researchers consider that a chronic radiation syndrome exists; however, the signs and symptoms are non-specific and do not present as a defined syndrome. In many places where these complaints have been reported, other environmental hazards exist, such as extensive environmental heavy metal contamination.

Effects of partial body exposure to radiation

In almost all partial body exposures, whether acute or chronic, the skin will be affected. Table 19.4 shows the severity of skin damage with increasing dose. The effects would only be seen in accident situations or where flagrant breaches of safety practices have occurred.[26] Depending on the type of exposure, deeper tissues may also be affected. Incidents where small sources have been carried in shirt pockets for short periods have given rise to exceptional doses (measured in hundreds of Gy) leading to serious necrotic lesions of the chest wall.

Table 19.4 *Effects of radiation on the skin*

Skin dose	Signs
0–100 mGy	Nil
100–400 mGy	Nil expected
400 mGy–4 Gy	Transient erythema expected within 3 days of exposure
4 Gy–8 Gy	As above followed by fixed erythema after variable atent period
	Temporary hair loss
8 Gy–15 Gy	Prompt erythema followed by vesiculation
	Permanent hair loss
>15 Gy	Severe vesiculation, tissue slough
	Very slow to heal
	Possible site of malignant change

STOCHASTIC EFFECTS

Carcinogenesis

Following irradiation a viable but modified somatic cell may retain its mitotic capacity and may result, after a prolonged and variable period, in the development of a malignancy. The cancers induced by radiation, with or without the contributions of other agents, are indistinguishable from those occurring 'spontaneously' or from other causes. Since the probability of cancer resulting from the radiation is related to dose, this type of effect of radiation can only be detected by statistical means in epidemiological studies carried out on exposed population groups. If the number of people in an irradiated group and the doses that they have received is known, and if the number of cancers eventually observed in the group exceeds the number that could be expected in an otherwise similar but non-irradiated group, the excess number of cancers may be attributed to radiation, and

the risk of cancer per unit dose may be calculated, i.e. the risk factor. The probability of causation can be ascribed based on radioepidemiological tables (see below).

A major source of information on the risk of radiation-induced cancer following whole body irradiation is the follow-up studies of the survivors of the atomic bombing in Hiroshima and Nagasaki in Japan in 1945.[27] Data have also been obtained for a number of tissues from other exposed human population groups, for example, tuberculosis patients who had high x-ray doses during treatments,[28–32] and from people exposed to nuclear weapons fallout in the Marshall Islands.[33] Risk estimates have also been developed for cancers of some individual organs, based on information on the effects of incorporated radionuclides, in miners exposed to radon and its decay products,[34] from employees exposed to radium in the luminizing industry,[35] and from patients given the x-ray contrast medium Thorotrast (thorium oxide).[36] Some of the available epidemiological data of second cancers, for example of the breast, in patients who have been irradiated for Hodgkin's disease[37,41] are far from ideal for calculating risk estimates because of the confounding influence of various chemotherapy and radiotherapy regimes. A further example is the significant increase in childhood (but not adult) thyroid cancer in Belarus, the Ukraine and the Russian Federation following the inhalation and ingestion of radio-iodines after the Chernobyl accident. It has proved difficult to reconstruct the thyroid doses and so the risk estimates are not yet robust. Furthermore the accuracy of the dosimetry involved in many of the large epidemiological studies is also a potential source of error and needs careful evaluation. Recent risk estimates are based largely on the Japanese bomb survivor data,[27] and one drawback to the use of these data for risk estimates at low dose and dose rates, is the contribution from neutron exposure. Estimates of the dose were revised in 1986[38] which along with the appearance of more cancers in the ageing survivors has led to a revision upwards of the risk estimates.

Information of this nature has been reviewed in BEIR,[39] in ICRP 60[5] and in the 1994 report of UNSCEAR.[40] These reports assess the risks of radiation-induced fatal cancer, based predominantly on data on the Life Span Study (LSS) of the atomic bomb survivors. Where risk factors are not available from the LSS they have been developed from the many other epidemiological studies. The risks have increased partly as a result of new estimates of tissue doses received by the Japanese population, because more cancers have appeared in the longer period of follow-up to 1990, and because different models have been used to predict the risk over a lifetime. However, there is uncertainty in how many cancers will arise in the future as over half of the Japanese cohort were still alive in 1990.

The research on the atomic bomb survivors in Japan

has shown that leukaemia appears first after whole body irradiation, with a latent period of 2 years and peaks at 6–7 years. Solid tumours begin to appear after about 10 years and their incidence continues to increase for several decades. No threshold is detectable and statistically significant increased risks exist at doses down to 50 mSv.[27] This is important for setting acceptable occupational dose limits (see below).

However, as discussed earlier, the cancer risks derived from such exposed groups are based largely on exposures to high doses delivered over a short period of time. In practice most people are exposed occupationally to low doses of radiation received over relatively long periods. On the basis of available information, therefore, UNSCEAR[6] and ICRP[5] have assessed that the risk factors obtained directly from observations at high doses and high dose rates should be reduced by at least a factor of two (UNSCEAR 2–10 and ICRP 2) to give more realistic risk factors for low doses and dose rates. The risk factor or lifetime fatality probability coefficient from ICRP for a reference population of both sexes and of working age is 4×10^{-2}/Sv for the sum of all fatal malignancies, i.e., a dose of 1 Sv in a working lifetime results in a 4% chance of a fatal cancer occurring[5] More recent epidemiological studies involving lower dose exposures from the UK National Registry for Radiation Workers have shown that the leukaemia incidence trend with dose is consistent with the ICRP risk estimates.[41]

Probability of causation

The concept of the probability of causation (PC) has been developed to answer the question: if a person has been exposed to ionizing radiation and subsequently develops a cancer, what is the probability that the cancer was due to the earlier exposure? The US National Institutes of Health[42] used earlier data on the Japanese atomic bomb survivors to compile tables on the probability of causation relating an individual's cancer to a prior radiation dose. This topic has also been reviewed recently by the International Atomic Energy Agency (IAEA).[43] In essence, the probability that a radiation dose to an organ of a person's body leads to the subsequent development of cancer there can generally be calculated as:

$$PC = \frac{ERR}{(1+ERR)}$$

where ERR is the excess relative risk associated with the exposure, i.e. ERR is the relative increase in risk, with the value 1 subtracted. For example, an ERR of 1 represents a doubling of the risk, relative to that in the absence of exposure. This gives a probability of causation of

$$PC = 1/(1 + 1) = 0.5$$

i.e. a 50% chance that the cancer was induced by radiation. The ERR can depend on a number of factors. Among them, the size of the radiation dose is very important. Generally the ERR varies in direct proportion to the dose, although in some circumstances the trend in risk with dose is more complex. For example, data on the Japanese survivors indicate that the risk of leukaemia varies not as a simple linear function of dose, but according to both linear and quadratic functions of dose. As well as dose, ERR can be affected by factors such as sex, the age at which the exposure occurred, and the time between exposure and the development of the disease. For example, for leukaemia and for many solid cancers, data from the Japanese survivors and other studies indicate that the ERR is greater for exposure in childhood than in adulthood. Also, the ERR for leukaemia tends to be higher soon after exposure than at later times whereas – at least for exposures in adulthood – the ERR of solid cancers is fairly stable over time. The degree to which the dose was protracted may also need to be taken in calculating the ERR, since various animal studies have suggested that, for a given total dose, radiation risks may be higher if received acutely rather than over a prolonged period.

For a given exposure scenario i.e. the size of the dose, the sex of the person exposed, the age of exposure, the time between exposure and the onset of disease, the degree of dose protraction), it is therefore possible using models such as those developed by the US BEIR V Committee[39] to derive an estimate of the ERR. This can then be used, via the approach described above to estimate the PC. However, in instances where the dose is not known or where there are differing views about its magnitude, the calculation can be reversed to obtain the dose required to produce a given value for PC. For example, it was explained earlier than a 50% probability of causation (i.e. a PC of 0.5) corresponds to an ERR of 1. For a given person and a likely time of exposure, it is then possible using a standard risk model to derive an estimate of the dose required to give such an ERR. This approach could be used to calculate the doses required to attain various values for the PC in individual employees who have cancer.

In the UK the nuclear industry has set up a no-fault compensation scheme based on PC calculations, to avoid unnecessary litigation and allow the current scientific risk factors to be used in a generous manner for those claiming a radiation-induced cancer.

Examples of probability of causation calculations[43]

It is essential to establish that the radiation exposure was work related and the exposure had a certain probability to cause the particular cancer. The cancer concerned should be known to be radiation inducible, for example, there is no evidence that chronic lymphatic leukaemia or Hodgkin's disease are induced by radiation.

It is important to establish that the latency period between exposure and cancer diagnosis is consistent with those accepted as a result of epidemiological studies of radiation-exposed populations. It takes at least 2 years for leukaemia and bone cancer and 10 years for all other cancers to clinically manifest after exposure. Therefore, a lung tumour diagnosed 5 years after exposure is unlikely to be radiation induced. The radiation exposure should normally be greater than that typically accumulated from natural background radiation. Radiation-induced cancer in tissues or organs other than those exposed would normally be excluded.

For the calculation of the probability of causation the following data should be known: age at exposure; gender; external and/or internal dose to the whole body or individual organs; dose estimation (where there is inadequate formal dosimetry); the diagnosis; age at diagnosis; and other major risk factors besides radiation (smoking, exposures to solvents, medical radiation exposures, chemotherapy, etc.).

The two examples below illustrate how the relative risk (RR) and hence the PC varies with age at exposure and time since exposure using the BEIR V leukemia model[39] Although in both cases the single acute dose received is 100 mSv, the PC ranges from 7% when the age at exposure is greater than 20 years and the leukaemia is diagnosed more than 30 years since exposure, to 78% when the age at exposure is less than 21 years and the leukaemia is diagnosed less than 16 years since the exposure.

Example 1

A male is diagnosed with leukaemia at the age of 68 years. He received a single, uniform acute radiation dose to the red bone marrow of 100 mSv at the age of 35 years. Using the BEIR V model,[39] and because the dose was received 33 years before diagnosis the probability of causation by radiation is 7%.

Example 2

In this case, a single acute dose of 100 mSv is received at the age of 20 years and a leukaemia is diagnosed at the age of 33 years. Now, because the age at irradiation is less than 21 years, and the time since exposure is only 13 years the probability of causation is 78%.

Hereditary effects

The other main late effect of radiation is the concept of hereditary damage and arises through irradiation of the germ cells. Ionizing radiation induces mutations which are frequently harmful in the germ cells or their precursors. The hereditary diseases that mutations may cause range from afflictions such as colour blindness or minor disorders of metabolism (e.g. disorders of amino acid metabolism) to serious defects which may cause early death or severe mental retardation (e.g. Down syndrome).

The study of genetic or hereditary effects caused by radiation is even more difficult than the study of cancer. However, no conclusive evidence for hereditary effects attributable to exposure to radiation has been found in human offspring.[6,44] Genetic and cytogenetic studies of the progeny born to the atomic bomb survivors in Japan have so far yielded no evidence of a statistically significant increase in severe hereditary defects.[45] Extensive studies made on experimental animals provide some information of the frequency with which genetic effects, including chromosome aberrations (numerical or structural) and mutations of genes (dominant and recessive), can be expected to occur.[46] The research so far suggests that the doubling dose for all genetic effects is around 1 Gy.

PARENTAL EXPOSURE AND OFFSPRING

Follow-up of the atomic bomb survivors and their offspring has not yielded evidence for a statistically significant excess of malignancy in those children conceived after exposure;[47] however, a study in the UK suggested a link between paternal occupational exposure to radiation at the Sellafield nuclear reprocessing plant (West Cumbria, UK) and leukaemia in the offspring.[48] The associations did not provide evidence of causality and more recently the UK Committee on the Medical Aspects of Radiation in the Environment (COMARE) has shown that occupational exposures to radiation are very unlikely to account for the excess of leukaemia in West Cumbria. Other agents such as infections and population mixing may be the cause.[49]

BIOLOGICAL BASIS FOR RADIATION EFFECTS

It is generally accepted that for carcinogenesis, the cellular DNA of the genome is the critical molecule. Damage to this molecule leading to cancer can be mediated through direct ionization by the radiation or by its indirect action in the formation of free radicals in the fluid in close proximity to the genome. This indirect effect accounts for about two-thirds of the biological effect in the case of low LET radiation, but the direct effect predominates with high LET radiation. Evidence is building that there are fragile sites unusually prone to breakage and rearrangement in DNA, which could explain particular sensitivities.

In some medical conditions, such as ataxia telangiectasia and Li-Fraumeni syndrome, there exist genetic defects in cell repair mechanisms which produce an increase in individual sensitivity to ionizing radiation. At high doses, cell death will predominate leading to organ malfunction, whose severity is dependent on the dose.

FACTORS INFLUENCING RADIOSENSITIVITY AND MODIFICATION OF EFFECTS OF EXPOSURE

Susceptibility to the carcinogenic effects of radiation is summarized in BEIR V,[39] and can be affected by a number of factors such as genetic constitution, sex, age, physiological state, smoking habits, drugs, and various other physical and chemical agents. The genetic basis of some diseases including increased cancer susceptibility is becoming clearer. For example, it has been shown that the full expression of ataxia telangiectasia, including enhanced cancer susceptibility, results from homozygous mutated genes on chromosome 11. In addition, the heterozygous carriers, who do not express the full-blown disease, are known to be subject to a higher cancer incidence, especially for breast cancer. This mutation is thought to act through inactivation of repair mechanisms.[50,51] The mechanisms through which these factors influence the radiosensitivity are, however, not fully understood. They depend on the particular type of cancer, the tissue at risk, and the specific modifying factor under consideration.

Cancer rates are highly age dependent and, in general, increase exponentially in older age-groups. The expression of radiogenic cancers varies with age in a similar way, so that the age-dependent increase in the excess risk of radiogenic cancer is conventionally expressed in terms of relative risk; that is, the increased risk tends to be proportional to the baseline risk in the same age interval. However, in some cases such as breast cancer, the change in the baseline cancer rate with age is more complicated. For lung cancer the situation is also not simple. Smoking and prolonged exposure to inhaled α-particle emitters interact synergistically and this is said then to be a multiplicative effect.

For lung cancer and most other non-sex-specific solid cancer, it is unclear how a person's sex affects the risk of radiogenic cancer. In general, baseline rates for such cancer in males exceed those in females, possibly because of increased exposure to carcinogens and promoters in occupational activities and life-style factors, such as increased smoking and consumption of alcohol. While sex-specific excess rates of cancer can generally be modelled adequately as being proportional to the corresponding sex-specific baseline rates; in many cases an additive excess risk model fits the data equally, that is, the number of radiation-induced cancer per unit dose is nearly the same in both sexes.

For example, as it is known, the carcinogenic process includes the successive stages of initiation, promotion and progression. The promotion phase, appears to be particularly sensitive to cigarette smoking.

SOURCES AND MAGNITUDES OF HUMAN EXPOSURE

Cosmic radiation

Cosmic rays come mainly from our galaxy and some come from outside it. They also may arise from the sun in bursts during solar flares. The numbers of cosmic rays entering the earth's atmosphere are also affected by the earth's magnetic field: more enter near the poles than at the equator. As they penetrate the atmosphere, they are gradually absorbed, so that the dose decreases as altitude decreases. The average annual dose from cosmic rays at ground level in the UK is about 0.25 mSv. The intensity of cosmic rays for a typical flying altitude is greater than on the ground and also varies with latitude.

γ-Rays from the earth

All materials in the earth's crust are radioactive. For example, uranium is dispersed throughout the soil and rock at various low concentrations around a few parts per million (ppm). Potassium-40 constitutes 120 ppm of the stable element, which in turn makes up 2.4% by weight of the earth's crust. The γ rays are emitted by the radionuclides in the earth and since building materials are extracted from the earth, they too are radioactive, and people are irradiated indoors as well as outdoors. Doses are affected by the geology of the area and the structure of the buildings, but the average dose from earth γ-rays in the UK is about 0.35 mSv in a year.

Radon

The average annual effective dose in the UK from radon decay products is estimated to be 1.3 mSv. There are pronounced variations about this mean, and in some dwellings the dose to the occupants was found to be more than two orders of magnitude higher (range 0.1–500 mSv). The indoor radon levels depend on the geology of the area and also building structures. Poorly ventilated properties or workplaces, e.g. mines, have higher levels (see Uranium, Chapter 7). Radon affected areas have been identified in Cornwall, Devon, Derbyshire, Northamptonshire and Somerset and in parts of Scotland and Northern Ireland.[52] The UK action level for radon in homes is 200 Bq/m^3. A lifetime exposure in dwellings at this level would lead to a 50% increase in fatal lung cancer. Among smokers and nonsmokers combined, about 6% of deaths in the UK are due to lung cancer. A lifetime exposure at the UK action level of 200 Bq/m^3 would increase the risk of fatal lung cancer from 6% to 9%. Many other parts of the world have higher radon levels (e.g. Finland and Germany).

Activity in diet

Other radionuclides from the uranium and thorium series are present in air, food and water, in particular lead-210 and polonium-210 which irradiate the body internally. Potassium-40 is taken into the body in the diet and is the major source of internal irradiation apart from radon decay products. A number of radionuclides, such as carbon-14, are created in the atmosphere by cosmic rays, and these also contribute to internal irradiation. The average annual dose from these sources of internal radiation in the UK is estimated to be 0.3 mSv in a year.

Total doses

The total dose from radiation of natural origin is, on average, about 2.2 mSv in a year in the UK. Differences in average doses from one locality to another may exceed 10 mSv in a year, and differences in individual doses may exceed 100 mSv in a year owing to the existence of dwellings with particularly high concentrations of radon.

Occupational exposures

Radiation is used in electricity generation (nuclear power), general industry (primarily for process and quality control), and for diagnostic purposes in medicine, dentistry and veterinary practice. Further, it is used as a research tool in colleges, universities and industry. All these processes result in occupational exposures to ionizing radiations and in the first half of the 1990s the total numbers of people working with ionizing radiations in the UK was about 40 000 in the nuclear power industry, and about 110 000 in general industry, health, defence and research. Some employees receive increased exposure to natural sources of radiation, the most notable being underground miners to radon and aircrew exposed to elevated levels of cosmic rays. About 100 000 employees are exposed to elevated levels of natural radiation.

Occupational doses

Legal controls (see below) require that the doses received by the more exposed employees are routinely assessed and records kept of their doses. These employees are often referred to as 'classified' persons. A significant proportion of the non-classified employees are also monitored, but the records for this group, who generally receive low doses anyway, are less comprehensive. Approximately every 4 years the National Radiological Protection Board, UK conducts a major review of the radiation exposure of the UK population, which along with public and medical exposure routes, also provides comprehensive data on all occupational exposure. The last such review was published in 1993 and related to data from 1991.[53] It is these data that are primarily quoted below.

As part of their regulatory controls the UK Health and Safety Executive (HSE) have established a Central Index on Dose Information (CIDI), which collates all the summary data from the dose records for classified persons and statistics are published annually.

In 1991, no worker in the nuclear power industry received doses in excess of the legal limit of 50 mSv a year but about seven workers received doses above 15 mSv. Most employees, however, received doses that are a relatively small fraction of the limit. The average dose in 1991 in the nuclear power industry was 1 mSv and the collective dose was 45 person Sv. The measure of the collective dose allows the employer and the regulators to assess whether the total dose for a site has remained static or been reduced and acts as a method of assessing the amount of sharing of dose. The more recent 1994 CIDI data shows a similar distribution. The averages and collective doses are about half of what they were during the 1980s.

The equipment used in general industry is normally well shielded and doses to employees are generally very low. One major exception is where radiographers in the construction and engineering industries are required to carry out their radiography *in situ* and appreciable doses, sometimes in excess of the limit, are received. Improvements in techniques and vigilance are being instituted to reduce these high doses. The average dose in general industry was 0.4 mSv in 1991, while for industrial radiographers it was 0.8 mSv; 97% did not exceed 5 mSv and less than 1% had doses over 15 mSv. The doses to those who work in medicine, dentistry and veterinary practices are generally low. In many cases monitoring is conducted more for the reassurance of staff than to fulfil statutory requirements. In 1991, about 99% of all medical employees received doses below 1 mSv and only 0.1% received more than 5 mSv. The overall average was 0.1 mSv.

In round terms, about 150 000 people in the UK are routinely monitored for occupational exposure to artificial sources of radiation. Their dose in 1991 was 0.5 mSv on average; 98% received doses below 5 mSv and less than 0.05% doses above 15 mSv. The CIDI data, which just cover classified persons, indicate that these low levels of exposure have been maintained. These data can be compared with those for 1987 when the average dose was 0.8 mSv with 95% receiving doses below 5 mSv and 1% doses above 15 mSv.

Occupational doses from natural radiation sources

The average annual dose to crew members of subsonic aircraft is estimated to be about 2 mSv. Higher dose rates are experienced by the crews of Concorde with the result that the annual doses are somewhat higher being between 2 and 3 mSv, but could be double this if the maximum hours were flown. The introduction to service of long-range aircraft has increased the potential for higher doses for subsonic flight crews, with the possibility of doses up to 5–6 mSv per year for some personnel.

Most coal mines are well ventilated with the result that coal miners are exposed to relatively low concentrations of radon daughters and the average dose in 1991 was about 0.6 mSv. The average radon daughter concentrations in non-coal mines, such as gypsum, tin and fluorspar mines, are generally higher and the average dose in 1991 was about 4.5 mSv.

In some parts of the UK, radon concentrations in buildings such as offices, schools and libraries are much higher than the national average. Tentative analysis indicates some 5000 premises with levels above that at which the Ionizing Radiations Regulations 1985 apply.[54] The average dose in 1991 was estimated to be 5.3 mSv with 5% of the employees exceeding 15 mSv. More attention is being given to this area because of the significance of the doses.

In round terms, some 100 000 people are considered to be exposed to elevated levels of natural radiation at work. The overall average dose in 1991 was 2.9 mSv with 2% receiving doses above 15 mSv.

Total occupational doses

The total collective dose to employees from both artificial and natural radiation in 1991 was about 430 person

Sv to which the nuclear industry contributes about 10%, defence 2%, general industry 3%, health 2%, coal mines 7%, natural radiation in workplaces other than mines 63% and aircrew 13%.

MEDICAL EXPOSURES

On average, individual doses to medical personnel are of the order of 1 mSv per year with values usually somewhat higher for radiologists and those involved in interventional radiological procedures. In nuclear medicine there is a need for protection against ingestion or inhalation during the production, analysis and administration of radio-pharmaceutical preparations. In some cases there can also be external exposure, as with technetium-99m, which can deliver substantial doses in very high dose rates to the hands of the operator if no protection is provided. The average doses here are of the order of 1–2 mSv per individual per year. Female nuclear medical technicians who are pregnant may be exposed above the special recommended dose limits if they continue their work for the duration of their pregnancy (see below).

RADIATION PROTECTION

Main principles of radiation protection are set out and promulgated by the ICRP in Publication 60.[5] They can be summarized as follows.

1 No practice involving exposure to radiation should be adopted unless it produces at least sufficient benefit to the exposed individuals or to society to offset the radiation detriment it causes. (Called 'justification of a practice'.)
2 In relation to any particular source of radiation within a practice, all reasonable steps should be taken to adjust the protection so as to maximize the net benefit, economic and social factors being taken into account. (Called 'optimization of protection'.)
3 Finally, a limit should be applied to the dose (other than from medical exposures) received by any individual as the result of all the practices to which he is exposed. (Called 'application of individual dose limits'.)

In simple terms, this framework is derived from three principles that apply to many human activities, and especially to medicine:

- the justification of a practice implies doing more good than harm;
- the optimization of protection implies maximising the margin of good over harm;
- the use of dose limits implies an adequate standard of protection even for the most highly exposed individuals.

These three principles overall avoid the possibility of deterministic effects and minimize the risk of stochastic effects in normal operations.

Protection against external irradiation

The general principles deployed in the workplace to keep external doses as low as reasonably practicable are to keep exposures as short as possible, keep as far away from the source as possible and wherever possible place shielding between the source and the employee. This simple concept of Time, Distance and Shielding is practised routinely in all clinical radiography departments with screens, lead aprons and special rooms for exposures.

Protection against external contamination

The use of protective clothing prevents contamination of the skin; however, loose contamination on such clothing will still irradiate the skin and so exposure times need to be strictly limited. Containment of contamination is essential wherever possible to prevent activities producing an inhalation hazard.

Protection against internal irradiation

The use of containment, such as with fume cupboards or glove boxes, is effective and is used at a level appropriate to the level of hazard. Work with α-emitting radionuclides presents a major hazard and these facilities require special detection systems for leaks to reduce the possibility of either inhalation or contamination of wounds.

LEGISLATION

In the UK the use of ionizing radiations at work is governed by the Ionizing Radiations Regulations 1985 (IRR85).[54] These regulations incorporate the guiding principles of the ICRP. Employees who are occupationally exposed to radiation and who are likely to receive 15 mSv in any one year are known as 'classified persons'. Those who are occasionally exposed to radiation by virtue of their employment and at levels below 15 mSv are known as 'non-classified persons.' The third category is the 'general public' and the dose limitation placed upon this category takes into consideration radiation doses from natural background. The following table (Table 19.5) shows the annual dose limits in mSv for the foregoing three categories.

An investigation level has been set at 15 mSv whole body dose for any classified person and, if exceeded, a local investigation is undertaken to establish whether all steps are being taken to keep radiation exposures as low as reasonably practicable (ALARP).

More recent changes now require an individual investigation for any classified person exceeding 75 mSv in any consecutive period of 5 years. In the future the dose limits will be revised to take account of increased knowledge of the radiation risk factors and the present acceptability of risk for occupational exposures. New European legislation is in place and this will lead to the enactment of new UK legislation at the turn of the century that will require exposures to be limited to no more than 100 mSv in any consecutive period of 5 years, i.e. effectively 20

Table 19.5 *Current UK annual dose limits (mSv)*[54]

Part of the body	Classified person	Non-classified person	General public
Whole body[a]	50	15	5
Any single organ or tissue	500	150	50
Hands, forearms, feet and ankles	500	150	50
Lens of the eye	150	45	15

[a]The dose limit in any 3-month interval for female employees of reproductive capacity is 13 mSv and for pregnant female employees is 10 mSv over the declared term of pregnancy.

mSv per year. This will equate to an annual risk of early death from radiation exposure at work of around 10^{-3} per annum.

MEDICAL ASPECTS

Classified persons are required to have health surveillance conducted by an appointed doctor formally appointed by the HSE under the IRR85.[54] In large organizations, this occupational health cover may include one or more occupational physicians, health physicists, occupational nurses, occupational hygienists and safety specialists, and the workers themselves. The routine health surveillance of persons occupationally exposed to ionizing radiations is no different from that for other groups exposed to other hazards. However, the physician will require special training, especially where radioactive contamination is anticipated.

It is emphasized that the statutory dose limits are set at levels well below those at which deterministic effects will occur and so no changes will be detectable by clinical examination, routine blood examination or special examinations, such as cytogenetic studies. For this reason routine medical examinations and investigations are not necessary. However, routine biological investigations, such as urine analyses, are sometimes performed for reassurance purposes.

HEALTH SURVEILLANCE

Employees should be medically examined prior to employment, and thereafter their medical fitness should be reviewed at periodic intervals (normally annually). The primary purpose of this medical surveillance is to assess the initial and continuing fitness of employees for their intended tasks. The nature of the periodic reviews will depend on the type of work that is undertaken. The frequency of examinations should normally be comparable with that of any other occupational health surveillance programme. Three situations may arise where special surveillance may be required:

- fitness for wearing respiratory protection devices;
- fitness for handling unsealed sources in the case of employees with skin diseases or skin damage;
- fitness of employees with psychiatric or psychological disorders.

Employees who wear respiratory protective equipment in the course of their radiation work, for example inside contaminated confined spaces, need to be checked periodically to verify their lung function. Employees with skin diseases, such as psoriasis, may need to be excluded from work with unsealed radioactive materials, unless the levels of activity are low and appropriate precautions are taken such as covering the affected parts of the body. However, there may be a need for periodic medical checks to ensure that unprotected areas have not become affected by the skin disease. In employees with psychiatric or psychological disorders, the primary concern is whether the employees could pose a danger to themselves or their colleagues, particularly in high radiation dose-rate areas and the handling of unsealed and portable sources.

There is no particular reason why employees who have previously been treated for malignant disease should be excluded from work with radiation if they are otherwise fit for the job. Any additional risk of radiation-related disease caused by future occupational exposure is likely to be small in comparison with the risks from the treatment with surgery, chemotherapeutic agents and/or radiotherapy. However, it may be necessary to restrict their employment in emergency teams where high doses in accident situations might be permissible, and essential when saving life.

Reassurance

Two types of employees may need special reassurance by the physician, sometimes supported by other medical specialists. These are:

- women who are, or may become pregnant;
- individual employees who have been or may have been exposed substantially in excess of the dose limits.

Once the physician or the management has been informed that a woman believes she is pregnant, arrangements may need to be made to change her conditions of work. The physician is often the best person to advise management on the need for any particular precautions or procedures to be adopted regarding the working conditions of pregnant women. The physician should also be able to inform the pregnant woman of the risks to her conceptus associated with her work and, in particular, reassure her on all the health issues. Pregnancy does not require a ban from working in designated areas or on handling radioactive sources, but does imply restriction where there is the potential for high dose exposures. Separate dose limits apply to pregnant persons.

In the case of accidental exposure or overexposure, the physician needs to liaise with the management and other safety specialists to ensure that all suitable arrangements for evaluating the scale of the exposure are undertaken. The medical aspects of the management of overexposed employees is dealt with below.

MEDICAL MANAGEMENT OF ACCIDENTALLY EXPOSED EMPLOYEES

As soon as an unexpected exposure is suspected, management should undertake an investigation to determine the dose to the employee. If a dose is established, an injury is sustained, or contamination occurs, then the appointed doctor or occupational health service should be informed.

EXTERNAL EXPOSURES

The majority of unexpected exposures are determined to be false alarms, such as the improper use of a dosemeter, and no further action is required. However, once the dose is deemed to have been received, the appointed doctor or occupational health service must be informed. The investigation should include the dose estimates from all types of available dosimetry. It is convenient to divide exposures into three categories of increasing doses:

Doses close to the dose limits
Normally, such doses do not require any special clinical investigations or therapy. The role of the occupational health personnel is to counsel the overexposed employee that the exposure is unlikely to produce adverse health effects.

Doses well above the dose limits
Where the exposure is significantly higher, but below the threshold for deterministic effects, the prime role of the occupational physician is to advise the employee of the risks. Then they need to determine whether biological dose indicators, such as, lymphocyte counts and chromosome aberration assays are needed to confirm the dose estimates. Normally, no further action is required other than counselling.

Doses at or above the threshold for deterministic effects
If the assessed external doses are around the threshold for deterministic effects, therapeutic action may need to be undertaken. In order to make this decision, the overexposed employee needs to be examined clinically and any abnormal findings or symptoms recorded. Haematological examination will need to be undertaken in order to monitor the clinical course of the overexposure. If the exposure is severe enough to lead to the acute radiation syndrome, early transfer to a designated hospital is essential. The occupational physician should institute the initial investigations and treatment of the early symptoms. Immediate life-threatening injuries such as fractures and burns, must be treated as a priority before transfer to a hospital.

The clinical management of such highly exposed individuals is dealt with below.

Internal exposures
Where the exposure is internal in origin (internal contamination), the employee should be removed temporarily from the workplace to prevent any further exposure, even when the dose is expected to be close to – but below – the dose limit. This action will allow more accurate dose estimates from sequential counting either of the body, an organ or body fluids.

High exposures may warrant interventional therapy to accelerate the excretion of radionuclides. Such therapeutic measures might include the administration of chelating agents to enhance the excretion of transuranic radionuclides, as for example in lead poisoning, forced diuresis for high doses from tritium intakes and pulmonary lavage for some inhaled plutonium compounds. For plutonium internal contamination intravenous administration of diethylene triamine pentoacetic acid (DTPA) will enhance excretion by chelation. Incidents involving radionuclides such as plutonium can only occur in specialist industries and they usually hold supplies of DTPA.

Medical procedures are not without risk and should only be undertaken when the expected benefit from saving the future dose from the incorporated radionuclide (committed dose) outweighs the risk of the intervention. Many of these therapeutic procedures would be undertaken only at a major hospital, for example lung lavage for a large inhalation of plutonium.

The occupational physician should be prepared to administer the first dose of chelating agents (such as DTPA for transuranic radionuclides) or give stable iodine (see below) for radio-iodine uptake.

External contamination
Where an employee has been externally contaminated, decontamination, by simple washing, should be under-

taken as quickly as possible. Significant skin contamination with β-emitting radionuclides can result in radiation burns if not treated quickly. It should be remembered that thermal burns could complicate skin decontamination and both may need to be treated simultaneously. The only justification for delay would be the immediate treatment of life-threatening physical injuries.

It is emphasized that a contaminated casualty will not represent a hazard to the physician or attending staff wearing standard medical dress, such as a gown, gloves and simple face mask.

Some radionuclides may be absorbed through the skin depending on their chemical form, and can lead to internal contamination. This is particularly true where skin contamination occurs with tritiated water and with some compounds of iodine and caesium.

Return to radiation work

Exposures which do not approach deterministic levels need not affect an employees fitness for further radiation work. An employee should be advised by the physician on the level of the increased risk for stochastic effects. Where their own actions contributed to an overexposure, consideration should be given by management to retraining before return to work. Return to work after internal contamination may be delayed until an adequate dose assessment has been made.

Where there is partial body overexposure which produces deterministic effects, for example, in industrial radiography where the source is handled producing skin and deep tissue hand damage, the employee should be advised on the future risks involved not only in radiation work (e.g. the stochastic risks), but also on future manual work involving exposure to cold and other physical agents, such as chemicals.

Medical records of overexposures

The medical record should be as complete as possible. It should contain details of all examinations, treatment and advice. It will also require copies of any dose reconstruction or assessment performed by health physics staff.

MEDICAL ASPECTS OF A MAJOR RADIATION ACCIDENT

The overall medical rôle will involve those responsible for the management and treatment of casualties, the provision of public health information, advice on the health hazards of ionizing radiation and the application of any public health countermeasures.

Treatment of casualties

It is likely that most non-essential personnel would be evacuated from a nuclear site as soon as an emergency was declared and before any serious release or irradiations could occur and so an accident, for example to a nuclear reactor, should not result in many casualties. At the Chernobyl accident, however, there was no warning and there were many casualties.[4] Casualties can be considered under three headings.

Conventional injury

These could arise from events, such as fires or steam leaks, or follow incidents and panic.

External irradiation

Personnel bringing the plant under control or attempting to save life, and injured individuals immobilized close to the reactor or plant could receive significant doses of whole body external radiation.

Contamination

Personnel exposed, either within the plant or in the open, to a radioactive cloud would become externally contaminated. In addition, the radioactive cloud, which could comprise fission products or actinides, could be swallowed and, without respiratory protection, inhaled with resultant internal contamination.

Radiation accident casualties, no matter what level their contamination, will not present a significant hazard to appropriately trained and equipped medical teams. Assessment of radiation exposure and contamination levels or actual decontamination procedures must *never* take precedence over lifesaving medical procedures.

Externally irradiated casualties

Following a nuclear accident, individuals suspected of being exposed to high doses of external penetrating radiation should be managed according to Table 19.6.

CONTAMINATED CASUALTIES

External exposure to contamination

Patients exposed to high levels of contamination may suffer the effects of skin irradiation from the β- and γ-emitting isotopes. This was a significant problem at Chernobyl mainly in those who were watch keepers on duty and in the emergency personnel (firefighters).[4] Skin lesions were also a serious problem in people contaminated by caesium in Goiânia, Brazil.[2] Overall medical management requirements for contaminated casualties are shown in Table 19.7.

Internal exposure to contamination

Once in the body, the hazards depend on the elements concerned – for example iodine to thyroid, radium and strontium to bone; the chemical form – for example tritiated water absorbed more rapidly than tritium gas; the solubility – generally soluble substances more hazardous than insoluble ones. Alpha emitters are the most hazardous isotopes when incorporated. Particle size is important in inhalation, smaller particles penetrating deeper into the lungs than larger ones and overall the stay time in body (effective half-life) which is determined by a combination of the radioactive decay or half-life ($t_{1/2}$ (physical)) and the biological half-life ($t_{1/2}$ (biol)):

$$\text{Formula: } t_{1/2}\text{ (effective)} = \frac{t_{1/2}\text{ (biol)} \times t_{1/2}\text{ (physical)}}{t_{1/2}\text{ (biol)} + t_{1/2}\text{ (physical)}}$$

Table 19.6 *Treatment of externally exposed casualties*

Type of exposure	Possible consequences	Treatment
Localized more often to hands	Localized erythema with possible development of blisters, ulceration and necrosis	Clinical observation and treatment Specialist advice may be sought
Total or partial body with minimal and delayed clinical signs	No clinical manifestation for 3 h or more following exposure Not life-threatening. Minimal haematological changes	Clinical observation and symptomatic treatment Sequential haematological investigations
Total or partial body with early prodromal signs	Acute radiation syndrome of mild or severe degree dependent on dose	Start treatment as above. Patient requires specialized treatment Full blood count and HLA typing are essential before transfer to a designated hospital if feasible
Total or partial body with thermal, chemical or radiation burns and/or trauma	Possible severe combined injuries, life-threatening	Treat life-threatening conditions Carry out actions as above and early transfer to a designated hospital

HLA: Human leucocyte antigen.

Table 19.7 *Treatment of externally contaminated casualties*

Type of contamination	Possible consequences	Treatment
Low-level intact skin which can be cleaned promptly	Unlikely; possible mild radiation burns	Decontaminate skin and monitor
Low-level intact skin where cleaning is delayed	Possible radiation burns; possible percutaneous intake of radionuclides	Specialist advice may be sought
Low level with thermal, chemical or radiation burns and/or trauma	Possible internal contamination	Specialist advice should be sought
Extensive with associated wounds	Likely internal contamination	Specialist advice should be sought
Extensive with thermal, chemical or radiation burns and/or trauma	Possible severe combined injuries and internal contamination	First aid, plus treatment of life-threatening injuries; early transfer to a designated hospital

The overall management aspects of treating internally contaminated patients are shown in Table 19.8 Examples for accelerating the decorporation of some isotopes in internally contaminated patients are shown in Table 19.9.

ADDITIONAL ASPECTS OF TREATMENT OF INTERNALLY CONTAMINATED CASUALTIES

Once radionuclides have been incorporated the treatment principles are to reduce absorption and deposition in critical organs (e.g. thyroid for iodine and bone for plutonium) and enhance excretion. Administration of stable iodine, which is normally in the form of potassium iodate tablets, may block significant uptake of radio-iodine in the thyroid gland but late administration does not enhance excretion. The normal dose of potassium iodate for an adult is 200 mg orally but the blocking efficacy depends on early administration (ideally when an accident is threatened and before a release

Table 19.8 *Treatment of internally contaminated casualties*

Type of exposure	Possible consequences	Treatment
Inhalation and ingestion of radionuclides insignificant quantity (activity)	No immediate	Specialist advice must be sought
Inhalation and ingestion of radionuclides significant quantity (activity)	No immediate	Nasopharyngeal lavage important Early transfer to a designated hospital is essential to enhance excretion of radionuclides
Absorption through damaged skin (see Table 19.7)	No immediate	Specialist advice should be sought
Major incorporation with or without external total, or partial body or localized irradiation, serious wounds and/or burns	Severe combined radiation injury	Treat life-threatening conditions and transfer to a designated hospital

Table 19.9 *Examples of treatments for internal contamination*

Isotope	Treatment
Iodine	Administration of stable iodine
Tritium	Forced diuresis
Plutonium	Chelating agents e.g. diethylene triamine pentaacetic acid (DTPA). May be given i.v. or as an aerosol inhalation
Caesium	Prussian blue given orally inhibits intestinal reabsorption

occurs) with approximately 50% effectiveness if administered 6 hours after the exposure.[55,56]

KEY FACTORS FOR HOSPITAL STAFF AND FACILITIES

Protection of medical staff

All paramedical and medical staff involved in the handling and treatment of contaminated patients should wear simple protective clothing consisting of overalls, surgical rubber gloves, boots or overshoes (operating theatre dress) and a face mask or respirator. A simple gown and mask would be adequate if other clothing was not available.

Designated treatment areas

Treatment areas should be clearly demarcated from adjacent clean areas and have adequate space to allow an initial triage and resuscitation and then space for decontamination and treatment. Wherever possible only decontaminated casualties should be allowed into the clean areas of the hospital. Monitoring of patients for radioactive contamination should take place at a suitable barrier between clean and dirty areas.

Areas designated to receive contaminated casualties must have an adequate water supply for decontamination and consideration should be given to control of ventilation systems to prevent spread of contamination.

BASIC PLAN FOR THE HANDLING OF CASUALTIES FOLLOWING A NUCLEAR REACTOR ACCIDENT

Reception centre

The plant operators and other personnel within the immediate vicinity will normally evacuate to a designated reception centre taking their casualties with them where possible in accordance with their detailed plans. These plans are usually required by the national legislation, such as the Ionizing Radiations Regulations in the UK[54] or recommended by the International Atomic Energy Agency. The initial medical triage should be undertaken by the most experienced medical staff member available, which could be a first-aider. This triage should identify any personnel requiring immediate despatch to a hospital without any radiation or contamination assessment.

Hospitals

Local plans to deal with accidents should include a designated hospital where radiation or contamination casualties should be taken. Where possible these should be National Health Service providing assistance within the National Arrangements for Incidents involving Radioactivity (NAIR) (applies to Great Britain [England,

Scotland, Wales] only). If the hospital designated to receive the radiation and contamination casualties is not the nearest accident and emergency unit, the local plan should also include the use of that unit to receive uncontaminated casualties. While the plan should include the transfer of radiation and contamination casualties to the specialized hospitals, it must also include instructions to direct casualties requiring immediate life-saving treatment to the nearest unit whatever the patient's radiation exposure status.

CLINICAL TREATMENT OF RADIATION INJURIES

Periodically, consensus treatment conferences on the treatment of radiation injuries have been held.[57,58] At the last held in Bethesda, USA in 1993[58] it was agreed that four main medical effects determined the treatment, which interlink: sepsis, marrow aplasia, gastrointestinal injury, and cutaneous injury. The consensus publication has an excellent summary for the treatment of radiation casualties. If conventional injuries are present then the patient is deemed to have a combined injury and the prognosis is worse. The World Health Organization (WHO) has set up a worldwide Radiation Emergency Medical Preparedness Assistance Network (REMPAN). Physicians who need advice or assistance should contact WHO at Geneva, who can then suggest suitable therapies and arrange for the nearest REMPAN Centre to give direct advice.

CLINICAL CARE OF RADIATION CASUALTIES

General

- Experience from many accidents has shown that the heterogeneous nature of the exposures tends to confound both the clinical and pathological picture so that estimating the scale of the radiation damage and exposure is difficult.
- The early treatment of conventional injuries is the main factor that determines survival in patients who have been accidentally irradiated.
- Casualties on admission can be classified into four treatment categories: mild, moderate, severe and lethal.
- Stating specific dose ranges for these categories is not possible, primarily because of the difficulty in converting an exposure to a meaningful tissue dose; however, equivalent whole body dose ranges would be <2 Gy, 2–5 Gy, 5–10 Gy and >10 Gy respectively.
- The most reliable prognostic guides for treatment in the early stage are the change in absolute lymphocyte counts and cytogenetics, levels of blood cells, which will give a good estimate of dose.
- The degree of radiation-induced marrow aplasia (reversible or irreversible) may not be known for days because of the uncontrolled nature of the exposure and the likelihood that it was non-uniform and heterogeneous.

- Assessment of the dose while important is secondary to the treatment.
- Reliable triage and good clinical care based on comprehensive biological data will ensure the best chance of recovery provided some critical stem cells survive the radiation exposure (see Table 19.10)
- Professional help may be necessary to treat psychological problems accompanying radiation accidents.

Sepsis

- The suppression of bone marrow activity will reduce the resistance to bacterial and viral infections.
- For febrile neutropenic casualties blood, urine and faecal samples for cultures need to be taken on admission.
- Patients need to be started on broad spectrum antimicrobials and these should be given until the patient is afebrile.
- Experience has shown that fungal lung infections can be the cause of late-deaths, when all the other radiation effects have been stabilized.
- Early use of antifungal agents and gamma globulin for viral infections is essential.

Marrow aplasia

- Following a suspected high radiation exposure, initial patient assessment should be based on dosimetric testing (biological, physical), daily full blood counts, viral titres (e.g. cytomegalovirus human immunodeficiency virus), human leucocyte antigen subtyping for possible bone marrow transplantation and the administration of haematopoietic growth factors (colony stimulating factors, such as G or GM-CSF) (see Table 19.10).
- Particular care is needed if the patient has other injuries, such as pulmonary infections, burns or smoke inhalation.
- Subsequent supportive therapy might include platelet transfusions particularly if surgery is indicated for other injuries. Other treatments might include the use of thrombopoietic drugs.
- Bone marrow transplants should only be given if an autologous donor is available.

Gastrointestinal

- Vomiting should be controlled by use of effective anti-emetics, e.g. ondansetron. This relaxes the gut and reduces mechanical damage of lining of the small intestine. Anti-emetics also help to reduce fluid loss.
- Diarrhoea should be treated with fluids and electrolytes and efforts should be made to improve host defences by appropriate nutritional support.

Cutaneous

- Remove all clothing as soon as possible, bathe very gently in lukewarm water, use acetic acid or ion exchangers if surface contamination is thought to be

Table 19.10 *Important laboratory samples to be taken*

Blood, approximately 20–30 ml for the following analyses:
- Full blood count
- Cytogenetic analysis (24 h after exposure is optimum time)
- Biochemical analysis (serum amylase)
- Analysis for radionuclide content

Urine
- Routine analysis
- Biochemical (creatinuria is a measure of tissue damage)
- Analysis for radionuclide content

Stools (for estimation of radionuclide contents)

soluble caesium, and only remove contamination mechanically from soles of feet or palms of hands.
- Later treatments might include use of topical creams, systemic acitretin and γ-interferon. These have been found to be helpful in treating the chronic skin damage seen in the Chernobyl firemen.

Combined injury

- Radiation injury is not immediately life threatening, initial care should address the associated conventional injuries, for example, thermal burns and wounds.
- After stabilization, radioisotope decontamination should be performed before emergency surgery, definitive care and treatment of radiation injuries.
- Collection of biological samples during the resuscitation stages will supplement the initial data collected during triage.
- Ideally, definitive care should immediately follow resuscitation.
- Management of soft tissue wounds requires alternative ways to close wounds, for example, biological wound coverings and skin grafts.
- Surgical correction of life-threatening and other major injuries should be carried out as soon as possible (within 36–48 hours); elective procedures should be postponed until late in the convalescent period (45–60 days) following haematopoietic recovery.
- Treatment of thermal burns should include early excision of potentially septic tissue and closure of the wounds, preferably by skin grafting.
- Radiation burns and thermal burns should be treated differently, especially when using surgery, which should be delayed in the case of radiation burns (see Table 19.7).

ACCIDENTS AND RADIATION RISK

In any radiation accident the workforce would take countermeasures to protect themselves. This would involve sheltering or considering evacuation. Similar actions may be necessary for the public. Workers and public would also be advised not to eat open foodstuffs. National authorities usually set the dosimetric criteria for taking these actions based on ICRP recommendations[59] in case of a nuclear power plant accident, where radio-iodines might be released and inhaled or ingested, reducing doses to the thyroid can be effective by taking stable iodine tablets (see above). Prophylactic iodine was issued to the workforce at Chernobyl and to most of the population in Poland immediately after that accident and no adverse side-effects were reported.[60,61] The failure to implement adequate early countermeasures against iodine contamination in the former Soviet Union in the immediate aftermath of the Chernobyl accident has resulted in over a 100-fold increase in the incidence of childhood thyroid cancer in the affected republics.[62] The Chernobyl accident showed that accident contingency plans need to be exercised regularly and that the decontamination of casualties needs to be carried out as soon as possible.[4]

Ionizing radiation is a highly emotive subject, and a radiation accident can cause widespread concern in a workplace. Individual perceptions of risk, knowledge of medical effects of radiation and the best methods of communicating these effects to people is important. The Chief Medical Officer at the Department of Health, UK, has made some tentative proposals on the language of risk.[63] Many facets of life affect perceptions, attitudes and behaviour. Changes in society also have affected attitudes and acceptability of different risks. Radiation risks from occupational exposures are low when compared with many other occupations or activities (Fig. 19.1). Determining acceptable levels of risk is central to the process of setting occupational and public dose limits. However, if the degree of risk that society is prepared to accept changes then the need for robust epidemiological and molecular biological studies to underpin the risk estimates and, *inter alia*, dose limits is emphasized.[64]

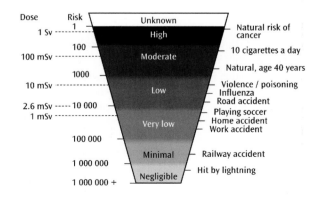

Figure 19.1 *Risks – on the state of the public health (1995).*

SUMMARY

Radiation is a fact of life. Natural radiation and radioactivity are all around us and humans have evolved in that environment. The man-made use of radiation in medicine and industry, and for nuclear power has shown that high doses are lethal and early (deterministic) effects are visible and can be life-shortening. Latent (stochastic) effects particularly cancer are well documented and risk estimates, based on the study of occupationally and medically exposed cohorts, are reasonably robust. Legislation to control radiation exposures at work by defining dose limits is based on these risk estimates. Occupational exposures below the dose limits will prevent deterministic effects and reduce the risk of stochastic effects to an acceptable level, although all doses should be kept as low as reasonably practicable. The acceptability of risk by the public may change.

REFERENCES

1 Berry RJ. The radiologist as a guinea pig: radiation hazards to man as demonstrated in early radiologists, and their patients. *J Roy Soc Med* 1986; **79**: 506–9.

2 International Atomic Energy Agency. *The Radiological Accident in Goiânia*. Vienna: IAEA, 1988.

3 World Health Organization. *Health Consequences of the Chernobyl Accident*. Scientific Report. Geneva: WHO, 1996.

4 Nuclear Energy Agency (OECD). *Chernobyl. Ten Years On. Radiological and Health Impact*. An appraisal by the NEA Committee on Radiation Protection and Public Health. Paris: NEA, 1996.

5 International Commission on Radiological Protection. 1990 Recommendations of the International Commission on Radiological Protection. Publication 60. *Ann ICRP* 1991; **21**(1–3).

6 UNSCEAR. *Sources, Effects and Risks of Ionising Radiation*. Report to the General Assembly with annexes. New York: United Nations, 1988.

7 Stather JW, Muirhead CR, Edwards AA, Harrison JD, Lloyd DC, Wood, NR. *Health Effects Models Developed from the 1988 UNSCEAR Report*. Report R226. National Radiological Protection Board Oxford: NRPB, 1988.

8 Mettler FA, Upton AC. *Medical Effects of Ionizing Radiation* 2nd edn. Philadelphia: W B Saunders Co, 1995.

9 Scott BR, Hahn, FF. (1985). Early and continuing effects. In: Evans JS, Moeller JW, Cooper DW eds. *Health Effects Models for Nuclear Power Plant Accident Consequence Analysis*. USNRC, NUREG/CR-4214 (SAND85–7185). Springfield, VA: NTIS.

10 Jones TD, Morris MD, Wells SM, Young RW. *Animal Mortality Resulting from Uniform Exposure to Photon Radiations*: calculated $LD_{50}s$ and a compilation of experimental data. ORNL-6338. Oak Ridge, Tennessee: Oak Ridge National Laboratory, 1986.

11 Evans JS, Abrahamson S, Bender MA, Boecken BB, Gilbert ES, Scott BR. *Health Effects Models for Nuclear Power Plant Accident Consequence Analysis*. USNRC NUREG/CR-4214. Rev. 2, Part I, ITRI-141, 1993.

12 International Atomic Energy Agency. *The Radiological Accident in San Salvador*. Vienna: IAEA, 1990.

13 International Atomic Energy Agency. *The Radiological Accident in Soreq*. Vienna: IAEA, 1993.

14 Trott K, Hermann T. (1991) Radiation effects on abdominal organs. In: Scherer E, Streffer C, Trott K eds. *Radiopathology of Organs and Tissues*. Berlin: Springer-Verlag, 1991.

15 Becciolini, A Relative radiosensitivities of the small and large intestine. *Advances in Radiation Biology* Vol 12. New York: Academic Press, 1987.

16 Andrews PLR, Davis CJ. The physiology of emesis induced by anti-cancer therapy. In: Reynolds DJM, Andrews PLR, Davis CJ eds. *Serotonin and the Scientific Basis of Anti-emetic Therapy*. Oxford: Oxford Clinical Communications, 1995.

17 Thomas RL, Storb R, Clift RA. Bone marrow transplantation. *N Engl J Med* 1975; **292**: 832.

18 International Commission on Radiological Protection. Non-stochastic effects of ionizing radiation. Publication 41. *Ann ICRP* 1984; **14**(3).

19 International Atomic Energy Agency. *Medical Handling of Accidentally Exposed Individuals*. Safety Series No. 88, Vienna: IAEA, 1988.

20 International Atomic Energy Agency. *International Conference on One Decade After Chernobyl: Summing Up the Consequences of the Accident*. Vienna: IAEA, 1996

21 International Commission on Radiological Protection. Effects of Developmental irradiation on the brain of the embryo and foetus. Publication 49. *Ann ICRP* 1986; **16**(4).

22 Otake M, Schull WJ, Yoshimaru H. *A Review of Radiation-related Brain Damage in Prenatally Exposed Atomic Bomb Survivors*. Report TR4-89. Hiroshima: Radiation Effects Research Foundation, 1990.

23 Bond VP, Fliedner TM, Archambeau JO. *Mammalian Radiation Lethality*. New York: Academic Press, 1965.

24 UNSCEAR. *Ionizing Radiation: Sources and Biological Effects: Annex K Radiation-induced Life Shortening*. Report to the General Assembly with annexes. New York: United Nations, 1982.

25 Smets E, Garssen B, Schuster-Utterhoeve A *et al*. Fatigue in cancer patients: A review. *Br J Cancer* 1993; **68**: 220–24.

26 Lloyd DC, Edwards AA, Fitzsimmons EJ *et al*. Death of a classified worker probably caused by overexposure to γ radiation. *Occup Environ Med* 1994; **51**: 713–8.

27 Pierce DA, Shimizu Y, Preston DL, Vaeth M, Mabuchi K. Studies of the mortality of atomic bomb survivors. Report 12, Part 1. Cancer: 1950–1990. *Radiat Res* 1996; **146**: 1–27.

28 Miller AB, Howe GR, Sherman GJ, Lindsay JP *et al*. Mortality from breast cancer after irradiation during fluoroscopic examinations in patients being treated for tuberculosis. *N Engl J Med* 1989; **321**: 1285–9.

29 Davis F, Boice JD, Hubre Z *et al*. Cancer mortality in a radiation exposed cohort of Massachusetts tuberculosis patients. *Cancer Res* 1989; **49**: 6130–36.

30 Boice JD, Engholm G, Kleinerman RA *et al.* Second cancer risk in patients treated for cancer of the cervix. *Radiat Res* 1988; **116**: 3–55.

31 Darby SC, Doll R, Gill SK, Smith PG. Long-term mortality after a single treatment course with X-rays in patients treated for ankylosing spondylitis. *Br J Cancer* 1987; **55**: 179–90.

32 Weiss HA, Darby SC, Doll R. Cancer mortality following X-ray treatment for ankylosing spondilitis. *Int J Cancer* 1994; **59**: 327–38.

33 Conrad RA, Paglia D, Larsen P *et al. Review of Medical Findings in a Marshallese Population 26 years after Accidental Exposure to Radioactive Fallout.* Report No. BNL 5161. Upton, New York: Brookhaven National Laboratory, 1980.

34 National Research Council, Committee on the Biological Effects of Ionizing Radiations, *Health Risks of Radon and Other Internally Deposited Alpha-emitters* (BEIR IV). Washington, DC: National Academic Press, 1988.

35 Baverstock K, Papworth D. The UK radium luminiser survey, In: Taylor D *et al.* eds. *Risks from Radium and Thorotrast.* BIR Report 21. London: British Institute of Radiology, 1989.

36 Van Kaick G, Wesch H, Luhrs H *et al.* The German thorotrast study-report on 20 years of follow up, In: Taylor D *et al.* eds. *Risks from Radium and Thorotrast.* BIR Report 21. London: British Institute of Radiology, 1989.

37 Bhatia S, Robison LL, Oberlin O *et al.* Breast cancer and other second neoplasms after childhood Hodgkin's disease. *N Engl J Med* 1996; **334**: 745–51.

38 Shimizu Y, Kato H, Schull WJ. Studies of the mortality of a-bomb survivors. 9. Mortality, 1950–1985: Part 2. Cancer mortality based on the recently revised doses (DS86). *Radiat Res* 1990; **121**: 120–141.

39 National Research Council Committee on the Biological Effects of Ionizing Radiations. *Health Effects of Exposure to Low Levels of Ionizing Radiation* (BEIR V). Washington, DC: National Academic Press, 1990.

40 UNSCEAR. *Sources, Effects of Ionising Radiation.* Report to the General Assembly with annexes. New York: United Nations, 1994.

41 Muirhead CR, Goodhill AA, Haylock GRE *et al.* Occupational radiation exposure and mortality: second analysis of the National Registry for Radiation Workers. *J Rad Prot* 1999; **19**: 3–26.

42 NIH publication 85–2748. *Report of the NIH Ad Hoc Working Group to Develop Radioepidemiological Tables.* Bethesda, MD, National Institutes of Health, US Department of Health and Human Services, 1985.

43 International Atomic Energy Agency. *Methods for Estimating the Probability of Cancer From Occupational Radiation Exposure.* IAEA-TECDOC-870. Vienna: IAEA, 1996.

44 UNSCEAR. *Sources and Effects of Ionising Radiation.* Report to the General Assembly with annexes. New York: United Nations, 1977.

45 Neel JV, Schull WJ, Awa AA *et al.* The children of parents exposed to atomic bombs. Estimates of the genetic doubling dose of radiation in humans. *Am J Hum Genet* 1990; **46**: 1053–72.

46 Sankaranarayanan K. Ionising radiation and genetic risks. IV Current methods, estimates of risk of Mendelian disease, human data and lessons from biochemical and molecular studies of mutations. *Mutat Res* 1991; **258**: 99–122.

47 Yoshimoto Y, Neel JV, Kato H, Makuchi K *et al.* Malignant tumours during the first two decades in the offspring of atomic bomb survivors. *Am J Hum Genet* 1990; **46**: 1041–52.

48 Gardner MJ, Snee MP, Hall, AJ *et al.* Results of a case control study of leukaemia and lymphoma among young people near Sellafield nuclear plant in West Cumbria. *Br Med J* 1990; **300**: 423–9.

49 COMARE Fourth Report. *The incidence of cancer and leukaemia in young people in the vicinity of the Sellafield site, West Cumbria: Further studies and an update of the situation since the publication of the report of the Black Advisory committee in 1984.* London: Department of Health, 1996.

50 Pippard EC, Hall AJ, Barker DJ, Bridges BA. Cancer in homozygotes and heterozygotes of ataxia telangiectasia and xeroderma pigmentosum in Britain. *Cancer Res* 1988; **48**: 2929–32.

51 Thacker J. Cellular radiosensitivity in ataxia telangiectasia. *Int J Radiat Biol* 1994; **66**: 587–96.

52 National Radiological Protection Board. *Radon Affected Areas: England, Wales.* Documents of the NRPB, Vol 7 No. 2. Oxford: NRPB, 1996.

53 Hughes JS, O'Riordan MC. *Radiation Exposure of the UK Population- 1993 Review.* National Radiological Protection Board Report No. R263. Oxford: NRPB, 1993.

54 Ionising Radiations Regulations 1985. SI 1333. London: HMSO 1985.

55 Rubery E, Smales E. *Iodine Prophylaxis following Nuclear Accidents: Proceedings of a Joint WHO/CEC Workshop, July 1988.* (Contains: WHO regional Office for Europe Guidelines for iodine prophylaxis). Geneva: WHO, 1990.

56 Kovari MD, Morrey ME. The effectiveness of iodine prophylaxis when delayed: implications for emergency planning. *J Radiol Prot* 1994; **14**: 345–8.

57 Browne D, Weisss JF, Mac Vittie TJ *et al.* (eds). *Treatment of Radiation Injuries.* New York: Plenum Press, 1990.

58 MacVittie TJ, Weiss JF, Browne D (eds). *Advances in the Treatment of Radiation Injuries. Advances in the Biosciences* Vol 94. Oxford: Pergamon, 1996.

59 International Commission on Radiological Protection. *Principles for Intervention for Protection of the Public in a Radiological Emergency.* Publication 63. *Ann ICRP* 1993; **22**(4).

60 Nauman J, Wolff J. Iodide prophylaxis in Poland after the Chernobyl reactor accident: benefits and risks. *Am J Med* 1993; **94**: 524–32.

61 HArrison JR, Paile W, Beaverstock KF. Public health implications of iodine prophylaxix in radiological

emergencies. In: *Proceedings of International Sympsium on Radiation and the Thyroid*. Cambridge UK: World Science, 1999: 455–63.

62 Williams ED, Becker D, Dimidchik S, Nagataki S, Pinchera A, Tronko ND. Effects on the thyroid in populations exposed to radiation as aresult of the Chernobyl accident. In: *International Atomic Energy Agency, International Conference on One Decade After Chernobyl: Summing Up the Consequences of the Accident*. Vienna: IAEA, 1996.

63 Calman KC. Cancer: science and society and the communication of risk. *Br Med J* 1996; **313**: 799–802.

64 Clarke RH. Managing radiation risks. *J Roy Soc Med* 1997; **90** 2: 88–92.

ADDITIONAL READING ON MEDICAL TREAMENT OF CASUALTIES

1 MacVittie TJ, Monroy R, Vigneulle RM *et al*. The relative biological effectiveness of mixed fission-neutron gamma radiation on the hematopoietic syndrome in the canine: Effect of therapy on survival. *Radiat Res* 1991; **128**: 529–36.

2 Peter RU. Chronic cutaneous damage after accidental exposure to ionizing radiation: the Chernobyl experience. *J Am Acad Dermatol* 1994; **30**: 719–23.

3 Powles R, Smith C, Milan S *et al*. Human recombinant GM-CSF in allogeneic bone-marrow transplantation for leukaemia. Double-blind, placebo-controlled trial. *Lancet* 1991; **336**: 1417–20.

4 Thierry D, Gourmelon P, Parmentier C, Nenot JC. Haematopoietic growth factors in the treatment of therapeutic and accidental irradiation-induced bone marrow aplasia. *Int J Radiat Biol* 1995; **67**: 103–17.

5 Wilson A. A Meeting Report (with extended abstracts): CEIR forum on the effects of cytokines on radiation responses. *Int J Radiat Biol* 1993; **63**: 529–40.

20

Non-ionizing radiation and the eye

MIKE BOULTON, DAVID H SLINEY

What is non-ionizing radiation?	419	Chronic light damage	429
Basic principles of vision	419	Damage by infrared and microwaves	430
Basic mechanisms of light damage in tissues	423	Protection against light damage	431
Light absorption by ocular tissues	424	Photosensitization	431
Ocular light damage	425	Conclusions	435
Acute light damage	426	References	435

Visual deterioration, whether through disease or excessive exposure to non-ionizing radiation (generally referred to as light damage), is often severely debilitating. Any reduction of normal vision which affects our everyday functions can place a considerable socioeconomic burden on the family and government agencies. Light damage, though less common in recent years due to improved protective measures and health and safety at work, can still result as a complication of occupation. Anyone believed to have suffered occupational light damage should be referred to a doctor for a medical opinion.

WHAT IS NON-IONIZING RADIATION?

The electromagnetic radiation spectrum has been divided into a number of frequency regions. The most useful divisions are between ionizing (x-rays, gamma (γ) rays and cosmic rays) and non-ionizing radiation (ultraviolet (UV) radiation, visible, infrared radiation, radiofrequency waves).[1] The division between ionizing and non-ionizing radiation is generally considered to be at wavelengths around 1 nm in the far UV region. Non-ionizing radiation is that part of the electromagnetic spectrum which does not have sufficient energy to ionize matter but can excite atoms by raising their outer electrons to higher orbitals, a process which may store energy, produce heat or cause chemical reactions (photochemistry). The wavelengths of non-ionizing radiation of major importance to the eye are grouped under the following headings:

- Ultraviolet   200–400 nm (wavelength)
- Visible   380–760 nm
- Infrared   760 nm–1 mm
- Microwave   1 mm–1 m

The natural, and major source, of these wavelengths is sunlight which has a broad emission ranging from far UV (200–280 nm) to far infrared (3000–10000 nm). However, it should be noted that the eye is not normally exposed to the far UV component of the spectrum since this solar component is blocked by the atmosphere. In addition to sunlight there is an ever-increasing amount of man-made candescent and incandescent sources which cover the full non-ionizing radiation spectrum. Details of the source and wavelength of non-ionizing radiation reaching the eye are given in Table 20.1.

BASIC PRINCIPLES OF VISION

Visual perception results from a series of optical and neural events; visible radiation arriving at the eye is focused by the cornea and lens creating a retinal image which is then converted by photoreceptors to nerve impulses which are conducted to the visual area of the cerebral cortex. The light pathway to the retina (consisting of cornea, aqueous, lens and vitreous) is almost completely transparent to all wavelengths of visible light (although transmission characteristics do vary with age).[2] In considering the basic principle of vision we will briefly describe the anatomy of the eye and phototransduction. A more comprehensive review of these areas can be acquired from a variety of general texts.[3–6]

Table 20.1 *The pathophysiology of optical radiation and the eye*

| Spectral domain | | Wavelength (nm) | Sources | | Absorption site | | Nature of damage |
Physical	Biological		Lasers	Others	Tissue	Location	
Far ultraviolet	Ultraviolet C	200–280	Excimer	Sunlight, Arc lamps, Germicidal lamps, Mercury lamps	Cornea	Epithelium	Photochemical photokeratitis corneal opacity —
Far ultraviolet	Ultraviolet B	280–315	Excimer	Sunlight, Sun lamps, Welding arcs	Cornea	Epithelium	Photochemical photokeratitis corneal opacity
		295–315			Lens	Epithelium Nucleus	Photochemical cataract
Near ultraviolet	Ultraviolet A	315–400	Excimer	Sunlight, UV-A sun lamps, Sunbeds	Lens	Epithelium Nucleus	Photochemical cataract —
Visible	Visible	400–780	Argon, Dyes, Helium-neon	Sunlight, Incandescent lamps, Fluorescent lamps	Retina	Pigment Epithelium	Thermomechanical Thermal Photochemical visual loss
			Krypton	Arc lamps		Haemoglobin	Thermal visual loss
						Macular pigment	Thermal visual loss
						Visual cells	Photochemical incidious visual loss colour vision problems accelerated ageing
Near infrared	Infrared A	780–1400	Gallium arsenide, Neodymium YAG	Sunlight, Arc lamps, Electric fires, Furnaces	Retina	Pigment epithelium	Thermal visual loss
					Iris, Lens	Pigment epithelium Nucleus	
Far infrared	Infrared B	1400–3000	Erbium	Sunlight, Furnaces	Cornea	Epithelium	Thermal corneal opacity aqueous flare
					Lens	Epithelium	Thermal cataract
Far infrared	Infrared C	3000–10,000	Carbon dioxide	Furnaces	Cornea	Epithelium	Thermal cataract

Modified from Ref. 2

Ocular anatomy

The eyeball is situated in the anterior part of the orbital cavity, towards the roof and to the temporal side. The eyeball is not completely spherical being made up of the segments of two spheres; the anterior segment, the transparent cornea, occupies about one-sixth of the whole surface while the opaque posterior segment, the sclera, occupies the remainder of the exterior surface. Anatomy textbooks classically consider the eye to consist of three layers; the fibrous tunic (cornea and sclera), the vascular or uveal tunic (choroid, ciliary body and iris) and the retina (neural retina and retinal pigment epithelium) (Fig. 20.1a). Within lie the internal media, aqueous humor, lens and vitreous. Since this chapter concentrates on ocular light damage the following description of ophthalmic anatomy will concentrate on those tissues which lie on the optic axis.

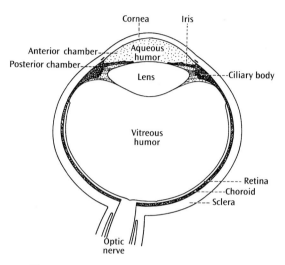

Figure 20.1a *Cross-section of an eyeball.*

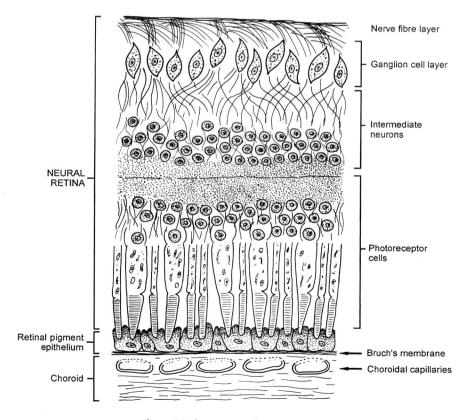

Figure 20.1b *Cross-section of the retina.*

CORNEA

Microscopically the cornea consists of five distinct layers:

1 the epithelium,
2 Bowman's layer,
3 the stroma,
4 Descemet's membrane,
5 the endothelium

The corneal epithelium

The corneal epithelium which is located at the front of the eyeball and is protected by the tear film, is a non-keratinized stratified epithelium five to six cells deep.

Bowman's layer

Bowman's layer is an acellular basement membrane consisting of interwoven collagen fibres which is located immediately beneath the epithelium. The membrane is about 10 μm thick and forms a strong attachment site for the basal cells of the epithelium.

The stroma

The stroma forms about 90% of the corneal thickness. This transparent, avascular, structure consists of between 200 and 250 flattened lamellae with each lamella consisting of collagen fibres lying parallel to one another and embedded in a glycosaminoglycan matrix. The lamellae are arranged in a definite pattern with collagen fibres in alternate layers often being at right angles to one another. Interspersed between the flattened lamellae are stromal fibroblasts (often referred to as keratocytes). The transparency of the cornea is dependent upon the thickness of the collagen fibres, their arrangement into parallel patterns and the constant separation between fibrils. Disease or trauma can cause the loss of regular stromal structure culminating in corneal opacification.

Descemet's membrane

This is a thin elastic basement membrane (8–10 μm thick) located between the stroma and the corneal epithelium.

The corneal endothelium

The corneal endothelium is a monolayer of flattened polygonal endothelial cells whose major role is to control the normal hydration of the cornea.

The cornea is avascular but is extensively innervated with nerve fibres derived from the ophthalmic division of the trigeminal nerve.

AQUEOUS

The aqueous is a colourless, transparent liquid whose composition includes protein, glucose, electrolytes and oxygen which is generated at the ciliary processes. The aqueous enters the anterior chamber via the pupil whence it supplies nutrients to the avascular cornea and lens and removes waste substances as it flows out of the anterior chamber into the canal of Schlemm.

LENS

The lens is a biconvex structure situated between the vitreous and the back of the iris. The lens is composed of three major parts:

1 An elastic capsule that envelops the entire lens;
2 the lens epithelium which is a monolayer of cuboidal cells which are attached to the posterior surface of the anterior capsule;
3 the lens fibres which constitute the majority of the lens and are high in the protein crystallin which provides the focusing power of the lens.

Opacification of the lens, usually resulting from the degeneration of the lens fibres, is referred to as cataract. The lens is held in position by radially arranged suspensory ligaments, termed zonules, which connect the ciliary processes and the lens capsule.

VITREOUS

The vitreous is a colourless, transparent gel which occupies the majority of the posterior chamber. It consists of 99% water, collagen fibrils, hyaluronan, soluble proteins and salts.

RETINA

The retina extends from the vitreous base towards the optic nerve covering the whole of the eye cup. It functions to capture an ocular light image and to transduce it into a pattern of electrical signals for processing into a visual image in the brain. The retina can be divided into two layers:

1 the neural retina;
2 the retinal pigment epithelium.

The neural retina

The neural retina contains three zones of neurons, named in the order which they conduct impulses, the photoreceptor cells, the intermediate neurons and the ganglion cells (Fig. 20.1b). The photoreceptor cells are located in the outer retina adjacent to the retinal pigment epithelium. Two types of photoreceptor are present, rods (specialized for vision in dim light and do not recognize colour) and cones (specialized for colour vision and visual acuity). The photoreceptors consist of an inner and outer segment and it is the outer segment, abutting the retinal pigment epithelium which contains the light-sensitive pigment rhodopsin. The inner segments project into the inner retina where they synapse with inner retinal neurons which in turn synapse with the retinal ganglion cells. The ganglion axons exit through the optic nerve head and send nerve impulses to the visual cortex. In addition the neural retina also contains supporting glial cells and the retinal vasculature.

The retinal pigment epithelium

The retinal pigment epithelium is a single layer of polarized hexano-cuboidal cells located beneath the neural retina and separated from the choroid by Bruch's membrane (Fig. 20.1b). These cells contain melanin (an absorber of stray light), form the outer blood retinal barrier (controlling the supply of nutrients to the photoreceptors) and maintain the integrity of photoreceptor outer segments by ingesting the spent tips of photoreceptor outer segments.

At the posterior pole of the eye, approximately 3 mm lateral to the optic disc, is a shallow depression in the retina which forms the centre of the macula. The macula is an oval yellowish area approximately 5.5 mm in diameter. The yellowish colouration of the macula is caused by the macular pigment which principally consists of the carotenoid xanthophyll. The fovea is a depression in the centre of the macula and is about 1.5 mm in dimater. The floor of this depression, about 0.35 mm in diameter, is called the foveola. The depressed area is formed by the nerve cells being displaced peripherally, leaving only densely packed photoreceptors in the centre. There are no blood vessels and no rod photoreceptor cells in the foveola, i.e. this is an all-cone region of the retina. The macula is anatomically adapted to permit light to have greater access to the photoreceptors than elsewhere in the retina and explains in part why this is the area of the most acute vision.

In addition, to the ocular structures which lie on the optical axis the eye is also made up of:

- the sclera – the outer, opaque, fibrous coat constituting the posterior 83% of the outer surface of the eye;
- the iris – a contractile diaphragm which forms a central aperture, the pupil, which controls the amount of light entering the eye and impinging on the retina;
- the ciliary body – an annular portion of the uvea extending from the ora serrata to the root of the iris which provides the necessary muscular changes for accommodation and produces the aqueous fluid;
- the choroid – predominantly a vascular structure whose principal function is to nourish the retinal photoreceptors and pigment epithelium; this tissue contains melanocytes whose melanin granules absorb light and xenobiotics.

Phototransduction

Within picoseconds after an image is formed on the retina photons are absorbed by the light-sensitive pigment rhodopsin, the chromophore is isomerized and the protein portion becomes activated.[7] The photoexcitation of rhodopsin triggers a rapid chain of molecular events within the photoreceptor outer segments which results in the closure of ion channels such that the receptor potential takes the form of a hyperpolarization and a decrease in the rate of neurotransmitter release. The generator potentials produced by the photoreceptor cells induce signals in both bipolar neurons and horizontal

cells which are transmitted as a partially processed excitatory visual signal to the ganglion cells. The ganglion cell axons connect via the optic nerve and optic chiasma to the visual areas located in the occipital lobes of the cerebral cortex.

BASIC MECHANISMS OF LIGHT DAMAGE IN TISSUES

While optical radiation is essential for visual perception it can also, given the appropriate conditions, produce tissue damage.[8] Such damage, although generally considered detrimental to visual function, can be of considerable therapeutic value if used appropriately. Radiation damage is thought to occur via at least one of three fundamental processes;[9] mechanical (or ionization), thermal and photochemical (Fig. 20.2). It should be noted that although this broad classification is used for simplicity, light damage often results from more than one of these processes through a continuum of photoinduced events.

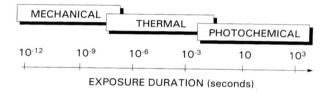

Figure 20.2 *The mechanisms of light-induced retinal damage related to exposure duration. Modified from Ref. 9.*

Mechanical damage

Mechanical damage results from extremely short wavelength light exposures (nanosecond or less) at high irradiance levels causing sonic transients or shock waves that mechanically disrupt the tissue.[9] The injury may be due to ionization where electrons are stripped from the outer orbitals of atoms resulting in a plasma. In the eye, such mechanical damage is normally associated with radiation originating from Q-switched or mode-locked lasers.

Thermal damage

Thermal damage can occur if incident energy is trapped or absorbed in a substrate molecule resulting in a significant increase in temperature. A rise in temperature of 10°C or more in the retina is considered sufficient to cause coagulative tissue damage.[10] Such damage usually occurs at longer wavelengths than for mechanical damage with exposure duration usually between 10^{-6} and 10^{-3}

seconds and is dependent on the absorption of light by specific chromophores.[9] The retina contains a number of chromophores which readily absorb visible light i.e. melanin, blood, xanthophyll and lipofuscin. Typical sources of thermal energy are xenon arc and laser photocoagulators, the extent of tissue damage being dependent on exposure time. The depth of penetration is dependent on wavelength e.g. optical radiation from argon lasers (457–524nm) is primarily absorbed at the retinal pigment epithelium while that from the krypton red (around 650nm) and diode lasers (790–830nm) is absorbed by the choroid as well as the retinal pigment epithelium.

Photochemical damage

This has been the most extensively studied form of light damage owing to its ability to cause damage under ambient conditions and its potential role in ocular pathologies (e.g. cataract and age-related macular degeneration). Photochemical damage is brought about by prolonged exposure (seconds to years) to the more energetic short wavelengths of light such as blue and UV which, when absorbed by a chromophore, lead to an electronic transition of the substrate to an excited state with a potential for causing tissue damage.[9]

Although photochemical damage is reported to occur in most ocular structures it has been most studied in the lens and the retina.[11] The interactions of endogenous, as well as exogenous, biomolecules with UV radiation has demonstrated that the major UV absorbers in the lens are free or bound aromatic amino acids as well as numerous age pigments and fluorophores.[11] Photochemical changes in the lens appear to be cumulative and certainly contribute to ageing changes and the development of cortical cataract.[12]

Retinal photochemical damage is currently classified as either type 1 or type 2 on the basis of animal studies.[9] Type 1 damage is caused by prolonged exposure (hours or days) to low irradiances which at threshold result in damage to the retinal photoreceptors. The action spectra of type 1 damage corresponds reasonably with the absorption spectrum of the visual pigments thus supporting the view that these pigments are the prime chromophores responsible for the generation of type 1 damage.[13] By contrast type 2 damage is considered to originate in the retinal pigment epithelium and appears to correlate with relatively higher retinal irradiances than for type 1 damage delivered over shorter time spans (seconds to minutes).[14] However, current evidence suggests that prolonged exposure to low retinal irradiances can result in cumulative damage similar to that of type 2 (see section on chronic light damage). Ham and colleagues measured the action spectrum of type 2 damage and reported that its sensitivity increased with decreasing wavelength,[15,16] a feature which led to this type of damage

being referred to as 'blue light damage'. Melanin in the retinal pigment epithelium has been proposed as the major chromophore although more recent evidence suggest that the age-pigment lipofuscin which accumulates within retinal pigment epithelium cells may be the primary chromophore in man.[17]

LIGHT ABSORPTION BY OCULAR TISSUES

Visual perception results from a response to visible radiation (400–780nm) reaching the retina. The light pathway to the retina is almost completely transparent to all wavelengths of visible light (although transmission characteristics do change with age). However, these 'transparent' tissues do have the ability to absorb varying amounts of non-ionizing radiation normally present in the environment.[2,11] Thus the various structures of the eye can also be considered as a consecutive series of spectral filters with each component absorbing exclusive wavelengths and preventing/reducing the likelihood of retinal photodamage (Fig. 20.3).[18] Table 20.1 provides details of spectral domain, wavelength, non-ionizing radiation sources, absorption site and type of light damage for different ocular tissues.

All non-ionizing radiation below approximately 295 nm is cut off by the cornea and does not reach the lens. The cornea is thus capable of absorbing the UV-C (100–280nm) and the short wavelengths in the UV-B between 280 and 295nm. It should be noted that the cornea is only exposed to UV-C from artificial non-ionizing radiation sources since this solar component is blocked by the atmosphere. The lens absorbs strongly in the long UV-B (300–315nm) and the full UV-A (315–400nm); appreciable irradiances of UV-B and UV-A reach the retina only in aphakic eyes. Both the cornea and the lens absorb in the infrared (1400–10000nm). Neither the aqueous nor the vitreous demonstrates any significant absorption of radiant energy under non-pathological conditions. Thus the light reaching the retina is the so-called 'visible component' of the electromagnetic spectrum (380–760nm). The most obvious absorber in the retina is the visual pigment which has a broad band absorption across the whole of the visible spectrum. In addition, the retina contains a number of chromophores which readily absorb visible light:

- the broad band absorbers melanin and lipofuscin – absorption increases with decreasing wavelength and thus these chromophores have been implicated in blue light damage to the retina.
- haemoglobin with absorption properties between 400 and 600nm
- macular pigment which strongly absorbs between 400 and 530nm – this spectral absorption may protect the macula from potential blue light damage.

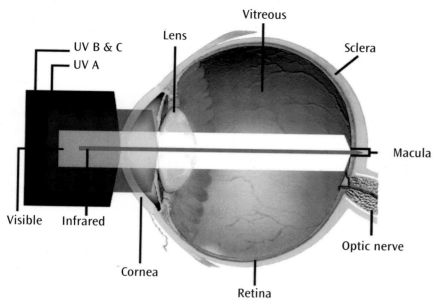

Figure 20.3 *The penetration/absorption of ultraviolet, visible and infrared radiation by the different structures of the eye. See colour plate section.*

It should be noted that the absorption characteristics of different ocular tissues vary with age, e.g. the yellowing of the lens increases its absorptive characteristics between 300 and 400nm with end absorptions extending to 500nm.

A final point that should be emphasized is that the combined refractive powers of the cornea and lens can increase the light intensity reaching the fovea.

OCULAR LIGHT DAMAGE

Although light is essential for vision its absorption by various tissues can result in tissue damage (Fig. 20.4). As discussed earlier, dependent on wavelength, irradiance energy and exposure duration, three different types of light damage can be identified; ionizing, thermal and photochemical. The damaging effect of non-ionizing

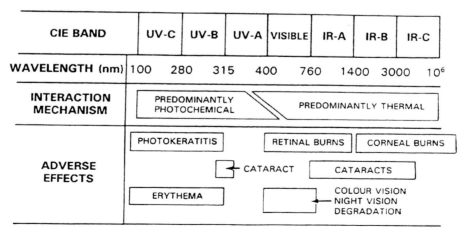

Figure 20.4 *International Commission on Illumination (CIE) spectral bands with their corresponding effects. The direct biological effects of optical radiations are frequency dependent. In the visible and infrared (IR) regions, the interaction mechanism is primarily thermal. In the ultraviolet (UV) region the interaction mechanism is predominantly photochemical, although thermal injury is also present. The biological effects for IR radiation are corneal burns and cataracts. The biological effects for visible radiation are retinal burns, cataracts, and degradation of colour or night vision. The biological effects for UV radiation are photokeratitis, cataracts, and erythema. UV-A and UV-B also cause skin cancer. Reproduced from Ref. 1.*

radiation can be broadly divided into acute and chronic depending on the immediacy of the response, type of damage and the ability of the damaged tissue to recover.

ACUTE LIGHT DAMAGE

Ultraviolet damage most commonly occurs in the superficial structures of the eye and is caused by excessive exposure to UV light (e.g. photokeratitis, photoconjunctivitis).[19,20] There is usually a latent period of up to 12 hours following UV exposure before damage to ocular tissues becomes apparent. The adverse effects of UV are related to the duration, intensity of the exposure and the degree of penetration (i.e. UV-A will reach the lens while the majority of UV-B is absorbed by the cornea). By contrast, light in the visible spectrum will usually affect the retina (e.g. solar retinopathy, welding arc maculopathy).[21] Infrared damage will be discussed in a later section.

Photokeratitis and photoconjunctivitis

The acute damage to ocular tissues by exposure to excessive UV is well documented and usually affects the corneal (photokeratitis) and conjunctival (photoconjunctivitis) epithelia. This damage is photochemical and is most commonly caused by exposure to UV-A, B and/or C. The acute inflammatory reaction of the superficial part of the cornea (and conjunctiva) to UV was originally termed 'photophthalmia'. One of its forms (snowblindness – photokeratitis) was first described in 1722, although the condition became more common and better recognized after the introduction of the electric arc furnace and lighting in 1879. Epithelial damage is observed within 8–12 hours of exposure. The photochemical changes induce a painful (foreign body sensation), red, photophobic profusely lacrimating eye with pronounced blepharism,[20,22] all manifestations of inflammatory keratoconjunctivitis (e.g. arc-eye, flash-eye, ophthalmia electra, snowblindness, exposure from sun lamp/sunbeds). Resolution takes 2–7 days depending on the severity of the burn and the patient may be advised to lubricate the eye with antibiotic ointment (e.g. chloramphenicol) and take analgesics during the recovery period which involves the proliferation and migration of healthy epithelium to replace the damaged cells.

Despite the normal use of protective goggles the most common industrial cause of damage is from welding arcs. It should be noted that damage can be cumulative; short exposures are additive within a period of 24 hours. Individuals receiving repeated exposure to UV radiation over extended periods (e.g. welders, those inhabiting snowy regions) can develop chronic blepharoconjunctivitis (with loss of elasticity of the conjunctiva and band degeneration of the cornea) as well as playing a role in the pathogenesis of pterygia, pinguecula and act as a trigger for recurrent corneal erosion.[23,24]

Ophthalmic instruments

Powerful light from ophthalmic instruments used for diagnostic and therapeutic purposes has been reported to cause iatrogenic phototoxicity in some patients.[25,26,27] To date there have been no confirmed reports of occupational risk from the use of these instruments in either the clinic or operating theatre. However, there is a potential occupational risk from ophthalmic lasers.[28] This is discussed in more detail below in the section on lasers.

Solar retinopathy

Solar retinopathy is a well recognized form of acute light damage caused by direct or indirect viewing of the sun.[20,21] Duke-Elder reports that solar retinopathy has been recognized since the time of the ancient Greeks;[29] Socrates advised that 'a solar eclipse should be only observed by looking at its reflection in water'. Galileo injured his eye while viewing the sun through his telescope. As detailed by De La Paz and D'Amico[21] the most common cause of solar retinopathy is the direct viewing of a solar eclipse but photic retinopathy has also been described in association with direct sun gazing by sunbathers and patients with psychotic disorders, religious festivals, military personnel and the use of hallucinogenic drugs such as lysergic acid diethylamide (LSD).

Retinal damage is considered to be photochemical since sunlight exposure is insufficient to raise the retinal temperature by 10°C provided macular choroidal blood flow is maintained.[30] The patient complains of blurred central vision immediately or soon after (usually within minutes) and the damage is usually, but not always, bilateral. The fundus presents initially with a yellow spot at the fovea which after several days changes to a reddish area with surrounding pigmentary change (Fig. 20.5). There is a marked drop in visual acuity with a central scotoma. By 2 weeks a red, well circumscribed lamellar hole (100–200μm diameter) often with a larger area of retinal pigment epithelium mottling is apparent. Visual acuity usually improves to near normal by 6 months although a slight-to-moderate loss in visual acuity may persist in some individuals. A very small central red spot may remain throughout life. Oral corticosteroids have been advocated as a treatment for acute lesions with severe visual loss but their efficacy remains unproven.

Welding arc maculopathy

Photic retinopathy may occur, due to photochemical damage by the blue light component of the welding arc, to individuals welding without goggles. In general,

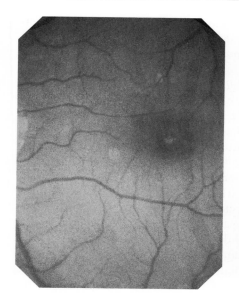
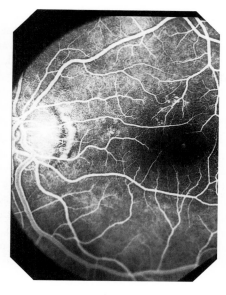

Figure 20.5 *Photographs of solar retinopathy. The fundus photograph shows pigmentary disturbance at the fovea and the angiogram confirms a focal window defect in the pigment epithelium at the fovea. Provided by Professor D McLeod, Manchester. See colour plate section.*

patients present with a decrease in vision which occurs immediately or soon after the injury; fundus appearance and visual recovery resemble those described for solar retinopathy[21,31] (see Chapter 9).

Laser

Laser is an acronym for Light Amplification by the Stimulated Emission of Radiation. Lasers are sources of non-ionizing radiation that can operate in the UV, visible and infrared region of the electromagnetic spectrum. The light emitted has a unique combination of spatial coherence (i.e. all the waves are in step), monochromaticity (one colour or narrow wavelength range) and usually high collimation. Furthermore, the emission may be continuous wave or pulsed for either long or short (Q-switched) duration.

The known effects of acute light damage to ocular tissues are exploited in preventive ophthalmology. Optical breakdown damage from Q-switched or mode-locked lasers are important procedures in iridotomy and posterior capsulotomy. Photoreactive keratectomy is now a standard procedure in Europe for the correction of refractive error less than 4 dioptres as well as becoming fashionable for the treatment of high myopia and is routinely undertaken using an Excimer laser emitting in the UV-C region of the spectrum.[32] Providing irradiance, exposure time, pulse rate and beam alignment are optimal the operation is successful, however, poor quality control can result in corneal fibrosis and opacification.[33] Argon, krypton and diode lasers are routinely used in retinal scatter photocoagulation to induce the regression of subretinal and preretinal vessels in conditions such as proliferative diabetic retinopathy.

Lasers are in common use both in the industrial (e.g. drilling, cutting, welding, communication) and military

(e.g. rangefinders, tactical target designators, night vision) settings and there have been numerous reports of accidental exposure resulting in immediate loss of central vision. Depending on the type of laser, damage occurs by either a thermal or mechanical mechanism.[34] In the case of retinal damage a gliotic scar develops and a paracentral or central scotoma may persist. Lasers are divided into four major classes depending on the potential safety hazard. These classes are defined by British Standard BS EN 60825 : 1992.

- Class 1 – non hazardous lasers; (i) the output is so low the laser is inherently safe or (ii) the laser is part of a totally enclosed system.
- Class 2 – low power visible continuous wave and pulsed lasers which, in the case of continuous wave lasers, are not hazardous within the blink reflex or aversion response (i.e. ≤ 0.25 seconds). Hazard can be controlled by relatively simple procedures (e.g. use of a beam stop and ensuring that beam paths are not at eye-level).
- Class 3 – Divided into A and B. A – low to medium power lasers where protection is still afforded by natural aversion responses but direct viewing with optical aids may be hazardous. B – medium power lasers where the viewing beam either directly or by specular reflection is hazardous, but diffuse reflections are safe.
- Class 4 – high power lasers which are not only a hazard from direct viewing and from specular reflections but also from diffuse reflections. The direct beam may also be a skin and fire hazard. Their use requires extreme caution.

Most laser accident experience comes from careless use of lasers in the research laboratory, with fewer in industry and military applications.[1,35–41] A review of the accident data suggests that at least one type of laser is responsible for the majority of accidental injuries that result in a significant visual loss: the Q switched neodymium: YAG (Nd:YAG) laser which emits invisible, near-infrared radiant energy at 1064 nm. Although a continuous wave (CW) laser causes thermal coagulation of tissue, a Q-switched laser having a pulse of only nanoseconds duration disrupts tissue by thermomechanical processes. A visible or near-infrared laser can be focused on the retina, resulting in a vitreous haemorrhage (Fig. 20.6). Despite macular injuries[42] and an initially serious visual loss, the vision of many patients recovers surprisingly well.[43,44] Others may have severe vision loss. Corneal injuries resulting from exposure to reflected laser energy in the far-infrared account for surprisingly few reported laser accidents. The explanation for this accident statistic is not really clear. However, with the increasing use of lasers operating at many new wavelengths, the ophthalmologist may see more accidental injuries from lasers. Not all laser incidents result in injury, and temporary visual effects are now also of concern.[45]

As discussed, the eye is particularly vulnerable to injury in the retinal hazard region from 400 nm at the short-wavelength end of the visible spectrum to 1400 nm in the near-infrared part of the spectrum.[1,2,46,47] In this spectral band, a collimated beam can be focussed to a 15–20 μm diameter retinal spot (i.e. much smaller than the diameter of a human hair). Because of the great brightness of a laser, its radiant energy can be greatly concentrated when focussed (e.g. upon the retina) compared with the rays from conventional light sources which are much less bright. The gain in beam irradiance from cornea to retina is approximately 100 000 times in the visible spectrum. Hence, a corneal beam irradiance of 1 W/cm² becomes 100 kW/cm² at the retina. Vision loss can vary from temporary after-images to a permanent blind spot (scotoma) or even total loss of vision in an eye.[1,43,48]

Diffuse reflections of laser beams are normally safe to view, since the energy is dissipated upon reflection into all directions and the resulting image on the retina is that of an extended source. However, under special conditions, it is a realistic possibility to produce a hazardous diffuse reflection.[49] This can result from a diffuse reflection of a Q-switched (1–100 ns) laser in the retinal hazard region. Colour contrast sensitivity can be reduced in ophthalmologists using argon blue green lasers for retinal photocoagulation.[28] After argon blue-green laser treatment sessions, sensitivity was reduced for colours lying along a tritan colour-confusion line for several hours. This acute effect was due to spectacular 'flashbacks' from the aiming beam off the surface of the contact lens. In addition a correlation has been made between the number of years of laser experience and a chronic reduction in tritan colour sensitivity. Appropriate safety procedures have now been introduced following this finding.

Exposure limits

Occupational exposure limits have been promulgated by a number of organizations (see list of Health and Safety directives at end of chapter). In the USA, both the American Conference of Governmental Industrial Hygienists (ACGIH) and the American National Standards Institute (ANSI) have produced a comprehensive set of exposure limits which apply for pulse durations of 1 ns to 30 ks (8 hours) for wavelengths from 180 nm in the ultraviolet (UV) to 1 mm in the extreme infrared. These exposure limits are virtually identical, although exposure limits are termed threshold limit values by ACGIH and maximum permissible exposure limits in the ANSI Standard Z-136.1.[50] On the international

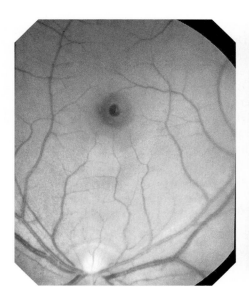 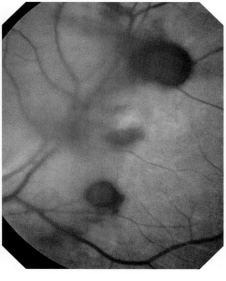

Figure 20.6 *Photographs of an accidental laser lesion causing a macular hole, a cuff of surrounding subretinal haemorrhage and choroidal bleeding into the surrounding vitreous. Provided by Professor A Bird, Moorfields Eye Hospital, London. See colour plate section.*

Table 20.2 *Selected occupational exposure limits for some common lasers*

Type of laser	Wavelength	Exposure limit
Argon-fluoride	193 nm	3.0 mJ/cm^2 over 8 h
Xenon-chloride	308 nm	40 mJ/cm^2 over 8 h
Argon ion	488, 514.5 nm	3.2 mW/cm^2 for 0.1 s
		2.5 mW/cm^2 for 0.25 s
Helium-neon	632.8 nm	1.8 mW/cm^2 for 1.0 s
		1.0 mW/cm^2 for 10 s
Helium-neon	632.8 nm	17 µW/cm^2 for 8 h
Neodymium-YAG	1064 nm	5.0 µJ/cm^2 for 1 ns to 100 µs
		5 mW/cm^2 for 10 s
Erbium glass	1540 nm	1.0 J/cm^2 for 1 ns–10 s
Erbium: YAG	2940 nm	10 mJ/cm^2 for 1–100 ns
Hydrogen-fluoride	2.7–3.1 µm	10 mJ/cm^2 for 1–100 ns
Carbon dioxide	10.6 µm	100 mW/cm^2 for 10 s to 8 h, limited area
		10 mW/cm^2 for > 10 s

Source: ACGIH EL

Note: to convert exposure limits in mW/cm^2, multiply by exposure time in seconds; e.g. the He-Ne or Argon EL at 0.1 s is 0.32 mJ/cm^2.

scene, the International Commission on Non-ionizing Radiation Protection (ICNIRP) published Guidelines for limits of human exposure to laser radiation in 1996. The basic resource used for the development of the laser exposure limits was the Environmental Health Criteria Document of the World Health Organization (1982). The International Electrotechnical Commission (IEC) and European guidelines are all similar to the ICNIRP, ACGIH, and ANSI exposure limits. Although the complete listing of all laser exposure limits is beyond the scope of this text, Table 20.2 provides a brief summary of some of the most commonly used limits.

Screening tests

Although not obligatory some employers undertake a pre-employment check of a potential employee's fundus appearance and visual acuity. This is largely for employer protection should an employee with a retinal lesion prior to working with a laser develop reduced vision and enter into litigation. Routine screening of employees is uncommon particularly since small or subthreshold lesions are difficult to detect; an individual will be aware of a large retinal lesion due to visual loss.

CHRONIC LIGHT DAMAGE

Chronic light damage has been clearly demonstrated in animal models but is difficult to prove in man; subclinical photodamage is believed to accumulate through a lifetime, eventually exceeding a threshold at which overt clinical damage is evident. However, to what extent such damage, particularly in the aged population, is primarily due to light exposure or other factors is open to debate. Furthermore, the major source of chronic light exposure has shifted dramatically over the last 50 years. Sunlight used to be the major non-ionizing radiation source; however, fluorescent lighting is now a common feature for many both at home and in the workplace. Furthermore, computers are now commonplace. Thus an increasing number of individuals are being exposed to non-ionizing radiation from visual display units in an environment of fluorescent lighting. Only time will tell if this change in lighting source will increase or reduce ophthalmic conditions attributable to chronic light exposure.

Sunlight

There are numerous epidemiological studies which have reported an association between chronic light exposure and cataract, pterygium, climatic droplet keratopathy and age-related macular degeneration.[20] The most detailed study of sun exposure and cataract was undertaken on 838 Chesapeake watermen in Maryland and a 60% increase in risk of cortical cataract with a doubling of cumulative sun exposure was noted.[51] This observation was subsequently supported by the smaller study undertaken by Bochow and colleagues.[52] Other less detailed studies have reported that the risk for posterior subcapsular cataract is slightly increased in persons with moderate and high light exposures.[12] Surprisingly, no association has yet been noted between light exposure and nuclear cataract. Severe cases of age-related macular degeneration have been shown to have received significantly greater exposures to either blue and/or full spectrum visible light over a 20-year period compared with controls especially in older subjects.[53] Thus high levels and chronic exposure of individuals to all or part of the visible light spectrum can manifest as ocular disease later in life.

Fluorescent lights

Many of the animal studies of light damage to the retina have employed fluorescent lamps, and this has given rise to concerns about human exposure to fluorescent lighting. It is important to recognize that the typical light exposure conditions for the test animals employed ring fluorescent lamps such that the animals (rats) could not look in any direction without seeing a bare fluorescent lamp. Under such conditions, where the luminance exceeded that of sunlight reflected from snow, retinal damage resulted after some days of exposure for 12 hours per day. Such conditions simply do not occur in human activity, where such a luminance would preclude seeing and result in almost continued 'bleaching' of the retinal pigment. It was necessary to dilate an animals's eyes in order to obtain this result in primates. There is no evidence of any detrimental effect in humans to date.

VISUAL DISPLAY UNITS

There is a large amount of literature on the viewing of visual display units and the suspected health hazards. Fundamentally, the research over the past two decades shows that whilst ergonomic (human-factor), refractive and visual comfort problems are real, there is no long-term adverse effect upon the visual system.[54,55]

DAMAGE BY INFRARED AND MICROWAVES

Infrared

Sources of infrared (IR) (which is normally invisible to the naked eye) include molten glass, furnaces, acetylene welding, the sun, various heating appliances, lasers (both commercial and opthalmic) and military weapons. IR-A damage is predominantly observed in the choroid, retina, iris and lens while the longer wavelength IR-B and IR-C are absorbed by the cornea and lens but do not reach the retina (Table 20.1). Specific sources of IR-B and IR-C are the erbium and carbon dioxide lasers respectively. Tissue damage is normally thermal, and in the case of the retina, largely irreversible.

Ocular damage from exposure to IR-A was common in workers involved with furnaces, molten glass or molten metals at temperatures over 1500°C. It was rec-

ognized as long ago as 1786 by Wenzel who observed that glass blowers had an increased incidence of cataract. Cataract formation appeared to be more common in the left eye probably due to the tendency for greater exposure to infrared on the left side as a result of common working practice.[56] It was calculated that the temperature of a human lens can increase by 9°C if the eye is exposed to molten glass at 1 foot (0.3048 m) distance for 1 minute.[57]

Infrared-induced cataract was 'prescribed' as an occupational disease in the UK in 1907 and the subsequent introduction of shields and goggles reduced the incidence of cataract in glass blowers dramatically such that in 1908 some 20% of workers had cataract whilst by 1945 only one case was reported in the UK in a whole year. Subsequently the bulk of glass production and foundry work has been mechanized, leaving only a small number of workers, especially in craft centres, at risk. However, a significant problem will still exist in developing countries where mechanisation and safety procedures are minimal.

Lens damage appears to be cumulative as a posterior cataract begins to develop after a decade or two of working near high intensity infrared sources. Cataract presents with a blurring of vision and associated lens opacities. Clinically the infrared cataract starts as a cobweb-like opacity which increases in size and density and develops into a saucer shaped posterior cataract.[58] The opacity will continue to grow and will ultimately form a complete opacity resembling a senile cataract. Treatment is by cataract extraction and intraocular lens implantation. Retinal damage often goes unnoticed since infrared is invisible and the retina has no pain receptors. However, pain may be experienced if the choroid is affected. Damage is thought to result from absorption of energy by melanin in the retinal pigment endothelium and choroidal melanocytes. This can result in a scotoma which, if at or near the fovea, can produce a profound loss of visual acuity. Examination may reveal localized areas of retinal oedema or patches of pigmentary disturbance, lesions often not appearing until 48 hours after exposure (fluorescein angiography can be used to identify burn areas not apparent by ophthalmoscopic examination). There is no recognized treatment for this condition.

Flash burns to the cornea may occur by the flashback of large artillery and by the flash of an atomic explosion. These burns which are a combination of infrared and ultraviolet are identical to those caused by other types of thermal exposure.[22] In most flash burns, the blink reflex protects the eyes from damage; however, in some instances the cornea is involved. The condition results in a painful eye which resolves within a few days. Treatment normally consists of topical antibiotics if epithelial defects and cycloplegia for discomfort. In more severe burns there is corneal thinning, neovascularization and scarring.

Microwaves

Microwave radiation is the high-frequency end of the radio-frequency region of the electromagnetic spectrum with a wavelength range of 1 mm to 1 m. Sources of microwaves include household ovens, radar, satellite communication, insect control appliances and surgical diathermy apparatus. It is unlikely that domestic appliances will pose a risk to the individual but military and civilian radar/communications workers may be at risk of exposure to dangerous levels of microwave radiation during service procedures near the antenna.[1] It has been hypothesized that in some tissues, especially the lens, repeated exposure causes cumulative damage and can manifest as cataract. However, evidence from chronic exposure animal and epidemiological studies have failed to confirm a direct correlation between microwave irradiation and cataract. Acute, accidental exposure of the eyes to microwave radiation may lead to skin burns, conjunctival infection and loss of corneal epithelium as well as stromal oedema and opacification. Epithelial loss can be managed with topical antibiotics (e.g. chloramphenicol or fuscidic acid) and cycloplegia (e.g. cyclopentolate) while topical steroids (e.g. prednisolone acetate) may also be considered if stromal damage and inflammation occur (indicated by corneal oedema and opacification). Exposure limits vary from approximately 1 to 10 mW/cm^2 in different standards and with animal ocular injury thresholds being in the order of 100 mW/cm^2.[59,60] More recent studies by Kues *et al.*[61] suggest that short-pulse exposures at 2.45 GHz may produce effects at lower average power densities. Individuals usually recover within 2 weeks although some stromal haze could persist for more than 12 months.

PHOTOSENSITIZATION

Photosensitizers, often given as drugs, can contribute to light-induced ocular damage.[8] Two groups of compounds, phenothiazides and psoralens, have been clearly identified as intraocular photosensitizing agents, capable of causing photochemical damage to the choroid, retina and lens in man as well as experimental animals. 8-Methoxypsoralen (8-MOP) is a typical example of such a photosensitizer which is used in the photodynamic therapy of psoriasis and other skin diseases.[62] Interaction between 8-MOP and the lens or retina results in the photobinding of the dye to these tissues. The phototoxic side effects of psoralen plus UV-A therapy (PUV-A) in patients on oral 8-MOP were evaluated in a large prospective study over 5 years. No significant dose-dependent increase in the risk of cataract formation was found in the group of patients receiving PUV-A therapy and using protective glasses constantly for 24 hours after therapy to block out UV-A and hence prevent photo-

binding. Lens opacities have been reported to occur within months in patients who did not use eye protection for 24 hours after PUV-A treatment.

PROTECTION AGAINST LIGHT DAMAGE

The eye is well adapted to protect itself against acute optical radiation (ultraviolet, visible and infrared radiant energy) injury from ambient sunlight. It is protected by a natural aversion response to viewing bright light sources that normally protects against injury from viewing sources such as the sun, arc lamps and welding arcs, since this aversion limits the duration of exposure to a fraction of a second (about 0.25 s). However, sources rich in ultraviolet radiation without a strong visual stimulus can be particularly hazardous. One can force oneself to stare at the sun, a welding arc or a snow-field and thereby suffer a temporary loss of vision, which in some cases may be permanent. In the industrial setting, when bright lights appear low in the field-of-view, the eye's protective mechanisms are less effective, and hazard precautions are particularly important.[63]

Safety standards

Safety standards for arc welding have long existed and specify eye protectors, curtains and barriers. Safety standards for lasers are also well developed world-wide; most following the general equipment and user guidance in IEC 825-1-1993. Lasers are grouped into several hazard classes and so labelled by manufacturers; the user then follows certain specified control measures based upon the laser class. However, standards for lamp safety are in their infancy. In North America, the Illuminating Engineering Society of North America (IESNA) issued photobiological safety standards for lamps and lighting system for the first time in 1996 and lamp groups are placed in risk groups somewhat similar to laser hazard classes.

Eye protector design and standards

The design of eye protectors for welding and other industrial optical sources (foundries, steel and glass manufacture, etc.) began at the beginning of this century with the development of Crooke's glass.[64] Eye protector standards which evolved later followed the general principle that since infrared and ultraviolet were not needed for vision, those spectral bands should be blocked as best as possible by the then currently available glass materials. Figure 20.7 illustrates the wide variety of design from spectacles to goggles and full-face welding helmets.

The empirical standards for eye protective equipment were tested in the 1970s and shown to have large safety

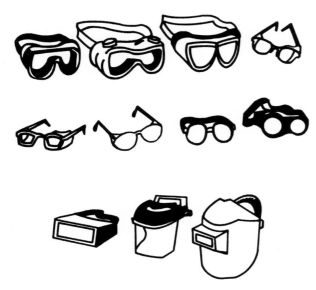

Figure 20.7 *Eye protectors. Eye protection for optical radiation hazards are produced in a variety of configurations from spectacles with and without sideshields to goggles, face shields and welding helmets. The choice of protector is dependent on the specification of the optical hazard together with local and national health and safety directives.*

factors for infrared and ultraviolet when the transmissions factors were tested against current occupational exposure limits, whereas the protection factors for blue light were just sufficient. Some standards requirements were therefore adjusted. Table 20.3 summarizes recommended eye protectors for different types of optical sources.

Laser protective eyewear was developed after occupational exposure limits had been established, and specifications were drawn up to provide the optical densities (a logarithmic measure of attenuation factor) that would be needed as a function of wavelength and exposure duration for specific lasers. Although specific laser eye protector standards exist in Europe, guidelines for laser eye protection are provided in the American National Standard ANSI Z136.1 and ANSI Z136.3 in the US.[30,65]

Human exposure limits

From knowledge of the optical parameters of the human eye and the radiance of a light source, it is possible to calculate irradiances (dose rates) at the retina. Exposure of the anterior structures of the human eye to ultraviolet radiation may also be of interest; and the relative position of the light source and the degree of lid closure can greatly affect the proper calculation of this ultraviolet exposure dose. For ultraviolet and short-wavelength light exposures, the spectral distribution of the light source is also important.

A number of national and international groups have recommended occupational exposure limits for optical radiation (i.e. ultraviolet, light, and infrared radiant energy) (see list of Health and Safety directives at end of chapter). Although most such groups have recommended exposure limits for UV and laser radiation, only one group has recommended exposure limits for visible radiation (i.e. light). This is the American Conference of Governmental Hygienists who, as previously mentioned, refer to its exposure limits as threshold limit values, and these are issued yearly, so there is an opportunity for a yearly revision. They are based in large part on ocular injury data from animal studies and from data from human retinal injuries resulting from viewing the sun and welding arcs. The threshold limit-values also have an underlying assumption that outdoor environmental exposures to visible radiant energy are normally not hazardous to the eye except when fixating the sun or in very unusual environments such as snow fields and deserts.

Optical radiation safety evaluation

Since a comprehensive hazard evaluation requires complex measurements of spectral irradiance and radiance of the source, or very specialized instruments and calculations, this is rarely done by industrial hygienists and safety engineers. Instead, the eye protective equipment is mandated by safety regulations in hazardous environments. Research studies have evaluated a wide range of arcs, lasers and thermal sources in order to develop broad recommendations for practical, easier-to-apply safety standards.

Protective filter materials

ULTRAVIOLET AND INFRARED PROTECTION

Almost all glass and plastic lens materials block ultraviolet radiation below 300 nm and infrared radiation at wavelengths greater than 3000 nm (3µm), and for a few lasers and optical sources, ordinary impact-resistant clear safety eyewear will provide good protection (e.g. clear polycarbonate lenses effectively block the 10.6 µm CO_2 wavelength). However, absorbers such as metal oxides in glass or organic dyes in plastics, must be added to eliminate UV-A and UV-B up to about 380–400 nm, and infrared beyond 780 nm to 3µm.[65] Depending upon the material this may be easy, or very difficult or expensive, and the stability of the absorber may vary somewhat. Filters that meet ANSI Z87.1 must have the appropriate attenuation factors in each critical spectral band.

FOUNDRY AND GLASS INDUSTRY EYEWEAR

Spectacles and goggles designed for ocular protection against infrared radiation generally have a light greenish

Table 20.3 *Selecting eye protection for intense optical radiation*

Type	Assessment	Protector type	Shade no no	Limitations	Not recommended
Welding electric arc	Shade based on visual comfort	Welding helmet	10–14	Protection from optical radiation directly related to filter lens density; Select the darkest shade that permits adequate task performance	Protectors that do not provide protection from optical radiation
Welding gas	Shade based on visual comfort	Welding goggle or welding face shield	4–8	Face shield can be worn over the primary protector	
Cutting			3–6		
Torch brazing			3–4		
Torch soldering	Shade based on visual comfort	Spectacles or Welding face-shield	1, 3–5	Face shield can be worn over the primary protector	
Glare	Shade based on visual comfort	Spectacle frontal protection	1–4	Shaded or special purpose lenses, as suitable	
Laser specified	Optical density as maximum laser exposure divided by exposure limit	Laser protective goggle or spectacle	Optical density units used	Choose filter lens based on comfort, optimal visual performance	Uncomfortable goggles, users fail to wear
RF/microwave	Psychological	Goggles made but not recommended	NA	NA	Not effective

Adapted from Ref. 63.   NA: not applicable.

tint, although the tint may be darker if some comfort against visible radiation is desired. Such eye protectors should not be confused with the blue lenses used in the steel and foundry operations where the objective is to visually check the temperature of the melt; these blue spectacles do not provide protection, and should only be worn briefly.[64]

FIREFIGHTING

Firefighters may be exposed to intense near-infrared radiation, and apart from the crucially important head and face protection, infrared attenuating filters are frequently prescribed. Here impact protection is also important.

ULTRAVIOLET RADIATION PROTECTION

A number of specialized UV lamps are used in industry for fluorescence detection and for photocuring of inks, plastic resins, dental polymers, etc. Although UV-A sources normally pose little real risk, these sources may either contain trace amounts of hazardous UV-B or pose

a disability glare problem (from fluorescence of the crystallin lens); UV filter lenses with very high attenuation factors are widely available to protect against the entire UV spectrum with either glass or plastic lenses. A slight yellowish tint may be detectable if protection is afforded to 400 nm. Of paramount importance in these types of eyewear (and for industrial sunglasses) is peripheral protection. Side-shields or wrap-around designs are important to protect against the coroneo effect (focussing of temporal, oblique rays into the nasal equatorial area of the lens (where cortical cataract frequently originates).

LASER EYE PROTECTORS

The objective of laser eye protective filters is to transmit as much visible light for seeing while at the same time blocking the laser wavelength(s) of concern. The protective factor used for laser eyewear is termed optical density (OD). The OD is a logarithmic expression for attenuation factor, e.g. a protection factor of 1000 (10^3) is an OD of 3.0, and a protection factor of one-million (10^6) is an OD of 6.0. Since most lasers emit powers or energies of the order of thousands to millions of times the maximum permissible exposure limit, optical densities of 4–6 are most typical. The ANSI standard Z136.1 *Safe Use of Lasers* provides detailed methods for determining the appropriate eyewear. Although some eyewear vendors and laser safety promoters have argued for very robust filters of coated glass to withstand extremely high beam irradiances of many kilowatts per cm^2, this is overkill, and polycarbonate laser protective lenses are quite adequate (the skin will be severely charred at much lower irradiances). Polycarbonate has superior burn-through characteristics[65] compared with other plastics and is also superior to all other lens materials for industrial impact protection.

At present, prescription lenses in laser filter materials are only available on a limited basis for glass lenses but there are a number of companies which supply cover goggles for laser protection. The Laser Institute of America, Orlando, Florida is a useful source of information on laser safety and laser eye protectors.

Welding filters

Infrared and UV radiation filtration is readily achieved in glass filters with additives such as iron-oxide, but the visible attenuation determines the shade number, which is a logarithmic expression of attenuation. Normally a shade 3–4 is used for gas welding (goggles), and 10–14 for arc welding and plasma arc operations (helmet protection required). The rule-of-thumb is that if the welder finds the arc to view, adequate attenuation is provided against ocular hazards. Supervisors, welders' helpers and other persons in the work area may require filters with a relatively low shade number (e.g. 3–4) to protect against welder's photokeratitis (arc-eye).[64] In recent years a new type of welding filter, the autodarkening filter has appeared on the scene. Regardless of the type of filter, it should meet ANSI Z87.1 and Z-49.1 standards for fixed welding filters specified for the dark shade.

AUTODARKENING WELDING FILTERS

Autodarkening welding filters represent an important advance in the ability of welders to produce consistently high-quality welds more efficiently and ergonomically.[66] Considering the total welding process, the welder formerly had to lower and raise the helmet or filter each time an arc was started and quenched. The welder had to work blind just prior to striking the arc. Furthermore, the helmet is frequently lowered and raised with a sharp snap of the neck and head which can lead to neck strain or more serious injuries. Faced with this uncomfortable and cumbersome procedure, some welders frequently initiate the arc with a conventional helmet in the raised position – leading to 'welder's flash' (arc-eye or photokeratitis). Under normal ambient lighting conditions, a welder wearing a helmet fitted with an autodarkening fil-

ter can see well enough with the eye protection in place to perform tasks such as aligning and fixturing the parts to be welded, precisely positioning the welding equipment and striking the arc. Then, in the most typical helmet designs, light sensors detect the arc flash and direct an electronic drive unit to switch a liquid crystal filter from a light shade to a preselected dark shade. The aforementioned drawbacks of fixed shade filters are largely eliminated by autodarkening filters which explains the widespread popularity of these newer systems.

Questions have frequently been raised whether there are hidden safety problems with the new autodarkening filters. For example, can afterimages (flash-blindness) result in impaired vision in the workplace? Do the new types of filters really offer equivalent or better protection than conventional fixed filters? The answer to the second question is Yes, but not all autodarkening filters are equivalent. Filter closure speeds and light and dark shade values vary, as does the weight of each unit. The temperature dependence of performance, variation of shade with electrical battery degradation, the 'resting state shade', and other technical factors vary depending upon each manufacturer's design. These are being addressed in new standards.

Since adequate filter attenuation is afforded by all systems, the single most important attribute specified by the manufacturers of autodarkening filters is the speed of filter switching. Current autodarkening filters vary in switching speed from 1/10th second (0.1s) to faster than 1/10 000th second (100 μs). Buhr and Sutter[67] have indicated a means of specifying the maximum switching time, but their formulation varies relative to the time-course of switching. Switching speed is crucial, since it gives the best clue to the really important (but unspecified) measure of how much light will enter the eye when the arc is struck compared with when wearing a fixed filter of the same working shade number. If too much light enters the eye for each switching during the day, the accumulated light energy dose produces transient adaptation and complaints about eye strain, etc. Current products with switching speeds of the order of 10 ms or less will provide adequate protection against photoretinitis. However, the shortest switching time of the order of 30–100 μs (0.03–0.1 ms) has the advantage of reducing 'transient adaptation' effects.[66,68] Transient adaptation is the visual experience caused by sudden changes in one's light environment which may be accompanied by discomfort, glare and temporary loss of detailed vision.

Simple check tests are available to the welder short of extensive laboratory testing. Suggest to the welder to simply look at a page of detailed print through each autodarkening filter. This will give an indication of its optical quality. Next, try striking an arc while observing it through each filter being considered for purchase. Fortunately, one can rely on the fact that light levels which are comfortable to view will not be hazardous. The UV radiation and IR filtration should be checked in the manufacturer's specification sheet to make sure that the unnecessary bands are filtered out. A few repeated arc strikings should give the welder a sense of whether discomfort will be experienced from transient adaptation, although a one-day trial would be best.

The resting or failure state shade number of an auto-darkening filter (e.g. if the battery fails) should provide 100% protection of the welder's eyes for at least one to several seconds. Some manufacturers use a dark state as the 'off' position and others use an intermediate shade between the dark and the light shade states. In either case, the resting state transmittance for the filter should be appreciably lower than the light shade transmittance to preclude a retinal hazard. In any case, the device should provide a clear and obvious indicator to the user when the filter is switched off or when a system failure occurs. This will ensure that the welder is warned in advance when the filter is not switched on or is not operating properly before beginning to weld. Other features, such as battery life, performance under extreme temperature conditions, etc. may be of importance to certain users.

CONCLUSIONS

Although technical specifications can appear to be somewhat involved for eye protectors against optical radiation sources, safety standards exist which specify shade numbers, and these standards provide a conservative safety factor for the wearer. However, should damage occur the recipient should be immediately referred to a doctor for a medical opinion.

REFERENCES

1 DeFrank J, Bryan P, Hicks C, Sliney D. Nonionizing radiation. In: Zatjchuk R ed. *Textbook of Military Medicine*. Office of the Surgeon-General, Department of the Army, 1993: 539–80.

2 Marshall J. Radiation and the ageing eye. *Ophthalmol Phys Opt* 1985; **5**: 241–63.

3 Hogan M, Alvarado J, Weddell J. *Histology of the Human Eye*. Philadelphia: WB Saunders Co, 1971.

4 Davson H. *Physiology of the Eye*. London: Macmillan Academic, 1990.

5 Saude T. *Ocular Anatomy and Physiology*. Oxford: Blackwell Scientific Publications; 1973.

6 Snell R, Lemp M. *Clinical Anatomy of the Eye*. Boston, Oxford: Blackwell Scientific Publications, 1989.

7 Berman E. *Biochemistry of the Eye*. New York: Plenum Press, 1991.

8 Lerman S. Light-induced changes in ocular tissues. In: Miller, ed. *Clinical Light Damage to the Eye*. New York: Springer Verlag, 1987: 183–215.

9 Mellerio J. Light effects on the retina. In: Albert D, Jakobiec F eds. *Principles and Practice of Ophthalmology: Basic Sciences*. Philadelphia: WB Saunders Co, 1994: 1326–45.

10 Mainster M, Sliney D, Belcher C, Buzney S. Laser photodistruptors, damage mechanisms, instrument design and safety. *Ophthalmology* 1983; **90**: 937–44.

11 Dillon J. The photophysics and photobiology of the eye. *J Photochem Photobiol B: Biol* 1991; **10**: 23–40.

12 Hankinson S. The epidemiology of age-related cataract. In: Albert D, Jakobiec F eds. *Principles and Practice of Ophthalmology: Basic Sciences*. Philadelphia: WB Saunders Co, 1994: 1255–66.

13 Noell W, Walker V, Kang, Berman S. Retinal damage by light in rats. *Invest Ophthalmol Vis Sci* 1966; **5**: 450–73.

14 Marshall J. The ageing retina: physiology or pathology. *Eye* 1987; **1**: 292–5.

15 Ham W, Mueller H, Sliney D. Retinal sensitivity to damage from short wavelength light. *Nature* 1976; **260**: 153–5.

16 Ham W. The photopathology and nature of the blue-light and near-UV retinal lesion produced by lasers and other optical sources In: Wolbarsht M ed. *Laser Applications in Medicine and Biology*. New York, Plenum Press, 1989: 191–246.

17 Rozanowska M, Jarvis-Evans J, Korytowski W, Boulton M, Burke J, Sarna T. Blue light-induced reactivity of retinal age pigment. *J Biol Chem* 1995; **270**: 18825–30.

18 Wolbarsht M. The function of intraocular color filters. *Fed Proc* 1976; **35**: 44–9.

19 Pitts D. The ocular effects of ultraviolet radiation. *Am J Optom Physiol Opt* 1978; **55**: 19–35.

20 Roh S, Weiter J. Light damage of the eye. *J Florida Med Assoc* 1994; **81**: 248–51.

21 De La Paz M, D'Amico D. Photic retinopathy. In: Albert D, Jakobiec F eds. *Principles and Practice of Ophthalmology: Basic Sciences* Vol 2. Philadelphia: WB Saunders, Co, 1994: 1032–7.

22 Parrish CM, Chandler JW. Corneal trauma. In: Kaufmann H, Barron B, McDonald M, Waltman S eds. *The Cornea*. New York, London: Churchill Livingstone, 1988: 599–646.

23 Zuclich J. Cumulative effects of near-UV induced corneal damage. *Hlth Phys* 1980; **38**: 833–8.

24 Mills B, Brown R, Saunders D. Non-ionising radiation and the eye. In: Raffle P, Adams P, Baxter P, Lee W eds. *Hunter's Diseases of Occupations* 8th edn. London: Edward Arnold, 1994: 387–400.

25 Mainster M, Ham W, Delori F. Potential retinal hazards. Instrument and environmental light sources. *Ophthalmology* 1983; **90**: 927–32.

26 Davidson P, Sternberg P. Potential retinal photoxicity. *Am J Ophthalmol* 1993; **116**: 497–501.

27 Azzolini C, Brancato R, Venturi G, Bandello F, Pece A, Santoro P. *Int Ophthalmol* 1995; **18**: 269–76.

28 Berninger TA, Canning C, Gunduz K, Strong N, Arden GB. Using argon laser blue light reduces ophthalmologists' color contrast sensitivity. Argon blue and surgeons vision. *Arch Ophthalmol* 1989; **107**: 1453–8.

29 Duke-Elder S. Radiational injuries. In: *System of*

Ophthalmology Vol 14, part 2. St Louis: CV Mosby, 1972 : 888–912.

30 Sliney D, Wolbarsht M. *Safety with Lasers and Other Optical Sources*. New York: Plenum Press, 1980.

31 Naidoff M, Sliney D. Retinal injury from a welding arc. *Am J Ophthalmol* 1974; **77**: 663–8.

32 McGhee C, Taylor H, Gartry D, Trokel S. *Excimer Lasers in Ophthalmology: Principles and Practice*. London: Martin Dunitz, 1997.

33 McGhee C, Ellerton C. Complications of excimer laser photorefractive surgery. In: McGhee C, Taylor H, Gartry D, Trokel S eds. *Excimer Lasers in Ophthalmology*: *Principles and Practice*. London: Martin Dunitz, 1997: 379–402.

34 Sliney D. Interaction mechanisms of laser radiation with ocular tissues, In: Count LA, Duchene A, Courant D eds. *First International Symposium on Laser Biological Effects*: *Lasers et Normes de Protection* Fontenay-aux-Roses Commissariat a l'Energie Atomique, Departement de Protection Sanitaire, 1988.

35 Boldrey E, Little H, Flocks M, Vassiliadis A. Retinal injury due to industrial laser *burns*. *Ophthalmology* 1981; **88**: 101–7.

36 Gabel V, Birngruber R, Lorenz B, Lang G. Clinical observations of six cases of laser injury to the eye. *Hlth Phys* 1989; **56**: 705–710.

37 Gibbons W, Allen R. Retinal damage from supra-threshold Q-switched laser exposure. *Hlth Phy* 1978; **35**: 461–9.

38 Henkes H, Zuidema H. Accidental laser coagulation of the central fovea. *Ophthalmologica* 1975; **171**: 15–25.

39 Liu H, Gao G, Wu D, Xu G, Shi L, Xu J, Hai H. Ocular injuries from accidental laser exposure. *Hlth Phys* 1989; **56**: 711–6.

40 Rathkey A. Accidental laser burn of the macula. *Arch Ophthalmol* 1965; **74**: 346–8.

41 Wolfe C. Laser retinal injury. *Military Med* 1985; **150**: 177–81.

42 Zweng H Accidental Q-switched laser lesion of human macula. *Arch Ophthalmol* 1967; **78**: 596–9.

43 Hirsch D, Booth G, Schockett S, Sliney D. Recovery from pulsed-dye laser retinal injury. *Arch Ophthalmol* 1992; **110**: 1688–9.

44 Sliney D. Ocular injuries from laser accidents. In: *Proceedings of Laser-inflicted Eye Injuries: Epidemiology, Prevention and Treatment*. San Jose, CA 1996: 25–33.

45 Mainster M, Sliney D, Marshall J, Warren K, Timberlake G, Trokel S. But is it really light damage? *Ophthalmology* 1997; **104**: 179–80.

46 Ham W, Mueller H, Wolbarsht M, Sliney D. Evaluation of retinal exposures from repetitively pulsed and scanning lasers. *Hlth Phys* 1988; **54**: 337–44.

47 Ham W, Ruffolo J, Mueller HGuerry, D. III: The nature of retinal radiation damage, dependence on wavelength, power level and exposure times. *Vision Res* 1980; **20**: 1105–11.

48 Baleshevich L, Zhokov V, Kirillov YL, Preobrazhenskiy P. Some incidents of eye damage by laser radiation. *Vestnik Oftal'mologii* 1981; **1**: 60–1.

49 Curtin T, Boyden D. Reflected laser beam causing accidental burn of retina. *Am J Ophthalmol* 1968; **65**: 188–9.

50 Wolbarsht M. Sliney D. Historical development of the ANSI Z136 laser safety standard. *J Laser Appl* 1991; **3**: 5–11.

51 Taylor H, West S, Rosenthal F, Munoz B, Newland H *et al*. Effect of ultraviolet radiation on cataract formation. *New Engl J Med* 1988; **319**: 1429–33.

52 Bochow T, West S, Azar A, Munoz B, Sommer A, Taylor H. Ultraviolet light exposure and risk of posterior subcapsular cataract. *Arch Ophthalmol* 1989; **107**: 369–72.

53 Taylor H, West S, Munoz B, Rosenthal F, Bressler S, Bressler N. The long-term effects of visible light on the eye. *Arch Ophthalmol* 1992; **110**: 99–104.

54 Yeow P, Taylor S. Effects of long term visual display terminal usage on visual factors. *Optom Vis Sci* 1991; **68**: 930–41.

55 Jackson A, Barnett C, Stevens A, McClure M, Patterson C, McReynolds M. Vision screening, eye examination and risk assessment of display screen users in a large regional teaching hospital. *Ophthalmol Vis Opt* 1997; **17**: 187–95.

56 Lydahl E, Glansholm A. Infrared radiation and cataract: differences between the two eyes of glassworkers. *Arch Ophthalmol* 1985; **63**: 39–44.

57 Goldman H. Genesis of heat cataract. *Albrecht Von Graefes Arch Klin Ophthalmol* 1933; **9**: 314–23.

58 Hanna C. Cataract of toxic ecology. In: Bellow J ed. *Cataract and Abnormalities of the Lens*. New York: Grune and Stratton, 1975: 217–24.

59 Lin R, Dischinger P, Conde J *et al*. Occupational exposure to electromagnetic fields and the occurrence of brain tumors. *J Occup Med* 1985; **27**: 413–9.

60 Sliney D, Stuck B. Microwave exposure limits for the eye: applying infrared laser-threshold. In: Klauenberg B ed. *Radiofrequency Standards* New York: Plenum Press, 1994: 79–87.

61 Kues HA. *Microwave Biological Effects Program Review*. Report JHU/APL, SR 90–2. Laurel MD, Johns Hopkins University Applied Physics Laboratory, April 1990.

62 Andley U. Photoxidative stress. In: Albert D, Jakobiec F eds. *Principles and Practice of Ophthalmology: Clinical Practice* Vol 2. Philadelphia: WB Saunders Co; 1994: 1032–7.

63 Vinger P, Sliney D. The prevention of sports and work related injury. *Issues Ocular Trauma* 1995; **8**: 709–21.

64 Sliney D, Freasier B. The evaluation of optical radiation hazards. *Applied Opt* 1973; **12**: 1–24.

65 Sliney D, Sparks D, Wood R. The protective characteristics of polycarbonate lenses against CO2 laser radiation. *J Laser Appl* 1993; **5**: 49–52.

66 Sliney D. A safety managers guide to the new welding filters. *Welding J* 1992; **71**: 45–7.

67 Buhr E, Sutter E. Dynamic filters for protective devices, In: Mueller G, Sliney D eds. *Dosimetry of Laser Radiation in Medicine and Biology* Vol IS-5, Bellingham, WA: SPIE 1989: 101–7.

68 Eriksen P. Time resolved optical spectra from MIG welding are ignition. *Am Ind Hyg Assoc J* 1985; **46**: 101–4.

69 Hemstreet H, Bruce W, Altobelli K, Stevens C, Connolly J.

Ocular Hazards of Picosecond and Repetitive Pulse Argon Laser Exposures. First Annual Report, February 1973-February 1974, San Antonio, TX, USAF Contract for School of Aerospace Medicine. Technology Inc/Brooks AFB, 1974.

HEALTH AND SAFETY DIRECTIVE REFERENCES

American Conference of Governmental Industrial Hygienists. *Threshold Limit Values and Biological Exposure Indices for 1996*. Cincinnati, OH: ACGIH, 1996.

American National Standards Institute. *Safety with Welding and Cutting*. ANSI Z49.1. Orlando, FL: ANSI, Laser Institute of America, 1980.

American National Standards Institute. *Safe Use of Lasers*. Z-1361–1986, Orlando, FL: ANSI, Laser Institute of America, 1986.

American National Standards Institute. *Eye and Face Protection*. ANSI Z87.1, Orlando FL: ANSI, Laser Institute of America, 1989.

American National Standards Institute. *Safety Use of Lasers*. ANSI Z136.1/3, Orlando, FL: ANSI, Laser Institute of America, 1993.

British Standards Organization. *Radiation Safety of Laser Products and Systems*. BS4803. London: BSI, 1984.

British Standards Organization. *Radiation Safety and Users Guide*. BS EN 60825. Milton Keynes: BSI, 1992.

Deutsche Institut fur Normung. *Radiation Safety of Laser Products*. VDE 0837. Berlin DIN/VDE, 1984.

Duchene AS, Lakey JRA, Repacholi MH (eds). *IRPA Guidelines on Protection Against Non-Ionizing Radiation*. New York: Macmillan, 1991.

Health Council of the Netherlands. *Acceptable Levels for Micrometer Radiation*. Rijswijk: Gezondheidsraad, 1979.

Illuminating Engineering Society of North America. *Photobiological Safety of Lamps and Lighting Systems*. ANSI RP27.1 and RP27.3. New York: IESNA, 1996.

International Electrotechnical Commission. *Radiation Safety of Laser Products, Equipment Classification, and User's Guide*. Document WS 825. Geneva: IEC, 1984 [with amendment, 1989, 1993].

International Non-Ionizing Radiation Committee, International Radiation Protection Association (IRPA). Guidelines for limits of human exposure to laser radiation. *Hlth Phys* 1985; **49**: 341–59; amended in: Recommendations for minor updates to the IRPA 1985 Guidelines for limits of exposure to laser radiation. *Hlth Phys* 1988; **54**: 573–5.

International Non-Ionizing Radiation Committee, International Radiation Protection Association (IRPA). *Guidelines for Limits of Human Exposure to Non-Ionizing Radiation*. New York: Macmillan, 1991.

Prevention Blindness America. *Caution: Battery on Board*. Schaumburg, IL:PBA, 1994.

Stuck BE, Lund DJ, Beatrice ES. *Repetitive Pulse Laser Data and Changes in the Maximum Permissible Exposure Limits*. Institute Report No. 58. San Francisco, CA: Letterman Army Institute of Research, Division of Non-Ionizing Radiation, 1978.

World Health Organization. *Lasers and Optical Radiation*. Environmental Health Criteria No. 23. Joint publication – Geneva: United Nations Environmental Program/The International Radiation Protection Association/WHO, 1982.

21

Extremely low frequency electric and magnetic fields

LEEKA I KHEIFETS

The nature of electric and magnetic fields	439	Magnetic resonance imaging	446
Acute effects in humans	440	Conclusions	446
Long-term health effects	440	References	447

Dedicated to Leonard Sagan, a free thinker and a friend

THE NATURE OF ELECTRIC AND MAGNETIC FIELDS

Electricity use has grown throughout the industrialized world since the first public power station began operating in London on 12 January 1882. Electricity is generated and usually transmitted as alternating current (ac) in North America at 60 cycles per second, or 60 Hertz (Hz), and in Europe and elsewhere at 50 Hz.

Electricity is generally considered safe, but it is not completely without hazard. For example, in the United States of America each year there are about 1100 deaths attributed to electric shocks. Approximately 75% of these deaths occur from unsafe operation of electrical appliances in the home and the remainder are from accidents in the workplace.[1] However, the subject of clinical treatment of electric shocks and burns resulting from direct contact with electrical conductors is beyond the scope of this chapter, which considers health effects postulated from exposure to electric and magnetic fields (EMF) associated with the delivery and use of electricity.

Electric and magnetic fields are ubiquitous. The magnitude of electric fields, measured in kV/m, is directly proportional to line voltage, while magnetic fields, measured in tesla (T) or microtesla (μT), are determined by the magnitude of the electric current. These fields are found around every electrical conductor, motor and appliance. Magnetic field exposure in the home occurs from the use of various appliances, house wiring, including current flow on the safety grounding system, and utility lines outside the home. In office buildings, computers and copy machines are common sources of magnetic fields. Power distribution facilities and large motors used to drive building air conditioning systems can also contribute significantly to the magnetic field environment. In factories high magnetic fields are encountered near large machines, electrical heating equipment and other high current-carrying devices.

Measurement of 50–60 Hz EMF is easily carried out with hand-held field meters. However, extreme variability of fields, both in space and time, makes exposure assessment and the use of exposure surrogates difficult. This difficulty is further complicated by the lack of knowledge regarding what aspects of exposure are biologically relevant and what might constitute a dose.

Average magnetic field exposures vary from 0.4 to 0.6 μT among electricians and electrical engineers to about 1.0 μT for power line workers. The highest average exposures are encountered by welders, some of whom are exposed to average levels of 3.7 μT. However, these exposure averages are often driven by a few high exposures. Geometric mean, as opposed to arithmetic mean, is not influenced by a few high measurements and is thus much smaller; it ranges from 0.2–0.3 μT for electricians and electrical engineers to 0.4 μT for power line workers. Welders experience a geometric mean of 0.6 μT. Although we have learned much about exposures in the electric utility industry, less is known about exposures in other industries.

ACUTE EFFECTS IN HUMANS

Electric fields can be detected as a slight tingling of the hair at field strengths of 5–10 kV/m. Electrical workers may also be affected by contact currents ('microshocks') which have sometimes been suggested as the source of certain effects in cells and tissues, such as chromosomal anomalies.[2] It should be noted, however, that there is no substantial evidence implicating microshocks as harmful beyond their nuisance effects.

There is evidence that certain animals and organisms (e.g. birds, bacteria) can detect and be guided by the earth's static magnetic field and very low frequency ac fields (<10 Hz). Humans cannot sense time-varying magnetic fields of 50–60 Hz except at very high field strengths (3–5 mT). At this field strength humans perceive visual flashes of light[3] known as magnetophosphenes, which are transient and are not thought to produce any permanent retinal lesions.[4]

In the past, exposures to ambient EMF have been thought to be without biologic effects. The first suggestion that exposures might be detrimental to one's health arose from Soviet Union studies in the early 1960s.[5] These studies focused on utility workers, particularly substation employees. Studies of these employees found an excess of such symptoms as sleeplessness, headache and upper respiratory distress. Investigations of the general health of electrical workers in several Western countries have failed to confirm these findings. Indeed, in health evaluations of electrical workers[6] and comparison groups, no differences were found based on the response to a survey questionnaire by persons on whom field measurements had been made.[7]

Some recent experimental evidence suggests that combined electric and magnetic fields can, under certain exposure conditions, produce physiologic effects in human volunteers. At the Midwest Research Institute in Kansas City, human heart rate and evoked cerebral potentials were observed to be slightly affected by exposures to EMF.[8] In these experiments, researchers used the following combinations of electric and magnetic fields: 6 kV/m and 100 mG, 9 kV/m and 200 mG, and 12 kV/m and 300 mG (1 mG or milligauss = $1/10^{-7}$ T). Such levels are found intermittently in some occupational environments. While these observations are preliminary and their possible health consequences obscure, they offer some evidence that there may be human responses to EMF.

LONG-TERM HEALTH EFFECTS

The suggestion that exposures to EMF could have long-term impacts on human health first arose in the 1970s. The health effects that have received the most attention are cancer, reproductive effects and neurobehavioural effects. The evidence linking these outcomes to EMF exposure is discussed below.

Cancer (see Chapter 39)

EPIDEMIOLOGICAL

The first publication linking EMF to human cancer appeared in 1979.[9] The paper reported an association between childhood cancer and presumed residential exposure to EMF, originating from neighbourhood power lines. This observation spurred a number of studies that examined the effect of occupational exposure to EMF and cancer.

The study of the hypothesized association of EMF exposure with human cancer has mostly continued to follow these two lines of investigation, i.e., cancer among children whose exposure to EMF is residential in origin, and cancer among workers in broadly defined 'electrical occupations' whose exposure to EMF presumably occurs at the workplace. Childhood leukaemia has been moderately associated with wire codes, a presumed surrogate for exposure to 60-Hz magnetic fields, but less consistently with measured fields.[10] Other studies of residential exposure and biological effects from EMF are largely negative so far. These studies are outside the scope of this review; for a detailed review of residential studies, see Ref. 11.

Occupational studies of EMF have employed several designs such as proportionate mortality, case-control and cohort analysis. The occupational groups studied included one or more of the following categories of workers: linemen, substation workers, welders, electricians, motion picture projectionists, electronic assemblers, and electrical engineers. Unfortunately, the definition of electrical workers in these studies is broad, varies considerably among investigations and does not always reflect a high EMF exposure.

A brief summary of the numerous studies investigating occupational EMF exposures and several cancers is presented below. Leukaemia and brain cancers have received the most attention although breast cancer is currently being examined in several ongoing studies, albeit with a focus on residential exposures. Also, occupational exposure to electric fields has re-emerged as an issue of potential importance.

Because of the large number of occupational studies of EMF and leukaemia and brain cancers, specific study references which have been included in meta-analyses are omitted below. Please refer to Refs 11 and 12 for a more detailed review of the literature.

LEUKAEMIA

The risks of leukaemia associated with exposure to EMF are generally low. Pooled analyses suggest an excess of all leukaemias, with a risk estimate of 1.18 (95% confidence interval 1.12–1.24);[11] risks were slightly higher for the various leukaemia subtypes (Fig. 21.1). Although most studies reported a small elevation in risk, the apparent lack of a clear pattern of exposure to EMF substantially detracts from the hypothesis that magnetic fields in the work environment are responsible for it. These findings were not sensitive to assumptions, influence of individual studies, weighting schemes, or modelling. Some evidence of publication bias was noted.[12]

Improvements in study quality have not clarified the relationship between occupational EMF exposure and leukaemia. While recent studies represent substantial improvements over earlier research, each has unique limitations. The most recent studies do not point to strong biases or confounding in the earlier studies. However, so little is known of the risk factors for adult leukaemia that confounding from an as yet unidentified risk factor remains a possibility. Also, the lack of an exposure-response relationship and the inconsistencies in results from different studies make it difficult to conclude that occupational EMF exposure is a risk factor for adult leukaemia.

BRAIN CANCER

Similarly, there is a small but significant increase in brain cancer risk associated with estimates of potential workplace magnetic field exposure: the relative risk = 1.21 (95% confidence interval 1.11–1.33).[13] While most studies reported a small elevation in risk, there was considerable heterogeneity in the results (Fig. 21.2). Pooled risk estimates (based on inverse variance weighted pooling) decreased over time (Fig. 21.3). The findings of this meta-analysis were not affected by inclusion of unpublished data, influence of individual studies, weighting schemes, or model specification.

Recent increased use of wireless communications has brought new concerns about biological effects of radiofrequency radiation. While it is well established that at higher power levels radiofrequency energy can produce deleterious effects, today's wireless communication systems employ a low-power modulated form of radiofrequency radiation, the effects of which are still uncertain.[14]

While some studies reported a slight elevation in risk for adult brain tumours among those in electrical

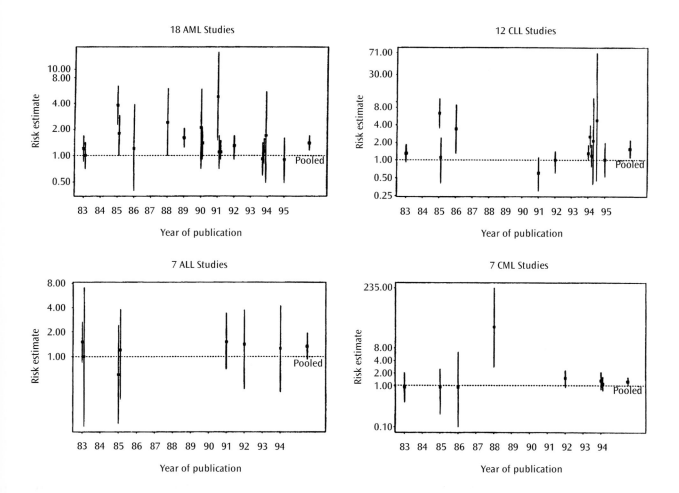

Figure 21.1 *Pooled and individual risk estimates with 95% confidence intervals for leukaemia subtypes. AML: acute myeloid leukaemia; ALL: acute lymphocytic leukaemia; CLL: chronic lymphocytic leukaemia; CML: chronic myeloid leukaemia.*

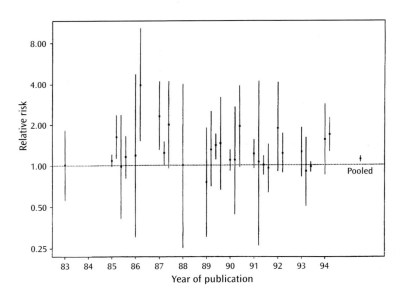

Figure 21.2 *Pooled and individual risk estimates, with 95% confidence intervals for brain cancer.*

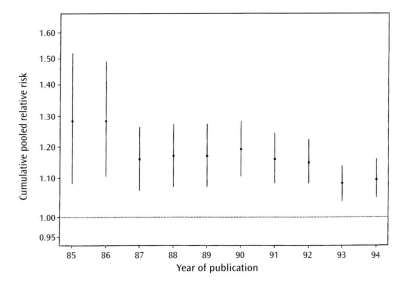

Figure 21.3 *Pooled risk estimates for brain cancer for each year.*

occupations, the lack of a dose-response relation in some studies and the lack of knowledge of other risk factors for brain tumours that could be confounding variables limit our ability to reach conclusions about the risks for adult brain cancer from occupational exposure to EMF.

BREAST CANCER

Numerous studies have examined cancer in electrical occupations, with many considering breast cancer as one of the outcomes. Male breast cancer is very rare and most of the studies were based on insufficiently large populations, so estimates of risk for male breast cancer often were not included in the tables of results unless an excess risk had been observed. This limitation makes it difficult to evaluate the risk of male breast cancer. Although several reports were suggestive of a positive association, the more recent large studies of electrical workers[15-17] did not identify any excess of male breast cancer (Fig. 21.4).

Few occupational studies of electrical workers included sufficient numbers of women to address the potential association between occupational EMF exposure and female breast cancer. Although some studies supported a possible association, others did not. Exposure assessment in some of these studies was poor and may have led to a significant amount of misclassification. Because the results of these studies are inconsistent, a possible association between breast cancer and EMF exposure remains speculative. Rigorous studies

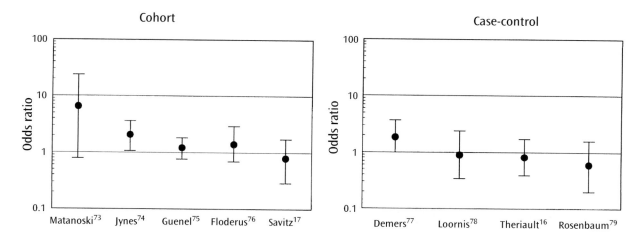

Figure 21.4 *Occupational exposure and breast cancer in men.*

examining occupational exposures and female breast cancer are yet to be done.

LUNG CANCER

Studies that have examined the possible association between electrical occupations or power-frequency magnetic field exposure and lung cancer have been largely negative. However, researchers at McGill University in Montreal and the Institut National de la Santé et de la Recherche Medicale in Paris[18] reported a positive relationship between presumed measures of high-frequency power system transient magnetic fields and incidence of lung cancer. They referred to this presumed exposure as pulsed electromagnetic fields (PEMF). Several follow-up analyses of existing data[19–21] tended not to confirm the findings. These follow-up analyses were limited in terms of exposure assessment and information on cigarette smoke, which is a potent lung carcinogen. The initial finding also suffers from several unresolved issues, particularly the fact that the exposure meter did not perform according to its intended specifications, so the actual characteristics of the detected fields are unclear. Also, although the investigators who reported the initial finding adjusted for smoking, the information on smoking, and thus the adjustment for it, is likely to have been incomplete. Further research on the occurrence of cigarette smoking in electrical occupations and better characterization of workplace PEMF exposures will help resolve this issue.

OTHER CANCER

Sporadic reports of elevated risks for other cancers, most notably malignant melanoma, have appeared in the literature, but none has been sufficiently strong or consistent to warrant further discussion here. However, cancers of the prostate, testis and pituitary gland could be of interest because of their roles in the production of hormones. Patterns of risk for these cancers in relation to jobs with exposure to magnetic fields remain largely unexplored.

ELECTRIC FIELDS

Magnetic, rather than electric, fields have been identified as the exposure of potential interest in most epidemiological studies. In addition to the plethora of well-known difficulties in measuring magnetic field exposures today and extrapolating them to workers who held similar jobs in the past, measuring electric field exposure presents unique difficulties. Electric fields are perturbed by conducting objects such as humans and their surroundings. The interaction of the subject with the field affects the reading of a field meter placed on the body. The field that is recorded by the instrument is therefore very dependent on where the device is worn, the posture of the subject, and the relative location of sources of fields. These variables make measurements of electric fields difficult to perform and interpret, often yielding relative, as opposed to absolute, values of exposure for different individuals.

Because most exposure assessments in occupational environments have focused on magnetic, rather than electric fields, little is known about the reliability and validity of electric field measurements. However, recent reanalyses[22,23] of the two cohorts of a large study of electrical workers in Canada and France[16] and of a study in Los Angeles County, USA[24] considered electric field exposure (the original focus of these studies was magnetic fields).

In the first reanalysis, Miller *et al.*[22] reported an association of all leukaemias and leukaemia subtypes (but not brain cancer) with increasing electric field exposures.

The primary effect occurred when both electric and magnetic field exposures were considered together. In contrast to these results, the second reanalysis[23] found no evidence of an increased risk of leukaemia but some evidence of an increased risk of brain tumours among utility workers exposed to electric fields. Finally, a limited reanalysis of data from Los Angeles County did not find an association between leukaemia and electric field exposures in a variety of occupations.[24]

Due to the inconsistency of results and the special difficulties in assessing electric field exposure, there is currently little research studying possible associations between electric field exposure and cancer.

SUMMARY OF EPIDEMIOLOGICAL RESEARCH

In summary, over 80 occupational studies have examined magnetic fields as a potential risk factor for a variety of cancers. A few of these studies also considered electric fields as a risk factor, and one investigated the combination of electric and magnetic fields appearing together. These studies have varied widely in the design, types of study subjects, methods of exposure assessment, outcomes considered and quality.

Among the many cancers and exposures examined, a consistent small increase in the risk of leukaemia and brain tumours in electrical workers has been noted. This finding appears to be replicated in several studies.

The likelihood of positive findings due to chance alone is difficult to evaluate. Many of the studies were not specifically designed to test the EMF hypothesis, but rather were secondary analyses of existing data collected for other purposes. Nevertheless, with many studies reporting some elevation in risk in occupational settings, chance alone seems to be an unlikely explanation for the reported associations.

Biases are undoubtedly present in many or all of the epidemiological studies. However, the magnitude and direction of biases in the studies of EMF are not well understood. These potential biases vary from study to study and over time some sources of bias have been largely eliminated, while others remain.

Electric and magnetic field exposure is an uncertain risk factor for the cancers studied, based on the small to modest elevation in risk reported in some studies, general lack of a dose-response relationship, possible uncontrolled confounding, and inconsistencies among the studies in specific cancers and exposures identified as most important.

Despite the large number of studies published, several endpoints have not been rigorously examined in a sufficient number of studies. As the methodology of studies has improved, estimates of risk have become lower, making it unlikely that a large risk is being missed. Nevertheless, a sufficient uncertainty about potential EMF involvement in cancer aetiology remains. Even a small risk associated with a ubiquitous exposure could have important public health consequences.

LABORATORY

As a whole, laboratory research does not support EMF exposure as a carcinogenic agent. Multiple studies have failed to show those cellular or tissue findings usually associated with the transformation of normal cells into neoplastic cells[25] For example, with certain rare exceptions, EMF has not been shown to be mutagenic,[26] clastogenic, or teratogenic, nor has any mechanism been established for weak to moderately strong fields.[27] There is contradictory evidence that gene expression is altered by exposure to weak magnetic fields. Several studies reported altered gene expression in the presence of weak magnetic fields,[28–30] while other, later studies, incorporating many improvements in study design, reported that no significant effect of magnetic field exposure could be detected.[31,32] Even when an effect is present it appears to be small (less than twofold enhancement).

The absence of laboratory evidence of EMF as a cancer-initiating agent has led to some speculation about and evaluation of EMF as a cancer promoter or progressor. There is some evidence that fields at relatively high levels (at or above 50 µT) can influence cell growth and signal transduction.[10] The few completed animal studies have been negative, with the possible exception of a mammary cancer study.[33,34] However, on reanalysis of a previously positive result, no association was observed.[35] Many more studies evaluating the possibility that EMF might promote or co-promote cancer are now in progress.[36]

Reproductive effects (see Chapter 40)

Reports of the effects of EMF on human reproductive outcomes are fewer than those of cancer. While there are a number of reports linking some forms of adverse reproductive outcomes to EMF exposure, more rigorous studies of residential exposure and use of electric blankets have not found an effect on reproductive outcomes such as miscarriages or intrauterine growth retardation. Among occupationally exposed populations, a variety of effects has been reported, including the following.

CONGENITAL MALFORMATIONS

There is only a single study of malformations among the offspring of males exposed to EMF. In 1983, Nordstrom et al.[37] used a written questionnaire to examine reproductive outcomes among Swedish workers employed in high-voltage switching facilities. The study reported an increase in a variety of malformations. Although no subsequent studies have been reported, a long-term prospective follow-up among Swedish utility workers is nearing completion.

Animal studies of possible teratogenic effects of EMF exposure have been conducted with electric and magnetic fields separately at several intensity levels. They have generally been negative.[38,39]

PARENTAL EXPOSURE AND BRAIN TUMOURS

Six case-control studies examined the occurrence of childhood brain tumours or neuroblastoma among the children of fathers whose work presumably exposed them to EMF.[40–45] As in most occupational studies, exposure assessment was based on job title. Elevated relative risks (above 2.0) reported in the first two studies were not confirmed in later studies (see Fig. 21.5). The predominance of positive findings in earlier reports could be due to selective reporting.

Some additional information regarding parental occupations and childhood brain tumours is provided by analyses of the childhood brain tumour studies of Feingold et al.[46] and Preston-Martin.[47] These studies further support the absence of an association.

PREGNANCY OUTCOMES AND VIDEO DISPLAY UNIT USE

The potential influence of occupational EMF exposure on reproduction has been examined among women working with video display units (VDUs). Initial concern was based on reports of several clusters of spontaneous abortions and congenital malformations among VDU operators. Subsequently, several epidemiological studies[48,49] provided very limited or no evidence of an association between VDU use and spontaneous abortion. A study by Goldhaber et al.[50] offered some evidence that extensive work with VDUs had a detrimental effect on pregnancy outcome. However, the results of this study did not show consistent increases in risk with either extent of VDU use or particular job categories. Moreover, both recall and information biases could explain the study findings. With the exception of a study by Schnorr et al.,[49] none of these investigations involved any measurements of fields produced by VDUs. The EMF exposures from VDUs in the Schnorr et al.[49] study were found to be similar to exposures encountered in the home.

Studies of congenital malformations among offspring of VDU operators have also been negative, although most of the studies were small and thus did not have the ability to detect small risks. Furthermore, laboratory studies and appropriate animal models employing VDU signals have not found adverse reproductive effects.

In summary, there is little evidence to implicate EMF exposure in adverse pregnancy outcomes. However, because of methodological problems such as the potential for omission of early miscarriages, recall bias, and the fact that the level of EMF exposure under study was not substantially different from the background level, additional studies designed to address these issues may be necessary to definitively resolve this question.

Neurobehavioural and neurodegenerative effects

A number of studies have focused on two categories of possible neurobehavioural effects in occupationally exposed populations: generalized neurasthenic effects and suicide. As a result of the early observations of Soviet scientists on depressive symptoms, several psychologists and industrial physicians conducted studies of such symptoms but found no effects.[7,8,51,52] Other investigators have examined suicide as a possible effect of EMF exposure and found no risk in an occupational cohort.[19,53]

Although the findings, to date, do not appear to provide evidence of neurobehavioural effects in humans, there is some evidence of behavioural effects in animal studies. For example, learning ability in laboratory animals exposed to EMF was impaired.[54] Furthermore, some evidence that EMF might influence the secretion of melatonin suggests that both neurobehavioural and circadian effects in occupationally exposed human populations deserve further evaluation.

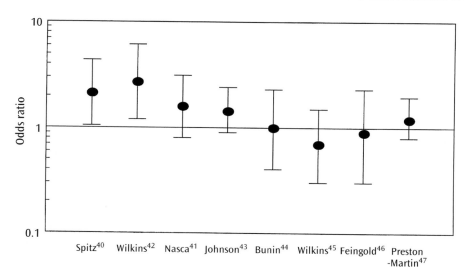

Figure 21.5 *Occupational exposure of parents, and brain cancer and neuroblastoma in children.*

Recently, a series of papers reported positive associations between occupations with presumed magnetic field exposure and Alzheimer's disease[55,56] and amyotrophic lateral sclerosis.[57] These investigators also suggested biological pathways that might be responsible for the associations.[57,58]

Additional support for the hypothesis that exposure to power-frequency magnetic fields is related to Alzheimer's disease and amyotrophic lateral sclerosis, but not to Parkinson's disease, was provided by Savitz *et al.*[59] The prior studies by Sobel *et al.*[55,56] reported that seamstresses and tailors had the highest risks, while Savitz *et al.*[59] focused on electric utility employees. Other investigators have reported possible associations between neurodegenerative illness and electric shock or work in electrical occupations.[60–62] Further research which includes better exposure assessment, more rigorous disease diagnosis and potential confounding due to electric shock and adjustment for occupational exposures to solvents should be considered.

MAGNETIC RESONANCE IMAGING

Magnetic resonance imaging devices are now widely used in clinical medicine (see Chapter 30). These imaging devices produce a time-varying magnetic field, a static field and radiofrequency fields. While the patient is exposed to all of these fields, technicians and other occupational personnel are exposed mostly to the static fields. Typical field strengths very close to the machine may be as high as 10 mT. Fields decrease to 1 mT at 3 metres from the machine where a technician may stand for a few minutes. Farther away at the operating console the technician is exposed to considerably lower field levels. From the available scientific data and the magnitude of measured fields, it is unlikely that the health of operators is affected by their exposure to these magnetic fields.[3,63] There are some contraindications for using MRI for individuals who have special implants or pacemakers,[64] or who have had operations involving metal aneurysm clips or metal sutures. In addition, caution is indicated for infants and for patients who are pregnant. Similar considerations apply to applicants seeking work as operators or researchers in magnetic fields.

In recent years, several national and international organizations have formulated guidelines to limit worker exposures to EMF. Among these are the International Radiation Protection Association/International Commission on Non-Ionizing Radiation Protection,[65] the American Conference of Governmental Industrial Hygienists,[66] the Comité Européen de Normalization Eléctrotechnique,[67] the National Radiological Protection Board in the United Kingdom,[68] and the Deutsches Institut für Normung-Verband Deutscher Elektrotechniker.[69] The rationale for all the guidelines is prevention of electrical stimulation by induced currents of electrically sensitive tissues in critical sites, for example, the heart and nervous system. None of the guidelines consider potential long-term effects, such as cancer.

All guidelines specify an induced current density of 10 milliamperes per square meter (mA/m^2) as the dose to tissue that should not be exceeded. Clear hazards are posed by exposures above $1000 mA/m^2$, which are estimated to be sufficient to disturb rhythmic cardiac function, such as extrasystole and ventricular fibrillation. There are few supporting data of possible adverse health effects at levels of induced current density between 100 and $1000 mA/m^2$.

The various guidelines are based on different biophysical models that employ different assumptions to estimate the relationship between external magnetic fields and induced currents.[70] Consequently, the models yield somewhat different magnetic field exposure limits (Table 21.1). The values given are for whole-body exposures. Several of the guidelines allow for 5 to 20 times higher exposure limits for limbs.[71]

CONCLUSIONS

A large body of epidemiological literature suggests an association between work in electrical occupations and cancer, particularly leukaemia and brain cancer. Nevertheless, there remains considerable uncertainty about the meaning of these associations because of the inadequate quality of exposure assessment, small elevations in risk, general lack of a dose-response relationship, possible uncontrolled confounding, and inconsistencies among the studies in specific cancers and exposures identified as the most important.

In addition, the laboratory evidence of a relationship is largely negative, although more research is underway. The data that are available do not meet the criteria of known carcinogenic agents; that is EMF does not function as either a mutagen or a complete carcinogen.

These conclusions are supported by those of the Report of an Advisory Group of the National Radiological Protection Board: *Electromagnetic Fields and Cancer*, chaired by Sir Richard Doll.[72] Excerpts of the conclusions of that committee are:

> In summary, the epidemiological findings that have been reviewed provide no firm evidence of a carcinogenic hazard from exposure of paternal gonads, the fetus, or adults to the extremely low frequency electromagnetic fields that might be associated with . . . work in the electrical, electronic, and telecommunications industries. . . . the findings to date can be regarded only as sufficient to justify formulating a hypothesis for testing by further investigation.

Table 21.1 *Occupational exposure guidelines for 60–Hz magnetic fields*

Organization	Exposure duration	Guideline exposure limit (mT)	External field to produce 10 mA/m² (mT)
ACGIH	Ceiling value	1	0.69
CENELEC	Work-day	1.3	1.3
DIN/VDE-89	Work-day	4.6	3.5
	Short-term (5min/h)	6.9	3.5
DIN/VDE-95	Work-day	1.1	3.5
	Short-term (2h/day)	2.1	3.5
Short-term	3.5 (1h/day)	3.5	
ICNIRP	Work-day	0.42	2.0
NRPB	Work-day	1.3	1.3

ACGIH: American Conference of Governmental Industrial Hygienists;
CENELEC: Comité Européen de Normalization Elécrotechnique;
DIN/VDE: Deutsches Institut Für Normung-Verband Deutscher Elektrotechniker

While the focus of another group, the National Academy of Science,[10] was on residential exposure, their general conclusions are relevant to our discussion. Their conclusions are:

> Based on a comprehensive evaluation of published studies relating to the effects of power-frequency electric and magnetic fields on cells, tissues, and organisms (including humans), the conclusion of the committee is that the current body of evidence does not show that exposure to these fields presents a human-health hazard.

Electricity use has spread throughout the industrialized world since the first public power station began operation. Today the developing nations look to electricity as a means of providing jobs and improving lifestyle. Yet concern over adverse health effects from electric and magnetic fields and from electric power delivery and use has risen since the 1960s. Much has been learned from the many years of research on EMF and the many studies that have been published to date. It is clear that EMF do not pose a large public health or occupational hazard. The widespread use of electricity justifies research designed to resolve the remaining uncertainties.

REFERENCES

1 Baker SP, O'Neill B, Karpf RS. *The Injury Fact Book*. Lexington, MA: DC Heath & Co, 1984: 149.

2 Nordenson I, Hansson-Mild K, Nordstrom S *et al*. Clastogenic effects in human lymphocytes of power frequency electric fields: *in vivo* and *in vitro* studies. *Radiat Environ Biophys* 1984; **23**: 191–201.

3 World Health Organization. *Magnetic Fields*. Environmental Health Criteria 69. UN Environmental Programme, International Labour Organization. Geneva: WHO, 1987.

4 Silny J. The influence threshold of the time varying magnetic field in the human organism. In: Bernhardt JH ed. *Biological Effects of Static and Extremely Low Frequency Magnetic Fields*. Munich: MMV Medizin-Verlag, 1986: 105–12.

5 Asanova TP, Rakov AI. *The State of Health of Persons Working in the Electric Field of Outdoor 400 and 500 kV Switchyards. Study in the USSR of medical effects of electric fields on electric power systems*. 78 CH01020-7-PWR. New York: The Institute of Electrical and Electronics Engineers, 1978. [*Gig Tr Prof Zabol* **10**: 50–2 (in Russian)].

6 Stopps GJ, Janischewskyj W. *Epidemiologic Study of Workers Maintaining HV Equipment and Transmission Lines in Ontario*. Montreal: Canadian Electrical Association, 1979: 123 pages.

7 Broadbent DE, Broadbent MPH, Male JC, Jones MRL. Health of workers exposed to electric fields. *Br J Ind Med* 1985; **42**: 75–84. [Correction in *Br J Ind Med* 1985; **42**: 357.]

8 Graham C, Cook MR, Cohen HD. *Immunological and Biochemical Effects of 60 Hz Electric and Magnetic fields in Humans*. Kansas City, MO: Midwest Research Institute. DOE-FC01-84-CE76246; 30 Jan 1990. Prepared for the US Dept of Energy, Office of Energy Storage and Distribution. Available from NTIS; Order No. DE90006671.

9 Wertheimer N, Leeper E. Electrical wiring configurations and childhood cancer. *Am J Epidemiol* 1979; **109**: 273–84.

10 National Academy of Science. *Possible Health Effects of Exposure to Residential Electric and Magnetic Fields*. Washington DC: National Research Council, National Academy Press, 1996.

11 Kheifets LI, Kavet R, Sussman SS. Wire codes, magnetic fields, and childhood cancer. *Bioelectromagnetics* 1997; **18**: 99–110.

12 Kheifets LI, Afifi AA, Buffler PA, Zhang ZW. Occupational

electric and magnetic field exposure and brain cancer: a meta-analysis. *J Occup Environ Med* 1995; **35**: 1327–41.

13 Kheifets LI, Afifi AA, Buffler PA, Zhang ZW, Matkin CC. Occupational electric and magnetic field exposure and leukemia: a meta-analysis. *J Occup Environ Med* 1997; **39**: 1074–91.

14 Lin JC. Health effects of radiofrequency radiation from wireless communication technology. In: *Advances in Electromagnetic Fields in Living Systems* Vol 2. New York: Plenum Press, 1997: 129–44.

15 Sahl JD, Kelsh MA *et al.* Cohort and nested case-control studies of hematopoietic cancers and brain cancer among electric utility workers. *Epidemiology* 1993; **4**: 104–14.

16 Theriault G, Goldberg M *et al.* Cancer risks associated with occupational exposure to magnetic fields among electric utility workers in Ontario and Quebec, Canada, and France: 1970–1989. *Am J Epidemiol* 1994; **139**: 550–72.

17 Savitz DA, Loomis DP. Magnetic field exposure in relation to leukemia and brain cancer mortality among electric utility workers. *Am J Epidemiol* 1995; **141**: 123–134.

18 Armstrong B, Theriault G, Guenel P, Deadman J, Goldberg M, Heroux P. Association between exposure to pulsed electromagnetic fields and cancer in electric utility workers in Quebec, Canada, and France. *Am J Epidemiol* 1994; **140**: 805–20.

19 Baris D, Armstrong BG, Deadman J, Theriault G. A mortality study of electrical utility workers in Quebec. *Occup Environ Med* 1996; **53**: 25–31.

20 Kelsh MA, Sahl JD. Mortality among a cohort of electric utility workers, 1960–1991. *Am J Ind Med* 1997; **31**: 534–44.

21 Savitz DA, Dufort V, Armstrong B, Theriault G. Lung cancer in relation to employment in the electrical utility industry and exposure to magnetic fields. *Occup Environ Med* 1997; **54**: 396–402.

22 Miller AB, To T, Agnew DA, Wall C, Green LM. Leukemia following occupational exposure to 60-Hz electric and magnetic fields among Ontario electric utility workers. *Am J Epidemiol* 1996; **144**: 150–60.

23 Guenel P, Nicolau J, Imbernon E, Chevalier A, Goldberg M. Exposure to 50-Hz electric field and incidence of leukemia, brain tumors and other cancers among French electric utility workers. *Am J Epidemiol* 1996; **144**: 1107–21.

24 Kheifets LI, London SJ, Peters JM. Leukemia risk and occupational electric field exposure in Los Angeles County. *Am J Epidemiol* 1997; **146**: 1–4.

25 Kavet R. EMF and current cancer concepts. *Bioelectromagnetics* 1996; **17**: 339–57.

26 Valberg PA, Kavet R, Rafferty CN. Can low-level 50/60-Hz electric and magnetic fields cause biological effects? *Radiat Res* 1999; **148**: 2–21.

27 McCann J, Dietrich F, Rafferty C, martin AO. A critical review of the genotoxic potential of electric and magnetic fields. *Mutat Res* 1993; **297**: 61–95.

28 Goodman R, Shirley-Henderson A. Transcription and translation in cells exposed to extremely low frequency electromagnetic fields. *Bioelectrochem Bioenerg* 1991; **25**: 335–55.

29 Blank M, Soo L, Lin H, Goodman R. Stimulation of transcription in HL-60 cells by alternating currents from electric fields. In: Blank M ed. *Electricity and Magnetism in Biology and Medicine* (*Review and Research Papers Presented at the First World Congress for Electricity and Magnetism in Biology in Medicine*), San Francisco, CA: San Francisco Press, 1993: 516–19.

30 Lin H, Goodman R, Shirley-Henderson A. Specific region of the *c-myc* promoter is responsive to electric and magnetic fields. *J Cell Biochem* 1994; **54**: 281–88.

31 Saffer JD, Thurston SJ. Short exposures to 60 Hz magnetic fields do not alter *myc* expression in HL60 or Daudi cells. *Radiat Res* 1995; **144**: 18–25.

32 Lacy-Hulbert A, Wilkins RC, Hesketh TR, Metcalfe JC. No effect of 60-Hz electromagnetic fields on *myc* or beta-actin in human leukemic cells. *Radiat Res* 1995; **144**: 9–17.

33 Beniashvili DS, Bilanishvili VG, Menabde MZ. Low-frequency electromagnetic radiation enhances the induction of rat mammary tumors by nitrosomethyl urea. *Cancer Lett* 1991; **61**: 75–9.

34 Loscher W, Mevissen M, Lehmacher W, Stamm A. Tumor promotion in a breast cancer model by exposure to a weak alternating magnetic field. *Cancer Lett* 1993; **71**: 75–81.

35 Mevissen M, Stamm A, Buntenkotter S, Zwingelberg R, Wahnschaffe U, Loscher W. Effects of magnetic fields on mammary tumor development induced by 7,12-dimethylbenz[a]anthracene in rats. *Bioelectromagnetics* 1993; **14**: 131–43.

36 McCann J, Kavet R, Rafferty CN. Testing electromagnetic fields for potential carcinogenic activity: a critical review of animal models. *Environ Hlth Perspect* 1997; **105**: 81–103.

37 Nordstrom SB, Birke E, Gustavsson L. Reproductive hazards among workers at high voltage substations. *Bioelectromagnetics* 1983; **4**: 91–101.

38 Chernoff N, Rogers JM, Kavet R. A review of the literature on potential reproductive and developmental toxicity of electric and magnetic fields. *Toxicology* 1992; **74**: 91–126.

39 Rommereim DN, Rommereim RL, Miller DL, Buschbom RL, Anderson LE. Developmental toxicology evaluation of 60-Hz horizontal magnetic fields in rats. *Appl Occup Environ Hyg* 1996; **11**: 307–12.

40 Spitz MR, Johnson CC. Neuroblastoma and paternal occupation, a case-control analysis. *Am J Epidemiol* 1985; **121**: 924–9.

41 Nasca P, Baptiste M, MacCubbin P *et al.* An epidemiologic case-control study of central nervous system tumors in children and parental occupational exposures. *Am J Epidemiol* 1988; **128**: 1256–65.

42 Wilkins JR, Koutras RA. Paternal occupation and brain cancer in offspring: a mortality-based case-control study. *Am J Ind Med* 1988; **14**: 299–318.

43 Johnson C, Spitz M. Childhood nervous system tumors: an assessment of risk associated with paternal occupations involving use, repair or manufacture of electrical and electronic equipment. *Int J Epidemiol* 1989; **18**: 756–62.

44 Bunin GR, Ward E, Kramer S, Rhee CA, Meadows AT.

Neuroblastoma and parental occupation. *Am J Epidemiol* 1990; **131**: 776–80.

45 Wilkins JR, Hundley VD. Paternal occupational exposure to electromagnetic fields and neuroblastoma in offspring. *Am J Epidemiol* 1990; **131**: 995–1007.

46 Feingold L, Savitz DA *et al*. Use of a job-exposure matrix to evaluate parental occupation and childhood cancer. *Cancer Causes Control* 1991; **3**: 161–9.

47 Preston-Martin S, Navidi W, Thomas D, Lee PJ *et al*. Los Angeles study of residential magnetic fields and childhood brain tumors. *Am J Epidemiol* 1996; **143**: 105–19.

48 Windham GC, Fenster L, Swan SH, Neutra RR. Use of video display terminals and the risk of spontaneous abortion. *Am J Ind Med* 1990; **18**: 675–88.

49 Schnorr TM, Grajewski BA, Hornung RW *et al*. Video display terminals and the risk of spontaneous abortion. *N Engl J Med* 1991; **324**: 727–33.

50 Goldhaber MK, Polen MR, Hiatt RA. The risk of miscarriage and birth defects among women who use visual display terminals during pregnancy. *Am J Ind Med* 1988; **13**: 695–706.

51 Knave B, Gamberale F, Bergstrom S *et al*. A cross-sectional epidemiologic investigation of occupationally exposed workers in high-voltage substations. *Scand J Work Environ Hlth* 1979; **5**: 115–25.

52 Baroncelli P, Battisti S, Chuccucci A *et al*. A health examination of railway high-voltage substation workers exposed to ELF electromagnetic fields. *Am J Ind Med* 1986; **10**: 45–55.

53 Baris D, Armstrong B. Suicide among electric utility workers in England and Wales (letter). *Br J Ind Med* 1990; **47**: 788–9.

54 Salzinger K, Frelmark S, McCullough M, Phillips D, Birenbaum L. Altered operant behavior of adult rats after perinatal exposure to a 60-Hz electromagnetic field. *Bioelectromagnetics* 1990; **11**: 105–16.

55 Sobel E, Davanipour Z, Sulkava R, Erkinjuntti T, Wikstrom J *et al*. Occupations with exposure to electromagnetic fields: a possible risk factor for Alzheimer's disease. *Am J Epidemiol* 1995; **142**: 515–24.

56 Sobel E, Dunn M, Davanipour Z, Qian Z, Chui HC Elevated risk of Alzheimer's disease among workers with likely electromagnetic field exposure. *Neurology* 1996; **47**: 1477–81.

57 Davanipour Z, Sobel E, Bowman JD, Qian Z, Will AD. Amyotrophic lateral sclerosis and occupational exposure to electromagnetic fields. *Bioelectromagnetics* 1997; **18**: 28–35.

58 Sobel E, Davanpour Z. Electromagnetic field exposure may cause increased production of amyloid beta and eventually lead to Alzheimer's disease. *Neurology* 1996; **47**: 1594–1600.

59 Savitz DA, Checkoway H, Loomis DP. Magnetic field exposure and neurodegenerative disease mortality among electric utility workers. *Epidemiology* 1998; **9**: 398–404.

60 Deapen DM, Henderson BE (1986): A case-control study of amyotrophic lateral sclerosis. *Am J Epidemiol* **123**: 790–9.

61 Schulte PA, Burnett CA, Boeniger MF. Neurodegenerative diseases: occupational occurrence and potential risk factors, 1982 through 1991. *Am J Publ Hlth* 1996; **86**: 1281–88.

62 Feychting M, Pedersen NL, Svedberg P, Floderus B, Gatz M. Dementia and occupational exposure to magnetic fields. *Scand J Work Environ Hlth* 1998; **24**: 46–53.

63 Stuchly MA, Lecuyer DW. Survey of static magnetic fields around magnetic resonance imaging devices. *Health Phys* 1987; **53**: 321–4.

64 National Institutes of Health. *Magnetic Resonance Imaging*. Consensus Statement Online, 26–28 Oct 1987; **6**: 1–31.

65 International Radiation Protection Association/International Commission on Non-Ionizing Radiation Protection. Guidelines on Limits of Exposure to Static Magnetic Fields. *Hlth Phys* 1994; **66**: 101–6.

66 American Conference of Governmental Industrial Hygienists. *TLVs and BEIs: Threshold Limit Values for Chemical Substances and Physical Agents, Biological Exposure Indices*. Cincinnati, OH: ACGIH, 1996.

67 Comité Européen de Normalisation Electrotechnique. *Human Exposure to Electromagnetic Fields, High Frequency (10 kH₃ to 300 GH₃)*. CENELEC Standard ENV 50166–2, Jan 1995, Brussels: CENELEC.

68 National Radiological Protection Board. *Restrictions on Human Exposure to Static and Time Varying Electromagnetic Fields and Radiation: Scientific Basis and Recommendation for Implementation of the Board's Statement*. Documents of the NRPB. 1993; **4**: 8–69.

69 Deutsches Institut fur Normung-Verband Deutscher Electrotechniker. *Safety in Electromagnetic Fields: Protecting People in the Frequency Range from 0 to 30 kHz*. Provisional Standard, DIN/VDE. Vol. 0848–4 A/3, 1995.

70 Bracken JD, Bailey WH, Su SH, Senior RS, Rankin RJ. *Evaluation of Occupational Magnetic-Field Exposure Guidelines*. EPRI TR-108113. Palo Alto, CA: Electric Power Research Institue, 1997.

71 International Commission on Non-Ionizing Radiation Protection. Guidelines for limiting exposure to time-varying electric, magnetic, and electromagnetic fields (up to 300 Ghz). *Hlth Phys* 1998; **74**: 494–522.

72 National Radiological Protection Board. *Electromagnetic Fields and the Risk of Cancer*. Report of an advisory group on non-ionizing radiation. London: HMSO, 1992; **3**: No. 1.

73 Matanoski G, Elliott E, Breyesse P. Electromagnetic field exposure and male breast cancer. *Lancet* 1991; **337**: 737.

74 Jynes J, Andersen A, Langmark F. Incidence of cancer in Norwegian workers potentially exposed to electromagnetic fields. *Am J Epidemiol* 1992; **136**: 81–8.

75 Guenel P, Radmark P, Andersen JB, Lynge E. Incidence of cancer in persons with occupational exposure to electromagnetic fields in Denmark. *Br J Ind Med* 1993; **50**: 758–64.

76 Floderus B, Jorngvist S, Stenlund C. Incidence of selected cancer in Swedish railway workers 1961–79. *Cancer Causes Control* 1994; **5**: 189–94.

77 Demers PA, Thomas DB, Rosenblatt KA *et al*. Occupational

exposure to electromagnetic fields and breast cancer in men. *Am J Epidemiol* 1991; **134**: 340–70.

78 Loornis DP. Cancer of breast among men in electrical occupations (letter). *Lancet* 1992; **339**: 1482–3.

79 Rosenbaum PJ, Vena JE, Zielezny MA, Michalek AM. Occupational exposure associated with male breast cancer. *Am J Epidemiol* 1994; **139**: 30–36.

Part **4**

Diseases related to ergonomic and mechanical factors

Repeated movements and repeated trauma affecting
  the musculoskeletal system   453
Back pain and work   477

Repeated movements and repeated trauma affecting the musculoskeletal system

KEITH PALMER, CYRUS COOPER

Shoulder problems	454	Osteoarthritis	464
Neck problems	456	Risk factors for work-related musculoskeletal disorders	467
Elbow problems	457	Identifying work-related musculoskeletal disorders	470
Tenosynovitis and peritendinitis	459	Preventing and managing work-related musculoskeletal	
Carpal tunnel syndrome	460	disorders	471
Chronic upper limb pain	461	Conclusions	472
Dupuytren's contracture	463	References	472
Other soft tissue rheumatic conditions	464		

Work-related musculoskeletal disorders are considered an important source of occupational morbidity. Estimates of the size of the problem and its human and economic costs vary, depending on case definition and the source of the statistics. However, it is believed to represent the largest category of work-related illness in Britain today. Data from the labour force survey of self-reported illness[1] suggest that nearly 900 000 Britons believe their musculoskeletal problems to have been caused or made worse by work: 74 000 of these complaints related to non-specific forearm pain.

Work-related musculoskeletal disorders comprise a heterogeneous group of disorders – some well defined, some ill-defined, whose natural history is for the most part poorly characterized. In some cases the debate concerns whether a recognized clinical entity is actually being described at all; in others it is the epithet 'work-related' that is contentious.[2]

Physicians are most likely to be concerned with the following questions:

1 Which upper limb and neck conditions may be caused or aggravated by work, and which conditions make work difficult to perform?
2 How can such cases be identified clinically, and how should they be managed?
3 Who is most at risk? And how can the risk be assessed?
4 What can be done to prevent such problems, and how effective is the intervention likely to be?

Information exists on some of these questions, and this chapter will attempt a synthesis of the available information. However, it will help the reader in interpreting this information to possess some overview of the areas of difficulty and controversy.

The apparently simple question: 'Which musculoskeletal problems are known to be work-related?' has proved surprisingly difficult to answer. It is necessary first to state the problem more precisely, for example, to distinguish between exposures that *cause* a condition, and those that *aggravate* or accelerate it; and to identify unambiguously the end-points of interest (discomfort or disability? accepted rheumatological and orthopaedic conditions or ill-defined regional pain disorders?). In assessing the individual complainant the clinician would then need to consider several issues that bear on the likelihood of injury or complaint:

- the background level of the disorder and its natural history in unexposed populations (how unusual is its presentation?);
- factors personal to the worker (such as age, sex, the individual's anthropometrics and physical strength, medical history, mental health and threshold for complaint);
- factors particular to the working environment (e.g. job tasks and ergonomic stressors, workplace psychosocial conditions);
- factors arising outside work (such as sport, housework and home craft activities).

The clinician might turn to the epidemiologist for further guidance, and would then find that these issues have been studied, to greater or lesser extent, but that knowledge is incomplete and that its interpretation would be carefully qualified. For example, in general terms, there are data on the prevalence and incidence of complaints in the community, and how these vary by age and sex,[3–6] many studies describe associations between job title and musculoskeletal complaint,[7] and many others report a link in working groups between mental well-being and upper limb complaint.[8] But the epidemiologist would point out that most surveys of work-related musculoskeletal disorders have been cross-sectional in design, and may therefore have suffered from the problem of selection bias (for example, those worst affected may have selected themselves out of employment and escaped observation, leading to an underestimate of the problem); also that this study design does not permit the time sequence of events to be observed and makes it harder to separate cause from effect. (For example, does the association between poor mental well-being and upper limb symptoms stem from a causal relationship, or do anxious and depressed workers simply complain more often than others about their aches and pains?) The epidemiologist would also point out that some studies are of pain reports rather than specific diagnoses, and that cross-comparison is hindered because diagnostic criteria have varied or been ill-defined; and he would say that it has proved difficult to grade the complex biomechanical workplace exposures that combine elements of force, frequency, repetition and movement and then vary them so thoroughly, so that in assessing causality there is scant information on dose-response relationships. The net result is that doctors entertain different views on the relationship between work and particular symptom patterns presenting to them.

Two broad groups of musculoskeletal disorders that may be related to work will be considered in this chapter: neck/upper limb pain (Table 22.1) and osteoarthritis. We describe for each principal disorder in turn, its epidemiology, the evidence for its apparent association with work, its clinical presentation and its management. Later in the chapter we consider aspects of detection and prevention.

SHOULDER PROBLEMS

The glenohumeral joint has a greater range of movement than any other joint, and this is permitted at the expense of stability. The glenoid fossa is shallow, the capsule is lax and there are no strong traversing ligaments. Stability therefore mainly depends on the muscles and tendons of the rotator cuff (supraspinatus, infraspinatus, teres minor and subscapularis), while the deltoid muscle provides a further mechanical support. The joint is pro-

Table 22.1 *Upper limb and neck conditions that may be work-related*[a]

Shoulder
Shoulder tendinitis
Rotator cuff tendinitis
Bicipital tendinitis
Shoulder capsulitis (frozen shoulder)

Neck
Cervical spondylosis
Thoracic outlet syndrome
Tension neck syndrome

Elbow
Lateral epicondylitis
Medial epicondylitis

Wrist and forearms
Tenosynovitis of the wrist
De Quervain's disease of the wrist
Carpal tunnel syndrome
Non-specific diffuse forearm pain

[a]Some authorities include ganglia, Dupuytren's contracture and trigger finger within the definition.

tected superiorly by an arch formed by the coracoid process, the acromion and the coracoacromial ligament.

Epidemiology

Fraying and tearing of the rotator cuff tendons, thickening of the bursae and proliferative changes of the synovium are common age-related phenomena. They are often asymptomatic in life, but may be discovered at post-mortem. However, shoulder pain is also fairly common in community prevalence surveys. Bergenudd *et al.*[5] reported that 14% of middle-aged men and women in a sample from Malmo, Sweden, had experienced shoulder pain lasting a day or more in the preceding month, and 3% had taken sick leave because of it in the preceding year. A study of 15 268 Stockholm residents reported a point prevalence of shoulder pain of 20% in subjects aged 40–74,[9] and Dimberg found that 13.1% of workers in an aeroengineering factory had current shoulder pain.[4] Complaints become more common with age, although the Stockholm data suggest a peak around ages 55–60.[9] In the younger age group there appears to be little difference in prevalence between the sexes, but in their 50s and thereafter men complain more commonly.[9]

Data on incidence derive principally from the National Morbidity Surveys in General Practice in England and Wales, a general practice based surveillance system which collects details of consultations in participating practices over a 1-year period. The 1981 survey indicated an annual incidence for all shoulder syndromes of 6.6 per 1000 practice-registered patients.[10] In the Stockholm survey, a subset of the cross-sectional respondents were interviewed and examined a year on, also providing incidence data: around 1–2.5% had developed a painful shoulder, which included clinically verified restricted movement.[9] The peak annual incidence rate occurred in the fifth decade and there was little difference between the sexes.

Occupational studies

Injury appears to arise because of regular impingement of a relatively hypovascular area of the cuff against the acromioclavicular arch, an event that may be aggravated functionally through superior migration of the humeral head in abduction and elevation, or by an acromial spur or degenerative acromioclavicular joint. Studies of blood flow in the supraspinatus muscle[11,12] and muscle fatigue[13] confirm the importance of postural risk factors in the development of shoulder disorders. Occupational studies have therefore concentrated on working groups who elevate the shoulder repeatedly or for sustained periods at work, such as crop production workers, assembly line and production workers.

Table 22.2 summarizes some of the findings. Although the risk estimates vary, most reports have concluded that there is good evidence of an association between overhead work and shoulder problems. It should be noted that these studies have mainly investigated the occurrence of rotator cuff tendinitis, (defined operationally as localized shoulder pain and tenderness over the humeral head[14]); the relation of other shoulder problems to work activity has not been examined in detail, although they may arise, co-exist, or become confused with tendinitis, and may certainly contribute to work incapacity when they occur. For this reason they are separately described below.

Clinical aspects

ROTATOR CUFF TENDINITIS

Rotator cuff tendinitis (most commonly an inflammation of the supraspinatus tendon) tends to have an insidious onset, causing a dull shoulder aching or discomfort in the absence of a trauma history. Nocturnal pain is a prominent feature. Pain is felt over the deltoid region, and difficulty is encountered in reaching up, in dressing and in overhead work.

On examination, there may be tenderness over the humeral head and greater tuberosity, and the diagnosis is confirmed by reproducing the pain in resisted movement of the affected tendon. Supraspinatus tendinitis causes discomfort on abduction with a painful arc occurring between 70 and 120° abduction.

Chronic rotator cuff tears are often found at autopsy,[21,22] and in life these tend to be associated with falls on the outstretched hand, as well as overuse, and are noteworthy clinically because of weakness and muscle wasting, and because of the inability to maintain abduction (a positive 'drop-off' sign).

Plain radiographs show evidence of calcification in the rotator cuff tendons in 8% of the asymptomatic population over the age of 30,[23] and sometimes cystic and sclerotic changes at the greater tuberosity insertion. Ultrasound and magnetic resonance imaging may be used to demonstrate rotator cuff tears, while arthrography will demonstrate full thickness tears.

CALCIFIC TENDINITIS

Calcific tendinitis often arises against a background of chronic shoulder pain on movement, and arises at the

Table 22.2 *Occupational studies of shoulder tendinitis*

Cases	Controls	Study Design	Relative Risk[a]	Source
Male shipyard workers and plate workers	Office workers	C	11–13	Herberts *et al.* (1984)[15]
Female packers	Female shop assistants	C	2.6	Luopajarvi *et al.* (1979)[16]
Male and female packers	Knitters	C	2.2	McCormack *et al.* (1990)[3]
Sewers	Knitters	C	2.4	
Board manufacturers	Knitters	C	2.1	
Garment workers	Health service workers	C	2.2	Punnett *et al.* (1985)[17]
Assembly workers	General population	C	3.4	Ohlsson *et al.* (1989)[18]
Female data entry workers	Other female office workers	C	0.54	Kuorinka *et al.* (1979)[19]
Male industrial workers with shoulder tendinitis	Age and workshop matched non-cases	CC	11[a]	Bjelle *et al.* (1979)[20]

[a] Relative risk for work with hands at or above shoulder level.
C: cross-sectional study. CC: case-control study.

site of rotator cuff injury and calcification; but it has a clinical pattern distinctive enough to be separately described. Pain is severe, localized to the deltoid area and quite abrupt in onset. Passive and active shoulder movements are greatly limited by pain and there is extreme tenderness over the humeral head. Radiographs reveal well-defined or fluffy calcium deposits in the affected tendon (usually the supraspinatus). The erythrocyte sedimentation rate and white cell count are normal. Acute calcific tendinitis is a self-limiting process, lasting 1–2 weeks. Sometimes it occurs spontaneously and not in apparent relation to injury.

BICIPITAL TENDINITIS

The long head of the biceps tendon tends to become inflamed as part of a more generalized shoulder problem (such as rotator cuff or adhesive capsulitis), rather than in primary overuse; however, it has occurred following weight lifting and may well arise occupationally from prolonged repetitive carrying.

Pain occurs over the anterior shoulder, radiates into the biceps and is felt in overhead work and in shoulder extension, abduction and rotation. Tenderness is usually found over the tendon as it passes through the bicipital groove. In Yergason's test[24] pain is provoked over the anterior inner shoulder in resisted active supination of the forearm with the elbow bent at 90 degrees.

SHOULDER CAPSULITIS (FROZEN SHOULDER)

The primary form of this condition is characterized by global restriction of glenohumeral movement in all planes in the absence of significant underlying joint disease. It is believed to affect 2–3% of the population[25] and onset nearly always occurs after the age of 40. Classically there are three phases in the natural history of the condition, each lasting several months: a painful shoulder (phase 1) becomes painful and stiff (phase 2), and then profoundly stiff with slow natural resolution (phase 3). A minority of patients (7–15%) have persistent functional difficulties afterwards.[26,27]

The onset is insidious, with pain in the deltoid area increasing gradually until sleep is disturbed. In the adhesive phase there is equal restriction of active and passive glenohumeral movement in a capsular pattern (external rotation more than abduction more than internal rotation). The aetiology of the condition is poorly understood and a particular relation with work has not been demonstrated thus far.

Management

The treatment of rotator cuff tendinitis is often difficult. Rest and modification of aggravating activities are necessary to prevent the problem becoming chronic. Initial treatment should be directed at reducing inflammation by means of physical therapy (for example ultrasound) and a non-steroid anti-inflammatory agent. If symptoms fail to settle within 3 weeks, a subacromial injection of corticosteroid is useful. Once pain has eased and normal shoulder movements have been restored, a muscle-strengthening exercise programme should be instituted, concentrating on rotator cuff exercises. Failure to respond to a conservative programme within a year or so is a reasonable indication for surgical repair of the rotator cuff and release of acromial impingement.

Many therapies have been tried to modify the natural history of adhesive capsulitis of the shoulder joint. The mainstay of treatment remains intra-articular corticosteroid injection during the early phase when pain is the most prominent clinical complaint. During the phase of movement restriction without pain, it has been difficult to demonstrate the efficacy of any modality of treatment (including injection therapy, physiotherapy and anti-inflammatory drugs). Carefully directed corticosteroid injections also comprise the mainstay of treatment for a number of other shoulder problems, including acromio-clavicular joint dysfunction, bicipital tendinitis and subacromial bursitis.

NECK PROBLEMS

Epidemiology

Neck pain is a common complaint. Prevalence rates of 9.5–13.5% have been reported in Finland:[6] while in the United Kingdom, Lawrence found that the point prevalence of neck–shoulder–brachial pain was 9% in men and 12% in women.[28] Westerling and Jonsson found an 18% prevalence in 2500 randomly selected adults.[29] The age-specific prevalence rate appears to rise until the sixth and seventh decades of life, and in Holt's survey[30] of working age men, recurrent neck stiffness occurred in a quarter of those under 30 and half of those over the age of 45.

Occupational studies

Neck complaints do appear to show an association with occupation, with lower incidence rates in office workers than in manual workers.[31] Four categories of neck problem have been particularly considered in surveys: cervical spondylosis, cervical syndrome, tension neck syndrome and thoracic outlet syndrome.

CERVICAL SPONDYLOSIS

This condition is characterized by degenerative changes in the intervertebral discs (particularly of the lower cervical spine) with the development of osteophytes and spurs. These changes are commonly accompanied by osteoarthritic change in the facet and neurocentral joints. The diagnosis of cervical spondylosis is often made on clinical grounds but can be made with certainty only by the finding of typical changes on radiographs of the cervical spine. Cervical spondylosis is common from middle adult life and onwards, so that by the age of 65 years nearly everyone (90%) will show radiographic evidence of the disease, irrespective of their occupational history. Some patients complain of stiffness, creaking and pain in the neck (which sometimes radiates to the occiput, shoulders and arms and is made worse by movement of the cervical spine), but many with similar radiographic evidence of disease do not. This lack of consistency between the symptoms and radiographic signs of cervical spondylosis can cause diagnostic difficulty. Some patients with no neurological symptoms but clear radiographic evidence of cervical spondylosis can, nonetheless be shown to have abnormal neurological signs arising from causally related disturbances of the spinal nerve roots or the spinal cord. For these various reasons surveys aimed at defining the extent and clinical significance of cervical spondylosis in different populations must be of limited value when based simply on the radiographic appearances of the cervical spine and (or) symptom questionnaires. Radiographically verified cervical spondylosis has been found to occur significantly more commonly in meat carriers, dentists and miners than other groups.[14]

CERVICAL SYNDROME

Cervical syndrome is said to be present when pain in the neck coincides with symptom radiation along the distribution of a spinal nerve root. Some authorities also require limitation of neck movement and pain provoked by test manoeuvres before making the diagnosis. Although separately defined, this syndrome most probably arises from nerve root entrapment secondary to degenerative changes in the cervical spine. There have been relatively few studies of cervical syndrome in the occupational setting, and no compelling evidence of work-related risk.

TENSION NECK SYNDROME

This condition is reported in Scandinavian and American studies of occupation, but is not described in standard text books of rheumatology and orthopaedics, and is not widely recognized in the UK. However, it most closely corresponds to a regional pain disorder of the neck–shoulder area. It has been defined as a constant feeling of fatigue or stiffness in the neck associated with other subjective symptoms (such as neck pain or headache) and tender spots, palpable hardenings and neck muscle tightness.[14] Such clinical patterns have been described in excess in assembly line workers,[32] data entry operators,[33] scissor makers,[19] lamp assemblers[34] and other groups, with reported risk ratios of 2.3–7.3. Various mechanisms have been suggested, including local muscle

ischaemia, disturbed muscular microcirculation and sensitized pain receptors, but no specific pathological lesion has been identified. It seems plausible that tasks involving dynamic loading and tension of the shoulder and neck muscles produce such symptoms, but less clear whether they constitute a defined, discrete work-related musculoskeletal disorder. (This may be a semantic point for occupational physicians who are interested in good ergonomic practice and worker comfort.)

THORACIC OUTLET SYNDROME

A constellation of neurological and vascular features ascribed to entrapment of the brachial nerve plexus and subclavian vessels by a cervical rib or congenital fibrous band. The frequency of this condition is highly contentious – some orthopaedic authors regard the syndrome as very rare in the general population, whereas others describe large panels of successfully treated patients.[35] A similar divergence of opinion exists in occupational medicine: some authorities have described high prevalences of the condition in assembly line workers (14–44%),[36] cash register operators (32%)[36] and plate workers (31%),[37] but by contrast a UK expert workshop of occupational physicians, rheumatologists and orthopaedic surgeons considered it so rare as to obviate the need for consensus definition. This is as well, as the many sensory motor and vascular symptoms ascribed to thoracic outlet syndrome do not permit a ready description of established diagnostic criteria.

Management

The management of cervical pain syndromes is predominantly non-surgical. Acute exacerbations of neck pain are managed with a soft cervical collar, an 8-week course of combined analgesic and anti-inflammatory therapy, and a physiotherapy programme. The physical therapy should include the use of heat pad, neck exercises, ultrasound/short-wave diathermy and massage. Traction and transcutaneous electrical nerve stimulation (TENS) are helpful in controlling brachial root irritation. Manipulative therapy and acupuncture may assist in selected resistant cases. The principal indication for structural imaging (magnetic resonance imaging or computed tomographic scanning) is objective neurological deficit; if severe foraminal encroachment or myelopathy is discovered, surgical decompression may become necessary.

ELBOW PROBLEMS

The elbow joint actually comprises a compound synovial joint with articulation between the ulnar notch and the trochlea of the humerus, and also between the radial head and the humeral capitellum. In consequence, a large variety of movements are possible, including flexion of 150°, pronation of 75–80° and supination of 85–90°. Apart from epicondylitis and olecranon bursitis, soft tissue problems of the elbow are uncommon.

Epidemiology

Epicondylitis is a pattern of pain at the origins of the extensors of the fingers and wrists on the lateral epicondyle (lateral epicondylitis), or at the origin of the flexors on the medial epicondyle of the humerus (medial epicondylitis). Lateral epicondylitis (tennis elbow) is about seven times more common than medial epicondylitis (golfer's elbow). The point prevalence of elbow pain has been reported at 11–13% in aeroengineering workers[4] and textile workers[3]; and in a population survey the period prevalence of elbow pain during the previous year was 7% in 40- to 50-year-olds and 14% in those over 50.[38] However, clinically verified epicondylitis is less common: among textile workers only 2% had tender as well as painful elbows,[3] and in a Swedish community survey, that included clinical examination, the prevalence in 31- to 74-year-olds was 2.5%.[9] Clinical epicondylitis reaches a peak prevalence and incidence in the fifth decade of life and becomes increasingly less common after the age of 50.[9] It more commonly affects the dominant hand. Although 40–50% of tennis players have the condition,[39] less than 5% of cases arise from the sport.[40]

Aetiology

Lateral epicondylitis is believed to arise principally from overexertion of the finger and wrist extensors – in repeated hand dorsiflexion or in alternating forearm pronation and supination.[40] In those cases coming to clinical attention there is often a history of unaccustomed, forceful, repetitive use.

However, the pathological lesion remains a point of debate, and there have been at least 25 suggested causes.[41] The most widely held theory is that macroscopic or microscopic tears occur between the common extensor tendon and the periosteum of the lateral humeral epicondyle[42] and such tears have been identified in surgical procedures[43] but not consistently enough to resolve the argument.[40]

Occupational studies

In three cross-sectional surveys comparing meat cutters, sausage makers and packers with workers in less strenuous jobs, Viikari-Juntura et al.[44] found that elbow symptoms were 1.6–1.8 times more common in the exposed groups, but the prevalence of clinically verified epi-

condylitis was identical (0.8%). Dimberg reported a higher prevalence in aircraft factory workers (7.4%), but found no difference between white and blue collar workers.[4] McCormack et al. described a relative risk of 1.5 in packers and sewers compared with knitters,[3] a moderate excess of clinical epicondylitis has been described in a cross-sectional survey of public gas and water workers with long-term exposure to strenuous elbow work,[45] and Lopajarvi et al. described a similar-sized effect when women packers were compared with non-cashier shop assistants,[16] but these differences are comparatively modest and the confidence intervals for the risk estimates were compatible with chance differences. By contrast with cross-sectional investigations, the sole incidence study, a comparison between sausage makers and meat cutters ('exposed') and office workers and supervisors ('unexposed'), reported a much higher risk ratio for epicondylitis (7.1–10.3) in the former group.[46] These discrepant findings may be reconciled if patients with exposed incident cases quit employment, leading to an underestimate of risk in the cross-sectional surveys, and further investigation is warranted to examine this possibility.

Clinical aspects

The hallmark of lateral epicondylitis is slow onset pain and tenderness over the lateral epicondyle. The pain is reproduced by resisted dorsiflexion of the wrist with the elbow extended. Grip is impaired, and this may limit working ability. In medial epicondylitis the pain and tenderness (which are medially located) are often less prominent; pain is reproduced over the medial epicondyle by resisted palmar flexion of the wrist. Investigations are generally unhelpful and unnecessary.

Management

Many treatments have been proposed, though not all have been validated. Placing the arm in a sling or plaster cast may help, but recovery often requires 6 weeks of immobility. A wrist splint (to prevent wrist dorsiflexion) sometimes provides symptomatic relief. Pulsed ultrasound has been shown to be efficacious[47] while up to 90% of subjects respond to local injection of corticosteroids. In resistant cases surgery may be required as a last resort. After conservative treatment, relapse is fairly common (18–50% within 6 months[48,49]), especially in manual workers such as mechanics and builders.[50] In a case series of 88 workers visiting an occupational health department,[51] splint therapy combined with indomethacin treatment was compared with cortisone therapy; neither duration of absence from work, nor recurrence rate differed between the treatment groups.

It is said that lateral epicondylitis resolves sponta-neously in 8–12 months,[41] but in one rheumatology clinic a majority of sufferers were still symptomatic at the 1-year stage.[50]

TENOSYNOVITIS AND PERITENDINITIS

There is some confusion in the literature about the appropriate terminology for this lesion. Some authors draw a distinction between inflammation of the tendon sheath of the wrist (tenosynovitis), the paratendon at the muscle-tendon junction rather further up the arm (peri-tendinitis), and the tendon itself (tendinitis); but such a distinction is not often drawn in the classification crite-ria adopted in occupational and community surveys. For this reason we use the terms interchangeably in this account.

Epidemiology

In the US National Health Interview, 20 per 1000 adults reported that a doctor had told them they had 'tendini-tis';[52] while in the UK Primary Care Study for 1981, the incidence of tenosynovitis, tendinitis, synovitis and bur-sitis combined was 10.9 per 1000 persons per year.[10] The incidence was more common in women than men at all ages and peaked in middle age.

Occupational studies

There have been several cross-sectional surveys of hand-wrist tendinitis in the workplace. Board manu-facturers, sewers and packers were all found to be at increased relative risk (odds ratios 3.9–8) compared with knitters;[3] a relative risk of 7.1 was described in assembly-line workers compared with shop assistants,[16] and in one study, jobs that combined high force and high repetition carried a 29-fold greater risk of ten-dinitis than those lacking such features.[53] One cohort study compared the incidence of hand–wrist tendinitis in packers and sausage makers with office workers and supervisors (packing and sausage making were deemed to entail work strenuous to the musculotendinous junction of the upper limb): risk ratios of 24–36 were reported.[46]

Clinical aspects

The tendons most frequently involved are the radial extensors of the wrist and the long abductor and short extensor of the thumb; the flexor tendons are affected far less often.

TENOSYNOVITIS OF THE WRIST (DE QUERVAIN'S DISEASE)

Tenosynovitis of the wrist (De Quervain's disease) is characterized by pain on movement, localized to the ten-don sheaths in the wrist and reproduced by resisted active movement. Pain is centred on the radial aspect of the wrist and thumb base and particularly aggravated in grasping and employing the pinch grip. Typically symp-toms appear following return to work after a long lay-off, or following a change to unfamiliar work requiring new, rapid movements. For example, many cases occurred in the 1940s when people were required as part of the war effort to undertake unaccustomed work in factories and in agriculture.[54]

Initially a dull aching is experienced, but continuation of the work can give rise to severe pain. In the classical case, a sausage-shaped swelling is present on the radial side of the lower part of the dorsal surface of the fore-arm, proximal to the radial styloid process. The swelling, which is generally about 4 cm long, is tender, and crepi-tus is often palpable and audible over it, sometimes extending up the forearm. Local redness and warmth may occur. In the less florid case the diagnosis may be confused with osteoarthritis of the thumb base, but radi-ological assessment assists in this differential diagnosis: in the absence of typical radiographic changes, the pres-ence of osteoarthritis at this site would be unlikely. In patients with persistant pain but with little or no objec-tive evidence of tenosynovitis, magnetic resonance imag-ing can be helpful in diagnosis and can provide clear evidence of the state of the tendons and their related syn-ovial sheaths.

The treatment consists of local heat, non-steroidal anti-inflammatory drugs, and wrist and thumb immobi-lization by thermoplastic splinting. In patients with severe or persistent pain, one or more local corticos-teroid injections can be helpful, giving complete and lasting relief in about 70% of patients. Surgical decom-pression of the first extensor compartment (with or without tenosynovectomy) is indicated in those with persistent symptoms lasting longer than 6 months.

TRIGGER FINGER

Trigger finger is the result of tenosynovitis affecting the flexor tendons of the finger or thumb. The consequent fibrosis and constriction impair the tendon's motion at the first annular pulley, which overlies the metacar-pophalangeal joint. The most common cause of trigger finger is said to be overuse of the hands in repetitive gripping activities. Management consists of modifica-tion of hand activity, local heat treatment, gentle exer-cises and non-steroidal anti-inflammatory drugs as required. One or more corticosteroid injections to the affected flexor tendons cure the majority of patients. Surgical transection of the fibrous annual pulley is rarely required.

The evidence of benefit in these various treatments usually relates to short-term improvement, and there is clearly a need to demonstrate their longer term benefit in controlled trials of adequate design. Such trials should reflect the occupational environment in which the pain syndrome developed and the effect of ergonomic interventions instituted during the trial period.

CARPAL TUNNEL SYNDROME

As it passes through the carpal tunnel into the wrist, the median nerve lies immediately beneath the palmaris longus tendon and anterior to the flexor tendons. Conditions that decrease the size of the carpal tunnel or increase the volume of structures contained within it, tend to compress the median nerve against the transverse ligament which bounds the tunnel's roof. Such circumstances can arise traumatically, congenitally, or due to systemic or inflammatory effects (for example diabetes mellitus, rheumatoid arthritis, acromegaly, hypothyroidism, pregnancy and tenosynovitis). In many patients median nerve entrapment at the carpal tunnel occurs for no obvious cause.

Epidemiology

The symptoms, signs and nerve conduction abnormalities of carpal tunnel syndrome can arise separately, or in combination. Estimates of prevalence and incidence therefore vary according to the chosen case definition. In a large Dutch population survey that took as its definition sensory disturbance in the median nerve distribution occurring at least twice a week, generally waking the patient from sleep, and associated with neurophysiological abnormalities, the point prevalence was estimated at 0.6% in men and 8% in women.[55] Clinically diagnosed carpal tunnel syndrome occurred with a prevalence of 1.1% in textile workers[3] and 2.1% in other industrial workers,[53] The crude incidence rate is reported to be one per thousand person-years in hospital diagnosed patients.[56,57] and around two per thousand person years in UK primary care (unpublished data from the Royal College of General Practitioners).

Obesity and short stature appear to be independent risk factors for carpal tunnel syndrome.[57,58] In case reports, pregnancy, the oral contraceptive pill, the menopause, hysterectomy and breast feeding have all been linked with the syndrome, although epidemiological evidence is contradictory. The condition is often bilateral, and symptoms tend to be worse in the dominant hand.

Occupational studies

The relation between carpal tunnel syndrome and worker activities has been investigated repeatedly. For example, a review by Hagberg et al.[59] in 1992 identified 15 cross-sectional studies and six case-control studies that met high-quality criteria for case ascertainment. In the cross-sectional studies, the prevalence of carpal tunnel syndrome between different occupational groups varied from 0.6% to 61%. Particularly high prevalences and odds ratios were reported in grinders,[60] grocery store workers,[61] frozen food factory workers[62] and platers.[63] The authors concluded that repetitive and forceful gripping were major risk factors for occurrence of the syndrome. Silverstein et al.[64] classified the occupation of 652 workers from seven different industries according to the degree of force and repetition required, and found, compared with low force–low repetition jobs, that both high force and high frequency increased the risk moderately (odds ratios 1.8 and 2.7 respectively), but that the combination of high force and high frequency resulted in an odds ratio of more than 15.

The strongest associations in case-control studies have been with use of vibratory tools, and with activities that frequently flex or extend the wrist (Table 22.3). The link with vibratory exposure has also been described in industry-specific surveys, notably among foresters,[65] and is now accepted for compensation purposes by the UK State Industrial Injuries Scheme. However, use of vibrating tools is often correlated with forceful repetitive work and it remains unclear whether the effect arises from the ergonomic aspects of vibratory tool use or from a more general effect of vibration on peripheral nerves.

It should be remembered that case-control studies, like cross-sectional surveys, are susceptible to well-recognized biases. The association with a particular exposure may be spuriously inflated by recall bias, or by the effect of disease on work (if the decision to consult relates especially to difficulty in getting the job done). In carpal tunnel syndrome investigations, however, the studies have been in broad agreement. Furthermore, it can be demonstrated experimentally that extreme flexion and extreme extension of the wrist increase the pressure in the carpal tunnel sufficiently to impair blood perfusion of the median nerve. The epidemiological and physiological investigations provide a coherent view of causation.

Clinical aspects

The history is typically one of gradual onset of numbness and tingling in the median nerve distribution of the hand. Strenuous use of the hand usually aggravates symptoms, although this may not become apparent until several hours after the activity. Night-time pain commonly disturbs sleep and patients often hang the affected

Table 22.3 *Case-control studies of carpal tunnel syndrome and its relation to work activities*

Exposure	Odds ratio	Source
Vibration		
Use of vibrating tools	7.0	Cannon *et al.* (981)[66]
Exposure for more than 20 years	4.8	Wieslander *et al.* (1989)[67]
Use of vibrating tools		
>10 h per week	14.0 ⎫	
1–10 h per week	3.2 ⎬	Voog *et al.* (1985)[68]
Flexed wrist		
20–40 h per week	8.7 ⎫	
8–19 h per week	3.0 ⎬	
1–7 h per week	1.5 ⎭	De Krom *et al.* (1990)[55]
Extended wrist		
20–40 h per week	5.4 ⎫	
8–19 h per week	2.3 ⎬	
1–7 h per week	1.4 ⎭	
Repetitive wrist movement		
>20 years	4.6 ⎫	Wieslander *et al.* (1989)[67]
1–20 years	1.5 ⎭	
Keyboard typist	3.8	Voog *et al.* (1985)[68]

hand over the side of the bed in an effort to gain relief. Pain is commonly referred to the forearm and arm which can lead to difficulty in diagnosis. Many sufferers also complain of progressive weakness and clumsiness in their hands and tend to drop things.

Tinel's test (percussion over the flexor retinaculum reproducing parasthesiae over the median nerve distribution) is positive in about three-quarters of sufferers, and Phalen's test (sustained complete flexion of the wrist for 1 minute producing symptoms over the median nerve distribution) is positive in a similar proportion.[69] In one large series, clinical impairment of sensation could be demonstrated over the median nerve in 25% of cases, and thenar atrophy in 20%.

The most important diagnostic test is nerve conduction. A slowed sensory nerve conduction velocity across the carpal tunnel and a prolonged distal motor latency support the diagnosis. Electrodiagnostic tests are often quoted as the gold standard, but even the most sensitive latency tests confirm no more than 90% of 'classical' clinical cases. Some patients with exposure to hand-transmitted vibration develop a median nerve neuropathy as well as a digital neuropathy. Distinguishing these two conditions can be difficult but is important.

Management

The specific treatment of carpal tunnel syndrome depends to a large degree on whether there is an identifiable cause of the entrapment. Conservative measures may suffice when symptoms are of short duration. Electromyographic determinations repeated over time may help the clinician determine the correct therapeutic approach. Other measures which are known to be of benefit include splinting, local corticosteroid injection, the use of anti-inflammatory drugs and, ultimately, surgical release.

CHRONIC UPPER LIMB PAIN

In describing upper limb disorders, different physicians have used a variety of terms in a variety of ways. For some, 'work-related upper limb disorders', 'cumulative trauma disorders' and 'repetitive strain disorders' are synonymous and describe collectively the full range of recognized and ill-defined disorders arising (or appearing to arise) from frequent, forceful overuse at work of the upper limb. For others, repetitive strain injury refers to a particular diagnosis made by exclusion: chronic upper limb pain ascribed to overuse at work, for which no clinical diagnosis can be made. Inevitably confusion has ensued, among doctors and especially in medical litigation.

The problem can be illustrated by reference to some typical cases that have attracted publicity. In 1981 an enquiry over upper limb complaints in an Inland Revenue office accepted that complaints such as lateral epicondylitis and tenosynovitis could sometimes arise from the use of the visual display unit. In December 1991, Judge Byre found in the High Court that two British Telecom keyboard operators had repetitive strain injury, that had been induced by the nature of the work (at least 10 000 depressions per hour with a bonus for higher totals), and long hours in constrained postures on defective seating (the complaints were diagnosed as tenosynovitis and epicondylitis); and in 1994 a legal secretary received an award for tenosynovitis provoked by periods of intense typing. By contrast, in 1993, Judge Prosser dismissed the complaints of a Reuter's journalist concluding that 'repetitive strain injury did not exist'. Such a ruling plainly does not disprove the existence of well-established entities like lateral epicondylitis and tenosynovitis and the debate is really on two different fronts: (a) how often such specific complaints can arise from work activity; and (b) whether there is a condition of chronic upper limb pain which presently defies clinical diagnosis and which may be caused by work. Information on these questions has been tainted by studies that have drawn no distinction between potentially dissimilar clinical end-points.

In this chapter we have attempted to draw a clearer distinction. The term repetitive strain injury in the text that follows refers to chronic upper arm pain for which no diagnosis can be made and which has been ascribed to occupational overuse.

Epidemiology

It has proved difficult to define the epidemiology of a condition for which no clear definition and no validated or accepted diagnostic criteria exist. Routinely collected statistics tend to involve umbrella classifications that make it hard to disentangle information on non-specific upper limb pain. However, in Australia the Bureau of Statistics separately codes compensation awards for injuries without explicit diagnosis ascribed to repetitive movement. Table 22.4 illustrates the variation in incidence rate of compensated repetitive strain injury between men and women, and by industry.[70] Overall, repetitive strain injury was more common in blue collar workers than in clerical workers. For men, the highest rates occurred in the manufacture of textiles, clothing and footwear, food and beverages. In women, very high incidence rates occurred in parts of the manufacturing sector.

Sequential data over the period 1980–1987 showed dramatic changes with time. The number of successful claims among women in 1984–1985 was five times greater than in 1980–1981, and that amongst men 50% greater. Hocking[71] reported on the Australian repetitive strain injury epidemic as it affected one large employer, the nationalized telephone operator Telecom Australia between 1981 and 1985. Nearly half of the 3976 reports within the company arose in telephonists, providing an incidence rate of 343 cases per thousand keyboard workers over the 5 years, compared with 284 per thousand in clerical workers, 116 per thousand in process workers and 34 per thousand in telegraphists. Women accounted for 83% of all reports; 16% of subjects had symptoms lasting for longer than 6 months and the cost of the epidemic was estimated at more than $15 million dollars.

Of course, the decision to lodge a complaint or to compensate a claim can be heavily influenced by local awareness, fuelled by media publicity. By the 1990s the compensation rate in Australia had declined to a more normal level. Similar transient epidemics have been seen in other countries and other time periods: in Japan, an epidemic of 'occupational cervicobrachial disorders' was reported between 1958 and 1982; and an epidemic of writer's cramp occurred among male clerks in the British Civil Service in 1830. In the Japanese outbreak, the workers who most frequently complained were typists and keyboard operators, punchcard operators and telephone operators (10–28% of people claimed to be affected in some of the occupational groups[72]). As a result the Japanese Ministry of Labour introduced guidelines that restricted working time at the keyboard to no more than 5 hours a day and the maximum number of key strokes to 40 000 per day, and this was followed by a fall in the frequency of complaints.[73] Another crop of upper limb complaints developed in the Inland Revenue Department of the British Civil Service in 1981.

Table 22.4 *Incidence rates of compensated repetitive strain injury by industry in Australia, 1985–86*

Industry	Male Incidence[a]	Female Incidence[a]
Manufacturing		
food, beverages	4.5	7.4
textiles, clothing, footwear	4.7	4.2
Public administration	3.9	4.8
Agriculture	3.1	1.7
Transport equipment	3.0	16.2
Basic metal manufacture	2.5	16.7
Finance, business services	0.2	3.0
Mining	0.5	1.5
Health services	0.3	1.2
All industries combined	1.4	2.6

[a] Per thousand person-years

The time variation in these various data sets suggests that psychosocial variables play an important part in the presentation and recognition of the condition, if not also in its development.

Clinical aspects

Miller et al.[74] have described a series of 200 consecutive patients referred for specialist opinion with suspected repetitive strain injury in whom no other specific diagnosis could be made. In 75% the onset of pain was gradual, beginning as localized distal pain but more diffusely spread by the time of clinic attendance. Nearly all of the patients described parasthesiae and 73% described subjective swelling of the limb. The dominant hand was more commonly affected, but bilateral disease was also common. Anxiety, irritation, mood change, fatigue and sleep disturbance were nearly always present. Clinical signs were generally absent although most of the patients described tenderness at multiple sites.

In this respect repetitive strain injury has many similarities with fibromyalgia, a chronic musculoskeletal disorder of uncertain cause characterized by chronic widespread pain and multiple tender points. Fibromyalgia sufferers also tend to complain of fatigue, sleep disturbance, stiffness and parasthesiae and the clinical similarity between these two conditions has led to the suggestion that repetitive strain injury is a fibromyalgia variant.[74,75] Fibromyalgia is fairly common, affecting around 1–2% of the population,[76,77] 5–8% of hospital attendees[78] and 14–20% of patients referred to a rheumatology clinic.[79,80] The diagnostic criteria of the American College of Rheumatologists requires the pain of fibromyalgia to be present for at least 3 months in all four quadrants of the body and axial skeleton, with tenderness at 11 of 18 defined examination points.[81] The key point of clinical distinction is that in fibromyalgia, pain and tender points occur in the trunk and lower limbs as well as in the arm, shoulder and neck.

It has been suggested that repetitive strain injury is a condition of pain amplification leading to abnormally low cutaneous pain threshold (allodynia), muscle stiffness and vasomotor changes. However, these ideas remain largely untested. Clinical observation suggests that personality, emotional state, health beliefs and psyche are important too, though their relative contribution is unclear. In Australia, the Occupational Repetitive Strain Injuries Advisory Committee of the New South Wales Government of Industrial Relations proposed a clinical grading scale for repetitive strain injury. Stage 1 was characterized by aching and tiredness occurring at work but settling overnight; in stage 2 disease, symptoms failed to settle overnight and disturbed sleep, a condition that could persist for several months. Finally, in stage 3 disease symptoms persisted at rest, prevented even light duties and were persistent over months or years. The

relation between this proposed clinical grading scheme and the various specific and non-specific disorders that may be encountered in practice remains unclear.

Management

These aetiological components translate into the current biopsychosocial approach to treatment. A structured rehabilitation programme including graduated exercises, behavioural approaches to pain control, analgesic medication and assistive devices such as short-term splinting, may achieve dramatic benefits in the small number of severely affected patients. In this subgroup there is otherwise a very low probability of returning to gainful employment.

DUPUYTREN'S CONTRACTURE

Dupuytren's contracture is a nodular proliferation of fibrous tissue of the palmar fascia which leads to contracture and permanent flexion of the fingers (especially the fourth and fifth fingers) of one or both hands.

Epidemiology

Dupuytren's contracture is a common condition. In northern Europe, for example, it affects about 10% of men aged over 65 years. The condition is more common in men than women, and the prevalence increases with age.[82]

The condition is frequently bilateral. In a recent case-control study the condition was found to be independently associated with cigarette smoking and alcohol consumption.[83] It is also known to be more common in patients with diabetes and those with epilepsy receiving anticonvulsant drugs (phenytoin).

Occupational studies

The relation between Dupuytren's contracture and acute or cumulative traumatic injury is controversial. Case reports exist of Dupuytren's contracture arising soon after an acute injury to the hand, such as a penetrating wound, crush injury or fracture,[84] although epidemiological studies have not been conducted so far to investigate the association more formally. The relation between Dupuytren's contracture and chronic cumulative trauma has been reviewed recently by Liss and Stock.[85]

Bennett[86] observed a standardized morbidity ratio of 1.96 for Dupuytren's contracture among bagging and packing plant workers compared with the expected age-adjusted prevalence from an earlier survey, and an odds ratio of 5.5 compared with workers from the local plant who did not undertake these activities; while Mikkelsen[87] reported a sex-adjusted odds ratio of 3.1% for heavy versus light manual work in a population-based sample from Norway. However, the literature is comparatively sparse.

The relation with use of vibrating tools has been investigated more extensively. Thomas and Clarke[88] observed that Dupuytren's contracture was twice as common in 500 men claiming vibration-inducted white finger than in 150 controls admitted to hospital for elective surgery. An Italian case-control study[89] reported an odds ratio of 2.3 (95% confidence interval (CI) 1.5–4.4) for exposure to vibration at work after adjustment for alcohol. In another Italian investigation, Bovenzi et al,[90] observed an increased frequency of Dupuytren's contracture among quarry drillers and stone carvers compared with stone workers who performed manual work but were not exposed to vibration (odds ratio 2.6, 95% CI 1.1–6.2). Other researchers, by contrast, have failed to observe such an association.[85]

In summary, there is some evidence that Dupuytren's contracture may arise from occupational activities and this evidence is strongest for exposure to hand-transmitted vibration. The relation between Dupuytren's contracture and other manual work is uncertain at present.

OTHER SOFT TISSUE RHEUMATIC CONDITIONS

Two other categories of complaint that may be related to repetitive physical activity are recognized (prescribed) for state compensation under the UK Department of Social Security's industrial injuries benefits provisions:

- cramp of the hand or forearm 'due to repetitive movements';
- the 'beat' conditions – subcutaneous cellulitis of the hand (beat hand) and subcutaneous cellulitis or bursitis of the knee (beat knee) or elbow (beat elbow).

Carpal tunnel syndrome in vibrating tool users and tenosynovitis are also prescribed.

WRITER'S CRAMP, TELEGRAPHIST'S CRAMP, TWISTER'S CRAMP OR CRAFT PALSY

This is said to be a condition of occupations that involve a great deal of handwriting, typing or other repetitive movement of the hand or arm. According to Department of Social Security examiners' guidelines it manifests as symptoms of spasm, tremor and pain in the hand or forearm brought about by attempts to perform a familiar repetitive muscular action and occurs in the absence of physical signs or detectable abnormalities on investigation. Many physicians would question whether such an entity exists as a defined disease. The time course and chronicity of disease is not clearly defined, and it would appear difficult in practice to distinguish this condition from transient occupational discomfort or chronic non-specific upper limb pain. Despite these uncertainties around 120 new cases undergo assessment each year for prescription purposes.

THE BEAT CONDITIONS

These conditions are a more clearly recognized group of disorders. Repeated use of picks, shovels and hand tools in miners, quarrymen and labourers has sometimes been associated with a subcutaneous cellulitis of the hand with associated pain, tenderness, redness and swelling (beat hand) which may leave some residual disability. A sterile bursitis (beat knee) may sometimes arise in work that entails prolonged kneeling, such as coal mining, plumbing or carpet fitting. A similar disorder may arise at the elbow (beat elbow), although its association with occupational activity has been less clearly defined. It is assumed in each of these conditions that repeated physical trauma, friction and pressure are causal factors. It is not known how commonly these complaints occur, but in 1995–1996 nearly 200 new claims were assessed by Department of Social Security Special Medical Boards in connection with them.

OSTEOARTHRITIS

Epidemiology and clinical features

Osteoarthritis is probably the most common joint disorder in the world. In Western populations, radiographic evidence of osteoarthritis occurs in the majority of people by the age of 65 years, and in about 80% of those aged 75 years and over.[91] The disorder is second only to ischaemic heart disease as a cause of work-related disability in men over 50 years of age.

Osteoarthritis is defined as focal loss of articular cartilage with variable subchondral bone reaction. There is incomplete concordance between these pathological features and radiographic or clinical characteristics of the disorder. However, the difficulties encountered in using a pathological definition for epidemiological studies of osteoarthritis have led to the widespread use of radiological and clinical markers. The radiographic features conventionally used to define the severity of osteoarthritis include joint space narrowing, osteophyte, subchondral sclerosis, cyst formation and abnormalities of bony contour. These radiographic features can be incorporated in rating scales at the commonly affected joint sites (for example the hand, knee, and hip), permitting standardized grading of disease severity.[92] The two clinical sequelae of osteoarthritis that are most relevant are joint pain and functional impairment.

The development of osteoarthritis at any joint site depends upon a generalized predisposition to the condition, and biomechanical abnormalities that act at specific joints[91,93] Individual risk factors that may be associated with a generalized susceptibility to the disorder include obesity, a family history and hypermobility. Those that reflect local biomechanical insults include trauma, abnormalities of joint shape and physical activity, including work.

Occupational studies

KNEE OSTEOARTHRITIS

The four major non-occupational risk factors for knee osteoarthritis are obesity, knee injury, meniscectomy and the presence of Herberden's nodes.[94] Evidence has accumulated in recent years that risk is also increased by work that entails prolonged or repetitive knee bending. These data fall into four categories:

1. comparisons of the prevalence of knee osteoarthritis in different occupational groups;
2. assessment of the risk of knee osteoarthritis in different occupations;
3. case-control studies in which general assessments of activity level in the workplace are compared in patients with knee osteoarthritis and controls;
4. more detailed case-control studies in which a history of specific activities in the workplace is obtained.

Observational studies on the prevalence of symptomatic or radiographic knee osteoarthritis in different occupational groups date back over 40 years (Fig. 22.1). Kellgren and Lawrence found, in 1952, that the prevalence of moderate to severe radiographic knee osteoarthritis was almost six times greater among miners than clerical workers.[95] Later studies in dockers and civil servants,[96] painters and concrete workers,[97] and shipyard workers and clerks,[98] all confirmed that the risk of knee osteoarthritis is greater among men involved in heavy manual labour.

These observations have been extended by a register-based Swedish cohort study,[99] in which the risk of knee osteoarthritis coming to arthroplasty in various occupational groups was compared with the baseline population risk. Men employed as fire-fighters, farmers and construction workers presented significantly more often for surgery. Among women, there was a significant excess among cleaners. The risk estimates for these occupations varied from 1.4 to 3.0. These observations accord with the findings of three case-control studies of knee osteoarthritis in the USA,[100] the Netherlands[101] and Sweden.[102] When workplace activity was classified as heavy or light, the patients in all of these studies were between two and three times more likely to have been engaged in heavy activity occupations before the occurrence of knee osteoarthritis. However, the risk estimates in all studies failed to attain statistical significance.

Perhaps the most compelling evidence linking knee osteoarthritis with occupational activity comes from two population-based surveys in the USA. In an analysis of cross-sectional data from the HANES I study,[103] radiographic osteoarthritis of the knee at ages 55 to 64 years was three times more common in people whose jobs were judged likely to entail knee bending; and in a follow-up study of 1400 men and women from Framingham,[104] the risk of radiographic knee osteoarthritis was highest in subjects whose earlier jobs were classed as both physically demanding and likely to involve bending of the knees.

In each of these studies, data on knee use in the workplace was obtained by extrapolation from job title rather than through direct questioning about workplace activity, but one British population-based case-control study of knee osteoarthritis examined specific occupational activities in some detail. Subjects with symptomatic knee osteoarthritis from a defined population in Bristol were compared with age and sex-matched controls who had no evidence of knee pain or radiographic abnormality.[105] A lifetime occupational history was obtained, as well as details of specific workplace physical activities (kneeling, squatting, stair climbing, walking, standing, heavy lifting, sitting and driving). The risk of symptomatic knee osteoarthritis (after adjustment for body mass index and the presence of Heberden's nodes) was significantly increased among men and women whose major previous occupation had entailed prolonged squatting (greater than 30 minutes daily), prolonged kneeling (greater than 30 minutes daily) and repeated stair climbing (greater than 10 flights daily). There was no increase in risk associated with prolonged walking, standing, sitting or driving. Regular heavy lifting (25 kg daily) was not independently associated with an increase in risk, but subjects whose occupations involved heavy lifting and repeated knee flexion in combination had a substantial increase in risk (Fig. 22.2) Jobs frequently reported by the subjects as involving squatting or kneeling included teaching and nursing in women and steel erecting, electrical maintenance, roofing and other construction work in men. It was estimated from the data that around 5% of all symptomatic knee osteoarthritis

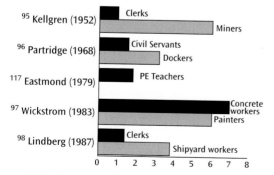

Figure 22.1 *Observational studies examining the prevalence of radiographic knee osteoarthritis among various occupational groups.*

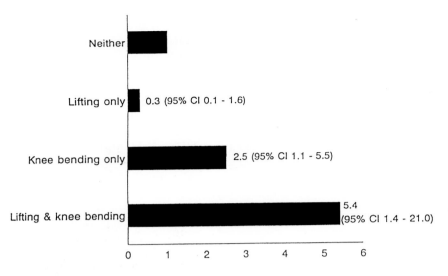

Figure 22.2 *Risk of knee osteoarthritis according to occupations involving heavy lifting and repetitive knee flexion. Data derived from a population based case-control study in Bristol.*

might result from occupations involving repetitive knee use. Extrapolation from the Framingham study suggests an even greater attributable risk.

HIP OSTEOARTHRITIS

The risk factor profile for hip osteoarthritis is somewhat different from that for knee osteoarthritis. There is a weaker association with obesity, hip injury and Heberden's nodes,[91,93] and a greater influence from developmental disorders of the hip joint, such as congenital dislocation of the hip, slipped upper femoral epiphysis and Perthes' disease.

Data on the relationship between specific work activities, such as heavy lifting, and the risk of hip osteoarthritis are not currently available. However, some studies have compared the occurrence of hip osteoarthritis with occupational title. Evidence is emerging that one such occupation – farming – is associated with high rates of the disorder.[106] Early studies from France, Norway and Sweden suggested that farmers had higher rates of total hip arthroplasty for osteoarthritis than other occupational groups. In a large Swedish cohort study, which included 250 000 people in the blue collar occupations[99] the relative risk for hip arthroplasty among farmers was 3.8 (95% CI 2.9–3.9). However, farmers may seek treatment more often than other occupational groups, not because they have a higher incidence of the disorder, but because they are more handicapped by it when it occurs. This issue may be addressed by population-based radiographic studies comparing the prevalence of hip osteoarthritis in farmers and other workers. In a British study[106] comparing men from a defined population aged 60–75 years who had always worked in farming with a group of controls who had spent their entire careers in clerical work, the prevalence of moderate/severe radiographic hip osteoarthritis (defined as a minimal joint space <1.5mm) was found to be 18% in the former group, compared with 2.4% in the controls. This gave a summary odds ratio for hip osteoarthritis among the farmers of 7.8 (95% CI 1.8–33.8), a risk estimate comparable with a Swedish study in which 15 000 agricultural workers were asked about previous hip radiography: 565 men and 151 women had had such examinations and the prevalence of hip osteoarthritis in male farmers was increased more than tenfold compared with the male population of similar age.

The precise risk factors for hip osteoarthritis in farmers have not been defined with certainty, and it is not known whether an excess risk also exists in other heavy manual workers, such as construction workers and labourers. In a second British case-control study,[107] the risk of hip osteoarthritis was found to be related to occupations that entailed regular heavy lifting (for example, the daily moving of weights greater than 25 kg by hand), prolonged standing and walking over rough ground; but the magnitude of risk associated with these exposures was much lower than that found in farmers, and further research is warranted.

Management

The goals of management in hip and knee osteoarthritis are to control pain, minimize disability, and educate the patient about the disorder and its therapy. The medical modalities of management currently available are shown in Table 22.5, and can be divided into non-pharmacological and pharmacological components.

The role of exercise in knee and hip osteoarthritis has been widely reviewed. Three randomized control trials in patients with knee osteoarthritis have demonstrated that strengthening of quadriceps musculature with isometric or isotonic exercises was associated with significant improvement in quadriceps strength, knee pain and

Table 22.5 *Medical management of patients with osteoarthritis of the knee or hip*

<u>**Non-pharmacological therapy**</u>
Patient education (self management programmes
    (e.g. Arthritis Self-Help Course))
Health professional social support (via telephone contact)
Weight loss (if overweight)
Physiotherapy
    range of motion exercises
    quadriceps strengthening exercises
    assistive devices for ambulation
Occupational therapy
    joint protection and energy conservation
    assistive devices for ADL
Aerobic exercise programmes

<u>**Pharmacological therapy**</u>
Intra-articular steroid injections
Analgesics (e.g. paracetamol, topical analgesics e.g. capsaicin
    and topical anti-inflammatory creams, non-steroidal
    anti-inflammatory drugs, opioid analgesics)

ADL: Activities of daily living

function, when compared with controls. Recent data suggest that exercise regimens, particularly those incorporating hydrotherapy, have similar benefits at the hip.

Proper use of a stick (in the hand contralateral to the affected knee or hip) reduces loading forces on the limb and is associated with decreased pain and improved function. In addition, patients may benefit from shoe inserts to correct abnormal biomechanic problems arising from angular deformity at the knees. Although trial data are not available, the wearing of shock absorbing shoes with insoles is believed to be of benefit. Finally, the use of lightweight knee braces may be helpful in patients with tibiofemoral disease, especially if complicated by lateral instability. Education also plays a central role.

Several studies have found that obesity is a major risk factor for the development and progression of knee osteoarthritis, and in one study, weight loss was associated with lower odds of developing symptomatic disease. Overweight patients with osteoarthritis of the lower limb joints, especially those being considered for arthroplasty, should be encouraged to participate in a comprehensive weight management programme, including dietary counselling and aerobic exercise.

Pain relief is the main indication for drug therapy in osteoarthritis. No drugs are available presently that reverse the structural or biochemical abnormalities of the disorder, but chondroprotective agents have been studied in animal models of osteoarthritis, and may become available in the future for human use.

Traditionally, non-steroidal anti-inflammatory drugs have been the agents of choice for pain relief. Recently however, because of concerns about their possible deleterious effects on articular cartilage metabolism, questions about the role of synovial inflammation in natural disease progression, and recognition of the greater risk of toxicity from prolonged therapy, the central role of these agents in the treatment of osteoarthitis has been questioned. Randomized controlled clinical trials suggest that anti-inflammatory agents offer no advantage over paracetamol in simple pain relief, whereas the adverse effects of paracetamol are substantially less than for long-term non-steroidal multi-inflammatory drug use, so paracetamol should be the analgesic agent of first choice in osteoarthritis. However, anti-inflammatory agents can be used in short courses among patients who have polyarticular disease with synovial inflammation.

In individuals with knee osteoarthritis who do not respond to oral analgesics, or who do not wish to take systemic therapy, topical analgesics or even capsaicin cream can be effective. Finally, patients who do not respond satisfactorily to these modalities may benefit from open or closed tidal knee irrigation with saline.

The response to surgical intervention in osteoarthritis of the hip and knee is dramatic. Pain is the most important single reason for surgery. When pain becomes intolerable or unmanageable by medical means, operative treatment should be considered. Other reasonable indications for surgery include progressive loss of movement, increasing deformity, complications such as sudden locking of the knee, and progressive disability and dependency.

RISK FACTORS FOR WORK-RELATED MUSCULOSKELETAL DISORDERS

A basic hypothesis exists that work-related musculoskeletal disorders are caused or aggravated by forceful, repetitive and awkward movements with insufficient rest or recovery time. The evidence from case reports, workplace surveys and formal epidemiological investigation points in this direction, although, as indicated earlier, evaluation is not straight forward. A variety of physiological, biomechanical and ergonomic investigations further underpin the hypothesis, so work-related musculoskeletal disorders have come to be described as repetitive strain injuries or cumulative trauma or overuse disorders. The mechanisms of injury are unclear, (and perhaps different for different outcomes), but it is generally felt that undesirable permutations of force, repetition, duration and posture contribute to disease onset.

Unfortunately work factors of this kind are only too common in industry. High productivity targets and machine pacing encourage highly repetitive actions of short cycle time with limited opportunity for respite; persistent static loading arises in jobs that involve prolonged standing, holding objects at arm's length and working above shoulder height for long periods; work in confined spaces often requires awkward postures that load joints asymmetrically and require prolonged kneeling or squatting. Other common work circumstances include ill-considered workstation, tool and task design, and the manipulation of heavy loads, sometimes under adverse conditions (such as a slippery or uneven footing). Figure 22.3 illustrates some typical situations.

The different risk factors often co-exist, and in practice it is difficult to disentangle their effects. Thus, undesirable forces matter because of the load they impose on muscles and the torques they impose on joints, but the outcome probably depends upon the degree and direction of loading (posture), its duration and its frequency, muscle fatigue and recovery times. The effort of work can be minimized by 'good' postures that allow as many strong muscles to contribute as possible, or exaggerated by 'bad' ones such as poor grip and ulnar or radial deviation of the wrist (which may reduce grip strength by up to 50%) – hence force and posture are inter-related. In general, avoidance of prolonged static loading is desirable, as high intramuscular tensions interrupt the blood supply and enforce anaerobic metabolism; but the problem is heightened if high forces are required, the posture is awkward or effort needs to be maintained for any length of time. Work by Monod and Scherrer[108] and Rhomert[109] indicates that effort that exerts 50% of the maximal force can last no more than a minute, while field studies suggest that loads of 15–20% at maximum will induce painful fatigue if kept up for days or months.

There are reasons for considering some occupational groups such as typists to be at special risk from these factors. The static loading of the neck and trapezius muscles in visual display unit workers has been reported to be 20–30% of the maximum voluntary contraction. Furthermore, the increasing use of a computer 'mouse' encourages typists to spend more time with their wrist in ulnar deviation and with their shoulder externally rotated.

The concurrence of risk factors matters particularly as they may act synergistically. The study of carpal tunnel syndrome by Silverstein et al. described earlier, provides an example of synergistic interaction between force and repetition: when either was present the risk increased about two to three times but when present together the risk of carpal tunnel syndrome was very significantly raised.[53]

Approaches to risk assessment and risk reduction take their cue from the putative risk factors, attempting to measure or control some combination of unwanted forces, repetitions and work positions. Many assessment methods have been attempted, though none has achieved primacy. Some techniques are time consuming, expensive and research-focused; others have been advocated for use in the workplace in assessment and planning of control measures.

Most elaborate are the video recording methods. These often employ pairs or panels of cameras providing alternative views of the work, with markers on the body (such as reflective spots or small lights) to provide measurement points. The results can be digitally encoded and analysed by computer, providing detailed spatial and temporal information on work postures and movements. Alternatively workers have worn electronic pendulum potentiometers and flexible lightweight tubes containing strain gauge strips that allow reconstruction of postures and movements – again computerized analysis is possible.

Static work activity has been assessed by mapping the various joint angles (for example, using photographs or goniometers); while static workloads and muscle fatigue have been investigated using electromyography. A high correlation has been shown between electromyographic activity and muscular force (for both static and dynamic activities), and muscle fatigue can be detected as an increase in the amplitude of the low frequency range of electromyographic activity. For research purposes, needle electrodes have been lodged in particular muscles, but in workplaces the technique has been adapted so that records can be obtained from surface electrodes.

These various analytical approaches enable biomechanical measurements of force, posture, frequency and duration to be compared with known human capability and the outcomes of health investigations. They further allow comparison across jobs, so that those expected to carry higher risk can be identified.

However, they require special expertise and skills. In occupational practice, simpler more rapid assessment techniques are required, and a number of systems have been proposed. In one of the earliest, the Ovako Working Posture Analysing System (OSWAS) method,[110] postures were observed and recorded using a six figure code during each stage of a representative task cycle. The first three digits represented a fairly crude description of trunk and limb postures; the fourth figure indicated the load or force employed, and the remainder were task designated. The procedure, which requires observer training and standardization, is to glance, look away and record it. For frequent activities the proportion of time in which particular postures are adopted and loads incurred can be estimated.

Other analogous scoring procedures exist for the upper limbs and neck, such as the Rapid Upper Limb Assessment (RULA) technique,[111] and these generally result in a risk score that is marked against advice on the urgency of corrective action. An alternative approach employs a risk factor check-list. Table 22.6 provides an example. In some cases it has been suggested that the priority for remedial action should be determined by the number of risk factors identified: the situation is clearly more complicated than this, but in the absence of better information this provides a convenient means for assembling an action plan.

In some cases these pragmatic tools have been tested empirically against levels of discomfort at work,[111] but at

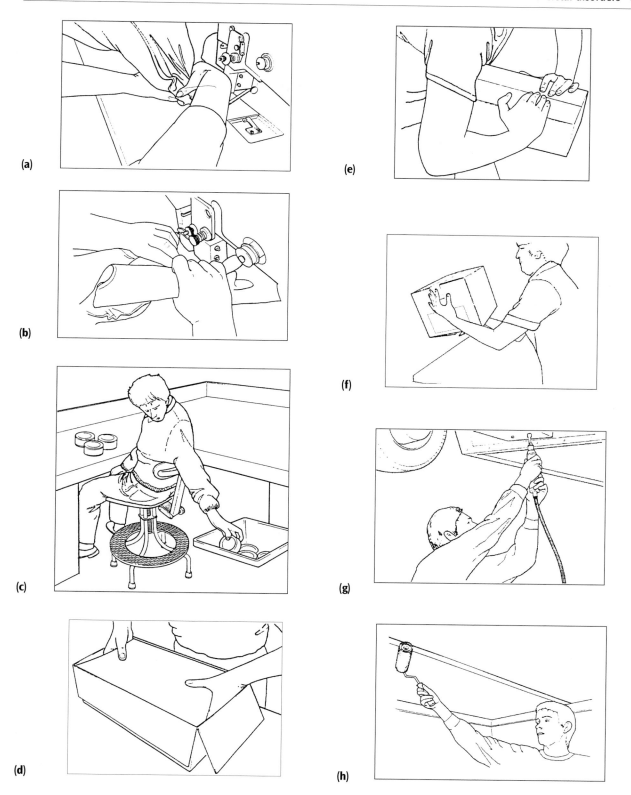

Figure 22.3 *Examples of some ergonomic risk factors in the workplace: (a, b): Some tasks requiring high force levels to be applied. (c-h) Some examples of static or awkward posture. Reproduced from Ref. 116, with permission from HMSO, London. Crown Copyright.*

Table 22.6 *Checklist for identifying work-related upper limb disorders*

Organizational factors
Is operator training thorough enough?
Is repetitive work arranged without a break or with compulsory overtime?
Do bonus systems encourage the exceedance of good working practice?

Task and equipment design factors
Applied forces
Is excessive force being used?
Are there static muscle loads?
Are forces applied with the joints at or near extremes of their range of movement?
Movements
Are the same movements repeated frequently?
Are they repeated rapidly?
Do they include forceful twisting or rotation of the wrist, movement of the wrist from side to side, highly flexed fingers and wrist, or upper limb motions beyond a comfortable range?
Postural factors
Are the arms raised high or outstretched at the shoulder?
Is the forearm held above the horizontal?
Is the upper arm held away from the vertical?
Do poor overall postures exist?
Duration of effort
Are tasks performed for long periods without relief?
Are short bursts of energetic work included in longer periods of activity?
Tool and equipment factors
Are women using tools designed for men?
Do the tools vibrate, without vibration dampening?
Do the tools impose shock loading upon the user?
Do the tools need to be held firmly to resist reaction torques?
Do tools have a jerking action?
Is considerable pressure required to hold/operate the tool?
Are the handles too large/too small/too short/too slippery to be gripped easily?
Do operators have to twist and turn to reach every-day items?
Do the operator's gloves affect grip or dexterity?

Personal and anthropometric factors
Do operators suffer from work or domestic stress?
Are operators at one or other of the extremes of height/reach/strength of the working population?

Environmental factors
Do levels of noise cause mental stress or interfere with communications?
Do lighting levels encourage awkward postures?
Do flickering lights and glare cause visual difficulties?
Does protective clothing constrain posture and affect grip?

Adapted from Ref. 116, with permission from HMSO, London. Crown Copyright.

present there no hard evidence concerning their predictive value for occurrence of work-related musculoskeletal disorders, and hence for the adequacy of the risk assessment produced. Nonetheless, they have evident attractions: they can be readily understood and applied, and facilitate attempts to prioritize remedial actions in an area where knowledge is far from complete.

IDENTIFYING WORK-RELATED MUSCULOSKELETAL DISORDERS

Work-related musculoskeletal disorders arise in the context of a background incidence of musculoskeletal complaint, in workers who do not always seek medical advice. In some cases (as in hip and knee osteoarthritis) they may present after retirement. Their multifactorial character and for some disorders their transience tend to impede detection. In clinical practice a high level of awareness is required if early recognition and intervention are to be achieved.

The starting point should be a knowledge of the occupations and tasks most likely to generate concern. Health professionals and safety managers should also be alert to the possibility of disease clustering. An 'outbreak' of apparently related symptoms in workers with a shared exposure suggests the need for wider investigation – for example, a health survey and a review of the work activity. The problem may be circumscribed, or bigger than first appreciated; and the process or materials may have changed, adding unrecognized risk to the job.

Many soft-tissue studies have used the Nordic questionnaire[112] as the basis of health enquiry. This simple self-completion questionnaire has been developed to standardize the data researchers collect and has been validated to some extent. It allows an estimate of the 1-week and 1-year period prevalences of limb and neck complaint (such as pain and interference with work), but further assessment would be required before making a clinical diagnosis. Other questionnaires of similar scope have been developed for use in surveys and screening, and some authors have given advice on analysing and interpreting the findings.[113]

PREVENTING AND MANAGING WORK-RELATED MUSCULOSKELETAL DISORDERS

Success in the prevention of work-related musculoskeletal disorders depends upon an informed assessment of risk; a sharing of information between medical personnel and employees, and a package of risk reduction measures, underpinned by suitable management systems for monitoring and enforcement.

A similar approach will help the affected worker to return to work, and to avoid a recurrent problem.

Preventive measures may include:

1 Advice and training, to ensure a higher risk awareness and better working practices.
2 An induction period, to allow new employees to start out at a slower pace than the established workforce.
3 Job rotation or job enlargement, to provide respite from work that requires repetitive monotonous use of the same muscles and tendons.
4 Rest breaks. These are often advocated as an alternative to job rotation, although little information exists on their value or the length that the break should be.
5 A rehabilitation programme, to ease affected workers back into productive work.
6 Redeployment, in recalcitrant and recurrent cases.
7 Task optimization. Better design of tools and equipment, and a better work layout make the task easier to perform. Often only a little thought is required to reduce work effort and to avoid undesirable working postures. Figure 22.4 illustrates, for example, how one tool and one task were redesigned to eliminate undesirable wrist and shoulder postures.

Work with visual display units in Great Britain now falls under the Health and Safety (Display Screen Equipment) Regulations 1992[114] which are based on the premise that use of visual display units is associated with musculoskeletal effects, visual fatigue and mental stress that can be controlled by simple ergonomic principles. Detailed

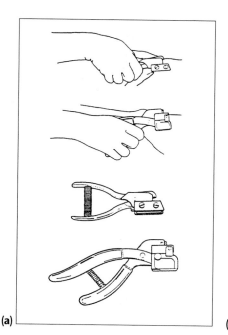

(a)

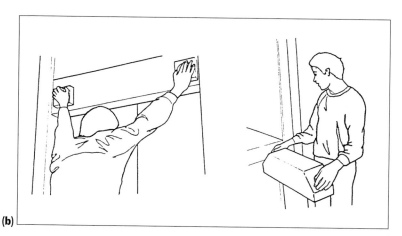

(b)

Figure 22.4 *Examples of some simple ergonomic solutions. (a) Redesigning the handles of a tool can lead to more comfortable hand positions and reduce the force required to do the job. (b) In this press operation repositioning of the control panel has eliminated the need for prolonged overhead work. Reproduced from Ref. 116, with permission from HMSO, London. Crown Copyright.*

guidance has been provided on the appropriate design of screens, chairs, desks, document holders and foot rests for work station users, as well as the need for frequent rest breaks.[115]

CONCLUSIONS

1 Work-related musculoskeletal disorders are common, and may be disabling.

2 They belong to one of two broad clinical categories: either to one of a number of specific diseases, or to one of a number of non-specific pain syndromes. Among the specific disorders, osteoarthritis of the hip and the knee are most important in the lower limb; while shoulder capsulitis and tendinitis, elbow epicondylitis, wrist tenosynovitis and carpal tunnel syndrome are important disorders of the upper limb. However, the relative contribution of specific and non-specific disorders to the overall burden of disease is not well described at present.

3 Two broad categories of risk factor are considered important in the causation of work-related musculoskeletal disorders: mechanical, and psychosocial. In addition, personal vulnerability and pain perception may play an important part. The relative contribution of these factors is likewise poorly characterized, and may perhaps differ between specific and non-specific disorders. Evidence exists for many health outcomes that adverse ergonomic factors pose a risk, but the role of psychosocial factors in the causation and presentation of disease is more problematic.

4 When assessing a patient with musculoskeletal complaints, the physician should always consider whether or not work may have caused or aggravated his condition; whether a rehabilitation programme could ease the patient's return to work; whether job modifications may be required, to mitigate against the risk of a recurrence; and whether the risk posed by existing work circumstances has been adequately assessed and controlled.

REFERENCES

1 Hodgson JT, Jones JR, Elliott RC, Osman J. *Self Reported Work Related Illness*. Sudbury: HSE Books, 1993.

2 Barton NJ, Hooper G, Noble J, Steel WM. Occupational causes of disorders in the upper limb. *Br Med J* 1992;**304**: 309–11.

3 McCormack RR Jr, Inman RD, Wells A, Berntsen C, Imbus HR. Prevalence of tendinitis and related disorders of the upper extremity in a manufacturing workforce. *J Rheumatol* 1990;**17**: 958–64.

4 Dimberg L. The prevalence and causation of tennis elbow (lateral humeral epicondylitis) in a population of workers in an engineering industry. *Ergonomics* 1987;**30**: 573–80.

5 Bergenudd H, Lindgarde F, Nilsson B, Petersson CJ. Shoulder pain in middle age. A study of prevalence and relation to occupational work load and psychosocial factors. *Clin Orthopaed* 1988;**231**: 234–8.

6 Makela M, Heliovaara M, Sievers K, Impivaara O, Knekt P, Aromaa A. Prevalence, determinants, and consequences of chronic neck pain in Finland. *Am J Epidemiol* 1991;**134**: 1356–67.

7 Hagberg M, Silverstein B, Wells R, Smith MJ, Hendrick HW *et al. Work-related Musculoskeletal Disorders (WMSDs): A Reference Book for Prevention*. Basingstoke: Taylor & Francis, 1995.

8 Bongers PM, De Winter CR, Kompier MAJ, Hildebrandt VH. Psychosocial factors at work and musculoskeletal disease. *Scand J Work Environ Hlth* 1993;**19**: 297–312.

9 Allander E. Prevalence, incidence and remission rates of some common rheumatic diseases or syndromes. *Scand J Rheumatol* 1974;**3**: 145–53.

10 Royal College of General Practitioners. *Third National Morbidity Survey In General Practice 1980–1*. Series MBS No. 1. London: HMSO; 1986.

11 Jarvholm U, Styf J, Suurkula M, Herberts P. Intramuscular pressure and muscle blood flow in supraspinatus. *Eur J Appl Physiol Occupat Physiol* 1988;**58**: 219–24.

12 Jarvholm U, Palmerud G, Karlsson D, Herberts P, Kadefors R. Intramuscular pressure and electromyography in four shoulder muscles. *J Orthopaed Res* 1991;**9**: 609–19.

13 Hagberg M. Electromyographic signs of shoulder muscular fatigue in two elevated arm positions. *Am J Phys Med* 1981;**60**: 111–21.

14 Hagberg M, Wegman DH. Prevalence rates and odds ratios of shoulder-neck diseases in different occupational groups. *Br J Ind Med* 1987;**44**: 602–10.

15 Herberts P, Kadefors R, Hogfors C, Sigholm G. Shoulder pain and heavy manual labour. *Clin Orthopaed* 1984;**191**: 166–78.

16 Luopajarvi T, Kuorinka I, Virolainen M, Holmberg M. Prevalence of tenosynovitis and other injuries of the upper extremities in repetitive work. *Scand J Work Environ Hlth* 1979;**5** (Suppl 3): 48–55.

17 Punnett L, Robins JM, Wegman DH, Keyserling WM. Soft tissue disorders in the upper limbs of female garment workers. *Scand J Work Environ Hlth* 1985;**11**: 417–25.

18 Ohlsson K, Attewell R, Skerfving S. Self-reported symptoms in the neck and upper limbs of female assembly workers. Impact of length of employment, work pace, and selection. *Scand J Work Environ Hlth* 1989;**15**: 75–80.

19 Kuorinka I, Koskinen P. Occupational rheumatic diseases and upper limb strain in manual jobs in a light mechanical industry. *Scand J Work Environ Hlth* 1979;**5**: 39–47.

20 Bjelle A, Hagberg M, Michaelsson G. Clinical and ergonomic factors in prolonged shoulder pain among

industrial workers. *Scand J Work Environ Hlth* 1979;**5**: 205–10.

21 Hazlett JW. Tears of the rotator cuff. *J Bone J Surg* 1971;**53**: 772.

22 Nixon JE, DiStefano V. Ruptures of the rotator cuff. *Orth Clin North Am* 1975;**6**: 423–47.

23 Boyle AC. Disorders of the shoulder joint. *Br Med J* 1969;**3**: 283–5.

24 Yergason RM. Supination sign. *J Bone J Surg* 1931;**13**: 160.

25 Lundberg BJ. The frozen shoulder. *Acta Orthop Scand* 1969;**119**: 1–59.

26 Reeves B. The natural history of the frozen shoulder syndrome. *Scand J Rheumatol* 1976;**4**: 193–6.

27 Binder A, Bulgen DY, Hazleman BL, Roberts S. Frozen shoulder: a long-term prospective study. *Ann Rheum Dis* 1984;**43**: 361–4.

28 Lawrence JS. Disc degeneration, its frequency and relationship to symptoms. *Ann Rheum Dis* 1969;**28**: 121–38.

29 Westerling D, Jonsson BG. Pain from the neck shoulder region and sick leave. *Scand J Soc Med* 1980;**7**: 131.

30 Holt L. The Munkfors investigation. *Acta Orthop Scand* 1954;Suppl 17.

31 Holt L. Frequency of symptoms for different age groups and professions. In: Hitsch C, Zotterman Y eds. *Cervical Pain*. New York: Pergamon Press, 1971: 17–20.

32 Amano M, Umeda G, Nakajima H, Yatsuki K. Characteristics of work actions of shoe manufacturing assembly line workers and a cross-sectional factor-control study on occupational cervicobrachial disorders. *Jap J Ind Halth* 1988;**30**: 3–12.

33 Hunting W, Laubli Th, Grandjean E. Postural and visual loads at VDT workplaces. I. Constrained postures. *Ergonomics* 1981;**24**: 917–31.

34 Onishi N, Namura H, Sakai K, Yamamoto T, Hirayama K, Itani T. Shoulder muscle tenderness and physical features of female industrial workers. *J Hum Ergol* 1976;**5**: 87–102.

35 Roos DB. Congenital anomalies associated with thoracic outlet syndrome. *Am J Surg* 1976;**132**: 771–8.

36 Sallstrom J, Schmidt H. Cervicobrachial disorders in certain occupations, with special reference to compression in the thoracic outlet. *Am J Ind Med* 1984;**6**: 45–52.

37 Toomingas A, Hagberg M, Jorulf L, Nilsson T, Burstrom L, Kihlberg S. Outcome of the abduction external rotation test among manual and office workers. *Am J Ind Med* 1991;**19**: 215–27.

38 Cunningham LS, Kelsey JL. Epidemiology of musculoskeletal impairments and associated disability. *Am J Publ Hlth* 1984;**74**: 574–9.

39 Gruchow HW, Pelletier BS. An epidemiologic study of tennis elbow. *Am J Sports Med* 1979;**7**: 234–8.

40 Goldie I. Epicondylitis lateralis humeri: A pathogenetical study. *Acta Chir Scand* 1964; **339**(Suppl): 119.

41 Cyriax JH. The pathology and treatment of tennis elbow. *J Bone Jt Surg* 1936;**18**: 921–40.

42 Cyriax JH. Diagnosis of soft tissue lesions. Treatment by manipulation, massage and injection. In: *Textbook of Orthopaedic Medicine*. London: Ballière Tindall, 1982.

43 Coonrad RW, Hooper RW. Tennis elbow: its course, natural history, conservative and surgical management. *J Bone Jt Surg Am* 1973;**55A**: 1177–87.

44 Viikari-Juntura E, Kurppa K, Kuosma E *et al.* Prevalence of epicondylitis and elbow pain in the meat-processing industry. *Scand J Work Environ Hlth* 1991;**17**: 38–45.

45 Ritz BR. Humeral epicondylitis among gas- and water-work employees. *Scand J Work Environ Hlth* 1997;**21**: 478–86.

46 Kurppa K, Viika RI, Juntura E, Kuomas E, Huuskonen M, Kivi P. Incidence of tenosynovitis or peritendinitis and epicondylitis in a meat-processing factory. *Scand J Work Environ Hlth* 1991;**17**: 32–7.

47 Binder A, Hodge G, Greenwood AM, Hazleman BL, Page Thomas DP. Is therapeutic ultrasound effective in treating soft tissue lesions? *Br Med J* 1985;**292**: 512–4.

48 Clarke AK, Woodland J. Comparison of two steroid preparation used to treat tennis elbow, using the hypospary. *Rheumatol Rehab* 1975;**14**: 37–49.

49 Nevelos AB. The treatment of tennis elbow with triamcinolone acetonide. *Curr Med Res Opin* 1980;**6**: 507–9.

50 Binder AI, Hazleman BL. Lateral humeral epicondylitis. A study of natural history and the effect of conservative therapy. *Br J Rheumatol* 1983;**22**: 73–6.

51 Kivi P. The etiology and conservative treatment of humeral epicondylitis. *Scand J Rehab Med* 1982;**15**: 37–41.

52 Kramer JS, Yelin EH, Epstein WV. Social and economic impacts of four musculoskeletal conditions. *Arthr Rheum* 1983;**26**: 901–7.

53 Silverstein BA, Fine LJ, Armstrong TJ. Hand wrist cumulative trauma disorders in industry. *Br J Ind Med* 1986;**43**: 779–84.

54 Thompson AR, Plewes LW, Shaw EG. Peritendinitis crepitans and simple tenosynovitis: a clinical study of 544 cases in industry. *Br J Ind Med* 1951;**8**: 150.

55 de Krom MCTFM, Kester ADM, Knipschild PG, Spaans F. Risk factors for carpal tunnel syndrome. *Am J Epidemiol* 1990;**132**: 1102–10.

56 Stevens JC, Sun S, Beard CM, OFallon WM, Kurland LT. Carpal tunnel syndrome in Rochester, Minnesota, 1961 to 1980. *Neurology* 1988;**38**: 134–8.

57 Vessey MP, Villard Mackintosh L, Yeates D. Epidemiology of carpal tunnel syndrome in women of childbearing age. Findings in a large cohort study. *Int J Epidemiol* 1990;**19**: 655–9.

58 de Krom MC, Knipschild PG, Kester AD, Thijs C, Boekkooi PF, Spaaris F. Carpal tunnel syndrome: prevalence in the general population. *J Clin Epidemiol* 1992;**45**: 373–6.

59 Hagberg M, Morgenstern H, Kelsh M. Impact of occupations and job tasks on the prevalence of carpal tunnel syndrome. *Scand J Work Environ Hlth* 1992;**18**: 337–45.

60 Nathan PA, Meadows KD, Doyle LS. Occupation as a risk factor for impaired sensory conduction of the median nerve at the carpal tunnel. *J Hand Surg (GB)* 1988;**13B**: 167–70.

61 Osorio AM, Ames R, Jones J. *Carpal Tunnel Syndrome Among Grocery Store Workers*. Berkeley, California: Californian Occupational Health Program, California Department of Health Services: Field Investigation FI-86-005, 1989: 61.

62 Chiang HC, Chen SS, Yu HS, Ko YC. The occurrence of carpal tunnel syndrome in frozen food factory employees. *Kaohsiung J Med Sci* 1990;**6**: 73–80.

63 Nilsson T, Hagberg M, Burstrom L, Lundstrom R. Prevalence and odds ratios of numbness and carpal tunnel syndrome in different exposure categories of platers. In: Okada A, Dupuis WTH eds. *Hand-Arm Vibration*. Kanozawa, Japan: Kyoei Press Co, 1990: 235–9.

64 Silverstein BA, Fine LJ, Armstrong TJ. Occupational factors and carpal tunnel syndrome. *Am J Ind Med* 1987;**11**: 343–58.

65 Bovenzi M, Zadini A, Franzinelli A, Borgogni F. Occupational musculoskeletal disorders in the neck and upper limbs of forestry workers exposed to hand-arm vibration. *Ergonomics* 1991;**34**: 547–62.

66 Cannon LJ, Bernacki EJ, Walter SD. Personal and occupational factors associated with carpal tunnel syndrome. *J Occup Med* 1981;**23**: 255–8.

67 Wieslander G, Norback D, Gothe CJ, Juhlin L. Carpal tunnel syndrome (CTS) and exposure to vibration, repetitive wrist movements, and heavy manual work: a case-referent study. *Br J Ind Med* 1989;**46**: 43–47.

68 Voog L, de Laval J, Ahlborg G, Holm Glad J. *Compression of the Median Nerve at the Wrist and Work, with Vibrating Tools* Report project 82-0545. Stockholm: Swedish Work Environment Fund, 1985.

69 Phalen GS. The carpal tunnel syndrome. *J Bone Jt Surg* 1966;**48A**: 211–28.

70 Gun RT. The incidence and distribution of RSI in South Australia 1980–81 to 1986–87. *Med J Aust* 1990;**153**: 376–80.

71 Hocking B. Epidemiological aspects of 'repetition strain injury' in Telecom Australia. *Med J Aust* 1987;**147**: 218–22.

72 Harris JE. *Repetition Strain Injury*. Proceedings of the Royal Australian College of Surgeons/Royal Australia College of Physicians Seminar Disability in the workforce. Sydney: RACS/RACP, 1984.

73 Ohara H, Aroyama H, Itani T. Health hazard among cash register operators and the effects of improved working conditions. *J Hum Ergol (Tokyo)* 1976;**5**: 31–40.

74 Miller MH, Topliss DJ. Chronic upper limb pain syndrome (repetitive strain injury) in the Australian workforce: A systematic cross-sectional rheumatological study of 229 patients. *J Rheumatol* 1988;**15**: 1705–12.

75 Wigley RD. Repetitive strain syndrome – fact not fiction. *N Z Med J* 1990;**103**: 75–6.

76 Hartz A, Kirchdoerfer E. Undetected fibrositis in primary care practice. *J Family Pract* 1987;**25**: 365–9.

77 Jacobsson L, Lindgarde F, Manthorpe R. The commonest rheumatic complaints of over six weeks' duration in a twelve-month period in a defined Swedish population. Prevalences and relationships. *Scand J Rheumatol* 1989;**18**: 353–60.

78 Muller W. The fibrositis syndrome: Diagnosis, differential diagnosis and pathogenesis. *Scand J Rheumatol* 1987;**16**: 40–53.

79 Yunus M, Masi AT, Calabro JJ *et al*. Primary fibromyalgia (fibrositis): Clinical study of 50 patients with matched normal controls. *Semin Arthr Rheum* 1981;**11**: 151–71.

80 Wolfe F, Cathey MA. Prevalence of primary and secondary fibrositis. *J Rheumatol* 1983;**10**: 965–8.

81 Wolfe F, Smythe HA, Yunus MB *et al*. The American College of Rheumatology 1990. Criteria for the classification of fibromyalgia. Report of the Multicenter Criteria Committee. *Arthr Rheum* 1990;**33**: 160–72.

82 Early PF. Population studies in Dupuytren's contracture. *J Bone Jt Surg* 1962;**44B**: 602–13.

83 Burge P, Hoy G, Regan P, Milne R. Smoking, alcohol and the risk of Dupuytren's contracture. *J Bone Jt Surg* 1997;**79B**: 206–10.

84 Hueston JT. Dupuytren's contracture and specific hand injury. *Med J Aust* 1960;**1**: 1084–5.

85 Liss GM, Stock SR. Can Dupuytren's contracture be work-related? Review of the evidence. *Am J Ind Med* 1996;**29**: 521–32.

86 Bennett B. Dupuytren's contracture in manual workers. *Br J Ind Med* 1982;**39**: 98–100.

87 Mikkelsen OA. Epidemiology of a Norwegian population. In: McFarlane RM, McGrouther DA, Flint MH eds. *Dupuytren's Disease: Biology and Treatment*. New York: Churchill Livingstone, 1990: 191–200.

88 Thomas PR, Clarke D. Vibration white finger and Dupuytren's contracture: Are they related? *J Soc Occup Med* 1992;**42**: 155–8.

89 Cocco PL, Frau P, Rapallo M, Casula D. Occupational exposure to vibrations and Dupuytren's disease: A case-control study. *Med Lav* 1987;**78**: 386–92.

90 Bovenzi M, Cerri S, Merseburger A *et al*. Hand-arm vibration syndrome and dose-response relation for vibration induced white finger among quarry drillers and stonecarvers. *Occup Environ Med* 1994;**51**: 603–11.

91 Cooper C. The epidemiology of osteoarthritis. In: Klipel J, Dieppe P eds. *Rheumatology*. New York: Mosby & Co, 1994: 7.3.1.–7.3.4.

92 Spector TD, Cooper C. Radiographic assessment of osteoarthritis: Whither Kellgren and Lawrence? *Osteoarthr Cartilage* 1993;**1**: 203–6.

93 Felson DT. Epidemiology of hip and knee osteoarthritis. *Epidemiol Rev* 1988;**10**: 1–28.

94 Cooper C, McAlindon T, Snow S *et al*. Mechanical and constitutional risk factors for symptomatic knee osteoarthritis: Differences between medial tibiofemoral

and patellofemoral disease. *J Rheumatol* 1994;**21**: 307–13.

95 Kellgren JH, Lawrence JS. Rheumatism in miners: part II x-ray study. *Br J Ind Med* 1952;**9**: 197–207.

96 Partridge REH, Duthie JJR. Rheumatism in dockers and civil servants: a comparison of heavy manual and sedentary workers. *Ann Rheum Dis* 1968;**27**: 559–68.

97 Wickstrom G, Hanninen K, Mattsson T, *et al*. Knee degeneration in concrete reinforcement workers. *Br J Ind Med* 1983;**40**: 216–9.

98 Lindberg H, Montgomery F. Heavy labour and the occurrence of gonarthrosis. *Clin Orthopaed* 1987; **214**: 235–6.

99 Vingard E, Alfredsson L, Goldie I, Hogstedt C. Occupation and osteoarthrosis of the hip and knee: A register-based cohort study. *Int J Epidemiol* 1991;**20**: 1025–31.

100 Kohatsu ND, Schurman DJ. Risk factors for the development of osteoarthrosis of the knee. *Clin Orthopaed* 1990; **261**: 242–6.

101 Schouten JSAG, Van den Ouweland FA, Valkenburg HA. A 12-year follow-up study in the general population on prognostic factors of cartilage loss in osteoarthritis of the knee. *Ann Rheum Dis* 1992;**51**: 932–7.

102 Bagge E, Bjelle A, Eden S, Svanborg A. Factors associated with radiographic osteoarthritis: Results from the population study 70-year-old people in Goteborg. *J Rheumatol* 1991;**18**: 1218–22.

103 Anderson JJ, Felson DT. Factors associated with osteoarthritis of the knee in the first National Health and Nutrition Examination Survey (HANES I). Evidence for an association with overweight, race, and physical demands of work. *Am J Epidemiol* 1988;**128**: 179–89.

104 Felson DT, Hannan MT, Naimark A *et al*. Occupational physical demands, knee bending, and knee osteoarthritis: Results from the Framingham Study. *J Rheumatol* 1991;**18**: 1587–92.

105 Cooper C, McAlindon T, Coggon D, Egger P, Dieppe P.

Occupational activity and osteoarthritis of the knee. *Ann Rheum Dis* 1994;**53**: 90–3.

106 Croft P, Coggon D, Cruddas M, Cooper C. Osteoarthritis of the hip: An occupational disease in farmers. *Br Med J* 1992;**304**: 1269–72.

107 Croft P, Cooper C, Wickham C, Coggon D. Osteoarthritis of the hip and occupational activity. *Scand J Work Environ Hlth* 1992;**18**: 59–63.

108 Monod H, Scherrer J. The work capacity of a synergic muscle group. *Ergonomics* 1965;**8**: 329–38.

109 Rohmert W. Problems in determining rest allowances. *Appl Ergonom* 1973;**4**: 158–62.

110 Karhu O, Kansi P, Kuorinka I. Correcting working postures in industry: A practical method for analysis. *Appl Ergonom* 1977;**8**: 199–201.

111 McAtamney L, Corlett EN. RULA: a survey method for the investigation of work-related upper limb disorders. *Appl Ergonom* 1993;**24**: 91–9.

112 Kuorinka I, Jonsson B, Kilborn A, et al. Standardised Nordic questionnaire for the analysis of musculoskeletal symptoms. *Appl Ergonom* 1987;**18**: 233–37.

113 Hagberg M, Silverstein B, Wells R *et al*. Health and risk factor surveillance for work related musculoskeletal disorders. In: *Work Related Musculoskeletal Disorders (WMSDs): A Reference Book for Prevention*. Basingstoke: Taylor & Francis, 1995: 213–45.

114 Health and Safety Executive *Health and Safety (Display Screen Equipment) Regulations 1992*. SI 1992/2792. London: HMSO, 1992.

115 Health and Safety Executive. *Display Screen Equipment Work*: *Guidance on Regulations (L26)*. London: HMSO 1992.

116 *Work-related Upper Limb Disorders: A Guide to Prevention*. H5(G) 60. London: HMSO, 1990.

117 Eastmond CJ, Hudson A, Wright V. A radiological survey of the hips and knees in female specialist teachers of physical education. *Scand J Rheumatol* 1979; **8**: 264–8.

23

Back pain and work

MALCOLM IV JAYSON

The magnitude of the back pain problem	477	Primary prevention of back pain	481
The causes of back pain	478	Secondary prevention of back pain	482
Examination and assessment	479	Conclusion	484
Risk factors for the development of back pain	480	References	484

Back pain is a remarkably common but also rapidly increasing cause of disability. Many workers develop back problems in association with their job or may lose time from work as a result of back pain. Often it is difficult to determine whether the work led to the development of back pain or the subject experienced symptoms in the course of undertaking physically demanding tasks.

This chapter will review our current understanding of the epidemiology of the problem, the causes of back pain and of back disability, risk factors for the development of back pain, primary prevention, secondary prevention including treatment, and the recognition and prevention of chronic disability.

THE MAGNITUDE OF THE BACK PAIN PROBLEM

It is important to distinguish between the symptoms of back pain and the disability that results. Back pain is extremely common. There has been little change in its prevalence over the years. In contrast there has been a dramatic increase in disability associated with back problems and it is this which is the major concern of industry today.

Back pain

Back pain is almost a universal experience. At any one time[1] an estimation of the prevalence of any type of back symptom in the preceding week is 42%. Our own studies of the prevalence of back pain lasting for 1 day or longer in the month preceding examination revealed a figure of 39%.[2] The lifetime prevalence is of the order of 60–80%.[3]

Back pain is experienced by people of all ages including children and the elderly. The peak prevalence appears to be in the age group 45–59 years.[1]

Most epidemiological surveys are restricted to back pain with little information about sciatica. The only critical examination for the prevalence of sciatica[4] led to estimates of the overall lifetime prevalence of true sciatica as 5.1% in men and 3.7% in women.

Most back episodes are short-lived with 90% settling and allowing return to work within 6 weeks.[3] However, many of these patients have residual and recurrent problems. The Office of Population Censuses and Surveys' (OPCS).[5] included questions on the duration of back pain and found that a significant proportion of people have continuing problems. In a prospective study persistent disabling pain was found in one-third of subjects in the year after an acute episode.[6] Croft et al.[7] found that in 20% of people who consulted their general practitioner because of back problems this was an exacerbation of a more chronic problem and in 8% it was part of a continuing problem. Biering-Sorenson[8] reported on the likelihood of recurrence in the 12 months following an acute back episode. The longer the time since the last attack the less the chance of recurrence.

Back disability

Interference with work because of back pain is remarkably common. In the OPCS survey[5] 11% of the UK population had their activities restricted by back pain during the previous 4 weeks and it has been calculated that 1.9% of all employed people lose at least 1 day from work in the previous 4 weeks including about 0.3% who are away from work for the entire period.[9] Walsh et al.[10] estimated a 1-year prevalence of work loss at 8.5% and an average duration of work loss of 1.3 days. Overall, the certified numbers of working days lost is of the order of 90 million working days per annum. This does not include self-certification for short periods of work loss. The total work loss has been estimated as 150 million work days per year. The rate of loss of work (Fig 23.1) appears to be increasing in exponential fashion.[9]

Most periods of loss of work are of very short duration but a small proportion of sufferers have prolonged periods away from work and may never return.[3] The longer the person is away from work the less are their chances of returning. Those away from work for a year have only a 25% chance of returning to employment and if away for 2 years only a 10% chance (Fig. 23.2).

In Western societies there has been a dramatic increase in disability benefits for working days lost for back sufferers. Data from the United Kingdom,[9] Sweden[11] and other countries have shown similar increases.

There are, however, signs that the back disability may have peaked. A recent study in North America[12] has shown a fall in annual rates of back pain together with a reduction in the annual claim costs.

The costs of back pain are staggering. The Clinical Standards Advisory Group[9] estimated the annual costs of back pain in the UK as £6 billion. In the USA it was esti-mated as between $50 and $100 billion.[13] Most back episodes are of short duration. There is, however, a small number of subjects with severe and cumulatively very expensive problems. Spengler et al.[14] estimated that 10% of all back injury claims were responsible for 79% of total back injury costs.

THE CAUSES OF BACK PAIN

Most back pain is due to simple mechanical problems in the spine. However, a small proportion arises as a consequence of other disorders. Every patient should be carefully assessed to ensure that important pathology is not missed.

The causes of back pain are classified as shown in Table 23.1. Mechanical problems predominate but in the majority of subjects it is not possible to make a specific diagnosis. Such patients are commonly labelled as having non-specific back pain.

Back pain may be acute, recurrent or chronic. Most acute episodes will resolve rapidly but there is always a risk of recurrence and in some patients this occurs in relation to relatively minor mechanical stresses. Only a small proportion develops chronic pain and disability

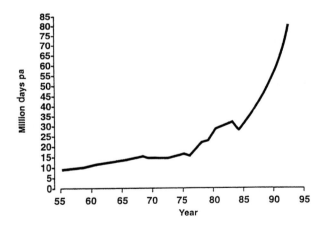

Figure 23.1 *The increase in British Sickness and Invalidity Benefit for back problems from 1955. Reproduced from Ref. 9, with permission of HMSO, London. Crown copyright.*

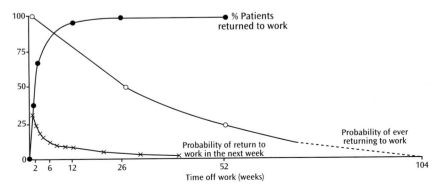

Figure 23.2 *The return to work and the probability of ever returning to work in patients with low back pain. Reproduced from Ref. 3, with permission.*

Table 23.1 *The causes of back pain*

Mechanical
Herniated intervertebral disc
Lumbar spondylosis
Spinal stenosis
Spondylolisthesis
Non-specific

Fibromyalgia

Inflammatory
Ankylosing spondylitis and related spondylarthropathies
Rheumatoid arthritis

Infective
Bacterial including tuberculosis

Metabolic
Osteoporosis
Paget's

Neoplastic
Primary
Secondary

Referred pain
Abdominal and pelvic disorders

Table 23.2 *Simple backache*

Age 20–55 years
Pain in lumbosacral region, buttocks and thighs
Pain is mechanical in nature – varies with physical activity and time
Patient is well
Prognosis is good; 90% recover within 6 weeks

Table 23.3 *Nerve root pain*

Unilateral leg pain worse than back pain
Pain generally radiates to foot or toes
Numbness and/or paraesthesiae in the same distribution
Signs of nerve root irritation – reduced straight leg raising which reproduces the pain.
Motor, sensory or reflex change limited to one nerve root
Prognosis reasonable – 50% recovery from an acute attack within 6 weeks

Table 23.4 *Red flag symptoms suggesting possible serious spinal pathology*

Age at onset less than 20 or over 55 years
Violent trauma – such as a fall from height or a road traffic accident.
Constant progressive non-mechanical pain
Thoracic pain
Patient systemically unwell or weight loss
Past history of cancer, HIV or other serious illness
Use of systemic corticosteroids
Misuse of drugs
Persistent severe restriction of spine movements
Structural deformity
Widespread neurological signs

HIV: Human immunodeficiency virus

Table 23.5 *Indications for emergency referral*

Difficulty with micturition
Loss of anal sphincter tone or incontinence
Saddle anaesthesia around anus, perineum or genitals
Widespread and progressive motor weakness in the lower limbs or disturbed gait

Nerve root pain may be due to herniation of an intervertebral disc. Experimental evidence suggests that disc prolapse occurs as a consequence of pre-existing degeneration with any stress on a weakened disc acting as a final precipitating event. Recovery is less good for nerve root pain than simple backache and a considerable proportion of patients have continuing problems.

If there is any evidence of a cauda equina syndrome such as widespread or advancing neurological signs or the development of bladder or bowel dysfunction an urgent neurosurgical opinion will be necessary (Table 23.5).

EXAMINATION AND ASSESSMENT

A careful clinical history is crucial. This should include the identification of any precipitating factors, the mode of onset of the problem and subsequent progress, the distribution of symptoms in the back and in the lower limbs, aggravation by physical activity or by rest and an assessment of interference with function supplemented by an enquiry into general health.

The physical examination should assess any pain behaviour as well as localizing signs in the back, abnormalities of straight leg raising and neurological signs in the lower limbs.

Investigations are unnecessary for the majority of patients. There is a poor correlation between imaging features of degenerative changes in the spine and the presence of symptoms. The increased details shown by

but it is this group who are responsible for most of the costs associated with back disability.

Acute episodes of back pain may be triaged into simple backache, nerve root pain and possible serious spinal pathology. Simple clinical assessment will identify these three groups (Tables 23.2, 23.3 and 23.4). If there is a red flag which may suggest serious underlying disorder, detailed investigations will be required.

Most patients have simple backache and in these, one generally does not make a specific diagnosis. Most will recover rapidly.

computed tomography and magnetic resonance imaging (MRI) scans frequently add to confusion. Jensen *et al.*[15] found abnormalities in 64% of asymptomatic subjects. Bulges were found in 52% of asymptomatic individuals and 76% of those with back pain and protrusions in 27% of asymptomatic subjects and 54% of those with back pain. The only MRI feature of diagnostic value was an extruded disc found in 1% of asymptomatic individuals but 26% of back pain sufferers. The significance of MRI changes in the intervertebral discs comes into even greater doubt when comparisons are drawn with asymptomatic subjects exposed to similar risk factors. Boos *et al.*[16] compared the appearances in a group of back pain patients and in symptom-free controls with similar age, sex- and work-related risk factors. Disc degeneration was found in 96% of back pain patients and 85% of asymptomatic individuals. The only finding which was statistically significant was nerve root compression which was found in 83% of patients and 22% of controls. The appearances of disc degeneration may therefore reflect normal ageing changes and the effects of physical activity but only bear a very weak relationship to the development of back pain.

Imaging investigations should not be performed for simple back ache. They are indicated when back problems have gone on for more than 6 weeks, if there is any evidence to suggest possible serious spinal pathology or if there are nerve root symptoms and surgery is being considered.

RISK FACTORS FOR THE DEVELOPMENT OF BACK PAIN

Risk factors may be individual and related to the patient, biomechanical related to the job and psychosocial.

Individual risk factors

Although common in both sexes and in all age groups back pain does appear slightly more frequently in women than men and in the age group 45–59 years.[2] There is, however, a further increase in older women possibly due to osteoporosis.[17] There also appear to be associations of back pain with tallness,[8] obesity, smoking and cardiovascular disease.[17,18] There is an association of back pain with numbers of children in the family. This appears to be related to child rearing rather than child bearing as this increased risk appears in men as well as women.[19]

There is contradictory evidence about whether physical fitness and muscle strength predict the risk for future back problems. Battie *et al.*[20] found that those with greater isometric lifting strength had a slightly increased risk of back injuries. On the other hand Battie *et al.*[21] did not find cardiovascular fitness was predictive of future

back injury reports. Mostardi *et al.*[22] tested isokinetic lifting strength in nurses but did not find that this predicted future back injuries.

The best predictor of future back problems is a history of back pain. In our own study,[23] those with a previous history of back pain had double the rate of new episodes than those with no previous back problems. Moreover, neck pain or pain in other musculoskeletal sites also increased the risk of a subsequent episode of back pain. A perception of poor general health and a variety of rather non-specific complaints such as claudication, restlessness or other trouble in the lower limbs, dyspnoea or cough, epigastric pain, stomach rumbling, fatigue, poor sleep, altered bowel consistency also predispose towards the later development of back trouble.[24]

In contrast, radiological abnormalities appear to be poor predictors of back problems.[25]

Biomechanical factors

There is an increased prevalence of back pain in those involved in heavy physical work. Commonly, however, it is difficult to determine whether this is a consequence of repeated physical stresses or the subject has constitutional back problems in which symptoms are experienced on undertaking forceful activities. Reviews describe associations with heavy physical work.[26,27] In particular high spine loading and awkward postures appear associated with back pain.[28,29] There appears to be an association of back pain with prolonged bending and twisting at work. Prolonged exposure to whole body vibration appears associated with back pain.[30] This may be particularly relevant to tractor drivers, users of earth moving equipment and other vehicle drivers. However, in a study of identical twins who were grossly different in terms of lifetime exposure to driving, no differences were found in MRI evidence of the development of disc degeneration.[31]

Frequently, acute back pain arises in relation to some sudden unexpected movement. The stress on the spine may not be great and it is difficult to determine whether this is the consequence of heavy work or alternatively a simple back episode in the patient with a vulnerable spine.

Psychosocial factors

There is increasing evidence that psychological risk factors are important in both predicting the development of back problems and in increasing the risk of the development of chronicity following an acute back episode. A prospective study of pre-employment environmental screening in the Boeing Aircraft Factory in Seattle[32] found that, apart from current or recent back problems, worker dissatisfaction with the job and in particular poor relations with the supervising officer was the only identifiable risk factor for the subsequent development of back pain. The study did not find a relationship between the physical demands of work and future back problems. In our own study in South Manchester[33] there was a significantly increased risk of future development of back pain in subjects free of back problems if there was evidence of psychological distress. The most distressed were 1.8 times more likely to develop a back problem than the least distressed. In particular, dissatisfaction with work, lower social status and perceived inadequency of income are independent risk features for the subsequent development of back pain.[34] In the Netherlands psychosocial work stresses were associated with musculoskeletal complaints including back pain.[35]

Once an acute episode of back pain has developed, psychological distress will predict a poor outcome. Factors such as poor coping strategies and catastrophizing when patients anticipate a poor outcome is in turn associated with a poor prognosis.[36] Premorbid factors including high levels of psychological distress, low levels of physical activity, smoking and dissatisfaction with employment as well as episode-specific factors such as duration of symptoms, pain radiating to the leg, widespread pain and restriction of spinal mobility between strains to predict the development of chronicity of symptoms[6] Early identification of psychological risk factors are important in recognizing subjects likely to develop chronic disability.

The National Advisory Committee on Health and Disability and Accident Rehabilitation and Compensation Insurance Association of New Zealand[37] have formally identified psychosocial 'yellow flags' which indicate when a person is at risk of developing long-term disability and work loss (Table 23.6). Early identification together with appropriate action at an early stage carries the best chance of avoiding long-term problems.

Table 23.6 *Yellow flag symptoms suggesting psychosocial risk factors for long-term disability and work loss*

Attitudes and beliefs about back pain
Pain behaviour
Compensation issues
Diagnosis and treatment factors
Emotional factors
Family factors
Work problems

PRIMARY PREVENTION OF BACK PAIN

Methods of preventing the development of back problems may be divided into pre-employment selection, teaching workers how to protect their backs and reducing the physical demands on the back.

Pre-employment screening

Pre-employment screening has frequently been suggested to try to reduce the risk of employing workers liable to develop back problems.[38-40] These screening efforts have included medical examinations, strength tests and other analyses of physical fitness and radiological examinations. In general they have not been effective in predicting those who will subsequently develop disabling low back pain.[25,38,41]

This approach does raise important ethical issues. The accuracy of prediction of future back problems is poor and many people may unnecessarily be excluded from work. The only effective predictor of future back problems is a previous history of back pain and in particular of periods of work loss due to back pain.

Training workers

Much effort goes into ergonomic training on the correct ways to lift, carry etc. There is an increased risk of back injury for nurses spending more time lifting or in bent or twisted postures.[42] Back training has become an act of faith but a study in nurses failed to show any value for training techniques in preventing back pain.[43] A large-scale randomized controlled trial of an educational programme to prevent work-associated low back injury in postal workers found no long-term benefits in rate of low back injury, the time away from work per injury, the median cost per injury, the rate of related musculoskeletal injuries or the rate of repeated injury after return to work despite the subjects' increased knowledge of pain behaviour.[44]

Exercise programmes appear to be of some value. In a controlled trial, nurses receiving exercise instruction developed fewer new episodes of back pain and less pain-related absenteeism than the group without the exercise regime.[45] Regular exercises at work may help to prevent back episodes but alternatively there may be a selection bias in that those with a back problem are less likely to undertake regular exercise.

Changing the work

Detailed ergonomic advice is provided to industry in an effort to reduce the risk of development of back pain. Measures suggested include:

- Avoiding hazardous manual handling operations as far as is reasonably possible; lifting aids may be appropriate.
- Making appropriate assessment of any hazardous manual handling operations which cannot be avoided.
- Reducing the risks of injury from these operations as far as is reasonably possible.

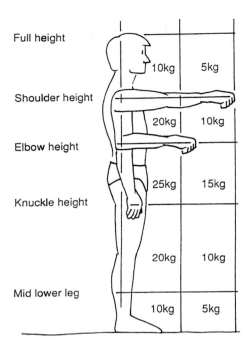

Full height

10kg   5kg

Shoulder height

20kg   10kg

Elbow height

25kg   15kg

Knuckle height

20kg   10kg

Mid lower leg

10kg   5kg

Figure 23.3 *Guidelines on weights that may be lifted. This diagram must be interpreted with caution. Reproduced from Ref. 44, with permission of HMSO, London. Crown Copyright.*

Guidance is often sought on the magnitudes of weight that may be lifted. This has proved a fallacious approach as much depends on the individual and the circumstances of any manoeuvre. The closer a load is held to the trunk the less the stress on the lumbar spine. In approximate terms holding a load at arm's length leads to five times the stress produced by the same load close to the trunk. Moreover, the further away the load from the trunk the less easy it is to control, so adding to the problem.

Guidelines about weights that may be lifted are therefore very crude as there is a wide range of individual physical capabilities even among fit and healthy people. There are no truly safe loads and back problems can develop in relation to quite trivial stresses. The levels shown in the accompanying diagram (Fig. 23.3) are thought to provide reasonable protection to nearly all men and between a half and two-thirds of women, assuming that the load is grasped by both hands, in reasonable working conditions, with the handler in a stable non-twisted body position and for relatively infrequent operations.[46]

Many episodes of pain arise with lesser movements. In these cases it is likely that the spine was vulnerable and at risk of developing problems.

SECONDARY PREVENTION OF BACK PAIN

Early treatment

Most acute back episodes resolve rapidly but a small proportion of patients have persistent problems and many will suffer recurrent episodes of back pain. The early management of acute back pain seems all important. Indeed it is likely that the seeds of chronicity are established within the first few weeks of onset of the problem. The traditional advice of long periods of bed rest until the back recovers appears likely to aggravate back problems and contribute towards the development of chronicity. In a study comparing treatment with 2 days of bed rest and 7 days of bed rest it was the former group who developed less disability and returned to work sooner.[47] A comparison was drawn between a normal period of bed rest, physiotherapy and maintaining normal activity. It was the last group who had the best results.[48]

In treating acute back ache of recent origin the patients are triaged into those with simple back ache, nerve root pain and possible serious spinal pathology. Most are in the first group. A small proportion have sciatica and may require specialist referral and if there is evidence of any serious underlying pathology or widespread neurological problems urgent investigations will be required.

In simple back ache the patients should stay at work if at all possible. If they have to stop work it should be for the shortest possible time and they should be encouraged to return to work as soon as possible. Bed rest should only be prescribed if absolutely essential and then for the shortest period of usually only 1 or 2 days. Analgesics such as paracetamol or ibuprofen are sufficient for the majority of patients. Above all it is important to maintain a positive outlook, to reassure the patients that the symptoms will remit and they should anticipate a full recovery.

The process of encouraging normal activity and minimizing the risk of long-term disability begins in the work place.[49] Employer-based strategies with an empathic approach, on-site symptom relief, one-to-one education in back care and maintaining contact with workers currently away from work lead to significant reductions in sickness absence.

Subacute backache

If the symptoms persist and do not resolve, early physical activation should be prescribed. This may take a wide variety of forms but may include mobilization and manipulation by physiotherapists, osteopaths or chiropractors. Manipulation has been a controversial subject but there now seems general agreement that it hastens the resolution of acute episodes of back pain. It is very doubtful whether it makes any long-term difference to the course of the problem.

Exercises should be recommended. These take a variety of forms including isometric, isodynamic, mobilizing and other exercises. There is no clear evidence that any one type is better than any other. If any particular exercise exacerbates the back pain this should be avoided but otherwise the most important part of the exercise programme appears to be physical activation. Commonly, I advise isometric exercises strengthening the abdominal muscles as these seem least likely to produce exacerbations of the problems. However, evidence comparing the different types of exercise remains controversial.

When symptoms persist for more than 6 weeks it is important to consider psychosocial confounding factors. Excessive distress, catastrophizing, excessive family involvement in the pain situation, work problems and medicolegal claims are all identified as indicating the risk of chronicity. If possible appropriate action should be taken at this stage. Simple reassurance may be all that is required. An aggressive work-conditioning rehabilitation programme combined with reassurance about the importance of returning to work appears effective in reducing morbidity and in improving the return to work rate.[50,51] A thorough clinical and physiotherapy examination educating the patient on the need to overcome the fear of activity, and reassurance about the importance of returning to normal function also appear effective.[52]

Recurrent back pain

Many patients have episodes of acute pain of short duration but make a full recovery between attacks. Sometimes they are able to identify specific precipitating events. If that is the case then these situations should be avoided.

In general, however, subjects require careful ergonomic advice. They should be taught how to lift and carry and avoid excessive stresses on the spine. Isometric exercise programmes are often prescribed although it is uncertain whether they make any specific difference other than give the patient confidence to return to activity.

Chronic back pain

A small proportion of subjects have persistent symptoms and become chronically disabled. In the first instance a careful clinical examination should be undertaken to ensure there is no other pathology which will require specific investigation and treatment. In particular it is important to exclude non-mechanical pathologies and to seek any evidence of nerve root problems which may suggest some form of surgical intervention.

The majority of patients have some evidence of degenerative disease of the lumbar spine. The correlation of imaging evidence of disc degeneration and the presence of back pain is poor and frequently it is difficult to relate the severity of symptoms to objective evidence of spine disease. In many of these patients secondary psychological factors have supervened, leading to chronic disability. This may be mediated by alterations of the central pain processing system within the spinal cord and brain. This is the subject of current ongoing research.

The management of these patients requires an initial careful assessment and includes medical, physical and psychological examinations. Based on these a treatment strategy may be planned.

Modalities that are used include:

1 *Careful selection of pain-relieving medication*
The choice of drugs should be related to the clinical features and underlying problems. Choices include:

- Simple analgesics such as paracetamol. These seem most helpful for patients with pure mechanical type pain aggravated by physical activity but relieved by rest.
- Anti-inflammatory drugs such as ibuprofen or diclofenac. These are used for patients who show an inflammatory type of response. In particular they are indicated in patients with stiffness and aching aggravated by rest and relieved by moving about. Such patients often have quite marked morning stiffness when they first wake up.
- Anti-spasmodics such as baclofen. These are used when there is a lot of muscle spasm.
- Serotonin antagonists such as amitriptyline. These seem helpful for patients with widespread pain and tenderness often associated with distress.
- Anti-epileptic drugs such as carbamazepine or sodium valproate. These are used for patients with neuralgic type pain who may describe electric shock type symptoms radiating into the lower limbs.

Careful consideration should be given to the formulation of the drug and the timing of administration so it is most effective when it is needed.

2 *Physiotherapy treatment with physical activation and encouragement to mobility*
Hydrotherapy may be a useful adjunct as it enables the severely disabled patient to exercise more comfortably.

3 *Various injection techniques are available*
These include local injection of tender points; epidural injections which seem more effective for sciatic pain than back pain; facet joint injections; and acupuncture. Transcutaneous Electrical Nerve Stimulation (TENS) is an electrical method of delivering acupuncture with the advantage that it can be administered by the patient. The specific benefits of these various injection techniques is in some doubt but many patients believe that they are very helpful and rely upon them.

4 *Functional restoration programmes*

A number of centres have established intensive courses of rehabilitation for the chronically disabled back pain patient. The elements of the programme include education on the structure and function of the back, the nature of pain, psychological counselling to reduce distress and progressive physical rehabilitation. Patients learn that inactivity aggravates the physical problems but at the same time have to learn pacing as many have unrealistic expectations and once they start to improve may do too much and then have a relapse. The first such programme, established in Dallas by Mayer et al.[53] reported an 87% rate of return to work against 41% in the control group. Interpretation of that study, however, was difficult as the selection for the programme was placed on the availability of funding from insurance companies. However, similar results were obtained by Hazard et al.[54] in Vermont. These programmes are very intensive and involve full-time treatment usually spread over 3-weeks. As a result they are extremely expensive and many have been discontinued through lack of adequate financial support. Our own approach at the present time is to triage the patients according to the levels of disability and psychosocial distress. For the most disabled patients we provide a 3-week inpatient programme in which there is an emphasis on psychological counselling as described above as well as physical rehabilitation. In contrast, for the patients in whom the physical problem predominates, treatment is on an outpatient basis and a 12-session programme has been developed. The results of this strategy are currently being assessed.

CONCLUSION

In recent years the requirement for heavy manual labour has decreased dramatically and there is increasing regulation in industry to protect workers. Despite this there has been a dramatic increase in disability associated with back pain. There has not been any significant change in the underlying pathological problems in the spine or indeed in the incidence of back pain. Rather it is the reaction of workers which has led to this dramatic increase in disability. Concerns by both employees and employers, family pressures, medicolegal problems and other psychosocial factors appear to be the principal causes of this dramatic change. Primary prevention such as pre-employment screening, ergonomic training and guidelines have only been of limited value. Secondary prevention seems more effective. Most important is the early management of back pain as the seeds of chronicity are sown within the first few weeks. Early physical activation with limited, if any, bed rest and return to work at the earliest possible stage appear fundamental. If the problem does not resolve, the patient should receive treatment from a physiotherapist, osteopath or chiro-

practor with the emphasis on physical rehabilitation and attention should be paid to possible psychosocial factors. Ergonomic advice and prevention of excessive stresses on the spine is important for those with recurrent back problems and for chronic back pain intensive rehabilitation programmes combining both physical rehabilitation and psychological counselling seem helpful. With this approach there is hope that the current back pain epidemic will be controlled.

REFERENCES

1 Rossignol M, Lortie M, Ledoux E. Comparison of spinal health indicators in predicting spinal status in a one-year longitudinal study. *Spine* 1993; **18**: 54–60.
2 Papageorgiou AC, Croft PR, Ferry S, Jayson MIV, Silman AI. Estimating the prevalence of low back pain in the general population. *Spine* 1995; **20**: 1889–94.
3 Waddell G. A new clinical model for the treatment of low back pain. *Spine* 1987; **12**: 632–44.
4 Heliovaara M, Impivaara O, Sievers K, Melkas T, Knekt P et al. Lumbar disc syndrome in Finland. *J Epidemiol Publ Hlth* 1987; **41**: 251–8.
5 Mason V. *The Prevalence of Back Pain in Great Britain.* London: HMSO, 1994.
6 Thomas EJ, Silman AJ, Croft PR, Papageorgiou AC, Jayson MIV, MacFarlane GJ. Predicting who develops chronic low back pain in primary care: a prospective study. *Br Med J* 1999; **318**: 1662–67.
7 Croft P, Joseph S, Cosgrove S, Jordan L, Papageorgiou A et al. *Low Back Pain in the Community and Hospitals.* A report to the Clinical Standards Advisory Group. Manchester: Arthritis and Rheumatism Council Epidemiology Research Unit and Rheumatic Diseases Centre, University of Manchester, 1994.
8 Biering-Sorenson F. Physical measurements as risk indicators for low back trouble over a one-year period. *Spine* 1984; **9**: 106–19.
9 Clinical Standards Advisory Group. *Epidemiology Review: The Epidemiology and Costs of Back Pain.* London: HMSO, 1994.
10 Walsh K, Cruddas M, Coggan D. Low back pain in eight areas of Britain. *J Epidemiol Commun Hlth* 1992; **46**: 227–30.
11 Nachemson A. Newest knowledge of low back pain: a critical look. *Clin Orthopaed Rel Res* 1992; **279**: 8–20.
12 Murphy PL, Violinn E. Is occupational back pain on the rise? *Spine* 1999; **24**: 691–7.
13 Frymoyer JW, Durrett CL. The economics of spinal disorders. In: *The Adult Spine: Principles and Practice* Vol. 8. Philadelphia: Lippincott-Raven, 1997;143–50.
14 Spengler D, Bigos SJ, Martin NA, Zeh J, Fisher L, Naachemson A. Back injuries in industry: a retrospective study. 1. Overview and cost analysis. *Spine* 1986; **11**: 241–51.
15 Jensen MC, Brant-Zawadzki MN, Obuchososki N, Modic MT,

Malkasian D, Ross JS. Magnetic resonance imaging of the lumbar spine in people without back pain. *N Engl J Med* 1994; **331**: 69–73.

16 Boos N, Reider R, Schade V, Spratt KF, Semmer N, Aebi M. The diagnostic accuracy of magnetic resonance imaging, work perception and psychosocial factors in identifying symptomatic disc herniations. *Spine* 1995; **20**: 2613–25.

17 Wright D, Barrow S, Fisher AD, Horseley SD, Jayson MIV. Influence of physical, psychological and behavioural signs on consultations for back pain. *Br J Rheumatol* 1995; **34**: 156–61.

18 Deyo RA, Bass JE. Lifestyle and low-back pain. The influence of smoking and obesity. *Spine* 1989; **14**: 501–6.

19 Silman AJ, Ferry S, Papageorgiou AC, Jayson MIV, Croft PR. Numbers of children as a risk factor for back pain in men and women. *Arthr Rheum* 1995; **38**: 1232–5.

20 Battie MC, Bigos, SJ, Fisher LD, Hansson TH, Jones MC, Wortley MD. Isometric lifting strength as a predictor of industrial back pain reports. *Spine* 1989; **14**: 851–6.

21 Battie MR, Bigos SJ, Fisher LD, Hansson TH, Nachemson AL *et al*. A prospective study of the role of cardiovascular risk factors and fitness in industrial back complaints. *Spine* 1989; **14**: 141–7.

22 Mostardi RA, Noe DA, Kovacik MW, Porterfield JA. Isokinetic lifting strength and occupational injury. A prospective study. *Spine* 1992; **17**: 189–93.

23 Papageorgiou AC, Croft PR, Thomas E, Ferry S, Jayson MIV, Silman AJ. Influence of previous pain experience on the episode incidence of low back pain: results from the South Manchester Back Pain Study. *Pain* 1996; **66**: 181–5.

24 Biering-Sorenson F, Thomson C. Medical, social and occupational history as risk indicators for low back pain in a general population. *Spine* 1986; **11**: 720–25.

25 Gibson ES. The value of pre-placement screening radiography of the low back. *Occup Med State Art Rev* 1988; **3**: 91–107.

26 Kelsey JL, Golden AL. Occupational and work place factors associated with low back pain. *Occup Med State Art Rev* 1988; **3**: 7–16.

27 Garg A, Moore JS. Epidemiology of low back pain in industry. *Occup Med State Art Rev* 1992; **7**: 593–607.

28 Marras WS, Lavender SPC, Leurgans SE, Rajulu SL, Allread WG *et al*. The role of dynamic three dimensional trunk motion in occupationally-related low back disorders: the effect of workplace factors, trunk position and trunk characteristics on risk of injury. *Spine* 1993; **18**: 617–28.

29 Punnett L, Fine LJ, Keyserling WM, Herrin GD, Chaffin DB. Back disorders and non-neutral trunk postures of automobile assembly workers. *Scand J Work Environ Hlth* 1991; **17**: 337–46.

30 Hulshof C, van Zanten BV. Whole body vibration and low back pain. *Int Arch Occup Environ Hlth* 1987; **59**: 205–20.

31 Battie MC, Videman T, Manninen H, Gill K, Pope M, Gibbons L. The effects of lifetime exposure to occupational driving on lumbar disc degeneration. *Int Soc Study Lumbar Spine* 1997; **46**(Abstr).

32 Bigos SJ, Battie MC, Spengler DM, Fisher LD, Fordyce WE et al. A prospective study of work perceptions and psychosocial factors affecting the report of back injury. *Spine* 1991; **16**: 1–6.

33 Croft PR, Papageorgiou AC, Ferry S, Thomas E, Jayson MIV, Silman AJ. Psychological distress and low back pain. *Spine* 1995; **20**: 2731–7.

34 Papageorgiou AC, Macfarlane GFJ, Thomas E, Croft PR, Jayson MIV, Silman AJ. Psychosocial factors in the work place – do they predict new episodes of low back pain? Evidence from the South Manchester Back Pain Study. *Spine* 1997; **22**: 1137–42.

35 Houtman ILD, Bongers PM, Smulders PGW, Kompier MAJ. Psychosocial stressors at work and musculoskeletal problems. *Scand J Work Environ Hlth* 1994; **20**: 139–45.

36 Burton AK, Tillotson KM, Main CJ, Hollis S. Psychosocial predictors of outcome in acute and subacute low back trouble. *Spine* 1995; **20**: 722–8.

37 National Advisory Council on Health and Disability and Accident Rehabilitation and Compensation Insurance Corporation of New Zealand. *Guide to Assessing Psychosocial Yellow Flags in Acute Low Back Pain: Risk Factors for Long-term Disability and Work Loss*. NZ. NACD, 1997.

38 Garg A, Moore JS. Prevention strategies and the low back in industry. *Occup Med State Art Rev* 1992; **7**: 629–40.

39 Halpern M Prevention of low back pain: basic ergonomics in the work place and the clinic. *Bailliére's Clin Rheumatol* 1992; **6**: 705–30.

40 Reimer DS, Halbrook BD, Dreyfuss PH, Tibiletti C. A novel approach to pre-employment worker fitness evaluation in a material handling industry. *Spine* 1994; **19**: 20 26–32.

41 Bigos SJ, Battie MC, Fisher LD, Hansson TH, Spengler DM, Nachemson AL. A prospective evaluation of pre-employment screening methods for acute industrial back pain. *Spine* 1992; **17**: 922–6.

42 Videman T, Nurminen T, Tola S, Kuorinka I, Vanharanta H, Troup JDG. Low back pain in nurses and some loading factors of work. *Spine* 1984; **9**: 400–4.

43 Harber P, Pena L, Hsu P, Billet E, Greer D, Kim K. Personal history, training and worksite as predictors of back pain of nurses. *Am J Ind Med* 1994; **25**: 519–26.

44 Daltroy LH, Iverson MD, Larson MG, Lew R, Wright E A controlled trial of an educational programme to prevent low back injuries. *New Engl J Med* 1997; **337**: 322–8.

45 Gundewall B, Liljeqvist M, Hansson T Primary prevention of back symptoms and absence from work: a propective randomised study amongst hospital employees. *Spine* **18**: 587–94.

46 Health & Safety Executive Manual Handling: *Guidance on Regulations*. London: HMSO, 1992.

47 Deyo RA, Diehl AK, Rosenthal M. How many days of bed rest for acute low back pain? A randomised clinical trial. *New Engl J Med* 1986; **315**: 1064–70.

48 Malmivaara M, Hakkinen U, Aro T, Heinrichs ML, Koskenniemi L *et al*. The treatment of acute low back pain-bed rest, exercise or ordinary activity? *New Engl J Med* 1995; **332**: 351–5.

49 Battie MC. Minimising the impact of back pain: Workplace strategies. *Semin Spine Surg* 1992; **4**: 20–8.

50 Agency for Health Care Policy and Research, Clinical Practice Guideline no.14. *Acute Low Back Problems in Adults: Assessment and Treatment*, Rockville MD: US Dept of Health and Human Services, 1994.

51 Lindstrom, I, Ohlund C, Eek C, Wallin L, Petersen L-E *et al*. The effect of graded activity on patients with subacute low back pain: a randomised prospective clinical study with an operant-conditioning behavioural approach. *Phys Ther* 1992; **72**: 279–90.

52 Indahl A, Velund L, Reikeraas O. Good prognosis for low back pain when left untampered: randomised clinical trial. *Spine* 1995; **20**: 473–7.

53 Mayer T, Gatchel R, Mayer H. A prospective two-year study of functional restoration in industrial low back injury: An objective assessment procedure. *JAMA* 1987; **258**: 1763–7.

54 Hazard RG, Fenwick JW, Kalisch SM, Redmond J, Reeves V *et al*. Functional restoration with behavioural support. A one-year prospective study of patients with chronic low-back pain. *Spine* 1989; **14**: 157–61.

Part 5

Diseases associated with microbial agents

Occupation and infectious diseases 489
Genetic modification and biotechnology 521

Part 3

Diseases associated with
microbial agents

24

Occupation and infectious diseases

JULIA HEPTONSTALL, ANNE COCKCROFT, ROBERT MM SMITH

Zoonoses	489	Rabies	499
Prevention and control	490	Streptococcosis	499
Occupational zoonotic infections	490	Toxoplasmosis	500
Food-borne zoonotic infections	493	Transmissible spongiform encephalopathies	500
Hantavirus infections	494	Zoonotic skin diseases	501
Hydatid disease	495	Other occupational infections	502
Leptospirosis	495	Health care workers and related occupations	502
Listeriosis	496	Laboratory research workers and animal handlers	512
Lyme disease	496	Infections associated with occupational travel	512
Newcastle disease	498	Others	514
Nipah virus infection	498	References	515
Q fever	498		

Infectious diseases remain a significant occupational hazard, although the organisms involved have changed over time. Infections that are largely only of historic interest in developed countries may remain very much an issue in developing countries, where 'new' infections are at least as much of a problem as in the developed world but may pass unrecognized because facilities for diagnosis and surveillance are lacking. Although it is true that many infections, particularly those caused by bacteria, fungi or parasites, are now treatable, this should not lead to complacency or lack of suitable precautions and preventive measures; witness the treatment problems of multidrug-resistant tuberculosis, hepatitis B and human immunodeficiency virus (HIV). Certain occupations continue to carry a significant risk of infections, either specific to the occupation or common in the general population but occurring at an increased rate in those with occupational exposure.

ZOONOSES

Zoonoses are infections that are transmissible from animals to man. The World Health Organization lists some 150 bacterial and viral zoonoses and about 60 parasitic zoonoses,[1] of which around 35 are known to occur in the United Kingdom.

In developed countries, many of the infections that used to be commonly transmitted from animals to man, such as bovine tuberculosis and anthrax, have disappeared or are now very uncommon. In other parts of the world, however, people live in close association with their domestic animals, often in conditions that provide opportunities for zoonotic infection.

Three main groups of workers are at risk of occupationally acquired zoonotic infection:

- those whose jobs involve direct contact with domestic or wild animals or their products – including farmers and agricultural workers, veterinarians, abattoir workers and slaughtermen, poultry workers, butchers and fishmongers, tanners, rodent trappers, zoologists and research laboratory workers;
- clinical laboratory workers, who may be exposed to specimens from infected patients;
- those whose work involves travel to higher prevalence areas; this group includes members of the armed forces and aid workers. Workers whose jobs may not at first appear to place them at risk may be incidentally exposed to infection, as, for example, a builder who undertakes the reconstruction of an aviary.

Prevention and control

Where practicable, employers should prevent the exposure of employees to health hazards. Most of the following discussion on prevention and control is relevant to people working directly with animals. The measures needed to protect laboratory workers from occupationally acquired infections have been outlined by the Advisory Committee on Dangerous Pathogens.[2]

Workers should be trained to avoid infection risks. Training should be appropriate to the employee's role, education and experience and should equip the employee to master a skill before encountering a hazard. Relevant training topics include: the safe handling of animals and animal products; the safe disposal of carcasses and animal waste; personal hygiene (including the importance of covering cuts and grazes promptly with waterproof dressings, of regular and correct hand washing, and of avoiding contact between unwashed hands and the mouth, eyes or face) and the appropriate use of personal protective equipment.

Goggles will protect the eyes; face shields will protect both the eyes and mucous membranes from splashes involving contaminated material. Overalls or work wear will help prevent contamination of street clothing. These should be changed when visibly soiled and laundered appropriately. Gloves provide a barrier protection for hands although they cannot protect against unintentional injuries from sharp implements. Nylon or steel mesh gloves may prevent injury during butchering. Knives and sharp implements should be handled and stored correctly.

Gloves, overalls and facemasks should be worn when slaughtering animals or dressing carcasses with thorough washing of hands and arms in soapy water after handling the animals or carcasses. Urine, faeces, blood and other body fluids should be washed from floors, work surfaces and other equipment and these areas disinfected using a 1:100 dilution of household bleach in tap water, peroxide at 5:100 or a saponified mixture of cresol and oil (Lysol®) at 1:100 dilution. Dust in lairage and slaughter areas should be kept to a minimum; manure should be removed promptly and yard facilities for livestock should, ideally, be away from human habitation

Reducing the prevalence of infection in reservoir species may reduce the risks to workers. In the UK, for example, test and slaughter policies in cattle herds have virtually eliminated the risks of bovine tuberculosis and brucellosis. Stock certification and stock vaccination (for example, against Newcastle disease) may also be useful. Effective quarantine measures minimize the risks of introducing new disease into established herds, flocks or colonies; quarantine periods should be long enough to allow the expression of any diseases present.

Vaccination may be indicated for specific groups of workers, for example, pre-exposure rabies vaccine for those working with animals in quarantine kennels, or anthrax vaccine for those working in hide-processing. Female workers in direct contact with animals (e.g. veterinary nurses and shepherdesses) may require specific advice on prevention of infection in pregnancy, particularly toxoplasmosis and chlamydiosis.

Health warning cards provide a means of giving advice and information to employees and should be carried at all times. They may also be useful in alerting medical practitioners to the possibility of a more serious infection whilst treating symptoms which may otherwise be attributed to more common ailments.

In recent years many farmers have diversified into the tourist/leisure industry by allowing public access to their farms. City or urban farms, animal sanctuaries, open rural farms and other educational and recreational facilities have become familiar features in many communities. The likelihood of members of the public becoming infected from the livestock or the farm environment appears to be small, but incidents have been reported with increasing frequency.[3] Cases of cryptosporidiosis, infection with *Escherichia coli* O157 followed by haemolytic uraemic syndrome, cowpox and orf have been reported. Farmers now need to consider health risks to visitors, especially vulnerable groups, such as young children and pregnant women, and the precautions necessary to protect them. Recommendations on these precaustions have been published.[4]

Occupational zoonotic infections

ANTHRAX

Anthrax is now uncommon in animals in countries that enforce strict quarantine laws and practise preventive vaccination.[5] It is caused by *Bacillus anthracis* and spread through its spores, which may be found in the carcasses of infected animals and in animal products such as wool, hair, hides, meat, skins, bones and bonemeal. Soil can become contaminated by the spores, which may survive for many years. Animal anthrax may also be spread by the use of infected animal feed.

Most human cases of anthrax (wool-sorter's disease) are now seen in Africa, the Middle East and southern Asia. It is usually contracted through contact with infected animals or contaminated animal byproducts. In the UK, where anthrax is now very rare, recently reported cases have occurred in people working directly or indirectly with animal products imported from epizootic regions. Those at occupational risk include veterinarians, farmers, slaughtermen, agricultural and rendering plant workers and workers in byproduct processing firms such as carpet factories, tanneries, fertilizer plants and bristle and brush manufacturers. Travellers to endemic countries who purchase items made of animal skin, hair or wool may also be at risk of exposure.

Cutaneous anthrax accounts for over 95% of cases, occurring when the infectious organism enters a cut or an abrasion. After an incubation period of 2–7 days, a small papule develops. This becomes vesicular, and over 24–48 hours, enlarges to form an ulcer with a characteristically black necrotic centre (an eschar), which is usually surrounded by considerable oedema, and accompanied by fever and local lymphadenopathy. In pulmonary anthrax, caused by inhalation of the organism, non-specific symptoms of an upper respiratory tract infection are followed by a rapid deterioration in respiratory function, severe breathlessness, prostration and shock. If untreated, the condition of pulmonary anthrax is rapidly fatal. The diagnosis of anthrax is made by culture of swabs of lesions, blood or sputum. Intestinal anthrax (acquired after eating infected meat) may also occur. Parenteral penicillin, to which the organism is highly sensitive, remains the treatment of choice for all forms of the disease.[6] Tetracycline may be used as an alternative in those allergic to penicillin.

In the UK, immunization is recommended only for workers at risk of exposure to the disease, such as those working in abattoirs or rendering plants and in wool or hide-processing plants, Environmental Health Officers, Meat Hygiene Inspectors and veterinarians. Hair, wool, hides and bonemeal should be sterilized or disinfected before processing. Control of dust and proper ventilation are essential facets of risk reduction in industries that handle raw animal fibres. Covering cuts or abrasions with waterproof dressings will reduce individual exposure to the risk of skin infection.

Anthrax is a prescribed disease (see Chapter 4).

BRUCELLOSIS

Around 500 000 cases of brucellosis are estimated to occur worldwide each year. The incidence varies widely. In some countries, including the UK, livestock are free from infection and infections in humans are likely to have been acquired abroad. Diagnosis is not difficult if the level of suspicion is high and the presentation is typical, but the varied and sometimes misleading manifestations of localized, subacute or chronic infection, mean that cases may be misdiagnosed.[7] Three species are of major importance:

Brucella abortus is found in cattle farming areas throughout the world. It has now been eradicated from cattle populations in some countries but continues to cause significant livestock losses and present significant human health risks in many less developed countries. Eradication schemes have more often been prompted by the substantial economic benefits of improved animal health than by the risks to human health. However, the substantial decline in the numbers of human cases in the UK, northern Europe, Japan and Israel is attributable to pasteurization of milk and milk products and to mass testing of cattle and slaughter of infected herds.

Brucella melitensis has a limited geographic distribution and is found primarily where intensive sheep and goat farming cultures exist. In Europe, *B. melitensis* is largely confined to the Mediterranean region and eastern Europe. Control programmes have greatly reduced the prevalence of this species in many countries, but no country has successfully eradicated the disease. Sheep, goats and their products remain the major source of infection, but *B. melitensis* has emerged as an important problem in cattle in some southern European countries and in Israel, Kuwait and Saudi Arabia.

Brucella suis is not found in pigs in the UK, but has been identified in pigs in the USA and in southern Europe. In countries in the Middle East, North Africa and Asia human infection is rare where pork is not part of the local diet. In some South American countries, especially Brazil and Colombia, *B. suis* biovar 1 has become established in cattle which are now more important than pigs as a source of human infection.[8] Other species may only present serious zoonotic hazards in a restricted number of countries.

Infection may be acquired through contact of the organism with the conjunctivae or abraded skin, by aerosol inhalation or by ingestion. Veterinary surgeons and farmers may become infected after exposure to vaginal discharges, placentae, or fetal membranes from infected animals; infection in abattoir workers may follow exposure to infected animal carcasses. Infection can also follow consumption of unpasteurized milk or milk products (e.g. sheep or goats cheese) from endemic areas; business travellers may therefore be at risk of infection. Clinical laboratory workers may be infected through exposure to clinical specimens or cultures; infection has occurred after misidentification of *Brucella* spp. as another, less pathogenic, species.[9] A laboratory-acquired infection with a recently isolated *Brucella* strain (G Fosten, pers. comm.), tentatively named *Brucella maris*, suggests that this type may be pathogenic for humans. Infection could result from occupational contact with infected seals or other marine mammals.

Results of serological surveys in high-risk groups suggest that perhaps a third of infections are subclinical. The incubation period ranges from 1 week to 7 months. Clinical features of infection are variable and include fever which is sometimes intermittent (undulant fever) and often accompanied by rigors, generalized aches and pains, headaches, anorexia and lassitude. The onset of the acute infection may be sudden, with high fever and rigors on the first day, or more insidious, the fever and malaise peaking after about 1–2 weeks. The acute illness usually resolves within 2–3 weeks, with or without treatment. Infection by any of the strains of *Brucella* may lead to chronicity, often associated with intense fatigue. The symptoms of chronic brucellosis, which may last for years, are often non-specific and include malaise, tiredness with little or no fever. Depression may also be prominent but it is important to recognize that in the absence of focal signs or unequivocal laboratory evidence of disease (other than persistence of antibodies in low titre) patients with neuropsychiatric symptoms are more likely to be suffering from primary depressive illness than chronic brucellosis. Localization of infection may become apparent at any time in the course of the disease.

No single physical sign is invariably present and fever is often absent even in patients whose symptoms have been present for several months. Splenomegaly, hepatomegaly and lymphadenopathy are most frequently observed in the first weeks of illness but are commonly absent. Transient skin rashes can occur. The spleen is sometimes also palpable in patients with more chronic illness.

Arthralgia is a common symptom of brucellosis and synovitis is among the most common forms of localization. The spine and knees are frequently involved. Spinal disease begins as an anterior spondylitis and may extend to involve the adjacent vertebral bodies, but in contrast to tuberculosis vertebral collapse is unusual. The lumbar spine is most frequently involved followed by the cervical and then the thoracic spines. Patients usually present with low back pain and other symptoms including fever, anorexia, apathy and depression. The pain, which may develop suddenly or insidiously, is usually aggravated by movement. An extradural inflammatory mass can develop and cause spinal cord compression. As with other bone infections, radiographs may show no abnormality until about 3 months after the onset of symptoms when evidence of bone destruction becomes apparent. Radioisotope bone scans may show abnormalities at an earlier stage. Osteitis can also involve long bones and bones of the hand. Synovial fluid from affected joints usually contains increased numbers of polymorphonuclear leucocytes and biopsies of the synovium can show non-caseating granulomata. Slight increases in serum transaminases and alkaline phosphatase are common but overt hepatitis is unusual. Non-caseating granulomata are commonly present in liver biopsies. Orchitis is relatively common. More serious manifestations of localized infection include meningitis, which may resemble tuberculous meningitis with a gradual onset and the development of cranial nerve palsies, endocarditis, and hepatic and splenic abscess.

Brucellosis is a prescribed disease (see Chapter 4).

Laboratory confirmation of the diagnosis, which may also indicate the source of the infection, is by serology and culture of the organism from blood, bone marrow, pus or infected tissue. A positive culture is diagnostic of infection as is the finding of a high antibody titre in a patient from a non-endemic area who gives a history of possible exposure. Blood cultures may take up to 6 weeks to become positive, so the laboratory must be forewarned of the possible diagnosis to prevent the culture from being discarded prematurely. Specialist interpretation of serological results may help to prevent the mislabelling of depressive illness as chronic brucellosis.

Drugs recommended for treatment, which may need to be prolonged, include tetracycline or doxycycline in combination with streptomycin or rifampicin. Cotrimoxazole has been used as an alternative and the organisms are also sensitive to aminoglycosides. Relapse may occur in around 10% of treated acute infections; it may be more common after shorter treatment regimens and after single drug therapy.[10–12] Combined medical and surgical treatment (e.g. for abscesses) may be required.

CHLAMYDIOSIS

Human infection due to *Chlamydia psittaci* occurs throughout the world, mainly affecting those exposed to infected psittacines (parrots, parakeets, cockatiels and budgerigars) or other birds (especially ducks, turkeys and pigeons) or to infected animals, especially sheep.

Avian chlamydiosis

Avian chlamydiosis occurs naturally in many wild and domestic birds. Human infection was first termed psittacosis, since it was acquired from psittacine birds. When non-psittacine birds are the source, the term ornithosis is used. Natural reservoirs include waterfowl, seabirds, shore and wading birds, pheasants and pigeons. Domestic birds may harbour the organism without showing any signs of infection. The International Animal Health Code and the EC Council directive 92/65/EEC lay down specific trade and import conditions for health certification and sourcing of psittacine birds. Transport stress may cause recrudescence in carrier birds; some, but not all, will develop symptoms during quarantine and be eliminated. Healthy carriers, however, probably present less of a hazard to human health.

Human infection follows inhalation of aerosols contaminated by infected avian faeces or fomites. Exposure may occur during evisceration of carcasses, or when handling pet birds or cleaning out birdcages. Serological surveys suggest that infection may often be subclinical or pass undiagnosed. Outbreaks have occurred in poultry processing workers, veterinarians and pet shop workers. Taxidermists may also be at risk.

The incubation period is usually 7–14 days but may range from 4 to 39 days. The onset of illness may be abrupt or insidious. Symptoms include headache, chills, fever and a non-productive cough. Chest signs may be limited, with little evidence of consolidation, but the chest radiograph will typically show evidence of interstitial pneumonitis with patchy or streaky shadowing. Extrapulmonary manifestations, including abdominal pain, vomiting, hepatitis, endocarditis and Stevens-Johnson syndrome may occur.[13,14] The infection may be more severe in the elderly. The diagnosis is confirmed by serological testing. Identification of the precise source of infection may be difficult as exposure may be from a single contact, from multiple sporadic contacts, or may be continual as in the case of breeders and carers. Colleagues or family members who may have been exposed to the same source of infection should be made aware of the need to report symptoms promptly. Tetracycline, doxycyline or erythromycin are the usual antibiotics of choice. Treatment should be continued for 12–14 days to reduce the possibility of relapse, which will require a second course of treatment.

Avian chlamydiosis is a prescribed disease (see Chapter 4).

Ovine enzootic abortion

Ovine enzootic abortion (OEA, or enzootic abortion of ewes, EAE) was first described in Scottish sheep in 1936 and recognized as a human pathogen in 1954.[15] It is now known to have a worldwide distribution. Infection in pregnant ewes causes abortion or the premature delivery of weak lambs. Large numbers of elementary bodies (an infectious cell type) are shed in fetal fluids and placentae from infected sheep. Sheep may excrete chlamydiae in the faeces and in fetal and placental products of subsequent pregnancies. Thus, sheep that are apparently healthy may be a source of infection. In the UK, over 80% of reported ovine cases occur in the lambing season between January and March, when the risk of human exposure is increased.

Human infection in pregnancy was first described by Giroud et al. in 1956.[16] Ovine chlamydiae probably possess a tropism for placental trophoblasts, which may explain the severity of the illness in pregnant women. Shepherdesses and farmer's wives may be exposed when delivering or bottle feeding infected lambs, and then develop a severe septicaemic illness which has a significant maternal and fetal mortality rate.[17] Women farm workers who are or may be pregnant should not participate in the lambing process.[18] The diagnosis should be considered in any pregnant woman who has been exposed to sheep, especially around lambing time, who presents with a severe febrile illness. Treatment, with parenteral erythromycin, should not await laboratory confirmation of the diagnosis, which is made by serology or by direct immunofluorescence of fetal or placental tissue.

A number of C. psittaci infections in other farm workers have been ascribed to contact with lambing or aborting ewes.[19] Infection is sporadic and no outbreaks have been reported. However, the widespread presence of antibodies to Chlamydia in sheep handlers without a history of associated disease suggests that many human infections are subclinical. Symptoms of a mild upper respiratory tract infection in workers handling sheep or sheep products should suggest the possibility of infection with C psittaci. Laboratory-acquired infection has

also been reported. Treatment is with tetracycline, doxycycline, or erythromycin.

Ovine chlamydiosis is a prescribed disease (see Chapter 4).

Food-borne zoonotic infections

All the enteric pathogens that have reservoirs in food, companion animals and exotic species of animals, birds or reptiles may be transmitted to humans where there is direct contact between humans and the natural host, or its faeces. Working on or visiting farms has been associated with the acquisition of infections with Salmonella spp., Campylobacter spp. and Cryptosporidium. Companion animals such as dogs and cats can act as a source of several pathogens, including Campylobacter spp., Salmonella spp. and Giardia spp. Exotic reptiles such as snakes and terrapins have also been associated with human cases of salmonellosis.

CAMPYLOBACTER

Occupationally related Campylobacter infections appear to be common in poultry workers, farmers and slaughtermen[20] and in kitchen workers handling poultry.[21] The majority of cases are sporadic; infection is most common in young adults.[22]

This acute enteric infection is of variable severity, and is characterized by diarrhoea, abdominal pain, malaise, fever and vomiting. In the severe form a prodromal state occurs which may last up to 2 days, during which the patient feels increasingly unwell and may develop a temperature of over 40°C. Occasionally this may be accompanied by confusion, delirium and rigors. Abdominal pain may precede the diarrhoea (typically watery or slimy, foul smelling and which may contain fresh blood), and be sufficiently severe to lead to an erroneous diagnosis of acute abdomen, needing laparotomy. Most infections, however, are self-limiting. As with other bacterial gastrointestinal infections, patients can develop a reactive arthritis which usually presents 1–2 weeks after the onset of illness, typically affects the sacroiliac joints or knees and can persist for several months. Erythromycin, if given early in the illness, may shorten the duration of diarrhoeal symptoms.

ESCHERICHIA COLI O157

The main reservoir of E.coli O157 is the intestine of healthy cattle. Consequently, beef is the human food source most likely to harbour the organism. E. coli O157 can also be present in milk, on fruit, or on vegetables that have come into contact with bovine faeces. It has been detected in around 3% of sheep at slaughter,[23] and there have been reports of detection in goats[24] and horses.[25] A detailed review of the pathogenesis, epidemiology, clinical features and diagnosis of *E. coli* 157 infection is given elsewhere.[26]

The infectious dose appears to be very low, and is probably less than 100 organisms. Humans usually become infected through the consumption of contaminated foods, particularly inadequately cooked minced beef (often in the form of beefburgers) and milk (unpasteurized or contaminated after pasteurization). Animal carcasses become contaminated through contact with intestinal contents at slaughter. Infection may also be spread by direct contact and person to person within families. Both outbreaks and sporadic cases have been linked microbiologically with the handling of animals, particularly cattle.

Symptoms range from mild diarrhoea to bloody diarrhoea (haemorrhagic colitis) and haemolytic uraemic syndrome (HUS) and are the effect of a verocytotoxin (VT) produced by the organism. Haemorrhagic colitis presents as bloody diarrhoea often accompanied by severe abdominal pain, usually without fever and only moderate dehydration; HUS is characterized by acute renal failure, haemolytic anaemia and thrombocytopenia. In Britain this is now the major cause of acute renal failure in children and HUS develops in up to 10% of patients infected with O157 VTEC. Some patients, usually adults, develop thrombotic thrombocytopenic purpura (TTP) in which the clinical features of HUS are seen together with neurological complications. The incubation period for O157 VTEC infection before the onset of diarrhoea can range from 1 to 14 days (median 3–4 days). Symptoms usually resolve within 2 weeks except in cases of HUS or TTP. Fatality rates ranging from 1 to 5% have been reported, with much higher rates in outbreaks involving the elderly. Treatment is essentially supportive. Administration of antimotility agents or narcotics may delay clearance of the pathogen, increasing toxin absorption[27] and the risk of developing HUS.

CRYPTOSPORIDIOSIS

Cryptosporidiosis is caused by a protozoan parasite, *Cryptosporidium parvum* whose main animal reservoirs are sheep, cattle, deer and goats.[28] It is acquired by ingestion of oocysts excreted in human or animal faeces, by drinking contaminated water or milk and by case-to-person contact. The oocysts, which are shed in large numbers by an infected host, are highly resistant, and can survive for months in cool, dark conditions in moist soil, or for up to a year in clean water. They are resistant to disinfectants commonly used domestically or in animal husbandry.

Infections may be asymptomatic. In normally healthy individuals cryptosporidiosis is usually characterized by an acute, self-limiting diarrhoeal illness, commonly of 2–3 weeks duration. In people who are immunosuppressed, including those with AIDS or malnutrition, the infection may cause severe and protracted illness.

Diagnosis is usually by microscopic examination of faecal smears stained by modified Ziehl–Neelsen (MZN).[29] There is currently no effective specific treatment; management is therefore essentially supportive. Patients may continue to excrete oocysts in low numbers after symptoms have resolved.

Hantavirus infections

Rodents (rats, harvest mice, voles, muskrats) are the natural reservoir of hantaviruses. A number of antigenically related but genetically distinct viruses have been recognized, including Hantaan, Seoul, Puumala, Prospect Hill, Dobraska, Black Creek Canal, Andes and Sin Nombre virus. Each has a different principal host species and its own geographic distribution.[30] Acutely infected rodents shed large amounts of virus in urine and excreta and subsequently continue to shed virus in lower quantities as a result of virus persistence. Birds, bats, cats and dogs have also been identified as vectors although their relevance to human infection is unclear.[31] Transmission to humans occurs mostly by inhalation of aerosolized infected rodent urine, saliva or excreta.

Groups at occupational risk include farmers, forestry workers, lumbermen, grain harvesters and those whose work brings them into close contact with rodents or their excreta (e.g. rodent trappers, plumbers, research laboratory workers). Two distinct clinical syndromes have been recognized: haemorrhagic fever with renal syndrome (HFRS), and hantavirus pulmonary syndrome (HPS).

HFRS was first described (as Korean haemorrhagic fever) in the English language literature when epidemics occurred in troops stationed in Korea. It is characterized by fever, headache and myalgia, followed by thrombocytopaenia, hypotension, shock, myocardial depression, acute tubular necrosis and renal failure. Studies to determine whether infection may cause chronic renal disease are in progress.

HPS was first described in the USA in 1993, and has since been reported from other countries, including Chile, Argentina and Paraguay. Initial respiratory symptoms, fever and myalgia are followed by acute respiratory distress, shock and myocardial depression, with a high case fatality rate.

HFRS occurs predominantly in Europe and Asia; HPS in the Americas. Milder forms of hantavirus infection occur, and the results of serological surveys of occupational risk groups suggest that many infections may be asymptomatic. Cases in Britain have been described as starting as an influenzal illness with prolonged pyrexia, headache and sore throat. There may be swelling of the face and neck followed by swelling of the hands and lower limbs with an erythematous rash.[32] Hantavirus infections can be confirmed only by serology.

Treatment of severe hantavirus infections is essentially

supportive; the use of antiviral treatment, with ribavirin, is being investigated. Intensive care support and dialysis for HRFS can reduce mortality rates to less than 5%. It may be difficult to distinguish HFRS clinically from leptospirosis; empirical antibiotic treatment of leptospirosis may be warranted while awaiting the results of serological tests for both infections. No hantavirus vaccine is available.

Hydatid disease (echinococcosis, hydatidosis)

Hydatidosis is caused by tapeworms of the genus *Echinococcus*. Two species, *E. granulosus* and *E. multilocularis*, are of importance. Both require two mammalian hosts; an intermediate host in which the cystic larval stage (metacestode) develops in the visceral organs and a definitive (final) carnivore host in which the adult develops in the small intestine to excrete free living eggs.

Hydatid disease in man is caused principally by infection with the larval stage of *E. granulosus*, which is distributed throughout Asia, Africa, South and Central America and the Mediterranean region. In many countries hydatidosis is more prevalent in rural areas where there is close contact between man and dogs and the various domestic animals which act as intermediate vectors. The disease has been the subject of successful eradication programmes in many sheep and cattle rearing countries.[33] A detailed clinical account of hydatid disease is given elsewhere.[34]

Sheep are the most important intermediate host, acquiring infection by grazing on pastures contaminated with infected dog faeces. Dogs are in turn infected by eating sheep meat and viscera containing viable cysts. Segments of the worm eliminated in dog faeces have been reported to migrate some distance from faecal matter over the vegetation before expelling eggs that subsequently adhere to it.[35] Man plays no role in the biological cycle but may help to perpetuate transmission by feeding infected meat to dogs. The infection is often acquired in childhood, but shepherds, and farmers who keep both sheep and dogs are at risk of infection. It may also be acquired by eating contaminated raw vegetables.

In the UK the incidence of the disease is highest in animals in sheep farming areas of Mid-Wales and Herefordshire, with documented foci in the Western Isles.[36,37] Elsewhere, cattle, camels and pigs may also act as intermediate hosts. Human infection is acquired by ingestion of eggs excreted in the faeces of infected dogs. Oncospheres released from the eggs penetrate the intestinal mucosa and, via the portal system, lodge in the liver, lungs, brain, eye, or other organs where the hydatid cysts form. The liver and lung are the organs most frequently involved. Cysts may take many years to produce clinical symptoms, though rapid development of illness may also occur. Asymptomatic infection occurs; cysts may be found only at autopsy or during surgery or clinical investigation for other reasons. Symptomatology depends on cyst size and location, the degree of compression caused, and on complications such as rupture, with the formation of daughter cysts and subsequent bacterial infection.

Most patients will have an eosinophilia. Calcification of the cyst wall may be visible radiologically, and the diagnosis may be confirmed by serology. It may be difficult to distinguish active infection from past infection; specialist advice should be sought, particularly if the patient is asymptomatic and the result is an unexpected finding. A detailed discussion of the value of the various serological tests used in diagnosis is given elsewhere.[34]

Surgery, which is sometimes difficult, is the treatment of first choice with supplementary chemotherapy using mebendazole or albendazole. Unfortunately, rupture of a cyst during enucleation is common and can cause immediate anaphylactic shock. Cysts can be sterilized before enucleation with the injection of a scolicide.[34]

Alveolar hydatid disease is caused by *Echinococcus multilocularis*, whose final and intermediate hosts are foxes and their rodent prey respectively. Throughout most of its range *E. multilocularis* is confined to sylvatic hosts and is therefore ecologically separated from man. In the Arctic region, for example, the arctic fox, wolves and dogs act as definitive hosts and humans may acquire infection from sledge dogs. Trappers and hunters may become infected after eating food contaminated by fox faeces. The cysts are multiloculate, and the condition is often inoperable.

Domestic cats have been found to be naturally infected in Japan, Canada and the USA; infected house mice have been found in the USA.[38] A human health problem could occur if a cycle of transmission were to develop in domestic cats and house mice. *Echinococcus multilocularis* has not been found in the UK in domestic pets or wild canids.

Important control measures include proper and rapid disposal of sheep carcasses; prevention of feeding raw offal to dogs and foxes; regular treatment of dogs with antihelminthics; quarantine of premises with infected livestock, meat inspection and effective disposal of offal at abattoirs.

Leptospirosis

Leptospirosis is caused by pathogenic serovars of the bacterial genus *Leptospira interrogans*. The genus has a wide distribution with over 200 known serovars in 23 serogroups, some of which are geographically specific. The three serotypes of most importance to humans are: Li serovar hardjo, which is common in cattle in the UK, Australia, New Zealand and the USA; Li icterohaemorrhagiae, whose principal reservoir is rats and is the agent of Weil's disease; and Li canicola which is adapted to dogs but may spread to cattle. The distribution of human disease is dependent on the local presence of carrier animals (wild animals, including rats, skunks and mongooses – and domestic animals, including dogs, cattle and pigs) and on local environmental conditions. Leptospires persist in the kidneys and genital tracts of carrier animals and are excreted in their urine and genital fluids. Survival outside the host is enhanced by warm, moist conditions. Globally, arid areas and deserts are not generally considered as potential endemic zones, as leptospires cannot survive in the environment. Human disease may follow the introduction of carrier species into newly irrigated areas, or changes in local farming practices. Areas with high rainfall and/or high levels of subsurface water will support leptospiral survival outside the host; hence monsoon areas are natural endemic zones.

Leptospirosis is an occupational disease in those who work brings them into close contact with carrier species. In the UK the groups at greatest risk include farmers, dairy workers and other agricultural workers, veterinary surgeons, abattoir, sewer, canal and fish workers. Safer working practices have considerably reduced the numbers of cases, and the infection is now less often associated with occupational exposure.[39] Elsewhere, people working in piggeries, in rice fields, on sugar or banana plantations, or in mining may be at risk.[40,41] Members of the armed forces may be exposed to risk during operations in jungle or swampy terrain. In temperate climates the incidence of leptospirosis is seasonal, increasing in early spring, peaking during the summer months, and declining with the onset of winter. Cyclical shifts have been recorded in serovar virulence, with accompanying changes in the severity of symptoms.

The infection is acquired by contact with an infected animal or urine containing viable leptospires or through contact with contaminated soil, food, water or implements. Laboratory acquired infection has been reported, and health care workers caring for patients have become infected.[42]

Leptospires gain entry by invading the mucous membranes, especially in the nasopharynx, and through abraded and water-softened skin. The incubation period is usually 5–14 days, but may vary from 3 to 30 days, depending on the route of infection, dosage and virulence of the organisms. The symptoms may be variable, and are not serotype specific. Typically, there is sudden onset of fever, headache, muscle pains and conjunctival injection with photophobia. Mild illness (as caused typically by serogroup hardjo) may last no more than 2–4 days and be difficult to diagnose. In more severe disease (often associated with serogroup icterohaemorrhagiae) petechial haemorrhage into the skin and mucous membranes, vomiting, severe myalgia, and the classic triad of meningitis, renal and hepatic failure may occur, as may myocarditis, pulmonary haemorrhage and uveitis. Chronic infection does not occur.

Laboratory confirmation, by serology or by visualization of leptospires direct or in cultured blood, cerebrospinal fluid or urine by dark ground microscopy, is required for diagnosis.

Mild infections will usually recover without specific treatment but antibiotic therapy, with penicillin, erythromycin or doxycycline, should be given to patients with suspected leptospirosis to prevent complications.[39] More severe infections may require intensive and specialized therapy, including correction of electrolyte and fluid imbalance and monitoring of cardiac and haematological function with dialysis if renal function deteriorates. The disease has a significant mortality, but provided that the patient survives the acute stage, complete recovery is usual.

Listeriosis

Listeriosis is caused by *Listeria monocytogenes*, a bacterium widely distributed in the environment, and unusual in that it can multiply slowly at refrigeration temperatures. Listeriosis is a common cause of sporadic abortion in cattle in the UK and is being isolated more frequently in veterinary investigations of ovine abortion.

Most cases of human listeriosis are sporadic. Although cases are usually associated with ingestion of contaminated foodstuff, the infection may also be acquired by direct contact with infected animals. Pustular dermatitis in veterinarians is often associated with *Salmonella* species but the same condition can also be caused by *Listeria*. Listeriosis in veterinarians and farmers attending animal abortions or stillbirths has been reported.[43] Listeriosis acquired in pregnancy can lead to infection of the fetus, resulting in abortion, stillbirth, neonatal sepsis or meningitis. Maternal infection is rarely severe and often asymptomatic, or presents with flu-like symptoms, including headache and backache.[44] In the immunosuppressed, the infection may present as septicaemia or meningoencephalitis.

The diagnosis is confirmed by culture of the organism from wound swab, blood or cerebrospinal fluid. Ampicillin, penicillin or erythromycin are the antibiotics usually recommended.[45]

Lyme disease

Lyme disease (Lyme borreliosis) is a spirochaetal infection caused by genospecies of *Borrelia burgdorferi*. It is transmitted by the bite of hard-bodied (ixodid) ticks. Vector ticks require shade, high humidity and ready access to vertebrate hosts in order to flourish. Leaf litter and bracken provide especially favourable microenvironments. In the USA for example, established tick populations are found in moist coastal or rural areas, particularly in mixed deciduous forests in the north eastern and north central regions. Lyme borreliosis has been documented in North America, Europe and northern Asia, congruent with the geographical distribution of ixodid ticks.

Lyme borreliosis is the most commonly diagnosed vector-borne disease in the USA, accounting for over 90% of all reported cases in 1991 (incidence rate 3.97 per 100 000). In England and Wales, reported cases have ranged from 20 to 180 per annum, with an average annual incidence rate of 0.34 per 100 000 over the period 1991 to 1997. The disease is an occupational hazard for shepherds, farmers, deerstalkers, foresters, abattoir workers and workers and those employed in the outdoor tourist and leisure industries (e.g. trek guides).

Infection may be acquired at any time of year but tick bites are more common in spring and summer, when human outdoor activity increases, and tick populations are at their most dense. Many human infections do not cause serious illness.[46] The bite itself is usually asymptomatic. The most common cutaneous sign of disease is erythema migrans, a characteristic annular rash which develops 7–10 days after the bite in 60–80% of cases (Fig. 24.1). It evolves over a period of days or weeks, spreading outwards from the site of the bite, and may be accompanied by local lymphadenitis and systemic upset. Other cutaneous manifestations (borrelial lymphocytoma, acrodermatitis chronica atrophica) may occur in cases infected in Europe and Asia.[47] Extracutaneous disease, affecting the joints, heart or nervous system, can occur up to 2 years after infection. Arthritis appears to be a more prominent feature of North American case series than neuritis or carditis; in Europe, the converse is true. An apparent fall in the frequency of late stage disease may reflect the widespread use of antibiotics to treat erythema migrans.

If a patient with erythema migrans presents in an area where Lyme borreliosis is endemic, the diagnosis should be made clinically. Otherwise, laboratory confirmation, by culture of the organism (from skin biopsy, other tissue samples, or blood) or serology (on blood, and cerebrospinal fluid if neurological disease is suspected) is necessary. In non-endemic areas, culture is more sensitive than serology for the diagnosis of erythema migrans. Serology remains the mainstay of laboratory confirmation of extracutaneous disease, but the results need interpreting with care, since the assays, though much improved, lack sensitivity and specificity. IgM antibodies to *B. burgdorferi* become detectable within 1–2 weeks of the first symptoms, but IgG responses may be delayed for many weeks.[48] False positive reactions to other spirochaetal infections (e.g. syphilis) may be encountered. False negatives may be found in early Lyme borreliosis and early antibiotic treatment may ablate the antibody response. Conversely, persistent IgG and IgM antibodies to *B. burgdorferi* do not necessarily represent persistent infection, but may represent false positive results.

Many infections resolve without treatment, but antibiotic therapy may speed the process and prevent disease progression. Erythema migrans is usually treated for 2 weeks with oral penicillin V, amoxicillin, tetracycline, doxycyline or cefuroxime axetil. Lyme arthritis is treated with a longer (4-week) course of oral doxycyline or amoxicillin, or with ceftriaxone for 2 weeks. Meningitis, radiculoneuritis, peripheral neuropathy, and encephalomyelitis are treated with 2–4 weeks of ceftriaxone, cefotaxime, or penicillin G. Up to 15% of patients may develop symptoms of a Jarisch–Herxheimer reaction, which should be treated symptomatically. Nonresponse to treatment is unusual, and should suggest the possibility of co-infection (for example, with *Babesia microti*, *Ehrlichia* spp, or tick-borne encephalitis).

Transmission of *B. burgdorferi* from an infected tick is unlikely to occur before 48 hours of attachment.[49,50] Furthermore, even in endemic areas, not all ticks will be infected. The risk of acquiring infection is below 5%. Routine antibiotic prophylaxis of asymptomatic bites is not recommended, since risk analysis has shown that the possible benefits are likely to be outweighed by the frequency of adverse reactions to the antibiotic. Exposure can be reduced by avoiding tick-infected areas, covering

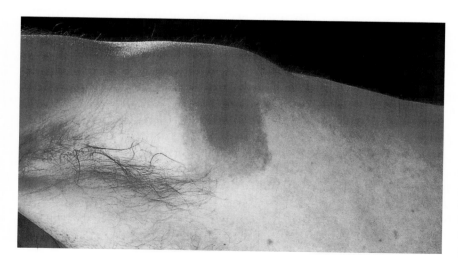

Figure 24.1 *Erythema migrans: the patient had been picnicking in an area known to be infested with* Ixodes ricinus, *the tick responsible for transmission of* Borelia burgdorferi. *See colour plate section.*

exposed skin, tucking trousers into footwear, and using tick repellents. Frequent skin inspection, which will allow early detection and removal of ticks, is also advisable. Recommendations for the use of a new Lyme disease vaccine have recently been published in the USA.[51]

Newcastle disease

Newcastle disease is caused by a paramyxovirus and affects both wild and domesticated birds. In poultry it produces a more severe infection with pneumonoencephalitis and subsequent economic losses. It has also become a zoonotic problem in racing pigeons.

Transmission to man is by direct inoculation of the eye or via the respiratory route. It causes a mild systemic illness with watering eyes and conjunctivitis. In at risk groups, which include poultry workers, veterinary workers, and pet shop staff, these symptoms should suggest a possible diagnosis, which can be confirmed by culture of conjunctival secretions for the virus or by serology. There is no specific treatment and symptoms usually resolve within a few days.

Nipah virus infection

Nipah virus is a paramyxovirus, first recognized in 1999 during investigation of cases of febrile encephalitis and respiratory illness among workers in Malaysia and Singapore who were exposed to pigs.[52] The incubation period ranged from 4 to 18 days; severe headache was the first symptom. In Malaysia nearly half of those with clinically apparent infection died. Infection is thought to be aquired through direct contact with body fluids of pigs in piggeries or abattoirs. A mass culling of pigs in outbreak areas may have halted the outbreak. The UK Advisory Committee on Dangerous Pathogens has assigned Nipah virus to Hazard Group 4 because of the relatively high mortality rate in human infections and the lack of effective treatment.

Q Fever

Q fever is caused by *Coxiella burnetii*. Infection in man occurs as the result of its inhalation, or through drinking inadequately pasteurized milk. The primary reservoir hosts for this rickettsial infection are ixodid and argasid ticks, which facilitate wildlife cycles in rodents, larger animals and birds. Arthropod faeces are a rich source of *C. burnetii*[53] although humans rarely acquire Q fever by exposure to them, or from arthropod bites.

First described by Derrick in Australia in 1937,[54] Q fever has since been found in all continents. The reservoirs of infection in Britain are probably sheep and cattle,[55] in which infection is usually asymptomatic but may cause abortion. *C. burnetii* is shed in vast numbers in infected products of conception, and human infection may be acquired when dealing with infected animals, or their contaminated bedding or litter. The organism can survive in dust and litter for several weeks. This unusual environmental stability facilitates the spread of infection (which may be wind-borne) and explains why many human cases have no history of direct contact with infected animals. However, outbreaks of infection have been described in abattoir workers, laboratory workers and wool handlers.

Serological surveys suggest that up to a half of all acute infections are asymptomatic. The incubation period may range from 7 to 40 days, varying with infective dose of the organism, the route of exposure and the age of the patient. The most commonly recognized presentation is of fever with an atypical pneumonia. The illness may be accompanied by severe sweating, shivering, myalgia, headache, backache, photophobia and reddened conjunctivae. The throat is often red and inflamed, though tonsillar exudate is not a feature. Single or multiple soft shadows are seen on chest radiograph, especially in the lower lobes, despite the absence of physical signs. Recovery usually takes 1–2 weeks, though atypical pneumonia can be rapidly progressive, leading to respiratory failure.[56] The liver is probably involved in all cases of acute Q fever and occasionally the acute infection may present as acute hepatitis; abnormal results of liver function tests are a more frequent finding. Liver biopsy shows cellular infiltration with diffuse granulomatous changes.

Months or years after the acute infection a small proportion of patients will develop signs of chronic *C. burnetii* infection. This usually presents as culture-negative endocarditis (often in patients with pre-existing valvular disease or a prosthetic valve), but may occasionally affect vascular grafts or aneurysms.[57]

Diagnosis is confirmed by serologic testing. In acute Q fever the phase II antibody titre is higher than the phase I antibody titre. In chronic Q fever the reverse occurs. Fournier *et al.*[58] found that a phase I titre of more than 1 : 800 was diagnostic of Q fever endocarditis.

Treatment with tetracycline or doxycycline is effective if given early in the acute infection. Rifampicin may also be effective, and some authors have suggested that quinolone compounds may be useful in Q fever meningoencephalitis as they penetrate the cerebrospinal fluid.[56] Q fever endocarditis requires prolonged antibiotic therapy, and some authorities recommend that treatment be continued indefinitely.[59] Replacement of the infected valve or prosthesis may be necessary. To prevent infection of the new valve, antibiotic therapy should continue after surgery and until clinical and biological signs have resolved and phase I antibody titres are lower than 1 : 200. Antibodies decrease very slowly and positive IgG titres may persist for many years.

In Australia a Q fever vaccine has been licensed for use in at-risk individuals in certain occupational groups. It is not available elsewhere.

Rabies

All warm-blooded animals are susceptible to rabies virus, which has reservoirs in a wide range of species including bats, cats, monkeys, foxes and mongooses. The virus occurs worldwide, except in some island countries, including the UK and Iceland. In most parts of the world, the main reservoirs are domestic or wild canines. The virus is excreted in the saliva of infected animals, and the neuroencephalitic effects of the virus may cause behavioural change, making an infected animal more likely to bite. The common vampire bat, which lives in colonies in caves, mines, trees and abandoned buildings, is another major reservoir of rabies in central and south America. The bat usually feeds on the blood of cattle, but may also feed on, and infect, humans. Infected insectivorous bats have been reported from Denmark, Germany, the Netherlands, France, Spain, Poland, Czechoslovakia and the states of the former USSR, but not from Switzerland or the UK, and fatal human cases of rabies following bat bites in Europe have been reported.[60] Veterinary surgeons, quarantine kennel staff, health care workers who care for rabies patients, laboratory workers in rabies endemic areas and groups such as zoologists, and archaeologists who plan to work in endemic areas may be at occupational risk of rabies.

The virus is transmitted by the bite of an infected animal, or, less commonly, by contact of infective saliva with mucous membranes or open wounds. Laboratory infection acquired by the respiratory route has been reported. Viral replication occurs initially – and asymptomatically – at the site of the inoculation; subsequently the virus travels via the nerve axons to the brain, which is followed by rapid replication, viral dissemination, and development of symptoms. The incubation period varies from 3 weeks to several months, and depends on the site and severity of initial exposure. Symptoms may begin with a mild flu-like illness, with fever, sore throat and headache and, characteristically, pain or tingling at the site of the bite – which will usually be long since healed and which may not be recalled except after specific questioning. Insomnia and general irritability are followed by more severe encephalitic symptoms, with severe agitation, convulsions, and pharyngeal spasms provoked by swallowing, or by the sight, or smell, of water. This phase is followed by paralysis, coma and death. The infection may be confirmed by viral culture, by histology (Negri bodies on corneal impression smears or skin biopsy), and by the finding of very high titres of rabies antibody on serologic testing. There is no specific treatment; sedation and intensive nursing care are required. Survival is very rare.

Control measures include control or destruction of stray dogs, immunization of domestic dogs and cats and immunization of foxes (and, potentially, other reservoir species) by using bait containing oral vaccine. The use of rabies vaccine in humans is the other mainstay of rabies prevention. The killed vaccine in use in the UK is produced in human diploid cells, and is safe and effective. It is used before exposure in those at high risk, or as prophylaxis after exposure (as five injections, intramuscularly, at days 0, 3, 7, 14 and 30), in combination with human rabies immunoglobulin. Those who work with rabies virus, who have animal contact in quarantine stations in the UK, who undertake field work outside the UK in potentially adverse conditions, or who may care for patients with rabies (including medical students going on elective to rabies endemic areas) should receive pre-exposure vaccine. This should also be considered for bat handlers,[61] and those (e.g. archaeologists) whose work may take them into bat caves abroad. Post-exposure prophylaxis is effective, but it is vital that it should be started as soon as possible after any contact with a mammal in a rabies endemic area which results in broken skin, or contact of animal saliva with an open wound.

Streptococcosis

The two species of streptococci of zoonotic interest are *Streptococcus suis* and *S. zooepidemicus*.

STREPTOCOCCUS SUIS

Streptococcus suis is part of the normal flora of the palatine tonsil of domesticated pigs, and may also be found in wild porcines. The majority of pigs over 6 weeks of age are inapparent carriers of infection; *S. suis* type II has also been isolated from cattle, sheep and goats. The organism has also been detected in the environment of piggeries and may survive at ambient temperatures for several days.

Human disease is usually found in those in direct contact with pigs or pork, and has also been associated with eating undercooked pork meat. However, human disease is rare, with estimates of fewer than 100 cases in total worldwide since it was first described in Denmark in 1965.[62] Cases reported from Holland, France, the UK, Hong Kong, Canada and New Zealand[63] have included infections in pig farmers, pork-pie factory workers, pork processing workers and machinery engineers.

Clinical features include skin infections, abscesses and thrombophlebitis. Typically, the illness consists of a primary skin wound with surrounding erythema and induration,[64] in association with septicaemia and a purulent penicillin-responsive meningitis. Ataxia and deafness occur in 50 to 75% of patients who develop meningitis, persisting in half the cases.[65] Lacerations of the skin of the hands and the arms may act as a portal of entry for the organism. Injuries, cuts or abrasions have been recorded as occurring 2–3 days before the onset of clinical disease. Transient or subclinical infections may be common. Diagnosis is based on isolation of the organism from pus, wound swab, cerebrospinal fluid or blood culture. Unless the laboratory is provided with an occupational history and asked to exclude the possibility of *S. suis* infection, minor skin and soft tissue infections may be diagnosed only as 'cellulitis' as many laboratories do not routinely use the antisera needed to speciate the organism. Treatment is with penicillin; however, even early parenteral treatment of meningitis may not prevent neurological deficit.

STREPTOCOCCUS ZOOEPIDEMICUS

Streptococcus zooepidemicus has a worldwide distribution and has been isolated from a wide range of mammals, particularly horses and cattle. Although contact with horses, and drinking unpasteurized milk from infected cattle have been considered to constitute risks, human infections (skin and soft tissue infection, sometimes aggressive, and pharyngitis) are rare.[66]

Toxoplasmosis

Toxoplasmosis is a protozoan infection common in both man and animals throughout the world. Cats are the definitive hosts for *Toxoplasma gondii* and the main reservoir of infection for man and other animals. Human infection is most often acquired through consumption of undercooked meat, and most infections are unlikely to have been occupationally acquired. However, since it may also be acquired by contact with cat faeces or contaminated soil, or through contact with infected pregnant ewes, their infected lambs or afterbirths, veterinary surgeons, farm workers and agricultural workers may be at risk of infection. A small number of infections are also known to have been acquired, mainly in veterinary surgeons, from needle-stick injuries whilst immunizing sheep with live vaccine.

Most human infections are asymptomatic; after primary *Toxoplasma* infection the parasite becomes latent. Symptomatic acute infection presents as a glandular fever-like illness, with fever, malaise, weakness, generalized lymphadenopathy, and mild hepatosplenomegaly. The infection is usually self-limiting in the immunocompetent. If primary infection occurs in pregnancy, however, the consequences for the fetus may be serious. The effects of congenital toxoplasmosis include spontaneous abortion, stillbirth, chorioretinitis, hepatosplenomegaly, hydrocephalus and mental retardation. The risk of fetal infection increases with gestational age at the time of maternal infection, but the earlier in pregnancy that infection occurs, the greater the extent of fetal damage. Maternal treatment may not reduce the risk of fetal infection, but may reduce the severity of fetal damage.

Reactivation of infection may follow loss of T-cell mediated immune surveillance in the immunocompro-

mised. Cerebral toxoplasmosis presents with headache, lethargy, and progressive confusion, with focal neurological signs.

Diagnosis is made by serological tests, including screening by microagglutination, detection of IgM antibody, and the Sabin–Feldman dye test. Specialist advice should be sought on the diagnosis and management of suspected primary infection in pregnancy. Treatment is usually with spiramicin or a combination of pyrimethamine and sulphadiazine, but is not usually required for uncomplicated acute infection. Dapsone and pyrimethamine may be used in the treatment of cerebral toxoplasmosis in the immunocompromised.

Transmissible spongiform encephalopathies

Bovine spongiform encephalopathy (BSE) is a transmissible spongiform encephalopathy (TSE) or prion disease. It is the most recently recognized member of a family of progressive, fatal neurological disorders of man and animals characterized clinically by behavioural changes and locomotor ataxia and microscopically by vacuolation of the nerve cells and ground substance of the brain and spinal cord. These diseases include scrapie in sheep and goats, chronic wasting disease (CWD) in deer and antelopes in wildlife collections, transmissible mink encephalopathy (TME) and in man, kuru, Creutzfeldt–Jakob disease (CJD) and the Gerstmann–Straussler–Scheinker syndrome (GSSS).[67]

BSE was first recognized in cattle in the UK in 1986. The common source epidemic, which peaked in 1993, was traced to contamination of meat and bone meal, a dietary supplement prepared for young animals from slaughterhouse offal. In the early 1980s, most rendering plants in the UK abandoned the use of organic solvents in the preparation of meat and bone meal. The epidemic has been thought to have been initiated by the presence of the scrapie agent (known in Britain for nearly 300 years) in meat and bone meal, and to have been amplified by the inclusion in meat and bone meal of recycled tissues from the infected cattle slaughtered before BSE was recognized as a clinical entity. However, recent characterization studies suggest that the prion strain that causes BSE is distinct from that of sheep scrapie.[68] The introduction of a ruminant feed ban in 1988, which prohibited the feeding of ruminant derived protein to ruminants, has probably terminated the epidemic. Comparison of data from the UK and relatively low incidence countries, such as Switzerland, suggests that the epidemic has been largely confined to the UK because of a unique combination of risk factors. These include the heavy feeding of meat and bone meal to dairy cattle; and changes in the rendering process used to prepare meat and bone meal.

The first cases of a new variant form of CJD (vCJD) were diagnosed in the UK in 1995.[69,70] The disease is phenotypically distinct from CJD: patients are younger;

depression is a prominent presenting symptom; neurological signs include cerebellar ataxia and involuntary movement, and the periodic complexes typical of sporadic CJD are not seen on electroencephalography.[71] There is, however, some clinical overlap, and it is not possible to distinguish vCJD from atypical sporadic CJD on the basis of clinical symptoms alone. Specialized neurohistological examination, of brain tissue, lymphoreticular tissue, or tonsil biopsy samples, is necessary for diagnosis.[72] The route of transmission remains unclear, but the agent that causes vCJD is indistinguishable from the agent that causes BSE. It is not yet clear how the numbers of cases of vCJD in the UK will evolve. A number of measures have been instituted to minimize the risk for disease transmission among animals and to humans. These include the ruminant feed ban, the compulsory slaughter and destruction of affected animals, the elimination of high risk organs such as brain, spleen and thymus from the animal and human food chains, a ban on mechanically recovered meat from bovine vertebral columns for human food and the removal of cattle older than 30 months and the heads of cattle older than 6 months from the food chain.

There is no clear evidence of occupational risk, but groups potentially at risk include workers in abattoirs, slaughterhouses and rendering plants, cattle farmers, neurosurgeons, pathologists and mortuary technicians. Advice on safe working practices and on instrument safety has been issued by the Advisory Committee on Dangerous Pathogens.[73]

Zoonotic skin diseases

COWPOX

Cowpox occurs only in Europe. It is a rare occupational human infection, usually resulting from contact with infected cattle or domestic cats, though wild rodents probably form the natural reservoir. In the UK, from 1975 to 1992, fewer than five laboratory-confirmed human cases were reported each year. Human infection is usually self-limiting but may be more severe in immunosuppressed patients. As the number of immunosuppressed patients who have never had smallpox vaccination rises, the incidence of severe cowpox infection may increase.[74] Infection is normally characterized by a single lesion followed by the development of vesicles and crusting, commonly resolving in about 4–6 weeks. Primary lesions are commonly found on the hand, forearm or on the face, and may be accompanied by malaise, pyrexia and local lymphadenopathy. Virus particles may be identified by electron microscopy in skin scrapings.

ERYSIPELOID

Erysipelothrix rhusiopathiae is widespread in the environment and carried by a variety of animal species. Infection in humans is caused by entry of *E. rhusiopathiae* through breaks in the skin. The commonest manifestation is a localized cellulitis ('fishmonger's finger'/'fish handler's disease') with, characteristically, a violaceous tinge, which spreads slowly outwards from the site of inoculation, usually on the hand or arm. People handling fish and other animals (fishermen, farmers, veterinary surgeons) or their products (fishmongers, butchers, poultry workers) are at risk. The infection is usually self-limiting but fever and systemic symptoms, including articular pain, may occur. Septicaemia and endocarditis have been reported, but are rare. The diagnosis may be made clinically, or by culture of the organism, ideally from a full thickness biopsy specimen taken from the outer edge of the violaceous area. *E. rhusiopathiae* is very sensitive to penicillin, which should be given parenterally to patients who are septicaemic. A cephalosporin, tetracycline, clindamycin or erythromycin are alternatives for patients allergic to penicillin. Changes in manufacturing processes, such as the use of plastic rather than bone buttons and the use of plastic rather than wooden fish boxes mean that human infection is now rare.[75]

MYCOBACTERIUM MARINUM

This fish pathogen causes discrete indolent but self-limiting granulomatous lesions in humans. Usually acquired from aquaria, it is sometimes known as 'fish tank granuloma'. Cases have also been reported in fish filleters. Lesions, usually on the hands, wrists or forearms, appear as small, tender, erythematous papules. These may later coalesce to form a nodule, which may become pustular. Lesions usually appear following cuts or abrasions, and will usually resolve spontaneously over a period of months.

ORF

Orf is a parapox virus infection important in sheep farming areas of the world, affecting those handling sheep, particularly those bottle feeding lambs in spring, or shearing or slaughtering sheep at other times.[76] Goats may also be a source of human infection. The virus causes scabby, granulomatous lesions on the lips of the young animals and on their mothers' teats. Human infection occurs following direct entry of the virus through abraded skin. After an incubation period of 3–7 days, a single maculopustular lesion surrounded by an erythematous rim develops at the site of virus entry, usually on the fingers, hands or forearm. The lesion dries and the crust will detach after 6–8 weeks leaving no scar. Secondary bacterial infection, causing local pain, cellulitis and lymphadenitis may occur and should be treated appropriately. Diagnosis is usually clinical, though it may be confirmed by electron microscopy of scab or vesicular fluid collected early in the course of infection. Recovered patients will have antibody to orf virus but there is anecdotal evidence that reinfection may occur.

Vaccination of animals with a live unattenuated viral vaccine protects them against the more severe forms of the disease, but may increase the risk of human infection.

RINGWORM

Fungal infections of keratinized tissue (skin, hair or nails) are usually caused by infections with the zoophilic dermatophytes. These include *Trichophyton verrucosum* (primarily from cattle, but also horses, pigs and sheep), *Microsporum canis* (from dogs and cats) and *Trichophyton mentagrophytes* (from other animals and rats) which are acquired by direct contact with an infected animal. Those at risk include farm workers, livestock handlers, veterinarians, stable workers and slaughterhouse workers. A rare cause of occupationally acquired ringworm is exposure to the geophilic species *Microsporum gypseum*, which may affect agricultural workers or gardeners. Lesions in humans are usually annular, beginning as red papules, which spread peripherally to form a ring with central scaling and a raised, red, active border. Lesions vary in size and may be single, multiple, or coalesce to give large, irregular patches. Characteristic green fluorescence under a Woods (UV) lamp may be diagnostic; culture or direct microscopic examination of hair, nail or scales may also be helpful. Topical treatment of limited skin infection with antifungals (e.g. clotrimazole) or Whitfield's ointment may be effective, but systemic treatment, with griseofulvin, oral ketoconazole, itraconazole or terbinafine is usually needed to eradicate infection involving the hair or nails. Specialist dematological advice may be needed as prolonged treatment may be necessary.

OTHER OCCUPATIONAL INFECTIONS

This section will consider in turn the main occupations at risk, and the infections associated with each occupation. The main occupational groups considered here are:

- Health care workers and people in related occupations.
- Laboratory workers.
- People whose work involves frequent travel or living abroad.
- Others.

Workers in almost any occupation may occasionally contract an infection as a result of their work, even if the occupation is not associated with a clearly recognized risk of infection, so the possibility that an infection may have been occupationally acquired should always be borne in mind.

Health care workers and related occupations

Health care professionals, ancillary workers and staff in health service laboratories have always been at risk of contracting infections from their patients. The spectrum of these infections has changed over time as a result of changes in the pattern of infectious disease in the general population and advances in immunization and exposure prevention. However, with the exception of smallpox none of the agents causing infections classically contracted by health care workers has been eradicated. A risk of infection, albeit small, remains, especially where lapses in exposure prevention occur. In developed countries there are regulations covering the control of exposure to infectious agents at work; for example in Europe there is the Biological Agents Directive, incorporated into the Control of Substances Hazardous to Health (COSHH) Regulations in the UK.[77]

The main infectious risks are considered in the following sections.

BLOOD-BORNE VIRUSES

The hepatitis viruses (particularly hepatitis B and C) and the human immunodeficiency virus (HIV) are important causes of occupational infectious disease, especially in health care workers. The occupational risk is increased because of the frequently long carrier phase when patients with undiagnosed infection are relatively well but nevertheless able to transmit infection.

Evidence of risk of infection in health care workers

Hepatitis B virus Viral hepatitis is a prescribed industrial disease in the UK in workers whose work activities expose them to frequent contact with blood and body fluids.[78] It is well recognized that hepatitis B can be transmitted via infected blood and other body fluids, either from those with acute infection or from individuals in the general population who have become virus carriers. Hepatitis B virus is usually transmitted by unprotected sexual intercourse, by sharing of blood-contaminated needles or injecting equipment between drug users, and by transmission from an infected mother to her child at birth. It may also be transmitted by transfusion of infected blood, particularly in countries where the prevalence of infection is high and resources for transfusion services are small, and by accidental exposure to blood and other body fluids. The transmission by blood exposure incidents is particularly relevant to occupational risk.

Surveys undertaken before hepatitis B vaccine became widely available show an excess of serological markers of hepatitis B infection in workers exposed to blood and body fluids. West[79] reviewed evidence from a number of seroprevalence studies in the USA and concluded that the overall risk to persons employed in health-related fields was four times that of the general adult population; physicians and dentists were at five to ten times the risk of the general population; groups with over ten times the risk included surgeons, clinical workers in dialysis units and mental handicap units, and laboratory workers having frequent contact with blood samples.

More recent studies have confirmed these findings.[80-83] Among 5813 Italian health care workers tested prior to hepatitis B immunization, 23% had markers of past or present hepatitis B infection, including 2% who were HBsAg positive.[84] A study from Stockholm of health care workers enrolling for hepatitis B immunization found a prevalence of hepatitis B markers of 4%, not greater than in the general population but related to age, duration of health care work and history of blood exposure incidents.[85] In the USA, hospital-based surgeons still show a significant rate of hepatitis B infection; 17% of 770 surgeons had markers of infection and 0.4% were HBsAg positive.[86] Risk factors for infection were non-vaccination and surgical practice for 10 years or more.

In the UK, in the 1970s and 1980s there was an excess rate of acute hepatitis B among health care workers compared with the general population. In 1975–9 the average annual rate for men in the whole population was 4 per 100 000 while health care workers had rates of up to 36 per 100 000.[87] In 1980–84 the average annual rate in men in the general population was 6 per 100 000 and again up to 37 per 100 000 among health care workers.[88] However, cases of acute hepatitis B acquired occupationally in the UK are now rare.[89] This is likely to reflect the results of the campaign to ensure hepatitis B immunization among health care workers; the few cases that did occur in the period of review were in workers who had not taken hepatitis B vaccine.

Even in countries where hepatitis B infection is endemic, and the background seroprevalence is high, there is evidence of additional occupational risk among health care workers. Among 234 dentists in the Philippines, the prevalence of markers of hepatitis B infection was found to be 58%, similar to the prevalence in the general population but increasing with the number of years in dental practice.[90] In Japan, a seroprevalence study found that over a third of hospital workers had evidence of previous hepatitis B infection, about the same as that in a group of healthy controls, but that the seroprevalence among nurses and surgeons was significantly higher than in other staff or the controls.[91] A study in Cairo revealed a higher prevalence of hepatitis B infection markers among non-professional staff (60%) than among doctors and nurses, presumably as a result of non-occupational infection in early life, but still found a relationship between infection markers and blood exposures and years of practice among the physicians.[92] In a recent serosurvey of health care workers in Belize, 29% had markers of past hepatitis B infection and 1% had detectable HBsAg. Prevalence of hepatitis B markers reached 57% in workers from one ethnic group.[93]

Occupations allied to health care may also carry a risk of hepatitis B infection. A serosurvey of 133 embalmers[94] found that they had hepatitis B infection markers at about twice the rate of a blood donor comparison group and commonly gave a history of needlestick injuries at work. A Canadian study reported that 13% of staff (and more than 20% of specialized teachers) in a day school for mentally handicapped children had markers of hepatitis B infection.[95] Emergency medical workers, such as emergency ambulance staff and paramedics, have been reported to have an increased risk of hepatitis B infection.[96-98]

However, other studies of groups of emergency workers and public-safety workers have not found an excess of hepatitis B infection markers. Morgan-Capner and Wallice[99] found no excess of hepatitis B markers among Lancashire ambulance personnel compared with blood donors; their subjects undertook both routine and emergency work. Studies of police officers,[100-102] prison officers[103] and firemen[104] have not documented an increased risk of hepatitis B infection.

Occupational hepatitis B infection has also been reported in professions unrelated to health care or the emergency services. Outbreaks of hepatitis B have been reported in butchers' shops,[105,106] apparently spread from infected employees to colleagues as a result of frequent cuts sustained at work. Studies have found an excess of hepatitis B infection among naval personnel and merchant seamen; this can be partly explained by work in a health care setting for some personnel but appears to be related mainly to para-occupational factors such as injecting drug use, unprotected sexual contact and tattooing performed in areas of high endemicity.[107-109]

Hepatitis C virus (HCV) Most serosurveys of health care workers have indicated that the prevalence of hepatitis C antibodies is low, and often not higher than in blood donor controls. Abb found hepatitis C antibodies in 8 of 738 health care workers (1%), compared with much higher seroprevalences among certain patient groups.[110] In another study, although only 0.58% of 1033 hospital employees had antibodies to hepatitis C this prevalence was significantly greater than the 0.24% of 2113 blood donor controls.[111]

Klein *et al.* found antibodies to hepatitis C among 2% of 456 dentists in New York compared with 0.1% of 723 controls; among a small group of oral surgeons the prevalence was 9%.[112] Dentists who had antibodies to hepatitis C reported more exposure incidents, and having treated more intravenous drug users in the previous month than did seronegative dentists. Among those dentists who had not been immunized against hepatitis B, 25% had anti-HBs. Some 6% of these had antibodies to hepatitis C, compared with only 2% among those who were anti-HBs negative. This suggests a common mode of transmission for the two viruses, though with a lower risk for hepatitis C.

More recent studies have confirmed the low prevalence of hepatitis C antibodies among health care workers and investigated risk factors. In Argentina, a survey of 439 health care workers found antibodies to hepatitis C by enzyme immunoassay in 1.6%.[113] In the Johns Hopkins Hospital in the USA, antibodies to hepatitis C were found in 0.7% of 943 health care workers and 0.4% of local blood donors.[114] Similarly in the UK, a study in a London teaching hospital among 1053 health care workers exposed to blood and body fluids found antibodies to hepatitis C in 0.28%, no higher than reported in blood donors in the same area.[115] Another UK study, from Nottingham, reported similar findings, with antibodies to hepatitis C in 0.2% of 1949 health care workers enrolled in a hepatitis B immunization programme.[116] Among 343 oral surgeons and 305 general dentists in the USA, 2% and 0.7% respectively were found to have antibodies to hepatitis C.[117] Hepatitis C infection was more prevalent in those who were older, had more years of practice and had serological markers of hepatitis B infection; but hepatitis C infection was much less common than markers of previous hepatitis B infection (8% in general dentists and 21% in oral surgeons). In serosurveys at 16 Italian hospitals, 2% of 3073 health care workers had antibodies to hepatitis C.[118] Infection was associated with previous acute hepatitis, blood transfusions, poor housekeeping and older age but not with occupational risk factors.

The occupational risk of hepatitis C is lower than that of hepatitis B. In a study of hospital-based surgeons in the USA, 0.9% of the 770 surgeons had antibodies to hepatitis C, compared with 17% who had markers of hepatitis B infection[86] and in a study of 3411 orthopaedic surgeons in the USA 13% without non-occupational risk factors had markers of HBV infection and 1% had HCV antibodies.[119] The prevalence of infection markers for both HBV and HCV was higher in older workers.

Human immunodeficiency virus (HIV) In contrast to hepatitis B and C, the studies that have examined the seroprevalence of HIV among health care workers have found a low seroprevalence and no evidence of an excess related to occupation; most health care workers with HIV will have acquired it non-occupationally. For example, in a study of orthopaedic surgeons in the USA, none of the 3267 surgeons without non-occupational risk factors had antibodies to HIV.[120] In six urban areas of the USA, only two of 8519 health care workers who had donated blood were HIV positive; information was not available on non-occupational risks.[121]

Types of exposure and risk of transmission in the health care setting

The most important means of transmission of blood-borne viruses in the occupational setting is by percutaneous exposure to infected blood, either by skin-penetrating injuries with blood-contaminated needles (needlestick injuries) or by cuts with scalpels or other sharp instruments contaminated with blood (sharps injuries). There is a lower risk of transmission associated with mucocutaneous exposure: blood contamination of eyes, mouth or broken skin. In addition, cases of hepatitis B, hepatitis C, and HIV transmission by skin-penetrating bites have been reported. Blood-borne viruses do not cross intact skin, and faeco-oral transmission does not occur.

Blood exposure is particularly common in surgery. Lowenfels *et al.* contacted surgeons in New York by letter or telephone and reported a median rate of puncture injuries of 4.2 per 1000 operating room hours, with 25% of the surgeons having injury rates of 9 or more per 1000 operating room hours.[122] Hussain *et al.* asked 18 surgeons in Saudi Arabia to record all accidental injuries during surgery and reported that sharps injuries occurred in 5.6% of operations.[123] An observational study of 1307 surgical procedures at San Francisco General Hospital revealed accidental blood exposures in 6.4% of procedures and percutaneous exposure to blood in 1.7%.[124] The risk of blood exposure was highest for procedures lasting more than 3 hours, when blood loss exceeded 300 ml, and for major vascular and gynaecological procedures. The authors believe that the lower rate of injuries in San Francisco may reflect greater attention to safe practices because of the high rate of HIV infection among the patients. However, in a more recent prospective observational study in four hospitals in the USA, sharps injuries were noted in 6.9% of procedures[125] and in the UK injuries were recorded by operating theatre staff in Glasgow at a rate of 1.6% per surgeon per operation, calculated to give 4.6% per operation overall.[126] Williams studied blood exposures in theatre staff during 6096 operations over a 6-month period;[127] sharps injuries occurred in 1.6% of operations. The risk of injury was increased with long procedures, high blood loss, major operations, wound closure with staples and the main surgeon wearing corrective spectacles. It was concluded that wearing spectacles could be a surrogate for increased age and reduced manual dexterity or that the spectacles themselves could be obscuring the operative field.

Blood exposures other than sharps injuries are also common in surgical practice. These include glove tears and perforations,[128–130] and eye splashes with blood and other body fluids.[131–133] Even minor suturing procedures undertaken in an accident and emergency department were found to be associated with one or more glove perforations in 11% of cases.[134]

The risk of blood exposures is not confined to surgery. Albertoni *et al.* found an overall rate of needlestick injuries over a 1-year period of 29% among 20 000 Italian health care workers interviewed in 1985; the rate was highest among surgeons (55%) and nurses (35%).[135] Collins and Kennedy have reviewed a number of studies of sharps injuries among groups of health care workers and compared the results in terms of needlestick injuries per 100 employee years for different occupational groups.[136] Nurses appear to suffer the highest number of injuries, even allowing for the number of nurses employed. A group of workers at particular risk are phlebotomists, who spend most of their working day using needles to gain access to veins.[137] Other groups at risk include domestic and portering staff, who are injured from improperly disposed needles and other sharp instruments, and laboratory staff. Relatively few injuries in reported studies occur to doctors. Sharps injuries and other blood and body fluid exposures have also been found to be frequent among embalmers.[138]

Surveys of routinely reported incidents must be interpreted with caution because of the high rate of underreporting, particularly among doctors. Some authors have attempted to quantify this underreporting.[139] Astbury and Baxter,[139] using questionnaire responses to estimate the incidence of sharps injuries and bites and scratches over the preceding year, found that only 5% of injuries had been reported by staff to the hospital Occupational Health service. The low (45%) response rate to their questionnaire may have biased their results. McGeer et al. reported a less than 5% reporting rate for sharps injuries among medical students, interns and residents in Toronto but they asked respondents to recall incidents occurring over several previous years, which may have led to inaccuracies.[140] A questionnaire study of 158 oper-

ating department staff at the Royal Free Hospital in London on reporting of needlestick injuries recorded 26 sharps injuries and 240 other blood exposure incidents during the preceding month; only 15% of the sharps injuries and none of the other blood exposures were reported to the occupational health department (or to anywhere else).[141]

Transmission risks

The risk of transmission of hepatitis B virus following a single needlestick from a source who is hepatitis Be antigen (HBeAg) positive may be as high as 30%.[142-144] The risk of transmission when the source is hepatitis B surface antigen (HBsAg) positive but HBeAg negative is much less, with studies reporting rates of transmission of between 1% and 6%[145] (see Table 24.1 for description of hepatitis B virus serology). The risk of hepatitis C transmission after an infected needlestick injury has been estimated more recently, since it became possible to test for hepatitis C antibodies. The risk is around 3%[146-148] ranging from 0 to 10% depending on the clinical status of the source patients and the tests used to identify infection in

Table 24.1 Serological markers of hepatitis B infection and immunity

Clinical situation	Serological markers					
	HBsAg	Anti-HBc	IgM	HBeAg	Anti-HBe	Anti-HBs
Very early acute infection	+	−	−	+/−	−	−
Acute hepatitis B	+	+	+	+/−	−	−
Hepatitis B carrier: higher infectivity	+	+	−	+	−	−
Hepatitis B carrier: lower infectivity	+	+	−	−	+/−	−
Recent past HBV infection	−	+	+	−	+/−	+/−
Distant past HBV infection	−	+	−	−	+/−	+/−
Vaccine induced immunity	−	−	−	−	−	+
True vaccine non-responder	−	(+)	−	−	−	−
False positive anti-HBc	−	+	−	−	−	−

HBsAg : Hepatitis B surface antigen
Anti-HBc : Antibody to hepatitis B core antigen (anti-core antibody)
Anti-HBc IgM : IgM antibody to hepatitis B core antibody (anti-core IgM antibody). Anti-HBc IgM lasts 3–6 months after an acute HBV infection
HBeAg : Hepatitis B e antigen
Anti-HBe : Antibody to hepatitis B e antigen (anti-e antibody)
Anti-HBs : Antibody to hepatitis B surface antigen (anti-surface antibody)

Table 24.2 Reported cases of occupational transmission of HIV up to December 1997

	USA	Europe (UK)	Rest of world	Total
Documented seroconversions (specific exposure incident)	52	32 (4)	11	95
Probable occupational infection (no lifestyle risks)	114	64 (8)	13	191
Total	166	96 (12)	24	286

From Ref. 149

the workers The overall risk of transmission of HIV after infected needlestick injuries has been extensively studied and is around 0.3%, markedly lower than for hepatitis B.[149] Up to December 1997 there were 95 documented HIV seroconversions after occupational exposures and a further 191 reported cases of probable occupational transmission.[149] Details are shown in Table 24.2

Some exposures may be of higher risk than others. A recent case control study suggested that factors increasing the risk of HIV seroconversion after a percutaneous exposure include: a 'deep' injury; the presence of visible blood on the instrument; procedures involving insertion of a device into an artery or vein; and exposure to a source patient who is terminally ill.[150] These are probably proxy measures for increased risks associated with exposure to a higher volume of blood and exposure to higher titres of HIV.

Clinical features in infected health care workers and risk of transmission to patients

The clinical features of infections with blood-borne viruses acquired occupationally by health care workers are essentially no different from the features of these infections acquired by any other means.

Hepatitis B Acute icteric hepatitis, sometimes fulminant, can occur 3–6 months after occupational exposure to the virus in non-immune workers, though only around a third of adults who become infected will develop clinically significant symptoms. In clinically apparent hepatitis, a prodromal illness with fever, nausea, anorexia and abdominal discomfort precedes the development of jaundice and dark urine. In some cases of acute hepatitis B infection, the first symptom may be urticaria or arthralgia. Reports of acute infections acquired occupationally in the UK are now rare.

Confirmation that a case of hepatitis is due to hepatitis B virus infection requires serological testing. The serology of hepatitis B virus infection is described in Table 24.1. This shows the pattern of hepatitis B markers found in different situations, including acute infection, natural immunity, the carrier state and immunity as a result of vaccination.

During the acute infection, supportive treatment is usually all that is required. Severe cases should be managed in specialist units. Sexual partners and other family and close contacts should be investigated and offered vaccination if they are non-infected and non-immune.

Fewer than 10% of adults with acute hepatitis B infection will fail to clear the virus and become carriers. The carrier state is indicated by *either* the detection of HBsAg on two occasions at least 6 months apart *or* the finding of HBsAg in the absence of anti-core antibody of IgM type (anti-HBc IgM). Those carriers who remain positive for HBeAg have much greater infectivity than those who clear the HBeAg but remain HBsAg positive. Treatment with antiviral drugs, such as α-interferon and other new agents, may sometimes be effective in helping to clear HBeAg.

Acutely or chronically infected health care workers who undertake exposure-prone procedures can transmit hepatitis B infection to their patients. An exposure prone procedure is one where there is a risk that the patient's open tissues may be exposed to the blood of a health care worker, as in surgery, dentistry and midwifery during complicated or instrumental deliveries. The risk of transmission depends on the types of procedure being performed, the role of the worker and the infectivity of the worker. In outbreaks associated with HBeAg positive surgeons, overall transmission rates have been around 5%, but transmission rates of 20% have been recorded in groups of patients undergoing longer and more complex procedures.[151] Recent evidence indicates that some health care workers who are HBsAg positive but HBeAg negative can also transmit hepatitis B to patients during exposure prone procedures, probably because of carriage of 'pre-core mutant' variants of hepatitis B virus, in which there is continuing viral replication even though HBeAg is not detectable in the blood.[152]

Hepatitis C It is now known that hepatitis C virus is the cause of a large proportion of cases of what was formerly called 'non-A non-B hepatitis'. Acute and even fulminant hepatitis can occur after occupational transmission of hepatitis C virus but is rare. The majority of infections will be anicteric, and many will be asymptomatic, occupational transmission being indicated by a rise in liver enzymes or by the detection of hepatitis C virus RNA or of antibody to hepatitis C virus on testing. Treatment with anti-viral drugs, especially if instituted early, may help to prevent the carrier state being established. In chronic hepatitis C virus carriers, there is sometimes a fluctuating hepatitis with 'yo-yo' transaminases. Sequelae can be serious, including cirrhosis, chronic liver disease and primary hepatocellular carcinoma.

Health care workers infected with hepatitis C can transmit the infection to patients during exposure-prone procedures.[153,154] The risk of transmission has not been quantified precisely, but, by analogy with the evidence on transmission to health care workers from needlestick exposures, it is likely to be substantially less than for hepatitis B (with HBeAg). Unlike hepatitis B there is no simple, relatively cheap, test marking 'higher infectivity' for hepatitis C.

Human immunodeficiency virus A seroconversion illness typically occurs about 4–6 weeks after the exposure. This is characterized by fever, generalized lymphadenopathy and a rash. Thereafter the infection is asymptomatic until an HIV-related illness or full-blown auto-immune deficiency syndrome (AIDS) occurs. The first AIDS-related illness in a young health care worker with undiagnosed HIV infection may be pneumonia due to *Pneumocystis carinii*. This may present with unexplained breathlessness on exertion or as failure of a chest infection to respond to common antibiotics. Immuno-compromised people with AIDS can develop a variety of bacterial and fungal infections, sometimes with opportunistic organisms and parasitic infestations. Oral candidiasis (thrush) can be the first clinical evidence of failing immunity. Tuberculosis is a particular problem, especially in areas with a high prevalence in the population. There is a risk of infection with atypical mycobacteria or with multidrug-resistant *Mycobacterium tuberculosis*. Modern combination antiretroviral therapy for HIV infection and primary prophylaxis against opportunistic infections have greatly improved the prognosis of HIV infection in developed countries, prolonging survival and delaying the onset of AIDS in people infected with HIV. The prognosis remains very poor in countries where this effective but expensive treatment is not available. Anyone with HIV antibodies is considered to be infectious through sexual contact or contact with their blood, but infectivity is higher at times when the level of virus in the blood is higher, for example during seroconversion and in the late stages of AIDS.

The potential for HIV infected health care workers to transmit to patients during exposure prone procedures is a cause of great concern, given the very serious consequences of such an occurrence. There are two reports of documented transmission from a health care worker to patients: a dentist in Florida,[155] and an orthopaedic surgeon in France.[156] The estimated risk of transmission to patients is much lower than for either hepatitis B or hepatitis C.

Management of infected health care workers

A health care worker may be found to have an infection with a blood-borne virus, either as a result of routine testing (see below), or by testing in relation to an illness or reported occupational exposure, or by testing during investigation of the source of infection in one or more infected patients. The recommendations about routine testing of health care workers for blood-borne viruses are under regular review.

In the UK all health care workers who undertake exposure-prone procedures are required to demonstrate that they are immune to hepatitis B as a result of immunization or that they are not HBeAg positive.[157] For the moment, those who are HBsAg positive but HBeAg negative can continue to practise exposure-prone procedures unless they are shown to have transmitted to patients, but this advice is likely to change. In the future, all health care workers who are HBsAg positive, or some of them considered more likely to transmit infection (perhaps on the basis of quantification of virus in the blood), may be barred from undertaking exposure-prone procedures. Medical schools in the UK do not admit medical students for training who are HBeAg pos-

itive and most do not admit those who are HBsAg positive, even if HBeAg negative.

Health care workers are not routinely tested for hepatitis C, and a worker found to be anti hepatitis C virus positive can continue to undertake exposure prone procedures unless shown to have transmitted to patients.[158] In light of reported transmissions from hepatitis C virus infected health care workers, this recommendation may change in the future.

For HIV, while screening of health care workers for infection is not a requirement, professional medical bodies in the UK require that health care workers who believe they might have been exposed to HIV (whether sexually, through injecting drug use, or occupationally) arrange to have a test to confirm their status.[159] Any UK health care worker found to be HIV infected must not undertake exposure-prone procedures.[160] Similar guidelines apply in other European countries and the USA.

It is recommended in the UK that if a health care worker who is infected with HIV has undertaken exposure-prone procedures, the patients concerned should be contacted and offered testing to confirm that they have not acquired HIV infection from the health care worker.[160] It is unlikely that infected patients will be identified in such 'look-back' exercises,[160] but it is considered that patients have the right to be informed even of this very small risk. There is similar guidance in the USA.

More general issues about fitness to work may arise in HIV infected health care workers and other people in jobs of high responsibility. These include concerns about their risk of acquiring infection if they become immunocompromised and about the effects of the neurological complications of HIV infection. The infection in most people, including health care workers, will have been acquired non-occupationally. The issues about HIV infection and fitness to work are considered in detail elsewhere.[161]

If a health care worker is found to be infected with a blood-borne virus, it is important to establish whether the infection is likely to be occupational, since they are eligible for certain financial benefits if this is the case. In the UK, since hepatitis B and hepatitis C are prescribed industrial diseases, what is needed is to show that the person is infected and that their work involves (or has involved) exposure to potentially infected blood, whether in the clinical setting or the laboratory. Although HIV infection is not a prescribed industrial disease, infected workers in the UK may be eligible for National Health Service Injuries Benefit if it can be shown that their infection is likely to be occupational in origin. For all blood-borne viruses, the most obvious way to demonstrate an occupational origin is to show seroconversion following an occupational exposure incident.

Prevention of infection with blood-borne viruses

Prevention rests mainly on reduction of the risk of exposure to blood or other infected body fluids. The most important risk is parenteral exposure so it is important to reduce the use of sharp instruments, develop safer techniques and types of equipment, and make proper use of suitable containers and systems for disposal of used sharp instruments.[162] In the laboratory setting the use of sharp instruments or equipment can be virtually eliminated. Suitable protective clothing prevents exposure of broken skin and the mucosa of the eyes and mouth. Although infection by aerosols is less of a risk (and probably not a risk at all for HIV), use of respirators or biological safety cabinets for laboratory work when blood aerosols are generated is recommended.[163]

There continues to be discussion about whether the best approach to prevention is to identify infected patients and specimens and take special precautions in these cases, or to assume that all patients and specimens could be infected and to take routine precautions to reduce blood exposures. The arguments for the two approaches have been set out elsewhere.[163] Where the prevalence of any of the blood-borne virus infections is high, such as in inner cities and developing countries, the argument for assuming infection in all cases and taking appropriate preventive measures (so-called 'universal precautions')[164] is strong. The level of precautions to be taken then depends upon a risk assessment of the procedure and the likelihood of blood contamination rather than a risk assessment of the patient.

However, not all occupational blood exposure incidents are preventable, and some will occur even where preventive measures have been well implemented. Other preventive strategies are available. For hepatitis B, the most infectious of the agents, there is fortunately an effective and safe vaccine. Immunization of all health care workers who may have contact with blood and body fluids is recommended.[162] Vaccines against hepatitis C and HIV have not yet been developed.

Around 90% of young, fit health care workers produce an adequate anti-HBs response to hepatitis B vaccine. Response rates are lower in males, smokers, older people and those who are immunosuppressed. Apparent non-responders (no or low level anti-HBs response) should be tested for evidence of hepatitis B virus infection. True non-responders, with no evidence of previous hepatitis B virus infection, should be informed they are not protected and strongly advised to report any occupational exposures to blood. Non-response to vaccine should not be considered a bar to employment as a health care worker in any capacity.

Once an exposure to infected blood has occurred, other measures can reduce the risk of infection in the worker. For hepatitis B, active immunization with the vaccine, using an accelerated course in those not previously immunized, is recommended.[165] Passive protection may also be provided using hepatitis B immunoglobulin (HBIG). However, HBIG gives incomplete protection and should be given in conjunction with the first dose or booster dose of vaccine; in workers who have failed to respond to the vaccine it is the only protection available. For hepatitis C, no effective post-exposure prophylaxis is available at present but follow-up to 6 months is recommended to check that transmission has not occurred.[166]

For HIV, recommendations about post-exposure prophylaxis have recently been revised in the UK[167] and USA.[168] A case-control study has suggested that the use of prophylactic zidovudine is associated with a reduced risk of HIV seroconversion after percutaneous (needlestick) exposure to HIV-infected blood.[169] By extrapolation from the effectiveness of combined antiretroviral therapy in established infection, current guidelines on post-exposure prophylaxis now recommend routine use of three antiretroviral drugs in the UK[167] or two, sometimes three in the USA[168] for 4 weeks after a significant occupational exposure to HIV. The recommended three drugs for post-exposure prophylaxis in the UK and USA are zidovudine, lamivudine and indinavir, with modification of this regime if the source patient is believed to have infection resistant to any of these drugs. The prophylaxis should be started as soon as possible after the exposure and preferably within 1 hour. The effectiveness of this regime in reducing the rate of seroconversion (in any case small) is unknown. However, experience of the combination drug regimes as prophylaxis in health care workers indicates that they are associated with significant side-effects in 50–90% of recipients.[169] Side-effects are severe enough to cause time off work in more than three-quarters of recipients. Follow-up for 6 months after exposure is necessary to rule out occupational transmission, as late seroconversion may occur.

Initiation of suitable post-exposure prophylaxis depends upon knowledge of the worker's immunity (for hepatitis B) and the source patient's infection status. Post-exposure testing of source patients for blood-borne virus infection is therefore important. Patients should be tested only with their consent and with appropriate pre-test discussion.[159] If approached sensitively, few patients will refuse testing. If immediate testing is not feasible, or the patient refuses testing, but there is a strong suspicion of infection, for example with HIV, then post-exposure prophylaxis should be considered.

Health care workers who have been involved in blood exposure incidents, especially when the source patient is known to be infected with a blood-borne virus, may understandably become extremely anxious. They should have access to timely, sympathetic and knowledgeable advice from an experienced designated physician (the occupational physician often takes on this responsibility). Giving accurate information and providing immediate and on-going support is an important, though not always recognized, part of the management of blood exposures at work.

Other workers may have occasional contact with blood or contaminated sharp instruments, for example emergency care workers, refuse workers, police, and prison officers. These workers should be trained to take appropriate precautions to reduce the risk of exposure to blood (especially sharps injuries) and should know how to obtain immediate post-exposure care. The need to offer them routine pre-exposure hepatitis B immunization is less clear cut, though this may be appropriate for selected subgroups. Arrangements should be made for them to have access to expert advice, and treatment if necessary, if they are involved in a blood exposure incident.

OTHER VIRUSES AS OCCUPATIONAL RISKS FOR HEALTH CARE WORKERS

Viral haemorrhagic fevers

Viral haemorrhagic fevers, caused by a range of viruses, are severe and potentially life-threatening diseases. They are endemic in Africa, parts of South America, and in rural eastern Europe and the Middle East. Cases in the UK are very rare and virtually always imported.

The infections are transmitted to humans by mosquito bite (yellow fever, dengue, Rift valley fever, Chikungunya); tick bite (Omsk haemorrhagic fever, Kyanasur Forest disease, Crimean Congo haemorrhagic fever); or through contact with virus excreted by infected rodents or other animal reservoir (the arenaviruses, including Lassa virus; Hantaan virus). However, only four of these infections are known to be readily capable of spreading from person to person, and thus present a potential risk of transmission to health care workers: Lassa fever, Crimean Congo haemorrhagic fever, Marburg disease and Ebola.

Crimean Congo haemorrhagic fever was first recognized in the USSR in 1944, and the virus isolated from the patients was subsequently shown to be identical to that isolated in 1956 from a sick child in Zaire. The virus is now known to be widely spread in Africa, central Asia, southern Europe, and parts of the Middle East, though there appear to be geographical variations in virulence, the disease being more severe in Asia than in Africa.[170] Lassa fever was first described in 1969 after three missionary nurses working in Lassa in north eastern Nigeria became seriously ill with an unknown infection, from which two died. The third nurse, who had cared for the other two, was flown to North America for treatment, and a new arenavirus was isolated from her serum, and subsequently from similar cases in Nigeria, and named Lassa virus.

Marburg virus takes its name from an outbreak of haemorrhagic fever among laboratory workers in Marburg, Germany in 1967. Workers in laboratories in Frankfurt and Belgrade also became infected. All 25 with primary infections had been in contact with organs, blood, or cell cultures from a batch of wild-caught African green monkeys from Uganda; six secondary cases occurred amongst those who had contact with

infected patients' blood. Small numbers of cases have since occurred in South Africa, Zimbabwe and Kenya.

Ebola haemorrhagic fever was recognized in 1976, when outbreaks of a new haemorrhagic fever, with a high case fatality rate and considerable secondary spread through blood contact, occurred simultaneously in Zaire and in the Sudan. Ebola virus has also been isolated from a zoologist working in Cote D'Ivoire who became accidentally infected while performing an autopsy on a chimpanzee found dead in the wild. After batches of monkeys were imported to the USA and Italy from the Philippines, some workers had serological evidence of asymptomatic infection, but there were no clinical cases among contacts.

The clinical illnesses are characterized by fever, haemorrhage and collapse, although serosurveys have suggested that subclinical and mild infections also occur. Mortality rates ranging from 3% (in a community outbreak of Lassa fever) to 66% (in hospitalized cases of Lassa fever) have been reported. Lassa fever tends to have a more insidious onset than Marburg or Ebola disease and can therefore be difficult to diagnose. The differential diagnosis of a fever in a patient who has been in rural West Africa within the last 3 weeks includes Lassa fever, typhoid fever and malaria. In Lassa fever there is usually fever and headache followed by pharyngitis, abdominal tenderness, sometimes with vomiting and diarrhoea and evidence of pleural effusion. There may be little or no evidence of haemorrhage other than some bleeding of the gums. Severe haemorrhage is unusual in Lassa fever but more common in Marburg or Ebola disease. Treatment is largely a question of providing intensive supportive care; antiviral drugs, such as tribavirin reduce the mortality of Lassa fever, especially if started early, and may also be helpful in Crimean Congo haemorrhagic fever, but have not been shown to influence the course of either Marburg or Ebola virus infection.

The viral haemorrhagic fevers pose a significant risk of infection to health care workers caring for cases and laboratory workers handling specimens from them. The main risk in the health care setting seems to be from direct contact with infected blood (for example by needlestick injury or contamination of broken skin or mucous membranes) but infection from droplet spread or blood aerosol cannot be entirely excluded. In the Ebola virus epidemic in the Sudan in 1979, it was reported that staff providing direct clinical care for ill patients had a five times higher risk of contracting infection than staff with less physical contact with the patients, and there were no cases of infection in staff who entered the room but had no physical contact.[171] Recent UK guidelines on the management and control of viral haemorrhagic fevers[170] advise that patients returning from abroad with a fever should be categorized on the basis of a risk assessment: area visited, clinical features and time of onset in relation to travel, household or occupational contact with known or suspected cases, or contact with potentially infected blood or body fluids. Any patient known or suspected to be suffering from a viral haemorrhagic fever, or in whom the diagnosis cannot immediately be excluded should be admitted to a specially designated high security infectious disease unit. Nearly all suspected cases will probably have malaria. The guidelines also cover the special precautions needed to obtain, transport, and examine laboratory specimens from a patient with a suspected viral haemorrhagic fever and the management of patients' contacts. The first investigation should always be to confirm or refute a diagnosis of malaria. If there is doubt, empirical treatment for malaria should be instituted.

Varicella zoster

Varicella zoster virus causes chickenpox (primary infection) and shingles (reactivation of previous infection). Health care workers who have not acquired immunity to varicella zoster as a result of childhood infection are vulnerable to contracting the infection from patients. Fortunately, more than half of health care workers give a history of chickenpox in childhood and have antibodies as a result, and antibodies are also detectable in most of those without a history of chickenpox.[172] Staff known to be susceptible (or not known to be immune) should not work with patients who have known or suspected chickenpox, disseminated zoster or shingles. Chickenpox in adults tends to be more severe than in children but the major concern is that health care workers who have chickenpox (who will have been particularly infectious in the 48 hours preceding the onset of the characteristic rash) may transmit the virus to susceptible patients. Health care workers with chickenpox should remain off work until there are no new lesions and the existing lesions have crusted and dried; those with shingles are also infectious and should similarly remain off work. Special measures are necessary for management of exposure to varicella zoster infection in susceptible health care workers who are immunosuppressed or pregnant, including consideration of the use of zoster immune globulin.[172]

Cytomegalovirus

Cytomegalovirus is found in many body tissues including blood, urine, breast milk, saliva and vaginal fluid. However, provided even the most basic infection control procedures are followed, any risk of transmission to health care workers from their patients is extremely small. Indeed, several studies have failed to show any excess of cytomegalovirus in health care workers with clinical contact compared with others with no clinical contact.[173] The most important consequence of cytomegalovirus in immunocompetent adults is its potential for fetal damage if acquired in pregnancy.

Rubella

Rubella infection (German measles) in children is usually a mild, self-limiting illness characterized by fever and a morbilliform rash. In adults, however, infection is more severe, with rash, fever, debility and prominent arthralgic symptoms in small joints. Maternal infection in the first 16 weeks of pregnancy, particularly if in the first trimester, causes severe fetal damage. Health care workers are unlikely to be at increased risk of rubella, especially since many countries now vaccinate infants as well as adolescents against rubella. However, many health care employers determine the rubella antibody status of both female and male new employees and vaccinate those who are found to be non-immune. This both protects the women workers of child-bearing age and prevents infections that could then be passed from the workers to pregnant women patients. The management of an undiagnosed morbilliform rash in a health care worker is simplified if she or he is known to be immune to rubella.

Parvovirus

Parvovirus B19 infection (which is not vaccine preventable) produces a febrile illness with a transient macular rash which may be mistaken for rubella. In adults, particularly women, it can cause arthropathy which is usually self-limiting, and fetal damage. Complications can occur in people with haemoglobinopathies and in those who are immunosuppressed. There is no specific treatment. Diagnosis is made serologically. Outbreaks in health care settings may necessitate ward closures to interrupt transmission.[175]

Herpetic whitlow or paronychia

These lesions on the fingers are due to direct contact with herpes simplex virus and used to be quite a common problem in health care workers. Diagnosis is by culture of virus from the lesions, electron microscopy or immunofluorescence. Contact with the mouth area, such as in mouth care or dentistry, with ungloved hands seems to be the major risk.[175]

OTHER INFECTIOUS RISKS FOR HEALTH CARE WORKERS

Tuberculosis

The clinical features of pulmonary tuberculosis include fever, weight loss, cough, malaise, night sweats and haemoptysis. The diagnosis should be considered in any health care worker who presents with such symptoms and no other apparent cause. Radiographs may be normal in early infection or show a rather diffuse bronchopneumonia but in more advanced cases there may be the more typical upper lobe pneumonia with cavitation. A recent study has confirmed that health care workers in the UK remain at increased risk of tuberculosis.[176]

Guidelines produced by the British Thoracic Society[177] cover pre-employment screening, protection of workers against infection (including the use of bacille Calmette-Guérin (BCG)) and safe working practices. The recom-

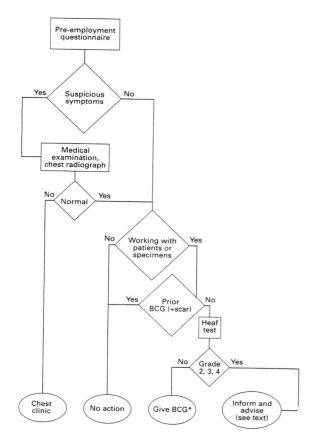

Figure 24.2 *Protection of health care workers against tuberculosis: recommendations for screening and immunization. Some units may prefer to repeat the Heaf test in older persons to detect a boosted reaction and avoid unnecessary BCG vaccination. Reproduced from Ref. 177.*

mendations for screening and immunizing staff are summarized in Fig. 24.2; BCG immunization is recommended in health care workers who are not tuberculin skin test positive as a result of previous BCG immunization. Guidance is also given on the management of health care workers who have a significant occupational exposure to tuberculosis, and of those who are infected with tuberculosis, regardless of source. Tuberculosis acquired through an occupation involving contact with sources of tuberculous material is a prescribed disease in the UK.

In the last 10 years, multidrug-resistant *M. tuberculosis* has become a problem, particularly in the USA. Occupational transmission to workers has been described.[178,179] Procedures such as sputum induction and aerosol treatments may increase the potential for transmission to patients and staff.[180] Workers and patients infected with HIV, or those who are immunosuppressed for other reasons are at greater risk.[181] Outbreaks have been associated with a high mortality (43–93%) and rapid progression of disease (median interval from diagnosis to death 4–16 weeks).[182]

In the USA, detailed guidelines for preventing transmission of *M. tuberculosis* in health care facilities were produced in response to several serious outbreaks of transmission of multidrug-resistant *M. tuberculosis*.[183] These include several levels of control: administrative controls to prevent exposing uninfected individuals to persons who have infectious tuberculosis; then engineering controls to reduce spread of infectious droplet nuclei, such as local exhaust ventilation, air flow control and air filtration; and finally the use of personal respiratory protective equipment in areas where there is still a risk of exposure to infection. The guidelines stress the need for early identification and treatment of patients with tuberculosis. Health care workers with HIV infection or other causes of immunosupression should be advised of the dangers of working with patients with tuberculosis, especially multidrug-resistant tuberculosis, and offered redeployment to other areas. Infection control guidelines for preventing the spread of tuberculosis in relation to HIV and multidrug-resistant tuberculosis have also been produced in the UK, designed to protect both other patients and health care workers.[183,184]

Scabies

This skin disease is caused by the mite *Sarcoptes scabiei*, and transmitted by close personal contact. The itchy rash characteristically presents on the fingerwebs, wrist and elbow flexures, and axillae but may sometimes present as a more widespread generalized dermatitis (Norwegian scabies). Linear burrows on the skin are present but will not always be visible, particularly if hypersensitivity to mite antigen has developed.

Nurses and other workers who provide physical care to patients are at risk. Cases are usually sporadic, but more extensive outbreaks have been described.[185] The use of gloves and gowns when handling patients who may have scabies is advisable. Treatment, of the patient and family members, is with malathion or permethrin, which should be applied to the whole body from the neck down and left for 24 hours. Benzyl benzoate can also be used, but often causes irritation and may need to be applied on up to 3 consecutive days.

Occasionally, strains of mites from infected pets can also cause a highly pruritic papular urticarial rash. In this case it is pet owners (and possibly veterinary surgeons) who are at risk, rather than health care workers.

Staphylococcal infections

Health care workers can become colonized with methicillin resistant *Staphylococcus aureus* (MRSA), carried in the nose, throat, axillae, perineum and on damaged skin. Such colonized workers pose a risk of transmitting to patients an infection which can be extremely difficult to treat and may be fatal in immunocompromised patients, including those who have undergone recent surgery. Even non-colonized health care workers can spread the infection between patients. Scrupulous attention to handwashing and to changing any barrier garments (gloves, aprons) between each patient is vital. Where a colonized worker has been detected as a result of an outbreak investigation, eradication of the organism may be attempted, but sometimes proves difficult to achieve. In rare cases, for example an infected cardiovascular surgeon or a nurse on the Intensive Care Unit, failure to eradicate MRSA may mean that they require long-term redeployment. Recent guidelines in the UK cover the prevention and management of MRSA outbreaks in hospitals and other institutions.[186]

Laboratory research workers and animal handlers

The infection risk to laboratory research workers will depend on the precise nature of the work in which they are engaged, and the techniques applied. Risk assessments of individual processes are necessary under the COSHH Regulations, and should result in the development, implementation and monitoring of safe standard operating procedures. Workers should carry a medical contact card which gives details of their work and provides the name of the doctor to be contacted if the worker develops an unexplained fever or other signs of infection. Workers seeking medical advice should always mention their occupation. Similarly, the doctor should always ask the patient about their work.

HUMAN IMMUNODEFICIENCY VIRUS INFECTION

At least three research laboratory workers worldwide have become infected by HIV after exposure while working with concentrated HIV.[149] Workers should have the same access to post-exposure prophylaxis and care as described above for clinical health care workers.

WORK WITH PRIMATES

Staff working with primates may be exposed to a number of infections, including herpes B virus, Marburg virus, human monkey pox, rabies, tuberculosis and enteric infections. Primates from reputable suppliers will, if wild caught, have been quarantined for 6 months and screened for these infections, although negative serological tests do not guarantee absence of infection. Primates for use in research which will involve human contact should, therefore, ideally have been bred in captivity and be herpes B virus seronegative. All primates should be regarded as potentially infective and handled with extreme care by trained staff. Suitable protective clothing should always be worn.

Infected animals shed herpes B virus from the oropharynx and genital tract; workers may acquire infection through bites or skin abrasions and subsequently develop a severe encephalomyelitis with a fatality rate of around 70%.[187,188] There is no evidence of asymptomatic infection in primate handlers.[189] Guidelines have been published for

the prevention and treatment of herpes B virus infections in exposed people.[188] Wounds should be gently irrigated with soap and water or normal saline. Antibiotic prophylaxis against oropharyngeal bacteria (including anaerobes) should also be given for bites. Aciclovir may be given as prophylaxis after an exposure to a source known or potentially infected with herpes B virus, and should also be used to treat any worker with suspected infection.

Infections associated with occupational travel

The risk to travellers will depend on the countries visited, the proportion of time spent abroad, and working and living conditions while abroad. The most important hazard for occupational travellers is non-infectious: injury, particularly in road traffic accidents. This is common and may often be fatal. There is good evidence that risk-taking behaviour abroad may differ from that at home; travellers should be counselled that unprotected sexual intercourse poses a clear risk of HIV and other infections and should be avoided.

MALARIA

Malaria is a major infectious risk for travellers. Around 2000 cases are imported into the UK each year, of which rather more than half are due to *Plasmodium falciparum*, which is the most serious of the four species of malaria parasite which cause disease in man, and is potentially fatal; *P. vivax*, *P. ovale* and *P. malariae* are less likely to cause life-threatening illness. Most malaria infections will have been acquired through being bitten by an infected mosquito, but transfusion acquired infection, transplacental transmission, and aquisition through needlestick exposure to infected blood are also well recognized. Prevention requires risk recognition; travellers should be encouraged to take measures to avoid being bitten by mosquitoes (appropriate clothing, insect repellents – used directly on skin or impregnated in wrist or ankle bands, mosquito nets, and insecticide sprays). They should comply with an appropriate chemoprophylactic regimen but should understand that there is no chemoprophylactic regime which is 100% effective. In choosing a regime, the risk of adverse reactions to any drug must be balanced against the risk of acquisition of disease.[190] Guidelines for the prevention of malaria in travellers from the UK have recently been revised,[191] and are regularly reviewed and updated. These contain up to date information about recommended chemoprophylaxis regimes by geographical area, and advice on the use of regimes for emergency self-treatment. The drugs most commonly used currently for prophylaxis include chloroquine, proguanil and mefloquine.

The incubation period for malaria varies depending on the species. Malaria due to *P. falciparum* usually presents either in the endemic area or within 2 months of leaving and typically 9–14 days after a bite from an infected mosquito. Malaria due to other species, particularly *P. vivax*, can take up to 12 months to present. Symptoms, especially in the early stages, are non-specific and include fever, headache, malaise and myalgia. The classically described fevers of specific periodicity associated with different species of malaria parasite are in practice rarely useful in diagnosis. It is important to have a high index of suspicion of malaria in anyone with an unexplained fever who has been in an endemic area. Particularly for falciparum malaria, sudden and catastrophic deterioration in clinical condition may occur resulting in death. Complications of malaria include pulmonary oedema, coma, fits, hypoglycaemia, anaemia, renal failure and abortion.[192] Widespread haemolysis can lead to haemoglobinuria, so called 'black water fever'. Falciparum malaria should be treated as a medical emergency. The diagnosis of malaria is made by identification of the parasite in thick blood films; specialist help may be needed for interpretation. A single negative film does not exclude the diagnosis, particularly in a first episode of malaria when severe symptoms can occur with a low parasitaemia and empirical treatment against *P. falciparum* may be appropriate.

The treatment regime depends on the known or suspected species of parasite and its likely sensitivities (depending on area of origin) as well as the severity of the clinical illness.[193] Expert advice should be sought about the appropriate treatment regime in each case. Chloroquine resistant *P. falciparum* is now so widespread that chloroquine should no longer be used for the treatment of falciparum malaria in the UK, although it remains the drug of choice for *P. malariae* and *P. ovale* and uncomplicated *P. vivax* infections. Additional treatment with primaquine is needed for infection with *P. vivax* and *P. ovale* to eradicate the hypnozoite stage of the parasite in the liver and prevent relapse. If this is not done, there is a risk of late relapse, which may occur years after the primary infection. Oral treatment can be used unless the patient is severely ill, confused or unconscious. Supportive care is an integral part of management and may include fluid replacement, management of fits, control of blood glucose, ventilation and renal dialysis.

TRAVELLER'S DIARRHOEA

In developed countries, *Campylobacter* sp. and salmonellae are the most common causes of infective diarrhoea. However, enterotoxin-producing strains of *E. coli* (ETEC) are the commonest cause of diarrhoea in travellers to less developed countries, where other infections which have a human, rather than an animal, reservoir are also more likely to be acquired. Diarrhoea caused by ETEC, shigellae, and *Giardia lamblia*, although unlikely to be life-threatening, may cause considerable morbidity, misery and loss of efficiency.

In theory, traveller's diarrhoea is wholly preventable if simple precautions are followed faithfully. These include eating only freshly prepared cooked food; washing and peeling all fruit; avoidance of salads and many seafoods, and treatment of all drinking water including that for ice in drinks. In practice, it may be difficult to follow this advice to the letter, especially for those who have little control over catering arrangements (e.g. delegates at an international conference). Some clinicians would advocate chemoprophylaxis with doxycycline, ciprofloxacin or trimethoprim for short trips to areas of poor hygiene; this might be justifiable in people who are susceptible to infection or who suffer from inflammatory bowel disease but this approach cannot be generally endorsed, especially given current concerns about increasing antimicrobial resistance.

Most cases of traveller's diarrhoea occur whilst the traveller is abroad, are self-limiting and are never investigated. Travellers can treat themselves effectively. They should be instructed on how to replace lost fluids using a suitable oral rehydration solution (proprietary packs are available but a homemade solution is equally effective). It is of course essential to make up the solution using clean water. Short-term use of a simple anti-diarrhoeal agent (such as loperamide) may be helpful, and where fever persists for more than 48 hours, self-treatment with short-course antibiotic therapy could be started. Appropriate agents would be trimethoprim or ciprofloxacin.

Travellers who have bloody diarrhoea should seek medical advice. Causes include infection with *Entamoeba histolytica*. (Clinical features are detailed in Ref. 194.)

Entamoeba histolytica can cause colitis of variable intensity; in the most severe cases all of the large bowel can be involved. Complications of amoebic colitis include peritonitis, pericolic abscess, colonic perforation, and profuse intestinal haemorrhage. In a significant proportion of cases, the first symptoms are those of an amoebic liver abscess, and a history of dysentry is then lacking. The principal symptoms include fever, hepatic and diaphragmatic pain, and weight loss. The abscess is usually solitary, and located in the right lobe of the liver; the precise anatomical location and extent is best defined by ultrasound and CT scans.

The diagnosis may be confirmed by microscopy and culture of faeces, bowel scrapings, or aspirate of a liver abscess. Patients usually respond to treatment with metronidazole or tinidazole; liver abscesses may sometimes need to be aspirated.

A few patients continue to have dysenteric symptoms despite successful treatment. These symptoms can last for several months. Many more patients develop irritable bowel syndrome which can also persist for many months.

Diarrhoeal symptoms that persist despite simple

measures require further investigation, including stool microscopy and culture. Blood cultures are appropriate in febrile patients. Symptoms beginning more than a week after travel or which persist for more than 10 days suggest the possibility of *Giarda lamblia* infection.

Acute giardiasis usually presents with watery diarrhoea of sudden onset which can be accompanied by anorexia, epigastric pain and weight loss. The stools are typically pale, frothy and foul smelling. Although spontaneous resolution usually occurs within a few weeks, in some patients the infection takes a more chronic course. Diarrhoea is then of variable severity ranging from the passage of a few bulky foul-smelling stools to more marked frequent diarrhoea. Many patients with chronic giardiasis develop intestinal malabsorption with steatorrhoea; acquired lactose intolerance is common. The diagnosis is usually confirmed by stool microscopy but when this is negative, trophozoites can be sought in duodenal aspirates obtained by endoscopy or in jejunal biopsy. Treatment with metronidazole or tinidazole is usually effective and restores small intestinal function to normal.

Food handlers who have suffered traveller's diarrhoea following a trip abroad should consult their occupational health department before returning to work.

HEPATITIS A

Hepatitis A virus is transmitted by the faeco-oral route, through close contact with an infected person or through contaminated food or water. Travel to countries of high or intermediate endemicity is a well recognized risk for infection. Other potential occupational risks include directly handling the virus in the laboratory, direct contact with untreated sewage, and direct contact with faeces of infected patients. After an incubation period of 2–6 weeks, symptoms of fever, anorexia, nausea, abdominal pain, pale stools, dark urine and jaundice develop. Disease severity is age-related; young children are usually asymptomatic or have non-specific symptoms of viral illness. Viral excretion is at a maximum towards the end of the prodromal period, in the 48 hours before the onset of jaundice. Hepatitis A infection cannot be distinguished from other causes of viral hepatitis by clinical examination alone; diagnosis is made by testing for specific IgM antibody to hepatitis A virus. The infection is usually self-limiting. There is no carrier state but full recovery may take 3–6 months. Treatment is largely supportive. The mortality rate is below 0.1% overall, but somewhat higher in those aged 45 years or over, and in those with pre-existing liver disease. Rarely, hepatitis A virus infection may appear to relapse; the mechanism underlying this is unclear.

Prophylaxis against hepatitis A infection is available.[172] Passive prophylaxis, with human normal immunoglobulin (containing antibody to hepatitis A virus) given shortly before travel, can provide protection against infection for up to 3 months, and is also used for post-exposure protection of family or household contacts of a case. More prolonged protection is provided by use of inactivated hepatitis A vaccine, which may be more useful for travellers likely to make frequent short trips to higher endemicity areas, or who will be travelling or living in such areas for longer periods. The prevalence of naturally acquired antibody to hepatitis A virus increases with age. In the UK – where the overall prevalence is gradually falling – testing for this (by detection of serum anti-hepatitis A virus IgG) prior to vaccination might be considered in those who have a past history of jaundice, those who were born outside the UK in areas of higher endemicity, and those aged 50 years or over.

Others

SEX WORKERS

Sex workers are clearly at risk of a variety of sexually transmitted infections and may, if their transactions involve sex for drugs rather than money, also be at risk of infective conditions associated with injecting drug use, including hepatitis C, abscesses and endocarditis. The risks may be reduced by the use of condoms, although this may be difficult to negotiate with clients.

Sex workers in the UK with local symptoms of a sexually transmitted infection will usually present to a genitourinary medicine clinic for treatment, where investigations for the full range of infections, including HIV, syphilis, gonorrhoea, hepatitis B and *Chlamydia trachomatis* should be undertaken. Those who present to other services may be less likely to disclose their occupation.

SEWAGE WORKERS

There is evidence that sewage workers are at increased risk of enteric infections including hepatitis A.[195,196] They are also at risk of leptospirosis (see pp. 495–496). The risks are mainly confined to those who come into contact with raw sewage,[197] and can be reduced by the use of protective clothing. Hepatitis A immunization may be appropriate for high-risk subgroups, such as those with more frequent contact with raw sewage.

ARCHAEOLOGISTS

Smallpox was officially declared to have been globally eradicated in 1980, but there is concern that viable virus could survive in corpses buried in permafrost or in cool dry crypts. Other viruses, including strains of influenza from previous pandemics, may also be able to survive in similar circumstances. Expert advice about the risks, and about protective equipment, should be taken before corpses are exhumed.[198]

REFERENCES

1 World Health Organization. *Zoonoses*. Second report of the Joint WHO/FAO Expert Committee. Technical Report Series No. 169. WHO Geneva 1959.

2 Advisory Committee on Dangerous Pathogens. *Categorisation of Biological Agents According to Hazard and Categories of Containment* 4th edn. Sudbury: HSE Books, 1995.

3 Dawson A, Griffin R, Fleetwood A, Barrett NJ. Farm visits and zoonoses. *Commun Dis Rep Rev* 1995;**5**:R81–6.

4 Department of Health, Central Office of Information. *While You are Pregnant: Safe Eating and How to Avoid Infection from Food and Animals*. London: HMSO, 1991.

5 Stein CD. Anthrax. In: Hull TG ed. *Diseases Transmitted from Animals to Man* 5th edn. Springfield IL: Charles C Thomas, 1963 : 82–125.

6 Turnbull PCB. Anthrax. In: Palmer SR, Lord Soulsby, Simpson DIH eds. *Zoonoses: Biology, Clinical Practice and Public Health Control*. Oxford: Oxford University Press, 1998: 3–16.

7 Young EJ. An overview of human brucellosis. *Clin Infect Dis* 1995;**21**:283–90.

8 Garcia-Carrillo C. Animal and human brucellosis in the Americas. *Paris OIE* 1990 : 287.

9 Peiris V, Fraser S, Fairhurst M, Weston D, Kaczmarski E. Laboratory diagnosis of infection: some pitfalls: *Brucella*. *Lancet* 1992;**339**:1415–16.

10 Hall WJ. Modern chemotherapy for brucellosis in humans. *Rev Infect Dis* 1990;**12**:1060–99.

11 Anza J, Corredoir J, Pallares R, Viladrich PF, Rufi G *et al*. Characteristics of and risk factors for relapse of brucellosis in humans. *Clin Infect Dis* 1995;**20**:1241–9.

12 Malik GM. Early clinical response to different therapeutic regimens for human brucellosis. *Am J Trop Med Hyg* 1999;**58**:190–1.

13 Caul EO, Sillis M. Chlamydiosis. In: Palmer SR, Lord Soulsby, Simpson DIH eds. *Zoonoses: Biology, Clinical Practice and Public Health Control*. Oxford: Oxford University Press, 1998: 53–65.

14 Crosse BA. Psittacosis: a clinical review. *J Infection* 1990;**21**:251–9.

15 Giroud P, Jadin J. Premiers resultats concernant le virus des Bashi isolé dans la provence du Kivu au Congo Belge. *Bull Soc Pathol Exot* 1954;**47**:578–88.

16 Giroud P, Roger F, Dumes N, Certaines avortements chez la femme peuvent être dus a des agents situés a côté du groupe de la psittacose. *Comptes Rendus Seanc Acad Sci* 1956; **242**:697–9.

17 Bloodworth DL, Howard AJ, Davies A, Mutton KJ. Infection in pregnancy caused by *Chlamydia psittaci* of ovine origin. *Commun Dis Rep CDR Weekly* 1987;**10**:3–4.

18 Beer RJS, Bradford WP, Hart RJC. Pregnancy complicated by psittacosis acquired from sheep. *Br Med J* 1982;**284**:1156–7.

19 Palmer SR, Salmon RL. Enzootic abortion in ewes: risks to humans. *Hlth Hyg* 1990;**11**:205–7.

20 Jones DM, Robinson DA. Occupational exposure to *Campylobacter jejuni* infection. *Lancet* 1981;**i**:440–1.

21 Hopkins RS, Scott AS. Handling raw chicken as a source for sporadic *Campylobacter jejuni* infections. *J Infect Dis* 1993;**148**:770.

22 Healing TD, Greenwood MH, Pearson AD. Campylobacters and enteritis. *Rev Med Microbiol* 1992;**3**:159–67.

23 Chapman PA, Siddons CA, Harkin MA. Sheep as a potential source of verocytotoxin-producing *Escherichia coli* O157 (letter). *Vet Rec* 1996; **138**:23–24.

24 Trevena WB, Hooper RS. Wray C, Willshaw GA, Cheasty T, Domingue G. Verocytotoxin-producing *Escherichia coli* O157 associated with companion animals. *Vet Rec* 1996;**138**:400.

25 Chalmers RM, Salmon RL, Willshaw GA, Cheasty T, Looker N *et al*. Vero-cytotoxin-producing *Escherichia coli* O157 in a farmer handling horses. *Lancet* 1997;**349**:1816.

26 Mead PS, Griffin PM. *Escherichia coli* O157 : 117. *Lancet* 1998;**352**:1207–12.

27 Tarr PI. *Escherichia coli* O157:H7: Clinical, diagnostic, and epidemiological aspects of human infection. *Clin Infect Dis* 1995;**20**:1–10.

28 Angus KW. Cryptosporidiosis in man, domestic animals and birds: a review. *J R Soc Med* 1983;**76**:62–70.

29 Casemore DP. Epidemiological aspects of human cryptosporidiosis. *Epidemiol Infect* 1990;**104**:1–28.

30 Peters CJ, Simpson GL, Levy H. Spectrum of hantavirus infection: haemorrhagic fever with renal syndrome and hantavirus pulmonary syndrome. *Ann Rev Med* 1999;**50**:531–45.

31 Bennett M, Hart CA. Hantavirus infection. *J Med Microbiol* 1994;**41**:71–3.

32 Pether JVS, Lloyd G. The clinical spectrum of human hantavirus infection in Somerset, UK. *Epidemiol Infect* 1993;**111**:171–5.

33 Gemmell MA, Roberts MG. Cystic echinococcus. In: Palmer SR, Lord Soulsby, Simpson DIH eds. *Zoonoses: Biology, Clinical Practice and Public Health Control*. Oxford: Oxford University Press, 1998: 665–688.

34 Radford AJ. Hydatid disease. In: Weatherall DJ, Ledingham JFG, Warrel DA eds. *Oxford Textbook of Medicine 3rd edn*. Oxford: Oxford University Press, 1996 : 955–9.

35 Gemmell MA, Johnstone PD. Factors regulating tapeworm populations: dispersion of eggs of *Taenia hydatigena* on pasture. *Ann Trop Med Parasitol* 1981;**70**:431–4.

36 Palmer SR, Biffin AHB, Craig PS, Walters TMH. Control of hydatid disease in Wales. *Br Med J* 1996;**312**:674–5.

37 McMarius DP, Smyth JD. Hydatidosis: changing concepts in epidemiology and speciation. *Parasitol Today* 1986;**2**:163–8.

38 Schantz PM. Migration of parasite captures parasitologists' attention. *JAMA* 1993;**202**:707–9.

39 Ferguson IR. Leptospirosis surveillance 1990–1992. *Commun Dis Rep Rev* 1993; :R47–8.

40 Everard CO, Ferdinand GA, Butcher LV, Everard JD. Leptospirosis in piggery workers in Trinidad. *J Trop Med Hyg* 1989;**92**:253–8.

41 Smythe L, Dohut M, Morris M, Symonds M, Scott J. Review of leptospirosis notifications in Queensland 1985 to 1996. *Commun Dis Intell* 1997;**21**:17–20.

42 Ratnam S, Seenivasan N. Possible hospital transmission of leptospiral infection. *J Commun Dis* 1998;**30**:54–6.

43 McLauchlin J, Low JC. Primary cutaneous listeriosis in adults: an occupational disease of veterinarians and farmers. *Vet Rec* 1994;**135**:615–7.

44 Newton L, Hall SM, Pelerin M, McLauchlin J. Listeriosis surveillance: 1990. *Commun Dis Rep Rev* 1991;**1**:R110–113.

45 McLauchlin J, Van der Mee-Marquet N. Listeriosis. In: Palmer SR, Lord Soulsby, Simpson DIH eds. *Zoonoses: Biology, Clinical Practice and Public Health Control.* Oxford: Oxford University Press, 1998: 127–140.

46 O'Connell S. Lyme disease in the United Kingdom. *Br Med J* 1995;**310**:303–8.

47 Nadelman RB, Wormser GP. Lyme borreliosis. *Lancet* 1998;**352**:557–65.

48 White DJ. Lyme disease. In: Palmer SR, Lord Soulsby, Simpson DIH eds. *Zoonoses: Biology, Clinical Practice and Public Health Control.* Oxford: Oxford University Press, 1998: 141–153.

49 Falco RC, Fish D, Piesman J. Duration of tick bites in a Lyme disease-endemic area. *Am J Epidemiol* 1996;**143**:187–92.

50 Piesman J. Transmission of Lyme disease spirochaetes (*Borrelia burgdorferi*). *Exp Appl Acarol* 1989;**7**:71–80.

51 Centers for Disease Control and Prevention. Recommendations for the use of Lyme disease vaccine: recommendations of the Advisory Committee on Immunization Practices (ACIP). *Morbid Mortal Weekly Rep* 1999;**48** (No. RR–7).

52 Centres for Disease Control and Prevention. Update: outbreak of Nipah virus – Malaysia and Singapore. *Morbid Mortal Weekly Rep* 1999; **48**: 335–7.

53 Williams JC, Sanches V. Q fever and coxiellosis. In: Beran GW ed. *Handbook of Zoonoses* Boca Raton FL: CRC Press, 1994 : 429–46.

54 Derrick EH. Q fever, a new fever entity: clinical features, diagnosis, and laboratory investigation. *Med J Aust* 1937;**2**:281.

55 Marmion BP, Stoker MGP. The epidemiology of Q fever in Great Britain. An analysis of the findings and some conclusions. *Br Med J* 1958;**ii**:809–16.

56 Marrie TJ, Raoult D. Q fever: a review and issues for the next century. *Int J Antimicrob Agents* 1997;**8**:145–61.

57 Raoult D, Raza A, Marrie TJ. Q fever endocarditis and other forms of chronic Q fever. In: Marrie TJ ed. *The Disease. Q fever*: Boca Raton FL: CRC Press, 1990 : 179.

58 Fournier P, Casalata JP, Habib G, Messana T, Raoult D. Modification of the diagnostic criteria proposed by the Duke endocarditis service to permit improved diagnosis of Q fever endocarditis. *Am J Med* 1996;**100**:629–33.

59 Marrie TJ. Q fever. In: Palmer SR, Lord Soulsby, Simpson DIH eds. *Zoonoses: Biology, Clinical Practice and Public Health Control.* Oxford: Oxford University Press, 1998: 171–85.

60 Communicable Disease Report. Bat brings rabies to Britain. *Commun Dis Rep CDR Weekly* 1996;**6**:205.

61 Communicable Disease Report. Management of bat bites. *Commun Dis Rep CDR Weekly* 1996;**6**:319.

62 Perch B, Kristjansen P, Skadhange KN. Group R Streptococci pathogenic for man. *Acta Pathol Microbiol Scand B* 1968;**74**:69–76.

63 Robertson ID, Blackmore DK. Occupational exposure to *Streptococcus suis* type 2. *Epidemiol Infect* 1989;**103**:157–64.

64 Walsh B, Williams AE, Satsangi J. *Streptococcus suis* type 2: pathogenesis and clinical disease. *Rev Med Microbiol* 1992;**3**:65–71.

65 Dupas D, Vignon M, Geraut C. *Streptococcus suis* meningitis. A severe noncompensated occupational disease. *J Occup Med* 1992; **34**:1102–5.

66 Edwards AT, Roulson MA. Milk-borne outbreak of serious infection due to *Streptococcus zooepidemicus* (Lancefield Group C). *Epidemiol Infect* 1988;**101**:43–51.

67 Ironside JW. Creutzfeldt-Jakob disease: the story so far. *Proc Roy Coll Physic Edinb* 1998;**28**:143–9.

68 Collinge J. Variant Ceutzfedlt-Jakob disease. *Lancet* 1999; **354**: 317–23.

69 Will RG, Ironside JW, Zeidler M, Cousens SN, Estibeiro K *et al.* A new variant of Ceutzfeldt-Jakob disease in the UK. *Lancet* 1996;**347**:921–5.

70 Brown P. Bovine spongiform encephalopathy [corrected] Creutzfeldt-Jakob disease [editorial]. *Br Med J* 1996;**312**:790–1.

71 Zeidler M, Stewart JE, Barraclough CR, Bateman DE, Bates D *et al.* New variant Creutzfeldt-Jakob disease: neurological features and diagnostic tests. *Lancet* 1997;**350**:903–7.

72 Hill AF, Butterworth RJ, Joiner S, Jackson G, Rosser MN *et al.* Investigation of variant Creutzfeldt-Jakob disease and other human prion diseases with tonsil biopsy samples. *Lancet* 1999;**353**:183–9.

73 Advisory Committee on Dangerous Pathogens. *Precautions for work with Human and Animal Transmissible Spongiform Encephalopathies.* London: HMSO, 1994.

74 Burton JL. Of mice, milkmaids, cats and cowpox. *Lancet* 1994;**343**:67.

75 Smith RMM. Erysipeloid. In: Palmer SR, Lord Soulsby, Simpson DIH eds. *Zoonoses: Biology, Clinical Practice and Public Health Control.* Oxford: Oxford University Press, 1998: 83–87.

76 Zimmerman JL. Orf. *JAMA* 1991;**266**:476.

77 Health and Safety Commission. *Biological Agents ACOP (control of biological agents): Control of Substances Hazardous to Health Regulations* London: Health and Safety Executive, 1994.

78 UK Benefits Agency. *If You Have An Industrial Disease:*

Industrial Injuries Disablement Benefit (NI 2, August 1989, revised October 1991). London: HMSO, 1991.

79 West DJ. The risk of hepatitis B infection among health professionals in the United States: a review. *Am J Med Sci* 1985;**287**:26–33.

80 Iserson KV, Criss EA. Hepatitis B prevalence in emergency physicians. *Ann Emerg Med* 1985;**14**:119–122.

81 McLean AA, Monahan GR, Finkelstein DM. Public health briefs: Prevalence of hepatitis B serologic markers in community hospital personnel. *Am J Publ Hlth* 1987;**77**:998–9.

82 Hadler SC, Doto IL, Maynard JE *et al*. Occupational risk of hepatitis B infection in hospital workers. *Infect Control* 1985;**6**:24–31.

83 Reingold AL, Kane MA, Hightower AW. Failure of gloves and other protective devices to prevent transmission of hepatitis B virus to oral surgeons. *JAMA* 1988;**259**:2558–60.

84 Petrosillo N, Puro V, Ippolito G and the Italian Study Group on Blood-Borne Occupational Risk in Dialysis. Prevalence of hepatitis C antibodies in health-care workers. *Lancet* 1994;**344**:255–6.

85 Struve J, Aronsson B, Frenning B, Forsgren M, Weiland O. Prevalence of hepatitis B virus markers and exposure to occupational risks likely to be associated with acquisition of hepatitis B virus among health care workers in Stockholm. *J Infect* 1992;**24**:147–56.

86 Panlilio AL, Shapiro CN, Schable CA, Mendelson MH, Montecalvo MA *et al*. Serosurvey of human immunodeficiency virus, hepatitis B virus, and hepatitis C virus infection among hospital-based surgeons. *J Am Coll Surg* 1995;**180**:16–24.

87 Polakoff S, Tillett HE. Acute viral hepatitis B: laboratory reports 1975–9. *Br Med J* 1982;**284**:1881–2.

88 Polakoff S. Acute viral hepatitis B: laboratory reports 1980–4. *Br Med J* 1986;**293**:37–8.

89 Collins M, Heptonstall J. Occupational acquisition of acute hepatitis B infection by health care workers in England and Wales, 1985–93. *Commun Dis Rep Rev* 1994;**4**:R153–5.

90 Lim DJ, Lingao A, Macasaet A. Sero-epidemiological study on hepatitis A and B virus infection among dentists in the Philippines. *Int Dental J* 1986;**36**:215–8.

91 Kashiwagi S, Hayashi J, Ikematsu H *et al*. Prevalence of immunologic markers of hepatitis A and B infection in hospital personnel in Miyazaki Prefecture, Japan. *Am J Epidemiol* 1985;**122**:960–9.

92 Goldsmith RS, Zakaria S, Zakaria MS *et al*. Occupational exposure to hepatitis B virus in hospital personnel in Cairo, Egypt. *Acta Trop* 1989;**46**:283–90.

93 Hakre S, Reyes L, Bryan JP, Cruess D. Prevalence of hepatitis B virus among health care workers in Belize, Central America. *Am J Trop Med Hyg* 1995;**53**:118–22.

94 Turner SB, Kunches LM, Gordon KF, Travers PH, Mueller NE. Public health briefs. Occupational exposure to human immunodeficiency virus (HIV) and hepatitis B virus among embalmers: a pilot seroprevalence study. *Am J Publ Hlth* 1989;**79**:1425–6.

95 Remis RS, Rossignol MA, Kane MA. Hepatitis B infection in a day school for mentally retarded students: transmission from students to staff. *Am J Publ Hlth* 1987;**77**:1183–6.

96 Kunches LM, Craven DE, Werner BG, Jacobs LM. Hepatitis B exposure in emergency medical personnel: prevalence of serologic markers and need for immunization. *Am J Med* 1983;**75**:269–272.

97 Pepe PE, Hollinger FB, Troisi CL, Heiberg D. Viral hepatitis risk in urban emergency medical services personnel. *Ann Emerg Med* 1986;**15**:454–7.

98 Valenzuela TD, Hook EW, Copass MK, Corey L. Occupational exposure to hepatitis B in paramedics. *Arch Intern Med* 1985;**145**:1976–7.

99 Morgan-Capner P, Wallice PDB. Hepatitis B markers in ambulance personnel in Lancashire. *J Soc Occup Med* 1990;**40**:21–2.

100 Peterkin M, Crawford RJ. Hepatitis B vaccine for police forces? *Lancet* 1986;**ii**:1458–9.

101 Morgan-Capner P, Hudson P. Hepatitis B markers in Lancashire police officers. *Epidemiol Infect* 1988;**100**:145–51.

102 Welch J, Tilzey AJ, Bertrand J, Bott ECA, Banatvala JE. Risk to Metropolitan police officers from exposure to hepatitis B. *Br Med J* 1988;**297**:835–6.

103 Radvan GH, Hewson EG, Berenger S, Brookman DJ. The Newcastle hepatitis B outbreak: observations on cause, management, and prevention. *Med J Australia* 1986;**144**:461–4.

104 Crosse BA, Teale C, Lees EM. Hepatitis B markers in West Yorkshire firemen. *Epidemiol Infect* 1989;**103**:383–5.

105 Gerlich WH, Thomssen R. Outbreak of hepatitis B at a butcher's shop. *Deutsch Med Wchenschr* 1982;**107**:1627–30.

106 Mijch AM, Barnes R, Crowe SM, Dimitrakakis M, Lucas CR. An outbreak of hepatitis B and D in butchers. *Scand J Infect Dis* 1987;**19**:179–84.

107 Dembert ML, A-Shaffer R, Baugh NL, Berg SW, Zajdowicz T. Epidemiology of viral hepatitis among US navy and marine personnel, 1984–85. *Am J Publ Hlth* 1987;**77**:1446–7.

108 Hyams KC, Palinkas LA, Burr RG. Viral hepatitis in the US navy, 1975–1984. *Am J Epidemiol* 1989;**130**:319–26.

109 Siebke JC, Wessel N, Kvandal P, Lie T. The prevalence of hepatitis A and B in Norwegian merchant seamen: a serological study. *Infection* 1989;**17**:77–80.

110 Abb J. Prevalence of hepatitis C virus antibodies in hospital personnel. *Int J Med Microbiol* 1991;**274**:543–7.

111 Jochen ABB. Occupationally acquired hepatitis C infection. *Lancet* 1992;**339**:304.

112 Klein RS, Freeman K, Taylor PE, Stevens CE. Occupational risk for hepatitis C virus infection among New York City dentists. *Lancet* 1991;**338**:1539–2.

113 Frider B, Sookoian S, Castano G, Rebora N, Gutfraind Z *et al*. Prevalence of hepatitis C in health care workers

investigated by 2nd generation enzyme-linked and line immunoassays. *Acta Gastroenterol Latinoamericana* 1994;**24**:71–5.

114 Thomas DL, Factor SH, Kelen GD, Washington AS, Taylor E, Quinn TC. Viral hepatitis in health care personnel at the Johns Hopkins Hospital. *Arch Intern Med* 1993;**153**:1705–12.

115 Zuckerman J, Clewley G, Griffiths P, Cockcroft A. Prevalence of hepatitis C antibodies in clinical health care workers. *Lancet* 1994;**343**:1618–20.

116 Neal KR, Dornan J, Irving WL. Prevalence of hepatitis C antibodies among health care workers of two teaching hospitals: who is at risk? *Br Med J* 1997;**314**:179–80.

117 Thomas DL, Gruninger SE, Siew C, Joy ED, Quinn TC. Occupational risk of hepatitis C infections among general dentists and oral surgeons in North America. *Am J Med* 1996;**100**:41–5.

118 Puro V, Petrosillo N, Ippolito G, Aloisi MS, Boumis E, Rava L and the Italian Study Group on Occupational Risk of Bloodborne Infections. Occupational hepatitis C virus infection in Italian health care workers. *Am J Publ Hlth* 1995;**85**:1272–5.

119 Shapiro CN, Tokars JI, Chamberland ME. Use of the the hepatitis-B vaccine and infection with hepatitis B and C among orthopaedic surgeons. The American Academy of Orthopaedic Surgeons Serosurvey Study Committee. *J Bone Jt Surg Am* 1996;**78**:1791–1800.

120 Tokars JI, Chamberland ME, Schable CA *et al*. A survey of occupational blood contact and HIV infection among orthopaedic surgeons. *J Am Med Assoc* 1992;**268**:489–94.

121 Chamberland ME, Petersen LR, Munn VP, *et al*. Human Immunodeficiency Virus infection among health care workers who donate blood. *Ann Intern Med* 1994;**121**:269–73.

122 Lowenfels AB, Wormser GP, Jain R. Frequency of puncture injuries in surgeons and estimated risk of HIV infection. *Arch Surg* 1989;**124**:1284–6.

123 Hussain SA, Latif ABA, Choudhary AAAA. Risk to surgeons: a survey of accidental injuries during operations. *Br J Surg* 1988;**75**:314–6.

124 Gerberding JL, Littell C, Tarkington A, Brown A, Schecter WP. Risk of exposure of surgical personnel to patients' blood during surgery at San Francisco General Hospital. *N Engl J Med* 1990;**322**:1788–93.

125 Tokars J, Bell D, Marcus R *et al*. Percutaneous injuries during surgical procedures. *Proceedings of the VII International Conference on AIDS, Florence, Italy*. 1991; Vol 2 : 83.

126 Camilleri AE, Murray S, Imrie CW. Needlestick injuries in surgeons: what is the incidence? *J Roy Coll Surg Edinb* 1991;**36**:317–8.

127 Williams S. Variables associated with the risk of blood exposures in operating theatres. MD Thesis, University of London, 1997.

128 Brough SJ, Hunt TM, Barrie WW. Surgical glove perforations. *Br J Surg* 1988;**75**:317.

129 Camilleri AE, Murray S, Squair JL, Imrie CW. Epidemiology of sharps accidents in general surgery. *J R Coll Surg Edinb* 1991;**36**:314–6.

130 Wright JG, McGeer AJ, Chyatte D, Ransohoff DF. Mechanisms of glove tears and sharp injuries among surgical personnel. *JAMA* 1991;**266**:1668–71.

131 Brearley S, Buist LJ. Blood splashes: an underestimated hazard to surgeons. *Br Med J* 1989;**299**:1315.

132 Porteous MJ Le F. Operating practices of and precautions taken by orthopaedic surgeons to avoid infection with HIV and hepatitis B virus during surgery. *Br Med J* 1990;**301**:167–9.

133 Hinton AE, Herdman RC, Timms MS. Incidence and prevention of conjunctival contamination with blood during hazardous surgical procedures. *Ann Roy Coll Surg Engl* 1991;**73**:239–42.

134 Richmond PW, McCabe M, Davies JP, Thomas DM. Perforation of gloves in an accident and emergency department. *Br Med J* 1992;**304**:879–80.

135 Albertoni F, Ippolito G, Petrosillo N, Sommella L, Di Nardo V *et al*. Needlestick injury in hospital personnel: a multicenter survey from central Italy. *Infect Control Hosp Epidemiol* 1992;**13**:540–4.

136 Collins CH, Kennedy DA. Microbiological hazards of occupational needlestick and 'sharps' injuries. *J Appl Microbiol* 1987;**62**:385–402.

137 Metler R, Ciesielski C, Ward J, Marcus R. HIV seroconversions in clinical laboratory workers following occupational exposure, United States. *VIIIth International Conference on AIDS; Amsterdam*. July 1992; PoC 4147.

138 Beck-Sague CM, Jarvis WR, Fruehling JA, Ott CE, Higgins MT, Bates FL. Universal precautions and mortuary practitioners: influence on practices and risk of occupationally acquired infection. *J Occup Med* 1991;**33**:874–8.

139 Astbury C, Baxter PJ. Infection risks in hospital staff from blood: hazardous injury rateas and acceptance of hepatitis B immunization. *J Soc Occup Med* 1990;**40**:92–3.

140 McGeer A, Sinor AE, Low DE. Epidemiology of needlestick injuries in house officers. *J Infect Dis* 1990;**162**:961–4.

141 Williams S, Gooch C, Cockcroft A. Hepatitis B immunisation and blood exposure incidents amongst operating department staff. *Br J Surg* 1993;**80**:714–6.

142 Hoofnagle JH, Seeff LB, Buskell Bales Z, Wright EC, Zimmerman HJ. Veterans Administration Study Group. Passive-active immunity from hepatitis B immunoglobulin. re-analysis ofa Veterans Administration Cooperative Study of needle-stick hepatitis. *Ann Intern Med* 1979;**91**:813–8.

143 Grady GF, Lee VA, Prince AM *et al*. Hepatitis B immune globulin for accidental exposures among medical personnel: final report of a multicenter controlled trial. *J Infect Dis* 1978;**138**:625–638.

144 Werner BA, Grady GF. Accidental hepatitis B surface

antigen positive inoculations. *Ann Intern Med* 1982;**97**:367–9.

145 Cockcroft A. Occupational aspects of hepatitis. In: Zuckerman AJ, Thomas HC eds. *Viral hepatitis – Scientific Basis and Clinical Management* 2nd edn London: Churchill Livingstone, 1998.

146 Kiyosawa K, Sodeyama T, Tanaka E *et al*. Hepatitis C in hospital employees with needlestick injuries. *Ann Intern Med* 1991;**115**:367–9.

147 Mitsui T, Iwano K, Masuko K *et al*. Hepatitis C virus infection in medical personnel after needlestick accident. *Hepatology* 1992;**16**:1109–14.

148 Puro V, Petrosillo N, Ippolito G and the Italian Study Group on Occupational Risk of HIV and other Bloodborne Infections. Risk of hepatitis C seroconversion after occupational exposure in health care workers. *Am J Infect Control* 1995;**23**:273–7.

149 PHLS AIDS & STD Centre at the Communicable Disease Surveillance Centre & Collaborators. *Occupational Transmission of HIV: Summary of Published Reports*, December 1997 edn. London: CDSC.

150 Cardo DM, Culver DH, Ciesielski CA *et al*. A case-control study of HIV seroconversion in health care workers after percutaneous exposure. *N Engl J Med* 1997;**337**:1485–90.

151 Heptonstall J. Outbreaks of hepatitis B virus infection associated with infected surgical staff. *Commun Dis Rep* 1991;**1**:R81–R85.

152 The Incident Investigation Teams and others. Transmission of hepatitis B to patients from four infected surgeons without hepatitis B e antigen. *N Engl J Med* 1997;**336**:178–84.

153 Esteban JI, Gomez J, Martell M, Cabot B, Quer J *et al*. Transmission of hepatitis C virus by a cardiac surgeon. *N Engl J Med* 1996;**334**:555–60.

154 Communicable Disease Report. Hepatitis C virus transmission from health care worker to patient. *CDR Weekly 5*: 30 June 1995.

155 Ciesielski C, Marianos D, Ou C-Y *et al*. Transmission of human immunodeficiency virus in a dental practice. *Ann Intern Med* 1992;**116**:798–805.

156 Lot F, Seguier JC, Fegueux S, Astagneau P, Simon P *et al*. Probable transmission of HIV from an orthopedic surgeon to a patient in France. *Ann Intern Med* 1999;**130**:1–6.

157 UK Health Departments. *Protecting Health Care Workers and Patients from Hepatitis B: Recommendations of the Advisory Group on Hepatitis*. London: HMSO, 1993.

158 UK Health Departments. *Protecting Health Care Workers and Patients from Hepatitis B*. Addendum (1996) under cover of EL(96)77. London: Department of Health, August 1993.

159 General Medical Council. *Serious Communicable Diseases*. London: General Medical Council, 1997.

160 UK Health Departments. *AIDS/HIV Infected Health Care Workers: Guidance on the Management of Infected Health Care Workers and Patient Notification*. London: UK Health Departments, 1998.

161 HIV infection and AIDS. In: Cox R Ed. *Fitness for Work* 2nd edn. Oxford: Oxford University Press, 1996.

162 UK Health Departments. *Guidance for Clinical Health Care Workers: Protection Against Infection with Blood-borne Viruses*. Recommendations of the Expert Advisory Group on AIDS and the Advisory Group on Hepatitis. London: UK Health Departments, 1998.

163 Cockcroft A, Walker P. For debate: testing patients for HIV antibodies is useful for infection control purposes. *Rev Med Virol* 1991;**1**:5–9.

164 Centers for Disease Control. Update: universal precautions for prevention of transmission of human immunodeficiency virus, hepatitis B virus and other blood borne pathogens in health care settings. *Morbid Mortal Weekly Rep* 1988;**37**:377–88.

165 Public Health Laboratory Service Hepatitis Subcommittee. Exposure to hepatitis B virus: guidance on post-exposure prophylaxis. *Commun Dis Rep Rev* 1992;**2**:R97–101.

166 Public Health Laboratory Service, Hepatitis Sub-Committee. Hepatitis C virus: guidance on the risks and current management of occupational exposure. *Commun Dis Rep Rev* 1993;**10**:R135–9.

167 UK Health Departments. *Guidance on Post-exposure Prophylaxis for Health Care Workers Occupationally Exposed to HIV*. London: Department of Health, 1997:PL/CO (97).

168 Centers for Disease Control and Prevention. Public health service guidelines for the management of health-care worker exposures to HIV and recommendations for postexposure prophylaxis. *Morbid Mortal Weekly Rep* 1998;**47**(No. RR-7):1–33.

169 Beekmann R, Fahrner R, Nelson L, Henderson DK, Gerberding JL. Combination post-exposure prophylaxis (PEP): a prospective study of HIV-exposed health care workers (HCW). [Abstract 481]. In: *Program and Abstracts of the Infectious Diseases Society of America 35th Annual Meeting*. Alexandria, VA: Infectious Diseases Society of America, 1997 : 161.

170 Advisory Committee on Dangerous Pathogens. *Management and Control of Viral Haemorrhagic Fevers*. London: HMSO, 1996.

171 Baron RC, McCormick JB, Zubeir OA. Ebola virus dissemination in southern Sudan: hospital dissemination and intrafamilial spread. *Bull WHO* 1983; **61**:997.

172 UK Health Departments. *Immunisation Against Infectious Disease*. London: HMSO, 1996.

173 Geberding JL, Bryant-LeBlanc CE, Nelson K *et al*. Risk of transmitting the human immunodeficiency virus, cytomegalovirus, and hepatitis B virus to health care workers exposed to patients with AIDS and AIDS-related conditions. *J Infect Dis* 1987;**156**:1–8.

174 Pillay D, Patou G, Hurt S, Kibbler CC, Griffiths PD. Parvovirus B19 outbreak in a children's ward. *Lancet* 1992;**339**:107–9.

175 Rosato FE, Rosato EF, Plotkin SA. Herpetic paronychia – An

occupational hazard of medical personnel. *N Engl J Med* 1970;**283**:804–5.

176 Meredith S, Watson JM, Citron KM, Cockcroft A, Darbyshire JH. Are healthcare workers in England and Wales at increased risk of tuberculosis? *Br Med J* 1996;**313**:522–5.

177 Joint Tuberculosis Committee of the British Thoracic Society. Control and prevention of tuberculosis in the United Kingdom: Code of practice, 1994. *Thorax* 1994;**4**:1193–200.

178 Centers for Disease Control. Nosocomial transmission of multidrug-resistant tuberculosis to health care workers and HIV-infected patients in an urban hospital – Florida. *Morbid Mortal Weekly Rep* 1990;**39**:718–22.

179 Centers for Disease Control. Nosocomial transmission of multidrug-resistant tuberculosis among HIV-infected persons – Florida and New York 1989–1991. *Morbid Mortal Weekly Rep* 1991;**40**:585–91.

180 Beck-Sagu C, Dooley SW, Hutton MD *et al*. Outbreak of multidrug-resistant Mycobacterium tuberculosis infections in a hospital: transmission to patients with HIV infection and staff. *JAMA* 1992;**268**:1280–6.

181 Pearson ML, Jereb JA, Frieden TR *et al*. Nosocomial transmission of multidrug-resistant Mycobacterium tuberculosis: a risk to patients and health care workers. *Ann Intern Med* 1992;**117**:257–8.

182 TB Infection-Control Guidelines Work Group. Guidelines for preventing the transmission of *Mycobacterium* tuberculosis in health-care facilities, 1994. *Morbid Mortal Weekly Rep* 1994;**43**:RR–13.

183 Interdepartmental working group on tuberculosis. *United Kingdom Recommendations for the Prevention and Control of HIV-related Tuberculosis and Drug-resistant, Including Multiple Drug-resistant, Tuberculosis*. Consultation Document. London: Department of Health, 1997.

184 Joint Tuberculosis Committee of the British Thoracic Society. *Chemotherapy and Management of Tuberculosis in the United Kingdom: Recommendations*. 1998.

185 Barrett NJ, Morse DL. The resurgence of scabies. *Commun Dis Rep Rev* 1993;**3**:R32–34.

186 Hospital Infection Society, Working Party Report. Revised guidelines for the control of methicillin resistant *Staphylococcus aureus. J Hosp Infect* 1998;**39**:253–90.

187 Holmes GP, Hilliard KJ, Kloutz KC *et al*. B virus (Herpes virus simiae) infection in humans: epidemiologic investigations of a cluster. *Ann Intern Med* 1990;**112**:833–9.

188 Holmes GP, Chapman LE, Stewart JA, Straus SE, Hilliard JK, Davenport DS. Guidelines for the prevention and treatment of B-virus infections in exposed persons. The B virus Working Group. *Clin Infect Dis* 1995;**20**:421–39.

189 Freifeld AG, Hilliard J, Southers J, Murray M, Savarese B *et al*. A controlled seroprevalence survey or primate handlers for evidence of asymptomatic herpes B virus infection. *J Infect Dis* 1995;**171**:1031–4.

190 Croft AMJ, Clayton TC, Gould MJ. Side effects of mefloquine prophylaxis for malaria: an independent randomised controlled trial. *Trans Soc Trop Med* 1997;**91**:199–203.

191 Bradley DJ, Fairhurst DC on behalf of an expert group of doctors, nurses and pharmacists Guidelines for the prevention of malaria in travellers from the United Kingdom. *Commun Dis Rev Rep* 1997;**7**:R138–52.

192 Warrell DA, Molyneux ME, Beales PF. Severe and complicated malaria. *Trans R Soc Trop Med Hyg* 1990;**84**(Suppl 2)

193 Winstanley P. Malaria: treatment. *J Roy Coll Phys Lond* 1998;**32**:203–7.

194 Knight R. Amoebiasis. In: Weatherall DJ, Ledingham JE, Warrel DA eds. *Oxford Textbook of Medicine* 3rd edn. Oxford: Oxford University Press, 1996;825–35.

195 Chriske HW, Abdo R, Richrath R, Braumann S. Risk of hepatitis A infection among sewage workers. *Arbeitsmed Sozialmed Praventivmed* 1990;**25**:285–7.

196 Skinhoj P, Hollinger FB *et al*. Infectious liver diseases in three groups of Copenhagen workers: correlation of hepatitis A infection to sewage exposure. *Arch Environ Hlth* 1981;**36**:139–43.

197 Brugha R, Heptonstall J, Farrington P, Andren S, Perry K, Parry J. Risk of hepatitis A infection in sewage workers. *Occup Environ Med* 1998;**55**:567–9.

198 Baxter PJ, Brazier AM, Young SEJ. Is smallpox a hazard in church crypts. *Br J Ind Med* 1998; **45**:359–60.

25

Genetic modification and biotechnology

ANNE M FINN, ALISTER J SCOTT, GREGG M STAVE

Development of biotechnology	521	Risk management of genetic modification work	530
Genetic modification	523	Health surveillance	532
Organisms used in biotechnology	523	Conclusion	533
Products and applications of biotechnology	524	References	534
Biotechnology processes and their health hazards	525		

The term 'biotechnology' has had many different meanings since its first use in 1919,[1] ranging from a branch of technology concerned with the development and exploitation of machines in relation to the various needs of human beings[2] to today's meaning, which is principally based on genetic modification. The definition is broad, but may be described as the use of biological processes for the production of goods and services, and for environmental management.[3,4] There is now a trend for the term to be used in the context of a specific industry, for example food biotechnology, pharmaceutical biotechnology and marine biotechnology. It is essentially a technology which integrates biology, microbiology, chemistry and biochemistry, as well as chemical and process engineering. Genetic modification is defined as the alteration of genetic material in a way that does not occur naturally by mating or natural recombination or both. This includes recombinant DNA techniques using viral or bacterial vectors, the direct introduction of DNA into any organism, e.g. by microinjection, and cell fusion or hybridization.

Biotechnology is widely employed in industry. The United Kingdom Chemical Industries Association estimated in 1994, that 30% of its member companies use biotechnology in three main areas: the production of novel feedstocks; more efficient manufacturing processes; and environmental remediation.[5] Many thousands of people are employed in the industry in roles ranging from molecular biologists and biophysicists to technical and non-technical staff. It is still growing rapidly and as it expands so does the range of biological, chemical and physical hazards to which employees are potentially exposed. The rate of change and development within the industry is also rapid, necessitating frequent revision of health, safety and environmental management of the potential risks surrounding rapidly changing processes.[6]

In general, the current consensus view is that 'biotechnology poses no risks that are fundamentally different from those faced by workers in other processing industries'.[7] Product hazards are deemed 'not likely to differ qualitatively from those encountered in other sectors of the pharmaceutical and chemical industries; the fact that the molecules . . . are the products of organisms rather than of synthetic catalysts will not alter their reactivity or toxicity'.[8] Risks from handling recombinant organisms may be considered to be no greater than those arising from handling unmodified pathogens.[9] Reports of illness or health effects attributable specifically to work with genetically modified microorganisms and recombinant DNA (rDNA) cells are rare.[10] Although exposure to these genetically modified microorganisms, biologically active products and processing chemicals constitutes a potentially serious risk to the health of employees, it is concluded that biotechnology processes are safe if practised with appropriate risk control measures in place.

DEVELOPMENT OF BIOTECHNOLOGY

Traditionally, biotechnology has been based on the purification and enhancement of the products of naturally occurring organisms through selection and mutation, in processes such as brewing and baking. Alcohol remains one of the main products of the biotechnology industry; not only ethanol, but also alcohol for industrial use.

In the last three decades the introduction of genetic modification has improved the yield and purity of products, and allowed the development of new ones. It has also enhanced the performance of traditional process organisms. In the 1950s, antibiotics and vaccines were produced using biotechnology methods, and in the 1960s, single cell protein as a source of food for animals and humans was developed. The early 1970s saw the development of recombinant DNA techniques. This had a major effect on biomedical research and diagnostics, on agriculture, and on food, chemicals and pharmaceutical manufacture.[11]

The first pharmaceutical products made were human insulin, somatostatin and growth hormone. Development since then has been in the area of pharmacologically active mammalian peptides, such as hormones, enzymes and antibodies. Biological response modifiers, such as the interferons and growth factors, such as epidermal growth factor, fibroblast growth factor and platelet derived growth factor have also been manufactured using biotechnology techniques. Tissue plasminogen activator was a successful product of the late 1980s which has been used extensively as thrombolytic therapy for coronary artery disease. Erythropoietin was developed for use in the treatment of anaemia secondary to renal disease and various clotting factors have also been produced. Table 25.1 shows a list of peptides, their host systems, and clinical indications.

There are many other industrial applications of biotechnology, including bacterial enzymes used in the manufacture of detergents, the treatment of leather, and the brewing and baking industries; fungal enzymes used in the preparation of fruit juices; and yeast enzymes in ice-cream manufacture. The water treatment industry also makes extensive use of biotechnology.

The increasing use of genetically modified organisms in laboratory research and large scale industrial processes resulted in concern about the potential health and environmental hazards of the organisms and their products. These concerns led to the introduction of legislative measures to ensure adequate control of any risks. The traditional applications of biotechnology have usually been within the scope of general health and safety law. In the UK, however, specific regulations made under the Health and Safety at Work Act 1974, the Genetically Modified Organisms (Contained Use) Regulations 1996, and the Environmental Protection Act 1990, the Genetically Modified Organisms (Deliberate Release) Regulations 1995, apply to work involving genetically modified organisms.

The UK regulations specify the following requirements:

1 To assess the risk to human health and the environment and to keep records.
2 To establish a local genetic modification safety committee to advise on risk assessments.
3 To classify organisms and operations.
4 To notify the Health and Safety Executive (HSE) of the intention to use premises for genetic modification work for the first time and of subsequent individual activities and, in some cases, to seek consent from the HSE.
5 To adopt controls, including suitable containment measures.
6 To inform the HSE of accidents involving genetically modified organisms.

Guidelines have been produced by the HSE[12,13] and the Department of Environment,[14] which give further information on procedures for risk assessment and control. Independent expert committees have been established to advise government in this complex area. In the UK, some techniques are exempt from the regulations, including mutagenesis, the construction and use of somatic hybridoma cells (for the production of monoclonal antibodies), plant cell fusion where the resultant organisms can be produced by traditional breeding methods and self cloning.

In the USA a number of government agencies are involved in the regulation of biotechnology, including the Food and Drug Administration, the Environmental Protection Agency, and the Department of Agriculture. Each agency has developed a wide range of guidance covering biotechnology. Additional guidance includes

Table 25.1 *Therapeutic or prophylactic products of biotechnology*

Protein	Date	Host system	Indication
Human insulin	1982	*E. coli*	Diabetes
Growth hormone	1985	*E. coli*	Hypopituitarism
Interferon-α	1986	*E. coli*	Hairy cell leukaemia
Hepatitis B surface antigen	1986	*S. cerevisiae*	Prevention of hepatitis B
Tissue plasminogen activator	1987	CHO	Myocardial infarction
Erythropoietin	1989	CHO	Anaemia of renal failure
Factor IX	1992	Hybridoma	Haemophilia B
Factor VIII	1992	CHO	Haemophilia A
Interferon-B	1993	*E. coli*	Multiple sclerosis

CHO: Chinese hamster ovary

guidelines for research involving recombinant DNA molecules,[15] and guidelines for biosafety in microbiological and biomedical laboratories.[16] The former constitutes regulatory guidelines for laboratory research which must be followed by organizations receiving federal funding, and the latter assigns biosafety levels to organisms and specifies the equipment and procedures to be used within each biosafety containment level.

GENETIC MODIFICATION

The development of organisms for use in biotechnology commonly involves the improvement of desirable properties, such as the level of production of a metabolite, as well as eliminating properties that are less useful. Such modification, either incidentally or deliberately as a control measure, may also reduce the ability of the organism to survive outside the bioreactor. Traditional methods for altering such characteristics include selection and mutation, either by chemical or by physical means.[17] Because mutagenesis is a random process, laborious and careful screening is necessary to isolate organisms with the required properties. An additional method for improving the process characteristics of organisms is hybridization; for example, by conjugation between closely related species or strains of bacteria, or by recombination between different mating types of yeast. Protoplast fusion offers an additional method of strain improvement, particularly between organisms of different species.

A specific example of hybridization is the formation of 'hybridomas' for the production of monoclonal antibodies. In this technique, antibody-producing cells from the spleen of an immunized animal (normally a rat or mouse) are fused with homologous myeloma cells and the resulting mixture of cell types grown in selective media. The fusion products are then screened to obtain clones of 'hybridoma' cells that produce useful amounts of antibody against the antigen used for the immunization. These clones are genetically identical and the resulting antibody will be a pure species, or 'monoclonal antibody'.

Much of the current interest in biotechnology is over the use of techniques to develop microorganisms that produce products coded for by genes from a wide variety of sources. Potential donor organisms include viruses, and eukaryotic microorganisms (i.e. microorganisms in which DNA is contained in a distinct nucleus) such as bacteria, plant and animal cells. Hormones and antibodies tend to be produced from animal cells, whereas biotechnology enzyme manufacturers, making components for polymerase chain reaction kits, might use a thermophilic microorganism, e.g. *Thermophilus aquaticus*, to produce the Taq enzyme. Virus donors include HIV (human immunodeficiency virus), whose DNA is used to make vaccines by expression in a heterologous organism.

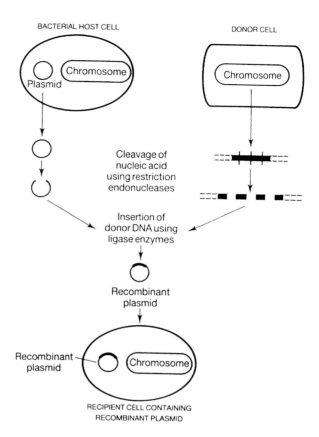

Figure 25.1 *Principles of genetic modification.*

DNA techniques were designed to locate and isolate the desired gene in the nucleic acid of a donor organism.[18] The selected gene is cleaved using restriction endonuclease enzymes (Fig. 25.1) and inserted into a vector capable of being inserted or incorporated into the recipient cell (either a circular piece of DNA termed a plasmid, or a virus). The 'new' gene is joined to the vector's nucleic acid using ligase enzymes. The vector can then be used to introduce the gene into the recipient or host cell, to which it is able to pass on the characteristics coded in the gene from the donor organism. Host species have included *Saccharomyces cerevisiae*, *Bacillus* spp. and *Streptomyces* spp., as well as *Escherichia coli*. Transfection is also used to produce recombinant organisms. This is another way of transferring genetic material without using plasmids or viruses.

ORGANISMS USED IN BIOTECHNOLOGY

These come from a wide range of taxonomic groups, including bacteria, fungi and viruses, as well as animal and plant cells. The most common organisms used for biotechnology medicines are animal cells and bacteria; however, fungi are still widely used in other industrial (i.e. non-pharmaceutical) processes. Viruses can carry and donate DNA and are most commonly used during vaccine production. Viruses are also used extensively as vectors in molecular biological research and in therapeutic delivery systems.

PRODUCTS AND APPLICATIONS OF BIOTECHNOLOGY

The various applications of biotechnology can be divided into five main categories: biomass production, metabolite production, recombinant DNA pharmaceutical production, transformation processes and enzyme production.

Biomass production

Biomass production involves the use of the organism itself as the product, usually for animal feed but in some cases as a human food product. Apart from the use of yeast cells in the baking industry, biomass production is often referred to in the UK as single-cell protein production. Examples include the use of *Fusarium graminearum* to produce Quorn® for human consumption and *Methylophilus methylotrophus* for the production of Pruteen® for animal feed.

Metabolite production

Metabolite production exploits the biosynthetic capabilities of organisms and has resulted in the establishment of many industrial processes. A metabolite is something that is produced during growth, stationary or even death phases of culture. Growth of an organism results in a range of metabolites being produced. Whether the desired metabolite will predominate depends upon the organism, its growth rate and the culture conditions used. The compounds produced may be either primary or secondary metabolites; or, in the case of a genetically modified organism, they could be 'foreign' or 'novel' metabolites introduced from another organism. Primary metabolites are compounds produced in the logarithmic growth phase when cells are growing at constant, maximal rate.

Compounds produced during this phase are either essential to the growth of the organism, such as amino acids, lipids and carbohydrates, or are byproducts of catabolism such as ethanol. Once the logarithmic growth phase has ceased, because either nutrients have been exhausted or toxic metabolites have built up, growth eventually stops and the culture enters the stationary phase. During the stationary phase, products termed secondary metabolites are produced which play no obvious role in cell growth and are usually specific to particular groups of organisms. Secondary metabolites include the antibiotics, alkaloids and some other molecules. Genetic modification has extended the range of metabolites that may be produced by microorganisms. For example, microbial cells may be developed with the ability to synthesize compounds normally associated with plant or animal cells, including hormones, growth factors, and proteins such as serum albumin.

Recombinant pharmaceutical products

Following the discovery of recombinant DNA in the early 1970s, within 4 years, genetically modified bacteria were being used to make human insulin, somatostatin and growth hormone. Since then the major thrust of recombinant DNA technology has been the production of rare mammalian peptides, which are pharmaceutically active hormones, enzymes, antibodies and biological response modifiers. Previously, these peptides were harvested from animal tissue. Large numbers of animals, and a significant amount of processing activity were required to produce tiny amounts of the desired substance. Now they can be made on demand, in bacterial or yeast culture and quality is easier to control. The problems associated with contamination of the product with infectious agents present in the host animal can be eliminated (e.g. the risk of transmission of the Creutzfeldt–Jakob disease agent from growth hormone derived from human pituitary glands). The proteins yielded are purer, and the process is more economical.

Examples of recombinant pharmaceutical products are human insulin, growth hormone, tissue plasminogen activator, erythropoietin, interferons and interleukins. Commonly used organisms are *E.coli, Bacillus subtilis, Saccharomyces cerevisiae,* and *Aspergillus niger.* Occasionally, the rDNA product differs slightly from the natural product but retains therapeutic activity, as with gamma interferon produced from *E.coli*.[19] In other cases, molecules or transformation steps can be added by the recombinant cell. Mammalian cells are frequently used and genes coding for reproductive hormones such as human chorionic gonadotrophin and luteinizing hormone have been cloned and expressed in such cells. As biotechnology progresses, some products currently made by mammalian cells may soon be made more cheaply using bacterial cells, e.g. human TPA (tissue plasminogen activator).[20] The qualities and specific activities of some peptides can be modified by adding various ingredients to the culture broth.[21] The peptides themselves can be changed by recombinant technology, e.g. by recombination of hybrid genes to produce proteins (analogues) with different but more desirable properties.

The pharmaceutical industry is also using this technology to research the amino acid sequence of naturally occurring bioregulatory proteins. This will allow the development of analogues which act as inhibitors or promoters of activity. Many vaccines are now produced using biotechnology. Genes can be cloned and expressed, which code for specific antigens of viruses, bacteria and parasites. An early example of this is the hepatitis B vaccine which utilizes yeast to produce hepatitis B surface antigen. Also, DNA from genetically modified vaccinia virus has been used to produce protective antigens for hepatitis B, rabies and malaria vaccines.[22]

Monoclonal antibodies (produced from a combination of myeloma cells and antibody-producing cells from the spleen of an immunized mouse) are used in diagnostic kits, in protein purification, and as therapeutic agents in cancer and organ transplant rejection. They have also been tested for use in septicaemia[23] and in rheumatoid arthritis, with disappointing results.

Recombinant DNA technology has also been applied to the production of antibiotics, and in the development of direct-acting gene therapies, e.g. for cystic fibrosis and rheumatoid arthritis. The 'normal' gene is administered to patients with the aim of incorporating this 'good' genetic material into cells to influence the course of the disease.

Transformation processes

Transformation processes involve the enzymic conversion of one compound into another. This may involve, for example, isomerization, oxidation, hydroxylation or dehydrogenation. Examples of transformation processes include the oxidation of ethanol into acetic acid and the production of steroids such as hydrocortisone or cortisone from plant steroids.

Enzyme production

Enzyme production involves the isolation of useful enzymes from organisms either to use in transformation processes or for other purposes. Examples include proteases from *Bacillus subtilis* which are used in the manufacture of biological detergents and pectinases from *Aspergillus* spp., used in drink manufacture. These applications of biotechnology can be divided into four different types of process:

1 non-aseptic processes using indigenous organisms such as in traditional wine production;
2 non-aseptic processes using specified inocula which include brewing and milk fermentation;
3 aseptic processes using specified inocula, as in antibiotic and single-cell protein production;
4 aseptic and contained processes using potentially hazardous organisms, such as vaccine production.

BIOTECHNOLOGY PROCESSES AND THEIR HEALTH HAZARDS

A typical industrial biotechnology process involves a number of stages: inoculum preparation (for processes using specific inocula); large-scale growth of the organism in a bioreactor; separation of the organism from its growth medium; and product recovery and purification. These stages are summarized in Fig. 25.2. The process may be

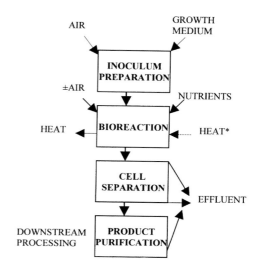

Figure 25.2 *A generalized schematic representation of a typical biotechnology production process. *Although cell growth is exothermic in mammalian cell culture, heat must still be added to maintain a high enough temperature for growth.*

Table 25.2 *Typical unit operations in downstream processing*

Downstream processing stage	Typical process alternatives
Harvesting	Centrifugation Filtration Flocculation Membrane separation
Product separation	Homogenization Solvent extraction Ultrafiltration Distillation Affinity chromatography Lysis
Product purification	Ion exchange Chromatographic separation Gel filtration Electrophoresis Fractional crystallization Precipitation
Product concentration	Precipitation Crystallization Evaporation Ultrafiltration

aerobic or anaerobic, depending upon the organism used, and may be carried out in bioreactors ranging from open pan vessels to highly enclosed systems that may require mechanical agitation or aeration. Downstream processing depends on whether the product is intracellular or extracellular. Intracellular product requires extraction whereas extracellular product is purified from spent medium (Fig. 25.3) and the health hazard and effluent issues may be quite different. Extraction of intracellular product generally requires that the cells are disrupted, usually by chemical lysis or by physical disruption such as homogenization. The potential for release of aerosols is greatest during disruption stages. The final processing stages are purification and concentration of the product, through some of the operations listed in Table 25.2. A typical biotechnology pilot plant is shown in Fig. 25.4.

Biotechnology processes may result in risk of exposure to biological, chemical, ergonomic, physical and other hazards.

Biological hazards

The organisms used in biotechnology processes present a number of potential hazards for consideration. These include infection, toxic effects, allergenic or other biological effects of the organisms or cells, its components or its naturally occurring metabolic products and other products expressed by the organism.[24–27] Occupational exposure may occur via inhalation, ingestion, inoculation or transmission through broken skin and mucous membranes.

The effect on health of exposure to an organism depends on the route of entry of the organism, its viability, transmissibility, dose received and immune status of the exposed individual. Most organisms used in industrial processes are unlikely to cause human disease or to cause significant harm to the environment. More risk may accompany the use of non-modified organisms than genetically modified microorganisms, which are often unable to survive outside the bioreactor. However, cases of ill-health amongst individuals involved in genetic modification work may not always be attributed to occupational exposure, leading to underreporting. Occupational infections are not always recognized as such, especially if the resulting disease or symptoms occur commonly in the community. Reports of ill-health associated with biotechnology processes are summarized in Table 25.3.

The biotechnology industry has experienced a good health and safety record. The current consensus is that the potential risks of rDNA research, development and manufacturing activities were overstated initially.[7] The hazards associated with this work are similar to those associated with the organisms, vectors, DNA, chemicals and physical apparatus being used. This is supported by the fact that studies designed to test the capacity of a host organism to acquire novel hazardous properties from DNA donor cells failed to demonstrate the existence of this potential hazard, and no illness attributed to infection with a genetically modified microorganism has been reported.

Possible human health hazards related to genetic modification work include:

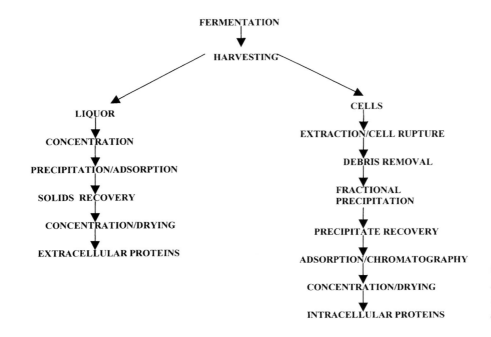

PURIFICATION OF FERMENTATION PRODUCTS

FERMENTATION

HARVESTING

LIQUOR

CONCENTRATION

PRECIPITATION/ADSORPTION

SOLIDS RECOVERY

CONCENTRATION/DRYING

EXTRACELLULAR PROTEINS

CELLS

EXTRACTION/CELL RUPTURE

DEBRIS REMOVAL

FRACTIONAL PRECIPITATION

PRECIPITATE RECOVERY

ADSORPTION/CHROMATOGRAPHY

CONCENTRATION/DRYING

INTRACELLULAR PROTEINS

Figure 25.3 *The various steps involved in purification of products from fermentation broth or cells.*[6]

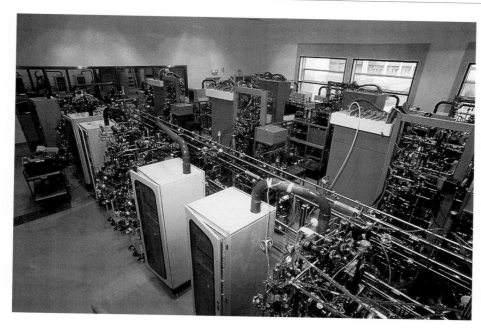

Figure 25.4 *Fermenters in a bioprocessing pilot plant. Courtesy of GlaxoWellcome Plc.*

Table 25.3 *Incidents of ill-health in biotechnology processes*

Organism	Process	Symptoms
Aspergillus penicillium[28]	Fermentation: citric acid production, Czechoslovakia	Bronchitis
Pseudomonas aeruginosa[29]	Downstream processing (centrifugation): enzyme isolation, UK	Flu-like symptoms Kidney/stomach pains
Methylophilus methylotrophus[30]	Fermentation/downstream processing: single-cell protein production, UK	Flu-like symptoms Conjunctivitis
Methylophilus methanolica[31]	Downstream processing (spray drying): single-cell protein production, Sweden	Flu-like symptoms Conjunctivitis
Aspergillus niger[32]	Fermentation/downstream processing: citric acid production, UK	Asthma. Respiratory symptoms
	Fermentation: citric acid production, USSR	Respiratory symptoms
Yeasts[33]	Fermentation/downstream	Asthma. Bronchitis
Streptomyces spp[34]	Downstream processing: single cell protein production, USSR antibiotic production, UK	Respiratory symptoms. Conjunctivitis

1 Exposure to a genetically modified microorganism resulting in infection or delivery of expressed biologically active molecules such as enzymes, hormones or toxins to target tissues.

2 Risk of transmissible spongiform encephalopathy from exposure to modified prion protein genes.

3 Exposure to cloned human genes that could lead to an immune response and subsequent autoimmune disorders.

4 Exposure to a gene product, leading to induction of an immune response, that could cause therapeutic complications if treatment with that product was required.

5 Respiratory sensitization related to exposure to

foreign proteins, with the possibility that inclusion bodies and fusion proteins may increase the risk of sensitization.

6   Exposure to cloned oncogenic sequences or genetically modified retroviruses that could pose a carcinogenic risk.

Special consideration should be given to work with DNA containing genes coding for potent toxins or for onco-genes. Theoretically, there is the possibility that the introduction of oncogenic sequences into a human, as a result of an occupational accident or cumulative expo-sure, could cause cell transformation and lead to tumour growth.[35] No cases of this have been reported. Particular concern has been raised about possible oncogene expo-sure through inhalation, since the newer potential thera-pies use airborne viruses such as adenovirus.

Much recombinant DNA work has used *E. coli* K12 as the recipient organism. Its modification demonstrates how many rDNA organisms are disabled so that they can no longer survive in the human host. Because *E. coli* K12 lacks certain surface antigens, the fimbriae which enable it to adhere to gut epithelial walls, resistance to lysis by serum complement, resistance to phagocytosis and part of an important liposaccharide, it is thus unable to colo-nize the human gut and is non-pathogenic as a result of these modifications.

Another potential source of biological hazard is cont-aminating organisms present in the culture. This may be of particular concern in animal cell cultures, where viruses (retro, simian, polyoma, herpes or hepatitis), mycoplasma and prions may exist as contaminants. Tasks involving potential aerosol generation or manipu-lation of sharps could expose the employee to a risk of potentially serious infection.

Toxic effects

Toxic effects may result from inhalation of Gram-nega-tive bacterial endotoxin.[36,37] The reaction may follow exposure to the dust of single-cell protein after it has been cultured in fermenters and subsequently dried in a spray drier. Workers exposed to the end-product as a result of inadequate protective measures can develop flu-like febrile reactions 4–12 hours later, with shivering, fever, tightness of the chest, aching limbs and cough. Blood tests reveal neutropenia followed by leucocytosis,[38] and a decline in forced expiratory volume in 1 second (FEV_1)[39] has been described. These symptoms may start during the evening or the night after a day's work but subside by the morning or over the next day. Acute symptoms of conjunctivitis, rhinitis or cough may start immediately after exposure. Sore red eyes with a persis-tent discharge have also been reported. Exposed workers can be found to have precipitating antibodies to the organism but the responses have been regarded as more likely to be due to endotoxin rather than an immunolog-

ical reaction to the organism. Endotoxin intolerance can develop on subsequent challenge.[40,41]

Inadequate protection against exposure to single-cell proteins (protein products developed for animal and human food, e.g. Mycoprotein) or enzymes, may result in allergic effects such as asthma[29–31,34,42–45] or contact der-matitis. Extrinsic allergic alveolitis can follow exposure to fungal spores. Type 1 immediate or anaphylactic response is a theoretical possibility after exposure to enzymes or antibiotics.[46]

The production of biologically active products such as hormones, interleukins and interferon is also potentially hazardous to workers either through direct effects on health or interference with existing disease treatment.

Chemicals

Although biological hazards are the primary focus of this chapter, it should be recognized that there are significant chemical hazards in the biotechnology industry. Potential chemical exposures may occur at many stages in the process.[47] There are differences in the type and vol-ume of chemicals encountered in a research and devel-opment environment and a production environment, and the levels of risk of exposure in each also vary due to differences in the way the chemicals are handled.

Growth media used in tissue cultures and fermenters consist mostly of water, inorganic salts, carbohydrates, amino acids, vitamins and other nutrients. Selective cell growth is supported by the addition of steroids, antibi-otics and anti-neoplastics e.g. methotrexate (Table 25.4), all of which pose a significant health concern, even at low

Table 25.4 *Tissue culture additives*[47]

Antibiotics
Chloramphenicol
Gentamicin
Rifampicin
Streptomycin
Tobramycin

Hormones
Dexamethasone
Growth hormones
Prednisone

Antineopastics and cytotoxins
Actinomycin
Adriamycin
Aminopterin
Bleomycin
Chlorambucil
Cyclophosphamide
Daunorubicin
Sodium azide
Vincristine

levels of exposure. Chronic low level exposure to antibiotics could lead to colonization with antibiotic-resistant organisms. It may also induce or activate drug allergy, which then becomes a problem when the employee is treated with that antibiotic at a later date. Process workers are at greater risk of exposure to chemical hazards than those involved in research scale work. Tasks involved in cell culture preparation including weighing out of chemicals, creating and agitating solutions and cleaning up spills all present a risk of exposure.

Extraction of nucleic acids from whole tissue or tissue culture is an important preliminary phase in virtually all biotechnology processes. Table 25.5 shows a list of solvents and precipitating agents used for these purposes. Trichloroacetic acid and perchloric acid are used commonly, the latter also being an explosion hazard. Dimethyl sulphate is widely used. Certain additives can be acutely hazardous, e.g. sodium azide used to suppress unwanted bacterial growth. Cyanide salts such as cyanogen bromide are used with the potential release of cyanide gas, and its attendant dangers.

High-pressure liquid chromatography is used for the identification of nucleic acid components and requires the use of toxic reagents.

Sequencing establishes the order of DNA pairs in a gene and can involve the use of toxic chemicals such as dimethyl sulphate and hydrofluoric acid. Gel electrophoresis involves the use of acrylamide but the risk of exposure can be reduced by using commercially prepared polyacrylamide gel or finished gel electrophoresis plates. Ethidium bromide, which is a mutagenic substance, is also added to electrophoresis gels.

Sterilizing agents such as formaldehyde are frequently used. Potent solvent detergents, driven through by pressurized steam, are used to sanitize lines in manufacturing facilities. If this is not used in an enclosed system, inhalation exposure may cause respiratory irritation.

Table 25.5 *Chemical solvents and extractants*[47]

Ammonium compounds	EDTA
2-Aminoethanol	Ethanol
Benzene	Ethers
Chloroform	Ethylene glycol
Carbon tetrachloride	Hydrazine
Chloral hydrate	Hydrochloric acid
Chromic acid	Formic acid
Chromium trichloride	Lithium compounds
Cyanogen bromide	2-Mercaptoethanol
Cyanogen chloride	Methanol
Cyclohexane	Naphthalene
Chlorodifluoromethane	Paraformaldehyde
Diisopropylethylamine	Phenylhydrazine
Dimethoxybenzidine dihydrochloride	Toluene
5-Bromo-4-chloro-3-indolyl phosphate *p*-toluidine	
Cobalt chloride hexahydrate	

EDTA: Ethylenediaminetetraacetic acid

Ergonomic hazards

Working environments where genetic modification work is conducted range from laboratory to manufacturing plant housing large bioreactors. Employees may also work in traditional office environments and processes are increasingly computer controlled. In addition, the role of scientists has changed to the extent that up to 30% of a bio-analyst's job may be carried out using a computer outside the traditional biological laboratory environment.

These working arrangements mean that employees are exposed to a variety of ergonomic hazards. The importance of a good ergonomic fit for staff using display screen equipment is well known. Less well appreciated is the ergonomic challenge presented by a laboratory environment. The design of safety cabinets may make it difficult to sit comfortably with a suitable work posture. Pipettes vary in weight and efficiency and do not suit all operators equally. Tasks in biotechnology labs are often repetitive, requiring accuracy and speed and are carried out while maintaining upper limbs in non-neutral postures. It is thus important to carry out an ergonomic assessment of these tasks, to minimize risks to health. The increasing trend to automate sample processing will help reduce ergonomic risks.

Media preparation involves a significant amount of material handling as sacks of powdered constituents are moved around, weighed, dispensed and added to solutions. The resulting liquids often have to be moved again to storage or to other parts of the plant. Manual handling risk assessment must be carried out, training delivered to handlers and recommendations adhered to. Despite the sophistication of the biotechnology industry, and the emphasis on biological and genetic modification risks, manual handling accidents and musculoskeletal ill-health are probably the leading causes of work-related ill-health in the industry.

Physical hazards

Another potential health hazard in biotechnology plants is noise, resulting in a risk of noise-induced hearing loss to exposed workers. The physical hazards of steam, heat, pressure and radiation, both ionizing and non-ionizing, must also be considered. It is still not uncommon for scalds to occur, as steam is used for sterilization of fermentation vessels and lines. Other physical hazards are combustion and explosion.

Mental stressors

Finally, this comprehensive list of hazards would not be complete without the inclusion of workplace stressors. Biotechnology employees are as susceptible as any other to mental health effects from exposure to excessive pressures at work, perhaps more than some, due to the rapid pace of change in their industry. There are the added fears and anxieties related to working with genetically modified organisms and substances which have the potential to cause lasting or heritable ill-health effects. The provision of information to staff is crucial to help allay these fears. The psychological aspects of lone working or shift working should also be considered.

Environmental considerations

To render process microorganisms non-viable and to inactivate other components, the waste stream may require treatment by physical, chemical or biological methods, or a combination of these. Effluent from biotechnology processes may include growth medium components, viable and non-viable organisms, suspended solids and waste water. It will also include such chemicals as inducers, solvents, detergents, cleaning agents, buffers and alkali and acids used for pH adjustment.

RISK MANAGEMENT OF GENETIC MODIFICATION WORK

The approach to the risk assessment of genetic modification work has focused on classification schemes that identify categories of microbiological hazard to human health and the environment, and schemes for assigning appropriate levels of containment and control measures to minimize risks. In the UK, the Genetically Modified Organisms (Contained Use) Regulations were amended in 1996 to implement the European Union directive on the contained use of genetically modified microorganisms.[12] This requires that all genetically modified microorganisms are classified into one of two hazard groups. The classification considers characteristics of the recipient or parental organism, the vector and insert, the insert DNA and the final microorganism.

Group I genetically modified microorganisms are those that are unlikely to cause disease to humans, animals and plants and adverse effects in the environment. Genetically modified microorganisms which do not fulfil the criteria for Group I are classified as Group II. Genetically modified microorganisms can be classified as Group II on environmental grounds, even if they do not pose a hazard to human health. The scheme also classifies operations into Type A or B according to the scale and purpose of the work. Genetic modification activities will be classified into four groups according to the containment level indicated by the risk assessment of the work. A similar classification scheme is operated in the USA.[15]

The procedure for risk assessment includes:

1 consideration of the predicted properties of the genetically modified microorganism to determine if there are any potential mechanisms by which it could represent a hazard to human health;

2 consideration of the likelihood that the genetically modified microorganism could actually cause harm to human health;
3 consideration of the nature of the work to be undertaken;
4 assignment of control measures to safeguard human health;
5 identification of hazards to the environment, assuming that the control measures required to safeguard human health have been applied, to determine the need for additional containment measures.

It is best if the risk assessment and conclusions about control measures are reviewed by a genetic modification safety committee, consisting of members with a range of relevant skills, to ensure that appropriate risk control decisions are made. Review by such a committee is a requirement in the UK under the Contained Use Regulations.

Specific systems exist for the assessment of risks to human health from genetically modified microorganisms. One such system, the Brenner Scheme,[13] has been practised in the UK since the 1970s and was originally developed to assess work that was almost entirely based on cloning into E. coli. The scheme involves assigning values (negative exponentials) to 'access' (the likelihood that the organism could enter and survive in a human), 'expression' (a measure of the level of expression of the cloned protein) and 'damage' (the potential for the expressed protein to cause harm). The values are multiplied to provide an index of hazard that then allows a provisional containment level to be assigned (Table 25.6). However, the scheme does not constitute a comprehensive risk assessment as it does not consider environmental risks, and there are some situations where the assessment is unreliable. It is also not applicable to the assessment of work with viral vectors.

It is important that the risk assessment relating to the genetically modified microorganism is considered in the wider context of all the hazards and risks associated with genetic modification work, so that appropriate risk management measures can be integrated. This involves including consideration of hazards arising from allergenic properties of the organism, toxic products expressed by the organism and chemical or ergonomic hazards related to the process.

Having identified and evaluated all the potential health

Table 25.6 *Brenner scheme hazard assessment and provisional containment levels*

Overall value	Provisional containment level
10^{-15} or lower	1
10^{-12} or lower	2
10^{-9} or lower	3
10^{-6} or lower	3 or 4
$> 10^{-6}$	4

and environmental hazards involved in the work, the sequence of tasks involved in the process should be reviewed to identify ways in which operator exposure or environmental release could occur. This should include assessment of both normal operating conditions and unplanned incidents such as spillages. The scale of work involved as well as the titre of microorganisms handled will influence the selection of control measures. The outcome of this assessment, combined with methods for assessing biological and other hazards involved in the process, will permit conclusions to be drawn about the combination of control measures required to minimize risks.

The control measures indicated will include some or all of the following: physical containment and segregation of work areas; general and local extract ventilation; work practices; organizational controls; operator training; and personal protective equipment. Although there are methods for monitoring for the presence of microorganisms in the work environment, there are no valid occupational exposure limits on which to base a judgement of adequacy of control. Relevant occupational exposure limits for other hazards should be observed. There may be a requirement to protect the product, particularly in the pharmaceutical and food industries, that may affect the methods of control selected.

There are schemes in the UK and USA which group control measures into four levels of containment with separate guidance for large- and small-scale operations.[13,16] Some examples of measures to contain small-scale work are given in Table 25.7.

The control measures applied should aim to protect a workforce of average susceptibility. However, it may be necessary to consider the need for additional measures for more vulnerable individuals or groups. Most of these can be addressed individually through a health surveillance programme, but the need to conduct a generic assessment of risks to female employees, in the event of pregnancy or a period of breast feeding, is a legal requirement in the UK. This requires consideration of special risks to mothers or their unborn or newborn baby, and conclusions to be drawn about any additional measures that would be indicated for such employees. Additional measures could include adjustments such as alterations to work arrangements, additional control measures or partial or complete removal from potential exposure.

Finally, an important aspect of the risk assessment process is effective communication of the hazards and risk control measures to the individuals who will perform the work. This ensures that individuals understand the work practices and procedures that must be followed to minimize health and environmental risks. It is advisable to extend risk communication activities to other employees who work alongside genetic modification activities. These employees have been shown to overestimate health risks.[48]

Table 25.7 *Examples of containment and control measures for small scale activities*

Containment and control measures	Containment level			
	1	2	3	4
Building/physical measures				
Workplace separated from other activities in the same building	No	No	Yes	Yes
Workplace maintained at an air pressure negative to atmosphere	No	No, unless mechanically ventilated	Yes	Yes
Input and extract air to be filtered using HEPA or equivalent	No	No	Yes, on extract air	Yes, on input and double (2 stage in series) on extract air
Workplace sealable to permit fumigation	No	No	Yes	Yes
Work practice measures				
Biohazard signs and level of work posted	No	Optional	Yes	Yes
Access restricted to authorized persons only	No	Yes	Yes	Yes
Laboratory to contain its own equipment	No	No	Yes, so far as is reasonably practicable	Yes
Viable material, including any infected animal, to be handled in biological safety cabinet or isolator or other suitable container	No	Yes, where aerosol produced	Yes, where aerosol produced	Yes (Class III cabinet)

HEPA: High efficiency particulate air

HEALTH SURVEILLANCE

Health surveillance was a prominent risk control measure in the past when the health risks arising from genetic modification were considered to be uncertain. National guidance in several countries promoted highly prescriptive health surveillance procedures, with a hierarchy of measures linked to categories of containment levels. However, with growing experience of occupational health outcomes showing little evidence of health problems related to genetic modification work,[6] it is clear that these traditional measures have been out of proportion to the risks to health.

The role of health surveillance has been revised in recently updated guidance, such as that produced by the Advisory Committee on Genetic Modification in the UK in October 1997.[13] The emphasis has been placed on determining appropriate health surveillance procedures based on a risk assessment of the likelihood of health effects resulting from exposure to all the potential hazards involved in genetic modification work. Health surveillance is likely to be appropriate when all of the following criteria are fulfilled:

1 an identifiable health effect may be related to exposure;
2 there is a reasonable likelihood that the disease or effect may occur under the conditions of the work;
3 there are valid techniques for detecting indications of the disease or health effect.

The purpose of any health surveillance programme could be to collect baseline information to assist in the identification of subsequent ill-health, identify health factors which are likely to increase vulnerability or susceptibility to exposure-related health effects or permit early detection of such effects. Additional aims could be to evaluate the efficacy of control measures or provide data for subsequent epidemiological study. There is also an opportunity to communicate health risks and to counsel employees about any health concerns.

Decision-making on the indications for, and content of, health surveillance programmes should be made by an occupational physician who is experienced in this field and who is involved with the organization's biological safety committee that has responsibility for reviewing risk assessments of genetic modification work. If health assessment procedures are indicated, an occupational health nurse can perform these and obtain advice from the occupational physician overseeing the programme.

Low risk genetic modification work

For work with genetically modified microorganisms that present no identifiable risk to human health, such as those classified as Group I in the European hazard classification scheme, it is unlikely that there will be any indication for health surveillance. However, health surveillance may still be appropriate if there are identifiable health effects related to an allergenic response to the genetically modified microorganism or to toxic effects from expressed products.

It may still be appropriate to conduct an initial health assessment to identify individuals who may be at greater risk because of pre-existing illness or an underlying medical condition. The aim of such an assessment would be to consider the need for additional control measures or to identify adjustments to allow the individual to carry out the work with tolerable control of health risks. The following factors may require special consideration:

1 relevant medical history such as a history of asthma or recurrent infections;
2 health problems which reduce the efficacy of barriers to infection such as disorders of the skin, respiratory tract and alimentary canal;
3 reduced immune competence;
4 treatment with antibiotics, in particular those used in the work, or systemic steroid therapy and other treatments that could increase susceptibility to infection.

Higher risk genetic modification work

Health surveillance may be indicated if there is likelihood that any of the following potential health hazards may result in exposure-related health effects:

1 infection, particularly with modified viruses which exhibit altered tissue tropism, reduced susceptibility to therapeutic agents or where conventional immunization would result in reduced protection;
2 oncogenic or tumorigenic sequences that could give rise to a risk of carcinogenisis if incorporated into human cells;
3 modified prion protein genes that could cause transmissible spongiform encephalopathy;
4 biologically active substances expressed by genetically modified microorganisms such as enzymes, hormones or toxins;
5 cloned human genes that may lead to an immune response and subsequent autoimmune disease;
6 substances that are asthmagens.

There is a range of health surveillance procedures that could be applied. Periodic enquiry about respiratory symptoms and lung function assessment would be an appropriate method of surveillance if occupational asthma were assessed to be a forseeable health effect. For lower risk situations, providing information about relevant symptoms and encouraging self-reporting may be all that is indicated.

Biological effect monitoring could be used to detect IgG antibody to the genetically modified microorganism in use, either to establish immune status prior to exposure, or to detect seroconversion after a period of potential exposure. Immunization may be indicated for work with certain organisms. In the past, immunization with smallpox vaccine was recommended for work with modified strains of vaccinia virus, but there would be few circumstances now when this would be indicated as a result of a risk assessment of work with this virus. Maintaining records of exposure may be an appropriate method of health surveillance for work with oncogenic sequences where there is likely to be a long latency period between exposure and possible carcinogenic effects.

Storage of serum samples

Long-term storage of serum samples taken prior to exposure as a baseline reference has been widely practised in the past. The idea was that if antibody responses relevant to the genetically modified microorganisms being handled were subsequently detected, the baseline sample could be tested for comparison. However, there are few circumstances when the health benefits to the individual justify conducting such an invasive procedure. The practice should be restricted to situations where consideration of the risk assessment for the work indicates a clear health or social benefit to the individual.

Possible indications include circumstances where immunological response to exposure to a genetically modified microorganism or an expressed product could cause confusion during diagnostic tests for infection with the same or a related microorganism. Examples include expressed HIV proteins, where antibodies to these proteins form the basis of serological tests for HIV infection. In general, there is only likely to be an indication for baseline serum storage when the current diagnostic tests would have difficulty distinguishing true infection from immunological response to a related protein, or acute from chronic infection states, and where such confusion could have substantial health or social consequences.

If serum storage is practised, then it is important that the purpose of the procedure is explained to the employee and informed consent obtained. It should be emphasized that the individual is only consenting to the sample being stored and that subsequent testing would only be conducted with the individual's express consent, even after the individual has left the organization where the sample is stored. A sample of approximately 5 ml of serum should be labelled to allow later identification of the donor and stored in a secure freezer at −20°C or below, with arrangements made for dealing with sample salvage in the event of freezer malfunction. The period of long-term storage before discarding the sample should be agreed with the donor. It is unlikely that there would be advantages in storing such samples for longer than 40 years.

Medical contact cards

In the past, issuing such cards to employees involved in genetic modification work with higher hazard genetically modified microorganisms was common practice. The purpose of the card was to alert other medical personnel to the possibility of occupationally acquired infection and provide details on how to contact someone at the employing organization who would be able to give the clinician information about relevant biohazards. As for other health measures, it would seem preferable to identify circumstances where this is indicated through consideration of the risk assessment for the work.

Health records

Health records should be maintained of all health assessments conducted as part of any health surveillance related to genetic modification work. Records that contain clinical information must be held in confidence by health care professionals.

Records of exposure may also be indicated for work which involves higher hazard microorganisms, prion proteins or oncogenic sequences where there is known to be a long latent period of many years between exposure and the onset of ill-health related to infection or carcinogenisis. These records should include personal identifying information, details of the nature of the hazards, the dates when the work started and finished and information that links the record to the relevant risk assessment and any exposure monitoring data. Such non-clinical records can be maintained by the employer. The records could also be used to provide retrospective information on health and related exposures for epidemiological investigation.

CONCLUSION

The clinician may be puzzled at the contrast between the complexities of biotechnology with its surrounding myriad of regulations and control measures and the dearth of data on ill-health in the scientists and production workers involved. The industry is perceived to have a good health record, but, to be able to demonstrate the absence of a problem or to provide early warning of an unforeseen health hazard in this novel and rapidly expanding technology, it will be important to ensure that health surveillance measures based on sound theoretical considerations, including epidemiological studies where appropriate, are maintained. The challenge for the future will be to ensure that any potential hazards to human health or the environment are controlled to the satisfaction of employees, health and safety professionals, regulatory authorities and, ultimately, the general public.

REFERENCES

1 Bud R. History of 'biotechnology'. *Nature* 1989; **337**: 10.

2 Simpson JA, Weiner ESC (eds). *Oxford English Dictionary*. Oxford: Clarendon Press, 1989.

3 Kennedy MJ. The evolution of the word 'biotechnology.' *Trends Biotechnol* 1991; **9**: 218–20.

4 Advisory Council on Science and Technology. *Developments in Biotechnology*. London: HMSO, 1990.

5 Anonymous. The biotechnology boom. *Eur Chem News Chemscope* 1994; **62**: 38–40.

6 Liberman DF, Ducatman AM, Fink R. Biotechnology: is there a role for medical surveillance? In: Hyer WC ed. *Bioprocessing Safety: Worker and Community Safety and Health Considerations*. Philadelphia: ASTM, 1990 : 101–10.

7 Miller H. Report on the World Health Organization Working Group on Health Implications of Biotechnology. *Recomb DNA Tech Bull* 1983; **6**: 65–6.

8 Landrigan PJ, Cohen ML, Dowdle W, Elliott LJ, Halperin W. Medical Surveillance of Biotechnology Workers: Report of the CDC/NIOSH Ad Hoc Working Group on Medical Surveillance for Industrial Applications of Biotechnology. *Recomb DNA Tech Bull* 1982; **5**: 133–8.

9 Frommer W, Kraeme P. Safety aspects in biotechnology: classifications and safety precautions for handling of biological agents e.g. genetically engineered micro-organism containment. *Drugs Made in Germany* 1990; **33**: 128–32.

10 Cohen R, Hoerner CL. Occupational health perspective: recombinant DNA technology – human gene therapy safety. *Biopharm Manufact* 1994; **7**: 28–38.

11 Demain AL. An overview of biotechnology. *Occup Med State Art Rev* 1991; 157–68.

12 Health and Safety Executive. *A guide to the Genetically Modified Organisms (Contained Use) Regulations 1992, as amended in 1996*. London: HMSO, 1996.

13 Health and Safety Executive. *Compendium of guidance from the Health and Safety Commission's Advisory Committee on Genetic Modification*. London: HMSO, 1997.

14 Department of Environment. *ACRE Guidance Note 7*. London: HMSO, 1996.

15 National Institutes for Health. *Guidelines for Research Involving Recombinant DNA Molecules*. Washington DC: Federal Register, 1994 (59FR34496).

16 Centres for Disease Control. *Biosafety in Microbiological and Biomedical Laboratories* 3rd edn. Washington DC: Government Printing Office, 1993.

17 Glover DM. *Gene Cloning: The Mechanics of DNA Manipulation*. London: Chapman and Hall, 1984.

18 Duffus JH, Brown CM. Health aspects of biotechnology. *Ann Occup Hyg* 1985; **29**: 1–12.

19 Rinderknecht E, O'Connor BH, Rodriguez H. Natural human interferon-γ: Complete amino acid sequencing and determination of site of glycosylation. *J Biol Chem* 1984; **259**: 6790–7.

20 Sarmientos P, Duchesne M, Denefle P *et al*. Synthesis and purification of active human tissue plasminogen activator from *Escherichia coli*. *BioTechnology* 1989; **7**: 495–501.

21 Knight P. The carbohydrate frontier. *BioTechnology* 1989; **7**: 35–40.

22 Brown F, Shild GC, Ada GL. Recombinant vaccinia viruses as vaccines. *Nature* 1986; **319**: 549–50.

23 Bone R. Why sepsis trials fail. *JAMA* 1996; **276**: 565–6.

24 Dutkiewicz J, Jabionski L, Olenchock SA. Occupational biohazards: a review. *Am J Ind Med* 1988; **14**: 605–23.

25 Lacey J, Crook B. Fungal and actinomycete spores as pollutants of the workplace and occupational allergen. *Ann Occup Hyg* 1988; **32**: 515–33.

26 Demain AL, Solomon NA. Industrial microbiology. *Scient Amer* 1981; **245**: 43–51.

27 World Health Organization. Health impact of biotechnology – report on a Working Group. *Swiss Biotech* 1984; **2**: 7–32.

28 Dunnil P. Biosafety in the large scale isolation of intracellular microbial enzymes. *Chem Ind* 1982; **22**: 877–9.

29 Topping MD, Scarisbrick DA, Luczynska CM, Clarke CE, Seaton A. Clinical and immunological reactions to *Aspergillus niger* among workers at a biotechnology plant. *Br J Ind Med* 1985; **41**: 312–8.

30 Mayers RW. Lack of allergic reaction in workers exposed to Pruteen (bacterial single cell protein). *Br J Ind Med* 1982; **39**: 183–6.

31 Ekenvall L, Dolling B, Gother C-J, Ebbinghaus L, Von Stedingk L-V, Wasserman J. Single cell protein as an occupational hazard. *Br J Ind Med* 1983; **40**: 212–5.

32 Caijka NA, Jakovskaja ME. Occupational fungal allergy and ways to detect it. *Gig Tr Prof Zabol* 1972; **16**: 32–5.

33 Rimmington A. *Release of Microorganism and Pollutants from Soviet Microbiological Facilities: the political and environmental fall-out*. Birmingham: University of Birmingham, 1989.

34 Horejsi M, Sach J, Tomasikova A, Med A, Blahnikova D *et al*. A syndrome resembling farmer's lung in workers inhaling spores of aspergillus and penicillin moulds. *Thorax* 1960; **15**: 212–7.

35 Burns PA, Jack A, Neilson F, Haddow S, Balmain A. Transformation of mouse skin endothelial cells *in vivo* by direct application of plasmid DNA encoding the human T24 *H-ras* oncogene. *Oncogene* 1991; **6**: 1973–8.

36 Burrell R, Ye Shu-Hua. Toxic risks from inhalation of bacterial endotoxin. *Br J Ind Med* 1990; **47**: 688–91.

37 Palchak RB, Cohen R, Ainslie M, Hoerner CL. Airborne endotoxin associated with industrial scale production of protein products in Gram-negative bacteria. *Am Ind Hyg Assoc J* 1988; **49**: 420–42.

38 Birch K. *The Role of Endotoxin Tolerance in Byssinosis*. Morgan town, WV: West Virginia University, 1983.

39 Pernis B, Vigliani EC, Cavagna C, Finulli M. The role of bacterial endotoxins in occupational disease caused by inhaling dusts. *Br J Ind Med* 1961; **18**: 120–9.

40 DeMaria TF, Burrell R. Effect of inhaled endotoxin-containing bacteria. *Environ Res* 1980; **23**: 87–97.

41 Lantz RC, Birch K, Hinton DE, Burrell R. Morphometric changes in the lung induced by inhaled bacterial endotoxin. *Exp Mol Pathol* 1985; **43**: 305–20.

42 Flindt MLH. Pulmonary disease due to inhalation of derivatives of *Bacillus subtilis* containing proteolytic enzyme. *Lancet* 1969; **i**: 1177–81.

43 Pepys J, Hargreaves RE, Longbottom JL, Faux J. Allergic reactions of the lungs to enzymes of *Bacillus subtilis*. *Lancet* 1969; **i**: 1181–4.

44 Newhouse ML, Tagg B, Pocock ST, McEwan AC. An epidemiological study of workers producing enzyme washing powders. *Lancet* 1970; **i**: 689–93.

45 Milne J, Brand S. Occupational asthma after inhalation of dust of the proteolytic enzyme, papain. *Br J Ind Med* 1975; **32**: 302–7.

46 Nava C. Allergy. In: Parmeggiani L ed. *Encyclopaedia of Occupational Health and Safety*. Geneva: International Labour Office, 1983; 124–6.

47 Ducatman AM, Columbis JJ. Chemical hazards in the biotechnology industry. *Occup Med State Art Rev* 1991; 193–225.

48 Health and Safety Executive. *An evaluation of the costs and benefits of the Genetically Modified Organisms (Contained Use) Regulations 1992*. Contract Research Report CRR 160/1998. Sudbury: HSE Books, 1998.

Part 6

Work and mental health

Bullying, post-traumatic stress disorder and
   violence in the workplace   539
Substance abuse and the workplace   557
Health and mental illness at work:
   clinical assessment and management   569
Shift work and extended hours of work   581

Work and mental health

26

Bullying, post-traumatic stress disorder and violence in the workplace

MAURICE LIPSEDGE

Bullying	539	Acknowledgements	554
Post-traumatic stress disorder	544	References	554
Violence at work	550		

It is recognized that a considerable amount of psychiatric morbidity and sickness absence is associated with aversive experiences in the workplace. The effects on the organization of losing employees because of bullying, post-traumatic stress disorder and violence in the workplace include labour turnover, recruitment and training of a replacement employee, lowered departmental morale and underproductivity of the team as well as the cost of repeated or long-term sickness absence. With increasing levels of violence in society as a whole, employees are exposed to the risk of physical abuse by clients, patients, customers, members of the public and indeed fellow workers. The employer's duty of care requires the workplace to be as safe as possible so that staff are protected from traumatic events. In addition, support and effective treatment have to be provided to employees who become the victims of abuse, accidents or violence.

BULLYING

CASE HISTORY 1

A 50-year-old senior telephone operator at a large City firm of accountants had been employed by the company for over 10 years and her sickness absence record had been satisfactory. She had worked very effectively until the appointment of a new manager responsible for the team of operators.

He was a young man who was immediately extremely critical of her. He would repeatedly rebuke her in public for alleged errors. She became increasingly distressed because the supervisor failed to give her unambiguous instructions or guidelines. She felt that she did not know how to cope with the situation because whatever action she took she was condemned. As a conscientious and previously reliable employee who was well regarded within the company, she now felt degraded and humiliated as a result of the repeated public disparagement. She began to feel 'like a nervous wreck'. She would weep frequently and she lost a stone in weight over a period of 4 months. Eventually she took protracted sick leave and was examined by the company's part-time medical advisor who wrote:

She can only cope with simple day-to-day activities if she can avoid dwelling upon what she believes was poor behaviour towards her by her employers. I conclude that she continues to suffer agitated depression with a marked phobic anxiety relating to any thought of return to work . . . I do not think she will respond to psychiatric treatment so I recommend that she be offered early retirement on the grounds of ill health . . .

Definitions of bullying at work

Bullying is defined as being repeatedly subjected to negative acts in the workplace in a situation where the victims feel unable to defend themselves due to a perceived or real imbalance of power between victim and persecutor. It is not bullying if two individuals of approximately equal 'strength' are in conflict or if the incident is an isolated event.[1] Bullying in the workplace is therefore an 'abusive interpersonal event'[2] which can consist of intimidation by unreasonable demands, intellectual belittling, putting down in front of others, repeated accusations of wrongdoing, being made the butt of jokes, being given 'the silent treatment', being talked to sarcastically or glared at and being the target of tantrums or swearing and being blamed for other employees' errors. According to Keashly and Trott[2] the primary aim of bullying is to undermine the other person in order to ensure compliance. Hostile verbal and non-verbal bullying behaviours include a sneering tone of voice, yelling at an employee for disagreeing, using derogatory names, engaging in explosive outbursts, intimidation by the use of threats, aggressive eye contact and humiliating the victim in front of others. Clearly, a single or even an occasional incident of this type cannot be regarded as systematic bullying.

Leymann[3] stipulates that this kind of behaviour can only qualify for the description of bullying if there is an incident occurring at least once a week over a minimum period of 6 months. At that intensity and frequency there is likely to be significant psychosocial damage. (In contrast to bullying, a single event of sexual harassment is sufficient to qualify legally for that description.) Rayner[4] regards these minimum frequencies and duration as too stringent and rightly emphasizes that it is the victim's perception of being bullied which is critical. The fear that the threshold for the definition of victimization might be pitched too low and cause frivolous or vexatious complaints was not supported by a study of sexual harassment on a university campus.[5] Over 88% of the women had been subjected to behaviour which could be defined as sexual harassment, but only 5.6% confirmed that they felt sexually harassed.

Victims of bullying might be distinguished by physical characteristics such as clumsiness, obesity, disability, hair colour or skin colour. One aspect of bullying is teasing. Etymologically, teasing has two roots, Anglo-Saxon 'tae-san' which means to tear to pieces (cutting the person down to size) and Norman French 'attiser' which means literally fuelling a fire, i.e. heating up the victim.[6]

Brodsky[7] who provided independent medical reports for the California Workers' Compensation Appeals Board, actually used the term 'harassment' when describing what we would now call bullying. He defined harassment as 'repeated and persistent attempts by one person to torment, wear down, frustrate or get a reaction from another' and describes the victims' reactions as 'subjective harassment' which is characterized by fear, intimidation and discomfort.

An early description of bullying at work is the account of male hostility to women working in non-traditional blue collar jobs.[8] The women were subjected to verbal teasing, practical jokes, social isolation (debarring women from lunch groups or refusing to talk to them) and excluding them from informal training about the job, thus reinforcing the stereotype that women cannot do non-traditional jobs.

Bullying at work was not systematically studied until the early 1980s. Bullying, both at school and in the workplace, has now been extensively researched in Scandinavia and to a lesser extent in the United States of America. The first important European paper was published in 1984 by the National Board of Occupational Safety and Health in Stockholm.[9] Scandinavian researchers prefer the word 'mobbing' to bullying since the latter has connotations of physical violence. 'Mobbing' refers to situations where an individual is persistently picked on or humiliated by supervisors, managers or fellow workers. The term is derived from the work of Konrad Lorenz, the ethologist, who used the word 'mobbing' to describe attacks by a group of small animals threatening a single larger animal. Originally the term 'mobbing' referred to group aggression but it now includes bullying in the sense of a single individual harassing another. According to Leymann,[3] bullying begins with a brief triggering situation (which has been little studied) which is followed by mobbing activities which are not in themselves necessarily indicative of aggression or expulsion from the social group. To meet the definition of mobbing or bullying the behaviour has to continue on an almost daily basis for a long period. The mobbing activities are summarized as 'aggressive manipulation' whose common denominator is the intention to 'get at a person or to punish them'. In contrast to school bullying where physical violence is predominant,[10] bullying at work is generally psychological and verbal.

Charlotte Rayner, who is one of the leading British academic researchers into adult bullying identifies the following categories of bullying behaviour:

1 threat to professional status such as belittling opinion;
2 threat to personal standing such as devaluing with reference to age;
3 isolation, for example, withholding information;
4 overwork, for example, by the imposition of impossible deadlines;
5 destabilization, for example, removal of responsibility on the one hand or setting up to fail on the other.[11]

The effects of bullying at work

Leymann[3] classifies the damage caused by bullying into:

1 the effects on society;
2 effects on the organization;
3 effects on the victim.

The overall impact of bullying is that victims feel harassed and their work is adversely affected.[12] Leymann[13] reported that between 10 and 20% of those who commit suicide in Sweden per year have a history of being bullied at work. Moreover, there are data from the Swedish National Board of Social Insurance for the year 1993 which indicate that between 20% and 38% of employees who take early retirement on health grounds have suffered from intensive bullying.[3] However, the individual victim may remain unproductively at the job because of fear of difficulty in finding a new one. Victims may adopt a posture of passive resistance in which they will only carry out duties that are regarded as absolutely necessary. In a study of patients who had experienced bullying in the workplace, consideration was given to four possible options or individual strategies, developed by victims of bullying, which might have an impact on their employer. These strategies were:

1 a reduction of commitment to work;
2 active problem solving;
3 remaining within the organization and passively hoping that things will improve;
4 leaving the job itself.

The two most common reactions were reduced commitment to the job or leaving the firm.[14]

Among children the emotional effects of bullying include a sense of degradation, humiliation, shame, intense anger and fear.[15] Victims might begin to believe in the abusive name-calling, thinking that names such as 'idiot' must be true otherwise they would have been able to cope with the bullying and that their inability to cope proves that they are indeed inferior. No systematic research has yet been carried out to examine the similarities between child and adult bullying but both forms of aggressive behaviour, carried out with the intention to cause pain, cover a wide spectrum from name-calling to the threat of violence to actual physical assaults (see for example Smith and Sharp,[16] and Randall[17]). The erosion of self-esteem and the shame of being unpopular in both children and adults, leads to difficulty in reporting the bullying due to a sense of helplessness, inadequacy, confusion, anxiety, tiredness, disorganization at work, lowered self-esteem and depression. The effects of exposure to derogatory and hostile behaviour include decreased pleasure in work, questioning one's skill on the job, reacting inappropriately to the bully, leaving the organization, reduced productivity, increased absenteeism and increased turnover of personnel.

Leymann[3] defines bullying and harassment at work as involving 'hostile and unethical communication, which is directed in a systematic way by one or a few individuals mainly towards one individual who, due to mobbing, is pushed into a helpless and defenceless position, being held there by means of continuing mobbing activities'. Leymann[3] has developed a typology of harassing communications which have five different effects on the victim. The first category which consists of repeated verbal attacks and threats has the effect of restricting the victim's ability to communicate. The second involves social isolation and exclusion ('being sent to Coventry') which curtails the victim's social contacts. The third involves gossip, ridicule or endless teasing and insults about a handicap or any conspicuous physical feature. These behaviours serve to undermine the victim's personal reputation. Criticising an individual's private life, or mocking a handicap or mannerism is psychologically the most damaging form of bullying, i.e. the one that correlates most closely with psychological ill health leading to absenteeism.[18] The fourth involves being deprived of work or constant denigration of performance or being given meaningless tasks which undermines the victim's professional competence. The final category consists of being deliberately exposed to physical danger with possible damaging effects on the victim's physical integrity and health. An example would be prison officers, police personnel or nurses in psychiatric secure settings, threatening not to come to the aid of an individual who is being attacked or actually failing to do so.

Leymann[3] describes how an individual who is attacked daily over a period of many months can be virtually immobilized by the experience. Some victims of bullying show the phenomenon of 'learned helplessness' originally described by Seligman and Maier.[19] In experimental studies, dogs which were given repeated electric shocks while restrained in a harness or subjected to loud noise or immersion in cold water eventually gave up trying to escape from the noxious stimuli. This syndrome of learned helplessness develops when laboratory animals are subjected to trauma and are deprived of the possibility of terminating the stress. When both these conditions apply, the animals become chronically distressed, apathetic and are unable to learn to escape from novel aversive situations. Some victims of bullying, exposed to repeated negative experiences, might fall into a comparable state of apathy and resignation and fail to make any constructive attempt to escape from persecution.

Clinically, the victims of workplace bullying might develop a variety of psychiatric disorders including depression and anxiety as well as psychosomatic conditions such as irritable bowel syndrome and myalgic encephalomyelitis (ME). They may submit certificates with vague diagnostic labels such as 'stress', 'burnout' or 'trauma'. Many victims may remain at work, however, and experience adjustment disorders which are defined as states of subjective distress and emotional disturbance which can interfere with social functioning and performance and which are a response to a stressful situation. The presenting symptoms include lowering of mood, anxiety and worry together with a feeling of inability to cope or plan ahead.

A general practitioner or occupational physician might suspect bullying or harassment at work when the patient presents with phobic anxiety focusing on the journey to work, especially when the individual appears to be relatively free of symptoms at weekends and/or during sickness absence, only to relapse when confronted with the prospect of returning to work. Although Rayner[11] found very low reported absence rates by the targets of bullying (which was attributed to the victims' fear of taking time off), others[20] report that 24% of bullying victims admit to using long-term sickness absence as a strategy to cope with victimization in the workplace.

It is always helpful to enquire about relationships with colleagues and with managers and whether the patient has a particular bête noire. Questioning has to be tactful because victims of bullying often feel ashamed. They are fearful of further intimidation and of being stigmatized as either a 'psychiatric case' or as a troublemaker. In the interests of fairness and to exclude the possibility of unfounded allegations, the occupational physician should seek written consent by the employee to discuss the problem with the Human Resources Department and to request further investigation. At times an independent member of management will have to be called in to sit in on discussions.

Failure to resolve the situation might lead to litigation on the basis of unfair dismissal or inappropriate premature retirement on grounds of ill health.[21] While the individual employee might be assisted by psychological treatment such as cognitive behaviour therapy and assertiveness training, the main emphasis has to be on addressing and resolving the underlying organizational causes. The behaviour of the bully has to be modified, and they may require counselling to provide insight into their habitual destructive behaviour with colleagues. Where more than one employee is affected this is often a clear indication of the need to explore the organizational factors.

Earnshaw and Cooper[22] suggest that bullying can cause post-traumatic stress disorder. However, the Diagnostic Statistical Manual (DSM-IV) criteria for post-traumatic stress disorder (309.81) require the individual to have experienced an event that is potentially life-threatening to themselves or in which they witnessed the death or serious injury of others. The victim's response must be one of intense fear, helplessness or horror. Protracted bullying, however distressing is not generally regarded as life-threatening.

Causes of workplace bullying: Personality and workplace factors

The victims of bullying have been described as conscientious, literal minded and unsophisticated with a tendency to be overachievers,[7] whereas, according to Adams[23] factors in the bully include sadism, narcissism and envy. While recognizing that psychopathic bullies are rarely found in the workplace, the English psychotherapist, Crawford tends to perceive bullies as individuals who are acting out their unresolved childhood conflicts in the workplace.[23] Scandinavian researchers eschew such psychoanalytic formulations and emphasize aspects of the work environment which appear to foster bullying. They have identified lack of leadership skills, insufficient work control and high levels of role conflict as providing a fertile ground for the development of workplace bullying. According to Vartia[24] the following features of the workplace are conducive to the development of bullying.

1 Lack of two-way communication between manager and employee causing poor flow of information.
2 An authoritarian way of resolving differences of opinion.
3 Lack of communication of the unit's tasks and goals.
4 Lack of autonomy and control of matters which directly affect the employees, i.e. an authoritarian organizational culture.

In workplaces characterized by lack of bullying there was better communication and discussion of matters of potential conflict and negotiation as opposed to an authoritarian mode of solving matters of disagreement. Conflict management is time-consuming and when there is little time available to solve the evolving conflict, the likelihood of escalation into bullying and mobbing is increased.[18] As regards the social climate of the workplace, Vartia[24] suggests that it is impossible to state at present whether bullying is the product or the cause of a strained, competitive, quarrelsome and sullen atmosphere at work. The same uncertainty about the direction of the casual arrow applies to the personality characteristics of the people involved in the bullying process. In fact there have been no systematic studies of the personality traits of bullies or indeed of their victims, and I believe that there are no specific personality features which might assist in the identification of a real or potential victim or bully.

Victims of bullying attribute the bullying to envy, a weak manager or supervisor, competition for advancement and competition for approval by the supervisor. Motives for bullying in the university setting include envy and competition for jobs and for status on the part of both the tormentor and the victim.[25] Rayner[11] has identified perceived bullies as being the managers or senior managers of the victims. The person doing the bullying is frequently in a line management position relative to the victim whereas in school children, most bullying is by the peer group.[26] Men and women are apparently equally capable of bullying. Whereas men rarely report being bullied by women, women themselves are as likely to be bullied by women as by men.

Toohey[27] found that bullied employees tended to be diagnosed as suffering from 'stress' so that the blame was located within the workers themselves rather than in the psychosocial work environment. Sometimes when bullying is investigated by personnel management, prior stigmatization might cause the situation to be misjudged and the victim might be identified as responsible for the situation in the first place.[3]

CASE HISTORY 2

A 50-year-old credit controller who had recently achieved promotion to managerial status was subjected to a campaign of harassment by a newly appointed employee who coveted her senior position. Her behaviour was continuously disagreeable and obstructive. She would make her manager feel uncomfortable by whispering her name to her colleagues, made malicious complaints to other managers about her, and made disparaging comments about her manager's ethnicity (she was Irish). After some months of continuous harassment the manager informed one of the directors but he failed to take any action and the goading and teasing continued. Eventually, the manager resigned from her supervisory position in the hope that the harassment would cease but it continued unabated. The bullying reached a crescendo when the target received an anonymous letter accusing her of having connections with the IRA and asking her whether her employees were aware of this. A few days later her coat, which was in the office cloakroom, was slashed. When the victim complained to her bosses about this she was accused of damaging it herself. Her own managers and the occupational physician described her as 'paranoid'. She developed a reactive depression and an anxiety state and eventually applied for early retirement on medical grounds. Before the bullying started, this employee had enjoyed perfectly satisfactory mental and physical health and had an excellent employment record.

Personal characteristics of the victim are often blamed rather than addressing the operational issues. In the UK, a bullying situation is often dismissed as a 'clash of personalities'. Bullying can lead to expulsion or extrusion, sometimes with the assistance of a medical label such as paranoia, depression or personality disorder. As in the case history offered by Leymann,[3] the mobbing process goes through four stages with an initial conflict which tends to escalate so that the harassed individual is subjected to hostile behaviour over a long period. Eventually management is forced to intervene and very often accepts the gossip and complaints about the victim from those colleagues who have themselves been doing the bullying. Finally the victim might escape into early retirement on grounds of ill health or into a new job with reduced status and a poor reference.

In the UK, Tim Field, the founder of the National Workplace Bullying Advice Line who was himself the victim of bullying at work, finds that about a fifth of his telephone callers are teachers and roughly a tenth are health care professionals and social workers.[28] (Health care professionals include nurses and general medical practitioners.) In 90% of cases, bullying involves a manager victimizing a subordinate, 8% peer on peer and 2% subordinate on manager. However, there could be a distortion in these figures as the Advice Line receives relatively few calls from shop-floor workers.[28] About 75% of the callers are female while over 50% of reported bullies are female which probably reflects the fact that teachers,

nurses and social workers have a higher than average percentage of female managers. Field writes 'Bullying demotivates, disenchants and alienates while bullying managers, who are loathed by the subordinates, run dysfunctional and inefficient departments'. He believes that people bullied at work 'live down' to the bully's expectations and spend increasing amounts of time covering their back in preference to working.[28] Leymann[3] concludes that mobbing does not occur because of abnormalities in the character of the protagonists and attributes bullying to poorly organized production and/or working methods and impotent or uninterested management. A secondary source of bullying is lack of organizational policies and practices for handling conflict situations. As a result a supervisor might choose sides or refuse to take action, i.e. denies that there is a conflict.[23] Leymann[3] suggests that employees who (understandably) lack the knowledge to analyse social stressors at work can become frustrated and begin to blame and victimize each other. The elements of behaviour involved in bullying are, taken in isolation, perfectly normal, interactive behaviour. However, when used very frequently and over a long period of time with the aim of harassing an individual, neutral items of social behaviour are transformed into dangerous communicative weapons.

Prevalence of workplace bullying

It is difficult to quantify the prevalence of bullying, harassment and mobbing because a tendency to either deny or minimize abuse is a way of surviving in an abusive environment.[29] Furthermore, people may be reluctant to admit to being a victim of bullying because it might give the impression that they are inadequate. Swedish and Norwegian research, following the work of Leymann, has shown incidence rates of 4–5% of employees being bullied at any one time. The average duration of reported bullying is 3 years.[3]

In Rayner's large scale survey of workplace bullying carried out at Staffordshire University the subjects were part-time students. The survey was anonymous and students were asked about the whole of their working lives. Only 1% of the sample refused to cooperate. To ensure a common broad definition of bullying the participants were given a vignette which provided an unequivocal illustration of interpersonal victimization in the workplace.[11] Rayner found bullying to be an extremely common phenomenon with approximately half of her 1137 respondents reporting that they had been bullied during their working lives at some point, while more than 75% of them had observed the phenomenon and over 25% had left their jobs because of the bullying. Rayner also found that a very high proportion of women who had experienced bullying reported that the person who harassed them had also harassed others.[11] The duration in Rayner's study ranged from under 6 months (42% of respondents) to over 2 years in 18% while 20% of the self-identified victims responded that they had been bullied at least once a week. Rayner speculates that bullying, which often coincides with a recent change in the job or change in manager tends to remit as the victim learns to adapt to the new work situation.[11] However, the fact that over 25% resigned because of bullying suggests that this is a far from trivial phenomenon in terms both of human suffering and economic cost.

Leymann's own study covered 2400 employees.[3] He found that 3.5% fitted the definition of victim of mobbing with men and women being equally affected. In Sweden, men were mainly mobbed by men and women by women but this is because of local conditions where the sexes tend to be segregated in the workplace. All ages were affected and in Sweden over 40% of the victims were subjected to attack by between two and four people. There appeared to be an overrepresentation of bullying in the educational setting, hospitals, child care centres and religious organizations.

A group of Norwegian workers[1] who have estimated the prevalence of bullying, define bullying and harassment as situations where a worker or a supervisor is systematically mistreated and victimized by fellow workers or supervisors through repeated negative acts. To be a victim of bullying, the individual has to feel inferior in defending themselves in the actual situation. The accumulated data from 14 different Norwegian questionnaire surveys with a total number of 7787 respondents showed that 8.6% of the respondents had been bullied at work during the previous 6 months with 1.2% reporting that bullying had occurred at least once a week. The highest prevalence of victimization occurred in male dominated organizations and large industrial organizations. Older workers were more at risk of victimization than younger workers while men were reported more often as bullies than women although men and women tended to be bullied at equal rates. These research workers speculate that work places with many employees have a higher frequency of bullying because smaller ones are more 'transparent' and there is a greater risk of being 'caught'.

Prevention of workplace bullying

Any measure that helps to increase the employees' control of their work through better job design can help to prevent mobbing.[30] These include a number of discussion and participation models with groups of employees having the power to influence the design of their own task and work conditions. Measures to increase social support of co-workers as well as training in coping strategies and assertiveness can also reduce interpersonal conflict at work. It has been demonstrated that poor work conditions reduce the social support of co-workers for each other.[31]

While there is no current legislation in the UK which specifically assists the victims of bullies who wish to resort to legal redress, the Dignity at Work Bill (1996) proposes to put bullying on the same footing as sex or race discrimination. Meanwhile, victims might resort to the Employment Protection (Consolidation) Act 1978 for a constructive dismissal or unfair dismissal or they might use the Health and Safety at Work Act 1974, if it can be demonstrated that psychiatric illness has been caused by the bullying. In those with personal injury which can be attributed to breach of care, the victim might resort to litigation under Section 2 of the Act which places a duty on employers to ensure the health (including mental health) of employees and to create a safe and healthy work environment. Thus, an employer who fails to take adequate steps to protect employees against bullying by their employees could be in breach of the Act. A residential care worker who had been 'sent to Coventry' and who had found it impossible to continue working successfully sued her employers for constructive dismissal.[32]

In the UK, the Littlewoods organization introduced a 'Promoting Dignity at Work' policy in 1994 which inter alia recognizes the commercial benefits of an anti-bullying policy. This is because bullying causes high absenteeism and sickness rates, a high staff turnover and low morale with poor work performance, sabotage, a poor company image and the need to replace staff. The Littlewoods organization makes managers responsible for ensuring that bullying does not occur and employ investigators trained to carry out formal investigations into allegations of bullying. Littlewoods have also introduced 'supporters' who are trained employees who can offer information and emotional support in confidence (and 'off the record') to assist victims of bullying. These approaches have been helpful in dispelling the myth that bullying is 'just a personality clash'.

Also in the UK, the Midland Bank provides another example of good practice in this field. In addition to a highly visible corporate policy on bullying and a trained team of investigators of any allegations of bullying, the Bank has placed bullying within the category of 'gross misconduct'.[33]

POST-TRAUMATIC STRESS DISORDER

Psychological disorder resulting from exposure to traumatic events was first recognized in military psychiatry. In the First World War the term 'shell shock' was coined while 'war neurosis', 'combat neurosis', 'combat fatigue' and 'battle exhaustion' were diagnostic labels used in the Second World War. Following the war in Vietnam the term 'post-traumatic stress disorder' was introduced by the American Psychiatric Association in 1980. This is now well recognized in civilian life and has been described in the survivors of natural disasters, major industrial and maritime accidents as well as in the victims of personal violence.

Both the American and the World Health Organization (WHO) diagnostic systems provide operational criteria for the nature of the provoking incident and the individual's response. The Diagnostic and Statistical Manual (DSM-IV) specifies very precisely the extreme nature of the traumatic incident and the emotional reaction of the subject.[34] The tenth edition of the International Classification of Diseases (ICD-10) similarly emphasizes that the traumatic event must be 'of an exceptionally threatening or catastrophic nature' and cites disasters, combat, a serious accident, witnessing violent death or being the victim of torture, terrorism or rape.[35]

The syndrome includes the persistent re-experiencing of the traumatic event in the form of recurrent intrusive and distressing recollections or dreams, attempts to avoid reminders of the trauma together with numbing of general responsiveness and symptoms of increased arousal including insomnia, irritability, poor concentration and hypervigilance. The survivor might become phobic of any situation which resembles the original traumatic event. While persistent re-experiencing of the trauma is *a sine qua non* for the diagnosis of post-traumatic stress disorder, this may take the form of images, thoughts, dreams or perceptions, but dreams do not necessarily occur in this condition. Furthermore, the content of the dreams and nightmares which follow exposure to trauma, while disturbing, may not be directly related to the events of the precipitating trauma. Since both diagnostic systems emphasize that the traumatic event has to be either 'an extreme traumatic stressor' (DSM-IV) or one 'of exceptional severity' (ICD-10), long-term harassment or bullying in the workplace does not fit the criterion of severity, even though bullying can undoubtedly lead to impaired psychosocial functioning. A useful diagnostic category for cases such as this might be prolonged duress stress disorder which is brought about by a series of unremitting though individually relatively less intense circumstances than the single overwhelming experience of great intensity of relatively short duration typically associated with post-traumatic stress disorder.[36] Prolonged duress stress disorder shows the characteristic clinical picture of post-traumatic stress disorder with intrusion, avoidance and arousal.

Frequently post-traumatic stress disorder co-exists with another psychiatric disorder, most commonly affective disorders, anxiety disorders, obsessive-compulsive disorder, antisocial personality and substance misuse.

Traumatic events, even of the most extreme type, do not invariably lead to mental disorder. It is recognized that post-traumatic stress disorder is only one among a variety of reactions which can follow exposure to an exceptionally traumatic event which is well outside the range of usual human experience. To what extent is the severity of the psychological reaction to severe trauma

determined by previous experiences and by previous morbidity? Volunteer fire fighters who were involved in an Australian bush fire tended to be more likely to develop chronic symptoms if they had had previous experience of adverse events[37] and there is evidence that rape victims with a previous psychiatric disorder tend to show a poorer initial adjustment and increased post-traumatic morbidity.[38,39]

CASE HISTORY 1

A combustion engineer was inspecting the back of a recently installed factory boiler. The engineer had just checked a gas control valve located to one side of the boiler when there was an explosion which knocked him about a metre backwards against a wall. The heavy metal burner in front of the boiler was detached by the force of the explosion and struck his colleague who was propelled a distance of 6–7 metres. The engineer saw the body of his colleague lying prone with a piece of the metal burner on top of him. The engineer managed to lift the burner off his colleague, who was unconscious. The engineer could see blood on his colleague's head and a contorted expression on his face. He himself suffered relatively minor flash burns and blistering but his colleague died shortly after the accident. For a few weeks afterwards and again for a few weeks before the inquest on his colleague, the engineer was troubled by frequent distressing intrusive recollections of the explosion and its immediate aftermath. He was also troubled by distressing dreams when he was reminded of the accident, despite his attempts to avoid thinking about it. He felt detached and remote from other people and he lost interest in his usual activities. He became irritable and prone to outbursts of anger. His concentration was impaired, he had difficulty in getting to sleep and was easily startled. When he met situations that reminded him of the accident he experienced rapid heart beat, sweating and shakiness. He avoided watching television programmes and actually had to leave the room if an accident or physical injuries were depicted. For some time after the accident he found it difficult to go near an industrial burner. He experienced 'survivor guilt' about his dead colleague. He felt unable to attend the funeral because he could not face the family. He frequently rehearsed the accident, speculating about alternative outcomes and about ways that the accident might have been prevented.

This engineer's traumatic experience fulfils the DSM-IV criteria for post-traumatic stress disorder i.e. he had witnessed an event that involved the actual death of the person who was in close proximity to him and he had also experienced the threat of death or, at the least, a threat to his own physical integrity. His immediate response to the accident involved intense fear, helplessness and horror. His survivor guilt was based on the irrational sense that his life was 'purchased at the cost of another.[40] Survivor guilt is derived from relief at not having died oneself, guilt for failing to save the victim, however irrational this might he, guilt that others might have died as the result of one's own actions, and guilt over being 'undeserving' of having been saved.[41]

CASE HISTORY 2

A man involved in the Piper Alpha oil rig fire in 1988 had clambered in semi-darkness over the bodies of his colleagues while escaping from the fire. He developed extremely severe post-traumatic stress disorder, and engaged in reckless behaviour including very fast driving and heavy alcohol consumption. He was tormented by grief and remorse, blaming himself irrationally for having survived at the expense of his comrades.

CASE HISTORY 3

A 60-year-old train driver was driving at standard line speeds in Kent. He had passed a signal which indicated that the way was clear for him to drive on to a single line in order to enter a tunnel. However, just before he entered the tunnel another signal changed unexpectedly from green to red. The driver responded by braking as fast as possible with his foot brake but the train sped into the tunnel and the driver imagined at that time that it was almost certain that a train was proceeding towards his own train on the single line. In the event the track was clear and on emerging from the tunnel he managed to stop his train on a double line. That night he consulted his GP who found that his blood pressure was very high. He found it difficult to sleep and ever since then has had a recurrent dream in which he is running along the road to reach a telephone box but his way is obstructed by a crowd of people who prevent him from reaching the telephone. He also has dreams of previous near-misses as well as dreams of the incident itself. He has lost his self-confidence and he has become fearful of crowds. He is so upset by any television programme that refers to the railways that he walks out of the room or changes the programme. He had been sensitized by an accident which had occurred 20 years previously when he was in charge of a runaway train whose brakes had failed when it was travelling at 60 miles an hour. The driver told me that he felt bitter and angry that there had apparently been no investigation of the faulty signal and that he had not heard from his managers although he had been on sick leave for some months. He had developed all the characteristic symptoms of post-traumatic stress disorder and he had undergone a change of personality. His wife contrasted his present 'zombie-like' with his previous personality as a 'happy-go-lucky person, a man's man, a do-it-all person'.

CASE HISTORY 4

An electricity worker who was close to an explosion at the bottom of a pit developed both post-traumatic stress disorder and a phobic anxiety state. He became phobic of electrical points and plugs to the extent that he was unable to change a lightbulb and would panic when his children went anywhere near the back of a television set.

Involvement in a second traumatic event might precipitate post-traumatic stress disorder in which the imagery and preoccupations are derived from the earlier traumatic experience, which has lain dormant until it is revived by the second trauma.

CASE HISTORY 5

A British Transport Policeman was involved in a serious and life-threatening road traffic accident. He developed post-traumatic stress disorder in which the dreams and recurrent distressing intrusive recollections featured images of a terrorist bomb explosion and its immediate aftermath which he had witnessed 'in real time' some years before as he was video-monitoring events on the concourse of a railway station.

Although most people exposed to a life-threatening traumatic event will experience intrusive recollections of the event for a few weeks, only a minority will experience symptoms for longer than about a month. Furthermore, a survivor may cope initially but might decompensate when later exposed to a new stressor.

CASE HISTORY 6

A vehicle maintenance engineer knocked down and killed an elderly pedestrian who wandered into the road. The incident revived intrusive memories of witnessing an individual committing suicide by jumping off a bridge and by the discovery of another person who had committed suicide by carbon monoxide poisoning.

The onset of post-traumatic stress disorder can be delayed by a matter of some years.

CASE HISTORY 7

A woman police officer began to be troubled 10 years later by distressing intrusive recollections of the sight of a dead baby in a mortuary when her own baby reached the same age.

The long-term prognosis of post-traumatic stress disorder has not yet been clearly established, but about 25% of rescuers involved in an oil rig disaster in the North Sea were still suffering from post-traumatic stress disorder nearly a year after the incident.[42] Long-term studies of Second World War prisoners of war have shown that about one-third of former prisoners still had significant residual symptoms.[43] O'Brien[44] cites other studies which demonstrate that at least 70% of severely abused Second World War and Korean War ex-prisoners of war were still suffering from post-traumatic stress disorder 40 years after their captivity.

However, in general only about 25% of individuals who are exposed to traumatic events develop the full blown post-traumatic stress disorder syndrome.[45] Are there specific features of traumatic events which increase the likelihood of developing post-traumatic stress disorder? Combat veterans who had been wounded were more likely to develop the disorder[46] while McFarlane[37] in his study of Australian fire fighters, found a similar relationship between physical injury and the development of post-traumatic stress disorder. Other studies, however, have reached the opposite conclusion, as in the survivors of a naval collision where less psychological disturbance was found among sailors who had been injured in the collision.[47] This was also the case with civilians exposed to bomb outrages in Northern Ireland where some of the non-physically injured survivors experienced survivor guilt in addition to post-traumatic stress disorder.[48]

The author's own clinical experience has been mixed, ranging from an iron foundry worker who was only slightly burnt by molten metal but who became intensely phobic of any event which remotely resembled the original incident such as steam rising from a boiling kettle, to a severely burnt electricity company worker who emerged apparently psychiatrically intact but whose colleagues, who were working nearby, and who were not physically injured, developed severe post-traumatic stress disorder with 'flashbacks', triggered off by sounds or odours which resembled what they had witnessed during the incident.

Weisaeth[49] who studied the survivors of an industrial explosion and fire at a paint factory, found that the incidence of an acute stress reaction was directly proportional to the proximity of the survivor to the centre of the explosion and conflagration. However, intensity of exposure to an overwhelming threat of death does not accurately predict post-traumatic stress disorder. This was the case with the Australian fire fighters dealing with a bush fire; nearly 50% believed that they were close to death, but only 27–32% developed post-traumatic stress disorder.[37] On the other hand, in situations where there is no direct personal threat, individuals might develop a significant level of symptomatology. Thus, 20% of police officers who had to handle bodies after an air crash developed post-traumatic stress disorder.[50] Such a reaction is not inevitable, however, and it is preventable.

In a study of the reactions of police officers to body-handling after the Piper Alpha oil rig disaster in 1988, investigators did not detect high levels of post-traumatic stress disorder or of psychiatric morbidity in the officers. The positive outcomes in these officers was attributed to their coping strategies and to major organizational factors.[51] Alexander and Wells[51] compared the reactions of police officers who had to search for and identify human remains after the oil rig disaster with a matched group of officers from the same force who had not had to carry out these duties. In the Piper Alpha disaster 167 men were killed. The officers were required to recover and prepare and help to identify 73 bodies which were recovered from the accommodation module of the oil rig which had lain at the bottom of the North Sea for 3 months. There was no detectable increase in psychiatric morbidity (as indicated by the officers' scores on the Hospital Anxiety and Depression Scale completed before and after body-handling duties), and there was no difference between the control group and the study group in terms of the number of sick days taken after completing the Piper Alpha exercise. The low morbidity was attributed to the managerial steps which were taken to reduce the likely impact of this traumatic experience. Powerful antidotes to the development of serious adverse psychological reactions included good team relationships, thorough preparation and high morale. A 3-year follow-up confirmed the lack of long-term psychiatric morbidity.[52]

Train drivers who inadvertently run down people who use the railway line as a means of committing suicide, frequently describe their feelings of impotence and helplessness as their engine bears down at great speed on the suicide victim. They are, of course, quite unable to stop the train in time to avoid colliding with the victim, whose face they can clearly see in the seconds prior to impact. The victim's facial features and expression are then visualized in distressing detail as part of flashbacks and dreams of the event. In his typology of railway suicides, Symonds[53] describes the 'train confronter' as an individual who stands on the railway line in the direct path of the train, confronting it in a characteristic pose with arms outstretched, facing towards the train: 'The driver of a fast train in open country saw [the suicide] walk on to a level crossing despite klaxon warnings. When the train, travelling at 90 mph, was 100 yards away the patient turned to face it'. There are approximately 90 incidents each year in which London Underground train drivers witness a train striking a person on the track. This is obviously a major, unexpected and violent event in the life of a train driver in whom over 16% develop post-traumatic stress disorder while nearly 40% of drivers interviewed a month after the incident had developed depression or phobic states. Previous experience of a similar incident is not invariably an important determinant of 'caseness'. This raises the possibility that in some cases a form of 'inoculation' or 'stress immunization' develops so that the driver uses coping strategies found helpful after the first incident.[54]

Predisposing factors for the development of post-traumatic stress disorder

There is still some uncertainty about whether the severity of the trauma or the pre-morbid psychological vulnerability of the individual involved is the more important factor in the cause of mental illness that follows an extremely traumatic event. Both DSM-IV and ICD-10 emphasize the central aetiological role of the traumatic event in the development of post-traumatic stress disorder. It has been assumed, on common sense grounds, that the magnitude of the stressor is the most important aetiological factor in the development of post-traumatic stress disorder. However, not all individuals exposed to stressors of overwhelming magnitude actually develop post-traumatic stress disorder.[55] Feinstein and Dolan[56] in their prospective study of 48 physically injured individuals, found no correlation between the severity of the stressor and the development of post-traumatic stress disorder. In his study of 469 Australian volunteer firemen, McFarlane[37] investigated the relative importance of the impact of the disaster, personality and ways of coping as determinants of post-traumatic morbidity. He found that neuroticism and a past history of treatment for a psychological disorder were better predictors of post-traumatic morbidity than the degree of exposure to the disaster or the losses sustained.

McFarlane[37] found that neither the nature and duration of the fire fighters' exposure to the fire nor their own bereavement and loss of property turned out to be the major determinant of post-traumatic morbidity. While these factors played a significant role in the immediate post-traumatic morbidity, chronic psychiatric morbidity was more likely to be associated with neuroticism and a history of previous psychiatric disorder. The Australian fire fighters' experience concurs with that of the survivors of an industrial accident where the prevalence of acute post-traumatic stress disorder was certainly influenced by the initial intensity of exposure but the 4-year prognosis was determined more by pre-accident psychological functioning than by the intensity of exposure to the explosion.[49] Pre-existing psychiatric disturbance increases the likelihood of long-term post-disaster morbidity.[49]

In a study of the survivors when a jet plane crashed into a hotel, a disaster which contained the elements of threat of injury or death, and exposure to horrific sights, together with suddenness, unexpectedness, unpreparedness and awareness of the loss of life, previous psychiatric disorder was also found to be a strong predictor of post-trauma psychopathology. However, in addition, those subjects who were most highly exposed to the trauma developed a higher level of psychopathology indicating that the severity of the traumatic experience also played a significant part.[57] Similarly, in a study of survivors of a North Sea oil rig disaster, both objective danger and neuroticism correlated with the development of an adverse psychological response.[58]

In summary, long-term outcome of psychological morbidity associated with an extreme stressor is better predicted by pre-disaster variables than by the nature of the victim's exposure or losses. Premorbid vulnerability is a more important cause of chronic post-traumatic morbidity than of acute disorder, and McFarlane[37] concluded that predisposing premorbid characteristics have a greater formative effect than features of exposure to the disaster itself.

The neuroendocrine basis of post-traumatic stress disorder

Post-traumatic stress disorder is caused by the complex interaction of the type of incident (e.g. man-made versus 'act of God'), severity and duration of the trauma, previous personality and psychiatric history, family history and post-traumatic experience. Research into the neuroendocrine substrate of post-traumatic stress disorder indicates that the intrusion symptoms (e.g. flashbacks) are associated with the potentiation of neural circuits after overwhelming stimulation and are due to sudden overactivity of noradrenaline with transient minor stimulation or remind.[44] Conversely, the avoidance symptoms (e.g. marked emotional detachment) develop against a background tonic state of chronic noradrenaline depletion due to inescapable shock.[44]

Treatment

Post-traumatic stress disorder can lead to considerable sickness, absence, and retirement on the grounds of ill health.

CASE HISTORY 8

> A gas company employee sustained burns when he sliced through an electric cable with a pneumatic drill equipped with a cutter. In addition to developing post-traumatic stress disorder he lost his professional self-confidence. Before the accident he had a reputation for being meticulous and careful. After the incident he felt inadequate and would blame himself. Previously he had tended to despise people who were less careful workers and he felt profoundly disappointed in himself. He had developed a moderately severe post-traumatic stress disorder but this remitted after a year. However, he resigned because he had lost his self-confidence.

Early crisis intervention as recommended by Lindemann[59] on the basis of his study of the survivors of the Coconut Grove disaster in Chicago where many people were burnt to death in a night-club, involves counselling aimed at helping the survivor to come to terms with their losses by ventilating their traumatic experiences. Survivors of extreme trauma have to re-evaluate their basic beliefs about the safety and predictability of their world, the dependability of other people and about the human condition in general.[60]

As yet there has been no large-scale controlled prospective study to evaluate the efficacy of early crisis interventions. Pending publication of such studies, it is now accepted that trauma victims might well benefit from an early counselling intervention even though the natural history of the disorder may be spontaneous resolution within a few months of the incident. Counsellors require supervision by more senior qualified counsellors than themselves or by counselling psychologists, and need support from peers or other mental health professionals.

In the occupational setting where counsellors are provided by management, they might become the target of resentment and hostility in situations where the employer is felt to be to blame for an accident by, for example, giving priority to productivity over considerations of safety. A widely used treatment is psychological debriefing in which people recently involved in a traumatic incident are encouraged, either individually or in a group setting to talk through their experience with an emphasis on both the emotional and the cognitive effects of the event.[61]

A definition of psychological debriefing is that it is a semi-structured intervention designed to prevent psychological sequelae following traumatic events by promoting emotional processing through the ventilation and normalization of reactions in preparation for possible future experience. There are two components to psychological debriefing: the ventilation of feelings about the event and a discussion of the signs or symptoms of a stress response with individual disclosure of emotions and personal revelation of symptoms. The aim is to facilitate the processing of information by enabling victims who have been subjected to the same traumatic event to process their experiences together in a group. There is ventilation of emotion, the generation of group support and the initiation of the grieving process. This allows for reconstruction of the event and encourages normalization of the experience and mobilization of further support if necessary.

The intention of the psychological debriefing exercise is to achieve integration of the disaster event into the life history of the worker. Intervention should take place within 24–48 hours of the disaster duty. During psychological debriefing there is detailed disclosure of expectations, facts, thoughts, sensory impressions and emotional reactions together with education about the stress response syndrome and guidance to assist coping for the future. Workers are encouraged to discuss their fears, anxieties and concerns including guilt, frustration, anger and ambivalence. The facilitator emphasizes the normality of the reactions. Debriefing can include a teaching phase about normal reactions to stress and it should be followed up by debriefing sessions several weeks later. A second type of intervention which is more cognitive than ventilatory, focuses on coping skills and cognitive restructuring with the encouragement of discussion of facts rather than feelings.

The Royal Air Force Wroughton post-traumatic stress disorder Rehabilitation Programme[62] comprises a 12-day structured inpatient course of group psychotherapy with follow-up sessions over a 1-year period. The main therapeutic approach is psychological debriefing. After 6 weeks follow-up in the RAF study there had been a highly significant global improvement in most subjects which was maintained over the follow-up period of 1 year. Busuttil et al.[62] reported anecdotally that most symptomatic improvements occurred on completing the personal account phase when there was a sudden reduction in arousal and flashbacks.

Because of the possibility of an adverse effect of psychological debriefing[63] there is a need for rigorous trials. In the first randomized controlled study of psychological debriefing with an assessment blind to the treatment received, 133 adult acute burn trauma victims were randomly allocated to treatment by psychological debriefing or a control group who received no intervention. At 13 months follow-up, 26% of the psychological debriefing group had post-traumatic stress disorder compared with only 9% of the control group. However, the active treatment group had higher initial questionnaire scores and more severe dimensions of burn trauma than the control group.[64] Other psychological treatments of the disorder are described by Joseph et al. in their comprehensive handbook.[65] They review the rationale of direct exposure therapies, cognitive therapy and eye-movement desensitization and reprocessing therapy. Randomized and/or controlled studies have shown that exposure, anxiety management training and cognitive therapy all improve post-traumatic stress disorder by 20–80%.[66]

Advice to victims and their families

It is useful to involve the survivor's family who will require education about acute stress disorder, otherwise they might find the victim's behaviour incomprehensible and alienating. One large UK employer (London Electricity plc) provides staff who have been exposed to a traumatic incident with a leaflet which provides information on immediate reactions to traumatic events and emphasizes the normality of such reactions for both the trauma victim and the family (see Fig. 26.1).

Dunning[67] devised a programme for reducing mental trauma which might result from service at the site of a disaster and emphasizes that intervention strategies aimed at achieving this must be devised before the event. He quotes Ivancevich et al.[68] who recommend a stress audit to monitor indicators of possible psychological trauma including chronic illness, changes in turnover, transfer, absenteeism and the performance of personnel

Trauma is an event that seriously threatens your safety. Examples of traumatic incidents:

- Being close to an explosion or a fire
- Involvement in a life-threatening accident
- Being the victim of a serious assault

The effects of trauma are normal responses that occur in normal people.
COMMON REACTIONS *DURING THE INCIDENT ITSELF* INCLUDE BOTH PSYCHOLOGICAL AND PHYSICAL FEELINGS.

Psychological Feelings
- Fear and panic
- Disbelief
- Feeling numb
- Confusion

Physical Feelings
- Rapid heart beat
- Sweating
- Shaking
- Nausea
- Breathing fast

COMMON REACTIONS THAT MIGHT OCCUR *FOR SOME DAYS AFTER THE INCIDENT*
Psychological and Emotional
- Fear, worrying and anxiety about further harm to oneself or to loved ones
- Feeling scared, miserable and tearful
- Feeling irritable, moody and bad tempered
- Feeling numb and unreal, remote or detached from other people
- Loss of interest in family, friends and in enjoyable activities
- Being jumpy and easily startled by sudden loud noises
- Avoiding reminders of the incident
- Feeling upset by TV programmes that show similar incidents
- Sudden life-like 'action replays' of the incident in your mind
- Feeling guilty or blaming yourself for the way you reacted during the incident
Physical
- Sleep problems
- Bad dreams
- Poor appetite
- Shakiness
- Sweating
- Tiredness
- Poor concentration
- Nausea
- Diarrhoea or constipation
- Loss of sex drive

Figure 26.1 *Leaflet issued by London Electricity plc expaining the immediate reactions to traumatic events. Reproduced with permission from Dr Margaret Samuel of the Occupational Health Department, London Electricity plc.*

as well as the state of union–management relations. The most common stressors reported by workers who have been involved in rescue and recovery operations are a sense of loss of control and feelings of vulnerability. He suggested that social support and group cohesion should be built into the response to disaster by maintaining work groups so that the same workers can remain together for the duration of the crisis.

Finally, tricyclic antidepressants and selective serotonin reuptake inhibitors may help to suppress flashbacks and nightmares, and reduce panic attacks in addition to their specific antidepressant effect.

VIOLENCE AT WORK

CASE HISTORY 1

A 40-year-old British rail booking office clerk was the victim of a robbery which occurred at her place of work. She was threatened with a sawn off, double barrel shotgun. The robber grabbed a woman passenger and held her as a hostage, placing the shotgun behind her ear. He ordered the railway clerk to open the office safe. At that point he held the gun to her own head. After handing over the money, the clerk and the other woman were bundled into the station lavatory by two of the gunman's accomplices. That night she was unable to sleep. Every time she closed her eyes she would relive the entire scene, like watching a video re-play of the robbery. The following day she wept fre-quently. She was tremulous and experienced panic attacks. As she had recognized the three robbers who had followed her home on two previous occasions, she felt extremely vulnerable since several weeks passed before they were arrested. Even after they had been sentenced she had an irrational fear of public places, especially post offices, banks and building societies because she knew that they were potential targets for robberies. She had also become phobic of returning to the station where the robbery occurred. She underwent a change of personality. She became morose and unso-ciable whereas previously she was a gregarious and fun-loving person. She blamed herself irrationally for events which had occurred during the robbery. She became reclusive, she lost her sex drive and she found it difficult to travel on public transport because of panic attacks. She became severely depressed and had thoughts of suicide. She began to drink heavily as a form of self-medication to help her sleep. She had a previous history of a severe depressive illness a few years prior to the robbery. It is known that a previous psychiatric history is one of the most important deter-minants of vulnerability to psychiatric disturbance after exposure to a life-threatening traumatic event.[57]

Despite intensive treatment with both potent antide-pressants and a programme of cognitive behavioural therapy, this booking clerk was still severely incapaci-tated by post-traumatic stress disorder and associated mood disturbance 3 years after the incident. She had moved to a different part of the country because she was afraid of reprisals. She remained virtually house-bound and continued to be phobic of any situation where another robbery might conceivably take place.

CASE HISTORY 2

A 35-year-old employee of a recently privatized utility who was employed as a customer services centre man-ager, was the victim of a series of relatively minor inci-dents. Over a period of 3 weeks a male customer had thrown a telephone at her; a woman client had grabbed hold of her and was threatening to hit her, and the employee had to be rescued by her manager. On another occasion when she was alone on the floor of the reception area, this employee was punched in the face. The following day another customer threw a chair at her. The employee attempted to take all these inci-dents in her stride but the last straw occurred when she was assaulted on a crowded train by an irate customer whose power supply had been cut off and who recog-nized her among the passengers. The employee became depressed and anxious and missed many months of work as a result.

Prevalence of violence at work

According to the North Western National Life Insurance company, between July 1992 and July 1993 nearly 25% of full-time workers in the USA were harassed, threatened or attacked on the job. Leading job categories in which employees are at risk of being assaulted include mental health workers, police, and security guards. In the USA murder is the leading cause of death in the workplace for women and the third most frequent cause for men.[69] A survey carried out by North Western National Life Insurance indicated that more than two million employ-ees may suffer physical attack at work each year in the USA and over six million are threatened at work.[69] According to the National Institute for Occupational Safety and Health an average of 15 people are murdered at work in the USA each week.[70] Reports of injury to American nurses from assaults by patients (including Accident and Emergency Department nurses and nurses involved in home care) exceed the rates of injury in con-struction work which is the country's most dangerous occupation.[71] In the UK too, National Health Service staff are three times more likely to be injured at work than industrial workers, principally because of attacks by violent patients.[72]

Psychological violence in the workplace is more com-mon than physical violence although it is known that physical aggression is often preceded by psychological violence.[73] It is also known that there is a significant amount of underreporting. Thus, five times more inci-dents occur at a psychiatric hospital than are actually reported.[74]

National Health Service staff have a 1 in 200 chance of major injury through wounding at work.[75] The highest risk of violence in the National Health Service is in spe-cific areas including Accident and Emergency, psychia-try, and community care.[72] One in four social workers are involved in a violent incident at work.[76] In the USA 9% of staff in two psychiatric units were suffering from post-traumatic stress disorder following assaults by patients[77] while in the UK over 8% of community psychiatric nurses had received physical injury in the previous 12 months.[78] In London, 7.6% of general medical practi-tioners had been assaulted over a 2-year period.[79]

Causes of violence at work

In the work-setting there might often be physical aggres-sion between strangers such as a nurse who is attacked by a patient or a relative in the Accident and Emergency Department or a ticket collector who is assaulted by a passenger, while in contrast there are accounts of bullied employees returning to the workplace to exact vengeance on their previous tormentors.

Common causes of workplace violence include a sense of being treated unfairly, being forced to wait, perceived intrusions into private life (e.g. searching personal questions to people with recent loss of self-esteem as in unemployment), racial or sexual prejudice, threatening attitudes from a colleague, an uncomfortable physical environment, use of alcohol or other central nervous system disinhibitors.[80]

Folger and Baron[81] in their definition of workplace aggression include violence, the spreading of negative rumours about individuals, and the withholding of information or resources needed by their targets. They believe that feelings of injustice play an important role in the genesis of aggression in the workplace.

With high levels of stress there is likely to be twice the rate of violence and harassment according to the North Western National Life Insurance study.[69] Job stressors which might contribute to the potential of workplace violence include ambiguous and conflicting role expectations, excessive work load, poor organizational communications, lack of job security and poor co-operation between employees.

Violence in the workplace occurs where there is an interaction between personal factors which include abuse of alcohol, a history of aggressive behaviour and recent loss of self-esteem, and work factors such as perceived injustice, job insecurity and electronic monitoring.[82] Alcohol abuse leads to violence at work because it increases the likelihood of a situation being 'misread' and impairs intellectual and verbal function.[83] If employees perceive themselves to be threatened at work in terms of the security of their jobs violence is more likely to occur. Barling[82] cites a number of workplace murders which were attributed to workers being passed over for promotion or laid off, believing that management actions were unfair and that there had been intimidating and inconsistent disciplinary procedures. Thus, perceptions of procedural injustice can precipitate violence.

Another factor identified by Barling[82] is intensive monitoring such as electronic monitoring which workers might regard as an invasion of privacy. Electronic monitoring is designed to increase the pace of work and to exert greater managerial control.[84] Barling predicts that being monitored electronically might increase the likelihood of workplace violence.

Baron and Neuman[85] in a study of several hundred employees at a number of different companies found a significant correlation between reported aggression and the magnitude of changes within the organization, including 'downsizing', redundancies and wage freezes. Barling[82] also identifies 'downsizing', mergers and restructuring and associated job insecurity as precipitants of workplace violence, partly because they induce feelings of powerlessness and loss of control. These feelings increase the likelihood of violence being resorted to as one possible means for regaining control.[86]

Folger and Baron[81] perceive workplace violence as the outcome of an interaction between an individual whose personality tends to predispose them to attribute malev-olence to others and one who believes that there has been a violation of fairness. Such a person may become intensely resentful and desire revenge. Thus, there is a complex interplay between a number of variables and conditions, and between personality features and workplace characteristics. Violence is more likely to occur in a setting where employees feel socially alienated by interpersonal conflict between colleagues or with supervisors and with a general feeling of powerlessness, i.e. lack of control over one's job which often occurs during a period of organizational change.

The effects of workplace violence

In considering workplace violence, it is important to take into account the perceptions and behaviour of secondary victims, such as employees who were not attacked themselves but whose vicarious exposure to the violence will affect their perceptions, fears and expectations.[82] They will feel increasingly vulnerable and their fear that they themselves might become primary victims will be enhanced.[87] In addition, the secondary victim will feel that they have lost personal control over what happens at work. Witnesses to assaults, e.g. psychiatric nurses, report heightened fear, anxiety, increased vulnerability and irritability as well as guilt about the injuries to the victim based on a perception that the witness should have intervened sooner.[88]

CASE HISTORY 3

A 30-year-old lecturer was talking to a group of students in a London college canteen. She heard an angry shout behind her and she was pushed downwards from behind by a male assailant (an aggrieved student) who forced her face downwards on to the table in front of her. The lecturer recalled thinking that if she resisted she might be stabbed as she knew that some of the students carried knives and one of her own students had actually come into the college with a gun. The group of students who were at the same table with her were terrified, silent and motionless. Her assailant intimidated her with shouted threats and abuse and then left before the security guard could be called. The lecturer became intensely anxious and was troubled by flashbacks. She was afraid of being alone at home while her husband was out at work and she had to seek refuge in her parents' home. She developed severe agoraphobia. She remained on sick leave for some months. She was informed that the college authorities had promised to install safety measures including tightening up security arrangements and the provision of a panic button on her desk, but in the event these arrangements were not made. Her condition was exacerbated by the fact that her teaching colleagues, who were mainly men, found it difficult to understand her fears and were unsympathetic.

The teacher's managers promised to relocate her in another building which she regarded as safer, but this did not materialize. Because of her continuing anxiety and fear of another assault, the lecturer resigned. Prior to the incident this lecturer had been a stable, well balanced individual with a high level of professional, political and social commitment as well as being active in local community politics, a union shop steward and a school governor. One of the reasons that the assault had such a profound effect on her personality was the sense of helplessness that she experienced when confronted and trapped by her assailant in the presence of her own students. As a committed teacher she had prided herself on her ability to set an example, to be in control and to 'lead from the front'. In the incident in which she was assaulted, this lecturer was overwhelmed by the superior physical strength of her assailant and she was unable to rely on her usual resourceful coping skills. Her sense of humiliation was subsequently compounded by the lack of constructive support shown by her employers.

Being the victim of an assault or serious accident threatens the three basic assumptions which are shared by most people and which underpin daily living:

1 belief in personal invulnerability;
2 perceiving the world as fair and predictable;
3 confidence in one's ability to cope with challenges.[60]

These assumptions are undermined and victims are forced to reconstruct this framework by which the world is judged because they no longer feel safe, the world has become unpredictable and potentially dangerous and they lose confidence in their professional ability together with self-blame. Victims become intensely aware of their relative helplessness and inability to control events. The positive aspect of self-blame is that the victim can regain a sense of control based on the belief that by changing their performance they can reduce the risk of being involved in a further incident.

When nurses are assaulted they find themselves in a position of divided loyalties between their professional duty to put their patients' needs first and attending to their own needs as a victim.[89] The immediate response of health-care professionals to an assault is a profound sense of helplessness which is enhanced by their knowledge that their professional responsibility requires them to control anger, to resist retaliating and to help and to assist their assailants in a therapeutic way.[90] This professional self-restraint might lead to an excessive degree of denial with an increased likelihood of protracted psychological stress.

Employees who can predict violence and are prepared to deal with it experience less negative outcomes than those who are unprepared. As Barling[82] points out 'Teachers do not expect to have to manage violent behaviour on the job, and they are often given no training on how to do so. Hence, a teacher who is slapped, shoved, pushed or even threatened by a student might experience workplace violence differently to a prison guard who is threatened or assaulted by an inmate'. The impact of a violent event has several characteristics which combine to determine the intensity of the impact. Thus, being the primary victim of extreme physical violence leads to the conviction that the employee has lost control within the organization and that violence is likely to recur in an unpredictable way.[82]

The psychological and psychosomatic effects of an assault on a member of staff include depression and anxiety, loss of confidence in one's professional competence, increased feelings of vulnerability, insomnia, nightmares and a variety of non-specific physical complaints, a tendency to increase the consumption of alcohol and cigarettes and phobic avoidance of reminders of the assault. Effects on work include loss of interest and motivation together with absenteeism.

The direct personal outcomes of workplace violence include negative mood, cognitive distraction and fear of violence with the risk of depression, post-traumatic stress disorder and psychosomatic disorders. The impact on the organization includes absence, resigning, emotional exhaustion, accidents and impairment of job performance. Workplace violence has been shown in systematic studies to have a negative effect on mood.[91] Furthermore, the stress associated with workplace violence increases arousal and impairs attention. Nurses who have been assaulted by patients report difficulties in concentrating on their work.[92] Whether the violence is experienced directly or vicariously, one of the major outcomes is fear of further violence. This in turn is associated with anxiety and psychosomatic symptoms. Fear of assault was found to be the most important source of work-related stress among a sample of bus drivers.[93] Anxiety and depression also have a disruptive effect on marriage and family life. Cognitive distraction might result in victims of violence being regarded as distant or being rejected by their families.[94] Finally, workplace violence affects commitment to the organization and leads to an increase in absenteeism and resignations as well as impairment of motivation and an increase in accidents.

Reducing the impact of violence at work

Cembrowicz and Ritter[79] in a chapter dealing with attacks on doctors and nurses provide helpful guidelines on the management of aggression and violent behaviour which have general application in the workplace. They enumerate non-verbal cues which provide warning signals of impending violence and they give guidelines on how to communicate with angry people including the use of non-provocative body language. The Royal College of Psychiatrists in a practical handbook entitled *The Management of Imminent Violence*[95] gives helpful advice on how to recognize the warning signs of violence as well as tactics for de-escalation.

Robb[96] makes specific recommendations for the management of staff who are assaulted in their workplace and points out that effective procedures can reduce the risk of staff developing post-traumatic stress disorder, demotivation and 'burnout'. After dealing with physical injuries, staff should undergo a structured and focused debriefing which takes place 48 to 72 hours after the incident. This session should be managed by a trained staff member who gives all the staff involved the opportunity to ventilate and to reconstruct what actually took place. Staff are encouraged to examine and acknowledge their emotional reactions and to provide mutual support. The group leader emphasizes the normality of the emotional reaction. Staff should be given advice on how to obtain further help if necessary. Robb emphasizes the importance of management being seen to be interested in staff well-being and of management being seen to be interested in staff well-being and safety.[96] Positive and committed supportive interventions by management can enhance the cohesion of the team.

The antecedents of violence include increased restlessness, pacing, increased volume of speech, erratic movements and refusal to communicate as well as obvious pointers such as verbal threats or gestures. The guidelines recommend that staff maintain an adequate distance, move towards a safe place avoiding corners, explain their intentions to the individual and to others, ensure that their own body language is non-threatening, engage in conversation and acknowledge concerns and feelings, ask for facts about problems and ask for any weapon to be put down rather than to be handed over.[95]

Although these guidelines[95] were developed with reference to incidents which occur on psychiatric wards and in mental health centres, the principles have a broader application to other workplace settings.

ACKNOWLEDGEMENTS

Thanks to Dr Doreen Miller for helpful advice and to Samantha Bland Rudderham for secretarial assistance.

REFERENCES

1 Einarsen S, Skogstad A. Prevalence and risk groups of bullying and harassment at work. *Eur J Work Organisat Psychol* 1996; **5**: 185–201.
2 Keashly L, Trott V. Abusive behaviour in the workplace: a preliminary investigation. *Violence Victims* 1994; **9**: 341–57.
3 Leymann H. The content and development of mobbing at work. *Eur J Work Organisat Psychol* 1996; **5**: 165–84.
4 Rayner C. Bullying in the workplace: the problem. In: *Strategies for Avoiding Bullying at Work: Litigation.* Conference held on 11 March 1997 at the (Scientific Society Lecture Theatre, London, organized by IBC UK Conferences Ltd.
5 Brooks L, Perot AR. Reporting sexual harassment: exploring a predictive model. *Psychol Women Quart* 1991; **15**: 31–47.
6 Pawluk CJ. Social construction of teasing. *J Theory Soc Behav* 1989; **19**: 145–67.
7 Brodsky C. *The Harassed Worker*. Lexington MA: DC Heath and Co, 1976.
8 O'Farrell B, Harlan SL. Craftworkers and clerks: the effect of male co-worker hostility on women's satisfaction with non-traditional jobs. *Soc Probl* 1982; **29**: 252–65.
9 Leymann H, Gustafsson A. Mobbing at work and the development of post-traumatic stress disorders. *Eur J Work Organisat Psychol* 1996; **5**: 251–75.
10 Olweus D. *Bullying at School: What We Know and What We Can Do*. Oxford: Blackwell, 1993.
11 Rayner C. The incidence of workplace bullying. *J Commun Appl Soc Psychol* 1997; **7**: 199–208.
12 Rayner C, Hoel H. A summary review of literature relating to workplace bullying. *J Commun Appl Soc Psychol* 1997; **3**: 181–91.
13 Leymann H. Sjalvmord till foljd av forhallanden i arbetsmiljon [Suicide and conditions at the workplace]. *Arbete manniska Miljo* 1996; **3**: 155–60.
14 Niedl K. Mobbing and well-being: economic and personnel development implications. *Eur J Work Organisat Psychol* 1996; **5**: 239–49.
15 Besag V. *Bullies and Victims in Schools*. Milton Keynes, Bucks: Open University Press, 1989.
16 Smith PK, Sharp S. *School Bullying*. London: Routledge, 1994.
17 Randall P. *Adult Bullying: Perpetrators and Victims*. London: Routledge, 1997.
18 Zapf D. Stress-oriented job-analysis of computerised office workers. *Eur Work Organisat Psychol* 1993; **3**: 85–100.
19 Seligman M. Maier S. Failure to escape traumatic shock. *J Exp Psychol* 1967; **74**: 1–9.
20 Zapf D, Knorz C, Kulla M. On the relationship between mobbing factors and job content, social work environment and health outcomes. *Eur J Work Organisat Psychol* 1996; **5**: 215–37.
21 Lipsedge M, Kearns J. Psychiatric disorders. In: Cox RAF, Edwards F C, MCallum R I eds. *Fitness for Work* 3rd edn. Cambridge: Cambridge University Press, 1998.
22 Earnshaw J, Cooper CL. *Employers Liability for Workplace Stress*. London: IPD, 1996.
23 Adams A. *Bullying at Work: How to Confront and Overcome It*. London: Virago Press, 1992.
24 Vartia M. The sources of bullying: psychological work environment and organisational climate. *Eur J Work Organisat Psychol* 1996; **5**: 203–14.
25 Bjorkqvist K, Osterman K, Hjelt-Back M. Aggression among university employees. *Aggress Behav* 1994; **20**: 173–84.
26 Whitney I, Smith PK. A survey of the nature and extent of bully/victim problems in junior/middle and secondary schools. *Educat Res* 1993; **35**: 3–25.
27 Toohey J. *Occupational Stress: Managing a Metaphor*. Sydney: Macquarie University, 1991.

28 Field T. *Bully in Sight: How to Predict, Resist, Challenge and Combat Workplace Bullying*. Didcot, Oxfordshire: Success Unlimited, 1996.

29 Randall T. Abuse at work drains people, money, and medical workplace not immune. *JAMA* 1992; **267**: 1439–40.

30 Resch M, Schubinski M. Mobbing: prevention and management in organisations. *Eur J Work Organisat Psychol* 1996; **51**: 295–307.

31 Marcelissen FH, Winnubst JA, Buunck B, DeWolff CJ. Social support and occupational stress: a causal analysis. *Spec Sci Med* 1988; **26**: 365–73.

32 Howard G. Beware! bullies at work. *Occup Hlth* 1991; **43**: 112–4.

33 Crabb S. Violence at work: the brutal truth. *People Mgmt* 1995; **1**: 25–7.

34 American Psychiatric Association, *Diagnostic and Statistical Manual of Mental Disorders* 4th edn. Washington DC: American Psychiatric Association, 1994.

35 World Health Organization. *The ICD-10 Classification of Mental and Behavioural Disorders*. Geneva: WHO, 1992.

36 Scott MJ, Stradling SG. Post-traumatic stress disorder without the trauma. *Br J Clin Psychol* 1994; **33**: 71–4.

37 McFarlane AC. The aetiology of post-traumatic morbidity: predisposing precipitating and perpetuating factors. *Br J Psychiat* 1989; **154**: 221–8.

38 Frank E, Turner SM, Stewart BD, Jacob M, West D. Past psychiatric symptoms and the response to sexual assault. *Comprehens Psychiat* 1981; **22**: 479–87.

39 Atkeson BK, Calhoun KS, Resich PA, Ellis EM. Victims of rape: reported assessment by depressive symptoms. *J Consult Clin Psychol* 1982; **50**: 96–102.

40 Lindy JB, Greenby L, Grace M, Titchner J. Psychotherapy with survivors of the Beverley Hills superclub fire. *Am J Psychother* 1983; **37**: 593–610.

41 Raphael B. *When Disaster Strikes: A Handbook for the Caring Professions*. London: Hutchinson, 1986.

42 Ersland S, Weisaeth L, Sund A. The stress upon rescuers involved in an oil rig disaster. *Acta Psychiatr Scand* 1989; **80** (Suppl 355): 38–49.

43 Kluznik JC, Speed N, Van VC, Magraw R. Forty-year follow-up of United States prisoners of war. Annual Meeting of the World Psychiatric Association, 1985, Athens, Greece. *Am J Psychiat* 1986; **143**: 1443–6.

44 O'Brien LS. *Traumatic Events and Mental Health*. Cambridge: Cambridge University Press, 1998.

45 Green BL. Psychosocial research in traumatic stress: an update. *J Traum Stress* 1994; **7**: 341–62.

46 Foy D, Sipprelle RC, Rueger DB. Aetiology of post-traumatic stress disorders in Vietnam veterans: analysis of premilitary, military and combat exposure influences. *J Consult Clin Psychol* 1984; **52**: 79–87.

47 Hoiber A, McCaughy B G. The traumatic after-effects of collision at sea. *Am J Psychiat* 1984; **141**: 70–3.

48 Bell P, Kee M, Loughrey GC, Curran PS, Roddy RJ. Post-traumatic stress in Northern Ireland. *Acta Psychiatr Scand* 1988; **77**: 166–9.

49 Weisaeth L. A study of behavioural responses to an industrial disaster. *Acta Psychiatr Scand* 1989;(Suppl 355) **80**: 25–37.

50 Davidson AD. Air disaster: coping with stress – a programme that worked. *Police Stress* (Spring) 20–2 (cited in Jones D R. *Am J Psychiat* 1985; **142**: 90–3).

51 Alexander DA, Wells A. Reactions of police officers to body-handling after a major disaster: a before and after comparison. *Br J Psychiat* 1991; **159**: 547–55.

52 Alexander DA. Stress among police body handlers: a long-term follow-up. *Br J Psychiat* 1993; **163**: 806–8.

53 Symonds RL. Psychiatric aspects of railway fatalities. *Psychol Med* 1985; **15**: 609–21.

54 Farmer R, Tranah T, O'Donnell I, Catalan J. Railway suicide: the psychological effects on drivers. *Psychol Med* 1992; **22**: 407–14.

55 March J. The nosology of PTSD. *J Anxiety Dis* 1990; **4**: 61–82.

56 Feinstein A, Dolan R. Predictors of post-traumatic stress disorder following physical trauma: an examination of the stressor criterion. *Psychol Med* 1991; **21**: 85–91.

57 Smith EM, North CS, McCool RE, Shea JM. Acute post-disaster psychiatric disorders: identification of persons at risk. *Am J Psychiat* 1990; **147**: 202–6.

58 Holen A. *A Long-term Outcome Study of Survivors from a Disaster. The Alexander Kielland Disaster in Perspective*. Oslo, Sweden: University of Oslo Publications, 1990.

59 Lindemann E. Symptomatology and management of acute grief. *Am J Psychiat* 1944; **101**: 141–8.

60 Janoff Bulman R, Frieze R. Theoretical perspective for understanding reactions to victimisation. *J Soc Iss* 1983; **39**: 1–17.

61 Dyregrov A, Mitchell JT. Critical incident stress debriefing. *Norweg J Psychol* 1988; **25**: 217–24.

62 Busuttil W, Turnbull GJ, Leigh AN, Rollins J, West AG et al. Incorporating psychological debriefing techniques within a brief group psychotherapy programme for the treatment of post-traumatic stress disorder. *Br J Psychiat* 1995; **167**: 495–502.

63 Raphael B, Meldrum L, McFarlane AC. Does debriefing after psychological trauma work? Time for randomised controlled trials. *Br Med J* 1995; **310**: 1479–80.

64 Bisson JI, Jenkins PL, Alexander J, Bannister C. Randomised controlled trial of psychological debriefing for victims of acute burn trauma. *Br J Psychiat* 1997; **171**: 78–81.

65 Joseph S, Williams R, Yule W. *Understanding Post-Traumatic Stress: A Psychosocial Perspective on PTSD and Treatment*. Chichester: Wiley, 1997.

66 Richards D, Lovell K. Behavioural and cognitive approaches. In: Black D, Newman M, Harris-Hendriks J, Mezey G eds. *Psychological Trauma: A Developmental Approach*. London: Gaskell, 1997.

67 Dunning C. Mental health sequelae in disaster workers: prevention and intervention. *Int J Ment Hlth* 1990; **19**: 91–103.

68 Ivancevich J, Matteson M, Richards E. Who's liable for stress on the job? *Harvard Bus Rev* 1985; **63**: 2.

69 Anfuso D. Workplace violence. *Personnel J* 1994; **73**: 66–77.

70 National Institute of Occupational Safety and Health,

Centers for Disease Control and Prevention. *Fatal Injuries to Workers in the United States, 1980–89; A Decade of Surveillance*. Washington, D C: US Department of Health and Human Services, 1993.

71 Lusk SL. Violence in the workplace. *J Am Assoc Hosp Nurses* 1992; **40**: 212–3.

72 Health and Safety Advisory Committee. *Violence to Staff. DHSS Advisory Committee on Violence to Staff Report*. London: HMSO, 1987.

73 VandenBos GR, Bulatao EQ (eds). *Violence on the Job: Identifying Risks and Developing Solutions*. Washington, DC: American Psychological Association, 1996.

74 Lion JR, Snyder W, Merrill GL. Underreporting of assaults on staff in a state hospital. *Hosp Commun Psychiat* 1981; **32**: 497–8.

75 Rowett C, Brakewell J. *Managing Violence at Work*. Windsor, Berks: Nelson, 1992.

76 Rowett CP. *Violence in Social Work*. Cambridge, UK: Institute of Criminology, 1986.

77 Caldwell ME. The incidence of PTSD among staff victims of patient violence. *Hosp Commun Psychiat* 1992; **43**: 838–9.

78 Whitefield W, Shelley P. Violence and the CPN: a survey. *Commun Psychiat Nurs J* 1991; **1**: 13–17.

79 Cembrowicz S, Ritter S. Attacks on doctors and nurses. In: Shepherd J ed. *Violence CE in Health Care: A Practical Guide to Coping with Violence and Caring for Victims*. Oxford: Oxford Medical Publications, 1994.

80 Hoad CD. Violence at work: perspectives from research among 20 British employers. *Secur J* 1993; **4**: 64–86.

81 Folger R, Baron RA. Violence and hostility at work: a model of reactions to perceived injustice. *Violence on the Job: Identifying Risks and Developing Solutions* In: VandenBos GR, Bulatao EQ eds. Washington DC: American Psychological Association, 1996.

82 Barling J. The prediction, experience and consequences of workplace violence. In: VandenBos GR, Bulatao EQ eds. *Violence on the Job; Identifying Risks and Developing Solutions*. Washington DC: American Psychological Association, 1996.

83 Cox T, Leather P. The prevention of violence at work: application of a cognitive behavioural theory. *Int Rev Indust Organisat Psychol* 1994; **9**: 213–46.

84 Lund J. Electronic performance monitoring: a review of research issues. *Appl Ergonom* 1992; **23**: 54–8.

85 Baron RA, Neuman JH. Workplace violence and workplace aggression: evidence on their relative frequency and potential causes. *Aggress Behav* 1996; **22**: 161–73.

86 Stuart P. Murder on the job. *Personnel J* 1992; **71**: 72–84.

87 Killias M. Vulnerability: towards a better understanding of a key variable in the genesis of fear of crime. *Violence Victims* 1990; **5**: 97–108.

88 Lanza ML. Violence against nurses in hospitals. In: VandenBos G R, Bulatao E Q eds. *Violence on the Job: Identifying Risks and Developing Solutions* Washington DC: American Psychological Association, 1996.

89 Lanza ML. How do nurses react to patient assault? *J Psychosoc Nurs Ment Hlth Serv* 1985; **23**: 6–11.

90 Mezey G, Shepherd J. Effects of assaults on health-care professionals. In: Shepherd J ed. *Violence in Health-Care*. Oxford: Oxford University Press, 1994.

91 Barling J, Kryl IP. Moderators of the relationship between daily work stress and mood. *Work Stress* 1990; **4**: 319–29.

92 Whittington R, Wykes T. Invisible injury. *Nursing Times* 1989; **84**: 30–2.

93 Duffy CA, McGoldrick AE. Stress and the bus driver in the UK transport industry. *Work Stress* 1990; **4**: 17–27.

94 MacEwen KE, Barling J. Type A behaviour and marital satisfaction: differential effects of achievement striving and impatience/irritability. *J Marriage Fam* 1993; **55**: 1001–10.

95 Royal College of Psychiatrists. *The Management of Imminent Violence: Clinical Practice Guidelines to Support Mental Health Services*. London: College Research Unit., RCP, 1998.

96 Robb E. Post-incident care and support for assaulted staff In: Kidd B, Stock C eds. *Management of Violence and Aggression in Healthcare*. London: Gaskell/Royal College of Psychiatrists, 1995: 140–62.

27

Substance abuse and the workplace

JONATHAN D CHICK

Definitions	557	Ingredients of successful treatment	563
Workplace problems related to alcohol	557	An occupation at risk: the medical profession	564
Work factors contributing to alcohol-related problems	559	Prevention	565
Identification of the problem drinker/drug addict	559	References	565
Management of substance abuse in the workplace	562	Additional reading	567

This chapter explores for clinicians the relation between substance abuse and health and performance at work. It also considers clinical management of substance abuse, company policies that may be available to help abusers and implications for the occupational physician. Numerous substances are abused, including cannabis, cocaine, opiates and benzodiazepines, but the most common is alcohol, which is the main focus of this chapter.

DEFINITIONS

Employees with a substance misuse problem can be defined as those whose regular or intermittent use of a substance or mix of substances repeatedly interferes with their work, or the work of others, their job performance or their ability to work, their relationships with colleagues or clients, or their health.

As in the general population, alcohol-related problems in the workplace can be considered as: heavy drinking, acute problems, chronic effects and dependence on alcohol. These overlap in different people in different ways (Fig. 27.1). Dependence is a state in which an individual experiences difficulty controlling the intake of the substance, and experiences withdrawal symptoms on reduction or cessation of intake. An affected person may move in and out of periods of dependence. The syndrome tends to be reinstated if, after a period of abstinence, the individual begins to use the drug again.

The terms 'drug addict', 'alcoholic' and 'alcoholism' are still widely used, and usually connote chronic excessive use of the substance, either regular or periodic (bout

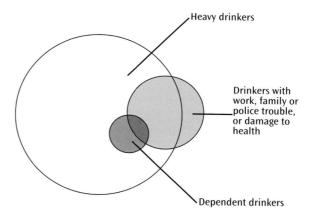

Figure 27.1 *The interrelation of heavy drinking, alcohol-related problems and dependence on alcohol.*

drinking); an admitted or an inferred difficulty in controlling when and how much is consumed; and usually experiencing or causing some problems.

WORKPLACE PROBLEMS RELATED TO ALCOHOL

Work competence and safety

The acute effects of alcohol are chiefly those of a central nervous system depressant, leading to impairment of reasoning, perception, reaction time, balance and coordination. In some drinkers, in the appropriate social setting, a transient disinhibition gives the feeling of enhanced interpersonal communication and well-being. This is partly due to culturally defined expectations. But in this state, decision making, operating machinery, driving and other skilled activities are compromised.

Surveys in Scotland have shown that 24% of company executives in a variety of organizations and 14% of manual workers in alcohol production industries admitted to occasional impaired work efficiency due to drinking in the preceding 6 months.[1] The dose-related effects of alcohol on motor/perceptual skills and judgment have been shown in American drivers.[2] A blood alcohol level of 60 mg/dl (produced by approximately two consecutive pints of beer–4 units) doubled the risk of involvement in an accident compared with drivers with no alcohol in the blood; levels of 100 mg/dl (7 units) and of 150 mg/dl (10 units) were associated with increased risk of 6 and 25 times respectively. Laboratory experiments show that risk-taking increases and perceptual decision-making skills begin to decline at blood alcohol levels as low as 25–50 mg/dl. After a major rail accident in California, a survey of drinking among railroad workers revealed that more than 33% of employees reported seeing a co-worker drinking on duty in the preceding year, 20% reported seeing a colleague too drunk to work.[3]

Workers seeking medical attention after an accident often refuse a blood alcohol test. Thus estimates of the role of alcohol in industrial accidents are very approximate. In an autopsy study of cases where the death certificate recorded 'injury at work', 9.2% were found to have a blood alcohol level of over 100 mg/dl; workers in the transport industry were the most commonly affected.[4] Diazepam was detected in 15.6% of cases, though the extent of its use in the local population of working age was not available for comparison.[4] An autopsy study of fatal occupational injuries in Maryland found that 11% of cases had a blood alcohol concentration of at least 80 mg/dl.[5] Since alcohol continues to be metabolized after death, these rates might underestimate the true prevalence.

Although heavy drinkers are most at risk of accidents at work, it is moderate drinkers who, because they are more numerous, account for most of the cases; hence 'the preventive paradox'.[1] Harm at work will be reduced if all employees reduce their alcohol consumption, not only the heaviest drinkers. When a port authority reduced availability of alcohol at lunchtime, it removed a peak of accidents in dock employees in the afternoon and reduced the overall rate of accidents.

Chronic heavy use of alcohol

Chronic heavy use of alcohol can lead to dementia, whose early signs are impaired problem solving, rigidity of thought, impaired recent memory and difficulty with spatial tasks. It is unlikely that cognitive damage occurs in 'social drinkers' (consumption below, say, 50 units per week[6] though, above 50 units per week, impairments of cerebral function have been detected in some studies by formal psychometric tests, even when they are not clinically obvious.[7]

Epilepsy

'Rum fits' were well known in the British Navy, and usually occurred 2–3 days after the ship left port. An analogous situation occurs now in oilrig workers. Oilrigs are alcohol-free zones to which workers return after 2 weeks on shore. In drinkers who develop chemical dependence an epileptic seizure can occur when alcohol consumption is reduced or ceases. Although this may be an immediate indication for change of job if machinery is involved, clinical experience shows that affected individuals do not have recurrence of fits if they maintain long-term abstinence from alcohol (or if, after some months of abstinence, they eventually resume drinking but keep consumption below, say, 10 units per week).

This may be the first presentation of alcohol dependence. Other investigations might be necessary to exclude other causes of late onset of fits. The electroencephalogram in alcohol dependence does not show epileptic foci.

Absenteeism

General practitioners are sometimes asked by drug or alcohol users for medical certificates to 'cover' absence from work actually spent seeking drugs or drinking, or recovering from the effects thereof. Clinicians should be aware of the typical pattern. Where weekend drinking is the culture, Monday morning is the most common day for alcohol-related absenteeism, usually because of hangover or gastrointestinal upset. If payday is on Thursday rather than Friday for the weekly paid staff, some drinkers will not appear for work on Friday. Such absenteeism is common even among those whose alcohol-related problems are not severe.

The study of Scottish company executives/alcohol production workers mentioned above[1] found that 4% of the executives and 23% of the workers admitted to being off work because of alcohol in the 2-year period before the survey interview. A higher than average medical consultation rate was noted in the 10 years that preceded a diagnosis of alcoholism in a sample of US Navy personnel.[8] Drinkers whose problems are sufficient to lead to attendance at an alcohol problem clinic have twice the sickness absenteeism rate of the general population.[9] In a French survey, problem drinkers were found to have four times the normal rate of absenteeism.[10] Sickness absence certificates covering alcohol-related absenteeism span a wide range of diagnoses, including gastritis, anxiety state, nervous disability and injuries.[9]

Mortality

Accidents are the most common cause of death, among young people.[2,11] The contribution of alcohol has been discussed above. Among new conscripts to the Swedish army (aged 18), those who admitted to drinking over 250 g of alcohol per week (30 units) had a mortality rate over the subsequent 15 years five times greater than the remainder. Accidents accounted for most of the deaths in those heavy-drinking young men.[12] (Although impulsive or risk-taking personality could be a confounder, alcohol is presumed in that study to have contributed, since heavy drinkers tend to remain at the heavy end of the drinking spectrum later in life.)

Longitudinal studies in surveyed populations find that alcohol intake reported at entry predicts excess deaths from cancer of the mouth, pharynx, larynx and oesophagus, and probably breast cancer in women.[13] Rates of death among heavy drinkers are also increased for cerebrovascular disease, liver disease, suicide and violence. This increased mortality commences with consumption as low as 4 units per day. However, in many studies abstainers had a higher mortality than light drinkers. Thus the mortality risk curve for alcohol consumption is J-shaped. Care has to be taken in interpreting these data because the group of 'abstainers' may include ex-drinkers (and often ex-smokers) who have commenced abstaining because of diagnosed illnesses such as heart disease, rather than being life-long abstainers. Moderate drinkers (1 to 3 units a day) may be people with better social adjustment and a healthier lifestyle than either abstainer or heavy drinkers, but even taking this into account the evidence is increasingly persuasive that moderate ethanol consumption protects against coronary artery disease.[14]

WORK FACTORS CONTRIBUTING TO ALCOHOL-RELATED PROBLEMS

Mortality rates from hepatic cirrhosis vary with occupational group and are highest in the alcohol manufacturing and retailing industries. Brewery workers were found to have a higher average intake of alcohol at recruitment than biscuit factory workers, but the brewery workers also increased their consumption to a greater extent during the next 2 years.[15] Thus both selective recruitment and exposure contribute to the alcohol-related risks in the brewing industry. Both may also be important in seamen (officers and crew) and fishermen, who have mortality rates for hepatic cirrhosis three or four times the average. Absence from home and family, and lack of a normal social and sexual life, are clear risk factors; they

may also contribute to the higher rates of cirrhosis in the armed services and the construction industry. In the latter occupation in England, recruitment of labourers from Ireland and Scotland is also relevant, because among them there is a higher proportion of heavy drinkers than among indigenous labourers.

Professions with higher risks include insurance, finance, law, journalism and medicine (see below). Freedom from supervision at work, high incomes and the emotionally demanding nature of their work have been proposed as reasons why these professions have increased rates of alcoholism. The culture at work presumably explains some of the journalists' problems, just as the business lunch routine and the after-business wine-bar have contributed to alcoholism among executives.

Other contributing factors

Clinicians assessing individual patients with alcohol and drug problems must consider the following factors outside the occupational sphere: other psychiatric disorder, to which substance misuse is secondary such as anxiety, phobic or panic disorder, and depressive illness; family history of alcohol or drug misuse; living alone; or death of a spouse. Divorce or legal separation from a spouse can, of course, be the cause or consequence of substance misuse.

IDENTIFICATION OF THE PROBLEM DRINKER/DRUG ADDICT

The workplace is often where an alcohol or drug problem is identified. Accidents, illnesses or a drink/drive conviction often make the diagnosis clear. Unreliable time-keeping, coming to work smelling of alcohol and (or) arguments with colleagues are earlier signs but are often missed. 'Denial' of the contribution of alcohol or drugs to such difficulties is common and such overt signs as shaky hands in the morning might wrongly be attributed to the tension of the morning business meeting. More often, it is because the individual evades any discussion that could implicate alcohol as the cause of his difficulties. The drinker or drug user is likely to perceive any discussion of his habit as one of moral disapproval: any comment about his behaviour is seen as an insult. Evasion of the issue may be skilled and colleagues at work may be misled or afraid of 'upsetting' the cantankerous employee, minimize the problem and cover up for him. Yet it is the manager at work who is best placed to intervene when an alcohol- or drug-related problem occurs.

Because alcohol has a legitimate and accepted role in Western society, the manager who confronts an employee about smelling of alcohol at work may be made to feel a 'killjoy' or 'wet blanket'. Managers may become more motivated to involve the personnel staff or occupational physician as soon as work performance is affected if they can be persuaded that early intervention for substance misuse can prevent later, more difficult and perhaps costly problems which might arise when the employee is involved in an incident – or tolerance of workmates finally evaporates.

The manager must, however, take a delicate and confidential approach. The manager's role is not the diagnosis of alcohol or drug problems but the assessment of work performance. He or she should firmly encourage the individual to consult the occupational physician or general practitioner, who should then deal with the patient with the usual care about confidentiality.

Any clinician assessing a patient with a drink problem should ask about comments or complaints from colleagues and managers at work as well as from those at home, and if disciplinary action has commenced, know what stage has been reached

When a health screening opportunity arises a useful questionnaire for alcohol screening is AUDIT (Alcohol Use Disorders Identification Test) developed by the World Health Organization (Fig. 27.2).[16] The test identifies problems with alcohol at an early stage as well as later cases of alcohol dependence.

Assessment

Within the confidential interview, the clinician discusses with the employee information he is given from management about performance and attendance. A full history, including a non-judgemental, objective enquiry into drinking patterns and drug use, is essential. The doctor goes over the past 7 days, work and leisure time, in detail to determine what and where drinking (or drug use) took place. A history of accidents at home, at work, on the road or at leisure should prompt enquiry about any relation to alcohol. The doctor should also obtain information from the family, because some individuals minimize their alcohol or drug intake and the problems caused.

THE ALCOHOL USE DISORDERS IDENTIFICATION TEST

Audit was developed by the World Health Organization to identify persons whose alcohol consumption has become hazardous or harmful to their health.

1. How often do you have a drink containing alcohol? |___|

(0) Never (3) 2 to 3 times a week
(1) Monthly or less (4) 4 or more times a week
(2) 2 to 4 times a month

2. How many drinks containing alcohol do you have on a typical day when you are drinking? |___|

(0) 1 or 2 (2) 5 or 6 (3) 10 or more
(1) 3 or 4 (3) 7, 8, or 9

3. How often do you have six or more drinks on one occasion? |___|

(0) Never (2) Monthly (4) Daily or
(1) < monthly (3) Weekly almost daily

4. How often during the last year have you found that you were not able to stop drinking once you had started? |___|

(0) Never (2) Monthly (4) Daily or
(1) < monthly (3) Weekly almost daily

5. How often during the last year have you failed to do what was normally expected from you because of drinking? |___|

(0) Never (2) Monthly (4) Daily or
(1) < monthly (3) Weekly almost daily

6. How often during the last year have you needed a first drink in the morning to get yourself going after a heavy drinking session? |___|

(0) Never (2) Monthly (4) Daily or
(1) < monthly (3) Weekly almost daily

7. How often during the last year have you had a feeling of guilt or remorse after drinking? |___|

(0) Never (2) Monthly (4) Daily or
(1) < monthly (3) Weekly almost daily

8. How often during the last year have you been unable to remember what happened the night before because you had been drinking? |___|

(0) Never (2) Monthly (4) Daily or
(1) < monthly (3) Weekly almost daily

9. Have you or someone else been injured as a result of your drinking? |___|

(0) No (4) Yes, during
(2) Yes, but not the last year
in the last year

10. Has a relative or friend or a doctor or another health worker been concerned about your drinking or suggested you cut down? |___|

(0) No (4) Yes, during
(2) Yes, but not the last year
in the last year

Record total of specific items here. |___|

If total > 8, alcohol problem very likely

CLINICAL SCREENING PROCEDURE

Record numerical score in the box at right.

TRAUMA HISTORY

Have you injured your head since your 18th birthday? |___|

(3) Yes (0) No

Have you broken any bones since your 18th birthday? |___|

(3) Yes (0) No

CLINICAL EXAMINATION

Code as follows:

(0) Not present (2) Moderate
(1) Mild (3) Severe

Conjunctival Injection |___|

Abnormal Skin Vascularization |___|

Hand Tremor |___|

Tongue Tremor |___|

Hepatomegaly |___|

GGT Values |___|
(0) Lower normal (0-30)
(1) Upper normal (30-50)
(3) Abnormal (50 or higher)

Record sum of individual items here. |___|

If total > 5, alcohol problem likely

Figure 27.2 *The Alcohol Use Disorders Identification Test.*

Clinical features

Intoxication with alcohol or sedatives may be recognized and, likewise, the fatuous giggling of cannabis intoxication. At physical examination, the heavy drinker may show excessive capillarization of the conjunctivae and skin of the cheeks and nose. Close examination of the tongue may reveal the smell of alcohol on the breath. In the dependent drinker, tremor of the tongue and mouth can be seen before it is visible in the outstretched fingers. Intoxication with sedatives may cause nystagmus. Opiates cause constriction of the pupils. There may be venepuncture marks. The drinker may have an enlarged liver, signs of parenchymal liver disease, cerebellar ataxia particularly affecting the gait, weakness of the proximal shoulder and pelvic girdle muscles or evidence of peripheral neuropathy.

Objective markers

DRUGS

Workplace urine screening

The UK Transport and Works Act 1992 has led to most operators of passenger transport systems in the UK introducing urine drug screening for operational staff. Police are empowered to test for alcohol and drugs in railway staff associated with a train accident. Similar legislation was passed in the USA in the 1980s and later Federal employees became subject to screening.

That safety is thereby improved has, however, proved difficult to demonstrate. For example, to assess the potential preventive impact of recruitment drug screening, the US Postal Service in Boston monitored industrial accidents, occupational injuries, disciplinary actions and turnover in 2537 new employees. Positive testing for cocaine in the urine at recruitment predicted a raised incident rate in the first and the second year of employment, but testing positive for cannabis was no longer predictive of incidents after the first year.[17] Perhaps cannabis users gradually change their lifestyle as they develop job responsibility. Interpretation of a positive result requires experience and sometimes further analysis.

Reliability of testing. Cannabis metabolites can be detected in urine several weeks after the last dose but only in very heavy regular users. Traces can be found for 3 or 4 hours after passive smoking. Eating biscuits containing poppy seeds can cause a trace of morphine to be found in urine. The concordance between urine analysis and self-reports of drug use in workplace samples tends to be low, suggesting that these detection methods should be regarded as complementary and not alternatives.

Hair analysis is rarely used. Hair grows about 1 cm per month. Drugs and their metabolites are absorbed into hair and can be extracted and measured, for example, by radioimmunoassay.[18] Evasion or manipulation of the results is easy with urine tests and very difficult with hair analysis. Hair analysis is generally only available through certain commercial laboratories. There is doubt about how accurately, if at all, hair analysis can distinguish between frequent and occasional use, and about whether the timing of use can be specified since drug metabolites might 'move along' the hair shaft.

Legal and ethical pitfalls. An employee's job could be threatened if a test is positive. Occupational physicians and physicians functioning as 'medical review officers' should be familiar with the recommendations given by The Faculty of Occupational Medicine (UK) in its Guidelines for Testing for Drugs of Abuse in the Workplace[19] or those of an experienced forensic toxicologist[20] which are:

1 if, at a recruitment examination or an examination at the request of the employer, blood or urine is to be tested for alcohol or drugs, informed consent must be obtained to collect and analyse the specimen, and to report the results to the employer;
2 employees should lists all medications currently taken;
3 the specimen is collected under supervision, to avoid adulteration or substitution, placed in a tamper-evident container and the steps to testing and recording of the result are audited (the 'chain of custody' must be observed);
4 it is good practice to divide the sample into two parts, for analysis at the employee's laboratory of choice if desired (the specimen cannot be deemed owned by the employer);
5 the employee will have the right to see the result;
6 the medical reviewer or occupational physician, in the view of Forrest,[20] 'cannot be exempt from the requirement to act in good faith in the best interests of the patients, even though paid by the employer . . .

Establishing a drug-testing programme. Before a drug-testing programme of any kind is announced in a company, the employer should be clear about its objectives. These may be public safety, employee safety, financial or information security, or improved performance and quality. The Faculty of Occupational Medicine[19] recommend that companies take legal advice before embarking on a programme. Testing may be in various circumstances, which also need specifying in advance, for example, pre-employment, in-house promotion or transfer, 'for cause' (i.e. if there has been unsatisfactory behaviour or performance, post-incident, 'periodic', during or after rehabilitation, or as part of a clinical assessment by the company physician).

Monitoring drug abuse treatment. Drug testing should not be an end in itself. It has a use in clinical decision making, for feedback to patients on progress, and for programme evaluation. However, for patients who are 'doing well' (e.g. complying with therapy, employed) detection of brief 'slips', if this leads the clinician to make a strong or punitive response, could be harmful overall.

ALCOHOL

The mean erythrocyte cell volume is greater than 98fl in 30% of men drinking over 50 units per week; serum γ-glutamyl transferase (GGT) is raised above 45 IU/litre in 70%, and in these drinkers rises and falls with changes in consumption.[21] If serum aspartate aminotransferase (AST) is also raised, the clinician can attach greater confidence to the diagnosis of alcohol abuse. Two abnormal findings are a stronger indication of heavy drinking than any single abnormality.

A promising test for excessive drinking, not yet in routine use but available in several laboratories, is the level in serum of carbohydrate-deficient transferrin (CDT). It may be elevated in primary biliary cirrhosis but is only rarely raised in other non-alcoholic liver disease and is not affected by medications.[22] Although sensitivity for detecting excessive drinking is only slightly greater for CDT than for GGT, specificity is much greater (i.e. fewer false positives).

An indirect method of screening for people in whom it might be clinically relevant to ask about drinking, is to ask about fractures or dislocations, head injuries, assaults or road traffic accidents since the age of 18. When sports injuries are excluded, it is found that people who answer 'yes' to two or more of the above, and then answer positively to the question 'have you been injured after drinking alcoholic beverages', are likely to have an alcohol problem.[23] A disguised questionnaire has been used for surveying a workforce to detect likely problem drinkers, but has had only limited research or practical use.[24]

MANAGEMENT OF SUBSTANCE ABUSE IN THE WORKPLACE

Intervention should occur early, before harm accumulates and dismissal or medical retirement needs to be contemplated. Substance misuse policies and treatment referral procedures have evolved over the last 30 years, first in North America. This is partly humanitarian and partly for financial reasons – it may be cheaper to encourage and allow the employee to have treatment than to put up with his behaviour or to dismiss him. Clinicians should be aware of the following policies even though it is only the occupational physician who is likely to be directly involved.

Workplace policies

The main statements in such policies are:

1 Alcohol or drug problems are to be regarded as a health matter, with the corollary that the employee is expected to pursue and comply with treatment.
2 If disciplinary action is indicated, it is postponed while the employee seeks treatment.
3 If sick leave is required for treatment, the firm will grant it.
4 (important for success of policies but not always written in) Information about compliance and success of treatment may be communicated from treatment agency to employer. Evidence of relapse visible at work should be passed to the treatment agency if the employee is still being dealt with under the policy.
5 The ultimate sanctions of disciplinary action or termination of employment on health grounds remain when all efforts at help have failed.

Some large companies in North America employ staff to run the alcohol and drug policy, and perhaps also to make assessments of drug and alcohol problems. Elsewhere the responsibility for the policy is with the personnel department or the occupational health and safety team; assessments are made by outside agencies including, in the UK, by the National Health Service. Guidance has been provided by the Health and Safety Executive.[25] It is important that clinicians clarify at the first interview whether such workplace policies exist, and especially whether point 4, above, is relevant to the particular patient.

Coercion? – ethics

It is generally regarded as ethical for a firm to dismiss an employee if there are clear grounds for dismissal, and the management has postponed dismissal to allow assessment and treatment of alcohol- or drug-related difficulties. This is regarded as 'constructive coercion'. It is not regarded as ethical for the employer to nudge an employee into medical assessment or treatment with the threat of dismissal if there are as yet no clear grounds for dismissal. Some firms require a medical examination, including evidence of healthy drinking habits and a normal serum GGT, to be one criterion for fitness for promotion. If this criterion is not met, an invitation to join the alcohol policy will follow.

Coercion? – efficacy

'Motivation to change' is one predictor of outcome of treatment for substance abuse. An ultimatum from the spouse or the threat of a serious physical illness will often influence motivation, as will an unequivocal statement from an employer. It is important that such statements are clear – that the obligations and intentions of the firm are delineated and that what is expected of the employee is spelt out. It is possible to do this in a way that is not felt by the employee as punitive.

Several North American studies have shown that the outcome of patients mandated into treatment from the courts or the workplace is no worse than the outcome of 'voluntary' patients. In the USA, physicians on probation because of drug or alcohol abuse have, in general, a better outcome than most populations of substance abusers. In part this may be due to their greater social resources, but may also be because a Licensing Board has had a role in their coming for treatment (see below).

When treating an employed substance misuser, if his or her problem is already known to the employer, it can sometimes improve the outcome of therapy to recommend such supervision by the employer or his nominee.

INGREDIENTS OF SUCCESSFUL TREATMENT

Perhaps the most important element is for the individual to enter a non-judgemental, objective relationship in which he can weigh up the advantages and disadvantages of continuing the alcohol or drug habit. Only then is it possible for him to make a firm decision to alter his habit and obtain support to stick to that decision.

It was common practice in North America, to offer the employee residential treatment with an emphasis on group therapy lasting 4–6 weeks. Controlled studies demonstrating the advantage of such relatively expensive treatment over outpatient care are lacking. However, specific psychological treatments such as marital counselling, anxiety management and social skills training have been shown to be effective. Alcoholics Anonymous has helped thousands of alcoholics, in many countries, and a stable fellow employee who is an AA member may be a great help in introducing a colleague. Narcotics Anonymous (NA), for drug abusers, can be found in some cities.

Psychotropic medication to reduce relapse may occasionally have a place if other psychiatric disorders are found to persist after the drug use has ceased.

Two compounds (naltrexone and acamprosate) are now licensed in several countries to help prevent relapse in newly abstaining alcoholics. Their neuropharmacological actions, while different from each other, are consistent with current knowledge of the neurotransmitter basis of dependence and relapse. The characteristics of patients most likely to respond are still to be specified.[26]

Medically assisted withdrawal

Withdrawal from alcohol can often be achieved as an outpatient or at home guided by the general practitioner or by a nurse. Ideally the patient is seen daily to monitor the dosage of the drug and to ensure that drinking is not continuing. Admission to hospital is appropriate if this fails, or if the individual is liable to severe withdrawal symptoms and lives alone. (A patient drinking 25 or more units per day may require 50 mg of diazepam or equivalent in the first 24 hours, reducing to zero over 5 days.)

Subjects can also withdraw from drugs as outpatients. With encouragement and perhaps the use of self-help groups, the older, socially stable, benzodiazepine user can often be treated by a very gradual reduction of the drug; the same is true for legally obtainable analgesics. The socially unstable young abuser often takes a very wide variety of substances, including alcohol, and discussion during a drug withdrawal regimen should include strategies of developing a different life style.

Medical aid for the opiate abuser who requests detoxification is necessary only if chemical dependence exists – often such abusers are only intermittent users and hope to obtain more drugs (sometimes to sell) by requesting detoxification. Treatment will consist of either substituting a reducing dose of oral methadone, with controls to check other continuing drug use, or attempting to reduce withdrawal symptoms with clonidine or lofexidine perhaps with a benzodiazepine to aid sleep. A specialist clinic should advise about appropriate doses. Ultra-rapid withdrawal by giving an opiate antagonist while the patient is unconscious under anaesthetic is possible but is rarely practised because of the risk of respiratory or circulatory failure. It requires full intensive care facilities, an experienced addiction specialist and an experienced anaesthetist. In such hands, the patient's discharge and return home after being prescribed naltrexone can be achieved in a few days.

Deterrent medication[26]

When an employee has been given his final warning, the treatment agency may suggest that he takes disulfiram supervised at work or at a clinic. The firm can know that day by day the employee is complying, if he is observed to swallow the tablets daily. The deterrent effect of this drug (i.e. its highly unpleasant alcohol interaction) functions only if it is taken regularly in sufficient dosage. Counselling on changing lifestyle during the disulfiram-induced abstinence is important in the prevention of relapse once the disciplinary period ends. Naltrexone can be used in the same way with an opiate abuser. Naltrexone blocks the rewarding mental effects of opiates rather than causing an aversive reaction, and, if taken regularly (perhaps three times per week), greatly reduces the risk of relapse. Some centres have successfully used this approach to help patients where there is a court or employment sanction.

Abstinence?

Early, not severely dependent, problem drinkers can sometimes resume problem-free drinking. Those with social supports (family and job) and without impulsive personalities and many social problems are the ones likely to succeed. Abstinence is the appropriate goal for most other alcohol and drug abusers. Among opiate addicts, there is a growing trend, because of AIDS (acquired immunodeficiency syndrome) prevention strategies, to offer maintenance oral methadone to reduce injecting. Such individuals may be able to perform satisfactorily at work, unless they are also using additional *ad hoc* street drugs, and not all treatment clinics can rule this out. Maintenance prescribing of benzodiazepine to benzodiazepine addicts is common, and many users continue functioning effectively at work, but should not drive vocationally or operate machinery because reaction time and cognitive function can be impaired.

When substance abuse has led to doubt about fitness to work in very critical posts, for example in the airline industry (pilots, traffic controllers) and medicine, random monitoring of breath, urine or blood tests contributes to good outcome.

Prognosis

In individuals who have reached criteria for dependence and/or have come for treatment, a period of abstinence from drugs or alcohol of less than a year has no prognostic value.[27] Abstinence for 1 year begins to indicate a good outcome. Individuals do best when they still have a job and a close relationship. In the emerging life-story of men who at some stage in their life abused alcohol, it can be seen that an abstinent period of 5 years is only very rarely followed by a relapse, but nevertheless can still occur.[28] It is clearly very difficult to decide whether or when an alcohol or drug misuser who has a highly responsible post, for example as a driver, pilot, ship's captain, or a surgeon should be allowed to resume that job. Monitoring is essential and might reasonably continue for up to 5 years, though practice varies and there are insufficient published data to be precise.

Vocational driving licences

In the European Union, and in many other countries, employees with an alcohol or drug problem are not permitted to have licences to drive large goods- or passenger-carrying vehicles. A minimum of several years (3 years in the UK) since cessation of treatment, and evidence of recovery, is required before renewal of the licence. The driver who develops a drug problem should declare this to the licensing authorities. Opiate addicts maintained on oral methadone and patients receiving regular benzodiazepines may not hold vocational licences in the UK and the European Community. It is a debated point whether such individuals may hold ordinary driving licences although studies of psychomotor performance in patients on a regular dose of methadone have not shown impairment.

Ordinary licence – The high risk offender scheme

On reapplication for an ordinary UK driving licence following disqualification for drink/driving; a driver must satisfy the Secretary of State for Transport's medical advisers that he or she is not, or never was, alcohol dependent, if (1) the blood alcohol at the time of the offence was 200 mg/litre or more; or (2) he or she refused the tests or (3) he or she has been disqualified more than once in 10 years.

AN OCCUPATION AT RISK: THE MEDICAL PROFESSION

In the UK, once a decade, tables are published of mortality by occupation. For the 1980s data for alcoholic cirrhosis deaths placed doctors higher in the league table than in the past two decades with a proportional mortality ratio (PMR) of 341 that is, over three times the expected, second only to publicans and bar staff (PMR 383). Doctors also have a higher than normal expectation of dying of other alcohol-related deaths including suicide, alcohol-related cancers and accidents.[29] Doctors are more frequently admitted to psychiatric hospital for treatment of alcoholism than others in the upper socioeconomic classes, though recently a trend has occurred in Scotland suggesting that younger doctors are not being admitted as frequently as in previous decades, which hopefully presages a reduction in the high alcoholism rates the profession has suffered.[30]

The Annual Reports of the UK licensing authority, The General Medical Council (GMC), show that alcohol and drug misuse, with or without other psychiatric disorders, is a common cause of unfitness to practise. From 1981 to 1993, 57 doctors with these diagnoses were processed. There are, of course, other doctors whose substance misuse does not become known to the GMC, although their family and professional life, and their health, is grievously harmed.

Stress in the medical profession has been more widely recognized in the 1990s than previously.[31,32] Personality features may have contributed both to the interest in medicine and a vulnerability to stress.[33] Stress can be a factor in substance misuse in doctors, but should not be too readily assumed to be the central issue. For some, addiction has simply begun as a great liking for a drug's euphoric effects. Medical student life in Western countries can involve heavy drinking. Later on, doctors not only have sufficient income to subsidise heavy drinking, but they also have relatively easy access to many other addictive substances. Anaesthetists are at particular risk of opiate misuse (oral or injected) or misuse of anaesthetics (sniffing) and may experiment to the point of dependence. Pharmacists and veterinarians are at higher risk, also because of relative availability of addictive drugs.

Helping a fellow physician[34,35]

Too often, work colleagues have maintained a blanket of secrecy, and the addiction is well advanced when help is eventually sought. Your friendship may be needed, but you may also need to take a firm even disciplinary stance to stimulate the misusing doctor to accept that there is a problem which needs attention. This requires courage and compassion, not covering up. If he or she is a work colleague, leave the treatment to a specialist. If the doctor makes no attempt to seek advice, then others who can bring some coercion to bear may need to be involved, for example the hospital managers, the appropriate section of the local health authority or, when none of these are relevant and fitness to practise is in question, the GMC or appropriate licensing board.

In helping a substance-misusing doctor, the dialogue should be as with an intelligent layman, without assuming he or she has special knowledge. Commence with the concerns that he or she has uppermost in the mind, using a non-judgemental style. Avoid secrecy. Be ready to set limits and prevent too early discontinuation of treatment. Beware too ready an acceptance of the view that 'stress' or 'depression' are the main issues: the main issue may be the substance-dependence itself, but this is not yet identified/accepted by the individual. It is easy to collude in a way that only postpones dealing with the dependence on the drug, that is, making a commitment to abstinence and following methods to achieve that. Monitor progress using objective markers such as breath, blood and urine tests. If matters have reached a point where the professional Licensing Board is involved, the Board's Health Screener is likely to require evidence that treatment is being followed and abstinence is being achieved before limitations on practice are rescinded.

Doctors tend to have a better outcome than other substance misusers, especially if they can resume work because then supervision can aid recovery.[36,37] Meeting with other doctors who are recovering from addiction is beneficial: in the UK, there is The Doctors' and Dentists' Group, c/o Medical Council on Alcoholism – Tel: 0207 487 4445. Also in the UK there is the National Counselling Service for Sick Doctors – Tel: 0207 935 5982, and the British Medical Association Stress Counselling Service.

PREVENTION

Limiting the availability of alcohol in the workplace is important and can reduce accidents; similarly, regulations about the taking of psychotropic drugs or alcohol at work or before coming to work can be helpful. A positive approach for heavy-drinking blue-collar workers included the provision of free hot lunches inside the plant to inhibit lunch hour and 'parking lot' drinking.[38]

Excessive drinkers, detected through general health screening services in the community and family practices, have been shown to respond favourably to fairly minimal medical intervention (such as occasional outpatient counselling and feedback about their serum GGT).[24,39–42] Over a 4-year follow-up, it has been possible to demonstrate a halving of days off work through sickness.[39] For such purposes, 'heavy drinking' has been defined as admitted consumption of over 21 units for women and over 35 units per week for men or an elevated serum GGT attributable to alcohol. There has been no published controlled study of early intervention in the workplace. Employee assistance programmes may aim to recruit problem drinkers early, but except in the USA where seeking help for personal problems is perhaps more accepted, self-referrals to these programmes are rare and managers still tend to refer only when impaired work performance is severe or chronic. Whether attempts to educate a worksite population in healthy lifestyle practices can result in a reduction in substance abuse problems at work, or in the number of abusers, has not been shown. It is notable that employee committees, when consulted about health promotion they would see as relevant, tend not to mention drugs or alcohol. They perceive organizational stressors as the most important: deadlines, unrealistic expectations, excessive supervision, inadequate supervision, poor feedback, harassment and the like.[43]

Health promotion in the workplace should be broad and look at links between personal health practices (eating, smoking, exercise, weight control, stress management) and factors at the workplace. Programmes should help participants to develop or regain a sense of control, efficacy and competence in their health practices, and to use support from family, friends and fellow workers if trying to change these. Such projects are most likely to be successful when the workforce is involved in their development. Didactic teaching that comes down from personnel departments or management is unlikely to succeed in individualistic Western society. A more successful approach might be the introduction of education projects initiated by the workforce to stimulate ideas on ways to help individuals cut down their drug or alcohol use.[43]

REFERENCES

1 Kreitman N. Alcohol consumption and the preventive paradox. *Br J Addict* 1986; **81**: 353–63.

2   National Highway Traffic Safety Administration, National Center for Statistics and Analysis. *Drunk Driving Facts*. Washington DC: NHTSA, 1988.

3   Seaman FJ. Problem drinking among American railroad workers. In: Hore B, Plant M eds. *Alcohol Problems in Employment*. London: Croom Helm, 1981: 118–28.

4   Lewis RJ, Cooper SP. Alcohol, other drugs and fatal work-related injuries. *J Occup Med* 1989; **31:** 23–8.

5   Baker S. Sankoff IS, Fisher RS *et al*. Fatal occupational injuries. *JAMA* 1982; **248:** 692–7.

6   Williams CM, Skinner AEG. The cognitive effects of alcohol. *Br J Addict* 1990; **85:** 911–18.

7   Dent OF, Sulway MR, Broe GA, Creasey H, Kos SC *et al*. Alcohol consumption and cognitive performance in a random sample of Australian soldiers who served in the second world war. *Br Med J* 1997; **314:** 1655–8.

8   Kolb D, Gunderson EKE. Medical histories of problem drinkers during their first twelve years of naval service. *J Stud Alcohol* 1983, **44:** 84–94.

9   Saad E, Madden J. Certificated incapacity and unemployment in alcoholics. *Br J Psychiat* 1976; **128:** 340–5.

10 Godard J. Alcohol and occupation. In: Hore B, Plant M eds. *Alcohol Problems in Employment*. London: Croom Helm, 1981: 105–17.

11 Report of the Chief Medical Officer of Health. *On the State of the Public Health in the Year 1990*. London: HMSO, 1991.

12 Andreasson S, Alleback P, Romelsjo A. Alcohol consumption and mortality among young men: longitudinal study of Swedish conscripts. *Br Med J* 1988; **296:** 1021–5.

13 Turner C, Anderson P. Is alcohol a carcinogenic risk? *Br J Addict* 1990; **85:** 1409–16.

14 Rimm EB. Alcohol consumption and coronary heart disease: good habits may be more important than just good wine. *Am J Epidemiol* 1996; **143:** 1094–8.

15 Plant M. Alcoholism and occupation: cause or effect? A controlled study of recruits to the drink trade. *Int J Addict* 1978; **13:** 605–26.

16 Seppä K, Makela R, Sillanaukee P. Effectiveness of the Alcohol Use Disorders Identification Test in occupational health screening. *Alcoholism Clin Exp Res* 1995; **19:** 999–1003.

17 Ryan J, Zwerling C, Jones M The effectiveness of preemployment drug screening in the prediction of employment outcome. *J Occup Med* 1992; **34:** 1057–63.

18 Magura S, Freeman RC, Siddiqui Q, Lipton DS. The validity of hair analysis for detecting cocaine and heroin use among addicts. *Int J Addict* 1992; **27:** 51–69.

19 Faculty of Occupational Medicine. *Guidelines for Testing for Drugs of Abuse in the Workplace*. London: Royal College of Physicians, 1994.

20 Forrest ARW. Ethical aspects of workplace urine screening for drug abuse *J Med Ethics* 1977; **23:** 12–17

21 Chick J, Kreitman N, Plant M. Mean cell volume and gamma glutamyl transpeptidase as markers of drinking in working men. *Lancet* 1981; **i:** 1249–51.

22 Litten RZ, Allen JP, Fertig JB. Gamma glutamyltrans-peptidase and carbohydrate – deficient transferrin: alternative measures of excessive alcohol consumption. *Alcoholism Clin Exp Res* 1995; **19**: 1541–6

23 Israel Y, Hollander O, Sanchez-Craig M. Booker S, Miller V *et al*. Screening for problem drinking and counseling by the primary care physician-nurse team. *Alcoholism Clin Exp Res* 1996; **20**: 1443–50.

24 Webb GR, Redman S, Hennrikus D, Rostas J, Sanson-Fisher RW. The prevalence and socio-demographic correlates of high-risk and problem drinking at an industrial worksite. *Br J Addict* 1990; **85**: 495–507.

25 Health and Safety Executive. *Drug Abuse at Work*: *A Guide to Employers*. IND(G)91L 6/90. London: HSE, 1990.

26 Chick J. Medication in the treatment of alcohol dependence. *Adv Psychiat Treatment* 1996; **2**: 249–57.

27 Yates WR, Reed DA, Booth BM, Masterson BJ, Brown K. Prognostic validity of short-term abstinence. *Alcoholism Clin Exp Res* 1994; **18**: 280–3.

28 Vaillant GE. A long-term follow-up of male alcohol abuse. *Arch Gen Psychiat* 1996; **53**: 243–9.

29 Drever F (ed) *Occupational Health: Decennial Supplement*. London: Office of Population Censuses and Surveys/Health and Safety Executive/HMSO, 1995: 72.

30 Harrison D, Chick J. Trends in alcoholism among male doctors in Scotland. *Addiction* 1994; **89**: 1613–17.

31 Ramirez AJ, Graham J, Richards MA, Cull A, Gregory WM. Mental health of hospital consultants: the effects of stress and satisfaction at work. *Lancet* 1996; **347**: 724–28.

32 Caplan RP. Stress, anxiety, and depression in hospital consultants, general practitioners and senior health service managers. *Br Med J* 1994; **309**: 1261–63.

33 Brooke D. Why do some doctors become addicted? *Addiction* 1996; **91**: 317–19.

34 Chick J. Doctors with emotional problems: how can they be helped? In, Hawton K, Cowen P eds. *Practical Problems in Clinical Psychiatry*. Oxford: Oxford University Press, 1992: 242–52.

35 Lloyd G. Supporting the addicted doctor. *Practitioner* 1990; **234**: 989–91.

36 Morse RM, Martin MA, Swenson WM, Niven RG. Prognosis of physicians treated for alcoholism and drug dependence. *JAMA* 1984; **251**: 743–6.

37 Shore JH. The Oregon experience with impaired physicians on probation: an 8 year follow-up. *JAMA* 1987; **257**: 2931–4.

38 Ames GM, Lanes GR. Heavy problem drinking in an American blue-collar population: implications for prevention. *Soc Sci Med* 1987; **25**: 949–60.

39 Kristenson H, Ohlin H, Hutten-Nosslin MB, Trell E, Hood B. Identification and intervention of heavy drinking in middle-aged men: result and follow-up of 24–60 months of long term study with randomised controls. *Alcoholism Clin Exp Res* 1983; **7**: 203–9.

40 Wallace P, Cutler S, Haines A. Randomised controlled trial of general practitioner intervention in patients with excess alcohol consumption. *Br Med J* 1988; **297**: 663–8.

41 Israel Y, Hollander O, Sanchez-Craig M, Booker S, Miller V *et*

al. Screening for problem drinking and counseling by the primary care physician-nurse team *Alcoholism Clin Exp Res* 1996; **20**: 1443–50.

42 Fleming MF, Barry KL, Manwell LB, Johnson K, London R, Brief physician advice for problem alcohol drinkers: a randomised controlled trial in a community based population. *JAMA* 1997; **277**: 1039–45.

43 Shain M. Worksite community processes and the prevention of alcohol abuse: theory to action. In: Giesbrecht N, Conley P, Denniston RW *et al*. eds. *Research, Action and the Community*: *Experiences in the Prevention of Alcohol and other Drug Problems*. US Dept of Health and Human Services OSAP Prevention monograph. Washington DC: US Government Printing Office, 1990: 106–12.

ADDITIONAL READING

1 Chick J, Cantwell R (eds). *Seminars in Substance Misuse*. London: Gaskell, 1994.

2 Ghodse H. *Drugs and Addictive Behaviour: A Guide to Treatment* 2nd edn. Oxford: Blackwell Scientific Publications revised, 1995.

3 Edwards G, Marshall J, Cook C. *The Treatment of Drinking Problems* 3rd edn. Oxford: Oxford University Press, revised, 1997.

28

Health and mental illness at work: clinical assessment and management

ERIC L TEASDALE, FRANCIS H CREED

Defining stress and occupational stress-related illness	570	Assessment of fitness to work	575
The incidence of stress-related illness	570	Raising awareness	576
The legal impact of stress on employers – statutory and civil	570	Assessing risks to employees	576
		Management of mental illness problems at work	577
The financial impact of stress on employers	571	Assessment and rehabilitation of employees returning to work after mental illness	577
Risk-factors for stress-related illness	571		
Pattern of referral	572	Provision of support for employees	578
Presentation of psychiatric disorder	572	Role of the occupational physician	578
Assessment	573	References	579
Detailed assessment of 'not coping'	573		

The World Health Organization defines health as a state of complete physical, mental, social and spiritual well-being. The spiritual angle has nothing to do with religion, it merely relates to the need we all have to be treated as individuals and to grow and develop during our adult life. Many of the 'physical' aspects of occupational health are now well understood, e.g. dermatitis, noise-induced hearing loss etc. Over the last 10–20 years the mental, social and spiritual sides of life have become much more prominent and are probably more difficult to understand and manage.

In the occupational or industrial setting, the emphasis on maintaining *mental* (as well as physical and social) well-being is essential to success. Occasional serious cases of mental illness must be recognized and managed appropriately. This should include the care of the individual who has a problem of substance abuse (e.g. alcohol or drugs of addiction), and the patient with a psychotic condition where prompt admission to hospital is required. In practice, however, the more common mental health problems encompass stress, anxiety and depression, and their manifestation in the workplace. The most frequent condition under the mental health umbrella is stress and much effort has been directed to this end.

Stress is a normal part of life and the challenge is to manage the pressures so that life is productive and enjoyable. Indeed stress itself is not an illness; rather it is a state. However, it is a very powerful cause of illness. Long-term excessive stress is known to lead to serious health problems. Unfortunately for some, the pressures cannot be managed (the individual may have little in the way of life skills) or, they may become overwhelming and unrelenting. The assessment of the individual patient requires critical scrutiny of the claim that work-related stress is responsible for the patient's symptoms; this requires detailed information about the patient's work – its nature and the working environment – as well as about the patient and symptoms. This inevitably leads the doctor to consider the global effects of working practices and the safety of other workers as well as the presenting illness.

Clinicians should recognize that the occupational physician is an invaluable resource in assessing the patient who complains of excess stress at work. He or she will be able to provide the clinician with information about the individual patient's previous work performance and sickness record, and also about the work situation – whether there really are excessive stresses and numerous health problems in that particular department. The occupational physician may also be able to modify the attitude of managers to the patient, negotiate part-time work and observe the patient in the work setting.

DEFINING STRESS AND OCCUPATIONAL STRESS-RELATED ILLNESS

Much is made of the difficulties in defining stress, and even more of defining occupational stress-related illness. This is reflected in the fact that there is no single agreed definition. Many would agree that a person experiences the negative effects of stress in the situation where there is a 'stimulus or environmental change of such intensity or duration that it taxes a person's adaptive capacity to the limit'.[1]

It is sometimes more helpful to think of pressure as the stimulus and stress or stress-related illness as possible consequences. There is general agreement that we all need some pressure to encourage us to perform well in all aspects of life, be they related to home or work. Although this is consistent with the view commonly expressed that 'some stress is good for you' clearly stress-related illness is not.

Stress has been described as 'a feeling of doubt about being able to cope, and stress management is aimed as much at modifying the perception of stress as at removing external stressors'.[2] This definition allows us to move forward in a workplace setting; raising awareness and modifying management perceptions of stress is often the biggest challenge for the health and safety advisor. Recognizing limitations in influencing external factors (such as family etc.) outside the workplace, which have a significant impact on the development of stress-related illness of individuals, is also an important realization. This allows the organization and its employees to focus on factors which they can influence for the common good.

THE INCIDENCE OF STRESS-RELATED ILLNESS

Mental illness is very prevalent in the working age community. In the United Kingdom, a survey by the Office of Population, Census and Surveys[3] confirmed that one in seven adults (aged 16–64) living in private households were suffering from some sort of mental health problem, such as anxiety or depression, in the weeks prior to interview. Although it is likely that the prevalence in a working population will be lower, as working populations are known to be made up of a healthier population than non-working groups (the 'healthy-worker effect'), mental ill-health clearly represents a significant burden to employers. The Health and Safety Executive (HSE) estimated that 80 million working days in a year were lost to employers in the UK as a result of mental disorders caused by stress.

In the Trailer to the 1990 Labour Force Survey, published by the HSE,[4] stress or depression caused, or made worse, by work was second only to musculoskeletal disorders as the most frequently cited cause of occupational ill-health. Occupational stress, or stress related to work, has been increasingly cited as a cause of morbidity. For workers, stress is often cited as a contributory factor to accidents, job dissatisfaction and illnesses such as coronary heart disease, alcoholism and hypertension. The inevitable conclusion of such data is that mental health problems will affect employees and businesses alike.

THE LEGAL IMPACT OF STRESS ON EMPLOYERS – STATUTORY AND CIVIL

In the UK, employers have been required to provide safe systems of work by the Health and Safety at Work etc Act since 1974. More recently, such obligations have been reinforced under the Management of Health and Safety at Work Regulations 1992 where employers are required to assess the risks of work activities and to take steps to minimize the realization of those risks to their employees. The Duty of Care includes providing help to members of staff such as measures to identify problems at an early stage and the means to deal with problems. For a small organization this may involve the family doctor, for larger establishments referral to an occupational health or counselling service may be appropriate. Of course, a good 'treatment' service should not be the only element in place. The working environment should be assessed and inappropriate stressors and the excessive demands and pressures on staff evaluated and, if prudent, reduced or removed.

The general requirements of statutory law have been tested in the civil courts in the UK. In the well-publicised case of *Walker v Northumberland County Council* (1994), an area social services officer succeeded in establishing that his employers were legally liable for his second nervous breakdown, and subsequent retirement on medical grounds.[5] Mr Justice Coleman held the employers to be in breach of their duty of care, by causing psychiatric injury by the volume or character of the work he was required to perform. In his judgement of the Walker case Mr Justice Coleman stated that:

> There has been little judicial authority on the extent to which an employer owes to his employees a duty not to cause them psychiatric damage by the volume or character of the work which the employees are required to perform. It is clear that an employer has a duty to provide his employee with a reasonably safe system of work and to take reasonable steps to protect him from risks which are reasonably foreseeable. Whereas the law on the extent of this duty has developed almost exclusively in cases involving physical injury to the employee as distinct from injury to his mental health, there is no

logical reason why risk of psychiatric damage should be excluded from the scope of an employer's duty of care or from the co-extensive implied term in the contract of employment.

However, Mr Justice Coleman did see difficulties for future cases and added:

> There can be no doubt that the circumstances in which claims based on damages are likely to arise will often give rise to extremely difficult evidential problems of foreseeability and causation. This is particularly so in the environment of the professions where the plaintiff may be ambitious and dedicated, determined to succeed in his career in which he knows the work is demanding, and may have a measure of discretion as to how and when and for how long he works, but where the character or volume of the work given to him eventually drives him to breaking point.

It is clear then that, under common law, where it is reasonably foreseeable that the risk of stress-induced ill-health is significant, the employer must take action under the duty of care that is imposed upon them.

As a result of this case, Mr Walker was awarded damages of £175 000. The true cost of this case to the employer is likely to have been in the region of £500 000, after taking into account legal costs, sick pay, management time expended and the costs of ill-health retirement.

In December 1996, the UK Disability Discrimination Act 1995 (DDA) became law. This act requires employees to make reasonable adjustments to working arrangements where they may cause a substantial disadvantage to the disabled person. Persons with a mental illness which is clinically well-recognized will be regarded as having a mental impairment for the purposes of the DDA. This highlights the importance of obtaining competent advice from an occupational health professional where a person has been or is thought to be suffering from a mental illness. Without such advice, employers may not be in the best position to judge whether they are required to make adjustments. The current focus on mental health risks in the workplace means that this area of disability law is likely to be one of continued legal development. It should be emphasized that personality disorders and problems of alcoholism are not included in the coverage of the DDA.

In the USA, Canada and Australia, Workers Compensation schemes exist. Claims for work-related illness (including mental illness) must be pursued by making application to the Boards which manage the arrangements. As this is not possible in the UK or other parts of the European Union, Civil claims must be brought.

It is of interest that in Australia, when national and local government employees are considered, that 5% of the total number of claims brought are for stress-related illnesses. These account for 20% of the budget reserved for claims of all types (personal communication, Professor C Cooper, Professor of Organizational Psychology, University of Manchester Institute of Science and Technology, UK).

THE FINANCIAL IMPACT OF STRESS ON EMPLOYERS

Estimates in surveys by the CBI[6] and the Department of Health suggest that up to 30% of sick leave in the UK is related to stress, anxiety or depression. The financial costs to employers are thought to be in the region of £3.7 billion each year.

For employers, stress has been cited as contributory to increased sickness absence, and reductions in quality and productivity. Costs are not just limited to those of sickness absence. For many organizations, mental health problems are the most common reason for early retirement on the grounds of ill-health. This represents a significant cost to the employer, not only in terms of pension benefits but also the costs involved in recruitment, retraining of staff and loss of experienced personnel.

For some employers, such as the emergency services, the hazardous nature of the work is recognized. Nevertheless, certain circumstances may be associated with an increased risk of post-traumatic stress disorder. In such situations, early provision of appropriate assessment, support and treatment can minimize its impact on employer and employee. In the UK, recent awards exceeding £1 million to police officers suffering mental trauma following the Hillsborough tragedy highlight the importance of effective prevention. (In this tragedy, which occurred at a football ground, many spectators were crushed to death when the crowd surged forwards against unyielding control barriers. The local police force not only witnessed the unfolding drama but were also heavily criticized for poor policing of the crowds.)

RISK FACTORS FOR STRESS-RELATED ILLNESS

Research carried out for the HSE into work-related stress shows that there are many factors, both inside and outside work, that are implicated in stress disorders. Relationships at home, job satisfaction, lifestyle, physical health, social status, working conditions and types of personality are all implicated.

First there are external stressors, which may be at work (night duty or increased workload because a colleague leaves and is not replaced) or which may occur at home (a recent bereavement or a disabled spouse).

Second, there are modifying factors, such as personality and social support, which determine whether the individual can cope with the stresses or whether illness occurs.

Some personalities are ill-suited to particular jobs. Obsessional personalities, for example, cannot cope with jobs that involve frequent different demands and rapid decision-making, and anxiety or depression occurs if demands at work are increased. On the other hand, many individuals can cope with increased demands at work provided they have adequate support at home and their health is generally good. The onset of psychological illness may reflect a reduction of support, for example marital separation, even when the job stresses remain constant.

Third, there are the symptoms themselves. These may be typical anxiety symptoms which occur only at work; avoidance of work may result. Close questioning will reveal exactly which situations (or people) within work are responsible. Alternatively, the symptoms of anxiety may occur at work *and* at home, and therefore be the result of a generalized anxiety disorder, depression or even hyperthyroidism. Faced with vague symptoms, the doctor must have a high index of suspicion for alcohol or drug misuse and for early dementia if these problems are not to be missed.

PATTERN OF REFERRAL

Definite psychiatric disorder, or less clearly defined psychological problems may be referred in different ways.

Referral by a third party

The patient may be referred directly from a manager at work or via the occupational physician. This may make assessment complicated if the patient is defensive and determined to prove that he or she is fit to continue working. The manager may have already clearly identified the patient as not performing adequately either as a result of direct evidence of declining performance, or as a result of excessive time off work (repeated short-term absences or long-term sick leave).

The patient may have broken down in tears at work, become involved in interpersonal difficulties or be accused of smelling of alcohol on one or more occasion. For more senior members of the staff, it may have been noticed that the individual is not forthcoming at meetings, expected promotions are not realized or a colleague fears that impaired concentration might mean an incorrect decision. In some jobs, e.g. air traffic controllers, doctors, firemen, there is a fear that impaired decision-making might harm others. The doctor's assessment regarding fitness to work is therefore crucial.

Self-referral

Individuals may refer themselves because they are concerned about some aspect of their own health and this is attributed to stress at work. In this case the patient may be motivated to present a firm case that work is to blame, making assessment of other areas of his life difficult. Alternatively, the patient may refer themselves for some 'routine' physical illness or be seen at a health check, during which the physician becomes aware that the patient is experiencing psychological difficulties, which affect work performance.

PRESENTATION OF PSYCHIATRIC DISORDER

The most common disorders which present are the neurotic disorders, most notably anxiety and depression, with obsessional, phobic and post-traumatic stress disorders being seen less commonly. The psychotic disorders are relatively rare but can cause a disproportionate amount of disturbance unless handled appropriately. They cause particular difficulties in the decision regarding fitness to work.

The patient with anxiety or depressive disorders may present with typical psychological symptoms, such as poor concentration, anxiety attacks, crying, feeling hopeless, impaired sleep. More commonly, however, such disorders present with somatic symptoms such as headaches, tiredness, back, chest and abdominal pains or vague bodily symptoms, that do not suggest any typical organic disease.[7] Alcohol and drug misuse may present with any of these symptoms and/or repeated time off work with gastrointestinal upset. These are dealt with separately in Chapter 27.

Post-traumatic stress disorder may present as a gradual decline in interest or performance at work, combined with anxiety, sleep disturbance, dreams and 'flashbacks', to a traumatic event which is outside of normal experience.[8] This condition should be diagnosed only when the individual has been involved in a particularly unpleasant incident such as rape or assault, or witnessed death in unpleasant circumstances, for example as a train-driver or a fire-fighter might do or as soldiers experience in military combat (see Chapter 26). The trauma does not relate to the 'ordinary' stresses of a hospital accident and emergency department or intensive care unit, though it may do so under exceptionally distressing circumstances; for example horrific burns to a child of the same age as that of a member of staff.

Dementia and other organic causes of declining performance are also important, presenting with impaired performance (e.g. increased mistakes, failure to adapt to new routines), loss of concentration or anxiety/depression. These conditions need to be differentiated, on the basis of detailed cognitive testing, from the much more common situation, where a middle-aged person, in the same job for many years, cannot adapt to new demands or equipment.

The usual detailed clinical assessment is therefore required.[9] It is important to assess whether the predominant symptoms, e.g. anxiety, depression, impaired concentration or memory are only observed in the work situation or are pervasive and affect the individual in all situations.

ASSESSMENT

A complete assessment must answer three questions:

1 Does the patient have a recognizable physical or psychiatric disorder?
2 Can work reasonably be blamed for the illness, either wholly or in part?
3 If the answer to question 2 is 'yes', can the work situation be modified to allow the person to continue working?

To do this the clinician might use a framework for assessment developed from a theoretical one.[10]

There are many ways of making an assessment but usually this is done indirectly by means of self-reported anonymous questionnaires of symptoms. These range from simple, but well validated, measures of psychological health to broad-ranging tools based on cliical assessment of affective and psychoneurotic behaviours such as anxiety and depression.

DETAILED ASSESSMENT OF 'NOT COPING'

If a patient is referred because they are 'not coping' at work, the assessment will begin with the patient's description of the problem. Specific enquiries must be made about anxiety, depression, alcohol abuse and dementia as follows:

Anxiety

- Does the patient suffer from somatic symptoms of anxiety such as palpitations, headache, backache, urinary frequency, diarrhoea or breathing difficulties?
- Does the patient feel tense, keyed up and on edge?
- Do frank panic attacks occur, which are extremely frightening to the patient and may have led to urgent medical treatment? If so, is the anxiety felt only at work or does it also occur at home? If only at work, are there specific situations or specific people that induce anxiety. These features can be identified by asking if there are days when the patient does not become anxious at work and then establish why. Does the patient experience anxiety symptoms at home, at the weekends and on holiday? If so, factors at home as well as work need to be explored.
- Are these symptoms accompanied by lack of concentration, impaired sleep and sexual difficulties suggesting a depressive illness?

Depression

Depression may also present with the somatic symptoms mentioned above. The patient may have been labelled as suffering from migraine, irritable bowel syndrome or asthma, so these 'diagnoses' need to be explored fully.

- Does the patient feel depressed or experience bouts of crying?
- Are sleep and appetite disturbed?
- Does the patient have difficulty concentrating at work and at home?
- Are there sexual difficulties?

Depressive illness is pervasive. If the patient feels depressed only at work this suggests that circumstances at work are responsible; these must be explored.

Long-term memory is usually assessed while taking the history. If the patient complains that the long-term memory is intact but short-term memory is impaired, care must be taken to distinguish between impaired attention and concentration, which might occur in depression from memory impairment itself.

Aids to clinical assessment include the Beck Depression Inventory,[11] which is completed by the patient in a few minutes and will give the clinician information on 20 symptoms of depression. These can be discussed with a patient and indicate the severity of depression. If the patient shows signs of depression it is always important to ask about suicidal ideas.

Alcohol abuse

The patient should be asked the following questions (CAGE questionnaire) to screen for alcohol abuse:[12]

- Have you ever felt you ought to cut down on your drinking?
- Have people annoyed you by criticising your drinking?
- Have you ever felt bad or guilty about your drinking?
- Have you ever had a drink first thing in the morning to steady your nerves or get rid of a hangover?

Dementia

Screening for dementia involves the following:

- Orientation in time, place, and person.
- Attention and concentration – can the patient say the months of the year in reverse order? or perform simple arithmetic – e.g. subtract 3 from 20 and continue subtracting 3 from each number in sequence (use a 'serial sevens': (100 minus 7) if appropriate)?
- Registration – can the patient repeat a series of digits immediately after the doctor has given them (e.g. telephone number)?
- Short term memory – can the patient learn a name

and address after one or two attempts and repeat it 1 and 5 minutes later?

Adjuncts to this clinical testing are the Minimental State[13] or Newcastle Scale.[14]

Stress at work or stress at home?

The following clinical examples indicate how external stresses, personality and psychiatric disorder interact.

INCREASED STRESS AT WORK/OBSESSIONAL PERSONALITY

A 47-year-old salesman developed anxiety attacks, impaired concentration and reduced sleep. These were worse at work, but also prominent during the weekends. He had obsessional traits in his personality and had previously been regarded as a conscientious and reliable worker, with very little time off sick. He had a good marriage and plenty of support from his wife; there were no crises or difficulties in his personal life that could account for the recent onset of anxiety and depressive symptoms. His symptoms had started when he was given a larger area for sales and a new boss who was critical of his careful approach to work; this led to several disagreements. Treatment of this man's anxiety and depressive symptoms by pharmacological and behavioural means were largely successful provided he did not return to work. Any attempt to return to work was accompanied by a major relapse of the symptoms – eventually he had to resign. This was supported on medical grounds. A more flexible personality might have been able to cope with the changes at work.

STRESS AT HOME

A senior nurse, highly regarded by her peers, ceased to work to her usual high standards following a reorganized work schedule. She complained bitterly about the change and on one occasion appeared tearful while discussing it with a colleague. She resented attempts to get her to seek medical advice feeling that she was being accused of professional incompetence. Eventually her employer persuaded her to see a psychiatrist in the hospital 'for an informal chat'. It transpired that she was coping with an elderly ill mother at home who required almost constant attention during her off duty time and who complained of being ignored as a result of the reorganized work schedule. This conflict was too much to bear and she became depressed. The answer to this problem lay not in a changed work pattern but in a restructuring of the support for the mother so the patient could lead her own life without feeling guilty about neglecting her mother.

DECLINING PERFORMANCE AT WORK

A 45-year-old executive developed asthma and neurological symptoms. The latter were initially diagnosed as multiple sclerosis, but further neurological opinion suggested post-viral fatigue. After being off work because of sickness for nearly 2 years, the patient was referred to a psychiatrist. This referral was resisted by the patient, who insisted that his problems were 'all physical' and accused the neurologist of dismissing his symptoms as being 'all in the mind'. In fact, the patient had symptoms attributable to his asthma, steroids and depression. Careful review of his history indicated that most of his absences from work were the result of fatigue, not asthma. Clinical testing did not reveal any evidence of dementia. The patient was asked to keep a daily record of his symptoms: his fatigue was generally less on Friday and Saturday and most pronounced on Sunday evening/Monday morning – the first clue of stress at work. A considerable personal difficulty had arisen between himself and a female member of staff, the diary later revealed that he could function quite well at work on those days when she was away from the office. However, there was also a marked marital problem, which also contributed to the depression.

These examples indicate that the clinician must carefully assess stresses at home and at work to determine those responsible for the current illness. This appears to contradict the thesis that certain occupations carry a high risk of psychiatric disorder.[10] The apparent discrepancy must be explained. First, self-administered questionnaires used in surveys[10] measure symptoms of psychological distress, whereas the clinical examples cited are concerned with more severe symptomatology amounting to definite psychiatric disorder. The latter is more frequently related to personal difficulties than the general stress of work. Second, the sections of the community that experience stress at work are also at increased risk of stress at home. This is related to social class. In a recent study of Civil Servants in the UK[15] low social class was associated with poor conditions at work (monotonous work, low control and low satisfaction) *and* at home – less social support, more life events and more financial difficulties. The last three are recognized risk factors for depression.[16] Thus, the apparent relationship between work stress and illness might be explained by a simultaneous association with difficult social conditions outside of work.

Nevertheless, the clinician is repeatedly faced with patients who attribute their symptoms to stress at work. There are several reasons for this. First, there is a natural tendency to find an explanation for symptoms – psychologists have called this 'effort after meaning'. Because work fills much of our time, it is easily made the scapegoat. Second, blaming work relieves the patient of responsibility for the symptoms, whereas facing up to a marital or family problem requires the patient taking action to change personal circumstances – blaming difficulties at work for a high alcohol consumption is one such example. Third, stress at work is a 'respectable' cause of symptoms compared with the stigmatizing label of psychiatric disorder, which carries the pejorative connotation of not being able to cope.

Clear history taking usually enables the clinician to isolate the principal stress responsible for the symptoms, and this often leads the patient to appreciate this as well. If not, the patient can be asked to keep a daily record of his symptoms and note the situations in which they intensify.

Certain aspects of the work environment are known to be stressful and are associated with a high sickness record. If these stresses cannot be reduced, because they are inherent to the work (as, for example, in the intensive care unit of a hospital), support to cope with them should be increased. One way this may be done is by regular discussion groups with an 'outsider', such as the hospital chaplain.[17]

The recognition of high-stress jobs is also brought to attention by the individual, as illustrated in the following:

A junior hospital doctor, referred because he was not coping with the very heavy work load, turned out to have an anxiety state consequent upon excessive caution and checking in his clinical work. This cleared with time off work, and it became clear that his personality was not suited to the stresses of acute clinical medicine.

He found a hierarchy of stressful jobs, drawn up by the occupational psychologist, invaluable in choosing alternative employment. The hospital also modified the job description of that particular post.

There is evidence that there are important stress factors in certain organic diseases as well as in the psychiatric or 'functional' disorders mentioned above. In a detailed study of heart disease, chronic work-related stress was more closely associated with ischaemic heart disease than was non-work stress.[18] Likewise two studies of peptic ulcer have shown that onset of the condition was related more closely to chronic ongoing 'goal frustration' than to acute stress.[19,20] Such stress involves striving to attain a goal that appears impossible to attain. Stress from this cause is more likely to be at work than at home.

ASSESSMENT OF FITNESS TO WORK

The various clinical examples quoted here illustrate the difficulty in assessing fitness to work when the illness is clearly related to stress. The attitude of management, the scope for modifying the work routine and a detailed

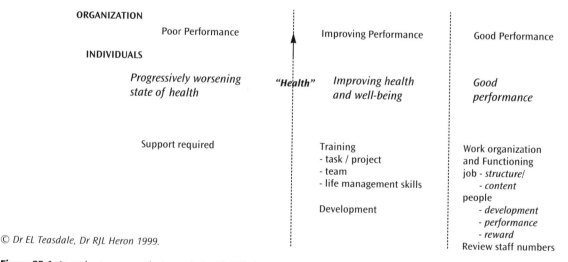

Figure 28.1 In order to ensure that people feel fulfilled and perform well for the organization for which they work, it is important that they are 'healthy' and their well-being is considered. There should be a focus on work organization and functioning with proper attention being paid to jobs, to the people who do the jobs in terms of their performance, being managed and their motivation being considered and reward being appropriate. This should be backed up with appropriate training and education so that staff are, or become, confident and competent. This should primarily revolve around the tasks and skills required e.g. assertiveness, team-building etc. Life management skills are important and training should be available. If both organization and training/education are fully addressed then staff should be 'healthy' and be able to perform effectively at their work place. However, many people run into problems from time to time and advice and support services should be available – perhaps by way of an Employee Assistance Programme (EAP). Much of this should be proactive to ensure the people have the skills to manage the complexity which is part and parcel of everyday life.

assessment of the patient's clinical state must all be determined before a decision can be made.

Occasionally the clinician is caught in 'crossfire' between a manager who firmly states that the patient is unfit for work and the patient themselves who provides an alternative and plausible interpretation of the difficulties presented by the manager. Reconciliation of these differing attitudes is not always possible in the short term, and the management might insist that the patient is ill and must be removed from work. In these circumstances the best solution sometimes is to take the person out of work to see if the symptoms settle. After a suitable interval, discussions can then recommence on possible modifications of the work routine which might allow the patient to return.

The prudent employer will ensure a framework so that those who suffer with mental illness can be helped and referred appropriately. There is also a need to have a comprehensive model of well-being (Fig. 28.1).

RAISING AWARENESS

A policy for mental health is not a 'stand-alone' initiative. It is an essential component of any workplace setting. It should address the pre-employment assessment situation and the support of employees during employment. The good 'health' of the organization is likely to promote effective working and employee well being.

Guidance issued by the Health and Safety Executive in 1998[21] advises employers to set in motion procedures to ensure that the problem is understood and that excessive stress is not seen as a personal problem, but an issue which managers, staff and the organization as a whole are committed to addressing. The guidance encourages staff to attend stress awareness and stress management courses, so that they are better able to handle the pressures they may encounter.

Publications from the UK Department of Health supporting the *Health of the Nation* initiative also refer to the importance of raising awareness about mental health in the workplace in order to help staff:

- recognize when something is wrong so they can get help for themselves or for their colleagues;
- take action to manage pressures which could lead to mental health problems.

ASSESSING RISKS TO EMPLOYEES

There is a great variation in individual susceptibility to the effects of stress. We all know how differently two people may react to any one stressful event. For example, after a bereavement, one relative may be unable to func-

tion at all and another seems to cope well. In assessing risks from work, employers are charged with taking reasonable steps to assess and manage workplace risks to health – be they physical (e.g. dermatitis or asbestos-related disease) or psychological (stress-related illness). Approaches adopted should identify major stresses, (for example, bullying, violence, lack of security or fear of redundancy) which might affect most people in a workplace. As such, risk assessment may be carried out at a number of levels:

Organizational level

At an organization level, a systematic approach to assessment and sensible management of risks can be adopted. In the UK, an HSE-funded research review, identified a number of potential risk factors for the development of occupational stress-related illness.[22] These include the following points:

1 Lack of control over the pacing of work.
2 Excessive periods of monotonous or repetitive work.
3 Uncertainty and constant change.
4 Lack of clear objectives
5 Inflexible and overdemanding work schedules.

Employee attitude surveys can be very valuable to elicit areas of concern which, when consistently reported, may reflect an underlying problem, for example, harassment, bullying or violence at work. Such surveys need not be stress questionnaires to provide the employer with valuable pointers for improvement. For example, equal opportunities surveys can highlight issues relating to working hours and the flexibility of working arrangements. Surveys of training needs can highlight skill deficits.

Job-type level

Risk assessments can be conducted at a job-type level. Ensuring that each job-type has an appropriate job description can improve clarity of role. Job descriptions may also contain details of the competencies required to 'do the job'. These are not 'what needs to be done' but the skills required, e.g. good communication skills and adaptability.

A logical next step from the clear job description with competency profile, is to identify the training needs for the individual who may be recruited into the particular role. Attention to these details is likely to lead to well-thought-out, 'do-able' jobs, and a reduction in the risks to the well-being of the individual as well as enhancing the performance of individuals in the role.

Personal level

Risk assessments can also be conducted at a personal level. The process of ensuring that you have a square peg in a square hole is to the mutual benefit of employee and employer. Recruiting against a well-described job, seeking evidence of job-related skills, or the ability to acquire them increase the chances of a good job-person fit.

With the advent of the Disability Discrimination Act (DDA) in the UK, there is more reason than ever for employers to assure themselves that they are matching their recruitment techniques to true job demands. The DDA also reinforces the importance of appropriate occupational health advice. The employer may be required to make reasonable adjustments for persons with disability. Competent advice from an occupational health physician can be invaluable in determining the individual limitations and the scope for making sensible adjustments. This can help the employer gain the skilled individual it requires and meet the requirements of the DDA, and improve the chances of a person with disability being accommodated in the workplace.

MANAGEMENT OF MENTAL ILLNESS PROBLEMS AT WORK

Neurotic illness

Problems of anxiety need to be carefully assessed to determine whether the problem can be managed at work. Referral to a clinical psychologist may be appropriate.

> A musician was referred because of failing to perform to the expected standard of the orchestra. Since the individual concerned had played satisfactorily for many years this decline might represent cognitive impairment or some form of stress reaction. The occupational physician excluded neurological disorder and referred the patient to a clinical psychologist for a) assessment of cognitive functioning and b) stress management. The former confirmed the absence of dementia. The latter involved isolating the situations which led to increased anxiety and getting the patient to use relaxation techniques in these situations.

Direct referral to a psychologist is appropriate for specific phobias, obsessional symptoms and anxiety in the absence of clinical depression. Referral to a psychologist is also indicated for assessment of possible cognitive impairment. The physician must perform any necessary medical investigations for possible underlying organic disease before referral. Definite depressive symptoms require treatment with antidepressants but more severe depression usually requires the help of a psychiatrist – even quite debilitating illness can be managed in the work situation.

> A 43-year-old medical records officer experienced a difficult bereavement when her son died suddenly. She experienced marked depression with ideas that she should join her dead son. There was much sympathy in the department and a general expectation that she required time off work but the psychiatrist thought it was best for her to continue working as this distracted her from her grief and she had the daily support of work colleagues. The occupational physician had to persuade management to allow this while recognizing that her work performance would be suboptimal for a period of weeks or months.

Schizophrenia

The presence of a serious mental illness, such as schizophrenia, does not necessarily debar the patient from employment. The prevalence of schizophrenia is much higher than is generally appreciated (1% lifetime risk), so in most large employing authorities there are likely to be several individuals who have, or have had, this illness. Such individuals may do very well if they have a job of a routine nature which is not too demanding.

Many employers would wish to employ a number of people with various disabilities including mental illness if this does not greatly impair the patient's ability to work.

It is the responsibility of the occupational physician, where there is one in post, to ensure that the patient is under psychiatric care and consents to free communication with the responsible psychiatrist. Problems may arise if the management put pressure on the individual to be more productive, for example through a financial or bonus scheme or to compensate for the absence of sick colleagues. A patient with a serious psychotic illness might react to such pressure by taking more time off work on sick leave because of their lower threshold to respond adversely to stress. Not infrequently, managers are unaware that the patient has a major mental disorder. In these circumstances, the occupational physician must explain in a general way that there is an underlying illness which makes it difficult for the individual to cope with the demands of extra work. Managers can become apprehensive if they know an employee has schizophrenia and the occupational physician has an important role in providing them with a sensible explanation of the problem.

ASSESSMENT AND REHABILITATION OF EMPLOYEES RETURNING TO WORK AFTER MENTAL ILLNESS

The high incidence of mental health problems in the UK and other developed countries means that every employer is likely to experience the situation of an employee being unable to attend work as a result of a mental health problem. Access to competent occupational health advice benefits the employer through the provision of advice about the likely timing of a return to work. In many cases, effective liaison with the employee's own doctor (with the employee's informed consent) can bring about a timely return to work. For the employee too, occupational health advice may promote a staged return to work as part of a rehabilitation programme, enabling them to return part-time and build-up to normal in a way that helps their return to full-health. It is worth remembering that the decision in favour of the plaintiff in *Walker v Northumberland County Council* was not made as a result of Mr Walker's first breakdown being caused by work. It was the fact that the employer, in the light of the knowledge of his first breakdown, did not take steps (e.g. provision of permanent and adequate support, alteration of working arrangements) to prevent its recurrence.

Many employees working for major organizations in the UK who have been absent from work through sickness for a significant time will be seen on their return to work at an occupational health centre. Such consultations, conducted within the bounds of employee confidentiality, can ensure that timely advice is given to management to enable the appropriate rehabilitation of the employee to their normal job wherever possible. They also provide an opportunity to identify any work factors which may be important in the management of the patient and their illness.

Rehabilitation policies that require the employee to be assessed by an occupational health professional on return to work after prolonged illness also provide the employer with an important opportunity to ensure compliance with the DDA.

PROVISION OF SUPPORT FOR EMPLOYEES

Over the past decade, counselling has become a growth industry, such that by the mid-1990s, around one-third of family doctor practices in the UK had someone who provided counselling. The evidence for the effectiveness of counselling services is inconclusive, although one study at least, showed that appropriate referral to psychotherapists for brief psychotherapy was as effective as general practitioner care for patients with emotional difficulties, and the patients preferred it.[23] Employers too have increasingly looked to counsellors and employee assistance programmes (EAPs) to address the issue of mental health in the workplace. In the UK, a 3-year study carried out at the University of Manchester School of Management highlighted the effectiveness of such programmes in helping individuals to cope with the pressures they faced. In the same study, EAPs were not shown to lead to any improvement in reduction of sources of stress.

The term 'employees assistance programmes' was originally introduced by the National Institute of Abuse and Alcoholism (NIAAA) in the United States of America during World War II to describe their occupational alcoholism programme. It was hoped that this term would render the service more acceptable. The employee assistance, or counselling programme, as we know it today, is largely a product of the 1960s; it now usually offers assistance to workers with personal problems of a more general nature. Minor psychiatric health problems may be prevented by trying to minimize the risk factors for becoming ill and by giving people the awareness and skills they need to improve their resistance to illness and cope with their busy lives.

Assistance programmes can certainly provide personal support for individuals in dealing with a wide variety of issues, home or work-oriented, affecting their mental well-being. Areas commonly addressed by EAPs include personal concerns which may arise from emotional distress, relationships, family worries, problems with alcohol and drugs and legal or financial concerns. They aim to minimize the impact of such concerns for the mutual benefit of employer and employee. In more proactive programmes they may also provide staff with access to training. They may be involved in courses such as 'coping skills' aimed at enhancing employee resilience, 'management of change' where an organization is undergoing restructuring, as well as training in traditional relaxation techniques. 'Balanced living' is a more recent area for provision of training whereby employees are encouraged to focus on strategies that enable them to balance home and work commitments. The aim is to enhance their own sense of well-being and to encourage more productive work practices. Providers of support services can also be very helpful in raising general awareness of mental health issues in the workplace.

The increase in use of EAPs has also highlighted the importance of seeking competent providers of service. In one report[24] the majority (76%) of EAP counsellors had satisfactory training and qualifications. However, 22% of counsellors involved in EAP work were not properly qualified, with 11% holding a basic Certificate in Counselling and a further 11% holding no formally recognized qualification in counselling. In the UK, organizations such as the British Association of Counselling (BAC) and the United Kingdom Council for Psychotherapy (UKCP) set rigorous criteria for counsellors who wish to register with them. Employers who wish to take on a counsellor can seek evidence for their registration as support of their professional competence to provide services.

ROLE OF THE OCCUPATIONAL PHYSICIAN

The occupational physician plays a crucial role in managing employees with mental illness. This is a unique position with responsibilities both to the individual patient and to the organization. These responsibilities need to be balanced at all times. The occupational physician also has an important role in liaison between the many different parties involved in the situation of employees with psychiatric disorders or psychological difficulties. Confidentiality is paramount throughout.

The final decision about whether a patient with a difficult clinical problem is fit to work also may have to rest with the occupational physician, who must take into account the patient's state of health and the situation in which the patient is to work. In reaching this decision, the occupational physician needs to be free to liaise with the psychiatrist and management to sort out arrangements that best serve the patient and their employer.

REFERENCES

1 Linford-Rees W. Stress, distress and disease. *Br J Psychiat* 1976; **128**: 3–18.

2 Editorial. Essence of stress. *Lancet* 1994; **344**: 1713–14.

3 Meltzer H, Gill B, Pettigrew M. *OPCS Survey of Psychiatric Morbidity*. Office of Population, Census and Surveys, 1994.

4 Health and Safety Executive. *Trailer to the 1990 Labour Force Survey*. London: HMSO, 1990.

5 Croner's Health and Safety at Work. Special Report. *Stress*. Issue 28, April 1997.

6 Sigman D. *Report by Confederation of British Industry* London: CBI, 1992.

7 Bridges KW, Goldberg DP. Somatic presentation of DSM III psychiatric disorders in primary care. *J Psychosomat Res* 1985; **29**: 563–9.

8 American Psychiatric Association. *DSM-III-R. Diagnostic and Statistical Manual of Mental Disorders* Washington, DC: APA, 1987.

9 Goldberg D, Benjamin S, Creed F. *Psychiatry in Medical Practice* London: Tavistock Publications, 1987.

10 Fletcher BC, Jones F. Stress at work. In: Raffle PAB, Adams PH, Baxter PJ *et al.* eds. *Hunter's Diseases of Occupations*

8th edn. London: Edward Arnold. 1994: 593–601.

11 Beck AT, Ward CH, Mendelson M, Mock JE, Erbaugh JK. An inventory for measuring depression. *Arch Gen Psychiat* 1961; **4**: 561–71.

12 Mayfield D, McLeod C, Hall P. The CAGE questionnaire – validation of a new alcoholism screening instrument. *Am J Psychiat* 1974; **131**: 1121–3.

13 Folstein MF, Folstein SE, McHugh PR. 'Mini-mental state'. A practical method for grading the cognitive state of patients for the clinician. *J Psychiat Res* 1975; **12**: 189–98.

14 Blessed C. Tomlinson BE, Roth M. The association between quantitative measures of dementia and of senile change in the cerebral grey matter of elderly subjects. *Br J Psychiat* **114**; 797–811

15 Marmot MC, Smith CD, Stansfeld S *et al.* Health inequalities among British civil servants: the Whitehall 11 study. *Lancet* 1991; **337**: 1387–9

16 Brown CW, Harris TO. *Social Origins of Depression*. London: Tavistock Publications, 1978.

17 Marteau L. The hospital – its staff and patients. In: Creed FH, Pfeffer J eds. *Medicine and Psychiatry: A Practical Approach*. London. Pitman, 1982.

18 Neilson E, Brown GW, Marmot M. Myocardial infarction. In: Brown GW, Harris TO eds. *Life Events and Illness* London: Guildford Press, 1989.

19 Craig TKJ, Brown CW. Goal frustration and life events in the aetiology of painful gastrointestinal disorder. *J Psychosomat Res* 1984; **128**: 411–21.

20 Ellard K, Beaurepaire J, Jones M, Piper D, Tennant C. Acute and chronic stress in duodenal ulcer disease. *Gastroenterology*, 1990; **99**: 1628–32.

21 Health and Safety Executive. *Help on Work-Related Stress – A Short Guide*. HSE Booklet, INDG281. 8, 1998.

22 Cox T. *Stress Research and Stress Management: Putting Theory to work*. HSE contract research report No. 61, 1993.

23 Highley JC, Cooper CL. Evaluating EAPs. *Personnel Rev* 1994; **23**: 46–59.

24 Highly-Marchington JC, Cooper CL. *An Assessment of Employee Assistance and Workplace Counselling Programmes in British Organisations*. HSE contract research report. No. 167, 1998.

29

Shift work and extended hours of work

GIOVANNI COSTA, SIMON FOLKARD, J MALCOLM HARRINGTON

Biological and social interference	581	Medical surveillance and preventive measures	585
Effects on health	582	The health effects of extended hours of work	587
Factors affecting tolerance	584	References	588

Shift work includes any arrangement of daily working hours that differs from the standard, and is aimed at extending the organization's operational time from 8 hours up to 24 hours per day, by means of a succession of different teams of workers. The shift systems adopted may have very different features – in particular: the duration of the worker's duty period (from 6 to 12 hours); the number of crews who alternate during the working day (two, three or four shifts); the presence and extension of night work; the speed (slow or fast) and direction (clockwise or counterclockwise) of the shift rotation; the regularity and length of the shift cycles; the start and finishing times of shifts; the interruption or not of weekends or Sundays (discontinuous or continuous shift rotas).

Shift work has increased progressively over recent decades, mainly for economic and production reasons, but also due to technological developments and to an increased demand for social services and leisure activities. It has recently been reported that 17.6% of European workers are involved in night work for at least 25% of their working time (21.4% of men, 11.8% of women),[1] while in the United States of America it has been estimated that one in five of non-agricultural workers are employed in shift work, 25% of whom are on night work.[2] According to most international directives and legislation, extended working hours are defined as those involving more than 48 hours work per week. This can occur on either day work or shift work due to either a high number of hours worked per day or a high number of days worked per week, or both. According to the Eurostat 1990 data, in the European Union 18.5% and 6.8% of employees usually work more than 40 hours and 48 hours per week respectively.[1]

Working at irregular hours or for extended periods can have negative consequences for health and well-being due to the stress derived from interference with psychophysiological functions and social life.

BIOLOGICAL AND SOCIAL INTERFERENCE

Circadian rhythms and psychophysical conditions

It is commonly accepted that work efficiency at night is not the same as during the day. Humans are diurnal creatures, synchronized on the 24 hour light/dark cycle, who are naturally awake and active during daylight and consequently resting and sleeping at night. This behaviour is determined by the regular oscillation of bodily functions (circadian rhythms), which in general show higher levels during the day and lower levels during the night. For example, body temperature, an integrated index of metabolic rate, decreases during the night when people are asleep down to a minimum of 35.5–36.0°C in the early hours of the morning, and increases during the waking day to reach a maximum (acrophase) of about 37.0–37.3°C at around 17.00 (5 pm). This rhythmicity is controlled by a strong endogenous oscillator (or body clock), located in the suprachiasmatic nuclei, and is influenced by environmental factors (synchronizers) such as work, activity, sleep, meals and, in particularly, light exposure.[2,3]

Night work forces the individual to change their normal sleep/wake cycle and to attempt to adjust to the nocturnal activity, by a progressive phase shift of circadian rhythms that may be more or less complete depending on the number of successive night shifts. However, circadian rhythms very seldom show a complete inversion, rather there is a flattening of their amplitude and desynchronization between them due to different extents of partial adjustment of the rhythms in the different variables. In general this is due both to the continuous rotation through the different shifts and to the fact that most individuals try to maintain a normal, day-oriented, social and family life during their free time and on rest days.

These disturbances of circadian rhythms may have negative effects on health and well-being. In the short term, people may suffer to a greater or lesser extent from symptoms similar to those of jet lag following transmeridian flights and characterized by feelings of fatigue, sleepiness, insomnia, digestive troubles, and reduced mental agility and performance efficiency (see Chapter 17). In the longer term such rhythmic disturbances may, often in combination with other factors, eventually result in the manifestation of a number of complaints and illnesses.[4,5,6]

Performance efficiency

Human error is often cited as an important factor in work accidents and may depend on sleep and sleep-related factors, as well as on circadian rhythms in alertness and performance capabilities. Alertness can be substantially reduced by irregularity of the individual's rest/activity pattern and by prolonged physical and mental effort, as can be experienced by long-haul pilots. In general, performance efficiency appears to parallel the circadian rhythm in body temperature, but it can peak earlier or later in the day depending on the demands of the task (e.g. physical, cognitive or memory-loaded), on the length of time that has elapsed since the individual concerned woke from their last proper sleep, and on the individual's general level of arousal and motivation.

The desynchronization of circadian rhythms in combination with the associated sleep deficit and fatigue may significantly impair work efficiency, particularly during the early hours of the morning, making the worker more vulnerable to errors. This pattern has been reported for many groups of shift workers including train and truck drivers, nuclear power workers, nurses, switchboard operators and seamen. A post-lunch 'dip' has also been noted which appears to be only partially dependent on the meal itself, and which may also reflect 12-hour or shorter ultradian rhythms in alertness and wakefulness superimposed on the 24-hour circadian cycle.[7,8]

In addition, sleepiness due to the truncation of sleep by an early start to the morning shift has been shown to cause a higher frequency of errors and accidents in train and bus drivers, while increased sleepiness and changes in electroencephalogram ultradian rhythms (bursts of alpha and theta power density) have been recorded on the night shift, indicating a high propensity for the workers concerned to fall asleep 'on the job'.[9]

Family and social life

People engaged in shift work or long working hours can face greater difficulties in their social lives since most family and social activities are arranged according to the day-oriented rhythms of the general population. In addition, Saturday and Sunday work may also interfere with the weekly rhythms of various social activities such as sports events, religious ceremonies, travel and entertainment. Shift workers thus face more difficulties in combining their time budgets (work hours, commuting and leisure times) with the complex organization of social activities, particularly when these require regular contacts and involve many people. Hence shift work can lead to social marginalization.[10]

Shift work and extended working hours may also hinder the already complex co-ordination of family timetables, with the extent of any such hindrance depending on factors such as family composition and duties (e.g. marital status, number and age of children, housework, second job and illnesses) and the organization of public services (e.g. school and shop hours and transports). Time pressure is a constant condition among those who have a high family burden (e.g. women with small children). These interferences may be further complicated when both partners have the same working conditions (i.e. as shift workers or with long working hours), and this can have negative effects on marital relationships, parental roles and their children's education. Complaints from shift workers about family and social difficulties are more frequent than those related to biological adjustment, and are often the main cause of shift work intolerance.

On the positive side, shift work can give more flexibility to those who enjoy solitary activities, and to those, and in particular women, who give a higher priority to family and domestic duties than to personal leisure. Consequently, shift work is popular with some workers since it provides them with greater opportunities to use daytime hours to meet their own particular needs (e.g. access to public offices), or simply allows them to enjoy longer spans of rest days between shift cycles. For this reason some shift systems based on a backward fast rotation (night–afternoon–morning) that include 'quick returns' (working two shifts in one day), and compressed working weeks (e.g. 3 or 4 days of 12 hours per day), are often preferred because of the longer spans of rest days despite the clear negative effects of such systems on sleep and performance efficiency.

EFFECTS ON HEALTH

Sleep, chronic fatigue and psychoneurotic troubles

Sleep is the main function that is disrupted by shift work. A reduction of sleep hours can often occur before morning shifts because of their early start time and between night shifts because the individuals concerned are trying to sleep when their body clocks expect them to be awake. Thus people may have difficulty both in falling asleep and remaining asleep during the day because they are at the wrong point within their circadian cycle, while often the environmental conditions (noise in particular) are also far from ideal.

Some interference with sleep quality also occurs, both for the day-sleeps between night shifts (in particular a reduction in stage 2 and REM (rapid eye movement) sleep) and for the truncated night sleeps before morning shifts (a reduction in REM sleep due to the early wake-up).[9,11] This interference in sleep quality can start within months of starting shift work and, if the shift work continues, can cause severe disturbances of sleep which may result in the occurrence of and favour psychological and nervous disorders, such as chronic fatigue, nervousness, persistent anxiety, and depression, which often require the administration of psychotropic drugs.[12] Such stress-related symptoms are frequently complained of by people working extended hours, particularly if associated with high work loads or monotonous, repetitive jobs. These symptoms may also act as a risk or aggravating factor for other psychosomatic complaints or diseases (i.e. gastrointestinal and cardiovascular).

Digestive disorders

Many shift workers complain of digestive disorders which may reflect on both the irregularity of meal timing and the poor quality of the food consumed, namely an increased consumption of pre-packed and caffeinated drinks. According to a number of studies carried out over the last 50 years some 20–75% of night and shift workers, as opposed to only 10–25% of day workers, complain of disturbances of appetite, irregular bowel movements and constipation, dyspepsia, heartburn, abdominal pains and flatulence. Many workers also develop more serious disorders such as chronic gastritis, gastroduodenitis and peptic ulcers.

The majority of 36 epidemiological studies, carried out in the last five decades and covering over 98 000 workers of various work sectors by means of different methods of investigations (see Ref.13 for a review), pointed out a prevalence of such disorders (from two to five times higher on average) among shift workers whose work schedule included night work (on permanent basis or rotating), in comparison with day workers or shift workers without night duty.

However, one has to consider that such psychosomatic disorders are quite common among the general population and recognize the influence of several factors, including in particular infections (*Helicobacter pylori*), family heritage and life styles; although these can be promoted or aggravated by shift work. In fact, shift work can act as a stress factor not only through the above-mentioned perturbations of the eating habits, but also through the conflicts between the endogenous biological rhythms and the external synchronizers, as well as by higher strain levels deriving from insufficient sleep and difficulties in family and social life.

Cardiovascular diseases

The stress associated with shift work and/or long working hours may have both direct and indirect adverse effects on the cardiovascular system. On the one hand, it is possible that increased secretion of catecholamines and cortisol, as stress mediators, affect blood pressure, heart rate, thrombotic processes, and lipid and glucose metabolism. On the other hand, some risk factors for cardiovascular diseases are associated with factors related to shift work such as less favourable living conditions, eating and sleeping disorders, and smoking. In recent years, a number of epidemiological studies have yielded data suggesting an association between shift work and cardiovascular diseases. More specifically it has been shown that there is (i) a higher prevalence of cardiovascular risk factors, of angina pectoris and hypertension among shift workers; (ii) a higher morbidity due to cardiocirculatory and ischaemic heart diseases with increasing age and shift work experience; and (iii) an increased relative risk of myocardial infarction in occupations with a high proportion of shift workers.[14,15] Furthermore, recent studies support the connection between shift work and cardiovascular disease although the mechanism for this effect, if real, is unknown.[16]

Accidents

As mentioned earlier there is some evidence that shift workers may be more prone to errors and work accidents, due to reduced vigilance and performance capabilities, than their day-working counterparts. However, this evidence is somewhat inconsistent with some studies reporting a higher overall incidence of injuries and accidents on the night shift while others show either no overall increase in incidence, but an increase in their seriousness (i.e. those requiring hospital treatment rather than first-aid at the place at work) at night, or even an increased overall incidence on day shifts.[13] These inconsistencies reflect many potentially confounding factors. Some of these factors concern differences in the work sector studied and jobs examined which may influence the relative risk of accidents, but the most important factors relate to the manner in which work is organized on the different shifts. Thus, for example, maintenance and supervision are often lower on the night shift. Furthermore long, 'easy' runs of a particular job may be saved for this less supervised shift. The day shift may also be augmented by permanent day workers, thus increasing the potential for accidents on the day shift due to the mixing of teams of workers. It is noteworthy that in the single study in which the *a priori* risk appeared to be constant across the 24-hour day, industrial injuries were higher on the night shift, and particularly so in the case of the more serious injuries incurred by workers whose job was of a self-paced nature.[17]

Further, a number of studies show that peaks in accidents at around 10:00–11:00 and 13:00–16:00 (3–4 pm) which probably reflect peaks in work activity since performance capabilities due to circadian rhythms should be relatively high at these times. There is, however, evidence that both long-working hours and an early start time to the morning shift may be associated with an increased accident risk. Thus it is clear that careful attention needs to be paid to the potential accident risk when considering work schedules and other organizational factors. Indeed, it should be noted that the nuclear incidents at Three Mile Island and Chernobyl, the Bophal disaster, and many air accidents including the Challenger space shuttle, all occurred during the night hours, while in each case shift scheduling and fatigue due to sustained operation have been cited as important contributory factors.[18]

Absenteeism

Absenteeism is a rather indirect indicator of health which confounds a number of factors relating to work organization, socioeconomic conditions, and the characteristics of the individual concerned. Nevertheless, a number of authors have cited the influence of some aspects of shift scheduling on absenteeism rates, including the speed of rotation, the amount of overtime, and the shift start and finish times.[19] It has to be admitted that, in addition to the selection of healthier workers for shift work, there are a number of reasons why shift workers may show a lower absenteeism rate despite a higher frequency of complaints and illnesses. These may include (i) a higher solidarity towards colleagues since an unexpected absence may cause more problems for shift handovers than for normal day work, (ii) a higher threshold in the perception, labelling and reporting of complaints and symptoms since shift workers more often accept them as part of the job (e.g. digestive and sleep disorders), and (iii) a higher punctuality rate since shift workers are less likely to have to travel to work during rush hours or to have problems accessing public offices during normal working hours.

Women's reproductive function

There is good reason to assume that shift work, and in particular night work, may be a particular problem for women's health. This follows both from the potential disruption of their hormonal cycles, and from the increased stress caused by the conflict between their irregular working schedules and their additional domestic duties, particularly so for those who are married and/or have children. Women night workers with children sleep less during the day between night shifts and complain more of cumulative fatigue. Further, women shift workers have been shown to have an increased prevalence of disturbances of the menstrual cycle, increased menstrual pains, higher rates of spontaneous abortion, more premature births and lower birthweights.[13,20]

Toxicological risk

Shift workers may be particularly susceptible to xenobiotics due to: (i) fluctuations in the environmental concentrations of pollutants and concomitant increase of the risk at certain times of day in connection with periodical phases of the work cycle; (ii) reduced interval between shifts, often down to as little as 8 hours, which may not be enough to eliminate the toxic substances from the body; (iii) pronounced circadian rhythms in the bodily functions involved in the metabolism and excretion of toxic substances (e.g., liver enzyme activity, renal function), and the detrimental consequences of their possible desynchronization (See Chapter 6). Thus the balance between the biokinetics of the substance and the chronoesthesy (or circadian susceptibility to chemical agents) of the biological system is more likely to be unfavourable at night when metabolic function is slowing down. Considerably more attention needs to be paid to the appropriate environmental threshold limit values for shift workers, as has been suggested for those working prolonged hours, and to improving biological monitoring so that better strategies for the control and protection of the workers can be developed.[21]

Mortality

There has been only one well-controlled study that has examined the mortality rates of shift workers compared with day workers having the same job and work experience. This was of 8603 male industrial workers over a period of 13 years and it found slightly more deaths in shift and ex-shift workers than would be expected from the national rates.[22] Although this overall effect was not statistically reliable, deaths due to arteriosclerotic heart disease showed a significant excess in shift workers under 60 years with 99 observed deaths against 79.9 expected. It is suprising that so little has been published on mortality but the Taylor and Pocock studies,[22] although rather old, are well conducted examples.

FACTORS AFFECTING TOLERANCE

It has been suggested that about 20% of workers leave shift work because they clearly cannot tolerate it, about

10% postively enjoy it, and the remainder tolerate it to a greater or lesser extent.[4] Indeed, it is abundantly clear that a number of moderating variables, including individual differences, situational factors and social conditions, may significantly influence both the short-term circadian adjustment to, and the longer-term tolerance of, night and shift work.[4,6] Thus, for example, ageing (over 45–50 years) is generally associated with a progressive intolerance due to a number of reasons; in fact, the physiological decline of psychophysical conditions is associated with a reduction of the amplitude of circadian rhythms and an increased proneness to internal desynchronization; besides, the decrease in the restorative efficiency of sleep and the reduced physical fitness may further weaken the capacity to cope with stressors related to shift work.[23]

Individuals who are 'morning types' generally face more difficulties in adjusting their circadian rhythms to night work compared with 'evening types' because of their earlier circadian phase position which may reflect a shorter endogenous periodicity. In contrast, 'evening types' may have greater problems in waking up sufficiently early for the start of the morning shift and may suffer from an even greater truncation of their night sleeps taken between morning shifts. Similarly individuals who have a small amplitude of their circadian rhythms may have a less stable circadian structure (i.e. show larger phase shifts) and be more prone to internal desynchronization. Indeed, there are a number of other personality traits and/or behavioural characteristics, such as neuroticism, rigidity of sleeping habits and the ability to overcome drowsiness, that may influence the degree of adjustment of circadian rhythms and hence have a potentially negative influence on the long-term tolerance of irregular work schedules.[24] In contrast, physical fitness can improve sleep, lessen fatigue and increase performance, and may thus increase tolerance to night work, as may a strong commitment to shift work since this is associated with more stable-sleep timings and other circadian behaviours.

Social factors such as family composition and support, social services and commuting times, can also have a prominent bearing on long-term tolerance to shift work. Further, working conditions can be very important, particularly in relation to work load, job satisfaction and the organization of shift schedules. Some of these factors are, of course, often difficult or impossible to change (e.g. age, personality traits or family), while others (for example shift schedules or personal behaviour) can be modified more easily to facilitate tolerance to shift work.

In addition, it must be admitted that many of the complaints and illnesses associated with shift work are not uncommon among the general population and it is important to recognize their multiple contributory factors such as genetic and family heritage, personality traits, lifestyle and social conditions. Thus shift work (as

well as extended work hours) has to be considered as one of many risk factors which may contribute to the development of these complaints and illnesses, and as one which is more likely to have contributed after prolonged exposure. This may explain the large differences between individuals in their adaptation to, or tolerance of, shift work that have been found in many epidemiological investigations.

One important confounding factor in this respect, is the process of self-selection which occurs in shift workers. Most of the epidemiological studies in this field have been cross-sectional and have considered a workforce from whom an unknown number of individuals may previously have quit shift work because of illness or social problems. Indeed, longitudinal studies have found it virtually impossible to follow up the same sample of shift workers over a prolonged period, due either to transfers to day work because of problems, or to multiple changeovers from shift work to day work during the working life. This can lead to a serious underestimation of the problems associated with shift work since the shift workers available for investigation are those who have not left for health or social reasons and hence will tend to be those who have succeeded in coping better with shift work. In contrast, studies of former shift workers may overestimate the complaints of shift workers on the whole.

Despite all this, there are sufficient data to conclude that shift work *per se* can be detrimental to circadian rhythms, sleep quality, work performance, safety and probably cardiovascular health.[25]

MEDICAL SURVEILLANCE AND PREVENTIVE MEASURES

Since shift and night work are risk factors for health and well-being, medical reviews need to be carried out with the aim of informing the workers concerned and giving them suggestions and guidelines on how best to cope with shift work, as well as that of detecting the early signs of any intolerance to night work.[26] The importance of this has been recently emphasized in international directives and recommendations. Thus the ILO Night Work Convention (No 171) and Recommendation (No 178) concerning Night Work (1990), and the European Directive 93/104 concerning 'certain aspects of the organization of working time', cover a number of specific measures for night workers, including health assessments before assignment to night work, at regular intervals thereafter, and in the case of any health complaints. They also state that night workers found to be unfit for night work for health reasons should be transferred, whenever possible, to day work. Moreover, the European Community Directive requires that the average working time per week, including overtime, should not exceed 48 hours, that there should be a minimum daily rest period of 11 hours, and that there should be an additional uninterrupted rest period of 24 hours per week. Some European countries (e.g. France, Germany, Austria, Portugal, The Netherlands and the UK) have already passed specific laws to conform to this directive on aspects of working time.

Medical reviews required in these laws are not easy to formulate but should be aimed at ensuring an appropriate screening of workers who are going to be engaged in shift work in the first place, and then ensuring that regular (e.g. annual) assessments of their continued suitability for night and shift work are conducted. With regard to the former, it must be emphasized that the ability to cope with a bad shift schedule should not be used to select shift workers. Our primary aim must be to design shift schedules that minimize the potentially harmful consequences and to develop appropriate compensative measures. In this manner, disturbances to circadian rhythms, the accumulation of a sleep deficit and any marked interference with family and social life would be avoided, such that most people should be able to cope with shift work without significant health impairment.

It would be totally unreasonable, and probably also uneconomic, to develop a medical surveillance scheme for people obliged to work on an unfavourable shift system since a better shift schedule would certainly have less negative effects, thus reducing health complaints and the need for medical control or intervention. The main guidelines for designing shift systems according to psychophysiological criteria are:[27]

- Night work should be reduced as much as possible (perhaps by increasing the number of crews).
- Quickly rotating shift systems (that change every 1, 2 or 3 days) are preferable to slowly rotating ones (changing every 5 or more days), since they interfere less with circadian rhythms and minimize the extent of any cumulative sleep deficit.
- Permanent night work does not seem to be acceptable for social reasons, unless the particular working conditions (e.g. where safety is paramount) require a complete adjustment to night work in order to guarantee optimal performance levels.
- Clockwise rotation (morning/afternoon/night) is preferable to the counterclockwise (night/afternoon/morning) since it avoids quick changeovers (e.g. morning and night shift on the same day) and allows longer rest periods after each shift for the immediate recovery from fatigue and sleep deficit. It also parallels the endogenous circadian rhythms that have been shown to have a period slightly longer than 24 hours in free-running experiments.
- Extended workdays (9–12 hours) should only be contemplated when the nature of the work, and the workload, are suitable (adequate breaks, no over-

time) and the shift system is designed to minimize (i) the accumulation of fatigue and (ii) toxic exposure, by minimizing the number of successive work days before a span of rest days.
- Early starts to the morning shift should be avoided in order to reduce the truncation of the previous sleep (REM phase in particular) and the consequently increased fatigue and risk of errors.
- Shift system should be as regular as possible, and include some free weekends with at least 2 consecutive days off, to allow people to plan and enjoy their leisure time more conveniently. It is also desirable to consider flexible working time arrangements in all shift systems.

However, it is also obvious that some complaints or illnesses may be a contraindication for shift work, particularly when it is associated with other stress factors such as heavy work, heat, noise, monotony, or high cognitive demands. Thus the occupational health team needs to carry out an evaluation of both the working conditions and the health status of the individuals before assigning people to shift and night work. In the light of various criteria and suggestions proposed by a number of authors and institutions it appears reasonable to propose the following six strategies for medical intervention.[4,20,28,29]

1 Consider exempting from night work all those suffering from severe complaints and disorders that could be connected to, or worsened by, shift work. The list that follows, is extensive and it is not possible to offer blanket guidelines capable of implementation in all circumstances. As in so many aspects of occupational health, it is the physician who must use careful judgement in the individual circumstance:

- chronic sleep disturbances;
- severe gastrointestinal diseases (e.g. peptic ulcer, chronic hepatic and pancreatic diseases);
- chronic heart diseases (e.g. myocardial infarction up to 12 months previously or with impaired heart function, angina pectoris, hyperkinetic syndromes and severe hypertension);
- brain injuries with sequelae and severe nervous disorders, and in particular chronic anxiety and depression, since they are often associated with a disruption of the sleep/wakefulness cycle and can be influenced by the light/dark periods;
- epilepsy requiring medication since seizures can be encouraged by sleep deficit and the efficacy of the treatment can be hampered by irregular wake–rest schedules;
- insulin-dependent diabetes, thyroid (thyrotoxicosis and hypothyroidism) and suprarenal pathologies, since they require regular drug treatment that is strictly connected to the activity/rest periods;

- chronic renal impairment, since the disruption of circadian rhythms can further impair renal functioning;
- malignant tumours, to avoid further stress and facilitate medical treatment;
- pregnancy, particularly if there is a known risk of miscarriage;

2 Evaluate carefully before assigning to night work people who are or who have:

- over 45 years of age, as it becomes more difficult to sleep at irregular hours;
- digestive troubles or chronic respiratory diseases (asthma and chronic obstructive bronchitis);
- alcoholism or other drug addictions;
- marked hemeralopia or defective vision impairment, which can make night work difficult or dangerous;
- women with small children (under 6 years),
- long-distance commuters.

3 Pay particular attention also to those who score high on scales of neuroticism, morningness or rigidity of sleeping habits. In contrast, some individual characteristics and preferences could be considered to predispose people towards shift work and might be used to assign to shift work those who might be expected to encounter less difficulty in coping with it on the basis of their psychophysiological adaptability, health and living conditions (see p. 585).

4 Regular health reviews can be undertaken using a self-administered health questionnaires, aimed at detecting early signs or symptoms of difficulty in adjustment, and consequently intolerance to night work, which may require prompt intervention at an organizational (e.g. change the shift schedule) and/or individual (e.g. improve coping strategies or transfer to day work) level. Such special considerations are sleeping times and problems, eating and digestive problems, psychosomatic complaints, drug consumption, housing and commuting problems, workload, and out-of-job activities. Standardized questionnaires or check-lists may be used in order to facilitate a comparison of the worker's health over the years. Further, the use of sleep logs, diaries of daily activities, some rhythmometric recordings (e.g. body temperature, performance) or hormonal dosages (e.g. cortisol, melatonin) may be helpful in evaluating the level of an individual's adjustment.

5 Physicians should also bear in mind that shift work can worsen some disorders (e.g. sleep, digestive or nervous complaints) which workers may have independently of shift work and hence hamper the efficacy of their pharmacological control, particularly when this requires a precisely timed administration and/or a stable life regimen, as is case for diabetes, hypertension, asthma, hormonal pathologies, epilepsy and depression.

6 The frequency of medical reviews should be set by the occupational physician and take into account factors concerning both the working conditions (e.g. shifts rotas, environmental conditions, workload, etc.) and aspects of the individual (e.g. age and health condition). Several authors have suggested the following: a second health check not later than 12 months after starting night work, followed by successive health checks at least every 5 years for those under 45 years of age, and then every 2–3 years for those over 45 years. These guidelines are somewhat arbritary and are not required in the UK, but may serve to focus on the need for health review.

Many authors have emphasized the importance of careful monitoring during the first year of assignment to night work since it is probable that the short-term problems of adjustment of circadian rhythms, including sleep, are the main cause of night work intolerance in the first year or two. In contrast, longer-term intolerance may be more related to other personal, working and social factors. At each review the individual's fitness for shift work should be re-evaluated if they complain of sleep, gastrointestinal, psychological or other related problems, or if they contracted any other illnesses that might hamper their psychophysical equilibrium and working capacity. Temporary exemption from night work should be considered in the case of transient health impairment or severe difficulties in family or social life.

One approach is to give workers information, suggestions and guidelines on how best to cope with night and shift work.[30] Counselling and training should be carried out at both an individual and group level and educational programmes should be set up. They should deal with improving self-help strategies for coping, and in particular in relation to sleep hygiene, eating behaviour, stress management, physical fitness, housing conditions, transport facilities and out-of-work activities.

In addition to the optimum design of shift schedules based on ergonomic criteria (above), countermeasures that can prove beneficial include: the reduction of night work and/or working hours, the introduction of additional rest breaks (for meals and naps), the addition of compensatory rest-days or holidays, the improvement of canteen and transport facilities, the improvement of social services – particularly for women shiftworkers (e.g. childcare facilities, extended school and shop hours), the transfer to day work after a certain number of years on night work; and last, but not least, early retirement.

THE HEALTH EFFECTS OF EXTENDED HOURS OF WORK

Most of this chapter has been devoted to a review of health effects and health management of shift work. This is a reasonable stance, because the majority of workers engaged in unsocial work conform to one shift pattern or another, and because most of the research effort on health effects has been concentrated on the shift worker.

The recent European Community Directive on Working Hours has, however, highlighted the need to look more closely at extended hours of work. This is generally taken to mean working longer than 48 hours a week. Such work situations can occur with so-called shop floor workers but increasingly this is a work issue for 'white collar' staff.

A recent review of the literature has concentrated on the health and safety problems of long working hours and has excluded reference to the shift work literature.[31] The main finding of the review is the dearth of evidence to confirm or refute health related problems of long working hours. For mental health disorders, some studies do address this health effect although the populations studied are often rather unique and therefore preclude extrapolation to the general. Overall, however, what data do exist tend to support the view that weekly hours which exceed 50 – often greatly in excess of this figure – are associated with increased occupational stress both in terms of subjective reports and behavioural responses.

For cardiovascular disorders, the problem of 'karoshi' – sudden unexplained deaths in relatively young (and almost exclusively Japanese) workers are anedoctal but have attracted much media attention. Studies of hours of work and cardiovascular disease are relatively few and most of them not recent. Any link between heart disease and hours of work appears not to be a straightforward one. Perhaps long working hours play an interactive or an exacerbating part with other occupational stressors. Current evidence is sufficient to raise concerns but the nature and size of the effects is currently unknown.[31]

Performance is undoubtedly affected by the length of the working day but most of the better evidence was gathered 50–100 years ago with little recent research to refute or support it. Currently available data are not robust enough to determine exactly how many hours people should be required to work if they are to remain safe and healthy. Herein lies a major need for fresh research and this should include in addition to the above areas, a thorough analysis of the effect of long working hours on fetal health. The increasing trend towards long working hours makes the resolution of these issues all the more urgent.

REFERENCES

1 Wedderburn A (ed). *Statistics and News*. Bulletin of European Studies on Time No 9. Dublin: European Foundation for the Improvement of Living and Working Conditions, 1996: 1–72.

2 US Congress, Office of Technology Assessment. *Biological Rhythms: Implications for the Worker*. OTA-BA-463, Washington, DC: US Government Printing Office, 1991: 1–249.

3 Folkard S, Waterhouse JM, Minors DS. Chronobiology and shift work: current issues and trends. *Chronobiologia* 1985; **12**: 31–54.

4 Colquhoun WP, Costa G, Folkard S, Knauth P. *Shiftwork: Problems and Solutions*. Frankfurt: Peter Lang, 1996: 1–224.

5 Harrington JM. *Shiftwork and Health: A Critical Review of the Literature*. London: HMSO, 1978: 1–28.

6 Waterhouse JM, Folkard S, Minors DS. *Shiftwork, Health and Safety. An Overview of the Scientific Literature 1978–1990*. London: HMSO, 1992: 1–31.

7 Monk TH, Folkard S, Wedderburn AI. Maintaining safety and high performance on shiftwork. *Appl Ergon* 1996; **27**: 17–23.

8 Monk T. Shiftworker performance. *Occup Med State Art Rev* 1990; **5**: 183–98.

9 Åkerstedt T. *Wide Awake at Odd Hours*. Stockholm: Swedish Council for Work Life Research, 1996: 1–116.

10 Colligan MJ, Rosa RR. Shiftwork effects on social and family life. *Occup Med State Art Rev* 1990; **5**: 315–22.

11 Tepas DI, Carvalhais AB. Sleep patterns of shiftworkers. *Occup Med State Art Rev* 1990; **5**: 199–208.

12 Cole RJ, Loving RT, Kripke DF. Psychiatric aspects of shiftwork. *Occup Med State Art Rev* 1990; **5**: 301–14.

13 Costa G. The impact of shift and night work on health. *Appl Ergon* 1996; **27**: 9–16.

14 Knutsson A, Akerstedt T, Jonsson BG. Prevalence of risk factors for coronary artery disease among day and shift workers. *Scand J Environ Hlth* 1988; **14**: 317–21.

15 Kristensen TS. Cardiovascular diseases and the work environment. A critical review of the epidemiologic literature on nonchemical factors. *Scand J Work Environ Hlth* 1989; **15**: 165–79.

16 Akerstedt T, Knutsson A. Cardiovascular disease and shift work (editorial) *Scand J Work Environ Hlth* 1997; **23**: 241–2.

17 Smith L, Folkard S, Poole CJ. Increased injuries on night shift. *Lancet* 1994; **344**: 1137–9.

18 Price WJ, Holley DC. Shiftwork and safety in aviation. *Occup Med State Art Rev* 1990; **5**: 343–77.

19 Fischer FM. Retrospective study regarding absenteeism among shiftworkers. *In Arch Occup Environ Hlth* 1986; **58**: 301–20.

20 Scott AJ, LaDou J. Shiftwork: effects on sleep and health with recommendations for medical surveillance and screening. *Occup Med State Art Rev* 1990; **5**: 273–99.

21 Goyal R, Krishnan K, Tardif R, Lapare S, Brodeur J. Assessment of occupational health risk during unusual work shifts: review of the needs and solutions of modifying environmental and biological limit values for volatile organic solvents. *Can J Publ Hlth* 1992; **83**: 109–12.

22 Taylor PJ, Pocock SJ. Mortality of shift and day workers 1956–68. *Br J Ind Med* 1972; **29**: 201–7.

23 Härmä M. Interindividual differences in tolerance to shiftwork: a review. *Ergonomics* 1993; **36**: 101–9.

24 Costa G, Lievore F, Caseletti G *et al*. Circadian characteristics

influencing interindividual differences in tolerance and adjustment to shiftwork. *Ergonomics* 1989; **32**: 373–85.

25 Harrington JM. Shift work and health – a critical review of the literature on Working Hours. *Ann Acad Med Singapore* 1994; **23**: 699–705.

26 Kogi K. Improving shift workers health and tolerance to shiftwork. *Appl Ergon* 1996; **27:** 1–8, 1996.

27 Knauth P. Designing better shift systems. *Appl Ergon* 1996; **27:** 39–44.

28 Koller M. Occupational health services for shift and night work. *Appl Ergon* 1996, 27: 31–7.

29 Rutenfranz J. Occupational health measures for night and shiftworkers. *J Hum Ergol* 1982; **11** (Suppl): 67–86

30 Wedderburn A. *Guidelines for Shiftworkers*. Bulletin of European Studies on Time No 3. Dublin: European Foundation for the Improvement of Living and Working Conditions, 1991; 1–56.

31 Spurgeon A, Harrington JM, Cooper CL. Health and safety problems associated with long working hours: a review of the current position. *Occup Environ Med* 1997; **54:** 367–375.

Part 7

Occupational lung disorders

Imaging in occupational lung disease 593
Work and chronic air flow limitation 607
Byssinosis and other cotton-related
  diseases 621
Occupational asthma 633
Extrinsic allergic alveolitis 653
Inorganic dusts 663
Problems from indoor air in non-industrial
  workplaces 709

30

Imaging in occupational lung disease

PAUL M TAYLOR

Chest radiography	593	Magnetic resonance	598
Computed radiography	594	Radionuclide studies	599
Computed tomography	595	Occupational lung diseases	599
High resolution computed tomography	595	International Labour Organization classification	603
Ultrasound	598	References	605

The developments in imaging technology that have occurred in the last two decades have provided valuable insights into the body's structure and function. Despite this the chest radiograph remains the primary, and in many cases the only, radiological investigation performed. The use of more complex imaging techniques often carries a financial and radiation penalty and these must be balanced against the expected benefit.

CHEST RADIOGRAPHY

Within a year of Roentgen's discovery of x-rays, chest radiography had been used as a diagnostic tool. The initial images of the chest were crude but progress was rapid and by the early part of the twentieth century the chest radiograph was a recognized part of clinical investigation. Its validity in occupational lung disease was established as a result of correlative radiological and pathological studies.

The principles of chest radiography are well known. The patient is positioned with the anterior chest placed against the cassette containing the film and the x-ray tube approximately 2 metres from the film. The film is exposed during maximum inspiration. Technical factors can radically alter the appearances of the resultant radiograph. The radiographer can alter the kilovoltage (kV) of the x-rays produced by the tube. Higher kV x-rays possess more energy and pass more easily through all tissues, producing a 'flatter' image with less intrinsic con-

trast. A high kV exposure may be preferred since it produces clearer images of the mediastinum and the overlying lung. However, this is at the expense of clarity of the ribs and intrathoracic calcifications. The converse occurs with a lower kV exposure.

Radiographic film also varies in quality. In order to reduce radiation dose to the patient, manufacturers have developed faster films which produce a similar level of radiographic density at a lower exposure to x-rays. This development, although desirable, is not without drawbacks and faster films may produce a coarser image. This is of particular importance in occupational disease where subtle alterations in the parenchymal pattern may be significant. The practical impact of these considerations is that in longitudinal studies of workers no effort should be spared in ensuring that exposure factors and film quality vary as little as possible.

Of equal importance to technical factors are patient variables involved in the radiograph and before any attempt is made at interpretation the observer should consider the following:

- Is the patient rotated? Rotation produces asymmetry in the size and density of the lungs. Rotation is assessed by noting the position of the medial ends of the clavicles with respect to the spinous processes of the thoracic spine.
- Has the patient achieved a satisfactory inspiration? A poor inspiration causes crowding of the basal lung markings, an increase in density of the lower zones of the lungs and enlargement of the cardiac silhouette.

These changes are often misinterpreted as basal fibrosis. In a normal inspiration the dome of the right hemidiaphragm should lie between the anterior ends of the 6th and 7th ribs.

- Is the film adequately penetrated? An overpenetrated film causes the lungs to appear dark with loss of normal vascular markings; often misinterpreted as 'emphysematous lungs'. Underexposure causes the lungs to appear pale; often misinterpreted as due to pulmonary infiltration. Penetration is difficult to assess objectively and depends upon body habitus. It may be necessary to take two films at different penetrations to demonstrate the lungs and mediastinum.

COMPUTED RADIOGRAPHY

Computed radiography (CR) forms part of the larger concept of digital imaging. The potential advantages of digital imaging are well described and include reduction in radiation dose, greater reproducibility of the image, the ability to manipulate and post-process the image and the facility to store the image using one of a variety of storage media. Computed radiography encompasses a variety of systems which are used to produce digital radiographic images. These systems may stand alone, with the digital image being printed onto a film to be handled in a similar way to a conventional radiograph, or they may form part of a picture archiving and communication system (PACS)[1] where digital images from several sources e.g. CR, ultrasound, angiography are stored, manipulated and distributed within the radiology department and beyond. The techniques of CR are still evolving but it is likely that within the next decade most radiology departments will have some form of CR system. Detailed descriptions of CR systems are available in several comprehensive reviews.[2–4]

Whatever CR system is used the appearance of the resulting image will differ from a conventional radiograph. In its most obvious form this is because the image is displayed on a monitor rather than on a transilluminated film. Even when the image is printed, differences persist and the explanation for this is seen in Figures 30.1 to 30.3.

As Fig. 30.1 shows the relationship between the x-ray exposure and the film density on a conventional radiograph is non-linear and cannot be altered.

Figure 30.2 shows a theoretical relationship between exposure and film density in a CR system. The linear relationship ensures a more consistent density to the image and greater reproducibility between exposures. However, it is possible to use the software in the system to manipulate the image. For example if some of the film appears insufficiently dense the curve can be modified as in Fig. 30.3.

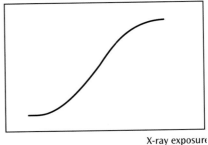

Degree of film blackening

X-ray exposure

Figure 30.1 *The relationship between the degree of blackening of the film and the amount of x-ray exposure for a conventional film. Note that the relationship is not linear and that at high or low exposure levels there is relatively little effect on the film for relatively large changes in exposure.*

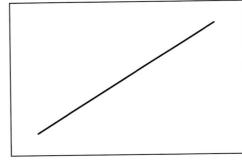

Degree of film blackening

X-ray exposure

Figure 30.2 *The theoretical relationship between the degree of blackening of the film and the amount of x-ray exposure for a CR system.*

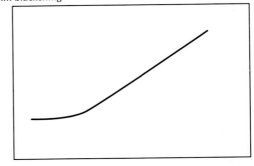

Degree of film blackening

X-ray exposure

Figure 30.3 *The possible relationship between the degree of blackening of the film and the amount of x-ray exposure for a CR system. The relationship between exposure and film blackening can be altered by the software in the system.*

In the context of occupational lung disease where early detection of subtle abnormality is important the software on the CR system should be optimized to permit this.

COMPUTED TOMOGRAPHY

The introduction of computed tomography (CT) into clinical practice was a milestone in radiological development.[5] First, it introduced computing into radiology thus laying the foundations for the development of digital imaging. Second, it established the utility of cross-sectional imaging as a method of displaying anatomy.

The initial CT scanners were suitable only for brain imaging with a small gantry aperture and long image acquisition times. By the late 1970s general purpose CT systems were available and the first reports of their use in the chest were published.[6,7] Now, CT has assumed an increasing role in thoracic imaging although the principles remain unchanged despite continuing technological development.

Within the CT gantry an x-ray tube rotates around the patient emitting a tightly collimated beam of x-rays. The x-rays emerging from the patient strike detectors and the data from these are fed to a computer. The computer calculates the attenuation of the beam by the patient's body to produce a matrix (typically 512*512) in which the attenuation value of each cell in the matrix is determined. The matrix is converted into an image by correlating the attenuation values with a grey scale in which the higher the attenuation value the brighter the shade of grey. Thus the image consists of many thousands of picture elements (pixels) each one of which represents the attenuation value of a small volume of tissue (voxel).

Because of the wide range of attenuation values and the limited number of shades of grey detectable by the human eye it is not practicable to display each attenuation value with a separate shade and a range of attenuation values must be selected (Fig. 30.4). The range chosen can be altered by changing the window width. A narrow window width ensures that tissues of slightly different attenuation are displayed as different shades of grey; this is suitable for demonstrating the mediastinal structures. A wider window is selected to demonstrate the lungs to accommodate the large range of attenuation present. Attenuation values above and below the chosen range appear white and black respectively. In addition to changing the window width, the window level can be altered. A low level is selected for predominantly low attenuation regions such as the lung and a high level for high attenuation structures such as bone.

Many other manipulations are possible including alterations of the processing algorithms to smooth or filter the image, reformation of the data in different planes and statistical analysis of the attenuation data.

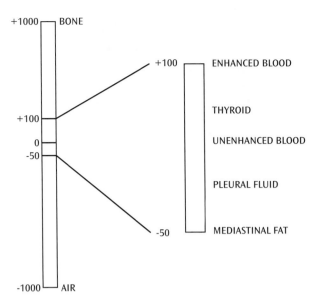

Figure 30.4 *The approximate attenuation values of structures within the thorax. Note the large possible range with clustering of values between −50 and +100 which necessitates the use of variable window settings.*

HIGH RESOLUTION COMPUTED TOMOGRAPHY

Introduced in the mid-1980s high resolution computed tomography (HRCT) of the lungs is now the preferred CT technique in the investigation of diffuse lung disease[8–10] (Figs 30.5a,b).

It differs from conventional CT in two key respects: section thickness and reconstruction.[11,12]

Section thickness

In conventional CT the sections are approximately 10 mm in thickness. In HRCT the sections are 1–2 mm thick. The beneficial effect of this is that partial volume averaging is reduced. Partial volume averaging occurs when a structure only partially fills a voxel. When the attenuation value for the voxel is calculated an average value is obtained lying between the true attenuation value of the structure and its background. As a result, small structures such as peripheral pulmonary vessels or small nodules can be 'lost' because they occupy only a small fraction of a voxel. By reducing slice thickness the voxels are made smaller and the percentage occupied by these small structures increases thus decreasing partial volume averaging. The disadvantages of thinner sections are twofold. First, if the section thickness is reduced from 10 mm to 1 mm ten times as many sections would be required to image the same volume of the body. In practice this is not a problem since the images are usually

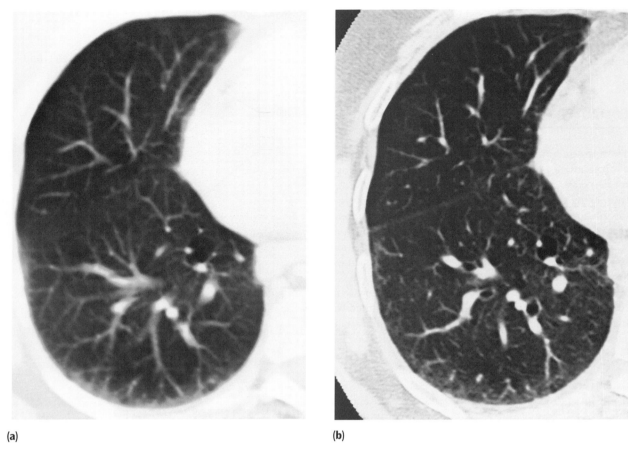

(a) (b)

Figure 30.5 *(a) A conventional CT section through the right lung. (b) An HRCT section through the right lung. This shows the greater clarity with which fine details, including the pulmonary vessels and bronchi, are seen compared with conventional CT.*

performed at 10 or 20 mm increments rather than contiguously. The second problem, inherent in all CT systems, is that reducing the section thickness decreases the signal:noise ratio. This makes the images appear rather 'noisy' with variations in pixel density even in homogenous body tissue. The problem can be overcome to some extent by altering the output of the x-ray tube.

Reconstruction algorithm

In calculating the attenuation values of the voxels the computer has to deal with biological heterogeneity of body tissue, statistical variation in x-ray output and other factors which produce variations in the calculated attenuation of ostensibly homogenous structures. To overcome this software, the computer smoothes these variations, reducing the differences between adjacent voxels. However, in heterogeneous tissues, such as the lung, smoothing results in loss of clarity of the margins of small structures. In HRCT a high spatial frequency processing algorithm is used which has little or no smoothing function.

HRCT techniques

In some centres HRCT images are targeted to the right and left lungs. Targeting means that only part of the body is displayed on each image resulting in each voxel being smaller, thus improving the resolution of the image. In practice the resolution gains are not large and extra time spent producing targeted images is rarely justified.

The majority of HRCT images are obtained with the patient supine during maximum inspiration. In the supine position due to the greater hydrostatic pressure the vessels in the posterior lung become distended and there is an increase in the extravascular fluid. This produces an increase in the attenuation of the posterior lung which can obscure underlying structural change. This is of particular importance in asbestosis since the posterior lung bases are the most frequently involved portions of the lung.

By turning the patient prone and repeating the sections the hypostatic changes are repositioned anteriorly. A period of 5–10 minutes is required for full reversal of these changes (Figs 30.6a,b). Failure to undertake this

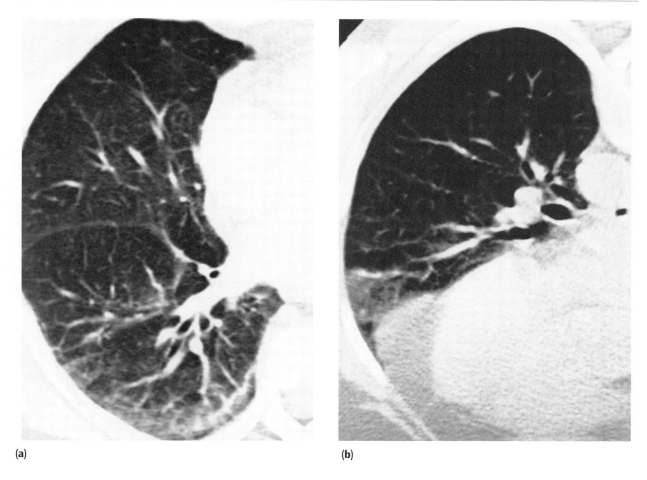

(a) (b)

Figure 30.6 *(a) An HRCT section obtained through the lung in a supine patient demonstrating marked hypostatic change in the posterior lung. (b) An HRCT section through the same patient obtained in the prone position demonstrating redistribution of the hypostatic changes to the anterior lung.*

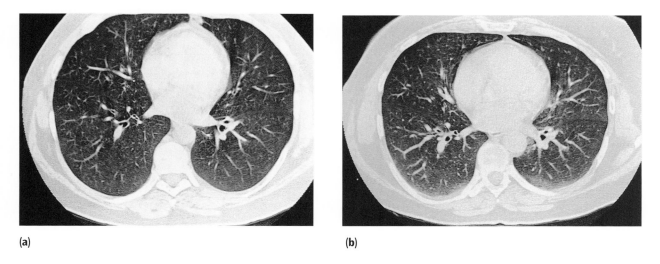

(a) (b)

Figure 30.7 *(a) An HRCT section obtained during maximum inspiration on a healthy subject. (b) An HRCT section obtained in the same subject during expiration. Note that in addition to the reduction in size of the thorax, the lung is of increased attenuation with accentuation of the normal gradient between the anterior and posterior lung.*

manoeuvre can result in fibrosis being obscured by the hydrostatic changes or normal lung being misinterpreted as abnormal.

Air trapping in the gas exchange spaces of the lungs is recognized to occur in several conditions including extrinsic allergic alveolitis.[13] It is difficult to detect air trapping on inspiratory scans but expiratory sections are helpful. On expiration the normal lung decreases in cross-section and increases in attenuation (Figs 30.7a,b). In regions of air trapping these changes fail to occur and they become highlighted against the normal lung (Figs 30.8a,b).

Enhancement of the mediastinal structures by intravenous contrast medium plays a key role in differentiating normal from abnormal structures, particularly lymphadenopathy. This is not usually required in patients with occupational lung disease but may be valuable in staging patients with occupationally induced bronchial carcinoma.

ULTRASOUND

Apart from the cardiovascular system, the applications of ultrasound in the thorax are limited by the inability of ultrasound to pass through the gas-filled lung. However, ultrasound has a role to play in imaging the pleura.[14] It is often difficult to differentiate pleural fluid from solid pleural masses on chest radiography, moreover the two can coexist. In addition, a CT can be difficult to interpret since the attenuation value of pleural fluid, particularly if it is haemorrhagic, may be similar to that of solid masses or atalectatic lung. Real time ultrasound usually allows detection and quantification of pleural fluid and is the most sensitive method of detecting small effusions. It can identify pleural masses and permits accurate percutaneous biopsy of lesions including mesothelioma.[15] Pleural plaques can be identified by ultrasound but CT is the preferred technique.

MAGNETIC RESONANCE

The ability of magnetic resonance (MR) to image in multiple planes with high intrinsic soft tissue contrast without using ionizing radiation has made MR an essential imaging tool in many areas of the body, particularly the neuraxis and skeleton.[16] Within the thorax it has an

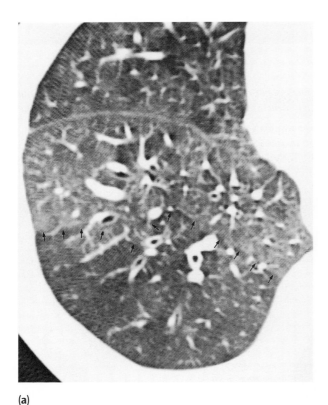

(a)

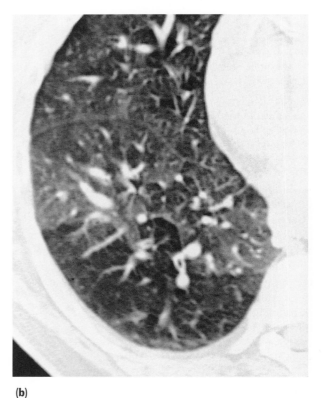

(b)

Figure 30.8 *(a) This is an HRCT section obtained during inspiration in a patient with extrinsic allergic alveolitis. The lungs are heterogeneous with areas of increased attenuation producing a 'ground glass' appearance. It is unclear if the area lying posteriorly, demarcated by the arrows, is normal lung or of abnormally low attenuation. (b) An expiratory HRCT section on the same patient. This shows that while much of the lung has decreased in size and increased in attenuation the posterior lung has remained largely unchanged thus confirming that air trapping is occurring in this portion of lung.*

established role in cardiovascular and mediastinal imaging.[17,18] The usefulness of MR in the lung is restricted for several reasons:[19]

1 MR primarily images protons. Within the lung the large amount of air produces a very low proton density.
2 The combination of air containing spaces and interlacing vessels produces inhomogeneity of the magnetic field.
3 There are physiological movements, in particular cardiac and respiratory motion which produce artefacts.

Despite these problems several studies have demonstrated the ability of MR to image patients with diffuse lung disease. It is likely that further developments in MR will be directed at improving our knowledge of pathophysiological events rather than replicating CT and providing structural data. In this context the high intrinsic soft tissue contrast of MR may enable the differentiation of active pulmonary infiltrates from more indolent fibrotic processes.

RADIONUCLIDE STUDIES

The most frequent radionuclide studies of the lung are ventilation/perfusion lung scans in patients with suspected pulmonary embolic disease. In occupational lung disease two other less frequently used techniques should be considered. Gallium-67 (^{67}Ga) is produced by cyclotron. When injected intravenously, ^{67}Ga is accumulated, by a variety of mechanisms, into inflammatory tissue including pulmonary inflammation. This accumulation occurs slowly and scans are obtained 1–3 days after the injection. Several inflammatory processes including drug-induced lung disease, sarcoidosis, fibrosing alveolitis and asbestosis have been shown to take up ^{67}Ga. As a result scans are sensitive but not specific.[20–22]

Technetium-99 m diethylenetriamine pentaacetic acid (Tc^{99}m DTPA) aerosols can be used to assess alveolar integrity. The patient inhales the aerosol and the lungs are imaged by the gamma camera. From the resultant images the rate of clearance of the radionuclide from the lungs is calculated. This is normally less than 4% per minute. Increased rates are seen in patients with a variety of conditions including extrinsic allergic alveolitis.[23] Higher rates of clearance are also seen in smokers and in respiratory infections.[24]

Although these techniques provide elegant demonstrations of pathophysiology their role in clinical management is limited. Structural changes are more clearly demonstrated by HRCT and conventional pulmonary function tests provide a more practical alternative in assessing functional impairment.

OCCUPATIONAL LUNG DISEASES

Coalworker's pneumoconiosis (see p. 682)

In addition to coal dust, miners frequently inhale quantities of silica dust from adjacent rock strata. The composition of the coal dust and the proportion of silica affect the radiological appearances of coalworker's pneumoconiosis (CWP) The prime radiological feature of CWP is the development of well defined, relatively discrete pulmonary nodules The nodules tend to spare the extreme lung bases and do not calcify.[25] Unlike pure silicosis, mediastinal and hilar lymph node enlargement do not occur. The size and clarity of the nodules are related to the composition of the dust, the profusion of the nodules is related to the degree of exposure.

COMPLICATED COALWORKER'S PNEUMOCONIOSIS

The defining process in the development of complicated CWP is the formation of areas of progressive massive fibrosis (see p. 684). Characteristically the lesions occur in the mid and upper zones of the lung and are frequently bilateral. They are ovoid or sausage shaped and enlarge over several years to reach several centimetres in diameter. The lesions rarely cavitate. In clinical practice the prime differential diagnosis is bronchial carcinoma which has an occurrence, even in miners, many times that of progressive massive fibrosis.

Silicosis

The appearances of silicosis (see p. 672) are not dissimilar to CWP.[26] However, the degree of fibrosis present in the lung is greater and as a result the nodules are larger, with less well defined margins and tend to become confluent. Hilar and mediastinal node enlargement occurs and the periphery of the nodes calcifies producing an

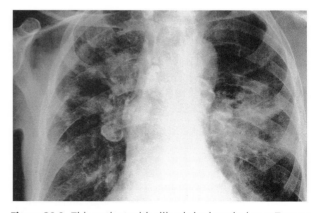

Figure 30.9 *This patient with silicosis had worked as a Terazzo floor worker for many years. Despite the radiographic changes he was only mildly incapacitated. Note the ill-defined, confluent pulmonary opacities and the eggshell nodal calcification.*

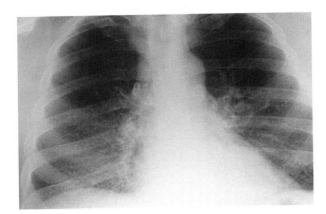

Figure 30.10 *Chest radiograph in a patient with sarcoidosis. The eggshell calcification at the right hilum had developed over a period of 6 years following the patient's initial presentation.*

eggshell appearance (Fig. 30.9). Silicosis is an uncommon condition and sarcoidosis is a more common cause of these appearances in clinical practice (Fig. 30.10). Progressive massive fibrosis occurs infrequently in silicosis.

Asbestosis

With the decline in coal mining in the UK asbestosis is now the most frequently encountered pneumoconiosis (see p. 686). The radiological features can be considered under three headings: pleural disease, pulmonary diseases and extrathoracic manifestations.

PLEURAL DISEASE

Pleural plaques are the most frequent radiological feature of asbestos exposure. They form well defined, rather angular densities which are most easily seen on the chest radiograph when they lie along the lateral chest wall or over the diaphragm since in these positions they lie tangential to the x-ray beam rather than *en face*. The plaques frequently calcify producing a holly leaf appearance (Fig. 30.11). The full extent of plaque deposition is most reliably assessed by CT[27] (Fig. 30.12). The appearance of plaques can be mimicked by subpleural fat deposits and prominent intercostal muscles[28] (Fig. 30.13). Pleural plaques are almost specific to asbestos exposure although they are occasionally seen in workers exposed to other silicates.[29]

Diffuse pleural thickening is much less common than pleural plaques[30] but is of greater significance since it encases the lung producing a restrictive functional abnormality. The thickening varies in thickness and has tapered, ill defined margins. Asbestos-induced pleural thickening uncommonly calcifies and this helps to differentiate it from thickening secondary to empyemas and haemothoraces (Fig. 30.14). As with pleural plaques the extent of pleural thickening is best assessed by CT.[31]

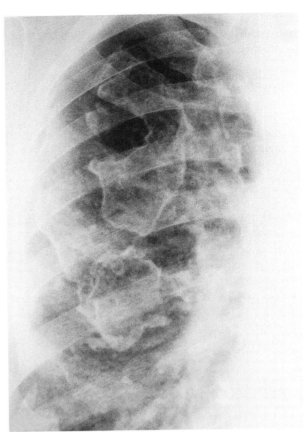

Figure 30.11 *Part of the chest radiograph in a patient with extensive 'holly leaf' pleural plaques. The patient had no pulmonary symptoms and had presented with a colonic carcinoma. This was a preoperative chest radiograph.*

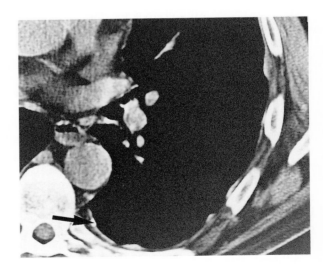

Figure 30.12 *Part of an HRCT study showing several small pleural plaques. Although there is a small area of calcification in one plaque, shown by the arrow, the majority are not calcified and, due to their small size, were not visible on the chest radiograph.*

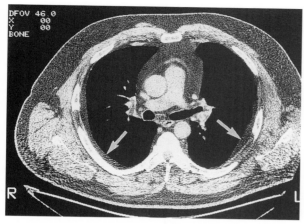

Figure 30.13 *This CT section shows extensive mediastinal and subpleural fat deposits (arrows) in an obese man. He had worked with asbestos in the past and, on the basis of a chest radiograph had been told he had bilateral pleural thickening. The CT clearly shows the 'thickening' to be due to fat. (Note that the density of this fat is similar to that of the subcutaneous fat surrounding the thorax.)*

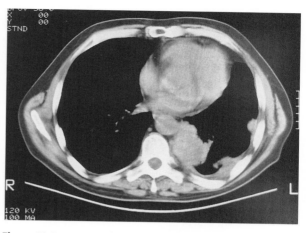

Figure 30.15 *A CT section on a patient with malignant pleural mesothelioma. The tumour is seen to encase the left lung with loss of volume of the hemithorax. Despite this the tumour has not involved any of the ribs. The diagnosis was confirmed by CT guided biopsy.*

Pleural effusions as a manifestation of asbestos exposure are indistinguishable radiologically from other pleural effusions. Although they are the most frequent radiographic manifestation of asbestos exposure in the first decade after the onset of exposure they are not common occurring in 3% of workers in one series.[32] Not uncommonly an effusion in an asbestos worker is secondary to an underlying bronchial carcinoma or mesthelioma.

Malignant mesothelioma is accompanied by a pleural effusion in approximately two-thirds of cases and this is often the main radiographic feature. The tumour itself forms a well defined lobular mass with tongues of tissue extending over the pleural surface producing a cuirass of tissue. The ribs appear crowded due the shrinkage of the underlying lung but rib destruction is an uncommon feature. The tumour can spread through the diaphragm. The features are often most easily appreciated on CT[33] (Fig. 30.15). Although biopsy can be obtained by CT or ultrasound guidance this is one of the few tumours which regularly seeds along the biopsy track and caution should be exercised. The main radiological differential diagnosis is of metastatic pleural tumour, particularly adenocarcinomas. Pleural thickening and thymic tumours, which have a predilection to extend into the pleura, can produce similar appearances.

PULMONARY DISEASE

The chest radiographic features of asbestosis are well described – a fine reticular basal shadowing producing loss of clarity of the cardiac silhouette. Increased public awareness and rigorous controls on asbestos use in North America and Europe have meant that patients are usually investigated when the extent of pulmonary fibrosis is mild, frequently before the radiographic features are visible. In the majority of these cases the radiological

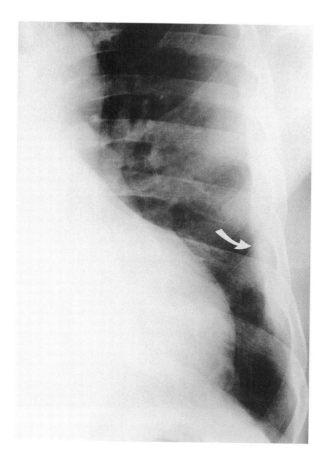

Figure 30.14 *Part of the chest radiograph of a patient with diffuse pleural thickening (arrow). This was confirmed by CT examination.*

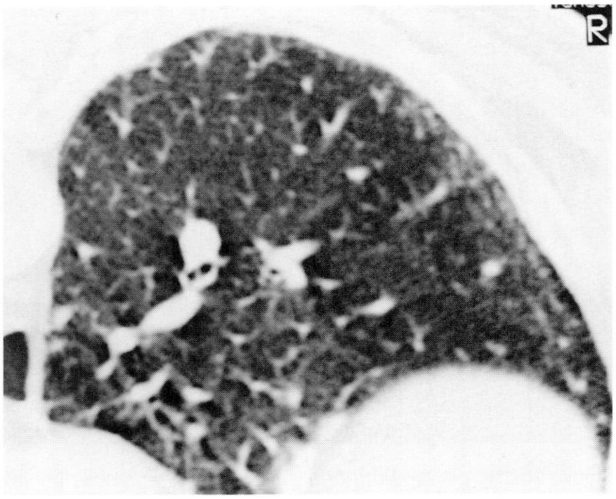

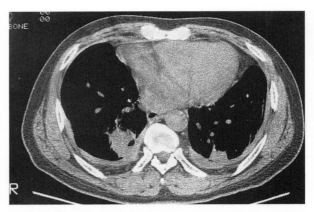

Figure 30.16 *A prone HRCT section in a patient with asbestosis. The patient, a shipyard worker had been exposed to asbestos over a 25-year period. The diffuse high attenuation area lying in the lung periphery is more extensive than that usually seen in such patients. It was present on sections obtained in the supine position and remains unchanged on this prone section. Physiological hypostatic change which can produce similar changes would be redistributed on turning the patient prone.*

Figure 30.17 *Bilateral pulmonary pseudotumours in a former asbestos worker. Both these lesions lie adjacent to areas of marked pleural thickening.*

changes are only seen on HRCT. In other parts of the world asbestos exposure is less regulated and chest radiographic signs of pulmonary fibrosis are more frequent.

The main HRCT features are ill defined areas of subpleural high attenuation, linear parenchymal band opacities due to fibrotic strands, peripheral reticulation and curvilinear subpleural densities[34,35] (Fig. 30.16). These features are most commonly encountered at the posterior lung base and for this reason prone HRCT sections are important to prevent them being obscured by hypostatic change. Although typical of asbestosis the features described are not specific and are seen in other fibrotic lung conditions, particularly cryptogenic fibrosing alveolitis.

Pulmonary pseudotoumour, also referred to as round atelectasis, is caused by a severe local inflammatory reaction occurring in the lung periphery adjacent to an area of pleural thickening. It produces a well defined rounded opacity, usually in the lower lobes and more commonly on the right.[36] (Fig. 30.17) The adjacent pulmonary vessels are shown on HRCT to be dragged into the mass producing a whorled appearance often described as the 'comet tail' or 'vacuum cleaner' sign.[37] Although round atalectasis is a well recognized feature of asbestos-related pleural disease, it is not specific for this condition.

Bronchial carcinoma occurring in patients with asbestosis has no distinguishing features from bronchial carcinoma occurring in other patients

although as in patients with fibrotic lung disease there is an increased incidence of synchronous and metachronous tumours.

EXTRATHORACIC MANIFESTATIONS

Extrathoracic malignancies, particularly of the digestive tract are known to be more frequent in asbestos workers than the general population. They have no differentiating features. The exception to this is peritoneal mesothelioma. This occurs almost exclusively after asbestos exposure. The tumour forms a dense cicatrizing mass which encases loops of small bowel and mesenteric vessels. Barium studies show areas of strictured bowel with fixity and loss of peristaltic activity. The tumour mass and any associated ascites are well seen on CT[38] (Fig. 30.18)

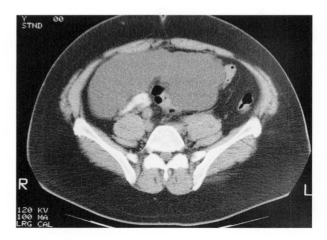

Figure 30.18 *This CT section shows peritoneal mesothelioma. The patient had presented with abdominal distension 3 years previously. The tumour had been resected but has recurred. The patient was from India where he had worked with asbestos for several years.*

Siderosis and stannosis (see p. 701)

Iron and tin are both inert dusts in that they do not excite an inflammatory reaction when they are inhaled. However, their radiological features are striking. Due to their high atomic number (Fe =26, Sn =50) they are both radiographically dense and produce a myriad of small high density nodules. The nodules of stannosis are often smaller but denser. The appearances can appear similar to other causes of miliary mottling such as miliary tuberculosis or miliary metastatic deposits; however, the density of the nodules should allow differentiation.

Extrinsic allergic alveolitis (see Chapter 34)

In its acute form extrinsic allergic alveolitis produces widespread ill defined opacities. These are almost invariably bilateral although the extreme lung bases and apices are often spared.[39] The opacities may not be particularly dense and produce hazy veiled appearance to the lungs, described as 'ground glass' opacification (Fig. 30.19). The opacities are fleeting and in a substantial proportion of patients the chest radiograph is normal at the time of presentation; HRCT shows abnormality more frequently than the chest radiograph and is particularly effective in demonstrating the ground glass opacities.[40]

Pleural effusions and nodal enlargement are uncommon and this helps differentiate the condition from infective pneumonias.

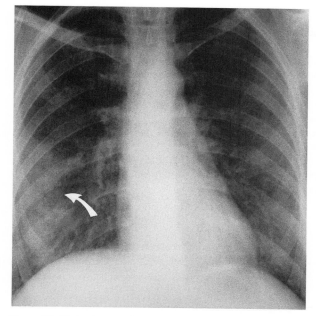

Figure 30.19 *A chest radiograph in a woman with extrinsic allergic alveolitis. There is fine, hazy opacification in the right lower zone (arrow) which resolved rapidly on admission to hospital. She had a budgerigar at home and her avian precipitins were strongly positive.*

In the chronic form of extrinsic allergic alveolitis, fibrosis develops, usually in the upper lobe. The radiological differentiation of this from other causes of upper zone fibrosis including sarcoidosis and tuberculosis may not be possible.

Zoonoses (see Chapter 24)

A wide variety of animal workers are at potential risk of contracting animal borne infections.[41] The most common are brucellosis, psittacosis and Q fever.

Brucella produces an acute pneumonic illness with areas of consolidation visible on the chest radiograph. Hilar and mediastinal lymph node enlargement occurs. In chronic brucellosis multiple bilateral nodular opacities are present and the appearances can resemble sarcoidosis.

Psittacosis and Q fever both produce pneumonic changes. The radiographic features are indistinguishable from other forms of pneumonia although Q fever may pursue a chronic course.

INTERNATIONAL LABOUR ORGANIZATION CLASSIFICATION

In 1930 the International Labour Organization (ILO) published a system for the classification of radiographs of the pneumoconioses. This has been revised on several occasions, most recently in 1980.[42] The system combines qualitative descriptions with qualitative assessments. In order to standardize the classification the ILO publishes a series of reference radiographs. In addition the ILO recommends the technical parameters which must be met by the radiograph to be classified. These parameters include the type of film used and the exposure of the film. In the USA radiologists and physicians wishing to apply the classification must attend a training programme to become accredited readers. This is recommended to reduce the well recognized problem of observer variation.[43] The effects of observer variability still obtain when conventional radiographs are compared with digitized images.[44] The aim of the classification is to standardize radiographic classification of the pneumoconioses, as such it can be used in research, epidemiological or statutory investigations but it is not a tool for routine clinical practice.

The classification exists in short and extended forms. There are five components which are considered and coded.

1 *Small opacities.* These are divided into regular and irregular opacities. The regular opacities are graded by size, the irregular opacities by width. The profusion of these opacities is then assessed. Using the short

Table 30.1 *ILO Classification – short form*

Feature	Code	Definition
Small opacities		
Rounded		
size	p	Up to 1.5 mm diameter
	q	1.5–3 mm diameter
	r	3–10 mm diameter
profusion	1	Few in number
	2	Numerous, lung markings visible
	3	Very numerous, lung markings obscured
Irregular		
type	s	Fine irregular or linear
	t	Medium irregular
	u	Coarse irregular
profusion	1	Few, lung markings visible
	2	Numerous, lung markings partially obscured
	3	Very numerous, lung markings totally obscured
Large opacities		
size	A	1–5 cm
	B	Larger than 5 cm but smaller than area of the right upper lobe
	C	Larger than the area of the right upper lobe
Pleural thickening	pl	Present
Pleural calcification	plc	Present
Additional symbols	ax	Coalescence of small rounded opacities
	bu	Bullae
	ca	Cancer of lung or pleura
	cn	Calcification in small pneumoconiotic opacities
	co	Abnormality of cardiac size or shape
	cp	Cor pulmonale
	cv	Cavity
	di	Marked distension of intrathoracic organs
	ef	Effusion
	em	Marked emphysema
	es	Eggshell calcification of hilar or mediastinal lymph nodes
	hi	Enlargement of hilar or mediastinal lymph nodes
	ho	Honeycomb lung
	kl	Septal (Kerley) lines
	od	Other significant disease. This includes disease not related to dust exposure
	pq	Uncalcified pleural plaque
	px	Pneumothorax
	rl	Rheumatoid pneumoconiosis (Caplan's syndrome)
	tba	Tuberculosis, probable active
	tbu	Tuberculosis, activity uncertain

form of the classification a 4-point profusion scale is used, a 12-point scale being employed in the extended form.

2 *Large opacities.* These are graded by size. They are usually few in number and profusion is not considered.

3 *Pleural thickening.* In the short form this is assessed as present or absent. In the extended form the position, thickness and extent of thickening are recorded for each hemithorax.

4 *Pleural calcification.* In the short form this is assessed as present or absent, whereas in the extended form observations are recorded regarding its side, site and extent.

5 *Additional features.* There is a list of additional features which are also coded.

The ILO classification (Table 30.1) was designed to be applied to chest radiographs; however, it can be applied to HRCT images. The results, although correlated, are not transposable since HRCT demonstrates higher sensitivity for most of the components (see p. 667).[45]

REFERENCES

1 Reynolds RA. Digital radiology and PACS. In: Grainger RG, Allison DJ eds. *Diagnostic Radiology: A Textbook of Medical Imaging*. London: Churchill Livingstone, 1997: 5–19.

2 Glazer HS, Muka MA, Sagel SS, Jost RG. New techniques in chest radiography. *Radiol Clin North Am* 1994; **32**: 711–29.

3 Fraser RG, Sanders C, Barnes GT, MacMahon H, Giger ML *et al*. Digital imaging of the chest. *Radiology* 1989; **171**: 297–307.

4 Aberle DR, Hansell D, Huang HK. Current status of digital projection radiography of the chest. *J Thorac Imaging* 1990; **5**: 10–18.

5 Ambrose J. Computerised transverse axial scanning (tomography). Part 2 – Clinical applications. *Br J Radiol* 1973; **46**: 1023–47.

6 Katz D, Kreel L. Computed tomography in asbestosis. *Clin Radiol* 1979; **30**: 207–13.

7 McLoud TC, Wittenberg J, Ferucci JT. Computed tomography of the thorax and standard radiographic evaluation of the chest – a comparative study. *J Comput Assist Tomogr* 1979; **3**: 170–80.

8 Nakata H, Kimoto T, Nakayama, Kido M, Miyazaki N, Harada S. Diffuse peripheral lung disease: Evaluation by high resolution computed tomography. *Radiology* 1985; **157**: 181–5.

9 Muller NL. Clinical value of high resolution CT in chronic diffuse lung disease. *Am J Roentgenol* 1991; **157**: 1163–70.

10 Padley SPG, Adler B, Muller NL. High resolution computed tomography of the chest: current indications. *J Thorac Imag* 1993; **8**: 189–99.

11 Mayo JR, Webb WR, Gould R, Stein MG, Bass I *et al*. High resolution CT of the lungs: An optimal approach. *Radiology* 1987; **163**: 507–10.

12 Mayo JR. High resolution computed tomography: Technical aspects. *Radiol Clin North Am* 1991; **26**: 1043–9.

13 Desai SR, Hansell DM. Small airways disease: Expiratory computed tomography comes of age. *Clin Radiol* 1997; **52**: 332–7.

14 Lipscombe DJ, Flower CDR, Hadfield JW. Ultrasound of the pleura: An assessment of its clinical value. *Clin Radiol* 1981; **32**: 289–90.

15 Chang DB, Yang PC, Luh KT, Kuo SH, Yuo CJ. Ultrasound guided pleural biopsy with Tru-Cut needle. *Chest* 1991; **100**: 1328–33.

16 Bradley WG, Bydder GM, Worthington BS. Magnetic resonance imaging: Basic principles. In: Grainger RG, Allison DJ eds. *Diagnostic Radiology: A Textbook of Medical Imaging*. London: Churchill Livingstone, 1997: 63–81.

17 Webb WR, Sostman HD. MR imaging of thoracic disease: Clinical uses. *Radiology* 1992; **182**: 621–30.

18 Mohiaddin RH, Longmore DB. Functional aspects of cardiovascular nuclear magnetic resonance imaging: Techniques and application. *Circulation* 1993; **88**: 264–81.

19 Mayo JR. Magnetic resonance imaging of the chest. *Radiol Clin North Am* 1994; **32**: 795–809.

20 Moiuddin M, Rockett J. Gallium scintigraphy in the detection of amiodarone lung toxicity. *Am J Roentgenol* 1986; **147**: 607.

21 Kramer EL, Sanger JH, Garay SM, Grossman RJ, Tiu S, Banner H. Radiology diagnostic implications of Ga[67] chest scan patterns in HIV seropositive patients. 1989; *Radiology* **170**: 671–6.

22 Hayes AA, Mullan B, Lovegrove FT, Ross AH, Musk AW, Robinson BW. Gallium lung scanning and broncho alveolar lavage in crocidolite exposed workers. *Chest* 1989; **96**: 22–6.

23 Bourke SJ, Banham SW, McKillop JH, Boyd G. Clearance of 99mTc DTPA in pigeon fanciers hypersensitivity pneumonitis. *Am Rev Respir Dis* 1990; **142**: 1168–71.

24 Minty BD, Jordan C, Jones JG. Rapid improvement in abnormal pulmonary permeability after stopping cigarettes. *Br Med J* 1981; **282**: 1183–6.

25 Stark P, Jacobson F, Schaffer K. Standard imaging in silicosis and coal workers pneumoconiosis. *Radiol Clin North Am* 1992; **30**: 1147–54.

26 Prendergrass EP. Silicosis and a few of the other pneumoconioses: Observations on certain aspects of the problem with emphasis on the role of the radiologist. *Am J Roentgenol* 1958; **80**: 1–41.

27 Friedman AC, Fiel SB, Fisher MS, Radiecki PD, Lev-Toaff AS, Caroline DF. Asbestos related pleural disease: A comparison of CT and chest radiography. *Am J Roentgenol* 1988; **150**: 269–75.

28 Sargent EN, Boswell WD, Ralls PW. Sub pleural fat pads in patients exposed to asbestos: Distinction from non calcified pleural plaques. *Radiology* 1984; **152**: 273–7.

29 Aberle DR, Gamsu G, Ray CS. Asbestos related pleural and parenchymal fibrosis: detection with high resolution computed tomography. *Radiology* 1986; **166**: 729–34.

30 Aberle DR, Gamsu G, Ray CS. High-resolution CT of benign asbestos-related diseases: clinical and radiographic correlation. *Am J Roentgenol* 1988; **151**: 883–91.

31 Aberle DR, Balmes JR. Computed tomography of asbestos related pulmonary parenchymal and pleural disease. *Clin Chest Med* 1991; **12**: 115–31.

32 Epler GR, McLoud TC, Gaensler EA. Prevalence and incidence of benign asbestos pleural effusion in a working population. *JAMA* 1982; **247**: 617–22.

33 Kawashima A, Libshitz H. Malignant pleural mesothelioma: CT manifestations in 50 cases. *Am J Roentgenol* 1990; **155**: 965–9.

34 Jones RN. The diagnosis of asbestosis. *Am Rev Respir Dis* 1991; **144**: 477–8.

35 Akira M, Yokoyama K, Yamamoto S, Higashihara T, Morinaga K *et al*. Early asbestosis: Evaluation with high resolution CT. *Radiology* 1991; **178**: 409–16.

36 Tylen U, Nilsson U. Computed tomography in asbestos pseudotumours and their relation to asbestos exposure. *J Comput Assist Tomogr* 1982; **6**: 229–37.

37 McHugh K, Blaquiere RM. CT features of rounded atelectasis. *Am J Roentgenol* 1989; **153**: 257–60.

38 Whitley NO, Bohlman ME, Baker LP. CT patterns of mesenteric disease. *J Comput Assist Tomogr* 1982; **6**: 490−6.

39 Cook PG, Wells IP, McGavin CR. The distribution of pulmonary shadowing in farmer's lung. *Clin Radiol* 1988; **39**: 21−27.

40 Hansell DM, Moskovic E. High resolution computed tomography in extrinsic allergic alveolitis. *Clin Radiol* 1991; **43**: 8−12.

41 Esposito AL. Pulmonary infection aquired in the workplace. *Clin Chest Med* 1992; **13**: 355−65.

42 International Labour Organization. *Guidelines for the use of ILO International Classification of Radiographs of the Pneumoconioses*. Geneva: ILO, 1980.

43 Amandus HE, Pendergrass EP, Dennis JM, Morgan WKC. Pneumoconiosis: inter-reader variability in the classification of the type of small opacities in the chest roentgenogram *Am J Roentgenol* 1974; **122**: 740−3.

44 Mannino DM, Kennedy RD, Hodous TK. Pneumoconiosis: comparison of digitized and conventional radiographs. *Radiology* 1993; **187**: 791−6.

45 Remy-Jardin M, Degreef JM, Beuscart R, Voisin C, Remy J. Coal workers pneumoconiosis: CT assessment in exposed workers and correlation with radiographic findings. *Radiology* 1990; **177**: 363−71.

31

Work and chronic air flow limitation

DAVID J HENDRICK

Historical background	607	Chronic obstructive pulmonary disease and agents known to induce occupational asthma	613
Uncertainties and controversies	608		
Cigarette smoking – confounding and interactions	608	Chronic obstructive pulmonary disease and occupational agents not known to induce occupational asthma	614
Pathophysiology and disease definitions	609		
Recognition of excess longitudinal decline in ventilatory function	610	Perspective in the population at large	616
		Conclusions	617
		References	617

The term chronic air flow limitation describes a diffuse reduction in airway calibre relative to the degree of lung inflation, which cannot be reversed by treatment. The 'fixed' nature of this obstruction is the cardinal feature of the disorder, which is more widely known as chronic obstructive pulmonary disease (COPD). Obstruction which responds partially but not fully to treatment implies there may be an asthmatic or acute bronchitic component to the disorder, of which the fixed component alone should be identified as COPD. Its importance lies with its tendency to progress and to cause a disabling, even life-threatening, loss of lung function.

HISTORICAL BACKGROUND

That COPD might arise as a consequence of the occupational environment is a matter of evolving interest and importance, and not a little controversy. The possibility of COPD of occupational origin, unassociated with complicated pneumoconiosis, first gained widespread acceptance as recently as the 1960s as a result of a series of investigations in cotton workers by Schilling and Bouhuys and their colleagues.[1,2] They suggested that byssinosis could be usefully classified into three distinct clinical grades. Workers who developed chest tightness and breathing difficulty only on the first working day of each week were said to have byssinosis grade 1; those who had similar symptoms on additional working days of the week, but who recovered fully away from the workplace, were said to have byssinosis grade 2; and

those who had symptoms of persisting respiratory disability were said to have byssinosis grade 3. Physiological studies indicated that byssinosis grades 1 and 2 were associated with reversible airways obstruction, while byssinosis grade 3 was associated with fixed airways obstruction. It was assumed that affected workers followed an orderly progression through these escalating grades. Cotton dust was consequently a potential cause of COPD, and byssinosis grade 3 was occupational COPD.

The specific effects of cotton dust are discussed in detail in the following chapter, and so cotton dust and byssinosis will be mentioned here only to provide a convenient historical focus for reviewing the claims and controversies which have arisen subsequently from many occupational environments concerning COPD.

Many (perhaps most) authorities would now regard byssinosis grades 1 and 2 as occupational asthma attributable to cotton dust. The physiological correlates (acute but reversible episodes of airway obstruction) are diagnostic of asthma, and the curious work-related periodicity of the symptoms (which had been considered particularly characteristic of byssinosis) has since been observed with many other types of occupational asthma. As with active asthma of any aetiology, airway hyperresponsiveness can be demonstrated to a variety of bronchoconstrictor agents at times when byssinosis grade 1 or grade 2 is active. If, then, byssinosis grades 1 and 2 are examples of occupational asthma, is occupational COPD (i.e. byssinosis grade 3) simply a consequence of occupational asthma? This is certainly plausible, since long-standing asthma of non-occupational origin often results in fixed airway obstruction, and many would consider chronic asthma to be one of a number of causes of COPD.

The relation of byssinosis grade 3 to byssinosis grades 1 and 2 may, however, be looked at from a different viewpoint to that adopted by Schilling and Bouhuys. The investigations which led to their grading classification were cross-sectional not longitudinal in structure, and this may pose problems over assumptions of causality. Grade 1 byssinosis was not, in fact, observed to progress to grade 3 byssinosis, and so it is entirely conceivable that byssinosis grade 3 is a fundamentally different disorder from byssinosis grades 1 and 2, albeit one which is also induced by occupational exposure to cotton dust. If this is so, byssinosis grade 3 could be regarded as the prototype for occupational COPD, and the question arises whether it is likely that cotton dust alone among occupational agents would have this effect on the airways?

Most of the cotton workers of the 1960s had been heavy cigarette smokers for many years, and doubts were expressed subsequently whether the confounding effect of this on the development of COPD (which was barely recognized in the 1960s) was adequately taken into account.[3] Although recent investigations have largely confirmed that COPD does arise as a consequence of occupational exposure to cotton dust independently of smoking,[4,5] this relationship remained uncertain for many years, and the confounding role of cigarette smoking has come to lie at the centre of current controversies.

UNCERTAINTIES AND CONTROVERSIES

The experience with the cotton industry consequently provides invaluable lessons for the assessment of occupational COPD, and for evaluating today's inevitable controversies. In essence they centre on whether an excess prevalence of COPD in a given working population can be attributed to smoking or non-occupational asthma rather than to the working environment; and whether, if the workplace is responsible, COPD arises independently of occupational asthma or as a direct consequence of it – or both (Fig. 31.1).

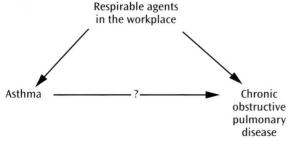

Figure 31.1 *Chronic obstructive pulmonary disease pathways. Adapted from Ref. 67.*

There is a further source of confusion – regular occupational exposure to respirable irritants commonly leads to mucus hypersecretion and to chronic productive cough (i.e. chronic bronchitis). In an occupational setting this is often termed 'industrial bronchitis'.[6] When chronic bronchitis develops coincidentally alongside asthma, the emergence of obstructive symptoms (wheeze, chest tightness, undue shortness of breath) is often attributed, not unreasonably, to COPD and to the cause of the productive cough. Mucus hypersecretion does not itself cause airway obstruction, however, and so obstruction when it does occur with chronic bronchitis has to be attributed to other pathophysiological processes – i.e. to asthma when obstruction is reversible, to COPD when obstruction is fixed, or to both when there are both reversible and fixed components.[7]

The possible presence of coincidental 'cryptogenic' asthma (an increasingly common disease at all ages in the population at large) may consequently simulate occupational COPD, just as asthma in smokers in a Chest Clinic setting may simulate smoking-induced COPD. This is particularly likely if industrial bronchitis (or smokers bronchitis) coexists. Cryptogenic asthma may also simulate occupational asthma because it is likely to worsen transitorily in the workplace if there are respirable irritants, and in some occupational settings (e.g. cotton mills) the development of occupational asthma is as plausible as the development of occupational COPD. If it is true that there are substantial differences in the prevalence of cryptogenic asthma from region to region, from population to population, and from birth cohort to birth cohort, as is now suggested, formidable difficulties must be expected in allowing for this if a given working population appears to show an excess of COPD.

CIGARETTE SMOKING – CONFOUNDING AND INTERACTIONS

The relative effects of smoking and occupation on COPD can only be assessed from meticulous epidemiological investigations where study populations include smokers and non-smokers, and workers with and without the relevant occupational exposure. There may be great difficulty in finding such a balanced population, and there may be great difficulty in avoiding bias in the exposure histories which are obtained. Most investigations of occupationally induced disease lead eventually to anxiety, anger, and claims for compensation in at least some of the study population; and once these arise memory tends to become unduly stimulated for the noxious nature of former workplace environments but paradoxically suppressed for estimates of former smoking consumption.

An important additional tendency is for those who are

best able to tolerate the heaviest levels of tobacco consumption to take on jobs with the most noxious occupational exposures (and vice versa), or for cultural or family influences to link smoking with recruitment to particular types of work. This inevitably confounds any potential effect of the work environment with that of smoking, and is illustrated in Table 31.1. Here the smoking habits of 15- to 16-year-old school leavers applying for a range of apprenticeships associated with three levels of exposure to noxious working environments (low, medium, high) are compared with established workers aged 19–26 years in the same trade groups.[8] The clear differences in current smoking prevalence seen between the occupational exposure groups of the workers can be observed also in the school leavers, though age exerts an additional effect and increases the prevalences in the older workers in all work-exposure categories.

Smoking is consequently likely to be associated with the very occupational environments which are themselves suspected of causing COPD. This may lead to two types of survival bias. First workers may leave the particular working environment if they develop smoking-induced COPD and the work becomes physically too demanding. This produces a surviving population of workers in whom the relative effect of any occupationally induced COPD may be exaggerated. Conversely, there may be a disproportionate loss of workers whose COPD is occupational in origin, thereby exaggerating in the survivors the effect of smoking and masking the effect of the workplace. Furthermore, those workers who are initially less able (or less willing) to tolerate noxious exposures will avoid the relevant working environments, and this will exert an additional bias on the selection of populations who work with the risk of developing occupational lung disease. These influences on worker selection make it particularly difficult to conduct reliable epidemiological studies among occupational populations, and to allow fully for the contributory effects to COPD from smoking. Thus investigators, regulating bodies, employers, and employees may be hard-pressed to recognize when 'excessive' longitudinal loss of ventilatory function in a working population is truly excessive once the idiosyncratic effect of cigarette smoking is taken into account. Full smoking histories are consequently essential in research, and should include a quantitative measure of cumulative consumption.

The issue is unduly complicated because only a minority of smokers (15–20%) appear to develop COPD (hence the idiosyncrasy) and because COPD in never-smokers is rare even in working populations with regular exposure to noxious occupational agents. This assumes the workers do not suffer from asthma. There is evidence, however, that when smokers additionally work with noxious respirable agents, COPD occurs with unusual frequency and/or severity. This implies an adverse interaction between smoking and the working environment. Recognizing such an interaction (i.e. the occurrence of COPD in excess of that to be expected through smoking alone and through the occupational environment alone) poses great difficulty for the investigator, largely because doubts over the accuracy of past smoking histories may invalidate, or at least weaken, the statistical analyses involved. There may be strong justification for such doubts. In a UK study of the population at large it was concluded that up to 7% of smokers and former smokers had described themselves incorrectly as never-smokers;[9] while in a US study of coal miners as many as 15% were said to be never-smokers despite records from earlier surveys which indicated they were regular smokers.[10]

PATHOPHYSIOLOGY AND DISEASE DEFINITIONS

Fixed airway obstruction may be a consequence of either intrinsic inflammatory/fibrotic disease of the intrathoracic airways, or of destructive disease of the parenchyma and interstitium of the lung (emphysema). With emphysema, airway obstruction and air trapping are associated additionally with impairment of gas transfer and loss of elastic recoil. It is this loss of elastic support to the smaller airways, whose walls are not supported by cartilage, which leads to airway collapse and obstruction (Fig. 31.2). This mechanism is seen in occupational COPD attributable to complicated pneumoconiosis. With the exception of cadmium-induced emphysema it appears to be an unusual mechanism for other types of COPD attributed to occupation, though it should be said that histological research into the matter is very limited.

With most types of COPD attributed to occupation,

Table 31.1 *Current or former smoking habits of apprentices compared with workers*

	No	Smokers %
Workers[a]		
low exposure	179	30
medium exposure	219	39
high exposure	284	58
School leavers[b]		
low exposure	53	9
medium exposure	126	21
high exposure	75	36

[1]Data taken from Ref. 8.
[a]Shipyard workers aged 19–26 years in trades with low, medium, and high levels of exposure to welding fume.
[b]School leavers aged 15–16 years seeking apprenticeships in the same trades.
The smoking prevalence trends across the welding fume exposure subgroups are highly significant in both the workers and the school leavers (p < 0.001).

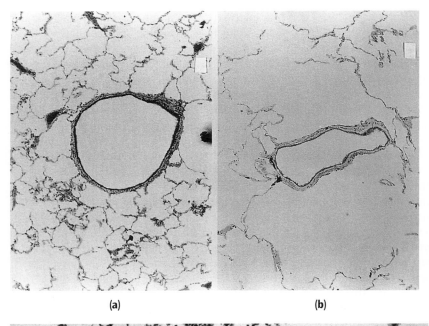

(a)   (b)

Figure 31.2 *Histology of a bronchiole and the surrounding parenchyma in (a) normal lung and (b) emphysema.*

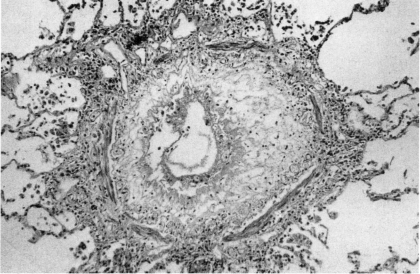

Figure 31.3 *Histology of a bronchiole and the surrounding parenchyma in obstructive bronchiolitis.*

lung function tests reveal no significant impairment of gas transfer compared with control data, implying that intrinsic disease of the airways is a more probable mechanism than emphysema. Extensive work with COPD attributable to smoking has suggested that the smaller unsupported airways again provide the most probable primary site for the obstruction to airflow, there being a mixed pathological picture of inflammation and fibrosis chiefly in and around the bronchioles. The disorder is more accurately described as an obstructive bronchiolitis, or bronchiolitis obliterans, than as a chronic obstructive bronchitis (Fig. 31.3). However, bronchial inflammation is often seen, especially when there is chronic productive cough. This is best regarded as an independent phenomenon, and is often unrelated to airflow limitation. The mechanism and primary site under-

lying COPD attributable to chronic asthma remain to be clarified, and so there is much to be said for using the diagnostic term COPD in a purely functional sense – i.e. to indicate fixed airway obstruction attributable to a variety of possible pathological processes.

RECOGNITION OF EXCESSIVE LONGITUDINAL DECLINE IN VENTILATORY FUNCTION

An epidemiological approach to estimating the rate of decline in ventilatory function offers the only practical means of identifying occupational causes of COPD in living populations. If the occupational contribution to COPD in a given workforce is relatively small and if

COPD itself is uncommon (often the case in populations subjected to 'healthy worker' and 'survivor' biases), the investigation of large numbers of subjects will be necessary if an occupational effect is to be shown convincingly. Such investigations are necessarily time-consuming and expensive. They must also be complex if modern statistical analyses using multiple regression techniques are to take adequate account of all the various factors which may independently influence the measured end point, i.e. the level of ventilatory function, or interact with environmental exposures of relevance. Otherwise there is the risk that these factors (e.g. age, height, race, gender, social grouping, changing body mass, smoking, viral infections, atopy, airway responsiveness) might be distributed unevenly between subgroups of the study population which differ also in the levels of exposure to the agent suspected of inducing COPD. If such unevenness occurs it might explain or exaggerate significant differences which appear otherwise to be a consequence of the occupational agent. Conversely, it might mask a true occupational effect in investigations which appear to give 'negative' results. The potential for such confounding is critical to the planning and analysis of investigations of this type.

Chronic obstructive pulmonary disease and cigarette smoking

From a series of pioneering epidemiological investigations of COPD attributable to cigarette smoking, Fletcher and colleagues showed during the 1960s that the majority of smokers appeared to experience no adverse effect on ventilatory function.[11] In the minority who were seen to be adversely affected, an excess annual decline in forced expiratory volume in 1 second (FEV$_1$) could be deduced from cross-sectional data (i.e. FEV$_1$ appeared to be excessively diminished in older subjects who had smoked). The magnitude of the apparent decline in FEV$_1$ with age (FEV$_1$ slope) was related to the level of smoking consumption. The mean annual decline among symptomatic smokers appeared to be approximately twice that of the non-smokers. The excess decline could be detected after as little as 5 years of regular smoking, and its cumulative dose-related effect was readily quantified by the degree of fixed airway obstruction evident already at the time of the initial measurement of ventilatory function.

A cohort of the men investigated cross-sectionally by Fletcher and colleagues (male transport and postal workers in London) were followed longitudinally, so that the actual annual changes in FEV$_1$ could be measured. The mean decline in FEV$_1$ (when standardized for height) was about 30 ml/year. The actual rates of decline were related to height, smoking and symptoms; and they appeared to increase a little with increasing age. The excess rate of decline in smokers ceased when they gave

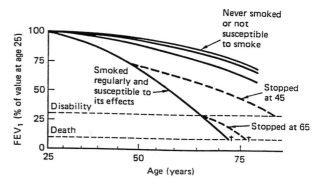

Figure 31.4 *Decline of FEV$_1$ with age: smokers vs non-smokers. (Reproduced from Ref. 66, where it was adapted from Ref. 11.)*

up the habit, but the damage already sustained was permanent (Fig. 31.4). A similar natural history is to be expected from any cause of COPD, though there will be much variability from individual to individual, and in some of those affected many exposure years will pass before the disease becomes evident.

Discrepancy between cross-sectional and longitudinal data

When data from the London transport workers were analysed from the initial cross-sectional study, regression of FEV$_1$ on age suggested a rather greater mean annual decline of 46 ml/year. That is to say, the differences in FEV$_1$ between the youngest and oldest participants in the initial study suggested that the mean annual decline in FEV$_1$, after allowing for differences in height, was about 1½ times the rate actually measured during the subsequent longitudinal phase of the investigation. The discrepancy was not readily explained at the time. It is a discrepancy which has since been recognized by a number of investigators. Those from Tulane University, New Orleans demonstrated a more striking discrepancy when estimating the annual decline in FEV$_1$ from a longitudinal study over 5 years of a normal population of males aged 30–58 years.[12] The cross-sectional data from each survey year indicated a mean decline of 40–50 ml/year with increasing age, once the effect of height was taken into account; while the mean of the actual longitudinal declines measured in each participant was of the order 15–20 ml/year (Table 31.2).

Thus cross-sectional data cannot be extrapolated to predict longitudinal change with any precision, and should not be compared directly with longitudinal data from other investigations. The discrepancy probably arises because subjects at the younger end of an age spectrum of, say, 20–60 years from a current cross-sectional investigation do not necessarily have the same mean FEV$_1$ as did those at the older end of the spectrum some 40 years earlier when they were of a similar young age. In

Table 31.2 *Age-related changes in ventilatory function: cross-sectional vs longitudinal data*

Cross-sectional regressions of mean FEV_1 against age:

1974	−42.6 ml/year
1975	−47.2
1976	−44.9
1977	−50.5
1979	−44.6

Mean of longitudinal regressions of FEV_1 against time:

1974 to 79 (5 years)	−12.4 ml/year
1975 to 79 (4 years)	−17.4

Reproduced from Ref. 12.
The investigation involved a 'normal' population of 52 adult cau-casian males, aged 30–58 years, of whom nine were current smokers, 16 former smokers, and 27 never-smokers. There were no relevant occupational exposures. Three subjects reported chronic cough, and seven undue breathlessness. The initial 1974 measurements were slightly less than those of 1975, possibly reflecting inexperience with spirometric manoeuvres, and so the period 1975–79 may provide a more accurate estimate of longitudinal change than 1974–79.

fact the currently young subjects are likely to have greater values of FEV_1 at a standardized young age, partly because they have larger lungs, and partly because they are less likely to have sustained respiratory diseases (e.g. tuberculosis, bronchiectasis) which impair ventilatory function. The difference in FEV_1 between younger and older subjects at the time of a cross-sectional study therefore exaggerates the true declines which were expe-rienced by the older subjects during the preceding years. Furthermore, the currently young subjects are likely to encounter less lung damaging insults as they age to 60 years, compared with subjects aged 60 years already. Thus mean longitudinal decline in lung function in pop-ulations is not wholly a consequence of increasing age

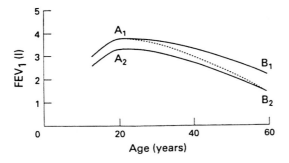

Figure 31.5 *Discrepant mean decline in FEV_1 from cross-sec-tional and longitudinal data.*
A1→B1 represents true (future) longitudinal decline in subjects currently aged 20 years.
A2→B2 represents true (completed) longitudinal decline in sub-jects currently aged 60 years.
A1→B2 represents apparent (current) decline using cross-sec-tional data from subjects currently aged 20–60 years. From Ref. 68.

and of cumulative exposure to cigarette smoke or occu-pational agents. It depends also on the cumulative bur-den of all damaging pulmonary insults throughout the ageing period (Fig. 31.5).

By using study subjects as their own 'controls' and avoiding the problems which arise from mismatching in cross-sectional studies (i.e. by eliminating between-worker variability), longitudinal studies are inherently more robust.[13] They may be unduly vulnerable to dimin-ishing participation rates, however, and this may intro-duce new risks of bias.

Other non-occupational factors of possible relevance

The study of London transport and postal workers use-fully showed that although intercurrent episodes of respi-ratory tract viral infection (i.e. episodes of acute bronchitis, exacerbations of COPD) caused significant reductions in ventilatory function, the effect was only temporary. Full recoveries to former levels of ventilatory function were noted within a few weeks, after which the rate of longitudinal decline returned to its usual level. Repeated viral infections do not therefore influence the assessment of occupational COPD from either cross-sec-tional or longitudinal studies, provided there are no acute infections at the time of study. Whether intercurrent episodes of acute bronchitis following brief exposure to toxic chemicals at work (e.g. gassing accidents) will prove to be equally benign is currently a matter of much specula-tion, concern, and on-going investigation. Major acci-dents which produce life-threatening pulmonary toxicity are recognized to cause bronchiolitis obliterans in a small proportion of survivors, though the majority of survivors appear to recover fully. A few develop asthma which may persist indefinitely and so pose a further pathway for the emergence of COPD. This complication of acute pul-monary toxicity has been termed 'reactive airways dys-function syndrome' (RADS) in North America.[14] The designation is possibly unhelpful since it suggests incor-rectly that RADS is a disorder which is somehow distinct from asthma.

Age, height, race and gender all exert important influ-ences on the measurement of ventilatory function, and it has recently been suggested that air pollution and increasing body mass during the course of a longitudinal investigation may also exert a potentially important (adverse) effect. The wide range of apparent individual susceptibility to COPD suggests the possible dependence on genetic factors, and there is supportive evidence for this especially from twin studies.[15,16] Genetically deter-mined atopy has not generally been found to influence COPD, but this depends on how COPD is defined and how vigorously an asthmatic contribution is excluded.

Analysis of the American multicentre Lung Health Study suggests that airway responsiveness (to methacholine) may prove to be almost as important as cigarette smoking in exerting an adverse influence on the rate of decline in ventilatory function.[17] If it is confirmed that a measure of asthmatic activity is relevant to predicting the development of COPD (a relationship enshrined in what became known as the 'Dutch hypothesis' of the 1970s and 1980s but was disputed thereafter), then factors of aetiological relevance to asthma may also need to be taken into account when studying COPD.[18,19] It may be useful therefore to consider the occupational agents which have been associated with COPD in two categories – those which are also believed to cause asthma and those which appear to have no asthmagenic properties.

CHRONIC OBSTRUCTIVE PULMONARY DISEASE AND AGENTS KNOWN TO INDUCE OCCUPATIONAL ASTHMA

Naturally occurring inducers of occupational asthma (See Chapter 33)

Respiratory disease in grain workers has been widely recorded since the eighteenth century and the time of Ramazzini. Grain dust has become a particularly well recognized cause of occupational asthma, though the precise causative agent (or agents) remains unclear. Storage mites, microbial contaminants, pesticides and fungicides, and even rodent urinary proteins have all been incriminated together with allergenic material derived from the grain itself. A number of investigators have produced impressive evidence that occupational exposure to grain dust may also lead to COPD, though none has suggested that this is a direct consequence of occupational asthma and most have found some inconsistencies among their data.[20,21]

The experience of Chan-Yeung and her colleagues in the port of Vancouver provides a useful illustrative example.[22] They followed port grain workers and control subjects working in civic centre posts between 1978 and 1990. After 6 years the annual rates for the decline in FEV_1 were significantly greater among the grain workers (−31 ml/year) than the controls (+4 ml/year), but when the smokers alone were compared little difference was noted between grain workers and controls (−36 ml/year vs −31 ml/year). In this particular investigation, therefore, the 'grain COPD effect' was seen largely in the non-smokers (in whom asthma was not satisfactorily excluded though atopy proved to be irrelevant), and it appeared to be of similar magnitude to the 'smoking COPD effect' in the control workers. Furthermore, its demonstration depended on there being an unusually small annual decline in FEV_1 (in fact there was a trivial increase) among the controls. After 12 years significant differences between grain workers and controls were no longer evident, but this may have been a consequence of

survivor bias or of the greatly diminishing levels of grain dust exposure during the course of the investigation. Not all investigators have found this COPD effect, and when it was observed it was generally more clear among the smokers than non-smokers.

With wood dust, a further common cause of occupational asthma, evidence for a COPD effect is less strong, but again there is evidence that smokers may be unduly susceptible to it. This is noteworthy in view of the curious 'protective' effect of smoking observed with occupational asthma attributable to western red cedar.[23] A similar protective effect in smokers, for which there are plausible immunological explanations, has been observed with extrinsic allergic alveolitis and sarcoidosis, and so should not be dismissed too hastily.[24,25]

Chemical inducers of occupational asthma

In Britain at present isocyanates seem to be the most common cause of occupational asthma, and isocyanate asthma continues to provide a typical example of asthma attributable to occupational chemicals (see Chapter 33). Not unnaturally isocyanate workers have provided a focus for investigations, of which there have been many, of possible occupational COPD. The results have been conflicting and have stimulated much controversy. A major multicentre surveillance programme in Britain revealed no hint of a COPD effect, while study of a single isocyanate producing plant in the USA suggested a crippling occupationally induced mean decline in FEV_1 exceeding 100 ml/year[26,27] Both investigations may have been flawed; the one because there was an implausibly low prevalence of occupational asthma (and possibly a major survivor bias), the other because the levels of ventilatory function observed initially were too well preserved for an excessive decline of such a degree to have been occurring before the investigation commenced.

Not surprisingly, reports of these investigations stimulated many others, and these have produced a spectrum of conclusions which is almost as wide. The 5-year investigation of Diem and colleagues of workers in a new toluene diisocyanate manufacturing plant included an extensive series of isocyanate exposure measurements, from which the workforce was usefully separated into categories of low-average cumulative exposure (≤ 68.2ppb-months) and high cumulative exposure (> 68.2 ppb-months).[28] The high exposure group did show a significantly greater annual decline in FEV_1 (−37 ml/year) than the non-smokers of the low exposure group (+1 ml/year), but it was not influenced by smoking. Smoking did, however, lead to a similar excessive decline in those with low levels of isocyanate exposure. Thus, the investigation suggested a modest excessive decline in FEV_1 as a consequence of

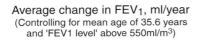

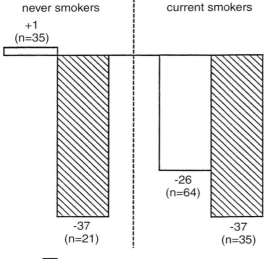

Average change in FEV₁, ml/year
(Controlling for mean age of 35.6 years
and 'FEV1 level' above 550ml/m³)

Figure 31.6 *Longitudinal loss of FEV, vs toluene diisocyanate (TDI) exposure. Compiled from data in Ref. 28. *ppb-months is the net result of multiplying the mean exposure in pints per billion (ppb) by the number of months over which the exposure is sustained.*

either isocyanate exposure or smoking, without there being any additive or multiplicative effects (Fig. 31.6). These conclusions differ from the general consensus, which does favour an interaction between smoking and the occupational environment, but they mirror those derived from the grain workers in the port of Vancouver. Interestingly, Diem and colleagues did attempt to identify asthmatics from their study population, and showed no weakening of the COPD effect when these workers were excluded from the analysis.

CHRONIC OBSTRUCTIVE PULMONARY DISEASE AND AGENTS NOT KNOWN TO INDUCE OCCUPATIONAL ASTHMA

Cadmium

Cadmium occupies an unusual place among occupational agents reported to cause COPD in that it appears to do so by causing emphysema. Occupational COPD attributable to non-focal emphysema seems otherwise to be confined to complicated pneumoconiosis. Cadmium-induced emphysema has not been without controversy, however, from the time of its first description in 1952.[29] For some years, doubts persisted as to whether smoking alone was responsible for the apparently excess prevalences of COPD noted among some, but not all, cad-

mium-exposed working populations.[30] More recent investigations involving long-term surveillance have provided more convincing evidence that cadmium does indeed cause emphysema.[31] Although cadmium is a trace component of cigarette smoke, cumulative exposures from smoking alone are not likely to approach those sustained occupationally. It seems improbable therefore that smoking-induced emphysema could be attributed to cadmium (see Chapter 7).

Mineral dusts

The mineral dusts (see Chapter 35) have provided perhaps the greatest opportunity for COPD controversy, even conflict.[32] Although airway obstruction was quickly recognized to be a feature of complicated pneumoconiosis and of its accompanying emphysema, COPD in the absence of complicated pneumoconiosis has generally been attributed to other, coincidental, disorders. High mortality rates from respiratory disease in some groups of miners led to early and intensive investigations of large numbers in many countries.[33–36] The outcome was the recognition that although complicated pneumoconiosis and occupational tuberculosis were associated with excess respiratory mortality and morbidity, the pattern of respiratory disease in miners was otherwise closely duplicated in their families and in suitably matched control populations.[37–40] It appeared to be related more to social circumstances (and particularly to smoking) than to the working environment.

The largest investigations have involved coal miners, principally because of the enormous populations employed over the years in the coal mining industry and partly because of political influence. In general, mean losses in ventilatory function attributable to coal dust exposure (rather than cigarette smoking) have been small or trivial in the absence of complicated pneumoconiosis, and because of the large numbers in many investigations these essentially negative findings have attracted high levels of confidence. Some investigations, however, have suggested that the COPD effect from coal dust might approach that of cigarette smoke.

The controversy has arisen because disabling levels of airway obstruction have been noted in a small minority of miners who claimed never to have smoked and who did not show evidence of complicated pneumoconiosis. They were found more prominently among retired miners, and protagonists have argued that this is to be expected in a job that did not readily tolerate any loss of physical fitness. Thus earlier reassuring epidemiological investigations of working coal miners were flawed by the industry's unusual susceptibility to the 'survivor effect'. Furthermore, a small mean loss in ventilatory function, which has not attracted much dispute, might be a consequence of large and disabling effects in a few miners rather than of small and clinically inconsequential losses in many. Antagonists have responded that smoking histories are notoriously unreliable in coal mining communities, and that if disabling losses of ventilatory function do occur they are more likely to be due to smoking (active or passive) or other non-occupational factors (perhaps asthma or the miners' penchant for breeding pigeons). Thus in one study 20% of miners who described themselves as light smokers were after death described by their relatives as heavy smokers;[41] and in another (quoted already) as many as 15% of miners, or their surviving families, claimed they had never smoked, having indicated in earlier surveys that they were regular smokers.[10]

The most recent detailed analyses of longitudinal data from UK and US coal mines did, like earlier cross-sectional investigations, provide evidence for a small excess decline in FEV_1, independent of pneumoconiosis and smoking, which was related to estimated cumulative levels of exposure to coal dust.[42–46] The decline in ventilatory function during the period of longitudinal surveillance could not, however, be related to the measured cumulative exposure during this time. The observed relationship lay with the cumulative exposure overall since employment began, and this was calculated from the measured levels during the study together with estimates of earlier levels using extrapolations. Because profound changes had occurred in both mechanization and ventilation within the mines, these estimates of cumulative exposure have been challenged. Furthermore, the estimated effects from coal dust, smoking, and increasing age have differed quite markedly between longitudinal and cross-sectional studies, and there is no clear consensus whether the coal dust effect is uninfluenced by smoking or is enhanced by it. This might be a consequence of co-linearity, since increasing age must be related to both cumulative exposure to coal dust and to cumulative consumption of cigarettes, thereby weakening the power of regression analyses to quantify the independent effect of any given variable. It has consequently been suggested that persisting controversies are not currently resolvable.[46] Nor are they ever likely to be, because exposure levels (hence risk) and the number of active coal miners (hence epidemiological power) have diminished too profoundly, and the optimal opportunity to demonstrate a COPD effect from coal dust has already passed.

The evidence overall nevertheless points to a COPD effect from coal dust. This has recently led to it becoming a prescribed industrial disease in Britain providing the claimant has worked underground for at least 20 years and severity is sufficient to reduce the FEV_1 by 1 litre from its predicted value (see Chapters 4 and 32).

A similar situation has arisen in South Africa, though strengthening evidence that respirable silica in gold mines might cause COPD was not published until after the introduction of state compensation in 1952.[47]

Again there has been controversy, some later investigations failing to provide clear confirmatory evidence of a silica-related loss of ventilatory function.[48,49] Other recent investigations (cross-sectional and longitudinal) have shown an excess of COPD in silica exposed workers which could not be attributed to smoking, but there was no clear relationship with intensity of exposure.[47,50,51] In one investigation silica and smoking appeared to exert effects of similar magnitude, while in another the influence of smoking on FEV_1 decline was approximately twice that of silica exposure. In the severe cases which led to death, an interaction between the two environmental factors seemed likely.

Welding fume (see Chapter 9)

Welding fume is conveniently considered separately from other mineral dusts, partly because the circumstances of exposure are rather different, partly because a possible COPD effect in welders is a matter of considerable topical interest, and partly because evidence of an additional asthmagenic effect in now emerging. Exposure to welding fume consequently brings the discussion full circle.

Consistent with the investigation of numerous workforces exposed regularly to respirable irritant or noxious dusts, vapours or fumes, many investigations of welders have demonstrated a clear excess prevalence of chronic productive cough (industrial bronchitis). Until recently none has found convincing evidence of an excess of airway obstruction implying, perhaps, that if there is a COPD effect it must be of relatively small degree.[52–54]

A small but significant COPD effect was the conclusion of a cross-sectional study of 607 shipyard workers carried out by Cotes and colleagues.[55] The workforce spanned an age range of 17–69 years. After allowing for age and height the trades associated with welding fume exposure showed a mean and significant overall loss in FEV_1 of 250 ml compared with the unexposed trades. This effect was noted only among the smokers. From the original study population, 487 were re-examined 7 years later.[56] Multiple regression analyses suggested that FEV_1 was declining at an annual rate of 16.2 ml for a 50-year-old non-smoking worker without occupational exposure to welding fume. The additional losses attributable to smoking and welding fume exposure were 17.7 ml/year and 16.4 ml/year respectively. Interactions were noted between welding fume and smoking, and between welding fume and atopy. There was no effect from welding fume on gas transfer. The longitudinal study consequently suggested that a mild COPD effect attributable to welding fume might also occur in non-smokers, but it confirmed that this effect was disproportionate in smokers. The further enhancement of the effect in atopic subjects provides a hint of an asthmatic component, and the lack of any effect on gas transfer suggests that COPD was not occurring as a consequence of emphysema.

A further hint that welding fume from mild steel might influence asthma (asthma is increasingly reported in stainless steel welders as a consequence of presumed chromium hypersensitivity) has emerged from work in a further shipyard.[57] Apprentices in various trades from the age of 16/17 years (when they left school) to 25/26 years (when they had completed 9 years work) were examined cross-sectionally. The investigation was focussed on methacholine tests to provide objective measurements of airway responsiveness.[58] Improving levels of airway responsiveness were associated with increasing age in apprentices without exposure to welding fume, but there was little age-related change in those with ambient exposure (shop floor trades not associated directly with fume generation), and airway responsiveness showed a small increase with age in the regular welders. The odds ratios for the estimated risk of having a positive methacholine test after 5 years work compared with the risk at 0 years are illustrated in Fig. 31.7. In essence the observations suggest that after 5 years of

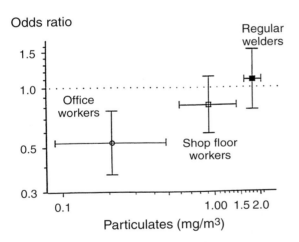

Figure 31.7 *Airway responsiveness vs welding exposure group. Odds ratios (+95% confidence intervals) for a positive methacholine test after working for 5 years. Reproduced with permission from Ref. 57.*

occupational exposure during the 1980s, when exposure levels were rigorously controlled, welding fume exposure led to a mean doubling of the level of airway responsiveness compared with that expected. This implies that of the regular welders with levels of airway responsiveness within the range consistent with active asthma, some 15–30%, depending on atopic status and smoking habits, represent an excess attributable to welding fume exposure.

PERSPECTIVE IN THE POPULATION AT LARGE

The relative risk posed to the general population by common allergens, outdoor air pollution, air pollution within the home, and respirable agents at work is a matter of increasing public concern, particularly with regard to the aetiology and progression of COPD and asthma. Both disorders are clearly dependent on changing patterns of life within developed countries, and so environmental factors must be of great relevance. It may be that many different respirable agents are capable of exerting an influence, and that in different individuals the measured COPD effects are due to different combinations of these agents (the 'multiple hit' hypothesis) together with some inherent susceptibility.

Recent investigations in the former East and West regions of Germany provide interesting comparisons within the developed world between an area of high smoking prevalence and relatively high outdoor air pollution from industrial emissions, and one of high domestic affluence.[59,60] It appears that COPD dominated in the former, and asthma in the latter; though in the more affluent societies there is greater not lesser outdoor pollution from vehicle exhausts. This is thought to be of relevance to asthma in Los Angeles where such pollution is persistently high and intermittently dramatically so, but a recent comparative study using measurements of airway responsiveness between an urban area with more modest exposure to vehicle exhaust (Newcastle upon Tyne, UK) and a rural area with low exposure (Cumbria and the English lake district) showed no difference.[61]

Further perspectives regarding the possible role of occupational exposures in the aetiology of COPD in the population at large can be seen from the results of an interesting epidemiological investigation of urban (Bergen) and rural (Hordaland) communities in western Norway.[62] A postal survey first sampled 5000 individuals from a total population of 250 000; and from the respondents an age stratified sample of 1500 was invited to undertake a more detailed investigation which included respiratory symptoms, smoking history, work history, and spirometry. In all, 1275 individuals participated. When COPD was defined from strict spirometric parameters alone ($FEV_1/FVC < 70\%$, and $FEV_1 < 80\%$ of predicted), smoking proved to be the only explanatory variable of clear relevance from multiple regression analyses.

When COPD was defined less stringently but more clinically from both objective spirometry ($FEV_1/FVC < 70\%$) and subjective symptoms (chronic productive cough together with undue breathlessness or wheeze), the odds ratios for participants reporting specific occupational exposure to aluminium, welding/metal fume, quartz or asbestos all increased to significant levels. So too did the odds ratio for heavy exposure to any source of occupational dust. An increased prevalence of COPD was also noted in the urban compared with rural communities, but this was attributable to the greater number of elderly individuals, who were affected disproportionately, living in the city of Bergen, Norway. The study population was consequently sufficiently large for subjective evidence of occupational productive cough to be demonstrated; but the excess prevalences of strictly defined airway obstruction, which were noted among certain groups of workers, did not reach conventional levels of statistical significance.

CONCLUSIONS

Evidence relating occupational environments to COPD is extensive but conflicting, and this inevitably stimulates controversy. Any summary is necessarily influenced by personal, biased, and possibly preconceived views; and so it should be emphasized that the following conclusions reflect a changing scene and a personal current interpretation of it. They also depend on additional, but often controversial, conclusions that COPD occurs with excessive prevalence in a number of other occupational settings, including paper pulping mills, printing, firefighting, and flour mills.[63-65]

- Some occupational environments are likely to exert a COPD effect.
- Its impact is likely to be less than that of smoking (perhaps much less), but will vary from industry to industry depending on potency and exposure level of the agent involved.
- Complex adverse interactions probably exist with smoking, and (presumably) with other environmental agents.
- Many environmental factors may be of relevance to its aetiology – the so called 'multiple hit' hypothesis.
- It is plausible that both asthmatic and non-asthmatic pathways play a role.
- It will be found rarely in the absence of either smoking or asthma.

REFERENCES

1 Bouhuys A, Heaphy LJ, Schilling RSF, Welborn JW. Byssinosis in the United States. *N Engl J Med* 1967; **227**: 170–5.

2 Schilling RSF, Vigliani EC, Lammers B, Valic F, Gilson JC. *A Report on a Conference on Byssinosis* (14th International Conference on Occupational Health, Madrid 1963). Int Congr Series No 62, Amsterdam: Excerpta Medica, 1963: 137–44.

3 Parkes WR. Occupational asthma (including byssinosis). In: *Occupational Lung Disorders*. London: Butterworth 1982: 445.

4 Glindmeyer HW, Lefante JJ, Jones RN, Rando RJ, Kader HMA, Weill H. Exposure-related declines in the lung function of cotton textile workers. Relationship to current workplace standards. *Am Rev Respir Dis* 1991; **144**: 675–83.

5 Glindmeyer HW, Lefante JJ, Jones RN, Rando RJ, Kader HMA, Weill H. Cotton dust and across-shift change in FEV_1 as predictors of annual change in FEV_1. *Am J Respir Crit Care Med* 1994; **149**: 584–90.

6 Morgan WKC, Seaton A. *Occupational Lung Disease.* Philadelphia: W B Saunders Co., 1984.

7 Ciba Guest Symposium. *Thorax* 1959; **14**: 286.

8 Hendrick DJ, Beach JR, Avery AJ, Dennis JH, Stenton SC. *An Epidemiological Investigation of Asthma in Apprentice (Shipyard) Welders*. A report to the Medical Research Council and Health and Safety Executive, 1994.

9 Wald NJ, Nanchahal K, Thompson SG, Cuckle HS. Does breathing other people's tobacco smoke cause lung cancer? *Br Med J* 1986; **293**: 1217–21.

10 Lapp NL, Morgan WK, Zaldivar G. Airways obstruction, coal mining and disability. *Occup Environ Med* 1994; **51**: 234–8.

11 Fletcher CM, Peto R, Tinker C, Speizer F. *The Natural History of Chronic Bronchitis and Emphysema*. Oxford: Oxford University Press, 1976.

12 Glindmeyer HW, Diem JE, Jones RN, Weill H. Noncomparability of longitudinally and cross-sectionally determined annual change in spirometry. *Am Rev Respir Dis* 1982; **125**: 544–8.

13 Becklake MR. Chronic airflow limitation: its relationship to work in dusty occupations. *Chest* 1985; **88**: 608–17.

14 Brooks SM, Weiss MA, Bernstein IL. Reactive airways dysfunction syndrome. Case reports of persistent airways hyperreactivity following high-level irritant exposures. *J Occup Med* 1985; **27**: 473–6.

15 Cohen BH, Diamond EL, Graves CG *et al.* A common familial component in lung cancer and chronic obstructive airways disease. *Lancet* 1977; **ii**: 523–6.

16 Redline S, Tishler PV, Lewitter FI *et al.* Assessment of genetic and non-genetic influences on pulmonary function: a twin study. *Am Rev Respir Dis* 1987; **135**: 217–22.

17 Tashkin DP, Altose MD, Connett JE, Kanner RE, Lee WW, Wise RA. Methacholine reactivity predicts changes in lung function over time in smokers with early chronic obstructive pulmonary disease. The Lung Health Study Research Group. *Am J Respir Care Med* 1996; **153**: 1802–11.

18 Van der Lende R. *The Epidemiology of Chronic Nonspecific Lung Disease*: Vol 1: *A Critical Analysis of Three Field Surveys of CNSLD Carried Out in the Netherlands*. Assen: Van Gorcum & Co, 1969.

19 Potsma DS, de Vries K, Koeter GH, Sluiter HJ. Independent influence of reversibility of air-flow obstruction and nonspecific hyperreactivity on the long-term course of lung function in chronic air-flow obstruction. *Am Rev Respir Dis* 1986; **134**: 276–80.

20 doPico GA, Reddan W, Flaherty D *et al.* Respiratory abnormalities among grain handlers: a clinical, physiologic and immunologic study. *Am Rev Respir Dis* 1977; **115**: 915–27.

21 Becklake MR. Grain dust and health. In: Dosman JA, Cotton DJ eds. *Occupational Pulmonary Disease in Grain Workers: Focus on Srain Dust and Health*. New York: Academic Press, 1980: 189–200.

22 Chan-Yeung M, Enarson DA, Kennedy SM. The impact of grain dust on respiratory health. State of the Art. *Am Rev Respir Dis* 1992; **145**: 476–87.

23 Chan-Yeung M, Lam S, Koerner S. Clinical features and natural history of occupational asthma due to Western Red Cedar (*Thuja plicata*). *Am J Med* 1982; **72**: 411–5.

24 Warren CPW. Extrinsic allergic alveolitis: a disease commoner in non-smokers *Thorax* 1977; **32**: 567–9.

25 Valleyre D, Soler P, Clerici C *et al.* Smoking and pulmonary sarcoidosis: effect cigarette smoking on prevalence, clinical manifestations, alveolitis, and evolution of the disease. *Thorax* 1988; **43**: 516–24.

26 Adams WGF. Long-term effects on the health of men engaged in the manufacture of tolylene diisocyanate. *Br J Ind Med* 1975; **32**: 72–8.

27 Peters JM, Murphy RLH, Pagnotto LD, Whittenberger JL. Respiratory impairment in workers exposed to 'safe' levels of toluene diisocyanate (TDI). *Arch Environ Hlth* 1970; **20**: 364–7.

28 Diem JE, Jones RN, Hendrick DJ, Glindmeyer HW, Dharmarajan V *et al.* Five-year longitudinal study of workers employed in a new toluene diisocyanate manufacturing plant. *Am Rev Respir Dis* 1982; **126**: 420–8.

29 Baader EW. Chronic cadmium poisoning. *Ind Med Surg* 1952; **21**: 427–30.

30 Leading article. Cadmium and the lung. *Lancet* 1973; **ii**: 1134–5.

31 Davison AG, Fayers PM, Newman Taylor AJ *et al.* Cadmium fume inhalation and emphysema *Lancet* 1988; **i**: 663–7.

32 Stenton SC, Hendrick DJ. Airflow obstruction and mining. In: Banks DE ed. The mining industry. *Occup6 Med State Art Rev* 1993; **8**: 155–70.

33 *The Registrar General's Decennial Supplement, England and Wales, 1951. Occupational mortality*, Pt II, Vol I, *Commentary*. London: HMSO, 1958.

34 Enterline PE. Mortality rates among coal miners. *Am J Publ Hlth* 1964; **54**: 758–68.

35 Atuhaire LK, Campbell MJ, Cochrane AL *et al.* Mortality of men in the Rhondda Fach 1950–80. *Br J Ind Med* 1985; **42**: 741–5.

36 Finkelstein M, Kusiak R, Suranyi G. Mortality among miners receiving compensation for silicosis in Ontario: 1940–75. *J Occup Med* 1982; **24**: 663–7.

37 Medical Research Council report. Chronic bronchitis and occupation. *Br Med J* 1966; **1**: 101–2.

38 Miller BG, Jacobson M. Dust exposure, pneumoconiosis, and mortality of coal miners. *Br J Ind Med* 1985; **42**: 723–33.

39 Foxman B, Higgins ITT, Oh MS. The effects of occupation and smoking on respiratory disease mortality. *Am Rev Respir Dis* 1986; **134**: 649–52.

40 Ortmeyer CE, Costello J, Morgan WKC *et al.* The mortality of Appalachian coal miners, 1963 to 1971. *Arch Environ Hlth* 1974; **29**: 67–72.

41 Cockcroft A, Seal RME, Wagner JC *et al.* Postmortem study of emphysema in coal workers and non-coal workers. *Lancet* 1982; **ii**: 600–3.

42 Love RG, Miller BG. Longitudinal study of lung function in coal-miners. *Thorax* 1982; **37**: 193–7.

43 Attfield MD, Hodous TK. Pulmonary function of US coal miners related to dust exposure estimates. *Am Rev Respir Dis* 1992; **145**: 605–609.

44 Marine WM, Gurr D, Jacobson M. Clinically important respiratory effects of dust exposure and smoking in British coal miners. *Am Rev Respir Dis* 1988; **137**: 106–12.

45 Soutar C, Campbell S, Gurr D, Lloyd M, Love R *et al.* Important deficits of lung function in three modern colliery populations. Relations with dust exposure. *Am Rev Respir Dis* 1993; **147**: 797–803.

46 Seixas NS, Robbins TG, Attfield MD, Moulton LH. Longitudinal and cross-sectional analyses of exposure to coal mine dust and pulmonary function in new miners. *Br J Ind Med* 1993; **50**: 929–37.

47 Hnizdo E. Loss of lung function asociated with exposure to silica dust and with smoking and its relation to disability and mortality in South African gold miners. *Br J Ind Med* 1992; **49**: 472–9.

48 Sluis-Cremer GK, Walers IG, Sichel HS. Ventilatory function in relation to mining experience and smoking in a random sample of miners and non-miners in a Witwatersrand town. *Br J Ind Med* 1967; **24**: 13–25.

49 Manfreda J, Sidwall G, Maini K, West P, Cherniack RM. Respiratory abnormalities in employees of the hard rock mining industry. *Am Rev Respir Dis* 1982; **126**: 629–34.

50 Hnizdo E. Combined effect of silica dust and tobacco smoking on mortality from chronic obstructive lung disease in gold miners. *Br J Ind Med* 1990; **47**: 656–64.

51 Cowie RL, Mabena SK. Silicosis, chronic airflow limitation, and chronic bronchitis in South African gold miners. *Am Rev Respir Dis* 1991; **143**: 80–4.

52 Barhad B, Teculescu D, Craciun O. Respiratory symptoms, chronic bronchitis, and ventilatory function in shipyard welders. *Int Arch Occup Environ Hlth* 1975; **36**: 137–150.

53 McMillan GHG, Pethybridge RJ. A clinical, radiological and pulmonary function case control study of 135 dockyard welders aged 45 years and over. *J Soc Occup Med* 1984; **34**: 3–23.

54 Simonato L, Fletcher AC, Andersen A, Anderson K, Becker N *et al.* A historical prospective study of European stainless steel, mild steel, and shipyard welders. *Br J Ind Med* 1991; **48**: 145–54.

55 Cotes JE, Feinmann EL, Male VJ, Rennie FS, Wickham CAC. Respiratory symptoms and impairment in shipyard welders and caulker/burners. *Br J Ind Med* 1989; **46**: 292–301.

56 Chinn DJ, Stevenson IC, Cotes JE. Longitudinal respiratory survey of shipyard workers: effects of trade and atopic status. *Br J Ind Med* 1990; **47**: 83–90.

57 Beach JR, Dennis JH, Avery AJ, Bromly CL, Ward R *et al.* An epidemiologic investigation of asthma in welders. *Am J Respir Crit Care Med* 1996; **154**: 1394–1400.

58 Beach JR, Young CL, Avery AJ, Stenton SC, Dennis JH. Measurement of airway responsiveness to methacholine: relative importance of the precision of drug delivery and

the method of assessing response. *Thorax* 1993; **48**: 239–43.

59 von Mutius E, Fritzsch C, Weiland SK, Roll G, Magnussen H. Prevalence of asthma and allergic disorders among children in united Germany: a descriptive comparison. *Br Med J* 1992; **305**: 1395–9.

60 Schlipkopter HW, Stiller-Winkler R, Ring J, Willer HJ. Impact of air pollution on children's health: results from Saxony-Anhalt and Saxony as compared to Northrhine-Westphalia. In: *Health and Ecological Effects*. Papers from the 9th World Clean Air Congress, Montreal, Quebec, Canada 1992. Pittsburgh: Air and Waste Management Association, 1992.

61 Devereux G, Ayatollahi SMT, Bourke SJ, Hendrick DJ. Effect of gender and geography on the prevalence of asthma symptoms and airway responsiveness (AR). *Am Rev Respir Dis* 1994; **4**: A915.

62 Bakke PS, Batse V, Hanoa R, Gulsvik A. Prevalence of obstructive lung disease in a general population: relation to occupational title and exposure to some airborne agents. *Thorax* 1991; **46**: 863–70.

63 Chan-Yeung M, Wong R, Maclean L *et al.* Respiratory survey of workers in a pulp and paper mill in Powell River, British Columbia. *Am Rev Respir Dis* 1980; **122**: 249–57.

64 Sparrow D, Bosse R, Rosner B, Weiss ST. The effect of occupational exposure on pulmonary function: a longitudinal evaluation of fire fighters and non fire fighters. *Am Rev Respir Dis* 1982; **125**: 319–22.

65 Kauffman F, Drouet D, Lellouch J, Brille D. Occupational exposure and 12-year spirometric changes among Paris area workers. *Br J Ind Med* 1982; **39**: 221–32.

66 Parkes WR. Chronic bronchitis, airflow obstruction and emphysema. In: Parkes WR ed. *Occupational Lung Disorders* 3rd edn. Butterworth-Heinemann, 1994: 223.

67 Becklake MR. Relationship of acute obstructive airways change to chronic (fixed) obstruction. *Thorax* 1995; **50**(Suppl): 516–21.

68 Hendrick DJ. Chronic and obstructive pulmonary disease (COPD). *Thorax* 1996; **51**: 947–55.

Byssinosis and other cotton-related diseases

CAC PICKERING

Prevalence studies	622	Pharmacological responses	627
Pathology	622	Smoking and byssinosis	627
Pathogenesis	622	Physical signs	627
Atopic status and bronchial		Chronic bronchitis	627
hyperreactivity	624	Prevention	628
Mortality and morbidity	625	Management	629
Clinical features	625	References	629

Respiratory disease associated with exposure to textile dusts was first recognized by Ramazzini amongst flax and hemp workers. The term byssinosis, which is derived from the Greek for flax, was first used by the Parisian physician A Proust in 1877.[1] Earlier in 1831 Kay, a Manchester physician, described cotton spinner's phthisis.[2] This condition was characterized by a work-related cough, which initially resolved on leaving the mill, later becoming more severe and persistent and associated with a sensation of uneasiness beneath the sternum. The first description of the symptom pattern now associated with byssinosis, that is respiratory symptoms most severe at the start of the working week, was given in 1845 by Mareska and Heyman.[3]

> All the workers have told us that the dust bothered them much less on the last days of the week than on the Monday and Tuesday. The masters find the cause of this increased sensitivity to be in the excesses of the Sunday, but the workers never fail to attribute it to the interruption of work which, they say, makes them lose, in part, their habituation to the dust.

Then in 1860 in response to concern about the high death rates from respiratory disease in some Lancashire towns, Greenhow[4] investigated the causes of this excess of pulmonary disease and described an asthma like-condition in cotton workers worse at the beginning of the working week and most severe on returning to work after a longer period away from work than a weekend. This syndrome is now generally referred to as byssinosis.[4] Subsequently byssinosis has been reported from most countries with a textile industry.[5–8] More recently the terminology relating to byssinosis has become complicated by the introduction of the terms acute and chronic byssinosis. Acute byssinosis referring to acute responses occuring in artificial cardrooms in subjects exposed to cotton dust or extracts of cotton dust for the first time. The relationship of this acute, fully reversible, response to the chronic changes which develop in cotton workers exposed to cotton dust for many years remains to be determined by prospective studies. It is likely that this acute response contributes to the high labour turnover which is seen in the first year of employment[9] in cotton spinning mills. Textile workers may also experience other acute symptoms (mill fever) on exposure to cotton, flax or hemp dust. Mill fever characteristically occurs following a worker's first exposure to cotton, flax or hemp dust. It consists of a fever with a non-productive cough, malaise and sneezing which usually lasts for a few hours, resolving despite continued exposure to dust.[10] It is thought that mill fever is due to endotoxins from Gram-negative bacteria contaminating the cotton.

PREVALENCE STUDIES

The prevalence of byssinosis amongst cotton workers depends on the quality and airborne concentration of cotton dust to which workers are exposed and to the duration of their exposure. The majority of prevalence studies have been cross-sectional in design and have thus been looking at 'survivor' populations and, therefore, likely to underestimate the true prevalence of this disease. The reduction in dust levels over the past 30 years has led to a fall in the prevalence of byssinosis. In the late 1950s in the United Kingdom the prevalence amongst male cardroom workers (coarse cotton) was 43% and in blowroom workers 66%.[11] By the 1970s the prevalence (combined) had fallen to 24%[12] and now the current overall prevalence of byssinosis in 30 Lancashire cotton mills is 4%.[13] The number of new cases developing under current working conditions in the UK is likely to be very small. In 1996 there were only four byssinotic claims for injury and disablement benefit under the Industrial Injuries Scheme in the UK.

In the USA similar prevalence rates have been found.[14] However, in some parts of the world (Australia) the prevalence of byssinosis has been found to be negligible, 1.1% (two of 176 employees) exposed at the time of the study to mean dust levels of between 0.14 mg/m³ to 0.25 mg/m³.[15] Earlier studies[16] revealed similarly low prevalence rates. In third world countries the prevalence of byssinosis remains high: Indonesia: 21.4–30%; Ethiopia: 24–43.2%; Sudan: 37% and India: 29.6–37.8%.

The prevalence of byssinosis has in past studies also been related to smoking habits, smokers having 1.4 times the frequency of byssinosis compared with non- or ex-smokers. The prevalence of byssinosis is also influenced by occupational group, being most frequent amongst Opening room operatives and cardroom workers (strippers and grinders) followed by drawframe tenters and least common amongst ring spinners.[17]

In flax workers the prevalence of byssinosis may also be related to occupational group, the dustiest jobs being associated with the highest prevalences.[18,19]

PATHOLOGY

No specific abnormalities have been described associated with byssinosis. Mucous gland hyperplasia and hypertrophy of smooth muscle have been described in upper and lower lobe bronchi, but not to a significant degree in segmental bronchi.[20] Emphysema was not a dominant feature. The finding of smooth muscle hypertrophy and mucous gland hyperplasia is of interest since it is a pathological finding in bronchial asthmatics rather than chronic bronchitis.[21] These pathological findings are consistent with physiological studies[22] in smoking and non-smoking byssinotics, the presence of emphysema and its severity being related to the cigarette smoking habits of the individual and unrelated to cotton dust exposure.

PATHOGENESIS

Despite the fact that byssinosis has been recognized for over 100 years the aetiology and pathogenesis remain obscure. The ability of textile fibres to produce byssinosis is determined by fibre type – cotton being the most potent, followed by flax, hemp and finally possibly sisal. Harvested cotton consists of a mixture of plant materials including leaves, bracts and stems; fibre; bacteria; fungi and other contaminants. An important fact is that the compounds which cause byssinosis are water soluble. The biological activity of cotton can be greatly reduced by either steaming[23] or washing[24] the cotton before processing. The particles of bract have attracted particular attention since aerosolization of extracts of bracts but not other plant components can cause acute symptoms similar to those of byssinosis[22] and will also release significant amounts of histamine from human lung tissue.[25] As cotton bract, specialized leaves at the base of the cotton flower, mature they become hard and brittle, shattering into small particles during harvesting and adhering to the cotton fibre. They comprise a major constituent of cotton dust in the mill. Many different compounds have been examined.

A number of different mechanisms have been proposed to explain the pathogenesis of byssinosis: immunological, bacterial endotoxin activity, non-immunological release of histamine and fungus enzymes.

Immunological mechanisms

The hypothesis that a specific immunological response is involved in the causation of byssinosis is appealing for a number of reasons. There is a time interval, usually of many years, between the development of symptoms and first exposure to cotton, compatible with a period of exposure prior to sensitization. In addition it is now a minority of workers who are affected by byssinosis. However, the majority of studies have failed to show convincing evidence of an immunological mechanism. Skin tests using cotton dust extracts failed to differentiate between normal, atopic and byssinotic subjects. The fact that 90% of normal subjects gave a late skin response suggests a non-immunological mechanism. In a further study[26] of groups of workers with byssinosis, asthma and chronic bronchitis, immediate skin responses and frequent late responses were demonstrated. Again the positive skin responses were not limited to those individuals with byssinosis.

Inhalation tests with textile allergens were also performed and positive reactions were obtained in only four of 39 subjects with byssinosis.

The total immunoglobulin E (IgE) levels in textile mill workers both with and without byssinosis show no difference between the subject groups and there is no relationship between the clinical grade of byssinosis and the level of IgE.[27] Because fungal antigens may play a part in the aetiology of byssinosis (see below), a study[28] of the antigenic composition of aqueous cotton extracts was made. It demonstrated a significant immune response directed against known fungal contaminants of cotton dust: *Alternaria tenuis*, *Aspergillus niger* and *Fusarium solani*.

There is at present no evidence that atopy plays a part in the aetiology of byssinosis. It would seem more likely that atopic mill workers develop IgE-mediated respiratory disease early in their employment and so select themselves out of the industry at an early stage.[29]

The finding of late skin responses raises the possibility of IgG-mediated pulmonary responses. Precipitating IgG antibody to cotton antigen is present in both cotton and non-cotton workers. Its titre is highest in grade 2 byssinotics, lower in non-byssinotic workers and lowest in unexposed subjects.[30,31] These elevated IgG antibody titres are probably markers of exposure to cotton dust rather than indicators of disease.

A condensed polyphenol (leucocyanidin) has been isolated from the bracts of cotton plants and used in inhalation studies in byssinotic and non-byssinotic subjects.[30] The challenge produced symptoms similar to those that they experienced in the mill without changes in lung function in five of six byssinotic subjects and in none of 11 non-byssinotic workers. A similar study[32] in a group of 29 byssinotic workers and 31 normal controls using the same polyphenol did not produce any significant differences in symptoms or pulmonary function changes between the two groups. Other *in vitro* experiments have shown that cotton mill dust can activate complement by the classical and alternative pathways[33] and demonstrated the release from rat fundal smooth muscle and cultured rabbit alveolar macrophages of prostaglandin F2 alpha.[34,35]

It is clear from these experimental studies that cotton dust is highly biologically active and capable of mediating an inflammatory response via a variety of different pathways.

Bacterial endotoxins

The presence of large quantities of Gram-negative bacteria in cotton mills was first reported by a Home Office Commission in 1932.[36] Ten years later the relationship between the grade of the cotton and the degree of contamination by Gram-negative bacteria was first described.[37] An endotoxin-like substance was identified in extracts from contaminated cotton and from the organism cultured from the cotton.

Subsequently, a role for endotoxin has been proposed in the aetiology of byssinosis.[38] The predominant species of Gram-negative bacteria found in cotton dust is of the *Enterobacter* genus and endotoxin is derived from the lipopolysaccharide cell wall. The relationship between the prevalence of byssinotic symptoms, dust concentrations and airborne Gram-negative bacteria[39] has been studied. The prevalence of byssinosis was shown to correlate better with concentrations of airborne bacteria than with dust concentrations. In a study[40] of millworkers with and without a history of byssinosis, who were challenged with varying levels of endotoxin and cotton dust in an experimental cardroom, a dose-response relationship was demonstrated between endotoxin levels, symptoms of byssinosis and mean group changes in forced expiratory volume in 1 second (FEV_1) in exposed workers. A dose–response trend between (FEV_1), the prevalence of byssinosis and current levels of endotoxin was also found in a study of Chinese cotton workers.[41] This study failed to show a significant relationship between current exposure to endotoxin and acute change in FEV_1.

Other studies have cast doubt on the role of endotoxin in the acute airway constrictor response. Healthy volunteers challenged with aqueous extracts of cotton bracts containing 0.086–50 µg/ml of endotoxin, showed no correlation between the severity of the airway constrictor response and the concentration of endotoxin. When endotoxin was almost completely eliminated from the extracts, airway responses were still greater than 60% of the responses seen with crude bract extract.[42] In a group of normal subjects, challenge tests using flax dust containing a known concentration of endotoxin produced an airway constrictor response whereas with pure endotoxin at an equivalent concentration there was no significant airways constriction.[43]

The non-immunological release of histamine

The release of pharmacological mediators such as histamine has been postulated as an explanation of the acute symptoms of byssinosis occurring on the first day back at work. Although histamine is found in the respirable fraction of cotton dust itself, the amounts present in the inhaled dust are considered too small to produce airways narrowing. The levels of blood histamine have been shown to be elevated in both flax and cotton workers within 2 hours of starting work, falling to pre-challenge levels by the second morning in all workers except those with grade II byssinotic symptoms. Cotton exposure produced significantly higher levels of blood histamine than exposure to flax. The concentration of the histamine metabolite, l-methyl-imidazole-4-acetic acid is increased in the 24 hour urinary specimens of control subjects challenged with cotton dust.

Nevertheless, the release of histamine alone does not explain the development of byssinosis, since histamine release is demonstrated in all those exposed, and immediate pulmonary responses occur on bronchial challenge with histamine, whereas byssinosis itself takes years to develop and immediate type responses during a working shift are usually not demonstrable.

Fungus enzymes

Cotton dust has a proteolytic enzyme activity, originating from contaminating microorganisms. Although it has been suggested that airborne enzyme concentrations in cotton dust correlate better than cotton dust itself with airway responses in cotton workers, there is a low incidence of byssinosis in some work situations (cotton willowing mills) where there are high enzyme levels.[44]

ATOPIC STATUS AND BRONCHIAL HYPERREACTIVITY

Because cotton dust may be highly contaminated by Gram-negative bacteria, endotoxin and fungi, it might be anticipated that atopic cotton workers would be unduly susceptible to the development of allergic respiratory disease from prolonged exposure to these agents. Some evidence suggests this. Cross-sectional studies of cotton workers have revealed a low prevalence of atopy (positive skin tests to common environmental allergens) compared with the prevalence in the general population. Only 15% of 30 workers in four cotton seed crushing mills had positive skin tests to two or more of ten common inhalant antigens. A similar percentage was found among 324 byssinotic subjects compared with 23.5% in an age- and sex-matched control population.[29] These figures suggest that the populations being studied are survivor populations from whom atopic subjects have selected out at an early age. In a study of the effect of atopy on the ventilatory decline across a working shift, the workers were divided into three dust exposure groups, in one of which (linter dust) there was a positive association between atopic status and large mean declines in FEV_1 and forced expiratory flow (FEF_{25-75}) across the working shift.

Atopic subjects frequently possess a degree of bronchial hyperreactivity which may be important in determining the bronchoconstrictor response to cotton dust. Cotton workers who develop constitutional bronchial asthma and known asthmatic subjects who enter a cotton mill tend to develop rapidly increasing airways obstruction and have to leave the mill at an early stage (personal observation).

It is surprising that so little research has been carried out on the effect of airways reactivity on the pulmonary responses of cotton workers considering its potential importance in determining the development of early respiratory disease and perhaps the degree of disability associated with byssinosis itself. The acute airways constrictor response to cotton bract extract in normal subjects was significantly greater to methacholine challenge than the non-responder group. The baseline measurements of pulmonary function were, however, significantly lower in the responder group than the non-responder group, offering another possible explanation for the difference between the two groups.[45] An earlier study, using histamine to measure airways reactivity, had failed to show any significant difference in airways reactivity between responders and non-responders to cotton bract extract challenge in another group of healthy subjects.

Studies of airways reactivity in byssinotic subjects have also given contradictory results. Histamine challenge studies, using two concentrations of histamine acid phosphate (0.03% and 0.1%). were performed on 26 cardroom workers, divided into two groups; one with pure byssinosis and a second with 'bronchitic byssinosis' (byssinosis with cough and sputum). The groups differed significantly in terms of their grades of byssinosis, length of exposure to cotton dust and their lung function, the bronchitic byssinotic group having higher grades of byssinosis, longer exposure to cotton dust and impaired lung function. There was a highly significant increase in airways reactivity in the bronchitic byssinotic group, nine of the 12 having falls in FEV_1 greater than 20% at a histamine concentration of 0.03%[46].

A second study, using a nitrogen washout method to estimate the bronchoconstrictive effect of inhaled histamine in control, asthmatic and byssinotic subjects, demonstrated a response to histamine at a concentration of 1 mg/ml or less in only two of 11 byssinotic subjects, in 10 of 13 asthmatic subjects and in none of 10 control subjects.[47]

The acute effect of cotton dust exposure on cotton workers[48] both with and without byssinosis, using a methacholine challenge to evaluate pre- and post-shift changes in airway reactivity, demonstrated an increase across the shift in 11 of the 16 byssinotic subjects. Baseline levels of airway reactivity were increased in the byssinotic subjects compared with the controls. A more recent study[49] was made of 85 cotton operatives with work-related symptoms and matched asymptomatic controls from the same mills. Of the symptomatic group, 23 were byssinotic and the remainder had work-related symptoms which did not conform to a diagnosis of byssinosis. Of the 23 byssinotics, 18 had increased airway reactivity, whereas 21 of 56 of the symptomatic non-byssinotic subjects and 14 of 84 of the asymptomatic subjects had increased airway reactivity. The byssinotic group thus had the highest levels of reactivity and the symptomatic non-byssinotics had an intermediate level. The distribution of atopy between the three groups did not differ significantly. It is interesting that in the byssinotic group the only factor differentiating responders from non-responders was the presence of bronchitic symptoms – a feature shown in the original paper.[46]

MORTALITY AND MORBIDITY

The long-term effects of exposure to cotton and flax dusts on lung function in textile workers both with and without byssinosis has recently become controversial. Early epidemiological studies in the UK suggested an excess morbidity and mortality amongst cotton workers. In 1909 a study of strippers and grinders from 31 mills showed a prevalence of an asthma-like condition varying between 74 and 91%[50] and it was noted that it was unusual for these men to remain in the cardroom beyond the age of 45. Twenty years later there were high death rates from respiratory disease amongst strippers and grinders when compared with ringroom and warehousemen. Surveys of cardroom workers 25 years further on revealed a prevalence of 14% of severe respiratory disease.

Mortality figures at that time are difficult to interpret as death was related to the last occupation of the workers and many individuals with respiratory disability left the industry to take up lighter jobs. Over the last 30 years there have been considerable improvements in working conditions in textile mills with marked reductions in dust levels. Several recent mortality studies have failed to demonstrate an increased mortality amongst textile workers or workers with byssinosis.[51,52] In a recent mortality study of a cohort of British workers initially identified between 1968 and 1970 both the total mortality and the mortality due to respiratory disease was less than expected in the whole study population although the respiratory disease mortality was raised in those who had initially reported byssinotic symptoms.[53]

There is accumulating evidence that even at low levels of exposure to textile dusts a small excess loss of lung function is demonstrable which may be greater in man-made fibre than in cotton workers. In a recent longitudinal study[54] of a large population of cotton and man-made fibre workers, with low cotton dust exposures (only 1% of the population had symptoms of byssinosis), a dose–response accelerated decline in FEV_1 and forced vital capacity (FVC) were observed in smoking cotton yarn workers (the highest exposure group) but not in non-smokers in the same work area or in workers in other cotton work areas. The declines demonstrated in current smokers were 41.2 ml/year at average dust exposures of 150 $\mu g/m^3$, 49.3 ml/year at 200 $\mu g/m^3$ and 57.4 ml/year at 250 $\mu g/m^3$. The accelerated declines in FEV_1 appear to be produced by a synergistic effect between cotton dust exposure and current smoking. An additional predictor of accelerated lung decline, was across-shift change in FEV_1. An unexpected and unexplained finding in this study was the demonstration of larger declines in lung function in the man-made fibre workers than in the cotton textile workers even after accounting for possible confounding factors.

A different approach, measuring the prevalence and incidence of disability pensions for respiratory and other diseases has been reported in a cohort of Finnish mill workers with a minimum exposure to cotton dust of 5 years. Both the prevalence and incidence of disability pensions were greater than expected, although there was no excess in standardized mortality ratios for respiratory diseases.[55]

The evidence suggests that exposure to cotton dust does cause a small, significant loss of lung function in textile workers, as a whole, and that a small subgroup (with byssinosis) develop respiratory disability with an associated excess mortality from respiratory disease. The presence of increased bronchial reactivity may be important in determining the presence of residual disability but any possible relationship with mortality is unknown.

CLINICAL FEATURES

Cross-sectional studies of textile spinning operatives have documented a variety of work related ocular and upper and lower respiratory tract symptoms on exposure to cotton and synthetic fibres.[56,57] These include ocular and nasal irritation, byssinosis, chronic bronchitis, persistent cough, non-byssinotic work-related chest tightness and work-related wheeze with work-related ocular (17.5%) and work-related nasal irritation (11%) being the most common symptoms complained of by both cotton and synthetic textile workers, with the prevalence being higher amongst cotton workers than synthetic fibre workers.

Acute byssinosis

The contribution that the symptoms of acute byssinosis (described in the introduction) make in the mills is not known. Artificial cardroom experiments suggest that approximately one-third of operatives exposed to cotton dust for the first time will experience a significant fall in lung function across the exposure period. Falls in FEV_1 exceeding 30% have been described after such experimental exposures.[58] One would anticipate that this would lead to a high labour turnover in the first year of employment. This has recently been documented in Finnish cotton spinning mills, where 10% of employees left within 2 weeks and 25% left within 3 months of taking up employment.[59] The across-shift changes demonstrated in the absence of symptoms[60] may represent one end of the spectrum of these responders.

Chronic byssinosis

The development of symptoms of byssinosis is rare in the first 5 years exposure to cotton, hemp or flax dusts and usually requires a period of dust exposure of between 20 and 25 years. The symptoms of byssinosis consist of chest tightness and breathlessness characteristically developing on the first day of the working week over the second half of the working shift and experienced most severely with the exertion of returning home in the evening. Other workers describe the very rapid onset of symptoms within 30 minutes of starting work, which may be most severe over the first half of the shift.[36] In all these workers their symptoms were most severe on the first working day. Roach and Schilling[61] devised a scheme for grading the clinical stages of byssinosis:

Grade 0: No symptoms of chest tightness or breathlessness on Mondays.

Grade 1/2: Occasional chest tightness on Mondays, or mild symptoms such as irritation of the respiratory tract on Mondays.

Grade 1: Chest tightness and/or breathlessness on Mondays only.

Grade 2: Chest tightness and/or breathlessness on Mondays and other days.

Later this was modified by substituting 'difficulty in breathing' instead of 'breathlessness' and adding a third grade:

Grade 3: Grade 2 symptoms accompanied by evidence of permanent respiratory disability from reduced ventilatory capacity.

Table 32.1 *WHO classification of byssinosis*

Classification	Symptoms
Grade 0	**No symptoms**
Byssinosis	
Grade B1	Chest tightness and/or short of breath on most of first days back at work
Grade B2	Chest tightness and/or short of breath on the first and other days of the working week
Respiratory tract irritation	
Grade RTI 1	Cough associated with dust exposure
Grade RTI 2	Persistent phlegm (i.e. on most days during 3 months of the year) initiated or exacerbated by dust exposure
Grade RTI 3	Persistent phlegm initiated or made worse by dust exposure either with exacerbations of chest illness or persisting for 2 years or more
Lung function	
1. Acute changes	
No effect	A consistent[a] decline in FEV_1 of less than 5% or an increase in FEV_1 during the work shift
Mild effect	A consistent[a] decline of between 5 and 10% in FEV_1 during the work shift
Moderate effect	A consistent[a] decline of between 10 and 20% in FEV_1 during the work shift
Severe effect	A decline of 20% or more in FEV_1 during the work shift
2. Chronic changes	
No effect	FEV_1[a] – 80% of predicted value[c]
Mild-to-moderate effect	FEV_1[b] – 60–79% of predicted value[c]
Severe effect	FEV_1[b] – less than 60% of predicted value[c]

[a]A decline occurring in at least three consecutive tests made after an absence from dust exposure of 2 days or more.
[b]Predicted values should be based on data obtained from local populations or similar ethnic and social class groups.
[c]By a pre-shift test after an absence from dust exposure of 2 days or more.

This clinical grading has been widely accepted and used for most epidemiological studies. It does, however, have shortcomings in that it does not take into account either the irritant effects of dust exposure or the lung function changes which may occur in asymptomatic workers. In order to try and address these deficiencies a classification has been proposed.[62] This classification grades byssinosis, respiratory tract irritation and acute and chronic lung function changes separately. Grade 1/2 byssinosis has been removed from the classification. This classification is shown in Table 32.1.

None of these classifications identifies which days of the working week are associated with most severe symptoms. Surveys of cotton workers reveal a group of workers experiencing chest tightness on each working day with no variation in severity across the working week.[57] The relationship between these symptoms and the classic symptoms of byssinosis is at present not clear.

It is generally thought that there is a progression through the clinical grades of byssinosis starting at grade 1/2 and, depending on their individual susceptibility and dust exposure, perhaps finishing as grade 3. This progression in individuals has yet to be demonstrated in prospective epidemiological studies. In some individuals the symptoms of byssinosis may remit, despite continued exposure to cotton dust.[17]

This study also demonstrated the presence of chest tightness in the absence of changes in FEV_1 and significant decrements in FEV_1 with no associated chest tightness. However, cotton workers with the greatest decrements in FEV_1 without byssinosis were the most likely to go on to develop byssinosis.[63]

PHARMACOLOGICAL RESPONSES

Various investigations have been carried out to evaluate the effect of drugs on the respiratory responses to cotton dust. Antihistamine and a bronchodilator reduce or prevent falls in FEV_1 across the working shift. Salbutamol is more effective than beclomethasone and disodium cromoglycate is the least effective in preventing symptoms and changes in ventilatory capacity.[64]

SMOKING AND BYSSINOSIS

Smoking habits have been shown to have an important potentiating effect on both the development of byssinosis and on the reduction in ventilatory capacity,[17,65] the prevalence of byssinosis being 1–4 times as frequent in smokers as non- and ex-smokers.[24] However, in recent studies in Egypt, Australia and England[17,66] no association was found between smoking habits and the prevalence of byssinosis.

PHYSICAL SIGNS

On physical examination there are no specific abnormalities associated with byssinosis. When physical signs are present they simply indicate the presence of airflow limitation.

Investigations

LUNG FUNCTION

The changes in lung function which are associated with byssinosis were not documented until 1958. There is a progressive decline in FEV_1 across the working shift in grades 1 and 2 byssinosis with the maximum decline occurring on the first day of the working week.

That does not imply that the level of airways obstruction improves over the remainder of the week. In a study of 25 carders made up of asymptomatic workers and grades 1/2 and 2 byssinotics, the greatest decline in FEV_1 occurred on the first day of the working week, but the mean FEV_1 was lowest towards the end of the week.[67] Serial peak expiratory flow rate (PEFR) measurements in grade 3 byssinotic cardroom workers may show a variety of patterns (Figs 32.1a,b associated with wide diurnal variations in PEFR consistent with a diagnosis of asthma. The measurement of mid-expiratory flow rates appears to be the most sensitive indicator of airways obstruction in cotton workers.[68,69] Gas transfer measurements were within normal limits when measured preshift in a small group of hemp, flax and cotton workers[69] and impairment of gas transfer, when present, appears to be related to an individual's past smoking habits rather than their exposure to cotton dust.[22]

RADIOLOGY

There are no specific abnormalities on the chest radiograph in byssinosis.

CHRONIC BRONCHITIS

Molyneux and Tombleson[70] first observed that bronchitis (mucus hypersecretion) occurred more frequently amongst cotton workers than man-made fibre workers. In a later study of 14 cotton mills and two man-made fibre mills[17] the prevalence of bronchitis ranged between 18.3 and 44.9% in cotton workers and 22.8 and 26% in man-made fibre workers. Although they demonstrated a positive trend between the prevalence of bronchitis and length of exposure in women, this was not present in men. In a recent study of 2991 textile workers[71] the prevalence of chronic bronchitis in workers over the age of 45 was more frequent amongst cotton workers and was significantly associated with cumulative cotton dust

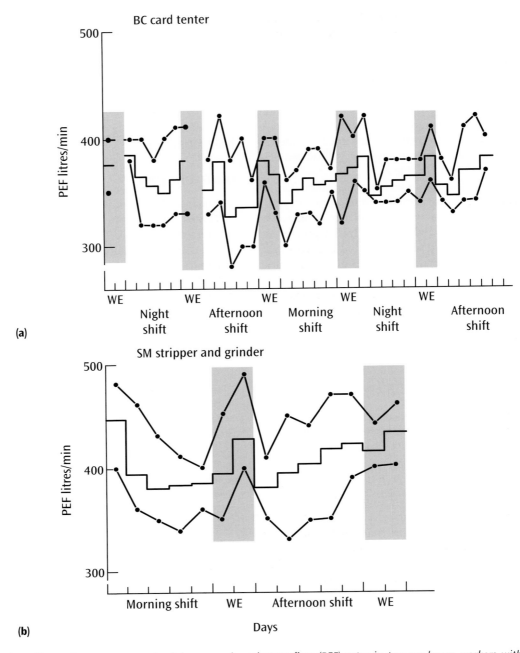

Figures 32.1a,b *Daily maximum, mean and minimum peak expiratory flow (PEF) rates in two cardroom workers with grade 3 byssinosis. WE: weekend.*

exposure. The diagnosis of chronic bronchitis was associated with a small, significant decrement in lung function. The effect of cotton dust exposure in a non-smoking cotton worker was the equivalent of light smoking in a man-made fibre worker.

In addition to chest tightness and breathlessness, byssinotics may also develop a productive or non-productive cough and wheezing. The prevalence of bronchitis (mucus hypersecretion), after allowing for age and smoking habits, is higher in byssinotics than non-byssinotics.

PREVENTION

The most important preventive measure is a reduction in dust levels. It has been calculated that approximately 10% of workers exposed to cotton dust for 40 years at a concentration of 0.5 mg/m³ will develop byssinosis.[72] Over the past 10 years there have been progressive reductions in cotton dust exposure levels in the USA such that now byssinosis is a rare disease. Attention is now focussed on preventing dust-related chronic decline in lung function. The results of the Tulane longitudinal study[60] suggest that to achieve this, smokers should be excluded from the high dust exposure areas (yarn manufacture) and that dust exposure should be reduced to approximately 100 µg/m³. This level is based on an area sampling technique. A comparison of area and personal sampling techniques[73] in cotton workers has shown a 7.8-fold difference in measurement between the two techniques in the opening processes. Personal sampling providing the higher levels of exposure. This difference becomes less in the later processes – 4.9 in carding, 4.2 in other cardroom processes, 1.4-fold difference in ring spinning, rising to 2.5 in winding. Since respiratory disease in cotton workers is predominantly in the early stages of processing this difference is highly significant in terms of setting exposure standards and has led to the setting of a personal exposure dust standard for cotton in the UK.

The preprocessing of cotton to prevent byssinosis has also been investigated. Cotton steaming reduced the biological activity and also the dust levels in the early stages of processing, although fine dust particles may then be released later in the manufacturing process, leading to an increased incidence of byssinosis in these work areas.[74]

MANAGEMENT

If the development of disability is to be prevented in workers who are experiencing symptoms of byssinosis they need to be identified early at a time when they have a low grade of byssinosis. In an ideal world their exposure to cotton dust should then cease either by their transfer to a mill handling pure man-made fibre or by their finding a new job. In practice new employment is difficult to find and the individual continues his or her exposure to cotton dust. This exposure should be kept to a minimum by using respiratory protection and by moving the worker to the least dusty work area. Finally their symptoms can be reduced by the regular use of prophylactic anti-asthmatic therapy (particularly inhaled steroids) and inhaled bronchodilators. This is a far from ideal solution to this occupational problem and the major emphasis of management should be on preventing exposure. Byssinosis is a prescribed disease (see Chapter 4).

REFERENCES

1 Proust A. *Traite d'hygiène publique et privée* Paris: Masson, 1877: 171–7.

2 Kay JP. Observations and experiments concerning molecular irritation of the lungs as one source of tubercular consumption; and on spinner's phthisis. *North Engl Med Surg J* 1831; **1**: 348–63.

3 Mareska J, Heyman J. Enquête sur le travail et la condition physique et morale des ouvriers employés dans les manufacturers de coton, à Gand. *Ann Soc Med Gand* 1845; **16**: 11 : 5, 199.

4 Greenhow H. *Third Report of the Medical Officer of the Privy Council. Sir John Simon.* 1861: 152.

5 Bouhuys A, Heaphy LJ Jr, Schilling RSF, Welborn JW. Byssinosis in the United States. *N Engl J Med* 1967; **277**: 170–5.

6 Gandevia B, Milne J. Ventilatory capacity changes on exposure to cotton dust and their relevance to byssinosis in Australia. *Br J Ind Med* 1965; **22**: 295–304.

7 Tsai SY. Study of byssinosis in cotton textile workers in Taiwan. *J Formosan Med Assoc* 1964; **63**: 10–15.

8 Morgan PGM, Ong SC. First report of byssinosis in Hong Kong. *Br J Ind Med* 1981; **38**: 290–2.

9 Koskela R-S, Klockars M, Jarvinen E. (Letter) *Br J Ind Med* 1991; **48**: 143–4.

10 Gill CIC. Byssinosis in the cotton trade. *Br J Ind Med* 1947; **4**: 48–55.

11 Schilling RSF, Hughes JPW, Dingwall-Fordyce I, Gilson JC. An epidemiological survey of byssinosis amongst cotton workers. *Br J Ind Med* 1955; **12**: 217–27.

12 Fox AJ, Tombleson JBL, Watt A, Wilkie AG. A survey of respiratory disease in cotton operatives. *Br J Ind Med* 1973; **30**: 42–53.

13 Cinkotai FF, Rigby A, Pickering CAC, Seaborn D, Faragher E. Recent trends in the prevalence of byssinotic symptoms in the Lancashire textile industry. *Br J Ind Med* 1988; **45**: 782–9.

14 Schrag PE, Coullett AD. Byssinosis in cotton textile mills. *Am Rev Respir Dis* 1970; **101**: 497–503.

15 Gun RT, Janckewiez C, Esterman A et al. Byssinosis: a cross-sectional study in an Australian textile factory. *J Soc Occup Med* 1983; **33**: 119–25.

16 Field GB, Owen P. Respiratory function in an Australian cotton mill. *Bull Eur Physiopathol Resp* 1979; **15**: 455–68.

17 Berry C, Molyneux MKB, Tomblesoy JBL. Relationships between dust levels and byssinosis and bronchitis in Lancashire cotton mills. *Br J Ind Med* 1974; **31**: 18–27.

18 Elwood PC, Pemberton J, Merrett JD, Carey GCR, McAuley IR. Byssinosis and other respiratory symptoms in flax workers in Northern Ireland. *Br J Ind Med* 1965; **22**: 27–37.

19 Noweir MH, El-Sadik YM, El-Dakhakhny AA, Osman HA. Dust exposure in manual flax processing in Egypt. *Br J Ind Med* 1975; **32**: 147–54.

20 Edwards C, Macartney J, Rooke C, Ward F. The pathology of the lung in byssinotics. *Thorax* 1975; **30**: 612–23.

21 Takizawa T, Thurlbeck WM. Muscle and mucous gland size in the major bronchi of patients with chronic bronchitis, asthma and asthmatic bronchitis. *Am Rev Respir Dis* 1971; **104**: 331–6.

22 Honeybourne D, Pickering CAC. Physiological evidence that emphysema is not a feature of byssinosis but is due to concomitant cigarette smoking. *Thorax* 1986; **41**: 6–11.

23 Imbus HR, Suh MW. Steaming of cotton to prevent byssinosis – a plant study. *Br J Ind Med* 1974; **31**: 209–19.

24 Merchant JA, Lumsden JC, Kilburn KH *et al.* Preprocessing cotton to prevent byssinosis. *Br J Ind Med* 1973; **30**: 247–57

25 Bouhuys A, Nicholls PJ. The effect of cotton dust on respiratory mechanics in man and in guinea-pigs. In: *Inhaled Particles and Vapours II.* Oxford: Pergamon Press, 1966: 75–84.

26 Popa V, Gavrilescu N, Preda N, Teculescu D, Plecias M, Cirstea M. An investigation of allergy in byssinosis: sensitisation to cotton, hemp, flax and jute antigens. *Br J Ind Med* 1969; **26**: 101–8.

27 Petronio L, Bovenzi M. Byssinosis and serum IgE concentrations in textile workers in an Italian cotton mill. *Br J Ind Med* 1983; **40**: 39–44.

28 O'Neil CE, Reed MA, Aukrust L, Butcher BT. Studies on the antigenic composition of aqueous cotton dust extracts. *Int Arch All Appl Immunol* 1983; **72**: 294–8.

29 Honeybourne D, Finnegan MJ, Pickering CAC. Does atopy matter in byssinosis? In: *New light On Byssinosis.* Cardiff: MRC Epidemiology Unit; 1985: 57–60.

30 Taylor C, Massoud A, Lucas F. Studies on the aetiology of byssinosis. *Br J Ind Med* 1971; **28**: 145–51.

31 Norweir MH. Studies on the etiology of byssinosis. *Chest* 1981; **79**: 62S–67S.

32 Edwards JH, Alzubaidy TS, Altikriti R, Bunni H. Byssinosis. Inhalation challenge with polyphenol. *Chest* 1984; **85**: 215–17.

33 Mundie TG, Boackle RJ, Ainsworth SK. *In vitro* alternative and classical activation of complement by extracts of cotton mill dust: a possible mechanism in the pathogenesis of byssinosis. *Environ Res* 1983; **32**: 47–56.

34 Mundie TG, Cordova-Salinas M, Bray VJ, Ainsworth SK. Bioassays of smooth muscle contracting agents in cotton mill dust and bract extracts: arachidonic acid metabolites as possible mediators of the acute byssinotic reaction. *Environ Res* 1983; **32**: 62–71.

35 Fowler SR, Ziprin RI, Elissalde MH, Greenblatt GA. The etiology of byssinosis – possible role of prostaglandin F_2 alpha synthesis by alveolar macrophages. *Am Ind Hyg Assoc J* 1981; **42**: 445–8.

36 *Report of the Departmental Committee on dust in cardrooms in the cotton industry.* London: Home Office, 1932: 1–96.

37 Schneiter R, Neal PA, Caminita BH. Etiology of acute illness among workers using low grade stained cotton. *Am J Publ Hlth* 1942; **32**: 1345–52.

38 Cavagna C, Foa V, Vigliani EC. Effects in man and rabbits of inhalation of cotton dust or extracts and purified endotoxins. *Br J Ind Med* 1969; **26**: 314–21.

39 Cinkotai FF, Whitaker CJ. Airborne bacteria and the prevalence of byssinotic symptoms in 21 cotton spinning mills in Lancashire. *Ann Occup Hyg* 1978; **21**: 239–50.

40 Rylander R, Haglind P, Lundholm M. Endotoxin in cotton dust and respiratory function decrement among cotton workers in an experimental cardroom, *Am Rev Respir Dis* 1985; **131**: 209–13.

41 Kennedy SM, Christiani DC, Eisen EA *et al.* Cotton dust and endotoxin exposure-response relationships in cotton textile workers. *Am Rev Respir Dis* 1987; **135**: 194–200.

42 Buck MG, Wall JH, Schachter EN. Airway constrictor response to cotton bract extracts in the absence of endotoxin. *Br J Ind Med* 1986; **43**: 220–6.

43 Jamison JP, Lowry RC. Bronchial challenge of normal subjects with the endotoxin of *Enterobacter agglomerans* isolated from cotton dust. *Br J Ind Med* 1986; **43**: 327–31.

44 Chinn DJ, Cinkotai FF, Lockwood MC. Airborne dust: its protease content and byssinosis in willowing mills. *Ann Occup Hyg* 1976; **19**: 101–8.

45 Schachter EN, Zuskin E, Buck MG, Witek TJ, Beck GJ, Tyler D. Airway reactivity and cotton bract-induced bronchial obstruction. *Chest* 1985; **87**: 51–5.

46 Massoud AE, Altounyan REC, Howell JBL, Lane RE. Effects of histamine aerosol in byssinotic subjects. *Br J Ind Med* 1967; **24**: 38–40.

47 Bouhuys A. Response to inhaled histamine in bronchial asthma and in byssinosis. *Am Rev Respir Dis* 1967; **95**: 89–93.

48 Haglind P, Bake B, Belin L. Is mild byssinosis associated with small airways disease? *Eur J Respir Dis* 1983; **64**: 449.

49 Fishwick D, Fletcher AM, Pickering CAC, Niven R, Faragher E. Lung function, bronchial reactivity, atopic status and dust exposure in Lancashire mill operatives. *Am Rev Respir Dis* 1992; **145**: 1103–8.

50 Collis EL. *Annual Report of Chief Inspector of Factories for 1908.* London: HMSO.

51 Berry G, Molyneux MKB. A mortality study of workers in Lancashire cotton mills. *Chest* 1981; **79**(Suppl): 11S–15S.

52 Elwood PC, Thomas HF, Sweetnam PM, Elwood JH. The mortality of flax workers. *Br J Ind Med* 1982; **39**: 18–22.

53 Hodgson JT, Jones RD. Mortality of workers in the British cotton industry in 1964–1984. *Scand J Work Environ Hlth* 1990; **16**: 113–20.

54 Glindmeyer HW, Lefante JJ, Jones RN, Rando RJ, Abdel Karder HM, Weill H. Exposure-related declines in the lung function of cotton textile workers. *Am Rev Respir Dis* 1991; **144**: 675–83.

55 Koskela R-S, Klockars M, Jarvinen E. Mortality and disability among cotton mill workers. *Br J Ind Med* 1990; **47**: 384–91.

56 Fishwick D, Fletcher AM, Pickering CAC, Niven R, Faragher E. Ocular and nasal irritation in operatives in Lancashire cotton and synthetic fibre mills. *Occ Environ Med* 1994; **51**: 744–8.

57 Fishwick D, Fletcher AM, Pickering CAC, Niven R, Faragher E. Respiratory symptoms and dust exposure in Lancashire cotton and man-made fiber mill operatives. *Am J Respir Crit Care Med* 1994; **150**: 441–7.

58 Castellan RM, Olenchock SA, Hankinson JL, Millner PD, Cocke JB, *et al.* Acute bronchoconstriction induced by cotton dust: dose-related responses to endotoxin and other dust factors. *Ann Intern Med* 1984; **101**: 157–63.

59 Koskela R-S, Klockars M, Jarvinen E. Mortality and disability amongst cotton mill workers. *Br J Ind Med* 1990; **48**: 143–4.

60 Glindmeyer HW, Lefante JJ, Jones RN, Rando RJ, Weill H.

Cotton dust and across-shift change in FEV₁ as predictors of annual change in FEV₁. *Am J Respir Crit Care Med* 1994; **149**: 584–90.

61 Roach SA, Schilling RSF. A clinical and environmental study of byssinosis in the lancashire cotton industry. *Br J Ind Med* 1960; **17**: 1–9.

62 Report of a World Health Organization study group. *Recommended health-based occupational exposure limits for selected vegetable dusts.* WHO Techn Rep Ser 684. Geneva: WHO, 1983.

63 Berry C, McKerrow CB, Molyneux MKB, Rossiter CE, Tombleson JBL. A study of the acute and chronic changes in ventilatory capacity of workers in Lancashire cotton mills. *Br J Ind Med* 1973; **30**: 25–36.

64 Fawcett IW, Merchant IA, Simmonds SP, Pepys J. The effect of sodium cromoglycate, beclomethasone dipropionate and salbutamol on the ventilatory response to cotton dust in mill workers. *Br J Dis Chest* 1978; **72**: 29–37.

65 Merchant JA, Lumsden JC, Kilburn KH *et al.* An industrial study of the biological effects of cotton dust and cigarette smoke exposure. *J Occup Med* 1973; **15**: 212–21.

66 Noweir MH, Noweir KH, Osman HA, Moselhi M. An environmental and medical study of byssinosis and other respiratory conditions in the cotton textile industry in Egypt. *Am J Ind Med* 1984; **6**: 173–83.

67 Merchant JA, Halprin GM, Hudson AR *et al.* Evaluation before and after exposure – the pattern of physiological response to cotton dust. *Ann NY Acad Sci* 1974; **221**: 38–43.

68 Merchant JA, Halprin GM, Hudson AR *et al.* Responses to cotton dust. *Arch Environ Hlth* 1975; **30**: 222–9.

69 Zuskin E, Valic F, Butkoyic D, Bouhuys A. Lung function in textile workers. *Br J Ind Med* 1975; **32**: 283–8.

70 Molyneux MKB, Tombleson JBL. An epidemiological study of respiratory symptoms in Lancashire mills 1963–1966. *Br J Ind Med* 1970; **27**: 225–347.

71 Niven R, Fletcher AM, Pickering CAC, Fishwick D, Warburton CJ *et al.* Chronic bronchitis in textile workers. *Thorax* 1997; **52**: 22–27.

72 Fox AJ, Tombleson JBL, Watt A, Wilkie AC. A survey of respiratory disease in cotton operatives. Part II Symptoms, dust estimations and the effect of smoking habit. *Br J Ind Med* 1973; **30**: 48–53.

73 Niven R, Fishwick D, Pickering CAC, Fletcher AM, Crank P. A study of the performance and comparability of the sampling response to cotton dust of work area and personal sampling techniques. *Ann Occup Hyg* 1992; **36**: 349–362.

74 Merchant JA, Lumsden JC, Kilburn KH, Intervention studies of cotton steaming to reduce biological effects of cotton dust. *Br J Ind Med* 1984; **31**: 261–74.

33

Occupational asthma

A J NEWMAN TAYLOR

Importance of occupational asthma	634	Investigation of causes of occupational asthma	643
Irritant-induced asthma	635	Outcome of occupational asthma	645
Causes of hypersensitivity-induced occupational asthma	636	Management of occupational asthma	646
Occupational asthma and allergy	640	Prevention of occupational asthma	646
Determinants of occupational asthma	641	Statutory compensation, UK	647
Diagnosis of occupational asthma	642	References	647

Asthma is usually defined as airway narrowing which is reversible over short periods of time, either spontaneously or as a result of treatment. This definition focuses on the variability of airway calibre which distinguishes asthma from other less reversible causes of airflow limitation, which are usually associated with chronic bronchitis and emphysema. A further cardinal characteristic of asthma is airway hyper-responsiveness – an increased responsiveness of the airways to non-specific provocative stimuli. Patients with hyper-responsive airways require smaller than normal doses of provocative stimuli, such as exercise or inhaled cold dry air, to provoke acute transient airway narrowing. These functional abnormalities used to define asthma are probably manifestations of a characteristic pattern of airway inflammation – desquamative eosinophilic bronchitis – with bronchial epithelial cell desquamation and mucosal infiltration by eosinophils and lymphocytes.

Occupational asthma is asthma initiated by an agent inhaled at work. Agents encountered at work may initiate or provoke asthma. Initiators of asthma induce asthma and cause airway inflammation and hyper-responsiveness. Provokers cause acute transient airway narrowing in individuals with pre-existing asthma, whose airways are hyper-responsive; they do not initiate asthma, cause airway inflammation or increase airway responsiveness (Table 33.1).

Initiators can induce asthma and cause airway inflammation as a result of toxic damage to the airway epithelium (irritant-induced asthma) or as the outcome of an acquired specific hypersensitivity response (hypersensi-

tivity-induced asthma). Toxic initiators include respiratory irritants such as chlorine and sulphur dioxide which cause airway inflammation by a direct toxic action on airway epithelial cells. Hypersensitivity initiators include inhaled proteins (such as animal excreta, flour and enzymes), other complex biological molecules (such as wood resin acids) and synthetic low molecular weight chemicals (such as isocyanates and acid anhydrides) which probably bind covalently to body proteins to form haptens. Airway inflammation occurs as the outcome of a hypersensitivity (probably allergic) response.

Provokers of acute airway narrowing may be physical, such as exercise and cold air inhalation, chemical such as sulphur dioxide, inhaled in subtoxic concentrations, and pharmacological such as histamine and methacholine. Avoiding exposure to an initiator can reduce the severity of asthma, airway inflammation and airway responsiveness; avoiding a provoker will reduce the frequency of provoked attacks, but not the magnitude of airway hyper-responsiveness.

Both initiators and provokers of asthma may be encountered at work. Cold air in storage rooms and outdoors, exertion and irritant chemicals may all provoke asthma in individuals with hyper-responsive airways. There is also evidence that the effects of different provokers on the airways can be additive. Asthma initiated by an irritant chemical inhaled in toxic concentrations has been described as 'reactive airways dysfunction syndrome' (RADS).[1] or 'irritant-induced asthma'. Irritant induced asthma may be distinguished from hypersensitivity-induced asthma by the absence of a latent interval.

Table 33.1 *Occupational asthma: initiators and provokers*

Irritant-induced	Hypersensitivity induced
Initiators	
Chemicals	**Proteins**
Chlorine	Enzymes
Ammonia	Animal urine proteins
Sulphur dioxide	Flour
	Latex
	Complex biological molecules
	Colophony
	Plicatic acid (Western Red Cedar)
	Antibiotics
	Low mol wt chemicals
	Isocyanates
	Platinum salts
	Acid anhydrides
Provokers	
Exercise	
Cold dry air	
Sulphur dioxide	
Inhaled histamine/methacholine	

Whereas hypersensitivity-induced asthma only develops several weeks or months from initial exposure to its cause, irritant-induced asthma and associated airway hyperresponsiveness develop within a few hours of a clearly identifiable exposure.

IMPORTANCE OF OCCUPATIONAL ASTHMA

The contribution of occupational causes to the prevalence of asthma is not known. Estimates in different countries have varied between 2 and 15%, but their basis has generally not been secure. In a recent community-based study of adults aged between 20 and 44 years in Spain, Kojevinas *et al.*[2] estimated the risk of asthma attributable to occupational causes (after adjustment for age, sex, residence and smoking) was between 5% (1 in 20) and 6.7% (1 in 15). The highest risks occurred in laboratory technicians, spray painters and bakers.

In the United Kingdom, information about the number of cases of asthma caused by agents inhaled at work and their relative importance has, until relatively recently, been confined to official statistics of compensation awarded under the Industrial Injuries Scheme. In Finland a register of occupational diseases, based on a legal requirement for doctors to report occupational diseases, was initiated more than 30 years ago. In the UK a national scheme – the Surveillance of Work Related and Occupational Respiratory Diseases (SWORD) – was set up in 1989 by Professor Corbett McDonald. This is a voluntary reporting scheme which has achieved almost complete coverage of chest physicians and a similar number (but unknown proportion) of occupational physicians.

The scheme provides estimates of case frequency by cause and of disease incidence by occupational group. In 1989 2101 cases of occupational lung disease were reported;[3] in 1992 a sampling scheme was introduced and the annual incidence estimated at 3500.[4] Asthma, which accounted for 28% of cases, was the single most common diagnostic category. Isocyanates have consistently been the most commonly reported cause accounting for 20% of cases; flour/grain dust, wood dust, solder flux and laboratory animals together accounted for the same proportion.

The overall annual incidence of occupational asthma during 1989 and 1990 was 22 per million working population.[5] The occupational sets with the highest incidence are shown in Table 33.2.

Comparison of the SWORD scheme with the Finnish register of occupational diseases indicate that the reported incidence of occupational asthma in Finland is appreciably higher than that reported to SWORD.[6] This is attributable, at least in part, to more complete ascertainment of cases by all physicians in Finland and is not limited to the specialists who report to SWORD.

The most common cause of occupational asthma in Finland is allergy to cow dander, a reflection of the high proportion of the population employed in agriculture and in close contact with their animals; the incidence of extrinsic allergic alveolitis, of which the most common

Table 33.2

Occupational set	Rate 10⁶/year
Coach and spray painters	658
Chemical processors	364
Plastics workers	337
Bakers	334
Metal treatment	267
Laboratory technicians and assistants	188

occupational cause is farmer's lung, is also many times higher in Finland than is reported to SWORD.

IRRITANT-INDUCED ASTHMA

Irritant-induced asthma (reactive airways dysfunction syndrome) is chronic asthma which persists after a single inhalation, usually of short duration, of a respiratory irritant in toxic concentrations. The diagnostic criteria for irritant induced asthma are set out in Table 33.3.

Most descriptions of irritant-induced asthma have been case reports and series. The original report described ten patients, none of whom had evidence of pre-existing respiratory disease.[1] All developed persistent asthma after a single exposure – usually a few minutes in duration, but in one case for 12 hours – to a variety of chemicals which included a spray paint containing ammonia, heated acid, floor sealant, uranium hexafluoride and smoke. The onset of respiratory symptoms occurred on average after 9 hours in all but three, in whom they developed immediately. The duration of symptoms to the time of follow-up ranged from 1 to 12

Table 33.3 *Criteria for the diagnosis of irritant-induced asthma*

- Absence of preceding respiratory complaints is documented.
- The onset of symptoms occurred after a single specific exposure incident or accident.
- The exposure was to a gas, smoke, fume or vapour that was present in very high concentrations and had irritant qualities.
- The onset of symptoms occurred within 24 hours after the exposure and persisted for at least 3 months.
- Symptoms were consistent with asthma – with cough, wheezing and dyspnoea predominating.
- Pulmonary function tests may show airflow obstruction.
- Appropriate challenge testing demonstrated increasing airway responsiveness.
- Other types of pulmonary diseases were excluded.

years; at follow-up all ten had increased airway responsiveness to inhaled methacholine and seven had evidence of airflow limitation.

Subsequent reports of irritant-induced asthma have documented asthma initiated by a single inhalation (in toxic concentrations) of several different chemicals which have included sulphur dioxide[7], toluene diisocyanate,[8] anhydrous ammonia fumes[9] and smoke (see Chapter 8).[10]

In general the cases reported of irritant-induced asthma have been highly selected and have not provided information on lung function prior to the relevant inhalation accident. One study[11] of hospital employees exposed to 100% acetic acid after a spill in a hospital laboratory, however, overcame these problems by:

1. studying a random sample of the exposed population;
2. demonstrating an exposure-response relationship between the estimated intensity of exposure, the prevalence of acute irritant symptoms and measured airway hyper-responsiveness: the risk of developing asthma was some tenfold higher in those most heavily, compared with those least, exposed to acetic acid following the spill;
3. partial validation of respiratory health before the inhalation accident by examination of pre-employment health questionnaires.

This study provides the most convincing evidence reported to date of the validity of 'irritant-induced asthma'.

During its first 5 years, 1989–1993, 904 cases of inhalation accidents (of 8586 newly diagnosed cases of ocupational lung disease) were reported to SWORD.[12] Taking account of the sampling scheme introduced in 1992, an estimated 250 inhalation accidents occurred in each of these years. A total of 85% of the agents responsible were chemicals, the most common being chlorine (13%), smoke/combustion gases (9%) and oxides of nitrogen (5%). The highest incidence occurred in metal and electrical processors (162/million/year) and chemical processors (75/million/year).

Physicians were asked by questionnaire about the outcome of 623 cases of inhalation accidents reported to SWORD during a 3.5-year period between 1990 and 1993.[13] Of the 383 cases where the occupational physician was aware of the diagnosis, 70% had recovered in 1 week and 75% returned to work within 1 week; 12% had symptoms for more than 1 month and a further 2% did not return to work. Eleven of 47 (23%) cases with persistent ill-health had developed asthma (i.e. 2.8% of the 383 inhalation accidents developed irritant-induced asthma). The agents responsible for these cases were in the main respiratory irritants which included chlorine, oxides of nitrogen, sulphur dioxide, ammonium, carboxylic acid and sodium fumes.

CAUSES OF HYPERSENSITIVITY-INDUCED OCCUPATIONAL ASTHMA

Many different agents encountered at work can stimulate a hypersensitivity response and cause asthma. The more prevalent causes are shown in Table 33.4.

Laboratory animals

Laboratory animal allergy is probably the most prevalent occupational health problem for those working in the pharmaceutical industry and in scientific laboratories. Some 32 000 persons have been estimated to work with laboratory animals in the UK and cross-sectional surveys have consistently found prevalence rates of laboratory animal allergy (LAA) of between 15 and 30%.[14,15] One survey found a prevalence of 44% of reported symptoms consistent with LAA and of 11% of LAA chest symptoms (shortness of breath, chest tightness, wheezing) in 138 pharmaceutical employees exposed at work to laboratory animals.[16] A prospective study estimated the incidence of allergy in the first year of work with animals was 15%, and of asthma 2%.[17]

Extracts of urine proteins of rats and mice elicit immediate skin test responses and when inhaled, provoke asthmatic reactions in sensitized workers. The important urinary proteins seem to be an $\alpha 2$ globulin and prealbumin in the rat and a prealbumin in the mouse, proteins excreted in high concentration by postpubertal male animals.[18]

The concentration of airborne urine proteins in animal laboratories is determined by the rates of their gen-eration and removal. In an experimental study Gordon et al. showed the concentration of rat urine protein had a log linear relationship with the number of rats in the study room and that airborne rat urine protein levels were reduced by decreasing stock density (the relationship of animal number of the volume of the room), the use of absorbent bedding and filter top cages.[19]

Grain dust

Grain dust is a complex mixture of grain, its disintegration products and organic constituents, whose composition depends upon whether the grain is encountered during harvesting or in storage. Several fungi which are saprophytic on growing and ripening grain, are released in large numbers during harvesting.

These include *Alternaria alternata* and *Cladosporium herbarum*, whose spores are released into the air by day, and *Didymella exitialis* whose spores are released into the air at night and after rainfall. During harvesting total airborne spore counts can reach $10^8/m^3$ of which some 75% are *C. herbarum* and 25% *A. alternata*. The spores are blown free by the wind with airborne concentrations maximal in dry windy weather. In contrast the spores of *D. exitialis* are expelled into the air after absorption of water and their airborne concentration is maximal in conditions of high humidity (and therefore during the night) and after rainfall.[20]

Inhalation of spores of *A. alternata*, *C. herbarum* and *D. exitialis* can stimulate immunoglobulin E (IgE) antibody production and cause asthma. The three fungi share several allergens.[21] In their study of Lincolnshire

Table 33.4 *Causes of occupational asthma*

	Proteins	Low molecular weight chemicals
Animal	Excreta of rats, mice etc; locusts, grain mites	
Vegetable	Grain/flour	Plicatic acid (Western Red Cedar)
	Castor bean	Colophony (pinewood resin)
	Green coffee bean Ispaghula latex	
Microbial	Harvest moulds Bacterial enzymes	Antibiotics, e.g. penicillins, cephalosporins
'Minerals'		Acid anhydrides Isocyanates Complex platinum salts Polyamines Reactive dyes

farmers Darke et al. found that nearly 25% reported symptoms consistent with asthma during the harvesting period.[22] Symptoms usually developed after several years of farm work and occurred particularly in those most heavily exposed to grain dust – drivers of combine harvesters and those working in grain bins or near grain driers and elevators.

The capacity of stored grain to support the growth of moulds and mites is determined primarily by its water content. Moulding occurs at water contents of between 10 and 15% and mites, which feed on moulds, grow at this water content. Grain stored with this content of water is liable to become infested with storage mites of which the most important in the UK are *Leptidoglycus destructor*, *Acaris siro* and *Glycyphagus domesticus*.

Inhalation of mites and their excreta can stimulate IgE antibody production and cause asthma.[23] In a study of Essex farmers, Blainey et al., found that nearly 20% had asthma which they considered to be caused by storage mites.[24] In a survey of Swedish farmers in Gotland, an island in the Baltic sea, Van Hage-Hamsten et al., estimated the prevalence of respiratory symptoms caused by storage mite allergy to be 6.2%.[25]

Flour

The incidence of occupational asthma in bakery workers was estimated to be one of the four highest of occupational groups reported to the SWORD surveillance scheme.[3] Cereal flour proteins and added fungal α-amylase seem the most important cause. Hendrick et al. studied two bakers with occupational asthma in whom inhalation of wheat and rye flour in one and wheat flour in the second provoked dual (early followed by late) asthmatic responses.[26] Skin testing with the same flours elicited immediate responses in both. Ingestion of uncooked flour provoked no adverse reactions. Baur et al., reported asthma, rhinitis and conjunctivitis associated with flour contact in 35 of 118 bakery and confectionery workers.[27] All 35 had specific IgE to wheat flour, of whom 33 had specific IgE to rye flour. In addition, 12 had specific IgE to fungal α-amylase (from *Aspergillus oryzae*), an important flour additive. Inhalation testing in four with the enzyme provoked immediate rhinitis or asthma.

In a cross-sectional study of a bakery in the UK, Musk et al. found that of 19% of 318 employees had work related nasal and 13% work related chest symptoms.[28] Both occurred more frequently among those currently employed in jobs with the highest dust concentrations. Measurable airway responsiveness to inhaled histamine was associated with exposure to highest dust concentrations at any time since starting employment in this bakery.

Enzymes

Enzymes are widely and increasingly used commercially for a variety of purposes. The incorporation of proteolytic enzymes into detergent powders is the most widely appreciated, but other uses include fungal α-amylase in the manufacture of bread, papain as a meat tenderiser and bromelain used as tenderizer and reaction booster in blood grouping laboratories. Enzymes are proteins and when inhaled can cause asthma. The risk of asthma occurs both in the enzyme producers and the manufacturers of products which incorporate them. Allergy to enzymes was reported in a small number of consumers using enzyme-containing detergents in Sweden and the United States of America during the early period of manufacture when powdered non-granulated enzyme products were marketed.[29,30] However, any important risk to consumers seems to have been markedly reduced since the introduction of granulated enzymes.[31]

The respiratory hazard of inhalation of proteolytic enzymes during detergent manufacture was initially reported in 1969.[32,33] Subsequent epidemiological studies in the UK,[34] USA[35] and Australia[36] demonstrated high rates of skin prick test responses and respiratory symptoms consistent with asthma. In a 7-year follow-up study of a detergent enzyme workforce exposed to *Bacillus subtilis* enzyme alcalase, Juniper et al.[37] showed a clear relationship between the development of a positive skin test reaction to alcalase with intensity of exposure and atopy.

Latex

Recognition of allergy to latex has increased greatly in recent years in the USA and Europe including the UK. The increasing incidence of latex allergy has followed the greatly increased use of rubber gloves by health care staff to reduce the risk of infection with human immunodeficiency virus (HIV) and hepatitis B and C viruses.

Latex is the milky sap of the tree *Hevea brasiliensis*. Raw latex is used in a variety of products which include surgical gloves, balloons, condoms and catheters. The allergens identified to date in latex have molecular weights of 14, 28 and 88 kD to which specific IgE in the serum of sensitized individuals binds. The majority of cases are probably sensitized by the inhalation of the dusting powder from the gloves which has adsorbed the latex proteins. Swanson et al.[38] found airborne concentrations of latex allergens of between 13 and 21 mg/m³ in areas of a hospital where rubber gloves were regularly used and between 0.3 and 1.8 mg/m³ in areas where they were rarely used. Thirty four cases of latex allergy were identified among 49 Mayo clinic employees investigated for possible latex allergy.[39] The majority of those affected were nurses and laboratory technicians; all had jobs which involved changing of latex gloves several times each day. Skin contact provoked urticaria and inhalation provoked rhinitis and asthma. A cross-sectional survey of latex allergy among 273 staff of a hospital in Belgium[40] found that 13 (4.7%) had an immediate skin test response to latex; all 13 had a history of contact urticaria, 12 of rhinitis and conjunctivitis and five of asthma. Inhalation tests with latex provoked an asthmatic response in seven (2.5%). A more recent cross-sectional survey of the employees of a general hospital in Ontario, Canada[41] found that 160 of 1351 participants (12.1%) had immediate skin test responses to an extract of latex. Patients with latex skin test responses were more likely to report work-related symptoms including urticaria (OR 6.3) and wheezy or whistling chest (OR 4.7). The prevalence of latex allergy was highest among laboratory workers (16.9%) and nurses and physicians (13.3%).

Latex allergy is of concern not only because of the subsequent risks of latex exposure at work, but also because of the high risk posed by subsequent exposure, often hidden, both to latex and to cross-reacting allergens in other substances. Rubber tree plants and weeping fig can provoke reactions in latex sensitive individuals, as can eating several foods including avocado, banana and chestnuts.[42] In the study of the hospital staff in Ontario 71 of 160 (44.4%) with a skin test reaction to latex also had a skin test response to one or more of the foods tested (avacado, banana, kiwi, potato, chestnut and cow's milk) as opposed to only 49 of 1166 (42%) of those who did not react to latex (OR 12.9).[41]

Natural latex is also a constituent of many rubber tyres and a recent study identified latex allergens present in airborne particles, presumably derived from degrading rubber tyres.[43] But, of greatest potential risk to the latex-sensitive individual, is contact with latex, often outside their place of work, which can provoke an anaphylactic reaction. Jaeger et al.[44] reported 70 patients with latex allergy, all health care workers, of whom 54% were nurses and technicians and 37% physicians or medical students. Four of these subjects had experienced anaphylactic reactions – provoked by glove contact in one case, a gynaecological examination in another, condom use in another and the use of rubber coated squash racket in the fourth. Because of the risk to latex sensitive individuals encountering latex from gloves worn by medical or nursing staff during an examination or operation, Bubak et al.[39] made specific recommendations for their protection (Table 33.5).

Wood dusts

Asthma can be caused by several different wood dusts, including cedar, mahogany, obeche and iroko. The best studied is Western Red Cedar (*Thuja plicata*), which is the most prevalent cause of occupational asthma in British Columbia. Asthma caused by Western Red Cedar was found in 4.1% of cedar mill workers[45] and 13.5% of those studied by Brookes et al.[46]

Table 33.5 *Specific recommendations for latex sensitive persons*

- Use vinyl gloves
- Use low protein non-powdered latex gloves
- Request that co-workers use vinyl or low protein non-powdered gloves
- Wear a medical identification tag
- Warn all health-care providers of sensitivity and ask them to eliminate or minimize use of latex

For persons with anaphylactic reactivity to latex
- Carry and know how to use an adrenaline-containing emergency kit

Gandevia and Milne reported six cases of asthma and four of rhinitis in patients working with Western Red Cedar dust. Inhalation testing in four with a water-soluble extract of Western Red Cedar provoked late and nocturnal asthmatic responses.[47] In a later study of 22 cases, Chan Yeung et al. found that asthmatic responses provoked by inhalation of water soluble extracts of Western Red Cedar could be reproduced by inhaled plicatic acid, a water soluble constituent unique to Western Red Cedar which is the major fraction (40%) of the non-volatile components of the wood.[48]

Colophony

Colophony is pinewood resin whose major use is as a solder flux in the electronics industry. Colophony fume which is generated during soldering is a complex mixture of resin acids and aldehydes, of which the most important is abietic acid.

Inhalation of colophony fume during soldering has been shown to provoke asthmatic responses in sensitized individuals.[49] In a cross-sectional survey of an electronics factory, where colophony was used as a soft solder flux, Burge et al. found that 22% of 446 shop floor employees had work-related respiratory symptoms compared with 16% of those working in other parts of the factory.[50] Some of those sensitized were not solderers but worked in the vicinity of others who soldered. Of the employees of this factory who had left during the 3½ years before the survey, a significantly greater proportion had worked on the factory floor than in other parts of the factory and this excess could largely be accounted for by those leaving with work-related respiratory symptoms.[51] In a survey of a factory which manufactured colophony flux cored solder Burge et al.[52] found the prevalence of work related respiratory symptoms to be related to measured atmospheric concentrations of colophony; 21% of those in the high exposure group had symptoms, but only 4% of the low exposure group.

Asthma caused by inhaled colophony has been reported, although considerably less frequently, in occupations not associated with electronic soldering. These have included a tool setter exposed to colophony as a constituent of an emulsified oil mist generated by the lathe on which it was used as a coolant,[53] a man exposed to unheated solid colophony while making a bitumen mixture[54] and a Hong Kong chicken plucker who dipped his chickens into heated liquid colophony prior to plucking them.[55]

Diisocyanates

Diisocyanates are bifunctional molecules used commercially to polymerize polyglycol and polyhydroxyl (polyols) compounds to form polyurethanes Because each diisocyanate molecule has two reactive isocyanate (NCO) groups, they link adjacent polyols to form a three-dimensional lattice. Diisocyanates also react with water to evolve carbon dioxide, a reaction exploited in the manufacture of flexible polyurethane foam. The urethane reaction is exothermic and the heat generated sufficient to evaporate diisocyanates with high vapour pressures, such as toluene (TDI) and hexamethylene (HDI). Diphenyl methane (MDI) and naphthalene (NDI) diisocyanates, whose vapour pressures are lower evaporate in significant amounts when heat is applied.

Polyurethanes have widespread applications and exposure to isocyanates occurs in many different occupations. These include the manufacture of flexible and rigid polyurethane foam, the application of two-part polyurethane paints by brush and by spray painting and in flexible packaging production where diisocyanates are used in inks and as laminating adhesives. It has been estimated in the USA that the use of polyurethanes reached 2.2 million tons by 1990 and that between 50 000 and 100 000 workers would encounter isocyanates in their work.

Inhaled diisocyanates have been reported to cause four different respiratory reactions.

1 Toxic bronchitis and asthma caused by isocyanate inhalation in toxic concentrations. Exposure to TDI in an atmospheric concentration of 0.5 ppm causes irritation of mucosal surfaces – eyes, nose and throat.[56] Persistent asthma and airway hyper-responsiveness following a single inhalation of TDI in toxic concentrations has also been reported.[8]
2 Bronchial asthma caused by sensitization to diisocyanates.
3 Accelerated decline of forced expiratory volume in 1 second (FEV$_1$). The rate of decline of FEV$_1$ in an isocyanate manufacturing plant workforce was similar in non-smokers with high cumulative exposures to TDI to the rate observed in smokers in both the high and low exposure groups. The rate in non-smokers with low cumulative exposure was not different from that expected for non-smokers. No

additive effect of TDI with smoking was observed.[57]
4 Extrinsic allergic alveolitis, which has been reported particularly in workers exposed to MDI[58] but also to HDI.[59]

Of these four, bronchial asthma caused by hypersensitivity to isocyanates has been the most frequently reported and is probably the most important both in terms of prevalence and morbidity. The most widely used isocyanates are TDI and MDI and they are the major causes of asthma, although with its increasing use in spray paints HDI has become a more prevalent cause.

A study of workers employed at a new TDI manufacturing plant identified 12 workers (some 4% of the total workforce) who had developed asthma during a 5-year period, nine developing in the first year of employment. The average exposure to TDI monitored by paper tapes was 0.002 ppm.[60] Half of the patients had been exposed to spills; six were maintenance workers, one a laboratory worker and only five were process workers. A cross-sectional study of a steel coating plant, where TDI had been introduced into process some years before, identified 21 cases of asthma out of a total of 221, which was probably an underestimate of the true number of cases.[61]

Inhalation tests with TDI have shown that asthmatic responses may be provoked in sensitized workers by very low atmospheric concentrations, in one report by 0.001 ppm.[62] Late asthmatic responses provoked by isocyanates are associated with the development of an increase in non-specific airway responsiveness[63] and cells recovered from bronchoalveolar lavage during a late asthmatic reaction provoked by TDI have an increased proportion of neutrophils, identifying an inflammatory response in the airways provoked by TDI.[64]

Acid anhydrides

Acid anhydrides are low molecular weight chemicals used industrially as curing agents in the production of epoxy and alkyd resins and in the manufacture of the plasticizer dioctyl phthalate. Epoxy and alkyd resins have widespread applications as paints, plastics and adhesives. Six acid anhydrides – phthalic (PA),[65] trimellitic (TMA),[66,67] tetrachlorophthalic (TCPA),[68] maleic (MA),[69,63] hexahydrophthalic[70] and himic[71] – have been reported to cause occupational asthma. Inhalation tests with the causal acid anhydride provoked asthmatic responses; specific IgE or IgG antibodies, or both, to the specific anhydride conjugated to human serum albumin were identified in the sera of the majority of cases, although this is less frequent with maleic than with the other anhydrides.

Zeiss et al. suggested that four separate clinical syndromes were caused by TMA,[67] for which they proposed separate immunological mechanisms: toxic airway irritation; immediate IgE mediated rhinitis and asthma; IgG mediated late asthma with systemic symptoms ('TMA flu'); and pulmonary haemorrhage–haemolytic anaemia syndrome as the outcome of antibody binding to circulating red blood cells and to pulmonary vascular cells. The distinction between 'immediate' and late 'asthmatic' reactions with flu and their different pattern of immunological response has not been consistently observed by others and it seems more likely that asthma caused by acid anhydrides, including TMA may be associated with specific IgE or IgG, or both, although specific IgE and IgG$_4$ seem to be more associated with asthma and IgG with exposure.[72] The pulmonary haemorrhage – haemolytic anaemia syndrome is real but rare.

It has been reported in those exposed to hot TMA fume and may be the outcome of a toxic reaction to inhalation of TMA in very high concentration rather than a hypersensitivity reaction. To date no cases have been reported in the UK.

Complex platinum salts (see Chapter 7)

The complex platinum salt ammonium hexachloroplatinate is an essential intermediate in the refining of platinum, a corrosion-resistant metal used as a catalyst and in jewellery. Allergy to platinum salts in refinery workers was first reported in 1945.[73] Subsequently inhalation of ammonium hexachloroplatinate was shown to provoke asthmatic responses and to elicit immediate skin test responses in sensitized individuals.[74]

The incidence of occupational allergy in the platinum refining industry was high in the UK in the mid 1970s. In a cohort study of 91 workers who entered employment in a platinum refinery in the years 1973 and 1974,[75] 22 developed respiratory symptoms and an immediate skin test response to ammonium hexachloroplatinate. The risk was greatest in the first year of employment and smoking was more important than atopy as a predictor of developing a positive skin test reaction.

OCCUPATIONAL ASTHMA AND ALLERGY

Occupational asthma fulfils the criteria for an acquired specific hypersensitivity response:
1 It occurs in only a proportion – usually a minority – of those exposed to its cause.
2 It develops only after an initial symptom-free period of exposure which is usually weeks or months but can be years.
3 In those who develop asthma, airway responses, both reduction in calibre and increase in non-specific responsiveness, are provoked by inhalation of the specific agent in concentrations which were previously tolerable and which do not provoke similar responses in others equally exposed i.e. in concentrations not toxic to mucosal surfaces.

These characteristics have stimulated a search for evidence of a specific immunological response to the causes of occupational asthma, both proteins and low molecular weight chemicals. Until recently, most attention has been directed towards the identification of specific IgE and IgG antibodies. In general, when demonstrated IgE and IgG$_4$ have been found in exposed populations to be associated with disease and total specific IgE with exposure. Specific IgE was associated with asthma and IgG with exposure in those working with laboratory animals[75] and specific IgE and IgG$_4$ with asthma and IgG with exposure to acid anhydride workers.[76]

Recent studies have suggested a central role for the T lymphocyte and in particular the TH$_2$ lymphocyte in the development of the eosinophilic bronchitis characteristic of asthma. Evidence for the involvement of T lymphocytes in occupational asthma was found in nine patients with isocyanate-induced asthma who had activated T lymphocytes and eosinophils in bronchial biopsy specimens.[77] Nonetheless, the IgE antibody–mast cell interaction is probably an important associated response dependent upon TH$_2$ lymphocyte stimulation and specific IgE remains a valuable marker of the immunological response associated with asthma caused by several agents inhaled at work.

Specific IgE antibody – inferred either from an immediate skin test response to a water soluble extract of the specific protein or hapten protein conjugate, or its identification in serum by radioallergosorbent test (RAST) – has been identified in patients with occupational asthma caused by inhaled proteins of animal, vegetable or microbial origin. These include the excreta and secreta of laboratory animals, small mammals,[18] and locusts,[78] wheat and rye flour,[79] and proteolytic enzymes.[80] Specific IgE has also been identified in the sera of patients with asthma caused by some low molecular weight chemicals, particularly acid anhydrides[81] and reactive dyes.[82] In a study to examine the determinants of allergenicity of low molecular weight chemicals, the properties of two β-lactam antibiotics were compared, clavulanic acid, which is not allergenic, and a carbapenam MM2283 which can cause asthma and stimulate IgE antibody production in man. The characteristics identified as relevant to allergenicity were (1) reactivity with body proteins, (2) hapten of single chemical structure, and (3) stability of the conjugate formed.[83]

Specific IgE antibody has been identified in only some 15% of cases of isocyanate-induced asthma. This may reflect the difficulties of working with reactive chemicals in *in vitro* systems or failure to prepare the relevant *in vivo* chemical-protein conjugate for the *in vitro test*. Reactants of the isocyanate water reaction are likely to form in the water-saturated respiratory tract which may bind to tissue proteins and form a number of different conjugates. Failure to find convincing evidence of a specific immunological response in cases of isocyanate-induced asthma has led to suggestions that it may be the outcome of a pharmacological rather than an immunological mechanism. In support of this, TDI was found to inhibit the *in vitro* stimulation of adenyl cyclase by isoprenaline in a dose-dependent fashion,[84] possibly by covalent binding of the isocyanate group to the membrane receptor, and suggested to provoke asthma by β-adrenoreceptor inhibition in those with pre-existing airway hyper-responsiveness. This, however, does not explain the well documented latent interval between exposure to TDI and the development of asthma and the failure of TDI to provoke asthma in patients with asthma and airway hyper-responsiveness from other causes.[85] Furthermore, inhalation of TDI induces an increase in non-specific airway responsiveness in sensitized individuals whose airway responsiveness in the absence of exposure has normalized[63] and fails to inhibit isoprenaline-induced tracheal smooth muscle relaxation.[86]

The development of molecular biological techniques and their application in identifying specific mRNA in T lymphocytes should provide a powerful tool to investigate further the immunological basis of these low molecular weight chemicals where evidence of associated IgE antibody for whatever reason, is not obtainable.

DETERMINANTS OF OCCUPATIONAL ASTHMA

Four separate factors have been reported to contribute to the development of occupational asthma in populations exposed to its causes: intensity of exposure, atopy, tobacco smoking and human leucocyte antigen (HLA) phenotype.

Exposure intensity

Although, in principle, the most directly amenable to control, exposure has until recently received the least attention, which in part has been due to the difficulty in measuring aeroallergen concentration. The development of inhibition immunoassays has now allowed this. Several recently reported studies have found evidence for a relationship between measured intensity of exposure and the prevalence of sensitization and asthma.

Cullinan *et al.*[87] found an exposure–response relationship between airborne rat urine protein concentration and the prevalence of both skin test reactions to rat urine protein and respiratory symptoms. Juniper *et al.*[37] in a study of a cohort of enzyme detergent workers, found the incidence of skin prick test responses to alcalase was greatest in those most heavily exposed. Coutts *et al.*[88] found the prevalence of work-related nasal and lower respiratory symptoms in pharmaceutical workers manufacturing tablets of cimetidine increased with increasing frequency of exposure during the working week. The prevalence of work-related respiratory symptoms and

airway hyper-responsiveness in bakery workers was greater in those who had ever worked in dustier conditions[89] and Burge *et al.*[90] found a gradient of work-related respiratory symptoms in relation to measured concentration of airborne colophony. Similarly Barker *et al.*[91] found the risk of a skin test response to trimellitic anhydride and work-related respiratory symptoms increased with increasing intensity of exposure.

Atopy

Atopy, defined in immunological terms as those who readily produce IgE antibodies on contact with environmental allergens encountered in everyday life, is commonly identified by the presence of one or more immediate skin prick test responses to common inhalant allergens (which in the UK include grass pollen, *D. pteronyssinus* and cat fur). The prevalence in workforces of atopy, defined in this way has been consistently reported as between 25 and 33%. Asthma and IgE antibody induced by several causes of occupational asthma have been reported to occur more commonly among atopic individuals. This association is best described for asthma caused by laboratory animals, *B. subtilis* enzymes and complex platinum salts.

Several studies have shown asthma to be some four to five times more prevalent in atopic than non-atopic laboratory animal workers.[92,93] In their cohort study of enzyme detergent workers, Juniper *et al.*[37] found the incidence of a skin test response to alcalase was greater among atopics at each level of exposure. Similarly Cullinan *et al.*[87] found atopy increased the risk of sensitization to rat urine proteins at each level of exposure. Dally *et al.*[94] found an increased incidence of skin prick test responses to ammonium hexachloroplatinate in atopics in a platinum refinery workforce. However, a subsequent study of the same population found smoking to be a more important risk factor.[95] For several causes of occupational asthma however, such as isocyanates and plicatic acid, atopics seem at no greater risk of developing asthma than non-atopics.

Tobacco smoking

Tobacco smoking has been reported to increase the risk of developing asthma and specific IgE antibody to several different causes of occupational asthma. Specific IgE antibody or an immediate skin test response has been found some four to five times more frequently in smokers than non-smokers exposed to tetrachlorophthalic anhydride,[96] green coffee bean and ispaghula[97] and ammonium hexachloroplatinate.[95] The risk of developing asthma is also increased, although less than for specific IgE. All seven cases of TCPA-induced asthma reported by Howe *et al.*[68] were cigarette smokers; smoking increased the risk of asthma in platinum refinery workers and snow crab processing workers[98] by some twofold. Smoking also interacted with intensity of exposure to increase the risk to sensitization to complex platinum salts in platinum refinery workers.[99] The greatest risk occurred in smokers in high exposure jobs; no cases occurred in non-smokers in low exposure jobs. The risk was similar and intermediate in non-smokers in high exposure and smokers in low exposure jobs.

The mechanism of this 'adjuvant' effect of tobacco smoking is unknown, but may be related to injury, whatever the cause to the respiratory mucosa, concurrently with inhalation of novel antigens. Inhaled tobacco smoke potentiated the IgE response to inhaled but not subcutaneous ovalbumin in an experiment in mice.[100] Other respiratory irritants can exert a similar effect. The proportion of cynomologus monkeys who developed asthma and a positive skin test after inhalation of complex platinum salts was increased in the animals who inhaled ozone concurrently.[102] Similarly, the frequency of IgE antibody production and airway responses provoked by inhaled ovalbumin were increased in a dose-dependent fashion in guinea pigs who inhaled sulphur dioxide concurrently with the sensitizing dose of ovalbumin.[102]

Human leucocyte antigen (HLA) phenotype

Recently the association of specific IgE antibody and asthma caused by agents inhaled at work and HLA Class II alleles has been investigated. Young et al.[103] in a case-referent study of acid anhydride workers found a significant excess of HLA-DR3 in cases with specific IgE to trimellitic anhydride (eight of 11 cases vs two of 14 referents:odds ratio 8.14) but not in cases with specific IgE to phthalic anhydride (two of 11 cases vs two of 14 referents). Bignon et al.[104] investigated HLA Class II alleles in cases of isocyanate-induced asthma. They found that allele DQB1*0503 and the allelic combination DQB1*0201/0301 were increased and the allele DQB1*0501 and DQA1*0101 – DQB1*0501 DR1 haplotype were significantly reduced in cases of isocyanate-induced asthma compared with unaffected isocyanate exposed workers. In a case-referent study of 111 platinum refinery workers Newman Taylor et al.[105] found that the risk of having developed an immediate skin test response to platinum salts was increased in HLA/DR3 positive and reduced in HLA/DR6 positive individuals. These associations were markedly stronger in those who had worked in 'low' rather than in 'high' exposure groups. At least for inhaled low molecular weight chemical haptens, HLA phenotype may be an important determinant of sensitization and asthma, which is possibly of more significance at lower levels of exposure.

DIAGNOSIS OF OCCUPATIONAL ASTHMA

Accurate and early diagnosis of cases of occupational asthma is important. Remission of respiratory symptoms and restoration of normal lung function including non-specific airway responsiveness, can follow avoidance of exposure to the specific initiating cause. Furthermore, chronic asthma is more likely to develop in those who remain exposed to the initiating cause after the onset of symptoms. However, avoidance of exposure frequently requires a change of work which, particularly in the present economic climate, can lead to loss of employment. Accurate diagnosis is also essential if those whose asthma is not occupationally caused are to avoid being advised unnecessarily to change or leave their work. The diagnosis of occupational asthma requires:

1 Differentiation of asthma from other causes of respiratory symptoms, in particular chronic airflow limitation and hyperventilation.
2 Differentiation of occupational cause from non-occupational asthma.
3 Differentiation of asthma initiated by an agent inhaled at work from pre-existing or incidental asthma exacerbated by non-specific irritants such as sulphur dioxide and cold air, inhaled at work.

The diagnosis of occupational hypersensitivity asthma is commonly suggested by the history. It usually occurs in an individual exposed at work to an agent recognized to cause occupational asthma and only develops after an initial symptom-free period when the patient has been exposed without symptoms to the concentrations which now provoke his asthma. Respiratory symptoms occur during the working week and may increase in severity as the week progresses, and improve during absences from work, at weekends or during holidays. The patient may also be aware of others who have developed similar respiratory symptoms at the place of work.

Non-specific stimuli provoke asthmatic reactions which usually occur within minutes of exposure to an irritant and resolve within 1–2 hours of avoidance of exposure. Where work-related respiratory symptoms are due to the provocation of asthma by a respiratory irritant encountered at work, the onset of asthma will often have preceded initial exposure to the irritant and the severity of asthma does not significantly improve when away from work. Non-specific irritants such as organic solvents which may have a characteristic and unpleasant smell, may also provoke a hyperventilation response when difficulty with breathing is associated with symptoms which are consequences of a low arterial pCO_2 such as tingling of the fingers, headaches and dizziness.

INVESTIGATION OF CAUSES OF OCCUPATIONAL ASTHMA

In the majority of cases a confident diagnosis of occupational asthma can be made from knowledge of exposure at work to a recognized cause of occupational asthma and a characteristic history. Where possible these should be supported by objective evidence, from serial measurements of peak expiratory flow (PEF), or immunological tests or both. Inhalation testing is reserved for occasions when the results of these investigations do not provide an adequate basis for advice about future employment.

Serial peak expiratory flow measurements

Asthma can be attributed with confidence to an agent inhaled at work where exposure to it in the work place reproducibly provokes airway narrowing. Repeated measurements of airway calibre, most conveniently made as PEF rates, need to be made during a period long enough to allow observation of the consistency of any changes and their relationship to periods at work. Measurements need to be made repeatedly during each day for a period of several weeks when the patient makes and records his own results. Such self-recording of PEF measurements is now widely used.

Patients are lent a peak flow meter and asked to record the best of three measurements of PEF made every 2 hours from waking to sleeping over a period of 1 month in the first instance.

To allow sufficient time for lung function to recover from exposure to an agent inhaled at work, it is helpful if the month includes a period away from work which is longer than a weekend, ideally a 1- or 2-week holiday. Self-recording requires patient compliance and honesty. The measurements may be conveniently summarized to show the maximum, minimum and mean peak flow measurements for each day (Fig. 33.1) and differences between periods at and away from work observed. This method of patient investigation has proved, in the hands of those experienced in its use, to be reliable and a relatively sensitive and specific index of occupational asthma.

Immunological investigations

The application of immunological tests in the investigation of occupational asthma has widened because of:

1 Identification of the nature and source of relevant allergens (e.g. the identification of laboratory animal urine) as a major source of allergenic protein allowing the preparation of immunologically relevant test extracts.
2 Preparation of hapten protein conjugates suitable for immunological testing (e.g. acid anhydride human

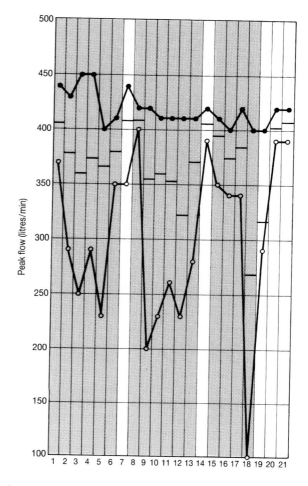

Figure 33.1 *Results of self-recorded serial peak flow measurements in a condom worker sensitive to* Lycopodium *spores. The best, worst and average peak flow rate are plotted for each day. The shaded areas are days at work, the unshaded areas days away from work. Record shows consistently worse peak flows during periods at work.*

serum albumin conjugates and reactive dye – human serum albumin conjugates).
3 Development of reliable methods for identification of specific IgE antibody in serum.

Extracts of several of the causes of occupational asthma can be used to elicit skin test reactions and to identify specific IgE antibody in serum. These include the *B. subtilis* enzyme, alcalase, urine proteins of laboratory animals, excreta of locusts, wheat and rye flour proteins, harvest moulds (including *Alternaria tenuis* and *Cladosporium herbarum*) and grain mites (such as *Acaris siro* and *L. destructor*). In addition, hapten protein conjugates, suitable for skin testing and identification of specific IgE antibody, have been prepared for acid anhydrides and reactive dyes. Complex platinum salts such as ammonium hexachloroplatinate can elicit immediate skin prick test responses without the need for conjugation to human serum albumin.

The value of such tests in the diagnosis of occupational asthma depends upon their sensitivity and specificity in populations exposed to the particular cause. Extracts of urine protein obtained from rats and mice have been shown in several studies to be a sensitive and relatively specific index of asthma, but not of rhinitis, conjunctivitis or urticaria.[15,16] Similarly, an immediate skin prick test response and specific IgE antibody identified by RAST, to extracts of locusts[78] and to conjugates of the acid anhydride, TCPA with human serum albumin[68] were associated with cases of asthma in exposed populations and not simply a reflection of exposure (see Chapter 2).

Inhalation tests

There are four major indications for inhalation testing in the diagnosis of occupational asthma.

1 Where the agent thought to be responsible for causing asthma has not previously been reliably shown to do so.
2 Where an individual with occupational asthma is exposed at work to more than one potential cause, and his future employment depends on knowledge of which one is responsible.
3 Where asthma is of such severity that further uncontrolled exposure in the work environment is not justifiable.
4 Where the diagnosis of occupational asthma remains in doubt after other investigations, including serial PEF and immunological tests, where appropriate, have been completed.

Inhalation tests undertaken solely for legal purposes are not justifiable and are not required for statutory compensation purposes.

Because they are potentially hazardous, inhalation tests with occupational agents should only be undertaken by those experienced in undertaking them who have adequate hospital facilities for continuous monitoring of patients for 24 hours after each test. Several facilities are now available in the UK.

The aim of an occupational type inhalation test is to expose the individual under single-blind conditions to the putative cause of his asthma in circumstances which resemble as closely as possible the conditions of his exposure at work. Wherever possible, atmospheric concentrations of the inhaled agent should be based on knowledge of the concentrations experienced at work and the physical conditions of exposure (e.g. size of dust particles, whether vapour or aerosol and temperatures to which the materials are heated), should be similar to those at work. The different methods used in inhalation tests depend primarily on the physical state of the test material. Soluble allergens, such as urine proteins of laboratory animals, are inhaled as nebulized extracts in solution. Volatile organic liquids such as TDI may be painted onto a flat surface in increasing concentrations on different days and the atmospheric concentration of evolved vapour measured with an appropriate monitor. Exposure to dusts such as antibiotics, complex platinum salts and acid anhydrides is made by tipping the test material, usually diluted in dried lactose, between two trays. The atmospheric concentration achieved is surprisingly reproducible and can be measured by use of a personal dust sampler.

Measurements of airway responses provoked by inhalation test should ideally include measurements of both changes in airway calibre and in non-specific airway responsiveness. Changes in airway calibre are most conveniently measured by regular measurements of forced expiaotry volume in 1 second (FEV_1) and forced vital capacity (FVC) or peak expiratory flow (PEF) before, and at regular intervals after the test, for at least 24 hours. Changes in airway responsiveness can be made by estimating the concentration of inhaled histamine or methacholine which provokes a 20% fall in FEV_1 (PC20) before the test and at 3 hours and 24 hours after the test. The changes in airway calibre and non-specific responsiveness observed are compared with those following a control challenge test, each test being made on a separate day (Fig. 33.2).

The patterns of change in airway calibre provoked by inhalation testing are distinguished by their time of onset and duration. Immediate responses occur within minutes and resolve spontaneously within 1–2 hours. Such reactions can be provoked by both allergic (e.g. grass pollen) and non-allergic (e.g. inhaled histamine or sulphur dioxide) stimuli. The response depends upon the concentration of the provoking agent and the degree of pre-existing non-specific airway responsiveness. Lone immediate responses (i.e. an immediate response not followed by a late response) are not usually associated with an increase in non-specific airway responsiveness. Late responses develop 1 or more hours after the inhalation test exposure, usually after some 3–4 hours, and may persist for 24–36 hours. Unlike the immediate response, late responses are often associated with an increase in non-specific responsiveness which can be identified 3 hours after the test prior to the onset of the late asthmatic response and less reliably 24 hours after the test.[47]

A dual response is an immediate response followed by a late response. Recurrent nocturnal responses may be provoked by a single inhalation test exposure with asthmatic responses occurring during several successive nights with partial or complete remission during the intervening days.[106] Such responses are almost certainly a manifestation of a provoked increase in non-specific airway responsiveness. The question to be answered from the results of an inhalation test is whether or not in the individual case the particular agent inhaled at work has induced asthma. The most reliable means of answering

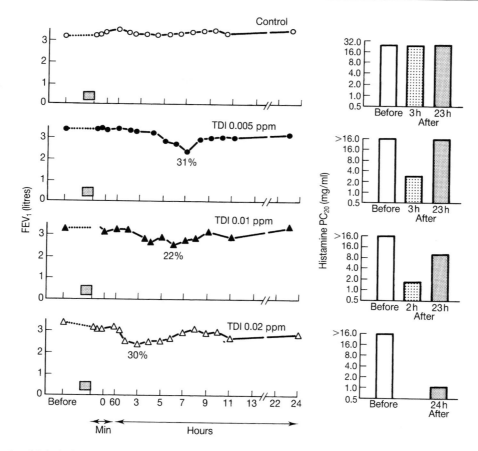

Figure 33.2 *Results of inhalation test with toluene diisocyanate (TDI) showing both FEV$_1$ and histamine PC20 before and during 24-hour period after test. Patient has a late asthmatic reaction provoked by TDI inhalation with associated reduction in histamine PC20 at 3 hours at lower exposures and at 24 hours at higher exposure concentrations.*

this question is to determine whether or not inhalation of the specific agent in concentrations to which exposure occurs at work reproducibly provokes a non-immediate asthmatic response and increases non-specific airway responsiveness. In such cases the specific agent can be considered to be the inducing cause in that particular individual. Non-specific irritants may provoke immediate responses in individuals with hyper-responsive airways, but do not provoke either an increase in non-specific airway responsiveness or a late asthmatic reaction. Agents which induce specific IgE antibody, however, may provoke lone asthmatic responses; in these cases inferences from the inhalation test result should take the immunological test into account.

OUTCOME OF OCCUPATIONAL ASTHMA

Asthma induced by an agent inhaled at work may become chronic, persisting for several years, if not indefinitely, after avoidance of exposure to its initiating cause. This seems particularly, although not exclusively, to occur with asthma caused by low molecular weight chemicals. Asthma caused by agents such as isocyanates, acid anhydrides, Western Red Cedar and snow crab has been reported to have persisted in over half of cases. Six cases of asthma caused by the acid anhydride TCPA were followed up 4 years after avoidance of exposure: all had chronic respiratory symptoms consistent with persistent airway hyper-responsiveness and a measurable histamine PC20 was present in the five in whom it was assessed. The rate of decline of specific IgE to a TCPA-human serum albumin conjugate during the period of avoidance of exposure was parallel in all six subjects and exponential with a half-life of 1 year, making it very improbable their continuing asthma was caused by further, albeit inadvertent exposure.[107]

In another study, 31 snow crab workers with occupational asthma, diagnosed by inhalation tests, were studied up to 5 years from their last exposure.[108] All denied exposure to crabmeat either by inhalation or ingestion. Respiratory symptoms persisted in all 31, of whom 26 had a measurable methacholine PC20. Although FEV$_1$ improved to within the range predicted during the first year of avoidance of exposure, PC$_{20}$ plateaued after 2 years and remained abnormal.

Chronic asthma in these cases is likely to be a manifestation of persistent airway inflammation which although initiated by the agent inhaled at work persists in its absence. Ten patients with TDI-induced asthma, who had continuing respiratory symptoms and airway hyper-responsiveness, were investigated 4–40 months from their last exposure.[109] Bronchial biopsies obtained from eight subjects showed basement membrane thickening with infiltration of the mucosa by eosinophils, lymphocytes and neutrophils; in four patients in whom airway responsiveness had not improved, the proportion of eosinophils in fluid recovered at BAL was increased, whereas this was the case in only one of five whose airway responsiveness had improved.

To date the only important determinant identified of persistence in occupational asthma is duration of exposure to the initiating cause after the onset of respiratory symptoms.

When examined, on average 4 years after avoidance of exposure, 60% of 136 cases of asthma caused by Western Red Cedar (*Thuja plicata*) continued to have asthma. The interval from onset of symptoms to diagnosis was on average 2½ years longer than in those whose symptoms had resolved.[110]

MANAGEMENT OF OCCUPATIONAL ASTHMA

Management advice for patients with occupational asthma has been greatly influenced by the results of studies of outcome of occupational asthma which have found evidence of continuing asthma and airway hyper-responsiveness despite many years avoidance of exposure to the initiating cause and in particular those studies such as of Western Red Cedar[110] and of azodicarbonamide[111] workers which have identified a relationship between the duration of symptomatic exposure and the risk of chronic asthma. The message from these studies has seemed to be clear: recognize occupational asthma as early as possible; identify its cause with reasonable certainty; avoid exposure as soon as possible. The importance of accurate identification of the specific cause cannot be overemphasized. Avoidance of exposure often involves relocation or loss of current employment. In the current economic situation, such a step without adequate reason could be the cause of considerable unnecessary hardship. Misdiagnosis of occupational asthma can be as hazardous for individual patients as missing the diagnosis.

Unfortunately, environmental changes, unless they involve substitution, are in general rarely able to reduce exposures sufficiently to prevent continuing airway responses in sensitized individuals. Venables and Newman Taylor examined the relationship between the concentration of TCPA in air and the provocation of

asthmatic responses in inhalation tests in four sensitive individuals. They observed a log linear relationship between the magnitude of late asthmatic responses and TCPA concentration, which passed through the origin, suggesting no threshold.[112]

Patients who develop occupational asthma in whom a specific cause is identified should be advised to avoid further exposure to the cause of their asthma. This seems particularly important where low molecular weight chemicals, such as isocyanates, plicatic acid or acid anhydrides, are the cause as these are particularly, although not exclusively, associated with the development of chronic asthma and airway hyper-responsiveness.

Avoidance of further exposure may require a change or loss of job, which for social or financial reasons, may not be possible. A change of occupation can be particularly difficult for highly trained individuals, such as experimental scientists whose livelihood depends on their knowledge and experience of working with laboratory animals.

Such individuals and others sensitized to biological dusts who are unable, at least in the short term, to change their job, should be advised to minimize organic dust exposure, and to wear respiratory protection, most conveniently laminar flow equipment, when in contact with the organic dust. In addition, background prophylaxis such as sodium cromoglycate can reduce the risk of the provocation of asthma by indirect allergen contact, as from dust on colleagues' clothing. Nonetheless, it should be emphasized that such measures are temporary and in the long term, the means should be sought to avoid exposure to the cause of asthma.

When an individual does remain in employment exposed to the cause of his asthma, either directly or indirectly, the effectiveness of relocation or of respiratory protection needs to be monitored. This can be conveniently done by serial self-recordings of peak flow to determine whether or not asthma persists and if so if it is work-related.

PREVENTION OF OCCUPATIONAL ASTHMA

Reduction in the incidence of occupational asthma will follow adequate control of exposure to its causes. Substitution of enzyme granules for powder in the manufacture of enzyme detergents was followed by a marked decrease in the incidence of allergy and asthma to subtilisins;[37] substitution of a different paint for one containing TDI halted an epidemic of asthma in a steel coating plant.[45] Measures to secure control of exposure to the majority of causes of occupational asthma have, however, been impeded by lack of knowledge of the nature of exposure–response relationships for sensitizing agents and inability to measure the concentration of airborne allergenic proteins.

Immunoassays to measure aeroallergen concentrations have been developed and, although they remain primarily a research tool, are being applied increasingly to occupational environments. The airborne concentration of urine proteins of rats and mice in animal laboratories has been the most extensively investigated; this reflects knowledge of the nature and source of the responsible allergens and the high prevalence of laboratory animal allergy. The steady state concentration of airborne allergens is determined by the ratio of rates of their generation and removal. The major factors influencing allergen generation are stock density (the number of animals per unit volume of the room) and working activities (e.g. cage cleaning and sweeping). The major determinants of allergen reduction are cage design, bedding type, ventilation, air filtration and humidity.[113]

Twiggs et al. estimated the concentration of airborne mouse urine allergens in an animal laboratory by RAST inhibition immunoassay. Airborne allergen concentrations varied between 1.8 and 825 ng/m^3 and were influenced by both stock density and level of work activity.[114] Gordon et al. in an experimental study found the concentration of airborne rat urine protein was directly related (in a log linear fashion) to stock density and was significantly reduced by the use of absorbent bedding and filter top cages.[19] Edwards et al. showed that increased ventilation rates and increased humidity in an animal laboratory appreciably reduced the concentration of airborne rat urine proteins.[115]

Juniper et al. reported the results of a 7-year follow-up of employers in an enzyme detergent factory during the years immediately after the introduction of granulation of the B. subtilis enzyme alcalase.[37] concentrations of both enzyme and total dust in the factory fell during the period of follow up: peak levels of total dust in 1969 and 1970 were 1200 µg/m^3, falling subsequently to levels which were consistently below 400 µg/m^3. In parallel with this the number of new employees who developed immediate skin test responses to alcalase fell from 29% in those who entered employment between 1969 and 1971 to 11% in those who joined between 1971 and 1973. Similarly the number who had to leave the factory because of the development of new respiratory symptoms fell from 50 between 1968 and 1971 to one each year in 1972–74.

Botham et al. reported the experience of a pharmaceutical company of the introduction of a code of practice, which included improved work practices and the use of approved respiratory protection to reduce airborne and inhaled animal allergen concentrations.[116] The changes in work practice were associated with a progressive reduction of some 66% in the rate of sensitization to animal urine proteins from about 30% before to 10% after the intervention.

The development of control measures which will significantly reduce the incidence of occupational asthma requires investigation of exposure–response relationships and of the effects of the interventions.

STATUTORY COMPENSATION, UK

Occupational asthma is a prescribed disease for 'employed earners'. The terms of prescription have recently been widened considerably. They now include asthma caused by exposure to 22 specified groups of agents as well as a 'z' category, which specifies 'any other sensitizing agent inhaled at work'. The current terms of prescription are shown in Table 33.6, below.

Table 33.6 *Current terms of prescription for asthma*

Exposure to
• Isocyanates
• Platinum salts
• Acid anhydride and amine hardening agents
• Fumes arising from the use of rosin as a soldering flux
• Proteolytic enzymes
• Animals including insects and other arthropods of their larval forms used for the purposes of research, education, in laboratories, pest control or fruit cultivation
• Dusts arising from barley, oats, rye, wheat or maize, or meal or flour made from such grain
• Antibiotics
• Cimetidine
• Wood dusts
• Ispaghula
• Castor bean dust
• Ipecacuanha
• Azodicarbonamide
• Glutaraldehyde
• Persulphate salts or henna arising from their use in the hairdressing trade
• Crustaceans or fish or products arising from these in the food processing industry
• Reactive dyes
• Soya bean
• Tea dust
• Green coffee bean dust
• Fumes from stainless steel welding
• Any other sensitizing agent inhaled at work

REFERENCES

1 Brookes SM, Weiss MA, Bernstein K. Reactive airways dysfunction syndrome (RADS): persistent asthma syndrome after high level irritant exposure. *Chest* 1985; **88**: 376–84.

2 Kojevinas M, Anto JM, Soriano JB, Tobias A, Burney P. The

risk of asthma attributable to occupational exposures. *Am J Respir Crit Care Med* 1996; **154:** 137–43.

3 Meredith SK, Taylor VM, McDonald JC. Occupational respiratory disease in the United Kingdom. *Br J Ind Med* 1991; **48:** 292–8.

4 Sallie BA, Ross DJ, Meredith SK, McDonald JC. SWORD '93. Surevillance of work-related and occupational respiratory disease in the UK. *Occup Med* 1994; **44:** 177–82.

5 Meredith S. Reported incidence of occupational asthma in the United Kingdom. *J Epidemiol Commun Hlth* 1993; **47:** 459–63.

6 Keskinen H. Registers for occupational disease. *Br Med J* 1991; **303:** 597–8.

7 Harkonen H, Nordman H, Korhonen O. *et al.* Long term effects from exposure to sulphur dioxide: lung function 4 years after a pyrite dust explosion. *Am Rev Respir Dis* 1983; **128:** 840–7.

8 Luo JCJ, Nelson K, Fischbein A. Persistent reactive airways dysfunction after exposure to toluene diisocyanate. *Br J Ind Med* 1988; **47:** 239–41.

9 Bernstein IL, Bernstein DI, Weiss M, Campbell GP. Reactive airways syndrome (RADS) after exposure to toxic ammonia fumes. *J All Clin Immunol* 1989; **83:** 173.

10 Mosain T. Prolonged asthma after smoke inhalation: a report of 3 cases and a review of previous reports. *J Occup Med* 1991; **33:** 458–61.

11 Kern DG. Outbreak of the reactive airways dysfunction syndrome after a spill of glacial acetic acid. *Am Rev Respir Dis* 1991; **144:** 1056–64.

12 Sallie BA, McDonald JC. *Circumstances, Severity and Outcome of Inhalation Accidents in the UK.* Proceedings of Tenth International Symposium on Epidemiology in Occupational Health. Como, 20–23 September 1994.

13 Sallie B, McDonald JC. Inhalation accidents reported to the SWORD surveillance project 1990–1993. *Ann Occup Hyg* 1996; **40:** 211–21.

14 Cockcroft A, Edwards J, McCarthy P, Andersson N. Allergy and laboratory animal workers. *Lancet* 1981; **ii:** 827–30.

15 Slovak AJM, Hill RN. Laboratory animal allergy: A clinical survey of an exposed population. *Br J Ind Med* 1981; **38:** 38–41.

16 Venables KM, Tee RD, Hawkins ER, Gordon DJ, Wale CJ *et al.* Laboratory animal allergy in a pharmaceutical company. *Br J Ind Med* 1988; **45:** 667–71.

17 Davies GE, Thompson AV, Niewola Z, Biurrows GE, Reasdale EL *et al.* Allergy to laboratory animals: a retrospective and prospective study. *Br J Ind Med* 1983; **40:** 442–9.

18 Newman Taylor AJ, Longbottom JL, Pepys J. Allergy to urine proteins of rats and mice. *Lancet* 1977; **ii:** 847–9.

19 Gordon S, Tee RD, Lowson D, Wallace J, Newman Taylor AJ. Reduction of airborne allergenic urine proteins from laboratory rats. *Br J Ind Med* 1992; **49:** 416–22.

20 Harries MG, Lacey J, Tee RD, Cayley JR, Newman Taylor AJ. *Didymella exitialis* and late summer asthma. *Lancet* 1985; **i:** 1063–6.

21 Tee RD, Gordon DJ, Newman Taylor AJ. Cross-reactivity

between antigens of fungal extracts studied by RAST inhibition and immunoblotting. *J All Clin Immunol* 1987; **79:** 627–33.

22 Darke CS, Knowelden J, Lacey J, Ward AM. Respiratory disease of workers harvesting grain. *Thorax* 1976; **31:** 293–302.

23 Ingram CG, Jeffrey IG, Symington IS, Cuthbert OD. Bronchial provocation studies in farmers allergic to storage mites. *Lancet* 1979; **2:** 1330–2.

24 Blainey AD, Topping MD, Ollier S, Davies RJ. Specific IgE to storage mites in Essex farmers. *Thorax* 1986; **41:** 251–2.

25 van Hage-Hamsten M, Johannson SGO, Hoglund S, Ptull P, Wyren A, Zetterstrom O. Storage mite allergy common in a farming population. *Clin All* 1985; **15:** 555–64.

26 Hendrick DJ, Davies RJ, Pepys J. Bakers asthma. *Clin All* 1976; **i:** 241–50.

27 Baur Z, Fruhmann G, Haug B, Rasche B, Reicher W, Weiss W. Role of *Aspergillus amyalse* in baker's asthma. *Lancet* 1986; **i:** 43.

28 Musk AW, Venables KM, Crook B, Nunn AJ, Hawkins R *et al.* Respiratory symptoms, lung function and sensitisation to flour in a british bakery. *Br J Ind Med* 1989; **46:** 636–42.

29 Belin L, Falsen E, Hoborn J, Ancre J. Enzyme sensitisation in consumers of enzyme containing washing powders. *Lancet* 1970; **ii:** 1153.

30 Zetterstrom O, Wide L. IgE antibodies and skin test reactions to a detergent enzyme in Swedish consumers. *Clin All* 1974; **4:** 273–80.

31 Zetterstrom O. Challenge and exposure test reactions to enzyme detergents in subjects sensitised to subtilisin. *Clin All* 1977; **7:** 355–63.

32 Flindt MLH. Pulmonary disease due to inhalation of derivatives of Bacillus subtilis containing enzyme. *Lancet* 1969; **i:** 1177–81.

33 Pepys J, Hargreave FE, Longbottom JL. Allergic reactions of the lungs to enzymes of *Bacillus subtilis*. *Lancet* 1969; **i:** 1181–4.

34 Newhouse ML, Tagg B, Pocock SJ, McEwan AL. An epidemiological study of workers producing enzyme washing powders. *Lancet* 1970; **i:** 689–93.

35 Weill H, Waddell LC, Ziskind M. A study of workers exposed to detergent enzymes. *JAMA* 1971; **217:** 425–33.

36 Mitchell CA, Gandevia B. Respiratory symptoms and skin reactivity in workers exposed to proteolytic enzymes in the detergent industry. *Am Rev Respir Dis* 1971; **104:** 1–12.

37 Juniper CP, How MJ, Goodwin BFJ, Kinshott AJC. *Bacillus subtilis* enzymes: a 7-year clinical epidemiologicla and immunological study of an industrial allergen. *J Soc Occup Med* 1977; **27:** 3–12.

38 Swanson MC, Bubak ME, Hunt L, Reed CE. Occupational respiratory disease from latex. *J All Clin Immunol* 1992; **89**A: 227.

39 Bubak ME, Fransway AW *et al.* Latex allergy in health care workers. *Mayo Clinic Proc* 1992; **67:** 1075–9.

40 Vandenplas O, Delurke JP, Everard G *et al.* Prevalence of occupational asthma due to latex among hospital

personnel. *Am J Respir Crit Care Med* 1995; **151**: 54–60.

41 Liss GM, Sussman GL, Deal K *et al*. Latex allergy: epidemiological study of 1351 hospital workers. *Occup Environ Med* 1997; **54**: 335–42.

42 Blanco C, Carrillo T, Queralto J, Cuevas M. Avacado hypersensitivity. *Allergy* 1994; **49**: 54–9.

43 Brock Williams Bulir MO, Weber RW. Latex allergens in responsible particulate air pollution. *J All Clin Immunol* 1995; **95**: 88–95.

44 Jaeger D, Kleinhans D, Czuppon AB, Baur Z. Latex specific proteins causing immediate type cutaneous nasal bronchial and systemic reactions. *J All Clin Immunol* 1992; **89**: 759–68.

45 Chan Yeung M, Vedal S, Cuss J, Maclean L, Ennarson D, Tse KS. Symptoms pulmonary function and bronchial hyper-reactivity in Western Red Cedar workers compared with those in office workers. *Am Rev Respir Dis* 1984; **130**: 1038–41.

46 Brookes SM, Edwards JJ, Appol A, Edwards FH. An epidemiologic study of workers exposed to Western Red Cedar and other wood dusts. *Chest* 1991; **80** (Suppl): 30–2.

47 Gandevia B, Milne J. Occupational asthma and rhinitis due to Western Red Cedar *(Thuja plicata)* with special reference to bronchial reactivity. *Br J Ind Med* 1970; **27**: 235–44.

48 Chan Yeung, Barton GM, Maclean L, Grzybowski S. Occupational asthma and rhinitis due to Western Red Cedar *(Thuja plicata)*. *Am Rev Respir Dis* 1973; **108**: 1094–102.

49 Fawcett IW, Newman Taylor AJ, Pepys J. Asthma due to inhaled chemical agents, fumes from 'Multicore' soldering flux and colophony resin. *Clin All* 1976; **6**: 577–85.

50 Burge PS, Parks W, O'Brien IM, Hawkins R, Green M. Occupational asthma in an electronics factory. *Thorax* 1979; **34**: 13–18.

51 Perks WH, Burge PS, Rehahn M, Green M. Work related respiratory disease in employees leaving an electronics factory. *Thorax* 1979; **34**: 19–22.

52 Burge PS, Edge G, Hawkins ER, White V, Newman Taylor AJ. Occupational asthma in a factory making flux cord solder containing colophony. *Thorax* 1981; **36**: 828–34.

53 Hendy MS, Beattie BE, Burge PS. Occupational asthma due to an emulsified oil mist. *Br J Ind Med* 1985; **42**: 51–4.

54 Burge PS, Wieland A, Robertson AJ, Weir D. Occupational asthma due to unheated colophony. *Br J Ind Med* 1986; **43**: 559–60.

55 So SY, Lam WK, Yu D. Colophony induced asthma in a chicken vendor. *Clin All* 1981; **11**: 395–9.

56 Henschler D, Assman W, Meyer K. Zurtoxikologie der toluylen diisocyanate. *Arch Toxicol* 1962; **19**: 364–87.

57 Diem JE, John RN, Hendrick DJ *et al*. Five-year longitudinal study of workers employed in a new toluene diisocyanate manufacturing plant. *Am Rev Respir Dis* 1982; **126**: 420–8.

58 Zeiss CR, Kanellaks TM, Bellone TD, Levitz D, Pruzansky JJ, Patterson R. Immunoglobulin E mediated asthma and hypersensitivity pneumonitis with precipitating antihapten antibodies due to diphenylmethane diisocyanate (MDI) exposure. *J All Clin Immunol* 1980; **65**: 347–52.

59 Malo J-L, Ouimet G, Cartier A, Lebitz D, Ziess CR. Combined alveolitis and asthma due to hexamethylene diisocyanate (HDI) with evidence of crossed respiratory and immunologic reactivities to diphenylmethane diisocyanate MDI. *J All Clin Immunol* 1983; **72**: 413–9.

60 Weill H, Butcher B, Charmarajan V *et al*. *Respiratory and Immunologic Evaluation of Isocyanate Exposure in a New Manufacturing plant*. (NIOSH technical report). DHHS (NIOSH) Publication no: 81–125. Cincinnati: US Department of Health and Human Services, 1981.

61 Venables KM, Dally MB, Burge PS, Pickering CAC, Newman Taylor AJ. Occupational asthma in a steel coating plant. *Br J Ind Med* 1985; **42**: 517–24.

62 O'Brien IM, Harries MG, Burge PS, Pepys J. Toluene diisocyanate induced asthma. Reactions to TDI, MDI, HDI and histamine. *Clin All* 1979; **19**: 1–6.

63 Durham SR, Graneek BJ, Hawkins R, Newman Taylor AJ. The temporal relationship between increases in airway responsiveness to histamine and late asthmatic responses induced by occupational agents. *J All Clin Immunol* 1987; **79**: 398–406.

64 Fabbri LM, Boschetto P, Zocca E, Melani G, Pivirotto F, Plebani M. Bronchoalveolar neutrophilia during late asthmatic reactions induced by toluene diisocyanate. *Am Rev Respir Dis* 1987; **136**: 36–42.

65 Maccia CA, Berstein IL, Emmett EA, Brookes SSM. *In vitro* demonstration of specific IgE in phthalic anhydride sensitivity. *Am Rev Respir Dis* 1976; **113**: 701–4.

66 Fawcett IW, Newman Taylor AJ, Pepys J. Asthma due to inhaled chemical agents – epoxy resin systems containing phthalic anhydride, trimellitic anhydride and triethylene tetramine. *Clin All* 1977; **7**: 1–14.

67 Zeiss CR, Patterson R, Pruzansky JJ, Miller MM, Resonberg M, Levitz D. Trimellitic anhydride induced airways syndrome: Clinical and immunologic studies. *J All Clin Immunol* 1977; **6**: 96–103.

68 Howe W, Venables KM, Topping MD, Dally MB, Hawkins R *et al*. Tetrachlorophthalic anhydride asthma: evidence for specific IgE antibody. *J All Clin Immunol* 1983; **71**: 5–11.

69 Topping MD, Venables KM, Luczynska CM, Howe W, Newman Taylor AJ. Specificity of the human IgE response to inhaled acid anhydride. *J All Clin Immunol* 1986; **77**: 834–42.

70 Moller DR, Gallagher JS, Benstein DI, Wilcox TG, Burroughs HE, Bernstein IL. Detection of IgE mediated respiratory sensitisation in workers exposed to hexahydrophthalic anhydride. *J All Clin Immunol* 1985; **75**: 663–72.

71 Bernstein DI, Gallagher JA, D'Souza L, Bernstein IL. Heterogeneity of specific IgE responses in workers

sensitised to acid anhydride compounds. *J All Clin Immunol* 1984; **74**: 794–801.

72 Forster H, Topping M, Newman Taylor AJ. Specific IgG and IgG$_4$ antibody to tetrachlorophthalic anhydride. *All Proc* 1988; **9**: 296.

73 Hunter D, Milton R, Perry KMA. Asthma caused by the complex salts of platinum. *Br J Ind Med* 1945; **2**: 92–8.

74 Pepys J, Pickering CAC, Hughes EG. Asthma due to inhaled chemical agents – complex salts of platinum. *Clin All* 1972; **2**: 391–6.

75 Venables KM, Dally MB, Nunn AJ, Stevens JF, Stephens R *et al.* Smoking and occupational allergy in a platinum refinery. *Br Med J* 1989; **299**: 939–42.

76 Platts Mills TAE, Longbottom J, Edwards J, Cockcroft A, Wilkins S. Occupational asthma and rhinitis related to laboratory animals: serum IgE and IgG antibodies to the rat urinary allergen. *J All Clin Immunol* 1987; **79**: 505–15.

77 Bentley AM, Maestrelli P, Fabbri LM, Menz G, Storz C *et al.* Immunohistology of the bronchial mucosa in occupational, intrinsic and extrinsic asthma. *J All Clin Immunol* 1991; **87**: 246 (abstr).

78 Tee RD, Gordon DJ, Hawkins ER *et al.* Occupational allergy to locusts: an investigation of the sources of the allergen. *J All Clin Immunol* 1988; **81**: 517–25.

79 Bjorksten F, Backman A, Jarvinen AJ, Savilahti EK, Syvanen P, Karkkaeinen T. Immunoglobulin E specific to wheat and rye flour. *Clin All* 1977; **7**: 473–83.

80 Pepys J, Wells ED, D'Souza M, Greenburg M. Clinical and immunological responses to enzymes of *Bacillus subtilis* in factory workers and consumers. *Clin All* 1973; **3**: 143–60.

81 Newman Taylor AJ, Venables KM, Durham S, Graneek BJ, Topping MD. Acid anhydrides and asthma. *Int Arch All Appl Immunol* 1987; **82**: 435–9.

82 Luczynska CM, Topping MD. Specific IgE antibodies to reactive dye-albumin conjugates. *J Immunol Meth* 1986; **95**: 177–86.

83 Edwards RG, Dewdney JM, Dobrzanski RJ, Lee D. Immunogenicity and allergenicity studies on two beta lactam structures, a clavam, clavulanic acid and carbapenam: structure activity relationships. *Int Arch All Appl Immunol* 1988; **85**: 184–9.

84 Davies RJ, Butcher BR, O'Neil CE, Salvaggio JE. The *in vitro* effect of toluene diisocyanate on lymphocyte cyclic adenosine monophosphate production by isoproterenol, prostaglandin and histamine. *J All Clin Immunol* 1977; **60**: 223–9.

85 Lozewicz S, Assoufi BK, Hawkins R, Newman Taylor AJ. Outcome of asthma induced by isocyanates. *Br J Dis Chest* 1987; **81**: 14–22.

86 Mackay RT, Brooks SM. Effect of toluene diisocyanate on beta adrenergeic receptor function. *Am Rev Respir Dis* 1983; **148**: 50–3.

87 Cullinan P, Lowson D, Nieuwenhuijsen MJ *et al.* Work-related symptoms, sensitisations and estimated exposure in workers not previously exposed to laboratory rats. *Occup Environ Med* 1994; **51**: 589–920.

88 Coutts II, Lozewitcz S, Dally MD, Newman Taylor AJ, Burge PS, Rogers JD. Respiratory symptoms related to work in a factory manufacturing cimetidine tablets. *Br Med J* 1984; **288**: 1418.

89 Musk AW, Venables KM, Crook B, Nunn AJ *et al.* Respiratory symptoms, lung function and sensitisation to flour in a British bakery. *Br J Ind Med* 1989; **46**: 636–42.

90 Burge PS, Edge G, Hawkins R, White V, Newman Taylor AJ. Occupational asthma in a factory making cored solder containing colophony. *Thorax* 1981; **36**: 828–34.

91 Barker RD, van Tongeren MJA, Harris JM, Gardiner K, Venables KM, Newman Taylor AJ. Risk factors for sensitization and respiratory symptoms among workers exposed to acid anhydrides: a cohort study. *Occup Environ Med* 1998; **55**: 684–91.

92 Slovak AMJ, Hill RN. Laboratory animal allergy: a clinical survey of an exposed population. *Br J Ind Med* 1981; **38**: 38–41.

93 Venables KM, Tee RD, Hawkins ER *et al.* Laboratory animal allergy in a pharmaceutical company. *Br J Ind Med* 1988; **45**: 660–6.

94 Dally MB, Hunter JV, Hughes EG *et al.* Hypersensitivity to platinum salts: a population study. *Am Rev Respir Dis* 1980; **4**: 120.

95 Venables KM, Dally MB, Nunn AJ *et al.* Smoking and occupational allergy in a platinum refinery. *Br Med J* 1989; **299**: 939–42.

96 Venables KM, Topping MD, Howe W, Luczynska CM, Hawkins R, Newman Taylor AJ. Interaction of smoking and atopy in producing specific IgE antibody against a hapten protein conjugate. *Br Med J* 1985; **290**: 201–4.

97 Zetterstrom O, Osterman K, Machado L, Johansson SGO. Another smoking hazard reused serum IgE concentrations and increased risk of occupational allergy. *Br Med J* 1981; **283**: 1215–7.

98 Cartier A, Malo J, Forest F *et al.* Occupational asthma in snow-crab proessing workers. *J All Clin Immunol* 1984; **74**: 261–9.

99 Calverley AE, Rees D, Dowdeswell RJ, Linnett PJ, Kielkowski D. Platinum salt sensitivity in refinery workers: incidence and effects of smoking and exposure. *Occup Environ Med* 1995; **52**: 661–6.

100 Zetterstrom O, Nordvall SL, Bjorksten B, Ahlstedt S, Sterlander M. Increased IgE antibody responses to rats exposed to tobacco smoke. *J All Clin Immunol* 1985; **75**: 594.

101 Biagini RE, Moorman WJ, Lewis TR, Bernstein IL. Ozone enhancement of platinum asthma in a primate model. *Am Rev Respir Dis* 1986; **134**: 719–725.

102 Riedel F, Kramer M, Scheibenbogen C, Rieger CHC. Effects of SO$_2$ exposure on allergic sensitisation in the guinea pig. *J All Clin Immunol* 1988; **82**: 527–34.

103 Young RP, Barker RD, Pile KD, Cookson WOCM, Newman Taylor AJ. The association of HLA-DR3 with specific IgE to inhaled acid anhydrides. *Am J Respir Crit Med* 1995; **151**: 219–21.

104 Bignon JS, Aron Y, Ju LT *et al*. HLA Class II Alleles in isocyanate-induced asthma. *Am J Respir Crit Care Med* 1994; **149:** 71–5.

105 Newman Taylor AJ, Cullinan P, Lympany PA *et al*. Interaction of HLA genotype and exposure intensity in IgE-associated sensitization. *Am J Respir Crit Care* 1999 (in press).

106 Newman Taylor AJ, Davies RJ, Hendrik DJ, Pepys J. Recurrent nocturnal asthmatic reactions to bronchial provocation tests. *Clin All* 1979; **9:** 213–9.

107 Venables KM, Topping MD, Nunn AJ, Howe W, Newman Taylor AJ. Immunologic and functional consequences of chemical (tetrachlorophthalic anhydride) induced asthma after 4 years of avoidance of exposure. *J All Clin Immunol* 1987; **80:** 212–8.

108 Malo JC, Carter A, Ghezzo H, Lafrance M, Cante M, Lehrer SB. Patterns of improvement in spirometry, bronchial hyper-responsiveness and specific IgE antibody levels after cessation of exposure in occupational asthma caused by snow-crab processing. *Am Rev Respir Dis* 1988; **138:** 807–12.

109 Paggiaro P, Bacci E, Pacetto P *et al*. Bronchoalveolar lavage and morphology of the airways after cessation of exposure in asthmatic subjects sensitised to toluene diisocyanate. *Chest* 1990; **98:** 536–42.

110 Chan Yeung M, MacLean L, Paggiaro PL. Follow up study of 232 patients with occupational asthma caused by Western Red Cedar (*Thuja plicata*). *J All Clin Immunol* 1987; **79:** 792–6.

111 Slovak AJM. Occupational asthma caused by a plastics blowing agent azodicarbonamide. *Thorax* 1981; **36:** 906–9.

112 Venables KM, Newman Taylor AJ. Exposure-response relationships in tetrachlorophthalic anhydride asthma. *J All Clin Immunol* 1990; **85:** 55–8.

113 Swanson MC, Agarwal MK, Yunginger JW, Reid CE. Guinea pig derived allergens: clincoimmunologic studies, characterization, airborne quantitation and size distribution. *Am Rev Respir Dis* 1984; **129:** 844–9.

114 Twiggs JT, Agarwal MK, Dahlberg MJ, Yunginger JW Immunochemical measurement of airborne mouse allergens in a laboratory animal facility. *J All Clin Immunol* 1982; **69:** 522–6.

115 Edwards RG, Beeson MF, Dewdney JM. Laboratory animal allergy: the measurement of airborne urinary allergens and the effects of different environmental conditions. *Lab Anim* 1983; **17:** 235–9.

116 Botham PA, Davies GE, Teasdale EL. Allergy to laboratory animals: a prospective study of its incidence and of the influence of atopy on its development. *Br J Ind Med* 1987; **44:** 627–32.

34

Extrinsic allergic alveolitis

A J NEWMAN TAYLOR

Farmer's lung	654	Clinical features	657
Bird fancier's lung	655	Diagnosis	658
Mushroom worker's lung	655	Outcome	659
Bagassosis	655	Management of the established case	659
Malt worker's lung	655	Cryptogenic fibrosing alveolitis	
Ventilation pneumonitis	655	and occupation	660
Pathology	656	Statutory compensation	660
Immunopathogenesis	656	References	661

Extrinsic allergic alveolitis, or hypersensitivity pneumonitis, is a granulomatous inflammatory reaction caused by a specific immunological response to various inhaled organic dusts – and possibly also to certain low molecular weight chemicals, which predominantly involves the peripheral gas-exchanging parts of the lung. It is one of several different patterns of inflammatory reaction in the lungs caused by inhaled organic dusts which include infections, such as psittacosis, so-called 'acute organic dust toxic syndrome' and allergic responses such as asthma and allergic alveolitis.

The number of causes of extrinsic allergic alveolitis is now long; some of the more important are shown in Table 34.1. It also includes the low molecular weight chemicals, isocyanates, which have been suggested to cause the disease, although the evidence for this is less secure than for the organic dusts.

The organic dusts which cause extrinsic allergic alveolitis fall into two major groups:

1 microbial spores which grow in vegetable matter such as hay, straw, grain, mushroom compost, wood bark and bagasse;
2 animal proteins both avian (in particular those derived from pigeons and budgerigars) and mammalian (bovine and pituitary extract).

The colourful names given to extrinsic allergic alveolitis caused by many of these different organic dusts reflect the varied occupational settings in which exposure to the particular cause occurs. The tissue response in the lungs and the clinical manifestations of the disease are essentially the same, whatever the cause.

The different causes of extrinsic allergic alveolitis share some important characteristics.

1 Their aerodynamic diameters are sufficiently small to allow penetration into and retention within the alveoli; the spores of *Micropolyspora faeni*, the major cause of farmer's lung, are about 1.9 microns (μ) diameter and those of *Aspergillus clavatus*, the cause of malt worker's lung, are about 3.5 μ diameter. (For comparison the diameters of harvest moulds such as *Alternaria alternata* and *Cladosporium herbarum* causes of asthma, are between 5 μ and 20 μ.)
2 Extrinsic allergic alveolitis usually occurs amongst those exposed in circumstances where the inhaled dose of organic dusts is very high. Spore counts in barns when bales of mouldy hay are opened suggest that up to 750 000 spores of respirable size may be deposited in the lungs during each minute of exposure.
3 The organic dusts (spores and animal proteins) which cause extrinsic allergic alveolitis are poorly degradable and able to persist in the lungs for long periods.

The number of reported causes of extrinsic allergic alveolitis is now considerable but many are uncommon.

Table 34.1 *Some causes of extrinsic allergic alveolitis*

Disease	Antigen source	Antigen
Organic dusts		
Farmer's lung	Mouldy hay, straw, grain etc.	*Micropolyspora faeni, Thermoactinomyces vulgaris*
Bird fancier's lung	Avian excreta and bloom	Avian serum proteins (probably IgA)
Bagassosis	Mouldy bagasse	*Thermoactinomyces sacchari*
Malt worker's lung	Mouldy maltings	*Aspergillus clavatus*
Mushroom worker's lung	Spores released during spawning	*? Thermophilic actinomycetes*
Maple bark stripper's lung	Bark removed from stored maple	*Cryptostroma corticale*
Ventilation pneumonitis	Contamination of air conditioning systems	Thermophilic actinomycetes
Chemicals		
	Polyurethane foam manufacture	Diisocyanates: toluene (TDI)
	Spray painting	Diphenylmethane (MDI)

Furthermore, the risk of many of the classical microbial causes of extrinsic allergic alveolitis has been considerably reduced by improved work practices. Malt worker's lung is now confined to maltings where the traditional 'open floor' method continues to be used; the introduction of mechanical spawning has reduced the risk of developing mushroom worker's lung; and bagassosis can be prevented by treating raw bagasse with propionic acid to inhibit moulding.

Farmer's lung and bird fancier's lung remain the most prevalent causes of the disease. Farmer's lung has been described in Europe, the United States of America and Australia, and seems likely to occur worldwide, wherever exposure to mouldy vegetable matter occurs. Even where farmers are able to ensure that hay is harvested and stored dry or have substituted silage for hay as cattle fodder, they can still encounter microbial matter from mouldy straw used for animal bedding and when grinding mouldy grain for animal feed. In addition, new working conditions can create unexpected hazards: air conditioning systems with reservoirs of heated water have provided the conditions in which thermophilic actinomycetes can grow and, primarily in North America cause farmer's lung in office workers – the inelegantly named 'ventilation pneumonitis'.

FARMER'S LUNG

Farmer's lung is the most prevalent occupational form of extrinsic allergic alveolitis. It is the outcome of an allergic response to thermophilic actinomycetes, in particular *Micropolyspora faeni* and *Thermoactinomyces vulgaris*, which mould vegetable matter in storage. Inhalation of spores and mycelial fragments typically occur when mouldy hay, straw or grain is handled in enclosed and poorly ventilated buildings, which can create spore clouds of up to 1600 million spores/m³.[1] Crops mould when they are harvested damp and stored with a high water content. Moulding generates heat, the maximum temperature achieved being dependent upon the water content of the hay. Stored with a water content of between 35% and 50% the temperature of the hay can reach between of 50°C and 65°C sufficiently high to permit the growth of thermophilic actinomycetes. This general relationship between water content, heating and microbial growth applies also to other crops and vegetable matter, such as straw, grain, bagasse and mushroom compost, which can support the growth of microorganisms whose spores cause extrinsic allergic alveolitis.

The prevalence of farmer's lung is related to local rainfall and to farming methods. In general, the disease is most prevalent in areas of high rainfall and where economic circumstances (as on small and undercapitalized farms) do not allow drying of crops before storage or the prevention of wetting during storage. The estimated prevalence of the disease will also vary with the criteria used to identify cases. The prevalence of the disease in Scotland as identified by questionnaire varied between 23 per 100 farm workers in East Lothian and 86 per 1000 in the wetter Ayrshire and Orkneys. The inclusion of only cases with serum precipitins to *M. faeni* reduced the prevalence to 43 per 1000 in Orkneys and 36 per 1000 in Ayrshire.[2]

Farmer's lung can be prevented by drying crops adequately before storage, by preventing their becoming damp and ensuring good ventilation during storage. To prevent significant moulding hay must be stored with a water content of less than 20%. The disease can also be prevented by the substitution of silage for hay. The addition of 1% propionic acid to grain before storage prevents moulding and therefore the rise in temperature necessary for growth of thermophilic organisms. Respiratory protection should be worn by farm workers when working with mouldy crops in conditions likely to generate spores into the air in high concentration and in particular by those who have experienced an attack of farmer's lung in the past.

BIRD FANCIER'S LUNG

Bird fancier's lung is caused by inhaled avian serum proteins, (probably immunoglobulin A (IgA) is most important), present in the birds' excreta and secreta, and in pigeons particularly the bloom from their feathers. It primarily occurs amongst individuals who breed and keep pigeons for racing and those who share their homes with caged birds, especially, although not exclusively, budgerigars. Protein-containing dust is disseminated into the air during the cleaning of pigeon lofts and budgerigar cages. Antigenic dust is also generated continuously by birds when active and inhaled by owners and others observing the birds in their cages.

Budgerigar fancier's lung has been described as the most important cause of extrinsic allergic alveolitis in Britain, with an estimated prevalence among current budgerigar owners of between 0.5% and 7.5%.[3] This is similar to the risk of farmer's lung among farm workers; the greater number of budgerigar owners in the community however suggests that alveolitis caused by budgerigars is the more common disease.

MUSHROOM WORKER'S LUNG

Mushroom worker's lung is caused by the inhalation of microbial spores generated during commercial mushroom cultivation. Mushrooms are cultivated commercially on compost, a mixture of wheat straw and fresh horse manure. After decomposition outdoors, the compost is heated indoors in boxes to 60°C at 100% humidity, conditions ideal for the growth of thermophilic organisms. After 5 days of these conditions mushroom spawn is added to the compost and mechanically mixed, generating large numbers of spores. The mushrooms are grown in sheds at a temperature of about 20°C and 90% humidity. After the mushroom crop is picked the spent compost is removed and dumped outdoors. Exposure to microbial spores primarily occurs during spawning, particularly when done by hand and during disposal of spent compost. The specific microorganisms responsible for the disease have not been identified with any certainty, but may be microbes growing in the compost, from the mushrooms or both.

The risk of developing mushroom worker's lung has decreased since the introduction of mechanical spawning.

BAGASSOSIS

Bagassosis is caused by the inhalation of *Thermoactinomyces sacchari*, a thermophilic microorganism which moulds bagasse. Bagasse is the fibrous cellulose residue of sugar which remains after the sugar has been extracted. Bagasse is used in the manufacture of several different materials which include paper and boarding. After sugar extraction, bagasse is stored in bales often outdoors. Storage with a water content in excess of 27% permits moulding, heat generation and the growth of thermophilic microorganisms including *T. sacchari*. Exposure to *T. sacchari* primarily occurs to those involved in the removal, opening and milling of bagasse. Moulding of bagasse can be prevented by treating fresh bagasse with 1% propionic acid. Bagassosis is now uncommon although sporadic outbreaks continue to be reported.

MALT WORKER'S LUNG

Malt worker's lung is caused by *Aspergillus clavatus*, a contaminant of barley to which maltmen in whisky distilleries may be exposed during malting. Barley is dried in hot air kilns, stored in silos for at least 8 weeks and dehydrated in steeping tanks with hypochlorite as a mild fungicide. In the traditional 'open floor' malting process the barley is then spread out on open floors and allowed to germinate. Heat is generated by respiration of the germinating barley, and the temperature maintained by regular turning and raking of the barley. Germination is stopped by putting the barley into a hot air kiln, in which the malt is dried and turned.

Exposure to *A. clavatus* spores occurs primarily to those turning barley on the malt floor and in the malt kilns. In modern maltings these processes have been partly or wholly mechanized and both exposure to *A. clavatus* and the risk of malt worker's lung have been greatly reduced.

'VENTILATION PNEUMONITIS'

Extrinsic allergic alveolitis also occurs in the inhabitants of air conditioned homes and among those working in air conditioned office blocks.[4] The majority of cases reported to date have occurred in the USA where the disease is caused by thermophilic actinomycetes growing in reservoirs of humidification systems where water recirculates at temperatures which are sufficiently high to permit their growth. The conditioned air acts as the vehicle of antigen dissemination. 'Ventilation pneumonitis', like other forms of extrinsic allergic alveolitis, can cause progressive pulmonary fibrosis. It should be distinguished from 'humidifier fever' which causes similar acute symptoms and changes in lung function. The symptoms of humidifier fever have a characteristic periodicity: they occur on the first day back at work after a weekend or holiday absence and improve despite continuing exposure during the working week. Furthermore, abnormalities on the chest radiograph and progressive pulmonary fibrosis do not develop in humidifier fever.[5] Humidifier fever is associated with humidification systems whose reservoir of water is cold. In general, ventilation pneumonitis is a disease associated with humidification systems where the water reservoir is hot and has been described in the USA. Humidifier fever is usually associated with cold water reservoirs, although three cases of extrinsic allergic alveolitis caused by contaminants of a cold water humidifier have been described in a printing works in the UK[6] (see Chapter 36).

PATHOLOGY

Knowledge of the pathological changes in the lungs in extrinsic allergic alveolitis is based on the appearances of biopsies obtained at various intervals from the onset of symptoms. The characteristic pathological finding is a granulomatous inflammatory response centred on the peripheral bronchioles, which extends peripherally into adjacent alveoli. The inflammatory exudate consists primarily of plasma cells and lymphocytes; macrophages and cells derived from them – epithelioid cells and giant cells – accumulate in foci, granulomata, within the bronchiolar and interstitial inflammation. Although the appearances of the granulomata are similar to those found in sarcoidosis, the bronchocentric nature of extrinsic allergic alveolitis and the formation of granulomata within areas of interstitial inflammation distinguish the granulomatous response in extrinsic allergic alveolitis from sarcoidosis.

With avoidance of exposure, the granulomata resolve in some 3–4 months. If avoidance of exposure occurs at a sufficiently early stage in the disease process the inflammatory response in the lungs can resolve. In other cases the inflammatory exudate may organize by fibrosis, causing irreversible damage to the lungs. The determinants of fibrosis are not clear, but it seems particularly to occur after repeated symptomatic exposures to the specific cause. For reasons which are unknown, fibrosis in allergic alveolitis, as in other granulomatous lung disease such as tuberculosis and sarcoidosis, predominantly involves the upper lobes causing lobar shrinkage and cyst formation.

IMMUNOPATHOGENESIS

Concepts of the immunological basis of extrinsic allergic alveolitis have undergone considerable change in recent years, particularly since the introduction of bronchoalveolar lavage, via the fibreoptic bronchoscope, has provided direct access to cells lining the lungs which may be participating in the immunological response.

The original hypothesis that extrinsic allergic alveolitis was the outcome of local complement-fixing immune complexes, formed between inhaled antigen and circulating antibody, deposited in the lungs was based on several observations: the presence of specific IgG antibodies (precipitins) in the sera of patients with extrinsic allergic alveolitis; the provocation by inhaled antigens of a late alveolar response with a time of onset and duration which paralleled the time course of the late oedematous skin reaction; and the finding of Ig and complement by immunofluorescence at the site of late skin responses[7] provoked in the skin and in lung tissue of patients with farmer's lung 36 hours after inhalation of *M. faeni*.[8] However, the explanation of extrinsic allergic alveolitis as an immune complex mediated response was unsatisfactory for two major reasons: granuloma formation, a characteristic component of the pathological response in extrinsic allergic alveolitis, was more typical of a T lymphocyte than immune complex dependent inflammatory reaction; also, depending on the sensitivity of the serum assay, IgG antibody could be detected in up to 50% of individuals without disease but exposed to causes of extrinsic allergic alveolitis.

The role of the T lymphocyte in extrinsic allergic alveolitis and the nature of the immunological response in the disease has been considerably clarified by the study of T lymphocytes recovered from the lungs by lavage. Incubation with pigeon serum of lymphocytes recovered by lavage from the lungs of a patient with pigeon fancier's lung stimulated their transformation.[9] The proportion of lymphocytes recovered at bronchoalveolar lavage, from patients with extrinsic allergic alveolitis, is, as in sarcoidosis, greatly increased above normal. Whereas in normal individuals some 85–90% of the cells recovered are macrophages, in sarcoidosis the proportion of lymphocytes may be increased to 50% and in allergic alveolitis to 60–70% or more. In sarcoidosis the ratio of CD4:CD8 (helper: suppressor) T lymphocytes is increased from the normal 1.5–2:1 to 5:1. In allergic alveolitis the ratio of CD4:CD8 ratio can be normal or low and CD8 T lymphocytes can comprise 40% and CD4 T lymphocytes 30% of the total lymphocytes recovered to give a CD4:CD8 ratio of less than one.[10]

The increase in the proportion of lymphocytes recovered at bronchoalveolar lavage and the reversed CD4:CD8 T lymphocyte ratio has, however, also been observed in healthy asymptomatic farmers and pigeon breeders. In one study of 28 farmers with increased bronchoalveolar lavage lymphocytes, none of 27, all of whom had remained on their farms, studied 2–3 years later, had developed farmer's lung.[11] The T-lymphocyte response in the lungs by itself is no more able to explain the disease than the presence of IgG antibody in serum.

The explanation may be found in two possibly connected observations.

First, pigeon fanciers with extrinsic allergic alveolitis have been found to differ from asymptomatic exposed individuals with similar increases in bronchoalveolar lavage lymphocytes in that they show a defect in antigen-specific T lymphocyte suppressor function.[12] This defect may allow inhaled allergen to provoke a T lymphocyte-dependent inflammatory response; in the asymptomatic person with bronchoalveolar lymphocytosis, translation of the immunological response into granulomatous inflammation may be inhibited by antigen-specific suppressor T lymphocytes.

Second, patients with extrinsic allergic alveolitis characteristically also have an increase in the number of mast cells recovered at bronchoalveolar lavage.[13] These could release vasoactive mediators which allow the passage of monocytes from the circulation into the lung. It is tempting to speculate that the recruitment of mast cells, possibly by T lymphocyte-derived interleukin 3 (IL3) is one of the important factors which enables translation of the immunological into the inflammatory response.

The risk of developing specific IgG antibody and allergic alveolitis in those exposed to its causes has been consistently reported to be lower in cigarette smokers than in non-smokers.[14,15] This seemingly unmerited protection may be a reflection of impaired alveolar macrophage function. Cigarette smoking has been found to inhibit the expression of the major histocompatibility 2 antigens on the cell surface of alveolar macrophages impairing antigen presentation to helper T lymphocytes.[16]

CLINICAL FEATURES

The clinical features of extrinsic allergic alveolitis, however caused, depend on the pattern of exposure to the cause and on variation in the severity and nature of the individual response. Two distinct but overlapping forms of clinical presentation can be distinguished: acute and potentially reversible and chronic irreversible.

Acute allergic alveolitis

Acute allergic alveolitis typically follows exposure to antigen in high concentration. Recurrent episodes of alveolitis follow intermittent exposures to antigenic dust in high concentration; progressive disease occurs in those continuously exposed to high concentrations of antigen. In a typical case of recurrent acute alveolitis, as in the farmer who feeds mouldy hay to cattle in a cowshed, symptoms do not occur during the period of exposure, but several hours later when breathlessness and flu like symptoms – fever, constitutional upset, muscle pains and headache – develop.

Considerable weight loss may also occur. The systemic symptoms can dominate the clinical picture. In the absence of further exposure to their cause, symptoms usually start to improve within 48 hours but may persist for a week or more before resolving completely. Where exposure is continuous the symptoms do not resolve but become increasingly severe. On examination during the acute episode, scattered inspiratory crackles and on occasions inspiratory squeaks may be heard over the lungs. In some cases, no abnormal sounds are audible. A variety of patterns of changes on the chest radiograph may develop during the acute disease. A ground glass pattern can occur, often difficult to detect unless a previous (or subsequent) radiograph is available for comparison. The generalized haze is associated with a loss of sharpness of outline of the vascular shadows, particularly in the lower lung zones. Micronodular (less than 3 mm) or nodular shadows, either widespread or more prominent in the lower zones may also occur (Fig. 34.1a). On occasions nodules can merge into larger areas of patchy consolidation. The chest radiograph appears normal in some cases. In the absence of antigen exposure these acute shadows can take 4–6 weeks or longer to resolve (Fig. 34.1b).

The important abnormalities of lung function in acute allergic alveolitis are a reduction in lung volumes and impairment of gas transfer. Total lung capacity (TLC) and residual volume (RV) are reduced as are vital capacity (VC) and forced expiratory volume in 1 second (FEV_1). The FEV_1/FVC ratio is maintained or increased. Both transfer factor for carbon monoxide (TLCO) and gas transfer coefficient (KCO) are reduced. Of these abnormalities the reduction in TLCO is the most sensitive indicator of disease. In addition the alveolar–arterial pO_2 gradient is increased at rest and widens with exercise. In severe cases pO_2 at rest may be sufficiently reduced for patients to be cyanosed; pCO_2 is normal or reduced. Lung function in patients with acute alveolitis generally improves during 4–6 weeks of avoidance of exposure, but can continue to improve for up to 6 months. During the acute illness the blood neutrophil count and erythrocyte sedimentation rate are usually increased.

Chronic allergic alveolitis

Chronic allergic alveolitis is distinguished from acute alveolitis by the development of irreversible pulmonary fibrosis. It may develop as the consequence of recurrent episodes of acute alveolitis or where antigen exposure has been in concentrations, often over a long period, insufficient to provoke acute respiratory or systemic symptoms but sufficient to cause progressive pulmonary damage. The commonly cited example of this pattern of presentation is the budgerigar fancier exposed to low concentrations of bird dust in his home who only comes to medical attention when pulmonary fibrosis has caused sufficient loss of respiratory reserve to cause symptoms.

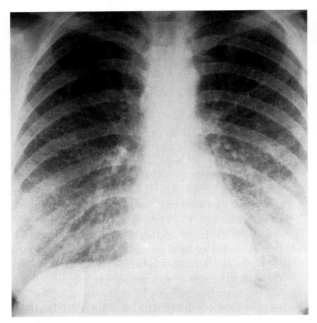

Figure 34.1a *Acute extrinsic allergic alveolitis in a woman occupationally exposed to horses. Widespread nodular shadowing on chest radiograph.*

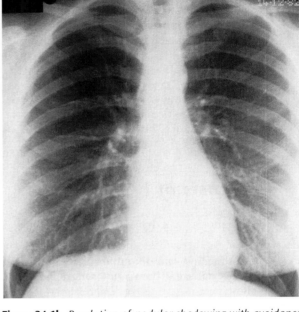

Figure 34.1b *Resolution of nodular shadowing with avoidance of further contact with horses.*

The dominant symptom of chronic allergic alveolitis is breathlessness on exertion. Other than weight loss which can be considerable, systemic symptoms are usually absent. On examination in contrast to cryptogenic fibrosing alveolitis finger clubbing is unusual; scattered inspiratory crackles and squeaks may be audible over the lungs. Chronic irreversible changes develop on the chest radiograph. Linear shadows, honeycombing and lung shrinkage occur, particularly in the upper lobes, with compensatory dilatation in the lower lobes (Fig. 34.2).

The abnormalities of lung function although similar to those in acute alveolitis, may improve little with avoidance of exposure to their cause, and can progress in its absence. Lung volumes – TLC, RV and VC – are reduced, FEV_1/FVC is maintained or increased and TLCO and KCO are reduced. The magnitude of the reduction in TLC and TLCO correlate with the profusion of abnormalities on the chest radiograph.[17] Arterial pO_2 is reduced and in severe cases patients are cyanosed; alveolar–arterial gradient is increased and widens on exercise. Pulmonary hypertension can develop in patients with widespread pulmonary fibrosis and patients may present at this stage of the disease.

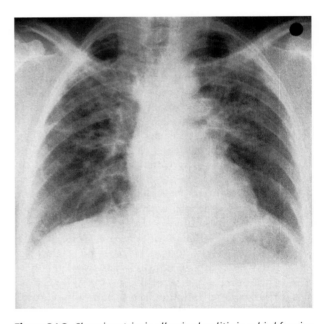

Figure 34.2 *Chronic extrinsic allergic alveolitis in a bird fancier. Changes in chest radiograph predominantly in the upper lobes which are shrunken and scarred.*

DIAGNOSIS

The diagnosis of extrinsic allergic alveolitis is based on:

1 Identification of a potential source of antigen in the patient's home or working environment.

2 Characteristic clinical, radiographic and functional changes of the disease.

3 Demonstration of precipitating antibodies (precipitins) in the patient's serum to the causal antigen.

The most important differential diagnoses in acute allergic alveolitis are acute febrile microbial respiratory illnesses which cause widespread shadows on chest radiograph. The important microbial respiratory illnesses are pneumonias caused by influenza virus, *Mycoplasma*, tuberculosis, psittacosis and Q fever; in the immunocompromised, *Pneumonocystis carinii* should as far as possible be excluded before starting treatment with corticosteroids. The diagnosis of acute allergic alveolitis is suggested by a history of recent exposure to a relevant organic dust, particularly if this has been associated with respiratory and systemic illness in the past. A potential antigen source is usually identifiable from the history. When the diagnosis seems likely but its cause not apparent, it is often helpful to visit the patient's home or place of work, when the patient's occupational physician and the Employment Medical Advisory Service can provide valuable advice.

Reduction in TLCO is the most sensitive functional abnormality in both acute and chronic farmer's lung; its reduction is closely correlated with the severity of changes on the chest radiograph. The chest radiograph and transfer factor are good indicators of the presence and severity of disease.

Serum precipitins are in general a more sensitive than specific index of extrinsic allergic alveolitis. In farmer's lung precipitins to mouldy hay, *M. faeni* or *T. vulgaris* are found in the serum of between 75 and 100% of cases during an acute episode, but in only about 50% after 2 years from the last acute episode and in only 33% of cases after 5 years.[18] On the other hand the majority of farmers who have serum precipitins do not have farmer's lung. In a random sample of Quebec dairy farmers 8.4% had serum precipitins but only four of the 56 with precipitins had farmer's lung.[19] The great majority of pigeon breeders with acute allergic alveolitis have been reported to have serum precipitins, as have some 15% of healthy breeders without disease.[20] Budgerigar fanciers with inhalation test diagnosed alveolitis were all found to have serum precipitins, but interestingly in the same report, none of a group of healthy exposed individuals.[21]

OUTCOME

The important long-term consequence of extrinsic allergic alveolitis is pulmonary fibrosis which can be disabling and shorten life. Because of its important economic consequences for farmers, the risk of developing disabling pulmonary fibrosis and the factors determining its occurrence have been particularly investigated. One large study followed up 144 patients for an average period of 15 years during which time some 10% died of causes associated with farmer's lung. Of those alive at the end of follow-up, some 40% had

radiographic evidence of chronic alveolitis, less than 25% had exertional dyspnoea, and about 33% reduced TLCO, the most sensitive index of impaired lung function in extrinsic allergic alveolitis. The development of disabling fibrosis particularly occurred in those with a history of recurrent (more than five) episodes of acute alveolitis. Continuing to farm, and disease of long duration were not associated with worse lung function. Provided adequate precautions were taken to minimize exposure to mouldy hay and other sources of thermophilic actinomycetes, the majority of farmers were able to remain on their farms without developing disabling pulmonary fibrosis.[22] The results of several other studies support this finding.

One study compared the outcome 5 years after an attack of acute farmer's lung in 24 farmers who had left their farms with 37 who had remained. Mean TLCO improved in those who had left their farms but not in those who remained. However, there was wide variation between subjects in both groups and the majority of farmers were able to continue to farm without developing disabling disease.[23] A similar follow-up study of 86 cases of farmer's lung in Finland found that lung function improves during the 6 months after an acute episode but that after 5 years there was no difference in lung function between the two-thirds who had continued to farm compared with those who had left. Corticosteroid treatment accelerated the rate of improvement following an acute attack, but did not produce any long-term improvement in lung function.[24]

MANAGEMENT OF THE ESTABLISHED CASE

The aims in management of cases of extrinsic allergic alveolitis are to ensure maximum restoration of lung function and to prevent the development of progressive pulmonary fibrosis. Acute cases should avoid exposure to the cause of their disease, until maximum restoration of lung function has occurred. Corticosteroids accelerate the rate of recovery but do not seem to provide additional long-term benefit.

Treatment with oral prednisolone in acute disease should be discontinued within 3–6 months. An initial dose of prednisolone of 1 mg/kg body weight should be reduced within 4–8 weeks to 20 mg on alternate days which can be continued for 3–4 months. The initial high dose prednisolone should be maintained until maximum resolution of the chest radiograph and sustained improvement in lung function are obtained. There is no evidence that long-term steroid treatment confers additional benefit. Occasionally, however, some patients develop a progressive fibrosing disease which should be treated with regular oral steroids supplemented when appropriate by an immunosuppressant, such as cyclophosphamide or azathioprine.

Long-term management is primarily based on avoidance of exposures which cause progressive pulmonary fibrosis. It is clear from the studies of farmers that only a minority develop disabling pulmonary fibrosis and the majority are able to continue to farm without this occurring. If a farmer wishes to continue in employment it is reasonable to support this provided a) he takes appropriate measures to minimize exposure to mouldy hay (including the use of effective respiratory protection, such as laminar flow equipment when handling stored hay, straw and grain) and b) lung function is monitored regularly, at the minimum before and after each winter season. Should lung function show progressive deterioration during the winter and incomplete resolution in the summer, he should be strongly advised against continuing farm work.

A similar approach may be taken with other occupational causes of extrinsic allergic alveolitis, where complete avoidance of exposure is only obtained at the expense of an individual's job. The situation is less clear with bird fancier's lung where an individual's employment is not dependent on keeping the bird. In this situation it seems more reasonable to advise avoidance of all further contact with birds. However, particularly in the case of pigeon fanciers, the birds may be the focus of a social life with which the individual is unwilling to part. In this situation it seems appropriate to apply the same rules as for occupational alveolitis: minimal exposure with the use of respiratory protection when exposed and serial measurement of lung function (in particular of gas transfer) to monitor the effectiveness of this strategy.

CRYPTOGENIC FIBROSING ALVEOLITIS AND OCCUPATION

Cryptogenic fibrosing alveolitis is characterized by inflammation and fibrosis of the gas exchanging parts of the lung. The term 'cryptogenic' implies that no cause can be identified. The condition is synonymous with 'idiopathic pulmonary fibrosis' by which the disease is known in the USA.

The prevalence of the disease, which occurs most commonly during the fifth and sixth decades, has been estimated at 6 per 100 000 adults and there is evidence that its incidence may have increased in recent years.[25]

Characteristically, patients with cryptogenic fibrosing alveolitis present with increasing shortness of breath on exertion, finger clubbing and inspiratory crackles audible at the bases of their lungs. Their chest radiographs show reticular or reticulonodular shadowing, which is predominantly basal in distribution; on computerized tomography (CT) the abnormal shadowing is seen to be predominantly subpleural in distribution. Lung function tests show evidence of small stiff lungs with impairment of gas transfer. The prognosis of the disease is poor with a median survival of 4 years from diagnosis.

Diffuse interstitial fibrosis of the lungs caused by inhaled asbestos (asbestosis) and cobalt (hard metal disease) share the same clinical characteristics, although they can usually be distinguished from cryptogenic fibrosing alveolitis; asbestosis in individuals occupationally exposed to asbestos by the associated presence of pleural plaques or thickening on the chest radiograph or CT; hard metal disease by giant cell transformation of Type 2 epithelial cells and alveolar macrophages (the latter by bronchoalveolar lavage).[26]

Two recent studies have suggested that cryptogenic fibrosing alveolitis might also be associated with other occupational exposures – in particular metal and wood dusts. Johnston et al.[25] found that mortality from cryptogenic fibrosing alveolitis tended to be higher in areas of England and Wales which traditionally had high levels of employment in manufacturing industries. The risk of cryptogenic fibrosing alveolitis was increased more than tenfold in those exposed to metal dust or who had worked with cattle and threefold in those exposed to wood dust.[27] These relationships were tested in a further case-referent study of hospital-based cases of cryptogenic fibrosing alveolitis with age- and sex-matched community-based referents, also living in the Trent region. Questionnaire-reported exposure to metal dust was greater in cryptogenic fibrosing alveolitis cases than referents – OR 1.68 (1.07–2.65) and also to wood dust – OR 1.71 (1.01–2.92). The estimated aetiological fraction of cryptogenic fibrosing alveolitis attributable to metal and wood dust exposure was some 20%.[28]

These observations are of great potential interest, but need to be repeated in other populations. The use of community-based referents for hospital-based cases of a respiratory disease, for which there are known occupational causes, has the potential for recall bias. Furthermore, the diagnosis of cryptogenic fibrosing alveolitis may have been applied to cases of hard metal disease in those exposed to metal dust and to asbestos in those exposed to wood dust (particularly among those working in the construction industry).

STATUTORY COMPENSATION (see Chapter 4)

Extrinsic allergic alveolitis is prescribed for 'employed earners' in certain occupations. These are defined as any job involving exposure to moulds or fungal spores or heterologous proteins by reason of employment in:

- agriculture, horticulture, forestry, cultivation of edible fungi or maltworking;
- loading or unloading or handling in storage mouldy vegetable matter or edible fungi;
- caring for or handling birds;
- handling bagasse.

'Employed earners' (i.e not the self-employed) who develop extrinsic allergic alveolitis as a consequence of employment in which they have been exposed to one of these groups of agents are entitled to certain benefits from the Department of Social Security (DSS). These include disablement benefit and reduced earnings allowance. Initial application is made to the local DSS office. Medical adjudication of each case is made by two doctors of the Medical Boarding Centre (Respiratory Diseases). Claimants have the right of appeal against the decision of the Medical Boarding Centre both on the question of diagnosis and the assessment of disablement to a Medical Appeal Tribunal.

REFERENCES

1 Lacey J, Lacey ME. Spore concentrations in the air of farm buildings. *Trans Br Mycol Soc* 1964; **47:** 547–52.

2 Grant IWB, Blyth W *et al*. Prevalence of farmer's lung in Scotland: a pilot survey. *Br Med J* 1972; **1:** 530–34.

3 Hendrick DJ, Faux JA, Marshall R. Budgerigar fancier's lung: the commonest variety of allergic alveolitis in Britain. *Br Med J* 1978; **2:** 81–4.

4 Banaszak EF, Thiede WH, Fink JN. Hypersensitivity pneumonitis due to contamination of air conditioners. *N Engl J Med* 1970; **183:** 271–6.

5 Newman Taylor AJ, Pickering CAC, Turner-Warwick M, Pepys J. Respiratory allergy to a factory humidifier contaminant presenting as a pyrexia of undetermined origin. *Br Med J* 1978; **2:** 94–5.

6 Robertson AS, Burge PS, Wieland GA, Carmalt MHB. Extrinsic allergic alveolitis caused by a cold water humidifier. *Thorax* 1979; **42:** 32–7.

7 Pepys J, Turner Warwick M, Dawson PC, Hinson KFW. Arthus (type 3) skin test reactions in man. Clinical and immunopathological features. In: Rose B, Richer M, Sehon A, Frankland SW eds. *Allergology*. Amsterdam: Excerpta Medica, 1968: 221.

8 Ghose T, Landrigan P, Killeen R, Dill J. Immunopathological studies in patients with farmer's lung. *Clin All* 1974; **4:** 119–29.

9 Schuyler MR, Thypen TP, Salvaggio JE. Local pulmonary immunity in pigeon breeder's lung. *Am Intern Med* 1978; **88:** 355–8.

10 Salvaggio J. Hypersensitivity pneumonitis. *J All Clin Immunol* 1987; **79:** 558–71.

11 Cormier Y, Belanger J, Laviolette M. Prognostic significance of bronchoalveolar lymphocytosis in farmer's lung. *Am Rev Respir Dis* 1987; **135:** 692–5.

12 Keller RH, Swartz S, Schlueter DP *et al*. Immunoregulation in hypersensitivity pneumonitis: phenotypic and functional studies of bronchoalveolar lavage lymphocytes. *Am Rev Respir Dis* 1984; **130:** 766–71.

13 Haslam PL, Dewar A, Butchers P, Primett ZS, Newman Taylor AJ, Turner-Warwick M. Mast cells, atypical lymphocytes and neutrophils in bronchoalveolar lavage in extrinsic allergic alveolitis. *Am Rev Respir Dis* 1987; **135:** 35–47.

14 Morgan DC, Smyth JT, Lister RW *et al*. Chest symptoms in farming communities with special reference to farmer's lung. *Br J Ind Med* 1975; **32:** 228–34.

15 Warren CPW. Extrinsic allergic alveolitis: a disease commoner in non-smokers. *Thorax* 1977; **32:** 567–9.

16 Laurence EC, Fox TB, Hall BT, Martin RR. Deleterious effects of cigarette smoking on expression of Ia antigens by human pulmonary alveolar macrophages. *Clin Res* 1983; **31:** 418a.

17 Cormier Y, Belanger J, Tardif A *et al*. Relationships between radiographic change, pulmonary function and bronchoalveolar lavage fluid lymphocytes in farmer's lung disease. *Thorax* 1986; **41:** 28–33.

18 Braun SR, do Pico GA, Tsiatsis A *et al*. Farmer's lung disease: Long-term clinical and physiological outcome. *Am Rev Respir Dis* 1979; **119:** 185–91.

19 Cormier Y, Belanger J, Durand P. Factors influencing the development of serum precipitins to farmer's lung antigen in Quebec dairy farmers. *Thorax* 1985; **40:** 138–42.

20 Barboriak JJ, Sosman AJ, Reed CE. Serological studies in pigeon breeder's disease. *J Lab Clin Med* 1965; **65:** 600–4.

21 Faux JZ, Wide L, Hargreave FE *et al*. Immunological aspects of respiratory allergy in budgerigar (*Melopsittacus undulatus*) fanciers. *Clin All* 1971; **1:** 149.

22 Braun SR, do Pico GA, and Tsiatsis A. Farmers lung disease: long-term clinical and physiologic outcome. *Am Rev Respir Dis* 1979; **119:** 185–91.

23 Cormier Y, Belanger J. Long-term physiologic outcome after acute farmer's lung. *Chest* 1985; **87:** 796–800.

24 Monkare S, Haahtela T. Farmer's lung – a 5-year follow up of eighty-six patients. *Clin All* 1987; **17:** 143–51.

25 Johnston I, Britton J, Kinnear W, Logan R. Rising mortality from cryptogenic fibrosing alveolitis. *Br Med J* 1990; **301:** 1017–21.

26 Davison AG, Haslam PL, Corrin B, Coutts II, Dewar A *et al*. Interstitial lung disease and asthma in hard metal workers; broncho-alveolar lavage ultrastructural and analytical findings and results of bronchial provocation tests. *Thorax* 1983; **38:** 119–28.

27 Scott J, Johnston I, Britton J. What causes crytogenic fibrosing alveolitis? A case control study of environmental exposure to dust. *Br Med J* 1990; **301:** 1015–7.

28 Hubbard R, Lewis S, Richards K, Johnston I, Britton J. Occupational exposure to metal or wood dust and aetiology of crytogenci fibrosing alveolitis. *Lancet* 1996; **347:** 284–9.

35

Inorganic dusts

PETER ELMES, ANNE COCKCROFT, BENOIT NEMERY

The lung's defences	663	Metal dusts and fumes	697
The pathogenesis of inorganic dust diseases	664	Pneumoconioses and specific interstitial lung disorders	
Investigation and diagnosis	665	caused by metals	700
Non-fibrous mineral dusts	672	References	704
Fibrous mineral dusts	686		

Medical writers of classical times recognized that certain occupations were associated with an increased risk of lung diseases, but considered that these were just severe versions of those prevalent in the population. This concept was accepted by mediaeval writers and reinforced by names such as 'miner's phthisis' and 'potter's asthma'. The Industrial Revolution in the latter part of the eighteenth and the first part of the nineteenth century brought about a great enlargement of the towns and cities in the United Kingdom and elsewhere in Europe with a shift of the population in from the countryside. Overcrowding, poverty, malnutrition and gross environmental pollution with smoke and fumes led to a great increase in respiratory deaths due to infection and this delayed the recognition of the many occupational lung diseases which the Industrial Revolution also created. The concept that occupation can cause specific lung diseases with a different pathology and clinical course from lung diseases arising in the general population has been developed during the last half century. More recently still, there has been a further recognition that certain occupational exposures can lead to an increased risk of lung diseases that occur commonly in the general population, such as chronic obstructive pulmonary disease and bronchial asthma. In the UK and other developed countries, this is now more of a problem than the specific occupational lung diseases, such as silicosis, although these remain a major concern in developing countries.

Research in the last 50 years has shown that most occupational lung disease is due to the inhalation of dust and fumes released into the air at work. This can affect not only the workers themselves but also bystanders or even family members, due to dust taken home on the clothes of workers. Dusts released into the air at work can also cause disease in people outside the workplace due to atmospheric pollution.

In this chapter the first two sections consider the lung defences against inhaled materials and how they fail and disease develops. The next section describes the investigation and diagnosis of inorganic dust diseases, in so far as they are common to many of the diseases. The remaining sections describe the different types of lung disease due to inorganic dusts: non-fibrous mineral dusts; fibrous mineral dusts; metal dusts and fumes.

Before considering individual dust-related lung diseases it is necessary to consider the lung defences against inhaled materials and how they fail.

THE LUNG'S DEFENCES

Protection against dust and aerosols is at four levels:

1 the upper airway filter;
2 the lower airway filter;
3 macrophage clearance to the airways;
4 macrophage segregation of dust particles and clearance via the lymphatics.

The upper airway filter

The hairs and the folds of the mucosa over the turbinates direct the airflow through the nose so that most particles over 15 μm diameter hit the surface and are carried in the mucus to the pharynx and swallowed. If the particles are irritant or cause an allergic reaction, running of the eyes and nose and sneezing often persuade the individual to get away from the dust. At work a certain tolerance may develop. People doing heavy work as well as a significant proportion of 'normal' people with nasal obstruction breathe through their mouths and bypass this protective mechanism.

The lower airway filter

The part of lower airways lined by mucociliary epithelium acts as a low resistance filter which removes nearly all of the particles down to about 5 μm and a proportion of those a bit smaller. Inflowing air throws the particles onto the mucus below the bifurcations. They are carried in the mucus back to the larynx, join the particles from the upper airways and are swallowed. Even during deep breathing (hard work) the external air does not reach beyond the mucociliary lined part of the airways, pushing ahead of it the air left in the airways at the end of the previous breath. For dust to get beyond the mucus clearance system it must remain in suspension during several breaths while mixing occurs between the incoming air and that remaining in the lung.

Dust landing on the mucociliary lining provokes secretion both by the goblet cells and by the submucosal seromucous glands. This aids clearance, but if the dust particles are irritant there is stimulation of nerve endings, causing cough, airways narrowing and outpouring of secretions. Prolonged exposure to irritants causes hypertrophy of the submucous glands and proliferation of the goblet cells further and further down the airways. This is the pathology of chronic bronchitis. Irritant exposures were a feature of the smogs that occurred in cities in the UK until 50 years ago, with high levels of particles and sulphur dioxide. Levels of pollutants are now much lower in UK cities but high levels are still found in cities in Eastern Europe and developing countries, where there is little or no control over industrial emissions. Exposures similar to those in city smogs may also occur to people in rural communities in developing countries, including women and children, as a result of cooking over smoky fires in poorly ventilated dwellings. There is now good evidence that this mucus hypersecretion (the diagnostic feature of chronic bronchitis) is not itself a cause of loss of lung function but is associated with it because many exposures (such as cigarette smoking) cause both.[1]

Macrophage clearance to the airways

Particles getting beyond the mucociliary system (i.e. the respirable or alveolar fraction of the inhaled dust), fall onto the lining of the alveolar ducts and alveoli and may be retained. But very small particles (less than 0.5 μm in diameter) sediment so slowly that only a proportion are caught in this way before being carried out again by the mixing of the alveolar air with clean inspired air. The alveoli that open directly off the terminal bronchioles, being encountered first, catch the bulk of the retained dust.

As soon as the dust settles it becomes coated with surfactant (inhaled dust stimulates type II cells to produce more surfactant). Macrophages move out from the wall and engulf the particles, some moving back in when fully loaded. Many of the dust particles are dissolved by lysosomal enzymes. When they are fully laden with insoluble material the macrophages migrate through the interstitium to the centres of the lobules. Here they enter the mucus-lined airway and are carried by the mucus to the larynx with the rest of the dust.

By this mechanism the lungs can clear most dust retained as a result of regular exposure at work up to about 4 mg/m³ of 'respirable' particles provided the macrophages are not damaged by the dust, by cigarette smoke or by atmospheric pollution outside the workplace. Above this level the system becomes overloaded and dust accumulates in the lung. One of the remarkable effects of the Clean Air Acts in the UK has been that the lungs of city dwellers in Britain can no longer be distinguished at a glance from the lungs of country dwellers. Before the Acts, a city dweller's lungs were black due to the accumulation of soot-laden macrophages around the centrilobular airways and out along the interlobular septa.

When the overload is very heavy then the type II and even the type I alveolar lining cells may take on a phagocytic role and help to pick up and remove dust gravitating onto them.

Macrophage clearance via the lymphatics

Failure of clearance of dust to the airways is usually a result of a combination of overload and some property of the dust which damages the macrophages. The cells die and the dust is picked up by other macrophages which attempt to carry it to the hilar lymph nodes either via the lymphatics in the interlobular septa and under the pleura or those along the blood vessels. Dust can get stuck along either route or in the hilar nodes, but some material can get carried on into the blood stream and end up in the spleen, bone marrow or even the Kupffer cells in the liver. Once it misses being carried out into the airways the dust cannot be removed from the body. Hence even low activity long half-life insoluble radioactive dust may be dangerous.

THE PATHOGENESIS OF INORGANIC DUST DISEASES

The 'bronchitis' changes in the mucociliary airways produced by inorganic dusts are minor compared with those produced by the organic dusts (see Chapters

32–34) and by cigarette smoking. The main effects of inorganic dusts are in the lung parenchyma, rather than the airways. The term pneumoconiosis should be used for all dust damage to the alveolar part of the lung, including the airways that have no mucociliary lining. By convention the term does not include bronchitis, asthma or the cancers. In many work situations exposure leads to a combination of different pathologies in each individual. The features of lung disease due to occupational exposure to inorganic dusts depend not only on the dust itself but also on other features of the individual, such as cigarette smoking, infection with tuberculosis, living in a heavily polluted city, and individual susceptibility.

There are several common features in the process of lung damage due to retained inorganic dusts. The timing and relative importance of these depends on the dust load and the toxicity of the particular dust. It can also be modified by other insults to the lung, such as cigarette smoking.

1   The lung is damaged when macrophages die and the system fails to clear the dust landing beyond the mucociliary system.
2   Where macrophages die, substances are released from the dying cells that provoke an inflammatory reaction. While initially reversible, if this process occurs repeatedly in the same site, permanent damage is done to the structure of the lung. The site of the damage is determined by how far the macrophages get before they die. In a few cases the macrophages die in the alveoli and the damage occurs there. But it is more usual for them to die in aggregations around the centrilobular bronchioles or along the lymphatics leading to the hilar lymph nodes either via the interlobular septa and the pleura or along the bronchovascular bundles.
3   The severity and form of the damage depends on the toxicity of the dust and the level of exposure. Prolonged high levels of exposure to dust of low toxicity may in the end produce the same amount of damage as lower-level, shorter exposure to a very toxic dust like quartz.
4   If the dust is of low toxicity the pathological process may halt after exposure. But for most dusts there is a progression (even if slow) of the pathology after exposure ceases, due to the continuing reaction to the retained dust.
5   The accumulation of dust in the phagocytic cells of the lung leads to release of inflammatory mediators from neutrophils and other cells.[2] The resulting migration and activation of leucocytes leads to proteolysis of fibronectin and subsequent laying down of fibrin, reticulin and even collagen. Evidence about the toxicity of mineral dusts at cellular level has suggested the involvement of reactive oxygen species (especially for silica),[3] the role of release of tumour necrosis factor[4] and the role of cytokine release from

macrophages.[5] The result is a mixture of tissue destruction and fibrosis and different features may predominate depending on the nature of the dust. With coal dust and other relatively low toxicity dusts, there is typically some fibrosis in the form of a nodule, or macule, around the terminal bronchiole with some mild surrounding centrilobular emphysema. This causes little problem unless it progresses to more marked fibrotic changes or to more severe emphysema, as happens in some cases with heavy coal dust exposure. Silica, a more toxic dust, causes a more severe fibrotic reaction, but still mainly in discrete nodules. Adjacent foci of scarring may link up to form masses, and blood vessel walls may become involved leading to thrombosis and patchy necrosis. Asbestos more typically leads to a more diffuse fibrotic reaction, giving a form of interstitial fibrosis. In some cases, immune mechanisms may be involved in the tissue reaction to retained dust and this is discussed below in relation to specific dusts.

INVESTIGATION AND DIAGNOSIS

The diagnosis of occupational lung disease may be delayed or missed altogether because it is not considered. Without a history of exposure the clinical features and radiographic appearances may be non-specific or suggestive of non-occupational disease.

Occupational history

Unlike diseases due to inhalation of organic dusts, most forms of pneumoconiosis do not cause immediate symptoms and most require prolonged exposure and have a long latency after first exposure. Therefore the cause must be sought in past occupations. A general job classification such as 'joiner' or 'fitter' is of no help without hearing what the worker actually did, what the industry was and what the dust conditions and the nature of the materials were.

The symptoms of bronchitis (persistent productive cough) may develop early but it is usually many years before the worker notices either symptoms or disablement from the underlying disease. Radiographic changes may not develop until 10–20 years after exposure starts and may appear and progress long after exposure ceases. By the time the breathlessness of the pneumoconiosis is noticed the radiographic changes are usually well advanced. In mild cases symptoms may be attributed by the worker to 'old age' and may indeed be due to falling respiratory reserve (ageing of the normal lung) rather than progression of the dust disease. In the case of the asbestos-related cancers the latent interval may average 40 years or more. Recent occupations are often unimportant but past and present smoking habits are always important.

Symptoms

Breathlessness on exertion is often the only symptom. Cough and sputum can occur due to the dust exposure itself but are frequently due to concomitant smoking. Complicated pneumoconiosis with cavitation of necrotic masses leads to the expectoration of large volumes of dirty material (once euphemistically called 'melanoptysis' in coal workers) and sometimes to serious haemoptysis. The cavities left behind may become secondarily infected, causing a cough productive of copious foul sputum, similar to bronchiectasis.

Pain is virtually never the result of pneumoconiosis: however, the chest tightness of a restrictive lesion (as seen in asbestosis or severe silicosis) can be mistaken for the 'tightness' of angina and has been reported as pain.

Signs

There are no physical signs in simple pneumoconiosis. They begin to appear as the disease becomes 'complicated'. Chest movement will be restricted a little if there is interstitial fibrosis or extensive pleural scarring which may also cause some dullness. Even the large masses of complicated pneumoconiosis before and after cavitation are usually not detectable on physical examination because they are relatively central and are surrounded by emphysematous lung.

Confluent fibrosis such as occurs in asbestosis is indistinguishable from other interstitial fibrotic lung disease and is associated with limited chest expansion, basal end-inspiratory 'dry' crepitations, cyanosis, polycythaemia and sometimes (but not always) clubbing of the fingers.

Investigations

Ordinary haematological and biochemical tests are of no value in pneumoconiosis as they become abnormal only in extreme situations. The erythrocyte sedimentation rate and the plasma angiotensin converting enzyme level may indicate the activity of the destructive lesion in the lung but have no diagnostic specificity. Tuberculin and Kveim tests, if positive, may indicate that the chest disease is tuberculosis or sarcoidosis, respectively, but there is no reliable way of distinguishing between beryllium pneumoconiosis and sarcoidosis in a worker with exposure to beryllium, except by performing a beryllium lymphocyte transformation test.

Examination of the sputum and bronchial lavage may yield confirmation of the occupational history in that the dust cells (dust-loaded macrophages) can be examined under the electron microscope and the nature of the dust identified. Asbestos bodies can be detected with the light microscope. They usually indicate amphibole exposure (which may be confirmed with the analytic electron microscope) and their profusion is a useful indication of the lung asbestos burden but is not necessarily indicative of active disease. The cell count in the lavage fluid is increased in various forms of pneumoconiosis but this is non-specific.

It is more difficult to define the place of lung biopsy especially now that fibreoptic bronchoscopy has made transbronchial biopsy readily available. The role of biopsy will be discussed for individual diseases. On the whole, because of the focal nature of dust diseases, percutaneous and transbronchial biopsy have proved disappointing for diagnosis because the biopsy may miss the foci of disease. To determine the precise nature of the dust and its relationship to the pathology may require sophisticated electron microscopy of material taken at thoracotomy. However, it is rarely justifiable to undertake a thoracotomy to obtain a biopsy for diagnostic purposes. Biopsies obtained by thoracoscopy are less invasive and may represent an acceptable alternative in selected patients. On the other hand, in modern pneumology, 'crystals' or 'fibres' are often found in lung biopsies obtained for diagnosing interstitial lung disease, and it is not always easy in such cases to assign a causal role to these materials, which may or may not be incidental.

Chest radiography (see Chapter 30)

Fortunately most patients with a chest complaint have a chest radiograph and it is at this stage that either the radiologist or the clinician may realize that the disease is occupational. Even then, because many occupational lung diseases have non-specific radiographic features, cases are missed. The radiograph is useful in the diagnosis of the individual case, although the degree of radiographic abnormality is poorly related to the pathological severity of disease or the loss of lung function for many dusts. Some dusts produce dramatic radiographic shadows with little or no loss of lung function. In simple coalworkers' pneumoconiosis the radiographic appearance of small, rounded opacities relates well to dust exposure but almost not at all to lung function. In asbestosis, the radiographic abnormality is a poor guide to the pathological severity of disease. However, the chest radiograph is of particular value for epidemiological purposes. Radiographic surveys combined with exposure, lung function and pathology information have helped to determine whether certain patterns of change are associated with particular occupations. This sort of research has also helped to establish the relationships between radiology, lung function and pathology in groups of workers.

THE ILO CLASSIFICATION OF RADIOGRAPHS OF THE PNEUMOCONIOSES[6]

During the last 50 years the International Labour Office (ILO) in Geneva has sponsored the development of a classification of the radiographic changes in pneumoconiosis which is used to describe the pattern and severity of the change in groups of workers. In principle, it is *not* intended as a method of diagnosis or of estimating the severity of an *individual* case. Despite many modifications, there remains a subjective element in how an individual reader classifies a particular film. The reading is also dependent on the quality of the film (in particular how dark or light it is). Films should be read in batches mixed with controls and 'trigger' films. The readings must then be subjected to statistical analysis to determine whether there is any relationship between radiographic changes and dust exposure measurements (or estimates of level of dust exposure). It is also possible to relate the radiographic changes to measurements of lung function in the population. Each batch of radiographs should be read independently by three trained observers and all the readings should be taken into account in the analysis. The readers should not be aware of any other information about the individuals whose films they read, to avoid bias. The method of reading is to compare each film with a set of standard films supplied by the ILO in Geneva. The results are recorded on a special form, an example of which is shown in Fig. 35.1. The brief description of the classification which follows indicates the range of changes that may be the result of dust exposure (see p. 603).

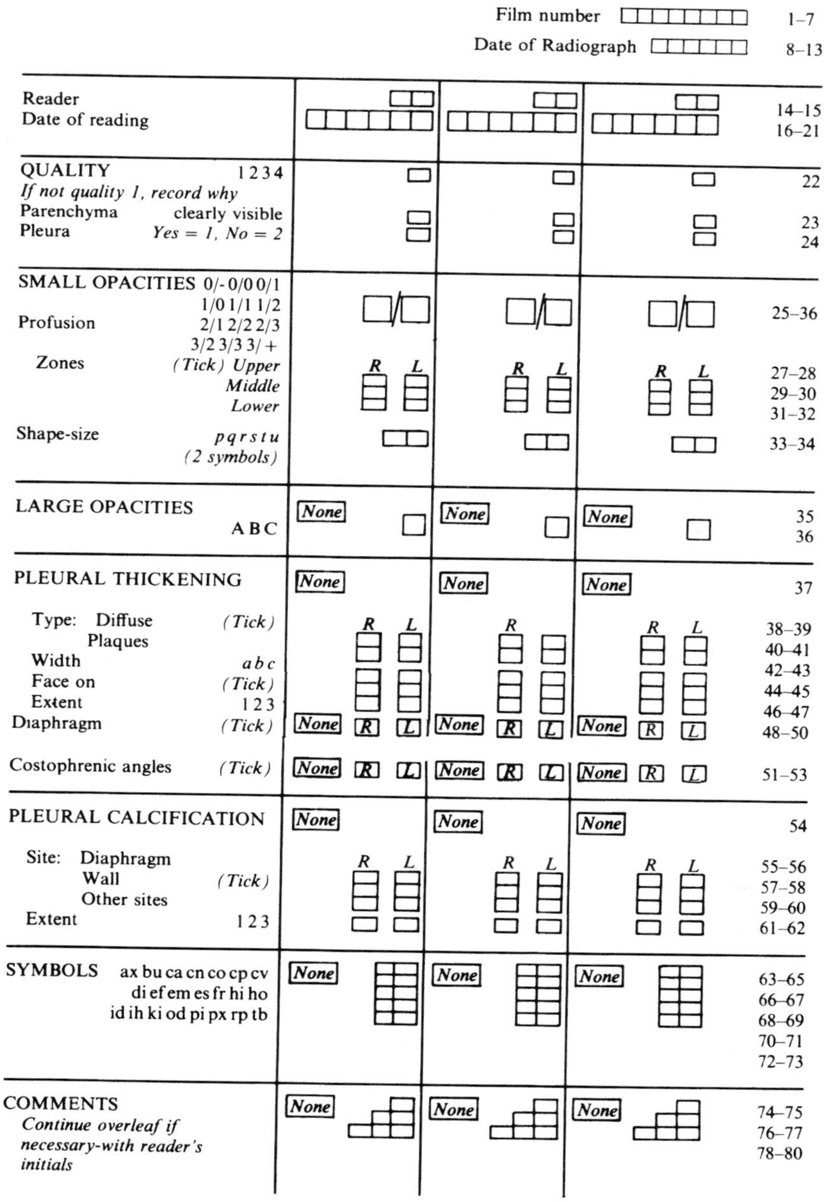

Figure 35.1 *Example of the form for recording the reading of chest radiographs to the ILO classification by three independent readers. (It is essential that no reader should know the readings of the other two until the reading is complete.)*

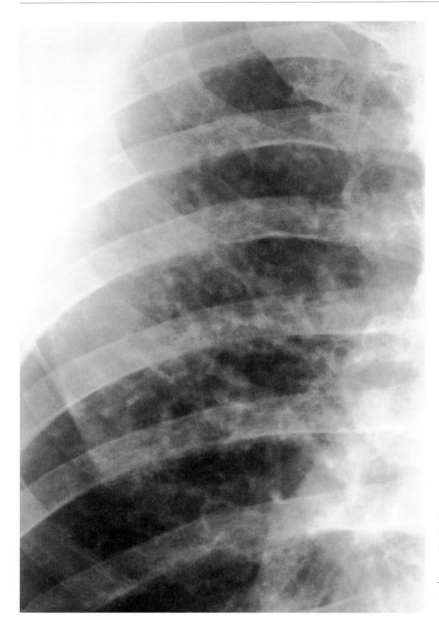

Figure 35.2 *Part of the right mid-zone of the standard ILO film 1/1, q/q 1980 (actual size) for comparison with Fig. 35.3. Middle-sized small rounded opacities, profusion sufficient to be definitely abnormal. (ILO International Classification of Radiographs for Pneumoconioses. Copyright 1980, International Labour Organization, Geneva.)*

Small opacities

The profusion of small shadows is recorded on a 12 point scale, by comparison with a set of four standards 0/0, 1/1, 2/2 and 3/3.[6] If the film being read is between two standards then the nearer standard is recorded first and the further second so that a film between 1/1 and 2/2 but nearer to 1/1 is recorded as 1/2. A completely normal film (clearer than the standard 'normal' film which is 0/0) is recorded as 0/– and one with more profuse shadows than 3/3 as 3/+ (Figs 35.2 and 35.3).

The size and shape of the small shadows is then recorded. The shadows, which may vary from just visible (about 1.0 mm) to about 5.0 mm, are graded into three by comparison with standards rather than by measurement. For rounded shadows, such as are seen in coal workers, these grades are p, q and r and for irregular shadows s, t and u. (Fig. 35.4). The dominant shape/size is recorded first and the next most dominant second.

Pleural thickening

The recording of pleural changes has given rise to much difficulty because of the variety of changes which may occur (especially as a result of asbestos exposure) and the difficulty of identifying and interpreting these on a simple chest radiograph. The classification divides the changes into discrete patches of thickening (plaques) and poorly defined areas (diffuse). The thickness, extent and distribution and the amount of calcification are recorded.

Symbols

This section is for recording other abnormalities seen on the radiographs that may influence the reading of changes due to dust. The symbols include fractures of

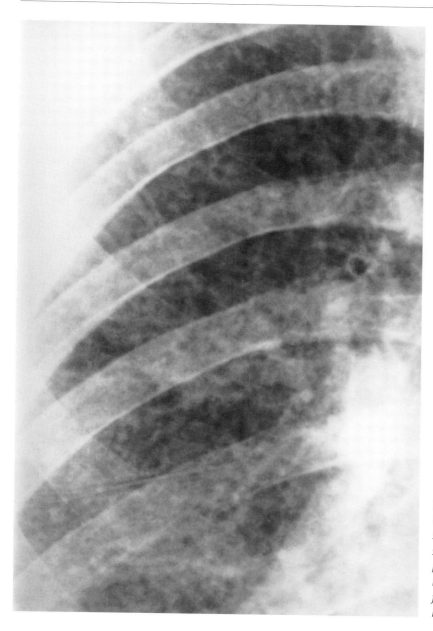

Figure 35.3 *Part of the right mid-zone of the standard ILO film 3/3, q/q 1980 (actual size) for comparison with Fig. 35.2. Same sized rounded opacities as in Fig. 35.2 but profusion nearly maximal. (ILO International Classification of Radiographs for Pneumoconioses, Copyright 1980, International Labour Organization, Geneva.)*

ribs (fr), cancer (ca) and tuberculosis (tb) as well as changes which may be part of the dust disease such as calcification of the small opacities (cn), rheumatoid pneumoconiosis (rp), bullae (bu) and emphysema (em).

Computed tomographic scanning

Computed tomographic (CT) scanning is not part of the normal diagnostic routine for the pneumoconioses. However, it can yield information not readily apparent on the chest radiograph. It is particularly useful for delineating the nature and extent of pleural changes, which is notoriously difficult based on a chest radiograph. It can also allow the extent of emphysema to be estimated quite accurately and the severity of interstitial

fibrosis to be gauged. A scoring system for high resolution CT scans, similar to the ILO classification of radiographs, has been described.[7]

Lung function tests

Lung function tests are used in two ways in inorganic dust diseases: to study exposed populations of workers and to follow individuals over time, in which case spirometry is the suitable measure; and to diagnose individual cases of lung disease, in which case a battery of tests and comparison with predicted values is useful.

FOR SURVEYS AND MONITORING

In spite of their lack of specificity the simple spirometric

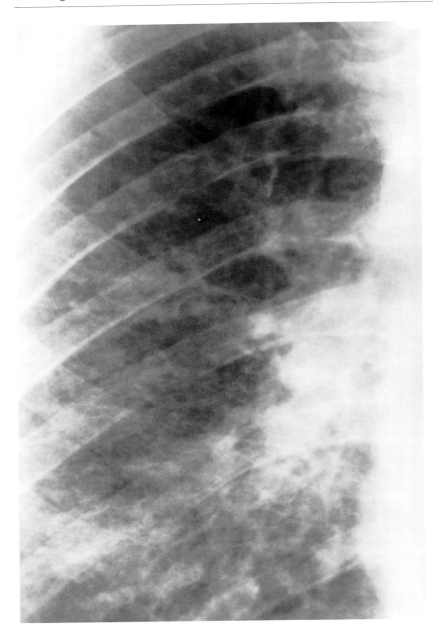

Figure 35.4 *Part of the right mid-zone of the standard ILO film 2/2, t/t (actual size). (ILO International Classification of Radiographs for Pneumoconioses. Copyright 1980, International Labour Organization, Geneva.)*

tests (forced vital capacity, FVC, and forced expiratory volume in 1 second, FEV_1) remain the most suitable tests for either cross-sectional surveys or long-term monitoring. Comparison with 'predicted' values for age, sex and height is not especially helpful. It may be appropriate to compare with non-exposed workers and to compare individuals with themselves over time. These tests are by no means the best measures of parenchymal lung disease and can be markedly affected by other conditions such as asthma and chronic obstructive pulmonary disease due to smoking. The reasons they have proved most useful are:

1   The equipment is cheap, easy to keep standardized and widely available.

2   The tests are easy to learn and not frightening for the subject so that reliable, repeatable readings can usually be achieved after a few minutes' practice. Repeat tests at 6-monthly or yearly intervals take less than 5 minutes.

3   It is easy to train technicians to do the test properly, maintain the apparatus and calculate the results. Modern spirometers often do the calculation automatically.

Electronic spirometers now widely available also give information about the whole of the flow-volume curve, allowing more sophisticated analysis of the curve to study dysfunction of the smaller airways. Unfortunately, the predicted results for the indices of small airways function from the flow-volume curve are much less reliable than the FEV$_1$ and FVC.

FOR DIAGNOSIS IN INDIVIDUAL CASES

In the diagnosis or assessment of the lung function deficit and disability in an individual case a wide range of tests can be useful. Simple pneumoconiosis with dust macules forming around the centrilobular airways may or may not show up on tests for small airways narrowing or compliance, depending on the severity. Early alveolar lesions or interstitial fibrosis should show up as a reduction in gas transfer capacity. In practice, damage at either level produces abnormalities in both types of test, and either can be used as a measure of loss of lung function. Both types of test have proved useful in the detection of early disease in relatively young workers. Increasing age increases the scatter of findings in the 'normal' population. Much of this can now be shown to be due to cigarette smoking (and in the past to urban atmospheric pollution). The high proportion of smokers amongst workers in dusty occupations means that these tests are of little diagnostic value in older individuals. The precise choice of test must be left to the laboratory as the technical accuracy of the test is very much dependent upon its frequency of use, the experience and skill of the technician and the availability of local standards for correcting for height, age and smoking.

When lung function tests are used in individual diagnosis it is useful to compare with the values predicted for age, height and sex, derived from large studies for normal individuals. The normal populations used usually do not include smokers. Predicted values derived from one population may not be applicable to another ethnic group and it is important to use the most appropriate predicted values for an individual.

Post-mortem examination

Histological examination of autopsy material and the study of the dust extracted from the lung after death have been major sources of information about the nature and causes of occupational lung disease in the last 100 years. Although chest physicians with special experience may have little difficulty with the diagnosis during

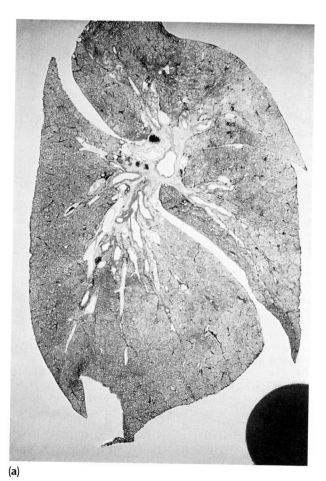

(a)

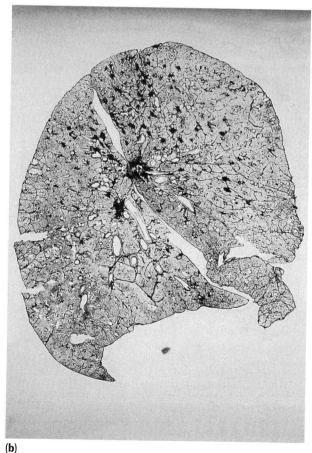

(b)

Figure 35.5 *(a) Gough paper-mounted whole lung section of a normal lung. (b) Gough paper-mounted whole lung section of a lung with dust macules of simple coalworker's pneumoconiosis.*

life, in the light of the occupational history, the chest radiograph and the pattern of lung function loss, still the diagnosis is often made by the pathologist on the basis of the post-mortem appearances and histology.

Until the last few years, because of the arrangements in the UK for the granting of widows' pensions, most compensated cases of occupational lung disease came to autopsy, providing a source of important information to further understanding of these conditions. Similar material has been available from South Africa but in many other countries difficulties in obtaining autopsy material have delayed the study of these diseases and made the administration of systems of compensation more difficult. There is no longer the same administrative requirement for an autopsy in the UK and so many fewer cases of suspected or confirmed ocupational lung disease now come to autopsy. Previous studies that compared post-mortem lung pathology with radiographic appearances and lung function during life would now be very hard to mount.

A special technique should be used for suspected cases of occupational lung disease because in an ordinary autopsy an overall view of the pathology is lost and considerable damage done to the detailed histology by dissecting and cutting the lung before it is fixed. Instead, the lungs should be removed *en bloc* with the trachea and with the parietal pleura still attached if it is adherent. Any tears in the visceral pleura should be oversewn and the lungs should be fixed in inflation via the trachea either with formol-saline or with formalin vapour. After fixation (which takes several days) the lungs should be cut in 1.0-cm thick slices and examined in detail before taking representative histological blocks. The slices may be recolourized with alcohol and photographed under water to provided a permanent record of the texture of the lung. Or they can be impregnated with gelatine and used to prepare 'Gough' paper mounted whole lung sections (Fig. 35.5).

NON-FIBROUS MINERAL DUSTS

This group of dusts is still an important cause of fatal lung disease in a number of developing countries where many workers are exposed to dangerous levels of dust in industry and particularly in mining, quarrying and civil engineering. There is a widely held view in developed countries that the risks are so well known and controlled by government regulation that the diseases no longer occur. However, this is not true; serious outbreaks continue to occur, such as one in the UK reported in 1991.[8] The SWORD reporting scheme (surveillance of work-related and occupational respiratory diseases) for occupational lung diseases in Britain indicates that these dusts account for about 400 of the 2400 new cases of occupational lung disease reported to the scheme annually.

Quartz dust is among the most toxic of the non-fibrous mineral dusts and can cause fatal disease after exposure for only a few months to concentrations not perceptible to the naked eye. Many mixed dusts produce disease due to their quartz content; any of them inhaled at levels above the lung clearance capacity for long enough will cause a pneumoconiosis and most will ultimately cause serious disease. In British industry only a limited variety of quartz-containing dusts are inhaled under dangerous conditions and only some of them are used enough in the UK and internationally to warrant specific mention in this chapter.

The pathology of silicosis and silicate dust pneumoconiosis was reviewed in some detail by an international panel of pathologists a decade ago and much of this is still relevant.[9]

Quartz and related dust

Silicosis results from the inhalation of one of the three crystalline forms of silicon dioxide. Quartz is by far the most common, the other two being cristobalite and tridymite. Workers may die of silicosis having retained as little as 1.0 g of pure quartz dust or less than 0.5 g of tridymite or cristobalite.

Glass is supercooled liquid silicon dioxide and if ground to a respirable dust can cause acute cell damage as can other forms of amorphous or resublimed silica. Such non-crystalline silica dusts dissolve fairly rapidly in the tissue and do not cause the progressive pulmonary disease produced by crystalline forms, although the dissolved silica may damage other tissues such as the kidney.

Quartz is found free as (silica) sand which is the residue left by the erosion of igneous rocks, like granite, in which the quartz crystals formed when larva cooled. Pure quartz is colourless but traces of metal in the melt have produced various gemstones such as citrine, cairngorm, etc. Quartz is very hard and is virtually insoluble in tissue fluids and in most acids and alkalis.

Much of the earth's crust is made up of the metal salts of silicic acid (silicates). Dust from these compounds can also damage the lung (silicatosis) but their mode of action and toxicity is not comparable to quartz; examples will be discussed later in this chapter.

TOXICITY

It is still not clear how apparently inert insoluble particles of quartz damage cells, although there is evidence of the involvement of cytokines[5] and oxygen radicals.[10] Freshly ground respirable particles will kill phagocytic cells in culture, and kill the cells lining the alveoli of experimental animals and of humans at high levels of exposure. At lower levels, especially when the quartz is diluted with an inert dust, the macrophages will take up a few active particles with the inert ones and survive long enough to move into the alveolar wall or to the centrilobular interstitium before dying. At greater dilution some of the quartz mixed in with the other dust will be cleared by the macrophages to the bronchial mucus escalator.

Resuspended quartz dust, such as that which blows off the Sahara desert, is relatively inert and much of it is cleared from the lung without causing damage. Similarly quartz mixed with metal oxides, as in iron ore mining, does not show the expected toxicity. Experimentally this has been shown to be due to the adsorption of a layer of the metal oxide onto the crystal. Experimental studies have since shown that these coatings, applied before inhalation, will delay the onset of fibrosis and reduce its severity, but that the coating is eventually lost and the particles become actively fibrogenic.[11]

In the hope that metals such as aluminium and some polymers might make quartz dust less toxic, such compounds have even been administered to workers who have already inhaled quartz dust in the hope that silicosis may be prevented or even cured. Long-term use of aluminium powder as a prophylactic inhalation in Canadian uranium miners was abandoned after 30 years because of lack of evidence of its efficacy. (Metallic aluminium powder has been shown to be fibrogenic in animals in the same size range as quartz (0.5–5 μm) and cases of pulmonary fibrosis have been reported from industry). Aluminium citrate given parenterally has been shown both in laboratory animals and on clinical trial in humans to reduce the severity of silicosis. However, the known toxicity of aluminium to the central nervous system probably precludes its long-term parenteral use (see Chapter 7).

ACUTE SILICOSIS

This is also known as 'silicotic alveolar proteinosis' or even 'silicotic alveolar lipoproteinosis'. High level exposure to active dust causes immediate damage in the alveolus with death of the type I and II alveolar lining cells as well as the macrophages. Protein fluid, followed by inflammatory cells, leaks from the capillaries into the alveoli, mingling with the surfactant. Resolution does not occur and the alveoli become obliterated with fibrous tissue. This acute alveolitis may present within weeks of the start of exposure. The first symptoms are breathlessness and dry cough which get gradually worse despite all treatment. The radiograph shows patchy pulmonary oedema but with the shadows gradually hardening and the affected areas shrinking. Lung function tests indicate a restrictive lesion with falling gas transfer leading to hypoxia and cyanosis. The disease is often fatal, sometimes within a few months, the prognosis being dependent on the amount of active dust already retained before the exposure stopped.

As there is no safe or effective treatment of this (or any other) form of silicosis, acute silicosis should never be allowed to occur in any country. There are documented incidents of large numbers of men dying of acute silicosis in the face of high, uncontrolled silica exposure in tunnelling.[12] It is still reported, for instance, where a small enterprise is set up to sand blast metal parts or to make silica flour without dust control.

The lesions of acute silicosis can also be seen in parts of the lung in cases of chronic active silicosis when the exposure has been high and recent. This intermediate disease is known as 'accelerated silicosis' and outbreaks of this condition continue to occur in Britain.[8]

CHRONIC (ACTIVE) SILICOSIS

This disease was once widespread in industrial countries. It is now uncommon in developed countries mainly due to the use of safer alternative materials. Where this is not possible (hard rock mining, tunnelling, etc.) the adoption of modern methods of dust control and the enforcement of international standards have minimized the risk. In developing countries many sources of risk still exist and the disease is still a major problem.

Symptoms are a late manifestation of the disease. By the time breathlessness is noticed or is sufficient to interfere with labouring work, the radiograph shows widespread change. The first shadows to appear are the medium to large size of small, rounded opacities (q or r on the ILO scale) and are either evenly distributed or more frequent in the upper zones. Hilar node enlargement is common. The histology of the lesions in the lung is diagnostic; they are discrete nodules made of concentric layers of dense collagen tissue with a core containing birefringent quartz particles. They seldom grow to more than 1 cm in diameter. Larger masses consist of a conglomeration of these nodules as do the enlarged hilar lymph nodes. The nodules first form in the centrilobular area and then along the lymphatics both to the pleura and the hilar nodes with lines of less organized fibrous tissue linking them together. In the absence of further exposure the nodules may become inactive and calcify from the periphery inwards. A similar phenomenon in the hilar nodes gives rise to the appearance of 'eggshell calcification' ('ec' in the ILO symbols). However, it may take 20–30 years for nodules to form, become quiescent and calcify; few workers with active silicosis live this long. A short period of relatively high exposure can give rise to hilar gland enlargement and nodules in the pleura with adhesions and pleural thickening before there is a build-up of nodules in the lung parenchyma.

The onset of breathlessness is usually due to the beginning of coalescence of individual nodules through the contraction of the linking fibrous bands. In the absence of complicating tuberculosis there may be a dry cough and no pain. A restrictive pattern is found on lung function testing with loss of gas transfer capacity. Eventually hypoxia and cyanosis occur, first on exercise and then at rest. Death is usually due to cor pulmonale.

There are usually no physical signs in the chest and clubbing is not a feature. Depending possibly on the presence of amorphous silica in the dust, severe silicosis may be associated with liver and renal damage.[13] The risk of lung cancer in association with silicosis is discussed below.

The accelerated form of silicosis can produce symptoms within a year of the start of exposure, when the lungs may show some of the features of acute silicosis, and when some deaths may occur within 5 years. In the last 50 years it has been uncommon in Britain to see radiographic changes starting before 10–20 years from first exposure and leading (in the absence of tuberculosis) to life-threatening lung impairment before the retiring age. The longer the interval between first exposure and the onset of symptoms, the slower they tend to progress and the greater the likelihood of the subject living to the retiring age and beyond. If the dust is relatively pure quartz, then little will be seen on the radiograph until the first nodules (r shadows) appear 5–15 years after first exposure. When there is heavy admixture of inert dust then a simple small opacity pneumoconiosis (p or q) may appear first. It is possible for workers exposed to quartz to leave their occupation after 5 or more years, free of symptoms, with a normal chest radiograph and lung function tests at that time, and then to develop classical silicosis and die of respiratory failure or complicating tuberculosis many years later.

CHRONIC (INACTIVE) SILICOSIS

Just as there is no clear distinction between acute and chronic (active) disease so there is none between chronic (active) and chronic (inactive). It is a matter of the level and duration of exposure. The presence of other dusts, cigarette smoking and environmental pollution outside the workplace can also modify the effect of the quartz.

When workers are exposed for many years to a dust which is occasionally contaminated with quartz or which contains, most of the time, a very small proportion, their pneumoconiosis will show mixed features. On the radiograph a simple pneumoconiosis with mainly p- and q-sized rounded opacities may be present after 20–30 years. A few workers may show r shadows in the upper zone and hilar gland enlargement. These r shadows may become more profuse, tend to coalesce to form irregular masses or they may remain static and calcify. The hilar nodes may show eggshell calcification without obvious r-sized parenchymal shadows ever appearing. In workers with a long exposure history and who show these mixed features it is unwise to give a good prognosis without following the case for at least 10 years after exposure has ceased. Histology of such lungs often shows silicotic nodules in various stages of development, some dating from early exposure and others arising more recently with scope for further development. Calcification is probably the only sure indication that a silicotic lesion is no longer active.

SILICOTUBERCULOSIS

When active tuberculosis is common in the community, many patients with silicosis develop a combined disease with an extremely poor prognosis and called 'silicotuberculosis'. This is now rare in developed countries but remains common in many developing countries. Conventional chemotherapy for tuberculosis may delay progression but patients can die with their infection still active in spite of chemotherapy that would eradicate the disease in patients without silicosis. Some years ago Westerholm[14] calculated that the risk of developing tuberculosis after the diagnosis of silicosis in Sweden was up to 15 times the risk for the general population. A study of mortality among silicosis claimants in California (cases from 1945 to 1975 followed from 1946 to 1991) found a grossly elevated mortality from tuberculosis among these silicotics.[15] The risk in the individual is related to the severity of the silicosis. It remains high for at least 15 years after the diagnosis of the silicosis and probably for a lifetime. The mechanism is unknown but *in vitro* studies indicate that macrophages are less able to engulf and kill tubercle bacilli when quartz dust is present. Silicosis causes damage to the lymphatic drainage of the lung which is important for the control of tuberculous infections; there may be an additional constitutional factor.

The detection of active tuberculosis in patients with early asymptomatic silicosis is not difficult because the onset of cough, sputum, night sweats, malaise and weight loss may be enough to bring the patient to the clinic. On the chest radiograph new soft upper zone shadowing should show up clearly against the pre-existing r-sized rounded opacities. A raised sedimentation rate and the presence of tubercle bacilli in the sputum confirm the diagnosis. The diagnosis is difficult in advanced silicotics, especially those who smoke, as they probably already have a cough, sputum and loss of weight. Confluent silicotic nodules in the upper zone with associated emphysema may mimic the appearance of cavities and make new infiltrates difficult to see on conventional radiographs. Confluent silicotic nodules (unlike the masses of progressive massive fibrosis in coal miners and those of Caplan's syndrome) rarely cavitate in the absence of tuberculosis. Haemoptysis and cavitation of the lung masses (confirmed by CT scan if possible) are strong indications of active tuberculosis. The organisms may be hard to identify on sputum smear or culture from the sputum and it is often necessary to treat such cases on suspicion, without microbiological confirmation of the diagnosis. Treatment is as for pulmonary tuberculosis (for example, following the British Thoracic Society guidelines in the UK). There is evidence that treatment should be more prolonged than for tuberculosis in the absence of silicosis.[16] It can be difficult to gauge effectiveness of treatment in the absence of organisms in the sputum, as the radiographic shadows may not regress.

Prevention of silicotuberculosis

Prevention of silicotuberculosis is difficult. The main risk of silicosis now is in developing countries where the general risk of tuberculosis is high and most of the population are exposed to the tubercle bacillus in childhood. Occupational exposure to quartz dust then carries the risk of reactivation of latent infection or new infection. The overcrowded and insanitary conditions prevailing for migrant workers in mine compounds contribute to the spread of the disease. In a developing country where most children are already Mantoux positive before they start breathing in quartz dust, there is obviously no point in giving BCG (Bacille Calmette-Guérin) when work starts. The use of BCG among Mantoux negative mine workers exposed to silica in Eastern Europe apparently had an *adverse* effect,[17] although a benefit was reported for copper miners in Africa.[18] It is not clear whether prophylactic chemotherapy, for example with isoniazid, for people with silicosis confers a benefit; in any case this is impractical in most developing countries where the majority of the cases now occur. Careful monitoring of silicotics is important, with treatment on suspicion of infection, even without microbiological confirmation.

SILICA EXPOSURE AND LUNG CANCER

The evaluation of the International Agency for Research on Cancer (IARC) in 1987 stated that there is 'limited evidence' for the carcinogenicity of crystalline silica to humans.[19] During the last decade a number of epidemiological studies of silica-exposed workers have addressed this issue. The issues included: whether it was the silica itself or some other associated exposure that was carcinogenic; whether the effects of smoking could be taken into account adequately; whether there was a dose–response relationship; and whether the risk was confined to those men who had silicosis or was also present in those with exposure but no evidence of silicosis. A recent review of the evidence concluded that there is an elevated risk of lung cancer among workers who have been exposed to silica; it is highest and most consistent in silicotics, who have received the highest doses.[20] The risk of lung cancer is increased when radiographic silicosis is present.[21] A recent study from Australia concluded there was no evidence that exposure to silica causes lung cancer in the absence of silicosis[22] and a study in Germany found no dose response with silica exposure in men without silicosis.[23] A study from South Africa[24] concluded that since those with the higher exposures are also those with silicosis, it is not possible to say if the increased risk of lung cancer is due to the silica exposure itself or to the silicosis (perhaps as a result of the lung scarring). A recent IARC monograph states that crystalline silica should be regarded as a probable human carcinogen.[24a]

It seems clear that silica exposure can cause lung cancer in humans, but there remains some doubt about the mechanism, whether due to genotoxicity or an indirect effect from the lung scarring of silicosis. A recent review has discussed the possible role of reactive oxygen species in silica-induced carcinogenesis.[25]

SILICOSIS AND ITS PREVENTION IN DIFFERENT OCCUPATIONS

Grinders

When the cause of lung disease in grinders (Fig. 35.6) was recognized as being due to their exposure to silica dust (for example knife grinders in Sheffield) the first move was to change from dry to wet working. The workers disliked the change and claimed it reduced their pro-

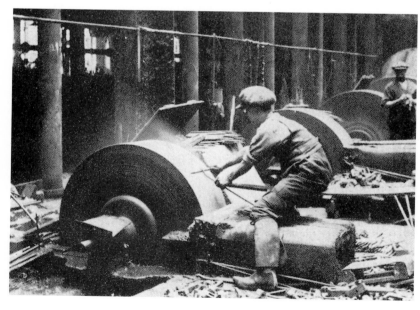

Figure 35.6 *Grinding with a sandstone wheel, wet working was not by itself sufficient to prevent silicosis partly because it was not accepted by the workers. Courtesy Platt Bros & Co. Ltd.*

ductivity and earnings. It was not completely successful and so sandstone or millstone grit grinding wheels were replaced by synthetic silicon carbide. Although harder than quartz, this produces a dust which is very much less fibrogenic and its use for grinding, etc. has virtually eradicated silicosis from this occupational group. As even silicon carbide dust can cause lung fibrosis, most of this work should still be done wet and exposure must be kept well below the limits for 'nuisance dusts'.

Masons and polishers

Wet working by itself appears to have been effective in controlling silicosis amongst monumental masons and men who polish granite and other quartz containing rock for architectural and decorative use. Failure to take precautions leads to accelerated disease.

In some traditional workplaces, materials like precious stones, jade and metals are polished with dangerous powders. Silicosis has been reported from a workshop where jade was polished (dry) using a mixture containing silica flour.[26] This could be avoided by using a non-fibrogenic polishing powder.

Miners

Hard rock mining for tin, gold, copper, etc. was another occupation early recognized as causing silicosis, and similarly the cutting of shafts and 'drivages' (passages or

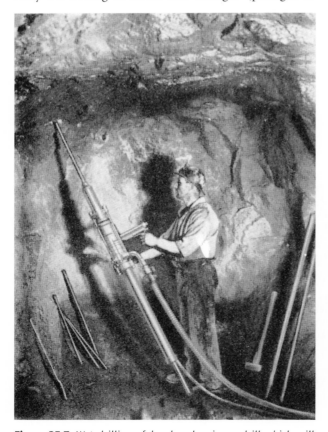

Figure 35.7 *Wet drilling of hard rock using a drill which will only rotate when the water running down the middle is turned on. Courtesy Mr T Holman.*

roadways) through hard rock to gain access to coal seams and other ores. Civil engineering tunnelling first for canals and then railways and now for motorways and underground railways, hydroelectric schemes, etc. are situations where the risk may vary from week to week depending on the strata encountered. The most important step was the introduction of hollow drills which could not be used without water flowing down the centre (Fig. 35.7). But in hard rock situations it is not possible to inject water into the rock face to prevent dust formation when charges are fired. This is dealt with by positive ventilation and waiting periods after shot firing to allow the dust and toxic fumes to be cleared by the ventilation before the workers go back in.

Pottery and refractory making

Silicosis was common in the UK area in Staffordshire known as the Potteries where the making of crockery and ceramics was concentrated. It resulted partly from the grinding of quartz-containing minerals like 'china stone' for mixing with the clay for making porcelain. But the main problem appears to have been the use of silica sand and silica flour as a parting medium to prevent the pots from sticking together or to the stands while they were being fired. Not only did the dust from applying the silica sand and flour cause silicosis but by the time firing was complete the quartz was converted to cristobalite and the workers handling the items after firing were at even greater risk. Refractory bricks for lining furnaces were made of silica sand and caused silicosis during manufacture and use when the lining of furnaces had to be renewed at regular intervals by digging out the old bricks (a very dusty job). The spent bricks contained cristobalite as well as quartz and fibres of mullite are also formed which may contribute to the lung damage. All these risks could be avoided by dust suppression but this is technically very difficult especially when cleaning the lining out of an old furnace. Better solutions may result from automation and changing to ingredients and parting media that are not fibrogenic.

Moulders and fettlers

Traditionally iron and brass were cast by pouring the metal into moulds formed of damp sand. When cool the mould was broken open, leaving some of the sand embedded in the surface of the metal. This was first knocked off with a hammer and chisel (fettled) and the surface finished by grinding. Both these processes released sufficient quartz dust to cause chronic active silicosis in a proportion of the workers. It was a slow, labour-intensive process and was replaced by sand blasting, which caused acute silicosis. The sand was replaced by steel shot but there was still the sand on the casting and silicosis still occurred. Even the replacement of silica sand as a main casting medium by less fibrogenic material such as 'green sand' has not completely solved this problem. If castings are to be cleaned in this manner the work has to be completely enclosed in a specially ventilated cabinet. High-precision casting such as is demanded of the light alloy components for the motor industry has moved towards the use of binders in the moulding medium and various separating agents to produce a clean smooth casting. Dust has been eliminated but silicosis has been replaced by occupational asthma because of the release of allergens when the hot metal is poured into moulds made with certain polymeric binders, etc.

DUST MONITORING FOR SILICA EXPOSURE

Most countries now accept the recommendations of the World Health Organization and the International Labour Office concerning the protection of workers exposed to dust containing crystalline silica and the use of personal as well as fixed samplers. When the dust contains more than 1% quartz it is recommended that dust measurements must be made regularly and work suspended if the safe limits are exceeded. In most countries these limits are expressed as time-weighted average values for an 8-hour shift and are best measured using a personal sampler fixed in the breathing zone of the individual while he works. For quartz the limits are usually about 0.1 mg/m^3 for respirable dust and 0.3 mg for total dust. The limits for cristobalite and tridymite are half this.

These limits have been decided upon by trial, error and negotiation rather than being strictly scientifically based. They take no account of the variation in toxicity between different quartz dusts or the effect of modifying materials in mixed dust exposures. Accurate dose response estimates are difficult because they are often based on poor, extrapolated exposure data. Nevertheless, if exposure to respirable dust is carefully limited to below 0.1 mg/m^3, silicosis is unlikely to occur. However, in many developing countries the legislative framework for exposure control is weak and enforcement is even weaker so high exposures continue to occur, with the inevitable associated morbidity and mortality.

MEDICAL MONITORING FOR WORKERS EXPOSED TO SILICA DUST

Because the exposure limits discussed above have a limited scientific basis and because in practice one cannot rely on the employer or the workforce to keep within them, medical monitoring of exposed workers is important. The following section outlines the sort of monitoring that is appropriate, recognizing that this may be difficult to achieve in developing countries. Not only can this be of benefit to individual workers by allowing them to cease exposure at an early stage of the disease, but it is also a means of double-checking the adequacy of control measures. Medical monitoring of the workers should never be used as an excuse for not controlling the exposure.

Ideally, workers should be screened for tuberculosis

before they start work and, in situations where the tuberculosis rate in the population is low, the Mantoux and BCG status should be recorded. A positive history or radiological evidence of past or present pulmonary tuberculosis are good reasons for advising against employment involving exposure to quartz. Previous dusty work or indeed any past chest disease which has given rise to radiographic changes are also contraindications for working with quartz because this would interfere with the early detection of changes due to silicosis. The initial examination should include an FEV$_1$ and FVC or similar reliable baseline measurement of ventilation. At follow-up examinations the cumulative dust exposure for each individual (where available), details of respiratory illnesses and changes in smoking habits should be added to the results of the routine examination, radiograph and ventilation tests.

The frequency of medical monitoring that is advisable will depend on the situation. When the dust monitoring and worker compliance are good then a chest radiograph, spirometry and a simple examination of the chest could be done perhaps every 5 years for the first 20 years and perhaps every 3 years from then on. In setting up monitoring of an established workforce which has experienced poorly controlled dust conditions in the past it may be advisable to examine them more frequently, perhaps even annually. Workers with a significant cumulative exposure, even if they have a normal chest radiograph and lung function at the time, should be offered continued follow-up after they leave or retire.

The development of radiographic changes suggestive of silicosis, especially if accompanied by an unexpected drop in ventilatory capacity, should lead to the worker being removed from dusty work and to a re-examination of the working conditions. The worker should be advised against further exposure to quartz in any employment, and acquainted with the procedure for claiming appropriate statutory benefit where such a scheme exists (see Chapter 4). The same applies to workers whose disease becomes manifest after they have ceased exposure or left employment. Consideration should also be given to some form of prophylaxis against tuberculosis.

Mixed dust containing quartz

SLATEWORKER'S PNEUMOCONIOSIS

The industry

The slate quarries and mines in North Wales supplied most of the slate for the roofing of factories and houses in Britain during the nineteenth century, and slate for export in large quantity. Because explosives and machines tended to shatter the slate and make it unsuitable for roofing or cladding, most of the work had to be done by hand. At its peak at the end of the nineteenth century the industry employed about 100 000 people in many small businesses. Since then the industry has dwindled because it could not compete with synthetic roofing and cladding material made close to the point of use.

Exposure

Slate is formed by the sedimentation of a mixture of finely divided mineral particles in layers onto a flat surface. The mixture varies from layer to layer and site to site. The North Wales slate contains mica, feldspar and anything from 15 to 35% crystalline quartz (other deposits may contain over 60%). A little puff of respirable dust is released every time the rock is split along the plane of cleavage (Fig. 35.8).

The pneumoconiosis was recognized over 100 years ago when 'silicosis' was diagnosed and attributed to the use of mechanical saws to cut slabs dry and the dry engraving of tombstones, etc. That work was often done in sheds and was very dusty. Because the problem was believed to have been solved by the introduction of wet working (Fig. 35.9), regulations that were introduced elsewhere did not require the monitoring of dust levels in this industry.

The disease

Up to the 1950s the high rate of chest disease in the slate-working areas of North Wales was attributed to tuberculosis. But a subsequent study[27] that included men who had left the industry found evidence of radiographic change and loss of lung function related to time spent in slate work. The jobs with most exposure were 'getting' of slate underground (as opposed to open quarrying) and 'dressing' of roof slates indoors.

The radiographic changes in slate pneumoconiosis are somewhat different from silicosis seen in other industries. The findings in North Wales were as follows.

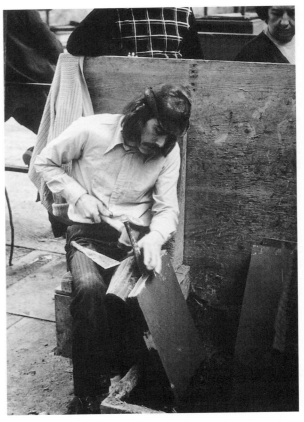

Figure 35.8 *Splitting slate by hand. A puff of dust is released as the sheets separate, creating a risk when done in a poorly ventilated shed but not at the open quarry face.*

Against a clear background or a low profusion of smaller rounded opacities (q or p), r shadows appeared in the upper zones in the older men. These sometimes

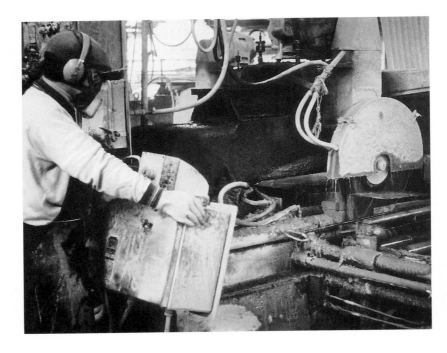

Figure 35.9 *Sawing slabs of slate for tombstones. When this process was converted to wet working about 100 years ago the problem of silicosis in slate workers was thought to have been solved.*

remained static and calcified and sometimes coalesced to form irregular massive shadows. The massive shadows were difficult to distinguish during life from cavitating tuberculosis because the associated emphysema looked like cavitation. There was sometimes patchy pleural thickening overlying the irregular coalescent masses in the upper zone or evidence of more extensive pleurisy. But the most unusual feature was the amount of bilateral hilar gland enlargement with eggshell calcification which was found even in some men with no radiological evidence of parenchymal disease. The lung dust burden at autopsy is high, perhaps 100 g per lung, and the proportion of quartz higher than in the inspired dust. The radiographic changes and pathology were those of a mixed dust pneumoconiosis with only part of the abnormality in the lung and the hilar nodes in the form of silicotic nodules.

The risk of tuberculosis in men with radiological slate pneumoconiosis seems to have been at least as high as that reported by Westerholm in silicotics in Sweden.[14] Many of the cases were treated with conventional courses of chemotherapy. Most of the deaths in recent years have been in men well past the retiring age and it is difficult to estimate the loss of life expectancy as this was a surviving population. Those with confirmed tuberculosis were not dying any younger than those without.

Prevention

Established methods of dust sampling with estimations of the quartz content of the respirable dust will confirm which jobs still present a hazard. Wet working, wherever possible, simple dust extraction and ventilation should be sufficient to render these safe.

Although the conditions in the North Wales slate industry do not present a serious health risk at present, slate dust is potentially dangerous. Silicosis has been reported[28] in small-scale slate pencil manufacture in India, where the workers, often teenagers, sawed pencils from blocks of slate containing up to 60% quartz. Gross disease and early deaths resulted.

KAOLIN PNEUMOCONIOSIS

The industry

Kaolin (china clay) is formed by the action of water on granite. In Cornwall in the UK the deposits of clay are still in the cone-shaped holes in the granite where they formed. They are associated with silica sand, mica, fluorspar and undegraded granite (china stone). In other parts of the world, such as in the southern USA, the clay was washed out of the granite and sedimented into layers of pure clay millions of years ago. Such pure deposits are sufficiently free of parent minerals that clay can be dug out, dried and sold without purification. But in the main Cornish industry the clay is extracted with high pressure hoses and the contaminating mica and silica sand removed by sedimentation before drying and mar-

keting as a fine powder. The level of contamination of the product by quartz and mica depends both upon the nature of the original deposit and the method of extraction. The exposure in one country may be quite different from that in others. Whereas, by the time it is handled dry, Cornish kaolin seldom contains as much as 1% of quartz (with up to 7% fluorspar and 6% mica), some of the 'ball clays' which are dried directly may contain up to 20% quartz.

The kaolin itself (kaolinite) is a multilayered particle made up of alternating plates of aluminium hydroxide and silicon oxide and is a powerful adsorbent. Nowadays more is used as a filler for paper than for making crockery. It is also used as a thickener for paints, as an ingredient of special plasters and as a medication for treating diarrhoea. In Cornwall a by-product of the industry was 'china stone'. Lumps of quartz-containing stone in the kaolin deposit were either shipped unground to the potteries for milling or were milled locally and added to the kaolin before it was sent to the potteries.

In the pottery industry any hazard from kaolin was swamped by the effect of silica. In Cornwall most of the workers lived well beyond the retiring age so that the occasional case of serious chest disease was attributed to tuberculosis, to silicosis from working in the tin mines or from milling 'china stone'. Early animal studies compared the effect of inhaled kaolin with inhaled quartz. The kaolin effect was described as minor with a reticulin reaction but no true fibrosis. As a result kaolin was classified as a nuisance dust.

The disease

An early survey by Sheers[29] described changes on the radiograph in men working with kaolin who had not had any obvious exposure to quartz. Kaolin workers develop an exposure-related simple pneumoconiosis similar to that seen in British coal miners. Even though the dust appears to have contained considerably less than 1% quartz, the simple rounded opacity change appeared earlier than for coalworkers. Men who had worked a lifetime in the dustiest jobs could reach category 2/2 change by retiring age. Although some coalescence is seen, calcification and hilar gland changes are rare. Progressive massive fibrosis is not now seen in working and recently retired men but has been found in men seeking compensation after leaving the industry in the past. The massive shadows tend to be smooth outlined, resembling those seen in coalworkers rather than those seen in silicotics.

Further detailed surveys of ventilatory capacity, respiratory symptoms, radiographic changes and exposure to kaolin have confirmed radiographic changes and a small loss of lung function related to exposure.[30,31] They have confirmed that the effects seen were mainly due to earlier, higher dust exposures and that men employed after 1971 in the Cornish china clay industry are unlikely to develop radiographic changes or lung function loss after a full working life in the industry.

Pathology

The pathology associated with kaolin exposure and the nature of the dust retained in the lung has been reported from a post-mortem study of 62 workers, some of whom had ground china stone.[32] The proportion of quartz in the lung dust was 1% or less in the pure china clay group and up to 45% in the mixed exposure group. Three types of pathological change were noted: nodular fibrosis similar to that seen in silicosis, related to high amounts of quartz in the lung dust; diffuse or interstitial fibrosis similar to that resulting from mica exposure; and massive lesions similar to those seen in coal workers and not showing the histological characteristics of either silicosis or rheumatoid pneumoconiosis.

Prevention

The adherence to the exposure limit for nuisance dust greatly reduced the risk of kaolin pneumoconiosis in the china clay industry.[30,31] More recently, in view of the evidence for an exposure-response effect on lung function and radiographs that made it possible to define a no-effect exposure level, a somewhat lower, specific exposure standard has been set for kaolin. The industry has continued to modify its processes to reduce exposures.

TALC

Talc is a form of magnesium silicate that has crystallized into thin plates which readily split and slide over each other. Powdered talc is used as a lubricant and parting medium in industrial processes varying from the moulding of tyres to the making of chocolate coated toffee bars. It is also used as a filler in heat-resistant ceramics, refractories and insulators. It is best known as the fine white powder used for powdering babies (and others) after bathing.

The disease

The quarrying and mining of talc and its subsequent milling to a powder have been known to be risk occupations for nearly a hundred years. The disease was described as disabling and affecting a high proportion of the workers with heavy dust exposure. Talc deposits are often contaminated with other minerals and at first it was assumed that the disease was really silicosis due to quartz in the ore, but radiographs showed a fine nodular pneumoconiosis with either rounded (p and q) or irregular opacities (s and t), unlike those usually seen in silicosis. The histology also showed a more diffuse granulomatous lesion with more interstitial fibrosis and few if any of the typical silicotic nodules.

Talc was the traditional coating for surgeon's gloves to prevent them sticking together during autoclaving. Unless carefully washed off at the beginning of an operation some was left in the wound. Granulomas filled with talc were recognized as the cause of intra-abdominal adhesions and similar late complications of opera-tion. In the 1950s talc was replaced by starch powder for surgical gloves.

In 1949 McLaughlin[33] described fibrous particles and coated fibres resembling asbestos bodies in a case of talc pneumoconiosis arising in the motor tyre industry. In the early 1960s when the full extent of the risks of asbestos was being explored, the situation with regard to talc was reviewed because some ore deposits were known to contain fibrous forms of calcium and magnesium silicates (tremolite, actinolite and anthophyllite) which were really forms of asbestos. Regulations were introduced in Britain to restrict the importation of talc for cosmetic use to material completely free of fibres. No such controls, however, were applied to talc for industrial purposes.

Epidemiological work in the USA clarified the situation. Talc from Montana, Texas and North Carolina is almost free from fibres and contains very little quartz. Heavily exposed workers showed a simple rounded opacity pneumoconiosis without significant loss of lung function although some develop disabling pleural changes. There was no increase in cancer.[34] Talc is also produced in New England where the deposits vary in their tremolite content. There was a variable incidence of disabling interstitial fibrosis leading to right heart failure in some workers and a simple non-disabling pneumoconiosis in others.[35] The evidence suggests that the severe disease is associated with fibre (tremolite, actinolite or anthophyllite) contamination and that this is also associated with an increase in both lung cancer and mesothelioma (see Chapter 39).

Prevention

Tremolite falls into the group of asbestos minerals for which the safe limits of exposure are too low to define. Therefore talc deposits containing respirable tremolite fibres should not be worked and talc from such deposits should not be used in industry. On the other hand, there appear to be adequate deposits of fibre-free talc and there is no reason why talc from these sources should not continue to be used for industrial and cosmetic purposes.

THE MICAS AND VERMICULITE

This family of silicates shares the same crystal structure (monoclinic with basal cleavage) which forms flat sheets like talc but often on a much larger scale. They are aluminium and potassium silicates with varying amounts of magnesium, iron, lithium and sodium, and have a number of geological names such as muscovite, biotite, phlogopite, etc.

The large transparent sheet material (mostly mined in India) was used as window glass in stoves, furnaces, etc. because of its heat resistance. Other sheet material was used as an insulator in the electrical industry and the waste material was ground and used instead of talc. Synthetic materials have replaced mica for most purposes except perhaps as a filler in iridescent paints and except in those countries where mica is produced, such as India and South America.

A benign simple pneumoconiosis has been reported in men mining and milling mica as well as the occasional more serious case. Because animal experiments have shown that mica dust produces no significant disease it seems likely that the disease in humans is due to contaminating minerals.

Vermiculite

Vermiculite is a poorly compacted form of mica which exfoliates to occupy more than ten times its original volume when heated. It is then used as an insulator for roof spaces, domestic stoves, etc. and in lightweight materials which combine fire resistance with insulation. Like the other micas, pure vermiculite does not appear to be a significant risk.

A cluster of mesotheliomas has been found round a commercial deposit of vermiculite in Montana, USA. Although the present product does not contain easily detectable quantities of tremolite, investigation has shown that sufficient tremolite fibre was released in the past to have caused primary lung cancers and mesotheliomas.[36] Not all vermiculite deposits are contaminated with fibrous tremolite.

This hazard can be eliminated by avoidance of those vermiculite deposits contaminated with fibrous tremolite in civil engineering operations as well as for commercial exploitation.

DIATOMITE (KIESELGAHR)

This is a soft rock or clay resulting from the dust deposition of dead plankton (diatoms) on the floors of lakes and shallow seas. It is of geologically recent origin so that the skeletons of the diatoms are still easily seen under the microscope. The main constituent is amorphous silica with some calcium, magnesium and aluminium silicates. Depending on how dry the deposit is, the extraction may or may not be dusty. Heat processing is carried out in two stages:

- Stage 1: Drying and burning off the residual organic content.
- Stage 2: Treatment at about 1200°C (calcining) which converts the amorphous silica to cristobalite (see p. 672).

Diatomite is milled and marketed as a fine powder either after stage 1 or 2. The stage 1 material is used in face powder, as an improver for heavy soils, as a filter aid and to clarify soft drinks. The stage 2 material can be used (dry) for polishing or in special plasters and cements and ceramics.

Serious progressive pneumoconiosis leading to respiratory failure and with a high risk of tuberculosis has occurred with exposure to diatomite.[37] Histology showed silicotic nodules in some cases but a more diffuse cellular reaction (similar to that found with talc) in others. Epidemiological investigations indicate that the serious risk comes from the calcined product. There may be a risk after stage 1 if this process is carried out at too high a temperature (above 600°C). Raw material and that dried at low temperature may cause a simple pneumoconiosis without loss of lung function or risk of tuberculosis.

Prevention

It is probable that serious disease would not occur if current nuisance dust and silica content standards were applied to the extraction of diatomite and the stage 1 type of drying and milling. But the high temperature calcining produces a product which contains too much cristobalite to be handled safely under commercial conditions. This form of processing should not be undertaken.

OTHER NON-FIBROUS CLAYS

The bentonites, montmorillonite, fuller's earth, etc.

This ill-defined group comprises mixtures of poorly crystallized and amorphous silicates of sodium, potassium, aluminium and magnesium. Some deposits were formed when fresh water with a high silica content ran into the sea and the silicates precipitated out. They are often contaminated by silts containing silica sand, etc.

They are used in many building materials and as drilling muds in oil exploration, etc. They also have adsorbent qualities which lead to their traditional use in cleaning raw wool (fulling). They are used in treating patients who have swallowed poisons or have diarrhoea, as a vehicle for pesticides, to prevent workers slipping on oil spills and as cat litter. They are nearly always marketed in a dry dusty state after kiln drying with or without calcining.

Because production and use are usually on a small scale, epidemiological data are scarce. Some operations seem to cause a simple pneumoconiosis, but more aggressive disease has been reported.[38] It is not clear whether the disease reported is due to the clay itself, to the contaminating crystalline materials or to the products of calcining. These cannot be regarded just as 'nuisance dusts'. Workers should be monitored and exposure controlled.

Gypsum, plaster of Paris

Gypsum is a hydrated calcium sulphate in microcrystalline form that is used in the building industry, especially in plaster board. Careful heating will drive off part of the water to produce 'plaster of Paris' which sets when mixed with sufficient water to return it to the fully hydrated state. Gypsum is found in many places and varies from rock (alabaster and selenite) to soft clay. Some deposits are contaminated with quartz and others contain elongated crystals likely to damage the lung. Such long crystals also form when gypsum is processed to make plaster board. Gypsum is mined, dried and sometimes 'calcined' before being milled and marketed in powder form. The mines may be open-cast or deep, the level of dust exposure and the quartz contamination vary considerably.

Gypsum is classified as a nuisance dust because workers survive many years of exposure without serious respiratory difficulty and animal studies using pure gypsum have failed to produce lung fibrosis. However, study of two English deposits has shown that a pneumoconiosis can occur.[39] A simple pneumoconiosis up to category 2/1 was seen with only minor loss of lung function; disability occurred in the most heavily exposed. Disease was more frequent in Sussex than in Nottinghamshire with similar exposure; but in Nottinghamshire there were pleural changes. The quartz content of the dust was higher in Sussex.

Coalworker's pneumoconiosis

HISTORY

The British coal mines (which employed at one time nearly a million men) first came under close investigation by the medical profession in the first part of the nineteenth century. Research has continued ever since, intensifying world wide in the last 50 years, but even in the last decade the precise nature of the disease and the components of dust responsible have been a matter of debate both in Britain and internationally.

Medical and social agitation about the air in the coal mines, the very long hours worked and the employment of women and children, led to improvements which included ventilation. This was effective and, by the end of the century, Scottish experts claimed that severe disabling disease had disappeared. Some men subsequently shown to have heavily pigmented lungs with small soft and even firm dust foci were not seriously disabled. Experts suggested that coal dust protected against tuberculosis. Coal mining came to be regarded as a *healthy* occupation especially when compared with metal mining and stone masonry. However, Collis[40] reported that respiratory symptoms ('bronchitis') were more common amongst the miners of South Wales and Lancashire. He linked this with the narrow seams, frequent faulting and therefore a greater amount of rock work in these fields.

Severe respiratory disease ('silicosis'), reported first from Somerset and then South Wales in the 1920s, was attributed to extra rock work in gaining access to new seams, deeper mines with more ventilation problems and the introduction of machines which raised the concentration of respirable dust. Undoubtedly the pressure to produce coal at all costs during the 1914–18 war had contributed to the increased health hazard, just as the 1939–45 war was to cause another increase.

By the 1950s[41] it was apparent that the amount and severity of the pneumoconiosis was mainly related to the total cumulative respirable dust exposure and that individual susceptibility and the exposure to quartz were important only in certain situations. It also seemed probable that disabling disease could be dramatically reduced if men showing the early changes of simple pneumoconiosis were removed from dusty work. The industry in the UK (by that time nationalized) set in motion measures that did indeed go a long way towards controlling the problem of coalworker's pneumoconiosis. These measures were:

1 Improved ventilation with standardized dust monitoring bringing the dust levels down progressively until in the UK they are now slightly below the current standard for nuisance dusts in industry with similar rules dealing with quartz levels above 1%. A great deal has been achieved by the improved design of cutting and other machines, reducing the impact speed and incorporating dust suppression with water.
2 Medical monitoring of all employees (surface as well as underground) so that those with early signs of chest disease can be moved to non-dusty work. Most reliance has been placed on good quality full-size chest radiographs read to the successively improved ILO classification (see p. 667). Action in the individual case is taken when the radiograph change reaches 2/2 or a large opacity appears.
3 Perhaps most important, a research scheme was set up in the UK to determine whether the measures were effective. It led to a tightening of the controls on dust by demonstrating continuing development of disease with previous levels of dust control. It also provided a large volume of data which have subsequently been analysed, mainly by the Institute of Occupational Medicine in Edinburgh, and led to important advances in understanding of the effects on the lung of exposure to underground coal mine dust.

SOURCES OF DUST

Workers in the coal-mining industry are exposed to a variety of mineral dusts besides coal.

Opening up a coal mine
To open up a coal mine, shafts and roadways must be driven though other strata which may contain hard rock with 75% or more of quartz. The silicosis which used to result from this in Britain was confined to the special gangs who did this work under contract. In other countries this work is done by men drawn from the coal face and returning to that work so that the risk of silicosis for face workers is greater than in the UK. During the lifetime of a mine similar rock work has to be done to reach new seams, to cross fault lines and to extend ventilation shafts and roadways. Even in the UK the practice varies as to whether this is done by men normally employed at the coal face or specialists in rock work.

Rock immediately above and below the coal seam

When the seams are 2 metres or more thick this rock is left undisturbed. One of the reasons that most mines in Britain are now not economic is because the seams are much thinner and frequently faulted so the rock must be cut above and below to allow the men and machines access to the coal (hard heading). All underground workers are exposed to this rock dust to some extent.

Rock within the coal seams

Coal was formed when forests were crushed under the weight of sedimentary rock. It therefore includes stones from the forest floor and from above. This is a source of rock dust exposure to surface and transport workers as well as those down the mine.

Dust can be produced at every stage from the coal face to the fuelling of the power station or domestic fire. The amount of dust depends on how the work is done, the engineering design of the machines and conveyors and the use of water and ventilation to deal with high risk areas.

The proportions of quartz and other mineral dusts vary from mine to mine and from job to job within a coal field and even more between different coal fields. The big differences are between countries where the work practices and the regulations controlling exposure are different. It is not surprising that doctors studying the disease in one area can disagree profoundly over the characteristics of the disease with their colleagues in other areas or countries.

Open cast coal mining

The exposure to dust in open cast mining is much lower than in underground mining. However, there is evidence that some workers in open cast coal mines develop radiological changes of pneumoconiosis, perhaps contributed to by the quartz content of the dust.[42]

SIMPLE COALWORKER'S PNEUMOCONIOSIS

This condition develops after relatively high cumulative exposures to underground coal mine dust, usually over a period of more than 20 years (see below). It has been a source of continuing controversy in the UK and internationally, with some people arguing that it is not associated with any respiratory disability unless the relatively rare complicated form of the disease is present. Others have presented convincing evidence of a loss of lung function related to cumulative dust exposure in coalworkers and ex-coalworkers without complicated pneumoconiosis,[43,44] which can be severely disabling in some men,[45] as a result of the associated chronic airflow limitation (mainly emphysema). During the last two decades, much evidence has accumulated in favour of the proposition that coal dust exposure can produce serious respiratory disability in the absence of complicated coalworker's pneumoconiosis, and this is now generally accepted. A recent review covers this in detail[46] and a summary of the main points is included below.

The features of simple coalworker's pneumoconiosis result from accumulation of dust in the lung parenchyma and the tissue reaction to that dust. Typically, the chest radiograph shows small, rounded opacities scattered through the lung fields. In the early stages there is little or no impairment of lung function. Pathologically, there are simple coal macules: collections of dust laden macrophages around the terminal bronchioles in the centre of the acinus, with a little surrounding centrilobular emphysema ('focal' emphysema).

If men are removed from dust exposure at this stage, very few will progress to complicated pneumoconiosis and most will not suffer respiratory impairment. However, even without further dust exposure, some men have a progression of disease. The opacities on the chest radiograph tend to become more irregular in shape,[47] an obstructive pattern of lung function loss occurs and the lungs pathologically show increasing emphysema and fibrosis around the centrilobular collections of dust-laden cells. The picture is often complicated by the effects of cigarette smoking but severe pathological emphysema can occur even in non-smoking coalworkers (or, more usually, retired coalworkers) with heavy dust exposure.[48] There is good evidence of an excess of pathological emphysema, including severe degrees, in coalworkers compared with non-coalworkers, taking smoking into account.[49] A study from the Institute of Occupational Medicine in Edinburgh was able to demonstrate a dose–response relationship between pathological emphysema and dust exposure in coalworkers.[50]

Research on the relationship between radiographic appearances, pathology and lung function in coalworkers has shown that small irregular opacities are better associated with emphysema and loss of lung function than small rounded opacities.[51] Findings based on data from the Pneumoconiosis Field Research scheme set up by British Coal have confirmed a relationship between small irregular opacities, as well as small rounded opacities, and cumulative dust exposure.[52]

The main cause of lung function loss and disability in men with simple coalworker's pneumoconiosis is emphysema, possibly with some associated fibrosis. Until relatively recently, the prevalent belief was that the emphysema was due to other factors, mainly cigarette smoking, and not related to the simple pneumoconiosis process. However, since 1993 emphysema and chronic bronchitis are prescribed diseases in coalworkers in the UK (see below and Chapter 31). Some argue that the emphysema is nevertheless a distinct process and not part of simple coalworker's pneumoconiosis. However, as both are due to the accumulation of dust in the lungs and the reaction to it, this is perhaps an unnecessary distinction.

Disability benefit and common law claims

Prior to 1993, Industrial Disability Benefit in the UK was payable to coalworkers with simple pneumoconiosis only if their chest radiograph showed at least category 2/2 profusion of small rounded opacities. The level of benefit was low since it was argued that the simple pneumoconiosis itself did not lead to disability. Sometimes a small amount of additional benefit was granted for concomitant emphysema and chronic bronchitis, but only if the radiograph showed the qualifying changes (category 2/2 rounded opacities). Severely disabled men were generally considered to be suffering the effects of cigarette smoking and men who claimed to smoke little or not at all were usually not believed.

Further evidence accumulated, and data were published allowing estimation of the effects of coal dust on loss of lung function in smokers and non-smokers separately.[53] Following a report of the Industrial Injuries Advisory Council (IIAC) in 1992, the benefit arrangements for coalworkers in the UK were revised to reflect the recognition of emphysema and chronic bronchitis as prescribed diseases in coalworkers. Chronic obstructive pulmonary disease is also compensated as an occupational disease in Germany. In the UK, coalworkers had to meet certain qualifying criteria: 20 years underground exposure, a loss of lung function (FEV_1) of at least one litre below the predicted value, and evidence of dust retention (category 1/1 changes on the chest radiograph). The UK arrangements were changed in 1996, after a review by the IIAC recommended removing the requirement for evidence of dust retention on the chest radiograph. The qualifying criteria of length of underground work and loss of ventilatory capacity remain. The new system has been criticized on the grounds that the radiograph is a better index of actual exposure and dust retention in the lungs than the length of time underground.[54]

Coalworkers with serious respiratory disability can claim compensation from their employer in court, alleging negligence. This has been uncommon in the UK and there was little chance of success while the official view was that coal dust exposure without complicated pneumoconiosis does not cause respiratory disability. With the prescription of chronic bronchitis and emphysema in coalworkers in the UK the situation has changed and in a recent case a number of coalworkers were awarded significant compensation payments.[55]

COMPLICATED COALWORKER'S PNEUMOCONIOSIS

This describes cases in which simple pneumoconiosis is complicated by additional (related) pathology. As a group, coalworkers do not have an increased risk of tuberculosis or lung cancer. However, coalworkers with high exposure to hard rock dust and the changes of silicosis are at increased risk of tuberculosis, and possibly also lung cancer. The pneumoconiosis 'complication' usually takes the form of large masses of solid tissue within the parenchyma, and is disabling. There are three main causes: coal mine dust itself, quartz encountered in coal mines, and dust plus rheumatoid disease.

Progressive massive fibrosis

The most frequent type of mass occurring in the lungs of coalworkers in Britain both in the early nineteenth century and again in the middle of this century is circumscribed, smooth in outline and a uniform black or dark grey. It is usually in the upper or middle zone, oval in shape, with the long axis parallel to the pleura and the outer surface initially 2 or 3 cm from the pleura. It is convex, the inner surface can be flattened or slightly concave and is clearly separate from the hilum. (Fig. 35.10). Size ranges from around 3 cm to over 10 cm long. The masses may appear singly or one in each lung and others may appear some years later. They may be missed (except in retrospect) for several years because each first shows as a faint but clearly defined area of increased density which becomes denser and slightly smaller as the years go by. Due to emphysematous change in the lung between the mass and the pleura they appear to move towards the hilum over time. They are not detectable on physical examination but are associated with a definite loss of lung function. The lung function loss is mainly obstructive, partly because the lesions distort and produce scar emphysema in the surrounding lung and partly because they usually occur on a background of heavy simple pneumoconiosis with associated emphysema.[56] Some loss of lung volumes can occur due to the space occupied by large progressive massive fibrosis masses.

After many years these masses may cavitate and yield, once or repeatedly, large quantities of material like black ink (melanoptysis) which is necrotic tissue and dust. Death may occur from aspiration of the black material or from associated haemoptysis, but this is uncommon. The cavity may shrink and cause no further trouble or become infected with fungi (to form a mycetoma) or with opportunistic mycobacteria. Both can be life shortening in spite of treatment and are indications for surgery if lung function permits. Infection with *Mycobacterium tuberculosis* is not a feature of straightforward progressive massive fibrosis and the lesions are not prone to malignant change.

Pathologically, before they cavitate the lesions are firm and rubbery with no definite capsule. On microscopic examination there is a lot of amorphous ground substance mixed with the dust and the ghosts of macrophages, but no collagen. At the periphery there are living macrophages and other mononuclear cells set in a reticulin network. The blood vessels within the mass show a low-grade inflammatory change leading to obliteration. The siting and shape of the mass suggest that the vascular occlusions are secondary. Immunoreactive cells and immune complexes are present in the lesions, espe-

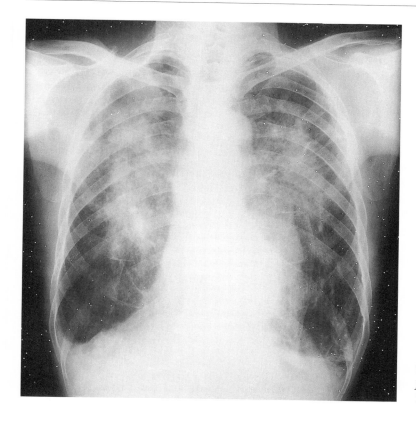

Figure 35.10 *Bilateral progressive massive fibrosis on the chest radiograph of a coalworker. There is emphysema in the lower lobes.*

cially around the periphery. It has been suggested that progressive massive fibrosis results at least in part from an immune reaction to dust in the hilar lymph nodes, with passage of activated material back into the lung parenchyma by invasion of bronchi or branches of the pulmonary artery.[57]

The incidence of progressive massive fibrosis has varied considerably between the British coalfields and also with time. There was a surge between 1930 and 1960, particularly in South Wales. Within a particular area the frequency is related to cumulative dust exposure, the amount of simple pneumoconiosis and the amount of quartz in the dust.[58,59] The frequency of progressive massive fibrosis in South Wales has been far higher than might be expected from dust exposure or the relative quartz concentrations. Retrospective dust and quartz exposure estimations have, however, been shown to be very inaccurate when applied to individual miners. Cases classified as progressive massive fibrosis may have included silicosis and rheumatoid pneumoconiosis, both of which may be difficult to differentiate from coalworker's progressive massive fibrosis without expert histology. It remains uncertain why progressive massive fibrosis was so common in the South Wales pits particularly.

Moving miners out of dusty work when they reach category 2/2 and the general reduction of the dust levels in the mines has produced a dramatic fall in the incidence of progressive massive fibrosis in the UK.

However, there is no real threshold and it can occasionally occur at low profusions of simple pneumoconiosis. A few men may develop it long after they have stopped being exposed to dust.[60] The risk rises steeply when radiographic changes of above category 2/2 are present, reflecting high cumulative dust exposure, especially if dust exposure continues.

Silicosis in coalworkers

The lesions of subacute or chronic silicosis have been seen in coal miners and men working in and around the pits. They can usually be traced to special exposure to quartz in work on shafts, drivages (passages and roadways), etc. and to coal face dust with an exceptional quartz content due to hard heading or to working rock contaminated coal. Coalworkers with these exposures may show larger, rounded (r) opacities in the lung fields, subsequently leading to confluent irregular massive shadows in the upper zones with pleural thickening, hilar enlargement, calcification of the parenchymal shadows and eggshell calcification of the hilar nodes. It is more common to see the features of coalworker's pneumoconiosis, with or without the more usual type of massive lesion, mixed with some of these features of silicosis or a few typical silicotic nodules may be found in the lung or hilar nodes at autopsy.

Rheumatoid pneumoconiosis

At the peak of the surge in progressive massive fibrosis cases in the mid-twentieth century, Caplan, working in

South Wales, noticed atypical shadows on the radiograph of coalworkers who also had rheumatoid arthritis.[61] The shadows could appear at any level of dust exposure, being relatively common in young miners with little or no simple coalworker's pneumoconiosis and with short exposure.

The lesions were round, 1–4 cm in diameter, and usually about 2 cm in from the pleura. There was no definite change in the surrounding lung so that they looked like secondary cancer deposits. They often remained the same size for months or years and then enlarged by perhaps 0.5 cm, sometimes at the same time as new lesions appeared. The clinical arthritis often developed later than the lung lesions and was relatively mild but the men were seropositive for rheumatoid factor. After perhaps 5 or 10 years the lesions sometimes cavitated (a brief flu-like illness followed by the coughing up of inky sputum often with haemoptysis which could be severe). The cavities that formed often closed and the lesions recavitated at intervals.

As they enlarged, lesions lying close together often used to form large lumpy masses which were difficult to distinguish from progressive massive fibrosis or confluent silicosis. The distinction could only be made histologically. It is not known whether the treatments given for rheumatoid arthritis affected the course of the lung lesions. The prognosis in the absence of further dust exposure depended on when the rheumatoid disease became inactive, but the risk of cavitation remained.

The histology of the early lung lesions showed the same regular arrangement of subacute inflammatory cells as rheumatoid nodules in other tissues. Older lesions showed central necrosis with new concentric layers of inflammatory reaction surrounding it. This layered pattern is so characteristic that rheumatoid lesions causing massive shadows or adding to the lesions produced by coal dust or quartz could be identified easily. Rheumatoid pneumoconiosis was not necessarily associated with the other lung lesions of rheumatoid arthritis.

Between one and two hundred cases of this syndrome were identified in South Wales. In the rest of Britain and indeed the rest of the world only isolated cases have been reported. It seems to have been a characteristic of South Wales and the physicians from that area have not reported any new cases since the early 1960s.

FIBROUS MINERAL DUSTS

Long, thin respirable particles (fibres), especially if more than ten times as long as they are thick, are very much more dangerous than other particles. A higher proportion of the inhaled dust is caught in the lung and little (if any) is cleared again. These elongated particles are carcinogenic if they remain in the tissue for long enough. By far the most important are the asbestos family. Their industrial use started in the 1870s and there has been increasingly awareness of the frequency and severity of the health hazards since 1930. The sequence of events relating increasing scientific and medical knowledge, public awareness and government regulation has been reviewed by Elmes.[62]

Asbestos minerals

These are compound metallic silicates which have crystallized as very long thin particles. Asbestos is not a specific mineralogical term and includes chrysotile which is structurally different from the rest which are the amphiboles. They all result from the leaching by water of siliceous minerals and recrystallization in the interstices of the parent rock. Therefore their metal content shows some variability within the limits set by the crystal lattices; the nomenclature is not very precise. Only four varieties of asbestos have been used commercially: chrysotile (white), crocidolite (blue), amosite (brown) and anthophyllite. However, a number of other amphiboles occur in a variety of commercially exploited minerals. They are all relatively inert to chemical attack, are poor conductors of heat and stand temperatures up to 300–400 C.

Exposure to asbestos occurs either in mining and milling, where there is exposure to other dusts as well as to the asbestos fibres, or in the end use of the material in various industries (see below). An important source of exposure in developed countries in recent years is in construction and building maintenance work, where workers are exposed to asbestos containing materials put in place years ago. Legislation in developed countries requires a high level of protection for workers in these industries when dealing with asbestos, but in practice the law is not always obeyed. In developing countries the legislative framework is often weak and enforcement even weaker.

CHRYSOTILE (WHITE ASBESTOS)

This is relatively abundant and easy to mine, producing bundles of soft flexible fibres up to several centimetres long. The longer fibres have been, and in some countries still are, used to make textiles and the shorter for reinforcing cement and plastics and for insulation, friction materials and filters. The fibres split up easily to smaller bundles and eventually to individual fibrils. Each fibril consists of double sheets of brucite ($Mg(OH)_2$) and silica (SiO_2) rolled up like a scroll around a small core of amorphous magnesium silicate and forming a curved tube between 25 and 50 nm in diameter. The brucite forms the outer surface; in acid conditions magnesium leaches out and the fibre disintegrates.

Chrysotile has always provided at least 90% of the asbestos in commercial use and is mined in large deposits in central Russia and Quebec in Canada.

Smaller deposits are mined in western Canada and the USA, in the Mediterranean basin, in southern Africa and in Australia. Some deposits, particularly those in the Mediterranean basin and a large one in western China, are associated with fibrous tremolite. This is less obvious in the Quebec deposits and it is not clear to what extent this has contaminated the chrysotile. Tremolite is a calcium magnesium silicate which crystallizes either as a platey talc (see p. 680) or as an amphibole fibre.

CROCIDOLITE (BLUE ASBESTOS)

Blue asbestos is mined in the North West Cape province of the Republic of South Africa and to a lesser extent in the Transvaal. Other deposits, notably one at Wittenoom in Western Australia, have been mined on a small scale. Crocodilolite is found in banded ironstone which also yields commercial iron ore which crocidolite may contaminate. It is the fibrous form of the sodium iron silicate riebeckite. The bundles of fibres are much shorter and stiffer than chrysotile and readily split to straight fibrils with a minimum diameter of about 100 nm. It is much more resistant to acid and has slightly higher heat tolerance but is not easily used for textiles unless supported by chrysotile. It was used where acid resistance was important and is still used in some countries to facilitate manufacture of large-diameter asbestos cement pipes.

AMOSITE (BROWN ASBESTOS)

Amosite is the commercial name for the fibrous grunerite (iron magnesium silicate), an amphibole mined in the Transvaal; similar deposits occur elsewhere but few are commercially viable. As mined, the fibres are coarse but split down to 100 nm in use. It is used in insulation and as a reinforcement for plastic tiles, etc. It is too harsh for some forms of machine processing and is seldom used in cement or textiles for that reason.

ANTHOPHYLLITE

This amphibole is the fibrous form of another iron magnesium silicate. It has been used mixed with clay for making pottery in Finland from prehistoric times and the same deposit was still worked until recently. Its properties are similar to amosite and it has ceased to have any commercial value. Its occurrence is widespread and occasionally causes environmental problems where it contaminates the soil and becomes airborne.

Diseases due to asbestos exposure: history and controversy

Asbestos was once regarded as safe and was handled like cotton or wool. Although cases of lung fibrosis were reported in the early part of this century they went unrecognized amongst the prevalent tuberculosis. As the volume of use and worker exposure increased, the num-ber of reports of lung disease increased. By the time Merewether and Price published their report in 1930[63] everyone was ready to admit that there was a problem. Under the worst conditions fibrosis was shown to develop within 5 years and death could occur within 15 years of first exposure. The risk was thought to be limited to the textile industry and to wherever bags were opened and the fibre blended dry.

Measures were then introduced to reduce the dust in factories in Britain and then other developed countries, but satisfactory methods of measuring fibre levels were not adopted for another 30 years. Lung fibrosis seemed to be reduced by the early regulations, but in the late 1940s another hazard was recognized. Over the previous 15 years individual cases of lung cancer had been reported in asbestos workers; the association was proved when Merewether[64] reported that men certified as suffering from asbestosis had a very high risk of dying with primary lung cancer. At that time it was 17% but by 1960[65] it was over 50%.

Pleural plaques were recognized as being associated with past exposure and causing no disability, but malignant diffuse mesothelioma of the pleura was a rare tumour which many experts would not accept as a clinical entity. In 1960 Wagner and colleagues[66] described a series of mesothelioma cases linked with exposure to crocidolite asbestos in the North West Cape Province of South Africa. The association between asbestos exposure and mesothelioma was confirmed in the asbestos user countries and in Britain and Europe mesothelioma became the marker for unexpected sources of exposure. The level of exposure sufficient to cause the tumour was apparently lower than that required to cause the other asbestos-related diseases.

Asbestos exposure and the diseases related to it have been, and still remain, a hotly debated topic. An important concern raised by organizations representing workers and society is that there was too long a delay between industry knowing of the dangers of asbestos exposure and acting to reduce the risk;[67,68] their case has been criticized by others.[69] Another continuing debate is about whether exposure to chrysotile on its own increases the risk of mesothelioma and lung cancer[70] or whether the risks found in some studies of chrysotile workers are due to the presence of amphiboles, especially tremolite. Is all asbestos dangerous enough to have it banned altogether, or is it safe to work with chrysotile under controlled conditions? A recent update of a cohort study of chrysotile miners and millers in Quebec[71] reported only small increases in the rate of lung cancer, stomach cancer and mesothelioma, mainly in men who had previous heavy exposure. While it is theoretically possible that chrysotile asbestos is not dangerous enough (in comparison with other forms of asbestos) to ban, its use is already banned in some countries and a ban on its use in most countries now seems inevitable. A further issue is whether the low fibre concentrations found in the air of some buildings lined with asbestos-boarding can, with prolonged exposure, increase the risk of mesothelioma. This leads onto the question of whether it is better to remove the asbestos, with all the expense and risk of exposure that entails, or to leave it *in situ*, contained in some way. In practice, a careful risk assessment of each case is required.

Features of asbestos-related diseases

ASBESTOS WARTS

When asbestos fibres get into the skin as a result of abrasion they provoke a low-grade inflammatory reaction with hyperkeratosis which eventually shells out, taking the fibres with it and leaving no scar.

PULMONARY FIBROSIS–ASBESTOSIS

Nowadays asbestos mines are kept wet and the dust exposure is low. In the mills, the ore is dried, crushed and the fibre separated by updraughts of air as the ore passes over vibrating screens. Even modern machinery is difficult to enclose and these mills are still dusty by comparison with manufacturing industry, but the dust is mainly rock dust and the fibre counts may be within current safety limits. The mine mill workers develop a simple rounded opacity pneumoconiosis before they develop the more serious lesions seen in the relatively pure fibre exposure which used to occur in secondary industry. With heavy pure fibre exposure the first change is the appearance of lower zone bilateral irregular opacities and, at about the same time, dry end-inspiratory crackles become audible in the axilla just above the diaphragm. A loss of transfer factor becomes apparent early although for survey purposes the FVC is a more dependable index of early change.

Radiography

The earliest radiographic changes are seen on CT scans (Fig. 35.11). They generally precede changes visible on the straight chest radiograph, the appearance of crepitations, the appearance of clubbing and the appearance of any change in respiratory function. The radiographic change may progress for a year or two, longer in smokers, after exposure ceases. It is not clear whether there is a difference between chrysotile and the amphiboles in this respect as some groups of subjects with exposure to crocidolite continue to show progression long after exposure ceases. If exposure continues the shadows become coarser (s to t or u), more profuse and extend further up the lung. There is a loss of volume and crowding of the airways in the lower zones, giving rise to the 'birch broom' appearance on the lateral view. The picture may be distinctive in young workers with short heavy exposure, but changes produced by ageing (especially in smokers) obscure it, making the diagnosis difficult in older men with long moderate exposure. More advanced changes of asbestosis, as they appear on the CT scan, are shown in Fig. 35.12.

The risk of small opacities and of pleural thickening in asbestos workers is increased if they are smokers.[72]

Pathology

The presence of asbestos bodies in the interstitium and alveoli used to be *the* sign of exposure. These bodies comprise an asbestos fibre coated with an amber layer of a ferritin-like substance containing iron and staining blue with the Prussian blue reagent. However, it turns out that these bodies are almost invariably formed on amphibole fibres over 20 μm long and underestimate the lung burden of the thinner fibres (over 5 μm long) which are thought to be the most toxic. Asbestos bodies fail completely as indicators of the presence of chrysotile. A truer estimate of the fibre load can be obtained by the examination of digests of the lung by optical microscopy but this fails to reveal the thinnest fibres or to distinguish between chrysotile, amphibole and anything else. Electron microscopy of the digests has been necessary to get a true picture of the relationship between mineral fibres and lung pathology, using energy dispersive x-ray analysis to identify the mineral.

In the early stages, fibres accumulate in those alveoli which open directly off the bronchioles. They penetrate the wall and produce a low grade inflammatory response followed by fibrosis. This causes thickening and some narrowing of the terminal airways which is picked up as a reduction of gas transfer and compliance on lung function testing. Fibres migrate away from these centrilobular foci into the interstitium between the alveoli and towards the pleura, causing extension of the low-grade inflammatory response and interstitial fibrosis.

The inflammation and interstitial fibrosis interferes with ventilation by making the lung rigid and leads to shrinkage of the affected area with honeycomb change. The change affects only the periphery of the lung and leaves the central part undamaged, but this normal lung is of little functional value as it is held immobile by the surrounding damage. Lavage of the airways in asbestosis will always yield increased numbers of polymorphs and other inflammatory cells and also asbestos fibres and bodies. Secondary infection of the honeycomb areas can accelerate the destruction of the lower part of the lung.

Clinical features

Asbestosis gives rise to no specific symptoms or signs apart from late inspiratory crepitations. These can also occur with other causes of interstitial fibrosis. The patient will complain of very gradually increasing breathlessness, but unless he is a smoker he will have no cough or sputum until the disease is very far advanced. Before this he may complain of tightness in the chest or inability to breathe in fully. That should not be confused with angina as it never amounts to pain of either pleu-

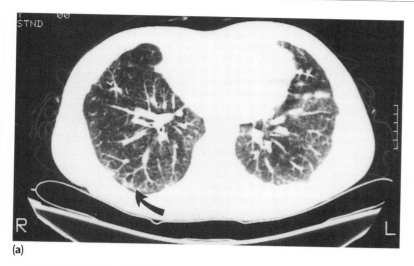

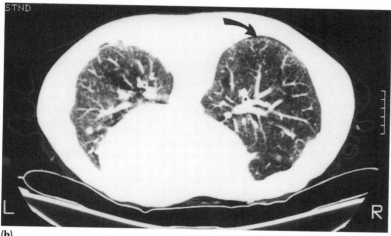

Figure 35.11 *(a) Supine CT shows fine reticular pattern of increased attenuation in the posterior peripheral one-third of the lung (arrow). This abnormality persists when the scan is repeated with the patient prone (b), confirming that it is early interstitial fibrosis (arrow) and not due to hypostatic effect. Courtesy Dr JE Adams.*

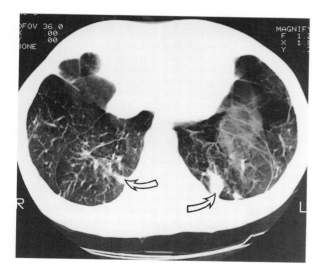

Figure 35.12 *CT of thorax. Advanced interstitial fibrosis. There are coarse and fine areas of increased attenuation in both lung bases with bullae, and 'round' atelectasis (arrows). Courtesy Dr JE Adams.*

ritic or anginal type. Spirometry shows a restrictive ventilatory defect, with a greater loss of FVC than FEV_1 and a high FEV_1/FVC ratio. There is a loss of compliance and a fall in gas transfer. This lung function pattern can be obscured by the concomitant effect of smoking causing a more marked fall in FEV_1 and a lowering of the FEV_1/FVC ratio due to emphysema. Clubbing is not a constant feature of fibrosis due to asbestos and may suggest either cryptogenic fibrosing alveolitis or primary lung cancer.

Asbestosis of sufficient severity to cause respiratory failure has become uncommon in Britain. The major cause of death in individuals with asbestosis is malignancy: primary lung cancer or mesothelioma. Berry[73] analysed cause of death among people certified as having asbestosis in the UK between 1952 and 1976 and found 39% of the deaths were from lung cancer (nine times the expected number of deaths occurred), 9% were from mesothelioma, and 20% were from asbestosis itself. Asbestosis is a prescribed disease in the UK and elsewhere (see Chapter 4).

PLEURAL PLAQUES

These are circumscribed areas of hyaline whorled fibrous tissue which appear on the surface of the parietal pleura, on the fibrous part of the diaphragm or on the pleura in the interlobar fissures. They do not appear on the free surface of the visceral pleura. They are 0.5–1.0 cm thick, have an abrupt margin and a shiny flat or slightly nodular concave surface. They are almost acellular but there are foci of chronic inflammatory cells in the subpleural connective tissue round their margins. They are usually elongated, lie along the axis of the ribs and have irregular edges sometimes likened to a holly leaf. They form first on the immobile part of the parietal pleura and although they may coalesce with plaques above and below in the paravertebral gutter and under the sternum, they do not interfere with the movement of breathing.

Pleural plaques probably take about 10 years to form and are at first difficult to see on the ordinary radiograph but easy to see with the CT scan (Fig. 35.13). They start calcifying after another 10 years, mainly near the edges, and eventually produce the unmistakable picture of bilateral pleural calcification. It is easy to mistake poorly calcified plaques for parenchymal lesions when reading chest radiographs without considering asbestos as the cause for the changes (Figs 35.14 and 35.15). Pleural plaques themselves are not a prescribed disease in the UK.

Plaques do not become malignant themselves. They are particularly common where the population is exposed from birth in an agricultural environment (anthophyllite in Finland and tremolite in eastern Europe, Greece and Turkey). Because they are seen in some chrysotile mining and user populations but not in others, this suggests that they may be due to contaminating tremolite rather than the chrysotile itself. They are associated with mesothelioma in some environments (south-east Turkey) but not in others (Finland and eastern Europe).

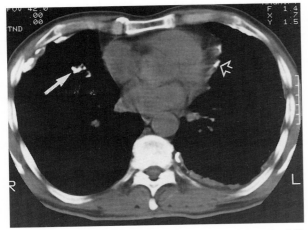

Figure 35.13 *CT scan of thorax. Pleural thickening and calcification in the left posterior paravertebral region and calcification in the pericardial (arrowhead) and right diaphragmatic (arrow) pleura. Courtesy Dr JE Adams.*

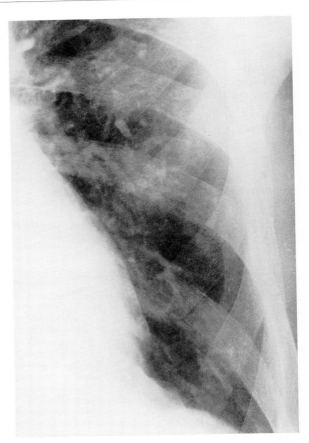

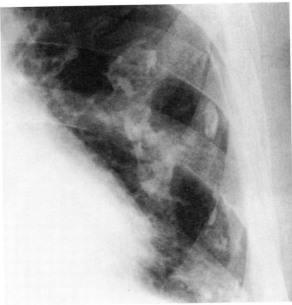

Figure 35.14 and 35.15 *The left lower zone of an asbestos insulation worker showing pleural plaques. The mottled calcification in the first film could easily be mistaken for a parenchymal lesion, but is obviously a plaque in the second.*

BENIGN PLEURAL EFFUSION

Asbestos exposure is related to the occurrence of pleurisy and effusions.[74,75] The effusions are sometimes blood-stained, often recurrent and bilateral, and sometimes without evidence of pulmonary fibrosis. The latent period between first asbestos exposure and pleural effusion is shorter than for other asbestos-related conditions: usually less than 20 years and sometimes less than 10 years. In one study pleural effusion was the most common asbestos-related abnormality within 20 years of first exposure.[75] Many of the effusions are symptomless and transient so their true incidence is probably higher than that reported from prevalence studies. One study reported an incidence of effusions from 0.7 to 9.2 per 1000 person-years with increasing degrees of asbestos exposure.

In florid cases a 'flu-like illness is followed by increasing breathlessness and discomfort in one side of the chest in an otherwise fit person. Laboratory tests show a raised sedimentation rate, a moderate leucocytosis and a serous fluid with polymorphs giving way to lymphocytes. The fluid is sometimes blood-stained, raising the worry of a mesothelioma. Diagnosis is based on a history of exposure (not always immediately obvious) and exclusion of other causes of effusion, particularly tuberculosis. Pleural biopsy specimens, especially those obtained with a needle, are often unhelpful. With or without the help of corticosteroids the fluid will absorb over a period of months, leaving a little pleural thickening which often disappears completely.

Progression of benign pleural effusions to diffuse pleural thickening or mesothelioma can occur.[74–76] Progression to mesothelioma is rare and the tumour may be co-incidental rather than a direct progression of the initial pathology. Pleural effusion is not a prescribed disease in asbestos exposed workers in the UK.

BILATERAL DIFFUSE PLEURAL THICKENING

Obliteration of one or both costophrenic angles with perhaps some thickening of the pleura over the diaphragm is relatively common with heavy asbestos exposure. As the thickening extends up the parietal pleura it may cause restriction of ventilation of the lower part of the lung. It also makes it difficult to see on the radiograph whether there is any parenchymal fibrosis present. Lung function tests are also inefficient in separating out the effects of bilateral pleural thickening and parenchymal fibrosis; both produce a restrictive ventilatory defect and reduction of gas transfer. High resolution CT scans make it possible to assess the pleura and parenchyma separately. A localized area of diffuse pleural thickening in the axilla, usually on both sides but not necessarily equally severe bilaterally, can occur either with or without evidence of asbestosis. These localized areas can have an irregular inner surface and raise the worry of mesothelioma. They cause no disability.

More extensive bilateral diffuse fibrosis immobilizes the lung and causes severe disability. It is a prescribed disease (see Chapter 4). It can occur as part of severe asbestosis or result from bilateral benign pleurisy. It is important to determine whether there is underlying parenchymal disease because in its absence these patients respond well to surgical stripping of the pleura. Surgery should not be attempted if there is asbestosis because the lungs will not re-expand or ventilate any better as a result of the operation.

PRIMARY CANCER OF THE LUNG AND LARYNX

Heavy exposure to a mixture of fibres, as used to occur in insulation work, caused an increase in lung cancer in smokers up to eightfold. Combined with heavy smoking this can shorten life expectation by 15 years.[77] There is evidence of synergy between asbestos exposure and smoking, such that smoking has a multiplicative effect on the lung cancer risk associated with asbestos exposure.[78] The risk from asbestos exposure becomes apparent at a level of exposure which can also cause minimal asbestosis. Fibre analysis suggests that it is the amphiboles which are principally responsible. In cases with lung cancer, the burden of fibres over 5 µm long by transmission electron microscopy is at least 30 million per dry gram.

Experimental studies indicate that it is probably the longer respirable fibres which are most active in causing pulmonary fibrosis and lung cancer. The fibrosis of asbestosis is little different from that seen in many other pneumoconioses that are not associated with a cancer risk. An obvious increase in the scar-related bronchoalveolar celled cancers has not been seen.

There is no way of distinguishing, either on clinical behaviour or pathology, between primary lung cancers induced by cigarette smoking, those due to asbestos and those due to other causes. Where there is evidence of asbestosis and/or bilateral diffuse pleural thickening and a prescribed occupation, lung cancer is a prescribed disease in the UK (see Chapter 4).

Clubbing of the fingers is often the first sign that a worker with established asbestosis is developing a primary cancer of the lung.

The prognosis of lung cancer is somewhat worse in a patient with asbestosis in that he or she may not tolerate surgical or other treatment because of the underlying disease. The ultimate prognosis is the same: very bad. Especially in view of the synergism between asbestos exposure and smoking all asbestos workers, whether they have asbestosis or not, should be persuaded to stop smoking.

Because carcinoma of the larynx is very uncommon in the general population and is related to both smoking and drinking, most small series have failed to show a significant risk in asbestos workers. However, as might be expected, some of the larger studies do show an increased risk.

MESHELIOMA

Because mesothelioma can result from comparatively short exposure to amphibole fibres, and because it has a mean latent interval of over 40 years, it is now and will remain the most important of the asbestos-related diseases. In most developed countries asbestos is the most frequent cause of mesothelioma. It has been estimated[79] that as a result of previous exposure to asbestos, the peak of annual male mesothelioma deaths in Britain will occur in around 2020; in the worst affected age cohorts mesothelioma may account for around 1% of all deaths. Mesothelioma can occur, rarely, without exposure to asbestos and most of these cases have no known cause. Cases not due to mineral fibre exposure can occur at any age, have a worse prognosis and occur with a frequency of about 1 per 2 million of the population per year in Western countries. Smoking does not seem to increase the risk of mesothelioma, with or without asbestos exposure.

Pathology

Pathologists were slow to accept that mesothelioma was a primary tumour and there are still difficulties in establishing the criteria for diagnosis. The opinion of three independent pathologists with special experience is sometimes needed in difficult individual cases.

The tumour arises from the mesothelium of one of the body's serous cavities, usually from the cells lining the parietal wall of the pleura. Where asbestos exposure has been heavy it can arise in the peritoneum or pericardium. Cases not due to mineral fibre exposure have a wider age range and more varied cell pattern but are difficult to distinguish from the fibre-induced ones in the individual case. The diagnosis is difficult because of the variable and complex cellular pattern which may be the result of the unusual derivation of these mesothelial cells.[80] There are two types of malignant cell and it is common to find one cell type in one area and the other in another. First are the cuboidal cells often lining clefts in fibrous tissue or forming tubulopapillary structures easily mistaken for adenocarcinoma. Second are the elongated sarcoma-like cells which merge into areas of collagen fibrosis and myxoma-like tissue. The tumour tends to remain confined to the serous cavity with superficial invasion of the chest or abdominal wall and sometimes invasion of the peripheral nerves. This invasion is characterized by a small cell inflammatory reaction and the laying down of more fibrous tissue so that the tumour may form a cuirass of tissue of almost cartilaginous consistency.

A serous or bloody effusion occurs in about two-thirds of cases, becomes loculated and is eventually replaced by fibrous tissue. The fluid does not contain exfoliated malignant cells throughout, nor is the presence or absence of hyaluronic acid a reliable diagnostic sign. The tumour spreads onto the visceral pleura or peritoneum and breaks through into the underlying tissue late in the course of the disease. It then usually shows the florid tubulopapillary type of growth. Secondaries may be widespread at death although they are seldom of clinical importance and are more cellular than the original pleural tumour. Extension into the mediastinum with involvement of the nodes and constriction of the oesophagus and great vessels may eventually lead to death in the pleural cases. Similar involvement of the gut can be fatal in peritoneal cases. Needle biopsy and even quite large open biopsies can be unreliable because of the patchy cell pattern. Immunochemical staining techniques (in particular those identifying some keratins) may be positive in 80% of cases, whereas the usual markers for squamous and adenocarcinoma are usually negative. Such techniques confirm the diagnosis when the cell pattern by itself is diagnostic, but may not help in difficult cases.

Clinical features

In pleural cases breathlessness is the symptom which usually brings the patient to the doctor. It may be of sudden or gradual onset and indicates the presence of a fairly large pleural effusion.[81] There may also be a feeling of discomfort or heaviness on the one side of the chest with patchy alteration in skin sensation and sweating. Symptoms may have been present for several weeks but the general health is usually well maintained.

On examination there are signs of an effusion and pleural thickening but the mediastinum eventually shifts towards the affected side, with crowding of the ribs but no palpable lymph nodes and only minimal clubbing. Aspiration can be difficult because of the toughness of the parietal tumour and repeated aspiration, needle biopsy and surgery all encourage the tumour to grow through the chest wall (Fig 35.16). The clinical diagnosis is often easy given an appropriate amphibole exposure and latent interval, the clinical picture described, the radiograph appearance of irregular tumour on the parietal wall (well seen after aspiration) and the absence of positive evidence of bronchial cancer. CT scans can be very helpful, even in the presence of fluid (Figs. 35.17 and 35.18).

Aspiration is justified to relieve breathlessness and sometimes provides diagnostic exfoliative cytology. Other forms of treatment including radical or palliative surgery with or without chemotherapy and/or radiotherapy have proved disappointing. Although the mean (untreated) survival from first diagnosis is about a year, many patients live for 5 or more years without treatment. When these long survivors receive various forms of treatment they are reported as treatment successes.

The outlook for the individual patient is always uncertain because death due to pulmonary embolism or infarction is common and the lingering death due to constriction of the lungs, mediastinal structures or the gut is uncommon. Pain, usually in the chest wall, can often be controlled with corticosteroids and anti-inflam-

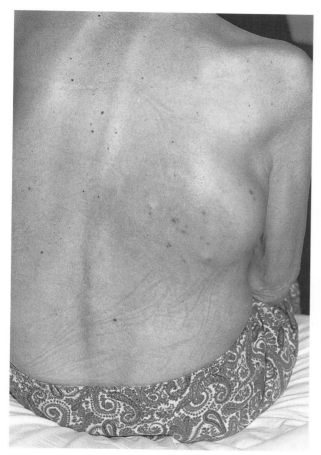

Figure 35.16 *Mesothelioma that has grown through the chest wall along the track of needles used to aspirate the pleural fluid.*

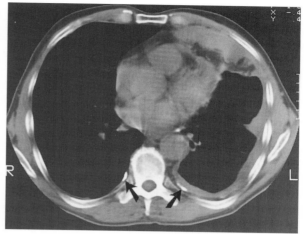

(a)

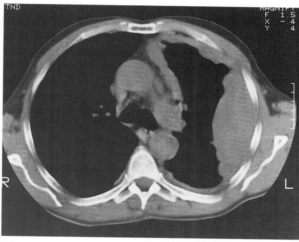

(b)

Figure 35.18 *Left mesothelioma: (a) pleural calcification in both paravertebral regions (arrows) and pleural thickening encasing lung; (b) higher CT section showing large lobulated pleural tumour mass in left thorax, but pleural thickening also encasing lung, with associated loss of volume of left hemithorax. Courtesy Dr JE Adams.*

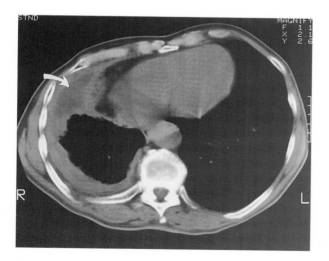

Figure 35.17 *Right mesothelioma. Marked loss of volume of right hemithorax with encasement of the right lung by a pleural mass. There is an associated low attenuation pleural effusion (arrow). There were calcified pleural plaques on other CT sections. Courtesy Dr JE Adams.*

matory drugs and it is wise not to embark on opiates in the early stages.

The distribution of peritoneal cases is uneven. In the 1960s about a quarter of the mesotheliomas reported from the East End of London and from Tyneside presented as peritoneal primaries, but elsewhere very few or none were found. They were usually associated with a history of exceptionally heavy exposure to amphibole (usually crocidolite) and showed more lung fibrosis than is usual for mesothelioma. The onset was insidious with vague abdominal discomfort, a change in bowel habit and some loss of weight. After weeks or months they would seek medical help by which time the abdomen would usually be swollen, with signs of free fluid or ill-defined masses or both. The masses were usually not hard enough to be obvious tumour because they comprised intestine, omentum, etc., stuck together by tumour. The histological diagnosis is difficult if the asbestos exposure is ignored and many cases were certified as peritoneal carcinomatosis with possibly an intestinal or an ovarian primary. It is very difficult to get an accurate estimate of the incidence of peritoneal mesothelioma but it appears to be less frequent as the generation who were exposed to high levels of crocidolite has died.

Compensation and disability benefit

Mesothelioma is a prescribed disease in the UK and elsewhere (see Chapter 4). There is a continuing increase in numbers diagnosed in the UK.[79] More than 90% are due to occupational exposure to amphibole asbestos. Western Europe is probably the same but the proportion appears to be lower in North America where proportionately less crocidolite and amosite has been used. All cases in the UK are assumed to be due to occupation and eligible for industrial injuries benefit under the government scheme, provided that the diagnosis is reasonably certain and there is a history of appropriate exposure. In many the diagnosis is not made until a full autopsy is carried out. All possible mesotheliomas should be reported to the coroner even when the patient or the relatives are unaware of significant exposure. Proof is provided by a lung fibre burden of amphibole. Significant exposure is deemed to have occurred when the electron microscope count is over a million amphibole fibres per dry gram using the digestion technique. Counts of up to 50 million amphibole fibres are commonplace in mesothelioma lungs.

Electron microscope analysis for fibre type is both expensive and not readily available. If ordinary light microscopy shows evidence of some asbestosis together with numerous asbestos bodies, that should be sufficient. Failing this, a high count of uncoated straight fibres by the light microscope digestion technique is accepted as proof. Only when these two tests yield doubtful answers is an electron microscope analysis essential. The studies by Pooley and his colleagues in American and British cases found no evidence that the chrysotile fibre load was any higher in the mesothelioma cases than the controls.[82]

With a mean latent interval of 40 years or more, few occupational cases are likely to occur below the age of 40. In the larger prospective studies (some with an incidence of tumour of over 20%) the earliest cases have been detected at about 25 years from first exposure. Isolated cases have been reported with what appears to be relevant exposure starting only 12 years before the onset of symptoms but exposures within 12 years of the onset of the tumour are unlikely to be the cause. There is the possibility that childhood cases could arise from maternal exposure.

OTHER CANCERS

Epidemiological studies of insulation workers both in the USA and Northern Ireland have shown an excess of cancers of the gastrointestinal tract. As a group these workers were exposed to a high dose of amphibole asbestos and had a marked loss of life expectancy due to lung cancer and mesothelioma. The raised incidence of gastrointestinal cancer did not contribute significantly to the loss of life expectancy but the risk was several times that of the general population. It is difficult to explain this finding against the many large follow-up studies of asbestos workers in other trades, with a lower average level of exposure, who have shown no increase in gastrointestinal cancers.

PATHOGENESIS OF ASBESTOS-RELATED DISEASES

A great many *in vitro* and animal studies have been undertaken, especially since the early 1960s. Results have been confusing and sometimes even misleading.

In vitro studies have failed to show the mechanism of fibre carcinogenesis and have not provided satisfactory tests for determining whether fibres are likely to cause either fibrosis or cancer. They do indicate that fibres shorter than 5 µm are unlikely to be dangerous.

Inhalation studies, carried out mostly on rats, indicate that at very high exposure all respirable fibres over 5 µm long cause lung fibrosis and some lung cancer. They also showed that, whereas the amphiboles and some other fibres survived indefinitely, chrysotile and some of the synthetic vitreous fibres had a half-life in the lung of only weeks or months. This may explain why chrysotile seems less carcinogenic in humans (from epidemiological studies), even though it is as carcinogenic as crocidolite in animal studies with high doses and insufficient time for clearance in the short animal life-span.[83]

It has proved very difficult to produce mesotheliomas by inhalation except with a particularly active sample of erionite. Most testing for induction of mesothelioma is done by intrapleural or intraperitoneal injection and indicates that it is the shape of the fibre rather than its chemistry that is important. Again the short survival of the fibre in the tissue does not interfere with carcinogenesis in the animal model. Similarly fibres too long to reach the pleura after inhalation can be shown to cause mesothelioma if put straight into the pleura.

The experimental work indicates that respirable fibres longer than 5 µm are dangerous because they are too long to be cleared by the macrophage and because they are capable (if they survive long enough) of causing lung fibrosis, lung cancer and mesothelioma. The longer fibres fail to reach the pleura so that it is those straight fibres in the size range 5–15 µm long and of the order of 0.1 µm thick which are most hazardous at low exposure because of the risk of mesothelioma.

EPIDEMIOLOGY OF ASBESTOS-RELATED DISEASES

Early studies showed a clear relationship between heavy exposure in the asbestos textile industry and the risk of asbestosis. When optical fibre counting was widely adopted it was possible to set a safety limit for asbestosis of 2 fibres per cm³. But as the incidence of asbestosis fell it became apparent that the more serious problems, of lung cancer and mesothelioma, did not fit the same model. Early on, the South Africans had reported that, despite high dust exposure in all mines and mills, lung cancer and mesothelioma were common in the North West Cape (crocidolite) but rare with Transvaal amosite (although asbestosis was common there). No lung cancers or mesotheliomas were reported from the Swaziland chrysotile mines. The same difference between crocidolite and chrysotile mines became apparent in Australia.

In Britain, North America and Germany there were several series reporting an increased risk of both lung cancer and mesothelioma resulting from apparently pure chrysotile exposure, for example among insulation workers.[84] The exceptionally high risk of mesothelioma due to pure crocidolite exposure was confirmed by the studies on military gas mask workers in Britain and Canada; this compares with the relative safety of the much dustier manufacture of civilian gas masks using chrysotile.[85] In one large friction material plant in Britain there was no evidence of an excess of cancer except for ten cases of mesothelioma which were associated with a special order of brake linings made with crocidolite.[86] All the other workers only used chrysotile.

Analysis of the size, shape and nature of mineral fibres in the lungs of workers and controls from many countries and industries has helped to explain the epidemiology. These analyses have indicated that tremolite may be the cause of lung cancer and mesothelioma in people exposed to chrysotile without added crocidolite or amosite. Tremolite is also the cause of environmental cases of mesothelioma in south-east Turkey, around the chrysotile mines in Cyprus and Corsica and the vermiculite deposits in Montana, USA. The mineralogy studies have been reviewed by Wagner and Pooley.[82]

Mesothelioma appears to be very rare in the former USSR where they use their own chrysotile, but has been reported from other East European countries where imported amphiboles have been used and there is an environmental tremolite problem.

PREVENTION OF ASBESTOS-RELATED DISEASES

The standard method of monitoring exposure is to count the fibres on a personal membrane filter using the optical microscope. The counts are reasonably accurate down to about 0.5 fibres/ml but very inaccurate at 0.1 and below.

The current exposure limit for chrysotile alone in the UK is 0.3 fibres/ml for a 4-hour average and 0.9 fibres/ml for a 10-minute period. For any other form of asbestos, alone or in mixtures (including mixtures with chrysotile), the limit is 0.2 fibres/ml averaged over 4 hours and 0.6 fibres/ml over 10 minutes. Most countries have adopted similar limits. The fibre counting method may not be sufficient for preventing mesothelioma from amphibole exposure (mainly because most of the relevant fibres are invisible to optical microscopy). It is logical to apply an optical standard for pure chrysotile while using some other test to ensure that there is no other form of asbestosis present. UK legislation and guidance requires the use of total protection suits (with external air supply) when amphiboles are present, for example when old insulation is being removed.[87]

In Scandinavia, Germany, France and the USA all asbestos usage is banned. A similar ban is likely to be applied in the UK in the near future. It is also logical to prevent the mining and use of all amphiboles. However, crocidolite or amosite are still mined in some countries. Some countries still allow the use of amphiboles, particularly in pressure pipes, while only applying the same protection standards as for chrysotile.

Monitoring workers who are or have been exposed to asbestos is of little value to the individual worker but is required by the safety authorities in most Western countries. This usually means routine full-size chest radiographs every 2 or 3 years and a simple physical examination and spirometry every year. The difficulties of maintaining constant standards of chest radiography and lung function testing have tended to prevent this monitoring from revealing whether or not the dust control is effective. Removal of the individual from exposure once changes have appeared is unlikely to reduce the risk of lung cancer or mesothelioma. In chrysotile mining and mine milling the monitoring is likely to detect simple pneumoconiosis due to serpentine rock dust rather than significant asbestosis unless the tremolite contamination is high.

Asbestos in buildings

'Passive' exposure to asbestos, as a result of the wearing of asbestos materials or insulation in buildings (public buildings, schools, sports centres, etc.), has often caused concern (in some cases extreme) in the occupants of these buildings. Except in very rare instances, the levels of asbestos found and, hence, the calculated risks of cancer have been extremely low for those simply doing administrative work or occupying such buildings. Exposure of custodial and maintenance workers in such buildings may nevertheless be significant, especially if the asbestos-containing boards and other materials are damaged. When asbestos is present in a building, a very careful evaluation of the degree of potential exposure must be carried out. This can be followed by methods of sealing-in the asbestos and, if necessary, an asbestos removal programme.[88]

OTHER NATURAL FIBRES

Zeolites

This group of commercially valuable minerals is formed by recrystallization from water which has percolated through deposits of volcanic ash. They are hydrated aluminium silicates with other metal ions within their open crystal lattice and act as catalysts, absorbents, etc. in the petrochemical industry, filters for sewage and water, water softeners, soil improvers and nitrogen adsorbers for oxygen concentrators. For most of these purposes non-fibrous zeolites with an amorphous or cuboidal crystal structure are used. They are even synthesized in this form with the precise characteristics needed for the particular use. They occur in many parts of the world where volcanic ash has been weathered for 100 million years or more. The deposits contain a mixture of volcanic glass and a variety of crystalline forms of zeolite. There are many different fibrous crystal forms but they are seldom present in sufficient quantity for commercial exploitation, some only occurring in geodes. However, one, erionite, has been found in large workable deposits in several places between the mountain ranges of the western USA and in the North Island of New Zealand.

The risk due to erionite was recognized from the studies of Baris[89] on the incidence of mesothelioma in scattered villages in Cappadocia in Turkey. Although the whole area consists of narrow valleys cut into the thick layer of volcanic luff with flat uplands in between, the incidence of mesothelioma varies from nil to over 50% of the adult population in villages within a few miles of each other. Only the villages where fine fibrous erionite is present are affected and the average age at death from mesothelioma is 45 years.

Experimental studies have not only confirmed that erionite fibres are very active in producing mesotheliomas but that this activity is very strongly size-dependent.[82] Future environmental exposure to erionite should be prevented, if necessary by moving populations, and commercial exploitation should be prevented completely.

The fibrous clays

In addition to those already mentioned in this chapter there is a group of clays and soft rocks which are used in the manufacture of quality tiles and ceramics. They are of special value because they consist of very fine fibre-crystals, mostly less than 0.1 μm in diameter and 5 μm long. However, many of the deposits contain a proportion of fibres long enough to cause mesothelioma and this has been confirmed by intrapleural studies in animals. It is not known how long these fibres survive in the lung.

The clays are often extracted damp and then dried, milled and marketed as a fine powder with or without calcining. Other uses are as adsorbents for insecticides, for mopping up oil spills and as cat litter. There is a wide range of potential exposure which is continuous only for small groups of workers and occasional for the rest. Little information about fibre exposure is available and what epidemiological information exists indicates pneumoconiosis with some high exposures but as yet no evidence of lung cancer or mesothelioma.

The main group are the aluminium silicates sepiolite, attapulgite, palygorskite and meerschaum, names which do not seem to correspond to different clearly defined minerals. The fibres break up easily and may not survive the normal milling procedure.

Wollastonite is a harder material mined mainly in the USA for use in the ceramics industry and as a filler to prevent cracking in cements, plasters and paints. It is a calcium silicate which formed into a mixture of platey and fibre like crystals. Again the commercial product is milled and contains few if any 'fibres' sufficiently long to cause concern. Problems may arise if the method of processing or use is changed to preserve the elongated crystals or if other deposits are exploited.

Synthetic mineral fibres

The health risks associated with the industrial use and consequent environmental contamination by asbestos have led to an increased production and use of man-made fibres to replace asbestos for insulation, filtration, fire protection, friction materials, etc. A number of structural similarities between some of these fibres and asbestos, as well as experimental data *in vitro* and in laboratory animals, have led to the legitimate concern that these asbestos substitutes may in fact be as hazardous as asbestos. Fortunately, this does not appear to be the case, although working with man-made fibre is not entirely free from health risks.[90,91]

The most common man-made (or manufactured or synthetic or artificial) fibres are vitreous fibres (MMVF), but there are also a number of other synthetic fibres, such as carbon/graphite fibres and silicon carbide fibres and whiskers, as well as synthetic polymers, such as Kevlar para-aramid fibres.

Also called (inappropriately) man-made mineral fibres (MMMF), MMVFs comprise glass fibres (glass wool, continuous glass filament and special purpose glass fibre), mineral wool (i.e. rock wool and slag wool) and refractory ceramic fibres. More than 80% of the total production of MMVFs is made up by the insulation wools (glass, rock and slag wool). They are obtained by melting glass (with stabilizers and modifiers or fluxes), rock (basalt, granite, slate, limestone), slag (from metallic ore refining) or kaolin clay (or combinations of alumina/silica often with zirconium), and producing fibres by rotary or other processes. Various materials are generally used as additives and the fibres are often held together with binders (e.g. phenol-formaldehyde resin). The size characteristics of MMVFs are such that their mean diameters exceed the sizes considered to be respirable (3 μm), except for refractory ceramic fibres and glass microfibres. In addition, airborne concentrations have been reported to be generally lower than 1 fibre/ml air during manufacture, although higher levels are possible during applications. Another reassuring feature of MMVFs compared with asbestos is that their biopersistence (durability) in the lung is much lower, again with the exception of refractory ceramic fibres.

Occupational (and residential) exposure to MMVFs is well known to lead to acute skin and eye irritation, as well as upper respiratory tract irritation. However, neither interstitial fibrosis nor chronic obstructive pulmonary disease have been demonstrated to result from exposure to them. Pleural changes have not been shown to occur either, except in the case of the more persistent refractory ceramic fibres, for which a recent study[92] of a cohort of production workers found a progressive relationship between plaques and cumulative exposure to refractory ceramic fibres, taking into account the possible exposure to asbestos. With regard to malignant lung disease, there is no evidence for an increased mortality from mesothelioma or bronchopulmonary cancer in workers producing MMVFs (with the possible exception of the early production stages of slag or rock wool), although it must be realized that there are still insufficient data on this subject with regard to refractory ceramic fibres.

The human health effects of fibres other than MMVFs are much less well studied. With the exception of silicon carbide fibres, which may lead to pneumoconiosis, no human disease has been reported following exposure to these fibres. However, an outbreak of interstitial lung disease (mainly non-specific interstitial pneumonia) has been recently described in workers exposed to microfibres made of nylon.[93] Nylon is not generally included among the man-made fibres, but like Kevlar, it is a synthetic fibre. This outbreak, as well as those that affected textile sprayers[94,95] are a reminder that in the right exposure circumstances severe lung disease may occur even with exposure to materials that are generally considered to be 'inert'.

METAL DUSTS AND FUMES

The subject of metal-induced lung diseases is complex, not only because there are so many different agents to be considered, but also because the conditions caused are quite diverse. Pulmonary diseases caused by occupational exposures to metals involve more than 'pneumoconioses'; they encompass almost the entire spectrum of respiratory conditions, ranging from acute inhalation injury to lung cancer, from airway disease to parenchymal disorders. The clinical experience and epidemiological understanding of metal-induced pulmonary disease is much less extensive than for silicosis, coal pneumoconiosis or asbestos-related disease. The topic is considered in more detail elsewhere.[96]

The toxicity of a metallic compound is heavily dependent on its physicochemical form, also called 'metal speciation'. Inhalation of metallic compounds does not necessarily lead to significant pulmonary damage. Lung disorders in workers occupationally exposed to metals are not always due to these metals, but may be due to cigarette smoking, concomitant exposure to silica (particularly in mining), asbestos, irritant gases (as in welding) and organic chemicals (such as solvents and isocyanates). Exposure to metals is not confined to metal mining or metallurgy, but may take place in almost every sector of industry, e.g. as paint pigments, as catalysts in chemical processes, as well as in the general or domestic environment.

It is customary to divide metals and their alloys into ferrous metals (iron and various types of steels) and non-ferrous metals. The first category is the most widely encountered and does not pose much specific respiratory hazard, whereas non-ferrous metals can cause a number of specific respiratory conditions.

Non-specific pulmonary disorders caused by exposure to metals: acute toxic effects

METAL FUME FEVER

Metal fume fever (see Chapter 9) is a non-allergic, influenza-like reaction following a single exposure to high concentrations of metal fumes. The syndrome consists of fever, chills, muscle pains and malaise, generally with relatively mild respiratory symptoms, and classically little or no radiographic or functional abnormalities, although this is not always the case. The symptoms usually begin at home a few hours after a heavy exposure to metal oxides and they subside spontaneously after 24 hours or a night's sleep. Peripheral leucocytosis is present during the acute illness, and recent studies using bronchoalveolar lavage have showed marked neutrophil infiltration and cytokine release in the lungs.[97]

Although metal fume fever is said to occur after exposure to the fumes of many different sorts of metals, it has been documented mainly following exposure to fumes of zinc (i.e. zinc oxide, ZnO) and to a lesser extent copper. Zinc fume fever commonly occurs, for example, after the smelting or thermal spraying of zinc without adequate exhaust, or after welding or flame cutting galvanized steel in a confined space. Workers at risk of metal fume fever are usually quite familiar with the condition; however, few cases come to the attention of physicians. No specific treatment is required, except preventive hygiene measures. Metal fume fever is said not to lead to sequelae, but this has not been adequately investigated.

ACUTE INHALATION INJURY

As indicated in Table 35.1, the inhalation of various metallic compounds can cause severe inhalation injury, involving the upper and/or lower respiratory tract. Depending on the agent and the intensity of exposure, the injury may manifest itself as rhinitis, laryngitis, tracheobronchitis or chemical pneumonitis and non-cardiogenic pulmonary oedema. Symptoms will, therefore, possibly include lacrimation, nose irritation with sneezing and bleeding, sore throat, hoarseness, cough, wheezing, chest pain or tightness, and dyspnoea. In severe cases the clinical picture may be that of the adult respiratory distress syndrome. When the deep lung is involved, respiratory distress is often delayed for several hours (without any alarming symptoms) until severe non-cardiogenic pulmonary oedema develops.

Table 35.1 *Non-exhaustive list of metallic agents described as possible causes of acute lung injury*

Oxides of cadmium (Cd), manganese (Mn), nickel (Ni), osmium (Os), vanadium (V), cobalt (Co), beryllium (Be)

Mercury (Hg) vapours

Zinc chloride ($ZnCl_2$) and other metal chlorides ($TiCl_4$, $SbCl_3$, $SbCl_5$, $ZrCl_4$, UF_6,)

Nickel carbonyl ($Ni(CO)_4$)

Hydrides (B_2H_6 or diborane, LiH, PH_3, AsH_3, SbH_3, . . .)

See also specific metals elsewhere in Chapter 7.

METAL OXIDES

Exposure to metal oxides (see Chapter 7) may result from the smelting, welding, flame-cutting or thermal spraying of pure metals or alloys, but sometimes also through direct exposure to dust particles (e.g. V_2O_5, MnO) or vapours (e.g. Os_3O_4). Inhalation injury may even occur with new technologies, such as those involving the thermal spraying of metals as shown by a recently described fatal case caused by spraying nickel.[98]

Cadmium

The best documented metallic agent causing toxic pneumonitis is cadmium. Cadmium is a by-product of the zinc and lead industry; it is used in metal plating and in special alloys; it is also used in the production of batteries, pigments, plastic stabilizers. Cadmium oxides may be liberated, often unknown to the worker, from the welding or burning of cadmium-containing alloys and cadmium-plated metal, from the use of hard solders, or from the smelting of zinc or lead (or scrap metal), which often contain significant levels of contaminating cadmium. It is important to distinguish acute toxic pneumonitis from simple metal fume fever.

Mercury

Acute pneumonitis after the inhalation of high quantities of mercury vapours has been described as a consequence of the refining of gold or silver (using amalgams) in confined spaces, which is often the case in the cottage industry, and after accidents involving mercury lamps.

Vanadium

Vanadium pentoxide (V_2O_5) may be present in significant quantities in slags from the steel industry (ferrovanadium) and, because some fuel oils contain high quantities of vanadium, in furnace residues from oil refineries or in soot from oil-fired boilers. Dust containing V_2O_5 may cause upper and lower airway irritation: rhinitis with sneezing and nose bleeds, pharyngitis, acute tracheobronchitis, with cough, wheeze and (possibly) airway hyperreactivity (boilermaker's bronchitis),[99] as well as possibly bronchopneumonia.

Zinc

Cases of adult respiratory distress syndrome, some with a protracted course, have been reported in military or civilian personnel accidentally exposed to smoke bombs which liberate zinc chloride ($ZnCl_2$).[100]

Other metallic agents

Accidental exposure, e.g. as a result of explosions, burst pipes or leaks in chemical plants, to antimony trichloride ($SbCl_3$) and pentachloride ($SbCl_5$), zirconium tetrachloride ($ZrCl_4$), titanium tetrachloride ($TiCl_4$), and uranium hexafluoride (UF_6) may also lead to inhalation injury. Nickel carbonyl [$Ni(CO)_4$] is a volatile liquid of very high toxicity for the lungs and brain. Acute inhalation may cause haemorrhagic pulmonary oedema.[101]

Lithium hydride (LiH), phosphine (hydrogen phosphide, PH_3, used as a doping agent for the manufacture of silicon crystals, or released from aluminium phosphide grain fumigants or zinc phosphide rodenticides), hydrogen selenide (SeH_3), and diborane (B_2H_5, used as high energy fuel) have also been reported to cause acute inhalation injury with, possibly, pulmonary oedema.[102]

Inhalation of the hydrogenated forms of arsenic (arsine, AsH_3) or antimony (stibine, SbH_3) can also be lethal as a result of fulminant hemolysis, which may sometimes manifest itself initially as dyspnoea, abdominal and lumbar pain and haemoglobinuria.

Chronic obstructive lung disease

There is good evidence that exposure to high concentrations of cadmium may cause pulmonary emphysema. This was demonstrated in a study of a large group of 101 workers and ex-workers from a cadmium alloy factory in England, in which a clear excess of functional and radiological signs of emphysema were found compared with appropriate controls.[103] The study found evidence of a dose–response relationship, with dose being estimated both by past hygiene measurements and by the internal (liver) cadmium burden. Other studies have found an increased mortality from non-malignant respiratory disease in cadmium-exposed workers.[104]

There have been many surveys of the prevalence of chronic obstructive lung disease in workers from the iron and steel industry, as well as among metal welders (see Chapters 9, 31). Although exposure in the iron and steel industry is mainly to iron-dust, many other metallic and non-metallic particulates (including silica and asbestos), as well as gases may be inhaled. During welding, even of steel, the plume is not so much composed of the metals being welded together, but of the materials which make up the electrode, the filler wire and the fluxes used. Despite the generally consistent finding of an increase in the prevalence of chronic bronchitis, as defined by questionnaire, among welders and steelworkers, the results regarding ventilatory function have been largely negative, inconclusive or showing only small effects.[105,106] However, because of the healthy worker effect and various methodological issues, one should not conclude from these studies that there are no specific work processes within these broad categories which entail a risk of significant obstructive respiratory impairment in susceptible subjects. Population studies indicate that there is an excess mortality[107] and morbidity[108] from non-malignant respiratory disease among steelworkers and welders. A longitudinal study of shipyard workers has shown a faster annual decline in FEV$_1$ in welders and caulker/burners than in controls.[109] In any case, the absence of certainty regarding the magnitude of the risk of chronic obstructive lung disease in welders and steelworkers should not lead to complacency about the need for adequate surveillance and prevention of dust exposure in these jobs, also because chronic obstructive lung disease is not the only risk incurred.

Cross-sectional studies have indicated an excess of chronic bronchitis and a loss of ventilatory function, sometimes mainly of FVC, associated with chronic exposure to beryllium, aluminium, cobalt (or hard metal), manganese, and titanium dioxide (TiO$_2$). This seems to be independent of the other respiratory diseases associated with some of these metals (see below). However, other surveys of workers exposed to these compounds have not reached the same conclusions, possibly because of differences in total dust, in concomitant exposures, or in population characteristics and study designs. The absence of demonstrable effects does not exclude the existence of a preventable health risk.

Bronchial asthma (see Chapter 33)

Several metals are known to be capable of causing bronchial asthma.[110] Metal-induced asthma is a particular case of an occupational asthma caused by agents of low molecular weight, a topic which is covered elsewhere in this book. In essence, the clinical characteristics of metal-induced asthma do not appear to be dissimilar from occupational asthma caused by other agents. With some metals (as in fact with some organic molecules),

alveolitis and asthma may co-exist, as has been described with cobalt. Other forms of metal-related occupational asthma are more likely to belong to the category of non-immunologic asthma, i.e. 'irritant-induced asthma' or 'occupational asthma without latency'.

The best known cause of metal-induced occupational asthma is that caused by complex platinum salts, which has mainly been described in workers from precious metal refineries. However, exposure to complex salts of platinum may also occur in the manufacture of catalysts, in photographic applications, and in electroplating. Platinum salts are extremely potent sensitizers and are generally considered to do so via IgE-mediated pathway. Palladium is another precious metal which may occasionally cause occupational asthma (see Chapter 7).

Nickel, chromium and cobalt are also potential causes of occupational asthma, although the number of reported cases is not high, certainly compared with the high prevalence of allergic sensitization of the skin caused by these metals. This may be partly due to differences in mechanisms of immunological sensitization, but there is probably also some degree of underdiagnosis. Patients with asthma caused by nickel or chromium often also have urticaria or allergic contact dermatitis. Significant exposure to hexavalent chromium occurs mainly in chromate production industries, in chrome plating, during stainless steel welding, but also in the building industry because cement generally contains small amounts of chromates, which is not only a frequent source of allergic contact dermatitis, but occasionally also an unsuspected cause of occupational asthma.[111]

Most cases of cobalt asthma have been described in relation to the manufacture or grinding of sintered hard metal, in which cobalt is used as a binder for tungsten carbide.[112,113] Coolants used in wet grinding of hard metal tools may contain a high concentration of dissolved (i.e. ionized) cobalt, thus leading to the paradox that wet grinding may be more 'harmful' than dry grinding.[114] Cobalt asthma has also been found in relation to the production of cobalt, the manufacture or use of cobalt pigments or additives, and in diamond polishers. It is possible that cobalt asthma is but an 'airway variant' of hard metal disease (see below) and there are occasional subjects who exhibit both asthmatic reactions and parenchymal involvement.

Pot room asthma is a peculiar form of occupational asthma described in aluminium smelters (see Chapter 7), who are exposed to the fumes evolving from the 'pots' in which aluminium ore is molten after addition of fluoride salts. Several clinical and epidemiological studies carried out mainly in the Norwegian aluminium industry,[115] but also elsewhere,[116] have described 'pot room asthma'. The exact causal agent of this form of asthma is not known and it probably does not involve allergic mechanisms. It seems more likely that pot room asthma is a form of irritant-induced asthma, with the irritants being most probably the fluorides present in the fumes.

Occupational asthma has also been reported as a result of exposure to aluminium fluoride salts.

There are rare reports[117] of asthma in subjects welding galvanized metal, with sensitization to zinc being postulated on the grounds of a positive bronchial challenge. Similarly, occupational asthma due to soldering fluxes containing zinc chloride has been described.[118] However, no immunological support for sensitization to zinc has been provided. It is conceivable that (some) individuals with non-specific bronchial hyperreactivity exhibit asthmatic reactions when they have a bout of metal fume fever. The possible presence of metals other than zinc should also be considered in such instances.

Exposure to vanadium, usually as vanadium pentoxide (V_2O_5), has been reported as a possible cause of occupational asthma. This exposure has been described in workers who maintain, clean or dismantle oil-fired boilers, because the fly ash produced by some types of fuel-oil may be very rich in vanadium (see above). From the available evidence it appears that this form of asthma essentially results from the strong irritation produced by V_2O_5 which may cause nasal ulceration and acute bronchitis (see above), with more or less lasting non-specific bronchial hyperreactivity as a result.

In addition to the specific causes of occupational asthma described above, welding is often mentioned as a cause of occupational asthma or as a risk factor of asthma.[119–121] It is not always clear whether these are cases of asthma from metal sensitization, 'irritant-induced' asthmas due to irritant gases, or work-related asthmas (see Chapter 9).

Lung cancer (see Chapter 39)

Several metallic compounds are proven lung carcinogens in humans,[122] they include radioactive metals (and their decay products) and non-radioactive metals. The increased incidence of lung cancer observed in uranium miners has been causally linked with the inhalation of radon daughters.[123] However, the underground mining of other compounds may also be associated with significant exposure to radioactivity, if there is insufficient ventilation of the radon which leaks from igneous rocks.[124] This factor has been implicated in the higher incidence of lung cancer seen in various groups of mineworkers, such as Swedish iron ore miners,[125] although it does not seem to play a role in the similarly increased lung cancer incidence of French iron ore miners.[126] Domestic radon gas exposure is also implicated in the causation of bronchial cancer.

Epidemiological and experimental studies have clearly established the carcinogenic risk of exposure to arsenic, chromates and nickel, at least to some of their chemical forms. Thus, the relationship of arsenic to increased lung cancer risk in copper smelting workers is unequivocal. This is also the case for other occupational exposures to arsenic, such as the manufacture or spraying of arsenical pesticides. A greatly increased risk of lung cancer has also been demonstrated for workers in the primary chromate production and in the chromate pigment industry. Epidemiological studies of the carcinogenic risk of exposure to chromium during metal plating or during stainless steel welding have been considered inconclusive. Occupational exposure to nickel compounds in nickel smelters and refineries is also unequivocally associated with an increase in cancer of the lung and the nasal sinuses.

Cadmium and beryllium have also recently been added to the possible causes of human lung cancer. There are also indications that cobalt exposure (particularly in the manufacture of hard metal)[127] may lead to a risk of lung cancer.

Studies of iron and steel foundry workers have consistently found an increased risk of lung cancer, but this may be due to the emission of polycyclic aromatic hydrocarbons as pyrolysis products of organic materials used.

PNEUMOCONIOSES AND SPECIFIC INTERSTITIAL LUNG DISORDERS CAUSED BY METALS

Recent epidemiologic surveys have revealed that subjects with 'idiopathic' lung fibrosis are more likely than controls to have been occupationally exposed to metals (and also to wood).[128] This means either that many patients receive a diagnosis of idiopathic lung disease because no good occupational and environmental history has been taken, or that some metals may play a hitherto unrecognized role in the causation of interstitial lung disease. It is reasonable to assume that both explanations are valid to some extent.

Documentation of exposure to metals may be obtained from the analysis of metal concentrations in blood or urine (or even hair or nails) taken for biological monitoring. In addition, elemental analysis may be carried out on bronchoalveolar lavage fluid, on biopsy tissue or on autopsy material. Both macroanalytical (or bulk) and microanalytical techniques may be applied. The former are destructive techniques which allow the detection, quantitation and/or characterization of the crystalline structure of inorganic elements. The latter techniques allow *in situ* analysis of individual cells and particles. Several sophisticated microanalytical techniques, coupled to scanning or transmission electron microscopy, exist: energy dispersive x-ray analysis (EDXA), particle-induced x-ray emission (PIXE), electron energy loss spectrometry (EELS) and laser microprobe mass analysis (LAMMA). These techniques have been successfully applied in both BAL fluid and lung biopsies, and databases are available with 'normal' values of inorganic particles.[129,130] Of course, the presence of a particular element, even in abnormally high quantities, does not in itself constitute proof that it is causally involved in the disease, but this information may be extremely useful to discover unsuspected past exposures or to document such exposures.

Siderosis

Of the metallic pneumoconioses the most frequent and best (although still poorly) studied is siderosis, which is caused by the inhalation of iron compounds. More than 90% of the total world production of metallic materials is in the form of steels and cast irons, and occupational exposure to iron is, therefore, extremely widespread. It occurs during iron (hematite) mining and related operations, during iron refining and at various stages in steelmaking, during welding, cutting and abrading of iron-containing materials, as well as during the manufacture or use of iron-containing abrasives (such as emery). Despite the large number of workers who are exposed to iron-containing dust, little research has been carried out in recent years regarding the pulmonary effects of occupational exposure to iron dust. Yet, in the past decade there has been a considerable interest in the possible role of iron in pulmonary diseases, because ferrous/ferric ions catalyse the Fenton reaction, whereby the very toxic hydroxyl radical (OH°) is produced.

There is a widespread belief that siderosis is only a 'radiological disorder' which manifests itself by the presence of small, very radiodense opacities with uniform distribution throughout the lungs, but without formation of conglomerates. With cessation of exposure the radiographic opacities may gradually disappear. Pure siderosis is not associated with respiratory symptoms or functional impairment, and does not predispose to tuberculosis. However, exposure to silica or asbestos is not uncommon in many jobs that involve exposure to iron, thus giving rise to mixed dust fibrosis ('siderosilicosis') or to asbestosis, with their associated morbidity. The view that the symptomatic interstitial fibrosis, which is sometimes found in welders ('welder's pneumoconiosis'), is simply siderosis with coexisting silicosis has been challenged on the grounds that the pulmonary silicon content of such cases did not differ from that of control lungs.[131] There are case reports of siderosis with significant fibrosis in welders.[105]

Aluminium lung

The existence of 'aluminium lung' has been the subject of some controversy. Indeed in view of the extensive industrial use of aluminium, parenchymal lung disease caused by exposure to this metal appears to be very uncommon, both at the stage of its production and during its use. On the basis of animal experimental data showing that aluminium counteracts the toxic effects of silica, inhalation of aluminium was proposed and even implemented (without real success, but also without apparent pulmonary adverse effects) for the prevention of silicosis and even for its therapy. Dinman[132] concluded that fibrosis only occurred in: workers who were heavily exposed to submicron-sized aluminium plates during the production of fireworks and explosives; and in workers involved in the smelting of bauxite for the production of Al_2O_3 (corundum) abrasive (Shaver's disease). The second group were perhaps also exposed to crystalline silica. An extensive review also concluded that pulmonary fibrosis was not a significant problem in aluminium smelter workers.[116] The conclusion is that exposure to aluminium dust does not pose an important risk of interstitial lung disease.

Nevertheless, the risk is not absent. Severe interstitial fibrosis was described in three workers (out of a workforce of about 1000 workers) who had been heavily exposed for 19–33 years mainly, but not exclusively, to Al_2O_3 in the production of abrasives.[133] There are reports of isolated cases of granulomatous lung disease, fibrosis and alveolar proteinosis in aluminium welders or polishers. The physical characteristics of the aluminium particles, notably their surface area, or even their possibly fibrous nature, have been suggested as important determinants of their bioreactivity and hence fibrogenicity.

Other metal pneumoconioses

Other rare 'benign' pneumoconioses include those caused by tin (stannosis), barium (baritosis), and antimony (antimoniosis). These pneumoconioses were described many years ago and few recent clinical and epidemiological data are available.

'Dental technician's pneumoconiosis' is an interstitial fibrosis of many potential origins,[134,135] including silica and beryllium,[136] but possibly also vitallium, an alloy consisting of chromium, cobalt and molybdenum.[137]

Although the synthetic abrasive silicon carbide or carborundum is not a metallic compound – in contrast to some other abrasives such as corundum (Al_2O_3) or emery (corundum with iron oxides) – it is worth mentioning that respiratory disease, including pneumoconiosis with fibrosis, has been associated with exposure to silicon carbide, during its manufacture or use.[138,139]

Beryllium lung

Berylliosis or chronic beryllium disease is relatively rare, but it has attracted considerable scientific attention because of its striking histologic and clinical resemblance to sarcoidosis.[140,141]

Apart from the extraction (as beryl ore) and primary refining industry, beryllium exposure is an occupational risk in several sectors of modern technological industries, such as aircraft and aerospace, electronics, computers and communications, where beryllium is utilized for its light weight, stability, hardness, lack of magnetic properties, and good electrical conductivity. Beryllium is mainly found in alloys (often with copper) or in ceramics. Beryllium exposure also occurs in the nuclear power industry, because it facilitates fission reactions of uranium and plutonium. Beryllium used to be present in fluorescent lights, but this is no longer the case. Unsuspected exposures to beryllium may take place during the refining of scrap metal, the machining or welding of non-ferrous alloys, and in dental laboratories.[136] The first manifestations of chronic beryllium disease may only occur long after exposure has ceased. Para-occupational exposure has also been described as a significant risk, not only in the older literature, when beryllium disease occurred in residents in the vicinity of beryllium refineries, but even very recently, when beryllium disease was diagnosed in the spouse of a beryllium production worker.[142]

High concentrations of beryllium fumes may cause a chemical pneumonitis, but modern exposures are mainly associated with chronic beryllium disease. This is characterized by diffuse pulmonary inflammation with formation of epithelioid non-caseating granulomas in the lung interstitium, mainly along the bronchovascular bundles, but also in the bronchial submucosa and subpleural regions, and in the intrathoracic lymph nodes. The pathology may also suggest extrinsic allergic alveolitis with more diffuse mononuclear cell infiltration. End-stage lung fibrosis with honeycombing may also be found, as well as conglomerate masses of granulomas and fibrosis.

As described by Newman[140] the presentation and clinical course of the disease are similar to those of sarcoidosis, with exertional dyspnoea of gradual onset, cough, and fatigue. However, asymptomatic hilar lymphadenopathy and pulmonary infiltrates, or ocular or skin lesions are not presenting features of chronic beryllium disease. Beryllium disease may also affect extrapulmonary organs, such as the lymph nodes, the skin (but there is no erythema nodosum), the salivary glands and other organs, although this is less frequently the case than in classical sarcoidosis, and no ocular or neurologic manifestations have been reported. Sarcoidosis and chronic beryllium disease cannot be distinguished from each other by radiology, pulmonary function testing, ordinary laboratory tests, or bronchoalveolar lavage fluid. The chest radiograph reveals diffuse parenchymal infiltrates of various types (reticular to nodular) and often also hilar lymphadenopathy. Functional impairment is variable with restrictive and obstructive patterns, as well as isolated reductions in gas transfer factor (DLCO) and alterations in gas exchange on exercise, even years before radiologic abnormalities are seen. Serum angiotensin converting enzyme actiivity may also be elevated. In the bronchoalveolar lavage fluid, lymphocyte numbers are increased and the CD4/CD8 ratio is markedly elevated. In principle, the treatment and prognosis of chronic beryllium disease are comparable with that of sarcoidosis, with some patients going into remission, but continuous steroid therapy is usually required (without always being effective) and progression to end-stage lung fibrosis is more frequent in chronic beryllium disease than in sarcoidosis.

Most recent advances in the field of chronic beryllium disease have been made with regard to its immunopathology. Beryllium has become the prime example of a small molecular weight antigen which can initiate, in susceptible individuals, a cell-mediated delayed-type hypersensitivity reaction in the lung. Although patch testing with beryllium was shown to be positive in patients with chronic beryllium disease in the early 1950s, it should now be standard practice to diagnose chronic beryllium disease by performing a beryllium-specific lymphocyte proliferation test. This test may be carried out in cells obtained by bronchoalveolar lavage or in peripheral blood lymphocytes. This *ex vivo* test is apparently highly specific, since lymphocyte proliferation does not occur in subjects without the disease, such as in ordinary sarcoidosis or extrinsic allergic alveolitis, and only rarely in exposed but non-diseased subjects. The test is also sensitive, particularly if it is performed on bronchoalveolar lavage fluid lymphocytes, although technical improvements have also rendered it sensitive when applied to blood lymphocytes.[143] The good positive and negative predictive value of the beryllium-specific lymphocyte proliferation test has led to its being proposed as a medical surveillance tool in beryllium exposed subjects.[144]

It has been shown that genetic factors (HLA-DPB1 glu 69 allele) determine, at least in part, the occurrence of a cell-mediated immunological reaction against beryllium.[145] This explains why chronic beryllium disease is not only found in the more highly exposed workers (such as machinists), but also in subjects with very low exposure, such as clerical workers in beryllium plants.[146] A recent study[147] has shown that sensitization occurred in workers exposed, during the machining of beryllia ceramics, to median levels of beryllium below 2 µg/m³, thus leading the authors to suggest that beryllium exposure should be kept as low as reasonably achievable.

Other interstitial lung disease with granuloma formation

Beryllium is not the only metal involved in causing sarcoid-like lung disease. Granulomatous lung disease has been attributed, mainly in case reports, to exposure to zirconium (Zr), during the manufacture of ceramic tiles[148] the welding of nuclear fuel rods[149] or lens grinding.[150] Exposure to titanium[151] and aluminium[152] are also said to have led to sarcoid-like lung granulomatosis.

Exposure to rare earth metals (or lanthanides), of which cerium (Ce) is the most abundant element, has also been associated with interstitial fibrosis in a small number of subjects.[153,154] Rare earths are essential components of carbon arc lamps used for photoengraving, and the majority of cases of this pneumoconiosis have been described in photoengravers. Deposits of rare earths have also been found, without radiologic abnormalities, in the lung of a movie projectionist.[155] Rare earths are also used in the fabrication and polishing of glass, where they have been associated with pneumoconiosis.[154,156] The presence of granulomatous interstitial alterations is mentioned occasionally, but this is not the case in most available pathologic descriptions of cerium-pneumoconiosis.

Hard metal lung disease – 'cobalt lung'

Hard metal (lung) disease (sometimes also called hard metal pneumoconiosis) is a specific form of interstitial lung disease, which may occur in workers as a result of exposure to cobalt-containing dusts during the manufacture or use of hard metal or diamond tools.[141,157] (Hard metal-induced bronchial asthma, which may coexist with interstitial disease in the same patient, is sometimes included in the clinical entity of hard metal lung disease, but usually the term hard metal lung disease is restricted to the parenchymal form of the disease).

Hard metal is a composite material composed mainly of tungsten carbide and varying amounts (5–25%) of cobalt, which functions as a binder. Besides tungsten carbide, other carbides (e.g. with tantalum, titanium, niobium) may also be used and small amounts of other metals (e.g. nickel, chromium) may also be present. Hard metals are also designated as sintered carbides or cemented carbides. (Sintering refers to a process by which a powder compact is converted into a solid polycrystalline material by pressing under specific conditions of temperature and pressure). Hard metals are mainly utilized in tools used for drilling, sawing, cutting, grinding or polishing various materials, such as stones, concrete, metals, wood, etc. In recent years, diamonds have also been increasingly used to make grinding tools or saw blades and here too, the binder used for the micro-diamond powder is cobalt, which makes up to 90% of the grinding surface. Although these diamond tools are not composed of 'hard metal', they pose a similar hazard (see Chapter 7).[158]

The highest exposures to cobalt dust take place during the various stages of the manufacture of hard metal or diamond tools. However, hazardous exposure to cobalt may also occur during the filing and re-sharpening of hard metal tools, particularly during wet grinding,[114] as well as during the polishing of diamonds with diamond-cobalt disks. Coating with hard metal by the detonation gun process and related operations may also give rise to significant exposure.[159] All these activities often take place in small or medium sized factories with poor hygiene conditions, and even in large plants, tool-sharpening is often not recognized as a significant health risk.

Hard metal lung disease shares many clinical features with hypersensitivity pneumonitis: the presentation may be that of a subacute alveolitis with fever, cough, dyspnoea and a clear exposure-related clinical course, while in other instances a more insidious course with progressive diffuse fibrosis may be found. Overt disease only occurs in a minority of exposed workers and those affected may be young subjects with only a short exposure. These features clearly point to a condition caused mainly by a specific, perhaps immunological, susceptibility, as opposed to a simple process of chronic accumulation of dust in the lungs, as in the classical mineral pneumoconioses. On the other hand, hard metal lung disease also exhibits characteristics which make it distinct from hypersensitivity pneumonitis caused by organic antigens. Thus, no precipitating antibodies are found in the serum and the lung pathology and cellular findings in the bronchoalveolar lavage fluid generally differ from those of hypersensitivity pneumonitis.

The most characteristic finding in the lungs, as well as in bronchoalveolar lavage, is the presence of numerous so-called 'bizarre' giant multinucleated cells with 'cell in cell' or 'cannibalistic' features. The latter feature, i.e. giant cell interstitial pneumonitis, is now considered pathognomonic for hard-metal disease.[160] However, these giant cells may be absent and histology may exhibit desquamation of numerous cells in the alveoli (desquamative interstitial pneumonitis), lymphoplasmocyte infiltration, and varying degrees of interstitial, mainly centrilobular fibrosis. Except for the possible presence of giant cells, bronchoalveolar lavage fluid findings are non-specific, with all cell types – macrophages, lymphocytes, neutrophils or eosinophils, and even mast cells – being possibly increased. The finding of the constituents of hard metal (usually only tungsten) in the bronchoalveolar lavage fluid or lung tissue is a useful indicator of (past) exposure, but there is no quantitative relation with disease.

The evolution of hard metal lung disease is variable, but cessation of exposure usually results in clinical improvement and good recovery, but some patients do progress to end-stage fibrosis. Although corticosteroids have been given, no proof of their efficacy has been given.

While the role of cobalt in the causation of interstitial lung disease in hard metal workers and diamond polishers is undisputed, exposure to cobalt alone does not appear to be sufficient to lead to parenchymal disease and fibrosis.[161,162] Thus, occupational exposure to even high levels of 'pure' cobalt dust is apparently not associated with interstitial lung disease[163] (although pure cobalt and cobalt salts may cause asthma).

The mechanisms for the pulmonary toxicity of cobalt have not yet been entirely elucidated. The relative rarity of the condition and the fact that it may arise after short and apparently low exposures plead for an important role of individual susceptibility. The known dermal and respiratory sensitizing properties of cobalt and some of the clinical features of the disease, including the recurrence of giant cell interstitial pneumonitis in a transplanted lung despite cessation of exposure,[164] favour immunological sensitization as a possible mechanism. However, unlike the situation with beryllium, no hard evidence for immunological sensitization to cobalt as a cause for 'cobalt lung' is available. Experimental data and the observation that oxygen administration may be detrimental in 'cobalt lung'[165] suggest that poor defence against oxidants may also be involved.

REFERENCES

1 Fletcher CM, Peto R. The natural history of chronic airflow obstruction. *Br Med J* 1977; **i**: 1645–8.

2 Rom WN. Relationship of inflammatory cell cytokines to disease severity in individuals with occupational inorganic dust exposure. *Am J Ind Med* 1991; **19**: 15–27.

3 Schins RP, Schilderman PA, Borm PJ. Oxidative DNA damage in peripheral blood lymphocytes of coal workers. *Int Arch Occup Environ Med* 1995; **67**: 153–7.

4 Schins RP, Borm PJ. Epidemiological evaluation of release of monocyte TNF-alpha as an exposure and effect marker in pneumoconiosis: a five-year follow-up study of coal workers. *Occup Environ Med* 1995; **52**: 441–50.

5 Vanhee D, Gosset P, Boitelle A, Wallaert B, Tonnel AB. Cytokines and cytokine network in silicosis and coal workers' pneumoconiosis. *Eur Resp J* 1995; **8**: 834–42.

6 International Labour Office. *International Classification of Radiographs of Pneumoconioses*. Revised 1980. Set of standard films and accompanying booklet. Geneva: ILO, 1980.

7 Al Jarad N, Wilkinson P, Pearson MC, Rudd RM. A new high resolution computed tomography scoring system for pulmonary fibrosis, pleural disease, and emphysema in patients with asbestos related disease. *Br J Ind Med* 1992; **49**: 73–84.

8 Seaton A, Legges IS, Henderson J, Kerr KM. Accelerated silicosis in Scottish stonemasons. *Lancet* 1991; **337**: 341–4.

9 Craighead JE, Kleinerman J. Silicosis and silicate committee, NIOSH. Diseases associated with exposure to silica and non-fibrous silicate minerals. *Arch Pathol Lab Med* 1988; **112**: 673–720.

10 Vallyathan V. Generation of oxygen radicals by minerals and its correlation to cytotoxicity. *Environ Hlth Perspect* 1994; **102**(Suppl 10): 111–5.

11 Le Bouffant L, Daniel H, Martin JC, Bruyere S. Effect of impurities and associated minerals on quartz toxicity. *Ann Occup Hyg* 1982; **26**: 625–32.

12 Cherniack M. *The Hawk's Nest Incident: America's Worst Industrial Disaster*. New Haven: Yale University Press, 1986.

13 Sluis-Cremer GK, Hessel PA, Nizdo EH, Churchill AR. Zeiss EA. Silica, silicosis and progressive systemic sclerosis. *Br J Ind Med* 1985; **42**: 838–43.

14 Westerholm P. Silicosis, observations on a case register. *Scand J Work Environ Hlth* 1980; **6**(Suppl 2): 1–86.

15 Goldsmith DF, Beaumont JJ, Morrin LA, Schenker MB. Respiratory cancer and other chronic disease mortality among silicotics in California. *Am J Ind Med* 1995; **28**: 459–67.

16 Lam CW. *Comparison of 6- and 8-month Chemotherapy in the Treatment of Silicotuberculosis*. Singapore: Proc Int Union against Tuberculosis, 1986.

17 Pramatarov I. Investigation of the incidence of silicosis and silicotuberculosis among BCG vaccinated underground workers in the Rodopsk mine basin. *Gig Tr Prof Zabol* 1965; **9**: 41–9.

18 Paul R. Silicosis in Northern Rhodesia copper mines. *Arch Ind Health* 1961; **2**: 96.

19 International Agency for Research on Cancer. Monographs on the evaluation of carcinogenic risks to humans: 42. *Silica and Silicates*. Lyon: IARC, 1987: 111.

20 Steenland K, Stayner L. Silica, asbestos, man-made mineral fibres and cancer. *Cancer Causes Control* 1997; **8**: 491–503.

21 Finkelstein MM. Radiographic silicosis and lung cancer risk among workers in Ontario. *Am J Ind Med* 1998; **34**: 244–51.

22 De Klerk NH, Musk AW. Silica, compensated silicosis and lung cancer in Western Australian goldminers. *Occup Environ Med* 1998; **55**: 243–8.

23 Ulm K, Waschulzik B, Ehnes H, Guldner K, Thomasson B et al. Silica dust and lung cancer in the German stone, quarrying, and ceramics industries: results of a case-control study. *Thorax* 1999; **54**: 347–51.

24 Hnizdo E, Murray J, Klempman S. Lung cancer in relation to exposure to silica dust, silicosis and uranium production in South African gold miners. *Thorax* 1997; **52**: 271–5.

24a International Agency for Research on Cancer. Monographs on the evaluation of carcinogenic risks to humans: **68**. *Quartz*. Lyon: IARC, 1997.

25 Shi X, Castranova V, Halliwell B, Vallyathan V. Reactive oxygen species and silica-induced carcinogenesis. *J Toxicol Environ Hlth Crit Rev* 1998; **1**: 181–97.

26 Ng TP, Allan WGL, Tsin TW, O'Kelly FJ. Silicosis in jade workers. *Br J Ind Med* 1985; **42**: 761–4.

27 Clover JR, Bevan C, Cotes JE et al. Effects of exposure to slate dust in North Wales. *Br J Ind Med* 1980; **37**: 152–62.

28 Saiyed HN, Parikh DJ, Ghodasara NB et al. *Development and Progression of Silicosis in an Indian Slate Pencil Manufacturing Industry: A Longitudinal Study*. Proc VI Int

Pneumoconiosis Conf 1983, Bochum. Geneva: ILO, 1984: 1959–75.

29 Sheers G. Prevalence of pneumoconiosis in Cornish kaolin workers. *Br J Ind Med* 1964; **21:** 21–25.

30 Ogle CJ, Rundle EM, Sugar ET. China clay workers in the south west of England: analysis of chest radiograph readings, ventilatory capacity, and respiratory symptoms in relation to type and duration of occupation. *Br J Ind Med* 1989; **46:** 261–70.

31 Rundle EM, Sugar ET, Ogle CJ. Analyses of the 1990 chest health survey of china clay workers. *Br J Ind Med* 1993; **50:** 913–9.

32 Wagner JC, Pooley FD, Gibbs A, Lyons J, Sheers G, Moncrieff CB. Inhalation of china stone and china clay dust: relationship between the mineralogy of dust retained in the lungs and pathological changes. *Thorax* 1986; **41:** 190–6.

33 McLaughlin AIG, Rogers E, Dunham KC. Talc pneumoconiosis. *Br J Ind Med* 1949; **6:** 184–94.

34 Gamble J, Griefe A, Hancock J. An epidemiological industrial hygiene study of talc workers. *Ann Occup Hyg* 1982; **26:** 841–59.

35 Dement JM, Zumwalde RD, Gamble IF *et al. Occupational Exposure to Talc Containing Asbestos.* DHEW (NIOSH) Publication No. 80–115. Washington DC: US Govt Printing Office, 1980.

36 Amandus HE, Wheeler R, Armstrong B, McDonald AD, McDonald JC, Sebastien P. Mortality of vermiculite workers exposed to tremolite. VI International Symposium on Inhaled Particles, BOHS, Cambridge 1985. *Ann Occup Hyg* 1988; **32**(Suppl 1): 459–67.

37 Clark WC, Cralley LJ. *Pneumoconiosis in Diatomite Mining and Processing.* US Dept of Health/Education and Welfare Public Health Service Publication No. 601. Washington DC: US Dept of Health 1958.

38 McNally WD, Trostler IS. Severe pneumoconiosis caused by the inhalation of fullers earth. *J Ind Hyg Toxicol* 1941; **23:** 118–26.

39 Oakes D, Douglas R, Knight K, Wusterman M, McDonald JC. Respiratory effects of prolonged exposure to gypsum dust. *Ann Occup Hyg* 1982; **26:** 833–40.

40 Collis EL. Industrial pneumoconioses with special reference to dust-phthisis. *Publ Hlth* 1915; **28:** 252, 292; **29:** 11,37.

41 Gilson JC, Hugh-Jones P. *Lung Function in Coalworker's Pneumoconiosis.* Medical Research Council Special Report Series No. 290. London: HMSO, 1955.

42 Love RG, Miller BG, Groat SK, Hagen S, Cowie HA *et al.* Respiratory health effects of opencast coalmining: a cross sectional study of current workers. *Occup Environ Med* 1997; **54:** 416–23.

43 Soutar CA, Hurley JF. Relation between dust exposure and lung function in miners and ex-miners. *Br J Ind Med* 1986; **43:** 307–20.

44 Seixas NS, Robins TG, Attfield MD *et al.* Exposure-response relationships for coal mine dust and obstructive lung disease following enactment of the federal Coal

Mine Health and Safety Act of 1969. *Am J Ind Med* 1992; **21:** 715–34.

45 Hurley JF, Soutar CA. Can exposure to coal mine dust cause severe impairment of lung function? *Br J Ind Med* 1986; **3:** 150–7.

46 Coggon D, Newman Taylor A. Coal mining and chronic obstructive pulmonary disease: a review of the evidence. *Thorax* 1998; **53:** 398–407.

47 Cockcroft A, Lyons JP, Andersson N, Saunders MJ. Prevalence and relation to underground exposure of radiological irregular opacities in South Wales coalworkers with pneumoconiosis. *Br J Ind Med* 1983; **40:** 169–172.

48 Lyons JP, Ryder RC, Seal RME, Wagner JC. Emphysema in smoking and non-smoking coalworkers with pneumoconiosis. *Clin Resp Physiol* 1981; **17:** 75–85.

49 Cockcroft A, Seal RME, Wagner JC, Lyons JP, Ryder R, Andersson N. Post-mortem study of emphysema in coalworkers and non-coalworkers. *Lancet* 1982; **ii:** 600–3.

50 Ruckley VA, Gauld JS, Chapman JMC, Davis JMG, Douglas AN *et al.* Emphysema and dust exposure in a group of coalworkers. *Am Rev Respir Dis* 1984; **4:** 528–32.

51 Cockcroft A, Berry G, Cotes JE, Lyons JP. Shape of small opacities and lung function in coalworkers. *Thorax* 1982; **37:** 765–9.

52 Collins HPR, Dick JA, Bennett JG *et al.* Irregularly shaped small shadows on chest radiographs, dust exposure, and lung function in coalworkers' pneumoconiosis. *Br J Ind Med* 1988; **45:** 43–55.

53 Marine WM, Gurr D, Jacobsen M. Clinically important effects of dust exposure and smoking in British coal miners. *Am Rev Respir Dis* 1988; **137:** 106–12.

54 Seaton A. The new prescription: industrial injuries benefits for smokers? *Thorax* 1998; **53:** 335–6.

55 Rudd R. Coal miners' respiratory disease litigation. *Thorax* 1998; **53:** 337–40.

56 Lyons JP, Campbell H. Relation between progressive massive fibrosis, emphysema and pulmonary dysfunction in coalworkers' pneumoconiosis. *Br J Ind Med* 1981; **38:** 125–9.

57 Seal RME, Cockcroft A, Kung I, Wagner JC. Central lymph node involvement and progressive massive fibrosis in coalworkers. *Thorax* 1986; **41:** 531–7.

58 Cochrane AL. The attack rate of progressive massive fibrosis. *Br J Ind Med* 1962; **19:** 52–64.

59 Jacobsen M, Maclaren WM Unusual pulmonary observations and exposure to coal mine dust: a case-control study: Inhaled Particles V. *Ann Occup Hyg* 1982; **26:** 753–65.

60 Maclaren WM, Soutar CA. Progressive massive fibrosis and simple pneumoconiosis in ex-miners. *Br J Ind Med* 1985; **42:** 734–40.

61 Caplan A. Certain unusual radiological appearances in the chest of coal-miners suffering from rheumatoid arthritis. *Thorax* 1953; **8:** 29–37.

62 Elmes PC. Conflicts in the evidence on the health effect

of mineral fibres. In: Liddell D, Millar K eds. *Mineral Fibres and Health*. Boca Raton: CRC Press, 1991: 322–35.

63 Merewether ERA, Price CW. *Report on the Effect of Asbestos Dust on the Lungs and Dust Suppression in the Asbestos Industry*. London: HMSO, 1930.

64 Merewether ERA. *Annual report of the Chief Inspector of Factories for the Year 1947*. London: HMSO, 1949: 79.

65 Buchanan WD. Asbestososis and primary intrathoracic neoplasms. *Ann NY Acad Sci* 1965; **132:** 507–18.

66 Wagner JC, Sleggs CA, Marchand P. Diffuse pleural mesotheliomas and asbestos exposure in the north western Cape Province. *Br J Ind Med* 1960; **17:** 260–71.

67 Castleman BI. Asbestos and cancer: history and public policy. *Br J Ind Med* 1991; **48:** 427–30.

68 Murray R. Asbestos and cancer: history and public policy. *Br J Ind Med* 1991; **48:** 430–2.

69 Greenberg M. Attitudes and opinions: asbestos and cancer. *Am J Ind Med* 1992; **22:** 263–5.

70 Liddell FDK. Magic, menace, myth and malice. *Ann Occup Hyg* 1997; **41:** 3–12.

71 Liddell FDK, McDonald AD, McDonald JC. The 1891–1920 birth cohort of Quebec chrysotile miners and millers: development from 1904 and mortality to 1992. *Ann Occup Hyg* 1997; **41:** 13–36.

72 Zitting AJ, Karjalainen A, Impivaara O *et al.* Radiographic small lung opacities and pleural abnormalities in relation to smoking, urbanization status, and occupational asbestos exposure in Finland. *J Occup Environ Med* 1996; **38:** 602–9.

73 Berry G. Mortality of workers certified by pneumoconiosis medical panels as having asbestosis. *Br J Ind Med* 1981; **38:** 130–7.

74 Robinson BWS, Musk AW. Benign asbestos pleural effusion: diagnosis and course. *Thorax* 1981; **36:** 896–900.

75 Epler GR, McLoud TC, Gaensler EA. Prevalence and incidence of benign asbestos pleural effusion in a working population. *JAMA* 1982; **247:** 617–22.

76 Edler JL. A study of 16 cases of pleurisy with effusions in ex-miners from Wittenoom Gorge. *Aust NZ Med J* 1972; **2:** 328–9.

77 Elmes PC. Relative importance of cigarette smoking in occupational lung disease. *Br J Ind Med* 1981; **38:** 1–13.

78 Saracci R. Asbestos and lung cancer: an analysis of the epidemiological evidence on the asbestos-smoking interaction. *Int J Cancer* 1977; **20:** 323–31.

79 Peto J, Hodgson JT, Matthews FE, Jones JR. Continuing increase in mesothelioma mortality in Britain. *Lancet* 1995; **345:** 535–9.

80 Herbert A. Pathogenesis of pleurisy, pleural fibrosis and mesothelial proliferation. *Thorax* 1986; **41:** 176–89.

81 Elmes PC, Simpson MJC. Clinical aspects of mesothelioma. *Q J Med* 1976; **179:** 427–49.

82 Wagner JC, Pooley FD. Mineral fibres and mesothelioma. *Thorax* 1986; **41:** 161–6.

83 Elmes PC. Chrysotile appears 'more dangerous' than amphiboles in animals but 'less dangerous' in humans. In: Liddell D, Miller K eds. *Mineral Fibers and Health*. Boca Raton: CRC Press, 1991: 328–30.

84 Selikoff IJ, Hammond EC, Seidman H. Mortality experience of insulation workers in the United States and Canada, 1943–1976. *Ann NY Acad Sci* 1979; **330:** 91–116.

85 Acheson ED, Gardner MJ, Pippard EC, Grime LP. The mortality of two groups of women who manufactured gas masks from chrysotile and crocidolite asbestos. *Br J Ind Med* 1982; **39:** 344–8.

86 Berry G, Newhouse ML. Mortality of workers manufacturing friction materials using asbestos. *Br J Ind Med* 1983; **40:** 1–7.

87 Health and Safety Commission. *Asbestos at work: Control of Asbestos at Work Regulations 1987 Approved Code of Practice* 2nd edn. London: HMSO, 1993.

88 Samet JM, Shaikh RA. Asbestos in buildings. In: Harber P, Schenker MB, Balmes JR eds. *Occupational and Environmental Respiratory Disease*. St Louis: Mosby, 1996: 321–9.

89 Baris YI, Sahin AA, Ozesmi M. An outbreak or pleural mesothelioma and chronic fibrosing pleurisy in the village of Karain/Urgup in Anatolia. *Thorax* 1978; **33:** 181–92.

90 De Vuyst P, Dumortier P, Swaen GMH, Pairon JC, Brochard P. Respiratory health effects of man-made vitreous (mineral) fibres. *Eur Respir J* 1995; **8:** 2149–73.

91 Lockey JE. man-made fibers and non-asbestos fibrous silicates. In: Harber P, Schenker MB, Balmes JR eds. *Occupational and Environmental Respiratory Disease*. St Louis: Mosby, 1996: 330–44.

92 Lockey J, Lemasters G, Rice C *et al.* Refractory ceramic fiber exposure and pleural plaques. *Am J Respir Crit Care Med* 1996; **154:** 1405–10.

93 Kern DG, Crausman RS, Durand KTH, Nayer A, Kuhn C. Flock worker's lung: chronic interstitial lung disease in the nylon flocking industry. *Ann Intern Med* 1998; **129:** 261–72.

94 Moya C, Anto JM, Taylor AJN. Outbreak of organising pneumonia in textile printing sprayers. *Lancet* 1994; **343:** 498–502.

95 Camus PH, Nemery B. A novel cause for bronchiolitis obliterans organizing pneumonia: exposure to paint aerosols in textile workshops. *Eur Respir J* 1998; **11:** 259–62.

96 Nemery B. Lung disease from metal exposures. In: Banks DE, Parker JE eds. *Occupational Pulmonary Disease – An International Perspective*. London: Chapman & Hall,

97 Blanc PD, Boushey HA, Wong H, Wintermeyer SF, Bernstein MS. Cytokines in metal fume fever. *Am Rev Respir Dis* 1993; **147:** 134–8.

98 Rendall REG, Phillips JI, Renton KA Death following exposure to fine particulate nickel from a metal arc process. *Ann Occup Hyg* 1994; **38:** 921–30.

99 Levy BS, Hoffman L, Gottsegen S. Boilermakers

bronchitis. Respiratory tract irritation associated with vanadium pentoxide exposure during oil-to-coal conversion of a power plant. *J Occup Med* 1984; **26:** 567–70.

100 Allen MB, Crisp A, Snook N, Page RL. 'Smoke-bomb' pneumonitis. *Respir Med* 1992; **86:** 165–6.

101 Zhicheng S. Acute nickel carbonyl poisoning: a report of 179 cases. *Br J Ind Med* 1986; **43:** 422–4.

102 Cordasco EM, Stone FD. Pulmonary edema of environmental origin. *Chest* 1973; 182–185.

103 Davison AG, Newman Taylor AJ, Darbyshire J *et al*. Cadmium fume inhalation and emphysema. *Lancet* 1988; **i:** 663–7.

104 Kazantzis G, Lam TH, Sullivan KR. Mortality of cadmium-exposed workers. *Scand J Work Environ Hlth* 1988; **14:** 220–3.

105 Billings CG, Howard P. Occupational siderosis and welders' lung: a review. *Monaldi Arch Chest Dis* 1993; **48:** 304–14.

106 Sferlazza SJ, Beckett WS. The respiratory health of welders. *Am Rev Respir Dis* 1991; **143:** 134–48.

107 Coggon D, Inskip H, Winter P, Pannett B. Lobar pneumonia: an occupational disease in welders. *Lancet* 1994; **344:** 41–83.

108 Valenton H, Smidt U *et al*. Chronic bronchitis and occupational dust exposure. Cross-sectional study of occupational medicine on the significance of chronic inhalative burdens for the bronchopulmonary system. *Deutsche Forschungsgemeinschaft Boppard, Germany:* Harald Boldt KG, 1978, 503pp.

109 Chinn DJ, Stevenson IC, Cotes JE. Longitudinal respiratory survey of shipyard workers: effectc of trade and atopic status. *Br J Ind Med* 1990; **47:** 83–90.

110 Bernstein IL, Brooks SM, Nemery B. Metals. In: *Asthma in the Workplace* 2nd edn. Bernstein IL, Chan-Yeung M, Malo JL, Bernstein DI eds. New York: Dekker, 1999.

111 De Raeve H, Vandecasteele C, Demedts M, Nemery B. Dermal and respiratory sensitisation to chromate in a cement floorer. *Am J Ind Med* 1998; **34:** 169–76.

112 Davison AG, Haslam PL, Corrin B *et al*. Interstitial lung disease and asthma in hard-metal workers: bronchoalveolar lavage, ultrastructural, and analytical findings and results of bronchial provocation tests. *Thorax* 1983; **38:** 119–28.

113 Kusaka Y, Yokoyama K, Sera Y *et al*. Respiratory diseases in hard metal workers: an occupational hygiene study in a factory. *Br J Ind Med* 1986; **43:** 474–85.

114 Sjögren I, Hillerdal G, Andersson A, Zetterström O. Hard metal lung disease: importance of cobalt in coolants. *Thorax* 1980; **35:** 653–9.

115 Kongerud J, Boe J, Soyseth V, Naalsund A, Magnus P. Aluminium potroom asthma: the Norwegian experience. *Eur Respir J* 1994; **7:** 165–72.

116 Abramson MJ, Wlodarczyk JH, Saunders NA, Hensley MJ. Does aluminum smelting cause lung disease? *Am Rev Respir Dis* 1989; **139:** 1042–57.

117 Malo JL, Cartier A. Occupational asthma due to fumes of galvanized metal. *Chest* 1987; **92:** 375–7.

118 Weir DC, Robertson AS, Jones S, Burge PS. Occupational asthma due to soft corrosive soldering fluxes containing zinc chloride and ammonium chloride. *Thorax* 1989; **44:** 220–223.

119 Wang ZP, Larsson K, Malmberg P, Sjögren B, Hallberg BO, Wrangskog K. Asthma, Lung function and bronchial responsiveness in welders. *Am J Ind Med* 1994; **26:** 741–54.

120 Vandenplas O, Dargent F, Auverdin JJ *et al*. Occupational asthma due to gas metal arc welding on mild steel. *Thorax* 1995; **50:** 587–8.

121 Beach JR, Dennis JH, Avery AJ *et al*. An epidemiologic investigation of asthma in welders. *Am J Respir Crit Care Med* 1996; **154:** 1394–400.

122 Cone JE. Occupational lung cancer. *Occup Med* 1987; **2:** 273–95.

123 Samet JM, Kutvirt DM, Waxweilen RJ, Key CR Uranium mining and lung cancer in Navajo men. *N Engl J Med* 1984; **310:** 1481–4.

124 Archer VE. Lung cancer risks of underground miners: cohort and case-control studies. *Yale J Biol Med* 1998; **61:** 183–93.

125 Radford EP, Renard SKG. Lung cancer in Swedish iron miners exposed to low doses of radon daughters. *N Engl J Med* 1984; **310:** 1485–94.

126 Mur JM, Meyer-Bisch C, Pham QT *et al*. Risk of lung cancer among iron ore miners; a porportional mortality study of 1,075 deceased miners in Lorraine, France. *J Occup Med* 1987; **29:** 762–8.

127 Moulin JJ, Wild P, Romazini S, Lasfargues G, Peltier A *et al*. Lung cancer risk in hard-metal workers. *Am J Epidemiol* 1998; **148:** 241–8.

128 Hubbard R, Lewis S, Richards K, Johnston I, Britton J. Occupational exposure to metal or wood dust and aetiology of cryptogenic fibrosing alveolitis. *Lancet* 1996; **347:** 284–9.

129 Abraham JL, Burnett BR, Hunt A. Development and use of a pneumoconiosis database of human pulmonary inorganic particulate burden in over 400 lungs. *Scann Microsc* 1991; **5:** 95–108.

130 Dumortier P, De Vuyst P, Yernault JC. Non-fibrous inorganic particles in human bronchoalveolar lavage fluids. *Scann Microsc* 1989; **3:** 1207–18.

131 Funahashi A, Schlueter DP, Pintar K, Bemis EL, Siegesmund, KA. Welders' pneumoconiosis: tissue elemental microanalysis by energy dispersive X-ray analysis. *Br J Ind Med* 1988; **45:** 14–18.

132 Dinman BD. Alumina-related pulmonary disease. *J Occup Med* 1988; **30:** 328–35.

133 Jederlinic PJ, Abraham JL, Churg A, Himmelstein JS, Epler GR, Gaensler E A. Pulmonary fibrosis in aluminum oxide workers. Investigation of nine workers, with pathologic examination and microanalysis in three of them. *Am Rev Respir Dis* 1990; **142:** 1179–84.

134 Rom WN, Lockey JE, Jeffrey LS *et al*. Pneumoconiosis and exposure of dental laboratory technicians. *Am J Publ Hlth* 1984; **74:** 1252–7.

135 Choudat D. Occupational lung disease among dental technicians. *Tubercle Lung Dis* 1994; **75:** 99–104.

136 Kotloff RM, Richman PS, Greenacre JK, Rossman MD. Chronic beryllium disease in a dental laboratory technician. *Am Rev Respir Dis* 1993; **147:** 205–7.

137 De Vuyst P, Van de Weyer R, Decoster A *et al.* Dental technician's pneumoconiosis. A report of two cases. *Am Rev Respir Dis* 1986; **133:** 316–20.

138 Peters JM, Smith TJ, Bernstein L, Wright WE, Hammond SK. Pulmonary effects of exposures in silicon carbide manufacturing. *Br J Ind Med* 1984; **41:** 109–114.

139 Funahashi A, Schlueter DP, Pintar K, Siegesmund KA, Mandel GS, Mandel NS. Pneumoconiosis in workers exposed to silicon carbide. *Am Rev Respir Dis* 1984; **129:** 635–40.

140 Newman LS. Beryllium disease and sarcoidosis: clinical and laboratory links. *Sarcoidosis* 1995; **12:** 7–19.

141 Newman LS, Maier LA, Nemery B. Interstitial lung disorders due to beryllium and cobalt. Schwartz MI, King TE Jr eds. *Interstitial Lung disease* 3rd edn. St Louis: Mosby, 1998: 367–92.

142 Newman LS, Kreiss K. Non-occupational beryllium disease masquerading as sarcoidosis: identification by blood lymphocyte proliferative response to beryllium. *Am Rev Respir Dis* 1992; **145:** 1212–4.

143 Mroz MM, Kreiss K, Lezotto DC, Campbell PA, Newman LS. Reexamination of the blood lymphocyte transformation test in the diagnosis of chronic beryllium disease. *J All Clin Immunol* 1991; **88:** 54–60.

144 Kreiss K, Wasserman S, Mroz MM, Newman LS. Beryllium disease screening in the ceramics industry. *J Occup Med* 1993; **35:** 267–74.

145 Richeldi L, Sorrentino R, Saltini C. HLA-DPB1 Glutamate 69: a genetic marker of beryllium disease. *Science* 1993; **262:** 242–4.

146 Kreiss K, Mroz MM, Zhen B, Martyny JW, Newman LS. Epidemiology of beryllium sensitization and disease in nuclear workers. *Am Rev Respir Dis* 1993; **148:** 985–91.

147 Kreiss K, Mroz MM, Newman LS, Martyny J, Zhen B. Machining risk of beryllium disease and sensitization with median exposures below 2 µg/m^3. *Am J Ind Med* 1996; **30:** 16–25.

148 Liippo KK, Anttila SL, Taikina-Aho O, Ruokonen EL, Toivonen ST, Tuomi T. Hypersensitivity pneumonitis and exposure to zirconium silicate in a young ceramic tile worker. *Am Rev Respir Dis* 1993; **148:** 1089–92.

149 Schneider J, Freitag F, Rödelsperger K. Durch Zirkonium-Einwirkung am Arbeitsplatz verursachte exogen-allergische Alveolitis (Nr.4201 BeKV). *Arbeitsmedizin Sozialmed Umweltmedizin* 1994; **29:** 382–5. (Abstract)

150 Bartter T, Irwin RS, Abraham JL *et al.* Zirconium compound-induced pulmonary fibrosis. *Arch Intern Med* 1991; **151:** 1197–201.

151 Redline S, Barna BP, Tomashefski JF Jr, Abraham JL. Granulomatous disease associated with pulmonary deposition of titanium. *Br J Ind Med* 1986; **43:** 652–6.

152 De Vuyst P, Dumortier P, Schandené L, Estenne M, Verhest A, Yernault JC. Sarcoidlike lung granulomatosis induced by aluminium dust. *Am Rev Respir Dis* 1987; **135:** 493–7.

153 Haley PJ. Pulmonary toxicity of stable and radioactive lanthanides. *Hlth Phys* 1991; **61:** 809–20.

154 Pairon JC, Roos F, Sébastien P *et al.* Biopersistence of cerium in the human respiratory tract and ultrastructural findings. *Am J Ind Med* 1995; **27:** 349–58.

155 Waring PM, Watling RJ. Rare earth deposits in a deceased movie projectionist. A new case of rare earth pneumoconiosis? *Med J Aust* 1990; **153:** 726–30.

156 McDonald JW, Ghio AJ, Sheehan CE, Bernhardt PF, Roggli VL. Rare earth (cerium oxide) pneumoconiosis: analytical scanning electron microscopy and literature review. *Modern Pathol* 1995; **8:** 859–65.

157 Cugell DW, Morgan WKC, Perkins DG, Rubin A. The respiratory effects of cobalt. *Arch Intern Med* 1990; **150:** 177–83.

158 Demedts M, Gheysens B, Nagels J *et al.* Cobalt lung in diamond polishers. *Am Rev Respir Dis* 1984; **130:** 130–5.

159 Figueroa S, Gerstenhaber B, Welch L, Klimstra D, Smith GJ, Beckett W. Hard metal interstitial pulmonary disease associated with a form of welding in a metal parts coating plant. *Am J Ind Med* 1992; **21:** 363–73.

160 Ohori NP, Sciurba FC, Owens GR, Hodgson MJ, Yousem SA. Giant-cell interstitial pneumonia and hard-metal pneumoconiosis. A clinicopathological study of four cases and review of the literature. *Am J Surg Pathol* 1989; **13:** 581–7.

161 Lison D, Lauwerys R, Demedts M, Nemery B. Experimental research into the pathogenesis of cobalt/hard metal lung disease. *Eur Respir J* 1996; **9:** 1024–8.

162 Lison D. Human toxicity of cobalt-containing dust and experimental studies on the mechanism of interstitial lung disease (hard metal disease). *Crit Rev Toxicol* 1993; **26:** 585–616.

163 Swennen B, Buchet JP, Stanescu D, Lison D, Lauwerys R. Epidemiological survey of workers exposed to cobalt oxides, cobalt salts, and cobalt metal. *Br J Ind Med* 1993; **50:** 835–42.

164 Frost AE, Keller CA, Brown RW *et al.* Giant cell interstitial pneumonitis. Disease recurrence in the transplanted lung. *Am Rev Respir Dis* 1993; **148:** 1401–4.

165 Nemery B, Nagels J, Verbeken E, Dinsdale D, Demedts M. Rapidly fatal progression of cobalt-lung in a diamond polisher. *Am Rev Respir Dis* 1990; **141:** 1373–8.

36

Problems from indoor air in non-industrial workplaces

P SHERWOOD BURGE

Legionella pneumophila	709	Allergic rhinitis	713
Extrinsic allergic alveolitis	711	Sick building syndrome	713
Humidifier fever	712	References	718
Asthma	713		

The non-industrial indoor environment, such as is found in offices and schools, has traditionally been regarded as safe. The discovery of legionnaires' disease, killing 29 conference delegates staying in a Philadelphia hotel in 1976, and the discovery of extrinsic allergic alveolitis, humidifier fever and asthma caused by humidification systems in office buildings has changed this perception. During the investigation of humidifier fever it became apparent that a much more common group of symptoms, now known as the sick building syndrome or building sickness, was present in office workers. Office workers have been studied as there are fewer confounding factors present in their working environment than in workers in schools, shops and hospitals, where similar diseases occur. This chapter will review these diseases.

LEGIONELLA PNEUMOPHILA

Legionellae are a group of bacterial microorganisms of the genus Legionella which grow at increased temperature and require special nutrients on culture plates for their growth (buffered charcoal yeast extract with 4 days incubation). These two factors delayed the discovery that these organisms were an important cause of lobar pneumonia.[1,2]

Retrospective analysis of stored serum samples has shown that pneumonia in the 1940s was caused by these organisms. A surveillance of the incidence of legionnaires' disease has been maintained by the Centre for Disease Control for England and Wales, based largely on laboratory reports (and has therefore depended on the enthusiasm of clinicians sending appropriate specimens) since 1980. Cases can be divided into those acquired during travel; those of non-travel clusters; those acquired in hospital (nosocomial); and sporadic cases. Travel-associated cases are the most common, acquired mostly from hotel hot water systems and account for 46% of all notifications (of these only 10% were from hotels in the United Kingdom). The majority of community-acquired cases were thought to be sporadic (see below) and account for 36% of reports; 10% of all notifications were from outbreaks in the community, and 8% were possibly or definitely acquired in hospitals. This latter group is the only one which has shown a sustained fall in incidence since 1980 (Fig. 36.1). The estimates of incidence of disease vary between 0.5 and 10.6 per million per year, with a mode of about 3 per million.[3] The epidemic cases occur with both indoor and outdoor air contamination. The type species, Legionella pneumophila, are found widely in nature in wet surroundings; they are, however, capable of colonizing cooling towers and hot water systems. Colonization of cooling towers is favoured when bacteria are disturbed from nearby soil during building work and ploughing. The organisms multiply in the warm water of the cooling tower and are spread in the form of an aerosol to the surrounding area. Most cases occur in those exposed outdoors, such as in the outbreak from the rooftop cooling towers at the British Broadcasting Corporation (BBC) building in London in 1988,[4] where there were 95 cases of pneumonia and three deaths. Deposition of the infected droplet nuclei is very patchy and depends on the air currents induced by the

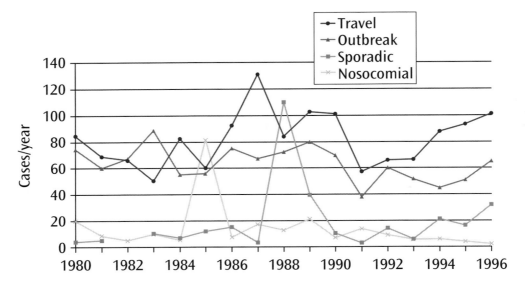

Figure 36.1 *Incidence of legionnaires' disease in the UK.*

surrounding buildings. The aerosol from cooling towers may enter the intake of air conditioning systems, distributing infected droplet nuclei around a building. This type of spread probably accounted for the outbreak at Stafford District General hospital in 1985 in which 101 cases occurred and 28 patients died,[5,6] and also the outbreak at the Glasgow Royal infirmary.[7] Both were made possible by the design of the air intake which was in a position where aerosol from cooling towers could enter.

There is evidence that many 'sporadic' cases of legionnaires' disease may be related to a common source. Bhopal and colleagues tested this hypothesis on the Scottish case data for 1978–1986.[8–10] To undertake these studies there needs to be a register of cases and of likely sources, particularly cooling towers. The risk of legionnaires' disease was related to the distance from the nearest cooling tower, with a relative risk of 3 for those within 500 meters compared with those more than 2 km away. They found that 28% of sporadic cases appeared to be related in time and place suggesting mini-outbreaks that had not been recognized at the time. When these clusters were excluded there still remained a significant relationship between incidence and distance from a cooling tower. The source of infection in sporadic cases may sometimes be in the patient's home. An ongoing study of domestic sources of legionellae from patients' homes has so far identified few homes with legionellae in the domestic hot water system (G Raw, pers. comm.).

Cooling towers must be maintained obsessionally to keep them safe, with regular cleaning and hyperchlorination (guidance notes are available from the UK Health and Safety Executive[11,12]). There is often insufficient supervision and training of those managing such systems. The compulsory notification of the presence of

cooling towers and evaporative condensers has allowed the recognition of their neighbourhood cases.[8,13] In Queensland, compulsory registration has resulted in fewer cases of legionnaires' disease. Following the Stafford District General Hospital outbreak in the West Midlands region of the UK, in 1985, air-cooled units have replaced evaporative cooling towers in all the region's hospitals. These require much less maintenance and cannot lead to aerosol emissions.

Hot water systems are the more usual source of legionellae in hotels and hospitals, where large volumes of hot water are used. Legionellae are killed by heating to over 60°C, as occurs in most small hot water systems. If water is drawn off before the water reaches 60°C, a particular problem with some calorifiers, or if the water cools in long blind loops of piping, or if the cold water supply is warmed by adjacent hot water piping, the possibility of legionella growth occurs. Some washer and jointing materials in taps, showerheads and piping also favour this.[14] *Legionella* infection derived from hot water systems usually results from aerosol spread from showers. Other outbreaks have resulted from jacuzzis and hotel fountains, which incorporate recirculated warm water. Humidifiers in air conditioning systems are unlikely sources as the water temperature is usually too low for legionella growth.

Legionnaires' disease is a lobar pneumonia, which in sporadic cases is indistinguishable from the more common pneumococcal pneumonia, and less common causes such as mycoplasma and Q fever. Legionnaires' disease tends to be associated with more confusion, more hyponatraemia and perhaps a poorer prognosis than other causes of lobar pneumonia. The diagnosis can be made by finding antigen in lung secretions or urine (diagnosis within a few hours), by positive culture taking about 5 days and needing special culture media, or by finding a fourfold increase in antibody after the infection. Positive titres are sometimes not achieved for a month after infection. As convalescent samples of blood are often not taken from patients who have recovered from pneumonia, and as culture and antigen detection are not widely available, many cases are likely to go undiagnosed. A number of other species of *Legionella* have been associated with pneumonia, the majority in immunosuppressed patients in hospital.[15]

There are no clinical trials of treatment of legionnaires' disease. Erythromycin used to be the treatment of choice, but has been replaced by ofloxacin or ciprofloxacin 800–1000 mg/day. Clarithromycin is probably superior to erythromycin, and rifampicin can be added to any regimen probably with benefit.[16]

There are substantial problems in assessing antibiotic sensitivities *in vitro*. Legionellae are intracellular organisms, standard cell-free culture media depend on the media used, and results do not correlate well with other methods of sensitivity testing. Infected microphage cell lines can be used to test intracellular sensitivities. In general there is a good relationship between intracellular sensitivity testing and clinical response, the main exception being gentamicin which works well in tissue culture but is inactive in animal models, which are the final way of sensitivity testing.

Positive titres of antibody against *Legionella* species are found in workers exposed to infected aerosol systems who do not develop pneumonia. The first confirmed outbreak occurred in a public health office in Pontiac, Michigan, USA, in 1968, and was called Pontiac fever. The attack rate was over 90%, the disease was short-lived with fever and a flu-like illness.[17] In retrospect this is probably a variety of humidifier fever. It is not clear why some subjects become infected with pneumonia and some develop the flu-like illness, but it is possible that Pontiac fever is caused by soluble antigen rather than viable whole organisms. A large number of staff in the Stafford District General hospital outbreak were exposed to the same aerosol system which resulted in the cases of pneumonia in patients. Only one member of staff fulfilled the case-definition for pneumonia; however, in nurses working regularly in the wards supplied by the contaminated cooling tower, 80% developed positive titres to legionellae, with about 30% of all the hospital staff sampled having titres of 1:16 or greater.[5,6] These workers reported no severe disease at the time, but in retrospect had a higher incidence of a flu-like illness at the time of the outbreak. A follow-up study of those with high titres suggests effects lasting some years after exposure.[18] An outbreak of Pontiac fever has also been caused by *Legionella feeleii* contaminating a water/oil emulsion used as a coolant in an engineering factory,[19] a situation where occupational asthma is more common.

EXTRINSIC ALLERGIC ALVEOLITIS

Extrinsic allergic alveolitis is occasionally caused by indoor air pollution (see Chapter 34). Banaszak first described extrinsic allergic alveolitis due to contamination of the indoor air in office workers in 1970, when four workers in an office building became ill.[20] The source of the alveolitis was warm water from the humidifier which was growing *Micropolyspora faeni* (the same organism responsible for most cases of farmer's lung). There have been several other outbreaks with similar causes, mostly related to home cool mist and furnace humidifiers,[21,22] and others where the exact cause is uncertain.[23,24] Other outbreaks have been attributed to *Thermoactinomyces vulgaris* and *Aspergillus fumigatus*,[25] which are also well recognized causes of extrinsic allergic alveolitis in other circumstances, particularly in farmers. Other implicated organisms include *Penicillium* species, particularly *Penicillium chrysogenum* and *Penicillium cyclopium*, *Aureobasidium pululans*, *Bacillus subtilis*, *Cephalosporium* species and *Sphaeropsidales* species. All of these grow preferentially in warm water. Cold water spray humidifiers may become contaminated with different organisms and at least one outbreak of allergic alveolitis was unrelated to thermophilic actinomyces.[26] In this outbreak the humidifier of a printing works, where the water was maintained at 15°C, became heavily contaminated with many microorganisms.

One outbreak in a textile works was found to be due to a previously unknown organism *Cytophaga allerginae*.[27] This organism was isolated from among 700 found in the humidifier as the one most likely to be the cause of the disease from serological testing. The antibodies were directed to an endotoxin produced by this organism, rather than the whole organism, which might explain the problems others have had in identifying specific organisms as the cause of disease. *Cytophaga allerginae* has some antigenic similarities to flavobacteria, with which it was originally confused.

Japan has been the centre of fairly widespread allergic alveolitis due to *Trichosporon cutaneum*, a fungus which grows particularly well in the wooden houses in the temperate and more tropical areas. Women who stay at home are affected twice as often as their men. Symptoms occur from May to October, giving it the name of (Japanese) summer type allergic alveolitis (hypersensitivity pneumonitis).[28] *Trichosporon cutaneum* is thermophilic preferring temperatures of 25–28°C. There are three serotypes with distinct antigens. Smokers have less disease as with other causes of extrinsic allergic alveolitis, those with human leucocyte antigen (HLA) DQw3 seem particularly susceptible. The disease is becoming less common, perhaps due to better housing.

HUMIDIFIER FEVER

The symptoms of humidifier fever are similar to those of extrinsic allergic alveolitis with fever, sweating, and aches in the limbs, sometimes breathlessness and wheeze. Again characteristically it starts 6–8 hours after exposure but continued exposure leads to tolerance. Attacks are usually worse following a break from work such as over the weekend and commonly occur on the first day of work only, although longer attacks may occur. There are no known long-term sequelae of humidifier fever and complete recovery is always thought to occur. The chest radiograph is always normal in this disease (nodular shadows occur in about half of the cases of extrinsic allergic alveolitis). It is unclear why some patients develop extrinsic allergic alveolitis and some humidifier fever. The same contaminated humidifier may give rise to both diseases. The precipitating antibodies in the blood are similarly positive in both diseases and again relate more to exposure than to the disease itself and are more common in non-smokers than smokers with the same exposure.[29] Many of the outbreaks have occurred in the printing industry, perhaps because such factories have been humidified for a long time and tend to have older humidifiers, partly perhaps because of the paper dust in the air which forms a good substrate for microbial growth.

Both humidifier fever and extrinsic allergic alveolitis can be reproduced in individuals by exposing them to extracts of the contaminated humidifier water.[26,30,31] An example of such a challenge is shown in Fig. 36.2 where the worker has kept a symptom diary following exposure to a control solution and to antigen from a humidifier on separate days. The challenges were repeated on two consecutive days; the figure shows that the reaction was much less on the second day than on the first day demonstrating that tolerance had developed. Most outbreaks of building-related extrinsic allergic alveolitis have resulted from exposure to aerosol systems from a mixed growth of a wide range of organisms, many of which have not been identified.[27,32] In some reports individual organisms have been thought to be the cause;[33] however, strict proof of this is usually lacking. There seem to be cross-reacting antibodies between the antigens from some, but not all, outbreaks. Most contaminated humidifiers contain amoebae as well as bacteria and fungi. The amoebae have been thought to be the cause of the symptoms on the grounds of antibody detection in affected individuals; however, antibody levels do not differentiate between those with and without disease, and are likely to be another example of cross-reacting antibodies, as the amoebae ingest the bacteria also present in contaminated humidifiers.[34] Currently, opinion as to the cause of humidifier fever is divided between individual organisms, and a soluble product (perhaps endotoxin) from these organisms. It is possible that disease which progresses with successive exposure, such as typical extrinsic allergic alveolitis, requires sensitization to particular and specific organisms, while disease that remits despite repeated exposure, such as humidifier fever, is less dependent on specific organisms, and may be due to toxins derived from the organisms.[35]

Occupants who do not develop allergic alveolitis or humidifier fever also develop precipitating antibodies in the blood directed against the relevant antigens. They are more a measure of exposure than disease. They can, however, be used as a method of biological monitoring to see if the source of the contamination has been controlled, as the levels decline after exposure ceases.

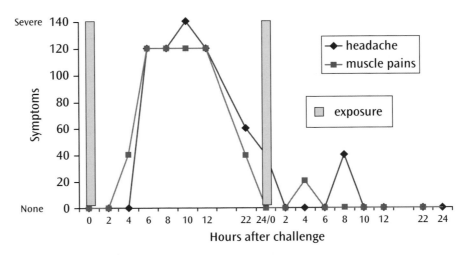

Figure 36.2 *An extract of water from the workplace humidifier was nebulized for 5 minutes each morning for two successive mornings, in a worker with humidifier fever. The record shows the results of hourly diary card assessments of symptoms. Following the first exposure headache and muscle pains start after 6 hours and resolve within 24 hours. There is no reaction on the second day showing that tolerance has developed.*

ASTHMA (See Chapter 33)

Asthma is sometimes due to indoor air pollution, mostly in office buildings with either humidifiers or chillers which have become microbially contaminated.[32] Solomon reported two cases due to contamination of home mist vaporizers with *Rhodotorula*.[36] Indoor plants in offices have caused outbreaks of occupational asthma, particularly in those who care for them, when up to 25% may become sensitized.[37] The Weeping Fig (*Ficus benjamina*) is most commonly involved; the antigen comes from the material secreted by the leaves, which is increased when humidity levels are low.[38] Spathe flowers (*Spathiphyllum walisii*) have also been implicated.[39] The materials used to clean buildings can cause occupational asthma, both in the cleaners themselves, and those exposed to the residues that were not present when the cleaning took place. Cleaners have been found to be at excess risk for occupational asthma from community-based surveys.[40,41] Individuals have been described with occupational asthma due to benzalkonium chloride,[42,43] amongst other cleaning materials. Many modern floor and surface cleaners now contain biocides, which leave residues capable of inhalation later.

ALLERGIC RHINITIS

Rhinitis may also be caused by microbial contamination of the indoor environment, and the other agents causing occupational asthma. Rhinitis is also a common symptom in the sick building syndrome; whether it is due to allergy or not is so far unknown

SICK BUILDING SYNDROME

The main symptoms comprising the sick building syndrome relate to the eyes, nose, throat and skin, together with what are often called general symptoms of headache and lethargy. All these symptoms are common in the general population, the distinguishing feature which makes them part of the sick building syndrome is their temporal relationship with work in a particular building. All but skin symptoms should improve within a few hours of leaving a problem building, dryness of the skin may take a few days to improve. The principal symptoms are as follows:

- *Lethargy*
  A general feeling of tiredness is often the most prevalent symptom.[44] It usually starts within a few hours of coming to work, and improves within minutes of leaving the building. A variant is more severe, with recovery taking some hours away from the building. Symptoms may be seasonal in northern climates, being worse in the winter months, suggesting a relationship with sunlight.
- *Headache*
  The typical headache is non-migrainous, and is often described as a pressure on the head. In Scandinavia an associated symptom of heavy headedness is often prevalent. The headache is rarely throbbing, usually being described as dull. It does not often occur over the face, making an association with rhinitis or sinus disease less likely.
- *Blocked nose*
  Eye, nose and throat symptoms are often grouped together as mucous membrane symptoms. The most common is the sensation of a blocked or stuffy nose. True rhinitis with sneezing and running of the nose is much less common. The latter are the typical symptoms of allergic rhinitis due to an inhaled allergen. Their lack makes an allergic mechanism for nasal blockage less likely.
- *Dry throat*
  A feeling of dryness of the throat, perhaps associated with increased thirst, is the next most prevalent mucous membrane symptom. It can be a particular problem in those who use their voice professionally, such as broadcasters or telephonists (these two groups often being housed in internal areas of buildings away from extraneous sources of noise).
- *Dry eyes*
  Although the least prevalent mucous membrane symptom, it can cause particular problems in those wearing contact lenses, who may not be able to use them throughout the day. Objective signs include reduced foam in the inner epicanthus, and increased tear-film break-up time.[45–47]
- *Dryness of the skin*
  Dryness of the skin is the most difficult symptom to elicit from questionnaires, which generally require a symptom to improve on days away from the building to be classed as a work-related symptom. The more prolonged recovery of skin dryness may lead to its under-recognition. There is a specific facial rash related to visual display unit (VDU) use which is very rarely identified, and may be related to precipitation of charged particulates onto the face.[48–50]

Causes of the sick building syndrome

Although there is a general agreement on the principal symptoms of the sick building syndrome, it does not necessarily imply that the causes for each symptom are the same, particularly as the mechanism underlying the symptoms are largely unknown. The ability of a study to identify a factor associated with a particular symptom requires a wide distribution of that factor between different workers. It is not therefore possible to identify a factor such as temperature to be associated with symptoms if all the workers studied come from areas with very similar ambient temperatures. Epidemiological studies can generally only detect an association of a factor with a symptom. Identifying that factor as causal is more difficult, and is favoured by consistency between different studies, the strength of the association, and a dose–response relationship. It is best confirmed by an experimental approach with blind alteration of that factor with independent monitoring of workers' symptoms. Such studies are in practice very difficult to achieve in the workplace; for instance it is very difficult to change the temperature, humidity or airflow individually without changing one of the other factors.[51] It is easy to jump to conclusions from worker interviews, as most workers attribute their symptoms to something they perceive in their environment. For instance many workers perceive the indoor air to be dry. There is, however, a very poor relationship between dryness of the air as perceived by an individual and the water content measured in the air.[52] It is likely that the perception of dryness in the air relates more to increased temperature and particulates in the air than to water content; one study showed a four-fold reduction in perceived air dryness following air filtration, without changing the water content of the air.[53] The situation in radiography departments is compounded by the belief that the problems are caused by chemicals in the developer. If the problem is assumed to be chemical contaminant, the measurement of very low levels of aldehydes and amines in the air can result in the environment being classed as satisfactory, whereas in reality the wrong measurements may have been made.

The symptoms of the sick building syndrome may be due to personal factors, individual exposures in the workplace, to organizational factors or to the building itself and its services.

PERSONAL FACTORS

Most studies find more symptomatic women than men, even after adjusting for the place in occupant hierarchy, which also shows more symptoms in those lower down the hierarchy.[44,54–56] The reasons for the sex difference are unknown. More important building occupants usually occupy less crowded areas of the office, which is better maintained, and have higher priority from building services personnel; these factors are likely to contribute to the reduced symptoms seen in managers.

ORGANIZATIONAL FACTORS

There are striking differences in the levels of stress and workload seen in the occupants of different buildings investigated in multibuilding studies. In particular, studies which have included both government and public sector buildings have shown increased symptoms in the public sector buildings.

One building has been investigated with both public sector and private sector occupants.[44] Both were similarly sick. Available evidence suggests that the differences are due to the poorer buildings occupied by the public sector and their less careful maintenance. There are several studies of different buildings occupied by the same employer. They show a wide range of symptoms between buildings which are sometimes interconnected, suggesting that the main determinant is the building and its maintenance[57] rather than the philosophy of management.

There are a number of individual exposures in the workplace which have been associated with symptoms, the most important are use of VDUs, paper use and cigarette smoke.

VISUAL DISPLAY UNITS

Several studies have shown a fairly weak but positive relationship between the number of hours spent working with a VDU and the symptoms of sick building syndrome. The mechanisms are unknown, but could relate to the lack of freedom experienced by a worker whose tasks and speed of work are determined by the computer rather than themselves. One study only found increased symptoms when working for 7 or more hours a day with a VDU,[58] in favour of such a mechanism; other studies have, however, shown an effect when the VDU is used for fewer hours.[54,59] There appears to be a rare but specific facial rash due to VDU use, perhaps due to precipitation of charged air particulates on the skin.[50]

PAPER

There is an association between the amount of paper handled and the symptoms of sick building syndrome in some studies, particularly those in low-technology government departments.[54] 'No carbon required' paper has also been associated with respiratory and dermal symptoms, perhaps due to release of the inks encapsulated on the back of the top sheets. This may be a particular problem during paper shredding.[60] Paper is a major contributor to the fibrous dust associated with symptoms in some studies.

CIGARETTE SMOKE

Cigarette smoke is the major preventable cause of indoor air pollution in office buildings where smoking is permitted. It is likely that smokers complain of less sick building syndrome symptoms than non-smokers (a variant of the healthy smoker effect). Non-smokers who work in a room with smokers have more symptoms than those working in a smoke-free environment.[61,62] The major source of environmental tobacco exposure in non-smokers is at work.[63] One study has shown a reduction of symptoms when smoking was stopped in the workplace.[64] Other studies have not shown an effect of cigarette smoke on symptoms; however smokers and non-smokers were not separated and the levels of exposure in the workplace were low.[65]

X-RAY CHEMICALS IN HOSPITALS

A postal survey of radiographers in New Zealand enquired about the frequency of 19 disorders in the previous year.[66] The most frequent were headache, sore eyes, lethargy, sore throat, nasal discharge and sinus problems. These are very similar to the common sick building syndrome symptoms, although they were attributed to darkroom fumes at the time. Glutaraldehyde is present in x-ray developer, and has been associated with eye, nose and throat irritation in endoscopy workers.[67] The working conditions in radiography departments can often be improved.[68] Glutaraldehyde has been shown to cause occupational asthma in radiography department staff, including a secretary who reacted to newly processed films.[69] In other situations constituents of the developer[70] or fixative[71] apart from glutaraldehyde have been implicated.

BUILDING FACTORS

After adjustment for the factors described above, the average number of work-related symptoms per building occupant (the building symptom index), still shows a four- to fivefold difference between good and bad buildings.[44] The building symptom index is stable over time, provided that proper sampling is used to avoid responder bias, and a sample size of about 100 is used.[57] In general, naturally ventilated buildings have fewer symptomatic occupants than those from air-conditioned offices,[44] despite measurements of air quality being better in the air-conditioned buildings. It seems that the major factors controlled by air-conditioning can have both positive and negative effects, the balance often being decided by post-design factors, particularly plant and system maintenance.[57] The main factors which have been studied include fresh air ventilation rates, temperature, humidity, dust and the microbial content of the air. Finding an association between these factors and symptoms does not, however, imply that altering that factor is likely to reduce symptoms. It is quite likely that all of them are surrogate makers of the underlying causes. Similar problems have been found in hospitals,[72,73] where the confounding factors of allergens such as latex, infected patients and a more mobile workforce present problems with epidemiological studies of sick building syndrome.

VENTILATION RATE

Increasing ventilation helps dilute pollutants generated by the building fabric, the office machinery and its occupants, but increases exposure to pollutants which may be generated by the ventilation system and its ducting. There are studies showing a relationship between ventilation rate and symptoms,[74] and others which fail to show a relationship.[74] Within air-conditioned buildings it is likely that low ventilation rates of less than 10 litres per second per person are associated with increased symptoms. Studies which have failed to show an effect of changing ventilation rate have generally included only values higher than this. Some studies have shown increased symptoms with increasing ventilation, suggesting that pollutants from the plant are the dominant cause in these cases.[75] This effect has also been shown in mechanically ventilated buildings without air-conditioning, particularly relating to skin and nasal symptoms.[76]

TEMPERATURE

Increasing symptoms with temperatures above 23°C has been one of the more consistent findings in Northern European studies.[54,57,77] There is, however, an association between increasing temperature, overcrowding and inadequate ventilation which makes it difficult to pinpoint the causative factor.

HUMIDITY

Many workers attribute their dry eyes, dry throat and blocked nose to their perception of dryness of the air. There is an association between the two during questionnaire studies; there is not, however, an association between the perception of air dryness and the water content of the air.[52] There is an association between the presence of a humidifier in the air-conditioning circuit and symptoms, rather than the reverse.[44] As with many other factors humidity can be good and bad. In parts of Scandinavia the humidity may be below 10% for the winter months, there is some evidence that increasing this to around 25% is associated with decreasing symptoms.[51] In more temperate climates the humidity indoors rarely falls below 25% and humidifiers in these circumstances can do more harm than good. Humidifiers in the ventilation circuit provide a place for microbes to flourish, and also provide a reason for adding biocides to humidified water. Many of these biocides are irritants or allergens in their own right, e.g. isothiazolinones,[78-80] glutaraldehyde,[69,81] chloramine,[82] chlorhexidine,[83] benzalkonium chloride[43] and chlorine.[84,85] Their addition to the water used for humidification will result in exposure to the building occupants.[79] There are so far no intervention studies investigating biocides in air-conditioning systems. They provide a plausible cause for the increased symptoms seen in systems containing a humidifier. In other areas dehumidifiers and chillers can be a potential problem. Water removed from the air can become stagnant and act as a reservoir for microbial growth in the air-conditioning system. Many chillers are situated in ceiling and wall spaces where maintenance is difficult. Microbial contamination of chiller condensate trays has caused asthma in one English office.

FRESHNESS OF THE AMBIENT AIR

There are no generally agreed methods of assessing the freshness of indoor air. Fanger has developed units of smell emission (the olf, defined as the smell emission derived from a standard non-smoking person having 0.7 baths per day) and perceived effect (the decipol, the smell in a 10 m³ room containing the standard man, ventilated with fresh air at 10 litres/second). Decipols are measured using a panel of trained sniffers.[86,87] They can be used to find the source of smells, such as sampling air before and after filters in the air supply ducting. He has shown that the building itself, its ventilation system, the contents such as carpets and furnishings, and its inhabitants, are all measurable sources. For instance the average smoker emits 6 olfs, against 1 for a non-smoker. There is an assumption that all smells are bad. This approach is leading to the quantification and hopefully the elimination of sources.

BACTERIA AND FUNGI

The role of indoor air microbial contamination in the aetiology of sick building syndrome is less clear than with alveolitis, humidifier fever and asthma. From an epidemiological point of view buildings with humidifiers and chillers have more problems than buildings without these.[44,88] There are few adequate studies of the relationship between microbial contamination with viable organisms and building sickness, but current evidence does not support a direct relationship between the two. British office buildings studied by Pickering showed that the average levels for all buildings were under 1000 colony forming units (cfu)/m³.[89] Within a group of air-conditioned buildings there was a positive correlation between the numbers of fungal (but not bacterial) colony forming units and building sickness. Outdoor air fungi, such as *Cladosporium* and *Alternaria*, predominate in naturally ventilated buildings, they are unlikely to have a role in sick building syndrome. The fungi found in indoor air are mostly derived from the incoming water.

Pickering and colleagues also studied a building with a clean room, the room being positively pressurized and supplied with air from high-grade filters. The microbial lode in the clean area (bacteria plus fungi) was 125 cfu/m³ compared with 400 cfu/m³ for the area supplied by the standard air conditioning system. Total dust levels were also halved in the clean area. Despite these changes the symptoms of sick building syndrome were if anything greater in the clean area.[89] The most likely explanation is that a soluble product, which requires the presence of water in the air-conditioning system, is the missing link (a similar situation to humidifier fever where the humidifier is clearly the usual source but the microbiology is equally confusing). An alternative explanation is that either there is a confounding variable that is not being measured, or that other agents associated

with humidifiers or chillers are the cause. Biocides are a possible link. They are not designed to be put into air-conditioning systems and subsequently inhaled (as apart from cooling towards where the biocide aerosol disperses in the outside air). Their use may result in widespread exposure to these agents via the ventilating system, and are therefore a potential cause for sensitization.[79,80]

Because of the problems in interpreting colony forming units, and because some outbreaks of disease occur with low viable organism levels, techniques of antigen detection in air have been developed. Reed and colleagues[90] found levels of antigen in air around 0.3 µg/m³ in working areas and 0.4 µg/m³ in ductwork in a factory with an outbreak of allergic alveolitis. Since antigens sometimes vary between outbreaks, a panel of relevant antigens and antibodies will be needed if these methods are to be used to monitor workplaces without identified problems.

The most appropriate method for control is to remove the sources of microbial growth from the building. The main source in buildings in the UK is from humidifiers and chillers. Once contamination of a humidifier has occurred it can be very difficult to eradicate. Reed *et al.*[90] treated a problem humidifier with a chlorinating agent, a slimicide and by regular cleaning. Antigen levels in the work place decreased from levels of up to 15 µg/m³ down to 0.06 µg/m³. No fresh cases of sensitization occurred once the antigen levels were reduced below 0.05 µg/m³ (and probably none below 0.2 µg/m³). Other outbreaks have not been controlled by cleaning and chlorination, and have required replacement of the water spray with steam humidification.[29] In this outbreak the initial antigen levels were between 1 and 10 µg/m³. Chillers are another possible source of problems; control rests with proper cleaning and maintenance. This requires good design so that the chillers are drained and the whole of the drip tray readily accessible for cleaning. Chillers sited in central plant rooms are much easier to service than chillers spread around the ceiling space, and wall cavities of peripheral offices. Control can often be achieved by better maintenance. The importance of design and maintenance has been recognized in the World Health Organization guidelines described below.[91]

1 The building and its heating, ventilation and air-conditioning systems should not produce biological contaminants which are introduced into the ventilation air. If biocides are unavoidable, they should be prevented from entering space which can be occupied.
2 Standards and building codes should ensure effective maintenance of ventilation systems by specifying adequate access paths, regular inspection and maintenance schedules.
3 In a building, in which occupants cannot effectively control the quality of ventilation air, an individual

who is responsible for this task should be identified to the occupants.

4 The maintenance personnel of public and office buildings should be given adequate training for routine inspection and maintenance for the building systems.

The American Conference of Government Industrial Hygienists has made the following recommendations for office buildings:

1 The sum of the total counts of fungae, bacteria (35°C) and thermophilic actinomycetes (55°C) should not exceed 10 000 cfu/m^3.

2 If the levels of *Bacillus* species and Gram-negative rods exceed 500 cfu/m^3, a building-associated source is presumed.

3 If any of the following exceed 500 cfu/m^3 remedial action is needed; *Staphylococcus*, *Streptococcus*, *Corynebacterium*, *Acinetobacter*, *Pseudomonas* or *Micrococcus* species.

4 Levels of *Actinomycetes* over 500/m^3 are considered high.

DUST

The first major multi-building study, the Copenhagen town hall study, showed an association between macromolecular dust and symptoms.[54] Most of these buildings were naturally ventilated. Poor cleaning, overcrowding and poor space management are factors associated with sick naturally ventilated buildings. The Copenhagen group have taken these investigation further and found associations between the Gram-negative bacterial content of the dust and symptoms; between the particulates and mucous membrane symptoms, between volatile organics desorbed from the dust and general symptoms, and between the macromolecular content of the dust and general symptoms.[92] One controlled study of office cleaning has shown a reduction in symptoms.[93] This intervention study involved weekly questionnaires, which can lead to diminishing reports of symptoms even where no intervention has been made. The above study, however, showed an increased benefit in the cleaned area which persisted for at least 2 months after cleaning.

By medical standards the symptoms of sick building syndrome are relatively trivial. Symptoms are generally more common and more problematical in the stressed, the unloved and in individuals who feel powerless to change their situation. There is a strong association between lack of control of the office environment and symptoms.[44] There is an association between environmental and job stress and symptoms.[58] The Dutch study showed that the strongest correlation with symptoms was the reporting of an inadequate system for dealing with environmental complaints.[55,94] The reduced symp-

toms seen in managers and men may be due to their greater success in getting the indoor environment to their liking. Good communication between workers, occupational health staff and building service managers and their plant staff is fundamental to improving existing sick buildings.

Economic consequences

The economic consequences of the sick building syndrome relate to the decreased or increased productivity resulting from the working environment, the costs of labour and the costs of providing the environment. These factors vary widely in different countries and environments. The costs of running a building consist of the building and equipment depreciation on invested capital plus operational costs. The economics have been worked out for an office building in Norway (Gaute Flatheim, pers. comm.). He calculated that doubling the outdoor ventilation rate and restricting the use of materials liable to offgas volatile organic compounds, results in insignificant changes in the total costs, which were dominated by the wages of the workforce (89.9% of the total costs, reducing to 89.3% with doubled ventilation). It would take only a very small increase in productivity or reduction in sickness absence to pay back the increased investment (Gaute Flatheim estimates this to be between 7 months and 2 years for his office building). Raw (evidence submitted to the UK parliamentary select committee on the environment) has also assessed the costs of sick building syndrome in a large government office with 2500 occupants, assuming 1 day of sickness absence per year attributed to sick building syndrome and 1 hour per month dealing with or complaining about the indoor environment.[95] At 1990 prices, the costs to the organization were £400 000 for one year.

Unfortunately it is very difficult to measure productivity in thinking office workers, and sickness absence has many determinants apart from the health of the worker. The British office environment study[44] included a question asking the worker how much they thought the office environment affected their productivity (on a 9-point scale from −40% to + 40%). Interestingly there were some workers who thought that the office environment increased their productivity. There was a clear linear relationship between the number of work-related symptoms of sick building syndrome and self-assessed productivity, suggesting that the 'disease' was the cause of the reduced productivity.[95] The study also showed a clear relationship between the type of building and the building symptom index. Those with an average of two (out of 10) work-related symptoms had a neutral effect on productivity. The majority of buildings with a building symptom index under two were naturally ventilated with cellular offices and substantial worker control of their environment.

Studies of sickness absence have shown variable results. Guberan in Switzerland[96] found increased sickness absence in a group moving from a naturally ventilated to an air-conditioned office. Moreover, most of the increased sickness absence was related to respiratory complaints. Studies of the relationship between ventilation type, sick building syndrome and sickness absence have been made in groups of workers employed by the same government department.[97] One group of workers moved from naturally ventilated offices to an air-conditioned headquarters building, the other group moved in the opposite direction. Sickness absence was collected prospectively. The differences in sickness absence were small, with 6 days per 100 workers per month less sickness absence in those working in naturally ventilated buildings (excluding sickness absence unlikely to be due to working in an office building such as operations, accidents and pregnancy). Sickness absence due to the sick building syndrome was also studied in the Dutch multibuilding cross-sectional study.[55] There were 34% fewer days off sick in workers who could control their own environment in their offices. Sickness absence was also higher in buildings with humidifiers.

A small study has shown improvement in both self-rated productivity and measured sickness absence in an office building retrofitted with an air filtration system fitted to each workstation, taking air from the room. It was fitted with both carbon and high efficiency particulate filters, and reduced the levels of particulates in the air.[53] The intervention area was compared with a control floor of the building. The questionnaire asked whether productivity was disrupted by poor air quality, rather than whether productivity was altered overall. There was a 61% reduction in certified sickness absence compared with a similar period the previous year, equivalent to a 3.1% increase in productive time per worker. A small control area was included on the intervention floor, where the furniture and fan unit was installed without the filtration system. Similar improvements in air quality assessment and symptoms were seen in this area, raising the possibility that the fan unit rather than the filtration were responsible for the improvement.

The current evidence suggests that individuals vary significantly in their requirements for indoor air quality, so that it is not possible to provide one environment that suits a large proportion of the workforce. Workers who are unable to alter environments which they find unsatisfactory are more likely to develop sick building syndrome. Their inability to improve their environment is a source of stress which can contribute to their symptoms, and perhaps to their reduced productivity.[59] The workers in a building are by far its most expensive commodity, looking after their environment as well as that needed for the mainframe computer is likely to be cost-effective.

REFERENCES

1 McDade JE, Shepard CC, Fraser DW, Tsai TF, Redus MA, Dowdle WR. Legionnaires' disease. Isolation of a bacterium and demonstration of its role in other respiratory disease. *N Engl J Med* 1977; **297**:1197.

2 Fraser DW, Tsai TR, Orenstein W, Parkin WE, Beecham JH, *et al*. Legionnaires' disease: description of an epidemic of pneumonia. *N Engl J Med* 1977; **297**:1189.

3 Bhopal RS. Geographical variation of legionnaires' disease: a critique and guide to future research. *Int J Epidemiol* 1933; **22**:1127–36.

4 Cunningham D. *Broadcasting House Legionnaires' Disease: Report of the Westminster Action Committee*. London: Environment Committee, Westminster City Council, 1988.

5 Badenoch J. *First Report of the Committee of Enquiry into the Outbreak of Legionnaires' Disease in Stafford in April 1985*. London: HMSO, CMD 9772, 1986: 1.

6 Badenoch J. *Second Report of the Committee of Enquiry into the Outbreak of Legionnaires' Disease in Stafford in April 1985*. London: HMSO, CMD 256, 1987.

7 Timbury MC, Donaldson JR, McCartney AC. Outbreak of legionnaires' disease in Glasgow Royal Infirmary: microbiological aspects. *J Hyg Camb* 1986; **97**:393–403.

8 Bhopal RS, Fallon RJ, Buist EC, Black RJ, Urquhart JD. Proximity of the home to a cooling tower and risk of non-outbreak legionnaires' disease. *Br Med J* 1991; **302**:378–83.

9 Bhopal RS, Diggle P, Rowlingson B. Pinpointing clusters of apparently sporadic cases of legionnaires disease. *Br Med J* 1992; **304**:1022–7.

10 Bhopal RS. Source of infection for sporadic legionnaires' disease: a review. *J Infect* 1975; **30**:9–12.

11 Health and Safety Executive. *Legionnaires' Disease*. London: HMSO, C180 1/87, 1987.

12 Health and Safety Executive. *The Control of Legionellosis Including Legionnaires' Disease*. London: HMSO, C100 5/93, 1993.

13 *The Notification of Cooling Towers and Evaporative Condensers Regulations* 1992 : 2225.

14 Niedeveld CJ, Pet FM, Meenhorst PL. Effect of rubbers and their constituents on proliferation of *Legionella pneumophila* in naturally contaminated hot water. *Lancet* 1986; **ii**:180–3.

15 Fang GD, Yu VL, Vickers RM. Disease due to the Legionellaceae (other than *Legionella pneumophila*). Historical, microbiological, clinical, and epidemiological review. *Medicine* 1989; **68**:116–32.

16 Edelstein PH. Antimicrobial chemotherapy for legionnaires' disease: a review. *Clin Infect Dis* 1995; **21**(Suppl 3):5265–76.

17 Glick TH, Gregg MB, Berman B, Mallison G, Rhodes WW, Kassanoff IRA. Pontiac fever. *Am J Epidemiol* 1978; **107**:149–60.

18 Lloyd RS, Guest D, Fairfax AJ. Prolonged lethargy in hospital staff after legionella infection. *Thorax* 1991; **46**:285P.

19 Herwald LA, Gorman GW, McGrath T, Toma S, Brake B *et al.* A new *Legionella* species, *Legionella feeleii* species *nova*, causes Pontiac fever in an automobile plant. *Ann Intern Med* 1984; **100**:333–8.

20 Banaszak EF, Thiede WH, Fink JN. Hypersensitivity pneumonitis due to contamination of an air-conditioner. *N Engl J Med* 1970; **283**:271–6.

21 Pestalozzi C. Febrile gruppenerkrankungen in einer Modellschreinerei durch Inhalation von mit Schimmelpilzen kontaminierien Befeuchterwasser (Befeuchterfieber). *Schweiz Med Wchschr* 1959;**27**:710–3.

22 Fink JN, Banaszak EF, Thiede WH, Barboriak JJ. Interstitial pneumonitis due to hypersensitivity to an organism contaminating a heating system. *Ann Intern Med* 1971; **74**:80–3.

23 Sweet LC, Anderson JA, Callies QC, Coates EO. Hypersensitivity pneumonitis related to a home furnace humidifier. *J All Clin Immunol* 1971; **48**:171–8.

24 Newman Taylor AJ, Pickering CAC, Turner-Warwick M, Pepys J. Respiratory allergy to a factory humidifier contaminant presenting as pyrexia of undetermined origin. *Br Med J* 1978; **ii**:94–5.

25 Jacobs RL, Andrews CP, Jacobs FO. Hypersensitivity pneumonitis treated with an electrostatic dust filter. *Ann Intern Med* 1989; **110**:115–8.

26 Robertson AS, Burge PS, Wieland GA, Carmalt MH. Extrinsic allergic alveolitis caused by a cold water humidifier. *Thorax* 1987; **42**:32–7.

27 Liebert CA, Hood MA, Deck FH, Bishop K, Flaherty DK. Isolation and characterization of a new Cytophaga species implicated in work-related lung disease. *Appl Environ Microbiol* 1984; **48**:936–43.

28 Ando M, Suga M, Nishiura Y, Miyajima M. Summer-type hypersensitivity pneumonitis. *Intern Med* 1995; **34**:707–12.

29 Finnegan MJ, Pickering CAC, Davies PS, Austwick PKC. Factors affecting the development of precipitating antibodies in workers exposed to contaminated humidifiers. *Clin All* 1985; **15**:281–92.

30 Stricker WE, Layton JE, Homburger HA, Katzmann JA, Swanson MC *et al.* Immunologic response to aerosols of affinity-purified antigen in hypersensitivity pneumonitis. *J All Clin Immunol* 1986; **78**:411–6.

31 Aro S, Muittari A, Virtanen P. Bathing fever epidemic of unknown aetiology in Finland. *Int J Epidemiol* 1980; **9**:215–8.

32 Burge PS, Finnegan M, Horsfield N, Emery D, Austwick P, Davies PS *et al.* Occupational asthma in a factory with a contaminated humidifier. *Thorax* 1985; **40**:248–54.

33 Kane GC, Marx JJ, Prince DS. Hypersensitivity pneumonitis secondary to *Klebsiella oxytoca*. A new cause of humidifier lung. *Chest* 1993; **104**:627–9.

34 Finnegan MJ, Pickering CAC, Davies PS, Austwick PKC, Warhurst DC. Amoebae and humidifier fever. *Clin All* 1987; **17**:235–42.

35 Rylander R, Haglind P. Airborne endotoxins and humidifier disease. *Clin All* 1984; **14**:109–12.

36 Solomon WR. Fungus aerosols arising from cold-mist vaporizers. *J All Clin Immunol* 1974; **54**:222–8.

37 Axelsson IG. Allergy to *Ficus benjamina* (weeping fig) in nonatopic subjects. *Allergy* 1995; **50**:284–5.

38 Axelsson IGK, Johansson SGO, Zetterstrom O. Occupational allergy to weeping fig in plant keepers. *Allergy* 1987; **42**:161–7.

39 Kanerva L, Makinen-Kiljunen S, Kiistala R, Granlund H. Occupational allergy caused by spathe flower (*Spathiphyllum wallisii*). *Allergy* 1995; **50**:174–8.

40 Ng TP, Hong CY, Goh LG, Wong ML, Koh KT, Ling SL. Risks of asthma associated with occupations in a community-based case-control study. *Am J Ind Med* 1994; **25**:709–18.

41 Kogevinas M, Anto JM, Soriano JB, Tobias A, Burney P. The risk of asthma attributable to occupational exposures. A population-based study in Spain. Spanish Group of the European Asthma Study. *Am J Respir Crit Care Med* 1996; **154**:137–43.

42 Bernstein JA, Stauder T, Bernstein DI, Bernstein IL. A combined respiratory and cutaneous hypersensitivity syndrome induced by work exposure to quaternary amines. *J All Clin Immunol* 1994; **94**:257–9.

43 Burge PS, Richardson MN. Occupational asthma due to indirect exposure to lauryl dimethyl benzyl ammonium chloride used in a floor cleaner. *Thorax* 1994; **49**:842–43.

44 Burge PS, Hedge A, Wilson S, Harris-Bass J, Robertson AS. Sick building syndrome; a study of 4373 office workers. *Ann Occup Hyg* 1987; **31**:493–504.

45 Franck C. Eye symptoms and signs in buildings with indoor climate problems ('Office eye syndrome'). *Acta Opthalmol (Copenhagen)* 1986; **64**:306–11.

46 Franck C, Skov P. Foam at inner eye canthus in office workers, compared with an average Danish population as control group. *Acta Opthalmol (Copenhagen)* 1989; **67**:61–8.

47 Franck C, Skov P. Evaluation of two different questionnaires used for diagnosing ocular manifestations in the sick building syndrome on the basis of an objective test. *Indoor Air* 1991; **1**:5–11.

48 Rycroft RJG. Low humidity and microtrauma. *Am J Ind Med* 1985; **8**:371–3.

49 Sundell J, Lindvall T, Stenberg B, Wall S. Sick building syndrome in office workers and facial skin symptoms amongst VDT-workers in relation to building and room characteristics. Two case-referent studies. *Indoor Air* 1994; **4**:83–94.

50 Carmichael AJ, Roberts DL. Visual display units and facial rashes. *Contact Derm* 1992; **26**:63–4.

51 Reinikainen LM, Jaakkola JJK, Helenius T, Seppanen O. The effect of air humidification on symptoms and environmental complaints in office workers. A six period cross-over study. *Indoor Air* 1990;**1**:775–80.

52 Anderson I, Lundquist GR, Proctor DF. Human perception of humidity under four controlled conditions. *Arch Environ Hlth* 1973; **26**:22–7.

53 Hedge A, Mitchell GE, McCarthy JF, Ludwig J. Effects of a furniture-integrated breathing-zone filtration system on

indoor air quality, sick building syndrome, productivity and absenteeism. *Indoor Air* 1993: 383–8.

54 Skov P, Valbjorn O. The sick building syndrome in the office environment; the Danish town hall study. *Environ Int* 1987; **13**:339–49.

55 Zweers T, Preller L, Brunekreef B, Boleij JSM. Health and indoor climate complaints of 7043 office workers in 61 buildings in the Netherlands. *Indoor Air* 1992; **2**: 127–36.

56 Sundell J, Lindvall T, Stenberg B. Associations between type of ventilation and air-flow rates in office buildings and the risk of SBS-symptoms among occupants. *Environ Int* 1994; **20**:239–51.

57 Burge PS, Jones P, Robertson AS. Sick building syndrome; environmental comparisons of sick and healthy buildings. *Indoor Air* 1990;**1**:479–83.

58 Hedge A, Burge PS, Robertson AS, Wilson S, Harris-Bass J. Work related illness in offices: a proposed model of the sick building syndrome. *Environ Int* 1989; **15**:143–58.

59 Hedge A, Erickson WA, Rubin G. Psychological correlates of sick building syndrome. In: Jaakkola JJK, Ilmarinen R, Seppanen O eds. *Indoor Air* 1993: 345–50.

60 Norback D, Wieslander G, Gothe CJ. A search for discomfort-inducing factors in carbonless copying paper. *Am Ind Hyg Assoc J* 1988; **49**:117–20.

61 Hedge A, Sterling TD, Sterling EM, Collett CW, Nie V. Indoor air quality and health in two office buildings with different ventilation systems. *Environ Int* 1989; **15**:115–28.

62 Robertson AS, Burge PS, Hedge A, Wilson S, Harris-Bass J. The relationship between passive cigarette smoke exposure in office workers and the symptoms of building sickness. In: Perry K, Kirk P eds. *Indoor and Ambient Air Quality* 1991; **1988**: 320–6.

63 Reynal A, Burge PS, Robertson AS, Jarvis M, Archibald M, Hawkin D. How much does environmental tobacco smoke contribute to the building symptom index? *Indoor Air* 1995; **5**:22–8.

64 Reynal A, Burge PS, Robertson AS, Jarvis M, Archibald M, Hawkin D. Estimated reduction in exposure to environmental tobacco smoke through removing smoking in the workplace. *Indoor Air* 1993 : 639–43.

65 Hedge A, Erickson WA, Rubin G. Effects of restrictive smoking policies on indoor air quality and sick building syndrome: a study of 27 air-conditioned offices. *Indoor Air* 1993 : 517–22.

66 Spicer J, Hay DM, Gordon M. Workplace exposure and reported health in New Zealand diagnostic radiographers. *Australas Radiol* 1986; **30**:281–6.

67 Norback D. Skin and respiratory symptoms from exposure to alkaline glutaraldehyde in medical services. *Scand J Work Environ Hlth* 1988; **14**:366–71.

68 Hewitt PJ. Occupational health problems in processing of X-ray photographic films. *Ann Occup Hyg* 1993; **37**:287–95.

69 Gannon PFG, Bright P, Campbell M, O'Hickey SP, Burge PS. Occupational asthma due to glutaraldehyde and formaldehyde in endoscopy and X-ray departments. *Thorax* 1995; **50**:156–9.

70 Trigg CJ, Heap DC, Herdman MJ, Davies RJ. A radiographer's asthma. *Resp Med* 1992; **86**:167–9.

71 Cullinan P, Hayes J, Cannon J, Madan I, Heap D, Newman Taylor AJ. Occupational asthma in radiographers. *Lancet* 1992; **340**:1477.

72 Nordstrom K, Norback D, Akselsson R. Influence of indoor air quality and personal factors on the sick building syndrome (SBS) in Swedish geriatric hospitals. *Occup Environ Med* 1995; **52**:170–6.

73 Nordstrom K, Norback D, Akselsson R. Subjective indoor air quality in hospitals- the influence of building age, ventilation flow, and personal factors. *Indoor Environ* 1995; **4**:37–44.

74 Mendell MJ, Smith AH. Consistent pattern of elevated symptoms in air-conditioned office buildings: a reanalysis of epidemiologic studies. *Am J Pub Hlth* 1990; **80**:1193–9.

75 Menzies RI, Tamblyn RM, Tamblyn RT, Farant JP, Hanley J, Spitzer WO. Sick building syndrome: the effect of changes in ventilation rates on symptom prevalence: the evaluation of a double blind experimental approach. *Indoor Air* 1990;**1**: 519–24.

76 Jaakkola JJK, Miettinen P. Ventilation rate in office buildings and sick building syndrome. *Br J Ind Med* 1995; **52**:709–14.

77 Jaakkola JJK, Heinonen OP, Seppanen O. Sick building syndrome, sensation of dryness and thermal comfort in relation to room temperature in an office building: need for individual control of temperature. *Environ Int* 1989; **15**:163–8.

78 Nagorka R, Rosskamp E, Seidel K. Air conditioning-assessment of humidification units. *Off Gesundh-Wes* 1990;**52**:168–73.

79 Rosskamp E. Air-conditioning plants- a health problem. *Bundesgesundhblad* 1990; **3**:117–21.

80 Clark EG. Risk of isothiazolinones. *J Soc Occup Med* 1987; **37**:30–1.

81 Curran AD, Burge PS, Wiley K. Clinical and immunological evaluation of workers exposed to glutaraldehyde. *Allergy* 1996; **51**:826–32.

82 Blasco A, Joral A, Fuente R, Rodriguez M, Garcia A, Dominguez A. Bronchial asthma due to sensitization to chloramine T. *J Invest All Clin Immunol* 1992; **2**: 167–70.

83 Waclawski ER, McAlpine LG, Thomson NC. Occupational asthma in nurses due to chlorhexidine and alcohol aerosols. *Br Med J* 1989; **298**:929–30.

84 Pickering CAC, Mustchin CP. 'Coughing water', bronchial hyperreactivity induced by swimming in a chlorinated pool. *Thorax* 1979; **34**:682–3.

85 Deschamps D, Soler P, Rosenberg N, Baud F, Gervais P. Persistent asthma after inhalation of a mixture of sodium hypochlorite and hydrochloric acid. *Chest* 1994; **105**:1895–6.

86 Fanger PO, Lauridsen J, Bluyssen P, Clausen G. Air pollution sources in offices and assembly halls, quantified by the olf unit. *Energy Buildings* 1988; **12**:7–19.

87 Fanger PO. Introduction of the Olf and Decipol units to

quantify air pollution perceived by humans indoors and outdoors. *Energy Buildings* 1988; **12**:1–6.

88 Finnegan MJ, Pickering CAC, Burge PS. Sick building syndrome; prevalence studies. *Br Med J* 1984; **289**:1573–5.

89 Harrison J, Pickering CAC, Finnegan MJ, Austwick PKC. The sick building syndrome, further prevalence studies and investigation of possible causes. *Indoor Air* 1987; **2**:487–91.

90 Reed CE, Swanson MC, Lopez M, Ford AM, Major J *et al.* Measurement of IgG antibody and airborne antigen to control an industrial outbreak of hypersensitivity pneumonitis. *J Occup Med* 1983; **25**:207–10.

91 World Health Organization. *Indoor Air Quality: Biological Contaminants*. WHO regional publications; European series no 3 Geneva: WHO, 1–54.

92 Gyntelberg F, Suadicani P, Nielsen JW, Skov P, Valbjorn O *et al.* Dust and the sick building syndrome. *Indoor Air* 1994; **4**:223–38.

93 Leinster P, Raw GJ, Thomson N, Leaman A, Whitehead C *et al.* A modular longitudinal approach to the investigation of sick building syndrome. *Indoor Air* 1990; **1**:287–92.

94 Preller L, Zweers T, Boleij JSM, Brunekreef B. *Gezondheidsklachten en klachten over het binnenklimaat in kantoorgebouwen*. Directoraat-General van de Arbeid 1990; S83:1–62.

95 Raw GJ, Leaman A. Further findings from the office environment study: productivity. In: *Proceedings of the 5th International Conference on Indoor Air Quality and Climate*. Ottowa 1990 : 231–6.

96 Guberan E, Dang VB, Sweetman PM. L'humidification de l'air des locaux previent-elle les maladies respiratoires pendant l'hiver. *Schweiz Med Wchenschr* 1978; **108**:827–31.

97 Robertson AS, Roberts KT, Burge PS, Raw GJ. The effect of change in building ventilation category on sickness absence rates and the prevalence of sick building syndrome. *Indoor Air* 1990;**1**:237–42.

Part **8**

Occupational diseases of the skin

Occupational diseases of the skin 725

37

Occupational diseases of the skin

RICHARD JG RYCROFT

Epidemiology	725	Non-eczematous occupational dermatoses	731
Clinical range	725	Contact urticaria	731
Contact dermatitis	726	Protein urticaria dermatitis	731
Irritant contact dermatitis	726	Oil folliculitis	731
Allergic contact dermatitis	727	Chloracne	732
Clinical diagnosis of occupational contact dermatitis	727	Leucoderma	732
Patch testing	728	Scleroderma-like diseases	732
Other investigations	729	Ulcerations	732
Treatment	729	Skin carcinomas	733
Prevention	730	Major occupations causing dermatoses	733
Prognosis	730	References	735

Notwithstanding the far earlier contributions of Celsus,[1] Agricola,[2] Paracelsus[3] and Ramazzini,[4] the history of modern occupational dermatology begins in 1915 with the first edition of the Englishman Prosser White's classic text,[5] followed in 1939 by those of the Dane Poul Bonnevie[6] and the North Americans Schwartz, Tulipan and Peck (and later Birmingham).[7] Since the Second World War, the major impetus has come from Europe[8] and, in particular, from Sigfrid Fregert in Southern Sweden.[9] Foussereau[10] and Zschunke[11] in Europe, and Adams[12] in the United States of America have since produced further major texts.

There is no universally accepted definition of an occupational skin disease (or dermatosis). Definitions vary according to the purpose for which they are framed. A broad definition is a dermatosis due wholly or partially to the patient's occupation. Occupation must be a major factor in stricter definitions,[13] and essential to causation in still stricter definitions.[14]

EPIDEMIOLOGY

Dermatoses are now generally reckoned as being less frequent only than musculoskeletal and stress conditions among occupational disorders. A 1995 self-reported survey in Great Britain led to an estimate of over 50 000 work-related conditions involving the skin.[15] Recent years' reports to EPIDERM and OPRA (Occupational physicians reporting activity) surveillance schemes in Great Britain suggest an annual rate rising towards 5000 new cases of occupational dermatoses seen by reporting dermatologists and occupational physicians when added together.[15] The annual costs of occupational dermatoses in the USA have been estimated at up to 1000 million dollars.[16] The cost to the working community is a human as well as a financial one, disablement from an occupational dermatosis sometimes approaching that from loss of a limb.[17] Many high-risk occupations have been identified in which the prevalence of occupational dermatoses rises as high as 15%.[18]

CLINICAL RANGE

While 90–95%[19] of occupational dermatoses are contact dermatitis, their clinical spectrum also includes contact urticaria, oil folliculitis, chloracne, leukoderma, scleroderma, ulcerations and epidermal carcinoma. Many substances that cause occupational dermatoses are also capable of causing respiratory and other disorders, for example rosin (colophony), chromate, formaldehyde, (meth)acrylates and organotins.[18] Psoriasis may be aggravated, or even initiated for the first time on the hands, by physical or chemical occupational irritants. Scabies, though rarely occupational, may mimic contact dermatitis (Fig. 37.1).

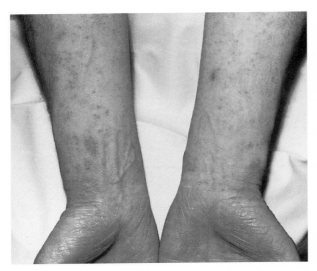

Figure 37.1 *Scabies mimicking contact eczema. See colour plate section.*

CONTACT DERMATITIS

Contact dermatitis is dermatitis caused by skin contact with external substances (Fig. 37.2). It is distinguished from endogenous (constitutional) dermatitis not by morphology or histopathology, but only by aetiology. The term dermatitis, as used above, is synonymous with the term eczema. Not only must dermatitis be divided into endogenous or contact (that is, exogenous), or a mixture of the two, but it must carefully be distinguished from clinically similar dermatoses, such as psoriasis and tinea. Practical experience is essential but can usefully be supplemented by reference to well-illustrated textbooks[20] and other helpful publications.[21]

To cause contact dermatitis a substance must first be capable of penetrating the superficial layers of the epidermis, known as the barrier layer. This is a paper-thin lipoprotein membrane, remarkably resistant to penetration, though vulnerable to substances of molecular weight below 1000. If a substance does penetrate to the living tissues beneath, it may then cause contact dermatitis by one of two mechanisms, contact irritation and contact sensitization (or contact allergy), which may go on to provoke irritant contact dermatitis and allergic contact dermatitis, respectively. Both forms of contact dermatitis may be morphologically indistinguishable from each other as well as from endogenous dermatitis. Because of their predominance as the site of occupational contact, the hands are involved in as much as 90% of occupational contact dermatitis.[22]

IRRITANT CONTACT DERMATITIS

A contact irritant is a chemical (or physical) agent capable of causing cell damage (cytotoxicity) if applied to the

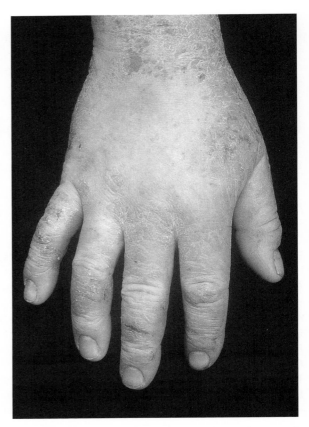

Figure 37.2 *Allergic contact dermatitis from chromate in cement. See colour plate section.*

skin for sufficient time and in sufficient concentration. The precise mechanisms of cytotoxicity are still not yet well defined, though they are already known to differ from one irritant to another.[23]

Acute (or strong) irritants are not usually so unprotected against at work as to cause irritant contact dermatitis, though their accidental spillage may cause chemical burns.[24] Occupational irritant contact dermatitis is usually caused instead by chronic (weak, mild or marginal) irritants, the damage from which is insidious and insensible but cumulative with time.[23] Chronic irritant contact dermatitis is often the result of more than one occupational irritant (multifactorial).

Individual susceptibility to chronic irritant contact dermatitis varies very widely, though still largely unpredictably.[23] One high-risk group that has been identified are subjects with a previous history of severe childhood eczema, particularly if this involved the hands.[25,26] Susceptibility to one irritant, however, does not necessarily imply susceptibility to another.[23] Variation in susceptibility to weak irritants results in chronic irritant contact dermatitis involving only a certain proportion of an exposed workforce, which rarely rises in practice above a third.[18]

Age of onset varies from one occupation to another, sometimes showing a bimodal curve, with those at both ends of working life seeming to be at higher risk than those in mid-career,[18] and other times increasing with age (or sometimes even apparently decreasing). Similarly, length of exposure prior to onset varies widely, depending both on the irritant and the degree of contact with it, but sometimes being years rather than, more commonly, months. Any apparent difference in susceptibility between the sexes arises from the different type of work that they do, rather than from any inherently increased susceptibility in either sex.[23]

The principal occupational irritants[18,23,27] may be grouped broadly into soaps and detergents, alkalis and acids, metalworking fluids (cutting oils), organic solvents, other petroleum products, oxidizing agents, reducing agents, animal and plant products, and physical factors, such as friction and low relative humidity, as well as desiccant powders. Common high-risk occupations for chronic irritant contact dermatitis[18,24] are catering, cleaning, construction, hairdressing, horticulture and floristry, metalworking, nursing, painting, printing, and vehicle maintenance and repair.

ALLERGIC CONTACT DERMATITIS

Though probably not as common as occupational irritant contact dermatitis, occupational allergic contact dermatitis is generally less amenable to subsequent prevention, because of the much smaller quantities of allergen that may sustain a contact dermatitis in a sensitized individual, compared with the quantities required of irritants. It may therefore become much more difficult to manage than irritant contact dermatitis.

A contact allergen (or contact sensitizer), after penetrating the barrier layer of the skin, is chemically reactive enough to provoke delayed, cell-mediated or Type IV allergy.[28,29] The first stage of this process is termed induction and, once initiated, takes around 7 days to be completed. After such time, further skin contact with that particular allergen results in the second stage of the process, called elicitation, that results in allergic contact dermatitis within from a few hours to a day or two, depending on both degree of contact and degree of sensitivity. Allergic contact dermatitis is usually morphologically indistinguishable from irritant contact dermatitis.

Sensitization may be induced after only one contact,[30] or after many contacts over a prolonged period. Occupationally, it is often induced after a few months of repeated contact, though sometimes it can occur after many years of well-tolerated contact, as with chromate sensitization in bricklayers.[18] There is a very wide individual variation in susceptibility to contact sensitization, and susceptibility to one allergen does not necessarily imply any general susceptibility to contact sensitization. Age and sex are not significant influences.

Knowledge of the mechanism of Type IV hypersensitivity has accumulated in the last three decades to a fascinating degree.[28,29] Allergic contact dermatitis depends primarily on the activation of specifically sensitized T cells, an untoward side-effect of a well-functioning immune system.

Induction of contact sensitization begins with the binding of allergen to major histocompatibility complex (MHC) class II molecules on the surface of allergen-presenting cells. These MHC class II molecules are present on Langerhans' cells within the epidermis, which migrate via the lymphatics to the paracortical areas of the regional lymph nodes. Here, T cells specifically recognize the allergen-class II molecule complexes and are activated to proliferate within the node, subsequently to be released into the circulation and enter the skin. The process of induction is then complete, having taken around 7 days.

Elicitation of allergic contact dermatitis then depends on allergen-presenting cells and specific T cells subsequently meeting in the skin and leading there to cytokine production. Release of such mediators results in the arrival of more T cells, thus further amplifying local mediator release. This leads to a dermatitic reaction, peaking after 1–2 days.

Several thousand contact allergens are now recognized.[31] Chromates, epoxy resins and hardeners, (meth)acrylates, formaldehyde and formaldehyde-releasers, other biocides (preservatives), and plants and woods are common occupational examples.[18,29] High-risk occupations include chemical and pharmaceutical manufacture, construction, dyeing, electronics, hairdressing, and tanning.[18]

CLINICAL DIAGNOSIS OF OCCUPATIONAL CONTACT DERMATITIS

Establishing the occupational causation of contact dermatitis can be far from straightforward.[32–34] The foundation remains a thorough dermatological and occupational history, coupled with a close examination of the whole skin. There are certain essential facts that form the basis of every such history.

The time of onset of the earliest signs

The shorter the history, the more likely is contact dermatitis. However, there is an important proviso to this general statement. Patients initially tend to underestimate the length of history, remembering the exacerbation that finally led them to seek medical advice rather than the original onset of the earliest signs. Many patients do not seek medical advice until they have had milder degrees of contact dermatitis for considerable periods. In Fregert's study,[9] 22% of cases of occupational contact dermatitis had a history of less than 1 month, yet 29% had a history of more than 1 year.

The primary site of onset

In occupational cases this is usually the hands.[22] In a few cases, the wrists, forearms, lower legs or face are the primary site. The covered areas of the trunk or feet are rare primary sites.[22]

The route and timing of any secondary spread

Local spread from one hand to the other and from the hands to the forearms commonly occurs, even in the absence of contact at such secondary sites.[35] Distant spread from the hands to the feet or to the face is more common in allergic contact dermatitis rather than irritant.[36] Photocontact dermatitis is rarely occupational but primarily involves the backs of the hands and face.

Atopy

Those with a history of severe childhood eczema, particularly if this involved the hands, are at higher risk as a group, of developing occupational irritant, though not allergic, contact dermatitis.[25,26]

Occupation

The essential questions that need to be asked of the patient are their occupational title, length of time in this job, and precisely what it involves them in doing. As exact a picture as possible must be acquired of the degree of skin contact, as well as simply the substances involved. Personally visiting the workplace and actually looking at the work being done can increase the understanding of a dermatitis problem.[18,32]

Work-relatedness

The question as to whether the dermatitis improves away from work and worsens on return to work is clearly fundamental, but can usefully be refined a little further. Primarily endogenous eczema may also show such a pattern, but occupational contact dermatitis usually shows greater and more consistent work-relatedness. Occupational allergic contact dermatitis tends to relapse more rapidly on return to work than does irritant contact dermatitis, and allergic may sometimes be slower than irritant to improve away from work. As occupational contact dermatitis of either type becomes chronic,

its initial work-relatedness tends to become increasingly less clear-cut.

Preventive measure

Attempts to prevent or remove skin contamination should be enquired about, as well as the amount of success achieved by such methods. Occupational contact dermatitis may sometimes be aggravated further by the irritancy of skin cleansers or allergy to protective gloves.

Fellow-workers

The involvement of a substantial proportion of working colleagues is more suggestive of irritant than allergic contact dermatitis. Patients' own assessments of the similarity of their workmates' dermatoses are, understandably, often unreliable, and a personal examination of any such additional cases is always to be recommended.[37]

PATCH TESTING

While there is no routine skin test to confirm the diagnosis of irritant contact dermatitis, patch testing is the only way of confirming the diagnosis of allergic contact dermatitis. The principle of patch testing is relatively straightforward, yet its reliability is highly dependent on the abilities of the person(s) carrying it out.

Patch testing is based on the dilution of potential contact allergens to below their threshold for either induction of contact sensitivity, or for contact irritancy under the conditions of the test, down to a level at which they nevertheless remain capable of an elicitation reaction in an already-sensitized patient.[29]

The appropriate dilution for patch testing varies widely from substance to substance. Its selection is crucial to the reliability of the test. Underdilution may result in a positive reaction in the absence of contact allergy (false-positive reaction), whereas overdilution may result in a negative reaction in the presence of contact allergy (false-negative reaction).

A set of 20–30 common allergens (standard series) and some additional series directed towards specific occupations are available commercially, but in occupational cases these will frequently need to be supplemented by patch tests to a patient's own contactants. It is here that dilutional errors are easily made. Reference sources are a guide to correct patch test dilution,[31] but there is no substitute for training and experience: even commercial patch test preparations may occasionally give false-positive or false-negative reactions.

Appropriate dilutions are occluded against the skin (Fig. 37.3), usually in shallow aluminium chambers and usually on the back, for either one or (more usually) two

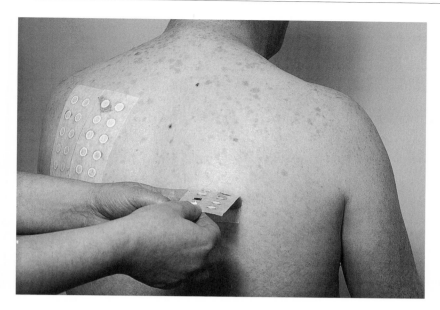

Figure 37.3 *Patch tests being applied. See colour plate section.*

days. Readings are made of any reactions that are present after removal of the tests and, preferably, again at between 3 and 7 days after application. The interpretation of such reactions requires trained skills.[18] Positive reactions also require further informed assessment of their relevance to the current dermatitis, which may involve substantial investigation of potential occupational sources.

OTHER INVESTIGATIONS

As well as patch testing, other special investigations may be required in order to make an accurate diagnosis. radio-allergosorbent testing (RAST) or prick testing may be indicated in contact urticaria and protein contact dermatitis (described later). Skin biopsy may be needed in certain other non-eczematous dermatoses.

Simple chemical tests for the identification of specific allergens, more advanced chemical analytical techniques, and methods for measuring the degree of skin contamination are reviewed in Refs 18 and 32. Such chemical elucidation has considerably advanced our understanding of contact sensitization by such occupational allergens as chromate, epoxy resin, phenol-formaldehyde resin and colophony.

In recent years, non-invasive measurement techniques have come to play an increasing role in contact dermatitis research,[29] including transepidermal water loss, skin reflectance and conductance, and laser Doppler flowmetry. As yet these have no routine applications in clinical dermatology.

In vitro tests for sensitization, such as the migration inhibition and lymphocyte transformation tests, are described in Ref. 29; but have not yet reached the level of reliability required to replace patch testing.

TREATMENT

The treatment of occupational contact dermatitis rests on the foundation of accurate diagnosis combined with partial or complete separation of the patient from the cause.

Acute contact dermatitis may sometimes require a period away from work, everything possible being done to minimize the length of any such period. Dermatological treatment is essentially the same as for any other acute eczema.[38] Hospital clinicians and general practitioners should be aware of the demoralization that can be produced by periods off work – even if only for a few weeks.

Chronic contact dermatitis, with certain exceptions indicated below, can usually be treated while the patient continues to work, even if this is in a temporary alternative location. Again, dermatological therapy is as for other chronic eczemas.[38]

Isolated uncomplicated allergic contact dermatitis may, however, respond so well to a permanent change of occupation that, if substitution of an allergen cannot be achieved,[39] this may become the best advice. Also, atopic individuals who find themselves with dermatitis from unavoidable irritants, such as in metalworking, hairdressing or catering, may be best advised to look for a permanent alternative.

Irritant contact dermatitis may often respond better to the regular use of emollients (moisturizers) than to potent topical corticosteroids, the latter being more likely to be needed in *allergic contact dermatitis*. In either type of contact dermatitis, secondary bacterial infection may require additional treatment with topical or systemic antibiotics.

PREVENTION

The prevention of occupational contact dermatitis[18] is based on the same hierarchy of measures as for other occupational diseases, usefully considered under the headings of reduction of exposure, reduction of the effects of exposure, and reduction of the effects of disease.

While substitution[39] will always remain the ideal exposure control, clinicians will more often find themselves involved in advising on personal protective equipment, and this largely in the form of gloves. Awareness is required here both that in some jobs gloves are either unsafe or impracticable, as well as that the choice of glove material can be crucial for certain substances.[18]

The effectiveness of 'barrier' creams remains controversial but data are beginning to accumulate on their role in preventing at least some of the effects of skin contact, particularly from irritants.[40] The benefit of emollient (moisturizer) application following skin cleansing is also beginning to receive some experimental support, again particularly with respect to irritants.[41]

The preventive role of pre-employment assessment[25] remains limited by our lack of reliable indicators of susceptibility, although a partial exception to this is that subjects with a history of severe childhood eczema are, as a group, more susceptible to skin irritation.[25,26] Such susceptibility does not appear to extend, however, to those with a history of only mucosal atopy (hay fever and asthma).

The primary objective in reducing the long-term effects of occupational contact dermatitis is to enable the patient to remain at work.[14] Clinicians should therefore strive to reduce periods of work absence to a minimum, with any unavoidable breaks in work being regularly monitored. Delay in diagnosis is a prime contributor to dermatological disability.[42]

PROGNOSIS

In his pioneering questionnaire study, Fregert[9] found that only 25% of his patients diagnosed as having occupational contact dermatitis had completely healed 2–3 years later: 50% still had intermittent symptoms, while as many as 25% still had continuous symptoms. Although 40% had changed their occupation, the change had not improved their prognosis. These considerations applied to irritant as much as to allergic contact dermatitis.

Wall and Gebauer[43] refined this study by increasing the number of patients followed up, examining the majority of these, and establishing more precisely what their change of job had entailed. More than half their patients still had their dermatitis to some degree. Again, around 40% had changed their jobs, but of these more than 25% had chosen new jobs in which the work environment further aggravated their skin. Of the 57% who were either in the same job or deemed to be still in the same type of occupation, as many as 68% were still symptomatic, whereas of the 43% who had changed to an entirely different work environment, from the dermatological point of view, only 37% were still symptomatic. Overall, 11.5% of the patients had an ongoing skin disease for which there was no identifiable present cause: this the authors termed 'persistent postoccupational dermatitis'.

Rosen and Freeman[44] took such studies still further by documenting improvement as well as complete healing, establishing improvement in 82% of those who changed duties within the same industry, 76% of those who changed industry altogether, and 61% of those who remained with the same duties in the same industry.

The main findings of all three of these major studies can be summarized as follows. The prognosis of occupational contact dermatitis severe enough to be referred to a dermatologist (known to have a special interest in occupational dermatoses) is one of persistence in more than half, though with improvement in around half of these. This applies to irritant as much as to allergic contact dermatitis. Appropriate occupational changes improve the prognosis for most, but around 10% of patients overall develop persistent postoccupational dermatitis. Chromate was the major allergen in all studies causing persistent postoccupational dermatitis, allergic contact dermatitis from plastics and resins having the best prognosis.[9]

Questionnaire studies of cutting fluid dermatitis (mainly irritant) have shown varying results. In a small study in Birmingham, UK, clearance was found in 45% of patients followed for up to 2.5 years after diagnosis: only one of 40 patients had been obliged to change their job.[45] In a larger such study in London, UK, of those who continued to work with water-based metalworking fluids, 78% had not healed after 2 years, and of those who had stopped working with soluble oils, 70% had still not healed 2 years after discontinuing contact; a generally poor prognosis was found whether or not such patients continued in their work.[46]

The prognosis for catering workers studied by Cronin[47] was also poor. Of 32 such patients followed up for around 2 years, 12 had been obliged to give up their work because of their contact dermatitis. Of the 19 who remained in catering only four healed completely; of the 13 who left, still only four healed.

The reasons for this generally poor prognosis, which applies to irritant as much as to allergic contact dermatitis, remained debatable. However, many less severe cases than those having to be referred to specialist dermatologists have a much better prognosis, as occupational physicians will be well aware. Also, even in such severe cases, dermatitis may become significantly more manageable after adequate investigation and treatment.

NON-ECZEMATOUS OCCUPATIONAL DERMATOSES

There are a number of non-eczematous skin disorders that, even together, constitute only a small minority of occupational dermatoses. Nevertheless, some have serious implications that demand their accurate diagnosis.

CONTACT URTICARIA

This is a wheal-and-flare reaction usually within 20–30 minutes of contact between certain substances and the skin surface (Fig. 37.4). It may be of immunological (allergic), non-immunological (irritant), or uncertain aetiology. The most frequent occupational cause currently is immunological (Type I) contact urticaria from natural rubber latex, the main at-risk

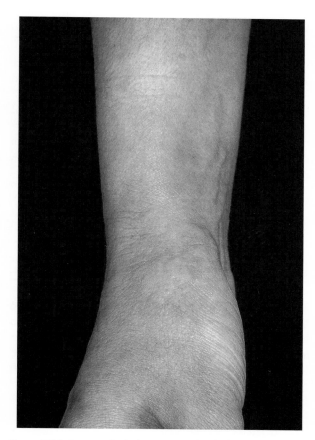

Figure 37.4 *Immunological contact urticaria from natural rubber latex gloves. See colour plate section.*

group being health care professionals who wear rubber gloves.[29,48] Clinical symptoms of Type I allergy to natural rubber latex may extend from contact urticaria, conjunctivitis and rhinitis, to asthma and anaphylaxis. Two major latex allergens have been identified, the important one for health care professionals being a soluble protein, hevein.[49] Cross-reacting proteins are present in many fruits and vegetables, including avocado, banana, sweet pepper, potato, kiwi fruit and tomato. Atopics are at greater risk. Latex allergens are adsorbed onto cornstarch glove powder, thus increasing airborne exposure: powdered natural rubber latex gloves should therefore no longer be used. Guidance is increasingly available as to how to control this problem, particularly in the health care setting.[50]

The most common other causes of occupational contact urticaria are foodstuffs,[29] which are considered below under protein contact dermatitis.

Confirmation of the diagnosis of immunological contact urticaria may be obtained by use tests, prick tests or RASTs, guided by clinical assessment of the extent and severity of symptoms.[29] Prick testing should never be conducted without appropriate resuscitation equipment to hand.

PROTEIN CONTACT DERMATITIS

Food handlers[29,51] and those working closely with animals may have hand dermatitis, either as well as or rather than contact urticaria, yet show positive prick tests or RASTs, rather than positive patch tests, to foodstuffs or animal products, a phenomenon first termed protein contact dermatitis in 1976.[52] The underlying allergic mechanism may depend on specific immunoglobulin-E being bound on the surface of epidermal Langerhans' cells.[53] Testing for Type I as well as Type IV allergy may therefore be required in chefs, animal laboratory technicians and veterinarians with hand dermatitis, as well as in the natural rubber latex glove wearers.

OIL FOLLICULITIS (OIL ACNE)

Petroleum oils exert a localized irritant effect on hair follicles, which causes a folliculitis of the hair-bearing skin of the backs of the hands, arms, thighs, abdomen, face and neck.[54] The primary lesions are open comedones ('blackheads'), causing mechanical blockage of the follicular openings (Fig. 37.5). Secondarily, inflammatory papules and pustules may develop. Metalworking machine operatives are the prime at-risk group, though adequate industrial and personal hygiene should nowadays make it rare. Those with previous cystic acne are more susceptible.

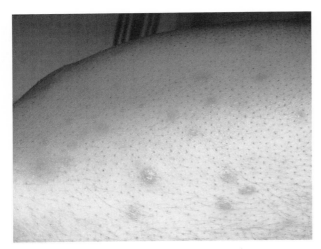

Figure 37.5 *Oil folliculitis. See colour plate section.*

CHLORACNE

This is both clinically and aetiologically distinct from oil acne. It might better be termed halogenacne, in that, as well as polychlorinated aromatic hydrocarbons of a highly specific molecular structure, brominated, iodinated and fluorinated homologues are also causal.[55] These uncommon chemicals, of which the dibenzodioxins are an example (see Chapter 12), may be encountered in pesticide manufacture, chemical disposal plants and, sporadically, in other chemical and pharmaceutical work.[56,57] Lesions are distributed typically over the temples, behind the ears and on the male genitals, and may spread to the trunk and limbs (Fig. 37.6). The primary lesions are open comedones and pale-yellow cysts. In

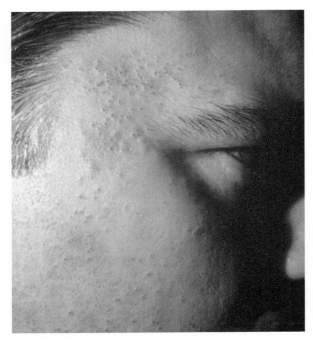

Figure 37.6 *Chloracne. See colour plate section.*

more severe cases, inflammatory lesions are also seen. The condition is notoriously chronic, even after complete removal of the cause, and may be extremely resistant to treatment.[57] Chloracne is always a symptom of systemic absorption[55] and may be associated with systemic morbidity.[58]

LEUCODERMA

Chemical depigmentation of the skin can arise occupationally from exposure either to various chemicals themselves or to their residues in products such as adhesives.[59] The chemicals responsible include phenols, catechols and hydroquinones.[60] Because of systemic absorption, white patches may appear well beyond sites of direct skin contact, thus closely mimicking idiopathic vitiligo. There are several possible explanations for the effects of such chemicals on the pigmentary system, their structures being very similar to melanin precursors.[60] Death of melanocytes results in depigmentation usually being permanent. Associated changes in liver function tests of uncertain significance have been reported.[61] Occupational leucoderma is a prescribed disease in its own right (see Chapters 4, 12).

SCLERODERMA-LIKE DISEASES

Vinyl chloride monomer, silica dust, organic solvents and epoxy resins have all been reported as associated with scleroderma-like conditions (see Chapter 8).[62] Exposure to vinyl chloride monomer has also caused acro-osteolysis and angiosarcoma of the liver in polymerization vessel cleaners, and miners exposed to silica dust may have associated silicosis (see Chapter 35). A more recent case was reported of a sclerodermatous syndrome following occupational exposure to herbicides.[63] The mechanism remains obscure: no cases have been observed in UK miners, for example.

ULCERATIONS

There are two main occupational causes of ulcerations, hexavalent chromium compounds and wet cement, in both cases the cause being toxic (irritant) rather than allergic. Chrome ulcers are mainly seen on the hands in those exposed to chromic acid in electroplating,[64] though regulation has generally made them rarer, and may occur from other sources, such as porcelain enamel paints.[65] Nasal septal ulceration, proceeding to perforation, may be associated (see Chapter 7).

Cement ulcers (or cement burns) are a rapid effect of wet cement trapped against the skin, for example by kneeling in it or by it entering footwear.[66] Symptoms may come on within an hour or two, the resulting ulceration then inexorably progressing and often requiring skin grafting. Precautions to avoid the occlusion of wet cement against the skin should be preventive, but inexperienced, amateur or heavily-exposed professional,[67] cement users may still be affected.

SKIN CARCINOMAS

Although now largely of historical interest,[68] except in outdoor workers from sun exposure, cancerous and precancerous skin lesions can still present, for example in elderly machine operatives exposed to cutting oils in the 1950s and 1960s, as well as sporadically from previously unsuspected causes.[69] The characteristic skin lesions are keratoses ('oil warts') and squamous cell carcinomata. They affect particularly the scrotum in machine operatives, and also commonly the hands and forearms, but rarely the face and neck. The carcinogens in mineral oils have been identified as polycyclic aromatic hydrocarbons. Solvent refining is considered to have reduced these to an adequately safe level, which epidemiological analysis of new cases has since begun to reflect.[70] Those occupationally exposed to polycyclic aromatic hydrocarbons in coal tar pitch may be similarly affected (see Chapter 7).

MAJOR OCCUPATIONS CAUSING DERMATOSES[18,32]

Agriculture[71]

Irritant contact dermatitis can arise from disinfectants and cleansers for milking equipment, and from diesel oil powering machinery. Allergic contact dermatitis is seen mainly from: rubber chemicals, including N-isopropyl-N'-phenyl-p-phenylenediamine (IPPD), in gloves, boots and milking equipment; plants, including Compositae (Asteraceae) such as the common weeds dandelion and thistle; pesticides; antibiotics in animal feeds and veterinary use; cobalt in fertilizers and animal feeds; other animal feed additives such as ethoxyquin and quinoxaline derivatives; and chromate in cement. Contact urticaria or protein contact dermatitis may be caused by animal hair and dander. Zoonoses include cattle ringworm and orf in sheep.

Catering[51]

Detergents, as well as fish, meat, fruit and vegetable juices, and dough, can all cause irritant contact dermatitis. Allergic contact dermatitis is caused mainly by onion and garlic, spices, formaldehyde and other preservatives, and rubber chemicals in gloves. Contact urticaria or protein contact dermatitis[52] is common from fish, shellfish, meat, fruit, vegetables, flour and flour improvers, and natural rubber latex in gloves. Candidal paronychia and viral warts also occur.

Chemical and pharmaceutical[72]

Irritants and sensitizers are specific to each process. Sensitization is often more common during research and development than in later full-scale production. Halogenated chemical intermediates are potent allergens. Inadvertent synthesis of new chloracnegens may result in sporadic outbreaks of chloracne.[57]

Cleaning[73]

Detergents and cleansers containing organic solvents, acids or alkalis are irritant. Rubber chemicals in gloves, formaldehyde and other preservatives, and fragrance chemicals cause allergic contact dermatitis. Contact urticaria and protein contact dermatitis arise mainly from natural rubber latex in gloves.[49] Candidal paronychia is also a problem.

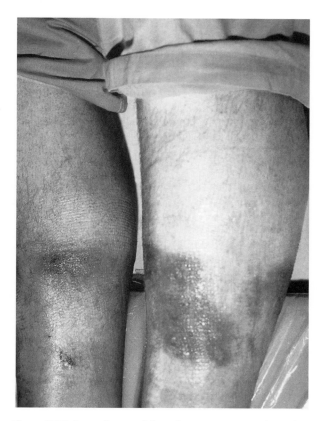

Figure 37.7 *Burns from quick-setting cement. See colour plate section.*

Construction[74]

Cement, fibreglass and wood preservatives can all cause irritant contact dermatitis, as well as mould oil in brickmaking. Cement burns are caused by wet cement trapped against the skin (Fig.37.7). Chromate (and cobalt) in cement, epoxy resin in special cements,[75] softwoods and hardwoods, and rubber chemicals in boots and sealing strips are the main allergens. Leptospirosis is an infectious hazard of open watercourses.

Electronics[76]

Soldering fluxes are a cause of irritancy, sensitization and contact urticaria. Warm dry air causes itchy dry skin. Epoxy resin and anaerobic acrylic sealants are other important sensitizers.

Fishing[77]

Irritant contact dermatitis arises from wet work, especially in the cold, friction, oils and fuels, and fish juice itself. The major sensitizers, apart from rubber chemicals in boots, are marine organisms, such as those responsible for Dogger Bank itch, and plants. Contact urticaria and protein contact dermatitis can also be caused by fish, marine organisms and plants.

Hairdressing[78]

Shampoos, permanent-wave solutions and bleaches are all irritant. The principal allergens are p-phenylenediamine (PPD) in hair dyes, glyceryl thioglycolate (GTG) in acid/pH balanced permanent-wave solutions, and formaldehyde or isothiazolinones as preservatives in hair gels and mousses. Contact urticaria or protein contact dermatitis can arise from ammonium persulphate in bleaches, as well as natural rubber latex in gloves.

Health care[79]

The main irritants are skin cleansers and disinfectants. Warm dry air in hospitals causes itchy skin dryness. Rubber gloves cause allergic contact dermatitis from their chemical content, and contact urticaria or protein contact dermatitis from their natural rubber latex.[48] Dentistry sensitizes to local anaesthetics, resins and catalysts. Orthopaedic surgeons run the risk of sensitization from acrylic cement. The cold sterilant glutaraldehyde has been a sensitization hazard in, for example, endoscopy units. Propacetamol is the latest in a long line of drugs to sensitize their handlers.

Horticulture and floristry[80]

Irritant contact dermatitis arises from wet work, friction from manipulating wire, handling bulbs, and certain plants such as *Dieffenbachia*, daffodils and spurges. Many other plants and flowers are sensitizers: *Primula obconica*, chrysanthemum, other Compositae (including common weeds), tulip and alstroemeria. Daffodils (and narcissi) may also sensitize. Dermatitis provoked by exposure to sunlight following contact with plants (phytophotodermatitis) occasionally occurs occupationally.[81] In the UK, the two main families of plants responsible are: the Apiaceae (Umbelliferae), including celery, parsley, parsnip and carrot, as well as giant Russian hogweed; and the Rutaceae, including rue. In hotter climates, the Moraceae (figs) and Leguminosae (pea) may also be causal. The level of phototoxic furocoumarins (psoralens) is increased in response to fungal disease. Tending plants in aquaria may result in *Mycobacterium marinum* infection. Rubber gloves may cause the same problems as in other occupations. Contact urticaria and protein contact dermatitis may also be caused by plants such as *Schlumbergera* cacti.

Metalworkers[82]

So-called 'soluble oils' are the major irritants, as well as organic solvents and aggressive skin cleansers. The irritancy of soluble oils may be increased by the overaddition of alkaline biocides. Both soluble oils and neat cutting oils also contain potential sensitizers, such as biocides (including formaldehyde-releasers) and tall-oil-based emulsifiers (which cross-react with colophony in the patch test standard series) in the former and epoxides in the latter. The usually trace amounts of nickel, cobalt and chromate in cutting oils rarely sensitize.

Mining[83]

Mineral dusts, oils and hydraulic fluids, and cement can all cause irritant contact dermatitis. Rubber chemicals in boots and chromate (and cobalt) in cement sensitize. Tinea pedis tends to be endemic, because of shared washing facilities at the surface, and may spread to the hands, among other areas. Scleroderma-like disease has been documented in miners in Eastern Europe and South Africa.

Office workers[84]

Low relative humidity may dry out the skin in air-conditioned offices, leading to intense pruritus and asteatotic eczema. Allergic contact dermatitis may arise from nickel (paper clips and staplers), rubber chemicals (rubber bands, thimbles and sponges) and colophony (paper size).

Painting[85]

Thinners (especially when used for skin cleansing), emulsion paints and wallpaper adhesives are irritant. Organotin compounds in antifouling paints for ships are highly irritant. Turpentine is now a sensitizer only in arts and crafts painters (e.g. porcelain). Other sensitizers include D-limonene (the 'citrus solvent'),[86] organocobalt paint driers, epoxy, acrylic and polyurethane resins, preservatives, such as chlorothalonil, in water-based paints, and triglycidyl isocyanurate (TGIC) in polyester powder paints.

Photographic processing[87]

Photographic processing chemicals include many sensitizers, such as metol (p-aminophenol) in black-and-white processing, and substituted para-phenylenediamines in colour developing (sometimes causing lichenoid eruptions). Rubber gloves cause the same problems as in other occupations.

Printing[88]

Irritant contact dermatitis arises from organic solvents and multifunctional acrylates in ultraviolet curing inks, lacquers and printing plates. Colophony is a sensitizer in paper size, rubber chemicals in offset printing roller blankets, formaldehyde or isothiazolinones as preservatives in gum arabic and fountain solutions, and multifunctional acrylates in the ultraviolet-curing products already referred to. Rubber gloves are also a source of sensitization.

Tanning[89]

Acids, alkalis, reducing and oxidizing agents are all irritant, while chromate, formaldchyde, glutaraldehyde, vegetable tannins, dyes and resins are potential allergens. Formaldehyde may also be a source of contact urticaria, in addition to rubber gloves. Anthrax remains a risk from hides from endemic areas.

Veterinary care[90]

Disinfectants may irritate. Rubber gloves, antibiotics and antimycotics, glutaraldehyde, and preservatives in rectal lubricants may all sensitize. Sources of contact urticaria and protein contact dermatitis include animal hair and dander, obstetric fluids and animal tissues, as well as rubber gloves. Zoonoses are clearly also a risk (see agriculture).

Woodworking[91]

Irritation may arise from certain hardwoods, wood preservatives, and formaldehyde resins in fibreboard and chipboard. Other woods (both soft and hard) are sensitizers, as may also be formaldehyde resins, and frullania and lichens may in addition sensitize forestry workers.

REFERENCES

1 Celsus AC. *De Re Medicina*. Florence, 1487.
2 Agricola AG. *De Re Metallica*. Basel, 1556.
3 Paracelsus T. *Von der Bergsucht*. Dilingen, 1567.
4 Ramazzini B. *De Morbus Artificum Diatriba*. Geneva, 1713.
5 White RP. *The dermatergoses or Occupational Affections of the Skin* 3rd edn. London: Lewis, 1928.
6 Bonnevie P. *Aetiologie und Pathogenese der Eczemkrankheiten*. Copenhagen: Busck, 1939.
7 Schwartz L, Tulipan L, Birmingham DJ. *Occupational Diseases of the Skin* 3rd edn. London: Kimpton, 1957.
8 Calnan CD. Dermatology and industry (Prosser White oration). *Clin Exp Dermatol* 1977;**3**:1–16.
9 Fregert S. Occupational dermatitis in a 10-year material. *Contact Derm* 1975;**1**:96–107.
10 Foussereau J, Benezra C, Maibach HI. *Occupational Contact Dermatitis*. Copenhagen: Munksgaard, 1982.
11 Zschunke E. *Grundriss der Arbeitsdermatologie*. Berlin: VEB Verlag Volk und Gesundheit, 1985.
12 Adams RM. *Occupational Skin Disease* 2nd edn. Philadelphia: WB Saunders Co, 1990.
13 Agrup G. Hand eczema and other dermatoses in South Sweden. *Acta Derm Venereol (Stockh)* 1969;**49**(Suppl):61.
14 Calnan CD, Rycroft RJG. Rehabilitation in occupational skin disease. *Trans Coll Med S Afr* 1981;**25**(Supplement Rehabilitation):136–42.
15 Health and Safety Commission. *Health and Safety Statistics 1996/97*. London: HSE, 1997.
16 Mathias CGT. The cost of occupational skin disease. *Arch Dermatol* 1985;**121**:332–34.
17 Burry JN, Kirk J. Environmental dermatitis: chrome cripples. *Med J Aust* 1975;**2**:720–1.
18 Rycroft RJG. Occupational contact dermatitis. In: Rycroft RJG, Frosch PJ, Menné T eds. *Textbook of Contact Dermatitis* 2nd edn. Berlin: Springer, 1995 : 341–400.
19 Mathias CGT. Occupational dermatoses. *J Am Acad Dermatol* 1988;**19**:1107–14.
20 Rycroft RJG, Robertson SJ. *A Colour Handbook of Dermatology*. London: Manson Publishing; 1999.
21 Calnan CD. Eczema for me. *Trans St John's Hosp Derm Soc* 1968;**54**:54–64.
22 Fregert S. *Manual of Contact Dermatitis* 2nd edn. Copenhagen: Munksgaard; 1981.
23 Wilkinson JD, Willis CM. Contact dermatitis: irritant. In: Champion RH, Burton JL, Burns DA, Breathnach SM eds.

Textbook of Dermatology 6th edn. Oxford: Blackwell Science, 1998 : 709–31.

24 Frosch PJ. Cutaneous irritation. In: Rycroft RJG, Menné T, Rycroft RJG eds. *Textbook of Contact Dermatitis* 2nd edn. Berlin: Springer, 1995 : 28–61.

25 Davies NF, Rycroft RJG. Dermatology. In: Cox RAF, Edwards FC, McCallum RI. *Fitness for Work. The Medical Aspects* 2nd edn. Oxford: Oxford University Press, 1995 : 102–12.

26 Coenraads P-J, Diepgen TL. Risk for hand eczema in employees with past or present atopic dermatitis. *Int Arch Occup Environ Hlth* 1998;**71**:7–13.

27 Rycroft RJG. Principal irritants and sensitizers. In: Champion RH, Burton JL, Burns DA, Breachnach SM eds. *Textbook of Dermatology* 6th edn. Oxford: Blackwell Science, 1998 : 821–60.

28 Scheper RJ, von Blomberg BME. Cellular mechanisms in allergic contact dermatitis. In: Rycroft RJG, Frosch PJ, Menné T eds. *Textbook of Contact Dermatitis* 2nd edn. Berlin: Springer, 1995 : 11–27.

29 Wilkinson JD, Shaw S. Contact dermatitis: allergic. In: Champion RH, Burton JL, Burns DA, Breachnach SM eds. *Textbook of Dermatology* 6th edn. Oxford: Blackwell Science, 1998 : 733–819.

30 Kanerva L, Tarvainen K, Pinola A, Leino T, Granlund H *et al.* A single accidental exposure may result in a chemical burn, primary sensitization and allergic contact dermatitis. *Contact Derm* 1994;**31**:229–35.

31 De Groot AC. *Patch Testing: Test Concentrations and Vehicles for 3700 Chemicals* 2nd edn. Amsterdam: Elsevier, 1994.

32 Rycroft RJG. Occupational dermatoses. In: Champion RH, Burton JL, Burns DA, Breachnach SM eds. *Textbook of Dermatology* 6th edn. Oxford: Blackwell Science, 1998 : 861–81.

33 Wilkinson DS. Some causes of error in the diagnosis of occupational dermatoses. In: Griffiths WAD, Wilkinson DS eds. *Essentials of Industrial Dermatology*. Oxford: Blackwell Science, 1985 : 47–57.

34 Freeman S. Diagnosis and differential diagnosis. In: Adams RM ed. *Occupational Skin Disease* 2nd edn. Philadelphia: WB Saunders Co, 1990 : 194–214.

35 Meneghini CL, Angelini G. Primary and secondary sites of occupational contact dermatitis. *Dermatosen* 1984;**32**: 205–7.

36 Dooms-Goossens A, Debusschere KM, Gevers DM, Dupré KM, Degreef HJ *et al.* Contact dermatitis caused by airborne agents. A review and case reports. *J Am Acad Dermatol* 1986;**15**:1–10.

37 Rycroft RJG. Occupational dermatoses in perspective. *Lancet* 1980;**ii**:24–26.

38 Wilkinson JD. The management of contact dermatitis. In: Rycroft RJG, Frosch PJ, eds. *Textbook of Contact Dermatitis* 2nd edn. Berlin: Springer, 1995 : 659–92.

39 Calnan CD. Studies in contact dermatitis. XXIII. Allergen replacement. *Trans St John's Dermatol Soc* 1970;**56**:131–8.

40 Frosch PJ, Kurte A, Pilz B. Efficacy of skin barrier creams (III). The repetitive irritation test (RIT) in humans. *Contact Derm* 1993;**29**:113–8.

41 Zhai H, Maibach HI. Moisturizers in preventing irritant contact dermatitis: an overview. *Contact Derm* 1998;**38**:241–4.

42 Pryce DW, Irvine D, English JSC, Rycroft RJG. Soluble oil dermatitis: a follow-up study. *Contact Derm* 1989;**21**:28–35.

43 Wall LM, Gebauer KA. A follow-up study of occupational skin disease in Western Australia. *Contact Derm* 1991; **24**:241–3.

44 Rosen RH, Freeman S. Prognosis of occupational contact dermatitis in New South Wales, Australia. *Contact Derm* 1993;**29**:88–93.

45 Grattan CEH, Foulds IS. Outcome of investigation of cutting fluid dermatitis. *Contact Derm* 1989;**20**:377–8.

46 Pryce DW, Irvine D, English JSC, Rycroft RJG. Soluble oil dermatitis: a follow-up study. *Contact Derm* 1989; **21**:28–35.

47 Cronin E. Dermatitis of the hands in caterers. *Contact Derm* 1987;**17**:265–9.

48 Turjanmaa K, Alenins H, Mäkinen-Kiljunen S, Reunala T, Palosno T. Natural rubber latex allergy. *Allergy* 1996; **51**:593–602.

49 Posch A, Chen Z, Raulf-Heimsoth M, Baur X. Latex allergens. *Clin Exp All* 1998;**28**:134–40.

50 Medical Devices Agency (UK). Device Bulletin 9601. *Latex Sensitisation in the Health Care Setting (Use of Latex Gloves)*. MDA London: 1996.

51 Cronin E. Dermatitis in food handlers. In: Callen JP, Dahl MV, Golitz LE, Schachner LA, Stegman SJ eds. *Advances in Dermatology* Vol 4. Chicago: Year Book, 1989 : 113–24.

52 Hjorth N, Roed-Petersen J. Occupational protein contact dermatitis in food handlers. *Contact Derm* 1976;**2**:28–42.

53 Lahti A. Immediate contact reactions. In: Rycroft RJG, Frosch PJ, Menné T, eds. *Textbook of Contact Dermatitis* 2nd edn. Berlin: Springer, 1995 : 62–74.

54 Rycroft RJG. Petroleum and petroleum derivatives. In: Adams RM ed. *Occupational Skin Disease* 2nd edn. Philadelphia: WB Saunders Co, 1990 : 486–502.

55 Tindall JP. Chloracne and chloracnegens. *J Am Acad Derm* 1985;**13**:539–58.

56 Poskitt LB, Duffill MB, Rademaker M. Chloracne, palmoplantar keratoderma and localized scleroderma in a weed sprayer. *Clin Exp Dermatol* 1994;**19**:264–7.

57 Scerri L, Zaki I, Millard LG. Severe halogen acne due to a trifluoromethylpyrazole derivative and its resistance to isotretinoin. *Br J Derm* 1995;**132**:144–8.

58 Zober A, Ott MG, Messerer P. Morbidity follow up study of BASF employees exposed to 2,3,7,8-tetrachlorodibenzo-p-dioxin (TCDD) after a 1953 chemical reactor incident. *Occ Environ Med* 1994;**51**:470–86.

59 Stevenson CJ. Environmentally induced vitiligo (leucoderma) from depigmenting agents and chemicals. *J Cut Ocular Toxicol* 1984;**3**:299–307.

60 Bolognia JL, Pawalek JM. Biology of hypopigmentation. *J Am Acad Derm* 1988;**19**:217–55.

61 James O, Mayes RW, Stevenson CJ. Occupational vitiligo

induced by p-tert-butylphenol. A systemic disease? *Lancet* 1997;**ii**:1217–9.

62 Black CM, Welsh KI. Occupationally and environmentally induced scleroderma-like illness: etiology, pathogenesis, diagnosis, and treatment. *Int Med Specialist* 1988; **9**:135–54.

63 Dunnill MGS, Black MM. Sclerodermatous syndrome after occupational exposure to herbicides – response to systemic steroids. *Clin Exp Derm* 1994;**19**:518–20.

64 Williams N. Occupational skin ulceration in chrome platers. *Occup Med* 1997;**47**:309–10.

65 Fleeger AK, Deng J-F. A case study of chromium VI-induced skin ulcerations during a porcelain enamel curing operation. *Appl Occ Environ Hyg* 1990;**5**:378–82.

66 Rycroft RJG. Acute ulcerative contact dermatitis from Portland cement. *Br J Dermatol* 1980;**102**:487–9.

67 Irvine C, Pugh CE, Hansen EJ, Rycroft RJG. Cement dermatitis in underground workers during construction of the Channel Tunnel. *Occup Med* 1994;**44**:17–23.

68 Cruickshank CND, Squire JR. Skin cancer in the engineering industry from the use of mineral oil. *Br J Ind Med* 1950; **7**:1–11.

69 Bowra GT, Duffield DP, Osborn AJ, Purchase IFH. Premalignant and neoplastic skin lesions association with occupational exposure to 'tarry' byproducts during manufacture of 4,4′-bipyridyl. *Br J Ind Med* 1982;**39**:76–81.

70 Waldron HA, Waterhouse JAH, Tessema N. Scrotal cancer in the West Midlands 1936–76. *Br J Ind Med* 1984;**41**:437–44.

71 Veien N. Occupational dermatoses in farmers. In: Maibach HI ed. *Occupational and Industrial Dermatology* 2nd edn. Chicago: Year Book, 1987 : 436–46.

72 Sherertz EF. Occupational skin disease in the pharmaceutical industry. *Derm Clin* 1994;**12**:533–6.

73 Nilsson E. Contact sensitivity and urticaria in 'wet' work. *Contact Derm* 1985;**13**:321–8.

74 Avnstorp C. Risk factors for cement eczema. *Contact Derm* 1991;**25**:81–8.

75 Van Putten PB, Coenraads PJ, Nater JP. Hand dermatoses and contact allergic reactions in construction workers exposed to epoxy resins. *Contact Derm* 1984;**10**:146–50.

76 Koh D, Foulds IS, Aw TC. Dermatological hazards in the electronics industry. *Contact Derm* 1990;**22**:1–7.

77 Ashworth J, Curry FM, White IR, Rycroft RJG. Occupational allergic contact dermatitis in east coast of England fishermen: newly described hypersensitivities to marine organisms. *Contact Derm* 1990;**22**:185–6.

78 Van der Walle HB, Brunsveld VM. Dermatitis in hairdressers (I). The experience of the past 4 years, II. Management and prevention. *Contact Derm* 1994;**30**:217–21, 265–70.

79 Lammintausta K. Hand dermatitis in different hospital workers who perform wet work. *Dermatosen* 1983; **31**:14–19.

80 Schmidt R. Plants. In: Adams RM ed. *Occupational Skin Disease* 2nd edn. Philadelphia: WB Saunders Co, 1990 : 503–24.

81 Lovell CR. *Plants and the Skin*. Oxford: Blackwell Science, 1993 : 86–95.

82 Pryce DW, White J, English JSC, Rycroft RJG. Soluble oil dermatitis: a review. *J Soc Occup Med* 1989;**39**:93–8.

83 Puttick LM. Skin disorders in the mining industry [dissertation]. London: University of London, 1989.

84 Rycroft RJG. Occupational dermatoses among office personnel. *Occup Med State Art Rev* 1986;**1**:323–8.

85 Högberg M, Wahlberg JE. Health screening for occupational dermatoses in house painters. *Contact Derm* 1980;**6**:100–6.

86 Karlberg A-T, Dooms-Goossens A. Contact allergy to *d*-limonene among dermatitis patients. *Contact Derm* 1997;**36**:201–6.

87 Rustemeyer T, Frosch PJ. Allergic contact dermatitis from colour developers. *Contact Derm* 1995;**32**:59–60.

88 Andrews LS, Clary JJ. Review of the toxicity of multifunctiional acrylates. *J Toxicol Environ Hlth* 1986;**19**:149–64.

89 Burrows D. Adverse chromate reactions on the skin. In: Burrows D ed. *Chromium: Metabolism and Toxicity*. Boca Raton: CRC Press, 1983 : 137–63.

90 Falk ES, Hektoen H, Thune PO. Skin and respiratory tract symptoms in veterinary surgeons. *Contact Derm* 1985; **12**:274–8.

91 Hausen BM. *Woods Injurious to Human Health. A Manual*. Berlin: Walter de Gruyter, 1981.

Part 9

Occupational cancer

Biological mechanisms and biomarkers   741
Clinical and epidemiological aspects   791

38

Biological mechanisms and biomarkers

STANLEY VENITT

Carcinogenesis as a multi-step process	741	Testing chemicals for genotoxicity and carcinogenicity	763
Evidence for the role of genetic change in carcinogenesis	742	Biomonitoring for carcinogen exposure in the workplace	767
Cancer as a genetic disease of somatic cells	747	Mechanisms of occupational carcinogens	775
Processes that are perturbed during carcinogenesis	747	Acknowledgement	779
Genes involved in the development of cancer	748	References	779
Mechanisms of invasion and metastasis	755		
Cancer susceptibility: germline *versus* somatic mutation of cancer genes	756		

The aim of this chapter is to review current knowledge of mechanisms of chemical carcinogenesis and to apply it to occupational carcinogenesis. Much of what is known about carcinogens and carcinogenesis arose from the recognition that certain forms of cancer were associated with exposure of workers to chemicals in the workplace. The first concise description of an association of specific cancer with an occupational exposure – soot – was made by Percival Pott, who, in 1775, described cancer of the scrotum as an occupational hazard in 'climbing boys' – who swept chimneys by climbing through them with brushes.

The widespread exposure of workers to pitch, soot, coal tar and later to shale-oil and mineral oil which ensued from the Industrial Revolution led to the idea that these complex mixtures must contain substances that could cause cancer, since skin cancer was common in workers exposed to these mixtures. The word 'carcinogen' was coined to describe a substance that could induce cancer. Further progress in discovering the chemical nature of carcinogens and the mechanism of carcinogenesis depended on the ability to produce cancer at will under controlled conditions. It was not until 1915 that two Japanese pathologists, Yamagiwa and Ichikawa, produced cancer experimentally by repeated and prolonged application of coal tar to the ears of rabbits. Fifteen years later a pure carcinogen was identified – a single substance of known chemical structure capable of producing cancer in laboratory animals. Kennaway and Hieger reported in 1930 that dibenz[a,h]anthracene caused skin cancer when applied to the backs of mice. It was soon shown that coal tar and similar mixtures contained many kindred chemicals, known collectively as polycyclic aromatic hydrocarbons. The discovery of these and a variety of other chemical carcinogens opened the way to the rational study of cancer in the laboratory.[1,2]

CARCINOGENESIS AS A MULTI-STEP PROCESS

Carcinogenesis proceeds in a series of steps.[3,4] Epidemiological studies of human cancer suggest a succession of five or six independent stages in carcinogenesis, each of which is rate-limiting. This has been reviewed extensively by Lawley.[5,6]

Lessons from experimental studies

Experiments in two-stage and three-stage carcinogenesis in animals supported the multi-step nature of carcinogenesis and led to the concepts of 'initiation', 'promotion' and 'progression' which have dominated this field of enquiry for many decades.[7] Although still widely used, the distinction between these stages has become increasingly blurred as knowledge has increased. Recognition that carcinogens fall into two distinct classes – agents that cause cancer by mutation (genotoxic carcinogens) and those that do not (non-genotoxic carcinogens) – has further complicated the terminology used in describing the multi-stage model of carcinogenesis. The terms genotoxic and non-genotoxic are themselves the subject of lively debate, as is the best way of distinguishing by experiment those chemicals that are genotoxic from those that are not.[8,9]

The distinction between non-genotoxic carcinogens and promoting agents is far from clear. It is important not to confuse the terms which have been used to describe the stages recognized in experimental carcinogenesis – initiation, promotion, progression – with those that describe the properties of particular substances that appear to elicit one or more of these stages. Classically, the term promotion is used to describe the process in which a chemical enhances the incidence of tumours when applied chronically and repeatedly after a single or brief treatment with an initiating agent. However, such promoting agents, although usually devoid of genotoxic activity, can themselves produce tumours after protracted dosing of rodents which have not been treated with an initiating agent.[10]

At the experimental level, an initiator is a mutagen. A promoter is an agent that enhances the yield of tumours in an animal exposed to a low dose of an initiator.[11,12] For example, tumours can be induced in the skin of mice given a single subcarcinogenic dose of a carcinogen such as 7,12-dimethylbenz[a]anthracene (which is metabolized to a mutagen) provided that this treatment is followed by repeated application of a second substance such as a phorbol ester which itself is not necessarily carcinogenic. The development of tumours can also be enhanced by other stimuli to cell proliferation, such as wounding and possibly lung fibrosis. Progression is a less well-defined concept and describes the development of malignant tumours from benign neoplasms – for example, the progression of benign adenomatous polyps in the colon to malignant colonic carcinoma.

Many carcinogens are 'complete' or 'solitary'; application of such an agent to an animal can induce the entire sequence of events necessary to produce a malignant tumour.[13]

Site-specificity of carcinogens

Certain chemical carcinogens induce tumours only at specific sites or at a limited number of sites.[14] This is known as organotropy. For example, aflatoxin-B_1 is specifically carcinogenic to the liver in several different mammalian species and 1,2-dimethylhydrazine induces colon cancer in mice and rats when given by subcutaneous injection. Organotropy is particularly characteristic of carcinogenic N-nitroso compounds. Tumours can be induced in different animal organs, depending on the chemical structure, the animal species, the route of administration and the frequency and timing of dosage. Organotropy is also characteristic of cancers induced by agents that affect hormone levels.

Differences in toxicokinetics and metabolism between

species play a major role in determining target sites for different carcinogenic chemicals. For example, the occupational carcinogen 2-naphthylamine is a potent human bladder carcinogen. It induces bladder tumours in non-human primates, dogs and Syrian hamsters. However, it is only weakly carcinogenic in the bladder in the rat, and in mice where it induces tumours only in the liver and lungs.[15]

Interaction of two or more carcinogens

Epidemiological studies of human populations and experiments with animals show that concurrent exposure to two carcinogens often results in a carcinogenic effect that is more than simply additive. The multiplicative effect of smoking and asbestos on lung cancer in people occupationally exposed to asbestos is a good example.[16]

EVIDENCE FOR THE ROLE OF GENETIC CHANGE IN CARCINOGENESIS

Carcinogenic substances fall into a wide range of chemical classes and vary greatly in terms of their potency, the range of tumours they induce and their modes of action. Nevertheless, many carcinogenic chemicals share one critical property with other tumour-inducing agents such as oncogenic viruses and ionizing and ultraviolet radiation – the capacity to provoke genetic change.

There is compelling evidence that cancer is a genetic disorder of somatic cells and can be triggered by the genotoxic action of carcinogens.[5,6,12,17] This 'somatic mutation' theory of carcinogenesis is now accepted as the best working hypothesis to explain the carcinogenic properties of most chemical and physical carcinogens. However, there are substances that while displaying no evidence of genotoxic activity, are nonetheless carcinogenic.

The idea that cancer is a genetic disorder of somatic cells dates at least as far back as 1914, with Boveri's observations of chromosomal abnormalities in neoplastic cells from human tumours. There is now abundant evidence that human cancer develops in a series of steps, that it originates in single cells and that mutational events play a central role in carcinogenesis.[12,18,19] The use of molecular analysis of the genetics of germline and somatic mutations in human cancer has revealed that mutations in 5, 6 or more genes can be identified during development of, for example, colorectal cancer (Fig. 38.1), lending further support for the multi-step, somatic mutation theory of cancer.[20]

Several strands of evidence support the idea that cancer arises as a genetic disorder of somatic cells and that instability of the genome plays a crucial role in carcinogenesis:[12,19,21]

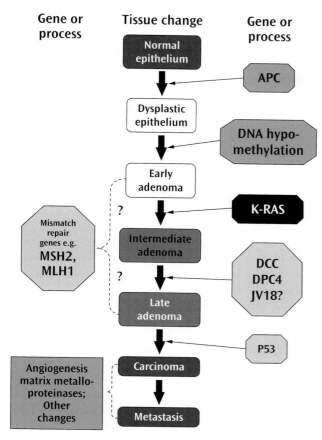

Gene or process | **Tissue change** | **Gene or process**

Figure 38.1 *(See colour plate section where this figure also appears in colour.) A genetic model for colorectal tumorigenesis, based on Ref. 20. 'Tissue changes' refers to the pathological changes that occur during the development of human colorectal cancer. 'Gene or process' refers to the genes or processes that are perturbed or changed during carcinogenesis. The genes depicted in pale blue are tumour-suppressor genes (see Table 38.2 for details). During carcinogenesis, tumour suppressor genes are inactivated by mutation and other genetic events that lead to the loss of both alleles. DCC, DPC4 and JV18 are candidate tumour-suppressor genes. K-RAS is an oncogene (Table 38.1) which requires point mutation in just one of its two alleles for its activation. DNA hypomethylation may allow inappropriate gene expression. Inactivation of mismatch repair genes increases the mutability of affected cells. The precise timing of mismatch-repair inactivation is unknown.*

- most carcinogens are genotoxic;
- genetically determined cancer-prone conditions exist in which there are deficiencies in DNA repair or increases in chromosomal fragility;
- non-random chromosomal anomalies occur in many type of human tumours;
- certain rare childhood tumours carry chromosomal rearrangements that in some cases are heritable;
- most human tumours are clonal in composition;
- many different tumours contain genes (activated oncogenes) that carry point mutations or whose

activity or quantity has been changed by chromosomal rearrangement or amplification;
- genes that suppress tumour formation (tumour-suppressor genes) can be inactivated by gene mutation and by structural and numerical chromosomal mutation.

These strands of evidence are considered in more detail below.

Mutagenic and DNA damaging effects (genotoxicity) of carcinogens

The ability to induce DNA damage and mutation is a characteristic shared by a very diverse range of physical and chemical carcinogens. Mutation is a heritable change in the amount or structure of the genetic material that results in a phenotypic change. This change may be expressed, for example, as a change in the structure of a protein that alters or abolishes its properties. Mutation occurs spontaneously or may be induced by physical and chemical agents.[22] Changes in the content or arrangement of information in DNA can occur in a variety of ways, and at several levels, ranging from a change in a single nucleotide within a codon, to changes in the number of complete chromosomes in a cell. Mutations are of three general types: point, chromosomal and genomic.[23–25]

POINT MUTATION

A point mutation is a change in the nucleotide sequence in one or a few codons, and can occur by base-substitution (one base is substituted by another) or by deletion or addition of one or more bases from or to one or more codons. Base-pair substitutions occur in two ways. In *transitions* one purine is substituted by another purine, or one pyrimidine is substituted by another pyrimidine (for example, adenine (A) by guanine (G), or thymine (T) by cytosine (C)). *Transversions* occur when a purine is replaced by a pyrimidine or vice versa (e.g. A by C; G by C). Additions or deletions change the reading frame of the DNA and are known as frameshift mutations.[23–25]

CHROMOSOMAL MUTATIONS

Chromosomal mutations are recognized as morphological changes in the gross structure of chromosomes, and are usually detected by microscopic examination of cells fixed and stained at metaphase. Chromosomal mutations result from breakage and reunion of chromosomal material during the cell cycle and include inversions (a length of chromosome is inserted back to front) and translocations (one section of chromosome becomes attached to another). The loss of DNA or its repositioning during these events may have dramatic consequences for gene expression, and in many cases chromosomal mutations are lethal to the affected cell or individual.

There is clear evidence that chromosomal mutations are of critical significance in carcinogenesis.[26]

GENOMIC MUTATION

Genomic mutation is a change in the number of chromosomes in the genome. The normal diploid genome is euploid and contains a complete set of chromosomes from each parent. Polyploidy occurs where the diploid genome is doubled or tripled. Loss or gain of a single chromosome is known as aneuploidy and may occur as a result of non-disjunction during cell division. Addition of one chromosome is trisomy; deletion of one chromosome is monosomy. Like chromosomal mutation, aneuploidy is regarded as an important element in the process of carcinogenesis.[27]

DNA DAMAGE

Throughout the course of evolution DNA has been subjected to wear and tear. This occurs endogenously, by errors during DNA replication, by slow hydrolysis in the aqueous environment of the cell, and by free-radical formation and aberrant methylation of DNA.[28] Exogenous mutagens also contribute: these include ultraviolet light, cosmic and terrestrial ionizing radiation, and a variety of chemicals such as polycyclic aromatic hydrocarbons produced by burning of organic matter. There are several consequences of DNA damage, including DNA-repair, mutation or cell death; DNA contains many potentially reactive sites and its structure can be modified in a number of ways.

Hydrolytic damage (reaction with water)

Spontaneous point mutations may occur by hydrolytic damage to DNA. This includes loss of bases and deamination of exocyclic amino groups.[28,29]

Adduct formation

Covalent binding of chemicals to DNA, with the formation of chemically stable products known as adducts, plays a major role in the mode of action of chemical mutagens and carcinogens and is a property common to a wide variety of otherwise disparate carcinogens.[5,30,31] Adducts range in size and complexity from simple alkyl groups (e.g. methyl, ethyl) to bulky multi-ring residues from chemicals such as polycyclic aromatic hydrocarbons and aromatic amines. Adducts can form links between adjacent bases on the same strand (intrastrand crosslinks) and can form interstrand crosslinks between each strand of the duplex.

Some chemicals known to be genotoxic, are intrinsically reactive and can form DNA adducts directly, either with DNA in solution in a test-tube, or with DNA in a living cell. These are called (ungrammatically) 'direct-acting' agents and include alkylsulphonic esters, epoxides, aromatic N-oxides, aromatic nitro compounds, lactones, alkylnitrosoureas and alkylnitrosamides. These are all electrophilic – they acquire electrons during chemical reactions. DNA contains many nucleophilic centres – atoms that donate electrons (e.g. N-2, N-7, O-6 atoms of guanine). DNA-adduct formation occurs mainly by the reaction of electrophiles with nucleophilic centres in DNA – the attraction and bonding of positive to negative.

METABOLIC ACTIVATION

Other chemicals are known as 'indirect-acting agents'. These are not electrophilic *per se*, but are converted to electrophiles by cellular enzyme systems. This is known as metabolic activation and is a normal biochemical activity of vertebrates. It provides for detoxification and elimination of potentially toxic substances that are generated by normal metabolism, or are absorbed from the diet, or as drugs, or as occupational chemicals or environmental contaminants. Enzymes with these functions fall into two main classes, 'phase I' and 'phase II'. Most phase I enzymes are members of the cytochrome P450 superfamily of enzymes – 'mono-oxygenases' – that carry out oxidative metabolism by inserting one atom of oxygen into a relatively inert and usually non-polar substrate. Cytochrome P450s catalyse the biosynthesis and degradation of many normal biochemical substrates. Phase II enzymes conjugate reactive intermediates formed by oxidative metabolism with endogenous molecules, such as glutathione, to polar, hydrophilic products that are readily excreted from cells.[32–35] This benign and necessary house-keeping activity is perverted to a more sinister course when a chemically inert and genetically inactive molecule is converted to a metabolite which can react with DNA.[30,36] A variety of carcinogens can be metabolized to reactive electrophiles. They include occupational carcinogens such as polycyclic aromatic hydrocarbons, aromatic amines, and alkyl and arylnitrosamines.[31]

DNA ADDUCTS AND MUTATION

In most cases, a single chemical will give rise to several different DNA adducts, depending on the number and nature of different metabolites formed from the given chemical and on the affinity of these metabolites with various atoms in the DNA molecule. Stereochemical and physicochemical constraints also play a part in determining the spectrum of DNA adducts formed by a given compound.[37]

The biological consequences of adduct formation depend to a large extent on the nature of the adduct and its precise location in the DNA molecule.[5,25,38] For example, a methyl group at the N-7 position of guanine (N7-G) is much less mutagenic than the same group at O-6 of guanine (O6-G), since the latter participates in hydrogen-bond formation during complementary base-pairing, whilst the former does not. However, a bulky adduct such as that formed by aflatoxin B_1 at N7-G is highly mutagenic, because it causes gross distortion of the DNA structure which seriously impairs hydrogen bonding. Adduct formation can lead to base-substitution, deletion and addition, and therefore to point mutation. For example, 7-methylbenz[a]anthracene *anti*-3,4-dihydrodiol 1,2-epoxide (the ultimate carcinogenic metabolite of 7-methylbenz[a]anthracene) reacts with DNA to form adducts mainly with the N-2 of guanine. In experiments using a plasmid of known DNA sequence, 94% of 77 base-pair substitution mutations were transversions involving guanine (GC to TA; GC to CG).[39] In contrast, the hepatocarcinogen dimethylnitrosamine is metabolized *in vivo* to an alkylating species that methylates DNA mainly at the O-6 position of guanine. Studies of mutation in bacteria injected intravenously into dimethylnitrosamine-treated rats and then recovered from their livers showed that GC to AT transitions predominated, as would be predicted from the disturbance of base-pairing engendered by methylation of O6-G.[40]

MUTATIONAL HOTSPOTS

Experiments of these types have also shown that the distribution of point mutations within a gene is not random, but occurs at 'hotspots' determined, *inter alia*, by the base sequence of the given gene and by the chemical structure and reactivity of the adduct-forming agent.[25] A strong link between a defined chemical carcinogen, its DNA adducts and human cancer has been established by a study of the distribution of benzo[a]pyrene-adducts along the *P53* gene in human cells treated with (±)-*anti*-7,8-dihydroxy-9,10-epoxy-7,8,9,10-tetrahydrobenzo[a]pyrene (BPDE), the ultimate carcinogenic metabolite of benzo[a]pyrene, which is an important carcinogenic component of cigarette smoke. This revealed strong and selective adduct formation with guanine in those three codons that comprise the major mutational hotspots in *P53* in human lung cancers.[41] Further studies revealed that biomethylation of cytosine at CpG dinucleotides (see p. 754) is the primary driving force for codon-specific adduct formation of this type.[42]

STRAND BREAKAGE

The sugar-phosphate DNA backbone can be cut in several ways. Adduct formation may modify the chemical structure of DNA such that strand breaks can occur, for example, by depurination and hydrolytic cleavage following alkylation of DNA. Physical agents such as x-rays can cause single and double strand breaks by engendering free-radical formation.[38]

FREE RADICALS

Free radicals are atoms or molecules that contain an unpaired electron and that seek out another electron to attain a more stable and less reactive state. A variety of agents can generate free radicals by several different

mechanisms. Of the many oxygen radicals encountered in biological systems, the hydroxyl radical is the most reactive, degrading any molecule within diffusion distance, and is considered to be the ultimate radical species responsible for damaging DNA. It causes breaks in the sugar-phosphate backbone, and can chemically modify DNA bases.[28,38,43] DNA damage induced by oxygen free-radical formation is believed to play a major part in the mechanisms underlying the carcinogenicity of several important occupational carcinogens, including chromium and nickel compounds and asbestos. These are discussed later.

DNA-INTERCALATION, TOPOISOMERASES AND CHROMOSOME DAMAGE

As well as forming DNA adducts by covalent binding, certain carcinogens, such as the antineoplastic drug doxorubicin, interact with DNA by intercalation. This is the physical binding of an agent such that it becomes wedged between the stacked bases of the DNA double helix. Intercalation alters a variety of DNA functions – for example, it can inhibit DNA and RNA polymerases. However, it is the effect of intercalation on topoisomerases that is of most interest as a mechanism leading to genotoxic and possibly carcinogenic effects.

Topoisomerases are mammalian enzymes that control the degree of coiling adopted by DNA molecules over and above the primary double helical configuration of native DNA. The coiled-coil structure allows enormous lengths of DNA to be packed into very small volumes. For example, a single human somatic cell contains about half a metre of DNA packed into a nucleus whose diameter is measured in microns.[44] A remarkable degree of topological management ensures that such huge lengths of DNA are replicated accurately and that gene expression and regulation are controlled in an orderly manner. Mammalian topoisomerase II makes transient double-stranded cuts in DNA. These allow coiled coils to relax and replicated domains to separate or to knots to untangle – a process known as decatenation. Substances that produce DNA breaks by interfering with topoisomerase II induce chromosomal aberrations that are independent of cell-cycle stage and are more typical of ionizing radiation than of carcinogens such as alkylating agents.

DNA repair

A wealth of evidence indicates that the response of the organism to DNA damage is just as important to the final outcome as the nature of the primary damage. The essence of a mutation is that it is a heritable change; the damage that causes a mutation must be fixed before it can be expressed in succeeding generations. The primary DNA damage (e.g. an adduct) is not of itself a mutation, but a pre-mutational lesion – a mutation waiting to happen.

A cell that has sustained DNA damage may respond in several ways. The cell might die; the presence of an adduct (e.g. a cross-link) may kill a cell by blocking DNA replication, or might prevent the synthesis of an essential protein by obstructing transcription of its mRNA. DNA damage also invokes apoptosis (programmed cell death), a process by which a cell commits suicide. When a cell dies, the possibility of mutation is eliminated, since there are no daughter cells to inherit the damage. Alternatively, a cell might repair the damage and restore its DNA to the pristine state it was in before it sustained the damage, in which case mutation will not occur, the repair being error-free. However, the fact that DNA damage does lead to somatic mutation in daughter cells implies that repair mechanisms can and do fail, allowing survival and cell division despite a burden of pre-mutational lesions. Several different types of DNA repair mechanisms have evolved which allow cells to remove or circumvent the effects of DNA damage. For an extensive review of DNA repair and mutagenesis see Ref. 38.

Genetically determined cancer-prone conditions

Defects in DNA-repair lead to genomic instability, which is characteristic of cancer cells.[22,45] Several rare inherited disorders are associated both with an increased predisposition to develop cancer and with DNA-repair deficiencies or increased chromosome fragility. For example, patients with the recessively inherited syndrome xeroderma pigmentosum are defective in DNA repair and develop multiple skin tumours when exposed to sunlight. Bloom's syndrome, Fanconi's anaemia and ataxia telangiectasia are all recessively inherited syndromes associated with an increased risk of cancer and chromosomal instability, and possibly DNA-repair defects.[46–48] Dominantly inherited mutations in genes involved in the maintenance of the genetic code during replication ('mismatch repair') confer increased risks of colorectal and other cancers, as described later.

Chromosomal anomalies and hereditary cancer

Karyotypic analysis of thousands of human neoplasms has shown that chromosomal aberrations in neoplastic disorders are of three kinds: (1) primary abnormalities, which are essential steps in establishing the tumour; (2) secondary abnormalities, which develop only after the tumour has developed, but which nevertheless may be important in tumour progression; and (3) cytogenetic 'noise', which is the background level of inconsequential aberrations that, unlike types 1 and 2, are randomly distributed throughout the genome.[49] Of 26 523 cases examined, 215 balanced and 1588 unbalanced recurrent aberrations were identified among 75 different neoplas-

tic disorders.[50] Usually the primary abnormalities are strictly associated with particular cancers and even with histopathological subtypes within a given cancer. Clonal chromosomal abnormalities are a feature of both benign and malignant neoplasms, although the abnormalities are often less severe in benign tumours. Many of the chromosomal abnormalities associated with neoplasia have been characterized at the molecular level, revealing previously unknown genes that are closely associated with carcinogenesis.[50]

Certain childhood tumours (e.g. Wilms' tumour, retinoblastoma, and neuroblastoma) bear chromosomal rearrangements and in some cases are heritable. Tumours developing in these rare circumstances tend to be bilateral or multiple and present very early in life. This suggests that cancers require for their development at least two mutations, one of them being transmitted via the gametes in hereditary cases.[51,52]

Clonal composition of tumours

One or more mutations in a single somatic cell will result in the production of a 'clone' – a cell population whose members all descend from that single mutant cell. If mutation is a critical step in carcinogenesis, it is expected that tumours should be clonal, i.e. descended from a single cell rather than from a cluster of cells. Examination of a variety of tumours from women heterozygous for a particular X-linked enzyme (the two alleles being chemically distinguishable) showed that of those tumours examined, the majority expressed only one of the two alleles.[53] This indicates that the tumours were homozygous, unlike the normal tissues which were heterozygous since they showed the expected X-inactivation mosaicism characteristic of normal women. Thus, the tumours were probably clonal in origin – powerful supporting evidence for implicating somatic mutation in the genesis of cancer.

More recent experiments have supported and extended knowledge of the clonal nature of human neoplasms. For example, Shibata et al.[54] observed differences between early and late mutational events in human colorectal carcinogenesis using a technique which allowed them to see how mutations in the c-K-ras oncogene were distributed among cells obtained from multiple regions of the same primary tumour. Seven adenocarcinomas and seven adenomas were selected for the presence of mutant c-K-ras oncogenes and histological transitions between normal and neoplastic tissue. This analysis revealed that in all seven adenocarcinomas and three of the seven adenomas c-K-ras mutations never extended into normal mucosa and were present in all neoplastic cells regardless of phenotypes. Further examination of two carcinomas for P53 mutations or loss of heterozygosity showed that these additional mutations were also present in all tumour cells, suggesting that the tumour arose from a single transformed clone. However, four other adenomas displayed heterogeneity, in that c-K-*ras* mutations were detected only in discrete portions. It was concluded that adenoma formation may include a stage in which multiple and genetically distinct neoplastic clones are present, while most carcinomas appear to have a homogeneous composition that results from the successful progression of one of these clones.

CANCER AS A GENETIC DISEASE OF SOMATIC CELLS

It is now accepted that cancer is a genetic disorder of somatic cells and that an accumulation of genetic changes underlies the process by which a normal cell can give rise to a cancer. The number and kinds of genes that have to be mutated in order to establish the full cancer phenotype is still under investigation and may vary from one type of cancer to another, but is probably at least two in inherited cancer predispositions, and not less than five or six in most types of sporadic cancer, as judged by interpretation of the relationship between age and incidence of various human cancers. For most sites the risk of cancer is proportional to the 4th to the 6th power of age, suggesting that four to six independent events are necessary for cancer to develop.[6,22]

Somatic mutation and clonal evolution

In the somatic-mutation model of cancer it is proposed that a single cell acquires a mutation in a regulatory gene that confers a selective growth advantage over its normal neighbours. This single cell divides to produce a clone of mutant offspring. The mutant clone expands by further cell divisions and one of its cells acquires a mutation in a second regulatory gene and thereby produces a clone carrying mutations in two regulatory genes. A cell in this doubly mutant clone then acquires an advantageous mutation in a third regulatory gene and produces a clone that is even more aberrant in its capacity for autonomous growth. This process of selective 'clonal evolution' continues until a clone appears that has accumulated enough mutant genes to enable it to express the full malignant phenotype.[17,55] As already mentioned, most cancers that have been examined are clonal in composition and their cells carry mutations in growth-regulatory genes, or have lost such genes. This supports the theory that clonal evolution driven by somatic mutation and Darwinian selection is a crucial mechanism in carcinogenesis.

Serial accumulation of independent mutations during carcinogenesis

Direct evidence for the serial accumulation of independent mutations in genes whose products mediate signal transduction, control the cell cycle, maintain genomic stability, mediate apoptosis and cellular senescence has been obtained from studies of the occurrence of mutations in successive histopathological stages that mark progression from normal tissue to a fully malignant tumour.[17,19,20] The best documented and widely quoted example is colorectal cancer, which appears to require for its development seven independent genetic events in the same cell lineage (Fig. 38.1). This illustrates the multi-step nature of carcinogenesis and gives a flavour of the complexity of the process. Similarly, consistent associations between mutations in specific regulatory genes and histopathological stages of carcinogenesis are seen in other cancers, including those of the skin, brain and stomach, cervix, breast, prostate, lung and lymphatic system.[19]

It is evident that carcinogenesis and mutation are closely linked, but what is the identity and nature of the particular genes that have to be altered or rearranged in order to provoke the induction of cancer? Recent discoveries – in particular the ability to find, isolate, sequence, manipulate, mutate and transfer genes to new hosts[56] – have made it possible to solve this problem. Of paramount importance is the recognition of families of genes that control the cell cycle and maintain genomic stability. Disturbance of the structure and function of these genes by mutation and chromosomal rearrangement at specific sites is causally related to carcinogenesis. This is not unexpected, since cancer is essentially a disease characterized by uncontrolled cell division and excessive proliferation, followed by migration and colonization of distant tissues and organs by malignant cells.

PROCESSES THAT ARE PERTURBED DURING CARCINOGENESIS

The cell cycle

The cell cycle consists of well-defined phases of activity that a cell must undertake in order to produce two daughter cells. In eukaryotes DNA replication occurs only during a discrete interval of the interphase known as the S ('S' for DNA synthesis) phase. Before and after the S-phase, cells are said to be in G_1 or G_2 ('G' for gap) and engage in growth and metabolic activity but not in chromosome replication. The G_2 period is usually followed by mitosis (M), and the sequence $G_1 \rightarrow S \rightarrow G_2 \rightarrow M$, followed by another G_1, is known as the cell cycle. There is also a stationary, or G_0, phase in which cellular metabolism shifts into a holding pattern. During cell division, cells pass through critical checkpoints. One is at the $G_1 \rightarrow S$ transition, where the cell is committed to replicate its DNA. Another is at $G_2 \rightarrow M$, where mitosis begins. Genes that control the cell cycle have been identified as specific targets for mutation in cancer and its precursor lesions.[12,18,19]

Senescence, immortalization, telomeres and telomerase

A critical stage in the life of normal cells is the development of senescence – the loss of a cell's ability to divide. This is not to be confused with apoptosis, which is an active process of cell death. In culture, normal cells undergo a limited number of divisions and then stop dividing, whereas cancer cell lines grow indefinitely. This escape from senescence is also referred to as 'immortalization'. One system that regulates senescence and prevents immortalization does so by maintaining the integrity of chromosome ends – 'telomeres'. Human telomeres consist of TTAGGG sequences tandemly repeated up to a thousandfold. They appear to have at least two functions.[57] The first is to protect chromosomes from recombination and loss. The second is to resolve the 'end-replication problem' which predicts the progressive and potentially catastrophic shortening of the 3′ end of DNA molecules over many cycles of replication, because DNA replication can proceed only in the 5′ to 3′ direction. This problem is overcome by telomerase, a ribonucleoprotein that makes, by reverse transcription, a DNA copy of its own telomere antisense sequence and fuses it to the 3′ terminus of the chromosome. By virtue of this second function, the telomere has a third function, namely as a mitotic clock. The number of divisions that normal primary human fibroblasts can undergo in culture is directly proportional to the initial length of their telomeres when placed in culture. The length of a telomere is determined by the number of cell divisions and by the presence or absence of telomerase; 50–200 telomeric nucleotides are lost at each cell doubling. Germ cells and stem cells express telomerase throughout life, but most somatic tissues do not. Somatic tissues lose telomere length progressively and, in culture, stop dividing when telomeres have become critically short; however, malignant cells and tumours re-express telomerase and escape from senescence. Immortal tumour cell-lines express telomerase and, of hundreds of human cancers examined, about 85% express telomerase activity. Thus, telomerase expression appears to be stringently repressed in normal human somatic tissues but is reactivated in cancer, suggesting that re-expression of telomerase coincides with immortalization, which is a crucial step in progression to malignancy.[57]

Genomic stability

Genomic stability goes hand in hand with cell-cycle control. In complex metazoan organisms DNA must be replicated with exquisite fidelity from one cell generation to the next, and each generation of cells must receive a complete and balanced set of chromosomes. This must happen during every cell cycle. Evolution has arranged that a cell destined to divide can survey its DNA for damage and can check whether it has produced, at metaphase, a spindle to which is attached an appropriate number of daughter chromosomes. The fidelity of the DNA code is checked and corrected by proofreading systems during and after DNA replication. Should the cell detect DNA damage or chromosomal anomalies, it can halt cell division and allow the DNA to be repaired, or it can decide to commit suicide by apoptosis or by other types of programmed death. If these surveillance and correction mechanisms are circumvented, and the cell reproduces itself it might well find a mutant clone that possesses growth advantages sufficient to allow it to escape the constraints under which its normal neighbours operate. Such clones may then undergo further mutation, selection and clonal evolution as described earlier. Some of the genes whose products engage in cell-cycle control and guard the integrity of the genome have now been identified and cloned, and have been found to be mutated in human cancers.

Such genes are often referred to as 'cancer genes'. This is a useful shorthand, but it must be borne in mind that a cancer gene is a mutant version of a normal gene and that proteins encoded by 'cancer genes' are abnormal or present in abnormal amounts, or are absent.

GENES INVOLVED IN THE DEVELOPMENT OF CANCER

Oncogenes

Oncogenes are mutant forms of a large family of genes – 'proto-oncogenes' – that control cell growth and proliferation.[18,19,58,59] Cellular proto-oncogenes were discovered following extensive studies of acutely transforming oncogenic retroviruses that induce cancers in vertebrates. More than 20 such viruses are known, each containing a specific oncogenic sequence, the viral oncogene – 'v-onc'. It is now evident that each viral oncogene was derived during evolution by transduction from a normal cellular counterpart, referred to as the cellular proto-oncogene (c-onc).[19] There are different classes of cellular proto-oncogenes (Table 38.1). Broadly speaking, their gene products drive cells through the cell cycle. Some code for growth factors. These are proteins that bind to cell surface receptors and by doing so, send signals to the interior of cells to switch on cell division. Others code for growth-factor receptors. These are complex protein molecules that straddle the cell membrane. The part of the molecule which is on the outer surface of the cell interacts with its specific growth factor and transfers signals across the cell membrane to the internal part of the molecule, which has enzymatic properties. This is known as signal transduction and allows cells to regulate their proliferation in response to specific growth factors. A third family of proto-oncogenes encodes membrane-bound proteins that also regulate cellular activity by signal transduction. The gene-products of the cellular proto-oncogenes mentioned so far act in the cytoplasm. A fourth family codes for proteins that act in the nucleus by controlling the transcription of specific messenger RNAs from DNA or the replication of DNA itself.

In cancers, only one of the two homologous proto-oncogene alleles in a diploid cell is mutated, and its gene product – a protein – acquires 'gain of function' – new and abnormal properties. Thus, oncogene mutations are 'dominant' at the cellular level, since their effects are exerted despite the presence in the cell of a normal homologous wild-type allele. Table 38.1 gives some examples of activated proto-oncogenes in human cancers. An example of the participation of oncogene acti-vation at an early stage in carcinogenesis is shown in Fig. 38.1. However, proto-oncogene activation may be important throughout carcinogenesis.

The link between mutation, proto-oncogenes and human cancer was made by the discovery that DNA extracted from a human bladder cancer could, when introduced into rodent fibroblasts growing in culture, transform a proportion of them to a state characteristic of malignancy; DNA from normal bladder cells could not.[60,61] The genetic change that led to the activation of the oncogene in the human bladder carcinoma cells was shown to be a single point mutation – a transversion of G to T. This substitution results in the incorporation of valine instead of glycine as the twelfth amino acid residue of ras-oncogene-encoded p21 protein. Thus, a

Table 38.1 *Examples of human cellular proto-oncogenes: the nature and location of their gene products (oncoproteins), their occurrence in cancer and their mode of activation*

Proto-oncogene	Activity of normal protein product	Type of tumour in which oncogene is activated	Activating event in cancer
ABL	Signal transduction: regulation of growth-factor stimulated cell proliferation	CML[a]	Chromosomal translocation (Ph chromosome)[b] containing chimaeric gene BCR/ABL
BCL2	Cell-death regulator: inhibits apoptosis	Lymphoid neoplasms; CLL[c]	Chromosomal translocation
HER2/erbB-/NEU	Signal transduction	Breast, ovary, bladder and stomach	Amplification
INT2	Growth factor	Breast, squamous head and neck	Amplification
MYC	Transcription factor: regulates gene expression and cell proliferation and differentiation	Burkitt's lymphoma Carcinoma of lung, breast and cervix	Increased expression by proviral insertion, chromosomal translocation, amplification
HRAS	Signal transduction	Carcinoma of colon, lung, pancreas; melanoma	Point mutations
KRAS	Signal transduction	Acute myelogenous and lymphoblastic leukaemia; carcinoma of thyroid; melanoma	Point mutations
NRAS	Signal transduction	Carcinoma of genitourinary tract and thyroid; melanoma	Point mutations
REL	Transcription factor: regulates gene expression in response to variety of primary and secondary pathogenic stimuli	Lymphoma, cutaneous T-cell leukaemia, lung carcinoma	Chromosomal translocation, amplification
MYB	Transcription factor: essential for normal haematopoiesis	AML,[d] CML, ALL,[e] T-cell leukaemias, colon carcinoma, melanoma	Amplification
RET	Signal transduction: may be involved in neuronal differentiation	Multiple endocrine neoplasia type 2A, 2B; familial medullary thyroid carcinoma	Dominantly-acting point mutations in the germline
		Papillary thyroid carcinoma	Chromosomal translocation

Compiled from information in Ref. 19.
[a] Chronic myelogenous leukaemia.
[b] Philadelphia chromosome.
[c] Chronic lymphocytic leukaemia.
[d] Acute myelogenous leukaemia.
[e] Acute lymphocytic leukaemia.

Table 38.2 *Examples of human tumour-suppressor genes, the functions of their gene products and their involvement in inherited and sporadic cancers*

Tumour-suppressor gene	Probable function/activity of normal protein product	Inherited susceptibility caused by germline mutation	Mode of inheritance	Sites at excess risk of cancer in carriers of germline mutations	Somatic loss or mutation in sporadic cancers
APC	Binds β-catenin May mediate cell adhesion and cell-cycle progression	Familial adenomatous polyposis	Autosomal dominant	Colon, duodenum	Colon, stomach, pancreas, oesophagus
ATM	Involved in cell-cycle control, DNA repair and recombination[64]	Ataxia telangiectasia	Autosomal recessive	Lymphoreticular system	T-cell prolymphocytic leukaemia[65,66]
BRCA1	Interacts with Rad51 protein (DNA) repair protein). Involved in DNA repair and cell-cycle control[67,68]	Familial breast and ovarian cancer	Autosomal dominant	Breast, ovary, prostate	None(?)
BRCA2	Interacts with Rad51 protein (DNA repair protein). May regulate DNA repair[67]	Familial breast (female and male) and ovarian cancer	Autosomal dominant	Breast, ovary, prostate, pancreas	None(?)
INK4A/MTS/p16	Cyclin-dependent kinase inhibitor; cell-cycle regulator	Familial cutaneous melanoma	Autosomal dominant	Cutaneous melanoma	Homozygous deletion is a common event in primary tumours, including ALL,[a] pancreas, brain, eosophagus, NSCLC,[b] bladder, pituitary
MLH1 MSH2 MSH3 MSH6/GTBP	Proteins involved in DNA mismatch repair. Proof-reading and maintenance of genomic stability	Hereditary non-polyposis colon cancer (Lynch syndrome, Muir-Torre syndrome)	Autosomal dominant	Colon, uterus, ovary, urothelium	Colorectal cancer
NF1	RAS-GTPase-activating protein; signal transduction	Peripheral (von Recklinghausen) neurofibromatosis	Autosomal dominant	Pheochromo-cytoma, malignant Schwannoma and fibrosarcoma	Benign neurofibromas

Continued

Table 38.2 – *cont*.

Tumour-suppressor gene	Probable function/activity of normal protein product	Inherited susceptibility caused by germline mutation	Mode of inheritance	Sites at excess risk of cancer in carriers of germline mutations	Somatic loss or mutation in sporadic cancers
P53	Transcription factor; cell-cycle regulator, promotes growth arrest and apoptosis, maintains genomic stability	Li-Fraumeni syndrome	Autosomal dominant	Breast, adrenal cortex, brain; sarcoma, leukaemia	Most types of human cancer
PTEN/MMAC1[c]	Protein tyrosine phosphatase; signal transduction[69]	Cowden disease[70,71]	Autosomal dominant	Breast, thyroid	Brain, prostate, kidney, breast[72,73]
RB1	Transcription factor; cell-cycle regulator	Familial retinoblastoma	Autosomal dominant	Retinoblastoma, osteosarcoma	Retinoblastoma, osteosarcoma, breast, prostate, bladder, lung, pancreas
VHL	(?) Signal transduction and/or regulation of cell–cell contacts	Von Hippel–Lindau disease	Autosomal dominant	Renal cell cancer, pheochromo-cytoma, CNS[d] haemangio-blastoma	Renal cell cancer
WT1	Transcription factor; may participate in normal genitourinary development	Wilms' tumour	Autosomal dominant	Embryonal renal neoplasia	Wilms' tumour
E-cadherin/CDH1	Transmembrane glycoprotein; mediates intercellular adhesion and morphogenesis	None known	Autosomal dominant	None known	Breast, endometrium, ovary

Compiled largely from information in Ref. 19. Other references are cited in the table.
[a] Acute lymphoblastic leukaemia.
[b] Non-small-cell lung cancer.
[c] Denotes synonyms for the some gene.
[d] Central nervous system.

single amino acid substitution was sufficient to confer neoplastic properties on the gene product of the human bladder *c-ras* oncogene.

This discovery led to an intensive search for other ways in which proto-oncogenes could be *activated* to states that would provoke malignancy. Several different activating mechanisms have been identified, all of which involve modifications to DNA structure or function. These are: point mutation within the oncogene; chromosomal rearrangement which results in creation of a new gene, part of which consists of sequences from the proto-oncogene; chromosomal rearrangement, which places a proto-oncogene next to an inappropriate promoter of mRNA transcription; addition of a strong promoter of mRNA transcription from a virus to an oncogene; increase in the number of copies of the proto-oncogene in the cell – this is called gene amplification. The first two mechanisms result in *qualitative* changes to proto-oncogenes – in effect, the creation of new genes which over-ride the functions of the normal genes they are derived from. The last three lead to *quantitative* changes – normal proto-oncogenes make abnormally high levels of their gene-products.

There is evidence that proto-oncogenes may also be activated during later stages in the carcinogenic process – promotion and progression – as well as in the phase of initiation, emphasizing the multi-step nature of carcinogenesis, and reinforcing the notion that the process requires a succession of mutagenic events rather than just one. Progression of human tumours to increasing malignancy is accompanied by increased levels of oncogene activation and expression.

Tumour-suppressor genes

Activation of proto-oncogenes by the various mechanisms described above is a dominant-like effect; the cell acquires genes or gene-products which over-ride or add to the genes or gene-products which are normally expressed. There are other classes of gene – tumour-suppressor genes – which are involved in carcinogenesis only when they are deleted or inactivated by mutation, loss or by epigenetic processes such as hypermethylation. Marshall[62] has reviewed the three lines of evidence (studies of cell hybrids; familial cancer; and loss of heterozygosity in tumours) that support the idea that neoplastic transformation involves genes that are negative regulators of growth – their loss of function by mutation provokes cell proliferation. In general, tumour-suppressor gene products participate in mechanisms that suppress or delay progress through the cell cycle or protect the integrity of the genome. Mutations that inactivate tumour-suppressor genes are recessive at the cellular level, since they exert their effects only in the absence of the gene product. There is a growing catalogue of tumour-suppressor genes;[19,63] Table 38.2 lists examples, with information on their possible functions and their occurrence in human cancers.[64–73] Figure 38.1 provides an example of the role of tumour-suppressor genes in colorectal carcinogenesis.

RETINOBLASTOMA AND THE *RB1* GENE

The first tumour-suppressor gene to be identified and cloned was the *RB1* gene. Individuals who develop the hereditary form of retinoblastoma inherit from one of their parents a deletion or mutation in a gene (the *RB1* gene) carried on chromosome 13. This is a heterozygous germ-cell mutation and is present in all the cells of the affected individual. The eye tumour that arises in early childhood develops when the second normal copy (allele) of the *RB1* gene is lost or mutated by somatic mutation (frequently by chromosomal rearrangement or loss of the normal chromosome). This suggests that the normal gene suppresses the development of the tumour. The loss of the second normal allele unmasks the absent

function of the first allele, resulting in the formation of a tumour.[63]

When introduced into retinoblastoma cells *in vitro*, the *RB1* gene restores normal growth control. A similar mechanism operates in osteosarcomas that develop as second tumours in retinoblastoma patients, and in hereditary forms of Wilms' tumour, where chromosome 11 carries the critical mutation. In the more common non-hereditary cases of these childhood cancers, it is proposed that the first mutation (equivalent to the germ-cell mutation in hereditary cases) is a recessive *somatic* mutation which is then followed by a second somatic mutation. This is thought to delete or inactivate the normal copy of the gene and allows expression of the first recessive mutation. Inactivation of the *RB1* gene has been observed in sporadic breast cancers, prostate cancers, about one-third of bladder cancers, and virtually all small-cell lung cancers, adding weight to the idea that this gene is a general tumour-suppressor gene.[63] Why expression of the wild-type *RB1* is ubiquitous in normal tissues, but only certain tumours contain mutant *RB1* genes remains to be answered. The protein encoded by the *RB1* gene, a phosphoprotein known as pRB1, is a negative regulator of cell growth. It represses the transcription of genes essential for cell division and, in concert with several other regulatory proteins, controls the timing of the cell cycle.[63]

THE *P53* GENE

The most widely studied tumour-suppressor gene is *P53*. Its gene product, p53, is a phosphoprotein that plays a central role in normal cell division, in differentiation and development, and in maintaining genomic stability. It possesses a variety of functions[63,64,74,75] including:

- preservation of genetic stability;
- induction of growth arrest in the G_1 phase of the growth cycle in response to DNA damage;
- induction of apoptosis following DNA damage;
- inhibition of growth of tumour cells *in vitro* and *in vivo*;
- control of spindle and centrosome function during mitosis.

Studies with mouse cells show that in addition to acting as a tumour-suppressor gene, *P53* can also behave as a dominantly acting oncogene if it undergoes a point mutation which causes amino acid changes at sites highly conserved during evolution. It is believed that this 'dominant-negative' activity results from complexing of a mutant monomer of the p53 protein with a wild-type monomer, this being sufficient to subvert normal function.[74] In addition to point mutations (discussed in more detail below), allelic loss, rearrangements and deletions of the *P53* gene have been detected in human tumours.

Germline mutations in the *P53* gene have been detected in families afflicted by the Li-Fraumeni syndrome – an autosomal dominant syndrome which confers a high risk of diverse cancers at many sites.[74] Affected families carry point mutations that cluster within a narrow region of the gene. As in other examples of germline mutations in tumour-suppressor genes, non-cancerous cells of affected individuals carry these mutations in the heterozygous state, that is, each cell contains what appears to be a normal allele and a mutant allele. Neoplasia is thought to result when the second, normal, *P53* allele is deleted by chromosome loss or by mitotic recombination.

This 'two-hit' inactivation of *RB1* and *P53* is now known to be characteristic of tumour-suppressor genes in general. The event that inactivates the first allele of a tumour-suppressor gene is almost invariably a point mutation or small deletion in the gene itself. The second event that knocks out the second allele may range from a point mutation to the loss of the entire chromosome. The eclectic nature of mutations in tumour-suppressor genes and their occurrence over a broad span of the gene stands in sharp contrast to the remarkable specificity of point mutations found in activated oncogenes such as *ras*, where mutations cluster at just three codons.[74,76] Thus, while many different and non-specific alterations in a suppressor gene such as *P53* or *RB1* can lead to destruction of its function, specific mutations that confer new properties on the gene product appear to be required for oncogene activation.[74]

Other genes that maintain genomic stability

MISMATCH-REPAIR GENES

As already mentioned, cancers usually display signs of genomic instability, manifested as chromosomal anomalies, gene amplification and aneuploidy. Mutation or loss of genes (e.g. *P53*) that maintain the stability of the genome is a common event in human cancer. Other genes inactivated in certain cancer predispositions are those that ensure that errors do not accumulate during DNA replication. Each cell division of a somatic diploid mammalian cell requires the accurate and timely distribution of 6×10^9 base pairs of DNA to each daughter cell. In long-lived species like *Homo sapiens*, this process must operate accurately and unremittingly over many decades. A change in just one base pair can be enough to cause mutation. DNA replication is remarkably accurate, with error frequencies of less than one mutation per billion base pairs per cell division. However, errors do occur but are corrected either by enzymes which 'proof-read' the nascent chain before it is elongated or by enzyme complexes that repair remaining mismatches caused by inappropriate base pairing between mother and daughter strands.[21,22,38,45,77]

The absence of genes for various components of this mismatch-repair system substantially increases the risk of mutation at each round of DNA replication. Germline mutations in such genes (e.g. *MLH1*, *MSH2*, *MSH3*, Table 38.2) predispose to hereditary non-polyposis colon cancer.[20] Every somatic cell in an individual with a germline mutation in one of these genes contains only one intact copy. Loss of this copy due to a second genetic accident results in a cell lineage with a greatly enhanced mutation rate and a high risk of acquiring further mutations that lead to cancer. Such cells are said to exhibit a 'mutator phenotype'. This 'two-hit' mode of inactivation qualifies mismatch-repair genes as tumour-suppressors. Hereditary non-polyposis colon cancer is one of the most common human genetic disorders, and accounts for between 2 and 4% of all colorectal cancer. The discovery that heritable defects in mismatch-repair are causally related to a common cancer is powerful evidence for the central role of mutation in the genesis of cancer. However, some argue that acquisition of a mutator phenotype is not necessary for carcinogenesis and that the 'normal' rate of spontaneous mutation combined with clonal selection is more important than an increased rate of mutation.[55,78]

POINT MUTATIONS IN THE *P53* GENE

Perhaps half of all cancers contain *P53* mutations. Although found throughout the gene, they occur with the greatest frequency in those regions of the gene which have been most highly conserved during evolution. At least four hotspots for mutation can be identified.[79–81] Crystallographic studies of the *P53* protein show that these hotspots are those that code for amino acids that bind the *P53* protein to its binding domain in DNA.[82]

It is possible to detect all of the six possible base-substitution mutations in the *P53* gene in fresh or archival specimens of human tumours. This, and the fact that *P53* mutation is so common among so many different kinds of cancer, makes it feasible to construct 'mutational spectra' in which the type and frequency of mutation can be plotted as a function of position within the gene for each type of cancer.[74,80,81,83,84] As at January 1997 over 6000 point mutations in *P53* in tumours and tumour cell-lines had been catalogued from the published literature. This database is now available through the Internet.[85] Analysis of the spectrum of mutations in the *P53* gene in different kinds of human cancers reinforces the importance of point mutations in carcinogenesis and offers intriguing clues about the aetiologies of different cancers.

Effect on mutation of biomethylation at CpG dinucleotides

Transitions at one particular hotspot – the CpG dinucleotide – contribute substantially to the *P53* mutational spectrum of many kinds of cancers. The cytosine residue in the dinucleotide CpG in DNA is frequently biomethylated to 5-methylcytosine during normal processing of DNA after its replication. Such biomethylation is characteristic of vertebrates and plays a crucial role in the control of gene expression.[86] However, by a cruel trick of nature, 5-methylcytosine residues can deaminate spontaneously to thymine, giving rise at the next DNA replication to TpG or CpA transitions. It is argued that these transitions represent spontaneous mutations and can be used as an index of endogenous mutation of a particular gene. Moreover, a fall in the proportion of CpG or CpA mutations may signal the effect of an exogenous chemical or physical mutagen.[24,83,87] All 46 CpG sites in exons (the expressed regions of genes) 5–8 of the *P53* gene are methylated, suggesting that this gene is particularly vulnerable to endogenous mutation.[88] As already mentioned (p. 745) BPDE (an important carcinogenic metabolite of cigarette smoke) selectively forms adducts with guanine in the three codons that comprise the major mutational hotspots in *P53* in human lung cancers,[41] and biomethylation of cytosine at CpG dinucleotides appears to be the major determinant of this codon-specific adduct formation.[42] Thus, biomethylation of CpG dinucleotides in DNA may influence the pattern of mutation of critical 'cancer genes' by exogenous carcinogens, as well contributing to the endogenous mutational burden.

Mutational spectra and environmental and occupational exposure to carcinogens

Analysis of the mutational spectra of genes such as *P53* that are intimately connected with the development of cancer in many different organs and tissues and which are large targets for physical and chemical insult, offer a promising approach to understanding the origin of human cancers. For example, mutational spectra obtained from a given tumour from patients with well-documented occupational exposures to carcinogens can be compared with spectra of the same genes from the same kind of tumour in patients with no history of occupational exposure. A pronounced shift from 'endogenous'-type mutations to those characteristic of DNA-reactive carcinogens would be powerful evidence that exposure to chemical carcinogens had indeed occurred. Evidence that those 'induced' missense mutations are of the same type as those produced by the suspect chemical in laboratory experiments *in vitro* or in appropriate animal models provide further support that occupational exposure had caused those cancers.

It is now routine to extract DNA from paraffin-embedded tissues, to amplify selected regions of a given gene by the polymerase chain reaction and to detect mutations in those regions. It is thus possible to detect mutations in specific genes in tissues that have been preserved in paraffin blocks for several decades.[89] The use of such techniques allow retrospective mutational analyses

of large numbers and varieties of normal and neoplastic tissues from well documented patients. Several such studies have been published and the term 'molecular epidemiology' has been coined to describe this and similar approaches to the aetiology of human cancer.[90–96]

P53 mutations related to specific carcinogenic exposures

Several environmental and occupational agents known to cause human cancers have been linked with characteristic *P53* mutations, some of which can be related mechanistically to the chemical nature of the exposure.[81] Some examples are given below.

AFLATOXIN B₁

A high proportion of human hepatocellular carcinomas associated with exposure to the potent liver carcinogen aflatoxin B_1 contain a mutation at codon 249 (AGG to AGT) which can be produced by incubating the *P53* gene *in vitro* with the ultimate metabolite of aflatoxin B_1.

ULTRAVIOLET IRRADIATION/SUNLIGHT

Skin cancers associated with exposure to sunlight have *P53* mutations at dipyrimidine sites that are usually G:C to A:T transitions, and also exhibit characteristic CC: TT to TT:AA mutations that would be predicted from experimental studies showing that ultraviolet irradiation causes adjacent pyrimidines in DNA to form chemical bonds with each other.

TOBACCO

In oral cancers, *P53* mutation correlates with a patient's tobacco and alcohol consumption; the mutational spectrum of lung cancers is dominated by G:C to T:A transversions. This spectrum can be explained by targeted DNA adduct formation by polycyclic aromatic hydrocarbons driven by 5-methylcytosine at CpG sites, as explained earlier.

VINYL CHLORIDE (see Chapters 8, 43)

Hepatic angiosarcomas in people with occupational exposure to vinyl chloride carry *P53* mutations almost exclusively at A:T base pairs. This is consistent with the mutational properties of vinyl chloride in experimental systems, and contrasts with the relatively infrequent G:C to A:T mutations in sporadic angiosarcomas. The majority of the missense mutations in the *P53* gene in hepatic angiosarcomas induced in rats with vinyl chloride involve A:T base pairs, suggesting that vinyl chloride-induces *P53* mutations in rats and humans by a common mechanism, namely formation of DNA etheno adducts.[97]

CHROMATES (see Chapter 7)

There is preliminary evidence that lung cancers in patients with occupational exposure to chromates carry specific *P53* mutations, namely G:C to AT coding-strand transversions at non-CpG sites.[98] However, this is based on just three patients, two of whom had been exposed to a variety of other potentially carcinogenic agents. Further studies using larger numbers of patients with well-defined exposures are clearly warranted. Moreover, the ever-present spectre of cigarette smoking – a potent cause of lung cancers and *P53* mutations – looms over all such studies, making their interpretation all the more problematic.

ASBESTOS (see Chapter 35)

This is true of a study in which asbestos exposure was linked with *P53* mutations in lung cancer.[99] These authors found that *P53* mutations occurred significantly more frequently in patients with a history of occupational exposure to asbestos, based on 3/60 (5%) patients without *P53* mutations *versus* 5/25 (20%) of those with *P53* mutations. Four of the five patients with asbestos exposure and *P53* alterations had G:C to T:A transversion mutations, and all three double mutations that were seen in the *P53* gene occurred in patients who smoked and had a history of asbestosis.

Factors other than adduct formation *per se* may play a role in the development of a particular mutational spectrum. For example, the rate of removal of damaged bases by excision-repair in mammalian genes depends strongly on the sequence context of the damaged base. Several of the mutational hotspots in the *P53* gene in skin cancer are likely to result from such an effect.[81]

Mutations in the *VHL* tumour-suppressor gene

Somatic mutations of the von Hippel–Lindau (*VHL*) tumour-suppressor gene have been implicated in the development of inherited and sporadic renal cell carcinomas (Table 38.2). An excess of renal cell carcinoma has been reported in men occupationally exposed to high and prolonged occupational exposures to trichloroethene (trichloroethylene), although this finding is controversial.[100] Trichloroethene is regarded by the International Agency for Research on Cancer as a probable human carcinogen.[101] Evidence for a causal relationship between the exposure and the cancer was therefore sought by looking for somatic mutations in the *VHL* gene in renal cell tumours from 23 patients with occupational histories of very high exposure to trichloroethene.[102] All 23 tumours examined showed aberrations of the *VHL* gene. Other studies of renal cell tumours from patients not exposed to trichloroethene have reported *VHL* mutation frequencies of 33–55%,

suggesting that *VHL* is a susceptible and specific target in trichloroethene-induced renal carcinogenesis. This study, on its own, does not constitute proof that trichloroethene induced those cancers in those men, but it does illustrate the way in which molecular studies may shed light on an epidemiologically-derived association between a specific exposure and a specific cancer. Whether studies of mutational footprints left by chemical carcinogens in genes such as *P53* and *VHL* will ever establish cause and effect at the level of an individual worker remains to be established but, given the uncertainties in assessing individual exposure over decades, and uncertainties introduced by other concomitant exposures, it is rather unlikely.

MECHANISMS OF INVASION AND METASTASIS

An accumulation of mutations in genes that control the cell-cycle and maintain genomic stability is essentially a description of carcinogenesis at the molecular and cellular level. It does not embrace the hallmark of cancer – metastasis – which is the spread of cancer from a primary tumour to distant sites in the body. Tumour cells must overcome a series of barriers in order to metastasise; they '. . . must detach from the primary tumour, invade the extracellular matrix and enter the circulation, survive in the circulation to arrest in the capillary bed, adhere to subendothelial basement membrane, gain entrance into the organ parenchyma, respond to paracrine growth factors, proliferate and induce angiogenesis, and evade host defences.[103]

Angiogenesis

A crucial step in tumour growth and metastasis is angiogenesis, the development of a new blood supply, since a primary tumour cannot grow beyond a volume of about 1 mm^3 without one. Metastases must also develop blood supplies in order to survive and grow. Over the past few years it has become recognized that tumours develop new blood supplies by aberrant angiogenesis pathways in which endothelial cells migrate into the tumour and divide much more rapidly than normal endothelial cells to produce leaky blood vessels.[103–106] These processes are thought to be triggered by an angiogenic switch in genetically unstable and evolving tumour clones. Tumours also secrete factors that inhibit angiogenesis of normal tissues and metastases. The balance of angiogenesis and anti-angiogenesis may help to explain tumour dormancy – the decades that elapse between the initiation of cancer and its florid metastatic presentation. A metastasis with a limited blood supply will have a high rate of apoptosis owing to the hostile hypoxic environment; angiogenesis will ameliorate these conditions, reduce apoptosis and allow further growth of the metastasis.[105] The genes and their protein products, such as the vascular endothelial growth factors A, B and C, that control angiogenesis are now being identified, leading the way towards a detailed understanding of the molecular mechanism of metastasis and the possibility of drugs that could control it.

Matrix metalloproteinases

Proteolysis of adjacent tissues is another essential step in metastasis and one family of proteolytic enzymes, the matrix metalloproteinases, is under intensive study in this regard.[104] These matrix metalloproteinases are secreted or transmembrane proteins that can digest components of the extracellular matrix and basement membrane. Sixteen matrix metalloproteinases have been identified and all require zinc for their catalytic function. matrix metalloproteinases are involved in normal and pathological matrix destruction in processes such as wound healing and connective tissue reconstruction. They also play a role in tumour progression. The number of different matrix metalloproteinases family members that are expressed tends to increase with progression of the tumour, and the relative levels of any individual matrix metalloproteinases family members

tend to increase with increasing tumour stage. Matrix metalloproteinases are produced either by tumour cells themselves or as a response of the host to the tumour. They are most abundant in tumours in which the basement membrane is breached and where there is evidence for local invasion and distant metastases. As well as promoting intravasation and extravasation (invasion and entry into and out of blood or lymphatic vessels) by breaking down physical barriers to metastasis, it is thought that matrix metalloproteinases may also play a role in regulating growth of tumours, at both primary and metastatic sites.[104]

A summary of the events that occur during carcinogenesis and the pathways that protect against it is given in Fig. 38.2.

CANCER SUSCEPTIBILITY: GERMLINE *VERSUS* SOMATIC MUTATION OF CANCER GENES

Mutations in genes involved in carcinogenesis can occur in germ cells (sperm or ova) or in somatic cells. Somatic mutations are passed from one cell generation to the next, whereas germline mutations are passed from parents to offspring. A germline mutation in a 'cancer gene' results in an individual who is heterozygous for that gene – every somatic cell contains one functional (wildtype) copy and one inactive (mutant) copy. Such an individual has a heritable predisposition to cancer, the site at increased risk being determined, *inter alia*, by the gene that is mutated and in some cases by the location and nature of the mutation within the gene. Cancer predisposition genes are mainly dominantly inherited tumour-suppressor genes (see Table 38.2) probably because the loss of function of the mutant allele is compensated for by the remaining wildtype allele, allowing normal development of the embryo. A somatic cell in an individual who is heterozygous for a cancer predisposition gene may lose its remaining functional copy by mutation or loss. Such a cell will then possess a selective growth advantage, since it can no longer produce the tumour-suppressing protein encoded by the tumour-suppressor gene. This 'second hit' is the trigger for the events leading to development of cancer in that individual (the 'first hit' is the germline mutation). Inherited disposition to cancer is estimated to account for between 1 and 5% of the total cancer burden, but its study contributes disproportionately to understanding the processes underlying carcinogenesis.

Genotype and phenotype

The cancer predisposition genes listed in Table 38.2 are highly penetrant, that is, most affected individuals will develop the cancer that is characteristic of the inherited genetic defect. However, even among these people, the

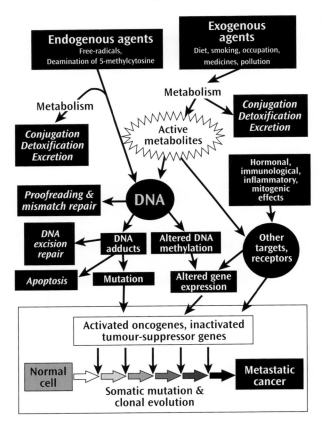

Figure 38.2 *(See colour plate section where this figure also appears in colour.) Pathways in carcinogenesis. The text in green boxes and the green arrows denote protective pathways and processes. The text in red boxes and the red arrows depict deleterious pathways and processes.*

relationship between the genotype (the mutation) and the phenotype (the clinical manifestation of cancer) can be very complex. This is not surprising, bearing in mind that other somatic mutations are required before cancer can develop. In some cases the phenotype is correlated with the position of the mutation within the gene. For example, in women carrying mutations in *BRCA1* or *BRCA2*, the risks of developing either breast or ovarian cancer are strongly related to the position of mutations within the gene.[107,108] In familial adenomatous polyposis the severity of polyposis depends to some extent on the position of the mutation in the *APC* gene. Moreover, patients with identical germline mutations in the *APC* gene can develop quite dissimilar patterns of extra-colonic neoplasia.[20] These complex relationships between genotype and phenotype in hereditary cancers suggest the intervention of modifying genes and of environmental factors (which may include occupational exposure) in the development of cancer.

Genotype, phenotype and environmental factors

The bulk of human cancer (probably 95%) is known by cancer geneticists as 'sporadic' and cannot be explained by genetic predispositions attributable to germline mutations of high penetrance. Rather, sporadic cancer is the outcome of a complex interplay between genetics, environment and the play of chance.[22] Although it is impossible, at present, to disentangle precisely the relative contributions that each of these factors makes to the risk of cancer in an individual or within a given population, the problem is susceptible to systematic analysis. Knudson[109] suggested that the population can be divided into four 'oncodemes' (a demographic unit with a peculiar sensitivity to a particular cancer), depending on the relative contributions of environment and genetics to the risk of cancer. The first oncodeme is *background*, in which cancer incidence is determined by random mutations in normal people. The second is *environmental* – cancer is caused by environmental carcinogens (chemicals, radiation or viruses, or combinations of these) in normal people. The third oncodeme is *environmental/genetic*, which is due to the effect of genetic susceptibility (e.g. defects in DNA, or genetic differences in carcinogen metabolism) on the response to carcinogens. The fourth oncodeme is *genetic*, in which genetic susceptibility is more important than spontaneous or environmentally induced events. This rare group includes two classes of people; those with enhanced rates of spontaneous mutation and chromosomal anomalies (e.g. Bloom's syndrome) and those with hereditary disposition to cancers such as retinoblastoma, Wilms' tumour and familial adenomatous polyposis.

Most human cancer probably occurs in oncodemes 2 and 3, since exposure to environmental carcinogens is difficult or impossible to avoid (so that oncodeme 1 is unlikely to exist in real life) and cancers that are due almost entirely to an inherited predisposition (such those caused by *APC*, *BRCA1* and *BRCA2*) are rare.

Pharmacogenetic polymorphisms and susceptibility to cancer

Oncodeme 3 includes genetic susceptibility to environmental carcinogens as a factor in determining risk of cancer. As well as including rare recessively inherited DNA-repair defects such as xeroderma pigmentosum and ataxia telangiectasia, it also includes much commoner genetically determined variations (polymorphisms) in genes whose products engage in metabolic activation of carcinogens.

What is a polymorphism?

Polymorphic alleles are defined as allelic variants of single genes that are present in more than 1% of the population. Metabolic polymorphisms (also known as pharmacogenetic polymorphisms) occur commonly in the human population, their effects being manifested by large differences in response to the same drug by different individuals.[110,111] There is a 10- to 200-fold range over which metabolic polymorphisms exert their effects,[112] suggesting that if this range were extrapolated directly to risk of human disease, at any given dose of drug or pollutant one person will be 10–200 times more sensitive to toxicity or cancer than another. Several metabolic polymorphisms have been linked to susceptibility to cancer (Table 38.3).[34,111–137]

As shown in the table these fall in two groups; those concerned with phase I metabolism (e.g. cytochrome P450s that oxidatively metabolise substrates to electrophilic, DNA-binding metabolites) and those (such as phase II enzymes like glutathione transferases and acetyltransferases) that conjugate electrophilic metabolites with nucleophilic substrates to form polar metabolites that are readily excreted. Before considering the evidence that cancer risk can indeed be influenced by pharmacogenetic polymorphisms, it is necessary to discuss the problems and pitfalls that have been encountered in such studies. Critical reviews of this topic can be found in Refs 112, 138 and 139.

Methods for detecting pharmacogenetic polymorphisms

In practice there are two methods for detecting metabolic polymorphisms. In the first (phenotyping) the phenotypic expression of the polymorphism is detected and quantitated by measuring in the urine the ratio of an unchanged drug of interest to a specific metabolite.

Table 38.3 *Metabolic polymorphisms with possible links to susceptibility to cancer in humans*

Gene product/usual name	Function	Gene	Examples of substrates and/or inducers	Polymorphic alleles thought to be associated with cancer	Approximate % population affected	Phenotypic effect of polymorphism on enzyme expression	Human cancer implicated
Aryl hydrocarbon hydroxylase receptor	Phase I Regulates CYP1As	AHR	Dioxin PAH[a]	ARH[H]	Caucasians 10%	Increased expression of CYP1As resulting in extensive metabolism (EM phenotype)	Lung (increased risk in ARH[H])[34]
Aryl hydrocarbon hydroxylase	Phase I Oxidative metabolism of PAH and other substrates to electrophiles	CYP1A1	PAH	MspI RFLP[b] m1/m2 m2/m2 exon 7 Ile-Val Val/val AA RFLP	Japanese 45% Scandinavians 20% Japanese 11% Scandinavians 1%[112] Japanese 31% Japanese 3.5%[113] African-Americans 17%[116]	Increased expression of CYP1A1 enzyme (EM phenotype)	Lung: discordant results, depending on ethnic group of study population, but results suggest increased risk in EM,[c] especially in Japanese smokers[34,111,113,114] No increased risk in African-Americans[115]
Debrisoquine hydroxylase	Phase I Oxidative metabolism of more than 30 drugs	CYP2D6	Anti-arrhythmics, monoamine oxidase inhibitors, β-blockers, anti-hypertensives (non-inducible, all substrates)	CYP2D6A CYP2D6B CYP2D6D CYP2D6E CYP2D6F	Caucasians 5–7% African-Americans 2% Orientals <1%	Null; absent protein resulting in poor rate of metabolism (PM phenotype)	Various cancers (e.g. lung, liver, gastrointestinal, leukaemia). No firm conclusions can be drawn[34,111]
Dimethyl-nitrosamine N-dimethylase	Phase I Oxidative metabolism of N-nitrosamines, benzene, ethanol	CYP2E1	N-nitrosamines, benzene, ethanol	PstI RFLP Rsa1 RFLP Dra1 RFLP	Distribution of various genotypes varies very widely between different ethnic groups	Variations in expression resulting differing rates of metabolism	Conflicting claims that certain rare genotypes influence susceptibility to lung cancer in various ethnic groups[117-123]

Enzyme	Function	Gene	Substrates	Polymorphism/mutation	Frequency	Effect	Clinical associations
NAD(P)H: quinone oxido-reductase	Phase I Functions as an antioxidant by acting as a 2-electron reductase that forms and maintains the antioxidant form of membrane-bound coenzyme Q. Activates or detoxifies quinones.[127]	NQO1	Quinones (e.g.) metabolites of benzene	NQO1[609] C→T mutation	Heterozygotes: African-Americans 34% Mexican-Americans 52%[124] — Homozygotes: African-Americans 5% Mexican-Americans 16%	Loss of enzyme in homozygotes	Conflicting claims that NQO1 variants are at greater or lesser risk of lung cancer than wild-type individuals[124,125] — Chinese subjects homozygous for NQO1[609] and with a rapid metabolizer CYP2E1 phenotype had a 7.6-fold increased risk of benzene poisoning compared with heterozygotes or wild-type subjects with slow CYP2E1 phenotype[126]
Glutathione S-transferases	Phase II Conjugation of glutathione with electrophilic substrates	μ GSTM1	Peroxidation products, phase I metabolites of PAH	GSTM1*0	Caucasians 50% African-Americans 28%[128]	Protein is absent; null homozygotes express no GSTM1 enzyme	Homozygotes said to suffer modest increases in risk of lung cancer (especially in smokers)[33,34,111,129] and of GI[d] bladder[130] and skin cancers[34,111]
		π GSTP1	Phase I metabolites of PAH	GSTP1b (GG genotype)	Caucasians 6.5%[131]	Homozygotes (GG) express low levels of GSTP1 enzyme	Homozygotes claimed to be at higher risk of bladder, testicular[131] and lung cancer[132]
		θ GSTT1	Monohalomethanes, solvents, ethylene oxide	GSTT1-null	Caucasians 16%–38% African-Americans 24%[128]	Protein is absent; null homozygotes express no GSTT1 enzyme[135]	Homozygotes at higher risk of MSD[f133] and BCC[134]
N-Acetyl-transferases	Phase II. Transfer acetyl group from acetyl coenzyme A to amine N of aromatic amines and hydrazines	NAT2	Aromatic amines, hydrazines, caffeine, dapsone	NAT2 M1 NAT2 M2 NAT2 M3; NAT2 M4 (found only in African-Americans)	Varies very widely by ethnic group e.g. Japan 6%, N. European 44–70%[111]	Homozygotes for combinations of 2 of these 4 alleles are slow acetylators	Caucasian homozygotes (slow acetylators) exposed to bladder carcinogens (occupational, or from smoking) have increased risk of bladder cancer.[130,136] Caucasian homozygotes have decreased risk of colorectal cancer (i.e. fast acetylators are at increased risk).[34,111] Postmenopausal female Caucasian homozygotes who smoke are claimed to be at higher risk of breast cancer[137]

[a] Polycyclic aromatic hydrocarbons.
[b] Restriction fragment length polymorphisms.
[c] Extensive metabulizer.
[d] Gastrointestinal.
[e] Myelodysplastic syndrome.
[f] Basal cell carcinoma.

Table 38.4 *Examples of the effect on cancer risk of interactions between metabolic polymorphisms*

Cancer site and study group	Details of study group	Main findings of study	Authors' conclusions	Ref.
Lung, 255 Japanese	170 population controls 85 patients with squamous-cell carcinoma of the lung	OR^a of 16.00 (3.8–68)^b for CYP1A1 Msp1/GST1-null OR of 41.00, (8.7–193.1) for CYP1A1 *Ile-Val*/GST1-null at a low level of cigarette smoking	Patients with CYP1A1 EM^c genotype (homozygotes for either Mspl or *Ile-Val*) developed cancer after smoking fewer cigarettes than lung-cancer patients with other genotypes. Cumulative cigarette consumption was lowest for patients with a combined CYP1A1 EM/GST1-null genotype. These patients had higher relative risks than those having a single susceptible gene. Susceptibility must be studied in relation to exposure levels	113
Bladder, 747 Germans	373 hospital controls 374 bladder cancer patients	NAT2; GSTM1, GSTT1, mEH^d and CYP1A1, 2C19, 2D6, 2E1 were analysed OR of 2.7 (1.0–7.4) for SA^e in heavy smokers OR of 1.6 (1.2–2.2) for GSTM1-null, independent of smoking and occupation OR of 2.6 (1.1–6.0) for GSTT1+/+ in non-smokers Two mEH polymorphisms were not associated with bladder cancer risk CYP2D6, 1A1 and 2E1 had no significant effects NAT2 SA and GSTM1-null showed no significant synergistic or antagonistic interactions	Molecular genetic analysis of a large sample demonstrated the increased bladder cancer risk of those who are deficient in NAT2 and GSTM1; the other traits proved to be of minor impact	130
Malignant and non-malignant pulmonary disease 145 Finnish asbestos insulators	69 had no pulmonary disorders 76 had asbestos-related pulmonary disorders including 24 with malignant mesothelioma	OR of 4.1 (1.1–17.2) for non-malignant pulmonary disease in asbestos-exposed group with GSTM1-null/NAT2 SA compared with asbestos-exposed group with GSTM1-non-null/NAT2 FA^f OR of 7.8 (1.4–78.7) for malignant mesothelioma in asbestos-exposed group with GSTM1-null/NAT2 SA compared with asbestos-exposed group with GSTM1-non-null/NAT2 FA	GSTM1-null individuals with a NAT2 slow-acetylator genotype exposed to high levels of asbestos appear to have enhanced susceptibility to asbestos-related pulmonary disorders including malignant mesothelioma	141
Bladder, 43 Egyptians	21 healthy controls 22 patients with schistosomal bladder cancer	OR of 7 (1.6–30.6) for bladder cancer in group with GSTM1-null genotypes compared with GSTM1+/+ genotypes OR of 14.0 (1.3–151.4) for bladder cancer in group with CYP2D6 EM/GSTM1-null genotypes compared with EM GSTM1+/+ genotypes OR of 8.4 (1.3–56) for bladder cancer in group with CYP2D6 EM/GSTM1-null genotypes compared with CYP2D6 PM^g/GSTM1+/+ genotypes	Genetic polymorphisms, especially in GSTM1 and CYP2D6 could play an important role as host risk factors for development of urinary bladder cancer among Egyptians	142

Basal-cell carcinoma (BCC), 345 British patients	Grouped for age, sex, skin type, hair colour, eye colour, smoking, occupation	OR of 2.24 for truncal BCC in GSTT1-null compared with GSST1+/+ OR of 2.86 (P = 0.038) for truncal BCC in CYP1A1 EM compared with CYP1A1 PM OR of 2.95 (P = 0.006) for truncal BCC in GSTT1-null/CYP1A1 EM compared with GSST1+/+/CYP1A1 PM	These data show a significant genetic influence on BCC site, and a significant interaction between GSTT1 and CYP1A1 genotypes	134
Lung, 472 Northwestern Mediterranean Caucasians (Catalonia, Spain)	120 healthy smokers, 192 blood donors from the general population, 160 lung cancer patients	No significant differences in frequencies of GSTM1-null or GSTT1-null between the cases and both control groups. 14.4% of the patients showed homozygous deletion of both GSTT1 and GSTM1 (12.5% among healthy smokers) (not significant)	Data suggest no potentiation between GSTM1 and GSTT1 null genotypes for lung cancer risk	143
Lung, 240 African-Americans 206 Mexican-Americans	132 African-American controls, 108 with lung cancer; 146 Mexican-American controls, 60 with lung cancer	Controlling for age, sex, race, and smoking, no significant association of GSTM1 or GSTT1 either trait with lung cancer was observed. Logistic regression showed an OR of 2.9 (p <0.04) for the association of lung cancer and the presence of both null polymorphisms compared with one (either GSTT1 or GSTM1) or no null genotype	These results suggest that there may be carcinogenic intermediates in cigarette smoke that are substrates for both the GSTT1 and GSTM1 enzymes, and that lung cancer risk is increased more than additively for individuals who have both GSTT1 and GSTM1 null polymorphisms	144

[a] Odds ratio.
[b] Values in parentheses indicate lower and upper 95% confidence intervals.
[c] Extensive metabolizer.
[d] Microsomal epoxide hydrolase.
[e] Slow acetylation, slow acetylators.
[f] Fast acetylator.
[g] Poor metabolizer.

The second, more recent technique (genotyping) employs molecular analysis of DNA using polymerase chain reaction. This became possible when several of the human genes involved in drug metabolism had been cloned and sequenced. Genotyping has placed pharmacogenetics on a sounder footing, but has not solved many of the problems connected with studies of the relevance of metabolic polymorphisms to cancer.

PHENOTYPING

Problems associated with phenotyping include the following.[139] It is invasive, requiring the administration of chemicals followed by urine collection and chemical analysis, with the possibility of errors due to variations in compliance due to poor tolerance to indicator drugs, storage and analysis. Different drugs can be used as markers for the same polymorphic trait, and thresholds for metabolic ratios that define the polymorphic trait have to be established before studies can be initiated. These variations in protocol make it difficult to compare different studies with each other. Metabolism of the indicator drug could be affected by other concomitant exposures, by age, and by lifestyle factors including diet, smoking and alcohol consumption. In case-control studies, the presence of cancer in the cases may affect metabolism of the indicator drug, as could other diseases in the controls.

GENOTYPING

Genotyping depends on the availability of relevant sequenced human genes and their polymorphic variants. Many of the drug-metabolizing enzymes are inducible (either by the compound of interest, or by other chemicals) and inducibility can be tissue-specific.[112] Conventional genotyping can detect only the presence or absence of a particular polymorphism – it is silent on the question of gene expression. Several polymorphisms are due to mutations in introns (non-coding DNA sequences) or other silent areas of DNA, raising the question of whether such genetic variations actually lead to changes in metabolic phenotype.

PROBLEMS OF STUDY DESIGN

Many of the problems in designing studies to measure the influence of pharmacogenetics on cancer risk in response to exposure to carcinogens are similar to those of epidemiological studies in general.[138] They include bias, confounding, choice of controls, insufficient statistical power, and the difficulties in establishing the nature and intensity of the exposure of interest while taking account of adventitious exposures. One problem peculiar to the epidemiological study of pharmacogenetics is the remarkable variation in the allele frequencies of several important pharmacogenetic polymorphisms in different ethnic groups, as illustrated in Table 38.3. For example, the *CYP1A1* m2/m2 extensive metabolizer trait is rare in Scandinavian and North American Caucasian populations, but is found in 11% of Japanese.[112] On the other hand, the proportion of slow *NAT2* acetylators is reported to be 44–70% in North Europeans compared with just 6% in Japanese.[111] It is therefore inappropriate to apply results obtained in one ethnic group to another.

Application of pharmacogenetics to occupational cancer

Knowing the extent to which genetic susceptibility contributes to an individual's risk of cancer might be important in the occupational setting, where, with few exceptions, exposure to noxious chemicals is restricted to levels believed to confer 'acceptable risks' on unselected populations of unknown susceptibility. However, before considering whether a worker's particular pharmacogenetic profile could or should be taken into account in a given occupational setting, a case must be made that certain polymorphisms can, in fact, decrease or increase the risk of cancer. Table 38.3 summarizes examples of studies (some of which have included subjects occupationally exposed to arylamines and to benzene) that have tackled this question and the topic is reviewed in Refs 34, 95, 111, 112, 138, 139.

As illustrated in Table 38.3, the picture that has emerged so far is by no means clear and few firm conclusions can be drawn as to the quantitative effects that metabolic polymorphisms have on cancer risk. The discordance in results between different studies of the same polymorphism is well illustrated in the extensive meta-analyses reported by d'Errico *et al.*[139] However, certain consistent trends are beginning to emerge. Even these must be regarded with some scepticism since they depend on a mixture of phenotyping and genotyping of heterogeneous groups of subjects, and causal associations have not been established.

Slow acetylators in Caucasian populations appear to be at increased risk (about 1.5-fold) of bladder cancer if exposed occupationally to bladder carcinogens, or are heavy smokers. But fast acetylators (especially meat-eaters[140]) are probably at increased risk of colorectal cancer, suggesting that the same polymorphism be detrimental or beneficial, depending on the nature of the exposure and the site of the cancer. Smokers with the *GSTM1* null genotype suffer about a 1.8-fold excess risk of lung cancer compared with *GSTM1*-plus smokers.

Individuals carry mixtures of different metabolic polymorphisms and genotyping makes studies of the effect on cancer risk of interactions between them feasible. Table 38.4 lists examples of such studies.[114–144] Of particular note with regard to occupational exposure is the increased relative risk (4.1) of pulmonary disease and mesothelioma (7.8) in slow acetylators who are *GSTMI*.[141] This study, and the studies that show that

Japanese smokers who are *CYP1A1* extensive-metabolizers and *GSTM1*-null are at substantially increased risk of developing lung cancer,[113,145] indicate that certain combinations of pharmacogenetic polymorphisms are more likely to confer substantially increased susceptibility to cancer than are single traits.

Although evidence that pharmacogenetic polymorphisms can modulate cancer susceptibility is beginning to emerge it is also clear that much more work needs to be done before screening workplace populations for these traits could be considered practicable or useful. Whether such an approach would ever be acceptable on ethical grounds will be referred to later. As far as the scientific basis of pharmacogenetics in cancer susceptibility is concerned, reviewers of this area of 'molecular epidemiology' have concluded that

> study designs are often immature and all the potential methodological flaws have not been assessed. [. . .]Such methodological problems must be properly addressed before any introduction of susceptibility tests in practice is considered.[138]

Raunio *et al.*[112] stated in 1995 that

> . . . no single genotypic marker in xenobiotic-metabolizing genes can be uneqivocally associated with cancer risk at present. The initial studies showing a substantially increased risk of developing lung cancer in individuals with combined high-risk *CYP1A1* and *GSTM1* genotypes[113,145] clearly suggest that inheritance of multiple altered alleles can contribute significantly to chemical carcinogenesis in humans. Future studies involving larger control and cancer populations, precisely and uniformly defined clinical classification of cancers and better exposure histories will undoubtedly lead to a more thorough understanding of the role of xenobiotic-metabolizing enzymes in cancer development.

Ethical issues in screening for genetic susceptibility to carcinogens

If it turns out, beyond peradventure, that individuals carrying certain pharmacogenetic polymorphisms are indeed particularly susceptible to known carcinogens, the ethical and legal implications of screening workers for cancer susceptibility genes must be addressed. Detailed consideration of these issues is beyond the scope of this chapter, but can be found in Refs 146–153. The need for such a debate is urgent, since it will not be long before the International Human Genome Project has completed the task of sequencing the entire human genome. Up-to-date information on this project is available on the Internet at the following web site: http://www.ornl.gov/TechResources/Human-Genome/home.html). Data on this scale will be useful only if there are methods for rapidly and accurately screening human

genes for mutations and polymorphisms. Such methods are already becoming available, in the form of DNA microchip technology.[154–159] Using techniques from the microelectronics industry and oligonucleotide synthetic chemistry, silica chips (about 1.6 cm²) can be prepared containing potentially hundreds of thousands of oligonucleotides of predetermined sequence.

A sample of fluorescently labelled DNA or RNA is applied to the chip, which is then interrogated for sequence information or gene expression using scanning confocal microscopy. It is estimated that the entire human genome could be accommodated on just ten chips. Thus, within the next few years it will be possible, rapidly and cheaply, to genotype individuals for mutations and polymorphisms in thousands of genes and to determine expression of specific genes in individual tissues. Puga *et al.*[160] describe novel approaches for harnessing this and related technologies to the discovery of genes, and their products, that determine susceptibility to environmental and occupational toxins (including carcinogens).

Genetic susceptibility to cancer involves genes other than those that determine pharmacogenetic polymorphisms. Table 38.2 lists several genes that confer greatly increased risk of certain cancers, by a variety of mechanisms. It is very likely that more genes of this highly penetrant type will be discovered, and that other cancer susceptibility genes, with lower penetrance but perhaps greater prevalence, also await discovery. The effect of such genes on susceptibility to occupational carcinogens is, at present, unknown. However, with the enormous speed at which genetic knowledge is expanding, and given the realistic probability of rapidly screening an individual's entire genome, such information may well be available sooner than some of us think. As Winston Churchill put it (in another context) 'This is not the end. It is not even the beginning of the end. But it is, perhaps, the end of the beginning'.

TESTING CHEMICALS FOR GENOTOXICITY AND CARCINOGENICITY

The idea that cancer is a genetic disorder of somatic cells is well founded and is now generally accepted. There is also little doubt that many carcinogens are carcinogenic *because* they are genotoxic. Determining whether a substance is genotoxic is therefore a useful guide to its potential carcinogenicity.

The first step in deciding whether a compound is genotoxic is to inspect its structure for sites – 'structural alerts' – that could react with DNA directly or after metabolism to electrophilic metabolites.[161,162] The accumulation of structure-activity data for a wide variety of chemical carcinogens has made looking for structural alerts feasible (Fig. 38.3). The compound under suspicion is tested for its ability to produce point mutations in bacteria, using the *Salmonella* test – also known as the Ames test[163-167] and assays for chromosomal aberrations in mammalian cells in culture.[26,168,169] Further tests for point mutations in mammalian cells *in vitro*[170,171] and chromosomal aberrations conducted *in vivo* may be also be required.[172-174] Additional data, for example, on DNA-adduct formation, may also be required. Extensive advice on the statistical evaluation of mutagenicity data can be found in Ref 175.

Experience shows that this strategy, though not perfect, will pick up most, if not all, genotoxic carcinogens[167,176-178] Many of the genotoxicity tests currently accepted by regulatory authorities were developed in the 1970s, and do not benefit from the enormous expansion in knowledge brought about by modern molecular biology and by improvements to instrumentation. However, this is now being remedied, and new tests are under development, using, for example, fluorescence *in situ* hybridization (FISH),[26,179] cell-lines genetically engineered to express human carcinogen-metabolizing enzymes,[180,181] single-cell gel electrophoresis ('comet assay'),[182-184] and transgenic animals using shuttle-vector systems.[185] A detailed compilation of modern methods for detecting DNA damage and mutations can be found in Ref. 186. Moreover, more information could be gained from existing assays – for example, mutational spectra can be assembled from DNA sequence analysis of mutants induced by known agents and isolated from bacterial and mammalian mutagenicity tests.[25]

Genotoxicity assays are now well established in the toxicological evaluation of chemicals, including those used in the workplace. If a chemical is found to be genotoxic it is reasonable to predict that it is carcinogenic. Unfortunately, however, the fact that a compound is not

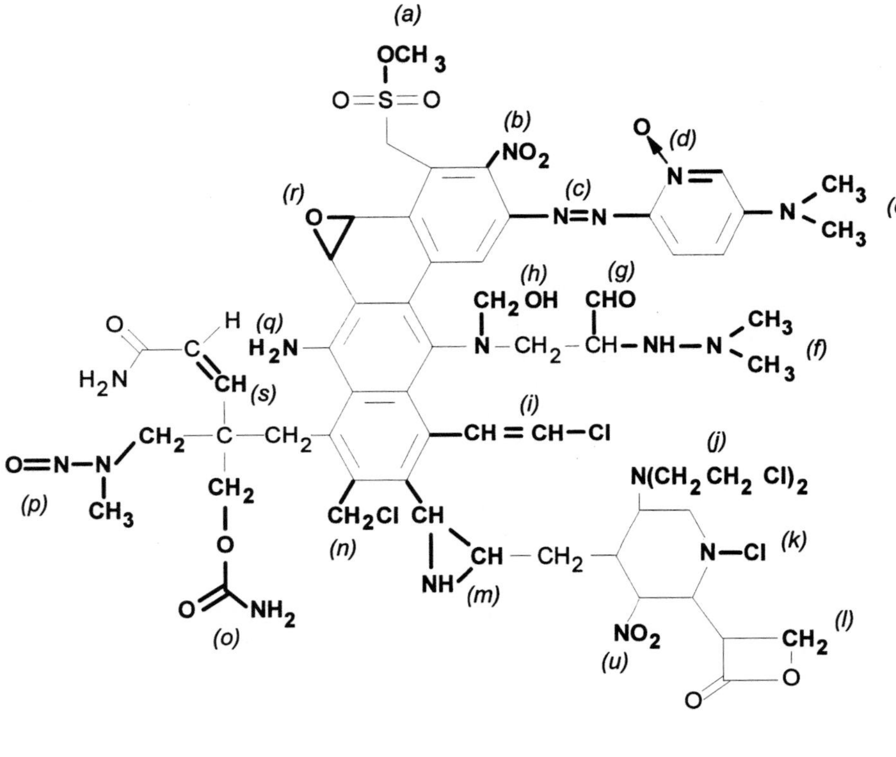

Figure 38.3 *Hypothetical organic molecule containing structural alerts (shown in bold and labelled in bracketed lower-case alphabeticals) to genotoxicity. Reproduced from Ref. 161, with permission. See this and previous references therein for a full discussion of the basis of this structure. The structural alerts are as follows: (a) alkyl esters of either phosphoric or sulphonic acids; (b) aromatic nitro groups; (c) aromatic azo groups, not per se but by virtue of their possible reduction to an aromatic amine; (d) aromatic ring N-oxides; (e) aromatic mono- and dialkylamino groups; (f) alkyl hydrazines; (g) alkyl aldehydes; (h) N-methylol derivates; (i) monohaloalkenes; (j) a large family of N and S mustards (β-haloethyl); (k) pchloramines. The N-chloramine substructure has not yet been associated with carcinogenicity, but potent genotoxic activity has been reported for it; (l) propiolactones and propiosultones; (m) aromatic and aliphatic aziridinyl derivatives; (n) both aromatic and aliphatic substituted primary alkyl halides; (o) derivatives of urethane (carbamates); (p) alkyl N-nitrosamines; (q) aromatic amines, their N-hydroxy derivatives and the derived esters; (r) aliphatic epoxides and aromatic oxides; (s) centre of Michael reactivity; (u) aliphatic nitro group, as present in tetranitromethane.*

genotoxic does not give assurance that it is not carcinogenic, as discussed below.

Non-genotoxic carcinogens

When tested in laboratory rodents, *genotoxic* carcinogens generally produce tumours in a number of different organs or tissues, in both sexes, in a range of strains and species, and often at doses lower than those that produce obvious organ-specific or general toxicity.[162,178]

However there is a substantial number of substances that, when tested in laboratory rodents, induce cancer in a single organ, sex or species, and when tested by the strategy described above, are found to be devoid of genotoxic activity. Such non-genotoxic carcinogens tend to produce neoplasms only at doses that evince organ-specific or generally toxic effects that are accompanied by cell proliferation (mitogenesis) in tissues or organs that are normally quiescent. Non-genotoxic carcinogens vary greatly in their chemical structure and biological effects, and include enzyme inducers, endogenous and synthetic hormones and hormone-modifying substances, and various chemically inert materials such as plastic films. Table 38.5 gives some examples of non-genotoxic carcinogens and the pathological and biochemical lesions associated with them.[187–193]

There is no general hypothesis to account for the mechanisms underlying non-genotoxic carcinogenesis. Instead, it is clear that a variety of quite different mechanisms must operate, each depending on the nature of the substance involved.[162] The only common factor linking otherwise disparate non-genotoxic carcinogens is their ability to stimulate sustained mitogenesis.[194] Studies are in progress to develop short-term tests for non-genotoxic carcinogens, with an emphasis on basing such tests on mechanistic models.[195]

Certain genotoxic agents may also exhibit properties that are more characteristic of non-genotoxic carcinogens. For example, formaldehyde, a well-characterized broad-spectrum genotoxin, induces squamous-cell carcinomas in the anterior nasal cavity of rats (but not

Table 38.5 *Some examples of mechanisms of non-genotoxic carcinogens established by experimental studies of rodents*

Species	Organ	Tumour	Accompanying pathology and/or biochemical disturbance	Examples of substances that produce the effects
Rat	Exocrine pancreas	Adenomas, carcinomas	Hyperytrophy, hyperplasia, atypical acinar cell foci	Unsaturated fat (corn oil); trypsin inhibitors (full-fat soya flour)[187]
Male rats that synthesize α_2-microglobulin	Kidney	Adenomas, carcinomas	Binding of α_2-microglobulin and accumulation in proximal-tubule lysosomes; tubular necrosis and proliferation	Unleaded gasoline; 2,2, 4-trimethyl pentane; D-limonene; 1,4-dichlorobenzene; isophorene[188]
Rats and mice	Kidney (renal cortex)	Clear-cell adenomas, carcinomas	Redistribution of systemic zinc, increased resorption of Zn by proximal tubules, tubular necrosis and proliferation	Nitrilotriacetates[188]
Female rats	Urinary bladder	Tumours of transitional epithelium	Hyperplasia, bladder ulcers, depletion of urinary Ca by free nitrilotriacetate	Sodium nitrilotriacetate[189]
Rats and mice	Liver	Hepatocellular hepatomas, carcinomas	Hepatocellular necrosis, cirrhosis, reparative hyperplasia	Carbon tetrachloride; chloroform; tetrachloroethylene; paracetamol[190]
Rats and mice	Liver	Hepatocellular carcinomas	Induction of peroxisome proliferation, increase in peroxidation hepatomegaly	Ciprofibrate; fenofibrate; nafenopin[190]
Rats	Liver	Hepatocellular carcinomas	Induction of a variety of mixed-function oxidases, hepatomegaly	DDT; polychlorinated biphenyls; hexacyclohexane; chlordecone; phenobarbitone, butylated hydroxytoluene[a190]
Rats or mice	Thyroid	Adenomas, carcinomas	Inhibition of thyroid hormone synthesis, or increase in their degradation; elevation in pituitary thyroid-stimulating hormone; goitrogenesis	Methylthiourea; ethylthiourea; aminotriazole; perchlorate[b191]
Rats	Fore-stomach	Papilloma, carcinoma	Reversible cellular proliferation in region where neoplasms arise	Butylated hydroxyanisole[192]
Beagle dogs	Mammary gland	Adeno carcinomas	Excessive hyperplasia	Progestagens or progestagen-oestrogen combinations[193]
Rats and mice	Pituitary; mammary gland	Adenomas, carcinomas	Inhibition of dopamine, release of prolactin, pituitary and mammary hyperplasia	Oestrogens; oestrogenic steroids[193]

[a] Rats only.   [b] Mice only.

mice) only after whole-body exposure to vapour at high doses for many months. Moreover, tumours develop only in areas of tissue that have sustained cell degeneration, necrosis and inflammation.[196]

If it is true that most, if not all, cancers develop as a result of an accumulation of somatic mutations, irrespective of the initial carcinogenic stimulus, an hypothesis to explain the molecular mechanisms by which non-genotoxic carcinogens induce cancer is required. The most widely canvassed theory states that dividing cells are more susceptible to mutation than are quiescent cells and that substances that are not genotoxic *per se* may nevertheless enhance mutagenesis by stimulating mitogenesis in cells which have suffered endogenous DNA damage.[197] Preston-Martin *et al.*[198] argue that there is substantial epidemiological evidence that mitogenesis is an important factor in certain human cancers.

Long-term animal tests for carcinogenicity

The idea that mitogenesis might be as important as mutagenesis has aroused much controversy, especially in the context of identifying and regulating environmental and occupational carcinogens. The argument centres on the conduct and interpretation of long-term carcinogenicity tests using rodents. By far the largest number of such tests have been conducted by the National Toxicology Program of the USA.[178] In these bioassays groups of rats and mice are subjected to lifetime administration of the test substance, usually by feeding, at the maximum tolerated dose – 'the highest dose of the test agent during the chronic study that can be predicted not to alter the animals' longevity from effects other than carcinogenicity'.[199] Ashby and Morrod[8] have encapsulated the problem by reference to three compounds shown to be carcinogenic in such tests. Glycidol is cited as an example of a typical genotoxic carcinogen. It is a directly-acting alkylating agent containing a structurally alerting epoxide group and is mutagenic to bacteria. It produces large increases in tumours at a variety of sites in both sexes of mice and rats, at both low and high doses. Tris(2-ethylhexyl)phosphate and butyl benzyl phthalate are examples of non-genotoxic carcinogens.

Neither compound contains a structural alert; nor are they mutagenic. Tris(2-ethylhexyl)phosphate produces tumours only at one site in one sex of one species – liver tumours in female mice. Butyl benzyl phthalate produces tumours of the haemopoietic system only in female rats and only at the maximum tolerated dose. It is thought that these last two compounds are detected as carcinogens because of the toxic effects they elicit specifically in rodents. The crux of the problem lies in the predictive value that can be attached to the results obtained with the two non-genotoxic carcinogens – do these bioassays predict a hazard to humans, or are they the result of mitogenic responses to sustained high doses?

Would such compounds present a hazard to rodents at lower, non-toxic doses approaching those experienced by humans? Would they cause human cancer at non-toxic levels?

The arguments for and against the continued use of carcinogenicity tests using the maximum tolerated dose approach in regulating involuntary exposure to environmental and occupational chemicals are now being displaced by the recognition that understanding how a given substance induces cancer in experimental animals is the most rational way of designing and using such tests in for evaluating hazard and risks to humans.[200,201] Such an approach is taken in the UK, where the distinction between genotoxic and non-genotoxic carcinogens is recognized in the regulation of carcinogens. The strategy is to identify a hazard and then to set an 'acceptable risk' based, where possible, on quantitative data.[176] The rule of thumb is that it is prudent to assume there is no threshold below which a genotoxic carcinogen will not be carcinogenic, and exposure limits are therefore based on 'acceptable levels'. Where there is convincing evidence that a carcinogen is devoid of genotoxicity, where animal experiments show a threshold dose for carcinogenicity, and where there is a plausible mechanistic explanation for the carcinogenic effect, 'no observable effect levels' can be set, which, with appropriate safety factors, can be used to set exposure limits.

Results of the National Toxocology Program carcinogenicity programme also raise questions about the ability of the *Salmonella* test to predict carcinogenicity. In a detailed analysis of that data base Ashby and Tennant[178] split the 301 chemicals tested for mutagenicity and carcinogenicity into 154 that contained structural alerts and 147 that did not. They came to the following conclusions:

- Most of the carcinogens that caused cancer in rodents, including most that induced cancer in both rats and mice and/or at multiple sites, contained structural alerts.
- Most of the structurally alerting chemicals were mutagenic; 84% of the carcinogens and 66% of the non-carcinogens. All 33 aromatic amino/nitro-type chemicals that were carcinogenic to both species were mutagenic. Thus, for structurally alerting chemicals, the *Salmonella* test assay showed high sensitivity and low specificity.
- Among the 147 non-alerting chemicals less than 5% were mutagenic, whether they were carcinogenic or not.

New methods for carcinogenicity testing – transgenic models

The present 'gold standard' test for carcinogenicity in laboratory animals is the 2-year National Toxicology Program bioassay described above. Apart from the controversy surrounding the conduct and interpretation of such tests, there are other reasons why results gained from them will diminish in the next few years. These include cost, issues of animal welfare and the requirement for information on mechanism. The International Conference on Harmonization of Technical Requirements for the Registration of Pharmaceuticals for human use is considering the number of species to be used when evaluating chemicals for carcinogenicity. Although these proposals will apply only to human pharmaceuticals, they have implications for the evaluation of chemicals in general for carcinogenicity. The basic scheme proposed comprises one long-term rodent carcinogenicity study, using rats, plus one other *in vivo* study that provides insight into carcinogenic mechanisms. Proposals for these include an initiation/promotion model, using hepatocarcinogenicity in rats, or a multi-organ model; transgenic mice, or a neonatal rodent model.

Several strains of transgenic mice are already available, including a *p53* +/– heterozygote and the TG.AC mouse, which carry a v-Ha-*ras* oncogene fused to the promoter of a globin gene, which makes it particularly sensitive to skin carcinogens.[202] Although mice genetically engineered to be highly susceptible to cancer will probably find an important place in carcinogenicity testing in the future, there are at present insufficient data to justify the use of any of the currently available models for routine testing.[203,204]

BIOMONITORING FOR CARCINOGEN EXPOSURE IN THE WORKPLACE

Monitoring body fluids or tissues for genotoxicity or for formation of protein or DNA adducts can be used for detecting exposure to and absorption of occupational carcinogens. This activity is a 'subspecies' of biomonitoring and overlaps with molecular epidemiology (e.g. studies of mutational spectra in tumours, pharmacogenetic polymorphisms and cancer susceptibility (see above). Reviews on biomonitoring as applied to environmental and occupational cancer can be found in Refs 90–93,95,96. A comprehensive and critical review of biomonitoring in cancer epidemiology, compiled under the auspices of The International Agency for Research on Cancer, is available in Ref 205 which contains recommendations that should be taken into account when designing future studies. Information on techniques is available in Refs 186 and 206.

Types of marker

Unlike traditional cancer epidemiology, which relies on collecting incidence and mortality data decades after the putative exposure, biomonitoring aims to prevent occu-

pational cancer by giving early warning of exposure (and in some cases, effect), long before cancer develops. Depending on the markers used, biomonitoring in this setting may provide several categories of information.[91,148] (1) internal dose, (2) biologically effective dose, (3) early pre-clinical biological effect or response, (4) susceptibility. In addition, useful insights into mechanism may be gained. The first three categories (1–3) reflect the temporal course of carcinogenesis, whereas (1, susceptibility) may operate at any or at all stages. As well as genetic susceptibility to cancer, there are other factors (e.g. smoking, diet, drugs, medicines and other diseases) that may influence an individual's susceptibility to the effects of occupational carcinogens. Examples of the first three categories of biomarkers are shown in Table 38.6, which also provides some examples of the studies that have been published in the 1990s using these methods.[207–254]

Table 38.7 gives some examples in which biomonitoring has been combined with markers of genetic susceptibility (pharmacogenetic polymorphisms).[255–265]

Specimens that can be used in biomonitoring

Monitoring human populations depends on a supply of samples of body fluids or tissues in amounts sufficient to allow reliable assay by the chosen method. Materials which meet this requirement and which comply with ethical and practical constraints include saliva, sputum, blood, urine, faeces and semen. Other materials that are relatively easy to collect include hair, and cells from buccal and nasal mucosa, exfoliated urothelial cells and lung cells from sputum. The sensitivity of techniques such as polymerase chain reaction (for mutational screening),[32]P-postlabelling (for detecting DNA-adduct formation) and fluorescence *in situ* hybridization (FISH) (for cytogenetic analysis) makes it practicable to use such specimens for biomonitoring. In practice, blood and urine are the most easily collected materials for biomonitoring, but suffer the drawback of not directly representing those sites (skin, lung, bladder) probably at greatest risk from occupational exposure.

Choice of method

The choice of biomonitoring method for any given exposure and workforce depends on many factors. For example, where there is potential exposure to one or two known chemicals, which can be measured, it would be logical to conduct hygiene measurements and to use markers of internal dose (e.g. urinary metabolites) for monitoring the workforce. If there are mixed, complex exposures, an eclectic marker of internal dose such as urinary mutagenicity could be used. This method is not without its problems but can yield useful information when used properly.[266]

Table 38.6 *Examples of the use of biomonitoring in occupational cancer*

Biomarker	Techniques required	Body fluid or tissue[a]	Interpretation	Examples of studies of occupational exposure			
				Exposure or occupation	Body fluid or tissue	Marker	Ref.
Markers of internal dose							
Xenobiotics or their products in body fluids	Analytical chemistry (e.g. HLPC,[b] GC,[c] MS,[d] immunochemistry)	Blood, urine	Absorption of xenobiotics or their metabolites, or excretion of DNA adducts, or products of oxidative DNA damage	Handling cytotoxic drugs	Urine	Cyclophosphamide, ifosfamide	207
				Handling cytotoxic drugs	Urine	Platinum	208
				Handling cytotoxic drugs	Urine	Thioethers	209
				Handling cytotoxic drugs	Urine	Thioethers, D-glucaric acid	210
				Diesel-exhaust (PAH)[e]	Urine	1-Hydroxypyrene	211
				Coke-oven workers (PAH)	Urine	1-Hydroxypyrene	212
				Filling stations attendants (benzene)	Urine	8-Hydroxyguanosine	213
				Handling cytotoxic drugs	Urine	Cyclophosphamide, ifosfamide platinum	214
Urinary mutagenicity (reviewed in ref. 215)	Bacterial mutation assays	Urine	Absorption, metabolism and excretion of mutagens	Handling cytotoxic drugs	Urine	Fluctuation test	209
				Handling cytotoxic drugs	Urine	Forward and reverse mutation	210
				Benzidine	Urine	Ames test	216
				Coke-oven workers	Urine	Ames test	217
				Variety of 'hazardous exposures'	Urine	Ames test	218
Markers of biologically effective dose							
Protein adducts (reviewed in ref. 219)	GC-MS of haemoglobin or albumin (protein, peptide, or amino acid) HPLC-fluorescence Immunochemistry	Blood	Absorption of compounds that are electrophilic or have been metabolized to electrophiles (surrogate for DNA adducts)	Coke-oven workers (PAH)	Blood	Hydroxyethylvaline adducts in Hb[f]	212
				Diesel-exhaust (PAH)[e]	Blood	Hydroxyethylvaline adducts in Hb	211
				Styrene, styrene oxide	Blood	Cysteine and carboxylic acid adducts in albumin and Hb	220
DNA adducts (reviewed in ref. 219)	Immunochemistry ^{32}P-postlabelling Physical methods (e.g. GC-MS, FLNS)[g]	Nasal mucosa Sputum (lung cells) Exfoliated urothelial cells Peripheral lymphocytes	Absorption of compounds that are electrophilic or have been metabolized to electrophiles that bind covalently to DNA	MbOCA[h]	Exfoliated urothelial cells	^{32}P-Postlabelling	221
				None (pilot study)	Nasal mucosa cells	^{32}P-Postlabelling	222
				Coke-oven workers (PAH)	Lymphocytes	^{32}P-Postlabelling	223
				Coke-even workers (PAH)	Blood plasma	Antibodies to benzo(a)pyrene DNA adducts	212
				Benzidine	Exfoliated	^{32}P-Postlabelling urothelial cells	224
				Greenhouse floriculturalists	Lymphocytes	^{32}P-Postlabelling	225
DNA-protein crosslinks	Selective extraction, precipitation after heat denaturation	Peripheral lymphocytes	Absorption of compounds that produce DNA-protein crosslinks	Metal are welders	Lymphocytes	DNA-protein crosslinks	226
				Welders, chrome platers	Lymphocytes	DNA-protein crosslinks	227
				Formaldehyde	Lymphocytes	DNA-protein crosslinks	228 (see comments in ref. 229)

Markers of early pre-clinical biological effect or response

Marker	Method	Cell type	Biological basis	Study population	Assay	Cell type	Ref.
DNA strand breaks	Alkaline elution	Peripheral lymphocytes	Absorption of compounds that produce DNA strand breaks	Coke-oven workers (PAH)	Alkaline elution	Lymphocytes	230
	Single-cell gel electrophoresis ('Comet') assay	Peripheral lymphocytes		Car paint sprayers	Alkaline elution	Lymphocytes	231
				Cytostatic drugs	Alkaline elution	Lymphocytes	232
				Styrene	Alkaline elution	Lymphocytes	233
				Benzene	Comet assay	Lymphocytes	234
				1,3-Butadiene	Comet assay	Lymphocytes	235
				Rubber industry	Comet assay	Lymphocytes	236
				Styrene	Comet assay	Lymphocytes	237
Somatic cell mutation (reviewed in refs 238, 239)	Haemoglobin variants	Erythrocytes	Absorption of compounds that produce somatic mutation	Chernobyl workers (ionizing radiation)	GPA variants	Erythrocytes	240
	Glycophorin A (GPA) variants	Erythrocytes		Uranium miners (radon progeny)	GPA variants / hprt mutations	Erythrocytes / Lymphocytes	241
	Mutations in T-cell receptor genes	Peripheral lymphocytes		Styrene	GPA variants	Erythrocytes	242
	Mutations in HLA-A locus	Peripheral lymphocytes		1,3-Butadiene	hprt mutations	Lymphocytes	235
	Mutations at hprt locus	Peripheral lymphocytes		1,3-Butadiene	hprt mutations	Lymphocytes	243
				Benzene	GPA variants	Erythrocytes	244
				Bus maintenance workers	hprt mutations	Lymphocytes	245
				Styrene	hprt mutations	Lymphocytes	237
				Styrene/dichloromethane	hprt mutations	Lymphocytes	246
				Handling cytotoxic drugs	hprt mutations	Lymphocytes	247
				Foundry workers (PAH)	GPA variants	Erythrocytes	248
				Ethylene oxide	hprt mutations	Lymphocytes	249
Chromosomal anomalies[i]	Metaphase analysis	Peripheral lymphocytes	Absorption of compounds that damage chromosomes and/or induce aneuploidy	Filling station attendants	SCE	Lymphocytes	250
	Micronuclei			Benzene and coke ovens	Micronuclei-FISH including aneuploidy	Buccal cells, lymphocytes	251
	Sister chromatid exchange (SCE)			Coke oven workers	SCE	Lymphocytes	230
	FISH[j]			Aircraft maintenance workers	SCE, micronuclei	Lymphocytes	252
				Filling stations attendants	Micronuclei	Lymphocytes	253
				1,3-Butadiene	Metaphase analysis, micronuclei	Lymphocytes	235
				Rubber industry	Micronuclei, SCE	Lymphocytes	236
				Benzene	Interphase FISH for aneuploidy	Lymphocytes	254
				Styrene/dichloromethane	SCE, micronuclei, metaphase analysis	Lymphocytes	246
				Ethylene oxide	SCE, micronuclei, metaphase analysis	Lymphocytes	249
				Handling cytotoxic drugs	SCE, micronuclei	Lymphocytes	209
				Handling cytotoxic drugs	SCE, micronuclei	Lymphocytes	214

[a] Includes only those readily available in an occupational setting. [b] High performance liquid chromatography.
[c] Gas chromatography.
[d] Mass spectrometry.
[e] Polycyclic aromatic hydrocarbons.
[f] Haemoglobin.
[g] Fluorescence line-narrowing spectroscopy.
[h] 4,4'-Methylene-*bis*(2-chloroaniline).
[i] Also includes assays where donors' cells are challenged *in vitro* with agents that can cause chromosomal anomalies.
[j] Fluoresence *in situ* hybridization.

Table 38.7 *Examples of studies of the effect of metabolic polymorphisms on various biomarkers thought to be relevant to cancer*

Ethnic groups (number in study)	Exposure or occupation	Site at risk of cancer	Polymorphisms examined (P, by phenotype or G, by genotype)[a]	Biomarker (method)	Tissue examined for biomarker	Results	Ref.
Caucasian (44) African-American (42) Asian (42) Total: 133	Smokers and non-smokers	Bladder	NAT-2 slow acetylator vs NAT-2 fast acetylator (P)	3-ABP-Hb and 4-ABP-Hb[b] adducts (GC-MS)[c]	Erythrocytes	Both adducts higher in smokers than in non-smokers. 3-ABP-adducts 2.5 times higher in slow acetylators than in fast acetylators, irrespective of smoking and ethnic group.	255
Caucasian (74) African-American (40) Asian (37) Total: 151	Smokers and non-smokers	Bladder	GSTM1-null vs GSTM+/+ (G) NAT-2 slow acetylator vs NAT-2 fast acetylator (P)	3-ABP-Hb and 4-ABP-Hb adducts (GC-MS)	Erythrocyte	Both adducts higher in smokers than in non-smokers. 4-ABP-adducts 1.6 times higher in GSTM1-null/slow acetylators than in GSTM1+/+/rapid acetylators, adjusted for ethnic group and smoking. GSTM1 and NAT independently contribute to ABP-adduct levels.	256
Caucasian (61) African-American (28) Oriental (1) Total: 90	Smokers and non-smokers	Lung	CYP1A1; EM vs PM[d] (G) CYPD6; EM vs PM (G) CYP2E1; (G) Dra1 DD vs CD (G) GSTM1-null vs GSTM+/+ (G)	7-methyl-dGMP[e] and PAH-dGMP[f] DNA adducts ([32P]-postlabelling)	Lung autopsy specimens	7-methyl-dGMP adducts found in all specimens. CYPD6 EM had 1.4 times more adducts then CYPD6 PM, but only in people with low tobacco-exposure. Slight differences between DD and CD genotypes. No differences with CYP1A1 polymorphisms. PAH-dGMP found in 10% of specimens. No data on adduct levels.	257
Caucasian (37) Hispanic (4) Other ethnic groups (6) Total: 47	Non-smoking fire-fighters	No specific site	CYP1A1 EM vs PM (G) GSTM1-null vs GSTM+/+ (G)	PAH-DNA adducts[f] (immunochemistry)	Peripheral blood lymphocytes	No significant associations between adduct levels and polymorphic genotypes	258
Not stated (78)	Smokers and non-smokers	No specific site	GSTT1-null vs GSTT1+/+ (G)	SCE induced in vitro by 6 μM 1,3-butadiene diepoxide (DEB)	PHA[g]-stimulated peripheral lymphocytes	0/60 DEB-resistant donors were GSTT1-null compared with 12/18 DEB-sensitive donors ($p < 0.001$). SCE in DEB-treated lymphocytes were 1.7 times higher in GSTT1-null than in GSTT1+/+. SCE in untreated lymphocytes were significantly higher in GSTT1-null than in GSTT1+/+.	259
Not stated (probably Finnish) (20)	19 current non-smokers, 1 smoker	No specific site	GSTT1-null vs GSTT1+/+ (G) GSTM1-null vs GSTM+/+ (G)	SCE induced in vitro by 5 μM 1,3-butadiene diepoxide (DEB)	PHA-stimulated peripheral lymphocytes	SCE in DEB-treated lymphocytes were 1.6 times higher in GSTT1-null than in GSTT1+/+. SCE in untreated lymphocytes were slightly higher in GSTM1-null than in GSTT1+/+. GSTM1 polymorphisms had no effect on background or DEB-induced SCE	260
						Results of this study confirmed in 7 subjects with repeated measurements over 55 months	261

Population (no.)	Site	Genotype comparison	Endpoint (method)	Tissue/sample	Results	Ref.
Not stated (probably Swedish) (69)	No specific site	GSTT1-null vs GSTT1+/+ (G); NAT-2 slow acetylator vs NAT-2 fast acetylator (G)	Non-polar bulky DNA adducts (^{32}P-postlabelling) hprt mutations (cloning assay)	PHA-stimulated peripheral lymphocytes	No difference in MF[b] between exposed and controls, but significant difference in adduct levels. MF and adduct level were highest in the most heavily exposed workers. Significant increase in MF with adduct level and with age. No significant difference in MF or in adduct level between the GSTM1-null and +/+ individuals, or between slow and rapid acetylators. Among the slow acetylators, there was a significantly higher adduct level in the GSTM1-null individuals vs GSTM1+/+ individuals.	245
Indians (48)	Bladder	NAT-2 slow acetylator vs NAT-2 fast acetylator (P and G)	BZD-DNA adducts[i] (^{32}P-postlabelling) Benzidine metabolites (GC-MS)	Exfoliated urothelial cells / Urine	4 DNA adducts were significantly elevated in exposed workers vs controls. The major adduct is N-acetylated and the only one significantly associated with total BZ urinary metabolites. Almost all urinary BZD-metabolites exposed workers were acetylated among slow, as well as rapid, acetylators. NAT2 activity was not associated with levels of any DNA adduct detected.	262
Italians (45)	No specific site	GSTM1-null vs GSTM1+/+ (G); GSTT1-null vs GSTT1+/+ (G); NAT-2 slow acetylator vs NAT-2 fast acetylator (G)	SCE, metaphase analysis for chromosomal aberrations, micronucleus formation	PHA-stimulated peripheral lymphocytes	Pesticide exposure had no effect on any of the cytogenetic endpoints.	262
Chinese (81)	Bladder	GSTM1-null vs GSTM+/+ (G)	BZD-DNA adducts[j] (^{32}P-postlabelling) Benzidine metabolites Urine (GC-MS) Urinary mutagenicity (Ames test on organic fraction)	Exfoliated urothelial cells / Urine	No overall increase in bladder cancer risk for the GSTM1-null genotype among 38 bladder cancer cases and 43 controls. GSTM1 genotype had no impact on urothelial cell DNA adduct and urinary mutagenicity levels in workers currently exposed to benzidine. Human GSTM1 did not conjugate benzidine or its metabolites.	263

Subjects:
- 47 Bus maintenance workers (exposure includes diesel exhaust, engine and other oils); 22 controls
- 15 controls, 18 benzidine-dye workers, 15 in benzidine manufacture
- 22 floriculturalists exposed to pesticides (sampled after low and high exposure)
- 43 benzidine-exposed controls, 38 benzidine-exposed bladder-cancer patients
- 15 unexposed controls 15 benzidine-dye workers 15 in benzidine manufacture

Continued

Table 38.7 – *cont.*

Ethnic groups (number in study)	Exposure or occupation	Site at risk of cancer	Polymorphisms examined (P, by phenotype or G, by genotype)[a]	Biomarker (method)	Tissue examined for biomarker	Results	Ref.
Finnish (100)	Iron-foundry workers exposed to PAH	No specific site	CYP1A1; EM vs PM (G) GSTM1-null vs GSTM+/+ (G)	PAH-DNA adducts (³²P-postlabelling) 1-hydroxypyrene	Peripheral lymphocytes Urine	DNA adduct levels were followed at 4 annual samplings, during which PAH exposure and DNA adducts decreased concomitantly. Exposure and adducts were related. Adduct levels correlated with urinary 1-hydroxypyrene, air benzo(a)pyrene, weekly working hours and daily cigarette consumption. GSTM1 or CYP1A1 genotypes had no clear effects.	264
Norwegians (435)	297 healthy controls 138 lung-cancer patients	Lung	GSTP1 AA or AG vs GSTP1 GG (G) GSTM1-null vs GSTM+/+ (G)	Non-polar bulky DNA adducts (³²P-postlabelling) (in 70 current smoking lung-cancer patients)	Peripheral lymphocytes	Patients had significantly higher frequency of the GG genotype and a lower frequency of AA than controls. GG patients had significantly higher adduct level than AA patients. In 135 patients and 342 controls, GSTM1-null genotype was associated with a slightly increased lung cancer risk. Patients with the combination GSTM1-null and AG or GG had significantly higher adduct levels than all other genotype combinations.	132
Italians (62)	32 controls, 30 flori-culturalists exposed to presticides	No specific site	GSTM1-null vs GSTM+/+ (G) GSTT1-null vs GSTT1+/+ (G)	Metaphase analysis for chromosomal aberrations (CA)	PHA-stimulated peripheral lymphocytes	No association between pesticide exposure and elevated frequencies of CA. Statistically significant increase in baseline CA in GSTM1-null smokers.	265

[a]Indicates whether polymorphism was determined by phenotype or by genotype.
[b]3-aminobiphenyl and 4-aminobiphenyl-haemoglobin adducts.
[c]Gas-chromatography and mass-spectrometry.
[d]Extensive metabolizers vs poor metabolizers.
[e]DNA adduct produced by metabolic activation of N-nitrosamines.
[f]DNA adduct produced by metabolic activation of polycyclic aromatic hydrocarbons.
[g]Phytohaemagglutinin.
[h]Mutant frequency.
[i]Benzidine-DNA adducts produced by metabolic activation of benzidine.

Of methods that detect the biologically effective dose, perhaps the most useful are those that measure adduct formation with protein of DNA.[219] Measurements of protein adducts in haemoglobin have revealed evidence of occupational exposure to ethylene oxide, styrene oxide, acrylamide and acrylonitrile.[219] ^{32}P-Postlabelling, which has produced data showing DNA adduct formation in white blood cells of workers in iron foundries, coke ovens and aluminium plants, and of bus drivers exposed to diesel exhaust, has some distinct advantages for biomonitoring.[219,267,268] It can detect extremely low levels of adducts ($1/10^{10}$) nucleotides) and data can be obtained from microgram (μg) quantities of DNA, making it applicable to human biopsy samples. It requires no prior knowledge of adduct precursors and can detect adducts resulting from exposure to complex mixtures and from electrophiles produced, for example, by free radicals. Its main disadvantage, which in part stems from its high sensitivity, is that it cannot identify adducts unless coupled with reference adducts of known identity. ^{32}P-Postlabelling is also very labour-intensive, requires highly skilled staff and high standards of radiological safety, and does not readily lend itself to automation. International trials are underway to determine the best ways of performing ^{32}P-postlabelling and to devise a set of standardized protocols, using a set of synthetic adduct standards.[268]

Detecting chromosomal aberrations in peripheral lymphocytes has been the most widely used method for biomonitoring for markers of early biological effect or response. As with ^{32}P-postlabelling, the damage that is detected using cytogenetic methods represents a collective footprint of exposure, and its detection does not require prior knowledge of the agents that caused the damage. With the advent of FISH and chromosome painting, the detection of chromosomal aberrations has gained a new lease of life.[179] Chromosome-specific repetitive probes enable the detection of aneuploidy and chromosome breakage in interphase cells. This allows increases in sample sizes and speeds up cytogenetic analyses. Techniques such as flow cytometry and image analysis could speed things up even more. Moreover, cytogenetic information can be obtained rapidly from cells, such as sperm and epithelial cells, which have previously been refractory to cytogenetic analyses. Chromosome painting is a rapid and efficient method for detecting and quantifying structural chromosomal aberrations in metaphase preparations. Of particular interest are stable translocations, which can be detected many years after their formation. Translocations are easily detected by chromosome painting and they may provide a sensitive biodosimeter to detect and quantify chronic occupational exposure to clastogenic agents.[179,269] Several examples of the use of FISH in biomonitoring for occupational exposures are given in Table 38.6.

Confounding factors

Advances of this kind cannot of themselves solve the abiding problems associated with biomonitoring studies in which the endpoints are intended to be early markers for hazard or risk of cancer. Cancer takes several decades to develop after the start of exposure, and some of the must common occupational cancers (lung, bladder and skin) also occur frequently in the general population as a result of exposures connected with lifestyle. This causes a high level of background 'noise' from which it is difficult to extract the 'signal' markers that distinguish occupational exposure from other exposures. Thus, one of the greatest obstacles to interpreting the results of biomonitoring is incomplete knowledge, in the given population, of the normal background levels of the chosen markers, and the influence of life-style habits on this background. The most serious confounder of occupational studies is the use of tobacco, especially cigarette smoking. For example, protein and DNA adducts are significantly higher in smokers than in non-smokers,[219] as is cytogenetic damage (chromosomal aberrations, sister-chromatid exchange and micronuclei),[16,270] and somatic mutations in peripheral lymphocytes[238] and erythrocytes.[242]

The possible confounding effects of diet must also be considered. For example, a study of fire-fighters showed that adduct levels in white blood cells correlated not with fire-fighting activity but with consumption of barbecued food, and the results of a study of military personnel extinguishing oil-field fires in Kuwait showed that their adduct levels were actually lower when on duty in Kuwait than when stationed at bases in Europe.[219] The principles underlying the use of these extremely sensitive methods are similar to those that govern epidemiological studies. In most cases subjects will be drawn from outbred human communities, will be genetically unique and will have created his or her own *milieu interieur*, for example, by choice of diet, whether to smoke, to consume alcohol or other drugs. Other factors, such as passive smoking, ill-health and living conditions, may also contribute to the background level of 'genotoxic noise'. Some of these factors may also explain the high inter-individual variation in signal seen in many of the biomarkers used in biomonitoring. This problem can be mitigated to some extent by using large numbers of subjects, but this increases the costs and complexity of studies, and may not be practicable where only a few workers are involved. Serial measurements in the same individuals over time is one method for overcoming the problem of small groups.

Another important factor to consider is age. There is a clear age-dependent increase in the frequency of *hprt* mutations[271] and chromosomal aberrations[270] in peripheral lymphocytes. Using chromosome painting to detect chromosomal aberrations (translocations and insertions), Tucker and co-workers[269,270,272,273] observed a curvilinear increase in aberrations with age, with a slow increase up to age 45–50, followed by a more rapid increase. Relative to the frequencies observed in cord blood, the frequencies of stable aberrations, dicentrics, and acentric fragments in adults aged 50 and over were elevated 10.6-fold, 3.3-fold, and 2.9-fold, respectively. The increase in genotoxic damage with age could result from a build-up of endogenous damage (caused, for example, by free-radicals) or by a progressive failure of DNA-repair against a fairly constant level of damage, or by a combination of both. Irrespective of the mechanism, these findings make it imperative to age-match controls and exposed groups very closely in epidemiological studies.

Are biomarkers predictive of cancer hazard and cancer risk?

The acid test of a biomarker intended to provide early warning of future cancer hazard is to show that it does indeed predict an excess risk in those groups in which it is elevated. Many of the biomarkers mentioned above and in Table 38.6 have not been available long enough to answer this question, bearing in mind that most cancers take several decades to develop from initiation to diagnosis. However, this is not the case for the detection of chromosomal aberrations in peripheral blood lymphocytes and two studies have been published in which this question has been addressed.

In a continuing prospective cohort study in Sweden, Finland, Norway and Denmark, 3182 subjects were examined between 1970 and 1988 for chromosomal aberrations, sister-chromatid exchange or micronuclei in peripheral blood lymphocytes. In order to standardize for interlaboratory variation, the results were trichotomized for each laboratory into three strata: low (1–33 percentile), medium (34–66 percentile), or high (67–100 percentile). A total of 85 cancers was diagnosed during 1970–1991. There was no significant trend in the standardized incidence ratio for frequencies of sister-chromatid exchange or micronuclei, but the data for these endpoints were too limited to allow firm conclusions. However, there was a statistically significant linear trend relating strata for chromosomal aberrations to subsequent cancer risk, with point estimates of the standardized cancer incidence ratio of 0.9, 0.7, and 2.1 for the three strata respectively. This study indicates that a modestly increased level of chromosome breakage appears to be a relevant biomarker of future cancer hazard.[274]

This finding has been corroborated in a historical cohort study of a group of 1455 subjects screened for chromosomal aberrations in peripheral blood lymphocytes over the last 20 years in Italy. Statistically significant increases in standardized mortality ratio (SMR) for all cancers were found in subjects with medium and high levels of chromosomal aberration in peripheral blood lymphocytes (SMR = 178.5 and SMR = 182.0, respectively) and in subjects with high levels of chromosomal aberrations for respiratory tract cancers (SMR = 250.8) and lymphatic and haematopoietic tissue neoplasms (SMR = 548.8). Significant trends in the SMRs were observed for these latter causes of death.[275]

Although both studies are based on relatively small numbers of cancers, they do support the hypothesis that an elevated frequency of chromosomal aberrations in a non-target tissue (peripheral blood lymphocytes) is predictive of future cancer hazard. However, this approach, as it stands, cannot specify the risk (which is a quantitative measure), or the site at which a cancer is likely to occur.

At present, there is no validated method for estimating quantitatively the risk of cancer using data obtained from biomonitoring. Such a method would be of great value in an occupational setting. Ehrenberg et al.[276] show that conventional epidemiological studies that use cancer incidence or mortality as the endpoint are about one thousand times too insensitive to detect and properly assess risk factors that do not occur in large excess in specifically exposed populations, but which are none the less unacceptable. These authors argue that this 'insensitivity gap' can be bridged by using protein and DNA adduct formation as an auxiliary tool in epidemiology and that quantitative estimates of risk could be made from such data, although, as always, much more work needs to be done.

Combining markers of exposure and early effect with markers of susceptibility

The availability of biomarkers for both exposure and early effects and markers of susceptibility (pharmacogenetic polymorphisms) has made it possible to study both types of marker in the same individual. Examples of such studies are shown in Table 38.7 and the topic has been reviewed in respect of the interaction of pharmacogenetic polymorphism, DNA adducts, smoking and diet.[277] This approach may help to define those individuals who are particularly susceptible to the genotoxic and carcinogenic effects of specific occupational exposures and may shed more light on mechanisms of occupational carcinogenesis. However, it is too early to say whether such studies will help in predicting future cancer risk. Their ethical basis will also require debate.[146–153,278]

Biomonitoring occupational exposure to antineoplastic drugs

Many of the problems connected with biomonitoring as a means for protecting against occupational cancer are exemplified by the case of the potential exposure of hospital personnel to antineoplastic drugs. Many of the drugs used in cytotoxic chemotherapy for cancer are established human carcinogens, and most of those that are not are probably carcinogenic to humans (Table 38.8). This is not surprising, since most of them are genotoxic, being designed to react with DNA or to interfere with the cell cycle.[279] Clearly there is a *prima facie* case for assuming that exposure of staff who administer such drugs to patients is a hazard and could pose a carcinogenic risk. However, answering that case by the use of biomonitoring of the type under discussion has not been wildly successful. Some of the more recent studies are listed in Table 38.6, and the topic has been recently reviewed.[280,281] The current position is probably best summed up by Baker and Connor:[281]

> There is little conclusive evidence of detrimental health effects from occupational exposure to cytotoxic drugs. Work practices have improved since the issuance of guidelines for handling these drugs, but compliance with the recommended practices is still inadequate. Of 64 reports published since 1979 on studies of workers' exposure to these drugs, 53 involved studies of changes in cellular or molecular endpoints (biological markers) and 12 described chemical analyses of drugs or their metabolites in urine (two involved both, and two reported the same study). The primary biological markers used were urine mutagenicity, sister chromatid exchange, and chromosomal aberrations; other studies involved formation of micronuclei and measurements of urinary thioethers. The studies had small sample sizes, and the methods were qualitative, non-specific, subject to many confounders, and possibly not sensitive enough to detect most occupational exposures. Since none of the currently available biological and analytical methods is sufficiently reliable or reproducible for routine monitoring of exposure in the workplace, further studies using these methods are not recommended; efforts should focus instead on widespread implementation of improved practices for handling cytotoxic drugs.

Notwithstanding this negative view of the biomonitoring efforts of a large body of investigators, it is probably true to say that the publication[282] that first reported that urinary mutagenicity resulted from occupational exposure to antineoplastic drugs drew widespread attention to the problem, and in doing so, stimulated the adoption of improved practices for handling cytotoxic drugs. A recent text[283] provides comprehensive information on practical methods for the safe administration of antineoplastic drugs.

MECHANISMS OF OCCUPATIONAL CARCINOGENS

Space does not permit a discussion of mechanisms underlying all occupational carcinogens. Instead, some examples are given that illustrate some of the problems involved in understanding how such a disparate collection of substances and exposures induce cancer.

Classical broad-spectrum genotoxic carcinogens

Of the 74 chemicals, mixtures or processes that are classified by the International Agency for Research on Cancer as proven human carcinogens, 38 are directly linked to occupational exposures (Table 38.8) Eleven more are cytotoxic anti-tumour drugs or immunosuppressants that could present an occupational hazard to medical and nursing staff. Forty one of the 54 probable human carcinogens (counting UVA, B and C as one occupational exposure) reviewed by IARC are also likely to be encountered in occupational settings, of which nine are antineoplastics or immunosuppressants. Of these 90 proven or probable human carcinogens, 71 (79%) are unequivocally genotoxic; for eight more there is limited evidence of genotoxicity (Table 38.8). Ionizing radiation is causally linked with occupational cancer and is unequivocally genotoxic.[284]

For this highly selected group of chemicals and exposures there is little doubt that genotoxicity is a reasonably accurate predictor of carcinogenicity. This is not surprising given that most industrial intermediates are selected precisely because they are reactive *per se* or are readily converted to reactive species by chemical means. Likewise, the antineoplastic drugs listed in Table 38.7 owe their cytotoxicity activity to their ability to react with DNA or interfere with its replication, transcription or translation, properties that also confer genotoxic potential.[279] Most of the agents listed in Table 38.7 react with DNA directly or following metabolic activation and induce point mutations and chromosomal anomalies. Included in this category are acrylonitrile, the alkylating agents, polycyclic aromatic hydrocarbons, mustard gas, vinyl chloride and vinyl bromide, the aromatic amines, the alkylating anti-tumour drugs and cisplatin. This list now includes benzene, which has recently been shown to induce point mutations at two different loci (in addition to other manifestations of genotoxicity) in Syrian hamster embryo cells in culture[285] and gene-duplicating (but not gene-inactivating) mutations at the glycophorin-A locus in bone marrow cells of Chinese workers exposed to high benzene levels.[244] Reviews of the mechanisms underlying benzene leukaemogenesis are available.[286,287]

It is likely that the substances mentioned above induce cancer because they are powerful broad-spectrum genotoxins capable of producing many of the somatic mutational events discussed in the preceding pages. Ruder, from the US National Institute for Occupational Safety and Health,[288] has tabulated those chemicals and exposures that the International Agency for Research on Cancer has classified as Class 1, 2A or 2B and for which

Table 38.8 *Classification of occupational carcinogens by presence or absence of genotoxic activity*

Chemical, process or exposure	Genotoxic[a]	Non-genotoxic[b]	Inconclusive or unknown[c]	IARC Monograph, volume; year[d]
Group 1: Carcinogenic to humans				
Potential industrial exposure				
4-Aminobiphenyl	+			**1** (Suppl 7) 1987
Arsenic and arsenic compounds[e]	±			**23** (Suppl 7) 1987
Asbestos	+			**14** (Suppl 7) 1987
Benzene	+			**29** (Suppl 7) 1987
Benzidine	+			**29** (Suppl 7) 1987
Beryllium and beryllium compounds[f]	±			**58**; 1993
Bis(chloromethyl) ether and chloromethyl methyl ether (technical-grade)	+			**4** (Suppl 7) 1987
Cadmium and cadmium compounds	±			**58**; 1993
Chromium[VI] compounds	+			**49**; 1990
Erionite	+		+	**42** (Suppl 7) 1987
Ethylene oxide[g]	+			**60**; 1994
Mustard gas (sulphur mustard)	+			**9** (Suppl 7) 1987
2-Naphthylamine	+			**4** (Suppl 7) 1987
Nickel compounds	+			**49**; 1990
Silica crystalline (inhaled in the form of quartz or cristobalite from occupational sources)			+	**68**; 1997
Solar radiation	+			**55**; 1992
Talc containing asbestiform fibres	+			**42** (Suppl 7) 1987
2,3,7,8-Tetrachlorodibenzo-para-dioxin[g]		+		**69**; 1997
Vinyl chloride	+			**19** (Suppl 7) 1987
Mixtures				
Coal tar pitches	+			**35** (Suppl 7) 1987
Coal tars	+			**35** (Suppl 7) 1987
Mineral oils, untreated and mildly treated	+			**33** (Suppl 7) 1987
Shale-oils	+			**35** (Suppl 7) 1987
Soots	+			**35** (Suppl 7) 1987
Wood dust	+[h]			**62**; 1995
Exposure circumstances				
Aluminium production	+			**34** (Suppl 7) 1987
Auramine, manufacture of	+			(Suppl 7) 1987
Boot and shoe manufacture and repair			+	**25** (Suppl 7) 1987
Coal gasification			+	**34** (Suppl 7) 1987
Coke production	+			**34** (Suppl 7) 1987
Furniture and cabinet making	+			**25** (Suppl 7) 1987
Haematite mining (underground) with exposure to radon	+			**1** (Suppl 7) 1987
Iron and steel founding	±			**34** (Suppl 7) 1987
Isopropanol manufacture (strong-acid process)			+	(Suppl 7) 1987
Magenta, manufacture of	±			**57**; 1993
Painter (occupational exposure as a)			+	**47**; 1989
Rubber industry	+			**28** (Suppl 7) 1987
Strong-inorganic-acid mists containing sulphuric acid (occupational exposure to)	+			**54**; 1992
Potential occupational exposure in nursing and medicine				
Azathioprine	+			**26** (Suppl 7) 1987
N,N-Bis(2-chloroethyl)-2-naphthylamine (Chlornaphazine)	+			**4** (Suppl 7) 1987
1,4-Butanediol dimethanesulphonate (Busulphan; Myleran)	+			**4** (Suppl 7) 1987
Chlorambucil	+			**26** (Suppl 7) 1987
1-(2-Chloroethyl)-3-(4-methylcyclohexyl)-1-nitrosourea (Methyl-CCNU; Semustine)	+			(Suppl 7) 1987
Cyclosporin	±			**50**; 1990
Cyclophosphamide	+			**26** (Suppl 7) 1987
Melphalan	+			**9** (Suppl 7) 1987
MOPP and other combined chemotherapy including alkylating agents	+			(Suppl 7) 1987
Thiotepa	+			**50**; 1990
Treosulfan	+			**26** (Suppl 7) 1987

Table 38.8 – cont.

Chemical, process or exposure	Genotoxic[a]	Non-genotoxic[b]	Inconclusive or unknown[c]	IARC Monograph, volume; year[d]
Group 2A: Probably carcinogenic to humans				
Acrylamide[i]	+			**60**; 1994
Acrylonitrile	+			**19** (Suppl 7) 1987
Benz[a]anthracene[i]	+			**32** (Suppl 7) 1987
Benzidine-based dyes[i]	+			(Suppl 7) 1987
Benzo[a]pyrene[i]	+			**32** (Suppl 7) 1987
1,3-Butadiene	+			**54**; 1992
Captafol[i]	+			**53**; 1991
para-Chloro-ortho-toluidine and its strong acid salts[i]	+			**48**; 1990
Dibenz[a,h]anthracene[i]	+			**32** (Suppl 7) 1987
Diethyl sulphate	+			**54**; 1992
Dimethylcarbamoyl chloride[i]	+			**12** (Suppl 7) 1987
Dimethyl sulphate[i]	+			**4** (Suppl 7) 1987
Epichlorohydrin[i]	+			**11** (Suppl 7) 1987
Ethylene dibromide[i]	+			**15** (Suppl 7) 1987
N-Ethyl-N-nitrosourea[i]	+			**17** (Suppl 7) 1987
Formaldehyde	+			**62**; 1995
4,4′-Methylene bis(2-chloroaniline) (MbOCA)[i]	+			**57**; 1993
Styrene-7,8-oxide[i]	+			**60**; 1994
Tetrachloroethylene			+	**63**; 1995
Trichloroethylene	+			**63**; 1995
1,2,3-Trichloropropane	+			**63**; 1995
Tris(2,3-dibromopropyl)phosphate[i]	+			**20** (Suppl 7) 1987
Ultraviolet radiation A, B, C[i]	+			
Vinyl bromide[i]	±			**39** (Suppl 7) 1987
Vinyl fluoride			+	**63**; 1995
Mixtures				
Creosotes	+			**35** (Suppl 7) 1987
Diesel engine exhaust	+			**46**; 1989
Non-arsenical insecticides (occupational exposures in spraying and application of)			+	**53**; 1991
Polychlorinated biphenyls		+		**18** (Suppl 7) 1987
Exposure circumstances				
Art glass, glass containers and pressed ware, (manufacture of)			+	**58**; 1993
Hairdresser or barber (occupational exposure as)	+[j]			**57**; 1993
Petroleum refining (occupational exposures in)	+			**45**; 1989
Potential occupational exposure in nursing and medicine				
Adriamycin[i]	+			**10** (Suppl 7) 1987
Azacytidine[i]	+			**50**; 1990
Bischloroethyl nitrosourea (BCNU)	+			**26** (Suppl 7) 1987
Chloramphenicol[i]	±			**50**; 1990
1-(2-Chloroethyl)-3-cyclohexyl-1-nitrosourea (CCNU)[i]	+			**26** (Suppl 7) 1987
Chlorozotocin[i]	+			**50**; 1990
Cisplatin[i]	+			**26** (Suppl 7) 1987
Nitrogen mustard	+			**9** (Suppl 7) 1987
Procarbazine hydrochloride[i]	+			**26** (Suppl 7) 1987

[a] + Solid evidence from *in vitro* and *in vivo* short-term tests and/or studies conducted in humans; ± a mixture of positive and negative data.

[b] + Substance is devoid of genotoxic activity as judged by absence of activity in a range of assays.

[c] + Lack of reliable data.

[d] Classifications from IARC Monographs on the Evaluation of Carcinogenic Risks to Humans, International Agency for Research on Cancer, Lyon. (See *An Updating of IARC Monographs Vols 1–42* in Suppl.7, 1987.)

[e] This evaluation applies to the group of compounds as a whole and not necessarily to all individual compounds within the group.

[f] Evaluated as a group.

[g] Overall evaluation upgraded from 2A to 1 with supporting evidence from other data relevant to the evaluation of carcinogenicity and its mechanisms.

[h] Organic extracts of beech.

[i] Overall evaluation upgraded from 2B to 2A with supporting evidence from other data relevant to the evaluation of carcinogenicity and its mechanisms.

[j] Many hair dyes are genotoxic.

there is any evidence of genotoxicity. For each chemical or exposure he has estimated the numbers of workers at risk of exposure in the USA. He concluded that:

Millions of workers in the United States alone are potentially exposed to chemicals already evaluated by IARC as being carcinogenic in humans, and millions more to probable and possible carcinogens. With thousands of unevaluated chemicals already in use, and with newly synthesized chemicals being put into commercial production at the rate of thousands yearly, clearly there is an urgent need for rapid evaluation of the risk of mutagenicity and carcinogenicity. There also is a need for additional epidemiologic studies focusing on chemicals currently classified by IARC in groups 2A and 2B, for which IARC has judged the epidemiologic evidence to date as insufficient or inconsistent and to which large numbers of workers are currently exposed.

Carcinogenic metals: chromate and nickel

Reviews of the genotoxicity of carcinogenic metals[289] and the possible role of oxidative damage in metal-induced carcinogenesis[290] are available. Of the four metals classified by the International Agency for Research on Cancer to be causally related to human cancer (Table 38.8), chromate and nickel have been studied extensively and are discussed in more detail below. Less is known about cadmium and arsenic.[289,290]

CHROMIUM (see Chapter 7)

Hexavalent chromium – which causes lung and sinonasal cancer in people engaged in chromate production, chromate pigment production and chromium plating – falls into the category of powerful broad-spectrum genotoxins. Various Cr[VI] compounds induce a variety of genotoxic effects, including DNA damage, point mutation, sister-chromatid exchange, chromosomal aberrations, aneuploidy, germline mutations, in a number of targets, including bacteria, fungi, insects and mammalian cells, in assays conducted *in vitro* and *in vivo*.[291]

It is generally accepted that Cr[VI] compounds, which, unlike Cr[III], readily cross cell membranes, are reduced intracellularly to Cr[III]. The process of reduction and the intracellular reactivity of reduced chromium species to cellular macromolecules, including DNA, are thought to be critical events in the mechanism of chromate genotoxicity and carcinogenicity.[292–299] Production of oxygen free-radicals is also thought to play a role in the genotoxicity of chromate.[293,300,301] The carcinogenicity of chromate in humans appears to be organotropic, being restricted to the lung and sinonasal cavity – sites close to the initial portal of entry. This suggests that there are mechanisms that limit its bioavailability to more distant sites. De Flora *et al.*[302] suggest that

sequestration of Cr[VI] by its extracellular reduction to Cr[III] plays a major role in its organotropy and have provided evidence for this by measuring the Cr[VI] reducing capacity of several human body fluids and tissues. They found that whole blood and red blood cells possess potent sequestering activity, and concluded that this explains why chromate is not a systemic toxicant, except at very high doses, and also explains why it is not carcinogenic at sites distant from its portal of entry. They also concluded that reduction by fluids in the digestive tract, (e.g. saliva) and gastric juice, and sequestration by intestinal bacteria in faeces, account for the poor intestinal absorption of Cr[VI]. The Cr[VI] that does escape reduction in the digestive tract will be detoxified in the blood of the portal vein system and then in the liver, which itself has potent reducing capacity.

These processes explain the low oral toxicity of Cr[VI] and its lack of carcinogenicity when introduced by the oral route or is swallowed following reflux from the respiratory tract. Poor oral toxicity has been supported by a study in which Cr[VI] absorption, distribution, and excretion was determined following oral exposure of five adult male volunteers to 5 and 10 mg Cr[VI]/litre (as potassium chromate) in drinking water administered as a single bolus dose or over 3 days, at 6-hour intervals. The results suggest that virtually all (>99.7%) of the ingested Cr[VI] was reduced to Cr[III] before entering the blood-stream.[303]

NICKEL (see Chapter 7)

Occupational exposure to nickel sulphate, and to combinations of nickel sulphides and oxides in the nickel refining industry, is causally related to lung and nasal cancer. Metallic nickel, nickel monoxides, hydroxides and crystalline nickel sulphides cause cancer in experimental animals.[304] The mechanism for nickel carcinogenesis remains an enigma, not least because of the variety of nickel compounds encountered in the workplace. There is no doubt, however, that Ni[II] compounds, usually at relatively high doses, are genotoxic, inducing DNA strand breaks and chromosomal aberrations in a variety of *in vitro* and *in vivo* assays.[289,304,305] There is considerable evidence, from *in vitro* studies[301] and *in vivo* studies[306,307] that nickel compounds owe their genotoxicity to the generation of oxygen free-radicals.

The problems of understanding nickel carcinogenicity have been addressed in a review by Oller *et al.*[308] in which they have combined relevant human, animal and *in vitro* data into a general model that may help to explain the different carcinogenic potentials of various nickel compounds. They identify two main components that could contribute to the development of lung cancer by exposure to certain nickel compounds. The first component comprises the heritable changes (genetic or epigenetic) caused by direct or indirect actions of nickel compounds. The second component is suggested to be the promotion of cell proliferation by certain nickel compounds. The authors emphasize the importance of recognizing the individuality of different nickel species in reaching regulatory decisions and the fact that different risk assessment considerations may apply for compounds that appear to produce immortality and cancer by genetic/epigenetic mechanisms (like nickel subsulphide), compounds that may present a threshold for the induction of tumours in rats (like high-temperature nickel oxide), or compounds that may only have an enhancing effect on carcinogenicity (like nickel sulphate).

Asbestos and man-made mineral fibres
(see Chapter 35)

Mechanisms whereby asbestos and man-made mineral fibres exert their carcinogenic effects have been subject to extensive review.[309] Asbestos is an example of a solid-state carcinogen (producing mesothelioma and lung cancer), as are man-made mineral (glasswool and ceramic) fibres, which induce cancer in animals and are possible human carcinogens.[310] The major determinants of the carcinogenic potential of mineral fibres are biological durability and persistence, length and diameter, and dose to the target organ.[310] Asbestos is a complete carcinogen – application of asbestos alone is sufficient to induce cancer.

How asbestos and other mineral fibres exert their carcinogenic effects is, at present, poorly understood. Based on evidence from studies of the physicochemical properties of such fibres, and biological and molecular studies of their effects, Kane[310] has put forward five hypotheses to explain the mechanisms underlying mineral-fibre carcinogenesis.

1 Fibres generate free radicals that damage DNA.
2 Fibres interfere physically with mitosis.
3 Fibres stimulate the proliferation of target cells.
4 Fibres provoke a chronic inflammatory reaction leading to the prolonged release of reactive oxygen/initrogen species, cytokines and growth factors in the lung.
5 Fibres act as co-carcinogens or carriers of chemical carcinogens to the target tissue.

Although there is evidence to support these various hypotheses, major gaps in knowledge still remain, especially with regard to studies in laboratory animals *in vivo* and in humans. In a Consensus Report[311] that considered the evidence, it was concluded that 'the available evidence in favour of or against any of the mechanisms leading to the development of lung cancer and mesothelioma in either animals or humans is evaluated as weak.'

ACKNOWLEDGEMENT

S Venitt has been funded by the Cancer Research Campaign and the Medical Research Council of the UK.

REFERENCES

1 Searle CE, Teale OJ. Occupational carcinogens. In: Cooper CS, Grover PL eds. *Chemical Carcinogenesis and Mutagenesis I. Handbook of Experimental Pharmacology* Vol 94/I. Berlin: Springer Verlag, 1990: 103–51.
2 Higginson J, Muir CM, Muñoz N (eds). *Human Cancer: Epidemiology and Environmental Causes*. Cambridge: Cambridge University Press, 1992: 577 pp.
3 Barrett JC. Mechanisms of multistep carcinogenesis and carcinogen risk assessment. *Environ Hlth Perspect* 1993; **100**:9–20.
4 Barrett JC. Role of mutagenesis and mitogenesis in carcinogenesis. In: Phillips DH, Venitt S eds. *Environmental Mutagenesis*. Oxford: Bios Scientific Publishers, 1995: 21–32.
5 Lawley PD. Basic concepts of carcinogenesis. In: Cohen RD, Lewis B, Alberti KGMM, Denman AM eds. *The Metabolic and Molecular Basis of Acquired Disease* Vol 1. London: Baillière Tindall, 1990: 44–73.
6 Lawley PD. Historical origins of current concepts of carcinogenesis. *Adv Cancer Res* 1994; **65**:17–111.
7 Foulds L. *Neoplastic Development* Vol. 1. London: Academic Press, 1969: 439 pp.
8 Ashby J, Morrod RS. Detection of human carcinogens. *Nature* 1991; **352**:185–6.
9 Ashby J. Determination of the genotoxic status of a chemical. *Mutat Res* 1991; **248**:221–31.
10 Hildebrand B, Grasso P, Ashby J *et al*. Validity of considering that early changes may act as indicators for non-genotoxic carcinogenesis. *Mutat Res* 1991; **248**:217–20.
11 Murray AW, Edwards AM, Hii CST. Tumour promotion: biology and molecular mechanisms. In: Cooper CS, Grover PL eds. *Chemical Carcinogenesis and Mutagenesis II. Handbook of Experimental Pharmacology* Vol 94/II. Berlin: Springer Verlag, 1990: 135–57.
12 Bishop MJ, Weinberg RA (eds). *Scientific American Molecular Oncology*. New York: Scientific American, Inc., 1996; 255 pp.
13 Pitot HC. Mechanisms of chemical carcinogenesis: theoretical and experimental bases. In: Cooper CS, Grover PL eds. *Chemical Carcinogenesis and Mutagenesis I. Handbook of Experimental Pharmacology* Vol 94/I. Berlin: Springer-Verlag, 1990: 3–29.
14 Dong Z, Jeffrey AM. Mechanisms of organ specificity in chemical carcinogenesis. *Cancer Invest* 1990; **8**: 523–33.
15 Garner RC, Martin CN, Clayson DB. Carcinogenic aromatic amines and related compounds. In: Searle CE ed. *Chemical Carcinogens* 2nd edn, Vol 1. ACS Monograph 182. Washington DC: American Chemical Society, 1984: 175–276.
16 International Agency for Research on Cancer. Monographs on the evaluation of carcinogenic risks to humans: 38. *Tobacco Smoking*. Lyon: IARC, 1986: 298–303.

17 Cavanee WK, White RL. The genetic basis of cancer. *Scient Amer* 1995 March: 50–7.

18 Yarnold JR, Stratton MR, McMillan TJ (eds). *Molecular Biology for Oncologists* 2nd edn. London: Chapman and Hall, 1996: 353 pp.

19 Hesketh R. *The Oncogene and Tumour Suppressor Gene Factsbook* 2nd edn. San Diego: Academic Press, 1997: 549.

20 Kinzler KW, Vogelstein B. Lessons from hereditary colorectal cancer. *Cell* 1996; **87**:159–70.

21 Venitt S. Genomic instability and cancer. In: Yarnold JR, Stratton MR, McMillan TJ eds. *Molecular Biology for Oncologists* 2nd edn. London: Chapman and Hall, 1996: 134–51.

22 Venitt S. Mechanisms of spontaneous human cancers. *Environ Hlth Perspect* 1996; **3**:633–7.

23 Goodenough U. *Genetics*. Philadelphia: WB Saunders College Publishing, 1984: 645 pp.

24 Cooper DN, Krawczak M. *Human Gene Mutation*. Oxford: Bios Scientific Publishers, 1993: 402 pp.

25 Glickman BW, Kotturi G, de Boer J, Kusser W. Molecular mechanisms of mutagenesis and mutational spectra. In: Phillips DH, Venitt S eds. *Environmental Mutagenesis*. Oxford: Bios Scientific Publishers, 1995: 33–59.

26 Parry EM, Parry JM. *In vitro* cytogenetics and aneuploidy. In: Phillips DH, Venitt S eds. *Environmental Mutagenesis*. Oxford: Bios Scientific Publishers, 1995: 121–39.

27 Parry JM, Parry EM, Bourner R *et al*. The detection and evaluation of aneugenic chemicals. *Mutat Res* 1996; **353**:11–46.

28 Lindahl T. Instability and decay of the primary structure of DNA. *Nature* 1993; **362**:709–15.

29 Lawley PD. Carcinogenesis by alkylating agents. In: Searle CE ed. *Chemical Carcinogens* 2nd edn, Vol 1. ACS Monograph 182. Washington DC: American Chemical Society, 1984: 325–484.

30 Singer B, Grunberger D. *Molecular Biology of Mutagens and Carcinogens*. New York: Plenum Press, 1983: 348 pp.

31 Cooper CS, Grover PL (eds). *Chemical Carcinogenesis and Mutagenesis I and II. Handbook of Experimental Pharmacology* Vols 94/I, 94/II. Berlin: Springer Verlag, 1990: 604, 467 pp.

32 Coles B, Ketterer B. The role of glutathione and glutathione transferases in chemical carcinogenesis. *Crit Rev Biochem Mol Biol* 1990; **25**:47–70.

33 Ketterer B, Christodoulides LG. Enzymology of cytosolic glutathione S-transferases. *Adv Pharmacol* 1994; **27**:37–69.

34 Nebert DW, McKinnon RA, Puga A. Human drug-metabolizing enzyme polymorphisms: effects on risk of toxicity and cancer *DNA Cell Biol* 1996; **15**:273–80.

35 Nebert DW, McKinnon RA, Puga A. Genetic differences in drug metabolism and cancer risk. *Proc Ann Meet Am Assoc Cancer Res* 1995; **36**:5.

36 Miller EC, Miller JA. Searches for ultimate chemical carcinogens and their reactions with cellular macromolecules. *Cancer* 1981; **47**:2327–45.

37 Osborne MR. DNA interactions of reactive intermediates derived from carcinogens. In: Searle CE ed. *Chemical Carcinogens* 2nd edn, Vol 1. ACS Monograph 182. Washington DC: American Chemical Society, 1984: 485–575.

38 Friedberg EC, Walker GC, Siede W. *DNA Repair and Mutagenesis*. Washington DC: ASM Press, 1995: 698 pp.

39 Bigger CA, Flickinger DJ, St. John J, Harvey RG, Dipple A. Preferential mutagenesis at G.C base pairs by the *anti* 3,4-dihydrodiol 1,2-epoxide of 7-methylbenz[a]anthracene. *Mol Carcinog* 1991; **4**:176–9.

40 Zeilmaker MJ, Horsfall MJ, van Helten JB, Glickman BW, Mohn GR. Mutational specificities of environmental carcinogens in the *lacl* gene of *Escherichia coli* H. V: DNA sequence analysis of mutations in bacteria recovered from the liver of Swiss mice exposed to 1,2-dimethylhydrazine, azoxymethane, and methylazoxymethanolacetate. *Mol Carcinog* 1991; **4**:180–8.

41 Denissenko MF, Pao A, Tang MS, Pfeifer GP. Preferential formation of benzo[a]pyrene adducts at lung cancer mutational hotspots in P53. *Science* 1996; **274**:430–2.

42 Denissenko MF, Chen JX, Tang MS, Pfeifer GP. Cytosine methylation determines hot spots of DNA damage in the human P53 gene. *Proc Natl Acad Sci USA* 1997; **94**:3893–8.

43 Vuillaume M. Reduced oxygen species, mutation, induction and cancer initiation. *Mutat Res* 1987; **186**:43–72.

44 Ross WE, Sullivan DM, Chow K-C. Altered function of DNA topoisomerases as a basis for antineoplastic drug action. In: De Vita VT, Hellman S, Rosenberg SA eds. *Important Advances in Oncology*. Philadelphia: JB Lippincott, 1988: 65–81.

45 Cheng KC, Loeb LA. Genomic instability and tumor progression: mechanistic considerations. *Adv Cancer Res* 1993; **60**:121–56.

46 Digweed M. Human genetic instability syndromes: single gene defects with increased risk of cancer. *Toxicol Lett* 1993; **67**:259–81.

47 Harnden DG. Inherited susceptibility to mutation. In: Phillips DH, Venitt S eds. *Environmental Mutagenesis*. Oxford: Bios Scientific Publishers, 1995: 61–81.

48 Li FP. Hereditary cancer susceptibility. *Cancer* 1996; **78**:553–7.

49 Mitelman F, Heim S. Chromosome abnormalities in cancer. *Cancer Detect Prev* 1990; **14**:527–37.

50 Mitelman F, Mertens F, Johansson B. A breakpoint map of recurrent chromosomal rearrangements in human neoplasia. *Nature Genet* 1997; **15** Spec No: 417–74.

51 Moolgavkar SH. Carcinogenesis models: an overview. *Basic Life Sci* 1991; **58**:387–96.

52 Little MP. Are two mutations sufficient to cause cancer? Some generalizations of the two-mutation model of carcinogenesis of Moolgavkar, Venzon, and Knudson, and of the multistage model of Armitage and Doll. *Biometrics* 1995; **51**:1278–91.

53 Fialkow PJ. Clonal origin of human tumors. *Biochim Biophys Acta* 1976; **458**:283–321.

54 Shibata D, Schaeffer J, Li ZH, Capella G, Perucho M. Genetic heterogeneity of the c-K-ras locus in colorectal adenomas but not in adenocarcinomas. *J Natl Cancer Inst* 1993; **85**:1058–63.

55 Tomlinson IP, Novelli MR. The mutation rate and cancer. *Proc Natl Acad Sci USA* 1996; **93**:14800–3.

56 Singer M, Berg P. *Genes and Genomes. A Changing Perspective*. California/Oxford: University Science Books/Blackwell Scientific, 1991.

57 Rhyu MS. Telomeres, telomerase, and immortality. *J Natl Cancer Inst* 1995; **87**:884–94.

58 Bishop JM, Hanafusa H. Proto-oncogenes in normal and neoplastic cells. In: Bishop JM, Weinberg RA eds. *Scientific American Molecular Oncology*. New York: Scientific American Inc, 1996: 61–83.

59 Pawson T. The biochemical mechanisms of oncogene action. In: Bishop JM, Weinberg RA eds. *Scientific American Molecular Oncology*. New York: Scientific American Inc, 1996: 85–109.

60 Reddy EP, Reynolds RK, Santos E, Barbacid M. A point mutation is responsible for the acquisition of transforming properties by the T24 human bladder carcinoma oncogene. *Nature* 1982; **300**:149–52.

61 Tabin CJ, Bradley SM, Bargmann CI *et al*. Mechanism of activation of a human oncogene. *Nature* 1982; **300**:143–9.

62 Marshall CJ. Tumor suppressor genes. *Cell* 1991; **64**:313–26.

63 Leis JF, Livingston DM. The tumour suppressor genes and their mechanisms of action. In: Bishop JM, Weinberg RA eds. *Scientific American Molecular Oncology*. New York: Scientific American Inc, 1996: 111–41.

64 Morgan SE, Kastan MB. *p53* and ATM: cell cycle, cell death, and cancer. *Adv Cancer Res* 1997; **71**:1–25.

65 Vorechovsky I, Luo L, Dyer MJ *et al*. Clustering of missense mutations in the ataxia-telangiectasia gene in a sporadic T-cell leukaemia. *Nature Genet* 1997; **17**:96–9.

66 Stilgenbauer S, Schaffner C, Litterst A *et al*. Biallelic mutations in the ATM gene in T-prolymphocytic leukemia. *Nat Med* 1997; **3**:1155–9.

67 Brugarolas J, Jacks T. Double indemnity: *p53*, BRCA and cancer. *p53* mutation partially rescues developmental arrest in *Brca1* and *Brca2* null mice, suggesting a role for familial breast cancer genes in DNA damage repair. *Nat Med* 1997; **3**:721–2.

68 Scully R, Chen J, Ochs RL *et al*. Dynamic changes of BRCA1 subnuclear location and phosphorylation state are initiated by DNA damage. *Cell* 1997; **90**:425–35.

69 Li DM, Sun H. TEP1, encoded by a candidate tumor suppressor locus, is a novel protein tyrosine phosphatase regulated by transforming growth factor beta. *Cancer Res* 1997; **57**:2124–9.

70 Nelen MR, van Staveren WC, Peeters EA *et al*. Germline mutations in the PTEN/MMAC1 gene in patients with Cowden disease. *Hum Mol Genet* 1997; **6**:1383–7.

71 Liaw D, Marsh DJ, Li J *et al*. Germline mutations of the PTEN gene in Cowden disease, an inherited breast and thyroid cancer syndrome. *Nature Genet* 1997; **16**:64–7.

72 Steck PA, Pershouse MA, Jasser SA *et al*. Identification of a candidate tumour suppressor gene, *MMAC1*, at chromosome 10q23.3 that is mutated in multiple advanced cancers. *Nature Genet* 1997; **15**:356–62.

73 Li J, Yen C, Liaw D *et al*. PTEN, a putative protein tyrosine phosphatase gene mutated in human brain, breast, and prostate cancer. *Science* 1997; **275**:1943–7.

74 Stratton MR. The *p53* gene in human cancer. In: Yarnold JR, Stratton MR, McMillan TJ eds. *Molecular Biology for Oncologists* 2nd edn. London: Chapman and Hall, 1996: 92–102.

75 Almog N, Rotter V. Involvement of p53 in cell differentiation and development. *Biochim Biophys Acta* 1997; **1333**:F1–F27.

76 Cooper CS. The role of oncogene activation in chemical carcinogenesis. In: Cooper CS, Grover PL eds. *Chemical Carcinogenesis and Mutagenesis II. Handbook of Experimental Pharmacology* Vol 94/II. Berlin: Springer Verlag, 1990: 319–52.

77 Minnick DT, Kunkel TA. DNA synthesis errors, mutators and cancer. *Cancer Surv* 1996; **28**:3–20.

78 Simpson AJ. The natural somatic mutation frequency and human carcinogenesis. *Adv Cancer Res* 1997; **71**:209–40.

79 Hollstein M, Shomer B, Greenblatt M *et al*. Somatic point mutations in the *p53* gene of human tumors and cell lines: updated compilation. *Nucleic Acids Res* 1996; **24**:141–6.

80 Greenblatt MS, Bennett WP, Hollstein M, Harris CC. Mutations in the *p53* tumor suppressor gene: clues to cancer etiology and molecular pathogenesis. *Cancer Res* 1994; **54**:4855–78.

81 Pfeifer GP, Holmquist GP. Mutagenesis in the *P53* gene. *Biochim Biophys Acta* 1997; **1333**:M1–M8.

82 Arrowsmith CH, Morin P. New insights into p53 function from structural studies. *Oncogene* 1996; **12**:1379–85.

83 Warren W, Biggs PJ, el-Baz M, Ghoneim MA, Stratton MR, Venitt S. Mutations in the *p53* gene in schistosomal bladder cancer: a study of 92 tumours from Egyptian patients and a comparison between mutational spectra from schistosomal and non-schistosomal urothelial tumours. *Carcinogenesis* 1995; **16**:1181–9.

84 Harris CC. p53 tumor suppressor gene: at the crossroads of molecular carcinogenesis, molecular epidemiology, and cancer risk assessment. *Environ Hlth Perspect* 1996; **104** (Suppl 3): 435–9.

85 Hainaut P, Soussi T, Shomer B *et al*. Database of *p53* gene somatic mutations in human tumors and cell lines: updated compilation and future prospects. *Nucleic Acids Res* 1997; **25**:151–7.

86 Bird A. The essentials of DNA methylation. *Cell* 1992; **70**:5–8.

87 Biggs PJ, Warren W, Venitt S, Stratton MR. Does a genotoxic carcinogen contribute to human breast cancer?

The value of mutational spectra in unravelling the aetiology of cancer. *Mutagenesis* 1993; **8**:275–83.

88 Tornaletti S, Pfeifer GP. Complete and tissue-independent methylation of CpG sites in the *p53* gene: implications for mutations in human cancers. *Oncogene* 1995; **10**:1493–9.

89 Cooper CS, Stratton MR. Extraction and enzymatic amplification of DNA from paraffin-embedded specimens. In: Mathew C ed. *Methods in Molecular Biology*. Vol. 9. *Protocols in Human Molecular Genetics*. Clifton, New Jersey: Humana Press, 1991: 133–40.

90 Hurst RE, Rao JY. Molecular biology in epidemiology. In: Schulte PA, Perera FP eds. *Molecular Epidemiology*. San Diego: Academic Press, 1993: 45–78.

91 Perera FP, Santella R. Carcinogenesis. In: Schulte PA, Perera FP eds. *Molecular Epidemiology*. San Diego: Academic Press, 1993: 277–300.

92 Schulte PA, Perera FP (eds). *Molecular Epidemiology*. San Diego: Academic Press, 1993

93 Schulte PA. A conceptual and historical framework for molecular epidemiology. In: Schulte PA, Perera FP eds. *Molecular Epidemiology*. San Diego: Academic Press, 1993; 3–44.

94 Perera FP. Molecular epidemiology and prevention of cancer. *Environ Hlth Perspect* 1995; **8**:233–6.

95 Perera FP. Molecular epidemiology: insights into cancer susceptibility, risk assessment, and prevention. *J Natl Cancer Inst* 1996; **88**:496–509.

96 Perera FP. Uncovering new clues to cancer risk. *Scient Amer* 1996; May: 40–6.

97 Barbin A, Froment O, Boivin S. *et al*. *p53* Gene mutation pattern in rat liver tumors induced by vinyl chloride. *Cancer Res* 1997; **57**:1695–8.

98 Harty CH, Guinee DGJ, Travis WD *et al*. *p53* Mutations and occupational exposures in a surgical series of lung cancers. *Cancer Epidemiol Biomarkers Prev* 1996; **5**:997–1003.

99 Wang X, Christiani DC, Wiencke JK *et al*. Mutations in the *p53* gene in lung cancer are associated with cigarette smoking and asbestos exposure. *Cancer Epidemiol Biomarkers Prev* 1995; **4**:543–8.

100 Henschler D, Vamvakas S, Lammert M *et al*. Increased incidence of renal cell tumors in a cohort of cardboard workers exposed to trichloroethene. *Arch Toxicol* 1995; **69**:291–9.

101 International Agency for Research on Cancer. Monographs on the evaluation of carcinogenic risks to humans: 63. *Dry Cleaning, Some Chlorinated Solvents and Other Industrial Chemicals*. Lyon: IARC, 1995: 75–158.

102 Bruning T, Weirich G, Hornauer MA, Hofler H, Brauch H. Renal cell carcinomas in trichloroethene (TRI) exposed persons are associated with somatic mutations in the von Hippel-Lindau (VHL) tumour suppressor gene. *Arch Toxicol* 1997; **71**:332–5.

103 Ellis LM, Fidler IJ. Angiogenesis and metastasis. *Eur J Cancer* 1996; **32A**:2451–60.

104 Chambers AF, Matrisian LM. Changing views of the role of

matrix metalloproteinases in metastasis. *J Natl Cancer Inst* 1997; **89**:1260–70.

105 Harris AL. Antiangiogenesis for cancer therapy. *Lancet* 1997; **349** (Suppl 2): SII13–5.

106 Bicknell R, Lewis CE, Ferrara N eds. *Tumour Angiogenesis*. Oxford: Oxford University Press, 1997: 381 pp.

107 Stratton MR. Recent advances in understanding of genetic susceptibility to breast cancer. *Hum Mol Genet* 1996; **5** Spec No: 1515–9.

108 Gayther SA, Mangion J, Russell P *et al*. Variation of risks of breast and ovarian cancer associated with different germline mutations of the *BRCA2* gene. *Nature Genet* 1997; **15**:103–5.

109 Knudson AGJ. Genetic oncodemes and antioncogenes. In: Harris CC ed. *Biochemical and Molecular Epidemiology of Cancer*. New York: Alan R Liss, 1986: 127–34.

110 Nebert DW. Role of genetics and drug metabolism in human cancer risk. *Mutat Res* 1991; **247**:267–81.

111 Smith G, Stanley LA, Sim E, Strange RC, Wolf CR. Metabolic polymorphisms and cancer susceptibility. *Cancer Surv* 1995; **25**:27–65.

112 Raunio H, Husgafvel-Pursiainen K, Anttila S, Hietanen E, Hirvonen A, Pelkonen O. Diagnosis of polymorphisms in carcinogen-activating and inactivating enzymes and cancer susceptibility – a review. *Gene* 1995; **159**:113–21.

113 Nakachi K, Imai K, Hayashi S, Kawajiri K. Polymorphisms of the CYP1A1 and glutathione S-transferase genes associated with susceptibility to lung cancer in relation to cigarette dose in a Japanese population. *Cancer Res* 1993; **53**:2994–9.

114 Xu X, Kelsey KT, Wiencke JK, Wain JC, Christiani DC. Cytochrome P450 CYP1A1 MspI polymorphism and lung cancer susceptibility. *Cancer Epidemiol Biomarkers Prev* 1996; **5**:687–92.

115 London SJ, Daly AK, Fairbrother KS *et al*. Lung cancer risk in African-Americans in relation to a race-specific CYP1A1 polymorphism. *Cancer Res* 1995; **55**:6035–7.

116 Crofts F, Cosma GN, Currie D, Taioli E, Toniolo P, Garte SJ. A novel CYP1A1 gene polymorphism in African-Americans. *Carcinogenesis* 1993; **14**:1729–31.

117 Uematsu F, Kikuchi H, Motomiya M *et al*. Association between restriction fragment length polymorphism of the human cytochrome P4501IE1 gene and susceptibility to lung cancer. *Jpn J Cancer Res* 1991; **82**:254–6.

118 Watanabe J, Yang JP, Eguchi H *et al*. An Rsa I polymorphism in the CYP2E1 gene does not affect lung cancer risk in a Japanese population. *Jpn J Cancer Res* 1995; **86**:245–8.

119 Persson I, Johansson I, Bergling H *et al*. Genetic polymorphism of cytochrome P4502E1 in a Swedish population. Relationship to incidence of lung cancer. *FEBS Lett* 1993; **319**:207–11.

120 London SJ, Daly AK, Cooper J *et al*. Lung cancer risk in relation to the CYP2E1 Rsa I genetic polymorphism among African-Americans and Caucasians in Los Angeles County. *Pharmacogenetics* 1996; **6**:151–8.

121 Hirvonen A, Husgafvel-Pursiainen K, Anttila S,

Karjalainen A, Vainio H. The human CYP2E1 gene and lung cancer: DraI and RsaI restriction fragment length polymorphisms in a Finnish study population. *Carcinogenesis* 1993; **14**:85–8.

122 El-Zein RA, Zwischenberger JB, Abdel-Rahman SZ, Sankar AB, Au WW. Polymorphism of metabolizing genes and lung cancer histology: prevalence of CYP2E1 in adenocarcinoma. *Cancer Lett* 1997; **112**:71–8.

123 Wu X, Shi H, Jiang H et al. Associations between cytochrome P4502E1 genotype, mutagen sensitivity, cigarette smoking and susceptibility to lung cancer. *Carcinogenesis* 1997; **18**:967–73.

124 Wiencke JK, Spitz MR, McMillan A, Kelsey KT. Lung cancer in Mexican-Americans and African-Americans is associated with the wild-type genotype of the NAD(P)H: quinone oxidoreductase polymorphism. *Cancer Epidemiol Biomarkers Prev* 1997; **6**:87–92.

125 Rosvold EA, McGlynn KA, Lustbader ED, Buetow KH. Identification of an NAD(P)H: quinone oxidoreductase polymorphism and its association with lung cancer and smoking. *Pharmacogenetics* 1995; **5**:199–206.

126 Rothman N, Smith MT, Hayes RB et al. Benzene poisoning, a risk factor for hematological malignancy, is associated with the NQO1 609C→T mutation and rapid fractional excretion of chlorzoxazone. *Cancer Res* 1997; **57**:2839–42.

127 Beyer RE, Segura-Aguilar J, Di Bernardo S et al. The role of DT-diaphorase in the maintenance of the reduced antioxidant form of coenzyme Q in membrane systems. *Proc Natl Acad Sci USA* 1996; **93**:2528–32.

128 Chen CL, Liu Q, Relling MV. Simultaneous characterization of glutathione S-transferase M1 and T1 polymorphisms by polymerase chain reaction in American whites and blacks. *Pharmacogenetics* 1996; **6**:187–91.

129 McWilliams JE, Sanderson BJ, Harris EL, Richert-Boe KE, Henner WD. Glutathione S-transferase M1 (GSTM1) deficiency and lung cancer risk. *Cancer Epidemiol Biomarkers Prev* 1995; **4**:589–94.

130 Brockmöller J, Cascorbi I, Kerb R, Roots I. Combined analysis of inherited polymorphisms in arylamine N-acetyltransferase 2, glutathione S-transferases M1 and T1, microsomal epoxide hydrolase, and cytochrome P450 enzymes as modulators of bladder cancer risk. *Cancer Res* 1996; **56**:3915–25.

131 Harries LW, Stubbins MJ, Forman D, Howard GC, Wolf CR. Identification of genetic polymorphisms at the glutathione S-transferase Pi locus and association with susceptibility to bladder, testicular and prostate cancer. *Carcinogenesis* 1997; **18**:641–644.

132 Ryberg D, Skaug V, Hewer A et al. Genotypes of glutathione transferase M1 and P1 and their significance for lung DNA adduct levels and cancer risk. *Carcinogenesis* 1997; **18**:1285–9.

133 Chen H, Sandler DP, Taylor JA et al. Increased risk for myelodysplastic syndromes in individuals with glutathione transferase theta 1 (GSTT1) gene defect. *Lancet* 1996; **347**:295–7.

134 Lear JT, Smith AG, Bowers B et al. Truncal tumor site is associated with high risk of multiple basal cell carcinoma and is influenced by glutathione S-transferase, GSTT1, and cytochrome P450, CYP1A1 genotypes, and their interaction. *J Invest Dermatol* 1997; **108**:519–22.

135 Pemble S, Schroeder KR, Spencer SR et al. Human glutathione S-transferase theta (GSTT1): cDNA cloning and the characterization of a genetic polymorphism. *Biochem J* 1994; **300**:271–6.

136 Okkels H, Sigsgaard T, Wolf H, Autrup H. Arylamine N-acetyltransferase 1 (NAT1) and 2 (NAT2) polymorphisms in susceptibility to bladder cancer: the influence of smoking. *Cancer Epidemiol Biomarkers Prev* 1997; **6**:225–31.

137 Ambrosone CB, Freudenheim JL, Graham S et al. Cigarette smoking, N-acetyltransferase 2 genetic polymorphisms, and breast cancer risk. *JAMA* 1996; **276**:1494–501.

138 Vineis P. Use of biomarkers in epidemiology. The example of metabolic susceptibility to cancer. *Toxicol Lett* 1995; **77**:163–8.

139 d'Errico A, Taioli E, Chen X, Vineis P. Genetic metabolic polymorphisms and the risk of cancer: a review of the literature. *Biomarkers* 1996; **1**:149–73.

140 Vineis P, McMichael A. Interplay between heterocyclic amines in cooked meat and metabolic phenotype in the etiology of colon cancer. *Cancer Causes Control* 1996; **7**:479–86.

141 Hirvonen A, Saarikoski ST, Linnainmaa K et al. Glutathione S-transferase and N-acetyltransferase genotypes and asbestos-associated pulmonary disorders. *J Natl Cancer Inst* 1996; **88**:1853–6.

142 Anwar WA, Abdel-Rahman SZ, El-Zein RA, Mostafa HM, Au WW. Genetic polymorphism of GSTM1, CYP2E1 and CYP2D6 in Egyptian bladder cancer patients. *Carcinogenesis* 1996; **17**:1923–9.

143 To-Figueras J, Gené M, Gómez-Catalán J et al. Glutathione S-transferase M1 (GSTM1) and Ti (GSTT1) polymorphisms and lung cancer risk among Northwestern Mediterraneans. *Carcinogenesis* 1997; **18**:1529–1533.

144 Kelsey KT, Spitz MR, Zuo ZF, Wiencke JK. Polymorphisms in the glutathione S-transferase class mu and theta genes interact and increase susceptibility to lung cancer in minority populations (Texas, United States). *Cancer Causes Control* 1997; **8**:554–9.

145 Hayashi S, Watanabe J, Kawajiri K. High susceptibility to lung cancer analyzed in terms of combined genotypes of P450IA1 and Mu-class glutathione S-transferase genes. *Jpn J Cancer Res* 1992; **83**:866–70.

146 Vineis P, Schulte PA. Scientific and ethical aspects of genetic screening of workers for cancer risk: the case of the N-acetyltransferase. *J Clin Epidemiol* 1995; **48**:189–97.

147 World Health Organization. Guidelines on ethical issues. In: *Medical Genetics and the Provision of Genetic Services World Health Organization, Hereditary Diseases Programme, 1995.* Geneva: WHO, 1995.

148 Van Damme K, Casteleyn L, Heseltine E *et al*. Individual susceptibility and prevention of occupational diseases: scientific and ethical issues. *J Occup Environ Med* 1995; **37**:91–9.

149 Schulte PA, Sweeney MH. Ethical considerations, confidentiality issues, rights of human subjects, and uses of monitoring data in research and regulation. *Environ Hlth Perspect* 1995; **103** (Suppl 3): 69–74.

150 Grandjean P, Sorsa M. Ethical aspects of genetic predisposition to environmentally-related disease. *Sci Total Environ* 1996; **184**:37–43.

151 Norseth T. Individual susceptibility to occupational toxicants: practical consequences for risk management. *Arch Toxicol Suppl* 1996; **18**:367–78.

152 Soskolne CL. Ethical, social, and legal issues surrounding studies of susceptible populations and individuals. *Environ Hlth Perspect* 1997; **105** (Suppl 4): 837–41.

153 Rothenberg K, Fuller B, Rothstein M *et al*. Genetic information and the workplace: legislative approaches and policy challenges. *Science* 1997; **275**:1755–7.

154 Chee M, Yang R, Hubbell E, *et al*. Accessing genetic information with high-density DNA arrays. *Science* 1996; **274**:610–4.

155 Hacia JG, Brody LC, Chee MS, Fodor SP, Colins FS. Detection of heterozygous mutations in BRCA1 using high density oligonucleotide arrays and two-colour fluorescence analysis. *Nature Genet* 1996; **14**:441–7.

156 McGall G, Labadie J, Brock P, Wallraff G, Nguyen T, Hinsberg W. Light-directed synthesis of high-density oligonucleotide arrays using semiconductor photoresists. *Proc Natl Acad Sci USA* 1996; **93**:13555–60.

157 Anonymous. To infinity . . . and beyond! *Nature Genet* 1996; **14**:367–70.

158 Marshall A, Hodgson J. DNA chips: an array of possibilities. *Nat Biotechnol* 1998; **16**:27–31.

159 Schafer AJ, Hawkins JR. DNA variation and the future of human. *Nat Biotechnol* 1998; **16**:33–9.

160 Puga A, Micka J, Chang CY, Liang HC, Nebert DW. Role of molecular biology in risk assessment. *Adv Exp Med Biol* 1996; **387**:395–404.

161 Tennant RW, Ashby J. Classification according to chemical structure, mutagenicity to *Salmonella* and level of carcinogenicity of a further 39 chemicals tested for carcinogenicity by the US National Toxicology Program. *Mutat Res* 1991; **257**:209–27.

162 Ashby J, Paton D. The influence of chemical structure on the extent and sites of carcinogenesis for 522 rodent carcinogens and 55 different human carcinogen exposures. *Mutat Res* 1993; **286**:3–74.

163 Maron DM, Ames BN. Revised methods for the *Salmonella* mutagenicity test. *Mutat Res* 1983; **113**:173–215.

164 Venitt S, Crofton-Sleigh C, Forster R. Bacterial mutation assays using reverse mutation. In: Venitt S, Parry JM eds. *Mutagenicity Testing. A Practical Approach*. Oxford: IRL Press, 1984: 45–98.

165 Gatehouse DG, Wilcox P, Forster R, Rowland IR, Callander RD. Bacterial mutation assays. In: Kirkland DJ ed. *Basic Mutagenicity Tests: UKEMS Recommended Procedures*. Cambridge: Cambridge University Press, 1990: 13–61.

166 Gatehouse D, Haworth S, Cebula T *et al*. Recommendations for the performance of bacterial mutation assays. *Mutat Res* 1994; **312**:217–33.

167 Zeiger E. Mutagenicity tests in bacteria as indicators of carcinogenic potential in mammals. In: Phillips DH, Venitt S eds. *Environmental Mutagenesis*. Oxford: Bios Scientific Publishers, 1995: 107–19.

168 Dean BJ, Danford N. Assays for the detection of chemically-induced chromosome damage in cultured mammalian cells. In: Venitt S, Parry JM eds. *Mutagenicity Testing. A Practical Approach*. Oxford: IRL Press, 1984: 187–232.

169 Scott D, Danford ND, Dean BJ, Kirkland DJ. Metaphase chromosome aberration assays *in vitro*. In: Kirkland DJ, ed. *Basic Mutagenicity Tests: UKEMS Recommended Procedures*. Cambridge: Cambridge University Press, 1990: 62–86.

170 Cole J, Arlett CF. The detection of gene mutations in cultured mammalian cells. In: Venitt S, Parry MJ eds. *Mutagenicity Testing. A Practical Approach*. Oxford: IRL Press, 1984: 233–73.

171 Clive D. Mammalian cell mutation assays. In: Phillips DH, Venitt S eds. *Environmental Mutagenesis*. Oxford: Bios Scientific Publishers, 1995: 201–18.

172 Adler I-D. Cytogenetic tests in mammals. In: Venitt S, Parry JM eds. *Mutagenicity Testing. A Practical Approach*. Oxford: IRL Press, 1984: 275–306.

173 Richold M, Ashby J, Bootman J, Chandley A, Gatehouse DG, Henderson L. *In vivo* cytogenetics assays. In: Kirkland DJ ed. *Basic Mutagenicity Tests: UKEMS Recommended Procedures*. Cambridge: Cambridge University Press, 1990: 115–41.

174 Heddle JA. *In vivo* assays for mutagenicity. In: Phillips DH, Venitt S eds. *Environmental Mutagenesis*. Oxford: Bios Scientific Publishers, 1995: 141–54.

175 Kirkland DJ (ed). *Statistical Evaluation of Mutagenicity Test Data*. Cambridge: Cambridge University Press, 1989.

176 Committee on Carcinogenicity of Chemicals in Food, Consumer Products and the Environment. *Guidelines for the Testing of Chemicals for Carcinogenicity*. Department Of Health. Report On Health and Social Subjects 42. London: Department of Health, 1991: 80 pp.

177 Committee on Mutagenicity of Chemicals in Food, Consumer Products and the Environment. *Guidelines for the Testing of Chemicals for Mutagenicity*. Department Of Health. Report On Health and Social Subjects 35. London: Department of Health, 1989: 99 pp.

178 Ashby J, Tennant RW. Definitive relationships among chemical structure, carcinogenicity and mutagenicity for 301 chemicals tested by the US NTP. *Mutat Res* 1991; **257**:229–306.

179 Eastmond DA, Rupa DS. Fluorescence *in situ* hybridization: application to environmental mutagenesis. In: Phillips DH, Venitt S eds. *Environmental*

Mutagenesis. Oxford: Bios Scientific Publishers, 1995: 261–90.

180 Crofton-Sleigh C, Doherty A, Ellard S, Parry EM, Venitt S. Micronucleus assays using cytochalasin-blocked MCL-5 cells, a proprietary human cell line expressing five human cytochromes P-450 and microsomal epoxide hydrolase. *Mutagenesis* 1993; **8**:363–72.

181 Crespi CL. Use of genetically engineered cells for genetic toxicology testing. In: Phillips DH, Venitt S eds. *Environmental Mutagenesis.* Oxford: Bios Scientific Publishers, 1995: 233–60.

182 Tice RR. The single-cell gel/Comet assay: a microgel electrophoretic technique for the detection of DNA damage and repair in individual cells. In: Phillips DH, Venitt S eds. *Environmental Mutagenesis.* Oxford: Bios Scientific Publishers, 1995: 315–39.

183 Singh NP. Microgel electrophoresis of DNA from individual cells. Principles and methodology. In: Pfeifer GP ed. *Technologies for Detection of DNA Damage and Mutations.* New York: Plenum Press, 1996: 3–24.

184 Collins AR, Dobson VL, Dusinska M, Kennedy G, Stetina R. The comet assay: what can it really tell us? *Mutat Res* 1997; **375**:183–93.

185 Forster R. Measuring genetic events in transgenic animals. In: Phillips DH, Venitt S eds. *Environmental Mutagenesis.* Oxford: Bios Scientific Publishers, 1995: 291–314.

186 Pfeifer GP (ed), *Technologies for Detection of DNA Damage and Mutations.* New York: Plenum Press, 1996: 441 pp.

187 Woutersen RA, van Garderen-Hoetmer A, Lamers CB, Scherer E. Early indicators of exocrine pancreas carcinogenesis produced by non-genotoxic agents. *Mutat Res* 1991; **248**:291–302.

188 Dietrich DR, Swenberg JA. Preneoplastic lesions in rodent kidney induced spontaneously or by non-genotoxic agents: predictive nature and comparison to lesions induced by genotoxic carcinogens. *Mutat Res* 1991; **248**:239–60.

189 Anderson RL. Early indicators of bladder carcinogenesis produced by non-genotoxic agents. *Mutat Res* 1991; **248**:261–70.

190 Grasso P, Hinton RH. Evidence for and possible mechanisms of non-genotoxic carcinogenesis in rodent liver. *Mutat Res* 1991; **248**:271–90.

191 Thomas GA, Williams ED. Evidence for and possible mechanisms of non-genotoxic carcinogenesis in the rodent thyroid. *Mutat Res* 1991; **248**:357–70.

192 Clayson DB, Iverson F, Nera EA, Lok E. Early indicators of potential neoplasia produced in the rat forestomach by non-genotoxic agents: the importance of induced cellular proliferation. *Mutat Res* 1991; **248**:321–31.

193 Neumann F. Early indicators for carcinogenesis in sex-hormone-sensitive organs. *Mutat Res* 1991; **248**:341–56.

194 Anonymous. Special Issue. Early indicators of non-genotoxic carcinogens. *Mutat Res* 1991; **248**:211–376.

195 Yamasaki H, Ashby J, Bignami M *et al.* Nongenotoxic carcinogens: development of detection methods based on mechanisms: a European project. *Mutat Res* 1996; **353**:47–63.

196 International Agency for Research on Cancer. Monographs on the evaluation of carcinogenic risks to humans: Vol 62. *Wood Dust and Formaldehyde.* Lyon: IARC, 1995: 217–362.

197 Ames BN, Gold LS, Willett WC. The causes and prevention of cancer. *Proc Natl Acad Sci USA* 1995; **92**:5258–5265.

198 Preston-Martin S, Pike MC, Ross RK, Jones PA, Henderson BE. Increased cell division as a cause of human cancer. *Cancer Res* 1990; **50**:7415–21.

199 Infante PF. Prevention versus chemophobia: a defence of rodent carcinogenicity tests. *Lancet* 1991; **337**:538–40.

200 International Agency for Research on Cancer. Consensus report. In: Vainio H, Magee P, McGregor D, McMichael AJ eds. *Mechanisms of Carcinogenesis in Risk Identification.* IARC Scientific Publications No 116. Lyon: IARC, 1992: 9–54.

201 EPA. *Proposed Guidelines for Carcinogen Risk Assessment.* Report No EPA/600/P-92003C. Washington, DC: Office of Research and Development, US Environmental Protection Agency, 1996.

202 Tennant RW, Spalding J, French JE. Evaluation of transgenic mouse bioassays for identifying carcinogens and noncarcinogens. *Mutat Res* 1996; **365**:119–27.

203 Ashby J, Paton D. Chemicals for evaluating the sensitivity and specificity of reduced/transgenic rodent cancer bioassay protocols. *Mutat Res* 1995; **331**:27–38.

204 Ashby J. Identifying potential human carcinogens – the role of genetically altered rodents. *Toxicol Pathol* 1997; **25**:241–3.

205 Toniolo P, Boffetta P, Shuker DEG, Rothman N, Hulka B, Pearce N (eds). International Agency for Research on Cancer. *Applications of Biomarkers in Cancer Epidemiology.* Scientific Publications No 142. Lyon: IARC, 1997: 318 pp.

206 Phillips DH, Venitt S (eds). *Environmental Mutagenesis.* Oxford: Bios Scientific Publishers, 1995: 403 pp.

207 Ensslin AS, Stoll Y, Pethran A, Pfaller A, Rommelt H, Fruhmann G. Biological monitoring of cyclophosphamide and ifosfamide in urine of hospital personnel occupationally exposed to cytostatic drugs. *Occup Environ Med* 1994; **51**:229–33.

208 Ensslin AS, Pethran A, Schierl R, Fruhmann G. Urinary platinum in hospital personnel occupationally exposed to platinum-containing antineoplastic drugs. *Int Arch Occup Environ Hlth* 1994; **65**:339–42.

209 Thiringer G, Granung G, Holmen A *et al.* Comparison of methods for the biomonitoring of nurses handling antitumor drugs. *Scand J Work Environ Hlth* 1991; **17**:133–8.

210 Newman MA, Valanis BG, Schoeny RS, Hee SQ. Urinary biological monitoring markers of anticancer drug exposure in oncology nurses. *Am J Publ Hlth* 1994; **84**:852–5.

211 Nielsen PS, Andreassen A, Farmer PB, Øvrebø S, Autrup H. Biomonitoring of diesel exhaust-exposed workers. DNA

and hemoglobin adducts and urinary 1-hydroxypyrene as markers of exposure. *Toxicol Lett* 1996; **86**:27–37.

212 Øvrebø S, Haugen A, Farmer PB, Anderson D. Evaluation of biomarkers in plasma, blood, and urine samples from coke oven workers: significance of exposure to polycyclic aromatic hydrocarbons. *Occup Environ Med* 1995; **52**:750–6.

213 Lagorio S, Tagesson C, Forastiere F, Iavarone I, Axelson O, Carere A. Exposure to benzene and urinary concentrations of 8-hydroxydeoxyguanosine, a biological marker of oxidative damage to DNA. *Occup Environ Med* 1994; **51**:739–43.

214 Ensslin AS, Huber R, Pethran A *et al*. Biological monitoring of hospital pharmacy personnel occupationally exposed to cytostatic drugs: urinary excretion and cytogenetics studies. *Int Arch Occup Environ Hlth* 1997; **70**:205–8.

215 Venitt S. The use of short-term tests for the detection of genotoxic activity in body fluids and excreta. *Mutat Res* 1988; **205**:331–53.

216 DeMarini DM, Brooks LR, Bhatnagar VK *et al*. Urinary mutagenicity as a biomarker in workers exposed to benzidine: correlation with urinary metabolites and urothelial DNA adducts. *Carcinogenesis* 1997; **18**: 981–8.

217 Gabbani G, Hou SM, Nardini B, Marchioro M, Lambert B, Clonfero E. GSTM1 and NAT2 genotypes and urinary mutagens in coke oven workers. *Carcinogenesis* 1996; **17**:1677–81.

218 Choi BC, Connolly JG, Zhou RH. Application of urinary mutagen testing to detect workplace hazardous exposure and bladder cancer. *Mutat Res* 1995; **341**:207–16.

219 Phillips DH, Farmer PB. Protein and DNA adducts as biomarkers of exposure to environmental mutagens. In: Phillips DH, Venitt S eds. *Environmental Mutagenesis*. Oxford: Bios Scientific Publishers, 1995: 367–95.

220 Yeowell OCK, Jin Z, Rappaport SM. Determination of albumin and hemoglobin adducts in workers exposed to styrene and styrene oxide. *Cancer Epidemiol Biomarkers Prev* 1996; **5**:205–15.

221 Kaderlik KR, Talaska G, DeBord DG, Osorio AM, Kadlubar FF. 4,4′-Methylene-bis(2-chloroaniline)-DNA adduct analysis in human exfoliated urothelial cells by ^{32}P-postlabeling. *Cancer Epidemiol Biomarkers Prev* 1993; **2**:63–9.

222 Flato S, Hemminki K, Thunberg E, Georgellis A. DNA adduct formation in the human nasal mucosa as a biomarker of exposure to environmental mutagens and carcinogens. *Environ Hlth Perspect* 1996; **104** (Suppl 3): 471–473.

223 Øvrebø S, Haugen A, Phillips DH, Hewer A. Detection of polycyclic aromatic hydrocarbon-DNA adducts in white blood cells from coke oven workers: correlation with job categories. *Cancer Res* 1992; **52**:1510–4.

224 Rothman N, Bhatnagar VK, Hayes RB *et al*. The impact of interindividual variation in NAT2 activity on benzidine urinary metabolites and urothelial DNA adducts in

exposed workers. *Proc Natl Acad Sci USA* 1996; **93**:5084–9.

225 Peluso M, Merlo F, Munnia A, Bolognesi C, Puntoni R, Parodi S. ^{32}P-Postlabeling detection of DNA adducts in peripheral white blood cells of greenhouse floriculturists from Western Liguria, Italy. *Cancer Epidemiol Biomarkers Prev* 1996; **5**:361–9.

226 Toniolo P, Zhitkovich A, Costa M. Development and utilization of a new simple assay for DNA-protein crosslinks as a biomarker of exposure to welding fumes. *Int Arch Occup Environ Hlth* 1993; **65**:S87–9.

227 Costa M, Zhitkovich A, Toniolo P, Taioli E, Popov T, Lukanova A. Monitoring human lymphocytic DNA-protein cross-links as biomarkers of biologically active doses of chromate. *Environ Hlth Perspect* 1996; **104** (Suppl 5): 917–9.

228 Shaham J, Bomstein Y, Meltzer A, Kaufman Z, Palma E, Ribak J. DNA-protein crosslinks, a biomarker of exposure to formaldehyde – *in vitro* and *in vivo* studies. *Carcinogenesis* 1996; **17**:121–5.

229 Casanova M, Heck HD, Janszen D. Comments on 'DNA-protein crosslinks, a biomarker of exposure to formaldehyde – *in vitro* and *in vivo* studies' by Shaham *et al*. *Carcinogenesis* 1996; **17**:2097–101.

230 Popp W, Vahrenholz C, Schell C *et al*. DNA single strand breakage, DNA adducts, and sister chromatid exchange in lymphocytes and phenanthrene and pyrene metabolites in urine of coke oven workers. *Occup Environ Med* 1997; **54**:176–83.

231 Fuchs J, Hengstler JG, Hummrich F, Oesch F. Transient increase in DNA strand breaks in car refinishing spray painters. *Scand J Work Environ Hlth* 1996; **22**:438–43.

232 Fuchs J, Hengstler JG, Jung D, Hiltl G, Konietzko J, Oesch F. DNA damage in nurses handling antineoplastic agents. *Mutat Res* 1995; **342**:17–23.

233 Walles SA, Edling C, Anundi H, Johanson G. Exposure dependent increase in DNA single strand breaks in leucocytes from workers exposed to low concentrations of styrene. *Br J Ind Med* 1993; **50**:570–4.

234 Andreoli C, Leopardi P, Crebelli R. Detection of DNA damage in human lymphocytes by alkaline single cell gel electrophoresis after exposure to benzene or benzene metabolites. *Mutat Res* 1997; **377**:95–104.

235 Tates AD, van Dam FJ, de Zwart FA *et al*. Biological effect monitoring in industrial workers from the Czech Republic exposed to low levels of butadiene. *Toxicology* 1996; **113**:91–9.

236 Moretti M, Villarini M, Scassellati-Sforzolini G *et al*. Biological monitoring of genotoxic hazard in workers of the rubber industry. *Environ Hlth Perspect* 1996; **104** (Suppl 3): 543–5.

237 Vodicka P, Bastlova T, Vodickova L, Peterkova K, Lambert B, Hemminki K. Biomarkers of styrene exposure in lamination workers: levels of O6-guanine DNA adducts, DNA strand breaks and mutant frequencies in the hypoxanthine guanine phosphoribosyltransferase gene in T-lymphocytes. *Carcinogenesis* 1995; **16**:1473–81.

238 Albertini RJ, O'Neill JP. Human monitoring for somatic mutations in humans. In: Phillips DH, Venitt S eds. *Environmental Mutagenesis*. Oxford: Bios Scientific Publishers, 1995: 341–66.

239 Olsen LS, Nielsen LR, Nexo BA, Wassermann K. Somatic mutation detection in human biomonitoring. *Pharmacol Toxicol* 1996; **78**:364–73.

240 Bigbee WL, Jensen RH, Veidebaum T *et al*. Biodosimetry of Chernobyl clean-up workers from Estonia and Latvia using the glycophorin A *in vivo* somatic cell mutation assay. *Radiat Res* 1997; **147**:215–24.

241 Shanahan EM, Peterson D, Roxby D, Quintana J, Morely AA, Woodward A. Mutation rates at the glycophorin A and HPRT loci in uranium miners exposed to radon progeny. *Occup Environ Med* 1996; **53**:439–44.

242 Bigbee WL, Grant SG, Langlois RG, *et al*. Glycophorin A somatic cell mutation frequencies in Finnish reinforced plastics workers exposed to styrene. *Cancer Epidemiol Biomarkers Prev* 1996; **5**:801–10.

243 Hayes RB, Xi L, Bechtold WE *et al*. hprt mutation frequency among workers exposed to 1,3-butadiene in China. *Toxicology* 1996; **113**:100–5.

244 Rothman N, Haas R, Hayes RB *et al*. Benzene induces gene-duplicating but not gene-inactivating mutations at the glycophorin A locus in exposed humans. *Proc Natl Acad Sci USA* 1995; **92**:4069–73.

245 Hou SM, Lambert B, Hemminki K. Relationship between hprt mutant frequency, aromatic DNA adducts and genotypes for GSTM1 and NAT2 in bus maintenance workers. *Carcinogenesis* 1995; **16**:1913–7.

246 Tates AD, Grummt T, van Dam FJ *et al*. Measurement of frequencies of HPRT mutants, chromosomal aberrations, micronuclei, sister-chromatid exchanges and cells with high frequencies of SCEs in styrene/dichloromethane-exposed workers. *Mutat Res* 1994; **313**:249–62.

247 Dubeau H, Zazi W, Baron C, Messing K. Effects of lymphocyte subpopulations on the clonal assay of HPRT mutants: occupational exposure to cytostatic drugs. *Mutat Res* 1994; **321**:147–57.

248 Perera FP, Tang AL, JP ON *et al*. HPRT and glycophorin A mutations in foundry workers: Relationship to PAH exposure and to PAH-DNA adducts. *Carcinogenesis* 1993; **14**:969–973.

249 Tates AD, Grummt T, Tornqvist M *et al*. Biological and chemical monitoring of occupational exposure to ethylene oxide. *Mutat Res* 1991; **250**:483–97.

250 Pitarque M, Carbonell E, Lapeña N *et al*. SCE analysis in peripheral blood lymphocytes of a group of filling station attendants. *Mutat Res* 1997; **390**:153–9.

251 Surrallés J, Autio K, Nylund L *et al*. Molecular cytogenetic analysis of buccal cells and lymphocytes from benzene-exposed workers. *Carcinogenesis* 1997; **18**:817–23.

252 Lemasters GK, Livingston GK, Lockey JE *et al*. Genotoxic changes after low-level solvent and fuel exposure on aircraft maintenance personnel. *Mutagenesis* 1997; **12**:237–43.

253 Pitarque M, Carbonell E, Lapeña N *et al*. No increase in micronuclei frequency in cultured blood lymphocytes from a group of filling station attendants. *Mutat Res* 1996; **367**:161–7.

254 Zhang L, Rothman N, Wang Y *et al*. Interphase cytogenetics of workers exposed to benzene. *Environ Hlth Perspect* 1996; **104** (Suppl 6): 1325–9.

255 Yu MC, Skipper PL, Taghizadeh K *et al*. Acetylator phenotype, aminobiphenyl-hemoglobin adduct levels, and bladder cancer risk in white, black, and Asian men in Los Angeles, California. *J Natl Cancer Inst* 1994; **86**:712–6.

256 Yu MC, Ross RK, Chan KK *et al*. Glutathione S-transferase M1 genotype affects aminobiphenyl-hemoglobin adduct levels in white, black and Asian smokers and nonsmokers. *Cancer Epidemiol Biomarkers Prev* 1995; **4**:861–4.

257 Kato S, Bowman ED, Harrington AM, Blomeke B, Shields PG. Human lung carcinogen-DNA adduct levels mediated by genetic polymorphisms *in vivo*. *J Natl Cancer Inst* 1995; **87**:902–7.

258 Rothman N, Shields PG, Poirier MC, Harrington AM, Ford DP, Strickland PT. The impact of glutathione S-transferase M1 and cytochrome P450 1A1 genotypes on white-blood-cell polycyclic aromatic hydrocarbon-DNA adduct levels in humans. *Mol Carcinog* 1995; **14**:63–8.

259 Wiencke JK, Pemble S, Ketterer B, Kelsey KT. Gene deletion of glutathione S-transferase theta: correlation with induced genetic damage and potential role in endogenous mutagenesis. *Cancer Epidemiol Biomarkers Prev* 1995; **4**:253–9.

260 Norppa H, Hirvonen A, Järventaus H, *et al*. Role of GSTT1 and GSTM1 genotypes in determining individual sensitivity to sister chromatid exchange induction by diepoxybutane in cultured human lymphocytes. *Carcinogenesis* 1995; **16**:1261–4.

261 Landi S, Ponzanelli I, Hirvonen A, Norppa H, Barale R. Repeated analysis of sister chromatid exchange induction by diepoxybutane in cultured human lymphocytes: effect of glutathione S-transferase T1 and M1 genotype. *Mutat Res* 1996; **351**:79–85.

262 Scarpato R, Migliore L, Hirvonen A, Falck G, Norppa H. Cytogenetic monitoring of occupational exposure to pesticides: characterization of GSTM1, GSTT1, and NAT2 genotypes. *Environ Mol Mutagen* 1996; **27**:263–9.

263 Rothman N, Hayes RB, Zenser TV *et al*. The glutathione S-transferase M1 (*GSTM1*) null genotype and benzidine-associated bladder cancer, urine mutagenicity, and exfoliated urothelial cell DNA adducts. *Cancer Epidemiol Biomarkers Prev* 1996; **5**:979–83.

264 Hemminki K, Dickey C, Karlsson S *et al*. Aromatic DNA adducts in foundry workers in relation to exposure, life style and CYP1A1 and glutathione transferase M1 genotype. *Carcinogenesis* 1997; **18**:345–50.

265 Scarpato R, Hirvonen A, Migliore L, Falck G, Norppa H. Influence of *GSTM1* and *GSTT1* polymorphisms on the frequency of chromosome aberrations in lymphocytes of smokers and pesticide-exposed greenhouse workers. *Mutat Res* 1997; **389**:227–35.

266 Venitt S. The use of short-term tests for the detection of genotoxic activity in body fluids and excreta. *Mutat Res* 1988; **205**:331–53.

267 Gupta RC. ^{32}P-postlabelling for the detection of DNA adducts. In: Pfeifer GP ed. *Technologies for Detection of DNA Damage and Mutations*. New York: Plenum Press, 1996: 45–61.

268 Phillips DH. Detection of DNA modifications by the ^{32}P-postlabelling assay. *Mutat Res* 1997; **378**:1–12.

269 Tucker JD, Preston RJ. Chromosome aberrations, micronuclei, aneuploidy, sister chromatid exchanges, and cancer risk assessment. *Mutat Res* 1996; **365**:147–59.

270 Tucker JD, Moore DH 2nd. The importance of age and smoking in evaluating adverse cytogenetic effects of exposure to environmental agents. *Environ Hlth Perspect* 1996; **104**(Suppl 3): 489–92.

271 Cole J, Skopek TR. International Commission for Protection Against Environmental Mutagens and Carcinogens. Working paper no. 3. Somatic mutant frequency, mutation rates and mutational spectra in the human population *in vivo*. *Mutat Res* 1994; **304**:33–105.

272 Tucker JD, Lee DA, Ramsey MJ, Briner J, Olsen L, Moore DH. On the frequency of chromosome exchanges in a control population measured by chromosome painting. *Mutat Res* 1994; **313**:193–202.

273 Ramsey MJ, Moore DH, Briner JF *et al*. The effects of age and lifestyle factors on the accumulation of cytogenetic damage as measured by chromosome painting. *Mutat Res* 1995; **338**:95–106.

274 Hagmar L, Brøgger A, Hansteen IL *et al*. Cancer risk in humans predicted by increased levels of chromosomal aberrations in lymphocytes: Nordic study group on the health risk of chromosome damage. *Cancer Res* 1994; **54**:2919–22.

275 Bonassi S, Abbondandolo A, Camurri L *et al*. Are chromosome aberrations in circulating lymphocytes predictive of future cancer onset in humans? Preliminary results of an Italian cohort study. *Cancer Genet Cytogenet* 1995; **79**:133–5.

276 Ehrenberg L, Granath F, Törnqvist M. Macromolecule adducts as biomarkers of exposure to environmental mutagens in human populations. *Environ Hlth Perspect* 1996; **104**(Suppl 3): 423–8.

277 Kaderlik KR, Kadlubar FF. Metabolic polymorphisms and carcinogen-DNA adduct formation in human populations. *Pharmacogenetics* 1995; **5** (Spec No:) S108–17.

278 Ashford NA. Monitoring the worker and the community for chemical exposure and disease: legal and ethical considerations in the US. *Clin Chem* 1994; **40**:1426–37.

279 Venitt S. Carcinogenic and genotoxic effects of antineoplastic agents. In: Plowman PN, McElwain TJ, Meadows AT eds. *Complications of Cancer Management* Oxford: Butterworth Heinemann, 1991: 27–54.

280 Sorsa M, Anderson D. Monitoring of occupational exposure to cytostatic anticancer agents. *Mutat Res* 1996; **355**:1–2.

281 Baker ES, Connor TH. Monitoring occupational exposure to cancer chemotherapy drugs. *Am J Hlth Syst Pharm* 1996; **53**:2713–23.

282 Falck K, Grohn P, Sorsa M, Vainio H, Heinonen E, Holsti LR. Mutagenicity in urine of nurses handling cytostatic drugs [letter]. *Lancet* 1999; **1**:1250–1.

283 Allwood M, Stanley A, Wright P eds. *The Cytotoxics Handbook* 3rd edn. Oxford: Radcliffe Medical Press, 1997.

284 Cardis E. Ionizing radiation. In: Higginson J, Muir CM, Muñoz N eds. *Human Cancer: Epidemiology and Environmental Causes*. Cambridge: Cambridge University Press, 1992: 167–78.

285 Tsutsui T, Hayashi N, Maizumi H, Huff J, Barrett JC. Benzene-, catechol-, hydroquinone- and phenol-induced cell transformation, gene mutations, chromosome aberrations, aneuploidy, sister chromatid exchanges and unscheduled DNA synthesis in Syrian hamster embryo cells. *Mutat Res* 1997; **373**:113–23.

286 Snyder R, Kalf GF. A perspective on benzene leukemogenesis. *Crit Rev Toxicol* 1994; **24**:177–209.

287 Smith MT. The mechanism of benzene-induced leukemia: a hypothesis and speculations on the causes of leukemia. *Environ Hlth Perspect* 1996; **104**(Suppl 6): 1219–25.

288 Ruder AM. Epidemiology of occupational carcinogens and mutagens. *Occup Med* 1996; **11**:487–512.

289 Hartwig A. Current aspects in metal genotoxicity. *BioMetals* 1995; **8**:3–11.

290 Kasprzak KS. Possible role of oxidative damage in metal-induced carcinogenesis. *Cancer Invest* 1995; **13**:411–30.

291 International Agency for Research on Cancer. Monographs on the evaluation of carcinogenic risks to humans: 49. *Chromium, Nickel and Welding. Lyon: IARC*, 1990: 49–256.

292 O'Brien P, Kortenkamp A. Chemical models important in understanding the ways in which chromate can damage DNA. *Environ Hlth Perspect* 1994; **102**(Suppl 3): 3–10.

293 Molyneux MJ, Davies MJ. Direct evidence for hydroxyl radical-induced damage to nucleic acids by chromium (VI)-derived species: implications for chromium carcinogenesis. *Carcinogenesis* 1995; **16**:875–82.

294 Kortenkamp A, Casadevall M, Faux SP *et al*. A role for molecular oxygen in the formation of DNA damage during the reduction of the carcinogen chromium (VI) by glutathione. *Arch Biochem Biophys* 1996; **329**:199–207.

295 Kortenkamp A, Casadevall M, Da Cruz Fresco P. The reductive conversion of the carcinogen chromium (VI) and its role in the formation of DNA lesions. *Ann Clin Lab Sci* 1996; **26**:160–75.

296 Mattagajasingh SN, Misra HP. Mechanisms of the carcinogenic chromium(VI)-induced DNA-protein cross-linking and their characterization in cultured intact human cells. *J Biol Chem* 1996; **271**:33550–60.

297 Dillon CT, Lay PA, Cholewa M *et al*. Microprobe X-ray absorption spectroscopic determination of the oxidation state of intracellular chromium following exposure of V79 Chinese hamster lung cells to genotoxic chromium complexes. *Chem Res Toxicol* 1997; **10**:533–5.

298 Stearns DM, Wetterhahn KE. Intermediates produced in the reaction of chromium(VI) with dehydroascorbate cause single-strand breaks in plasmid DNA. *Chem Res Toxicol* 1997; **10**:271–8.

299 Liu KJ, Shi X, Dalal NS. Synthesis of Cr(IV)-GSH, its identification and its free hydroxyl radical generation: a model compound for Cr(VI) carcinogenicity. *Biochem Biophys Res Commun* 1997; **235**:54–8.

300 Bagchi D, Hassoun EA, Bagchi M, Muldoon DF, Stohs SJ. Oxidative stress induced by chronic administration of sodium dichromate [Cr(VI)] to rats. *Comp Biochem Physiol C Pharmacol Toxicol Endocrinol* 1995; **110**:281–7.

301 Lloyd DR, Phillips DH, Carmichael PL. Generation of putative intrastrand cross-links and strand breaks in DNA by transition metal ion-mediated oxygen radical attack. *Chem Res Toxicol* 1997; **10**:393–400.

302 De Flora S, Camoirano A, Bagnasco M, Bennicelli C, Corbett GE, Kerger BD. Estimates of the chromium(VI) reducing capacity in human body compartments as a mechanism for attenuating its potential toxicity and carcinogenicity. *Carcinogenesis* 1997; **18**:531–7.

303 Kerger BD, Finley BL, Corbett GE, Dodge DG, Paustenbach DJ. Ingestion of chromium(VI) in drinking water by human volunteers: absorption, distribution, and excretion of single and repeated doses. *J Toxicol Environ Hlth* 1997; **50**:67–95.

304 International Agency for Research on Cancer. Monographs on the evaluation of carcinogenic risks to humans: 49. *Chromium, Nickel and Welding.* Lyon: IRAC, 1990: 257–445.

305 Zhuang ZX, Shen Y, Shen HM, Ng V, Ong CN. DNA strand breaks and poly (ADP-ribose) polymerase activation induced by crystalline nickel subsulfide in MRC-5 lung fibroblast cells. *Hum Exp Toxicol* 1996; **15**:891–7.

306 Kasprzak KS, Jaruga P, Zastawny TH *et al.* Oxidative DNA base damage and its repair in kidneys and livers of nickel(II)-treated male F344 rats. *Carcinogenesis* 1997; **18**:271–7.

307 Dally H, Hartwig A. Induction and repair inhibition of oxidative DNA damage by nickel(II) and cadmium(II) in mammalian cells. *Carcinogenesis* 1997; **18**:1021–6.

308 Oller AR, Costa M, Obserdorster G. Carcinogenicity assessment of selected nickel compounds. *Toxicol Appl Pharmacol* 1997; **143**:152–66.

309 Kane AB, Boffetta P, Saracci R, Wilbourn JD (eds). *Mechanisms of Fibre Carcinogenesis.* International Agency for Research on Cancer, Scientific Publications No 140. Lyon: IARC, 1996: 135 pp.

310 Kane AB. Mechanisms of mineral fibre carcinogenesis. In: Kane AB, Boffetta P, Saracci R, Wilbourn JD eds. *Mechanisms of Fibre Carcinogenesis.* International Agency for Research on Cancer, Scientific Publications No 140. Lyon: IARC, 1996: 11–34.

311 Anonymous. Consensus report. In: Kane AB, Boffetta P, Saracci R, Wilbourn JD eds. *Mechanisms of Fibre Carcinogenesis.* International Agency for Research on Cancer, Scientific Publications No 140. Lyon: IARC, 1996: 1–9.

39

Clinical and epidemiological aspects

J MALCOLM HARRINGTON, P BOFFETTA, R SARACCI

Historical perspective	791	The clinical approach	805
The burden of occupational cancer	793	Occupational carcinogenic agents and processes	813
Clinical assessment procedures and the occupational factor	794	Attribution of cancer risks to occupational causes	813
Compensation for the cancer patient	796	Prevention	817
The scientific basis for establishing occupational causality	796	References	818
The epidemiological approach	797		

The topic of occupational cancer has become so vast that it is difficult to envisage encompassing even a cursory account in two chapters. Whilst biological mechanisms of carcinogenesis are dealt with in Chapter 38, this chapter reviews the clinical and epidemiological aspects of the subject.

For this purpose, it is necessary to start – in true Donald Hunter fashion – with a short historical perspective. In the context of occupational cancer there is no doubt that a review of the historical development of knowledge in this area provides considerable insight into the current state of affairs. The lessons which should have been learnt must provide a basis for future effective prevention.

The study of occupational cancer has both clinical and epidemiological aspects. For the clinician, an attempt is made to review the more important sites of occupational cancer in the light of the patient's clinical presentation and occupational history. Epidemiological method is reviewed as well as its advantages and shortcomings in promoting knowledge about workplace carcinogens.

Interaction between occupation and other factors in initiating or promoting cancer are discussed and this leads naturally to the topic of attributability. The degree of occupational attributability, where available, provides a sound basis for setting priorities for prevention.

HISTORICAL PERSPECTIVE

Cancers in general

Malignant neoplasms are today distinguished from benign neoplasms by certain broad qualitative attributes[1] such as: progression, often infiltrative and destructive new growth, cellular atypism, polymorphism and metastases as well as the process of transformation of normal cell to malignant cell. In the second century AD, Galen described, under the term 'cancer', a variety of benign and malignant tumours as well as some non-neoplastic conditions such as erysipelas. Nevertheless, it is clear from studies of prehistoric remains that humans have long been subject to neoplastic growth. Indeed, dinosaurs of the Cretaceous period were known to have haemangiomata, so neoplastic disease is probably older than the human species.[2] Certainly all animal species appear to be capable of developing cancer, though the focus of most scientific accounts has, naturally, centred on humans.

The neoplastic process, however, did not begin to be understood until cellular structure could be visualized following the invention of the microscope. The overthrow of the theory that humour imbalance was the basis of cancer is generally attributed to Virchow (1821–1902). Thereafter, germ theories held sway until the end of the last century when incontrovertible human evidence for chemical carcinogenesis provided the impetus to return to animal models in order to study the malignant process in greater detail. Human observations began with – and to a large extent continue to come from – studies of workplace exposures.

Early observation of occupation-related cancer

Although many accounts of occupational cancer start with Percival Pott's description in 1775 of chimney sweeps' scrotal cancer, there is good reason to go back further, even though the earlier accounts are less clear cut and do not necessarily propose the link between occupation and cancer.

In this context, occupational cancers may well have been occurring in the metal mines of Central Europe for a thousand years. In 965, silver was discovered near Goslar and mining began in the Herz mountains. Discoveries of other precious metals in Bohemia and Silesia in the thirteenth century led to a thriving industry supplying the European market with the raw materials for currency. The classic description of this mining process arose from the observations of Agricola (1494–1555) who in 1526 was appointed physician to the mining town of Joachimstal. His book *De Re Metallica* was apparently completed in 1550 but not published until the year after his death.[3] Although the book contains unparalleled accounts of the mediaeval mining process as well as brilliant ideas for improving mine ventilation, it also contains descriptions of the lung diseases that affected and killed the miners. He speaks of the dry mines where the dust is 'stirred and beaten up by digging [which] penetrates into the windpipe and lungs and produces difficulty in breathing and implants consumption in the body'. Whilst a considerable portion of this lung pathology was perhaps silicotuberculosis, the fact that these mines have subsequently yielded radioactive ores (they were the source of Marie Curie's pitchblende) suggests that some at least of the lung disease was cancer induced by the inhalation of radon and radon daughters.

Agricola's description of occupational disease was restricted to miners whilst Ramazzini's *De Morbis Artificum* published in 1713 provided the first broad-based account of many occupations and their effect on human health.[4] Surprisingly, Ramazzini gave little indication of cancer in his patients – perhaps in part due to the widespread ignorance of the process and to adherence to galenic medicine. Nevertheless, in his chapter on wetnurses, he expands on the 'sympathy' of the uterus and the breast, noting that breast tumours are 'found in nuns more than any other women'. This he attributes to celibacy, thus invoking a 'lifestyle' cause for cancer.

A further lifestyle cause for cancer and the first to attribute a link with tobacco was noted in 1761 by John Hill, a London physician. He noted a high incidence of cancer of the nasal passages in tobacco snuff users.

Chemical carcinogenesis, and in particular the occupationally induced variety, was firmly established by Percival Pott even though he had no concept of the underlying process. His description of scrotal cancer in postpubertal chimney sweeps was followed by descriptions of other benign and malignant skin tumours in workers exposed to tar and paraffin (1875), shale oil (1876), tar, pitch and mineral oil (1892), pitch dust (1912) and mule spinner mineral oil (1922).

These early descriptions of occupationally related cancer associated with exposure to complex hydrocarbons led to experimental confirmation when in 1915 Yamagiwa and Ichikawa succeeded in inducing skin cancer in rabbits by painting their ears with coal tar. The advent of fluorescence spectroscopy then provided the opportunity for the Kennaways in 1924 to identify the first carcinogenic hydrocarbon as 1, 2, 5, 6-dibenzanthracene.

Whilst the polynuclear aromatic hydrocarbons were generating considerable interest as skin carcinogens, other clinical observations of dyestuffs workers were suggesting a link between bladder cancer and the aromatic amines. The first description, like so many instances in occupational medicine, came from the astute observations of clinicians. In this case Rehn, in 1895, described three cases of bladder cancer in a group of 45 workers who were involved in the preparation of fuchsine. Further reports from Germany, Britain and North America implicated other aniline dye preparation processes and the search for the specific offending amines was underway. Some of the most potent aromatic amines causing bladder cancer were confirmed by the classic epidemiological studies of Case and his co-workers[5] in the 1950s in which they showed that 2-naphthylamine and benzidine were human carcinogens in the manufacturing industry whilst in the user industry – in this case rubber manufacture – 2-naphthylamine was a contaminant in the antioxidant (see also p. 229).

Although the early accounts of polynuclear aromatic hydrocarbon exposure identified the first chemical carcinogens, the discovery of the carcinogenic potential of aromatic amines provided an additional advance in the knowledge of chemical carcinogenesis. That is, that an organ distant from the point of first contact could bear the main force of the carcinogenic effect. The carcinogenic influence is, therefore, greatest where the exposure is most prolonged and most intense.

In the same year that Rehn described his three occupational bladder cancers, Roentgen discovered x-rays, and 3 years later the Curies isolated radium. Radiation-induced dermatitis and skin carcinomata were noted in experimental scientists within the first few years of the twentieth century. Marie Curie and her daughter died of leukaemia whilst early radiologists succumbed to skin carcinomatosis. Bone sarcomata were induced in laboratory animals exposed to ionizing radiation in 1910, and by the 1930s these tumours were being described in the female workers using radium-226 and mesothorium to paint luminous dials. The inventor of the luminous paint, Dr von Sochocky, died of aplastic anaemia in 1928. Meanwhile, the inhalation of radioactive isotopes both in mines and in laboratories was linked to excess death rates for lung cancer. The splitting of the nucleus of uranium-235 in 1939 led the way to nuclear power and further opportunities to study the effects of ionizing radiation in inadvertent exposure at research facilities and deliberate exposure for the populations of Hiroshima and Nagasaki (see Chapter 19).

By the 1930s, a further lung carcinogen was being mooted. Effects from asbestos exposure appeared not to be restricted to lung fibrosis. Case series of asbestosis patients were noted to have an 18% frequency of lung cancer, and in the following two decades, peritoneal mesotheliomata were noted in asbestosis victims in London and in children who played on crocidolite mine tailings in South Africa[2] (see Chapter 35).

The current situation

Thus, within a lifetime of Rehn's discovery of the carcinogenic properties of aromatic amines, a number of chemical and physical agents were noted to be human carcinogens. Not all the list are occupational agents but the stimulus for much experimental work and further epidemiological studies has come from clinical observation of patients noted to have relevant workplace exposures. It would be otiose to continue the historical perspective through a description of all the other known or highly suspect workplace carcinogens but it is important to emphasize certain features of occupational cancer which have relevance in the wider areas of cancer studies. They are:

1 The discovery of occupational carcinogens has been the major influence in stimulating experimental research; some occupational carcinogens represent important models for the investigation of mechanisms of carcinogenesis in humans.
2 These occupational carcinogens provided the first good evidence that clearly defined agents can induce cancer in humans.
3 Such cancers tend to develop at sites where the action of the carcinogen is most prolonged and intense.
4 Cancer prevention is possible with the removal or strict control of workplace exposure to identified agents.
5 Although most occupationally induced cancers are indistinguishable histopathologically from non-occupational cancers at the same site, the gathering of a good occupational history can be the lead necessary to make the connection.

The last 30 years have seen great changes in the scientific and public attitudes towards cancer in general and occupational cancer in particular. The rise of epidemiology as an investigative tool has led to many published studies of working populations and their exposure to real (or imagined) carcinogens. With the public's increased awareness of such techniques, and their growing faith in the ability of these techniques to answer vital causation questions, has come the epidemiologists' concern that such studies are not as accurate or incontrovertible as the public perceive them to be. Such studies are, however, the ultimate test of clinical suspicion which in many cases remains the primary source of new information on carcinogenic risk. In other cases, the carcinogen entails a small increase in risk of one or several common neoplasms: this makes it impossible to detect clinically and requires the evidence to accumulate from repeated epidemiological studies.

Industry, for its part, has markedly reduced workplace exposures to suspect chemical and physical agents – either voluntarily or under pressure from regulatory agencies. Such reduced exposures, combined with the fact that a working population is rarely exposed to a single suspect agent, makes the task of the modern epidemiologist even more difficult. Matters will get worse in this context as the workforce of the next century becomes more mobile and multi-skilled. In addition, there is a growing tendency for large industrial undertakings to contract out the dirtiest job on site. The epidemiologists task of tracing exposed populations demands more and more multi-site, international cohorts in order to assess large enough groups for study.

The increasing tendency to resort to litigation does not bode well for balanced epidemiological studies. The legal process tends to accept lower levels of proof than that which would satisfy the epidemiologist. A good example is the current spate of litigation over residential exposures to electric and magnetic fields – including the use of mobile phones – whilst the scientific stance for both residential and occupational exposure to such sources of non-ionizing radiation provides no clear evidence of causal link to human cancer.

THE BURDEN OF OCCUPATIONAL CANCER

Cancer represents a public health problem of major proportions worldwide but particularly so in developed countries. As economically developing nations come to grips with infant mortality, cancer as an essentially middle- to old-age disease will increase in importance in these countries as well. This burden of cancer has been estimated for 18 major cancers and for all cancers in each of 24 geographical areas for the year 1985 based mainly on cancer registry data.[6]

In that year, it is estimated that 7.6 million cases of cancer occurred (excluding skin cancer). For both sexes combined, stomach cancer accounts for 9.9% of the total but the incidence is declining. Lung cancer, the most common tumour in men and in both genders combined, is still increasing. For males, lung cancer represents 17.6% of the total, whilst for women it is the fifth most common tumour with 5.8% of the total, the commonest tumour being cancer of the breast (19.1%). The percentages for lung cancer are even higher (22.2 and 7.1% respectively) for developed countries. A parallel estimate of cancer mortality suggests that 5.1 million people died of cancer, worldwide in 1985.

Whilst the cancer mortality rates for Western Europe have stabilized or in some cases fallen in recent years, the trend is disturbingly upwards in the countries of central Europe and the newly independent states of the former USSR.[7]

Complete elimination of all cancers would produce a gain in life expectancy at birth of 2.5 years (similar calculations for coronary artery disease would be 6 years). A better estimate of the effect of cancer might be obtained by considering the average numbers of years of life lost by the 20% of the population who develop cancer. In this case the loss is 16.0 years.[1] The economic impact of this must combine direct medical care costs with the indirect costs of loss of productive life, etc. Direct costs alone absorb some 5% of national health care costs in developed countries and a similar percentage of research costs.

Prevention of cancer is thus a vital human and economic goal. The part that occupation plays in this is limited but crucial. It is common practice to view cancer causation in terms of the percentage of all cancers due to specific causes. Doll and Peto[8] estimated that in a country such as the USA, cigarette smoking accounted for some 30%, diet might account for 35% and occupation about 4% (with 'acceptable limits' of 2–8%). If one applies these figures to the worldwide burden of cancer, the evaluation of the number of cancers attributable to occupational exposure is in the region of about 110 000 per year worldwide.[9]

The elimination of occupational cancers would not have the enormous impact of eliminating tobacco as a cause but these workplace exposures are, at least theoretically, more controllable than the 'lifestyle' factors. One should consider also that the burden of occupational cancer is not evenly distributed in society, rather it affects mainly male blue collar workers.

In short, the worldwide burden of cancer is large and growing. The occupational factor is modest but could be effectively diminished by preventive measures that are available. Their implementation is governed mainly by the technological cost and the perceived societal need for the products. Preventive strategies are discussed later in the chapter.

CLINICAL ASSESSMENT PROCEDURES AND THE OCCUPATIONAL FACTOR

The recognition of work-related factors is vital in the effective diagnosis, treatment and prevention of ill-health. Occupational diseases are most likely to be suspected by those closest to the patient or the workplace. This could be the workers themselves, though this is more likely to be the case for illness of short latency such as asthma and dermatitis. Cancer, with its long latency – induction often extending to two or three decades – is less likely to be recognized as work-related by the employee unless previous local instances have conditioned them to look for it and/or the agent responsible has a high carcinogenic potential.

It is the clinician of first or second referral who has to take this responsibility. In view of the limited number of trained occupational physicians, the doctor consulted by the worker is likely to be a family doctor or a hospital consultant who has had little or no training in occupational medicine.

Given that occupation accounts for all or part of the tumour process in 5% of cancers, physicians should contemplate occupation as a possible aetiological factor each time they see a new case of cancer. The rarity of the tumour may be the intellectual stimulus needed to consider workplace causes. It was occupational physicians at an American tyre manufacturer who were alerted to the carcinogenic potential of vinyl chloride monomer because of four cases of the extremely rare angiosarcoma of the liver in their workforce. However, it was an ear, nose and throat surgeon who first realized that woodworking was the common factor in her small series of rare adenocarcinoma of the ethmoid sinus.

A patient with a common tumour such as lung cancer presents greater diagnostic difficulty. Nevertheless, many urothelial surgeons are now aware that occupation should be investigated when dealing with bladder cancer, where the occupational attributability can be as high as 20%. Similarly, it is our experience that haematologists commonly consider occupation when reviewing the possible causes of adult leukaemia, particularly the myeloid varieties.

The identification of work-related medical problems depends most importantly on the occupational history. Physical examination and special investigations may lead to a suspicion of a workplace agent as the cause of the disease but, ultimately, it is essential to obtain a thorough occupational history. A sentence or two in the family and social section of the medical history is not good enough.

The standard texts in occupational medicine have sections on the information that needs to be elicited in a good occupational history. This book on occupational diseases is no exception (see Chapter 1). From the point of view of occupational cancer it is essential that this enquiry of 'work relatedness' goes back far enough in the patient's life to be sure of including relevant exposures. That means at least 20 years and sometimes as many as 40.

Three examples seen by us perhaps might illustrate the point:

Example 1

A 70-year-old man was admitted to hospital for a cardiological assessment following symptoms likely to be due to coronary artery disease. At routine examination on the ward, the junior member of the medical team undertook the 'standard' clinical history and proceeded to the physical examination. She, quite properly, did not restrict the physical assessment to the cardiovascular system and, as a result, discovered an indolent ulcer on the patient's scrotum. Further enquiry revealed that the patient's family doctor had been treating this lesion with emollient creams for over 2 years, without success. The examining physician, working in an area of the country where scrotal cancer was no rarity then turned again to the occupational history. The question: 'What is your job?' received the answer: 'I am retired'. She persisted (rightly) 'Yes, but what did you do before you retired?' The reply gave the answer: 'I was a multispindle lathe operator for 30 years.' The patient's mineral-oil-induced scrotal cancer was excised the following day. Fortunately, in this case, the junior doctor was not put off by the 'retired' answer, and, equally fortunately, the patient had an uncomplicated work history which gave the occupational link straight away. Detailed questioning may be required, as the second case demonstrates.

Example 2

A 65-year-old women was admitted to hospital with breathlessness and chest pain. A pleural effusion was clinically detectable and a pleural tap revealed a blood stained fluid which on microscopy was found to contain mesothelioma cells. In this case the suspicion of an asbestos-related aetiology was readily apparent but as a 'housewife' the exposure history appeared to be lacking. There began a painstaking review of the patient's life experiences. Finally, a crucial fact emerged. For a brief period of her early married life she was employed outside the home. She had worked during the Second World War for a short time and, for 6 months of that time, had filled gas masks with a 'blue fibrous material' 40 years before the onset of her symptoms of pleural mesothelioma.

Example 3

A third case – again of scrotal cancer highlights a further area for the clinician. Whilst working as a part time occupational physician for a small engineering company, one of us saw an employee for a routine post-sickness absence medical. At that consultation the employee stated that he was well but asked for the form from 'the Social Security' to be completed so that he 'would get money'. The form – for Industrial Injuries Disability –

stated that the man had under gonesurgery for scrotal cancer. In this case the diagnosis and treatment in the individual case was complete. What was now needed was a review of workplace practices for others at potential risk in the multispindle lathe section of the factory. On inspection, conditions were not good: there was poor hygiene for both skin and lung exposure to oils and oil mist, no formal policy for personal protection and no health surveillance for skin pathology.

These cases illustrate the importance of three aspects of a good clinical history:

- the suspicion that occupation might be of aetiological relevance;
- the need for a thorough lifetime review of those occupations;
- the need for *somebody* to consider others potentially at risk in the workplace.

Recognition of the importance of the first two aspects may not solve the problem even if occupation is the cause of the cancer. That is because patients may not know the relevant chemical (or physical) agents to which they were exposed or they may know them only by trade names or even nicknames. Second, the job titles used by patients may shed no light on the exposure issues and, finally, even if the employing company was known, it is possible that it has ceased to trade by the time of the enquiry. Use of certain chemicals is a problem but employment in the chemical manufacturing industry compounds these difficulties. Whilst the final product may be known and the exposures well documented, the range and the complexity of possible exposure to intermediates can be staggering and may defy analysis even by the company's chemists. A fourth example might illustrate this point:

Example 4

A chemical company manufacturing a range of pesticides noted, in the course of its sophisticated and extensive health surveillance programme, that some workers had developed skin lesions reminiscent of solar keratoses. Cursory statistical analysis suggested that the risk for these workers of developing these premalignant skin lesions was in excess of what might be expected. A thorough review of the manufacturing process, the worker exposure profiles and the intermediates involved suggested that certain plant improvements would eliminate some suspect agents and greatly diminish worker exposure to others. Action was prompt and health surveillance stepped up. A decade later, further cases of keratosis were noted – some in plant operatives who had never worked with the old process. The disturbing message was that the previous plant review had either failed to reduce exposure to the putative carcinogen(s) or, more likely, and more disturbing, those suspect agents were not the cause of the keratosis. The problem here is not ignorance nor incompetence but the sheer complexity of the chemical process with hundreds of organic chemicals, alone or in combination, being potential sources of risk and exposure.

In such cases, the clinician has every reason to fail to find an aetiological agent, but, for every case like that, there are many more where a simple careful account of workplace experience can pay dividends. Details of model occupational history proformas are described elsewhere (see Chapter 1) but one practical point is worthy of reiteration. It is our experience that occupational history taking can be a complex and time-consuming business and one which the busy clinician might be tempted to avoid in the face of lengthening outpatient queues. We provide the patient with an occupational history questionnaire in advance of the consultation. The patient then brings the completed proforma to the clinic where details can be checked and omissions rectified. Further enquiries of previous employers may be necessary but at least the basic information can be confirmed at the first consultation.

In summary, the difficulties of identifying occupational factors in relation to cancer in the clinical setting are:

- Ignorance of the risk by the worker – or management.
- Failure of the clinician to consider an occupationally related aetiology – for that patient or for others at risk in the same workplace.
- Diversity of chemical nomenclature.
- Variable degrees of worker exposure to single or complex chemical mixtures.
- Movement of workers between jobs, work areas or industries.
- Failure to record previous occupations to the current (or last) one.
- Long latency-induction times for cancer.
- Job obsolescence.
- Company closure.
- Busy clinical workload.

COMPENSATION FOR THE CANCER PATIENT

Whilst compensation for acquired disease is not of prime concern to the clinician, it is an aspect of the clinician–patient interaction that should be considered. Indeed, patients or their relatives – especially next of kin in the case of cancer patients who die – may wish to seek some financial compensation for their loss.

For the clinician this is a difficult area but one where some idea of processes and options should be known. If the particular cancer and the relevant occupation are listed in the national list of compensatable diseases (in the UK, the Department of Social Security has a list of 60 or so Prescribed Diseases, of which some are occupational cancers) State compensation may be available as a form of pension. This can be claimed through the Social Security offices and no fault is required to be proved against an employer. Indeed, court action is obviated in this system although the 'sums involved' are not great (see Chapter 4).

The alternative approach of suing the employer in the courts may, if successful, result in large sums of money but the plaintiff has to prove negligence – an extremely difficult procedure even where clear-cut links exist between the cancer type and the occupation of the patient.

Whilst clinicians may baulk at becoming embroiled in complex legal cases, they should be aware of the state compensation scheme and have access to up-to-date lists of compensatable diseases and the means whereby patients or their relatives can process their claim.

In recent years there have been attempts to formalize the use of results of epidemiological studies to derive an estimate of the probability that an individual cancer is caused by a given exposure or exposure circumstance, such as employment in a hazardous industry.[10] These methods are relatively straightforward when the cases to compensate belong to the same group of workers included in the investigation from which risk estimates are derived: the extrapolation across occupational groups, and even more across industries and occupations, on the other hand, relies on assumptions that may strongly influence the final decision on whether a given case deserves compensation.

THE SCIENTIFIC BASIS FOR ESTABLISHING OCCUPATIONAL CAUSALITY

Nothing in science can be proved conclusively. The process of approaching 'the truth' is the currency of scientific method. The object is to observe, develop hypotheses based on those observations, test those hypotheses and replace those refuted with stronger hypotheses that require further testing, and so on. Nevertheless, in a practical world, decisions on health matters are often matters of life or death. Thus a time comes when action is called for despite the fact that absolute truth remains elusive. Bradford Hill's excellent article on the differences between cause and association[11] also stated:

> All scientific work is incomplete – whether it is observational or experimental. All scientific work is liable to be upset or modified by advancing knowledge. That does not confer upon us a freedom to ignore the knowledge we already have, or to postpone the action that it appears to demand at a given time.

Epidemiology is not an exact science but its currency is human beings. Human beings are the only truly valid study model for human disease although other methods may assist in pointing to aetiological agents. Figure 39.1 outlines the process of establishing causality whilst the weight given to each in reaching a decision is typified by the approach used in the International Agency for Research on Cancer (IARC) Monographs (see p. 802). Suffice it to say here that clinical suspicion figures prominently – particularly in the early stages of the process.

An even earlier approach which sometimes bears fruit is the question of chemical similarity. Certain 'families' of chemicals act in similar ways, and the aromatic amines are a good example (Fig. 39.2). The link between 2-naphthylamine and benzidine with bladder cancer was established in the 1950s. The chemical similarity with 4-aminobiphenyl was noted by an astute occupational physician working in the British chemical industry. He prevailed upon the company to abandon the chemical, then at an advanced stage in research and development. No bladder cancers from this chemical occurred in the UK but did so in the USA where it was already in full production. Methylene-*bis*(2-chloroaniline) (MbOCA) is structurally related to 4-aminobiphenyl and is probably carcinogenic to humans but the epidemiological data are inadequate. It is, however, carcinogenic to animals at various sites. Oral administration of MbOCA to dogs has induced tumours of the bladder.

Animal studies involving long-term bioassays as well as short-term mutagenicity testing are described in Chapter 38. The problem of species variation precludes clear-cut extrapolation to humans. However, biological indicators of exposure and effect – so-called molecular (or biochemical) epidemiology – does offer the possibility of a halfway house between animal studies and human epidemiology. Epidemiology frequently requires decades of exposure before valid health effects can be assessed. The molecular epidemiology approach can be invoked earlier where measurement of the putative carcinogen or a metabolite could be assayed in exposed populations. Furthermore the products of such reactions might be assessed by measuring DNA or protein adducts or early cytogenetic change. Such techniques are in their relative infancy and their use in studies designed to epidemiological standards – that is with a sound population base – is only just beginning. Nevertheless, such techniques could provide earlier clues of carcinogenic potential than full scale epidemiological studies and have greater species validity than some older animal bioassay procedures (see Chapter 38). Molecular epidemiology is undoubtedly becoming an important research tool.

The ultimate question to be asked, of course, is whether a given exposure causes human cancer. For this question to be adequately addressed, there is necessarily recourse to epidemiological studies. Whatever the shortcomings of the methods, there is no substitute for such data.

Ideally, the whole process will lead not only to an estimate of excess risk but also a dose–response relationship for specific agents and site-specific tumours which would aid preventive action and regulatory control. There are, however, few known carcinogens for which good quality risk assessment data exist.

This introductory section has attempted to trace the development of knowledge on occupationally related carcinogens up to the present. It has emphasized the unique contribution of the clinical approach in discovering new carcinogens (or old ones in new guises). Thereafter a variety of techniques may be used to confirm or refute the notion that the agent is a human carcinogen. In this process, for all its shortcomings, there is no substitute for the good quality, well constructed epidemiological study of exposed working populations.

```
Chemical                          in vivo
similarity        Studies  <
                                  in vitro

        Clinical observation

Human epidemiology  ←→  Molecular
   Exploratory            epidemiology

        Analytical

        Risk assessment

        Preventative action
```

Figure 39.1 *Establishing occupational carcinogenicity.*

THE EPIDEMIOLOGICAL APPROACH

Epidemiological studies

The primary aim of the epidemiological approach in the context of this chapter is the qualitative and quantitative definition of cancer risks from environmental hazards in the workplace. Subsidiary aims are the monitoring of the effects on cancer incidence, of changes in the working

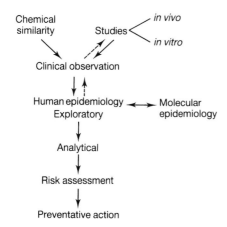

Figure 39.2 *Some occupational bladder carcinogens.*

environment (such as those following the adoption of hygiene standards) and the evaluation of the benefits of secondary prevention measures – for example, of cytological screening programmes for the early detection and treatment of occupational cancers. Complementary to the clinical approach, which investigates health and disease in working individuals, epidemiology studies health and disease, including cancer, in working populations. A grasp of the key principles underpinning the epidemiological approach is needed by any reader of the current epidemiological literature on occupational cancer as it appears in occupational medicine and general medical journals. A general account of epidemiological method is found in Chapter 3.

For the more methodologically orientated reader, an excellent presentation of occupational epidemiology methods can be recommended.[12] Further reading for those with some grounding in statistics can also be proposed.[13]

Exploratory studies

Exploratory epidemiological studies, also designated as descriptive or hypothesis generating, provide clues to the occupational aetiology of cancers. The strength of the clue derived from clinical case reports, the most basic form of exploratory studies, varies with the frequency of both the exposure and the disease. For instance, if two or more isolated cases of a common cancer – say colon – are reported following exposure to a widely distributed agent (i.e. electromagnetic fields), the most likely explanation is just chance or coincidence with no special meaning. However, if the cases are reported from a presumably small group of subjects exposed, the association is less likely to be purely coincidence. This holds particularly when the reported disease is a well identified and uncommon one such as oat cell carcinoma after exposure to bis(chloromethyl) ether,[14] liver angiosarcoma after vinyl chloride exposure,[15] mesothelioma following asbestos exposure[16] or erythroleukaemia following benzene exposure.[17,18] Even more suggestive of a non-chance association is a series of consecutive cases reported by a single centre such that a rough estimate of the exposed population can be attempted and an expected number of cancers computed to be compared with the observed one: this was possible for some early clinical series of leukaemia cases in benzene-exposed workers.[17] One step further, a quantitative or semi-quantitative relation may emerge between the intensity of exposure and, for instance, time between first exposure and appearance of clinical cancer. In an early group of seven cases of liver angiosarcoma in workers exposed to vinyl chloride the length of stay in high exposure jobs was roughly inversely related to the interval until discovery of the tumour.[19]

Other types of exploratory epidemiological studies

include analysis of cancer incidence or mortality patterns in time and space.

The marked time variations (rise and decline) of scrotal cancer prompted the search for parallel variations in other occupational exposures, such as to pitch and tars.[18] Cross-sections in time, for instance in the years around a census, of cancer mortality (and, more rarely, incidence) by site and occupational groups are routinely computed and published for England and Wales[20] and several other countries or areas. They can provide useful, though very basic, aetiological pointers, which can be reinforced if consistency is found in time and between countries or areas of enhanced rates for an occupational group.

Spatial analysis may also allow geographical areas with high rates of cancers to be earmarked, possibly related to occupational exposures as, for example, with 'hotspots' of mesotheliomas often detected in coastal sites with harbours and shipyards. More systematically, correlations may be explored between cancer rates by geographical areas and variables reflecting the prevalence of occupational exposures in the same areas. An important requirement for this analysis is that there should be sufficient variation in both rates and prevalence of exposures between the different geographical units and as little variation as possible within each unit.

In addition, other factors beyond those investigated should not show too much variation, for example accuracy of cancer registration or death certification, and the geographic units should be sufficiently large to provide stable rates. This was achieved in some correlation studies within the USA where cancer rates were related to several indicators of industrial concentration, adjusting for other demographic, socioeconomic and occupational indices, finding, for example, an association between elevated cancer rates and concentrations of paper, chemical, petroleum and transportation industries.[21] As for the clinical case reports, exploratory epidemiological analyses of time and space patterns of cancer rates can only offer useful pointers to aetiological factors, without allowing, in general, clear and firm conclusions to be drawn about the reality or otherwise of causal links. This task is left to analytical epidemiological studies aimed at estimating the magnitude and establishing the meaning, causal or non-causal, of an excess observed risk of cancer in subjects occupationally exposed to a physical, chemical or biological agent.

Analytical studies

COHORT STUDIES (see also Chapter 3)

In the analytical cohort study, workers are followed up in time, and their health experience in terms of occurrence of new cases of cancer or of cancer deaths is observed and compared in relation to different types and levels of workplace exposures. The historical cohort study is, to date, the most often employed for the investigation of occupational cancer, and can be conducted within the comparatively short time (a few months or, more often, a few years) required to sort out the documentation identifying each cohort member and their exposure history (as available) and to ascertain their vital status and, when applicable, the cause of death or the occurrence of a cancer. There is not much point in setting up a cohort study unless one has, based on prior information, reasonable confidence that a high follow-up rate, at the very least 90% and ordinarily between 95 and 100%, will be achieved. Lower follow-up rates would usually make the results of the study difficult or impossible to interpret with any clarity, as the workers lost to follow-up may be dissimilar from those traced, and include a disproportionately high (or disproportionately low) number of cancers.

A further important feature is the ability to document exposure in the past for each worker: this implies that an accurate and complete history of the exposures prevailing at the worksite at each point in time in the past does exist and that it can be matched to an existing and complete record of the job history of the worker.

It is rare that these two series of time-related events are fully available and one might often be forced to classify crudely the workers into overall 'high', 'medium' or 'low' rank of exposure or simply by their length of employment. In a cohort study one can directly express the results in terms of incidence or mortality rates of a cancer (e.g. lung cancer rate per 100 000 person-years in various exposure groups); comparisons can then be made in terms of 'relative risks' – i.e. of the ratios of rates for the different groups. Often in occupational studies internal comparisons, subdividing the worker population by category of exposure, are complemented by external comparisons of the worker population with the general population of the same sex and age at a given point in time. Often when internal comparisons are inadvisable because of a lack of adequate information on individual exposure history, external comparisons may be the only feasible ones. It is customary to compute the results of external comparisons in the form of standardized mortality ratio (SMR) or standardized incidence ratio (SIR) for various cancers, expressing the mortality or incidence rate of the worker population (adjusted for the effects of age and sex) as a percentage of that of the general population.

An important point in this analysis is that appropriate consideration must be given to the time element: standardized mortality ratios should be calculated separately for successive intervals of time of observation so that an effect such as a cancer, which is likely to occur late after onset of exposure, can be detected. Also, during the first years after start of work, employed populations often exhibit mortality rates that are, for several causes of death, lower than the corresponding mortality in the general population, i.e. SMRs lower than 100. This effect

('healthy worker effect') tends to disappear with time and reflects the conditions of health of subjects capable of enrolling for work, which are better than the condition of the general population, burdened by a proportion of ill people.

In cohort studies in which the reconstruction of the past history of exposure for each worker may be feasible but very cumbersome, as may happen when dealing with a cohort of several tens of thousands, one may resort to a sampling approach within the cohort. If, for example, lung cancer is the site of interest, or it has been shown to exhibit a high SMR in an initial overall analysis, the lung cancer cases and a suitable number of controls from the cohort, usually matched on such criteria as age and sex, are selected and their detailed exposure histories reconstructed. This may reduce the workload by one or more orders of magnitude and make feasible a study with good standards of quality in the data extraction.

CASE-CONTROL STUDIES (see also Chapter 3)

The cohort-based subsampling represents just a subtype of a more general study design, the case-control (or case-referent) study which is also currently being used to investigate occupational as well as other exposures.

The most critical aspect of a community-based case-control study is the choice of the controls. Ideally they should represent a random sample from the same population from which the diseased cases originated. However, this population may be difficult to delineate except when all newly diagnosed cases of a cancer in a given area can be studied, as when cancer registry cases are used. The controls can then be drawn at random (usually stratifying for age and sex) from the population of the area. Yet even this initially random sample may end up being a non-randomly selected sample; for example, because a sizeable proportion of the selected subjects refuse to participate in the study.

Another critical aspect of case-control studies is that a selective bias in recalling exposures may easily creep in because the extent of exposure is often based on interviewing patients (or their relatives) and controls (or their relatives). For instance, patients with lung cancer may be more prone to recall past exposure to dusty environments than healthy controls. A related bias may exist when the interviewer, usually unconsciously, exerts a different level of effort to elicit recall of exposure events among cases and controls: this type of bias can be reduced if interviewers are 'blind'; for example, interviewing the subjects before a final diagnosis is established. In the minority of situations in which interview data can be supplemented or even replaced by other sources of information (documents of past exposures in factories) this type of bias may be eliminated.

Given the peculiar structure of the case control study, which starts from the disease and goes backwards to explore exposures, no direct estimates of mortality or incidence rates are possible – in contrast with cohort studies. However, unbiased estimates of their ratios can be obtained ('odds ratios' estimating, under certain general conditions, the relative risks), so that relative risks for a cancer among exposed and unexposed subjects can be estimated from case-control studies.

The proportional mortality study can be regarded as a particular variant of the case-control study. For example, the proportion of workers in a dyes factory who died of bladder cancer is compared with the same proportion in the general population of the same sex and age, the results being usually expressed as a ratio (proportional mortality ratio or PMR). These results are relatively easy to obtain as they require information only on deceased workers (and not on a whole cohort) but may turn out to be very misleading: in fact, a high proportion of bladder cancer among the workers may derive from a real excess or simply from a deficit in the other causes of death. The best way of performing this type of study is to carry it out as a proper case-control study, comparing the exposure frequency (to dyes) among all bladder cancer deaths (workers plus general population) with the frequency among deaths due to a restricted number of other causes of death presumably unrelated to the exposure.

Interpreting the epidemiological evidence

From an occupational and public health viewpoint the major strength of the epidemiological approach derives from its ability to document and quantify the size of the actual burden of cancers arising from specified conditions or workplace exposure. The corresponding and major drawback is that, in order to be counted, the cases (or deaths) of cancer must already have occurred and therefore the method is applicable only to hazardous conditions that have escaped, for whatever reason, adequate control. Similarly, and from a scientific viewpoint, epidemiology is the only approach that can provide direct evidence of the carcinogenic role of an occupational exposure; but the interpretation of this evidence, particularly when small proportionate increases in risk are concerned, is not exempt from uncertainties, mostly stemming from the non-experimental nature of epidemiological investigations of free-living human groups. In all instances in which an excess risk of cancer, expressed as a relative risk higher than 1, has been observed among workers exposed to an agent, the question arises of whether this reflects a truly causal role of the agent or, instead, the play of chance, of other factors (confounders) or of some systematic error (bias) introduced into the investigation at the stage of its design, conduct or analysis.

THE ROLE OF CHANCE

To assess the role of chance, assistance is usually sought in a formal procedure of statistical inference. Often this leads to the calculation of confidence limits, at the 90 or 95% levels of confidence, for the observed relative risk: if the interval bound by the limits includes the null value of 1, which corresponds to no excess risk with respect to the expectation, it is likely that the observed excess is due to chance fluctuations alone.

THE ROLE OF CONFOUNDING FACTORS

The possibility that other causal confounding agents, occupational or non-occupational, may have been at work may present a more difficult problem. The difficulty is greatest when, information being available on other agents present in the workplace, they turn out to be so closely associated with the agent of primary interest that no procedure of statistical adjustment can separate the effects of each agent. This may happen, for instance, when several pesticides are used together in a given formulation, when polycyclic hydrocarbons or protective insulation asbestos are present in environments where combustion processes take place, whatever the other more specific materials involved, or when a few tremolite asbestos fibres occur together with the bulk of chrysotile fibres. The difficulty is less severe when the association of the confounder with the agent of interest is presumably not so tight, even when (somewhat paradoxically) the information on the confounder itself is poor or not available. For instance, information is rarely available on occupational exposures incurred by workers prior to or after employment in the industry under study; and information is almost always missing on non-occupational confounders, typically tobacco smoking.

This has sometimes led to the wrong contention that excesses of lung cancer, or of other tobacco-related cancers, in groups of workers are uninterpretable in the absence of smoking history. In fact, it can be algebraically demonstrated that if a relative risk for lung cancer of, say, 2 has been observed in a group of workers exposed to an inorganic dust (compared with the unexposed), the confounding by tobacco smoking can wholly explain away the risk only if the relative risk for lung cancer due to tobacco smoking is equal or higher than 2. This is usually true even for modest smokers; and, simultaneously that the smoking habit is twice as frequent or more among the exposed workers than among the unexposed (often represented by the general population), ordinarily a highly unlikely situation. This example illustrates the more general principle that only strong confounders, which are also very tightly associated with the exposure, can entirely explain away an excess of risk of, say, 50% or more (i.e. a relative risk of 1.5).

The situation would be more complex if an interaction were to occur between tobacco smoke and the dust, but again this poses a major problem of interpretation only if the dust acts in the presence of tobacco smoke, a type of interaction theoretically conceivable but up to now never actually observed for any agent.

THE ROLE OF BIASES

Finally, no general quantitative principle is applicable to biases of various kinds that may have crept into the study. For example, if exposed and non-exposed cohorts are followed up with different intensity of diagnostic ascertainment, substantial biases can be introduced in the comparison between the two groups. Whether this can then explain away an observed elevated relative risk can be assessed only in the light of the specific features of a study by evaluating, for each type of bias, the likelihood of its existence, its direction and the likely maximum size. Merely invoking the possibility of a bias as an explanation is a sterile exercise which does not lead to any advancement in understanding the results of the study.

NEGATIVE STUDIES AND NO EFFECT THRESHOLDS

Problems arise not only in interpreting a 'positive' study which has shown an increased relative risk but also in interpreting a 'negative' study which has not demonstrated any such increase. Chance, confounding and bias may in fact have the effect of obscuring an actual causal association and need to be ruled out as explanations for a negative study in which the divergence of the relative risk from 1 is within the limits of chance expectation (e.g. the confidence interval around the relative risk covers 1). For example, if a relative risk of 1.4 has been observed with 95% confidence limits of 0.8 and 2.6, only values lower than 0.8 or greater than 2.6 can be confidently excluded, while the true relative risk may lie anywhere between these two limits. In particular, if the primary concern is with the possible elevation in numbers of people exposed to an agent, such a study cannot exclude that a true relative risk is somewhere between 1 and 2.6. This means that a good negative study is one with a very narrow confidence interval around the value of 1 (the width of this interval can be reduced, all other things being equal, by enlarging the sample size). Confidence in a negative result is enhanced when several independent studies, made under different circumstances, are in agreement. Also, a negative study is relevant only to the levels of exposure within or below (but not above) the range of those actually observed.

Furthermore, where long-term effects are concerned a negative study is relevant only if sufficient time has elapsed from first exposure to the agent. Experience with human cancers with known aetiology suggests that the period from first exposure to a carcinogenic hazard to development of clinically observed cancer may sometimes be relatively short (e.g. for acute ionizing irradiation at high doses and leukaemia) but is usually in the order of decades and may even exceed 30 years. Particular caution should be exercised especially by occupational physicians before embarking on studies of small groups exposed to a known carcinogen (say, asbestos) in order to verify whether under the local conditions of exposure any excess risk has occurred: this small-sized study has a high likelihood of ending up with inconclusive results and even with false reassurance.

A special aspect of negative studies concerns the possibility of identifying a level of exposure below which no excess risk of cancer occurs; namely, a population 'threshold'. Near zero excesses such as one extra case of cancer per 100 000 or per million exposed workers over a lifetime are wholly beyond what can be detected and measured by epidemiological studies. Hence, attempts at identifying population thresholds have to rely on extrapolation of risks at low levels of exposure as observed at much higher levels of exposure. The very existence of a population threshold assumes some carcinogenic mechanism translating into an exposure response (risk) relationship that is non-linear in the low exposure range, an assumption most often questionable. Furthermore, the imprecision inherent in the fitting and extrapolation of the exposure-response curve may make it impossible to decide the issue of whether a theoretically assumed threshold is actually identifiable. In general, one is on safer ground in determining, with a given degree of confidence, the excess risk, however minute, associated with a given level of exposure.

New developments in epidemiology

Advances in the epidemiological identification of carcinogenic hazards, and in quantifying their cancer risks, depend on improvements in measurement of exposure and on refinements of biological end-points. Strategies for sampling and measuring pollutants currently present in the working environment are being devised that are capable of generating measurements usable not only, or not primarily, for the purpose of compliance control but also for epidemiological investigations. As, however, full monitoring of all agents present in a workplace is inconceivable, the problem of estimating in the future past exposures to pollutants now unsuspected as carcinogenic will remain. Thus, techniques for reconstructing past exposure are also currently the subject of active methodological research.[22,23]

Many agents currently suspected to be occupational carcinogens are likely to be less potent than classical carcinogens identified in the past via epidemiological studies. This leads to the need for large scale studies, that can often be performed only as international consortia. Such international multicentric studies present special challenges in terms of comparability of information collected on exposure and outcome.

Biological measurements of carcinogens or of their products of transformation in the body represent an important area of current research[24] (see Chapter 38).

Addition compounds (adducts) of carcinogens, such as benzo[a]pyrene or ethylene oxide, with DNA macromolecules or with proteins (haemoglobin) are starting to permit a molecular dosimetry capable of markedly reducing misclassification of exposure of workers and of increasing the sensitivity of epidemiological studies. In particular, biological markers of exposure should be able to measure a biologically effective dose, resulting from the interplay of external exposure, metabolic activity and sensitivity to damage of macromolecules (e.g. DNA adduct repair activity). The main problem remains the current rarity of markers capable of reflecting long-term exposures over months, years or decades. At the other end of the spectrum, which ranges from exposure to clinical cancer, the molecular biology characterization of cancers – for instance through activated proto-oncogenes – introduces a further dimension in the subtyping of cancers (besides histology, cytology, immunology) which might allow the singling out of specific subtypes aetiologically related to given exposures, thus again easing the sensitivity of the epidemiological tool. Other limitations of these oddments is the specificity, sensitivity, variability and duration of persistence in blood, urine etc., and what the background values might be. More speculatively, should some critical molecular lesions be clearly identified as an obligatory early step, leading with high probability to cancer, it might allow replacement of the actual observation of the clinical disease by the observation of such lesions, markedly shortening the time-scale of an epidemiological study.

Identifying occupational carcinogenic hazards: the IARC monographs programme

Epidemiology is a key component in the process of identification of carcinogenic hazards carried out since 1972 by the IARC programme on the Evaluation of Carcinogenic Risks to Humans.[25] Single physical, chemical or biological agents, complex mixtures, occupational exposures and industries for which some suspicion of carcinogenicity has been raised on various grounds are evaluated by the programme. The epidemiological evidence available from all published, or at least publicly accessible, studies on the exposure under investigation is evaluated by an expert working group, summarized and synthesized in one of four categories:

- *sufficient evidence* when the working group considers that a causal relationship has been established between the exposure and human cancer;
- *limited evidence*, when a causal interpretation is considered as credible, but chance bias or confounding could not be ruled out with reasonable confidence;
- *inadequate evidence*, when the available studies are of insufficient quality, consistency or statistical power to permit a conclusion regarding the presence or absence of a causal association;

- *evidence suggesting* lack of carcinogenicity, when there are several adequate studies covering the full range of levels of exposure that humans are known to encounter which are mutually consistent in not showing a positive association between the exposure and any studied cancer at any level of observed exposure.

The evidence so rated for human carcinogenicity is ultimately combined with the evidence of carcinogenicity in experimental animals, separately evaluated and rated, plus whatever supporting evidence is available (e.g. genetic effects in short-term tests) to provide an overall evaluation. This leads to a final classification of exposures into one of four groups:

- *group 1*: carcinogenic to humans;
- *group 2*:
  A: probably carcinogenic to humans (while sufficient evidence in animals, in the absence of or with inadequate human evidence, qualifies);
  B: possibly carcinogenic to humans (limited evidence in humans alone qualifies);
- *group 3*: not classifiable as to carcinogenicity to humans;
- *group 4*: probably not carcinogenic to humans (limited epidemiological evidence supported by sufficient evidence of lack of carcinogenicity in animals qualifies).

As a general rule exposures, occupational or otherwise, in group 2 should be regarded as if they entail a risk of cancer for humans, and actions minimizing them ought to be taken. A complete and updated list of such exposures to 1990 is found in a recent IARC publication.[2] The IARC evaluations (more than 700 agents have been examined up to now) represent a widely accepted scientific basis for the process of risk assessment. However, they cover only the first step, namely qualitative hazard identification. The second step, quantitative risk estimation, is built on the foundations of the first by national or international committees and regulatory agencies.

Tables 39.1 and 39.2 present the agents and occupational exposures for which sufficient evidence of carcinogenicity in humans is available. In the following paragraphs a few illustrative examples are briefly presented of how and how far the epidemiological approach has gone in identifying occupational carcinogenic hazards.

Three examples of established occupational carcinogenic hazards are asbestos, vinyl chloride and painting.

ASBESTOS[2,16,20,26–28]

The first modern description of a pathology (fibrosis) associated with exposure to the naturally occurring crystalline fibres of asbestos, in its different varieties, goes back to the beginning of the century, soon after the start of the mining and the exploitation of the mineral on an industrial scale. The first cases of pulmonary carcinomas superimposed on asbestosis were reported in the mid 1930s. The first clear epidemiological evidence of an increased risk of lung cancer from exposure to asbestos (in a textile industry) came, in the early 1950s, from a historical cohort study in a British factory, where 11 cases of lung cancer against an expectation of less than 1 were observed. Subsequently (by the end of the 1960s), it was shown that the lung cancer excess, in many circumstances of exposure to asbestos fibres, reflected an interactive effect of asbestos and tobacco smoking.

Mesothelioma of the peritoneum and pleura has been shown to occur following both environmental and occupational (mining) exposure to crocidolite in South Africa and was subsequently shown to occur also after exposure to other varieties of asbestos (see Chapter 35). Several studies have also indicated increased risks for cancer of the larynx whilst a few indicate an elevated risk for gastrointestinal cancers. Although the risk of both lung cancer and mesothelioma have been documented for all main varieties of asbestos (chrysotile – the most widely used variety – amosite and crocidolite), several issues still remain open. For example, data are inadequate for quantitative comparisons on a fibre by fibre basis, and on a mass basis, between the potency of different fibres in respect of lung cancer and mesotheliomas. For chrysotile and lung cancer, and taking into account the very substantial sources of uncertainty in the past exposure measurement, a simple linear relationship (with no threshold) has been proposed as the best summary of available data: 1 (fibre/ml) × year being estimated to produce an increase in the SMR of 1%.

At the mechanistic level the issue of whether lung cancer can occur only in association with fibrosis is periodically revamped, but in part the question depends on how finely one defines fibrosis. More important, at least for lung cancer there is some evidence that for subjects occupationally exposed for short periods the relative risk increase peaks at 15–19 years from first exposure and then declines to some extent, suggesting a possible late benefit from discontinuation of exposure. Some salient features emerge from the long 'epidemiological history' of asbestos in the working environment. First, there was a substantial lag between the first clinical case reports of cancers (in the mid 1930s) and the epidemiological evidence (mid 1950s), which led to an even longer delay in taking cancer into account when establishing hygiene standards. Second, the large volume of studies on a variety of exposed workers – such as miners and millers, textile workers, shipyard workers, including replicated cohort studies in several countries, which have contributed substantive evidence on the carcinogenic role of asbestos (and mineral fibres in general) – prompted methodological developments in occupational epidemiology and played a central role in demonstrating the need to prevent occupational cancers as well as the effectiveness of exposure controls. Third, and notwithstanding this mass of data, there is a residual substantial uncertainty in the quantitative exposure-response relationships, which is in part likely to persist forever, as in any case the information accruing from a longer follow-up of worker cohorts is limited by the mediocre quality of past exposure measurements (while today exposure levels have been lowered and should, hopefully, produce no detectable effects).

VINYL CHLORIDE[2,14,15,18,25,26,29,30]

Vinyl chloride is the basic monomer for the production of polyvinyl chloride (PVC), a widely used plastic material. After animal experiments clearly showed, in the early 1970s, the carcinogenicity of vinyl chloride, a strong suspicion arose of a vinyl chloride-related aetiology of a few cases of liver angiosarcomas which had already been recorded in highly exposed polymerization workers (see Chapter 8). Subsequently, a large number of epidemiological studies has substantiated this causal association. Reduction of exposures by one or often more orders of magnitude were implemented rapidly in many countries in the mid to late 1970s (Fig. 39.3); also, no cases of angiosarcoma have apparently been reported in a worldwide registry in workers exposed for the first time after 1969. Recently an updated multicentric follow-up of cohorts in Europe has demonstrated for liver angiosarcomas a clear relationship with cumulative exposure to vinyl chloride as well as a steady increase of the risk with time since first exposure. Although lung cancer, lymphosarcomas and brain tumours have been reported in excess in some studies from North America, the evidence for this increase appears inconsistent, particularly for lung cancer.

The vinyl chloride case is notable on three accounts. First, it shows how experimental evidence can initiate the process of hazard identification and control. Second, the exposure levels in the working environments were rapidly and drastically reduced, a good example of what can be achieved with appropriate technology; and it is striking that the fading out of angiosarcoma registrations parallels at least in part the period of low exposure. Third, it marked in the mid 1970s the renewed impulse to occupational epidemiology studies, specifically in the cancer area, which is still operative. 'Poisoning' by vinyl chloride is a prescribed disease in the UK (see Chapter 4).

PAINTING[31]

The evidence of a possible excess of cancer among automobile and construction painters accumulated slowly on the basis of exploratory studies and of cohort studies. Despite the absence of a striking excess for any type of cancer, the body of evidence that painters are at increased risk of lung cancer, and that the increase can

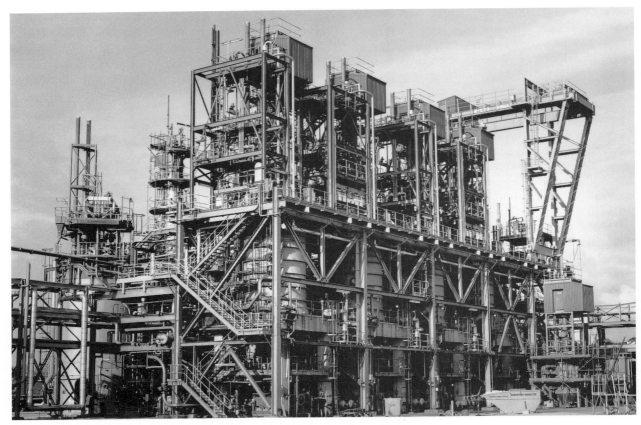

Figure 39.3 *A modern totally enclosed vinyl chloride monomer manufacturing plant.*

not be explained by differences in tobacco smoking, continued to grow during the 1970s and the 1980s. In particular, there were three cohort and more than ten case-control studies that evaluated lung cancer risk among painters in different countries: all of them consistently reported a 30–100% increase in risk. The evidence of other cancer sites, such as bladder, oesophgus and stomach, is far less consistent.

On the one hand, the lack of an obvious lung carcinogen to which painters are exposed made the interpretation of the evidence problematic. Possible candidates were salts of heavy metals such as chromates and organic solvents; exposure to asbestos and crystalline silica may also occur. On the other hand, the consistency and the strength of the findings allowed to rule out chance, bias and confounding as plausible explanations of the observed association, leading towards a conclusion of causal relationship. It is plausible that different carcinogenic agents caused an excess of lung cancer in different groups of painters.

This example illustrates how epidemiological evidence may slowly accumulate to identify a carcinogen or a circumstance entailing exposure to carcinogens. Furthermore, it shows how 'modern' occupational carcinogens cause small increases in the risk of common cancers, and require a large body of knowledge to accu-

mulate over decades in order to identify them. However, it also shows the potential of occupational epidemiology to clarify aetiological links, even when they are relatively weak.

Two examples of presumptive occupational carcinogenic hazards are man-made vitreous fibre (MMVF) and formaldehyde.

MAN-MADE VITREOUS FIBRE[32,33]

In contrast to the naturally occurring and crystalline asbestos for which they represent a substitute in a number of applications, MMVF are amorphous and synthetically produced inorganic fibres. Evidence from animal experiments has shown that some varieties of MMVF could, when injected directly into the pleura or peritoneum of rodents, elicit mesothelioma. This has promoted extensive epidemiological research over the last 15 years focused in particular on the question of whether any excess of respiratory diseases (chronic pneumoconiosis and lung cancer) would occur in workers exposed to MMVF (Fig. 39.4). These studies have included more than 50 000 workers in the producing industry in North America and Europe followed up within historical cohort studies investigating the possible effects of the

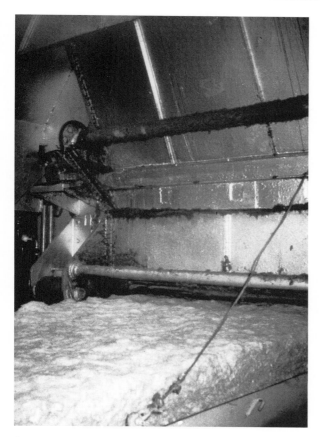

Figure 39.4 *Man-made mineral fibre production. Rock wool plant.*

main types of fibres, namely glass fibres (continuous filament and glass wool) as well as slag wool and rock wool (see Chapter 35). The results have not shown any increase in mortality or cancer incidence throughout almost all segments of the MMVF-producing industry, though the number of workers followed up for more than 30 years is still not large.

An excess of lung cancer has been observed after 30 years of follow-up of workers involved in the production of slag wool and rock wool (the two not being separated). The excess could not be ruled out on the basis of likely confounding and biases and it supports the inference that MMVF, at least as present in the environmental conditions of the past slagwool/rock-wool production, may indeed have played a role in the causation of lung cancer. The limitation of the current epidemiological evidence stems mainly from the small number of events (lung cancer) observed and the lack of reliable estimates of past MMVF exposure.

FORMALDEHYDE[34–36]

This chemical, widely used in industry and commercial products, has been shown in bioassay to cause nasal tumours in rats (see Chapter 11). Over 30 reports from epidemiological studies on formaldehyde have been published and included in recent reviews. The studies include both cohort investigations of professional workers, anatomists, pathologists and embalmers and studies of industrial workers at a variety of chemical plants, exposed to formaldehyde. For lung cancer some small excess appeared to be inconsistent between and even within studies, particularly with respect to the relationship with duration and level of exposure, making it difficult to attribute them to exposure to formaldehyde. Excesses have been observed for nasopharyogeal cancer in two cohort and three case-control studies and for nasal cancers in two studies. Some other studies were negative but they had small power to detect increases in such a rare type of tumour. On the other hand, in some of the positive studies an exposure response gradient was apparent. These findings, jointly with the consideration that nasal and nasopharyngeal cancers occur at direct contact sites of formaldehyde (a highly reactive compound at the level of the first encountered respiratory mucosae), make a causal explanation plausible. Still, the epidemiological evidence is limited essentially by the consideration that the role of confounders, especially other particulars (e.g. wood in some studies), cannot at present be completely ruled out.

THE CLINICAL APPROACH

Whilst considerable attention is given in other chapters of this book to the clinical presentation and management of occupational diseases, such an approach is unlikely to be so helpful here. As a general rule, cancers that are of occupational origin are not distinguishable from non-occupational cancers whether in clinical features, natural history, pathological findings or other special investigations. A patient with lung or bladder cancer due to occupational factors will be diagnosed in the same way and using the same procedures as one without occupational factors. Where distinguishing features are relevant, they will be cited in the text.

However, one feature which has been noted with a number of occupationally related tumours is the possibility that the occupational cancer may present earlier than the non-occupational varieties. Thus a patient aged 45 years with bladder cancer or one in his 30s with lung cancer – particularly if there is no history of tobacco consumption – should heighten the suspicion of the clinician that this might be an occupationally related tumour. For rarer tumours such as angiosarcoma of the liver, pleural or peritoneal mesthelioma and nasal sinus cancer, for example, the occupational causes may outweigh the chances of finding such a tumour from other causes – known or unknown. The clinician thus needs to be aware of these varieties and their close links with occupation.

The next question is what to include and what to leave out and whether to classify tumours by site and agent or to list the agents relevant to the site. For the first we will concentrate on the more common tumours in clinical practice but also include rarer ones where the occupational component is particularly relevant. This approach is followed in this section of the chapter in which attention is not necessarily given to all occupational agents capable, or presumably capable, of causing cancer at a given site, but rather is focused on those likely to be of more practical impact for the clinician, either for their frequency or for the problems they pose in ascertaining exposure or both. On the second point, an attempt is made to include the known workplace carcinogens, with a note on their target organs for neoplastic effects. This includes both single agents and, when the precise identification of single agents has not yet proved possible, complex mixtures or industrial processes. For the interested reader, Alderson's encyclopaedic book on occupational cancer[37] is worth reviewing. It is rather old now but there is no more recent book of equivalent scope.

Finally, two practical points about investigating a patient with suspected occupational cancer. First, these investigations can be very time consuming. Not only is it necessary to obtain a detailed lifetime occupational history in order to clarify whether a workplace factor is responsible for the tumour – and, if so, which one(s) – but it is also necessary to ask about workmates who may have a similar disease. In our experience a patient with an occupational disease is rarely, if ever, an isolated finding. Few patients are uniquely exposed at work and thus a case of occupational cancer should be assessed to be, in effect, the index case of what might turn out, on further enquiry, to be a cluster of cases.

The second point is that the clinician should, if possible, acquire information about the worksite either directly from the occupational health service or, if this is not possible or not sanctioned by the patient, make enquiries from the employer about the job and about any other relevant workplace exposures which might cast some light on the suspected association with occupation. Whilst textbooks may help here, much useful assistance can be gained from talking to the local representatives of the national government agency responsible for health and safety at work. In the UK this is the Employment Medical Advisory Service of the Health and Safety Executive. They might confirm the clinical suspicion or the enquiries may stimulate their investigations, locally and nationally, for further cases in similar workplaces. Where available, academic departments of occupational health serve a similar function and should be capable of providing the clinician with a second opinion on the case, as well as literature searches for published evidence of occupational risks for that cancer site in addition to information on whether the suspect agent or process has been reported to be linked with tumours at that site.

Your case might be yet another example of an occupa-

tional cancer already extensively reported in the specialist literature. It might, however, be the first case.

Specific tumour sites

RESPIRATORY SYSTEM

Numerically, lung cancer is the most important tumour to present to the clinician. It is the most common malignancy in men, and its association with tobacco consumption requires no further emphasis here. It is important to note, however, that certain workplace exposures that cause respiratory tumours may act additively or even synergistically with cigarette exposure. Further details of this effect are described in the section **The role of interactions** (p. 814). In particular, asbestos and cigarette consumption is, perhaps, the best known example of interaction in occupational health, as the two agents have a multiplicative effect on the risk of developing lung cancer.

Although the clinician might seem to be looking for a needle in a haystack when contemplating occupational factors for yet another lung cancer case, it is worth noting that estimates for occupational attributability vary between 0.6 and 40%, depending on the place, and the time.[38] Of the occupational exposures, the most potent agents are probably asbestos fibres and the chloromethyl ethers.

For the clinician, the presenting features of lung cancer are all too well known and the confirmatory investigations usually demonstrate extensive and often inoperable spread at the time of diagnosis. The prognosis is frequently poor. Histopathologically, 90% of all lung carcinomata are covered by four main categories: squamous, small cell, large cell and adenocarcinoma. Attempts to tease out a relationship between histopathology and putative lung carcinogens have not proved particularly successful but some pointers are available from the authoritative review of Ives et al.[39] For example, adenocarcinoma or small cell carcinoma predominate in beryllium-exposed cases, whilst small cell types are in excess in uranium miners and in patients with exposure to bis(chloromethyl) ether.

Recent reviews of occupational lung carcinogenesis,[40–42] suggest that there are a number of proven causes that can be determined from the literature:

- *Individual agents*
Arsenic compounds
Asbestos
Bis(chloromethyl) ether
Beryllium compounds
Cadmium compounds
Chromium[VI] compounds
Crystalline silica
Ionizing radiation
Mustard gas

Nickel compounds
Radon and its decay products

- *Complex mixtures*
Coal tars
Coal-tar pitches
Soots
Tobacco smoke, including environmental tobacco
   smoke

- *Exposure circumstances*
Aluminium production
Coal gasification
Coke production
Iron and steel founding
Isopropyl alcohol manufacture
Painting

Such a list is less extensive than many but even as it stands it begs some questions. Arsenic exposure these days can occur in smelting metalliferous ores or manufacturing certain pesticides. As for nickel, it is in nickel refining that the excess risk of lung (and nasal sinus) cancer has been observed. The precise compound has not been fully elucidated but the available evidence points to the carcinogenicity of nickel sulphate and of the combination of nickel sulphides and oxides encountered in the nickel refining industry (see Chapter 7). However, an exhaustive review of the processes, feedstock and procedures at the Clydach nickel refinery in South Wales over a 70-year period suggests that the main culprit in the lung and nasal cancer excess might be nickel arsenide. For chromium, it appears that the sparingly soluble hexavalent chromium compounds are the culprits and, of these, the pigments, strontium, calcium and zinc chromate seem to be the most potent. Some recent evidence of excess lung cancer in chrome platers[43] suggests that chromic acid may be carcinogenic to humans as well. Ionizing radiation exposure also subsumes many studies of underground miners of metalliferous ores where relevant exposure is probably related to radon gas. These include uranium, haematite and exposures in tin mining.

The interest in the carcinogenicity of the chloromethyl ethers (which are of importance in the production of ion exchange resins), is out of proportion to their incidence. These chemicals seem to be particularly potent lung carcinogens, producing symptomatic neoplastic change in as short a latency period as 10–15 years, and with relative risks for heavily exposed workers as high as 20-fold. Their apparent association with small cell carcinoma has already been noted. (Lung cancer due to exposure to bis(chloromethyl) ether is a prescribed disease) (see Chapter 4).

Polynuclear aromatic hydrocarbons are well known lung (and skin) carcinogens and their presence in soot, tar, pitch and petroleum product exhaust fumes provides a potential opportunity for a wide variety of workplace exposures. The relevant worksites include gas retort and coke oven processes (see Fig. 39.5), the steel industry, the printing industry, aluminium refining sites, iron and steel foundries as well as the motor vehicle transport industry and possibly the rubber industry. Chimney sweeping has re-emerged as an occupation at risk of cancer, as recent studies in Sweden[44] and Denmark[45] have shown a lung cancer excess in chimney sweeps. Welders are potentially exposed to a wide variety of gases and fumes, including nickel, chromium (VI) and nitrogen oxides.[46]

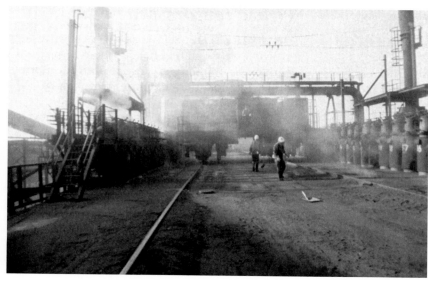

Figure 39.5 *Topside coke oven workers.*

Other agents or processes suspected of causing lung cancer include:

- *Agents*

Acrylonitrile
Antimony compounds
Chlorinated toluenes
Cobalt compounds
Diesel engine exhaust
Formaldehyde
Inorganic strong acid mists (containing sulphuric acid)
Man-made vitreous fibres
Vinyl chloride monomer
Welding fumes

- *Exposure circumstances*

Butchering
Vineyard working
Pulp and paper manufacture

A few examples from these lists illustrate some interesting clinical points. The evidence for beryllium being a lung carcinogen rests largely on the excess risk associated with relatively short (1–5 years) exposure and a latency period of two decades. Some authorities doubted the biological relevance of such short exposures but it appears that these exposures were short because the affected individuals developed acute berylliosis. The exposures would therefore have been high and the inhaled dose, if not readily removed, could have lain there long enough to induce neoplastic change.

The question of formaldehyde is more vexed. There is no doubt that formaldehyde is a respiratory tract irritant and that it is a rat respiratory carcinogen by the inhalational route. Nevertheless, a review of the human epidemiological studies provides no conclusive proof of carcinogenicity. The International Programme on Chemical Safety (IPCS) review in 1989[35] sums up the situation succinctly:

> The available human evidence indicates that formaldehyde does not have a high carcinogenic potential. Given the relative rarity of tumours in the biologically plausible area of the upper respiratory tract and the widespread past occupational exposures to formaldehyde in various work situations, it can be concluded that formaldehyde is, at most, a weak human carcinogen.

Silicosis is dealt with in Chapter 35, but recent research has raised the spectre of lung cancer excess in silica-exposed workers. More precisely, the excess seems to be found in silicotics but not in silica-exposed workers without silicosis. Whether this simply reflects an average higher exposure to silica among the silicotics the role of fibrosis or itself as an intermediate stage in the causation of cancer remains unclear.

Of equal concern to industry in general has been the assertion that acid mists can give rise to lung cancer.[47] The excess exists after adjusting for smoking but no trend with duration of exposure was found. Previous studies have suggested a link with laryngeal cancer. The importance here lies in the widespread industrial exposure associated with acid mists – particularly sulphuric acid.

Finally, mention must be made of the controversy surrounding the carcinogenic potential of the asbestos substitute products such as synthetic mineral fibres, which is discussed in greater detail on p. 802. For the clinician, it may well emerge that a worker with a history of using the newer insulation material was, in a previous job, using the older insulation products – namely, asbestos. This may even apply to those engaged in manufacture rather than use.

Many of the above assertions on occupations are disputed and the arguments revolve around the quality of the human epidemiological studies. Nevertheless, the clinician has plenty of occupational aetiologies to consider even when contemplating the cause of a common tumour predominantly associated with cigarette smoking.

Consideration of the rest of the respiratory system also provides evidence of occupational cancer risks. The pleural mesotheliomata need little further comment here but is it worth noting that there is no evidence that man-made vitreous fibres cause this malignancy. Nasal sinus cancer has also been associated with workplace exposure. Classically this was noted in the 1950s in nickel refiners who had worked at the Clydach plant in South Wales before certain process changes occurred in the late 1920s. Mention has been made earlier of the risk of ethmoid sinus cancer in furniture makers in Buckinghamshire. This study led to a major epidemiological exercise involving data linkage in the Oxford region. A further cluster of mixed cell type, mixed-site sinus cancers, emerged in the Northampton area, thus leading to the assertion that leather goods manufacture – in particular, boots and shoes – carried a risk of neoplasia. For neither the furniture nor the shoe industry has a specific carcinogen been identified but the evidence for wood workers points mainly towards hard wood dust (Figs 39.6, 39.7).

For laryngeal cancer there are the well known associations with smoking and alcohol – and, as previously noted, probably with strong inorganic acid mists. Asbestos exposure is also thought by many to be a risk factor for laryngeal malignancy.

DIGESTIVE SYSTEM

Emphasis here will be placed on the occupational neoplastic risks for stomach, liver and pancreas. For the stomach, the main clinical epidemiological features of note are the falling incidence of the condition in developed countries, which has been linked to better nutrition. Nitrosamines which are proven and potent animal carcinogens have been linked to human exposure in that the secondary amines in fish and preserved meat and vegetables could be converted to nitrosamines by gastric hydrochloric acid. For strictly occupational exposures, no clear evidence emerges of links to stomach cancer. A number of large-scale, multi-site cancer studies have sometimes shown links with lead exposure, coal mining and the rubber industry (? linked to dust exposure) but the evidence is not convincing. Recent studies[48] have sug-

gested a link between strong mineral acid mists and aerodigestive cancers (that is, lip, tongue, larynx, pharynx). This finding is biologically plausible given the earlier studies showing an excess risk of laryngeal cancer associated with sulphuric acid mists.

For the liver, hepatitis B and C viruses and aflatoxins (see Chapters 24, 43) have been shown to be risk factors for hepatocellular carcinoma. Among the occupational exposures that are suspected to cause hepatocellular carcinoma are polychlorinated biphenyls and trichloroethylene: the available evidence, however, does not allow firm conclusions. The rare angiosarcoma is known to be associated with exposure to vinyl chloride monomer as well as arsenic and the use of thorium dioxide (Thorotrast®) in biliary tract radiography of earlier days.

For the pancreas, occupational exposures associated with cancer include studies of chemists and also radiologists. In the latter case, the excess risk appears to be for those exposed before 1929. This cohort effect may thus be a legacy of earlier, less well controlled workplace exposures although the absence of such a finding from other large scale studies of workers exposed to ionizing radiation weakens the assertion that this physical agent alone was the responsible carcinogen. Among the chemical agents suspected to cause pancreatic cancer are some chlorinated organic solvents and chlorinated pesticides, including DDT (dichlorodiphenyltrichloroethane).

Occupational exposures have rarely been implicated in colorectal cancers. There has, however, been a recent flurry of interest in whether workers in the polypropylene production industry could be at increased risk. However, earlier cluster reports appear not to be confirmed on further review.[49] Intriguingly, a recent report suggests a tentative association between colorectal cancer

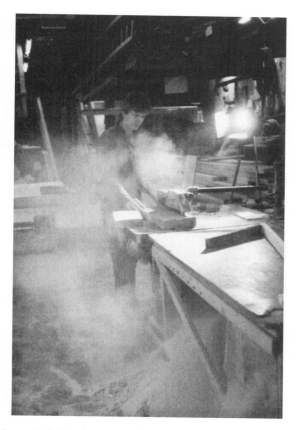

Figure 39.6 *Circular saw cutting hardwood – before exhaust ventilation.*

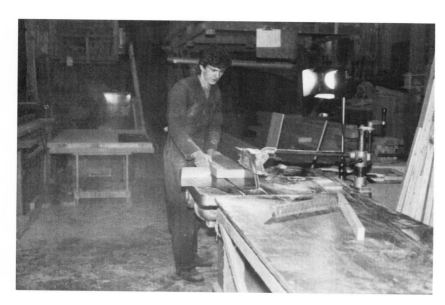

Figure 39.7 *Circular saw cutting hardwood – after exhaust ventilation.*

and the manufacture of the antiknock agent, tetraethyl lead.[50] One of the few established risk factors of colon cancer, however, is lack of physical activity: since occupation is one of the main determinants of physical exercise in adult populations, it can be indirectly implicated in the causation of this neoplasm.

THE SKIN

Skin cancer associated with occupation was the earliest of the observations in occupational health to show a clear-cut neoplastic risk. Exposures to mixtures of polynuclear aromatic hydrocarbons produce, in the main, squamous cell or basal cell tumours. An association with ultraviolet light, particularly in fair-skinned people, has also been noted in studies of outdoor workers.

The situation with malignant melanoma is particularly interesting. An association with fair skin and naevi is well known.[51] There is, however, no doubt that this is one of the few malignancies that is showing a true increase in incidence rate in recent years. Geographical epidemiological studies also reveal a link here with sunlight for Australia, the USA and Canada but for Europe the picture is less clear. For example, the Nordic countries and Switzerland have higher incidence rates than France or Italy.[2] The explanation almost certainly lies in recreational or intermittent exposure to sunlight and this is supported by a strong social class gradient in risk, with higher rates among the non-manual, professional classes. There is now some suggestion that melanoma mortality has plateaued in Australia.[52] A new slant on this contention comes from a recent study of US Navy personnel[53] where the highest rates were in the 'indoor' personnel and the lowest rates in those with jobs requiring time to be spent both indoors and outdoors. The authors suggest that there is a protective role associated with brief regular exposure to sunlight due to the possible influence of vitamin D as a factor in suppressing the growth of malignant melanoma.

An Anglo-Swedish study[54] of nearly 4000 cancer registration cases noted the highest risks in the higher socioeconomic groups, which may be associated with greater opportunities for travel for the more affluent. Interestingly, the highest incidence ratios were found for airline pilots, raising the twin aetiological factors of travel to hot countries and in-flight ultraviolet irradiation, though the latter is supposedly unlikely in view of the cockpit shielding.

A new slant on the role of ultraviolet light in the causation of cutaneous malignancy is the finding in several studies of a higher incidence of non-Hodgkin's lymphoma in individuals diagnosed earlier to have a skin cancer. This might explain the association of agricultural work and an increased incidence of this lymphoma variety and the mechanism may be one of immune suppression by ultraviolet light.[55]

BRAIN

Brain tumours show a bimodal frequency distribution with a small peak in childhood and a second, larger, peak in the seventh decade. The majority of adult malignant tumours are astrocytomata or undifferentiated glioblastomata. Mortality rates are rising in developed countries but this may be, at least in part, due to improved accuracy of certification.

Occupational factors have been invoked in recent years. Reviews[56,57] suggested that both professional and manual occupations had been reported to be at increased risk. These include; laboratory workers, petrochemical plant workers and embalmers.

Certain, possibly multiple, chemical exposures may be common features. These include certain organic solvents, as well as ionizing radiation.

Recent additions to this list might include lead[58] but the greatest interest of late has centred around the possibility that electric fields or magnetic fields (or both) from residential or occupational exposure might be associated with an increased risk of brain tumours. Thorough reviews of residential exposure studies[59] and meta-analysis of the brain cancer risks from occupational exposures[60] have failed to resolve the issue. Studies subsequent to these reviews have not clarified this putative risk.[61]

URINARY BLADDER (see Chapter 12)

Bladder cancer is the eighth most common malignancy in men, accounting for about 5% of all cancers world wide. The highest incidences are in white populations in North America and north-western Europe. The majority are transitional cell tumours. Early detection of the tumours has greatly improved the survival rates although incidence rates are continuing to rise. Tobacco consumption is the main lifestyle risk factor in Western countries.

Lung cancer and bladder cancer are among the few occupational cancer sites for which there have been serious attempts at estimating occupational attribution.[62] Depending upon the study and the degree of stringency applied to the attributability, the range is 2–24% with most estimates around 20%. The industries that figure most prominently are rubber (Figs 39.8 and 39.9), dyestuffs (Fig. 39.10) and gas. Other industries identified as carrying an excess risk but not necessarily of the same order include textiles, leather, painting and construction work.[63]

The specific carcinogens that figure most prominently are the aromatic amine benzidine based dyes such as 2-naphthylamine, benzidine, 4-aminobiphenyl and the curing agent 4,4'-methylene bis(2-chloroaniline) as well as unknown (complex) mixtures associated with the manufacture of auramine, and the manufacture of magenta. Other suspect dyestuff carcinogens[64] include p-chloro-o-toluidine, 3, 3'-dichlorobenzidine and o-diani-

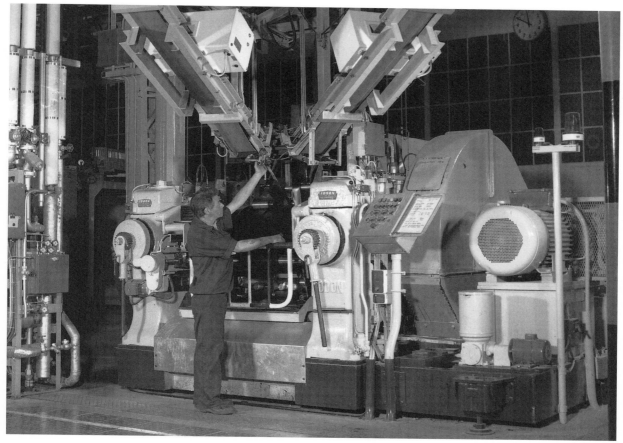

Figure 39.8 *Rubber tyre production – a modern two-roll mill fed from an extruder.*

sidine. There are many more for which animal carcinogenicity is proven but for which human data are not available (see p. 229).

From a clinical point of view, bladder cancer due to occupation frequently occurs 10–15 years earlier than in the general population and some researchers have postulated that occupation-related bladder cancer may have a different natural history with, possibly, a greater incidence of carcinoma *in situ*.[65] Such an observation, if true, provides an opportunity to screen exposed workers at an early stage. The arguments continue to rage, however, on the value of urinary cytology in improving the final prognosis.[66]

One final point: the link between tobacco consumption (presumably polynuclear aromatic hydrocarbons (PAH) exposure) and bladder cancer has led investigators to look at other workplace sources of combustion gases, soots and pitch-tar volatiles. Such work has shown an excess of bladder cancer in truck drivers, chimney sweeps and dry cleaners.[67] The evidence is particularly strong for linking PAH exposures in aluminium pot room workers with bladder cancer.[68,69]

HAEMOPOIETIC SYSTEM

Tumours of the blood-forming organs make up a complex group in which frequent changes in the nomenclature seem to add to the complexity. Ionizing radiation is associated with non-lymphocytic leukaemia, multiple myeloma and non-Hodgkin's lymphoma. The last-named disease has also been associated with phenoxy acid herbicides, some chlorinated organic compounds such as trichloroethylene, tetrachloroethylene and polychlorinated biphenyls and, more recently, with solar ultraviolet radiation.[55] The main occupational exposures with any degree of certainty of neoplastic effect are, however, associated with leukaemia.

Leukaemia

Except for the excess risk of myelogenous leukaemia noted with exposure to ionizing radiation (see Chapter 19), the best established workplace exposure is from benzene.[70–72] (*Note*: Benzene should not be confused with benzine which is another name for petrol.) There is no doubt that benzene causes acute myelocytic leukaemia – it may also cause other varieties. What is in question is the potency of that effect which, of course, influences the workplace exposure limits which should be enforced to ensure a 'safe' concentration. Substitution by another chemical is not an option in most circumstances given the central role that benzene plays in most of the aromatic organic chemical and petroleum production industries. Workplace exposures identified as being

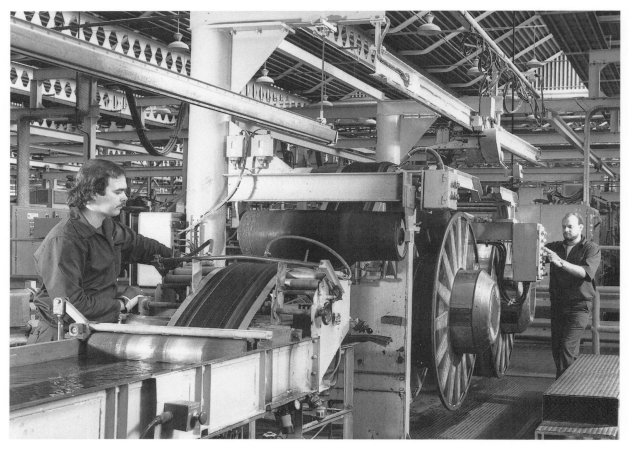

Figure 39.9 *Tyre thread with extrusion, cooling and wind-up in sequence.*

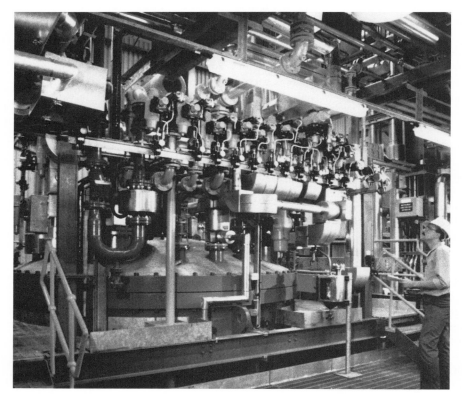

Figure 39.10 *A modern totally enclosed dyestuff plant.*

associated with a leukaemia risk – at least in the past – include much of the petrochemical industry. A variety of other chemicals have been implicated as possible leukaemogens. Apart from the antineoplastic drugs the most frequently cited chemicals are styrene, butadiene, epichlorhydrin and ethylene oxide. The source studies are often small, however, or the workplace exposures are confounded by benzene.

Of special interest is the consistent finding of an increased risk of leukaemia associated with 'electrical' occupations.[73] Whilst electricians, telephone, radio and telegraphic staff are potentially exposed to a number of volatile solvents and resins, much interest has now centred on the possible role of electromagnetic field exposure in the leukaemogenic process (see Chapter 21). These relationships have been studied extensively in the past few years. Improved exposure assessments and control of confounding factors has enhanced the quality of the latest studies. Nevertheless, a recent review suggests that although these studies provide some support for the hypothesis of an association between magnetic field exposure and adult leukaemia, especially for chronic lymphocytic leukaemia, inconsistencies within and between the studies weaken the evidence, and no firm conclusion can be reached at present.[74]

The investigation of a possible occupational aetiology for the leukaemia patient can frequently be a difficult one. In our experience, whilst the disease is in no doubt, the exclusion of cytotoxic drug exposure as well as benzene and ionizing radiation provides little opportunity for further progress. An attempt by one of us to look into the possible volatile exposures that might face a telephone engineer produced a bewildering array of organic chemicals with little or no evidence from literature searches for any link with the disease. Nevertheless, the patients are frequently younger than many with occupationally associated cancers and the failure to identify a causative agent is frustrating for the physician and harrowing for the patient.

Conclusions

It should be evident from this account that a search for occupational factors is worth pursuing for many of the more common cancers even though, for some, lifestyle factors are the predominant aetiological agent. For others, workplace exposures may be of particular relevance whilst the possibility of interaction between lifestyle and occupational factors may need to be considered. From the patient's point of view there may be considerable relief in knowing that there is a specific cause for the cancer – whatever the prognosis might be. For the physician, such a discovery will mean further enquiries of the patient's workmates and a search for similar exposures elsewhere. This could lead to an earlier diagnosis in subsequent cases, with the possibility, at certain sites, of a better prognosis. In any event, the discovery of a new workplace carcinogen would lead to the possibility of preventing further generations from harmful exposure.

OCCUPATIONAL CARCINOGENIC AGENTS AND PROCESSES

Tables 39.1 and 39.2 summarize, in our view, the current state of knowledge for known human carcinogens with a strong occupational component. Table 39.1 lists the chemicals or processes considered to be of proven carcinogenic potential. Table 39.2 lists the occupations recognized as presenting a carcinogenic risk to employees.

For some of the processes no specific agent has been identified. For the process, or agent, the human target organs of known (or suggested) importance are listed. Ascertaining that a patient has worked in an industrial process listed here should prompt the clinician to enquire if the patient has worked with any of the agents mentioned in these tables.

Other published lists may be longer (or shorter). Ours is based on Volume 1–70 of the IARC Monograph series published between 1971 and 1999.

ATTRIBUTION OF CANCER RISKS TO OCCUPATIONAL CAUSES

Global and local estimates

As indicated on p. 794, currently the most widely accepted estimates of the proportion of all cancers attributable to occupational exposures range from about 2 to about 8% for a typical industrially developed country such as the USA, these percentages being dependent not only on the frequency of cancers actually caused by occupational exposures but also on the frequency of cancers due to other causes such as tobacco smoking, alcohol or diet. Also, these figures refer to the whole population. They carry the implication that in the 20% or so of the population in which the occupationally related cancers are almost exclusively concentrated (manual workers aged 20 and over, in mining, agriculture and industry broadly defined, numbering 31 million out of a total US population of 158 million aged 20 and over),[75] as much as one cancer in every five may be attributable to exposure in the workplace. However, what the law regards as cancer related to occupation markedly varies even within industrialized countries[76] and certainly there is a wide variation in the medical recognition and in the (under) reporting of occupational cancers. These global population estimates of the fraction of cancers caused by occupational exposures are indirect generalizations derived by combining the proportions of cancers at different sites presumptively

Table 39.1 *IARC list of group 1 carcinogens (1999) (Vols 1–70)*

Chemicals and mixtures	Industrial processes	Medicinals	Other
4-Amino biphenyl	Aluminium production	Azathioprine	Aflatoxins
Arsenic and arsenic compounds	Auramine (manufacture)	N,N-Bis(2-chloroethyl) ether	Alcohol
Asbestos	Coal gasification	2-Naphthylamine	Betel nut (with tobacco)
Benzene	Coke production	Chlorambucil	Solar radiation
Benzidine	Haematite mining (underground, with radon exposure)	Cyclosporin	Tobacco
BCME		Cyclophosphamide	
Beryllium and beryllium compounds	Iron and steel founding	Melphalan	
CMME	Isopropyl alcohol manufacture (strong acid process)	Methyl CCNU	
Cadmium and cadmium compounds		MOPP	
Chromium compounds (hexavalent)	Magenta (manufacture)	Myleran	
Coal tar pitches	Painting	Oestrogens (some steroidal and non-steroidal)	
Coal tars	Rubber industry	Oral contraceptive (combinations)	
Dioxin (TCDD)	Wood (furniture and cabinet making)	Phenacetin (in analgesic mixtures)	
Erionite	Boot and shoe manufacture	Tamoxifen[a]	
Ethylene oxide		Thiotepa	
Inorganic acid mists (strong) containing sulphuric acid		Treosulfan	
Mineral oils (untreated and mildly treated)			
Mustard gas			
2-Naphthylamine			
Nickel compounds			
Radon (and its decay products)			
Shale oils			
Silica (crystalline)			
Soots			
Talc (containing asbestos)			
Vinyl chloride			

[a] Tamoxifen also exerts preventive activity.
BCME: Bis(chloromethyl) ether.
CMME: Chloromethyl methyl ether.
TCDD: 2,3,7,8-tetrachlorodibenzo-p-dioxin.
Melthyl CCNU: 1-(2-chloroethyl)-3-(4-methylcyclohexyl)-1-nitrosurea.

attributable to occupational factors on the basis of selected epidemiological studies. A more pertinent and direct approach has been subsequently applied to bladder and lung cancer by reviewing systematically all available and informative published studies and calculating the attributable proportions for each of them.

What this analysis has shown is that there is a substantial variability in the percentages of cancers at these two sites which can be attributed to occupational exposures. For instance, as noted on p. 806, for lung cancer (based on 16 mostly case-control studies in five countries in western Europe and North America)[38] the proportion varies widely from less than 1% to 40% for some of the general populations resident in the areas where the studies were located. Clearly it appears that the estimates

are strictly time- and place-dependent and certainly do not represent the true proportion of lung cancer due to occupational exposures in the general population at national level. This high variability, reflecting the local variability of occupational exposures, demands great caution when interpreting any estimate at the level of the general population of whole countries or large regions.

The role of interactions

In the presence of interactions between causative agents, a proportion of cancers will need to be attributed to both of the interacting agents, thus making the theoretical total of all attributable proportions greater than 100%; if

Table 39.2 *Occupations recognized as presenting a carcinogenic risk*

Industry	Occupation	Site of tumour	Likely carcinogen
Agriculture, forestry, fishing	Farmers, seamen Vineyard workers	Skin, lip Lung, skin	Ultraviolet light Arsenical insecticides
Mining Arseniferous ores	Iron ore miners Tin Asbestos	Lung, skin Lung Lung, bone marrow Lung, pleura and peritoneum	Arsenic compounds Radon decay products Radon decay products Asbestos
Talc; Mining Milling	Uranium miners	Lung Lung	Talc containing asbestiform fibres Radon decay products
Petroleum	Wax pressmen	Scrotum	Polynuclear aromatics
Painting	Painter	Lung, ? bladder	?
Metal	Aluminium production Copper smelting Chromate production Chromium plating Ferrochromium production Iron/steel production/ founding Nickel refining Pickling operations	Bladder, ? lung Lung, ?sino-nasal Lung, ?sino-nasal Lung Lung Lung Sino-nasal, lung Larynx, lung	Polynuclear aromatics Arsenic Chromium (VI) compounds Chromium (VI) compounds Chromium (VI) compounds Benzo[a]pyrene, ? others Nickel compounds Acid mists
Transport	Shipyards	Lung, pleura and peritoneum	Asbestos
Chemicals	BCME and CMME production Vinyl chloride production Isopropyl alcohol (manufacture by strong acid method) Chromate pigment production Dye manufacture and users Auramine manufacture Poison gas manufacturers Inorganic acid mists (strong) containing sulphuric acid	Lung Liver Paranasal sinuses Lung, sino-nasal Bladder Lung Larynx, lung	BCME, CMME Vinylchloride monomer ? Acid mists Chromium (VI) compounds Aromatic amines Mustard gas Sulphuric acid
Pesticides	Arsenical pesticides	Lung	Arsenic compounds
Gas production	Coke plant workers Gas retort house workers	Lung Lung, bladder	Benzo[a]pyrene Benzo[a]pyrene, naphthylamines
Rubber	Rubber manufacture Calendering, tyre curing and tyre building Cable makers, latex producers	Lymphatic and haemopoietic systems, Bladder Lymphatic and haemopoietic systems Bladder	Benzene Aromatic amines Benzene Aromatic amines

Continued

Table 39.2 – *cont.*

Industry	Occupation	Site of tumour	Likely carcinogen
Construction maintenance	Insulators, demolition engineers	Lung, pleura and peritoneum	Asbestos
	Painters	Lung	?
Leather	Boot and shoe makers	Sino-nasal, leukaemia	Leather dust, benzene
Wood pulp and paper	Furniture makers	Sino-nasal	Wood dust
Electric/ electronics	Engineers	Bone marrow, brain	? Fluxes, ?? Electromagnetic fields
Health-care industry	Pharmaceutical manufacturers	Bone marrow	Cytotoxic drugs
	Pharmacists Nurses, Radiologists/ radiographers	Bone marrow	Ionizing radiation
	'Patient carers'	Hepatoma Kaposi's sarcoma Non-Hodgkin's lymphoma	Hepatitis B & C HIV
	Sterilization unit	Lymphatic and haemopoietic systems	Ethylene oxide

BCME: Bis(chloromethyl) ether.
CMME: Chloromethyl melthyl ether.
HIV: Human immunodeficiency virus.

the actual total today falls short of even 100% it is because of our present ignorance of the causes of a sizeable fraction of cancers. This is particularly relevant when considering the relative effectiveness of removing (or reducing) exposure to one or two (or more) jointly acting agents. For instance, in a large cohort study of insulation workers in the USA and Canada[77] the following lung cancer mortality rates (per 100 000 person-years) were observed: 11.3 for subjects exposed to neither asbestos nor tobacco smoke; 58.4 for those exposed to asbestos; 122.6 for those exposed only to tobacco smoke; and 590.3 for subjects exposed to both agents. Owing to the multiplicative interaction of asbestos and smoking, the group exposed to both agents had the highest lung cancer rates, greatly in excess not only over those not exposed to either agent but also over those exposed only to asbestos (the excess rate in the latter group is 47.1, while it is 590.3, i.e. 12.5 times greater, in the group exposed to both agents). Superficially it could be concluded that, since smoking is by far the dominant factor, its removal will be correspondingly far more effective as a preventive measure than asbestos removal. However, this is not true. In fact, if smoking is removed, the fraction (or percentage) of the excess rate removed will be $[(590.3-47.1)/590.3] \times 100 = 92.0\%$, and if asbestos is removed $[(590.3-111.3)/590.3] \times 100 = 81.1\%$. This means that smoking removal is more effective than asbestos removal, but only $92.0/81.1 = 1.13$

times, and not 12.5 times, more effective, as it superficially appeared. The result is not surprising if one considers that the bulk of the effect in subjects exposed to both agents is the result of their positive interaction and is thus removed whichever of the two agents is eliminated; relative to the total effect the fraction due to interaction is $92.0 + 81.1 - 100.0 = 73.1\%$.

Thus, whenever a positive interaction occurs between two (or more) hazardous exposures, there is a greater possibility of effective prevention; the effect of the joint exposure can be attacked in two (or more) ways, each requiring the removal or reduction of one of the exposures; moreover, the larger the size of the interaction relative to the total effect, the more these ways of attack tend to become equal in effectiveness.

Besides asbestos, interactions have been demonstrated between tobacco smoking and several other agents such as arsenic, nickel and ionizing radiation.[78] Most of these interactions are formally multiplicative (namely, the relative risk due to the combined exposure equals the product of the relative risks due separately to each of the agents) or between multiplicative and simply additive. The consequence of multiplicative interaction is that when the relative risk due to one or both the individual agents is low, as might happen under well controlled hygiene conditions, the contribution of the interaction will be unimportant in respect of the contributions of the two agents separately. For instance, if the relative risk due to an occupational exposure is 1.5 and that due to smoking is 10, only 20% of the total effect will be due to the interaction. A much lower and virtually negligible fraction will apply, for instance, to the interactions of environmental tobacco smoke, which in itself may increase the lung cancer risk in those passively exposed by 1.3–1.5. Interactive effects also complicate the attribution of cancers in an individual rather than in a population, a problem of importance in compensation cases; formally probabilistic procedures of causal attribution to each agent are well described in the specialized literature.

PREVENTION

Prevention may be primary or secondary. For primary prevention to be a practical proposition, it is necessary to know of the existence of proven aetiological agents and, then, to know that separation of humans from exposure to the agent is feasible. Secondary prevention usually means early detection of the disease process, and, most important, presumes that early detection will lead to an improved prognosis following treatment.

In this context, there are examples of two regulatory actions that should help. In the UK there is a Code of Practice on Carcinogens in the Control of Substances Hazardous to Health Regulations (1994), whilst in Europe, the sixth 'daughter' Directive (90/394/EEC) concerns some workplace carcinogens – others will doubtless follow.

Primary prevention

In theory, all occupational cancers are preventable in that they result from workplace exposure. All that is required to prevent the disease is elimination of the exposure. Thus, ban the offending agent. In practice, this is less straightforward, for a number of reasons:

1 The exposure may be defined only in terms of a very complex mixture of, for example, chemicals, or as a whole industrial process or even as a section of an industry or a large occupational category ('painters'). This may make it difficult to envisage, apart from general hygiene measurements (often effective in themselves), what more targeted control procedures one could adopt.

2 The substance/process may be perceived to be of great societal importance. Benzene would be a good example here. It is the basic building block for so much of the aromatic organic chemical industry that its 'exclusion' from industry is difficult to conceive. It is also a natural ingredient of fossil fuels and thus would be difficult to eliminate even if the desire to do so were prevalent.

3 The substance has substitutes but substitution is either expensive or the substitutes themselves are not without risk. Asbestos is undoubtedly a major cause of occupational cancer. Some of the more hazardous (amphibole) varieties have been largely excluded from commercial use but chrysotile asbestos has a combination of valuable properties not easily found in synthetic substitutes. Moreover, these substitutes (MMVF) may not be without risk, it appears, partly because of filament size – particularly so for the vitreous varieties where temperature resistance goes hand in hand with persistence in body tissues and fluids and the latter property may be a risk factor for carcinogenesis.

4 The agent itself is of limited economic importance but its presence in an economically important industry is difficult to control. Radon exposure in metalliferous mining serves as an example here: effective control of radon exposure is extremely difficult yet the need to mine for metals in these environments remains.

Nevertheless, the principle remains that reduction of, substitution of, or, ideally, elimination of the known workplace carcinogens would be of great public health importance. The lesson of vinyl chloride monomer shows that exposure to a vital chemical agent can be reduced sufficiently to eliminate a relevant tumour – even if one doubts in theory that a 'threshold' exposure exists. In other cases, such as 2-naphthylamine, purer ingredients or effective substitutes have been formed, thereby reducing workplace-related disease and death. Where exposure, albeit at a reduced level, must continue, efforts should be made to shorten the duration of exposure. Indeed, when all else fails, it has been argued that it may then be a lesser evil to expose more people for shorter periods than fewer people for longer periods, despite the dubious morality of such a practice. It is important to remember that the results of prevention may take decades to be seen. This depends not only on the carcinogenic potential of the agent and the dose/time factor but also on the stage in the carcinogenic process at which the agent acts. The earlier the action, the earlier the effect of reduction of exposure will be recorded.

So far we have concentrated in this section on action against known carcinogenic agents or processes (IARC group 1). We should also consider group 2. For some of these compounds it will never be possible to get the incontrovertible evidence necessary to raise the category to 1. Some degree of uncertainty will remain. Action should not necessarily be delayed. Certainly group 2A agents should be treated as though they entail a cancer risk and preventive action taken accordingly. The higher the degree of uncertainty (as moving from group 2A to group 2B) about a cancer risk, the greater will be cost and feasibility considerations when contemplating control levels of worker exposure.

Secondary prevention

Primary prevention, although ideal, will never in the real world be the answer in every case. Therefore, secondary prevention in the form of early detection of human effect needs to be involved as well (not instead of). On the face of it, the earlier the neoplastic process is detected, the easier it should be to cure the patient. In practice this is not so clear cut. This is not the place to discuss the general question of screening nor to describe in detail the attributes of a good screening test. For this the reader is referred to a review article by Miller.[79] Suffice it to say that, for some cancer sites, screening is effective in leading to better cure/survival rates, whilst for others the case is either not yet proven or, to date, shown to be ineffective. The list below summarizes the current position for some of the more common occupational tumours.

Screening
- *Effective*
  Skin

- *Questionable*
  Bladder

- *Ineffective*
  Lung
  Liver

In summary, the whole purpose of detecting cancer is to cure or prevent other cases of cancer. Discovery of new workplace-related cancers by clinical acumen and the establishment of causative factors by epidemiological study provides the firm scientific basis for vigorous preventive action. Treating the cause of cancer has variable success. Eliminating a known cause ensures that, at least for the future, the need for treatment is obviated.

REFERENCES

1 Saracci R. Neoplasms. In: Holland WW, Detels R. Knox G eds. *Oxford Textbook of Public Health* Vol 3. Oxford: Oxford University Press 1991: 189–208.

2 Tomatis R (ed) *Cancer. Causes, Occurrence and Control*. International Agency for Research on Cancer, Scientific Publications No 100. Lyon: IARC, 1990.

3 Agricola G. *De Re Metallica* (1556) trans. Hoover HC, Hoover LH. New York: Dover Publications, 1950.

4 Ramazzini B. *De Morbis Artificum* (1713) trans. Wright WC. Chicago: University of Chicago Press, 1940.

5 Case RAM, Hosker ME, McDonald DB, Pearson JT. Tumours of the urinary bladder in workmen engaged in the manufacture and use of certain dyestuff intermediates in the British chemical industry. 1. The role of aniline, benzidine, alphanaphthylamine and beta-naphthylamine. *Br J Ind Med* 1954; **11**:75–104.

6 Parkin DM, Laara E, Muir CS. Estimates of the world-wide frequency of sixteen major cancers in 1980. *Int J Cancer* 1985; **41**:184–97.

7 World Health Organization. *Concern for Tomorrow's Future*: Health and Environment in the WHO European Region. WHO European Centre for Environment and WHO WISS. Stuttgard: Vertng and Ges. 1995.

8 Doll R, Peto J. *The Causes of Cancer*. Oxford: Oxford University Press, 1981.

9 Boffetta P. *Estimate of the Number of Cases of Cancer Attributable to Occupational Exposures*. Proceedings of WHO/ILO Expert Panel Group. Lyon: International Agency for Research on Cancer 1997.

10 Armstrong B, Theriault G. Compensating lung cancer patients occupationally exposed to coal tar pitch volatiles. *Occup Environ Med* 1996 **53**:160–7.

11 Hill AB. The environment and disease: association or causation? *Proc R Soc Med* 1965; **58**:295–300.

12 Hernberg S. *Introduction to Occupational Epidemiology*. Michigan: Lavris Publishers Inc, 1992.

13 Checkoway H, Pearce NE, Crawford DT. *Research Methods in Occupational Epidemiology*. New York: Oxford University Press, 1989.

14 International Agency for Research on Cancer. Monographs on the evaluation of carcinogenic risks to humans: 4. *Some Aromatic Amines, Hydrazine and Related Substances, N-nitroso Compounds and Miscellaneous Alkylating Agents*. Lyon: IARC, 1974.

15 International Agency for Research on Cancer. Monographs on the evaluation of carcinogenic risks to humans: 7. *Some Anti-Thyroid and Related Substances, Nitrofurans and Industrial Chemicals*. Lyon: IARC, 1974.

16 International Agency for Research on Cancer. Monographs on the evaluation of carcinogenic risks to humans: 14. *Asbestos*. Lyon: IARC, 1977.

17 Vigliani EC, Saita ST. Benzene and leukaemia. *N Engl J Med* 1964; **271**:872–6.

18 Swerdlow AJ. Effectiveness of primary prevention of occupational exposures on cancer risk. In: Hakama M, Beral V, Cullen JW, Parkin DM eds. *Evaluating Effectiveness of Primary Prevention of Cancer*. International Agency for Research on Cancer, Scientific Publications No 103. Lyon: IARC, 1990: 23–56.

19 Heath CW, Falk H Jr, Creech JL. Characteristics of cases of angiosarcoma of the liver among vinyl chloride workers in the United States. *Ann N Y Acad Sci* 1975; **246**:231–6.

20 Registrar General Office of Population Censuses and Surveys. *Registrar General's Decennial Supplement for England and Wales. Occupational Mortality. 1931; 1951; 1961; 1970–72, 1979–80 and 1982–90*. London: HMSO, 1938, 1958, 1971, 1978, 1995.

21 Blot WJ, Fraumeni IF Jr. Geographic patterns of lung cancer: industrial correlations. *Am J Epidemiol* 1976; **103**:539–50.

22 Smith TJ, Stewart PA Herrick RF. Retrospective exposure assessment. In: Harrington JM, Gardiner K eds. *Occupational Hygiene* 2nd edn. Oxford: Blackwell Science, 1995.

23 Boffetta P, Saracci R (eds). *Proceedings of the Conference on Retrospective Assessment of Occupational Exposures in Epidemiology: Occupational Hygiene* 1996, **1–3**:1–208.

24 Schulte PA, Perera FP (eds). *Molecular Epidemiology, Principles and Practice*. New York: Academic Press, Inc, 1993.

25 International Agency for Research on Cancer. Monographs on the evaluation of carcinogenic risks to humans: 1–70. Lyon: IARC, 1972–1999.

26 Selikoff IJ, Lee DHK. *Asbestos and Disease*. New York: Academic Press, 1978.

27 Doll R. Peto J. *Effects on Health of Exposure to Asbestos*. London: Health and Safety Commission 1985.

28 Bignon J, Peto J, Saracci R (eds). *Non-occupational Exposure to Mineral Fibres*. International Agency for Research on Cancer, Scientific Publications No 90. Lyon: IARC, 1989.

29 International Agency for Research on Cancer. Monographs on the evaluation of carcinogenic risks to humans. *Overall Evaluations of Carcinogenicity: An Updating of IARC Monographs Vols 1–42*, Suppl. 7. Lyon: IARC, 1987.

30 Simonato L, L'Abbé KA, Andersen A *et al*. A collaborative study of cancer incidence and mortality among vinyl chloride workers. *Scand J Work Environ Hlth* 1991; **17**:159–69.

31 International Agency for Research on Cancer. Monographs on the evaluation of carcinogenic risks for humans: 47. *Some Organic Solvents, Resin Monomers and Related Compounds, Pigments and Occupational Exposures in Paint Manufacture and Painting*. Lyon: IARC, 1989.

32 International Agency for Research on Cancer. Monographs on the evaluation of carcinogenic risks for humans: 43. *Man-made Mineral Fibres and Radon*. Lyon: IARC, 1988.

33 Boffetta R, Saracci P, Anderson A, Bertazzi PA, Chang-Claude J *et al*. Cancer morality among man-made vitreous fibre production workers. *Epidemiology* 1997; **8**:259–68.

34 International Agency for Research on Cancer. Monographs on the evaluation of carcinogenic risks for humans: 62. *Wood Dust and Formaldehyde*. Lyon: IARC, 1995.

35 International Programme on Chemical Safety (IPCS). *Formaldehyde. Environmental Health Criteria* 89. Geneva: World Health Organization, 1989.

36 Blair A, Saracci, R. Stewart PA, Stayner LT, Hayes RB, Shy C. Formaldehyde exposure and cancer: review of the epidemiologic evidence. *Scand J Work Environ Hlth* 1990; **16**:381–93.

37 Alderson M. *Occupational Cancer*. London: Butterworth, 1986.

38 Vineis P, Simonato L. Proportion of lung and baldder cancers in males resulting from occupation: a systematic approach. *Arch Environ Hlth* 1991; **46**:6–15.

39 Ives JC, Buffler PA, Greenberg DS. Environmental association and histopathologic patterns of carcinoma of the lung. The challenge and dilemma in epidemiological studies. *Am Rev Respir Dis* 1983; **128**:195–209.

40 Harrington JM, Levy LS. Lung cancer. In: Parkes WR ed. *Occupational Lung Disorders* 3rd edn. London: Butterworth-Heinemann, 1993.

41 Boffetta P, Saracci R. Occupational factors of lung cancer. In: Hirsch A, Goldberg M, Martin J-P, Masse R eds. *Prevention of Respiratory Diseases*. New York: Marcel Dekker, 1993: 37–63.

42 Steenland K, Loomis D, Shy C, Simonsen N. Review of occupation lung carcinogens. *Am J Ind Med* 1996 **29**:474–90.

43 Sorahan T, Burges DCL, Hamilton L, Harrington JM. Lung cancer mortality in nickel/chromium platers, 1946–1995. *Occup Environ Med* 1988; **55**: 236–42.

44 Gustavsson P, Gustavsson A, Hogstedt C. Excess of cancer in Swedish chimney sweeps. *Br J Ind Med* 1988; **45**:777–81.

45 Hansen E Mortality from cancer and ischemic heart disease in Danish chimney sweeps: a five year follow up. *Am J Epidemiol* 1983; **117**:160–4.

46 Lauritsen JM, Hansen KS. Lung cancer mortality in stainless steel and mild steel welders: A nested case control study. *Am J Ind Med* 1996 **30**:383–91.

47 International Agency for Research on Cancer. Monographs on the evaluation of carcinogenic risks for humans: 54. *Occupational Exposures to Mists and Vapours from Strong Inorganic Acid and Other Industrial Chemicals*. Lyon: IARC, 1992.

48 Coggon D, Pannett B, Weild G. Upper aerodigestive cancer in battery manufacture and steel workers exposed to mineral acid mists. *Occup Environ Med* 1996; **53**:445–9.

49 Legast H, Tomenson J, Stringer DA. Polypropylene production and colorectal cancer: a review of the epdiemiological evidence *Occup Med* 1995; **45**:69–74.

50 Fayerweather WE, Karns ME, Nuwayhid IA, Nelson TJ. Case control study of cancer risk in Tetra ethyl lead manufacturing. *Am J Ind Med* 1997; **31**:28–35.

51 Dennis LK, White E, Lee JAH, Kristal A, McKnight B, Odland P. Constitutional factors and sun exposure in relation to Nevi: a population based cross-sectional study. *Am J Epidemiol* 1996; **143**:248–56.

52 Giles GG, Armstrong BK, Burton RC, Staples MP, Thursfield VJ. Has mortality from melanoma stopped rising in Australia? An analysis of trends between 1931 and 1994. *Br Med J* 1996; **312**:1121–5.

53 Garland FC, Garland CF, White MR, Shaw E, Gurham ED. Occupational sunlight exposure and melanoma in the US Navy. *Arch Environ Hlth* 1990; **45**:261–7.

54 Vagero D, Swerdlow AJ, Beral V. Occupation and malignant melanoma: a study based on cancer registration data in England and Wales and in Sweden. *Br J Ind Med* 1990; **47**:317–24.

55 Bentham G. Association between incidence of non Hodgkins lymphoma and solar ultraviolet radiation in England and Wales. *Br Med J* 1996; **312**:1128–31.

56 Thomas TL, Waxweiler RJ. Brain tumours and occupational risk factors. *Scand J Work Environ Hlth* 1986; **12**:1–15.

57 Brem S, Rozental JM, Moskal JR. What is the etiology of human brain tumours? A report on the first LEBOW Conference. *Cancer* 1995; **76**:709–13.

58 Anttila A, Heikkila P, Nykvri E, Kauppinen T, Fukkala E,

Herberg S, Hemminki K. Risk of nervous system cancer among workers exposed to lead. *J Occup Environ Med* 1996; **38**:131–6.

59 National Research Council. *Possible Health Effects of Exposure to Residential Electric and Magnetic Fields*. Washington DC: National Academic Press, 1996.

60 Kheifets Li, Afifi AA, Buffler PA, Zhang ZW. Occupational electric and magnetic field exposure and brain cancer. A meta analysis. *J Occup Environ Med* 1995; **37**:1327–41.

61 Harrington JM, McBride DI, Sorahan T, Paddle GM, van Tongeren M. Occupational exposure to magnetic fields in relation to mortality from brain cancer among electricity generation and transmission workers. *Occup Environ Med* 1997; **54**:7–13.

62 Vineis P, Simonato L. Proportion of lung bladder cancers in males resulting from occupation: a systemic approach. *Arch Environ Hlth* 1991; **46**:6–15.

63 Porrus S, Aulent V, Donato F, Boffetta P, Fazioli R *et al.* Bladder cancer and occupation: a case control study in Northern Italy. *Occup Environ Med* 1996; **53**:6–10.

64 Oellet-Hellstrom R, Rench GD. Bladder cancer incidence in arylamine workers *J Occup Environ Med* 1996; **38**:1239–47.

65 Cartwight RA. Screening workers exposed to suspect bladder carcinogens. *J Occup Med* 1986; **28**:1017–19.

66 Schulte PA, Ringen K, Hemstreet GP, Ward E. Occupational cancer of the urinary tract. *Occup Med* 1987; **2**:85–107.

67 Steineck G, Plato N, Norell SE, Hogstedt C. Urothelial cancer and some industry-related chemicals: an evaluation of the epidemiologic literature *Am J Ind Med* 1990; **17**:371–91.

68 Ronneberg A, Anderson A. Mortality and cancer morbidity in workers from a aluminium smelter with pre-baked carbon amodes – Part III – cancer morbidity. *Occup Environ Med* 1995; **52**:250–4.

69 Tremblay C, Armstrong B, Theriault, Brodeur J. Estimation of risk of developing bladder cancer among workers exposed to coal tar pitch volatiles in the primary aluminium industry. *Am J Ind Med* 1995; **27**:335–48.

70 Austin H, Delzell E, Cole, Benzene and leukaemia. A review of the literature and a risk assessment. *Am J Epidemiol* 1988; **127**:419–39.

71 Landrigan PJ, Benzene and blood: One hundred years of evidence. *Am J Ind Med* 1996; **29**:225–6.

72 Savitz DA, Andrews KW. Review of the epidemiologic evidence on benzene and lymphatic and haeompoeitic cancers. *Am J Ind Med* 1997; **31**:287–95.

73 Fear NT, Roman E, Carpenter LM, Newton R, Bull D. Cancer in electrical workers: an analysis of cancer registrations in England 1981–1987. *Br J Cancer* 1996; **73**:935–9.

74 Feychting M. Occupational exposure to electromagnetic fields and adult leukaemia: a review of the epidemiological evidence. *Radiat Environ Biophys* 1996; **35**:237–42.

75 International Labour Organization. *1982 Yearbook of Labour Statistics*. Geneva: ILO, 1982.

76 Carnevale F, Montesano R, Partensky C, Tomatis L. Comparison of regulations on occupational carcinogens in several industrialised countries. *Am J Ind Med* 1987; **12**:453–73.

77 Hammond EC, Selikoff IJ, Seidman H. Asbestos exposure, cigarette smoking and death rates. *Ann N Y Acad Sci* 1979; **330**:473–90.

78 Saracci R, Boffetta P. Interactions of tobacco smoking with other causes of lung cancer. In: Sanet IM ed. *Epidemiology of Lung Cancer*. New York: Marcel Dekker, 1994: 465–93.

79 Miller AB. Fundamental issues in screening. In: Schottenfield D, Fraumeni JF eds. *Cancer Epidemiology and Prevention*. Philadelphia: WB Saunders Co., 1982.

Part 10

Reproduction and work

Workplace exposures and reproductive effects   823

Workplace exposures and reproductive effects

SUSAN M BARLOW, ANTHONY D DAYAN, ISABEL K STABILE

Normal reproduction	823	Pregnancy: the embryo and fetus	830
Gametogenesis	824	Postnatal exposures	832
The susceptibility of endocrine control processes	825	Investigation of complaints of effects on reproductive capacity	833
Postnatal development	825	Epidemiological investigations of the work force	834
Relationships between human and animal reproduction	825	Maintaining records	834
Reproduction and its uncertainties	826	Reliability of end points	834
Vulnerable stages in reproduction	827	Extrapolation of experimental data to people	836
Workplace agents interfering with human reproduction	828	Safefuarding reproductive health in the workplace: responsibilities and ethics	836
Germ cell mutation	828		
Male sexual behaviour and fertility	829	Conclusions	837
Female fertility	830	References	837
Pregnancy: enhanced toxicity to the mother	830		

Interference with the reproductive capacity of men and women may not be the first aspect which comes to mind when occupational health professionals consider the range of possible effects of exposures to chemical and physical agents in the workplace. Similarly, the family physician, obstetrician or gynaecologist investigating patients with abnormal reproductive function or adverse pregnancy outcomes may overlook the possible contribution of workplace exposures. This is understandable given the few situations in which workplace exposures have been clearly demonstrated to have affected reproduction. Whether this is a reflection of the true situation or indicative of underascertainment of causal links is not known. However, infertility and adverse pregnancy outcomes are relatively common and affected individuals may ask for authoritative advice about whether or not their work may be affecting them in this way. This chapter aims to provide the necessary background for developing such advice.

NORMAL REPRODUCTION

In man, no less than in other species, successful reproduction is the culmination of a lengthy and surprisingly chancy process (Fig. 40.2). Much may be known about the anatomy of the organs involved, and about many of the neural and endocrine systems that control the complex process of reproduction, but considerable scientific ignorance and many popular misconceptions still remain about this important aspect of human life, especially about details of the controls over successful gametogenesis, fertilization and implantation, and about the subsequent intrauterine development, postnatal development and maturation. The full reproductive cycle commonly extends over 18 or more years, from the original blastocyst to the development of a sexually capable member of the succeeding generation (Fig. 40.1). Given the length of the entire cycle from the conception of one human through to successful pregnancy and child rearing by that person's own children (Fig. 40.1), it will be appreciated that there are many points at which toxic effects may occur and that the capacity of epidemiologi-

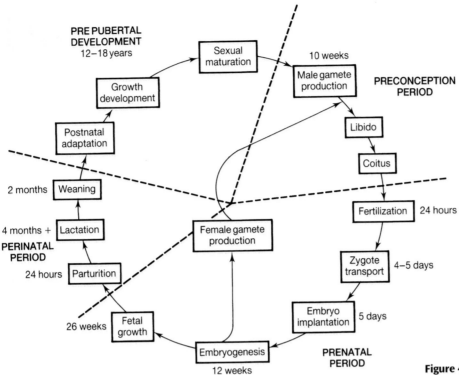

Figure 40.1 *The reproductive cycle.*

cal and clinical investigative procedures to cope with such extended processes remains limited.

The reproductive cycle can be divided into four distinct phases, all of which are susceptible to interference by occupational factors. Reproductive damage can range from effects that are immediately apparent (e.g. miscarriage due to heavy metal poisoning – to effects that may be latent for several decades (e.g. the late neurological sequelae in the succeeding generation of women poisoned by organic mercury compounds (see Chapter 7). During this generation-long reproductive cycle there are inevitably periods of heightened sensitivity to chemical and other occupational hazards, particularly during the meiotic divisions of gametogenesis and in embryogenesis. For general information on the processes involved in normal performance of human reproduction and the effects of chemicals upon them the reader is referred to reviews elsewhere.[1-7]

GAMETOGENESIS

In males gametogenesis commences at puberty, when testicular stem cells, which have remained quiescent since organogenesis, resume proliferation to produce spermatogonia. The spermatogonia then enter meiosis to produce primary and then secondary spermatocytes over a period of approximately 40 days. Spermiogenesis consists of the comparatively rapid transition from sec-

ondary spermatocytes to spermatids, which takes a further 20 days. This is followed by spermiation and finally capacitation, a maturation involving plasma membrane changes which endow fully matured sperm with the ability to fertilize. Three stages of this process are particularly sensitive to environmental factors that can cause oligospermia. The first is the initial mitotic divisions of spermatogonial development; the second and the most sensitive is during the meiotic divisions; the third is during spermiogenesis. Ultimately, the production of an ejaculate capable of fertilization is dependent upon the normal function of hormone-producing Leydig cells and of Sertoli cells, the integrated function of peripheral neural and vascular systems and a psychological component from the central nervous system.

In females, in contrast, gametogenesis commences in embryonic life as the germ cell syncytium develops via mitosis to primordial oocytes, which then enter the first meiotic division, and some of which continue development into the first few months of postnatal life to produce primordial follicles. The number of oocyte-containing primordial follicles is therefore fixed shortly after birth, and, although they are relatively damage resistant, subsequently there is only the potential to select against damaged oocytes rather than replace them. This normal selection process reduces the 5–7 million oocytes present during fetal life to approximately 400 000 at menarche.

Coincident with the onset of puberty, and in response to increasing pulsatile gonadotrophin concentrations, the second phase of folliculogenesis occurs, resulting in the cyclical growth of cohorts of primary and later antral follicles, one of which ultimately becomes the dominant, preovulatory or graafian follicle. Both the meiotic divisions of developing oocytes have phases of arrested growth. The first, which lasts for many years, extends from perinatal life until follicular development at puberty. The arrest in the second meiotic division occurs from early in graafian follicle development until the ovulated oocyte reaches the oviduct. The most sensitive period for damage to the developing oocyte occurs during preovulatory follicular growth and coincides with the completion of the initial meiotic division and the start of the second division.

In both sexes premeiotic damage to the germ cell DNA is most significant, as it carries a risk for the entire reproductive life span, whereas postmeiotic effects persist for only a limited period after exposure.

THE SUSCEPTIBILITY OF ENDOCRINE CONTROL PROCESSES

The various peptide and steroid hormones controlling reproduction act via conventional receptor-mediated mechanisms, which are correspondingly sensitive to anything that will cause an increase or decrease in the circulating hormone levels. Sources of variation include the normal rhythmical rise and fall in circulating gonadotrophin-releasing hormone (GnRH), follicle-stimulating hormone (FSH) and luteinizing hormone (LH) levels that are essential for the onset (menarche) and continuation of menstrual cycling in the female and the attainment of puberty in the male. They are also sensitive to pharmacological agonism or antagonism at the receptor, or up- or down-regulation of the numbers of receptors and the mechanisms coupling them to their specific effect. Production of the steroid hormones depends on a complex interplay of multiple sequential enzymatic steps; in the female they are synthesized in ovarian follicular stromal cells, resulting in the release of oestrogens and progesterone, and similarly androgens are produced by testicular Leydig cells. Control of function in the end organs of the genital tract, in the secondary sex organs and of behaviour are similarly mediated via gonadotrophin and steroid hormone sensitive receptors, which are susceptible to the same types of pharmacodynamic and toxicodynamic activities, including specific interference with each step in the sequential processes of sex steroid synthesis.

Endocrine control of developmental processes may be particularly susceptible to disruption. Adverse trends in human male reproductive health have been observed in some countries or regions and it has been hypothesized[6–11] that they may be related to increased exposure of the male fetus to environmental oestrogens, interfering with normal feedback mechanisms for gonadotrophic and testicular hormones. Effects observed include increases in testicular cancer, reduced sperm quality and possible increases in congenital anomalies (cryptorchidism, hypospadias) of the male reproductive tract.[12] These probably all have their origin during fetal development and might be expected to occur if exposure to oestrogenic substances was high. This, together with the observation that similar abnormalities (though not testicular cancer) have been seen in the sons of women exposed to the powerful synthetic oestrogen, diethylstilboestrol (DES) during pregnancy, provide the basis for the hypothesis. However, not all the relevant aspects of developmental physiology are presently understood and the proposal that there has been a general increase in exposure of the human population to environmental oestrogens (via food) in recent years is entirely speculative.

POSTNATAL DEVELOPMENT

The effect of prenatal exposure on postnatal development and behaviour is an emerging area of concern. Studies in Japan reported that prenatal exposure to methyl mercury could be linked to impaired co-ordination when the children reached school age, even though there were no obvious structural malformations at birth. Prenatal exposure to polychlorinated biphenyls has also been claimed to be associated with neurological (see Chapter 12) and behavioural effects in some children up to 6 years of age.[13] Unfortunately, it is far easier to propose ominous hypotheses about postnatal effects than to gather the information that will establish whether such an effect has really occurred. One should therefore evaluate critically and objectively any such claimed effect to ascertain its veracity.

One potential, but little investigated, effect of occupational exposure to chemicals is an alteration of the normal developmental pattern of enzyme expression.[12] Experimental studies have shown that exposure in utero to some drugs or industrial chemicals such as methyl mercury can affect fetal gluconeogenesis and alter levels of enzymes such as cytochrome P450s, which are responsible for the metabolism of steroids and some vitamins.[12,14]

RELATIONSHIPS BETWEEN HUMAN AND ANIMAL REPRODUCTION

Fortunately few occupational reproductive hazards have been directly demonstrated in humans and therefore many of the data on reproductive hazards in the workplace derive from animal studies. This introduces the uncertainties of cross-species extrapolation into any attempt to provide clinical advice.

Details of the reproductive hazards identified in conventional animal experiments have been comprehensively reviewed.[15–17] The major differences between the reproductive processes of animals and man must be borne in mind when attempting to assess human hazard even though the processes have overriding similarities.

The following brief summary identifies major features that should be considered when assessing experimental data from a clinical perspective. Most animal species are polytocous, whereas multiple births in humans are rare. In humans the hypothalamic control of GnRH and pituitary FSH, LH and prolactin secretion differs from that of common laboratory species. The oestrous cycle of rodents is only 4–6 days long and it has a brief secretory or luteal phase as, in the absence of copulation, the corpus luteum degenerates within about 24 hours of ovulation. In rodents, the survival and implantation of early blastocysts appear to be far more common than in humans, where a 90–95% loss is normal. There are also differences between rodents and humans in placental structure and function. For example, the rodent placenta has fewer layers and there are species differences in the duration and relative importance of histiotrophic *versus* haemotrophic nutrition. In addition, the first 10 days of pregnancy in the rodent are sustained by pituitary prolactin secretion rather than by oestrogenic stimulation from the corpus luteum.

Significant differences in pharmacokinetics between humans and animals may also exist. For instance, both dinitrotoluene and 1,3-dinitrobenzene have been widely used industrially and are potent testicular toxins in laboratory animals.[18] Happily, in the cases studied so far, occupationally exposed workers appear to have developed methaemoglobinaemia rather than any impairment of reproductive capacity, which is attributed to species differences in kinetics.[18] Conversely, there is some evidence that humans can be more sensitive than laboratory animals to reproductive hazards, as the doses of 1,2-dibromo-3 chloropropane or methyl mercury required to produce reproductive toxicity in animals are several times higher than those to which affected humans were exposed. Such sensitivity in the male may be related to the fact that human males produce only 5–20% of the numbers of sperm per gram of testis compared with most other species.[6,10]

Of all the types of reproductive hazard, effects during pregnancy, especially teratogenesis, have gained most public attention. Although male-mediated teratogenesis can occur in rodents[10] there is no clear evidence so far that it occurs in humans. Even in male survivors of atomic bombs and in patients who have received high doses of gonadal radio- or chemotherapy for malignant disease, there has been no convincing demonstration of increased adverse outcomes to pregnancies they have fathered (see Chapter 19). The absence of such a finding should not, however, be taken as indicating that humans have a greater ability to resist or repair damage to germ cells.

REPRODUCTION AND ITS UNCERTAINTIES

The relative improbability of reproductive success must be appreciated before deciding whether the reproductive capacity of a worker may have been affected by exposure to a toxic substance or to a physical insult. The quantitative rate of successful reproduction will vary from place to place, depending on such general aspects as nutrition and endemic infections in the community and other factors outside the remit of occupational health. There are also the vital physiological factors that affect fertility considered here as the capacity of an adult man and woman to produce a fetus, which the healthy mother successfully carries through pregnancy to birth and subsequently through to weaning. That covers many distinct stages, each of which has its own natural failure rate, and each of which may be influenced by occupational exposure.

In Western society, about 0.5–1.0% of couples exhibit irreversible infertility and some 10–20% experience an unexpected delay in conception, i.e. failure to achieve pregnancy within 2 years.[19] The chance on any given occasion of a successful pregnancy, even in Britain and the USA today, is surprisingly low[20] for a variety of reasons (Fig. 40.2), especially chromosomal abnormalities.[21] Also, about 6% of live births carry chromosomal and

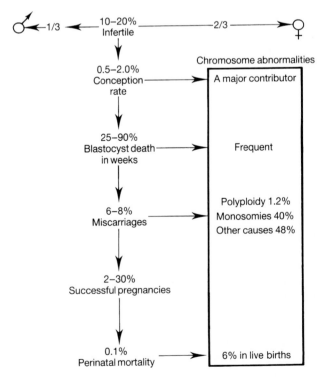

Figure 40.2 *The improbability of successful reproduction in the normal human.*

anatomical defects, many of which have a permanent effect on well-being.[21]

It will be seen that there are many uncertainties about the reproductive process, and that it may be difficult quantitatively to confirm or deny complaints or fears about harmful effects, even once the social and medical problems of investigating such matters have been overcome.

The following sections will show that, as reproduction is a dynamic process extending from gamete formation in the parents to maturation of their children, the detection and prevention of toxic and physical hazards extend over a much wider time frame and a much broader physiological framework than most other branches of preventive medicine. A toxic effect may be manifested close to the time of exposure, as is common to the effects of many substances, or years later, when the reproductive system is put to the ultimate test of successful procreation. A defect may be produced during gametogenesis (e.g. a mutation), which becomes overt only in the succeeding generation, or, as with transplacental carcinogenesis, the proximate toxicity occurs *in utero* but its ultimate expression does not appear until the subsequent adulthood; for example, maternal exposure to diethylstilboestrol producing vaginal tumours in the female due to an effect on the genital anlagen in the developing fetus. The search for and identification of

effects on reproduction pose difficult medical problems and their prevention creates unique problems.

VULNERABLE STAGES IN REPRODUCTION

The complexity of the physiological stages involved in successful reproduction gives a clue to the wide range of end points within the reproductive process which may be vulnerable to physical and chemical agents found in the workplace (Fig. 40.3). The investigation of potential human reproductive hazards may need to encompass preconceptional exposure of males and females as well as pregnancy itself and lactation. A wide range of studies is usually undertaken (mainly in animals) to investigate the potential risks of agents in the workplace.[22] Conversely, when adverse effects on reproduction are seen in individual patients, or more particularly in groups of workers, the possibility of an occupational cause must be borne in mind. The ability of single agents to bring about differing effects on the offspring, ranging for example from fetal death to postnatal behavioural changes, should also alert the general or occupational physician to the need to integrate clues about adverse events across the reproductive spectrum, rather than focus solely on single end points, such as abortion or congenital malformation.

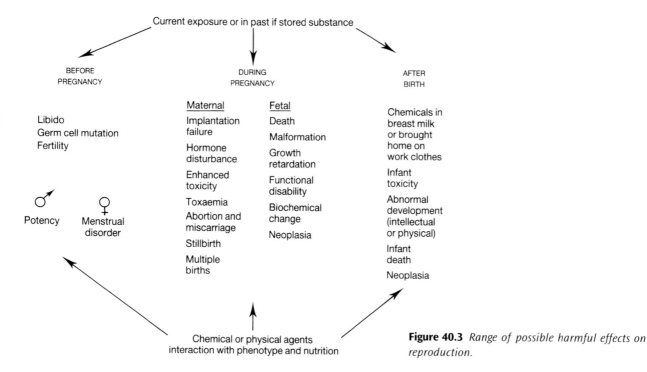

Figure 40.3 *Range of possible harmful effects on reproduction.*

WORKPLACE AGENTS INTERFERING WITH HUMAN REPRODUCTION

Animal studies reviewed elsewhere[5,11,15–17,23,24] have demonstrated the potential for toxicity of workplace agents to all of the stages of reproduction in males and females mentioned in Fig. 40.1. Human data from epidemiological studies and case reports are much more rare, and few, unequivocal examples of agents affecting each of the many stages of reproduction are available (Table 40.1[11,13–15,23,25–35] and Table 40.2). Reproductive outcome in relation to occupation remains a difficult and poorly studied area, and confirmatory studies are needed for most of the effects reported. There are, however,

examples of known hazards to human reproduction and some of these are discussed below. References are to reviews, rather than original sources, wherever possible, in which the interested reader will also find information on agents other than those mentioned here.

GERM CELL MUTATION

As explained earlier, agents causing germ cell mutation are more likely to affect males than females when exposure occurs during adulthood. Lethal mutations in sperm DNA have been recognized for a long time. However, the possibility that agents might interfere with

Table 40.1 *Examples of chemicals associated with human reproductive hazard following occupational exposure*

Agent	Males	Females
Drugs		
Anaesthetic gases[23]	Unknown ?Increased minor malformations in offspring	Abortion ?Fetal growth retardation, stillbirth, malformation
Cytotoxic drugs[32,35]	Unknown	Abortion, malformation
Stilboestrol[14,31]	Gynaecomastia, loss of libido, impotence	Infertility
Industrial chemicals		
2-Ethoxyethanol[34]	Oligospermia, abnormal sperm morphology	Unknown
Lead[27,28,87]	Oligospermia, abnormal sperm morphology, decreased sperm motility	Reduced fertility, abortion, stillbirth, neonatal death
Manganese[15]	Reduced libido, impotence	Unknown
Mercury (inorganic)[15,29,30]	Unknown	Menstrual disorders ?Abortion, malformation, stillbirth
Polychlorinated biphenyls[13,15]	Unknown	Minor malformation, fetal growth retardation, stillbirth, postnatal death Concentrates in milk
Pesticides		
Carbaryl[15]	Abnormal sperm morphology	Unknown
Chlordecone (Kepone)[15]	Oligospermia, reduced sperm motility, abnormal sperm morphology	Concentrates in milk
Chloroprene[15]	Reduced sperm motility, abnormal sperm morphology	Unknown
1,2-Dibromo-3-chloropropane[11,23]	Oligospermia, azoospermia	Unknown
2,4-Dichlorophenoxyacetic acid (2,4-D)[25]	Reduced sperm motility, abnormal sperm morphology	Unknown
Ethylene dibromide[26]	Oligospermia, reduced sperm viability and motility, altered sperm morphology	Unknown
Solvents		
Carbon disulphide[23]	Oligospermia, impotence, abnormal sperm morphology	?Menstrual disorders, abortion, premature birth

?: Questionable effects.

Table 40.2 *Causes of oligospermia/azoospermia*

Occupational

Dibromochloropropane
Chlordecone (Kepone)®
Lead

Non-occupational

Infections e.g. mumps
Pharmacological agents e.g. cytotoxic drugs,
    diethylstilboestrol, contraceptive pills
Ionizing radiation
Alcohol
Heat

DNA there, whilst the sperm retained its capacity to fertilize the ovum and produce a viable but damaged conceptus, has been less well recognized. The outcome of such events might be malformation, or functional or even malignant change in the offspring. If the effects are severe, the offspring may die *in utero* and/or be aborted. Some, however, may survive gestation with abnormalities that are evident at birth or which develop postnatally.

In addition to the well known effects of agents that cause dominant mutations in sperm that are lethal to the developing embryo and fetus, animal studies during the last decade[10] have shown the potential for certain agents, such as cytotoxic drugs and x-irradiation, to cause malformations and tumours in offspring following paternal exposure prior to conception.[36] Studies have claimed to show effects from occupational exposure of the father to lead (abortions, tumours in offspring),[15,28] vinyl chloride (increased fetal death),[16] hydrocarbons (tumours in offspring)[16] and anaesthetic gases (abortions, malformations).[11] However, many of the studies are significantly flawed, in some cases because of bias, the small number of subjects studied, or failure to exclude confounding factors. It may prove particularly difficult to draw firm conclusions about human effects in this area of reproductive toxicity because animal evidence indicates that only a very small proportion of offspring derived from exposed sperm may have a malformation or malignancy. Extremely large epidemiological studies would therefore probably be required to detect such small effects.

MALE SEXUAL BEHAVIOUR AND FERTILITY

Occupational exposure to oestrogens, carbon disulphide, chlordecone, chloroprene, boric acid, manganese and lead have all been reported to cause loss of libido and/or impotence.[7,11,15,16,37] However, the reports are mostly based on studies of only a few workers and are open to criticism, particularly because of the strong psychogenic influences on libido and potency and the lack of objective measures of assessment. Nevertheless, other known effects of high exposure to the above agents on hypothalamic and gonadal hormones (e.g. inorganic lead, oestrogens, carbon disulphide) or on neurological function (e.g. chlordecone, manganese, organic lead) increase the likelihood that they do indeed have the capacity to affect libido and potency. A further feature of agents reported to affect libido and potency is that a number of them have also been reported to affect sperm count, motility and morphology (see Table 40.1). Thus, signs and symptoms that may alert the worker to a potential problem, and may lead him to consult an occupational physician may be indicative of more fundamental effects on spermatogenesis which would be revealed only by laboratory investigation. However, the converse is also true: some agents may have substantial effects on spermatogenesis in the absence of any interference with libido or potency.

A chemical of the latter type provides perhaps the most striking and best investigated example of adverse effects on human reproduction. The pesticide dibromochloropropane (DBCP) has resulted in sterility, reduced sperm count and other evidence of testicular damage in men involved in the manufacture or agricultural use of DBCP; as a result, it is no longer made or used. The problem was first brought to light in 1977, 20 years after it came into use, not by clinicians or epidemiologists but by exposed workers themselves. Men involved in DBCP formulation in a Californian plant noticed that a number of them were experiencing difficulty in fathering children. Five of them underwent voluntary examination and were found to be oligospermic or azoospermic.[16]

In subsequent years, further reports from the USA and Israel, covering larger numbers of men, confirmed and extended the original finding[11,25,38] identifying three categories of affected workers: initially oligospermic with an increase in sperm count over time; initially azoospermic but with some later recovery in sperm count; and initially azoospermic with no recovery up to 11 years after cessation of exposure.[25,38] It is of interest to note that similar adverse effects on the testes were reported in rats, rabbits and guinea-pigs in the 1960s and 1970s prior to the first reports of effects in human,[16] and as a result DBCP was not manufactured or used in some countries, such as the UK.

Effects on sperm count, motility or morphology have also been reported in humans for other chemicals (see Table 40.1). With the exception of ionizing radiation and heat, both of which adversely affect male fertility at high exposures, few physical agents have been studied for reproductive effects in humans. A single study of occupational exposure to lower doses of ionizing radiation in Japanese radiologists suggested decreased fertility.[36]

FEMALE FERTILITY

Disorders of menstrual function do not always imply adverse outcomes on reproduction. Nevertheless, they may be caused by hormonal imbalances in the hypothalamic–pituitary ovarian axis and thus serve as useful indicators of endocrine effects which may also impair fertility or ability to maintain pregnancy. Disorders of menstruation include alterations in the length of the menstrual cycle, in menstrual flow, and an increase in painful menstruation.

Menstrual disturbances have been reported in association with such occupations as the manufacture of aniline dyes, electrical insulation products, rubber products and shoes, in-flight attendants, and following occupational exposure to formaldehyde, mercury, tetrachloroethylene and trichloroethylene.[11,16,22,39–41] Most studies of menstrual function carried out so far suffer from severe limitations, which make interpretation difficult, and any changes that may occur do so against a background of high variability in the cycle. Nevertheless, the possibility that an occupational factor may have influenced menstruation always warrants further investigation in exposed workers and the working environment.

PREGNANCY: ENHANCED TOXICITY TO THE MOTHER

The increased vulnerability of the embryo and fetus to toxic hazards is frequently highlighted in discussions of pregnant women at work. A less familiar consideration is the possibility that the pregnant woman herself may be at risk of enhanced toxic responses in comparison with other adults, and this may be in addition to already existing sex differences between non-pregnant adult females and males. One such agent is benzene for which there is a higher rate of uptake and longer persistence in the body in non-pregnant women compared with men.[16]

Exposure to benzene now should be low, but at the beginning of the twentieth century, when chronic benzene poisoning did occur, particular problems of vaginal bleeding and haemorrhagic complications of pregnancy were noted, alongside the usual symptoms of purpuric skin spots and bleeding from the nose and gums. The occurrence of vaginal bleeding was frequently associated with progression to severe and fatal complications of benzene poisoning.[16] It would be reasonable to assume that any agent causing bleeding or anaemia would pose an added risk to pregnant women (see Chapter 44).

The pioneering work of Hardy in assembling a register of beryllium poisoning cases in the middle of this century revealed that pregnancy was probably a precipitating factor in fatalities. In a total of 95 fatal cases of poisoning in women, 63 were in association with pregnancy.[16] Clearly, chronic berylliosis may be exacerbated by pregnancy.

Of chemicals to which women are more likely to be exposed nowadays, mercury, formaldehyde, styrene, superphosphate and organochlorine pesticides have all been reported to increase the incidence of toxaemia,[16] but the studies are poorly reported and difficult to interpret.

PREGNANCY: THE EMBRYO AND FETUS

The literature on possible adverse effects of workplace agents on the embryo and fetus is much more extensive than that covering other aspects of reproduction. Yet as far as humans are concerned, there have been no agents which, at the levels normally encountered in the workplace, have been as striking in their effects as DBCP in men, and none associated with a high probability of adverse outcome, such as was seen with the drug thalidomide, where most of the women who took it at the critical period of pregnancy gave birth to a malformed child. High exposures to lead[42] or carbon monoxide[16] are known to have severe effects on the embryo and fetus, but such exposures should not now be encountered in the workplace.

In this section, therefore, some frequently investigated workplace agents, about which pregnant women are often concerned, will be mentioned. However, the selection should not be taken to imply that they are necessarily the agents to which the embryo and fetus are most vulnerable. Comprehensive sources of information on a wide range of chemicals in pregnancy are to be found elsewhere.[7,15–17,43] It should be borne in mind that only about 5% of fetal malformations appear, at present, to be related to environmental causes, none of which is directly occupational, while in most cases the causes are unknown (Table 40.3).[44]

Mercury (see Chapter 7)

There is extensive information, reviewed elsewhere,[45] on the adverse effects of organic mercury on the central nervous system of the human embryo, fetus and infant, as a consequence of environmental disasters in which methyl and ethyl mercury have entered the food chain. Less

Table 40.3 *Aetiology of fetal malformations*[44]

Cause	%
Autosomal chromosome aberration	2
Gene mutation	5
Identifiable environmental agents	5
Sex chromosome aberration	8
Multifactorial causes	20
Unidentified causes	60

extensively studied is inorganic mercury to which women may be occupationally exposed in ore smelting, fluorescent lamp manufacture and dentistry. A study of dentists, dental assistants and dental technicians in Poland has shown increases in spontaneous abortion, stillbirth and congenital malformation (spina bifida) rates, which were significantly associated with total mercury levels determined in scalp and pubic hair.[31] Another, larger, study of 8157 infants born to dental workers in Sweden found no increased risk for prenatal survival, low birth weight or congenital malformations.[46] Specifically there was no increased risk of spina bifida which was seen in the Polish study. It is possible that the handling of amalgam has differed between the two countries, and exposures were said to have been reduced substantially in Sweden during the last 20 years.[46] Thus, the data on pregnancy in workers exposed to mercury remain inconclusive.

Solvents (see Chapter 12)

Studies covering a wide range of work involving solvents have fairly consistently reported an increased incidence of spontaneous abortions.[47,48] Defects of the central nervous system, palate and urinary tract have also been reported to be elevated in some studies. Specific solvents and the industries covered in these studies include styrene, toluene, xylene, tetrachloroethylene (dry-cleaning), viscose rayon manufacture, plastics and rubber (tyre and footwear) manufacture, pharmaceutical and chemical laboratories, and microelectronics manufacture (toluene, xylene, glycol ethers, strong acids and gases) as well as groupings of workers from different industries with general solvent exposure.[16,49–58] The incidence of low birth weight has also been studied and this is of particular interest since animal studies have shown reduced fetal body weight to be the principal effect.[16] However, to date no significant effect on birth weight has been shown in women exposed to solvents.[54,58,59] Thus, the evidence as a whole strongly suggests an adverse effect, that is spontaneous abortion, but the information on other aspects of pregnancy is inconclusive.

Anaesthetics and drugs (see Chapter 8)

Following the initial report from the USSR in 1967 of an increased rate of spontaneous abortions in women anaesthetists, numerous retrospective epidemiological studies have been carried out.[60] Most studies found an increase in spontaneous abortions (one-and-a-half to threefold) and some an increase in congenital malformations (one- to threefold) in pregnancies of female operating room and dental personnel. Increases in stillbirths and low birth weight were also reported in some studies. However, the validity of these earlier studies has been seriously criticized on methodological grounds, so there

is no generally agreed view about the occurrence or importance of the risk to humans. More recent studies have focused on the possible role of nitrous oxide as the reproductive toxicant in anaesthetic gases, surveying occupational groups, some members of which have high exposure to nitrous oxide. One study showed increased time to pregnancy and increased risk of sponaneous abortion among more highly exposed dental assistants[61] and another study showed increased time to pregnancy among more highly exposed midwives.[62]

Four studies of doctors and nurses administering antineoplastic drugs have found significant increases in fetal loss and/or congenital malformations.[33,55] These findings, together with work showing that such staff may excrete mutagens when handling these drugs, indicate the importance of handling cytotoxic agents with extreme care,[63] and that, whenever possible, pregnant women or women intending to become pregnant should avoid handling such drugs.

Leather workers

An increased risk of perinatal deaths, particularly from congenital malformations and macerated stillbirths, was reported in the offspring of leather workers in the UK.[55] A subsequent study in Canada confirmed an excess of stillbirths, but this time without defects, and no increase in spontaneous abortions or congenital malformations.[64] A retrospective analysis of UK data did not show any excess of stillbirths or neonatal deaths.[65]

Radiation (see Chapter 19)

The effects of medical and diagnostic radiation range from congenital malformations – particularly those of the central nervous system, including microcephaly and mental retardation, after high pelvic exposures – to an increased incidence of abnormal karyotypes in spontaneous abortions, and an increased incidence of childhood cancers, particularly leukaemias, after lower exposures.[2] However, radiation exposures in the workplace are much lower. The effects of occupational exposure to low doses were studied in a small group of women working in Swedish hospitals and showed a small but statistically non-significant increase in congenital malformations among x-ray workers.[66] Recommended exposure levels for pregnant women are generally 10% of the upper limits recommended for non-pregnant workers, which should be sufficient protection for the fetus. However, some workers may receive irregular exposure to radiation at a time when they are unaware they are pregnant.

Adverse pregnancy outcomes have been reported from eastern Europe in women working with microwaves, and a significant excess of congenital malformations and perinatal deaths has been reported in physiotherapists working with short-wave or microwave diathermy equipment.[67–69] The effects of microwaves on pregnancy in animals seem largely related to the heating effect of intense radiation. The power density and wavelengths of non-ionizing radiation encountered in the workplace vary considerably, depending on the source, with low power, short wavelength radiation penetrating only a short distance into tissues.

Visual display units

Weak electromagnetic radiation ranging from high to very low frequencies is also emitted from visual display units (VDUs) and there has been intense discussion of possible effects among VDU operators, which has generated much anxiety, following the first report in 1979 of a cluster of abnormal pregnancy outcomes. Since then, at least 20 further clusters of spontaneous abortions and/or congenital defects have been reported.

Electromagnetic radiation emitted from VDUs is rarely above background levels except at the extremely low frequency end of the range. VDU screens may also hold a static charge. Animal research on the biological effects of such magnetic fields has produced equivocal results with no suggestion of effects on pregnancy at the low levels found in association with VDUs. Stress and ergonomic factors, such as prolonged sitting in one posture, have also been suggested for investigation in VDU users.

A number of epidemiological studies have been completed in which congenital defects, abortions, perinatal deaths and low birth weight were studied. The epidemiological evidence to date does not support the suggestion that there is a relationship between adverse pregnancy outcome and VDU use,[55,70–75] although, due to limitations of several of the studies, the possibility of small effects cannot be completely ruled out. One can safely conclude, however, that, if there are any adverse effects, they are not as common as the extrapolation from the reports of clusters of pregnancy failures has led many to believe and it is impossible to ascribe any particular type or profile of abnormalities to exposure to VDUs during pregnancy.

Physical factors

The effects of noise and vibration have been investigated to a limited extent and associations reported with increased risk of threatened or spontaneous abortion, pregnancy-induced hypertension, abnormal labour and low birth weight.[32,36,66] However, such effects have not been observed in all studies and some were seen only when noise exposure was combined with shift work.[43,48] Heavy lifting, other physically tiring work, standing, long hours, irregular hours, shift work and extremes of heat and cold have all been reported to be associated with adverse outcomes such as spontaneous abortion, stillbirth, premature delivery, low birth weight and congenital malformations.[24,48,55,75,76] However, there are also conflicting finding of no effects on some of the above parameters, exemplifying the problems of small epidemiological studies in this area.

The effects of non-chemical hazards on human reproduction are summarized in Table 40.4.[24,36,43,48,66,67,69,75,76]

POSTNATAL EXPOSURES

Infants may be exposed via workplace agents brought into the home on work clothes, such as has occurred with lead in the past. However, the most common and most significant route for infant exposure to chemicals is

Table 40.4 *Non-chemical occupational hazards associated with adverse effects on reproduction*

Agent	Males	Females
x-Rays[36,66]	?Reduced fertility	?Developmental toxicity ?Teratogenicity
Microwaves[67,69]	Unknown	?Teratogenicity ?Perinatal deaths
Noise[43]	Unknown	?Abortion ?Fetal growth retardation
Vibration[67]	Unknown	?Menstrual disorders
Physically tiring work	Unknown	Amenorrhoea
Strenuous exercise[24,48,75,76]		?Abortion ?Stillbirth ?Teratogenicity ?Fetal growth retardation

?: Questionable effect.

via breast milk. Such intakes may be additional to exposures that have already occurred *in utero* by transfer of the same chemical across the placenta. However, in the case of fat-soluble chemicals such as organic solvents, organochlorine pesticides, polychlorinated biphenyls (PCBs), exposure via the breast milk can be considerable, with milk being a major route of excretion of maternal body burdens, which may have been built up over years prior to the first lactation.[77] In the case of certain highly fat-soluble organochlorine pesticides and PCBS, average cumulative intakes by women from the diet alone mean that infant intakes from breast milk exceed the recommended acceptable daily intakes set by a number of national and international bodies.[78,79] In women also occupationally exposed to PCBs, levels in breast milk are even higher.[80] Children born to women exposed to abnormally high levels of PCBs and dibenzofurans in the diet due to accidental contamination of cooking oil,[13,16] have shown dark, greyish-brown staining of the skin, gums and nails which faded slowly (see Chapter 12). All were underweight and some died. They also showed developmental delays and behavioural abnormalities. However, the possible effects of occupational exposure on postnatal development have not been investigated.

A single case report of jaundice in a baby that was breast-fed by a mother who paid regular lunchtime visits to her husband in the dry-cleaning establishment where he worked, is illustrative of the ready passage of tetrachloroethylene into breast milk.[16] This and the PCB story suggest that, in cases where women are occupationally exposed to highly fat-soluble compounds, their breast milk should be analysed for the chemicals and, if necessary, they should be cautioned against breast-feeding.

INVESTIGATION OF COMPLAINTS OF EFFECTS ON REPRODUCTIVE CAPACITY

The first and very difficult task is to establish the exact nature of the complaint: loss of libido or erectile inadequacy in the male, loss of libido or menstrual irregularity in the female, or true loss of fecundity in either sex, etc. Disentangling the true concern from the social overlay and confusion of popular rumours can be taxing but is essential. How much further the occupational physician may take the investigation will depend on the relationship with the family doctor and general medical consultant services. It is an area of human biology that needs to be handled with particular sensitivity and which greatly benefits from experience. Procedures for the investigation of males and females complaining of infertility have been proposed; a general approach to the detection of effects on reproductive capacity of workers has been described,[81,82] and a detailed, possibly idealized scheme for the investigation of reproductive functions

has been proposed.[83] The complexity and intrusiveness of those procedures and the requirement for sophisticated clinical and laboratory facilities make them best suited for application in specialized clinics. The primary roles of the occupational health worker here are to be alert to the possibility of effects associated with employment and to ensure appropriate referral of workers who appear to be infertile.

It is necessary to consider whether there may be a real effect associated with work, or whether non-occupational factors may be involved. This will require balancing evaluation of exposure to chemical and physical agents, and what is known about their effects, against other social and general medical factors, including social behaviour, nutrition and background disease, as well as taking into account the high background rates for certain adverse reproductive events, such as spontaneous abortion.[88]

Concern about a reproductive risk may be raised by a worker because of a personal reproductive problem, because of anxiety about substances or physical factors to which he or she is exposed, or, more generally, because of anecdotal information about reproductive outcomes relating to the locality or the occupation. Formal epidemiological surveillance findings in a register or, more commonly, unexpected clustering of an abnormality common to several workers are further ways in which concerns may present.

The immediate concerns of the individual are likely first to require taking a particularly searching personal history to determine the nature of the perceived problem, and whether it may have a factual basis, followed by clinical examination and appropriate laboratory studies. If an effect related to work is confirmed, or appears to be likely, full exploration of its underlying cause is necessary, which is likely to involve collaboration with specialists in occupational health and hygiene, the Health and Safety Executive in Britain and the employer and trade unions.

Formal epidemiological surveillance of other exposed subjects at that and other sites will be essential to determine who has been affected, to reinforce understanding of the responsible agent and as a basis for counselling about any long-term effects on parents and children. Action will involve stopping exposure to the harmful circumstance; specific therapy for the affected individual may not be available, depending on the nature of the toxic effect. Specialists will have to decide whether a lower exposure level will be safe so that effective preventive and control measures can be devised.

General schemes for the clinical investigation of the reproductive system in affected individuals have already been noted.[83] It is essential to relate the investigation to the pattern of the observed disorder and its probable cause. In the male, studies are generally based on the examination of semen for volume, chemical composition, sperm number, motility and the proportions of particular morphological abnormalities. Assay of circulating androgens, FSH and LH has been less useful, except when a specific defect has been suspected. In the female, the primary points for investigation are commonly the hormonal regulation of the menstrual cycle in terms of cyclical variation in FSH, LH and oestrogen levels, followed by evidence of appropriate changes in ovarian morphology (ultrasound examination), cyclical bursts of GnRH release and prolactin levels. Abnormal liveborn children or abortuses can be examined for chromosomal complement or teratogenic effects. The overall appearance of an abnormal fetus or baby, or a specific defect, may give a clue to the nature and timing of any external influence. These evaluations of the reproductive process must be accompanied by investigation of the history and pattern of sexual activities.[84] At the same time, a searching assessment of the workplace and of the exposure there to chemical and physical agents should be made by appropriate specialists. All these investigations of individuals entail detailed questioning about intimate personal matters and intrusive laboratory studies. The need for them must first be clearly accepted by all involved.

EPIDEMIOLOGICAL INVESTIGATIONS OF THE WORKFORCE

Epidemiological approaches have an important role to play in identifying reproductive hazards.[85] They cannot be reviewed here in detail, but a discussion of some practical aspects may be useful, including the reliability of the more readily available end points for evaluating reproductive function and an outline of the types of records that can be compiled about the workforce.[86,87] The latter may alert the occupational health physician to a possible hazard and so lead to referral of workers for general medical advice, as well as keeping a record for any subsequent epidemiological investigation (see Chapter 3).

MAINTAINING RECORDS

The nature of the questions that need to be asked in order to compile useful background records on reproductive function in the workforce requires awareness of the sensitivity of the information that will be gathered. It is important to prepare the ground thoroughly before embarking on such an exercise. The workforce needs to be fully informed and fully involved at every stage; the necessary co-operation will not be forthcoming unless there is a clear understanding of the reasons for such records being kept, assurance of individual confidentiality of records, a mechanism by which the workforce receives regular updates in anonymous form of what the

records show (whether good or bad news), ready access to occupational health staff and perhaps external medical services for consultation by concerned individuals, and an assurance that any potential reproductive problems discovered in the workforce will be openly followed up.

If such a programme is accepted by the workforce, the following types of information may be gathered by questionnaire, interview or from personal diaries. Menstrual function may be followed by asking women to keep diaries recording the onset and cessation of bleeding, together with some assessment of the amount of bleeding and any pain during menstruation. The latter may be entirely subjective or some guidance on a scoring system may be given. Fertility may be assessed by ascertaining the numbers of pregnancies in women workers or the wives of male workers in the current and previous employments, time intervals between onset of unprotected intercourse and recognized conception (time to pregnancy), and failure to conceive after 1 year of unprotected intercourse (defined as infertility). Events during pregnancies and the outcomes of pregnancies can include spontaneous abortion (although early ones often pass unrecognized), induced abortion, pregnancy-related illness such as hypertension or toxaemia, duration of gestation, fetal death, stillbirth, live birth, birth weight, postnatal death, congenital malformations, childhood cancer and developmental problems. The accuracy of some of the above information may be particularly questionable if it is obtained from male workers rather than their wives. Similarly, if information is obtained retrospectively, the accuracy of recall by either sex will deteriorate over time and there is likely to be better recall of adverse events by workers who suspect or know they may have been exposed to a reproductive hazard.[87]

All these data should be correlated with information about the job done, the associated exposure to chemical and physical factors[88] (including non-specific stresses), and more general information about health, nutrition and life style (smoking, drinking habits, etc.). Ethnic and cultural factors should also be taken into consideration.

RELIABILITY OF END POINTS

The most accurate index of impaired fertility is the measurement of time to conception.[81–83,87,89] However, recall problems may make this an unreliable measure for retrospective studies and its usefulness in prospective studies has yet to be demonstrated in the occupational setting.

Infertility and impaired fertility in both sexes may be ascertained retrospectively as the relatively simple measure of the number of pregnancies occurring over the relevant part of a couple's reproductive lifetime in comparison with controls. Such information may readily be obtained by questionnaire. However, it should be borne in mind that spontaneous abortions before 6–8 weeks of gestation will generally pass unrecognized. Hence, fertility ascertained in this way may reflect not only failure of fertilization but also early embryonic losses.

Modifications of this method have been developed in the USA using live birth rates rather than pregnancy rates and were successfully validated with DBCP workers. Live birth rates of exposed employees are compared with expected live birth rates derived from national probabilities specific for birth cohort, age, parity and race. The ratio of observed to expected birth rates is termed the standardized fertility ratio (SFR) or standardized birth ratio (SBR), analogous to the standardized mortality ratio. SFRs/SBRs may then be compared in exposed *versus* non-exposed workers or in pre-exposure periods *versus* post-exposure periods in the same workers, though the latter may well carry a built-in bias towards a positive finding because of lower maternal age and parity in the pre-exposure period. When the method was applied to one plant which produced DBCP from 1955 to 1976, it showed that significant reductions in SFRs would have become evident at least 18 years before the time when the DBCP problem actually became apparent[90] (see p. 829). This technique, however, may be insufficiently sensitive to detect small effects on fertility.

The most frequently used method for assessing chemical effects on males has been to study the characteristics of semen.[6,83,91] The method is non-invasive and has the power to detect effects in smaller groups than those generally necessary to show effects on fertility by questionnaire methods. However, persuading workers to participate is not easy, and the difficulties involved in carrying out and interpreting such studies are considerable. Sperm count, motility and morphology and scoring double Y bodies (signifying chromosomal non-disjunction) have all been used, and the significance and status of these tests are discussed elsewhere.[92–94] The methods have undoubtedly proved their worth in detecting effects of occupational exposures on the male, and clinical studies have shown that reductions in sperm count and motility and increases in abnormal sperm shapes are correlated with impairment of fertility and possibly with increased spontaneous abortions. However, no studies to date have correlated semen quality with the full reproductive histories of workers.

Studies of gonadotrophic hormones (FSH, LH and testosterone) have not proved to be particularly useful in general surveillance. In those instances where hormonal changes have been seen they have usually been associated with profound alterations in spermatogenesis.

Turning to pregnancy outcome, it is possible to utilize available surveillance systems, which routinely collect data on live birth parameters (birth weight and sex ratio) and on events such as spontaneous abortions requiring hospitalization, stillbirths, congenital malformations,

infant mortality and childhood cancer. Such registry data have the advantage of offering large sample sizes and have been used to test particular hypotheses about occupational influences and also, less robustly, to generate hypotheses about causation. Whilst the recording of sex, birth weight or stillbirth may be fairly complete and reliable, there are major problems, for example, in under-reporting of congenital malformations and the quality of the occupational data is often poor. The uses and limitations of such surveillance data have been discussed elsewhere.[71,72]

The use of questionnaires and interviews has the advantages of better ascertainment of occupation and exposure, but generally imposes constraints on sample size and raises questions about the reliability of the information obtained on pregnancy outcomes. For example, comparisons of interview or questionnaire results with information obtained from research or hospital records of reproductive events have revealed both over-reporting and under-reporting, particularly of spontaneous abortions.

In addition to the sources of bias common in epidemiological work (see Chapter 3), there are a number of possible biases that are peculiar to the study of occupational influences on reproduction. The nature of some of these and possible ways of overcoming them are discussed elsewhere.[87] One in particular deserves mention here, the infertile worker effect, as this is the opposite of what we are more used to considering in occupational epidemiology, i.e. the 'healthy worker effect'. In the absence of children, women are more likely to stay in paid employment; thus those in work are likely to be less healthy in reproductive terms than those not in work. Similarly, dilemmas in the choice of study design, which are familiar in any epidemiological survey, may require especially careful consideration in studies of reproduction and occupation.[89] For example, in a cohort study, should the pregnancies occurring during exposure be compared with pregnancies occurring in the same women either before or after they were exposed? Alternatively should the controls be matched women working elsewhere?[95] In a case-control study, say of births with abnormalities of the central nervous system should controls be women with normal pregnancy outcomes or a referent group with a different type of malformation?

Finally, gathering accurate exposure data always presents difficulties in occupational research, but when reproductive outcomes are being investigated the exposure triggering the adverse event may be relatively brief, with a short latency period between exposure and reproductive failure. Thus both acute and chronic exposures may be relevant. Moreover, when single types of reproductive outcome are studied, the familiar proof of cause and effect in toxicology, namely an increasing dose–response relationship, may not be apparent because related adverse events in the continuum of reproductive casualties have not been ascertained.

EXTRAPOLATION OF EXPERIMENTAL DATA TO PEOPLE

A problem throughout occupational toxicology is the extent to which findings in animal experiments or from *in vitro* systems can be extended to humans.[96,97] The major physiological differences are referred to earlier in this chapter.

In the field of reproduction toxicology, the usual cautions apply about relating exposure to dose, if possible using toxicokinetics and metabolic data to compare the concentration of the ultimate toxicant at the putative target site, or at least in the blood, and always taking account of known species differences.

The overall similarities between humans and laboratory animals are much stronger than the differences, so qualitative extrapolation of hazard is reasonable, unless there are known specific differences in toxicokinetics or response mechanisms. It is properly cautious to assume that a reproductive effect seen in animal experiments will be manifested in humans at an appropriate dose level, unless there is clear evidence that its mechanism or pathogenesis depends on processes that have been excluded in human tissues – absence of an important enzyme, a qualitative difference in the nature of the stimulus for a receptor, etc.

In the case of teratogenicity, several-surveys have supported the broad analogy that defects produced in animals are likely to occur in man,[98,99] although the exact nature of the teratogenic abnormality may differ in different species. It may be assumed, too, that the other phases of the reproductive cycle will show parallel susceptibility. In terms of general physiological processes, humans may react at 2–10% of the effective dose in animals. It is this relationship that underlies the common convention of applying an arbitrary safety limit of 1/500 to an animal teratogen; that is, if the 'no observed effect level' (NOEL) in an animal test is x mg/kg body weight, it is commonly assumed that an effectively safe exposure in a pregnant woman will be up to (x/500) mg/kg body weight. Use of the NOEL and a large additional safety factor will provide a considerable margin of protection.[98,99]

This is a useful working rule, because it does not involve any assumption about the slope of the dose–response relationship, or even whether there is a threshold of dose below which an effect will not occur anyway. Whether it is too cautious is left to the proponent of the substance to demonstrate, a conservative and therefore defensible regulatory position.

For disorders of the other phases of the reproductive cycle, there is much less evidence about the rules supporting extrapolation from animal tests to humans. In general, a substance that appears to act directly on the seminiferous epithelium, or on androgen receptors or androgen synthesis, should be accepted as a human risk and appropriate precautions advised. Substances that act by indirect, endocrine pathways cannot be regarded in the same way, because controls via the hypothalamus and anterior pituitary to the Leydig and Sertoli cells, and on adrenal androgen synthesis, are more species specific. This is well known in pharmacology, if less often appreciated in toxicology; for example, dopamine agonists in the rat cause excess release of prolactin and testicular atrophy and galactorrhoea, whereas humans exhibit none of these actions or only minimal galactorrhoea even during high-dose conventional therapy with these agents, such as certain neuroleptic drugs.

Toxicokinetic factors may sometimes be important, as the blood–testis and the placental barriers afford some hindrance to the permeation of substances from the blood stream into the testis and fetus, respectively. However, they are not absolute barriers and they change with time, so interspecies prediction must consider these processes, too.

Overall, it remains a prudent approach to regard any effect confirmed in animals as likely to occur in humans at some dose-level, and then, pragmatically, to evaluate case by case the evidence about dose, metabolism and mechanism.

SAFEGUARDING REPRODUCTIVE HEALTH IN THE WORKPLACE: RESPONSIBILITIES AND ETHICS

The objective should be to ensure that work does not harm individuals or their enjoyment of their sex life and the ability to produce a family. In the present context, it is necessary to protect the reproductive health of pregnant women at work, that of men and women prior to procreation and of women who have resumed work while continuing to breast-feed.

The practical problems of identifying and evaluating hazards and of investigating concerns expressed by those exposed through employment have already been discussed. Protection and surveillance at work are mainly the concern of specialists in occupational health and hygiene, but experts in general medicine and in the other fields of endocrinology, obstetrics, paediatrics and psychiatry also have responsibilities in this area. Whenever a patient with a relevant complaint is seen, it is important to consider whether it might have an occupational basis; this applies equally, say, to women anxious about impaired fertility (or multiple births), to men complaining about reduced libido, or to parents asking about clusters of abnormalities in babies. The scanty evidence does not suggest that work is a major source of reproductive harm, but facts are few and prudence demands vigilance by every physician, whether consulted by an individual woman or those professionally involved in surveillance of groups of people.

The general medical consultant may become involved in other aspects of reproductive hazards than investigating, treating and counselling individual workers. Social changes and better understanding of equity and justice mean that many more women work and that job discrimination based on gender has become illegal. The consequences for employment – for example, differential risks for men and women, policies about leave for pregnancy and child rearing – involve specialized understanding of industrial practices and law,[99,100] but they may also raise broader questions about the acceptability of jobs in relation to their physical and psychological stresses. Sexual activity and reproduction are such sensitive areas of life that concerns about them may sometimes extend from the occupational specialist to the general physician. The latter must first be quite certain that the nature of the concern has been clearly expressed, and that its relationship to work has been clarified, before offering any comments on more general implications for health. Combining prudence, caution and equality is difficult but essential.

Another way in which general physicians may become involved with reproduction toxicity is in counselling a woman who has been exposed to a suspect or potential teratogen while pregnant. Such counselling should not be undertaken without first discussing the risk with an expert in teratology. With a few exceptions, one would not predict a high risk of an adverse outcome in a woman who has not shown any other signs of toxicity.

Some practical approaches to the protection of reproductive health in the workplace have recently been discussed.[101,102]

CONCLUSIONS

Reproductive hazards in the workplace are, happily, rare although, with changing work practice and the synthesis of approximately 5000 new chemicals per year, there are no grounds for complacency. Experience has shown that the most potent occupational reproductive hazard was reported by the workforce rather than detected by occupational health screening, and so complaints that occupational factors are adversely affecting reproduction should be assiduously investigated. Irreversible effects, especially, on the fetus, generate most emotion and suspicion of a link to occupational hazard, but on epidemiological and experimental evidence so far the likelihood of an aetiological relationship has been very small.

Overall, reproduction involves the most intimate, sensitive and emotive aspects of life. We must strive to avoid toxic risks to any stage of this complex process, and we should do so with proper respect for the privacy and autonomy of the individual, whilst still being aware of every citizen's responsibilities to the community.

REFERENCES

1 Mattison DR. Reproductive toxicology. *Prog Clin Biol Res* 1983; **117**:1–396.
2 Dixon RL (ed). *Reproductive Toxicology*. New York: Raven Press, 1985: 1–350.
3 Mattison DR, Plowchalk DR, Meadows MJ, Aljuburi AZ, Gandy J, Malek A. Reproductive toxicity: male and female reproductive systems as targets for chemical injury. *Med Clin North Am* 1990; **74**:391–411.
4 Thomas JA. Toxic responses of the reproductive system. In: Klaassen CD ed. *Casarett and Doull's Toxicology* 5th edn. New York: McGraw-Hill, 1996: 547–81.
5 Olsham AF, Mattison DR. *Male-mediated Developmental Toxicity*. New York: Plenum Press, 1994.
6 Paul M. Occupational reproductive hazards. *Lancet* 1997; **349**:1385–8.
7 Sharpe RM, Skakkebaek NE. Are oestrogens involved in falling sperm counts and disorders of the male reproductive tract? *Lancet* 1993; **341**:1392–5.
8 Toppari J, Larsen JChr, Christiansen P *et al*. Male reproductive health and environmental xenoestrogens. *Environ Hlth Perspect* 1996; **104**:741–803.
9 Slotkin TA, Kavlock RJ, Cowdery T *et al*. Functional consequences of perinatal methyl mercury exposure. *Toxicol Lett* 1986; **34**:231–45.
10 Leridon H. Sterilité et hypofertilité. In:Henry-Suchet J, Mintz M, Spira A eds. *Recherches Recentes sur l'Epidemiologie de la fertilité*. Paris: Masson, 23–32.
11 Whorton MD, Follart DE. Mutagenicity, carcinogenicity and reproductive effects of dibromochloropropane (DBCP). *Mutat Res* 1983; **123**:13–30.
12 Snell K, Ashby SL, Barton SJ. Disturbances of perinatal carbohydrate metabolism in rats exposed to methylmercury *in utero*. *Toxicology* 1977; **8**:277–83.
13 Rogan WJ, Gladen BC, Hung K-L *et al*. Congenital poisoning by polychlorinated biphenyls and their contaminants in Taiwan. *Science* 1988; **241**:334–6.
14 Council on Environmental Quality. *Chemical Hazards to Reproduction*. Washington DC: US Government Printing Office, 1981.
15 Barlow SM, Sullivan FM. *Reproductive Hazards of Industrial Chemicals*. London: Academic Press, 1982.
16 John JA, Wroblewski DJ, Schwetz BA. Teratogenicity of experimental and occupational exposure to industrial chemicals. In: Kalter H ed. *Issues and Reviews in Teratology*. New York: Plenum Press, 1984: 267–324.
17 Rickert DE, Butterworth BE, Popp JA. Dinitrotoluene: acute toxicity, oncogenicity, genotoxicity, and metabolism. *CRC Crit Rev Toxicol* 1984; **13**:217–34.
18 Male-mediated Fl abnormalities. *Mutat Res.* 1990; **229**: 103–246. (Special issue; Anderson D ed.)
19 World Health Organization. *Principles for Evaluation of Health Risks to Progeny Associated with Exposure due to*

Chemicals During Pregnancy. Environmental Health Criteria No 30. Geneva: WHO, 1984: 1–177.

20 Biggers JD. *In vitro* fertilization and embryo transfer in human beings. *N Engl J Med* 1981; **304**:336–42.

21 Department of Health. *Guidelines for the Testing of Chemicals for Mutagenicity*. London: HMSD, 1989: 1–99.

22 Sullivan FM, Watkins WJ, van der Venne MT (eds). *The Toxicology of Chemicals* – Series Two: *Reproductive Toxicology* Vol 1: *Summary Reviews of the Scientific Evidence*. Luxembourg: Office for Official Publications of the European Communities, 1993.

23 Sever LE. Epidemiological evidence for toxic effects of occupational and environmental chemicals on the tests. In: Thomas JA, Colby HD eds. *Endocrine Toxicology* 2nd edn. Washington DC: Taylor and Francis, 1997: 287–326.

24 Armstrong BG, Nolin AD, McDonald AD. Work in pregnancy and birth weight for gestational age. *Br J Ind Med* 1989; **46**:196–9.

25 Lerda D, Rizzi R. Study of reproductive function in persons occupationally exposed to 2,4dichlorophenoxyacetic acid (2,4-D). *Mutat Res* 1991; **262**:47–50.

26 Ratcliffe JM, Schrader SM, Steenland K, Clapp DE, Turner T, Homung RW. Semen quality in papaya workers with long-term exposure to ethylene dibromide. *Br J Ind Med* 1987; **44**:317–26.

27 Lancranjan I, Popescu HI, Savanescu O *et al.* Reproductive ability of workmen occupationally exposed to lead. *Arch Environ Hlth* 1975; **30**:396–401.

28 Angle CR, McIntire MS. Lead poisoning during pregnancy. *Am J Dis Child* 1964; **108**:436–9.

29 De Rosis F, Anastasio SP, Selvaggi L, Beltrame A, Moriani C. Female reproductive health in two lamp factories: effects of exposure to inorganic mercury vapour and stress factors. *Br J Ind Med* 1985; **42**:488–94.

30 Sikorski R, Juszkiewicz T, Paszkowski T, Szprengier-Juszkiewicz T. Women in dental surgeries: reproductive hazards in occupational exposure to metallic mercury. *Int Arch Occup Environ Hlth* 1987; **59**:551–7.

31 Harrington J. Occupational hazards of formulating oral contraceptives. *Arch Environ Hlth* 1978, **33**:12–15.

32 Stucker I. Risk of spontaneous abortion among nurses handling antineoplastic drugs. *Scand J Work Environ Hlth* 1990; **16**:102–7.

33 Tannebaum TN, Coldberg RJ. Exposure to anaesthetic gases and reproductive outcome. *J Occup Med* 1985; **27**:659–68.

34 Ratcliffe JM, Schrader SM, Clapp DE, Halperin WE, Turner TW, Hornung RW. Semen quality in workers exposed to 2-ethoxyethanol. *Br J Ind Med* 1989; **46**:399–406.

35 McDonald AD. Work and pregnancy. (Editorial.) *Br J Ind Med* 1988; **45**:577–80.

36 Kitabatake T. Sterility in Japanese radiological technicians. *Tohoku J Exp Med* 1974; **112**:209–12.

37 Florack EI, Zielhuis GA, Rolland R. The influence of occupational physical activity on the menstrual cycle and fecundability. *Epidemiology* 1994; **5**:14–18.

38 Olsen GW, Lanham JM, Bodner KM, Hulton DB, Bond GG.

Determinants of spermatogenesis recovery among workers exposed to 1,2-dibromo-3-chloropropane. *J Occup Med* 1990; **32**:979–84.

39 Zielhuis GA, Gijsen R, van der Gulden JWJ. Menstrual disorders among dry-cleaning workers. *Scand J Work Environ Hlth* 1989; **15**:238.

40 Lemasters GK, Hagen A, Samuels SJ. Reproductive outcome in women exposed to solvents in 36 reinforced plastics companies. I. Menstrual dysfunction. *J Occup Med* 1985; **27**:490–4.

41 Iglesias R. Disorders of the menstrual cycle in airline stewardesses. *Aviat Space Environ Med* 1980; **51**:518–20.

42 Rom WN. Effects of lead on the female and reproduction. a review. *Mt Sinai J Med* 1976; **43**:542–52.

43 World Health Organization. *Women and Occupational Health Risks*. European Reports and Studies 76. Copenhagen: WHO, 1983.

44 Fraser FC. Relation of animal studies to the problem in man. In: Wilson JC, Fraser FC eds. *Handbook of Teratology* Vol 1. New York: Plenum Press, 1977: 75–96.

45 Koos BJ, Longo LD. Mercury toxicity in the pregnant woman, fetus and newborn infant. *Am J Obstet Gynecol* 1976; **126**:390–409.

46 Ericson A, Kallén B. Pregnancy outcome in women working as dentists, dental assistants or dental technicians. *Int Arch Occup Environ Hlth* 1989; **61**:329–33.

47 Pastides H, Calabrese EJ, Hosner DW, Harris DR. Spontaneous abortion and general illness symptoms among semiconductor manufacturers. *J Occup Med* 1988; **30**:543–51.

48 Holmberg PC, Hernberg S, Kurppa K, Rantala R, Riala R. Oral clefts and organic solvent exposure during pregnancy. *Int Arch Occup Environ Hlth* 1982; **50**:371–6.

49 Goulet L, Thériault G. Association between spontaneous abortion and ergonomic factors. A literature review of the epidemiologic evidence. *Scand J Work Environ Hlth* 1987; **13**:399–403.

50 Huel G, Mergler D, Bowler R. Evidence for adverse reproductive outcomes among women microelectronic assembly workers. *Br J Ind Med* 1990; **47**:400–4.

51 Blomqvist U, Ericson A, Kallén B, Westerholm P. Delivery, outcome for women working in the pulp and paper industry. *Scand J Work Environ Hlth* 1981; **7**:114–18.

52 Roman E, Beral V, Pelerin M, Hermon C. Spontaneous abortion and work with visual display units. *Br J Ind Med* 1992; **49**:507–12.

53 Lindbohm M-L, Hemminki K, Kyyrönen P, Kilpikari I, Vainio H. Spontaneous abortions among rubber workers and congenital malformations in their offspring. *Scand J Work Environ Hlth* 1983; Suppl **2**:85–90.

54 Lemasters GK, Samuels SJ, Morrison JA, Brooks SM. Reproductive outcomes of pregnant workers employed at 36 reinforced plastic companies. II. Lowered birth weight. *J Occup Med* 1989; **31**:115–20.

55 Ng TP, Foo SC, Yoong T. Risk of spontaneous abortion in workers exposed to toluene. *Br J Ind Med* 1992; **49**:804–8.

56 Cordier S, Ha M-C, Ayme S, Goujard J. Maternal occupational exposure and congenital malformations. *Scand J Work Environ Hlth* 1992; **18**:11–17.

57 Olsen J, Hemminki K, Ahlborg G *et al*. Low birth weight, congenital malformations and spontaneous abortions among dry-cleaning workers in Scandinavia. *Scand J Work Environ Hlth* 1990; **16**:163–8.

58 Olsen J, Rachootin P. Organic solvents as possible risk factors of low birth weight. *J Occup Med* 1983; **25**:854–5.

59 Colls BM. Safety handling of cytotoxic agents: a cause for concern by pharmaceutical companies? *Br Med J* 1985; **291**:1318–19.

60 Wyrobek AJ, Watchmaker G, Gordon L, Wong K, Moore D, Whorton D. Sperm shape abnormalities in carbaryl-exposed employees. *Environ Hlth Perspect* 1981; **40**:255–65.

61 Rowland AS, Baird DD, Shore DL, Weinberg CR, Savitz DA, Wilcox AJ. Nitrous oxide and spontaneous abortion in female dental assistants. *Am J Epidemiol* 1995; **141**:531–8.

62 Ahlborg G, Axelsson G, Bodin L. Shift work, nitrous oxide exposure and subfertility among Swedish midwives. *Int J Epidemiol* 1996; **25**:783–90.

63 Rowland AS, Baird DD, Weinberg CR, Shore DL, Shy CM, Wilcox AJ. Reduced fertility among women employed as dental assistants exposed to high levels of nitrous oxide. *N Engl J Med* 1992; **327**:993–7.

64 Golding J, Adelstein P. Leather close up work: a possible hazard to reproduction. *Br Med J* 1985; **290**:1986.

65 Hunt VR. The physical environment. *Work and the Health of Women*. Boca Raton: CRC Press, 1979: 61–95.

66 Baltzar B, Ericson E, Kallén B. Pregnancy outcome among women working in Swedish hospitals. *N Engl J Med* 1979; **300**:627–8.

67 Kallén B. Delivery outcome among physiotherapists in Sweden: is non-ionizing radiation a fetal hazard? *Arch Environ Hlth* 1982; **37**:81–4.

68 Taskinen H, Kyyronen P, Hemminki K. Effects of ultrasound, shortwaves, and physical exertion on pregnancy outcome in physiotherapists. *J Epidemiol Commun Hlth* 1990; **44**:196–201.

69 Ouellett-Hellstrom R, Stewart WF. Miscarriages among female physical therapists who report using radio- and microwave-frequency electromagnetic radiation. *Am J Epidemiol* 1993; **138**:775–86.

70 Bergqvist U. Visual display terminals and health. *Scand J Work Environ Hlth* 1984; **10** (Suppl 2): 1–87.

71 *Proceedings of the International Scientific Conference on Work with Visual Display Units, Stockholm 1986*. Stockholm: Elsevier, 1987.

72 World Health Organization. *Visual Display Terminals and Workers Health*. Geneva: WHO, 1987.

73 Blackwell R, Chang A. Video display terminals and pregnancy: a review. *Br J Obstet Gynaecol* 1988; **95**:446–53.

74 Nurminen T, Kurppa K. Occupational noise exposure and course of pregnancy. *Scand J Work Environ Hlth* 1989; **15**:117–24.

75 Axelsson G, Rylander R, Molin I. Outcome of pregnancy in relation to irregular and inconvenient work schedules. *Br J Ind Med* 1989; **46**:393–8.

76 Ahlborg G, Bodin L, Hogstedt C. Heavy lifting during pregnancy – a hazard to the fetus? A prospective study. *Int J Epidemiol* 1990; **19**:90–7.

77 Jensen AA. Chemical contaminants in breast milk. *Residue Rev* 1983; **89**:1–120.

78 Rogan WG, Bagniewska A, Damstra T. Pollutants and breast milk. *N Engl J Med* 1980; **302**:1450–3.

79 Sikorski R, Paszowski T, Radomanski T, Niewiadowska A, Semeniuk S. Human colostrum as a source of organohalogen xenobiotics for a breast-fed neonate. *Reprod Toxicol* 1990; **4**:17–20.

80 Yakushiji T, Watanabe I, Kuwabara K, Tanaka R, Kashimoto T, Kumita N. Postnatal transfer of PCBs from exposed mothers to their babies: influence of breast-feeding. *Arch Environ Hlth* 1984; **39**:368–75.

81 Joffe M. Time to pregnancy: a measure of reproductive function in either sex. *Occup Env Med* 1997; **54**:285–95.

82 Joffe M, Villard L, Li Z *et al*. A time to pregnancy questionnaire designed for long term recall: Validity in Oxford England. *J Epidemiol Commun Hlth* 1995; **49**:314–9.

83 Stijkel A, van Eindhoven CJ, Bal R. Drafting guidelines for occupational exposure to chemicals: the Dutch experience with the assessment of reproductive risk. *Am J Ind Med* 1996; **30**:705–17.

84 Working PK. *Toxicology of the Male and Female Reproductive System*. New York: Hemisphere Publishing, 1989.

85 McDowall ME. The epidemiological identification of reproductive hazards. In: Chamberlain C ed. *Pregnant Women at Work*. London: Royal Society of Medicine/Macmillan Press, 1984; 73–85.

86 Polednak AP, Janerich DT. Uses of available record systems in epidemiologic studies of reproductive toxicology. *Am J Ind Med* 1983; **4**:329–48.

87 Joffe M. Biases in research on reproduction and women's work. *Int J Epidemiol* 1985; **14**:118–23.

88 Winder C. Reproductive and chromosomal effects of occupational exposure to lead in the male. *Reprod Toxicol* 1989; **3**:221–33.

89 Selevan SC. Design considerations in pregnancy outcome studies of occupational populations. *Scand J Work Environ Hlth* 1981; **7**(Suppl 4): 76–82.

90 Levine RJ, Blunden PB, DalCorso D, Starr TB, Ross CE. Superiority of reproductive histories to sperm counts in detecting infertility at a dibromochloropropane manufacturing plant. *J Occup Med* 1983; **25**:591–7.

91 Wyrobek AJ, Gordon LA, Burkhart JG *et al*. An evaluation of human sperm as indicators of chemically induced alterations of spermatogenic function. *Mutat Res* 1983; **115**:73–148.

92 Wyrobek AJ. Methods for evaluating the effects of environmental chemicals on human sperm production. *Environ Hlth Perspect* 1983; **48**:53–9.

93 Schrader SM, Ratcliffe JM, Turner TW, Hornung RW. The use of new field methods of semen analysis in the study of occupational hazards to reproduction: the example of ethylene dibromide. *J Occup Med* 1987; **29**:963–6.

94 Schenker MB, Samuels SJ, Perkins C, Lewis EL, Katz DF, Overstreet JW. Prospective surveillance of semen quality in the workplace. *J Occup Med* 1988; **30**:336–44.

95 Sheikh K. Choice of control population in studies of adverse reproductive effects of occupational exposures and its effect on risk estimates. *Br J Ind Med* 1987; **44**:244–9.

96 Roloff MV (ed.) *Human Risk Assessment: The Role of Animal Selection and Extrapolation*. London: Taylor and Francis, 1987: 1–282.

97 Tardiff RC, Rodricks JW (eds). *Toxic Substances and Human Risk*. New York: Plenum Press, 1987: 1–445.

98 Brown NA, Fabro S. The value of animal teratogenicity testing for predicting human risk. *Clin Obstet Gynecol* 1983; **26**:467–77.

99 Hemminki K, Vineis P. Extrapolation of the evidence on teratogenicity of chemicals between humans and experimental animals: chemicals other than drugs. Teratogenesis *Carcinog Mutagen* 1985; **5**:252–318.

100 Kloss D. *Occupational Health Law*. London: B&P Professional Books, 1991.

101 Stijkel A, Reijnders L. Implementation of the precautionary principle in standards for the workplace. *Occup Environ Med* 1995; **52**:304–12.

102 Sullivan FM. The European Community Directive on the classification and labelling of chemicals for reproductive toxicity. *J Occup Environ Med* 1995; **37**:966–9.

Part 11

Other systemic effects of workplace exposures

Nephrotoxic effects of workplace exposures	843
Neurotoxic effects of workplace exposures	867
Hepatotoxic effects of workplace exposures	881
Haemopoietic effects of workplace exposures:	
anaemias, leukaemias and lymphomas	901

41

Nephrotoxic effects of workplace exposures

GORDON M BELL, HOWARD J MASON

Heavy metals	843	Bismuth and copper	853
Lead	844	Crystalline silica	853
Cadmium	849	Organic solvents and renal disease	854
Mercury	851	Case reports and experimental studies	855
Uranium	853	Mechanisms of solvent-induced nephrotoxicity	858
Chromium	853	Acknowledgement	859
Beryllium	853	References	859
Arsenic	853		

In the UK the annual incidence of new patients requiring renal replacement therapy (RRT) is between 80 and 120 per million population depending on demographic variables.[1] After commencing dialysis the treatment of each new patient costs the exchequer around £25 000 per year with a greater personal cost to the patient and his family.

In the United States of America glomerulonephritis, glomerulosclerosis and interstitial nephritis account for up to 47% of all cases requiring RRT.[2] While immunological and vasculopathic associations with such nephropathy are well recognized, occupational factors may also be relevant. In this regard the nephrotoxicity of heavy metals has been studied for a long time while more recent evidence links occupational organic solvent exposure with various kidney diseases.

This chapter reviews the renal effects of such workplace exposures.

HEAVY METALS (see Chapter 7)

Metals are probably the oldest toxic materials known to man. Lead usage may have begun more than 4000 years ago when supplies were obtained as byproducts of silver smelting. Indeed Hippocrates in 370 BC is credited with the first description of abdominal colic in a man who extracted metals. However, many of the metals of workplace concern today are only recently known to man. In 1817 cadmium was first recognized in ore containing zinc carbonate. Approximately 80 of the 105 elements in the periodic table are regarded as metals, 30 or so of which form compounds reported to produce toxicity in humans and of these only 10 are known to be nephrotoxic. The renal toxicological profile of metals such as indium and tantalum, which are used increasingly in newer industries such as microelectronics, is unknown. With present day occupational and environmental standards, the acute and overt renal effects (such as acute renal failure) associated with exposures to lead and mercury are now uncommon. While there must be a full understanding of these well-recognized acute problems, conceptually what we now regard as the toxic effect of metals continues to broaden into the more subtle, chronic effects or long-term nephrotoxicity. In this respect, cause and effect may not always be obvious and allocating blame to particular agents can be difficult especially when there are small repeated exposures to one or more substances. Physicians interested in these nephrotoxic effects need to have an understanding of the metabolism of metals including any renal cellular effects, and to recognize factors that might influence toxicity. Although treatment is clearly an important topic, prevention of toxicity through public health and worksite programmes, which include raising workers' awareness and adherence to control measures is of equal or perhaps greater importance. Increasingly, emphasis should be focused on the detection of early and possibly reversible biochemical indicators of toxicity, such as renal tubular dysfunction in cadmium toxicity.

Lead

Lead use and indeed lead poisoning date back to ancient times (see Chapter 7). Gout, which was thought to be common among the wealthy classes of seventeenth and eighteenth century Europe was probably due in large part to the adulteration or contamination of lead in wine.[3] Clinical and epidemiological observations in Europe, Australia and the USA have now made it clear that environmental or occupational lead exposure can lead to chronic renal failure and excess renal death.[3-7] Government regulation now limits most occupational lead exposure, but isolated cases of renal disease are still reported in certain industries (Table 41.1) where lead or its compounds are used. Furthermore, there is currently increasing pressure from many regulatory authorities worldwide to reduce occupational exposure limits. Non-occupational exposures such as the leaching of lead by weakly acid fluids from hand-crafted pottery are occasionally noted and serve to stress the importance of a careful history in all cases of renal disease of unknown cause.[4]

Four clinical manifestations of lead nephropathy are described:

1 Acute lead nephropathy resulting from short-term but massive lead absorption. This is associated with abdominal colic, encephalopathy, peripheral nephropathy, anaemia and renal tubular damage presenting as Fanconi syndrome.
2 Chronic slowly progressive renal failure. This results from accumulating lead absorption from a recognized occupational source and then often without overt symptoms of toxicity.
3 Hypertension arising from prolonged low level exposure to environmental or occupational lead. This area of interest is more controversial.
4 The presence of early markers of disturbed renal tubular function: the relevance of these findings to the development of more chronic renal dysfunction is unknown.

ACUTE LEAD NEPHROPATHY

This is uncommonly seen in adults, but children with lead encephalopathy develop a proximal renal tubular defect (Fanconi syndrome) which is characterized by aminoaciduria, phosphaturia and glycosuria. Both these conditions occur as a result of repeated ingestion of inappropriate materials e.g. lead paint chips.[8] As with other forms of Fanconi syndrome, vitamin D resistant rickets may develop and appears to be rapidly reversed following chelation therapy.[9] This renal tubular disorder is found in the presence of blood levels of lead usually in excess of 150 μg/dl (7.24 μmol/litre) and has been induced experimentally in animals fed dietary lead.[10] The renal histological appearances in both children and

Table 41.1 *Industries using lead*

Smelting, refining, alloying and casting
Battery manufacture
Jewellery manufacture
Glass making
Manufacture of pigments and colours
Glazes and transfers in the pottery industry
Manufacture of inorganic and organic lead compounds
Shipbuilding repairing and breaking
Demolition industry
Painting of buildings and vehicles
Scrap industry
Vehicle radiator repair
Cable coverings manufacture
Use of lead alloys e.g. manufacture of solder and on firing ranges
Metal reclamation industry

experimental animals is of the development of acid-fast intranuclear inclusions in proximal tubular epithelial cells.[11] These inclusion bodies consist of a lead protein complex;[12] mitochondrial changes and cytomegaly also occur.

Removal of lead by chelation therapy reverses both the tubular reabsorptive defect and removes the inclusion bodies.[13] However, chronic tubular interstitial nephritis, which is similar to the chronic lead nephropathy seen in adults, may develop several decades later.[5] When lead is absorbed excessively, it is deposited mainly in the skeleton from which it is slowly released once exposure ceases. This gradual release of lead over many years may contribute to this delayed nephrotoxicity.[6]

CHRONIC LEAD NEPHROPATHY

The chronic syndrome, which is more commonly associated with high occupational exposure, is characterized histologically by progressive renal interstitial fibrosis, dilatation of the tubules, and atrophy of tubular cells Fig. 41.1. These changes are accompanied by a reduction in glomerulofiltration and azotaemia. Typically, renal failure is evident only after years of excessive lead absorption and is then frequently associated with hypertension and/or gout[14-16] Non-occupational causes have also been identified. These include the childhood lead poisoning which was the result of licking off the sweet tasting lead paint from the painted, wooden verandas of Queensland houses; the high prevalence of chronic nephritis was confirmed in the 1950s.[17] A high incidence of chronic nephritis has also been observed in some Serbian villages situated near the river Kolubara which was associated with the chronic ingestion of flour contaminated with lead.[18] Renal dysfunction was also found in 280 subjects from 136 Scottish households living in houses in which the drinking water contained lead in excess of 100 μg/dl[19] Whether the susceptibility to lead-induced kidney dam-

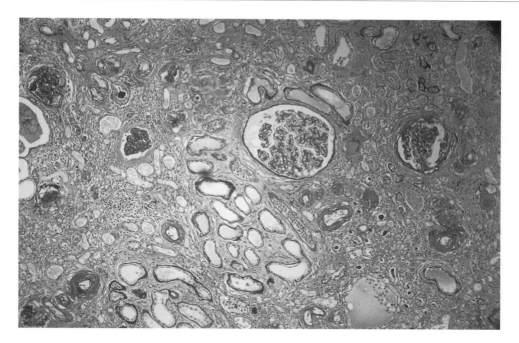

Figure 41.1 *Autopsy section of a kidney of a patient exposed to lead in childhood through eating lead-based paint. The features are those of a marked focal interstitial fibrosis with focal tubular atrophy. Photograph kindly provided by Dr J Searle of the Brisbane Hospital, Brisbane, Australia.*

age is related to genetic polymorphism in the enzyme 5-aminolaevulinic acid dehydratase (ALA-D), which may be associated with interindividual differences in the metabolism of lead and toxicity from lead storage,[20] remains unknown.

Most studies on the relationship between lead exposure and renal failure have been performed in occupational cohorts. A recent review has outlined the weaknesses of some of these studies.[21] Thus, in epidemiological studies, the relationship between lead exposure and the development of renal failure is often largely circumstantial. Several other aspects remain unclear – namely: relative and absolute risk, other concomitant risk factors, duration of exposure necessary for toxicity and occasionally even diagnostic criteria. The studies selected for inclusion here are, nonetheless, both scientifically satisfactory and interesting. Table 41.2 reviews some of the most important studies.[22–36] After two decades of investigating ways of trying to prevent lead nephropathy through the identification of possible early markers of nephrotoxicity, it is germane to note that in Africa the adverse consequences of poor worksite and personnel control measures are still seen among workers exposed to lead.[22]

High exposure to lead which is associated with blood levels of lead probably in excess of 80 µg/dl can induce kidney toxicity characterized by an acute phase involving tubular damage and a chronic phase involving both tubular changes and interstitial fibrosis. Although kidney toxicity has not been thoroughly investigated in occupationally exposed groups, the available studies provide no clear evidence of chronic lead-induced renal damage or functional changes at blood levels of lead below 60 µg/dl. Some studies suggest an association between low levels of occupational exposure and changes in renal function such as renal tubular enzymuria and abnormalities of prostanoid metabolism, but the importance of these changes to the long-term development of nephrotoxicity is unknown.

General descriptions of the effects of lead on the kidney in rodent models are described elsewhere,[10,37] and the structural and functional changes are broadly similar to those seen in human studies. At high exposure levels (producing blood concentrations of 60–125 µg/dl), similar but more severe morphological changes occur, including glomerulosclerosis in occasional animals. Furthermore, the cellular bioavailability and toxicity of lead can be influenced by high affinity lead binding proteins in rat kidneys.[38] Whether similar mechanisms operate in the human kidney and if they can influence cellular toxicities is unknown.

MORTALITY, HYPERTENSION AND CHRONIC RENAL FAILURE

Several mortality studies (Table 41.3)[39–46] indicate excess deaths due to renal disease among cohorts of workers exposed to lead but methodological problems related to

Table 41.2 *Occupational cross-sectional studies of the relationship between lead exposure and renal dysfunction*

Blood lead levels (or alternative)	Renal observations	Ref.
>100 µg/dl	Renal biopsies showed evidence of moderate-to-severe nephropathy in approx 50% of subjects	Radosevic[23]
>60 µg/dl	15% of subjects had renal impairment	Lilis et al.[24,25]
71–138 µg/dl	Renal biopsies of 7 shipyard workers, moderate-to-severe severe nephropathy in long-term exposed	Cramer et al.[26]
Range 50–105 µg/dl	17% of subjects had renal impairment	Baker et al.[27]
Range 20–98 µg/dl+ 'positive' EDTA chelation test	13% of subjects had renal impairment	Wedeen et al.[28]
Mean level 64 ± 16 µg/dl	33% had renal impairment	Pinto de Almeida[29]
Range 34–98 µg/dl	No evidence of renal impairment but elevated uNAG and significant correlation with blood lead levels	Verschoer et al.[30]
Range 3–80 µg/dl	Weak correlation between urinary lead excretion and blood urea and creatinine. uNAG increased in 'higher' exposed group.	Ong et al.[31]
Mean level 51 µg/dl 'exposed' group	No difference in wide variety of markers of renal dysfunction in exposed compared with control group range 40–75 µg/dl	Gennart et al.[32]
Mean level 48 µg/dl range 36–65 µg/dl	uNAG increased, urinary eicosanoids and sialic and excretion increased. Significant correlations of above with blood lead levels	Cardenas et al.[33]
Mean level 43 µg/dl	Baseline GFR increased in exposed group but no difference in GFR response to oral protein load test	Roels et al.[34]
Mean level 30 µg/dl. Range 4–66 µg/dl	uNAG only increased in those with recent elevation in blood lead level	Chia et al.[35]
Range 30–69 µg/dl	uNAG, uβ2 microglobulin levels increased; no difference in creatinine clearance	Kumar et al.[36]
Range 60–270 µg/dl	Evidence of severe lead toxicity with renal failure, gout and anaemia. Lack of worksite and personal protection	Ankrah et al.[22]

Conversion factor µmol/litre: µg/dl ÷20.72; uNAG: urinary *N*-acetyl-β-D-glucosaminidase; GFR: glomerular filtration rate; EDTA: ethylenediaminetetraacetic acid

Table 41.3 *Mortality due to renal disease in cohorts exposed to lead*

Cohort (n)	Mortality due to renal dysfunction	Number of patients with renal dysfunction	Ref.
7032	EM	21	Cooper and Gaffey[39]
241	EM	21	McMichael and Johnson[40]
1898	EM	19	Malcom and Barnett[41]
57	EM	3	Davies[42]
4519	EM	20	Cooper et al.[43]
2300	EM	8	Cooper et al.[43]
1987	EM	9	Selevan et al.[44]
437	NEM	2	Gerhardsson et al.[45]
2276	NEM	11	Fanning[46]

NEM: no excess mortality; EM: excess mortality.

the numbers of cases observed and the selection of controls or census data from the general population may limit their value.[47] Similarly, the role of lead in the genesis of renal hypertension is the subject of controversy. Nonetheless some mortality studies suggest that hypertensive cardiovascular disease is a more frequent cause of death amongst lead workers than among the general population.[15,46,48,49] Batuman et al.[15] studying lead mobilization using ethylenediaminetetraacetic acid (EDTA) reported a possible role for lead in hypertension associated with renal failure. While lead may contribute to a hypertensive effect, in some studies[50–52] doubts have been raised about the magnitude of this postulated dose–response curve,[48,53–56] It is possible that genetic factors may modulate the intracellular cation response to circulating lead levels[57–59] and adjust vasomotor responsiveness.[60] Patients who develop gout after the onset of renal failure have been shown to excrete excessive amounts of lead in the urine after the infusion of EDTA.[16] This finding has led to the suggestion that the development of gout in advanced renal failure should prompt clinicians to consider the patient's past or indeed current exposure to lead.

While a clinical study suggested that smoking, alcoholism and a history of lead exposure with increased amounts of mobilizable lead were contributory factors to the development of end-stage renal failure,[61] a case control study found that exposure to lead was not significantly greater in patients with end-stage renal disease.[62]

One interpretation of these studies is that in some subjects lead from previous exposure may well contribute towards progression of their renal disease. Whether the EDTA chelation test is of much value in identifying the possible role of lead in patients with chronic renal failure is unresolved. The pharmacokinetics of EDTA may well be different in renal failure because EDTA is normally excreted in the urine by glomerular filtration. In these circumstances excretion of EDTA is delayed with the effect that the serum concentration integrated over the duration of the test will be greater than normal.[16] The presence of increased bone turnover from secondary hyperparathyroidism might also expose more lead-containing bone surfaces to the effects of the chelating agent,[16] but the observed increases in mobilizable lead are unlikely to be explained simply on the basis of a pharmacokinetic artefact or the presence of metabolic bone disease.[61]

DIAGNOSIS

From the above data it would appear that the diagnosis of lead nephropathy can be problematic. In acute lead intoxication the diagnosis can be straightforward if the clinician has taken a full occupational history, is aware of the relative exposure risk and has identified the level of protection from worksite exposure. Concomitant blood and neurological sequelae are not detailed here but blood lead levels below 80 µg/dl would be incompatible

with lead nephropathy in the acute phase (below 40 µg/dl in children). Fortunately the condition is now rarely seen in children in the UK due to the removal of lead from paint and an increase in the environmental awareness of the dangers of lead.

With known chronic lead exposure, blood levels of lead greater than 60 µg/dl have been shown to be associated with chronic lead nephropathy but the blood level is inadequate for the detection of excessive body burdens after exposure has ceased. The biological half-life of lead in blood approximates to 2 weeks, whilst that of the lead retained in bone, which accounts for about 95% of the total body burden, is more than 10 years. Therefore, in comparison with blood lead the levels of lead in bone reflect cumulative exposure. Current practice suggests that previous lead absorption is best assessed by the EDTA lead immobilization test, as chelatable lead correlates well with bone lead concentrations[6,63] (Fig. 41.2).

The EDTA test is performed in adults by parenteral administration of 3 g of Ca Na₂ EDTA over 4–12 hours with subsequent urine collection over 1–4 days. A dose of 20–30 mg/kg is generally used in children. Neither the dose nor the route of administration (intravenous or intramuscular) appears to critically modify the normal response. In renal failure, however, (plasma creatinine > 1.5 mg/dl) the urine collection should be extended to 3–4 days. Children (when corrected to 1.73m² body sur-

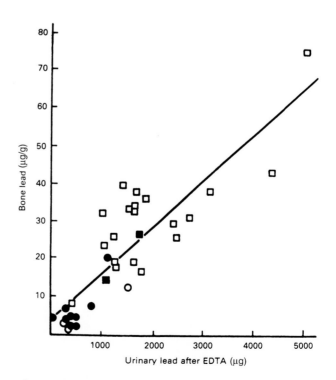

Figure 41.2 *Relation between EDTA lead immobilization tests and transiliac bone lead in 35 at-risk patients, including 22 lead workers (r = 0.87). Reproduced from Ref. 63 with permission.*

face area) and adults without unusual lead exposure excrete up to 650 µg (3.14 µmol).[49,64–65] The degree of renal failure that precludes interpretation of this test is not clear but one would be concerned about its use in patients with a plasma creatinine of more than 600 µmol/litre (approximately 7 mg/dl).

Tibial K x-ray fluorescence is a safe non-invasive and accurate technique at estimating bone lead levels at concentrations normally associated with lead-induced interstitial nephritis (Fig. 41.3). This may well replace the chelation test in future. Bone lead provides more direct information on cumulative lead absorption than either blood lead levels or chelatable lead. The characteristic K x-ray fluorescence records the calcium content of the region of bone under study and also permits measurement of the lead/calcium ratio. Whole body radiation during the half hour test is equivalent in most instances to background radiation absorbed over 10 hours.[65]

MANAGEMENT

The adage that prevention is better than cure was never more apt than when applied to lead nephropathy. Indeed this disorder is one of the few renal diseases that is preventable. While acute lead nephropathy can be treated effectively by chelation therapy,[64] there is no evidence that such treatment can improve renal function in patients with lead-induced interstitial nephritis[66] in whom the plasma concentration of creatinine is more than 3 mg/dl. The partial remissions which occur with treatment in symptomatic lead workers may reflect

reversal of acute renal lesions superimposed on the irreversible component of chronic lead nephropathy.

Most reports suggest that there is increased responsiveness of the renin system in subjects with lead nephropathy.[67] However, decreased aldosterone secretion is noted occasionally.[68] In these circumstances chronic volume depletion with hyporeninaemic hypoaldosteronism can contribute to the renal dysfunction. As in other situations, renal function can improve with correction of volume depletion.[68]

While lead can be removed from the body by chelation therapy, the potentially adverse long-term effects of this treatment in patients with renal failure are not known. The same can be said for the newer and therapeutically promising chelating agents such as dimercaptopropane sulphonate, dimercaptosulphonic acid and dimercaptosuccinic acid.[69–71]

Examples of primary prevention include minimizing industrial exposure by environmental controls and protection, and the avoidance of absorption from deteriorating lead-based paints and contaminated industrial sources. Fortunately, removal of lead from paints has been carried out in many countries.

Acute plumbism with Fanconi syndrome can be reversed by chelation therapy. In patients with more chronic renal disease the decision to embark on chelation therapy is more difficult and has to be tailored to the individual patient. When there is no evidence that established interstitial fibrosis or tubulopathy is being improved by chelation therapy, continuing a therapeutic trial may be of little value. Further information could be obtained by repeated chelation testing or by *in vivo* K x-ray fluorescence assessment.

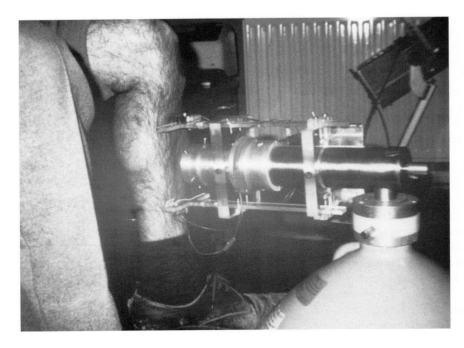

Figure 41.3 In vivo *measurement of tibial bone lead by x-ray fluorescence.*

Cadmium (see Chapter 7)

The use of cadmium in industry grew steadily after its discovery in 1817 by Strohmeyer. The first three cases of acute poisoning by cadmium were reported in 1858 by the Belgium physician, Sovet, in workers using silverware polishes containing cadmium carbonate. The clinical syndrome of cadmium nephrotoxicity with renal impairment and proteinuria was described by Friberg in 1948 following reports from Stephens in 1930 and Hardy and Skinner in 1947. Further studies in Italy, Japan, Sweden and the UK confirmed these observations and defined the proteinuria as tubular in origin.[72,73]

While used to a much lesser extent than previously, cadmium is still used on a significant scale in the production of alkaline batteries, to make industrial pigments, in electroplating, in special welding techniques and as a component in special metal alloys. While the acute absorption of as little as 10 mg of cadmium as dust or fumes may induce a severe gastrointestinal disturbance followed by pulmonary oedema, chronic low dose exposure can lead to proximal renal tubular reabsorptive defects which are characterized by low molecular weight proteinuria, aminoaciduria and renal glycosuria.[74] Urinary calculi can rarely result from the associated hypercalciuria and distal renal tubular acidosis and osteomalacia can also occur. There is increasing evidence that continued low-grade cadmium exposure can result in progressive renal failure. Because of these adverse renal effects, efforts have been made recently in Europe and the USA to reduce the usage of cadmium, for example by its substitution in specialized products like solders and pigments.

METABOLISM AND TOXICITY

Cadmium is not an essential element and it seems likely that cadmium ions are taken up through calcium channels.[75] As many cadmium salts are barely soluble it is estimated that only 5% of any oral dose of cadmium is absorbed in the body[76] but cadmium oxide fumes are readily absorbed through the lungs. Most cadmium is absorbed by inhalation and once in the body the biological half-life is tens of years with accumulation in the liver and kidney. This cadmium accumulation in the liver induces the synthesis of a special low molecular weight binding protein, metallothionein.[77]

The exact mechanism of cadmium toxicity is unknown. In acute animal experiments vacuolization and lysosomal changes in the renal tubule cells have been described.[78] Radioactively labelled cadmium is associated with membrane fractions[79] which can thus impair ion movements and energy systems. This toxicity probably depends on the initial overwhelming of the ability to induce intracellular metallothionein within target issues, thus reinforcing the concept of a threshold renal cadmium concentration.

While the urinary excretion of low molecular weight proteins such as retinol binding protein and β2-microglobulin is proportionally much more increased than that of high molecular weight proteins, significant increases in the urinary excretion of albumin, transferrin and IgG are observed in cadmium-exposed workers.[80] Low molecular weight proteins are taken up preferentially by the proximal renal tubule, and their increased urinary excretion with cadmium exposure can be explained in terms of cellular damage at this site.[80,81] Nonetheless, it is important to stress that irreversible decrements in glomerular filtration rate (GFR) have been found in those with tubular proteinuria.[82–83]

Experimental studies in animals suggest that in addition to the renal tubular dysfunction, cadmium may enhance the glomerular filtration of proteins through a depletion of the glomerular polyanion involving sialic acid and its charge.[81,84–86] Furthermore, occupational exposures to cadmium may induce subtle changes in glomerular permeability as shown by the increased urinary excretion of transferrin and albumin which may precede the onset of proximal tubular impairment.[87]

That cadmium may interfere with glomerular structure or function, is also supported by the finding of circulating antibodies to laminin (a glycoprotein present in the glomerular basement membrane) in both workers[88] and experimental animals.[89]

DIAGNOSIS OF RENAL DYSFUNCTION

The salient feature of cadmium nephrotoxicity is tubular dysfunction. Proteinuria is preceded by the increased excretion of small molecular weight proteins such as retinol binding protein (RBP) or β2-microglobulin with aminoaciduria, glycosuria, phosphaturia and calcium wasting.[74,82,90–93] For screening purposes RBP should be used in preference to β2-microglobulin because this protein is unstable in acid urine. Blood cadmium concentration falls rapidly after acute exposure and is therefore seldom used as the sole marker of acute toxicity. However, in subjects with a past history of high chronic exposure blood cadmium levels may increasingly reflect body burden rather than current exposure.[94]

In newly exposed workers the concentration of cadmium in blood increases linearly to reach a plateau at about 4 months.[95] In workers currently exposed to cadmium, blood cadmium levels are mainly a reflection of the uptake of the metal over the preceding few months. After removal from exposure the respective contributions of current exposure and body burden are progressively reversed and in former cadmium workers with high levels of cadmium in tissues the influence of body burden becomes more prominent.[96] Thus in excessive acute exposures urinary cadmium levels may be high, but generally urinary cadmium is an indicator of cumulative body burden. Above renal cortical levels of

100–300 μgCd/g, increases in urine cadmium may be found which arise either through renal losses or failure to reabsorb filtered low molecular weight cadmium complexes because of renal tubular dysfunction[96–97] The non-invasive technique of *in vivo* neutron activation analysis can afford more diagnostic precision without the need for biopsy analysis of cadmium,[96–97] but this remains a research technique not yet widely available.

However, in workers moderately exposed to cadmium and in the general population the urinary excretion of cadmium (expressed in terms of creatinine or as 24-hour output) is a reliable indicator of the body burden of cadmium[72,93] and urinary cadmium is better correlated with duration of exposure than blood cadmium. However, in Belgium it has been found that the urinary excretion of cadmium progressively increases with age in parallel with the body burden until the age of 50–60 years. These difficulties in interpreting blood and urinary cadmium have recently been reviewed.[98] The measurement of metallothionein in the urine of cadmium workers provides similar information to the determination of urinary cadmium.[98–100]

CLINICAL SYNDROMES

Cadmium-induced renal calcium wasting associated with a painful bone disease (osteomalacia) and pseudofractures was recognized in Japan in the 1950s. This was attributed to river water contamination of the food chain by an industrial effluent containing cadmium. The disorder locally known as 'itai-itai' or (ouch-ouch) disease mainly affected post-menopausal women. Renal complications of this syndrome included hypercalciuria, Fanconi syndrome, reduced GFR and occasional hypotension. In the population studied, low molecular weight proteinuria and β2-microglobulinuria correlated with renal dysfunction.[101] Hypertension was absent even in the presence of renal failure which in some of those affected continued to progress even after cessation of exposure. Interstitial nephritis was the histological picture observed in the limited material available. Concomitant clinical features in the most severely affected women were a waddling gait, short stature, osteomalacia, anaemia and lymphopenia.[101–103]

Epidemologic data do not support an association between blood or urinary cadmium levels and blood pressure.[104] Earlier mortality studies designed to evaluate the long-term effects of cadmium have yielded conflicting results.[105] Nonetheless, tubular interstitial nephritis was observed in 23 occupationally exposed and 26 environmentally exposed individuals in whom autopsy tissue or renal biopsy specimens were examined.[74] These findings taken together with further investigations[98,106,107] and the long-term follow-up of 'itai-itai' disease in Japan[102,103,108] serve to strengthen the link between exposure to cadmium and the development of chronic interstitial renal disease. Most recent studies suggest that this

renal tubular damage is irreversible and associated with a progressive dose-related decrease in GFR even many years after the end of exposure.[109] It is a matter for concern that tubular dysfunction may appear in environmentally exposed subjects at lower cadmium body burdens than previously anticipated.[109] These reports support earlier data that the finding of low molecular weight proteinuria (which may occur when the cadmium in urine exceeds 10 nmol/mmol creatinine (10 μg/g creatinine)) should be regarded as a significant adverse effect of exposure because the renal tubular damage is irreversible and associated with a worsening of the age-related decline in GFR.[82,90]

For these reasons the emphasis of the management of occupational exposure to cadmium has shifted to defining the most acceptable level of exposure and in the identification of the most sensitive markers of early tubular dysfunction. In this regard an integrated index of occupational exposure (years of exposure x the prevailing blood level of cadmium) has been proposed as one way of studying renal outcome.[110] Data from this and other studies [111] confirm the validity of the current recommended health based units for occupational exposure of blood levels of cadmium of 10 μg/litre and of urine cadmium of 10 μg/g of creatinine (10 μmol/mol creatinine). Recent data suggest that at the worksite the permissible exposure limits (PEL) for cadmium in air should not exceed 5 μg/m³ in order to protect workers from both lung cancer and kidney dysfunction over a working lifetime.[112]

The potential for early intervention and prevention of progressive nephropathy is therefore important in cadmium-exposed workers. Two recent investigations compared the relative sensitivity of urinary markers of cadmium nephrotoxicity.[109,113] In contrast to lead and mercury, cadmium was found to induce a broad spectrum of effects on the kidney and produced significant alterations in the amounts of almost all the potential indicators of nephrotoxicity that were measured in the urine. These indicators included low and high molecular weight proteins, kidney-derived antigens or enzymes, prostanoids and various biochemical indices such as glycosaminoglycans and sialic acid. Dose-related effect and response relations could be established between most of these markers and the urinary excretion and blood levels of cadmium. Three main thresholds could be identified, the first at around 2 μg of cadmium/g creatinine mainly associated with biochemical alterations, the second at around 4 μg of cadmium/g creatinine for high molecular weight proteinuria and some tubular antigen excretion and the third at around 10 μg of cadmium/g creatinine for low molecular weight proteins and other indicators. On this basis, the recent recommendations by the American Conference of Governmental Industrial Hygienists (ACGIH) of 5 μg of cadmium/g creatinine in the urine for occupational exposure appears justified.[113] The very early interference with production of prostanoids at a threshold level of 2 μg of cadmium/g of creatinine merits further investigation.

TREATMENT

After confirming the presence of early renal tubular dysfunction, the most important aspect of the management of cadmium nephrotoxicity is the removal of the subject from further exposure. While experimental studies in animals show that Ca Na[2] EDTA given simultaneously with cadmium results in the prompt excretion of the cadmium chelate, in humans this chelating agent has little effect once cadmium has been complexed with metallothionein.[114] Concomitant osteomalacia may be alleviated by calcium and vitamin D[115] but this can be a problem in patients with associated urinary calcium wasting disease. Whether zinc-metallothionein compounds are safe and will afford protection from cadmium-induced nephropathy as has been suggested from animal studies[116] will require further investigation.

Mercury (see Chapter 7)

Most of the occupational health problems caused by mercury arise through its use in its elemental form. The high vapour pressure of elemental mercury results in potential exposure whenever the metal is used or handled. The effect of body heat on contaminated clothing is sufficient to result in high exposures. Although the skin is not a barrier to mercury, absorption mainly occurs by inhalation. Mercury readily crosses biological membranes and is rapidly oxidized to divalent mercury in the blood and within cells; bronchial damage followed later by neurological disease being the classical pattern of toxicity.[117]

Mercury is mined in Russia, China and Almaden, Spain. Large-scale usage of elemental mercury occurs in the chloralkali industry, although this is decreasing as newer technology takes over and provides other means for producing chlorine and sodium hydroxide. Elemental mercury is widely used in temperature and pressure measuring equipment, and in the manufacture of fluorescent and discharge lamps. Amalgams are used in dentistry. Occupationally, exposure to elemental mercury is more widespread than exposure to mercury compounds but generally there has been a reduction in the usage of mercury in the Western hemisphere over the last two decades.

Although mercury salts are widely used as toxins in experimental models of acute renal failure, their role in human renal disease is limited to industrial or accidental exposure (Fig. 41.4). Biotransformation to the organic salts such as methyl, ethyl and phenoxyethyl mercury may occur in industrial and agricultural processes.[118] After exposure, these organomercurials can accumulate in proximal renal tubular cells where toxicity is determined by the intracellular interactions with sulphydryl groups, lysosomes and phospholipid membranes.[118] This tubular toxicity has been associated with increased leakage of tubular antigens and enzymuria[119] and

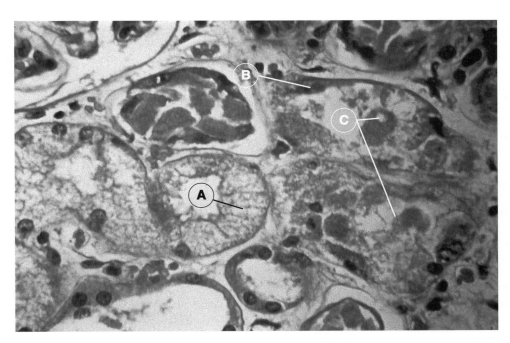

Figure 41.4 *Renal biopsy of acute tubular necrosis occurring in a patient secondary to mercury toxicity. The renal tubular cells show varying stages of degeneration from frothy vacuolated cytoplasm (A) to loss of nuclei in tubular cells with dark pyknotic nuclei (B). Shedding of cells is seen into the tubular lumen with tubular cell casts surrounded by epithelial cells (C). Photograph kindly provided by Dr A R Morley of Newcastle University, Newcastle, UK.*

biochemical alterations including decreased excretion of some eicosanoids and glycosaminoglycans with lowering of urinary pH.

Mercurous chloride (Hg$_2$ Cl$_2$, calomel) is relatively non-toxic and was widely used as a medicine until the twentieth century. In contrast, mercuric chloride (Hg Cl$_2$, corrosive sublimate) which has a relatively high vapour pressure and water solubility, is highly nephrotoxic and continues to be used experimentally to create animal models of acute renal tubular necrosis. Similar toxicity is produced by both the phenyl and methoxymethyl mercuric salts.[120] The biological half-life of inorganic mercury retained within the kidney is approximately 2 months.[121]

Reversible proteinuria was a well known feature in workers when mercury exposure was greater than 50 µg/m³. Currently the diagnosis of mercury-induced renal disease depends on a known exposure plus renal dysfunction, as many workers exposed to mercury have enhanced urinary mercury excretion without adverse renal effects.[122] However, blood mercury levels below 9 µg/l (45 nmol/litre) or urine levels below 36 µg/g creatinine (20 µmol/mol creatinine) have been established in the UK by the Health and Safety Executive as values unlikely to be injurious to health, including renal effects. Similar health guidance values have been established for urine mercury in the USA (35 µg/g creatinine) but higher values, currently under review, pertain in Germany (200 µg/litre or approximately 200 µg/g creatinine).

'Unexposed' reference ranges depend on the dietary intake of mercury especially from fish e.g. in Sweden such normal blood mercury values have been reported to be as high as 13 µg/litre (65 nmol/litre).[123]

However, an increased prevalence of proteinuria has been found in cross-sectional studies among exposed workers.[119,124-6] All authors have reported increased urinary enzymuria indicating an effect on the renal tubules.[119,127-130] These reported effects have generally been small and may be reversible with cessation of exposure,[131] but the long-term clinical significance of these findings is as yet unclear.

CLINICAL STUDIES

Autopsy studies have shown that mercury from dental amalgam may result in increased amounts of mercury in the renal cortex to almost nine times the normal range and up to 433 ngHg/gram of cortex, but no adverse effects were identified from this source of exposure.[132] Accidental or suicidal ingestion of as little as 0.5 g of mercuric chloride leads to typical oliguric acute renal failure with proximal tubular necrosis (Fig. 41.4). The clinical picture in the first few days is dominated by gastrointestinal haemorrhage due to erosive gastritis.[121] The prognosis for renal recovery is excellent with renal replacement and supportive therapy.[133] The administration of intravenous BAL (British anti-Lewisite: 2–3

dimercaprol) in the first 24–48 hours and before the development of oliguria may limit the extent of the renal failure.[118]

Nephrotic syndrome (albuminuria > 2.5g/day) has been reported sporadically following exposure to elemental and organic mercury.[134,135] In children the use of mercurial ointments or powders has been associated with the development of acrodynia or pink disease but in the occupational setting the association of mercury exposure and nephrotic syndrome has been described infrequently. Nonetheless, in some individuals mercury may be a triggering agent for immune reactions leading to proteinuria. In those cases where renal disease does develop membranous nephropathy is the form most commonly observed but minimal change nephropathy and anti-glomerular basement membrane (GBM) antibody mediated disease have also been described.[135] An increased prevalence of circulating anti-GBM antibody of the antilaminin variety has been reported in male workers exposed to mercury vapour.[136] More recent studies have suggested that anti-DNA antibodies and total IgE may be involved in this process as their circulating concentrations are positively associated with the concentration of mercury in both urine and blood.[119]

Fortunately, withdrawal from the exposure leads to disappearance of the proteinuria in humans and experimental animals.[137] While the immunopathological mechanism of the renal response in humans is not clear, in rats the renal lesion involves immune complex deposition, with anti-GBM antibodies, complement and polyclonal B cell activation.[138] The lack of a dose-response curve to the development of renal disease in both humans and animals suggests that this is an, as yet, undefined idiosyncratic response.

In 1956 an outbreak of chronic methyl mercury poisoning occurred in several hundred adults who ingested contaminated fish from Minamata Bay in Japan.[139] The dominant clinical feature of 'Minamata disease' was neurological disorder, but the renal manifestations were minor with low molecular weight proteinuria but no albuminuria or renal failure was recorded.[139]

TREATMENT AFTER CESSATION OF THE EXPOSURE

After cessation of exposure, BAL is an effective chelator for the treatment of acute inorganic mercury poisoning. Up to 5 mg/kg is given initially by the intramuscular route, followed by 2.5 mg/kg twice-daily for 10 days. In patients with acute renal failure the chelate can be effectively removed by haemodialysis. In chronic poisoning removal of the patient from the source of exposure is more appropriate as BAL is then of doubtful value. Therapeutically more potent and less toxic metal binding agents such as 2, 3 dimercapto-1-propane-sulphonic acid (sodium salt) are promising but require further study.[140]

Uranium (see Chapter 7)

While uranium has been used in animal models of experimental renal failure there are limited data on its nephrotoxicity in man. As in the case of lead, uranium is known to be deposited in bone but clinical nephrotoxicity has been largely confined to subjects employed in the development of the atomic bomb (the Manhattan project) during the Second World War.[141]

The uranyl ion circulates bound to transferrin, and is freely filtered at the glomerulus as the bicarbonate complex. This complex breaks down to UO_2^{2+} which then binds to proteins and phospholipids in the proximal renal tubule, where it has a half-life of approximately 1 week. The acute tubular necrosis produced in animal models is thought to be similar in aetiology to that seen in the men who worked on the Manhattan project, but chronic renal failure due to uranium has not been reported. Rats given uranyl nitrate subcutaneously develop intrarenal microcysts 8 weeks after injection.

A worksite hazard study of renal toxicity in uranium mill workers identified significantly increased urinary excretions of β2-microglobulin, catalase and alkaline phosphatase compared with non-exposed controls.[142] However, these increased urinary outputs remained within the accepted normal range and the clinical significance of these findings is unclear as many of these men had urine uranium levels in excess of the acceptable limit of 30 μg/litre (126nmol/litre). However, the nephrotoxic limit and the annual limit on intake for natural uranium have recently been questioned.[143]

Chromium (see Chapter 7)

Like other heavy metals chromium is selectively taken up by the proximal renal tubule and occasional cases of acute tubular necrosis following massive absorption have been described. Although chronic renal failure attributable to long-term exposure to chromium has not been described, low molecular weight proteinuria with increased urinary excretions of β2-microglobulin and retinol binding protein has been reported in chromium workers.[144] A urine threshold of 10 μg chromium/g creatinine (32 μmol/mol creatinine) has been suggested for nephrotoxicity after the finding of proximal tubular enzymuria in workers exposed to ferrochromium.[145] However, others[146] found no effect on the urinary excretion of transferrin, albumin or retinol binding protein in platers exposed to hexavalent chromium and in whom urine chromium levels were less than 19 μg/g creatinine (61 μmol/mol creatinine).

Beryllium (see Chapter 7)

A syndrome similar to sarcoidosis is induced by the long-term effects of beryllium exposure.[147] The features

in common include pulmonary fibrosis, hypercalcaemia and hypercalciuria. The cause of the hypercalcaemia is likely to be the same as that found in sarcoidosis and other granulomatous diseases, namely through the excessive extrarenal production of 1,25-dihydroxy vitamin D, but this is unproven. Renal complications such as interstitial nephritis may develop but are uncommon.

Arsenic (see Chapter 7)

Acute renal tubular necrosis can develop after exposure to arsine gas. Arsine is a powerful haemolytic agent and inhalation is soon followed (within a few hours) by acute circulatory collapse and haemolysis which are accompanied by haemoglobinuria, jaundice and abdominal pain.[148–150] Acute renal tubular necrosis presents within a few days. Haemodialysis is required for renal support, and removal of the arsenic haemoglobin complex by exchange transfusion may be lifesaving. Chronic renal failure can persist if the patient survives the acute illness. Similarly persistent renal disease has been described following ingestion of illicitly distilled spirits (moonshine) contaminated with arsenic.[151]

Bismuth and copper (see Chapter 7)

Acute tubular necrosis has been described after the use of bismuth therapeutically[152] and after self-poisoning with copper sulphate.[153] However, neither metal has been observed to be nephrotoxic in the occupational environment.

Crystalline silica (see Chapter 35)

Exposure to crystalline silica is through inhalation of quartz and related dust in mines and quarries and other sites (Fig. 41.5). Kallenberg has recently reviewed the occurrence of different forms of primary renal disease in patients exposed to silica[154] after initial reports had suggested such an association.[155] The development of systemic vasculitis and necrotizing glomerulonephritis have been reported more recently in association with silicosis.[156,157] Indeed antinuclear and other autoantibodies occur frequently with silicosis suggesting a possible link between environmental factors and the immunopathogenesis of the kidney disease.[158]

Case-control studies have recently suggested an association between exposure to silica and the development of Wegener's granulomatosis, a form of systemic vasculitis.[159] Previous studies had identified a possible link between occupational silica exposure and the development of end-stage renal failure but no specific data were available to relate exposure to patients with particular forms of renal disease.[160]

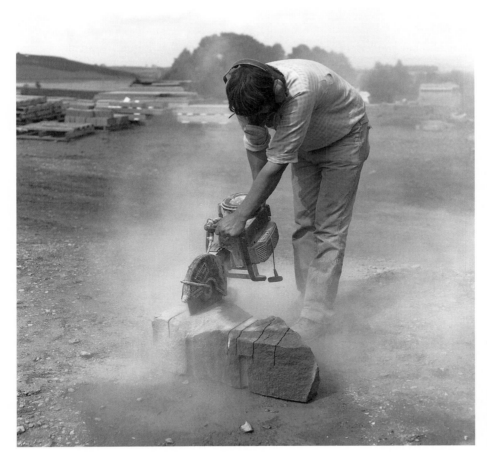

Figure 41.5 *A stone cutter wearing respiratory protective equipment during potential exposure to silica dust.*

To further substantiate the association between silica (cystalline silicon dioxide) and renal disease Kolev and associates[161] described focal glomerulonephritis in 23 of 45 patients with advanced pulmonary silicosis. Others[162] have described the autopsy findings of 17 patients with pulmonary silicosis, seven of whom had histological evidence of a focal segmental glomerulonephritis. Some patients with silicosis have been found to have slightly increased urinary excretions of either albumin, retinol binding protein and N-acetyl-β-D-glucosaminidase (NAG) and then without evidence of renal impairment.[163,164]

Furthermore, similar changes in renal function have recently been described in workers exposed to silica but without clinical evidence of silicosis.[165] In addition to these minor changes in renal function, a cohort study from the USA demonstrated an increased standardized mortality ratio for nephritis and nephrosis in man-made mineral fibre workers.[166] Thus epidemiological data suggest that silica exposure is associated with an increased risk for renal disease. Whether this is through a direct nephrotoxic effect or through stimulation of an autoimmune process will require further study.[154]

ORGANIC SOLVENTS AND RENAL DISEASE

Although the nitro, amino or chloro-derivatives of benzene have a known association with uroepithelial tumours (see Chapters 12, 39),[167] there is now a considerable body of evidence suggesting a role for organic solvent exposure in the development of non-neoplastic renal diseases.[168] The term 'organic solvent' refers to hydrocarbons such as aliphatic, alicyclic, aromatic, halogenated hydrocarbons (carbon tetrachloride, trichloroethylene) and the commonly abused solvents toluene and xylene. Hydrocarbons are often used as solvents in industrial manufacturing practices because of their lipid solubility (Fig. 41.6). Solvents are absorbed through the lungs, skin and gastrointestinal tract,[167,169] and are metabolized usually by cytochrome P450-dependent enzymes present in the liver, kidneys, lungs and other tissues.[170] Solvents are known to be neurotoxicants, affecting both the peripheral and central nervous systems.[171] Occupational exposure to hydrocarbons with resulting nephrotoxicity may explain the preponderance of male patients in dialysis programmes for end-stage renal failure.[172]

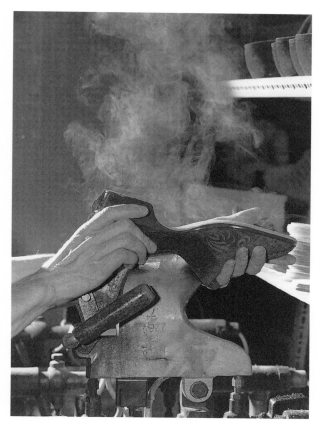

Figure 41.6 *Solvent fumes during shoe manufacture.*

Case reports and experimental studies

Case reports describe an association between organic-solvent exposure and the development of acute tubular necrosis;[168] chronic tubulo-interstitial damage[173] and different types of glomerulonephritis and Goodpasture's syndrome.[174–178] In parallel with these clinical observations, experimental studies in animals have identified organic-solvent exposure as a factor in the development of both tubular[179,180] and glomerular lesions.[178,181–185] Thus glomerular lesions similar to those found in Goodpasture's disease have been induced in rats exposed to petroleum vapours,[178] and the nephrotic syndrome with severe glomerulonephritis and renal impairment, which is not dependent on either deposition of fibrin or coagulative mechanisms, has been induced in rats fed *N,N′*diacetylbenzidine (*N,N′*-DAB).[182] Similarly, mesangial proliferative glomerulonephritis and tubulo-interstitial disease, which again did not appear to be mediated by glomerular deposits of antigen–antibody complexes, has been described in rats after the administration of carbon tetrachloride.[185]

CASE-CONTROL STUDIES

The majority of case-control studies from different research groups have reported a significantly greater exposure to organic solvents in patients with glomerulonephritis compared with control groups,[186–196] and have demonstrated substantial evidence in favour of a role for chronic solvent exposure in the development of various types of glomerulonephritis such as proliferative glomerulonephritis, membranous glomerulonephritis, post-strepococcal glomerulonephritis or rapidly progressive glomerulonephritis. Among the six studies in which estimated relative risks were either reported or calculable, there was a 2.8–8.9 fold increase in risk for the development of glomerulonephritis among solvent-exposed individuals.

The evidence presented in some of the older studies may be criticized on one of the following grounds: (i) the unsatisfactory nature of the control group; (ii) the possible bias of the unblinded interviewers; (iii) the failure to consider recall bias; (iv) failure to define a credible measure of solvent exposure; and (v) the diversity of glomerular disease patterns.

The most recent studies have addressed these criticisms. In one study[196] exposure to solvents was assessed blindly by telephone interview and questionnaire in patients with end-stage renal disease due to biopsy-proven primary glomerulonephritis and in whom there was no evidence of systemic disease. Their solvent exposure was compared with that of closely matched control groups of normal subjects and patients with other forms of kidney disease. Solvent-exposure scores derived from the results of the blind questionnaires were significantly higher in the patients with primary glomerulonephritis than the normal subjects and the internal control group. Moreover, more detailed assessment of the type of solvent exposure in patients with glomerulonephritis compared with normal controls showed significantly greater exposure scores in the patients to petroleum products, greasing/degreasing agents and paints/glue and a resulting estimated relative risk of developing glomerulonephritis with each type of solvent exposure respectively of 15.5, 5.3 and 2.0 times greater than normal. Furthermore in patients with primary glomerulonephritis the solvent exposure score was related to their serum creatinine concentration at the time of presentation suggesting a dose-effect relationship (Fig. 41.7). There was no significant difference in tobacco and alcohol consumption among subjects in the different groups, and it was concluded that occupational exposure to organic solvents may play an important role in the development of primary glomerulonephritis.

In a similarly carefully designed study, the role of solvent exposure was investigated in the development of diabetic nephropathy.[197] Exposure scores to solvents were significantly greater in patients with incipient (microalbuminuria) and overt (macroalbuminuria) diabetic nephropathy than those with no clinical evidence of nephropathy ($r = 0.4$, $p < 0.01$) suggestive of a dose-effect relationship also in patients with diabetic nephropathy. The one conclusion of this study suggested that solvent exposure may possibly play a role in the development and progression of diabetic nephropathy in patients with insulin-dependent diabetes mellitus (IDDM).

SOLVENTS AND PROGRESSION OF RENAL FAILURE

Three further studies have previously demonstrated that the prevalence of glomerulonephritis increases with the intensity and duration of antecedent solvent exposure.[189,191,192] Furthermore, an association between intensity of exposure and the severity of renal failure in patients with primary glomerulonephritis has been described.[196] (Fig. 41.7) Likewise, accelerated progression of renal failure in patients with glomerulonephritis and continued heavy solvent exposure has been reported.[198,199] More recently, a cohort study specifically investigated the role of solvent exposure in the progression of renal failure in patients with primary glomerulonephritis.[200] The results of this study suggested that patients with primary glomerulonephritis and progressive renal failure have greater solvent exposure and worse renal impairment at presentation than those with stable or improving renal function. Moreover, the patients with declining renal function were more likely to have had continued occupational solvent exposure following the diagnosis of glomerulonephritis. They were also more likely to have persistent heavy proteinuria and to develop hypertension than those without progressive renal failure. Tubular damage, as suggested by biochemical parameters of increased tubular enzymuria and low molecular weight proteinuria, was also significantly worse in the patients with progressive renal failure which indicates that this defect also played a part in the progression of

their renal disease. This study highlights an additional important role for continued solvent exposure in the progression of renal failure in patients with primary glomerulonephritis.

Histological evidence of tubulo-interstitial damage in primary glomerular disorders appears to correlate with severity of renal impairment and can predict the future outcome of renal disease.[201] The relationship between solvent exposure and morphological parameters of tubulo-interstitial damage was recently carefully examined in 59 patients with biopsy proven primary glomerulonephritis.[202] Solvent-exposure correlated significantly with both relative interstitial volume, an index of tubulo-interstitial damage, and serum creatinine, a marker of kidney function. Furthermore solvent-exposure scores were significantly greater in patients with progressive renal failure compared with those with stable or improving renal function, suggesting a close and possibly causal relationship between occupational organic solvent exposure and progressive renal failure in patients with glomerulonephritis.

CROSS-SECTIONAL STUDIES

The rarity of glomerulonephritis in the general population makes a prospective cohort analytic study of solvents in exposed populations logistically impossible.[203] Cross-sectional studies comparing parameters of renal dysfunction in solvent-exposed and matched non-exposed workers is feasible and the few such studies performed suggest an association between solvent exposure and renal damage.[204–211] Thus in one study,[204] workers exposed to moderate amounts of styrene, toluene and a mixture of mainly aromatic compounds were found to have slight but significantly increased urinary excretions of erythrocytes, white/tubular epithelial cells and albumin compared with a non-exposed group. Likewise, workers mainly exposed to aliphatic and acyclic hydrocarbons were shown to have increased proteinuria and tubular enzymuria (lysozyme and β-glucuronidase) in the absence of albuminuria, findings which were indicative of tubular rather than glomerular dysfunction.[205] In a study of 20 000 workers the prevalence of proteinuria was found to be higher in those exposed to hydrocarbons than in those who were not.[206] A significant shift of the cumulative frequency distribution of the urinary albumin concentration towards higher values has also been shown in workers exposed to styrene.[207]

Two other studies have used more sensitive markers of kidney damage. In one,[208] male oil refinery workers with exposures to hydrocarbons below the current USA threshold limit values, were found to have significantly higher urinary excretions of albumin and (brush border) renal tubular antigen and a higher prevalence of circulating anti-laminin antibodies than a non-exposed group. In the other, the study population was classified into heavy, moderate and low hydrocarbon exposure

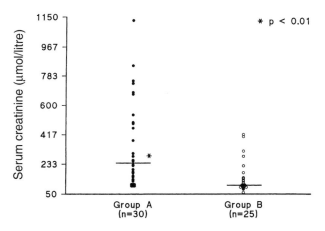

Figure 41.7 *Serum creatinine (μmol/litre) in patients with primary glomerulonephritis with heavy (group A) and moderate to low (group B) hydrocarbon exposure at the time of their presentation. Bar indicates mean and *indicates the level of significance. Reproduced from Ref. 196, with permission of Oxford University Press.*

groups (based on retrospective lifelong hydrocarbon-exposure scores using a method similar to that used in a recent study[196]) and the findings were compared with those of a control group.[209] The control group was unsatisfactory because 50% of the controls had a past history of heavy metal exposure. Despite introducing this bias, the workers exposed to hydrocarbons were found to have an increase in the urinary excretion of glycosaminoglycans (a marker of glomerular basement-membrane damage) and fractional albumin clearance.[209] The latter effect may have been secondary to an interaction between hypertension and hydrocarbon exposure.

Further studies have suggested that this interaction was significantly associated with abnormal proteinuria, an increased serum laminin concentration, albumin excretion rate and NAG activity. Furthermore exposure to hydrocarbons seemed to accelerate the age-dependent decline in kidney function.[210] This contrasts with earlier studies from the same group suggesting that long-term moderate exposure to solvents did not entail a significant nephrotoxic risk.[211]

Similarly two recent studies yielded contrasting conclusions about renal function in subjects occupationally exposed to perchloroethylene. In one,[212] no association could be found between exposure and renal outcome in workers exposed to perchloroethylene in dry cleaning shops. In the other, the findings were consistent with both glomerular and tubular dysfunction in workers exposed to low levels of perchloroethylene in dry cleaning (Fig. 41.8) and indicated that solvent-exposed workers, especially dry cleaners, may need to be monitored for the possible development of chronic renal disease.[213]

In view of the ongoing controversy in this area of nephrology we undertook one further such cross-sectional study in car manufacturing plant workers exposed to various solvents at their worksite.[214] The paint sprayers

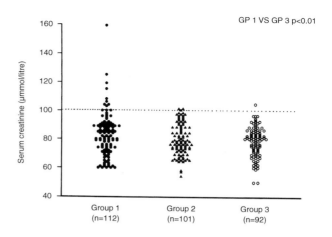

Figure 41.9 *Dottogram of serum creatinine levels in three groups of workers in a car plant. Group 1 (paint sprayers) had a significantly different distribution from group 2 (transmission shop workers) and group 3 (body shop workers). Evidence of renal impairment was present in 11% of group 1. The dotted line represents the upper reference limit derived from external controls. Reproduced from Ref. 214 with permission from Oxford University Press.*

exposed to paint-based solvents had a significantly higher prevalence of renal impairment than the other groups (Fig. 41.9) and a higher prevalence of abnormal total proteinuria and enzymuria than controls. Workers exposed to petroleum-based paints had a significantly higher prevalence of abnormal proteinuria, transferrinuria, tubular proteinuria and enzymuria but albuminuria was similar in all groups. These results suggested that chronic solvent exposure may be associated with both clinical and subclinical renal dysfunction.

Recently we have found evidence of endothelial activation and early basement-membrane disturbance resulting in autoantibody production as suggested by depressed serum laminin (marker of basement-membrane turnover) and elevated autoantibodies to laminin and Goodpasture's antigen (markers of anti-GBM antibody-mediated disease) in individuals occupationally exposed to paint and petroleum-based solvents[215] (Fig. 41.10).

Unfortunately there are no follow-up data on the renal outcome of these subjects. However, a recent study[216] of a matched cohort of paint sprayers from a different car plant suggested that the proximal tubule damage mentioned above may be reduced by improved respiratory and skin protection at the worksite.

COHORT STUDIES

A cohort study involves a sample of a population exposed to solvents who are compared with an age- and sex-matched cohort of unexposed individuals who are then followed for an outcome assessment such as

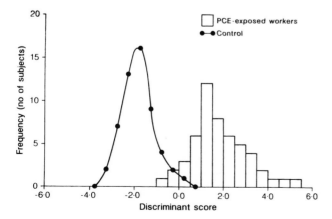

Figure 41.8 *Distribution of workers exposed to perchloroethylene (PCE) and matched controls classified on the basis of 13 selected early markers of renal damage. According to discriminate function 87% of subjects were correctly classified (χ^2 69.9, 13df, p<0.001). Reproduced from Ref. 213 with permission.*

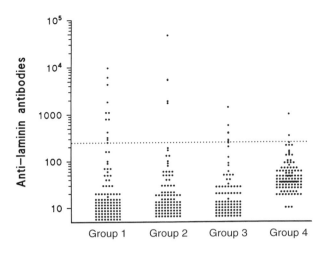

Figure 41.10 *Distribution of levels of serum anti-laminin antibodies in three groups of workers in a car plant (group 1 paintsprayers, group 2 transmission workers, group 3 body shop workers and group 4, normal external controls). In group 1 there was approximately a sixfold increase in the proportion of subjects with anti-laminin antibody results compared with controls. Reproduced from Ref. 215 with permission from Oxford University Press.*

mortality due to renal failure (see Chapter 3). Such studies may offer valuable information in the investigation of the association between solvent exposure and glomerulonephritis. However, the diagnostic categories of 'nephritis and nephrosis' or 'genitourinary diseases' are

likely to be invalid representations of renal mortality. Thus in four large cohort studies of solvent-exposed workers the risk of death (standardized mortality ratios) from renal causes was lower than otherwise expected in occupationally exposed cohorts.[217–220] The basic assumption for mortality studies is that the toxic effects are lethal. Such studies cast little light upon possible slight-to-moderate effects of exposure. Furthermore, the outcomes of 'register studies' are always difficult to interpret: diagnostic criteria may vary between and even within studies and the exposures are often vaguely or too generally defined. This may partly be explained by the influence of the well documented 'healthy worker effect' on non-cancer mortality frequently observed in occupational cohorts.[221] Moreover, mortality studies do not take into consideration those workers who take early retirement on health grounds (e.g. patients with end-stage renal failure requiring dialysis treatment), although the medical condition may eventually account for the individual's death.

Mechanisms of solvent-induced nephrotoxicity

The mechanism underlying solvent-induced glomerulopathy remains speculative despite solvents being well recognized tubulotoxins in both clinical and experimental settings.[179,215,222] Glomerulonephritis appears to be mainly an immune-mediated disease and there is experimental and clinical evidence of an immunosuppressive potential of various solvents.[223,224] Experimentally,

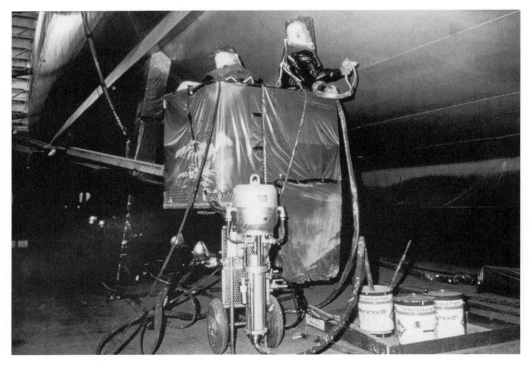

Figure 41.11 *Boat paint sprayers with protective equipment and using air fed masks.*

solvent exposures have induced glomerular lesions in the presence of concomitant tubulo-interstitial injury.[176,181–185,225–226] It is therefore possible to speculate that in susceptible individuals low-grade tubular damage from chronic exposure to solvents may provoke local autoimmunity by releasing either sequestered or altered tubular and basement-membrane antigens (antibodies to proximal tubular antigens, laminin, Goodpasture's antigens) (Fig. 41.10) with activation or damage of the overlying endothelium[227] which results in the development of glomerulonephritis.[215] Autoimmunity may be favoured by the immunosuppressive effects of solvent exposure.[223,224] Furthermore, carbon tetrachloride nephrotoxicity can be inhibited by whole body irradiation exposed at each injection,[228] favouring the role of primary tubular damage and local autoimmunity in the pathogenesis of solvent-induced glomerulopathy.

An alternative hypothesis is that potentially glomerulotoxic immune factors arise independently of solvent exposure and that solvents merely facilitate the deposition of these mediators of immune damage in renal tissue.[229] However, occupational exposure to solvents is widespread and glomerulonephritis and tubular interstitial disease are infrequently seen, which could suggest the operation of possible genetic or idiosyncratic factors in this association. In this regard we have recently reported significant differences in the genetic make-up of subjects with membranous nephropathy associated with occupational hydrocarbon exposure. Using analysis of the extracted DNA from patients' leucocytes, we found an increased prevalence of null enzyme activity for both the mu isoenzyme of glutathione S transferase (GST) and fast acetylator status of N-acetyl transferase (NAT-2) in subjects with membraneous nephropathy associated with hydrocarbon exposure.[230] Further studies are required in this area to investigate genetic links with occupational exposure. If corroborated there are considerable implications for occupational hydrocarbon exposure, worksite protection and the monitoring of such exposed subjects. With improved means of reducing exposure to solvents in occupational settings (Fig. 41.11) the risks should gradually reduce. Should further genetic associations be identified, however, then ethical issues regarding workforce screening and genetic suitability for employment in solvent-related industries may prove more difficult questions.

ACKNOWLEDGEMENT

The section on organic solvents (pp. 854–859) is an abbreviated, amended and updated version of a chapter: Organic solvents and renal disease, by M Yaqoob and GM Bell, In: *Horizons in Medicine No. 6* Royal College of Physicians, published by Blackwell Science Ltd in 1995, and appears with permission of the publisher.

REFERENCES

1 *Treatment of Adult Patients with Renal Failure*. London: The Renal Association and Royal College of Physicians, 1997.

2 *US Renal Data System Annual Report*. Bethesda, Maryland, USA: NIH, NIDDK, 1993.

3 Ritz E, Mann J, Stoeppler M. Lead and the kidney. In: Grunfeld J P, Bach J F, Gosnier J, Funck-Bretano J L eds. *Advances in Nephrology*. Chicago: Mosby Year Book 1988: 241.

4 Klein M, Namer R, Harpur E. Earthenware containers as a source of fatal lead poisoning. *N Engl J Med* 1970; **283**: 669–72.

5 Emmerson BT. Chronic lead nephropathy. *Kidney Int* 1973; **4**: 1–5.

6 Inglis JA, Henderson DA, Emmerson BT. The pathology and pathogenesis of chronic lead nephropathy occurring in Queensland. *J Pathol* 1978; **124**: 65–76.

7 Bennet WM. Lead nephropathy (clinical conference). *Kidney Int* 1985; **28**: 212–20.

8 Chisolm JJ. Harrison HC, Eberlern WR *et al*. Aminoacidura, hypophosphatemia and rickets in lead poisoning. *Am J Dis Child* 1955; **89**: 159–68.

9 Agency for Toxic Substances and Disease Registry. *The Nature and Extent of Lead Poisoning in Children in the United States. A Report to Congress*. Atlanta: US Dept of Health and Human Services, Public Health Service, 1988.

10 Goyer RA, Leonard DL, Bream PR *et al*. Aminoaciduria in experimental lead poisoning. *Proc Soc Exp Biol Med* 1970; **135**: 767.

11 Goyer RA. Environmentally related disease of the urinary tract. *Med Clin North Am* 1990; **74**: 377–89.

12 Schumann GB, Lerner SI, Weiss MA *et al*. Inclusion bearing cells in industrial workers exposed to lead. *Am J Clin Pathol* 1980; **74**: 192–6.

13 Goyer RA, Wilson MH. Lead inclusion bodies: results of ethylenediaminetetraacetic acid treatment. *Lab Invest* 1975; **32**: 149–56.

14 Batuman V, Maesaka JK, Habbad B, Tepper E, Landy E, Wedeen RP. The role of lead in gout nephropathy. *N Engl J Med* 1981; **304**: 520–23.

15 Batuman V, Laudry E, Maesaka JK, Wedeen RP. Contribution of lead to hypertension with renal impairment. *N Engl J Med* 1983; **309**: 17–20.

16 Behringer D, Craswell P, Mohl C, Stoeppler M, Ritz E. Urinary lead excretion in uraemic patients. *Nephron* 1986; **42**: 323–9.

17 Henderson DA. The aetiology of chronic nephritis in Queensland. *Med J Aust* 1958; **1**: 377–86.

18 Danilovic V. Chronic nephritis due to ingestion of lead contaminated flour. *Br Med J* 1958; **1**: 27–28.

19 Campbell BC, Beattie AD, Moore MR, Goldberg A, Reid AG. Renal insufficiency associated with excessive lead exposure. *Br Med J* 1977; **1**: 482–85.

20 Rabinowitz MB, Wetherill GW, Kopple JD. Kinetic analysis of lead metabolism in healthy humans. *J Clin Invest* 1977; **58**: 260–70.

21 Nuyts GD, Daelemans RA, Jorens PG, Elseviers MM, Van de Vyver FL, De Broe ME. Does lead play a role in the development of chronic renal disease? *Nephrol Dial Transplant* 1991; **6**: 307–15.

22 Ankrah NA, Kamiya Y, Appiah-Opong R, Akyeampon Y, Addae MM. Lead levels and related biochemical findings occurring in Ghanaian subjects occupationally exposed to lead. *East Afr Med J* 1996; **73**: 375–79.

23 Radosevic Z, Saric M, Beritic T, Knezevic J. The kidney in lead poisoning. *Br J Ind Med* 1961; **18**: 222–30.

24 Lilis R, Gavrilescu N, Nestorescu B, Dumitriu C, Roventa A. Nephropathy in chronic lead poisoning. *Br J Ind Med* 1968; **25**: 196–202.

25 Lilis R, Fischbein A, Eisinger J *et al*. Prevalence of lead disease among secondary lead smelter workers and biological indicators of lead exposure. *Environ Res* 1977; **14**: 255–85.

26 Cramer K, Goyer RA, Jagenburg R, Wilson MH. Renal ultrastructure, renal function, and parameters of lead toxicity in workers with different periods of lead exposure. *Br J Ind Med* 1974; **31**: 113–27.

27 Baker EL, Landrigan PJ, Barbour AG *et al*. Occupational lead poisoning in the US: Clinical and biochemical findings related to blood levels. *Br J Ind Med* 1979; **36**: 314–22.

28 Wedeen RP, Mallik DK, and Batuman V. Detection and treatment of occupational lead nephropathy. *Arch Intern Med* 1979; **139**: 53–7.

29 Pinto de Almeida AR, Carvalho FM, Spinola AG, Rocha H. Renal dysfunction and lead exposure (letter). *Am J Nephrol* 1987; **7**: 455–58.

30 Verschoer M, Wibowo A, Herber R, Hemmen JV, Zielhius R. Influence of occupational low-level lead exposure on renal parameters. *Am J Ind Med* 1987; **12**: 341–51.

31 Ong CN, Endo G, Chia KS, Phoon HY. Evaluation of renal function in workers with low blood lead levels. In: Fao V, Emmett EA, Maroni M *et al*. eds. *Occupational and Environmental Chemical Hazards*. Chichester: Ellis Harwood Limited 1987; 327–33.

32 Gennart JP, Bernard A, Lauwerys R. Assessment of thyroid, testes, kidney and autonomic nerve system in lead exposed workers. *Int Arch Occup Environ Hlth* 1992; **64**: 47–9.

33 Cardenas A, Roels H, Bernard AM *et al*. Markers of early renal changes induced by industrial pollutants. II Application to workers exposed to lead. *Br J Ind Med* 1993; **50**: 28–36.

34 Roels H, Lauwerys R, Konigs J, Buchet JP, Bernard A *et al*. Renal function and hyperfiltration capacity in lead smelter workers with high bone lead. *Occup Environ Med* 1994; **51**: 505–12.

35 Chia KS, Mutti A, Tan C *et al*. Urinary *N*-acetyl-B-D-glucosaminidase activity in workers exposed to inorganic lead. *Occup Environ Med* 1994; **51**: 125–29.

36 Kumar BD, Krishnaswamy K. Detection of occupational lead nephropathy using early renal markers. *J Toxicol Clin Toxicol* 1995; **33**: 331–5.

37 International Programme on Chemical Safety. *Lead. Environment Health Criteria*. Geneva: World Health Organization, 1989.

38 Fowler BA, Duval G. Effect of lead on the kidney: roles of high affinity lead-binding proteins. *Environ Hlth Perspect* 1991; **91**: 77–80.

39 Cooper WC, Gaffey WR. Mortality of lead workers. *J Occup Med* 1975; **17**: 100–07.

40 McMichael AJ, Johnson HM. Long term mortality profile of heavily exposed lead smelter workers. *J Occup Med* 1982; **24**: 375–78.

41 Malcolm D, Barnett HAR. A mortality of lead workers 1925–1976. *Br J Ind Med* 1982; **39**: 404–10.

42 Davies JM. Long-term mortality study of chromate pigment workers who suffered lead poisoning. *Br J Ind Med* 1984; **41**: 170–78.

43 Cooper WC, Wong O, Kheifet S. Mortality among employees of lead battery plants and lead producing plants, 1947–1980. *Scand J Work Environ Hlth* 1985; **11**: 331–45.

44 Selevan SG, Landrigan PJ, Stern FB, Jones JH. Mortality of lead smelter workers. *Am J Epidemiol* 1985; **122**: 673–83.

45 Gerhardsson L, Lundstrom NG, Nordberg G, Wall S. Mortality and lead exposure: a retrospective cohort study of Swedish smelter workers. *Br J Ind Med* 1986; **43**: 707–11.

46 Fanning D. A mortality of lead workers 1926–1985. *Arch Environ Hlth* 1988; **43**: 247–51.

47 Nuyts GD, Daelemans RA, Jorens PG *et al*. Does lead play a role in the development of chronic renal disease. *Nephrol Dial Transplant* 1991; **6**: 307–15.

48 Sharp DS, Becker CE, Smith AH. Chronic low-level lead exposure. Its role in the pathogenesis of hypertension. *Med Toxicol* 1987; **2**: 210–32.

49 Wedeen RP. Occupational and environmental renal diseases. *Current Nephrol* 1988; **11**: 65–106.

50 Pirkle JL, Schwartz J, Landis JR, Harlan WR. The relationship between blood lead levels and blood pressure and its cardiovascular risk implications. *Am J Epidemiol* 1985; **121**: 246–58.

51 Harlan WR. The relationship of blood lead levels to blood pressure in the US population. *Environ Hlth Perspect* 1988; **78**: 9–14.

52 Pocock SJ, Shaper AG, Ashby D, Delves HT, Clayton BE. The relationship between blood lead, blood pressure, stroke and heart attacks in middle aged British men. *Environ Hlth Perspect* 1988; **78**: 23–30.

53 Parkinson DK, Hodgson MJ, Bromet EJ, Dew MA, Connell MM. Occupational lead exposure and blood pressure. *Br J Ind Med* 1987; **44**: 744–48.

54 Elwood PC, Davey-Smith G, Oldham PD, Toothill C. Two Welsh surveys of blood lead and blood pressure. *Environ Hlth Perspect* 1988; **78**: 119–122.

55 Gartside PS. The relationship of blood lead level and

blood pressure in NHANES 11: additional calculations. *Environ Hlth Perspect* 1988; **78**: 31–4.

56 Mahaffey KR, Annest JL, Roberts J, Murphy RA. Natural estimates of blood lead levels, 1976–1980, association with selected demographic and socioeconomic factors. *N Engl J Med* 1982; **307**: 573–79.

57 Wedeen RP. Blood lead levels, dietary calcium and hypertension. *Ann Intern Med* 1985; **102**: 403–4.

58 Weiler E, Khalil-Manesh F, Gonick H. Effects of lead and natriuretic hormone on kinetics of sodium-potassium-activated adenosine triphosphatase: possible relevance to hypertension. *Environ Hlth Perspect* 1988; **78**: 113–18.

59 Batuman V, Dreisbach A, Chun E, Naumoff M. Lead increases the red cell sodium-lithium countertransport. *Am J Kidney Dis* 1989; **14**: 200–3.

60 Kopp SJ, Barron JT, Tow JP. Cardiovascular actions of lead and relationship to hypertension: a review. *Scand J Work Environ Hlth* 1985; **11**: 15–19.

61 Koster J, Erhardt A, Stoeppler M, Mohl C, Ritz E. Mobilisable lead in patients with chronic renal failure. *Eur J Clin Invest* 1989; **19**: 228–33.

62 Steenland NK, Thun MJ, Ferguson CW, Port FK. Occupational and other exposures associated with male end-stage renal disease: a case control study. *Am J Publ Hlth* 1990; **80**: 153–59.

63 Van de Vyver FL, D'Haese PC, Visser WJ *et al*. Bone lead in dialysis patients. *Kidney Int* 1988; **33**: 601–07.

64 Chisolm JJ, Mellits ED, Barrett MB. Inter relationships among blood lead concentration, quantitive daily ALA-U and urinary lead output following calcium EDTA. In: *Effects and Dose: Response Relationships of Toxic Metals* Nordberg GF ed. Amsterdam: Elsevier, 1976: 416–33.

65 Rosen JF, Markovitz ME, Bijur PE *et al*. K-Line x-ray fluorescence of cortical bone lead compared with Ca Na$_2$ EDTA test in lead toxic children. Public Health Implications. *Proc Natl Acad Sci USA* 1989; **86**: 685–89.

66 Germain MJ, Braden GL, Fitzgibbons JP. Failure of chelation therapy in lead nephropathy. *Arch Intern Med* 1984; **144**: 2419–20.

67 Campbell BC, Meredith PA, Scott JJC. Lead exposure and changes in the renin-angiotensin-aldosterone system in man. *Toxicol Lett* 1985; **25**: 25–32.

68 Ashouri OS. Hyperkalaemia distal renal tubular acidosis and selective aldosterone deficiency. Combination in a patient with lead nephropathy. *Arch Intern Med* 1985; **145**: 1306–07.

69 Aposhian HV. DMSA and DMPS water soluble antidotes for heavy metal poisoning. *Ann Rev Pharmacol Toxicol* 1983; **23**: 193–97.

70 Graziano JH, Lolacono NJ, Meyer P. Dose response study of oral 2,3 dimercaptosuccinic and in children with elevated blood lead concentrations. *J Paediatr* 1988; **113**: 751–57.

71 Twarog T, Cherian MG. Chelation of lead by dimercapto-propane sulfonate and a possible diagnostic use. *Toxicol Appl Pharmacol* 1984; **72**: 550–56.

72 Friberg L, Piscator M, Nordberg GF, Kjellstrom T. *Cadmium in the Environment* 2nd edn. Cleveland: CRC Press, 1994.

73 Lauwerys R, Bernard A, Roels HA, Buchet JP, Viau C. Characterisation of cadmium proteinuria in man and rat. *Environ Hlth Perspect* 1984; **54**: 147–53.

74 Kjellstrom T. Renal effects. In: Friberg L, Elinder CA, Kjellstrom T *et al*. eds. *Cadmium and Health: Toxicological and Epidemiological Appraisal* Vol 2. Boca Raton: CRC Press, 1986.

75 Nordberg GF, Kjellstrom T, Nordberg M. Kinetics, dose and Metabolism, other toxic effects. In: Friberg L, Elinder CG, Kjellstrom T *et al*. eds. *Cadmium and Health: A Toxicological and Epidemiological Appraisal* Vol 2. Boca Raton: CRC Press, 1986.

76 Vahter M, Berghing M, Lind B, Jorhem L, Slorach S, Friberg L. Personal monitoring of lead and cadmium exposure: a swedish study with special reference to methodological aspects. *Scand Work Environ Hlth* 1991; **17**: 65–74.

77 Shaikh ZA, Smith LM. Biological indicators of cadmium exposure and toxicity. *Experientia* 1984; **40**: 36–43.

78 Squibb KS, Pritchard JB, Fowler BA. Cadmium-metallothionein nephropathy. Relationships between ultrastructral biochemical alterations and intracellular binding. *J Pharmacol Exp Ther* 1984; **229**: 311–21.

79 Nordberg GF, Jin T, Nordberg M. Subcellular targets of cadmium nephrotoxicity: cadmium binding to renal membrane proteins in animals with or without protective metallothionein synthesis. *Environ Hlth Perspect* 1994; **102**: 191–94.

80 Bernard A, Buchet JP, Roels H, Masson P, Lauwerys R. Renal excretion of proteins and enzymes in workers exposed to cadmium. *Eur J Clin Invest* 1979; **9**: 11–22.

81 Bernard A, Lauwerys R, Ouled-Amor A. Loss of glomerular polyanion correlated with albuminuria in experimental cadmium nephropathy. *Arch Toxicol* 1992; **66**: 272–78.

82 Roels HA, Lauwerys R, Buchet JP, Bernard Am, Vos A, Oversteyns M. Health significance of cadmium-induced renal dysfunction: a five year follow up. *Br J Ind Med* 1989; **46**: 755–64.

83 Jarup L, Persson B, Edling C, Elinder CG. Renal function impairment in workers previously exposed to cadmium. *Nephron* 1993; **64**: 75–81.

84 Bernard AM, Ouled AA, Lauwerys R. Decrease of erythrocyte and glomerular membrane negative charges in chronic cadmium poisoning. *Br J Ind Med* 1988; **45**: 112–15.

85 Bernard AM, Ouled AA, Cardenas A, Lauwerys R. Validity of the alcian blue binding test as an indicator of red blood cell and glomerular membrane negative charges. *Nephron* 1989; **52**: 184–85.

86 Cardenas A, Bernard AM, Lauwerys R. Disturbance of sialic acid metabolism by chronic cadmium exposure and its relation to proteinuria. *Toxicol Appl Pharmacol* 1991; **108**: 548–58.

87 Bernard AM, Roels H, Cardenas A, Lauwerys R. Assessment of urinary protein/transferrin as early markers of cadmium nephrotoxicity. *Br J Ind Med* 1990; **47**: 559–65.

88 Bernard AM, Roels HR, Foldart JM, Lauwerys R. Search for anti-laminin antibodies in the serum of workers exposed

to cadmium, mercury vapour or lead. *Int Arch Occup Environ Hlth* 1987; **59**: 303–09.

89 Bernard A, Lauwerys R, and Gengoux R *et al.* Anti-laminin antibodies in Sprague Dawley and Brown Norway rats chronically exposed to cadmium. *Toxicology* 1984; **31**: 307–13.

90 Roels H, Djubgang J, and Buchet JP *et al.* Evolution of cadmium induced renal dysfunction in workers removed from exposure. *Scand J Work Environ Hlth* 1982; **8**: 191–200.

91 Elinder CG, Edling C, Lindberg E, Kaejedal BC, Veslerberg. Beta-2- microbulinaemia among workers previously exposed to cadmium: follow up and dose response analysis. *Am J Ind Med* 1985; **8**: 553–64.

92 Friberg L. Cadmium and the kidney. *Environ Hlth Perspect* 1984; **54**: 1–11.

93 Friberg L. In: Friberg L, Elinder CG, Kjellstrom T, Nordberg GF, eds. *Cadmium and Health: A Toxicological Epidemiological Appraisal Vol 1*. Boca Raton CRC Press, 1986: 1–6.

94 Verschour M, Herber R, Van Hemmen J, Wibowo A, Zeilhuis R. Renal function of workers with low level cadmium exposure. *Scand J Work Environ Hlth* 1987; **13**: 232–38.

95 Lauwerys R. *Cadmium in Man.* In: Webb M ed. *Chemistry, Biochemistry and Biology of Cadmium*. Amsterdam: Elsevier/North Holland. 1979, 433–45.

96 Roels H, Lauwerys R, Buchet JP *et al. In vivo* measurement of liver and kidney cadmium in workers exposed to this metal. *Environ Res* 1981; **26**: 217–40.

97 Roels H, Lauwerys RR, Dardenne AN. The critical level of cadmium in the human renal cortex: a re-evaluation. *Toxicol Lett* 1983; **15**: 357–60.

98 Bernard A, Roels H, Buchet JP, Cardenas A, Lauwerys R. Cadmium and health: the Belgian experience. In: Nordberg GF, Herber RFM, Alessio L eds. *Cadmium in the Human Environment: Toxicity and Carcinogenicity*. Lyons: International Agency for Research on Cancer, 1992, 15–33.

99 Chang CC, Lauwerys R, Bernard A, Roels H, Buchet JP, Garvey JS. Metallothionein in cadmium exposed workers. *Environ Res* 1980; **23**: 422–28.

100 Roels H, Lauwerys R, Buchet JP, Bernard A, Garvey JS, Linton HJ. Significance of urinary metallothionein in workers exposed to cadmium. *Int Arch Occup Environ Hlth* 1983; **52**: 159–66.

101 Nogawa K. Biologic indicators of cadmium nephrotoxicity in persons with low level cadmium exposure. *Environ Hlth Rep* 1984; **54**: 163–69.

102 Kido T, Nogawa K, Honda R *et al.* Long term observation between renal dysfunction and osteopenia in environmentally cadmium exposed subjects. *Environ Res* 1990; **51**: 71–82.

103 Kido T, Nogawa K, Ischizaki M *et al.* Long term observation of serum creatinine and arterial blood PH in persons with cadmium induced renal dysfunction. *Arch Environ Hlth* 1990; **45**: 35–43.

104 Geiger H, Bahner U, Anderes S *et al.* Cadmium and renal hypertension. *J Hum Hypertens* 1989; **3**: 23–7.

105 Anderson K, Elinder CG, Hogstedt C *et al.* Mortality among cadmium and nickel exposed workers in a Swedish battery factory. *Toxicol Environ Chem* 1984; **9**: 53.

106 Kawada T, Koyama H, Suzuki S. Cadmium, NAG activity and β_2 microglobulin in the urine of cadmium pigment workers. *Br J Ind Med* 1989; **46**: 52–55.

107 Thun MJ, Osorio AM, Schober S *et al.* Nephropathy in cadmium workers-assessment of risk from air borne occupational cadmium exposure. *Br J Ind Med* 1989; **46**: 689–97.

108 Tsuchiya K. Health effects of cadmium with special reference to studies in Japan. *IARC Sci Publ* 1992; **118**: 35–49.

109 Jarup L, Persson B, Elinder CG. Decreased glomerular filtration rate in solderers exposed to cadmium. *Occup Environ Med* 1985; **52**: 818–22.

110 Jakubowski M, Razniewska G, Halatek T, Trzcinka-Ochocka M. Integrated index of occupational exposure to cadmium as a predictor of kidney dysfunction. *IARC Sci Pub* 1992: 319–24.

111 Toffoletta F, Apostol P, Ghezzi T, Baj A, Cortona G, Rizzi L, Alessio L. Ten-year follow-up of biological monitoring of cadmium exposed workers. *IARC Sci Pub* 1992, 107–11.

112 Thun MJ, Elinder CG, Friberg L. Scientific basis for an occupational standard for cadmium. *Am J Ind Med* 1991; **20**: 629–42.

113 Roels H, Bernard AM, Cardenas A *et al.* Markers of early renal changes induced by industrial pollutants III. Application to workers exposed to cadmium. *Br J Ind Med* 1993; **50**: 37–48.

114 Friberg L. Edathamil calcium-disodium in cadmium poisoning. *Arch Ind Health* 1956; **13**: 18.

115 Blainey JD, Adams RG, Brewer DB *et al.* Cadmium induced osteomalacia. *Br J Ind Med* 1980; **37**: 278–84.

116 Dorian C, Klaassen CD. Protection of zinc-metallothionein (ZnMT) against cadmium-metallothionein-induced nephrotoxicity. *Fundam Appl Toxicol* 1995; **26**: 99–106.

117 Wedeen RP. Were the hatters of New Jersey 'Mad' *Am J Ind Med* 1989; **16**: 225–33.

118 Wedeen RP. Renal diseases of occupational origin. *Occup-Med* 1992; **7**: 449–63.

119 Cardenas A, Roels H, Bernard AM *et al.* Markers of early renal changes induced by industrial pollutants I. Application to workers exposed to mercury vapour. *Br J Ind Med* 1993; **50**: 17–27.

120 Magos L, Sparrow S, Snowden R. The comparative renal toxicology of phenyl mercury and mercuric chloride. *Arch Toxicol* 1982; **50**: 133–39.

121 Clarkson TW, Hursh JB, Sager PR *et al.* Mercury. In: Clarkson TW, Friberg L, Norberg GF, Sager PR eds. *Biological Monitoring of Heavy Metals*. New York: Plenum Press, 1988: 199–247.

122 Joselow M, Goldwater LJ. Absorption and excretion of mercury in man. *Arch Environ Hlth* 1967; **15**: 155.

123 Langworth S, Elinder CG, Sundquist KG, Vesterberg O.

Renal and immunological effects of occupational exposure to inorganic mercury. *Br J Ind Med* 1992; **49**: 394–401.

124 Foa V, Caimi L, Amante L *et al*. Patterns of some lysosomal enzymes in the plasma and of proteins in urine of workers exposed to inorganic mercury. *Int Arch Occup Environ Hlth* 1976; **37**: 115–24.

125 Buchet JP, Roels H, Bernard A, Lauwerys R. Assessment of renal function of workers exposed to inorganic lead, cadmium or mercury vapour. *J Occup Med* 1980; **22**: 741–50.

126 Roels H, Lauwerys R, Buchet JP *et al*. Comparison of renal function and psychomotor performance in workers exposed to elemental mercury. *Int Arch Occup Environ Hlth* 1982; **50**: 77–93.

127 Stonard MD, Chanter BV, Duffield DP, Nevitt AL, O'Sullivan JJ, Steel GT. An evaluation of renal function in workers occupationally exposed to mercury vapour. *Int Arch Occup Environ Hlth* 1983; **52**: 177–89.

128 Roels H, Gennart JP, Lauwerys R, Buchet TP, Malchacre J, Bernard A. Surveillance of workers exposed to mercury vapour: validation of a previously proposed biological threshold limit value for mercury concentration in urine. *Am J Ind Med* 1985; **7**: 45–71.

129 Barregard L, Hultberg B, Schutz A, Sallsten G. Enzymuria in workers exposed to inorganic mercury. *Int Arch Environ Hlth* 1988; **61**: 65–9.

130 Ehrenberg RL, Vogt RL, Smith AB *et al*. Effects of elemental mercury exposure at a thermometer plant. *Am J Ind Med* 1991; **19**: 495–507.

131 Elligsen DG, Barregard L, Gaarder PI, Huetberg B, Kjuus H. Assessment of renal dysfunction in workers previously exposed to mercury at a Chloralkali plant. *Br J Ind Med* 1993; **50**: 881–7.

132 Nylander M, Friberg, Lind B. Mercury concentrations in the human brain and kidneys in relation to exposure from dental amalgam fillings. *Swed Dent J* 1987; **11**: 179–87.

133 Gerstner HB, Huff JE. Selected case histories and epidemiological examples of human mercury poisoning. *Clin Toxicol* 1977; **11**: 131.

134 Kazantzis G, Schiller KFR, Asscher AW, Drew RG. Albuminuria and the nephrotic syndrome following exposure to mercury and its compounds. *Q J Med* 1962; **31**: 403–18.

135 Tubbs RR, Gerhardt GD, McMahon JT. Membranous glomerulonephritis associated with industrial mercury exposure. *Am J Clin Pathol* 1981; **77**: 409–13.

136 Lauwerys R, Bernard A, Roels H *et al*. Anti-laminin antibodies in workers exposed to mercury vapour. *Toxicol Lett* 1983; **17**: 113–6.

137 Druet P, Bernard A, Hirsch F. Immunologially mediated glomerulonephritis induced by heavy metals. *Arch Toxicol* 1982; **50**: 187.

138 Goldman M, Baran D, Druet P. Polyclonal activation and experimental nephropathies. *Kidney Int* 1988; **34**: 141–50.

139 Iesato K, Wakastin M, Wakashin Y. Renal tubular dysfunction in Minimata disease. Detection of renal tubular antigen and β_2 microglobulin in the urine. *Ann Intern Med* 1977; **86**: 731–37.

140 Torres-Alanis-O, Garza-Ocanas L, Pineyro-Lopez A. Evaluation of urinary mercury excretion after administration of 2, 3 dimercapto-1-propane sulfonic acid to occupationally exposed men. *J Toxicol Clin Toxicol* 1995; **33**: 717–20.

141 Dounce AL. The mechanism of action of uranium compounds in the animal body. In: Voegtlin C, Hodge HC eds. *Pharmacology and Toxicity of Uranium Compounds* Vol 1. New York: McGraw-Hill, 1949: Ch 15.

142 Thun MJ, Baker DB, Streeland K, Smith AB, Halperin W, Berl T. Renal toxicity in uranium mill workers. *Scand J Work Environ Hlth* 1985; **11**: 83–90.

143 Su Lu, Fu-Yao Zhao. Nephrotoxic limit and annual limit on intake for natural U. *Hlth Phys* 1990; **58**: 619–623.

144 Wedeen RP, Qian LF. Chromium-induced kidney disease. *Environ Hlth Perspect* 1991; **92**: 71–4.

145 Wang X, Qin Q, Xu X, Xu J, Wang J *et al*. Chromium-induced early changes in renal function among ferrochromium-producing workers. *Toxicology* 1994; **90**: 93–101.

146 Nagaya T, Ishikawa N, Hata H, Takahashi A, Yoshida I, Okamoto Y. Early renal effects of occupational exposure to low-level hexavalent chromium. *Arch Toxicol* 1994; **68**: 322–24.

147 Stoeckle JD, Hardy H, Weber AL. Chronic beryllium disease. Long-term follow-up of sixty cases and selective review of the literature. *Am J Med* 1969; **46**: 545–61.

148 Muehrcke RO, Pinani CL. Arsine-induced anuria: A correlative clinicopathological study with electron microscopic observations. *Ann Intern Med* 1968; **68**: 853–66.

149 Fowler BA, Weissberg JB. Arsine poisoning. *N Engl J Med* 1974; **291**: 1171–74.

150 Gilberson A, Varizi ND, Mirahamadi K *et al*. Haemodialysis of acute arsenic intoxication with transient renal failure. *Arch Intern Med* 1976; **136**: 1303.

151 Gerhardt RE, Crecelis EA, Hudson JB. Moonshine related arsenic poisoning. *Arch Intern Med* 1977; **140**: 211–13.

152 Randall RE, Osheroff RJ, Bakerman S *et al*. Bismuth nephrotoxicity. *Ann Intern Med* 1972; **77**: 481–82.

153 Dash SC. Copper sulfate poisoning and acute renal failure (editorial). *Int J Artif Organs* 1989; **12**: 610.

154 Kallenberg CGM. Renal disease–another effect of silica exposure. *Neph Dial Transplant* 1995; **10**: 1117–19.

155 Saldanha S, Rosen VJ, Gonick HC. Silicon nephrotoxicity. *Am J Med* 1975; **59**: 95–103.

156 Arnalich F, Lahoz C, Picazo ML *et al*. Polyarteritis nodosa and necrotizing glomerulonephritis associated with long-standing silicosis. *Nephron* 1989; **51**: 544–47.

157 Neyer U, Woss E, Neuweiler J. Wegener's granulomatosis associated with silicosis. *Nephrol Dial Transplant* 1994; **9**: 559–61.

158 Boll NJ, Stankus RP, Hughes J *et al*. Immune complexes

and autoantibodies in silicosis. *J Allergy Clin Immunol* 1981; **68**: 281–85.

159 Nuyts GD, Van Veem E and DeVos A *et al*. Wegener's granulomatosis is associated to exposure to silicon compounds: a case-control study. *Nephrol Dial Transplant* 1995; **10**: 1162–65.

160 Steenland WK, Thun MJ, Ferguson CW, Port FW. Occupational and other exposures associated with male end-stage renal disease: a case controlled study. *Am J Publ Hlth* 1990; **80**: 153–59.

161 Kolev K, Doitschinov D, Todorov D. Morphologic alterations in the kidneys by silicosis. *Med Lav* 1970; **61**: 205–15.

162 Slavin RE, Swedo JL, Brandes D, Gonzales-Vitale JC, Orsornio-Vargas A. Extrapulmonary silicosis: a clinical, morphological and ultrastructural study. *Hum Pathol* 1985; **16**: 393–412.

163 Ng TP, Ng YL, Lee HS, Chia KS, Ong HY. A study of silica nephrotoxicity in exposed silicotic and non-silicotic workers. *Br J Ind Med* 1992; **49**: 35–37.

164 Boujemaa W, Lauwerys R, Bernard A. Early indicators of renal dysfunction in silicotic workers. *Scand J Work Environ Hlth* 1994; **20**: 180–83.

165 Hotz P, Gonzalez J, Siles E, Trujillano G, Lauwerys R, Bernard A. Subclinical signs of kidney dysfunction following short exposure to silica in the absence of silicosis. *Nephron* 1995; **70**: 438–42.

166 Marsh GM, Enterline PE, Stone RA, Henderson VL. Mortality among a cohort of US man-made mineral fiber workers: 1985 update. *J Occup Med* 1990; **32**: 594–604.

167 Andrews LS, Snyder R. Toxic effects of solvents and vapors. In: Amdur MO, Doull J, Klaassen CD eds. *Casarett and Doull's Toxicology: The Basic Science of Poisons*. New York: Pergamon Press, 1991: 681–721.

168 Yaqoob M, Bell GM. Organic solvents and renal disease. In: Holgate S ed. *Horizons in Medicine No 6*. Oxford: Blackwell Science 1995: 206–17.

169 Pederen LM. Biological studies in human exposure to and poisoning with organic solvents. *Pharmacol Toxicol* 1987; **3**: 1–38.

170 Clayton GD, Clayton EE eds. *Industrial Hygiene and Toxicology*. New York: Wiley, 1981: Vol 26; 1982: Vol 27.

171 Seaton A. Organic solvents and the nervous system: time for reappraisal. *Q J Med* 1992; **84**: 637–69.

172 Finn R, Harmer D. Aetiological implications of sex ratio in glomerulonephritis. *Lancet* 1979; **i**: 1194.

173 Navarte J, Saba SR, Ramirez G. Occupational exposure to organic solvents causing chronic tubulo-interstitial nephritis. *Arch Intern Med* 1989; **149**: 154–59.

174 Anderson K. Acute nephritis due to turpentine absorbed by the skin. *Br Med J* 1912; **3**: 881.

175 Cagnoli L, Cassanova S, Pasquali S, Donini U, Zucchelli P. Relationship between hydrocarbon exposure and the nephrotic syndrome. *Br Med J* 1980; **280**: 1068.

176 Beirne GJ, Brennan JT. Glomerulonephritis associated with hydrocarbon solvents. *Arch Environ Hlth* 1972; **25**: 365–69.

177 Daniell WE, Couser WG, Rosenstock L. Occupational solvent exposure and glomerulonephritis. *JAMA* 1988; **259**: 2280–83.

178 Klavis G, Drommer W. Goodpasture's syndrome and the effects of benzene. *Arch Toxicol* 1970; **26**: 40–55.

179 Bruner RH. Pathological findings in laboratory animals exposed to hydrocarbon fuels of military interest. In: Mehlman MA, Hemstreet III CP, Thorpe JJ, Weaver NK eds. *Renal Effects of Petroleum Hydrocarbons*. Princeton, New Jersey: Princeton Scientific Publishers, 1984, 133–40.

180 Halder CA, Warne TM, Hatoum NS. Renal toxicity of gasoline and related petroleum naphthas in male rats rats. In: Mehlman MA, Hemstreet III CP, Thorpe JJ, Weaver NK eds. *Renal Effects of Petroleum Hydrocarbons*. Princeton, New Jersey: Princeton Scientific Publishers, 1984: 73–88.

181 Dunn TB, Morris HP, Wagner BP. Lipaemia and glomerular lesions in rats fed diets containing N-N diacetyl and tetramethyl-benzidine. *Proc Soc Exp Biol Med* 1956; **91**: 105–7.

182 Harman JW, Miller EC, Miller JA. Chronic glomerulnephritis and nephrotic syndrome induced in rats by N, N-diacetylbenzidine. *Am J Pathol* 1952; **28**: 529.

183 Harman JW. Chronic glomerulonephritis and nephrotic syndrome induced in rats with N, N-diacetylbenzidine. *J Pathol* 1970; **104**: 119–128.

184 Zimmerman SW, Norbach DH. Nephrotoxic effects of long-term carbon tetrachloride administration in rats. *Arch Pathol Lab Med* 1980; **104**: 94–9.

185 Zimmerman SW, Norbach DH, Powers K. Carbon tetrachloride nephrotoxicity in rats with reduced renal mass. *Arch Pathol Lab Med* 1983; **17**: 264–69.

186 Zimmerman SW, Groehler K, Beirne GJ. Hydrocarbon exposure and chronic glomerulonephritis. *Lancet* 1975; **ii**: 199–201.

187 Lagrue G, Kamalodine T, Hirbec G, Bernaudin JF, Guerero J, Zhepova F. Rôle de L'Inhalation de substances toxique dans la genese des glomerulonephritis. *Nouv Presse Med* 1977; **6**: 3609–13.

188 Ravnskov U. Exposure to organic solvents – a missing link in post-streptococcal glomerulonephritis. *Acta Med Scand* 1978; **203**: 351–56.

189 Ravnskov U, Forsberg B, Skerfving S. Glomerulonephritis and exposure to organic solvents. A case control study. *Acta Med Scand* 1979; **205**: 575–79.

190 Finn R, Fennerty AG, Ahmad R. Hydrocarbon exposure and glomerulonephritis. *Clin Nephrol* 1980; **14**: 173–75.

191 Ravnskov U, Lundrstrum S, Norden A. Hydrocarbon exposure and glomerulonephritis. Evidence from patients' occupations. *Lancet* 1983; **ii**: 1214–16.

192 Bell GM, Gordon ACH, Lee P *et al*. Proliferative glomerulonephritis and exposure to organic solvents. *Nephron* 1985; **40**: 161–65.

193 Harrison DJ, Thompson D, MacDonald MK. Membraneous glomerulonephritis. *J Clin Pathol* 1986; **39**: 167–71.

194 Sesso R, Stolley PD, Salgada N, Pereora AB, Ramos OL. Exposure to hydrocarbons and rapidly progressive

glomerulonephritis. *Brazilian J Med Biol Res* 1990; **23**: 225–33.

195 Steenland NK, Thun MJ, Ferguson CW, Port FK. Occupational and other exposures associated with male end-stage renal disease: a case control study. *Am J Publ Hlth* 1990; **80**: 153–59.

196 Yaqoob M, Bell GM, Percy D, Finn R. Primary glomerulonephritis and hydrocarbon exposure: a case-control study and literature review. *Q J Med* 1992; **83**: 409–18.

197 Yaqoob M, Patrick AW, McClelland P *et al*. Occupational hydrocarbon exposure and diabetic nephropathy. *Diabet Med* 1994; **11**: 789–93.

198 Bell GM, Doig A, Thompson D, Anderton JL, Robson JS. End-stage renal disease associated with occupational exposure to organic solvents. *Proc EDTA-ERA.* 1985; **22**: 725–29.

199 Ravnskov U. Influence of hydrocarbon exposure on the course of glomerulonephritis. *Nephron* 1986; **42**: 156–60.

200 Yaqoob M, Stevenson A, Mason H, Bell GM. Hydrocarbon exposure: additional factors in the progression of renal failure in primary glomerulonephritis. *Q J Med* 1993; **86**: 661–67.

201 Cameron JS. Tubular and interstitial factors in the progression of glomerulonephritis. *Paediatric Nephrol* 1992; **6**: 292–303.

202 Yaqoob M, King A, McClelland P, McDicken I, Bell GM. Relationship between hydrocarbon exposure and nephropathology in primary glomerulonephritis. *Nephrol Dial Transplant* 1994; **9**: 1575–79.

203 Churchill DW, Fine A, Gault MH. Association between hydrocarbon exposure and glomerulonephritis: an appraisal of the evidence. *Nephron* 1983; **33**: 169–72.

204 Askergren A, Allgen LG, Bergstrom J. Studies on kidney function in subjects exposed to organic solvents I. Excretion of albumin and beta-2-microglobulin in the urine. *Acta Med Scand* 1981; **209**: 472–83.

205 Franchini I, Cavartorta A, Falzoi M, Lucertini S, Mutti A. Early indicators of renal damage in workers exposed to organic solvents. *Int Arch Occup Environ Hlth* 1983; **52**: 1–9.

206 Brochard P, De Palmas J, Martini M, Blondet M, Lagrue G. *Étude de la prevalence des proteinuries dipistées chez des sujets exposé professionellment aux solvants.* XXI International Congress Occupational Health. Dublin. September 1984.

207 Lauwerys R, Bernard A, Viau C, Buchet JP. Kidney disorders and haematotoxicity from organic solvent exposure. *Scand J Work Environ Hlth* 1985; **11**(Supp I): 83–90.

208 Viau C, Bernard A, Lauwerys R *et al*. A cross-sectional survey of kidney function in oil refinery employees. *Am J Ind Med* 1987; **11**: 177–87.

209 Hotz P, Pilliod J, Berode M, Rey F, Boillat MA. Glycosaminoglycans, albuminuria and hydrocarbon exposure. *Nephron* 1991; **58**: 184–91.

210 Hotz P, Thielemans N, Bernard A, Gutzwiller F, Lauwerys R. Serum laminin, hydrocarbon exposure and glomerular damage. *Br J Ind Med* 1993; **50**: 1104–10.

211 Vyskocil A, Popler A, Skutilova I *et al*. Urinary excretion of proteins and enzymes in workers exposed to hydrocarbons in a shoe factory. *Int Arch Occup Environ Hlth* 1991; **63**: 359–62.

212 Solet D, Robins TG. Renal function in dry cleaning workers exposed to perchloroethylene. *Am J Ind Med* 1991; **20**: 601–14.

213 Mutti A, Alinovi R, Bergamaschi E *et al*. Nephropathies and exposure to perchloroethylene in dry cleaners. *Lancet* 1992; **340**: 189–93.

214 Yaqoob M, Bell GM, McGregor AJ, Mason H, Percy DF. Renal impairment due to hydrocarbon exposure. *Q J Med* 1993; **86**: 165–74.

215 Stevenson A, Yaqoob M, Mason H, Pai P, Bell GM. Biochemical markers of basement disturbances and occupational exposure to hydrocarbons and mixed solvents. *Q J Med* 1995; **88**: 23–8.

216 Pai P, Stevenson A, Mason H, Bell GM. Occupational hydrocarbon exposure and nephrotoxicity: a cohort study and literature review. *Postgrad Med J* 1998; **741**: 225–228.

217 Rushton L, Anderson MR. An epidemiologic survey of eight refineries in Britain. *Br J Ind Med* 1981; **38**: 225–34.

218 Kaplan SD. Update of a mortality study of workers in petroleum refineries. *J Occup Med* 1986; **28**: 574–76.

219 Morgan RW, Kaplan SD, Gaffey WR. A general mortality study of production workers in the paint and coatings manufacturing industry. *J Occup Med* 1981; **23**: 13–21.

220 Divine BJ, Barron V, Kaplan SD. Texaco mortality study I. Mortality among refinery, petrochemical and research workers. *J Occup Med* 1985; **27**: 445–47.

221 Fox AJ, Collier PF. Low mortality rates in industrial cohort studies due to selection for work and survival in the industry. *Br J Prev Soc Med* 1976; **30**: 225–30.

222 Streicher HZ, Gabow PA, Moss AH, Kono D, Kaehny WD. Syndromes of toluene sniffing in adults. *Ann Intern Med* 1981; **84**: 758–62.

223 Ravnskov U. Possible mechanisms of hydrocarbon associated glomerulonephritis. *Clin Nephrol* 1985; **23**: 294–98.

224 Bekesi JG, and Holland JF, Anderson HA *et al*. Lymphocyte function of Michigan dairy farmers exposed to polybrominated biphenyls. *Science* 1978; **199**: 1207–09.

225 Glassock RJ, Edginton TS, Watson JI, Dixon FJ. Autologous immune complex nephritis induced with renal tubular antigen. *J Exp Med* 1968; **127**: 573–87.

226 Shibita S, Yokoyama M. Nephritogenic glycoprotein. *Nephron* 1990; **55**: 152–58.

227 Nishikawa K, Guo YJ, Miyasaka M *et al*. Antibodies to intercellular adhesion molecule 1/lymphocyte function – associated antigen 1 prevent cresent formation in rat auto-immune glomerulonephritis. *J Exp Med* 1993; **177**: 667–77.

228 Ogawa M, Mori T, Mori Y *et al*. Study on chronic renal

injuries induced by carbon tetrachloride: selective inhibition of the nephrotoxicity by irradiation. *Nephron* 1992; **60**: 68–73.

229 Yamamoto T, Wilson CB. Binding of anti-basement membrane after intratracheal gasoline instillation in rabbits. *Am J Pathol* 1987; **126**: 497–505.

230 Pai P, Hindell P, Stevenson A, Mason H, Bell GM. Genetic varients of microsomal metabolism and susceptibility to hydrocarbon – associated glomerulonephritis. *Q J Med* 1997; **90**: 693–8.

42

Neurotoxic effects of workplace exposures

PK THOMAS, MICHAEL J AMINOFF

Acrylamide	868	Organophosphate and carbamate insecticides	873
Allyl chloride	868	Organochlorine pesticides	874
Carbon disulphide	868	Pyrethroids	874
Carbon monoxide	869	Styrene	874
Dimethylaminoproprionitrile	869	Toluene	875
Ethylene oxide	870	Solvent mixtures	875
Hexacarbon solvents	870	Trichloroethylene	875
Metals	871	Wartime exposure	876
Methyl bromide	872	References	877

Increasing numbers of chemical agents are being introduced into the occupational environment, and many of these agents are liable to produce neurotoxic effects manifested either as neurobehavioural changes or neurological deficits affecting cognition, motor control, sensation or autonomic function. Either the central or the peripheral nervous system, or both, may be damaged. This chapter will consider the main agents that have been implicated in the setting of workplace exposure. These may affect workers involved in the manufacture of potentially neurotoxic substances and those subject to industrial, agricultural, horticultural, or military exposure.

The assessment of neurotoxic effects poses a variety of problems, particularly with regard to the detection of mild or subclinical neurobehavioural disturbances related to chronic low-dose exposure or following a single episode of acute toxicity. Structured psychometric tests for investigating possible cognitive impairment are sensitive to focal disturbances in individual cortical regions. Potential confounding factors during testing, such as fatigue or exposure to alcohol and psychotropic drugs, have to be considered. This also applies to the use of the electroencephalogram (EEG) and event-related evoked potential studies. For disturbances of motor function, quantitative tests of muscle strength and of coordination, body sway, and balance are sometimes useful. Quantitative sensory testing may be helpful; a variety of modalities can be examined, including vibration and discriminative tactile sensibility, cold and warm thermal thresholds, and heat pain thresholds. Quantitative evaluation of autonomic (mainly cardiovascular) function is now a well-established procedure. Many of these tests are laborious and time-consuming, but less elaborate tests suitable for use in the field have been devised for some assessments.

Peripheral nerve function can be analysed using nerve conduction tests which assess function both in motor and sensory fibres. The sensitivity of measurements of motor and sensory nerve conduction velocity, in particular the former, is substantially greater than that for evoked muscle action potential and sensory nerve action potential amplitude. Strict temperature control during testing is vital. For the comparison of exposed workers with control subjects, the selection of appropriate control subjects is important. The use of sedentary office workers as controls for manual workers, for example, has led to erroneous conclusions, as manual workers frequently accumulate abnormalities of nerve conduction during their occupation as a consequence of repeated minor trauma or the development of subclinical entrapment neuropathies. Neuromuscular transmission and muscle function can be assessed by quantitative electromyography (EMG), but such testing is technically demanding.

Epidemiological studies involving case-control observations again demand scrupulous care in the selection of appropriate control subjects. For neurobehavioural observations, careful matching for age, sex, ethnic group and educational background is necessary. With these multiple problems in establishing a causal relation between exposure to a particular neurotoxic agent and the occurrence of symptoms in a workforce, it is understandable that conflicting reports may arise, particularly as individual variations in susceptibility may complicate the issue. Animal experiments are not always informative because of interspecies differences but may be crucial in clarifying the mechanism of action of toxic substances.

ACRYLAMIDE

Acrylamide polymers are used to separate solids from aqueous solutions in certain industries, and are constituents of adhesives and certain products such as cardboard and moulded parts (see Chapter 11). The monomer, but not the polymer, is neurotoxic. Exposure typically occurs by inhalation or cutaneous absorption during the manufacture of the monomer or in the polymerization process. Acrylamide is also used for grouting in mines and tunnels; for this purpose, liquid monomer is pumped into the soil, where polymerization occurs after the addition of various catalysts, rendering the soil waterproof. Intoxication has occurred occasionally in workers involved in such grouting operations.[1] Occupational exposure may result in an encephalopathy, with confusion, hallucinations, poor concentration, drowsiness, and other changes, depending on the duration and severity of exposure. A length-dependent sensorimotor neuropathy also occurs and is typically associated with hyperhidrosis and redness and exfoliation of the skin[2,3] and occasionally with urinary retention. Cerebellar disturbances may be conjoined.[4] Numbness of the feet is usually the earliest symptom. The tendon reflexes are lost at an early stage.

The neuropathy is arrested and may slowly reverse after discontinuation of exposure, but residual deficits – including sensory ataxia – are common. Histopathological studies show a distally predominant accumulation of neurofilaments in axons, and distal axonal degeneration in both the peripheral and central nervous systems. There is little secondary demyelination. On electrophysiological examination, maximal motor conduction velocity is normal or only slightly reduced, but compound muscle action potentials may be small and dispersed, with a prolongation in the distal motor latency.[2] These changes have been attributed to degeneration and subsequent regeneration of the distal parts of the motor axons. In keeping with an axonopathy, sensory nerve action potentials are reduced or absent[2,5] and this is the preferred electrophysiological means of monitoring workers who are at risk of developing the disorder.

More sophisticated electrophysiological studies have revealed that sensory fibres are more vulnerable than motor fibres, and large fibres more vulnerable than small ones;[6] function is disturbed especially in the short, intra-

muscular segment of the large-diameter stretch receptor afferent axons from gastrocnemius.[7] Experimental studies have also indicated that sudomotor dysfunction occurs later than motor involvement and reflects damage to postganglionic sympathetic efferent nerve fibres.[8]

The recommended airborne exposure limit (threshold limit value, TLV) in the United States of America is 0.3 mg/m[3]. Myers and Macun[9] described the occurrence of acrylamide neuropathy in workers in a small factory in South Africa who were exposed to varying levels of acrylamide while manufacturing polyacrylamide flocculants. Logistic regression showed dose–response relationships of exposure with symptoms, abnormal sensation, weakness, gait disturbances, and cutaneous abnormalities. Acrylamide-related abnormalities occurred in 67% of those with exposure exceeding the recommended exposure level of National Institute of Occupational Safety and Health (NIOSH), compared with lesser exposure.

The encephalopathy and mild peripheral neuropathy resolve following cessation of exposure to acrylamide, but recovery is incomplete in patients with severe neuropathies. There is no specific treatment to hasten recovery.

ALLYL CHLORIDE

Allyl chloride, a chlorinated hydrocarbon, is used in the manufacture of epichlorohydrin which is employed for the manufacture of epoxy resins. It is also used in the production of glycerine insecticides and in the synthesis of polyacrylonitride. The occurrence of a mixed motor and sensory neuropathy has been described in workers exposed to allyl chloride[10] and a central-peripheral distal axonopathy has been reproduced experimentally in mice.[11] A multifocal intra-axonal accumulation of neurofilaments preceded axonal degeneration.

CARBON DISULPHIDE (see Chapter 8)

Carbon disulphide has been used as a soil fumigant, in the manufacture of viscose rayon and cellophane films, in the cold vulcanization of rubber, in perfume production, and as a component in certain varnishes and insecticides. It has also been used as a solvent for rubber, wax resins, various oils and certain other chemicals. Toxicity may result from inhalation, ingestion and possibly skin contact, and is not confined to the nervous system. The TLV in the USA is 30 mg/m[3] (10 parts per million: ppm) (see Chapter 11).

Inhalation exposure to concentrations above 400 ppm leads to narcosis. An encephalopathy may result from acute high exposure, with headache, irritability, uncontrollable anger, disrupted sleep, memory disturbances, mood swings, mania, depression, suicidal tendencies, confusion, and other psychiatric manifestations.[12,13] Such symptoms may follow subacute exposure to levels in the order of 300 ppm, but are common also when workers are exposed chronically to concentrations averaging between 40 and 50 ppm; they are not to be expected at concentrations below 20 ppm.[14] Minor intellectual, affective, or motor changes may only be revealed by neuropsychological testing.[15]

Long-term exposure to carbon disulphide may lead to a variety of behavioural or psychiatric disturbances,[13] to extrapyramidal findings such as cogwheel rigidity, bradykinesia, or dyskinesia, and to pyramidal deficits such as a pseudobulbar palsy. The pupillary and corneal reflexes may be lost,[12] a retrobulbar optic neuropathy sometimes develops, and funduscopic examination may reveal a characteristic retinopathy with microaneurysms and punctate haemorrhages.[16] In addition, there may be clinical or subclinical evidence of polyneuropathy.[17–19] The neuropathy develops after exposure to levels of 100–150 ppm for several months or to lower levels for several years. It is histologically similar to the neuropathy produced by n-hexane, with focal axonal swellings and accumulations of neurofilaments.

There is no specific treatment for the neurological complications of carbon disulphide intoxication, but further exposure must be prevented and general symptomatic measures may be helpful.

CARBON MONOXIDE (see Chapter 8)

Carbon monoxide (CO) is an odourless, colourless gas derived from the incomplete combustion of carbon-containing materials. The noxious effects are the result of hypoxia. It binds tenaciously to haemoglobin to form carboxyhaemoglobin (COHb) and also impairs the dissociation of oxyhaemoglobin so that tissue hypoxia is greater than for a comparable degree of anaemia. It also binds to myoglobin, cytochrome oxidase, cytochrome P450, catalases and peroxidases. Elimination of carbon monoxide is increased by breathing pure oxygen or, more rapidly, by hyperbaric oxygen. Some is eliminated by conversion to carbon dioxide (CO_2).

Carbon monoxide poisoning may occur as a result of occupational exposure. In a series studied by Smith and Brandon,[20] 10% of the cases were related to industrial exposure, mainly in miners, garage employees and gas workers.

The consequences of acute exposure are highly variable.[21] Cognitive or behavioural dysfunction is evident in most cases. Disorientation, excitement, apprehension or depression are seen in about 25% of patients. Impaired consciousness is seen in about 66%, ranging from lethargy, through stupor to coma. Affected individuals may show tremor, spasticity, rigidity, dyskinetic move-

ments, exaggerated or depressed tendon reflexes and extensor plantar responses. Respiratory depression can lead to death. Garland and Pearce[22] drew attention to the occurrence of localized neurological signs, including evidence of focal cortical dysfunction. Generalized epileptic seizures may be observed in the first or second week after intoxication.

Delayed deterioration was first noted by Grinker.[23] Following a period of partial or apparently full recovery, after an interval of 2–3 weeks on average, a relapse occurs, sometimes abrupt in onset, with confusion, psychotic behaviour, focal cortical dysfunction and often an extrapyramidal syndrome of rigid parkinsonian type. These features may persist or subsequently improve.

Peripheral nerve involvement has been described. Sometimes this has been focal or multifocal, presumably related to a combination of hypoxia and compression. A neuropathy with paranodal changes has been produced experimentally in rats.[24]

Pathologically the central nervous system changes are typical of hypoxic/ischaemic damage, with focal or laminar necrosis of the cerebral cortex and neuronal loss in the hippocampus, cerebellar cortex and substantia nigra. Bilateral necrotic lesions of the globus pallidus are particularly characteristic.[25] White matter lesions also occur, both diffuse and focal. The delayed deterioration is often associated with a diffuse subcortical leukoencephalopathy, but this is also seen in cases without a biphasic course and the pathology in patients with delayed deterioration after anoxia may be confined to grey matter.[26]

Treatment of acute carbon monoxide poisoning consists of removal from the carbon monoxide containing atmosphere, the administration of oxygen, with hyperbaric oxygen if available, and supportive measures including treatment of the metabolic acidosis.

Adverse effects of chronic low level carbon monoxide exposure are questionable. Stewart[27] concluded that visual perception was possibly marginally impaired at carboxyhaemoglobin levels of 5% but that cognitive function and the performance of complex motor tasks were not altered unless concentrations exceeded 10%.

DIMETHYLAMINOPROPRIONITRILE

Dimethylaminoproprionitrile (DMAPN) has been used, along with acrylamide, in a grouting mixture. This combination is known to have caused peripheral neuropathy. It was then incorporated as a catalyst in the production of polyurethane foams. After its introduction in 1976–77 an unusual neuropathic syndrome developed in exposed workers.[28] This began with difficulty with micturition and was followed by erectile impotence and sensory symptoms in the feet and hands. These symptoms were accompanied by insomnia and fatiguability. Examination showed distal sensory loss in the limbs and also in sacral dermatomes, slight distal weakness and depressed ankle jerks. Gradual recovery ensued but urinary and sexual dysfunction sometimes persisted. Exposure had probably occurred by inhalation. Dimethylaminoproprionitrile toxicity was unusual as autonomic involvement is uncommon in toxic neuropathies. Nerve biopsy showed loss of both myelinated and unmyelinated axons.

ETHYLENE OXIDE

Ethylene oxide (EtO) has been employed to sterilize heat-sensitive products such as operating gowns used by hospital personnel and patients (see Chapter 8). Its byproduct ethylene chlorohydrin (EtC) is considered to be highly toxic. Chronic exposure to ethylene oxide and ethylene chlorohydrin has been reported to lead to peripheral neuropathy and mild cognitive impairment in operating department nurses and technicians,[29] although disposable operating gowns and drapes are now widely used. It has also been suggested that residual ethylene chlorohydrin in dialysis tubing after sterilization could contribute to the polyneuropathy encountered in patients receiving chronic haemodialysis.[30] It is known that neuropathy can be produced by exposure of rats to ethylene oxide.[31] This is a central-peripheral distal axonopathy.

HEXACARBON SOLVENTS (see Chapter 11)

Methyl n-butyl ketone and n-hexane

Methyl n-butyl ketone is a solvent that has been used in the manufacture of vinyl and acrylic coatings and adhesives, and in the printing industry. In 1975, Allen and associates[32] reported on an outbreak of polyneuropathy among workers in a plant producing plastic-coated and colour-printed fabrics. The temporal onset and cause of the outbreak correlated with exposure to methyl n-butyl ketone, which had recently replaced methyl isobutyl ketone, and new cases failed to appear after its elimination from the work place. It has since become apparent that exposure via inhalation or skin contact to only small traces (a few ppm) of methyl n-butyl ketone is sufficient to lead to a neuropathy in exposed workers.[33]

n-Hexane is a solvent used in various paints, lacquers and printing inks. It is also widely used in the rubber industry and in glues, and exposure occurs in workers involved in manufacturing shoes or sandals, laminating processes and cabinet finishing. Exposure leads to an insidiously progressive, distal, sensorimotor polyneuropathy, sometimes accompanied by visual impairment (due to optic neuropathy or maculopathy[16]) or facial numbness.[34] Tendon reflexes may show only mild changes. There is marked slowing of nerve conduction velocity and terminal motor latency in addition to signs of denervation in affected muscles and small or absent sensory nerve action potentials. The neuropathy results from a disturbance of axonal transport, and is associated with giant, multifocal axonal swelling with accumulation of axonal neurofilaments, and with distal degeneration in both peripheral and central axons accompanied by secondary demyelination.[35]

n-Hexane and methyl n-butyl ketone are metabolized to 2,5-hexanedione, the agent responsible predominantly for their neurotoxic effects. Acute exposure by inhalation to these hexacarbon solvents produces a pleasurable sense of euphoria, together with headache, unsteadiness, hallucinations, and mild narcosis.[36] The inhalation for recreational purposes of certain glues has been associated with the development of the same sensorimotor polyneuropathy described above.[37]

The neurological deficit progresses for some months after occupational or recreational exposure is discontinued, and examination may show evidence of minor pyramidal dysfunction in addition to the neuropathy. Multimodality evoked potential studies have provided confirmatory evidence of central involvement at different levels of the nervous system (cord, brainstem, and cerebral hemispheres) in workers exposed to n-hexane.[38]

Methyl ethyl ketone

Methyl ethyl ketone is a solvent used in paints and lacquers, printer's ink, and certain glues. Occupational exposure to methyl ethyl ketone has been monitored by measuring its concentration in the air of the working environment and also by determination of urinary levels at the end of a work-shift. It was present with methyl n-butyl ketone in the mixture of chemicals that led to the outbreak of neuropathy referred to earlier. It has also been present with n-hexane in a number of compounds that have been inhaled for recreational purposes, with resulting development of a neuropathy. It is generally believed that methyl ethyl ketone does not itself cause a peripheral neuropathy but that it may facilitate its development when exposure occurs to other hexacarbon solvents.[39–41]

Chronic occupational exposure to methyl ethyl ketone through both skin contact and inhalation has been associated in a single graphics worker with the development of multifocal myoclonus, ataxia and a postural tremor that resolved over 1 month after exposure to the work environment was discontinued.[42] Other similarly exposed workers were not affected, suggesting that individual susceptibility was an important factor. Ataxia and tremor have also been reported, together with dysarthria, cognitive changes, headaches and respiratory difficulties, in a labourer after acute exposure to a mixture of methyl ethyl ketone and toluene while spray-painting equipment in an enclosed, unventilated garage.[43]

METALS (see Chapter 7)

Aluminium

Although a progressive encephalopathy with neurofibrillary degeneration can be produced experimentally in susceptible animals by the administration of aluminium salts, the only established neurotoxic effect of aluminium in man is dialysis encephalopathy.[44] This occurred in individuals who had been on haemodialysis for several years because of end-stage renal failure. A progressive fatal encephalopathy developed with dementia, speech disturbances, myoclonus and focal and generalized seizures. It was associated with markedly elevated blood and brain aluminium concentrations. There was no characteristic neuropathology and, in particular, neurofibrillary degeneration of Alzheimer type was not present. Uptake of aluminium into the brain was probably enhanced by elevated parathormone levels.

Workplace exposure to aluminium is not a definite hazard, but miners exposed over the course of years in northern Ontario to inhalation of aluminium particles to reduce pulmonary silicosis do display a dose-related cognitive decline.[45]

Arsenic

Inorganic arsenic poisoning may occur industrially in workers engaged in the smelting of copper and lead ores, or because of drinking water from wells adjacent to mines containing ores rich in arsenic. Chronic exposure leads to gastrointestinal symptoms including anorexia, vomiting and diarrhoea from mucosal irritation, and skin changes such as melanosis, keratoses and cutaneous malignancies. The predominant neurological complication is a peripheral neuropathy. This usually begins with distal sensory symptoms, often painful, in the lower limbs and then in the hands. Distal weakness follows. Most clinical descriptions of neuropathy are of cases following acute exposure.[46,47] Nerve biopsy has shown axonal loss,[48] although the occurrence of acute demyelinating neuropathy following arsenic ingestion has been reported.[49] Acute poisoning can be treated with 2,3-dimercaptopropane sulphonate (DMPS). The DMPS-arsenic complex probably has a lower penetration into the central nervous system than dimercaprol (British Anti-Lewisite; BAL) and may result in lower acute and residual toxicity.

Lead

Poisoning with lead is primarily related to inorganic lead compounds. Lead is widely employed industrially and excessive exposure may therefore occur in a broad range of occupations, including smelting, metal foundry work, battery manufacture and repair, demolition and ship-breaking, the manufacture of paint pigments and polyvinylchloride (PVC), and storage tank construction and repair. Absorption is both by ingestion and inhalation, although it can occasionally occur through the skin. Within the body, lead is distributed between the blood, mainly in erythrocytes, a relatively labile component in the general tissues including the brain, and a more stable fraction in bone. At the cellular level, it is concentrated in nuclei and mitochondria.

The clinical manifestations differ between children and adults but this discussion will be confined to the latter. Acute or subacute lead encephalopathy is less common in adults, but it can be superimposed on chronic intoxication. Early features are mental confusion and reduced alertness. This progresses, with continued exposure, via increasing obtundation to stupor and coma, often accompanied by focal or generalized seizures. Examination may reveal papilloedema and extensor plantar responses. Loss of tendon reflexes can indicate a concomitant neuropathy and sometimes provides a valuable clue to the diagnosis.

Pathologically, the brain may show few changes or may be seen to be swollen, with vascular congestion and perivascular exudates. Histologically, there may be white matter oedema. Scattered necrotic neurons may be detected, sometimes with focal atrophy and gliosis, particularly in the cerebellum, indicative of more chronic pathology.[50]

Lead neuropathy is predominantly motor in type, manifested by bilateral finger and wrist drop and bilateral foot drop. The older literature drew attention to the occurrence of focal weakness in muscle groups that were frequently used, such as those at the wrist in painters. In more severe cases, weakness of proximal muscles develops. Distal sensory loss may occur, but is less prominent. The tendon reflexes are depressed or lost. Other signs of chronic lead intoxication may be present.

The pathological changes in the peripheral nerves are poorly characterized. Although experimental animal studies have demonstrated widespread demyelination,[51] the available evidence in man, both from nerve conduction studies and nerve biopsies[52] indicates an axonopathy.

The mechanism of lead neurotoxicity is not understood. It is considered to bind competitively to sulphydryl groups and to displace divalent ions such as calcium, but the effect of this on cell function is unclear. It is also not established how far lead encephalopathy depends upon a disturbance of the blood–brain barrier and how much to a direct toxic effect on neurons and glia.

Acute lead encephalopathy is treated by supportive measures, together with dexamethasone for cerebral oedema and chelation of lead with dimercaprol; DMPS may be preferable. The management of lead neuropathy merely requires removal from the source of exposure and the provision of orthotic appliances while recovery is awaited. This is usually satisfactory. There is no good evidence that chelation affords any additional benefit.

Manganese

Manganese is included in a variety of metal alloys and has been used as an anti-knock agent to replace lead in petrol. Industrial exposure occurs in manganese miners and cases have been reported from several countries, in particular Chile[53] and Taiwan. Absorption is by dust inhalation.

The initial signs of neurotoxicity are usually behavioural and cognitive changes, including disturbed compulsive behaviour, and with headache. These are followed by motor problems, predominantly of an extrapyramidal nature, with facial impassivity, dysarthria, muscle rigidity and hypokinesia, dystonia and tremor. Pathologically, neuronal loss is evident in the globus pallidus and substantia nigra pars reticulata and, to a lesser extent, in the subthalamic nucleus and the striatum.[54] The parkinsonian features and dystonia show little response to levodopa. Observations in experimentally intoxicated monkeys confirmed predominant damage to the globus pallidus.[55] It was suggested that the parkinsonism is caused by interference with pathways downstream to the nigrostriatal pathway.

Mercury

Intoxication with inorganic mercury has mainly occurred as a result of industrial exposure, either from dust inhalation or ingestion from contamination of the hands with mercury compounds. In former years this was encountered in the hat making industry.[56] A large outbreak was reported from an Italian factory in 1949.[57] The clinical picture was dominated by tremor and personality change, but muscle weakness was also described, together with cutaneous erythema. Adequate information as to the pathological changes in the nervous system is not available.

Poisoning with organic mercury compounds had long been recognized as an occasional industrial hazard, but intoxication with methyl mercury achieved prominence with the large outbreak in Minamata Bay in Japan in the 1950s.[58] This was the result of the discharge of industrial effluent into the sea and the consumption of contaminated fish. The nature of the condition was recognized from its resemblance to the cases described by Hunter and Russell.[59] The initial neurological features were usually sensory, with tingling and numbness in the hands and sometimes the tongue, followed by progressive constriction of the visual fields leading to blindness. Hearing loss was frequent. Limb weakness and ataxia were prominent but tremor was less evident than in poisoning with inorganic mercury.

The pathological changes in the nervous system were described by Hunter and Russell[59] and were similar in the Minamata Bay cases. Atrophy and neuronal loss were seen in the cerebral cortex, particularly in the occipital region, and in the cerebellum, together with glial cell proliferation. Degenerative changes were also observed in the peripheral nerves.

Extensive experimental studies have been undertaken in an attempt to establish the mechanism of neural damage. It is clear that the effects of mercury on the nervous system are complex and they are not yet fully understood. They include blood–brain barrier dysfunction, disruption of protein synthesis, interference with the glycolytic pathway and mitochondrial respiratory chain function, intracellular protein denaturation and breakdown of cell membranes. They have been reviewed by Chang.[60]

Tellurium

This metal is mainly derived from copper refinery slimes but is also obtained during the mining of a variety of other metals. It gave its name to Telluride, Colorado, where Butch Cassidy carried out his first bank robbery. It has multiple industrial uses including incorporation in alloys, the colouration of glass, ceramics and metalware, in the manufacture of thermoelectric devices and in the production of rubber. Industrial exposure is predominantly through the lungs by the inhalation of volatile tellurium compounds. Intoxication can be acute or chronic, but both result in a characteristic garlicky odour to the breath, dryness of the mouth and a metallic taste, headache, dizziness, drowsiness and gastrointestinal symptoms. Hypohidrosis, rashes and a bluish skin discolouration may occur. Spontaneous recovery takes place.

Interesting neurological phenomena have been produced experimentally in animals. These consist of congenital hydrocephalus,[61] cerebral lipofuscinosis[62] and a paralytic demyelinating neuropathy that recovers by remyelination despite the continued administration of tellurium, suggesting selective Schwann cell vulnerability at a critical period of development.[63] No human counterparts of these phenomena are known.

METHYL BROMIDE

Methyl bromide has been used as a fumigant, fire extinguisher, refrigerant and insecticide (see Chapter 8). Because of its high volatility, dangerous concentrations may accumulate in work areas and inhalation then leads to neurotoxicity. Clinical manifestations depend on dose and duration of exposure. Acute poisoning produces convulsions, pulmonary oedema, hyperpyrexia, coma, and death. Other neurological manifestations of acute toxicity include psychosis,[64] affective changes, ataxia, tremor and myoclonus.[65–66] Seizures may also occur following exposure to low concentrations,[67] as may headache, nausea, dysarthria, confusion, hyperreflexia and visual abnormalities.[68]

Long-term exposure has been associated with a polyneuropathy[68,69] that may occur in the absence of systemic symptoms.[70] Paraesthesiae in the feet are followed by symmetric, distal sensory and motor deficits and areflexia. Gait ataxia may be conspicuous. Recovery to a variable extent occurs over the 3–9 months following withdrawal from exposure. Visual disturbances and optic atrophy have also been reported.[71]

Cavanagh[66] has related methyl bromide intoxication to altered glycolysis and pyruvate oxidation. The peripheral manifestations have been attributed to a distal axonopathy that reflects the altered metabolism of the neuronal perikaryon or an alteration of axonal transport.

A latent period of several hours or even 1 or 2 days may occur after exposure before the onset of symptoms, and victims may die without awareness that exposure to the odourless, colourless gas has even occurred.[72] Chloropicrin is a common additive that leads to conjunctival and mucosal irritation, thereby warning of inhalation exposure to methyl bromide. Symptoms of toxicity may occur at a bromide level in the order of 3 mg/ml. With levels over 5 mg/dl, mental changes may lead to careless handling of the chemical by fumigators, and thus to even greater exposure.[73]

In the past, chelating agents, haemoperfusion, and N-acetylcysteine[65] have been advocated for therapy, but their efficacy is uncertain. Otherwise, treatment is symptomatic and supportive.

ORGANOPHOSPHATE AND CARBAMATE INSECTICIDES (see Chapter 10)

There are a large number of organophosphate compounds, which are used mainly as pesticides or herbicides. They inhibit acetylcholinesterase, leading to acute cholinergic toxicity with both central and neuromuscular manifestations. Symptoms include weakness, nausea, salivation, lacrimation, headache, and bronchospasm with mild poisoning. With more severe intoxication, there may also be diarrhoea, bradycardia, tremor, chest pain, cyanosis, convulsions, pulmonary oedema, and, eventually, coma. Death occurs from respiratory or cardiac failure unless treatment is instituted promptly. This involves administration of pralidoxime, 1 g intravenously, together with atropine 1 mg subcutaneously every 30 minutes until sweating and salivation settle. If there is no obvious benefit, a second dose of pralidoxime can be administered intravenously. If this too is unhelpful, it may be necessary to infuse pralidoxime, titrating the dose against clinical response, and giving atropine every 20–30 minutes until benefit follows.

Carbamate insecticides, like organophosphorus compounds, inhibit cholinesterases but their duration of action is much shorter as the carbamate–enzyme complex dissociates spontaneously.[74] The symptoms of intoxication resemble those of organophosphate poisoning but are usually less severe. Treatment with atropine may be required but the use of oximes is usually not necessary.

A constellation of symptoms resembling those of influenza are common in farmers exposed to organophosphate sheep dips and is referred to as 'dippers' flu'. It immediately follows a dipping session and consists of headache, dizziness, coryzal symptoms, and myalgia that clear after 1–2 days. It may represent mild organophosphate toxicity although this is not established.

Senanayake and Karalliede[75] described an intermediate syndrome that may follow acute toxicity or at times occurs without any preceding illness. It is characterized by mainly proximal limb weakness and, sometimes, cranial nerve involvement. It develops within 1–4 days of exposure and recovers in 2–3 weeks. Although the precise mechanism is uncertain, it is due to a disturbance of neuromuscular transmission.[76]

Some 2–3 weeks after acute exposure to certain organophosphates, a neuropathy, organophosphate-induced delayed polyneuropathy, may develop. The interval between exposure and symptom-onset relates in part to the dose and nature of the exposure. The initial complaint is often of cramping muscle pain in the legs, and distal numbness and paraesthesiae may also occur. The legs then become progressively weaker, and after a few days similar symptoms and signs may develop in the upper limbs. The tendon reflexes are depressed. Sensory abnormalities are often relatively inconspicuous, but may be severe. The clinical deficit is therefore that of a distal, symmetric, predominantly motor polyneuropathy affecting the lower limbs more than the upper limbs. In severe cases, patients become quadriplegic. Minor pyramidal deficits may also be noted, especially as functional recovery occurs in the peripheral nerves,[77,78] and are important with regard to the prognosis for functional recovery.[79]

Electrophysiological studies reveal findings typical of an axonal neuropathy, with partial denervation of affected muscles and a reduced interference pattern on needle examination, normal or only slightly reduced maximal motor conduction velocities, and small compound muscle action potentials with somewhat delayed distal motor latencies. Histopathology confirms a distal axonopathy.[80,81]

Organophosphate–induced delayed polyneuropathy only occurs following exposure to certain organophosphates, such as tricresylphosphates, mipafox, leptophos, trichlorphon, trichlornate and methamidophos.[82,83] These organophosphates inhibit an enzyme, neuropathy target esterase (NTE), to produce the delayed neuropathy. More specifically, the neuropathy is initiated by the phosphorylation of NTE in nervous tissue. Neurotoxicity occurs with the loss of a group attached to the phosphorus, leaving a negatively charged phosphoryl group attached to the protein (so-called 'aging'). Inhibition of NTE without subsequent aging, as occurs with carbamates, for example, does not lead to the development of neuropathy. The precise pathogenesis of the neuropathy is uncertain. It seems unlikely to relate to impaired axonal transport or to defective protein synthesis.[84,85] The physiological role of NTE in the nervous system is unknown. Measurement of lymphocyte NTE has been used to monitor chronic occupational exposure to various organophosphates. There is no specific treatment to prevent the occurrence of the neuropathy.

The possibility of chronic effects following acute exposure to organophosphates remains controversial. Largely anecdotal reports have described residual sequelae.[84–86] Nevertheless, several case-control control studies have indicated that behavioural and neurological dysfunction, including EEG and EMG abnormalities, may be detectable.[87–90] The possible occurrence of chronic sequelae in the absence of episodes of acute toxicity is less well established. This question has arisen in the UK particularly in relation to repeated organophosphate exposure during sheep dipping. Again there are anecdotal reports of such effects, but these are difficult to assess because of a lack of adequate documentation of the organophosphate exposure and because exposure may also have occurred to various other pesticides and solvents. Several studies employing control groups of varying suitability have reported neurobehavioural deficits, and impairment of vibration sense and two-point tactile discrimination[91–95] whereas others have obtained negative results.[96,97] Further epidemiological and controlled neurobehavioural and neurophysiological studies are required.

ORGANOCHLORINE PESTICIDES

The chlorinated hydrocarbons constitute a wide range of chemicals[98] and include the organochlorine insecticide dichlorodiphenyltrichlorethane (DDT), now no longer in use, and others such as aldrin, dieldrin and lindane. They are only slowly degraded and persist for long periods in animals and in the environment. One member of this group, chlordecone (Kepone®) was responsible for a major episode of industrial exposure in 1975 at a manufacturing plant in Hopewell, Virginia, and also environmental contamination through the James River which feeds into Chesapeake Bay.[99] Workers developed a neurological illness characterized by 'nervousness', opsoclonus, tremor, clumsiness for manual activities and mild gait ataxia.[100] Slight memory impairment was noticed. Slow but sometimes incomplete recovery occurred. Benign intracranial hypertension was observed in a small proportion of cases. Absorption was by inhalation of dust. The mechanism of neural damage was not established (see Chapter 10).

PYRETHROIDS

Synthetic pyrethroids were introduced as insecticides in the wake of the withdrawal of DDT. They act on voltage-dependent sodium channels resulting in a prolonged sodium current during membrane excitation, particularly in sensory nerve fibres. This leads to repetitive firing and ultimately membrane depolarization with block of excitation. Occupational exposure in man can lead to the occurrence of paraesthesiae, especially in the face and hands, presumably from repetitive activity in sensory fibres.[101] Massive exposure can result in more severe toxicity. With treatment by supportive measures, recovery is good (see Chapter 10).

STYRENE

Styrene is used in the manufacture of reinforced plastic and certain resins (see Chapter 12). It is used especially in the construction of fibreglass-reinforced plastic boats and other articles, and significant occupational exposure may occur by contact and by inhalation. Exposure is often estimated using biological indices that are not specific for styrene, such as urinary mandelic acid or phenylglyoxylic acid concentration. Environmental measures of styrene may not reflect biological levels because there is considerable variation in styrene uptake and metabolism, depending on personal activities. Thus both environmental and biological measures are required when exposure to styrene is being considered. Occupational exposure is typically not restricted to styrene but also involves exposure to cleansing solvents and other chemicals, thereby complicating the interpretation of any disturbances that may arise in the work place.

Concerns about the neurotoxicity of styrene have been underscored by its high lipid solubility. Acute changes in cognition, behaviour, or level of consciousness occur at certain concentrations, but concerns regarding its safety in an industrial setting relate primarily to chronic, low-level exposure. A number of studies have been held to suggest that abnormalities in reaction time and psychomotor performance are induced by styrene at levels approaching current exposure standards, which range between 20 and 50 ppm in many countries. Following a critical analysis of this literature, Rebert and Hall[102] found that this contention was unjustified, relating to misinterpretation of the data or to type I statistical errors, or that confounding factors had invalidated the various studies. Indeed, no compelling evidence could be found by these authors of persisting neurological sequelae to long-term, low-level styrene exposure.

The inadequacies of these various studies merit

emphasis. Rebert and Hall[102] noted that in many the documentation of exposure was poor and that the number of subjects studied was often very low when subgroups were considered, as when stratifying by level of exposure. Confounding factors were often problematic, demographic data and job characterization were usually incomplete, no attempt was made to validate self-reports of drug and alcohol use, and details of medication use were sparse. The potential effects of exposure to other chemicals were often neglected or minimized. Rarely was mention made of blind procedures. A variety of statistical shortcomings were also conspicuous, including probable violation of certain statistical assumptions. The incidence of statistical significance was often overestimated because it was based on comparisons of non-independent measures and on multiple comparisons. In addition to these concerns, there was no general consistency in the literature and no clear indication of causal factors or biological mechanisms that might account for any real effects of styrene.

TOLUENE

Toluene is a solvent in paints and glues. It is also used to synthesize benzene, benzoic acid, nitrotoluene, and other compounds. Exposure may occur in workers involved in laying linoleum or spraying paint, and in the printing industry (see Chapter 12).

The effects of exposure are primarily neurobehavioural. Chronic, high exposure may lead to cognitive changes, pyramidal tract findings, cerebellar ataxia, brainstem or cranial nerve disturbances, and tremor.[103] Bilateral visual loss from optic neuropathy has been described[104] as also has ocular flutter or dysmetria and opsoclonus.[105] Cognitive abnormalities are characterized by disturbances of attention, memory, and visuospatial function. Apathy and a flat affect are common. Cerebral magnetic resonance imaging may show diffuse abnormalities of the cerebral white matter, the degree of which correlates with neuropsychological impairment.[106] Diffuse cerebral atrophy and symmetric lesions in the basal ganglia and cingulate gyri have also been reported.[107]

The level and duration of exposure necessary to produce clinical evidence of neurotoxicity is uncertain, and it is not clear what neurobehavioural effects are produced by long-term, low-level exposure. Exposure to toluene at a level of 125 ppm may produce no neurological symptoms.[108,109] although minor abnormalities may be present on neurobehavioural studies.[110] At levels of 250 ppm there may be insomnia, nervousness, and intermittent stupor. A peripheral neuropathy does not occur with toluene.

SOLVENT MIXTURES

Prolonged, low-level, occupational exposure to mixtures of organic solvents occurs commonly, for example in house painters. Such exposure is reported to cause an encephalopathy or 'organic brain syndrome' characterized primarily by disturbances of memory, concentration, and attention, and by changes in personality. However, the studies that form the basis of such claims generally fail to stand up to rigorous scientific scrutiny.[111–114] These studies, which have originated mainly from Scandinavia, are primarily epidemiological in nature. Objections to them include concerns that other factors, such as alcohol or drug/medication use or the lingering effect of acute exposure to solvents, may have been responsible for the encephalopathic features that were described. In addition, precise details concerning work conditions and extent of probable exposure to solvents were often not obtained or provided, or there was an overreliance on subjective recall in determining the severity and duration of exposure. Moreover, factors known to influence the neuropsychological tests used to document the presence of an encephalopathy, such as educational background, age, stress, and cultural factors, were not taken fully into account in certain uncontrolled studies. The use of controls from other workplace settings may have led to bias when comparisons were made. This is especially important when test and control populations differ in educational or other factors that may have been responsible for their original choice of occupation or if one group is prone to certain occupationally related non-toxic disorders such as anxiety syndromes.

This is well exemplified by the study of Gade and associates[115] in which 20 solvent-exposed workers, mostly painters, were re-examined 2 years after they had originally been diagnosed with a chronic toxic encephalopathy.[116] Their performance on neuropsychological testing was unchanged, but the previous impression of significant cognitive decline could not be substantiated when comparison was now made to a non-exposed control group and allowance was made for the influence of age, educational background and level of intelligence.

The existence of a chronic encephalopathy characterized solely by cognitive, affective and personality changes in those exposed for long periods to low-levels of organic solvents remains uncertain. No definite causal relationship has been established and the underlying mechanism for such an association is elusive.

TRICHLOROETHYLENE

Trichloroethylene was once used as an anaesthetic agent (see Chapter 12). It is now used as a de-waxer, degreaser, and drycleaner, and in paint removers and glues. Inhalation exposure to levels in the order of 50 to 200 ppm have led to changes in reaction time and performance on psychological tests in some but not other studies. With increasing exposure in an occupational setting, complaints of headache, fatigue, irritability, nausea and dizziness are common. Facial hyperaesthesia and masticatory weakness may result from dysfunction of the trigeminal nerve; other cranial nerves, such as the facial, optic and oculomotor, may also be affected. An autopsy study has shown fibre degeneration in the trigeminal nerve.[117] The reason for the susceptibility of the cranial nerves is unknown. At levels of exposure below 40 ppm, there is no convincing evidence of significant or long-term disturbances of cognitive function.

Vacor®

Ingestion accidentally or deliberately of *N*-3-pyridomethyl-*N*-*p*-nitrophenylurea (PNU) in the form of Vacor®, a rodenticide, has led to the acute onset of a rapidly progressive distal axonopathy with conspicuous dysautonomia. Symptoms commence within hours of intoxication. Limb weakness, cranial neuropathy, areflexia, and urinary retention are typical, with marked impairment of blood pressure regulation. Pancreatic necrosis leads also to diabetes mellitus. Variable neurological recovery occurs over several months.

An abnormality of fast axonal transport in somatic and autonomic nerves has been held to account for the axonopathy, but its precise basis is uncertain.[118]

WARTIME EXPOSURE

Agent Orange and the Vietnam War

Over a 10-year period during the war in Vietnam, American forces sprayed millions of gallons of herbicides to strip vegetation that might conceal or provide sustenance for opposition forces. The preparation known as Agent Orange was used most commonly; more than 11 million gallons of Agent Orange were used before spraying was discontinued in 1971 because of concerns about long-term safety. Over the years since then, public concern has increased about the potential health hazards of exposure to Agent Orange. In addition to numerous scientific studies, various governmental reports have been published that bear on the issue.

Agent Orange contained 2,4,5-trichlorophenoxyacetic acid, and one of its contaminants was 2,3,7,8-tetrachlorodibenzo-*p*-dioxin (or TCDD) (see Chapter 12). It has now become apparent that exposure to the major herbicides used in Vietnam or to TCDD is associated with the development of Hodgkin's or non-Hodgkin's lymphoma, soft-tissue sarcoma, chloracne, and porphyria cutanea tarda and perhaps also of certain other neoplastic disorders.[119] Attention here is confined to the potential neurotoxicity of these agents.

The literature is voluminous but much of it is methodologically flawed. Careful analysis of it has revealed no compelling evidence of an association between Agent Orange exposure and the development of cognitive or neuropsychological disorders or of chronic peripheral neuropathy.[119,120] Anecdotal reports suggest that peripheral neuropathy may develop acutely or subacutely following occupational exposure to herbicides,[121–123] although the possibility cannot be excluded that the neuropathy in these cases related not to the exposure but to other factors, such as development of the Guillain-Barré syndrome. There are no data on the development of an acute neuropathy following Agent Orange exposure in Vietnam.

Exposure of the local population to dioxin followed the chemical explosion that occurred in an industrial plant at Seveso in Italy, but there did not appear to be an increased risk of acute neuropathy[124] and the prevalence of peripheral neuropathy several years after the accident was not increased among those with heavy exposure to dioxin.[125,126]

Gulf War syndrome

A proportion of both male and female US and UK military personnel who took part in the Gulf War in 1990–91 began reporting debilitating symptoms soon after their return when the conflict ended (see Chapter 8). Commonly reported complaints included fatigue, memory impairment, difficulty in concentrating, sleep disturbances, headaches, and muscle and joint pains. These symptoms thus had a considerable degree of overlap with the chronic fatigue syndrome (see Chapter 2). A variety of possible toxic explanations have been entertained, including exposure to pesticides and chemical warfare agents, pyridostigmine, bromide, oil well fires and smoke and petroleum products. Haley and Kurt[127] in a cross-sectional epidemiological study on self-reported exposure to combinations of potentially neurotoxic chemicals identified three syndromes: impaired cognition, confusion-ataxia and 'arthroneuromyopathy'. They concluded that some individuals may have sustained delayed chronic effects from exposure to combinations of chemicals that inhibit butyrylcholinesterase and neuropathy target esterase. Jamal *et al.*[128] detected mild abnormalities of nerve conduction and cold thermal sensory threshold testing in a small group of UK military personnel who had served in the war. These two studies require replication. A US Government report[129] concluded that although some veterans clearly have service-connected illnesses, the evidence does not support a causal link with toxic exposure. In the UK, a review of 284 self-selected veterans with symptoms that they related to service during the Gulf War[130] concluded that these could be subdivided into five groups: minor physical illness (the most frequent category), major physical illness, post-traumatic stress disorder, other psychiatric conditions, and the chronic fatigue syndrome. No unique cluster of symptoms could be identified.

REFERENCES

1 Kesson CM, Baird AW, Lawson DH. Acrylamide poisoning. *Postgrad Med J* 1977; **53**:16–17.

2 Fullerton PM. Electrophysiological and histological observations of peripheral nerves in acrylamide poisoning in man. *J Neurol Neurosurg Psychiat* 1969; **32**:186–92.

3 Garland TO, Patterson MWH. Six cases of acrylamide poisoning. *Br Med J* 1967; **4**:134–8.

4 He F, Zhang S, Wang H *et al*. Neurological and electroneuromyographic assessment of the adverse effects of acrylamide on occupationally exposed workers. *Scand J Work Environ Hlth* 1989; **15**:125–9.

5 Takahashi M, Ohara T, Hashimoto K. Electrophysiological study of nerve injuries in workers handling acrylamide. *Int Arch Arbeitsmed* 1971; **28**:1–11.

6 Sumner AJ, Asbury AK. Acrylamide neuropathy: selective vulnerability of sensory fibers. *Arch Neurol* 1974; **30**:419.

7 Sumner AJ, Asbury AK. Physiological studies of the dying-back phenomenon: muscle stretch afferents in acrylamide neuropathy. *Brain* 1975; **98**:91–100.

8 Navarro X, Verdu E, Guerrero J, Buti M, Gonalons E. Abnormalities of sympathetic sudomotor function in experimental acrylamide neuropathy. *J Neurol Sci* 1993; **114**:56–61.

9 Myers JE, Macun I. Acrylamide neuropathy in a South African factory: an epidemiologic investigation. *Am J Ind Med* 1991; **19**:487–93.

10 He FS, Lu BQ, Zhang SC, Dong SW, Yu Y, Wang BY. Chronic allyl chloride poisoning. An epidemiology, clinical, toxicological and neuropathological study. *Giorn Ital Med Lav* 1985; **7**:5–15.

11 He F, Jacobs JM, Scaravilli F. The pathology of allyl chloride neurotoxicity in mice. *Acta Neuropathol* 1981; **55**:125–33.

12 Davidson M, Feinleib M. Carbon disulfide poisoning: a review. *Am Heart J* 1972; **83**:100–14.

13 Huang CC, Chu CC, Chen RS, Lin SK, Shih TS. Chronic carbon disulfide encephalopathy. *Eur Neurol* 1996; **36**:364–8.

14 Putz-Anderson V, Albright BE, Lee ST *et al*. A behavioral examination of workers exposed to carbon disulfide. *Neurotoxicology* 1983; **4**:67–78.

15 Hanninen H. Psychological picture of manifest and latent carbon disulphide poisoning. *Br J Ind Med* 1971; **28**:374–81.

16 Striph GG, Miller NR. Neurotoxicology of the visual system. Part 2: Clinical evidence and concerns. In: Bleecker ML ed. *Occupational Neurology and Clinical Neurotoxicology*. Baltimore: Williams and Wilkins, 1994 : 172–86.

17 Seppäläinen AM, Tolonen MT. Neurotoxicity of long-term exposure to carbon disulfide in the viscose rayon industry: a neurophysiological study. *J Scand Work Environ Hlth* 1974; **11**:145–53.

18 Peters HA, Levine RL, Matthews CG, Chapman LJ. Extrapyramidal and other neurologic manifestations associated with carbon disulfide fumigant exposure. *Arch Neurol* 1988; **45**:537–40.

19 Chu CC, Huang CC, Cheng RS, Shih TS. Carbon disulfide-induced polyneuropathy in viscose rayon workers. *Occup Environ Med* 1995; **52**:404–7.

20 Smith JS, Brandon S. Acute carbon monoxide poisoning: 3 years experience in a defined population. *Postgrad Med J* 1970; **46**:65–70.

21 Meigs JW, Hughes JPW. Acute carbon monoxide poisoning. An analysis of one hundred cases. *Arch Indust Hyg Occup Med* 1952; **6**:344–53.

22 Garland H, Pearce J. Neurological complications of carbon monoxide poisoning. *Q J Med* 1967; **36**:445–55.

23 Grinker RR. Über einen Fall von Leuchtgasvergiftung mit doppelseitiger Pallidumer weichung und schwer Degeneration des tieferen Grosshirnmarklagers. *Zeit Ges Neurol Psychiatr* 1925; **98**:433–54.

24 Grunnet ML, Petajan JH. Carbon monoxide induced neuropathy in the rat. Ultrastructural changes. *Arch Neurol* 1976; **33**:158–63.

25 Lapresle J, Fardeau M. The central nervous system and carbon monoxide poisoning. II. Anatomical study of brain lesions following intoxication with carbon monoxide (22 cases). *Prog Brain Res* 1967; **24**:31–74.

26 Dooling EC, Richardson Jr EP. Delayed encephalopathy after strangling. *Arch Neurol* 1976; **33**:196–9.

27 Stewart RD. The effect of carbon monoxide on humans. *J Occup Med* 1976; **18**:304–9.

28 Pestronk A, Keogh J, Griffin JG. Dimethylamino-proprionitrile intoxication: a new industrial neuropathy. *Neurology* 1979; **29**:540–9.

29 Brashear A, Univerzagt FW, Farber MO, Bonnin JM, Garcia JE, Grober M. Ethylene oxide neurotoxicity: a cluster of 12 nurses with peripheral and central nervous system toxicity. *Neurology* 1996; **46**:992–8.

30 Windebank AJ, Blexrud MD. Residual ethylene oxide in hollow fiber hemodialysis units is neurotoxic in rats. *Ann Neurol* 1989; **26**:63–8.

31 Ohnishi A, Inoue N, Tamamoto T, Murai Y, Hori H *et al*. Ethylene oxide neuropathy in rats. Exposure to 250 ppm. *J Neurol Sci* 1986; **74**:215–21.

32 Allen N, Mendell JR, Billmaier DJ, Fontaine RE, O'Neill J. Toxic polyneuropathy due to methyl n-butyl ketone: an industrial outbreak. *Arch Neurol* 1975; **32**:209–18.

33 Bos PMJ, de Mik G, Bragt PC. Critical review of the toxicity of methyl n-butyl ketone: risk from occupational exposure. *Am J Ind Med* 1991; **20**:175–94.

34 Yamamura Y. n-Hexane polyneuropathy. *Folia Psychiatr Neurol Jap* 1969; **23**:45–57.

35 Spencer PS, Schaumburg HH. Central-peripheral distal axonopathy: the pathology of dying-back neuropathies.

In: Zimmerman H ed. *Progress in Neuropathology* Vol 3. New York: Grune and Stratton, 1976 : 276–85.

36 Spencer PS, Couri D, Schaumburg HH. n-Hexane and methyl n-butyl ketone. In: Spencer PS, Schaumburg HH eds. *Experimental and Clinical Neurotoxicology*. Baltimore: Williams and Wilkins, 1980 : 456–75.

37 Korobkin R, Asbury AK, Sumner AJ, Nielsen SL. Glue-sniffing neuropathy. *Arch Neurol* 1975; **32**:158–62.

38 Chang Y-C. Neurotoxic effects of n-hexane on the human central nervous system: evoked potential abnormalities in n-hexane polyneuropathy. *J Neurol Neurosurg Psychiat* 1987; **50**:269–74.

39 Saida K, Mendell JR, Weiss HS. Peripheral nerve changes induced by methyl n-butyl ketone and potentiation by methyl ethyl ketone. *J Neuropath Exp Neurol* 1976; **35**:207–25.

40 Altenkirch H, Stoltenburg G, Wagner HM. Experimental studies on hydrocarbon neuropathies induced by methyl-ethyl-ketone (MEK). *J Neurol* 1978; **219**:159–70.

41 Abou-Donia MB, Hu Z, Lapadula DM, Gupta RP. Mechanisms of joint neurotoxicity of n-hexane, methyl isobutyl ketone and O-ethyl O-4-nitrophenyl phenylphosphonothioate in hens. *J Pharmacol Exp Ther* 1991; **257**:282–9.

42 Orti-Pareja M, Jimenez-Jimenez FJ, Miguel J, Montero E, Cabrera-Valdivia F *et al*. reversible myoclonus, tremor, and ataxia in a patient exposed to methyl ethyl ketone. *Neurology* 1996; **46**:272.

43 Welch L, Kirschner H, Heath A, Gilliland R, Broyles S. Chronic neuropsychological and neurological impairment following acute exposure to a solvent mixture of toluene and methyl ethyl ketone (MEK). *J Toxicol Clin Toxicol* 1991; **29**:435–45.

44 Alfrey AC, Le Gendre GR, Kaehny WD. The dialysis encephalopathy syndrome. Possible aluminum intoxication. *N Engl J Med* 1976; **294**:184–8.

45 Rifat SL, Eastwood MR, Crapper B, McLachlan DR, Corey PN. Effect of exposure of miners to aluminum powder. *Lancet* 1990; **336**:1162–5.

46 Jenkins RB. Inorganic arsenic and the nervous system. *Brain* 1966; **89**:479–98.

47 Le Quesne PM, McLeod JG. Peripheral neuropathy following a single exposure to arsenic. *J Neurol Sci* 1977; **32**:427–51.

48 Ohta M. Ultrastructure of sural nerve in a case of arsenic neuropathy. *Acta Neuropath* 1970; **16**:233–40.

49 Greenberg SA. Acute demyelinating neuropathy with arsenic ingestion. *Muscle Nerve* 1996; **19**:1611–3.

50 Pentschew A. Morphology and morphogenesis of lead encephalopathy. *Acta Neuropath* 1965; **5**:135–60.

51 Fullerton PM. Chronic peripheral neuropathy produced by lead poisoning in guinea pig. *J Neuropath Exp Neurol* 1966; **25**:214–36.

52 Buchthal F, Behse F. Electrophysiology and nerve biopsy in men exposed to lead. *Br J Ind Med* 1979; **36**:135–47.

53 Schuler P, Oyanguren H, Maturawa V, Valenzuela A, Creuz E *et al*. Manganese poisoning. Environmental and medical study at a Chilean mine. *Indust Med Surg* 1957; **26**:167–73.

54 Barbeau A, Inque N, Cloutier T. Role of manganese in dystonia. In: Eldridge R, Fahn S eds. *Advances in Neurology* Vol 14. New York: Raven Press, 1976.

55 Shinotoh H, Snow BJ, Hewitt KA, Pate BD, Doudet D *et al*. MRI and PET studies of manganese-intoxicated monkeys. *Neurology* 1995; **45**:1199–204.

56 Neal PA, Jones RR. Chronic mercurialism in the hatter's fur-cutting industry. *JAMA* 1938; **110**:337–51.

57 Vigliani E, Baldi G. Una insolita epidermia di mercurialismo in une fabbrica de capelli di fetro. *Med Lav* 1949; **40**:65–72.

58 Kurland LT, Faro S, Sielder H. Minimata disease: the outbreak of a neurological disorder in Minamata, Japan, and its relationship to the ingestion of seafood contaminated by mercury compounds. *World Neurol* 1960; **1**:370–81.

59 Hunter D, Russell DS. Focal cerebellar atrophy in human subject due to organic mercury compounds. *J Neurol Neurosurg Psychiat* 1954; **17**:235–44.

60 Chang LW. Mercury. In: Spencer PS, Schaumburg HH eds. *Experimental and Clinical Neurotoxicology*. Baltimore: Williams and Wilkins. 1980;508–26.

61 Garro F, Pentschew A. Neonatal hydrocephalus in the offspring of rats fed during pregnancy nontoxic amounts of tellurium. *Arch Psychiat Nervenkrank* 1964; **206**:272–85.

62 Duckett S, White R. Cerebral lipofuscinosis induced with tellurium: electron dispersive x-ray spectroscopy analysis. *Brain Res* 1974; **73**:205–14.

63 Lampert P, Garro F, Pentschew A. Tellurium neuropathy. *Acta Neuropath* 1970; **15**:308–17.

64 Zatuchni J, Hong K. Methyl bromide poisoning seen initially as psychosis. *Arch Neurol* 1981; **38**:529–30.

65 Hustinx WNM, van de Laar RTH, van Huffelen AC, Verwey JC, Meulenbelt J, Savelkoul TJF. Systemic effects of inhalational methyl bromide poisoning: a study of nine cases occupationally exposed due to inadvertent spread during fumigation. *Br J Ind Med* 1993; **50**:155–9.

66 Cavanagh JB. Methyl bromide intoxication and acute energy deprivation syndromes. *Neuropath Appl Neurobiol* 1992; **18**:575–8.

67 Rathus EM, Landy PJ. Methyl bromide poisoning. *Br J Ind Med* 1961; **18**:53–7.

68 De Haro L, Gastaut JL, Jouglard J, Renacco E. Central and peripheral neurotoxic effects of chronic methyl bromide intoxication. *Clin Toxicol* 1997; **35**:29–34.

69 Cavalleri F, Galassi G, Ferrari S, Merelli E, Volpi G *et al*. Methyl bromide induced neuropathy: a clinical, neurophysiological, and morphological study. *J Neurol Neurosurg Psychiat* 1995; **58**:383.

70 Kantarjian AD, Sattar AS. Methyl bromide poisoning with nervous system manifestations resembling polyneuropathy. *Neurology* 1963; **13**:1054–8.

71 Chavez CT, Hepler RS, Straatsma BR. Methyl bromide optic atrophy. *Am J Ophthalmol* 1985; **99**:715–9.

72 Collins RP: Methyl bromide poisoning: a bizarre neurological disorder. *Calif Med* 1965; **103**:112–6.

73 Drawneek W, O'Brien MJ, Goldsmith HJ, Bourdillon RE. Industrial methyl-bromide poisoning in fumigators. *Lancet* 1964; **2**:855–6.

74 Ballantyne B, Marrs TC. *Organophosphates and Carbamates*. Oxford: Butterworth-Heinemann. 1992.

75 Senanayake N, Karalliede L. Neurotoxic effects of organophosphorus insecticides: an intermediate syndrome. *N Engl J Med* 1987; **316**:761–3.

76 Sedgwick EM, Senanayake N. Pathophysiology of the intermediate syndrome of organophosphate poisoning. *J Neurol Neurosurg Psychiat* 1997; **62**:201–2.

77 Senanayake N. Tri-cresyl phosphate neuropathy in Sri Lanka: a clinical and neurophysiological study with a three year follow up. *J Neurol Neurosurg Psychiat* 1981; **44**:775–80.

78 Morgan JP, Penovich P. Jamaica ginger paralysis: forty-seven-year follow-up. *Arch Neurol* 1978; **35**:530–2.

79 Vasilescu C. Triorthocresyl phosphate neuropathy. *Arch Neurol* 1979; **36**:455.

80 Bouldin TW, Cavanagh JB. Organophosphorous neuropathy. I. A teased-fiber study of the spatio-temporal spread of axonal degeneration. *Am J Pathol* 1979; **94**:241–2.

81 Bouldin TW, Cavanagh JB. Organophosphorous neuropathy. II. A fine-structural study of the early stages of axonal degeneration. *Am J Pathol* 1979; **94**:253–70.

82 Lotti M, Becker CE, Aminoff MJ. Organophosphate polyneuropathy: pathogenesis and prevention. *Neurology* 1984; **34**:658–62.

83 Lotti M. A key step forward in understanding the pathogenesis of organophosphate polyneuropathy. *Hum Exp Neurotoxicol* 1995; **14**:69–70.

84 Gershon S, Shaw FH. Psychiatric sequelae of chronic exposure to organophosphorus compounds. *Lancet* 1961; **1**:1371–4.

85 Wadia RS, Sadagopan C, Amin RB, Sardesai HV. Neurological manifestations of organophosphorus insecticide poisoning. *J Neurol Neursurg Psychiat* 1974; **37**:841–7.

86 Weinbaum Z, Schenker MB, O'Malley MA, Gold EB, Samuel SJ. Determinants of disability in illnesses related to agricultural use of organophosphates (OPs) in California. *Am J Ind Med* 1995; **28**:257–74.

87 Savage EP, Keefe TJ, Mounce LM, Heaton RK, Lewis JA, Burcar PJ. Chronic neurological sequelae of acute organophosphate pesticide poisoning. *Arch Environ Hlth* 1988; **43**:38–45.

88 Rosenstock L, Keifer M, Daniell EW, McConnell R, Claypoole K. Chronic central nervous system effects of acute organophosphate pesticide intoxication. *Lancet* 1991; **338**:223–7.

89 McConnell R, Keifer M, Rosenstock L. Elevated quantitative vibro-tactile threshold among workers previously poisoned with Methamidiphos and other organophosphate pesticides. *Am J Ind Med* 1994; **25**:325–33.

90 Steenland J, Jenkins B, Ames RG, O'Malley M, Chrislip BA, Russo J. Chronic neurological sequelae to organophosphate pesticide poisoning. *Am J Publ5. Hlth* 1994; **84**:731–6.

91 Levin HS, Rodnitsky RL, Mick DL. Anxiety associated with exposure to organophosphate compounds. *Arch Gen Psychiat* 1976; **33**:225–8.

92 Maizlish N, Schenker M, Weisskfoff C, Seiber J, Samuels S. A behavioral evaluation of pest control workers with short term, low level exposure to the organophosphate Diazinon. *Am J Ind Med* 1987; **12**:153–72.

93 Stephens R, Spurgeon A, Calvert IA, Beach J, Levy LS, Harrington JM. Neuropsychological effects of long term exposure to organophosphates in sheep dip. *Lancet* 1995; **345**:1135–9.

94 Stokes L, Stark A, Marshall E, Narang A. Neurotoxicity among pesticide applicators exposed to organophosphates. *Occup Environ Med* 1995; **52**:648–53.

95 Beach JR, Spurgeon A, Stephens R, Heafield T, Calvert IA, Harrington JM. Abnormalities in neurological examination among sheep farmers exposed to organophosphate pesticides. *Occup Environ Med* 1996; **53**:520–5.

96 Ames RG, Steenland D, Jenkins B, Chrislip D, Russo J. Chronic neurologic sequelae to cholinesterase inhibition among agricultural pesticide applicators. *Arch Environ Hlth* 1995; **50**:440–3.

97 Rodnitzky RL, Levin HS, Mick DL. Occupational exposure to organosphosphate pesticides. *Arch Environ Hlth* 1995; **30**:98–103.

98 Evangelisia De Duffard AM, Duffard R. Behavioral toxicology, risk assessment, and chlorinated hydrocarbons. *Environ Hlth Perspect* 1996; **104** (Suppl 2):353–60.

99 Cannon SB, Veazey Jr JM, Jackson RS, Burse VW, Hayes C, Straub WE, Landigan PJ, Liddle JA, Epidemic kepone poisoning in chemical workers. *Am J Epidemiol* 1978; **107**:529–37.

100 Taylor JR, Selhorst JB, Calabrase VP. Chlordecone. In: Spencer PS, Schaumburg HH eds. *Experimental and Clinical Neurotoxiciology*. Baltimore: Williams and Wilkins. 1980;407–21.

101 Vijverberg HP, Van den Bercken J. Neurotoxicological effects and mode of action of pyrethroid insecticides. *Crit Rev Toxicol* 1990; **21**:105–26.

102 Rebert CS, Hall TA. The neuroepidemiology of styrene: a critical review of representative literature. *Crit Rev Toxicol* 1994; **24**:S57–S106.

103 Hormes JT, Filley CM, Rosenberg NL. Neurologic sequelae of chronic solvent vapor abuse. *Neurology* 1986; **36**:698–702.

104 Keane JR. Toluene optic neuropathy. *Ann Neurol* 1978; **4**:390.

105 Lazar RB, Ho SU, Melen O, Daghestani AN: Multifocal

central nervous system damage caused by toluene abuse. *Neurology* 1983; **33**:1337–40.

106 Filley CM, Heaton RK, Rosenberg NL. White matter dementia in chronic toluene abuse. *Neurology* 1990; **40**:532–4.

107 Ashikaga R, Araki Y, Miura K, Ishida O. Cranial MRI in chronic thinner intoxication. *Neuroradiology* 1995; **37**:443–4.

108 Antti-Poika M, Juntunen J, Matikäinen E, Suoranta H, Hanninen H, Seppäläinen AM, Liira J, Occupational exposure to toluene: Neurotoxic effects with special emphasis on drinking habits. *Int Arch Occup Environ Hlth* 1985; **56**:31–40.

109 Juntunen J, Matikäinen E, Antti-Poika M, Suoranta H, Valle M. Nervous system effects of long-term occupational exposure to toluene. *Acta Neurol Scand* 1985; **72**:512–7.

110 Foo SC, Jeyaratnam J, Koh D. Chronic neurobehavioural effects of toluene. *Br J Ind Med* 1990; **47**:480–4.

111 Grasso P, Sharratt M, Davies DM, Irvine D. Neurophysiological and psychological disorders and occupational exposure to organic solvents. *Food Chem Toxicol* 1984; **22**:819–52.

112 Grasso P, Neurotoxic and neurobehavioral effects of organic solvents on the nervous system. *Occup Med* 1988; **3**:525–39.

113 Errebo-Knudsen EO, Olsen F. Organic solvents and presenile dementia (the painters' syndrome). A critical review of the Danish literature. *Sci Total Environ* 1986; **48**:45–67.

114 Lees-Haley PR, Williams CW. Neurotoxicity of chronic low-dose exposure to organic solvents: a skeptical review. *J Clin Psychol* 1997; **53**: 699–712.

115 Gade A, Mortensen EL, Bruhn P. 'Chronic painter's syndrome'. A reanalysis of psychological test data in a group of diagnosed cases, based on comparisons with matched controls. *Acta Neurol Scand* 1988; **77**:293–306.

116 Arlien-Soborg P, Bruhn P, Gyldensted C, Melgaard B. Chronic painters' syndrome: chronic toxic encephalopathy in house painters. *Acta Neurol Scand* 1979; **60**:149–56.

117 Buxton PH, Hayward M. Polyneuritis cranialis associated with industrial trichlorethylene poisoning. *J Neurol Neurosurg Psychiat* 1967; **30**:511–8.

118 Watson DF, Griffin JW. Vacor neuropathy: ultrastructural and axonal transport studies. *J Neuropathol Exp Neurol* 1987; **46**:96–108.

119 Institute of Medicine. *Veterans and Agent Orange Health Effects of Herbicides Used in Vietnam*. Washington DC: National Academy Press, 1994.

120 Institute of Medicine. *Veterans and Agent Orange, Update* Washington DC: National Academy Press, 1996.

121 Goldstein NP, Jones PH, Brown KR. Peripheral neuropathy after exposure to an ester of dichlorophenoxyacetic acid. *JAMA* 1959; **171**:1306–9.

122 Berkley MC, Magee KR. Neuropathy following exposure to a dimethylamine salt of 2,4-D. *Arch Intern Med* 1963; **111**:133–4.

123 Todd RL. A case of 2,4-D intoxication. *J Iowa Med Soc* 1962; **52**:663–4.

124 Filippini G, Bordo B, Crenna P. Relationship between clinical and electrophysiological findings and indicators of heavy exposure to 2,3,7,8-tetrachlorodibenzo-p-dioxin. *Scand J Work Environ Hlth* 1981; **7**:257–62.

125 Barbieri S, Pirovano C, Scarlato G, Tarchini P, Zappa A, Maranzana M. Long-term effects of 2,3,7,8-tetrachlorodibenzo-p-dioxin on the peripheral nervous system. Clinical and neurophysiological controlled study on subjects with chloracne from the Seveso area. *Neuroepidemiology* 1988; **7**:29–37.

126 Assennato G, Cervino D, Emmett EA, Longo G, Merlo F. Follow-up of subjects who developed chloracne following TCDD exposure at Seveso. *Am J Ind Med* 1989; **16**:119–25.

127 Haley RW, Kurt TL. Self-reported exposure to neurotoxic chemical combinations in the Gulf War. A cross-sectional epidemiologic study. *JAMA* 1997; **277**:231–7.

128 Jamal G, Hansen S, Apartopoulos F, Peden A. The 'Gulf War syndrome'. Is there evidence of dysfunction in the nervous system. *J Neurol Neurosurg Psychiat* 1996; **60**:449–51.

129 Presidential Advisory Committee on Gulf War Veterans' Illnesses. *Final Report*. Washington. DC: US Government Printing Office, 1996.

130 Coker WJ. A review of Gulf War illness. *J Roy Nav Med Serv* 1996; **82**:141–146

43

Hepatotoxic effects of workplace exposures

THOMAS W WARNES, SANJIV K JAIN, ALEXANDER SMITH

Patterns of toxic liver injury	882	Specific occupational hepatotoxins	890
Treatment	886	Conclusions	895
Mechanisms of liver toxicity in model		Acknowledgements	895
hepatotoxins	887	References	895

A variety of classifications of hepatotoxic agents exists in the medical and toxicological literature based variously on the source and chemical nature of the toxicant,[1-3] the type of liver pathology produced[4,5] or on the toxic mechanisms involved.[6,7] In this chapter we will approach hepatotoxicity from a more practical, clinical viewpoint, in order to both increase the index of suspicion in the diagnosis of these conditions and to give the practising clinician guidelines to the assessment and management of hepatotoxicity and an outline of some contributory factors which may exacerbate liver damage.

The liver is the first organ after the gut exposed to ingested chemicals, toxins and drugs and its rich blood supply ensures that agents absorbed through the lungs and skin also reach the liver quickly and at high concentrations. It is thus easily injured by direct exposure to these agents. In addition, many xenobiotic compounds are actively removed from the bloodstream by the liver and detoxified by hepatic metabolic processes. However, in the course of detoxification, some are metabolized into even more toxic substances[7] including free radicals.[8]

Occupational liver disease may occasionally present after an acute incident at work and in these circumstances, diagnosis and identification of the toxic agent is relatively straightforward. In general, however, the diagnosis of occupational liver disease is rare in clinical practice and likely to be difficult. The patient may present with general symptoms of liver dysfunction or alternatively, an individual health check or routine workplace screen may have provided the initial clue to liver disease. However, the large functional reserve of the liver allows most cases of occupational liver injury to go undetected during many years of chronic exposure or until long after exposure has ceased and thus advanced liver disease may already be present and the occupational aetiology may be missed. Even when an occupational cause is suspected, it is usually difficult to quantify the level of exposure to a specific toxin, particularly when, with routine safety measures in place, exposure may have occurred in unpredictable ways such as machine breakdown, during cleaning of machinery, or as a result of accidental leakage.

It should be appreciated, furthermore, that abnormal liver function tests are found quite commonly in the general population not exposed to industrial chemicals.[9] The most common cause of abnormal liver function tests in the general population of Western countries is hepatic steatosis associated with obesity.[10,11] Gilbert's syndrome is present in 5% of the population[12] and is diagnosed by the finding of indirect hyperbilirubinaemia in the absence of haemolysis. Serum γ-glutamyl transpeptidase may be a sensitive indicator of hepatotoxicity since it is a marker, among other things, of liver microsomal enzyme induction, but it is essentially non-specific.[9] Following the initial detection of an abnormality in liver function, a non-invasive screen should be carried out, including ultrasound scan of the liver, together with appropriate blood tests (Table 43.1 and Fig. 43.1). These should permit diagnosis of metabolic, autoimmune and viral liver disorders, and if these have been excluded, then workplace exposure to chemicals needs to be carefully considered and liver biopsy may be required.

Table 43.1 *Non-invasive screening of an individual with abnormal liver function tests*

History	Workplace, environmental exposure	
	Alcohol, drug ingestion	
	Previous medical history	Hepatitis, Jaundice
	Family history	Autoimmune disorders
		Liver or autoimmune disorders
Ultrasound scan	Steatosis	
	Chronic liver disease	
	Extrahepatic biliary obstruction	
	Infiltration	
	Venous abnormalities	Portal hypertension
	Tumours	Portal or hepatic vein occlusion
Immunology	Smooth muscle antibody	
	Anti-nuclear factor	Autoimmune hepatitis type 1
	Liver/kidney microsomal	
	antibody	Autoimmune hepatitis type 2
	Antimitochondrial antibody	Primary biliary cirrhosis
Biochemistry	Serum iron; Ferritin	Haemochromatosis
	Iron binding capacity	
	Serum caeruloplasmin	Wilson's disease
	α1-Antitrypsin	α1-Antitrypsin deficiency
	αFetoprotein	Hepatoma
Viral screen	Hepatitis A antibody, IgM	Acute type A hepatitis
	HBsAg	
	HB core antibody, IgM	Acute type B hepatitis
	HB core antibody, IgG	Chronic type B hepatitis
	HCV antibody	
	HCV-RNA by PCR	Type C hepatitis

Chemicals and toxins can produce a wide spectrum of clinical presentations ranging from mildly abnormal liver function tests in asymptomatic patients, to fulminant liver failure. The liver has only a limited number of ways of responding to chemical insults: these include steatosis, acute or chronic hepatitis, hepatocellular necrosis, cirrhosis, veno-occlusive disease, non-cirrhotic portal hypertension and hepatic neoplasia. Chemical compounds may have both hepatotoxic and carcinogenic potential. No classification of chemically induced hepatotoxicity is entirely satisfactory, since the response of the liver depends upon the dose, duration and route of the exposure as well as on differing sensitivities of individuals to the particular chemical. Alcohol and drugs such as anti-epileptics as well as other chemicals such as dichlorodiphenyltrichloroethane (DDT), all increase hepatic microsomal enzyme activity and are degraded by specific cytochrome P450 isoforms. These agents can therefore increase the damage produced by hepatotoxins such as carbon tetrachloride[13] which are activated by the cytochrome P450 system.[7] In animals, repeated exposure to combinations of carbon tetrachloride and other agents, such as phenobarbitone and acetone, reliably produce cirrhosis,[14] and in some cases, hepatoma. Other drugs which the patient may be taking (e.g. cimetidine) may inhibit the cytochrome P450 system,[7] with sec-

ondary effects on the metabolism of chemical hepatotoxins. Phenothiazines (chlorpromazine, promazine and promethazine) have also been shown to inhibit the effect of carbon tetrachloride, possibly by membrane stabilization.[15]

The physician must therefore have a high index of suspicion regarding chemicals and toxins in the genesis of liver dysfunction and must be aware of the occupations which present a risk in this respect (Table 43.2), together with the wide range of industrial chemicals, elements and toxins which have been reported to produce hepatotoxicity (Table 43.3). This list is not exhaustive but serves to indicate the wide range of substances which must be considered.

PATTERNS OF TOXIC LIVER INJURY

Acute injury

This may produce hepatocyte damage or cholestasis. Major elevations of the serum transaminase levels with marginal elevation of alkaline phosphatase, are consistent with cytotoxic injury. Hepatomegaly may be present but clinical signs of acute liver injury may be marginal, or similar to those found in symptomatic

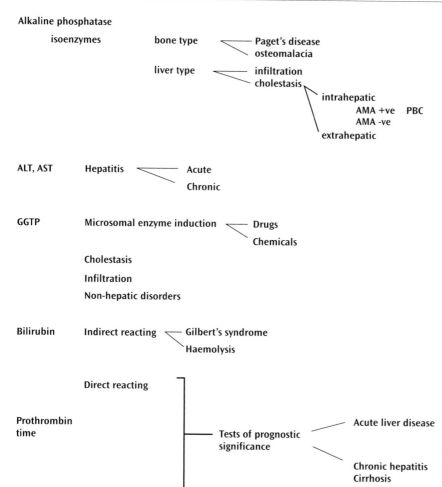

Alkaline phosphatase

isoenzymes — bone type — Paget's disease
osteomalacia

liver type — infiltration
cholestasis

intrahepatic
AMA +ve   PBC
AMA -ve

extrahepatic

ALT, AST   Hepatitis — Acute
Chronic

GGTP   Microsomal enzyme induction — Drugs
Chemicals

Cholestasis

Infiltration

Non-hepatic disorders

Bilirubin   Indirect reacting — Gilbert's syndrome
Haemolysis

Direct reacting

Prothrombin
time

Tests of prognostic
significance — Acute liver disease

Chronic hepatitis
Cirrhosis

Albumin

Figure 43.1 *Disorders producing abnormal liver function tests (ALT). AST: aspartate transaminase; GGTP: γ-glutamyl transpeptidase.*

viral hepatitis. Clinically, cholestasis presents with pruritus, jaundice and elevation of the serum alkaline phosphatase and γ-glutamyl transpeptidase, with a much less impressive elevation of serum transaminase levels. The morphological findings are those of intracellular accumulation of bile or of canalicular bile deposits. Mixed hepatocellular and cholestatic forms of liver injury may be found, for example, that produced by exposure to 4,4'-methylenedianiline[16] (diaminodiphenylmethane) a compound used in industry as an epoxy resin hardener, in the preparation of isocyanates, in the production of polyurethane and as an antioxidant in latex rubber. It was first identified as a liver toxin during an epidemic outbreak of jaundice in 84 inhabitants of the English town of Epping who had eaten bread baked with contaminated flour (see Chapter 12).[17] Jaundice was accompanied by elevation of serum alkaline phosphatase and transaminase levels. Needle biopsies showed cholestasis and hepatocellular damage. Recovery was rapid in most patients and none died. Re-exposure to methylene dianiline may cause recurrence of hepatitis but the mechanism of action has not been extensively studied.[18]

Acute cytotoxic injury is indicated by steatosis and necrosis and these are often encountered together, for instance after intoxication with carbon tetrachloride. Yellow phosphorus steatosis may be microvesicular or macrovesicular,[19] or mixed; the type of steatosis is frequently characteristic for a number of chemicals. The chemical injury can also be classified according to its localization, since zonal damage often occurs in parallel with the activity of enzymes which mediate the metabolic activation of the chemical to the toxic metabolite. Thus, carbon tetrachloride and dimethylnitrosamine produce centrilobular necrosis because cytochrome P450 is more abundant in Rappaport zone 3 (the centrizonal area).[20] It has been suggested[21] that yellow phosphorus may produce periportal fibrosis, but this claim has not been substantiated.

Acute liver injury may result in hepatic failure and death. However, if the patient recovers from the acute attack, the prognosis is good since complete recovery usually occurs.

Table 43.2 *Occupations associated with hepatotoxicity*

Aircraft industry	Manufacture and maintenance	Beryllium alloys
	Fuel handling	Kerosene
	Machine degreasing	See below
Car industry		Triorthocresyl phosphate
	Machine degreasing	See below
	Paint spraying	See below
Chemical industry	Acetone recycling	Acetone
Laboratory work	Acrylic fibre production	Acrylonitrile, Dimethylacetamide
	Fruit paper production	Biphenyls
	Chlorine/acetaldehyde production	Mercury vapour
	Chemical production	Allyl chloride
		Benzidine/β naphthylamine
		Benzene
		p-tert Butylphenol
		Dimethylformamide
		2,4,5-Trichlorophenol (TCP)
Dry cleaning		Tetrachloroethylene
Machine degreasing		Trichloromethane (chloroform)
		1,1,1-Trichloroethane
		Trichloroethylene
Environmental	Contaminated wheat	Hexachlorobenzene
	Contaminated bread	Methylenedianiline (Epping jaundice)
	Contaminated rice oil	Polychlorinated biphenyls (Yusho incident)
	Contaminated rapeseed oil	Toxic oil syndrome (Spain)
	Vinyl chloride in environment	Vinyl chloride
	Contaminated wells	Arsenic
Electrical industry	Capacitor/transformer manufacture	Polychlorinated biphenyls (PCBs)
	Semiconductors	Selenium
Epoxy resin application		Methylenedianiline
		2-Nitropropane
Firework production		Phosphorus
GRP plastics manufacture		Styrene
Horticulture/Gardening/ Pesticide production	Pesticide use	Carbamate insecticide (Isolan®)
		Chlordecone (Kepone®)
		Dichlorodiphenyltrichloroethane (DDT)
		γ-Hexachlorocyclohexane
		MCPA (2-methyl-4-chlorophenoxyacetic acid)
		Mucochloric acid
		Malathion
		Paraquat
		Pyramin
	Soil disinfection	Bromomethane (methyl bromide)
Metal production/use	Beryllium ore reduction	Beryllium
	Fluorescent lamp manufacture	Beryllium
	X-ray tube manufacture	Beryllium
	Gold melting	Cadmium
	Chromium plating	Chromium
	Copper smelting/refining /working	Copper (plus contaminants arsenic cadmium, iron, sulphur, zinc)
	Nickel alloy production	Nickel
Munitions work		TNT (trinitrotoluene)
	Manufacture or disposal	
Neoprene application		Polychloroprene
Nursing		Cytostatic agents

Table 43.2 – cont.

Painting		1,2-Dichloroethane
		2-Nitropropane
		Xylene
Pharmaceutical industry		Trichloromethane (chloroform)
Plastic and rotogravure industry		Toluene
PVC production		Vinyl chloride
Refrigeration/air conditioning		Chloromethane (methyl chloride)
Rocket industry		1,2-Dimethyl hydrazine
Rodent control		Phosphorus
Shoemaking		Toluene
Styrene polymerization		Styrene
Wine industry	Vintners	Arsenic
	Vineyard spraying	Bordeaux mixture (copper sulphate)
		Insecticide sprays (arsenic)

Table 43.3 *Chemicals associated with liver disease*

Haloalkanes
Carbon tetrachloride
Tetrachloroethane
Trichloromethane (chloroform)
Tetrachloroethylene
Toluene

Nitroparaffins
Nitromethane
Nitroethane
Nitropropane

Nitroaromatics
Trinitrotoluene
Nitrobenzene

Metals/metalloids
Copper
Arsenic/Arsine
Beryllium
Yellow phosphorus
Cadmium
Selenium
Chromium
Mercury
Nickel

Pesticides and herbicides

Polychlorinated biphenyls

Vinyl chloride

Cytostatic agents

Phthalate esters

Chronic injury

Occasionally, long-term sequelae of acute intoxication eventually result in chronic liver disease, though this is much more commonly found after repeated or long-term exposure to chemicals. Chronicity is manifest by the presence of fibrosis in the liver. This is a consequence of the activation and transformation of hepatic stellate (Ito) cells into collagen-producing myofibroblasts. This activation can be induced by a number of factors such as free radicals and cytokines.[22] Cirrhosis is frequently the end-result with fibrous tissue disrupting the functional anatomy of the organ. The cirrhotic patient may be asymptomatic, or may present with hepatic decompensation associated with bleeding varices, ascites or encephalopathy. Cirrhosis has been reported after chronic exposure to arsenical pesticides[23] and to halogenated aliphatic hydrocarbons such as carbon tetrachloride and chloroform.

Vascular lesions

Non-cirrhotic portal hypertension has been reported after exposure to vinyl chloride[24,25] and inorganic arsenicals[26,27] and usually presents with bleeding from gastric or oesophageal varices. Liver function tests may be normal or minimally disturbed. Splenomegaly, if present, is detected clinically and confirmed on ultrasound. The wedged hepatic vein pressure in such cases is either normal or only slightly raised, whilst the splenic pulp pressure is markedly elevated, indicating presinusoidal portal hypertension.

The histology shows enlargement and thickening of the portal vein branches with perisinusoidal fibrosis. In some cases, activation and proliferation of sinusoidal cells is seen. The liver histology closely resembles that found in idiopathic portal hypertension (Banti's syndrome) suggesting that this syndrome may sometimes result from unrecognized toxic injury. Occasionally, peliosis hepatis is seen in chemical liver injury, particularly with vinyl chloride. Both peliosis hepatis and non-cirrhotic portal hypertension can progress to hepatic angiosarcoma and this progression is well documented in vinyl chloride workers.

Malignant change

A wide range of chemicals has been shown to induce primary liver tumours in animal studies, but in humans, a causal relationship between primary liver tumours and previous exposure to a specific chemical has been shown convincingly for only a few compounds. Primary liver cancer is seen in association with arsenic[28] and vinyl chloride exposure,[29] but less commonly than angiosarcoma. Such tumours may present with right upper quadrant pain and weight loss. The diagnosis is made on abdominal ultrasound scan and confirmed on computed tomography scan, hepatic angiography and ultrasound guided liver biopsy. Serum α-fetoprotein levels may be normal or raised. Dioxin has been shown to be a potent hepatocarcinogen in animal studies[30] and it has also been implicated in man,[31] although firm evidence is difficult to obtain.

Disturbances in porphyrin metabolism

Porphyrias can be acquired or can result from inborn metabolic errors of haem synthesis and they are characterized by increased urinary excretion of porphyrins or their precursors. Porphyria cutanea tarda (PCT) usually presents with photosensitive skin lesions including bullae, hypertrichosis and hyperpigmentation, together with increased uroporphyrin excretion in the urine. Constitutional PCT is inherited in an autosomal dominant fashion and is characterized by a deficiency of uroporphyrinogen decarboxylase (UROD) in the liver, erythrocytes and other tissues, with a secondary elevation of 5-aminolaevulinic acid synthetase (ALAS). Clinical presentation is precipitated by liver cell damage most often due to alcohol, oestrogens or hepatitis C; iron deposition in the liver is an important cofactor.

Acquired PCT occurs when UROD, particularly the liver enzyme, is inhibited by ingested agents. An outbreak of PCT in Turkey between 1956 and 1960 followed ingestion of bread contaminated with the fungicide hexachlorobenzene.[32] Three to four thousand people from several distinct genetic populations were affected, suggesting that there was no inherited predisposition. The time interval from ingestion to initial symptoms was about 6 months; these included weakness, loss of appetite and sensitivity to sunlight. A small number of patients were treated with ethylenediaminetetraaceticacid (EDTA), a heavy metal chelator, with reversal of skin symptoms and signs.[33,34] Exposure to vinyl chloride,[35] methyl chloride,[36] hexabromobenzene and polybrominated and polychlorinated biphenyls[37] may also cause acquired PCT. In animal studies, 2,3,7,8-tetrachlorodibenzo-p-dioxin (TCDD), is the most por-phyrinogenic substance known.[38] Following an explosion at a chemical plant near Seveso in Italy in 1976, the nearby population were exposed to TCDD. A brother and sister who were exposed to low levels developed overt PCT. They were part of a large family of 66 members who were also exposed but showed no evidence of PCT. In these two siblings PCT developed on the background of a predisposing genetic defect resulting in UROD deficiency in erythrocytes and thus increased susceptibility to porphyria.[39] Thirteen of 60 other exposed individuals (22%), not of the same family, developed coproporphyrinuria; UROD levels in erythrocytes were not decreased.[37] In the two patients with PCT, treatment with chloroquine resulted in remission of symptoms.[40]

Diagnosis of PCT depends on the finding of a characteristic isomeric distribution of porphyrins in the urine, stool and to a lesser extent plasma. Analyses are best done in a specialized laboratory using the sensitive and specific technique of high pressure liquid chromatography. Normal urine porphyrin content is 70% coproporphyrin (70% of which is isomer III), and 15% uroporphyrin (90% isomer I) with the remainder being 5-, 6-, and 7-carboxylate porphyrins (all mostly isomer III). In PCT, urine contains mostly uroporphyrin (predominantly isomer I) and 7 carboxylate porphyrin (isomer III), 6- carboxylate porphyrin is mostly type III, whilst 5-carboxylate porphyrin and coproporphyrins are present as equal amounts of isomers I and III. These proportions hold for both familial and acquired PCT, although, with hexachlorobenzene, more uroporphyrin III is present. Porphyrin excretion in faeces is increased, particularly isocoproporphyrin, and consists predominantly of type III isomers. The profile of porphyrins in plasma is similar to that in the urine. Total urinary porphyrins in patients exposed to chlorinated hydrocarbons without overt disease show no increase compared with controls but the pattern of porphyrin distribution may be abnormal, indicating subclinical disease (PCT type A).[41]

Conventional treatment for porphyria is venesection. Inhibition of UROD by TCDD is prevented by an iron deficiency state. Venesection should be continued until urinary porphyrin concentration falls below 0.5 mg/litre.

TREATMENT

Identification of the offending chemical, and removal of the patient from it is the most important measure in treatment of acute hepatotoxicity. However, if the patient presents with symptoms of chronic liver injury, it is unlikely that exposure has been continuous and it may have been many years in the past.

Specific treatments or antidotes to hepatotoxins encountered in the workplace have been proposed but few are of proven value (Fig. 43.2). Patients who develop acute liver failure, or complications of chronic liver disease, should be referred for specialized care in a Liver

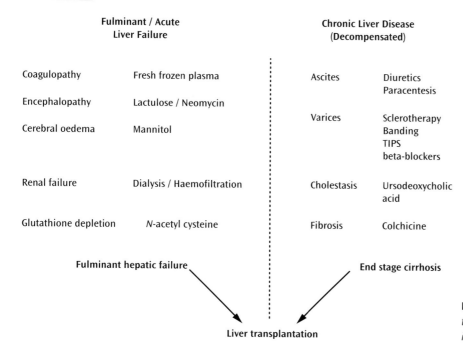

(a) Specific therapies of unproven value

Arsenic   Dimercaprol [77]
Copper   Penicillamine [73]
Carbon tetrachloride   Prostacycline [52]
Porphyria: dioxin   Chloroquine [40]
Chlordecone (Kepone®)   Cholestyramine [93]

(b) Non-specific

Fulminant / Acute
Liver Failure   Chronic Liver Disease
                                         (Decompensated)

Coagulopathy   Fresh frozen plasma   Ascites   Diuretics
                                                                Paracentesis

Encephalopathy   Lactulose / Neomycin   Varices   Sclerotherapy
                                                                Banding
Cerebral oedema   Mannitol   TIPS
                                                                beta-blockers

Renal failure   Dialysis / Haemofiltration Cholestasis   Ursodeoxycholic
                                                                acid

Glutathione depletion N-acetyl cysteine   Fibrosis   Colchicine

Fulminant hepatic failure   End stage cirrhosis

Liver transplantation

Figure 43.2 *Treatment of occupational liver diseases. TIPS: Transjugular intrahepatic portal–systemic shunt.*

Unit. Management will generally be supportive and is aimed at detecting and addressing specific problems as they arise. Liver transplantation is an option for both acute or chronic liver disease, including malignancy, which is refractory to medical therapy.

MECHANISMS OF LIVER TOXICITY IN MODEL HEPATOTOXINS

The different processes resulting in hepatotoxicity can be illustrated by considering hepatotoxic mechanisms for four agents which are relatively well understood: carbon tetrachloride, vinyl chloride, hexachlorobenzene and TCDD. Whilst the dangers of these particular agents are now well appreciated and their use has been restricted and stringent controls applied, patients exposed in the past may still present with chronic problems. An understanding of the mechanisms established for these agents may also help in understanding how other established and novel hepatotoxins produce their effects.

Carbon tetrachloride

The various mechanisms resulting in carbon tetrachloride hepatotoxicity have been extensively studied in the experimental animal[6,7] (Fig. 43.3). Initially, direct lipid solvent injury to the hepatocyte and mitochondrial membranes produces altered cellular function. In adipose tissue, solvent effects lead to increased mobilization of triglyceride stores which then contributes to fat accumulation within the liver (steatosis) (see Chapter 11).

A secondary effect, occurring after 3 hours of exposure to carbon tetrachloride (CCl_4), involves metabolic activation of CCl_4 by the cytochrome P450 system to the trichlorethyl radical ($\cdot CCl_3$) and then to the trichloromethylperoxy radical ($\cdot OOCCl_3$) in the presence of molecular oxygen.[42] The initial liver injury is centrizonal, due to the location of the cytochrome P450 enzyme. These free radicals derived from carbon tetrachloride initiate a chain reaction of lipid peroxidation within the endoplasmic reticulum by hydrogen abstraction from unsaturated fatty acids. Hepatic fibrogenesis leading to fibrosis and cirrhosis, may be triggered either directly by free radical-induced hepatocyte damage leading to activation of Kupffer cells, and activation of stellate cells by cytokines or may be triggered by secondary activation of hepatic stellate cells by lipid peroxidation products such as malondialdehyde or 4-hydroxy nonenal.[22,43] Concomitant with, and/or subsequent to lipid peroxidation, other destructive processes occur in the endoplasmic reticulum. Carbon tetrachloride acts as a

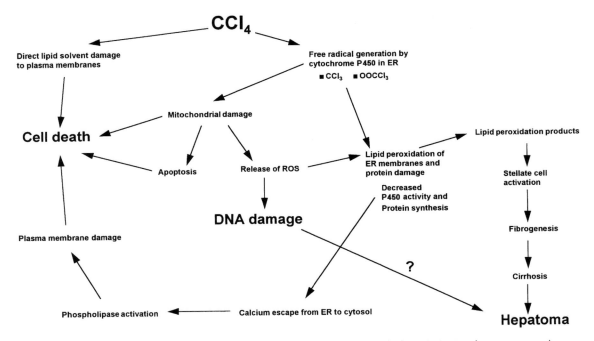

Figure 43.3 *Mechanisms of carbon tetrachloride hepatotoxicity. ER: endoplasmic reticulum; ROS: reactive oxygen species.*

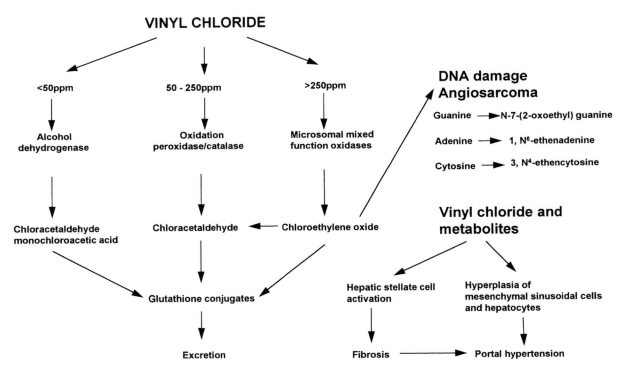

Figure 43.4 *Mechanisms of vinyl chloride hepatotoxicity.*

suicide substrate for cytochrome P450 leading to loss of enzyme activity. Damage to the rough endoplasmic reticulum also leads to decreased protein synthetic activity. Fat accumulation leading to steatosis is partly due to this decrease in protein synthesis, especially reduced syn-

thesis of very low density lipoproteins, which leads to a failure of the lipid export mechanism.[44,45]

Microsomal Ca^{2+}-ATPase, the pump responsible for sequestration of Ca^{2+} into the endoplasmic reticulum, is damaged by oxygen free radicals. Consequently the intracellular free Ca^{2+} concentration is raised, thus activating a number of proteolytic enzymes including phospholipases which are capable of propagating membrane disturbance at distant sites, and endonucleases which give rise to DNA strand breaks.[46]

Vinyl chloride (see Chapters 8, 39)

Vinyl chloride metabolism occurs via different pathways depending on the level of exposure (Fig. 43.4) At concentrations of less than 50 parts per million (ppm), vinyl chloride is metabolized by alcohol dehydrogenase to produce chloroacetaldehyde and monochloroacetic acid, whilst at levels of more than 50 ppm, oxidation occurs by the peroxidase-catalase system to chloroacetaldehyde and at concentrations of more than 250 ppm it is metabolized by microsomal mixed function oxidases to chloroethylene oxide. Vinyl chloride and its reactive metabolites bind covalently to hepatic glutathione and are then hydrolysed and excreted in the urine as conjugates of cysteine. Both vinyl chloride and its metabolites produce hyperplasia of mesenchymal sinusoidal lining cells in the liver and spleen and also hyperplasia of hepatocytes. Hepatic stellate cell activation results in fibrosis and the end result is splenomegaly and portal hypertension. The metabolite chloroethylene oxide damages DNA bases, and is thought to play a key role in the development of angiosarcoma.

Hexachlorobenzene

Hexachlorobenzene (Fig. 43.5) provides an excellent illustration of the mechanisms by which hepatic toxins may disturb haem synthesis and thereby produce acquired porphyria (see Chapter 12). This compound inhibits hepatic uroporphyrinogen decarboxylase and coproporphyrinogen oxidase and causes secondary coproporphyrinuria which may progress to uroporphyrinuria and to porphyria cutanea tarda. The $\cdot O^2$ radical may be involved in inhibition of uroporphyrinogen decarboxylase.[47]

Dioxin

2,3,7,8-Tetrachlorodibenzo-p-dioxin (TCDD) is the most fully investigated member of the very large polychlorinated dibenzo-p-dioxin family and is the most toxic synthetic compound known.[31] These compounds do not occur naturally but are now ubiquitous in the environment (see p. 232). They are produced as contaminants during a variety of industrial synthetic reactions such as the production of chlorinated phenols, during incineration of municipal and hospital wastes, from petrol and other fossil fuel combustion and during a host of other industrial processes. Dioxins are lipophilic and therefore accumulate in adipose tissue, skin, liver and breast milk in mammals and have an extremely long half-life of between 5 and 8 years in man. Known to be

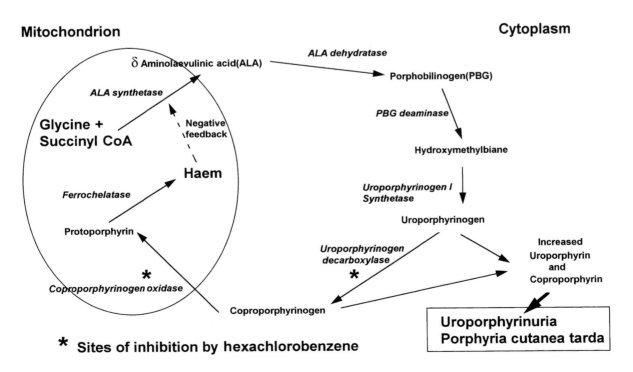

Figure 43.5 *Disturbance of haem synthesis by hepatotoxins.*

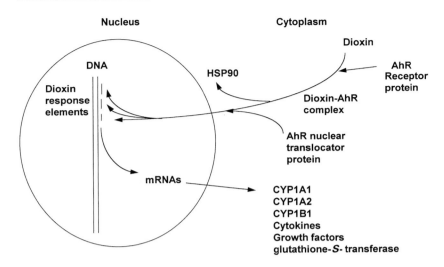

Figure 43.6 *Proposed mechanisms of dioxin hepatotoxicity.*

immunotoxic and teratogenic, TCDD affects the gut, liver, skin and kidneys. Acute toxicity produces chloracne and death following a period of wasting. In chronic low dose studies (as low as 0.1 μg/kg/day) TCDD acts as a potent carcinogen in many organs, including the liver.

Much is known about the mechanisms of TCDD toxicity but many aspects remain uncertain.[31] On entering the cell, TCDD binds to a specific aryl hydrocarbon (dioxin) receptor (AhR) (Fig. 43.6). Binding of dioxin releases heatshock protein 90 (HSP90) from the complex which can then bind an AhR nuclear translocator protein (Arnt). This allows the complex to enter the nucleus and interact with dioxin response elements (DREs), specific base sequences in the cell genome.[48] Binding to these sequences triggers expression of a number of genes including several cytochrome P450 genes and other enzymes.[49] The mechanisms by which activation of these gene products result in the clinical problems associated with dioxin toxicity is still poorly understood although effects on intracellular calcium levels, cytokine expression, and effects on oestrogen expression have all been proposed. Differences in the affinity of the AhR for dioxin in different species probably account for the enormous range (3000-fold) of sensitivity to dioxin in different species.

In laboratory animals, it is well established that dioxin is a potent hepatocarcinogen[30] which can both initiate and promote carcinogenesis and produce cancers with exposures as low as 0.001 μg/kg/day. While TCDD does not itself modify DNA it is a very effective tumour promotor, increasing cell turnover and fixing DNA defects which clonally expand to tumours. Initiation may arise following Ca[2+]-triggered endonuclease DNA damage[46] or alternatively, free radical-induced DNA damage.

World concern over dioxin contamination was triggered by the Seveso incident in July 1976 when an explosion in an Italian chemical factory heavily contaminated the surrounding countryside and population. Bird-life in the area was wiped out. Human problems initially

appeared to be limited to chloracne, but long-term follow-up studies have shown an increased incidence of a variety of cancers, including hepatocellular carcinoma.[31]

SPECIFIC OCCUPATIONAL HEPATOTOXINS

The solvent controversy

Most industrial plants and businesses use solvents in one form or another. Evidence regarding their hepatotoxicity is conflicting. Abnormalities in liver function tests and histology have been reported in chemical industry workers and painters exposed to solvents, but these studies lacked controls. The situation is further complicated by the fact that workers may be exposed to multiple agents.[50]

Haloalkanes (see Chapter 11)

CARBON TETRACHLORIDE (TETRACHLOROMETHANE)

Industrial accidents account for most cases of carbon tetrachloride poisoning, the usual mechanism being the inhalation of fumes in a poorly ventilated environment. As little as 5 ml can produce histological evidence of hepatic necrosis. Within hours of an acute exposure, initial symptoms of headache, dizziness, confusion and blurred vision are found and these are followed by nausea, vomiting and diarrhoea.[51] Evidence of liver damage occurs 24–48 hours after exposure with tender hepatomegaly, increasing jaundice and a bleeding diathesis. In severe cases, ascites and coma can result. Death due to liver disease usually occurs within 10 days of the onset of symptoms. The liver disease can last for 3 weeks, before recovery occurs, which in survivors, is rapid. The laboratory findings include marked elevation of the serum transaminase levels. Serum bilirubin rapidly rises, due to hepatocyte necrosis, haemolysis, destruction of the cytochrome P450 enzymes and decreased renal excretion of bilirubin. Liver histology shows centrilobular necrosis and steatosis.

Treatment is supportive. In the experimental animal, carbon dioxide-induced hyperventilation has been shown to increase the pulmonary elimination of volatile hydrocarbons and to prevent carbon tetrachloride toxicity. Prostacycline (prostaglandin I_2) is hepatoprotective, even when given 24 hours after intoxication.[52] The mortality rate from carbon tetrachloride poisoning is 10–25%, most deaths occurring from renal failure. Hepatic causes of death account for 25% of the total, and occur in the first week after intoxication. If the patient survives, recovery is usually complete, but hepatic fibrosis and cirrhosis can ensue.

TRICHLOROMETHANE (CHLOROFORM)

This chemical was used in the community as a spot cleaning agent and formerly as an anaesthetic when death due to hepatic necrosis was occasionally reported.[53] Exposure is by inhalation. Some workers exposed daily for 12–48 months to moderately high levels of trichloromethane developed liver disorders. Subjects with pre-existing liver disease may be more sensitive to the effect of trichloromethane. Possible clinical presentations include jaundice, hepatomegaly and 'transaminitis' and cirrhosis is a possible sequel.

TRICHLOROETHANE

The most important isomer is 1,1,1-trichloroethane (methylchloroform) which is used extensively as an industrial degreasing agent. Experimental hepatotoxicity has been demonstrated in mice.[54] In man, presentation may be with ascites and hepatosplenomegaly whilst the liver biopsy may show fibrosis, perivenular sclerosis of the central vein and subacute hepatic necrosis.[55] Occupational exposure has been associated with cirrhosis. Patients with pre-existing chronic liver disease may be more sensitive to liver injury following exposure to very high levels of trichloroethane.

TETRACHLOROETHANE

This chlorinated hydrocarbon solvent is no longer used because of its hepatotoxicity, identified as a result of heavy exposures to workers in the First World War when it was used as 'dope' in aeroplane manufacture.[5] Absorption was mostly by inhalation, though occasionally by ingestion and skin absorption. Low grade exposure produced hepatomegaly and a few patients became jaundiced. If the patient is removed from the contaminated environment, the liver recovers rapidly but continued exposure can produce jaundice, hepatomegaly and ascites together with fulminant hepatic failure and subacute hepatic necrosis, both of which may be fatal.[56] The

overall mortality rate was approximately 17%. The histology was similar to that found with carbon tetrachloride and included centrizonal necrosis, steatosis and bile duct proliferation. If exposure is prolonged, the patient may die of subacute hepatic necrosis often followed by post-necrotic fibrosis.[53]

TRICHLOROETHYLENE

Trichloroethylene is used in the dry cleaning industry and is structurally similar to vinyl chloride. Severe liver injury can be seen in individuals who have sniffed solvents; they may develop raised serum transaminase levels associated with acute hepatic and renal failure.[57] Liver disease is rarely caused by occupational exposure, though fatal addiction at work may occur,[58] and acute hepatic failure has been described with degreasing. The liver histological changes include fatty liver, fibrosis and centrilobular necrosis, many of which have the potential for recovery after withdrawal from exposure.

TETRACHLOROETHYLENE

This is probably the least hepatotoxic of the chlorinated hydrocarbons used as dry cleaning agents. Accidental exposure can produce depression of the central nervous system, followed by hepatic and renal damage. Serum bilirubin, transaminases, and alkaline phosphatase may be elevated; a variety of liver lesions has been described including acute hepatitis, and centrilobular necrosis.[59–61] Diagnosis is dependent on the history, supported by a chloroform-like odour of the solvent, which may be detected on the patient's breath for several hours after exposure. Repeated vapour exposures to high concentrations of tetrachloroethylene have produced hepatitis in experimental animals.

NITROPARAFFINS

Nitromethane, nitroethane, 1-nitropropane and 2-nitropropane are used extensively in industry as solvents. Hepatotoxic effects may be underdiagnosed because 2-nitropropane is rarely used alone as a solvent and any toxicity is usually blamed on other chemicals. This chemical can produce acute liver failure.[62] Histology shows centrilobular necrosis, bile duct proliferation, cholestasis, steatosis and a mild inflammatory infiltrate in the periportal areas.[63] In one report,[64] two construction workers applied epoxy-resin coating to a water main in an underventilated underground vault; no protection was provided for their respiratory tracts or skin. One died of fulminant hepatic failure; the other survived.

TOLUENE

Acute hepatocellular injury, with reversible renal failure, has been reported in a glue sniffer.[65] However, in a controlled study of car painters exposed to toluene, no increased hepatotoxicity was seen compared with controls.[66]

CHLORINATED NAPTHALENES

A number of cases of acute yellow atrophy of the liver have occurred in workshops in which chlorinated naphthalenes were used to impregnate electrical equipment. The average time of exposure varied from 4 to 6 months. The presentation is with general malaise followed by jaundice, associated with anorexia, dizziness, weight loss, vomiting and upper abdominal pain. Liver changes include necrosis, fibrosis and regeneration which may be associated with acute enterocolitis together with pancreatitis. Hepatic decompensation was revealed by the presence of jaundice, ascites and oedema. Many patients who survived the acute insult developed subacute hepatic necrosis or macronodular cirrhosis.[67,68]

NITROAROMATICS (see Chapter 12)

Trinitrotoluene produced a considerable amount of hepatotoxicity in munitions workers in the First and Second World Wars, with an incidence of hepatotoxicity ranging from <0.01 to 5%.[69] Since this time, the incidence of liver damage has been markedly decreased by improvement in industrial techniques. Absorption is largely through the skin, but inhalation, ingestion or mucus membrane exposure, may also result in significant absorption. The toxic mechanism is unclear but may be related to the production of a toxic intermediate. There appears to be a marked individual difference in susceptibility to the hepatotoxic effects of trinitrotoluene. After a latent period of 2–4 months during the exposure period, the patient develops anorexia, weakness, nausea, vomiting and abdominal pain with hepatomegaly and jaundice. Some patients go on to develop fulminant hepatic failure, which may be fatal in up to 25%. Others develop subacute hepatic failure with ascites and portal hypertension. These symptoms may be accompanied by extrahepatic manifestations, including rash, aplastia anaemia and methaemoglobinaemia. Some patients who survive chronic exposure may go on to develop macronodular cirrhosis.[70,71]

Metals and metalloids (see Chapters 7, 41)

COPPER

With acute poisoning, jaundice due to liver injury and haemolysis occurs on the second or third day in about 25% of patients. Elevated transaminases and hepatomegaly are also features.

Liver granulomas containing copper have been found in vineyard workers exposed to an antifungal spray called Bordeaux mixture which contained a 1–2% aqueous copper sulphate solution.[72] The commonest hepatic abnormality was a raised serum alkaline phosphatase;

hepatomegaly was present in 40% and one of seven patients biopsied had hepatic granulomata. Other features described in chronic occupational copper toxicity in vineyard sprayers include proliferation of Kupffer cells, fibrosis, cirrhosis, portal hypertension and one case of angiosarcoma. Whilst copper can be demonstrated in the liver histochemically, the gold standard for the diagnosis of liver disorders associated with increased hepatic copper is direct biochemical estimation by neutron activation analysis.

Acute copper toxicity is managed by gastric lavage to remove copper. Although penicillamine, a heavy metal chelator, is extremely effective in Wilson's disease,[73] there is no evidence that it is of benefit in acute copper poisoning.

ARSENIC

An outbreak of arsenic-induced liver disease in beer drinkers was reported from Manchester, UK in 1900,[74] where the severity of the liver disease was proportional to the amount of arsenic in the beer. However, occupational exposure to arsenic has been most common in the production and use of pesticides. Up to 1942, when the use of these insecticides was banned, there was a significant incidence of cirrhosis in grape workers and vintners.[23] Exposure was in the form of oral ingestion via insecticide sprays and dust, which also led to high levels of residual arsenic in the wine. Occupational and environmentally induced liver disease secondary to arsenic exposure is exclusively chronic. Associated clinical features include pigmentation with spotty melanosis of the skin and hyperkeratoses of palms of hands and soles of feet with tumours of the skin and other sites.[75]

Both organic and inorganic arsenicals cause necrosis of hepatocytes, injure sinusoidal and endothelial cells, and may cause obliteration and thrombosis of intrahepatic portal vein radicals. Although the number of cases of chronic liver disease in German vintners declined after 1942, the incidence of arsenical cirrhosis at autopsy continued to rise until the early 1950s due to the persistent effect of arsenic in the tissues, though alcoholism was likely to be a compounding factor in many cases.[23] Four patients with severe liver damage due to arsenic poisoning in the Mosel vintners died of cirrhosis but milder forms of arsenic liver damage underwent healing with some degree of periportal scarring.[23] Chronic arsenic exposure can produce a variety of different patterns of liver injury, including steatosis, cirrhosis, non-cirrhotic portal hypertension, angiosarcoma[76] and primary liver cancer. The liver function tests in liver damage due to chronic arsenic poisoning are frequently normal, though bromosulphophthalein retention may be present. Scalp hair arsenic levels may be raised and skin biopsy sometimes shows marked hyperkeratosis typical of chronic arsenic poisoning. On the other hand, analysis of tumour, liver, hair and other organs and tissues in a patient dying of haemangioendothelial sarcoma due to arsenic poisoning showed no significant traces of arsenic.[76] In one case of non-cirrhotic portal hypertension, arsenic content on percutaneous liver biopsy, measured by neutron activation analysis, was markedly increased at 28 μg/g (normal being <0.25 μg/g dry liver).[26] The value of treatment with dimercaprol, a heavy metal chelator, is uncertain.[77]

Environmental arsenic poisoning has reached massive proportions in recent years in West Bengal and Bangladesh.[78] In an effort to supply clean drinking water to rural villages, thousands of tube wells have been sunk to allow use of subsurface water. Unfortunately, natural arsenic concentrations in this groundwater can reach very high levels and it is reported that over 220 000 people are now suffering from arsenic-related diseases. It is estimated that up to 90 million people in these areas are at risk. A number of internet websites have been set up to provide information on this massive problem.

BERYLLIUM

Beryllium poisoning can produce a spectrum of hepatic abnormalities[79] including hepatomegaly, focal or centrilobular necrosis, and granulomata which mimic those found in sarcoidosis, and contain beryllium.[80]

PHOSPHORUS

Acute poisoning is usually from suicidal intent, but hepatotoxicity from the manufacture of firecrackers has been reported.[81] Histological changes include steatosis and necrosis[5] whilst, in the long-term, fibrosis may develop.[21] Diagnosis depends on the detection of a characteristic garlic odour on the breath, with phosphorescence of the stool.

CADMIUM

A wide spectrum of hepatotoxic effects, ranging from minor abnormality in liver function tests to necrosis or cirrhosis are found.[82] Increased hepatic cadmium concentrations have been implicated in the pathogenesis of cryptogenic liver disease in Japan.[83] Occupational hepatotoxicity has been noted in gold melting.

SELENIUM

At low concentrations selenium is an essential trace element. At higher concentrations, acute hepatotoxicity can occur from accidental ingestion or inhalation of selenium dioxide or hydrogen selenide, resulting in steatosis.[84] In large quantities, and with chronic exposure, selenium can produce cirrhosis and, possibly, hepatic neoplasia.[85] In contrast, low plasma selenium levels are found in alcoholic liver disease[86,87] possibly resulting in oxidant stress, since glutathione peroxidase, an important factor in anti-oxidant defence, requires selenium as a co-factor.

CHROMIUM

Chronic occupational exposure produced hepatotoxicity in a chromium plating factory. Toxic hepatitis was accompanied by mild-to-moderate abnormalities in liver function tests.[88]

Pesticides and herbicides

This section includes herbicides, insecticides and fungicides which have different chemical structures and toxicities. The common pesticides associated with hepatotoxicity are DDT, methoxychlor, chlordane, heptachlor, aldrin, dieldrin, lindane and chlordecone. The evidence that they are hepatotoxic or hepatocarcinogenic in humans is conflicting. Acute hepatotoxicity has been reported after rare accidental ingestion of large amounts of DDT[89] whilst centrizonal necrosis and hepatic failure after a single dose of 6 g of DDT has occurred. However, despite massive production, there is little evidence from the literature of poisoning. Only minor elevations of aspartate amino transferase and reductions in bromosulphophthalein excretion have been recorded. Hepatic mixed function oxidase is induced by DDT and may result in production of hepatotoxic and hepatocarcinogenic metabolites from parent chemicals or drugs already in the environment or body.[90,91] Carcinogenicity in humans has been debated for years. However, no study has shown a definite risk of cancer in humans and the carcinogenic role of pesticides in the experimental animal is also disputed.

CHLORDECONE

Chlordecone (Kepone®), was detected in high concentrations in samples of blood, adipose tissue and liver from factory workers at a manufacturing plant in Virginia, USA.[92,93] Many of the exposed factory workers had hepatomegaly and some had splenomegaly. Liver function tests were usually normal and liver biopsy showed only non-specific changes. For 2 or 3 years after exposure ceased, there was no pesticide in the tissues, the liver and spleen were of normal size and the liver histology was normal.[94] Animals exposed to chlordecone develop liver cell injury and neoplastic changes[95,96] but the ultimate effects of exposure in humans are unknown. Cohn et al.[93] reported on the use of cholestyramine to accelerate elimination of chlordecone following industrial exposure and toxicity.

CHLOROPHENOXY HERBICIDES

In experimental animals, there is only minor evidence of hepatotoxicity[97] and the major effect on the liver appears to be induction of mixed function oxidases of the hepatic microsomes. Hepatotoxic effects have been attributed to 2,4,5-trichlorophenoxyacetic acid but this toxicity is probably due to contamination with 2,3,7,8-tetrachlorodibenzo-*p*-dioxin. A major concern is a possible synergistic hepatotoxicity from two or more synthetic chemicals. Despite concurrent exposure to multiple organochlorine compounds, workers engaged in the manufacture or handling of mixtures of pesticides seldom manifest hepatotoxic effects.[98]

PARAQUAT

Paraquat (1,1'dimethyl 4,4'dipyridylium dichloride) is a powerful herbicide. Accidental ingestion of as little as 2 g can produce shock, renal failure, pulmonary oedema and jaundice.[99,100] Toxicity may occur as a result of skin exposure or ingestion. Liver histology shows congestion with centrilobular necrosis, acidophilic bodies, steatosis, injury to the interlobular bile ducts and cholestasis. There may be two phases of hepatotoxicity; first, hepatocellular injury and then after 2 days, cholangiocellular damage.[100] Biochemical findings include raised serum bilirubin, transaminases and alkaline phosphatase.

Polychlorinated biphenyls

Skin absorption of polychlorinated biphenyls (PCBs) in workers in the electrical manufacturing industry is followed by hepatic metabolism resulting in induction of the cytochrome P450 system and ALAS[4,101–104] which may lead to porphyria (Fig. 43.5). Abnormal liver function tests have been reported in workers exposed to PCBs[105,106] but these reports have been poorly controlled and lack histology. Raised γ-glutamyl transpeptidase levels in serum may persist for up to 2 years after handling PCBs.[107] In general, raised enzyme levels correlate with serum PCB concentrations; PCBs can produce hepatocellular carcinoma in animals.[101] It is not clear whether they are direct carcinogens or whether carcinogenicity is associated with the metabolites, produced by cytochrome P450. Two cases of hepatoma have been reported in autopsy examinations of patients from the Yusho epidemic in Japan.[108] Over 1600 people were affected after consuming rice oil accidentally contaminated with PCBs.[109,110] The major features were chloracne, conjunctivitis, neuropathy and oedema of the eye lids, whilst jaundice developed in 11%.[111] Porphyria has also been reported.[112] Epidemiological studies of the long-term effects of PCBs in humans have failed to show a significant increase in deaths from cirrhosis or hepatoma, but the long-term consequences of exposure are not known.

Vinyl chloride (see Chapters 8, 39)

This halogenated aliphatic hydrocarbon is structurally similar to trichloroethylene. Severe acute exposure

(more than 8000 ppm) produces hepatic necrosis 24–48 hours after exposure, associated with raised serum transaminases and γ-glutamyl transpeptidase levels.[5] Recovery is usually rapid and fulminant hepatic necrosis is rare. Histology shows isolated necrosis of hepatocytes with occasional polymorph infiltrate. Chronic exposure to vinyl chloride monomer may lead to hepatic fibrosis and non-cirrhotic portal hypertension. Liver function tests may be normal and liver biopsy findings unremarkable. In other patients, hepatic fibrosis is more marked, with extensive capsular and subcapsular fibrosis and portal fibrosis extending into the parenchyma and into the wall of portal vein branches.[113] Peliosis hepatis is occasionally seen. Non-cirrhotic portal hypertension, including nodular regenerative hyperplasia, has been reported and may be a precursor to angiosarcoma. The latter has a latent interval of up to 30 years from first exposure to the development of the tumour. By 1993, 173 cases had been documented in 14 countries[114] but with the introduction of industrial measures designed to minimize exposure (in the UK, the 1975 Code of Practice) the risk has been controlled and it is likely that, in the long term, there will be a steady decline in incidence of this tumour. However, UK experience[25] of the 20 cases diagnosed up to 1994, demonstrates that the annual incidence shows, at the moment, no sign of decreasing (Fig. 43.7). The authors have calculated, based on duration of manufacture, age range and number of workers exposed and maximum latency of angiosarcoma that a further 11–14 cases are likely to present. This study is also interesting in that all 20 of the UK cases of angiosarcoma came from only two of the seven factories in the UK producing vinyl chloride monomer. In the 2 years since the publication of this

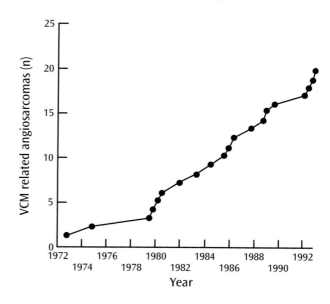

Figure 43.7 *UK cumulative total of vinyl chloride monomer (VCM)-related angiosarcomas 1974–1995. Reproduced from Ref. 25 with permission from the BMJ Publishing Group.*

paper only two further cases have been diagnosed by this group (pers. comm.). These findings may suggest a latent period of around 20 years.

The clinical features are those of a rapidly enlarging malignant liver tumour, though serum levels of α-feto-protein (a tumour marker associated with hepatocellular carcinoma) are normal. Metastases are unusual, but the prognosis is poor, the mean survival from presentation to death being 3.5 months (range 1.5–13). Most patients die from hepatic failure, though death from intraperitoneal haemorrhage may occur. Vinyl chloride monomer workers also have an increased incidence of hepatocellular carcinoma especially if they are infected with the hepatitis B virus; serum α-fetoprotein is frequently raised in such cases.[115] Stringent exposure/restrictions are essential for vinyl chloride monomer workers, but the value of screening with routine liver function tests is controversial; they may be of value in predicting hepatic fibrosis, but are of limited use in predicting angiosarcomas. Other screening tests advocated have included determination of fasting serum bile acids or low dose indocyanine green clearance and measurement of urinary coproporphyrin excretion; none of these is widely used.

Methyl bromide

Methyl bromide is known to be hepatotoxic in both humans and animals. In one report,[116] intoxication simulated Reye's syndrome but the liver histology merely showed hepatocyte swelling and sinusoidal congestion (see Chapter 8).

Cytostatic agents

Personnel working in oncology units may develop insidious liver disease after chronic handling of cytostatic drugs including neomycin, vincristine, cyclophosphamide, doxorubicin, 5-fluorouracil and methotrexate.[117] Absorption is percutaneous or by inhalation. A free-radical based mechanism for the formation of active metabolites may explain the hepatotoxicity of some of these agents. Nurses handling these drugs can develop raised levels of gamma glutamyl transpeptidase and alkaline phosphatase, whilst liver histology may show portal hepatitis, fibrosis and steatosis.[118] Increased mutagenicity in the urine of nurses handling these drugs has also been demonstrated.[119]

Phthalate esters

Both dioctyl phthalate and its isomer di-(2-ethyl hexyl) phthalate are plasticizers, which may be hepatotoxic[120,121] and hepatocarcinogenic[122,123] in the animal model. However, there is no conclusive evidence for hepatotoxicity in humans.

CONCLUSIONS

In clinical practice, overt liver disease due to workplace exposure to hepatotoxins is rare. However, it is probably underdiagnosed and may be significantly more common than generally reported. Exposure is often difficult to quantify, and may occur some time prior to presentation of the liver disease. Furthermore, multiple agents may be implicated, making the actual toxic substance difficult to identify. Multiple agents which are themselves minimally toxic may act synergistically to produce injury. Safety procedures should be in place in the work environment which implies that reports of toxicity only occur when these measures break down and exposure becomes uncontrolled.

A number of difficulties complicate the diagnosis of occupational liver disease. The finding of abnormal liver function tests is relatively common in the general population, and elevations of serum γ-glutamyl transpeptidase are non-specific, whilst the interpretation of abnormal results can be complicated by the fact that alcoholism and drug ingestion may be denied. In addition, liver histology may be suggestive, but is never diagnostic, of occupational exposure to hepatotoxins.

Finally, proof of hepatotoxicity, even following acute exposure, is difficult to obtain. It would require liver biopsy following the insult to quantify damage; the demonstration of recovery following removal of the hepatotoxin; and, most difficult, the demonstration (preferably including re-biopsy), of recurrence following re-exposure. In practice, these requirements are rarely, if ever, fulfilled.

In chronic liver disease, even when known causes are excluded, perhaps around 20% of cases remain cryptogenic. In these, we are left to consider the possibilities of a novel, currently undiagnosable virus or occupational exposure to a hepatotoxin. Clearly, the latter is only likely to be diagnosed by a well informed clinician who maintains a high index of suspicion.

ACKNOWLEDGEMENTS

We wish to acknowledge the assistance of Dr FI Lee and Dr PM Smith for their helpful discussions on the hepatotoxicity of vinyl chloride and for their permission to reproduce a figure from their recent paper[25] (reproduced as Fig. 43.7). We also wish to acknowledge the assistance of Dr R Ede, of Hope Hospital, Salford, for his advice on aspects of porphyrin metabolism and analysis.

REFERENCES

1 Kahl R. Appendix 2: Liver injury in man ascribed to non-drug chemicals and natural toxins. In: McIntyre N, Benhamou JP, Bircher J, Rizzetto M, Rodes J eds. *Oxford*

Textbook of Clinical Hepatology. Oxford: Oxford University Press, 1991.

2   Levy LS, Lee WR. Aliphatic chemicals In: Raffle PAB, Adams PH, Baxter PJ, Lee WR eds. *Hunter's Diseases of Occupations* 9th edn. London: Arnold, 1994.

3   Tar-Ching AW. Aromatic chemicals In: Raffle PAB, Adams PH, Baxter PJ, Lee WR eds. *Hunter's Diseases of Occupations* 8th edn. London: Arnold, 1994.

4   Pond SM. Effects on the liver of chemicals encountered in the workplace. *Western J Med* 1982; **137**: 506–14.

5   Gitlin N. Clinical aspects of liver disease caused by industrial and environmental toxins. In: Zakin D, Boyer TD eds. *Hepatology: A Textbook of Liver Disease* 3rd edn. Philadelphia: W B Saunders Co, 1996.

6   Kahl R Toxic Liver injury. In: McIntyre N, Benhamou JP, Bircher J, Rizzetto M, Rodes J eds. *Oxford Textbook of Clinical Hepatology*. Oxford: Oxford University Press, 1991.

7   Dahm LS, Jones DP. Mechanisms of chemically induced liver disease. In: Zakim D, Boyer TD eds. *Hepatology: A Textbook of Liver Disease* 3rd edn. Philadelphia: WB Saunders Co, 1996.

8   Dianzani MU. The role of free radicals in liver damage. *Proc Nutr Soc* 1987; **46**: 43–52.

9   Goddard CJR, Warnes TW. Raised liver enzymes in asymptomatic patients: investigation and outcome. *Dig Dis* 1992; **10**: 218–26.

10 Hultcrantz R, Glaumann H, Lindberg G, Nilsson LH. Liver investigation in 149 asymptomatic patients with moderately elevated activities of serum aminotransferases. *Scand J Gastroenterol* 1986; **21**: 109–13.

11 Van Ness MM, Diehl AM. Is liver biopsy useful in the evaluation of patients with chronically elevated liver enzymes? *Ann Intern Med* 1989; **111**: 473–8.

12 Owens D, Evans J. Population studies on Gilbert's syndrome. *J Med Genet* 1975; **12**: 152–6.

13 Hasumura Y, Teschike R, Lieber CS. Increased carbon tetrachloride hepatotoxicity and its mechanism, after chronic ethanol consumption. *Gastroenterology* 1974; **66**: 415–22.

14 Proctor E, Chatambra K. High yield of micronodular cirrhosis in the rat. *Gastroenterology* 1982; **83**: 1183–90.

15 Zimmerman HJ, Mao R, Israsena S. Phenothiazine inhibition of carbon tetrachloride cytotoxicity *in vitro*. *Proc Soc Exp Biol Med* 1966; **123**: 893–8.

16 Kopelman H, Scheuer PJ, Williams R. The liver lesion of the Epping jaundice. *Q J Med* 1966; **35**: 553–64.

17 Kopelman H, Robertson MH, Sanders PG, Ash I. The Epping jaundice. *Br Med J* 1966; **1**: 514–6.

18 Bastian PG. Occupational hepatitis caused by methylenedianiline. *Med J Aust* 1984; **141**: 553–5.

19 Diaz-Rivera RS, Collazo PJ, Pons ER, Torregrosa MV. Acute phosphorus poisoning. *Medicine* 1950; **29**: 269–98.

20 Slater TF. Necrogenic action of carbon tetrachloride in the rat: a speculative mechanism based on activation. *Nature* 1966; **209**: 36–40.

21 Greenburger NJ, Robinson WL, Isselbacher KJ. Toxic hepatitis after the ingestion of phosphorous with subsequent recovery. *Gastroenterology* 1964; **47**: 179–83.

22 Britton RS, Bacon BR. Retinoids and oxyradicals in fibrogenesis: therapeutic implications. In: Arroyo V, Bosch J, Bruguera M, Rodes J eds. *Therapy in Liver Disease and the Physiological Basis of Treatment*. Barcelona: Massoni SA, 1997: 163–71.

23 Lüchtrath H. Cirrhosis of the liver in chronic arsenical poisoning of vintners. *Germ Med* 1972; **2**: 127–8.

24 Smith PM, Crossley IR, Williams DMJ. Portal hypertension in vinyl chloride workers. *Lancet* 1976; **ii**: 602–4.

25 Lee FI, Smith PM, Bennett B, Williams DMJ. Occupationally related angiosarcoma of the liver in the United Kingdom, 1972–1994. *Gut* 1996; **39**: 312–8.

26 Morris JS, Schmid M, Newman S, Scheuer PJ, Sherlock S. Arsenic and non-cirrhotic portal hypertension. *Gastroenterology* 1974; **64**: 86–94.

27 Chainuvati T, Viranuvatti V. Idiopathic portal hypertension and chronic arsenic poisoning. Report of a case. *Dig Dis Sci* 1979; **24**: 70–3.

28 Jhaveri SS. A case of cirrhosis and primary carcinoma of the liver in chronic industrial arsenical intoxication. *Br J Indust Med* 1959; **16**: 248–50.

29 Evans DMD, Jones Williams W, Kung ITM. Angiosarcoma and hepatocellular carcinoma in vinyl chloride workers. *Histopathology* 1983; **7**: 377–88.

30 Huff J, Lucier G, Tritscher A. Carcinogenicity of TCDD: experimental, mechanistic and epidemiological evidence. *Ann Rev Pharmacol Toxicol* 1994; **34**: 343–72.

31 Whysner J, Williams GM. 2,3,7,8-Tetrachlorodibenzo-p-dioxin: mechanistic data and risk assessment; gene regulation, cytotoxicity, enhanced cell proliferation and tumour promotion. *Pharmacol Ther* 1996; **71**: 193–223.

32 Schmid R. Cutaneous porphyria in Turkey. *N Engl J Med* 1960; **263**: 397–8.

33 Peters H, Cripps D, Göcmen A, Bryan G, Ertürk E, Morris C. Turkish epidemic of hexachlorobenzene porphyria. *Ann N Y Acad Sci* 1987; **514**: 183–90.

34 Cripps DJ, Peters HA, Gocmen A, Dogramici I. Porphyria turcica due to hexachlorobenzene: a 20–30 year follow-up study on 204 patients. *Br J Dermatol* 1984; **111**: 413–52.

35 Doss M, Lange C-E, Veltman G. Vinyl chloride-induced hepatic coproporphyrinuria with transition to chronic hepatic porphyria. *Klin Wochenschr* 1984; **62**: 175–8.

36 Chalmers JNM, Gillam AE, Kench JE. Porphyrinuria in a case of industrial methyl chloride poisoning. *Lancet* 1940; **i**: 806–8.

37 Doss MO. Porphyrinurias and occupational disease. *Ann NY Acad Sci* 1987; **514**: 204–18.

38 Goldstein JA, Hickman P, Bergman H, Vos JG. Hepatic porphyria induced by 2,3,7,8-tetrachloro dibenzo-p-dioxin in the mouse. *Res Commun Chem Path Pharmacol* 1973; **6**: 919–28.

39 Doss MO, Sauer H, von Tiepermann R, Colombi AM. Development of chronic hepatic porphyria (porphyria cutanea tarda) with an inherited uroporphyrinogen

decarboxylase deficiency under exposure to dioxin. *Int J Biochem* 1984; **16**: 369–73.

40 Strick JJTWA, Janssen MMT, Colombi AM. Incidence of chronic hepatic porphyria in an Italian family. *Int J Biochem* 1980; **12**: 879–81.

41 Kappas A, Sassa S, Anderson KE. The porphyrias. In: Stanbury JB, Wyngaarden JB, Fredrickson DS, Goldstein JL, Brown MS eds. *The Metabolic Basis of Inherited Disease* 5th edn. New York: McGraw-Hill Book Co, 1983.

42 Recknagel RO, Glende EA, Britton RS. In: Meeks RG, Steadman D, Bull RJ eds. *Free Radical Damage and Lipid Peroxidation in Hepatotoxicology*, Kiderminster: Telford Press, 1991.

43 Britton RS, Bacon BR. Role of free radicals in liver disease and hepatic fibrosis. *Hepato-Gastroenterology* 1994; **41**: 343–8.

44 Recknagel RO. Carbon tetrachloride hepatotoxicity. *Pharmacol Rev* 1967; **19**: 145–208.

45 Judah JD, McLean AEM, McLean EK. Biochemical mechanisms of liver injury. *Am J Med* 1970; **49**: 609–16.

46 McConkey DJ, Aw TY, Orrenius S. Role of Ca 2+-mediated endonuclease activation in chemical toxicity. In: Dekant W, Nawmann H-A eds. *Tissue Specific Toxicity: Biochemical Mechanisms*. London: Academic Press, 1992.

47 De Matteis F. Role of iron in the hydrogen peroxide-dependent oxidation of hexahydroporphyrin (porphyrinogen): a possible mechanism for the exacerbation by iron of hepatic uroporphyria. *Mol Pharmacol* 1988; **33**: 463–9.

48 Dennison MS, Fisher JM, Whitlock JP. The DNA recognition site for the dioxin-Ah receptor complex. *J Biol Chem* 1988; **263**: 1722–4.

49 Pratt WB. The role of the hsp-90 based chaperone system in signal transduction by nuclear receptors and receptor signalling via MAP kinase. *Ann Rev Pharmacol Toxicol* 1997; **37**: 297–324.

50 Døssing M, Ranek L. Isolated liver damage in chemical workers. *Br J Ind Med* 1984; **41**: 142–4.

51 Nielsen VK, Larsen J. Acute renal failure due to CC14 poisoning. *Acta Med Scand* 1965; **178**: 363–74.

52 Divald A, Uihelyi A, Jeney K *et al*. Hepatoprotective effects of prostacyclins on CC14-induced liver injury in rats. *Exp Molec Pathol* 1985; **42**: 163–6.

53 Willcox W. Toxic jaundice. *Lancet* 1931; **ii**: 57–63.

54 McNutt NS, Amster RL, McConnell EE, Morris F. Hepatic lesions in mice after continuous inhalation exposure to 1,1,1-trichloroethane. *Lab Invest* 1975; **32**: 642–54.

55 Texter EC Jr, Grunow WA, Zimmerman HJ. Massive centrizonal necrosis of the liver due to inhalation of 1,1,1-trichloroethane (Abstract). *Gastroenterology* 1979; **76**: 1260.

56 Gurney R. Tetrachloroethane intoxication: Early recognition of liver damage and means of prevention. *Gastroenterology* 1943; **1**: 1112–26.

57 Baerg RD, Kimberg DV. Centrolobular hepatic necrosis and acute renal failure in 'solvent sniffers'. *Ann Intern Med* 1970; **73**: 713–20.

58 James WRL. Fatal addiction to trichloroethylene. *Br J Ind Med* 1963; **20**: 47–9.

59 Meckler LC, Phelps DK. Liver disease secondary to tetrachloroethylene exposure, a case report. *JAMA* 1966; **197**: 662–3.

60 Stewart RD. Acute tetrachloroethylene intoxication. *JAMA* 1969; **208**: 1490–2.

61 Hughes JP. Hazardous exposure to some so-called safe solvents. *JAMA* 1954; **156**: 234–7.

62 Hine CH, Pasi A, Stephens BG. Fatalities following exposure to 2-nitropropane. *J Occup Med* 1978; **20**: 333–7.

63 Skinner JB. The toxicity of 2-nitropropane. *Ind Med* 1947; **16**: 441–3.

64 Harrison R, Letz G, Pasternak G, Blanc P. Fulminant hepatic failure after occupational exposure to 2-nitropropane. *Ann Intern Med* 1987; **107**: 466–8.

65 O'Brien ET, Yeoman WB, Hobby JAE. Hepatorenal damage from toluene in a glue sniffer. *Br Med J* 1971; **2**: 29–30.

66 Kurppa K, Husman K. Car painter's exposure to a mixture of organic solvents: Serum activities of liver enzymes. *Scand J Environ Hlth* 1982; **8**: 137–40.

67 Flinn FB, Jarvik NE. Actions of certain chlorinated napthalenes on the liver. *Proc Soc Exp Biol Med* 1936; **35**: 118–20.

68 Flinn FB, Jarvik NE. Liver lesions caused by chlorinated napthalene. *Am J Hyg* 1938; **27**: 19–27.

69 McConnell WJ, Flinn RH. Summary of twenty-two trinitrotoluene fatalities in World War II. *J Med Hyg Toxicol* 1946; **28**: 76–82.

70 Livingston-Learmouth A, Cunningham BM. Observations on the effects of trinitrotoluene on women workers. *Lancet* 1916; **ii**: 261–4.

71 Martland HS. Trinitrotoluene poisoning. *JAMA* 1917; **68**: 835–7.

72 Pimentel JC, Menezes AP. Liver granulomas containing copper in vineyard sprayer's lung. *Am J Respir Dis* 1975; **111**: 189–95.

73 Sherlock S, Dooley J. *Diseases of the Liver and Biliary System* 10th edn. Oxford: Blackwell Science, 1997: 417–25.

74 Kelynack TN, Kirkby W, Delépine S, Tattersall CH. Arsenical poisoning from beer drinkers. *Lancet* 1900; **i**: 1600–3.

75 Cowlishaw JL, Pollard EJ, Cowan AE, Powell LW. Liver disease associated with chronic arsenic ingestion. *Aust N Z J Med* 1979; **9**: 310–3.

76 Regelson W, Kim U, Ospina J, Holland JF. Hemangioendothelial sarcoma of liver from chronic arsenic intoxication by Fowlers solution. *Cancer* 1968; **21**: 514–22.

77 Eagle H, Magnusson HJ. The systemic treatment of 227 cases of arsenic poisoning (encephalitis dermatitis, blood dyscrasias, jaundice, fever) with 2,3 dimercaptopropanol (BAL). *Am J Syph* 1946; **30**: 420–41.

78 Kumar S. Widescale arsenic poisoning found in South Asia. *Lancet* 1997; **349**: 1387.

79 Sneddon IB. Berylliosis: a case report. *Br Med J* 1955; **1**: 1448–50.

80 Prine JR, Brokeshoulder SF, McVean DE *et al.* Demonstration of the presence of beryllium in pulmonary granulomas. *Am J Clin Pathol* 1966; **45**: 448–54.

81 Marin GA, Montoya CA, Sierra JL, Senior JR. Evaluation of corticosteroid and exchange transfusion treatment in acute yellow phosphorous intoxication. *N Engl J Med* 1971; **284**: 125–8.

82 Singhal RL, Merali Z, Hrdina PD. Aspects of the biochemical toxicology of cadmium. *Fed Proc* 1976; **35**: 75–80.

83 Sumino D, Hayakawa D, Shibata T *et al.* Heavy metals in normal Japanese tissues. Amounts of 15 heavy metals in 30 subjects. *Arch Environ Hlth* 1975; **30**: 487–94.

84 Schellman B, Raithel HJ, Schaller KH. Acute fatal selenium poisoning. *Arch Toxicol* 1986; **59**: 61–4.

85 Diplock AT. Metabolic aspects of selenium action and toxicity. *CRC Crit Rev Toxicol* 1976; **4**: 219–26.

86 Korpela H, Kumpulainen J, Luoma PV, Arranto AJ, Sotaniemi EA. Decreased serum selenium in alcoholics as related to liver structure and function. *Am J Clin Nutr* 1985; **42**: 147–51.

87 Dworkin B, Rosenthal WS, Jankowski RH, Gordon GG, Haldea D. Low blood selenium in alcoholics with and without advanced liver disease. *Dig Dis Sci* 1985; **30**: 838–44.

88 Pascale LR, Sheldon S, Waldstein MD *et al.* Chromium intoxication with special reference to hepatic injury. *JAMA* 1952; **149**: 1385–9.

89 Smith NJ. Death following accidental ingestion of DDT. *JAMA* 1948; **136**: 469–71.

90 Fouts JR. Interaction of chemicals and drugs to produce effects on organ function. In: Lee DHK, Koten P eds. *Multiple Factors in the Causation of Environmentally Induced Disease.* New York: Academic Press, 1972.

91 Mitchell JR, Gillette JR. Drug-chemical interactions as a factor in experimentally induced disease. In: Lee DHK, Koten P eds. *Multiple Factors in the Causation of Environmentally Induced Disease.* New York: Academic Press, 1972.

92 Taylor JR, Selhorst JB, Houff SA *et al.* Chlordecone intoxication in man. 1. Clinical observations. *Neurology* 1978; **28**: 626–30.

93 Cohn WJ, Boylan JJ, Blanke RV *et al.* Treatment of chlordecone (Kepone) toxicity with cholestyramine: results of a controlled clinical trial. *N Engl J Med* 1978; **298**: 243–8.

94 Guzelian PS, Vranian J, Boylan JJ *et al.* Liver structure and function in patients poisoned with chlordecone (Kepone). *Gastroenterology* 1980; **78**: 206–13.

95 Anonymous. Report on carcinogenesis assay of technical grade chlordecone (Kepone). *Am Ind Hyg Assoc* 1976; **37**: 680–1.

96 Eroschenko VP, Wilson WO. Cellular changes in the gonads, livers and adrenal glands of Japanese quail as affected by the insecticide Kepone. *Toxicol Appl Pharmacol* 1975; **31**: 491–504.

97 Rip JW, Cherry JH. Liver enlargement induced by the herbicide 2,4,5-trichlorophenoxyacetic acid (2,4,5-T). *J Agric Food Chem* 1976; **24**: 245–50.

98 Deichmann WB, MacDonald WE. Organochlorine pesticides and liver cancer deaths in the United States, 1930–1972. *Ecotoxicol Environ Safety* 1977; **1**: 89–110.

99 Bullivant CM. Accidental poisoning by paraquat: report of two cases in man. *Br Med J* 1966; **1**: 1272–3.

100 Mullick FG, Ishak KG, Mahabir R *et al.* Hepatic injury associated with paraquat toxicity in humans. *Liver* 1981; **1**: 209–21.

101 Kimbrough RD. The toxicity of polychlorinated polycyclic compounds and related chemicals. *CRC Crit Rev Toxicol* 1974; **2**: 445–98.

102 Nicholson WJ, Moore JA. Health effects of halogenated aromatic hydrocarbons. *Ann N Y Acad Sci* 1979; **320**: 1–730.

103 Alvares AP, Fischbein A, Anderson KE, Kappas A. Alterations in drug metabolism in workers exposed to polychlorinated biphenyls. *Clin Pharmacol Ther* 1977; **22**: 140–6.

104 Alvares AP, Kappas A. The inducing properties of polychlorinated biphenyls on hepatic mono-oxygenases. *Clin Pharmacol Ther* 1977; **22**: 809–16.

105 Maroni M, Colombi A, Cantoni S, Ferioli E, Foa V. Occupational exposure to polychlorinated biphenyls in electrical workers. I. Environmental and blood polychlorinated biphenyls concentrations. *Br J Ind Med* 1981; **38**: 49–54.

106 Maroni M, Colombi A, Arbosti G, Cantoni S, Foa V. Occupational exposure to polychlorinated biphenyls in electrical workers. II. Health effects. *Br J Ind Med* 1981; **38**: 55–60.

107 Fischbein A. Liver function tests in workers with occupational exposure to polychlorinated biphenyls (PCBs): comparison with Yusho and Yu-Cheng. *Environ Hlth Perspect* 1985; **60**: 145–50.

108 Kikuchi M. Autopsy of patients with Yusho. *Am J Ind Med* 1984; **5**: 19–30.

109 Kuratsune M. An epidemiological study on 'Yusho' poisoning. *Fubuoka Acta Medica* 1969; **60**: 403–10.

110 Kuratsune M, Yoshimura T, Matzusaka J *et al.* Epidemiologic study on Yusho, a poisoning caused by ingestion of rice oil contaminated with a commercial brand of polychlorinated biphenyls. *Environ Hlth Perspect* 1972; **1**: 119–26.

111 Urabe H, Koda H, Asahi M. Current state of Yusho patients. *Ann N Y Acad Sci* 1979; **320**: 273–6.

112 Seki Y, Kawanishi S, Sano S. Mechanisms of PCB-induced porphyria and Yusho disease. *Ann N Y Acad Sci* 1987; **514**: 222–34.

113 Marsteller HJ, Lebach WK, Muller R *et al.* Chronic liver lesions in PVC (polyvinyl chloride) producing workers. *Dtsh Med Wochenschr* 1973; **98**: 2311–4.

114 Forman D, Bennett B, Stafford J, Doll R. Exposure to vinyl

chloride and angiosarcoma of the liver: A report of the register of cases. *Br J Ind Med* 1985; **42**: 750–3.

115 Du C-L, Wang JD. Increased morbidity odds ratio of primary liver cancer and cirrhosis of the liver among vinyl chloride monomer workers. *Occup Environ Med* 1998; **55**: 528–32.

116 Shield LK, Coleman TL, Markesbery WR. Methyl bromide intoxication: neurologic features, including simulation of Reye's syndrome. *Neurology*, 1977; **27**: 959–62.

117 Knowles RS, Virden JE. Handling of injectable antineoplastic agents. *Br Med J* 1980; **2**: 589–91.

118 Sotaniemi EA, Sutinen S, Arranto AJ, Sutinen S, Sotaniemi KA *et al.* Liver damage in nurses handling cytostatic agents. *Acta Med Scand* 1983; **214**: 181–9.

119 Falck K, Grohn P, Sorsa M *et al.* Mutagenicity in urine of nurses handling cytostatic drugs. *Lancet* 1979; **i**: 1250–1.

120 Reddy JK, Warren JR, Reddy MK Lalwani ND. Hepatic and renal effects of peroxisome proliferators: biological implications. *Ann NY Acad Sci* 1982; **386**: 81–110.

121 Moody DE, Reddy JK. Serum triglyceride and cholesterol contents in male rats receiving diets containing plasticizers and analogues of the ester 2-ethoxyethanol. *Toxicol Lett* 1982; **10**: 379–83.

122 Warren JR, Lalwani ND, Reddy JK. Phthalate esters as peroxisome proliferator carcinogens. *Environ Hlth Perspect* 1982; **45**: 35–40.

123 Kluwe WM, Haseman JK, Douglas JF, Huff JE. The carcinogenicity of dietary di-(2-thoxyethyl) phthalate (DEHP) in Fischer 344 rats and B6C3F mice. *J Toxicol Environ Hlth* 1982; **10**: 797–815.

Haemopoietic effects of workplace exposures: anaemias, leukaemias and lymphomas

ANTHONY YARDLEY-JONES, ATHERTON GRAY

Structure and function of the haemopoietic system	901	Hodgkin's disease and non-Hodgkin's lymphoma	909
Clinical evaluation	903	Work-related issues resulting from treatment of	
Anaemias	905	haematological disease	910
Leukaemia and myelodysplasia	908	References	912

The haemopoietic system is characterized by the rapid proliferation of three cell types which govern the delivery of oxygen to the tissues, the body's defence against infection and the maintenance of haemostasis. It is a system with a key physiological role and a high cell turnover which makes it very sensitive to the influence of haematotoxic agents. In developed countries many of the well-recognized causes of occupationally related disease, such as lead, benzene and ionizing radiation, are declining in incidence. However, in an increasingly complex globalized economy, with a migratory workforce operating in countries which have differing legislative controls, such diseases may still occur and it is important that an awareness of the effect of these exposures is maintained. Furthermore the advent of new industries and processes carries the potential for producing substances with hitherto unrecognized haemopoietic effects.

In recent years there have been extraordinary advances in the understanding of the molecular and genetic triggers of haematological diseases and these have allowed diagnoses to become more precise and treatments more focused. Treatment outcomes have improved and more patients, including those with occupational exposures, now have the option of returning to work. There is a need therefore to understand the issues concerning the long-term effects of some treatments and their impact on fitness for work. For all of these reasons the haemopoietic effects of workplace exposures are considered in this chapter as a distinct group.

STRUCTURE AND FUNCTION OF THE HAEMOPOIETIC SYSTEM

Stem cells and progenitor cells

The bone marrow stem cell has the capacity to renew itself as well as to produce progeny which will develop into mature cells. Stem cells are pluripotent which means that they are capable of forming colonies of progenitor cells (colony forming units or CFU) which are multilineage (Fig. 44.1). As a consequence it is not surprising that such a complex and rapidly proliferating system is sensitive to toxic effects at various stages. For example inorganic lead and benzene exert their haemotoxic effects on erythropoesis and progenitors respectively whilst ionizing radiation has the ability not only to damage dividing cells but also resting cells including stem cells.

Regulation of haemopoiesis

As the bone marrow precursor cells (stem cells and progenitors) mature they lose the capacity for self-renewal but increase their degree of differentiation before each cell division. It has been estimated that there are approximately 20 cell divisions in the maturation pathway and that one stem cell division is capable of producing one million mature blood cells. This is controlled by a complex array of interacting auxiliary cells, growth factors and extracellular matrix within the bone marrow stroma. The haemopietic growth factors are glycoproteins which regulate the proliferation, differentiation and function of the blood cells. They act only at specific

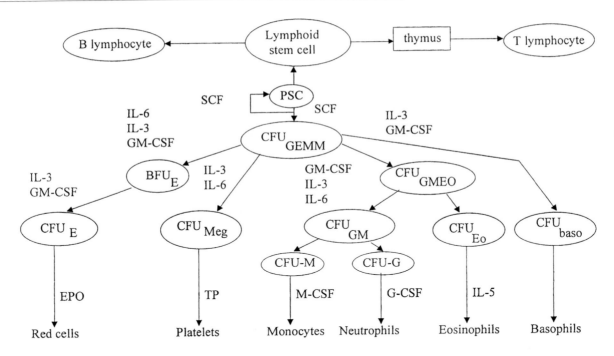

Figure 44.1 *Maturation of haemopoietic cells. A simplified diagram of the maturation of haemopoietic cells from the pluripotent stem cell (PSC). CFU: colony forming unit; BFU: burst-forming unit; GEMM: mixed granulocyte, erythroid, monocyte, megakaryocyte; E: erythroid; MEG: megakaryocyte; GM: granulocyte, monocyte; Eo: Eosinophil; baso: basophil. Haemopoiesis is regulated by a family of glycoprotein growth factors with overlapping function and multiple sites of production. IL: interleukin; CSF: colony stimulating factor; EPO: erythropoietin; TP: thrombopoietin; SCF: stem cell factor.*

phases of cell maturation and either singly or in combination control the direction and rate of precursor cell differentiation. Many of them have now been cloned and are available for clinical use.

Red cell metabolism

Red cells transport oxygen from the lungs to the tissues and carbon dioxide in the opposite direction. To fulfil these functions the erythrocyte is a deformable, biconcave disc, devoid of a nucleus and mitochondria. It generates energy as adenosine triphosphate (ATP) by the anaerobic glycolytic (Embden–Meyerhof, EM) pathway and generates reducing power as reduced nicotinamide-adenine dinucleotide (NADH) by the same pathway and as reduced nicotinamide-adenine dinucleotide phosphate (NADPH) by the hexose monophosphate (HMP) shunt.

The role of the erythrocyte in oxygen carriage continuously exposes it to the risk of oxidative injury from endogenous substances (e.g. hydrogen peroxide, H_2O_2) and exogenous oxidant drugs and chemicals. To counteract oxidant stress the red cell has an array of protective antioxidants and redox defence mechanisms. These are largely a group of enzymes and co-factors catalysing reduction steps. Haemoglobin is readily oxidized to methaemoglobin in which the ferrous iron (Fe^{2+}) is converted to the ferric state (Fe^{3+}) rendering the molecule

incapable of oxygen transport. The majority of methaemoglobin is reduced by methaemoglobin reductase utilizing NADH derived from the EM pathway and hereditary deficiency of this enzyme is associated with methaemoglobinaemia. Of lesser physiological significance is another methaemoglobin reductase which uses NADPH for its activity but hereditary deficiency of this enzyme does not lead to methaemoglobinaemia. Methaemoglobin-generating chemicals such as aniline and nitrobenzene have a tendency to overwhelm the erythrocyte's ability to reduce methaemoglobin to haemoglobin (Fig. 44.2).

A more important function of NADPH is as co-factor for glutathione reductase which maintains protein function by reduction of sulphydryl (-SH) groups whether the protein is haemoglobin, enzyme or membrane. Glucose-6-phosphate dehydrogenase (G6PD) working in the HMP shunt is the only source of NADPH in red cells. Deficiency of NADPH results in the inefficient recycling of glutathione and, therefore, suboptimal protection against peroxide and slow reduction of abnormal disulphides. The red cells are therefore unusually susceptible to added stress imposed by oxidant chemicals.

As molecular oxygen undergoes successive reductions, a number of reactive species e.g. superoxide, hydrogen peroxide and hydroxyl radicals are generated. These have strong oxidizing potential and unless they are scavenged by enzymes in the red cells such as superoxide dismutase,

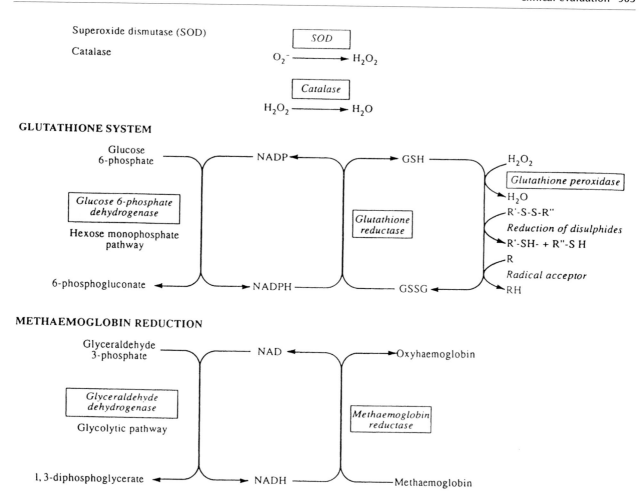

Figure 44.2 *Principal reactions in the erythrocyte for the reduction of oxidized compounds. O_2^-: superoxide; NADPH: reduced nicotinamide adenine dinucleotide phosphate; GHS: reduced glutathione; GSSG: oxidized glutathione.*

catalase and glutathione reductase, they may cause oxidative denaturation of haemoglobin, enzymes and other proteins as well as membrane damage through lipid peroxidation. Which of these is the most important in damaging erythrocyte function depends on the type and origin of the oxidant stress and on the nature of the failure in reducing antioxidant protective mechanisms.

All of these defences against oxidant damage can be compromised by either congenital deficiency or impaired function of the relevant enzymes. Strong oxidizing agents such as drugs and chemicals, however, may easily overwhelm these mechanisms resulting in oxidative haemolysis.

CLINICAL EVALUATION

History

The occurrence of haematological disorders such as leukaemia, aplastic anaemia or haemolytic anaemia should alert the physician to the possibility of a causal

occupational factor even though the pathological and clinical manifestations are in the main indistinguishable from those of non-occupational diseases. Diagnosis and management depend on a clear understanding of the exposure history and the associated mechanism of toxic injury. The latent interval between the onset of exposure and the clinical expression of disease may be many years, in which case the causal relation might well be overlooked. Acute conditions such as haemolysis are likely to be due to recent exposures whereas myelodysplasia and leukaemia may develop from exposures in previous workplaces. It is important, therefore, that the occupational history encompasses both current and all previous employments.

Exposure dose is important but can be difficult to quantify. Information on the use of personal protection (equipment and clothing) and general environmental control measures are essential in establishing whether a causal relation exists or not. Non-occupational environmental factors such as the domestic or recreational use of pesticides and metals and the abuse or misuse of solvents may also be relevant and should be recorded.

The history may also reveal the presence of pre-existing haematological conditions such as G6PD deficiency and methaemoglobin reductase deficiency which, though coincidental, may increase susceptibility to oxidizing chemicals. Current medication should also be understood – as, for example, diuretic therapy may temporarily relieve the symptoms of increasing anaemia and corticosteroids produce a spurious leucocytosis in the peripheral blood. The clinical expression of haematological disease may therefore be masked or modified.

Symptoms and signs

The clinical features of particular haematological disorders are the same irrespective of their underlying cause and are predominantly determined by the blood cell lines which are affected. Symptoms and signs of anaemia infection and bruising or bleeding suggest a significant reduction in the number of circulating red cells, white cells and platelets respectively. In cases where more than one cell line is affected, overlapping symptomatology can be expected. For example, pancytopenia arising as a result of marrow hypoplasia, myelodysplasia or leukaemia, may produce a combination of anaemia, infection and spontaneous bruising. Neutropenia is usually associated with bacterial infections (staphylococci, streptococci and coliforms) of the throat, skin and lungs. Lymphopenia or disorders of T and B cell function are more often associated with viral, parasitic and fungal infections.

Physical examination may show the presence of anaemia, superficial or systemic infection, bruising and in haemolytic states a mild degree of jaundice. None of these features, however, is pathognomonic of occupationally related disease. Certain occupational exposures may give rise to more specific physical signs, the detection of which should suggest the underlying diagnosis. These include central cyanosis caused by methaemaglobinaemia (nitrobenzene, aniline, aromatic amines); a blue line on the gingival margins (lead); peripheral neuropathy (arsenic, lead); plantar-palmar hyperkeratosis and transverse lines (Mee's lines) in the nail bed (arsenic); acneiform eruptions (organochlorine compounds).

Laboratory investigation

As with anaemias in general, those caused by workplace exposures can be microcytic, normocytic or macrocytic. Lead poisoning characteristically produces a microcytic or normochromic anaemia while haemolytic anaemias can be be either normocytic or slightly macrocytic depending on the degree of reticulocytosis. Hypoplastic and myelodysplastic anaemias usually show a degree of macrocytosis. In general, the reticulocyte count should increase in response to anaemia and do so in proportion to its severity. This is particularly so when erythroid hyperplasia has had time to develop as in chronic haemolysis. Failure of the reticulocyte count to increase in response to anaemia indicates impaired erythropoiesis. Investigation of haematological disorders is not discussed in detail, but examination of the blood film might reveal abnormalities which provide a clue to the underlying cause. Basophilic stippling of red cells (Fig. 44.3) can be evidence of lead exposure, although the degree of stippling does not correlate with the body burden of lead (see opposite under **Ineffective erythropoiesis**). Heinz bodies (Fig. 44.4) and other red cell inclusions are seen in haemolytic states associated with

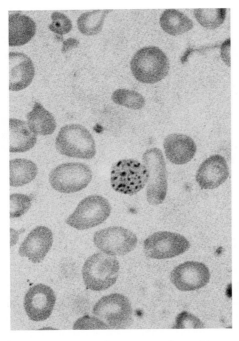

Figure 44.3 *Basophilic stippling. From Ref. 61 with permission. See colour plate section.*

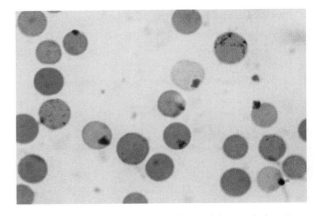

Figure 44.4 *Heinz bodies. From Ref. 62 with permission. See colour plate section.*

oxidant chemicals (aniline, naphthalene, nitrobenzene, nitrites and chlorates). These inclusions represent intracellular deposits of globin and are also found in inherited haemoglobinopathies.

ANAEMIAS

Haemolytic anaemia

Haemolysis may be defined as that condition where the rate of red cell destruction is accelerated. The bone marrow normally responds to this change by increasing red cell production (erythroid hyperplasia), and theoretically this response can compensate for the excessive red cell destruction, even when the lifespan of the circulating cells is reduced from the normal 120 days to as few as 15–20 days. Anaemia develops when this compensatory mechanism fails to match the rate of haemolysis.

Where haemolysis is attributable to occupational exposures, the clinical features are dependent on the agent and the route, duration and dose of the exposure. Haemolytic anaemia may develop insidiously over a period of weeks or months, in which case pallor and mild jaundice may be the first indication of illness. The anaemia may be asymptomatic due to cardiovascular adjustments and if there is also a significant degree of methaemoglobinaemia central cyanosis can be a feature. In its most acute form intravascular haemolysis develops which produces circulatory collapse, oliguria, haemoglobinuria, dyspnoea and generalized aching pains, especially in the loins and limbs.

Mechanisms of haemolysis

The most common mechanism of red cell damage is oxidative attack which can be directed at the membrane of the red cell, the globin chains of the haemoglobin molecule or the haem group. The chemical may act as an oxidizing agent itself or it may interact with oxygen to form free radicals or peroxides. These are capable of oxidizing haem-bound ferrous iron to ferric iron with the formation of methaemoglobin which cannot serve as an oxygen carrier. This is a potentially reversible step but if the oxidant stress is severe, the globin chains may denature and precipitate as inclusions known as Heinz bodies (Fig. 44.4). These inclusions have an affinity with the red cell membrane which becomes damaged. Lipid peroxidation may also disrupt the integrity of the membrane. The damaged cells are then destroyed or fragmented in the reticuloendothelial system by the process of extravascular haemolysis. If the oxidant stress is greater there may be rapid red cell destruction with the clinical picture of intravasular haemolysis.

Acute haemolysis is known to follow exposure to arsine, a highly toxic gas produced by the contact of acid with metals containing arsenic. Processes such as galvanizing, etching, soldering and lead plating may lead to occupational exposure. Stibine, trinitrotoluene and naphthalene may also cause a haemolytic anaemia. Commercial divers, tunnel workers and other individuals exposed to hyperbaric oxygen have rarely been shown to have evidence of haemolysis. A case of haemolysis has been reported, following exposure to 2 ATA (atmospheres absolute) of oxygen for 26 minutes. However, no haemolysis was detected in subjects exposed to 2.8 ATA of oxygen for 90 minutes.[1,2] In practice haemolysis does not seem to be an important consideration for those required to be exposed to hyperbaric oxygen as part of their work commitment.

Individuals with G6PD deficiency have an increased susceptibility to oxidant chemicals. This diagnosis should be sought in any patient with acute haemolysis or recurrent haemolysis and especially where there is the likelihood of occupational exposure to these agents. Such individuals must avoid further exposure to oxidant chemicals, even though the exposure might be well within the relevant occupational exposure control values.

METHAEMOGLOBINAEMIA

Substances with the ability to induce the oxidation of the haem group leading to the formation of methaemoglobin include the aniline dyes, aromatic amines, nitro-substituted benzene compounds and organic and inorganic nitrites and nitrates (see Chapter 12). Methaemoglobin formation by itself does not necessarily lead to premature red cell destruction as evidenced by the absence of haemolysis in patients with methaemoglobinaemia induced by nitrites.

Some chemicals which produce methaemoglobinaemia have additional toxic effects which dominate the clinical presentation, for example methaemoglobinaemia produced by paraquat[3] is almost trivial in comparison with its effects on the lungs and other organ systems.

Ineffective erythropoiesis

LEAD

Chronic exposure to inorganic lead primarily affects erythropoiesis producing a combination of anaemia and bone marrow erythroid hyperplasia, an association best described by the term ineffective erythropoiesis. The anaemia can be either microcytic or normochromic or mixed. Polychromasia may be noted on the blood film associated with slight elevation in the reticulocyte count and red cell survival is shortened. These are all features of haemolysis and reflect the inhibitory effect of lead on erythrocyte maturation and damage to the red cell membrane. The severity of the anaemia is poorly correlated with the degree of lead exposure but is rarely seen at blood lead levels below 60 µg/100 ml in occupationally exposed groups (pers. comm. D Gidlow, Associated Octel). The anaemia of chronic lead exposure is characteristically persistent, unlike that of acute lead poisoning (see Chapters 2, 7).

The bone marrow usually shows erythroid hyperplasia and may also be sideroblastic (ineffective erythropoiesis), but erythroid hypoplasia is also occasionally described.

Basophilic stippling (Fig. 44.3) of red cells may be prominent but it is not always found and correlates poorly with blood lead levels, haemoglobin level and clinical symptoms. It is unusual when blood lead levels are below 80–100 µg/100 ml. With improved controls of current occupational exposures this marker of lead poisoning is now a rare feature in the peripheral blood. In general haematological parameters are neither sensitive nor specific in relation to blood lead levels.[4]

The mechanism of lead-induced anaemia involves reduced red cell production (ineffective erythropoiesis) as well as reduced red cell survival (haemolysis) (see Chapter 7). The pathogenesis of the ineffective erythropoiesis is complex and not completely understood. 5-Aminolaevulinic acid (ALA) dehydratase is the enzyme most affected by lead, but the majority of the enzyme steps in the human biosynthetic pathway are inhibited by lead to some degree. The haemolytic component is due to both lead-induced structural alterations in the red cell membrane and impaired erythrocyte pyrimidine 5′-nucleotidase deficiency. Under normal conditions this enzyme plays a prominent role in the clearage of residual nucleotide chains that persist in the cell after nuclear extrusion. Deficiency, whether in the acquired or the congenital form, is usually associated with the presence of basophilic stippling which has been shown to result from the deposition of aggregates of ribosomal RNA. The accumulation of nucleotides inhibits the HMP shunt and this accelerates the rate of haemolysis. Lead may also impair globin chain synthesis. In view of its multiplicity of effects on the red cell it is interesting that anaemia is a late sign of lead intoxication.

Biological effect monitoring techniques utilize the increase in substrate concentrations such as urinary ALA and erythrocyte protoporphyrin to measure exposure. The general reduction in occupational exposures to the metal in developed countries has meant that patients with lead toxicity now more commonly present with other non-haematological manifestations.

Hypoproliferative anaemia

Hypoproliferative or aplastic anaemia is defined by the presence of a peripheral blood pancytopenia, a hypocellular marrow and the absence of abnormal cells in either (Figs. 44.5a,b). The cause of the bone marrow failure lies in the pluripotent stem cells but in some cases and at certain stages of the disease one of the cell lines may be more severely affected than the others. Among the chemical and physical agents associated with aplastic anaemia

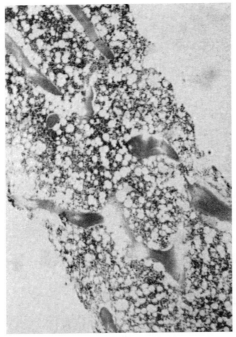

(a)

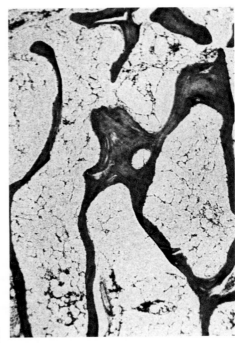

(b)

Figure 44.5 *(a) Normal and (b) hypoplastic marrow. From Ref. 62 with permission. See also colour plate section.*

are those which invariably cause aplasia given a sufficient dose (benzene, ionizing radiation) and those which only do so occasionally (arsenicals, gamma-benzene hexachloride and other insecticides, glycol ethers, carbon tetrachloride). Hair dye containing paratoluenediamine and closely related compounds have been linked to several case reports of aplastic anaemia in non-occupationally exposed individuals having used the dye 2–3 weeks prior to the onset of symptoms.[5] In such case studies it is difficult to be certain whether the dye was the aetiologic factor. Considering the widespread use of hair dye containing the compound, this complication is likely to be an idiosyncratic one.

BENZENE

Benzene is volatile and readily absorbed by inhalation or through dermal contact. It was formerly used as a solvent in a wide variety of manufacturing processes involving leather, rubber, paint spraying and removing, dry cleaning, printing, batteries, linoleum and metal plating (see Chapter 12). Benzene itself is no longer used as a commercial solvent having been replaced by non-aromatic organic solvents but it is still used in some chemical processes and is present in coal derivatives and petroleum fractions and distillates. Insecticides are often applied in petroleum based media and in these cases the precise component which is causative in the development of aplastic anaemia (the insecticide or solvent) is often unclear.

The haematological effects of benzene exposure vary widely between individuals and abnormalities may appear within weeks of exposure or only after many years. The most common haematological abnormality developing after chronic exposure to benzene is pancytopenia. This may be associated with a broad spectrum of marrow appearances from hypercellular through normal to hypocellular. There may also be dysplastic changes. Dysplastic features may herald the evolution of myelodysplasia and acute leukaemia. Acute myeloid leukaemia is the type of leukaemia that is usually associated with benzene exposure and may develop without prior marrow suppression.

The association of benzene with aplastic anaemia has been known about for nearly a century but in countries where there are strict controls and substitution for other solvents has occurred, this is now rarely seen (see Chapter 12). Cases may still occur in developing countries. The incidence of haematological problems increases with the dose and duration of exposure. Chronic exposure is more likely than acute poisoning to promote leukaemogenesis. Analysis of epidemiological studies suggests that there has to be a critical average concentration of benzene (> 20 ppm) together with exposure for several years (> 6 years)[6] before the increased risk of acquiring acute myeloid leukaemia becomes evident (see p. 908 under the heading:

LEUKAEMIA AND MYELODYSPLASIA). Frequent short-term exposures at high levels (> 100 ppm) may result in transient blood changes (leucocytosis, polymorphocytosis) with no apparent long-term effects. In contrast repeated low-dose exposure above 20 ppm[7,8] results in cytopenias (anaemia, leucopenia and thrombocytopenia). The role of occasional high exposures in addition to long-term chronic exposures in the risk of developing acute myeloid leukaemia is a difficult area to explore given the lack of detail in historical occupational history data. Although removal of such individuals from a benzene-containing environment usually results in the disappearance of such peripheral blood abnormalities over a period of months, the long-term risk of aplasia or leukaemia is not known.

OTHER AGENTS

There have been several case reports implicating the organochlorine lindane as a cause of aplastic anaemia, agranulocytosis or bone marrow hypoplasia.[9,10] However, lindane exposure was only confirmed in two of the cases. There have been no reported cases following therapeutic use where dermal absorption was documented[11] and epidemiological studies have not shown any association.[12] This suggests that blood dyscrasias following exposure to chlordane, lindane and DDT may be an idiosyncratic response (see Chapter 10).

There have been a number of case reports over the last 60 years suggesting that exposure to ethylene glycol mono methyl ether, (methoxyethanol or methyl cellosolve) can give rise to bone marrow hypoplasia in humans, some of which were occupationally exposed.[13–16] In virtually all cases there were concomitant exposures to other solvents and exposure concentrations were either unknown or uncertain. However, animal studies have shown that this solvent can reduce the cellularity of the marrow and the concentration of peripheral blood leucocytes, erythrocytes and platelets.[17,18] Currently there are few industrial applications although it is still used by the semiconductor industry in photoresistor/developer solvents.

Ionizing radiation

This is radiation that penetrates tissues and generates secondary ionizations. It includes neutrons, α-particles, electrons, x-rays and γ-rays. It may be further classified into particles with high linear energy transfer which do not penetrate deeply but generate relatively high levels of ionization and waves with low linear energy transfer such as x-rays and γ-rays which penetrate more deeply but generate less ionization (see Chapter 19). Bone marrow is the most sensitive tissue to radiation exposure and with increasing doses thereafter the gastrointestinal tract, skin, lungs and other tissues become affected. The severity of the injury is dependent on the type, quality, dose, dose rate and tissue distribution of the radiation. Radiation-induced bone marrow aplasia is now an uncommon occupational hazard owing to stringent controls of exposure and health surveillance procedures in the nuclear industry and in radiological medicine. Accidental exposure does, however, still occur.

Uniform whole-body irradiation with 1–10 Gy of low linear energy transfer radiation produces pancytopenia predisposing the recipient to infections and bleeding usually 2–4 weeks after the exposure. In human bone marrow the total number of nucleated cells is reduced at day 1 by 10–20% after 1–2 Gy, by 25–30% after 3–4 Gy, by 50–60% after 5–7 Gy and by a maximum of 80–85% after 8–10 Gy. Resistant cells such as macrophages, stromal cells, vascular endothelium and some mature granulocytes and eosinophils remain.[19] Doses exceeding 30 Gy damage the marrow microenvironment such that it can no longer sustain haemopoiesis.

In many radiation accidents, the exposure may be difficult or impossible to quantify but such information is vital in planning management especially if bone marrow transplantation is required. In this respect, the behaviour of haematological parameters can be useful in dosimetry estimations. The peripheral blood lymphocyte count is the most sensitive index of radiation injury and its fall is directly related to the whole body radiation dose up to doses of about 3 Gy. Neutrophils show an initial increase over the first few days after irradiation, then a dose-related fall. Between 10 and 15 days after a dose of 2–5 Gy, there is a second rise due to recovering haemopoiesis from precursor cell populations, followed by a second decline to about day 25. The time-course for platelet loss is similar to that for granulocytes but usually there is no second rise. The severity of the thrombocytopenia is also a measure of the exposure dose.

Figure 44.6 shows data from accident cases, depicting the average time-courses for suppression and recovery of neutrophils, lymphocytes and platelets in man following irradiation.

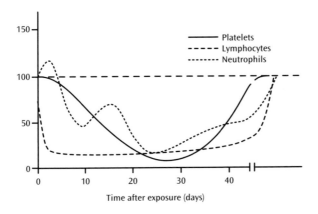

Figure 44.6 *Effects of ionizing radiation on blood counts. Redrawn from Ref. 63 with permission.*

Approximately 3 weeks after irradiation patients become symptomatic as a result of the reduction in blood cell components. Where the radiation dose is less than 4–5 Gy, it is possible to support the individual with the use of blood and platelet transfusions and to treat infection with antibiotics appropriate to the pathogens isolated or suspected. Despite these measures, most victims (as found following the explosion at the Chernobyl nuclear power plant) receiving more than 5 Gy will not survive long enough for marrow function to recover.[20] This is not solely due to the marrow aplasia but reflects the other injuries the patient may have suffered such as trauma, burns, inhalational effects, diarrhoea, fluid and electrolyte depletion. Bone marrow transplantation is the logical treatment of choice for this group of patients but is fraught with difficulties. These include the poor prognosis conferred by multiorgan damage, the inability to perform histocompatibility testing due to lymphocytopenia, the lack of compatible donors for most patients and the requirement for further immunosuppressive conditioning. As a result this modality of therapy is only available to a minority of victims.

LEUKAEMIA AND MYELODYSPLASIA

Ionizing radiation

The causal relationship between leukaemia and ionizing radiation is well documented and much of the risk estimates are based upon the incidence of acute myeloid leukaemia and myelodysplasia among the survivors of the Nagasaki and Hiroshima atomic bombs in 1945. There was also an increased incidence of chronic myeloid leukaemia with expression of the classical Philadelphia chromosome marker.[21]

The association of low level occupational exposures was established in studies on pioneering radiologists and radiation scientists[22] and led to changes in radiographic procedures (see Chapter 19). Significant numbers of excess leukaemias – acute myeloid leukaemia, chronic myeloid leukaemia and acute lymphoblastic – have been reported in medical radiation workers in China during 1950–1985.[23] The possibility that leukaemia and lymphoma could result from low level exposures to waste products from nuclear power plants has received some attention recently in the UK following the finding of geographic clusters of these diseases around such plants. Careful case-control studies did not suggest an obvious link but a hypothesis has been advanced that DNA damage to sperm may be aetiologic. This is based on the finding that the cases were concentrated among children whose fathers were 40 or more years old and had been exposed to more than 100 milliSievents (mSv) more than 6 months before conception of their children.[24] However, this has not been confirmed by a recent study[25] and the link remains controversial.

Non-ionizing radiation

There is considerable debate regarding the possibility that the very low frequency waves of electromagnetic fields such as those around electricity power lines,[26] household[27] and workplace appliances[28] may have leukaemogenic effects. The profusion of population variables make such studies difficult to carry out and small effects may be present without being detectable. In addition no clear distinction was made between the effects of electrical and magnetic fields. There is a view that whilst the risk may be small the populations at risk are large. Animal studies have not been helpful in elucidating any causative mechanisms and further studies are required (see Chapter 21).

BENZENE

Since the first suggestion in 1928 that benzene may be associated with leukaemia several epidemiology studies have established that there is a specific causal relationship between the development of acute myeloid leukaemia and chronic exposure to benzene (see Chapter 21).[29–32]

The metabolism of benzene is complicated and gives rise to several reactive metabolites both in man and experimental animals which interact with a number of highly complex biological processes. The quantity of benzene metabolites produced is the result of a subtle interplay of oxidation and conjugation pathways and distribution of enzyme systems in the liver and other organs, as well as relative rates of perfusion in different organs and different species.[33] Experimental studies *in vivo* and *in vitro* suggest that the timing, duration and concentration of exposure to benzene metabolites (hydroquinone, catechol and muconaldehyde) are important independent factors in predicting potential leukaemogenic effects.[34–36] Furthermore, it has been shown that a greater number of these metabolites result from short-duration, high-level rather than from long-duration, low-level exposures.[37]

The metabolites can cause chromosomal aberrations or deletions that can alter the regulation and function of gene expression and cell proliferation in the marrow. In addition they can interact with several interleukin genes (IL-3, IL-4, IL-5), granulocyte macrophage-colony stimulating factor (GM-CSF) and other regulatory genes resulting in myelosuppression or modification to bone marrow proliferation. Such modification is a critical step in recently proposed models of human leukaemogenesis.[38,39]

It is speculated that such effects may also play a role in the acute myeloid leukemia induced by benzene in humans.[38,39,40] The relationship of acute myeloid leukaemia to benzene exposure bears some similarity to therapy-induced or secondary leukaemias in clinical practice and may indicate similar mechanisms of causation. Chromosomal aberrations involving chromosomes 5 and 7, either alone or in combination with other changes, are found in most patients with therapy-related myelodysplastic syndrome prior to the development of overt[41] acute myeloid leukaemia and similar characteristic chromosomal aberrations have been found in some patients with benzene-induced leukaemia that were cytogenetically monitored from shortly after the onset of symptoms through a pre-leukaemic phase and until death.[42] A cytogenetic analysis of therapy related myelodysplasia/acute myeloid leukaemia, *de novo* acute myeloid leukaemia and refractory anaemia patients has revealed a critical region at band (5q31) that was deleted in all patients.[43,44]

Genes for several haemopoietic growth factors (IL-3, IL-4, IL-5, IL-9, M-CSF, GM-CSF) and growth factor receptors are located on the 5q chromosomal region and the loss or truncation of one of these genes or the inactivation of a suppressor gene in the region may play a role in the pathogenesis of these myeloid disorders. In other words there may be a common mechanism with respect to benzene-related, and secondary acute myeloid leukaemia[38,39] Epidemiological studies suggest that benzene concentrations of at least 20–25 ppm experienced over years, are necessary for the appearance of acute myeloid leukaemia in exposed individuals. In the past, refinery workers have been a target population for such effects but recent studies[45,46] have shown no consistently elevated risks in relation to acute myeloid leukaemia. This may be explained by lower levels of exposure.

OTHER AGENTS

There have been consistent reports of an increased risk of leukaemia in other occupational groups such as electrical workers, printing workers and workers in the rubber industry.[47–50] There is no indication of the agent that might be involved in these reports but there is some speculation that benzene which was used as a solvent, especially in the rubber industry, might have been one of the factors.

An excess prevalence of leukaemia has been reported in individuals with exposures to ethylene oxide.[51] However, there were exposures to several other substances thought to be responsible for confounding the results. Subsequent studies have not shown any excess risk.[52]

HODGKIN'S DISEASE AND NON-HODGKIN'S LYMPHOMA

Several studies have indicated an increased risk of Hodgkin's disease in woodworkers with tasks ranging from the manufacturing of furniture to the installing of fences.[49] Eight of the studies showed an increased risk, although the studies involved different methods and were carried out in three countries. However, the consistency of the results would suggest that association is unlikely to be due to chance, but no specific factor in terms of causative agent linked the studies.

Studies in farm workers have suggested an increased incidence of non-Hodgkin's lymphoma.[53] It has been speculated that possible farm risks would include elevated exposures to pesticides, agricultural chemicals, organic and inorganic dust, zoonotic pathogens and sunlight. The agricultural factor most prominently linked with non-Hodgkin's lymphoma has been exposure to phenoxyacetic acid herbicides[54,56] or insecticides.[54] There have been reports that suppliers of pesticides have increased chromosome rearrangements that may relate to the increased risk of non-Hodgkin's lymphoma.[57] Limited experimental data from human studies suggest that pesticides can cause thymus atrophy and suppressed T cell activity.[58] Organophosphate pesticides are known to inhibit serine esterases, which are important in T cell and natural killer cell cytolytic activity and may play an important role in lymphomagenesis through an immunosuppressive mechanism.[59]

Finally, fungicides and fumigants have also been associated with increased risks of non-Hodgkin's lymphomas.[60] A recent study[61] has strengthened the hypothesis in relation to exposure to phosphated insecticides by showing a dose-response relationship which was also suggested for stannates, carbamates, chlorinated compounds and for DDT. Exposures to such a variety of chemicals make the identification of a causative agent extremely difficult. Nevertheless the frequency with which such an association has been reported justifies a high index of suspicion.

WORK-RELATED ISSUES RESULTING FROM TREATMENT OF HAEMATOLOGICAL DISEASE

Major advances in the treatment of aplastic anaemia, acute leukaemia and lymphoma (whether due to occupational exposures or not) have meant that many more patients are being cured and are thus potentially able to return to work. This raises important questions of what is a safe working environment for such patients and what physical or mental limitations might they experience. As greater numbers of successfully treated patients are followed for longer periods of time, medical and social problems associated with the impact of the disease or its treatment have become apparent.

With improved medical technologies, it is likely that more people with chronic haematological or oncological diseases contracted through workplace exposures will enjoy improved therapy and be able to return to work. It is to be hoped that employers and their occupational health advisers will match the achievement with flexible and enlightened support and rehabilitation schemes.

Case study 1: Pancytopenia

A 56-year-old ex-patriate plant manager at an overseas petrochemical refinery had a routine executive medical examination. He was asymptomatic and physical examination was normal. The results of the full blood count were as follows: haemoglobin 12.8 g/dl, mean corpuscular volume (MCV): 100 fl, white cell count: 5.5, neutrophils: 1.5, lymphocytes: 2.0, monocytes: 1.5, eosinophils: 0.5 (all $\times 10^9$/litre) and platelets: 115 $\times 10^6$/litre. He was given a copy of the results for his general practitioner and advised to make an appointment on his next visit home in 4 weeks time. The repeat full blood count showed identical results. In addition, it was commented that the blood film showed a mild pancytopenia and some dysplastic neutrophils. He was referred for a haematological opinion.

His current job was manager of a distillation plant at a refinery in the Far East. His career since leaving school had been in the oil refining business and he had had several jobs overseas. One of his first jobs was as a maintenance fitter with frequent exposures to hydrocarbon solvents whilst carrying out routine and emergency repairs. He recalled a project about 20 years previously which lasted several weeks and involved work on a plant using mainly benzene. The refinery was in the tropics where he worked in enclosed areas, stripped to the waist. Little attention was given to personal protection and he was often breathing in an atmospheric heavily contaminated with various hydrocarbons. He had to have frequent rest periods to recover from acute inhalational effects.

Further investigations showed normal B12, folate and iron levels. Renal and liver function tests were also normal. In view of the persisting pancytopenia a bone marrow aspirate was performed and this showed hyperplasia with reduced numbers of megakaryocytes, dysplastic erythropoiesis and a blast count of 15% (normal < 5%).

The diagnosis was myelodysplasia (French–American British (FAB) classification: refractory anaemia with excess of blasts). Cytogenetic analysis of the marrow showed a complex karyotype and a clonal deletion of the long arm of chromosome 5. During subsequent follow-up the blood counts continued to decrease over a period of 12 months and he required regular blood transfusions to maintain the haemoglobin. Leukaemic blasts appeared in the peripheral blood and the bone marrow showed progression to acute myeloid leukaemia. There was no response to intravenous chemotherapy and he died following an intracranial haemorrhage 6 months after diagnosis.

COMMENTARY

This case illustrates the association between myelodysplasia, acute myeloid leukaemia and exposure to benzene. There continues to be debate about the risk posed by low-level exposures but here acute high-level exposures occurred over a period of a few weeks. Both inhalational and dermal exposure was reported and no protective measures were taken. It would have been valuable to know whether any of the high exposures had any short-term effects on the haemopoietic system such as pancytopenia or marrow hypoplasia although the history was not suggestive of this.

The marrow showed evolution from myelodysplasia to acute myeloid leukaemia with characteristic biological and clinical features. These features are not diagnostic of benzene-related leukaemogenesis and are shared with other secondary leukaemias such as those following chemotherapy. They are:

1 the long latent period lasting many years;
2 the complex chromosomal abnormalities particularly involving loss or interstital deletions of chromosomes 5 and 7;
3 the low remission rate in response to chemotherapy;
4 the poor prognosis.

Case study 2: Haemolytic anaemia

During the summer vacation, a 23-year-old, final year medical student presented to his general practitioner on a Friday evening with vague flu-like symptoms, headaches and a dry cough. He was a keen athlete and had noticed a decrease in his exercise tolerance over the previous week. Physical examination was unremarkable other than a comment in the general practitioner's notes that he looked 'pale and grey'.

The young man was told that it was probably a viral infection and was asked to return if there was no improvement in his symptoms. He felt better over the weekend but the symptoms returned the following week and he noticed a consistent change in the colour of his urine. His partner, who was a nurse, thought that he looked slightly jaundiced, especially at the end of the day. He also felt increasingly tired and had several bouts of shivering.

The general practitioner confirmed the clinical impression of mild jaundice and requested a urine test and some haematological and biochemical investigations. The student was told to stay off work because of the possibility of infectious hepatitis or mononucleosis. After 48 hours his symptoms had improved. The investigations showed a haemoglobin count of 10.1g/dl, MCV: 102fl, platelets: 395, white blood cell count: 8.5×10^9/litre and normal differential count. The blood film was reported as showing polychromasia and increased numbers of irregularly contracted cells. Reticulocyte count was 4.5%;

direct antibody test was negative; haptoglobins were reduced. Bilirubin 45 µm/litre with normal enzyme activities and normal renal function. The urine contained increased amounts of urobilinogen and urinary haemosiderin was detected on microscopy of the urinary deposit. Methaemoglobin levels in the blood were significantly raised.

On further questioning the young man admitted he had taken a part-time job during his current vacation as laboratory assistant in a small chemical company. His main task was cleaning glassware in a washroom adjacent to the main laboratory with occasional deliveries to the pilot plant where the bulk of the glassware originated. He said the room was hot with little in the way of ventilation. Protective respiratory equipment and gloves were available but he had not received any information or training in their use. He was unaware of what the chemicals were although the odour from the glassware was unpleasant. He had noticed small residues of a viscous chemical in the glass containers. Skin contamination had occurred because of the high volume of washing that had been required recently.

Contact with the Health and Safety Officer of the company revealed that the pilot plant was investigating a novel hallogenated aniline compound. The health and safety data sheet revealed that the compound was likely to cause blood problems by inhalation or dermal exposure and warned of the specific risk of methaemoglobinaemia and haemolysis.

COMMENTARY

This case highlights the importance of all personnel involved in the handling of toxic substances being fully informed of the risks and safety procedures. This includes not only regular employees who are directly involved with the primary handling but also casual staff and those who may be involved in cleaning and disposal. Whilst the substance was labelled as hazardous on the containers from the manufacturers and full-time employees were aware of the risks, health and safety checks had not identified the individual illustrated in this case in its risk assessment.

The blood tests showed the pattern of increased red cell destruction (hyperbilirubinaemia, increased urinary urobilinogen, reduced haptoglobins, polychromasia, reticulocytosis) with evidence of intravascular haemolysis (haemoglobinuria, haemosiderinuria). The direct antibody test excluded an immunological mechanism of the increased red cell destruction and the presence of methaemoglobinaemia was consistent with oxidative haemolysis.

The patient's symptoms recovered completely within 4–5 days and his haematology profile had resumed its normal characteristics after 10 days. The medical student continued with his studies and took an interest in toxicology.

REFERENCES

1 Mengel C E, Kann H E, Haeyman A, Metz E. Effects of *in-vitro* hyperoxia on erythrocytes. II. Haemolysis in a human after exposure to oxygen under high pressure. *Blood* 1965; **25:** 822–9.

2 Bradley M E, Vorosmati J. Haematological changes resulting from hyperbaric oxygenation in divers and non-divers. *Aerospace Med* 1968; **39:** 493–7.

3 Ng L L, Naik R B, Polak B. Paraquat ingestion with methaemoglobinaemia treated with methylene blue. *Br Med J* 1982; **284:** 1445.

4 Zielhuis R L. Dose-related relationships for inorganic lead. *Int Arch Occup Hlth* 1975; **35:** 1–18.

5 Hopkins J E, Manoharan A. Severe aplastic anaemia following the use of hair dye: report of two cases and review of literature. *Postgrad Med J* 1985; **61:** 1003–5.

6 Schnatter A R, Nicolich M J, Bird M G. Determination of leukemogenic benzene exposure concentrations: refined analyses of the pliofilm cohort. *Risk Analysis* 1996; **16:** 833–4.

7 Kipen H M, Cody R P, Crump K S, Allen B C, Goldstein B D. Haematologic effects of benzene: a 35-year longitudinal study of rubber workers. *Toxicol Ind Hlth* 1988; **4:** 411–30.

8 Chang I W. Study on the threshold limit value of benzene and early diagnosis of benzene poisoning. *J Cath Med Coll* 1972; **23:** 429–34.

9 Vodopick H. Erythropoietic hypoplasia after exposure to gamma benzene hexachloride. *JAMA* 1975; **234:** 850–1.

10 Loge J P. Aplastic anemia following exposure to benzene hexachloride (lindane). *JAMA* 1965; **193:** 110–4.

11 Morgan D P, Stockdale E M, Roberts R J *et al*. Anemia associated with exposure to lindane. *Arch Environ Hlth* 1980; **35:** 307–10.

12 Samuels A J, Milby T H. Human exposure to lindane: clinical hematological and biochemical effects. *J Occup Med* 1971; **13:** 147–51.

13 Donley D D. Toxic encephalopathy and volatile solvents in industry. *J Ind Hyg Toxicol* 1936; **18:** 571.

14 Parsons C E, Parsons M E. Toxic encephalopathy and granulopenic anaemia due to volatile solvents in industry: report of two cases. *J Ind Hyg Toxicol* 1938; **20:** 125.

15 Greenburg H, Mayers M R, Goldwater L J, Burke W J, Moscowitz S. Health hazards in the manufacture of 'fused collars'. *J Ind Hyg Toxicol* 1938; **20:** 134.

16 Ohi G, Wegman D H. Transcutaneous ethylene glycol mono ethyl ether poisoning in the work setting. *J Occup Med* 1978; **20:** 675.

17 Miller R R, Ayres J A, Calhoun L L, Young J T, McKenna M J. Comparative short-term inhalation toxicity of ethylene glycol monomethyl ether. *Toxicol Appl Pharmacol* 1981: 368.

18 Barbee S J, Terrill J B, De Sousa D J and Conway C C. Subchronic inhalation toxicology of ethylene glycol mono ethyl ether in the rat and rabbit. *Environ Hlth Perspect* 1984; **57:** 157.

19 International Atomic Energy Agency. *Manual on Radiation Haematology*. Vienna: IAEA, 1971.

20 Champlin R. Bone marrow aplasia due to radiation accidents: pathophysiology, assessment and treatment. *Baillière's Clin Haematol* 1989; **1:** 69–82.

21 Preston D L, Kusumi S, Tomonaga M *et al*. Cancer incidence in atomic bomb survivors. 3. Leukemia, lymphoma and multiple myeloma, 1950–1987. *Radiat Res* 1994; **137** (Suppl): S68–97.

22 Doll R S. Hazards of ionising radiation: 100 years of observations on man. *Br J Cancer* 1995; **72:** 1339–49.

23 Wang J-X, Inskip P D, Boice J D J, Li B-X, Zhang J-Y, Fraumeni J F J. Cancer incidence among medical diagnostic X-ray workers in China, 1950 to 1985. *Int J Cancer* 1995; **72:** 1339–49.

24 Gardner M J *et al*. Results of case-control study of leukaemia and lymphoma among young people near Sellafield nuclear plant in West Cumbria. *Br Med J* 1990; **300:** 423.

25 Draper G J, Little M P *et al*. Cancer in the offspring of radiation workers: a record linkage study. *Br Med J* 1997; **315:** 1181–8.

26 Miller A B, To T, Agnew D A, Wall C, Green L M. Leukemia following occupational exposure to 60-Hz electricity and magnetic fields among Ontario electric utility workers. *Am J Epidemiol* 1996; **44:** 50–60.

27 Li C Y, Theriault G, Lin R S. Epidemiological appraisal of studies of residential exposure to power frequency magnetic fields and adult cancers. *Occup Environ Med* 1996; **53:** 505–10.

28 Milham S Jr. Increased incidence of cancer in a cohort of office workers exposed to strong magnetic fields. *Am J Ind Med* 1996; **30:** 702–4.

29 Aksoy M, Erdem S, Dincol G. Leukemia in shoe-workers exposed chronically to benzene. *Blood* 1974; **44:** 837–41.

30 Rinsky R A, Smith A B, Hornung R, Filloon T G, Young R J *et al*. Benzene and leukemia: an epidemiologic risk assessment. *N Engl J Med* 1987; **316:** 1044–50.

31 Austin H, Delzell E, Cole P. Benzene and leukemia: A review of the literature and a risk assessment. *Am J Epidemiol* 1988; **127:** 419–39.

32 Paustenbach D J, Price P S, Ollison W, Blank C, Jernigan J D *et al*. Reevaluation of benzene exposure for the pliofilm (rubberworker) cohort (1936–1976). *J Toxicol Environ Hlth* 1992; **36:** 177–231.

33 Yardley-Jones A, Anderson D, Park D V. The toxicology of benzene and its metabolism and molecular pathology in human risk assessment. *Br J Ind Med* 1991; **48:** 437–44.

34 Green J D, Snyder C A, LoBue J, Goldstein B D, Albert R E. Acute and chronic dose/response effect of benzene inhalation on the peripheral blood, bone marrow, and spleen cells of CD-1 male mice. *Toxicol Appl Pharmacol* 1981; **59:** 204–14.

35 Toft L, Olfsson T, Tunek A. Toxic effects on mouse bone marrow caused by inhalation of benzene. *Arch Toxicol* 1982; **51:** 295–302.

36 Luke C A, Tice R R, Drew R T. The effects of exposure regimen and duration on benzene-induced bone marrow damage in mice II. *Mutat Res* 1988; **203:** 273–95.

37 Bois F Y, Paxman D G. An analysis of exposure rate effects for benzene using a physiologically based pharmacokinetic model. *Regulat Toxicol Pharmacol* 1992; **15:** 122–36.

38 Irons R D. Benzene toxicology and leukemogenesis. *Proc Ann Winter Meeting, Washington – The Toxicology Forum* 1997; **22:** 379–88.

39 Irons R D, Stillman W S. The process of leukemogenesis. *Environ Hlth Perspect* 1996; **104:** 1239–46.

40 Snyder R, Kalf G. A perspective on benzene leukemogenesis. *Crit Rev Toxicol* 1994; **24:** 177–209.

41 Koeffler H F, Rowley J D. Therapy-related acute nonlymphocytic leukaemia. In: Wiermik P H, Canelloe, G P, Kyle R A, Schiffer C A, eds. *Neoplastic Diseases of the Blood.* New York: Churchill Livingstone, 1984: 357.

42 Van den Berghe H, Louwagie A, Broechaert-van Orshoven A, David G, Verwilhen R. Chromosome analysis in two unusual malignant blood disorders presumably induced by benzene. *Blood* 1979; **53:** 558.

43 Rowley J D, Golomb H M, Vardiman J W. Nonrandom chromosome abnormalities in acute leukaemia and dysmyelopoietic syndrome in patients with previously treated malignant disease. *Blood* 1981; **58:** 759.

44 Le Beau M M, Albain K S, Larson R A *et al.* Clinical and cytogenetic correlations in 63 patients with therapy-related myelodysplastic syndromes and acute non-lymphocytic leukaemia. Further evidence for characteristic abnormalities of chromosomes Nos 5 and 7. *J Clin Oncol* 1986; **4:** 325.

45 Rushton L, Romaniuk H. A case-control study to investigate the risk of leukemia associated with exposure to benzene in petroleum marketing and distribution workers in the United Kingdom. *Occup Environ Med* 1997; **54:** 152–66.

46 Schnatter A R, Armstrong T W, Nicolich M J, Thompson F S, Huebner W W *et al.* Risk of lymphohematopoietic malignancies and quantitative estimates of benzene exposure in Canadian marketing/distribution workers. *Occup Environ Med* 1996; **53:** 773–81

47 McDowall M. Leukaemia mortality in electrical workers in England and Wales. *Lancet* 1983; **i:** 246.

48 Coleman N, Bell J, Skeet R. Leukaemia incidence in electrical workers. *Lancet* 1983; **i:** 982–3.

49 Alderson M. *Occupational Cancer.* London: Butterworth 1986; 108–9.

50 Wolf P H, Andjelkovic D, Smith A, Tyroler H. *J Occup Med* 1981; **23:** 103–8.

51 Hogstedt C, Aringer L, Gustavsson A. Epidemiologic support for ethylene oxide as a cancer-causing agent. *JAMA* 1986; **225:** 1575–8.

52 Currier M F, Carlo G L, Poston P L *et al.* A cross-sectional study of employees with potential occupational exposure to ethylene oxide. *Br J Ind Med* 1984; **41:** 492–8.

53 Blair A, Zahn S H. Cancer among farmers. *Occup Med* 1991; **6:** 335–54.

54 Cantor K P, Blair A, Everett G *et al.* Pesticides and other agricultural risk factors for non-Hodgkin's lymphoma among men in Lowa and Minnesota. *Cancer Res* 1992; **52:** 2447–55.

55 Hoar S K, Blair A, Holmes F F *et al.* Agricultural herbicide use and risk of lymphoma and soft-tissue sarcoma. *JAMA* 1986; **256:** 1411–17.

56 Zahm S H, Weisenburger D D, Babbitt P A *et al.* A case-control study of non-Hodgkin's lymphoma and the herbicide 2, 4-dichlorophenoxyacetic acid (2, 4-D) in Eastern Nebraska. *Epidemiology* 1990; **1:** 349–56.

57 Garry V F, Danzl T J, Tarone R *et al.* Chromosome rearrangements in fumigant appliers: possible relationship to non-Hodgkin's lymphoma risk. *Cancer Epidemiol Biomarkers Prev* 1992; **1:** 287–91.

58 Thomas P T, Busse W W, Kerfvleit N I *et al.* Immunologic effects of pesticides. In: Baker S R, Wilkinson C R eds. *The Effects of Pesticides on Human Health. (Advances in Modern Environmental Toxicology XVIII)* N J, Princeton: Princeton Scientific Publishers. 1990; 261–95.

59 Newcombe D S. Immune surveillance, organophosphorus exposure and lymphomagenesis. *Lancet* 1992; **339:** 539–41.

60 Hoar Zham S, Blair A. Pesticides and non-Hodgkin's lymphoma. *Cancer Res* 1992; **52:** 5485s–8s.

61 Nanni O, Amadori D, Lugaresi C, Falcini F, Scarpi E *et al.* Chronic lymphocytic leukaemias and non-Hodgkin's lymphomas by histological type in farming-animal breeding workers. *Occup Environ Med* 1996; **53:** 652–7.

62 Linch DC, Yates AP, Watts MJ (eds). *Colour Guide to Haematology.* Edinburgh, London: Churchill Livingstone, 1996.

63 Ballantyne B, Marrs T, Turner P. *General and Applied Toxicology* Vol. 2. 1993; Macmillan Press Ltd.

Appendix

Diseases of occupations – a short history of their
   recognition and prevention   917

APPENDIX

Diseases of occupations – a short history of their recognition and prevention

TIM CARTER

The factory system: master, servant and poverty	919	Impact of war	924
Miners, lungs and measurement	920	Modern industrial experience	924
Public opinion, politics, regulation and inspection	921	Conclusion: the meaning of occupational health	925
International collaboration	923	References	925

Bernardino Ramazzini (1633–1714) (Fig.1), who practised in the cities of Northern Italy, is often described as the father of occupational medicine. In 1713 he published a treatise *De Morbis Artificum Diatriba* (Fig.2)[1] in which he described the diseases of a wide range of trades, applying clinical acumen to his observations, for instance noting the different characteristics of skin ulceration in freshwater and sea fishermen. He not only described many conditions but also made practical proposals for prevention such as good ventilation and protective clothing. But he was not merely a curious doctor he was also deeply concerned about the ethics of harm from work:

> Medicine, like jurisprudence, should make a contribution to the well-being of workers and see to it that, as far as possible, they should exercise their callings without harm. So I for my part have done what I could and have not thought it unbecoming to make my way into the lowliest workshops and study the mysteries of the mechanical arts.

And he added the keystone of occupational medicine to medical practice:

> When a doctor visits a working-class home he should be content to sit on a three-legged stool, if there isn't a gilded chair, and he should take time for his examination; and to the questions recommended by Hippocrates, he should add one more – What is your occupation?

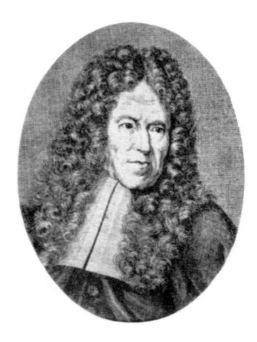

Figure 1 *Bernardino Ramazzini (1633–1714).*

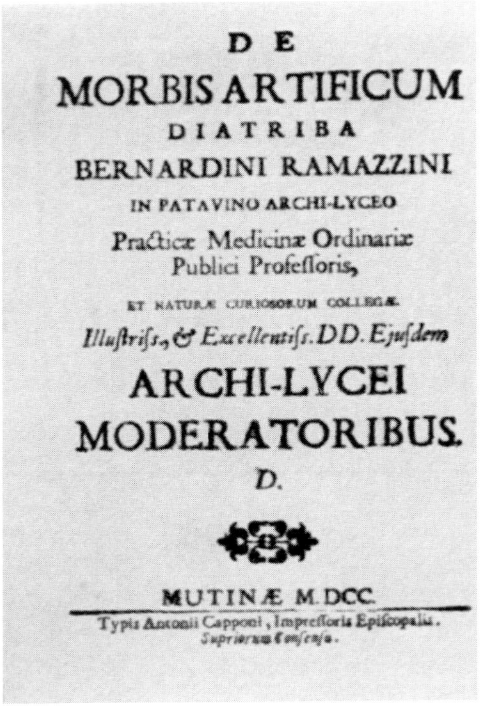

DE MORBIS ARTIFICUM DIATRIBA BERNARDINI RAMAZZINI IN PATAVINO ARCHI-LYCEO Practicæ Medicinæ Ordinariæ Publici Professoris, ET NATURÆ CURIOSORUM COLLEGÆ Illustriss, & Excellentiss. DD. Ejusdem **ARCHI-LYCEI MODERATORIBUS.** D.

MUTINÆ. M.DCC. Typis Antonii Capponi, Impressoris Episcopalis. Superiorum Consensu.

Figure 2 *Title page of first edition of Ramazzini's treatise:* De Morbis Artificum Diatriba, 1713.

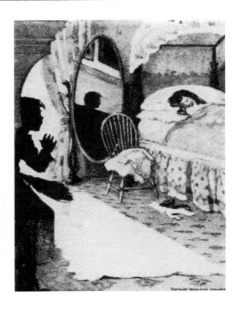

Figure 3 *Tom, the climbing boy, in Charles Kingsley's* Water Babies, *1863 (after Jessie Wilcox Smith).*

In Britain a risk was posed by one of the earliest technical innovations. Smoke and what we would now know as pollution of the indoor environment was greatly reduced by the introduction of the domestic chimney. Shortage of wood in London led to the importation of 'sea coal' by boat, mainly from Tyneside in the North East of England. Soot in chimneys posed a fire risk and had to be removed. Chimneys were often built with many bends in them which prevented sweeping from the ends. So sweeps employed 'climbing boys' – usually paupers who were bound to them as apprentices – to sweep from within the flues. It was an appalling job and one which later spearheaded reforms in both children's employment and building regulations. Percival Pott, a London surgeon, described scrotal cancer in climbing boys in 1775, the first record of an occupational cancer:

> ... when they get to puberty become liable to a most noisome, painful and fatal disease ... in the inferior part of the scrotum, where it produces a superficial, painful, ragged, ill-looking sore, with hard and rising edges: the trade call it a soot wart.

It reveals much about the lack of public concern for children and occupational risk that Kingsley wrote the children's book about climbing boys *Water Babies* nearly a hundred years after Pott's description (Fig.3). It was only in 1875, after a lifetime of campaigning, that the famous reformer Lord Shaftesbury secured effective prohibition.

For those commanding soldiers and sailors away from their home bases, the effectiveness of the unit or crew depended on good health. Early long-distance voyages such as those of Magellan and Drake around the world in the sixteenth century had huge morbidity and mortality from scurvy, caused by a diet deficient in vitamin C from fresh fruit and vegetables. Similar problems arose in winter armies, besieged towns and among explorers. The losses preoccupied the Royal Navy and James Lind, a naval surgeon, carried out the first carefully designed clinical trial in the history of medicine to investigate its causes publishing his *Treatise on Scurvy* in 1753. His findings were rapidly adopted by James Cook, the explorer and navigator who insisted that his crew ate fruit or drank juices. The naturalist Joseph Banks, who sailed with him and later became President of the Royal Society recorded:

> About a fortnight ago my gums swelled and some small pimples rose on the inside of my mouth which threatened to become ulcers ...

He took lemon juice

> The effect of this was surprising. In less than a week my gums became as firm as ever.

The Navy was slower to act, but in 1795 lemon or lime juice was included in ships' stores. In consequence, during the Napoleonic wars in the first two decades of the nineteenth century, the British navy had far less scurvy than their French counterparts.[2]

Thus, in pre-industrial conditions, some technologies and working conditions that led to harm were recognized. Certain diseases linked to them were identified.

Some risks were controlled but others were ignored – mainly because of their social, political and economic consequences – and the benefits of prevention were occasionally visible.

THE FACTORY SYSTEM: MASTER, SERVANT AND POVERTY

Between 1760 and 1830, major changes took place in British society and many of these were subsequently replicated worldwide. Stability and prosperity in the mid-eighteenth century led to improvements in agriculture and in transport, both by the building of toll roads and the excavation of canals, and in technology. The productivity of fabric manufacture rose with new spinning and weaving machines and then with new sources of power – at first water but later steam – as the prime movers rather than human and animal muscle.

A consequence of this was concentration of the means of production and wealth generation in the hands of a few – the capitalists, while an increasing proportion of the population worked for them in return for a wage – labour.

Traditional cottage industries, especially wool cloth manufacture, were severely disrupted by powered spinning and weaving. This and raised agricultural productivity meant that labour was abundant. Jobs were now in mills, which employed hundreds of hands and where the owners sought to minimize the costs of production by driving down pay and employing cheap labour such as women and children (Fig.4).

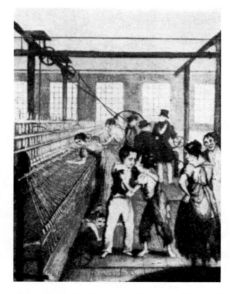

Figure 4 *Child labour in the textile factories. The well dressed visitors contrast with ragged apprentices. Note the small child crawling under the self-acting spinning mule. (From* The Life and Adventures of Michael Armstrong, the Factory Boy *by Frances Trollope, 1840.)*

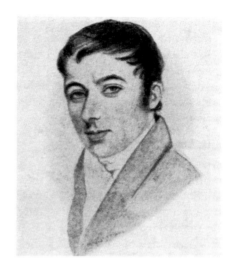

Figure 5 *Robert Owen.*

Attitudes to the health of textile mill workers varied widely. Some owners, such as Robert Owen in New Lanark (Fig.5) built model communities for their workers, either from idealistic motives or as in the case of the great Yorkshire capitalist Titus Salt to control the workforce and improve productivity. Other mills like Quarry Bank in Cheshire engaged doctors and provided schooling. Many owners regarded labour as a replaceable commodity and did nothing, except to panic if infections such as typhus broke out in the mill, which could spread to their families and damage their business. While injuries from powered but unguarded machinery were common and infections and malnutrition took their toll, specific diseases associated with the work were not at first noted.

One notable exception to this lack of interest in the effects of the Industrial Revolution on health is found in the work and writings of Charles Turner Thackrah (1795–1833), commonly identified as the founder of occupational medicine in Britain (Fig.6). His interest in occupational diseases may have been sparked by personal contact with Robert Owen. During his short life, which ended with his death from tuberculosis, probably contracted as a medical student, Thackrah studied and wrote about the diseases in the working population of Leeds. Not only was he an astute observer but he made extensive use of quantitative information to compare mortality in town and country and between different trades. In his book: *The Effects of the Principal Arts, Trades and Professions, and of Civic States and Habits of Living, on Health and Longevity, with Suggestions for the Removal of many of the Agents which produce Disease and shorten the Duration of Life* his writing lives up to his title and provides a vivid picture of life in 1830.[3] He also conveyed a social message about the practicality of prevention:

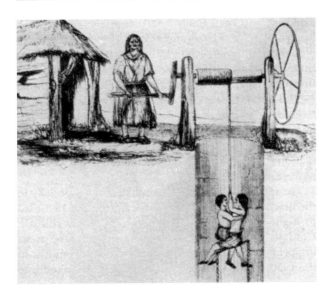

Figure 10 *Children in a mine: one of the pictures which shocked Victorian England.*

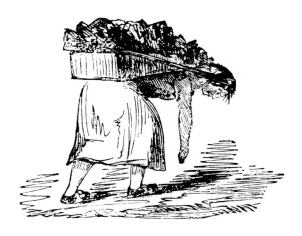

Figure 12 *In Scotland women were used to carry coal in baskets on their backs.*

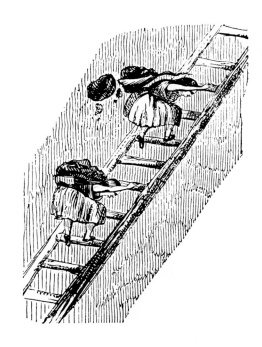

Figure 13 *In some cases girls of 6 were found carrying half a hundredweight of coal up a ladder.*

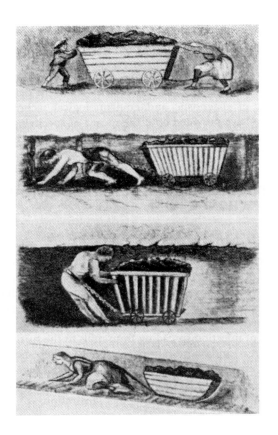

Figure 11 *Children hauled trucks of coal and women almost naked were harnessed like horses to coal trucks.*

In the first two decades of the century there were a number of attempts to regulate working conditions, but these were ineffective as they relied on local action. However, in 1833 The Factory Act, which applied to powered textile mills, led to the appointment of four inspectors with nationwide powers of entry and prosecution. Their initial priorities were the hours of work and education of children, and accidents. They had the power to appoint doctors to assist them and used them initially to assess age and to investigate injuries. During the century the Act was modified to include a wider range of workplaces, including a number, such as lead works and match factories that had specific health problems. At times, the political climate supported their work, but there were periods when the interest of manufacturers in free and unfettered trade led to their powers being curtailed.

For most of the century diseases from work did not receive much attention. There were far bigger problems with the infectious diseases that were prevalent in towns and not yet prevented, while there was a strong strand of fatalism about trade diseases among those at risk. Campaigners such as Florence Nightingale[5] pointed to the harm done by poor air in workplaces and the health and economic benefits of action:

> And yet the master is no gainer. His goods are spoiled by foul air and gas fumes, his own health and that of his family suffers, and his work is not so well done as it would be were his people in health … And the time will come when it will be found cheaper to supply shops, warehouses and workrooms with pure air than with foul air.

However, it was not until the 1880s when the germ theory of disease had led to better prevention of infections that the control methods introduced were seen as models for prevention of other diseases, such as those from work. A series of Dangerous Trade committees were set up for the Factory Department and studied problems such as lead poisoning in manufacture and in glazing,

phosphorus poisoning in match making and anthrax in the hair, hide and wool industries. They studied the diseases, who was harmed and why, as well as the scope for control by regulation and improved work practices. Some successes were achieved but it became apparent that there were important gaps in knowledge and that more reliable data on disease incidence was essential if progress was to be monitored.

In 1898 Thomas, later Sir Thomas, Legge was appointed as the first Medical Inspector of Factories (Fig.14). From then until 1926 he played a major part in characterizing occupational diseases,[6] setting up surveillance schemes for them and championing the introduction of rational and effective controls. His most long-lasting campaigns were on lead poisoning and on anthrax. On lead, the best means of control depended on the route by which lead entered the body. Using both observation and experiment, Legge demonstrated that inhalation of dust was the main route. Hence, control was a matter of dust suppression and regulations were introduced to secure this. Success was most easily achieved in the white lead pigment industry where manufacturers accepted that process changes and better hygiene were inevitable if they were to stay in business. By contrast, where lead glazes were used on ceramics, and incidentally resulting in many women exposed to an increased risk of abortion, progress was slow. Manufacturers were unwilling to use less technically desirable alternatives or to change processes until a technical development in the form of low solubility lead glazes became available. Progress with prevention was monitored by using the network of appointed doctors set up in the previous century to undertake regular examinations of lead workers and by requiring all doctors to notify cases of poisoning. It was lead that resulted in Legge's resignation from his post in 1926, when Britain refused to ratify an International Labour Office Convention, which Legge had earlier negotiated with government support, prohibiting lead from interior house paints.

INTERNATIONAL COLLABORATION

Working conditions that led to the recognition of diseases of occupations were present in many countries by the end of the nineteenth century.[7] Britain's early industrialization had simply led to some action in advance of other countries. But the result, as Hunter claimed, was that occupational medicine was born in Britain. Nevertheless, important work on lead poisoning had been undertaken in France by Tanquerel des Planches (1839) and later by Meillere, as well as by Teleky in Germany and Alice Hamilton in USA – resulting in regulations on prevention and on compensation for harm. The latter was part of the much wider social security

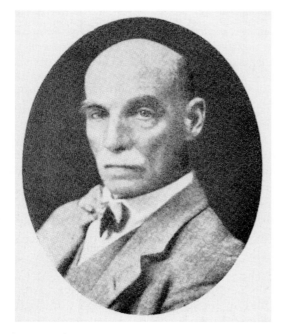

Figure 14 *Sir Thomas Morison Legge, 1863–1932, the first Medical Inspector of Factories, 1898.*

arrangements first introduced in Germany by Bismarck. Experts communicated internationally and began to meet to review problems. Alice Hamilton (1869–1970) was the first physician to devote herself to research in occupational medicine in the USA, where as well as being a pioneer in occupational hygiene and occupational epidemiology, she was also seen as a leading social reformer.

Certain diseases had an important international dimension. Anthrax from infected animals anywhere in the world was transported to the places where wool, hair and hides were processed. Studies by Legge and others identified the relative risk of different products and, although international action to disinfect wool before it was transported was never achieved, import and disinfection regimes were set up in many user countries to reduce risks. There was collaboration on such measures and the spreading of knowledge about how to treat cases most effectively. Ankylostomiasis (hookworm) became an endemic infection in some mines and in the early Alpine tunnelling projects; it was then carried by miners to infect other mines. There was collaborative international investigation and the provision of below-ground latrines to break the infective cycle by stopping faecal contamination of mine water, and this became a widespread regulatory requirement.

The foundation of the Permanent Commission for Occupational Health in Milan in 1906 was the public expression of international professional collaboration and it became an important means of exchanging information between countries. Legal strength was added with the formation of the International Labour Office in 1919. Through its legal instruments of conventions and its recommendations it has been able to influence the prevention of certain occupational diseases worldwide.

IMPACT OF WAR

International conflict on a larger scale than ever before has also been a feature of the twentieth century. This has had an important influence on the prevention of occupational diseases, not least because of the need to avoid the loss of war production through illness in war industries. The First World War (1914–18) was characterized by a number of major outbreaks of industrial disease. A solvent, tetrachloroethane, for dopes (laquers) used to treat the fabric wings of aircraft caused fatal liver damage both in Britain and Germany. Alternatives were found – and both combatants were aware of the other's experience through scientific channels. The production of trinitrotoluene (TNT) and other explosives in Britain and France was nearly halted by poisoning in munitions workers. Detailed medical supervision and the automation of shell filling were rapidly introduced to remedy the problem. In the Second World War (1939–45) indus-

trial risks were better controlled, but blackouts to protect against aerial bombing, for example, often led to poorly ventilated factory air. Women were counted upon to occupy jobs vacated by fighting men. Donald Hunter studied solvent and aluminium dust exposure – the latter because of reports of problems in German aircraft factories – but failed to find significant disease.

MODERN INDUSTRIAL EXPERIENCE

Many specific conditions where the link between exposure and disease were obvious, such as poisonings, infections and diseases such as accelerated silicosis, were to a greater or lesser extent controlled by 1950. Interest was moving from not only protecting, but also improving the health of the working population. But technology was changing ever faster and new, more latent, risks, especially from chemicals, were emerging. Analysis of these diseases with long latency, such as occupational cancers, required extending clinical observation to include epidemiological methods, especially for elucidating the role of occupational factors in disease causation and for developing exposure-response relations. In the United Kingdom, the medical statistician Sir Austin Bradford Hill had a seminal influence on the use of epidemiological methods in medicine, while Richard Schilling[8] was a notable occupational physician and teacher, who promoted the role of epidemiology in investigating occupational disorders. Notable early studies in the 1950s were by Sir Richard Doll on lung cancer in gas workers and bladder cancer among dyestuff and rubber factory workers by Robert Case. In the USA, studies by Irving Selikoff in the 1960–70s were leading to greater understanding of the asbestos-related diseases. Undoubtedly, occupational epidemiology came of age in 1973, when following leads from laboratory animal studies, human cases of the rare tumour angiosarcoma of the liver were identified in workers exposed to vinyl chloride monomer. The chemical industry was stunned that a chemical widely used in plastics (PVC) manufacture and believed to be safe could turn out to be carcinogenic. Epidemiological studies were rapidly set up and proved to be essential in delineating the risk and in determining whether the chemical also caused increases in the incidence of common cancers of such sites as the lung and brain.

Much of the identification and characterization of the diseases of occupations that are currently of concern, such as non-specific skin, lung, musculoskeletal and mental health conditions, has leant heavily on the epidemiological comparisons required to define non-specific conditions. In addition, long-term follow-up into retirement and death has been needed to assess the scale of chronic conditions.[9] These changes have had an important impact on the regulation of occupational disease prevention.[8–10] Occupational epidemiological studies are also influencing public policy in other directions – for example, the setting of air quality standards, which for some pollutants relies heavily on data from exposed cohorts of workers.

More recently, manufacturing and trade have become an integrated global network. This is seen most clearly in the development of multinational companies and in the worldwide licensing of technologies. It has resulted in more rapid sharing of information on risk (as in the example of cancer in vinyl chloride monomer workers) and other benefits include the international organization of epidemiological and toxicological studies. The less welcome effects of globalization include the move of industries with harmful effects to those countries where the regulatory controls are weakest and the export of old and dangerous equipment, products which fail to meet stringent regulatory requirements, and toxic waste to the same locations. Partly to counter this, international controls on chemicals and, in particular, pesticides have been introduced to attempt to reduce the transfer of risk.

CONCLUSION: THE MEANING OF OCCUPATIONAL HEALTH

The history of diseases of occupations and their prevention has been an interplay between technology, science and medicine and the expectations of society. Prevention of occupational diseases has also forged advances in occupational health provision, with unions and government regulations (e.g. Health and Safety at Work Act 1974 in the UK and The Occupational Safety and Health Act 1970 in the USA) having played a key part. Major improvements in protection have been made and there is scope for yet further improvements. Yet simply preventing diseases has not made work a fulfilling activity for many people. Current concerns about the health of those at work focus on a 'biopsychosocial' model, where risk factors outside work such as poor mental health may play an important part in exacerbating harm from work, or in reducing performance.[10] The detailed understanding of particular risks and diseases forms the subject of this book, but the move away from the control of serious specific diseases in well defined dangerous trades to the management of non-life threatening conditions that occur widely, and which may also have causes outside work, has led to a progressive shift in emphasis during the twentieth century.

Ramazzini's injunction to ask the question 'What is your occupation?' remains the key to occupational health practice, but it is now again being asked in terms of the whole person and not just in terms of specific risks, trades and diseases.

REFERENCES

1 Ramazzini B. *Diseases of Workers*. [Translation of *De Morbis Artificium* 1713 text.] New York: Hafner, 1964.

2 Porter R (ed.) *The Cambridge Illustrated History of Medicine*. Cambridge: Cambridge University Press, 1996.

3 Thackrah CT. *The Effects of Arts, Trades, and Professions on Health and Longevity* 1832. Reprint. London: WH Smith /Longman, 1989.

4 Rosen G. *A History of Miners Diseases*. New York, 1943.

5 Nightingale F. *Notes on Nursing*. London: Duckworth, 1859.

6 Legge TM. *Industrial Maladies*. Oxford: Oxford University Press, 1934.

7 Proceedings of First International Conference *The History of Occupational and Environmental Protection, Rome 1999*. Oxford: Reed Elsevier (in press).

8 Schilling RSF. *A Challenging Life*. London: Canning Press, 1998.

9 McDonald C. *Epidemiology of Work Related Disease*. London: BMJ Publishing, 1995.

10 McCaig R, Harrington M (eds.) *The Changing Nature of Occupational Health*. Sudbury: HSE Books, 1999.

Index

Page numbers in **bold** refer to the principal discussions; those in *italic* refer to tables.
The index is in letter-by-letter order, whereby spaces, hyphens and diagonal slashes are ignored.

abattoir workers
 anthrax 490
 brucellosis 491
 Campylobacter infections 493
 leptospirosis 496
 Lyme disease 497
 Q fever 498
 ringworm 502
 zoonoses 489
Abbeystead, methane incident 138
abdomen, gas in 362
abdominal discomfort, in lead
  poisoning 86, 87
abdominal disorders, as cause of back
  pain *479*
abdominal muscles, isometric exercises
  483
abdominal pain
 paraquat poisoning and *201*
 pesticide exposure and *200*
Aberdeen, sewer workers 137
abietic acid 638
abortion, enzootic in ewes 493
abortion, spontaneous 835
 anaesthetic gases associated with
   167, 831
 drugs associated with 831
 mercury and 831
 over- and under-reporting 835
 in semiconductor industry 172
 solvents causing 831
 visual display unit operators 445,
   832
abrasives, prescribed diseases due to
  54
abrasives production, aluminium lung
  and 701
abscesses, brucellosis 492
absenteeism
 alcohol-related 558–9
 shift work 584
absorption, of chemicals **68**, 221
 dermal 72, 77
 inhalation 71–2
 prevention 223
 rate 69
absorption, of metals 82
ABS rubber/plastics 237, 253, 264
abuse, *see* bullying; violence at work
acamprosate 563

Acaris siro 637, 643
acceleration
 in flying 365–6
 negative 366
acceleration atelectasis 363, 366
Access to Health Records Act 1990 58–9
Accident Compensation Scheme (New
  Zealand) 38
accidents 37, 38
 alcohol-related 558, 559
   preventive paradox 558
 shift work 583–4
 see also aircraft: accidents
acclimatization
 divers 347, 351
 heat 335, 337
 high altitudes 390, 391, *394*
acetaldehyde *224*, **245–6**
 carcinogenicity 245
 characteristics and uses 245
 clinical manifestations 245
 management 246
 metabolism/biochemical effects 245
acetazolamide, altitude sickness *387*,
   389, 391, 392, *394*
acetic acid 249
 production 245
acetone *247*
 cirrhosis due to 882
 as hazardous DIY material *6*
 occupational diseases caused by (EC
   schedule) *43*
 recycling, hepatotoxicity *884*
acetonitrile (methyl cyanide) 145
acetylacetone *247*
2-acetylaminofluorene, nitrogen
   oxidation 75
acetylation 76
acetylators, fast/slow 68
acetylcholinesterase (AChE) inhibition
   204–5, *205*
 by organophosphates 873
N-acetyl cysteine, as treatment for liver
   disease 887
acetylene (ethyne) 169, 239
 see also alkynes
N-acetylglucosaminidase, biological
   effect monitoring *19*
N-acetyl-β-D-glucosaminidase (NAG) 21,
   94, 95

acetylsalicylic acid, in decompression
   illnesses 355
acetyltransferase 76
N-acetyltransferases (NAT1 and NAT2)
   21
 metabolic polymorphisms with
   cancer susceptibility links *759*
aciclovir 512
acid anhydrides
 occupational asthma due to *634*,
   636, 639–40, 642, *647*
 see also specific acid anhydrides
acid anhydride workers, occupational
   asthma in 642
acid chlorides 236
acid mists 156
 aerodigestive cancers 809
 inorganic, carcinogenicity *814*
 lung and laryngeal cancer 808, *815*
 paranasal sinus cancer *815*
acid nitriles, formula and examples
   224
acidosis, metabolic 223
 methanol poisoning 241, 242
acid rain 155
Acinetobacter spp., in office buildings
   717
acitretin, radiation casualties 415
acneiform eruptions 904
acoustic impairment, benzene causing
   262
acoustic trauma 294
acquired immune deficiency syndrome,
   see AIDS
Acrilan 253
acrodermatitis chronica atrophica 497
acrodynia 852
acro-osteolysis 170, 732
acrylamide *224*, **250–1**
 acrylamide monomer poisoning 250
 carcinogenicity 250
 characteristics and uses 250
 clinical manifestations 250–1
 exposure limits 868
 genotoxicity 250, *777*
 management 251
 metabolism/biochemical effects 250
 neurotoxic effects 251, 868
acrylamide monomer poisoning, as
   prescribed disease due to *50*

acrylate glues, as hazardous DIY
        material 6
acrylates, dermatitis 735
acrylic emulsions, as hazardous DIY
        material 6
acrylic sealants 734
acrylonitrile (vinyl cyanide) 145, *224*,
        253
    carcinogenicity 253
    characteristics and uses 253
    clinical manifestations 253
    genotoxicity *777*
    hepatotoxicity *884*
    lung cancer 253
    management 253
    metabolism/biochemical effects 253
    occupational diseases caused by (EC
        schedule) *43*
acrylonitrile-butadiene-styrene, *see* ABS
        rubber/plastics
actinolite 680
Actinomyces, in office buildings 717
actinomycetes, thermophilic *654*, 654,
        655, 659
actinomycin, as tissue culture additive
        528
activated charcoal, *see* charcoal,
        activated
active noise reduction (ANR) 368
Acts of Parliament, *see individual Acts
        of Parliament*
acupuncture 457
    back pain 483
acute mountain sickness (AMS) **383–
        96**
    carbonic anhydrase inhibitors 391,
        392
    exercise *vs* rest 392
    incidence 383–4
    infection and 390
    on Mauna Kea *387*
    predisposition 388
    at risk groups 388–9
    treatment 391–4
    see also altitude sickness
adaptation, cold 328
addition compounds of carcinogens,
        see DNA adducts
adduct formulation, *see* DNA adducts
adenine 743
adenomas, non-genotoxic carcinogen
        mechanisms *765*
adenomatous polyposis 757
    familial, susceptibility and germline
        mutation *750*
adenosine triphosphate (ATP) 229, 902
S-adenosylmethionine (SAM) 229
adhesions, intra-abdominal 680
adhesive capsulitis 456
adhesives
    depigmentation due to 732
    as hazardous DIY material 6
adjudicating authorities, compensation
        schemes 39
adrenal cortex
    biotransformation capability *73*
    cancer risk and germline mutations
        751

adriamycin
    genotoxicity *777*
    as tissue culture additive *528*
adult respiratory distress syndrome
        (ARDS) 132
Advisory Committee on Dangerous
        Pathogens, UK 490, 498, 501
Advisory Committee on Genetic
        Modification, UK 532
Advisory Committee on Pesticides, UK
        197
aerodontalgia 362
aeroengineering workers, elbow pain
        458
aerosol cans, 1,1,1-trichloroethane
        (methyl chloroform) in 231
aerosol propellants 154
aerosols
    definition 124
    particle size 72
    sulphuric acid 156
aflatoxin-B₁ 742
    P53 gene mutations 754
African box wood (*Gonioma kamassi*)
        poisoning, as prescribed disease
        50
afterdamp 137
age
    confounding variable in carcinogen
        exposure monitoring 773–4
    contact dermatitis onset 726–7
    effect on biological monitoring 20
    metal absorption from
        gastrointestinal system 82
    and radiogenic cancer 406
Agent Orange 274
    neurotoxic effects 876
age-related hearing loss 290, 295
aggression, *see* bullying; violence at work
agranulocytosis
    nitrous oxide causing 168
    occupations/agents causing *4*
Agricola, Georgius 792, 920
agricultural workers/occupations
    anthrax 490
    carcinogenic risk in *815*
    dermatoses in 733
    infections **489–502**
    non-Hodgkin's lymphoma in 810
    prescribed diseases *49*
    zoonoses **489–502**
    see also farmers/farm workers
agrochemicals **195–219**
AIDS (acquired immune deficiency
        syndrome) 506–7
    cryptosporidiosis in 494
    see also HIV infection
aid workers, zoonoses 489
air
    cold and dry, provoking occupational
        asthma *634*
    composition *135*
    indoor, monitoring, *see* indoor air;
        indoor air pollution
    pollution, *see* air pollution
    rarefied, prescribed diseases due to
        46
    see also compressed air

air arc gouging, prescribed diseases due
        to *47*
air conditioning, hepatotoxicity in *885*
air-conditioning systems
    clean room 716
    cooling towers 709, 710, 711
    legionnaires' disease and 710
    sick building syndrome and 715
    ventilation pneumonitis and *654*,
        654, 655
aircraft
    accidents 374–5
        birdstrikes 370
        chemicals at crash sites 374
        medical factors 377
        post-traumatic stress disorder 548
        protection in 375
        during training 375
    ejection seats 375
    Fighter Index of Thermal Stress (FITS)
        333
    in-flight attendants, menstrual
        disturbances 830
    pressure loss 364
    pressurized cabins 364–5
    Public Health (Aircraft) Regulations
        1979 379
    see also decompression sickness
aircraft factory workers, elbow
        problems 458
aircraft industry, hepatotoxicity in *884*,
        891
aircrew
    clothing 367, 368
    fitness for flight 362, 372, 377–8
    medication approval algorithm 378
    natural radiation dose 407
    therapeutic drug use 378
    see also airline pilots
airline passengers
    deep vein thrombosis 379
    fitness for flight 379
    with medical conditions 379
    smoke hoods 375
airline pilots
    alertness 582
    drinking culture 374
    guidance documents for 13
    skin cancer 813
    see also aircrew
air monitoring 15
    carbon dioxide levels 139, 140
    oxygen levels 139
air pollution 125
    carbon monoxide 125, 144
    chlorine 128, 148
    dioxin exposures (Seveso incident)
        274–5, 876, 886, 890
    from fires 129–31
    fluorinated hydrocarbons 154
    in Germany, East *vs* West 616
    hydrogen chloride 149
    hydrogen fluoride 150
    hydrogen sulphide, New
        Zealand/Mexico 161
    indoor, *see* indoor air pollution
    inorganic dust disease and 665
    lead 83

major releases 126–8
methyl isocyanate release, Bhopal
    123, 165, 584
neighbourhood cases, beryllium
    disease 103
nitrogen dioxide 125
nuclear reactor incidents 131
ozone 158
sulphur dioxide 125, 155
sulphur trioxide 156
toxic gases 123–4, 126–9
    see also gases; and specific gases
ventilatory function and 612
see also environment
air quality standards 125, 127, 144
air sickness 372–3
    adaptation 372–3
    prevention and treatment 372–3
    symptoms 372
air trapping, in extrinsic allergic
        alveolitis 598
air travel, spread of disease 379
airway
    changes in calibre, occupational
        asthma 644
    chronic air flow limitation 607–19
    hyperresponsiveness
        asthma 633, 634, 646
        in byssinosis 607
        see also bronchial hyperreactivity
    inflammation 633
    narrowing 633, 643
    in organic dust disease 664–5
    in protection from dusts 663–4
    reactivity, in cotton workers 624
    see also respiratory tract
airway constrictor response 623, 624
air workers 361
akinesia, in manganese poisoning 108
ALA, see 5-aminolaevulinic acid
ALAD, see 5-aminolaevulinic acid
        dehydratase
alanine aminotransferase (ALT) 226,
        251
    abnormal liver function tests 883
albendazole 495
albumin 849, 856
    increased excretion in cadmium
        workers 94
alcalase 637, 641, 643, 647
alcohol
    abstainers, mortality 559
    abuse, see alcohol abuse
    acute effects 557–8
    aircrew 374
    avoidance
        in heat acclimatization 335
        in thermal illness prevention 337
    blood alcohol levels, work
        competence and safety 558
    chronic heavy use 558
        see also alcohol abuse; alcoholism
    cobalt toxicity and beer 106
    as confounder in mortality
        interpretation 559
    dependence 557
    effect on biological monitoring 20
    epilepsy associated with 558

'heavy drinking' 565
hypothermia and previous alcohol
        intake 331
industrial accidents and 558
neurotoxic effects of exposures
        modified by 867
objective markers 562
reproductive hazards 829
Scottish surveys 558
screening, AUDIT (Alcohol Use
        Disorders Identification Test)
        560
styrene excretion affected by 265
in superficial frostbite 328–9
in trichloroethylene exposures, effect
        234
xylene metabolism affected by
        264
alcohol abuse 557
    absenteeism 558–9
    abstinence after 563
    accidents and 558, 559
        preventive paradox 558
    assessment 560
    CAGE questionnaire 573
    carbon tetrachloride hepatotoxicity
        228
    clinical features 561
    coercion? ethics and efficacy 562–3
    consent to tests 561
    contributing factors 559
    counselling 563
    deterrent medication 563
    driving licences
        high risk offender scheme 564
        vocational 564
    employee assistance programmes
        565
    identification 559–62
    management in the workplace
        559–60, 562–3
        constructive coercion 562–3
    mortality 559
    prevention 565
    prognosis 564
    screening 562
    successful treatment 563–4
    and violence at work 552
    withdrawal 563
    work competence and safety 557–8
    work factors contributing to
        problems 559
    workplace policies 562
    workplace problems related to
        557–9
alcohol dehydrogenase 76, 241
Alcoholics Anonymous (AA) 563
alcoholism 557
    Medical Council on Alcoholism,
        Doctors' and Dentists' Group
        565
    professions associated with 559
alcohols 239–43
    classification 239–40
    examples and formulae 224, 239,
        239–40
    see also alcohol; butanol; methanol;
        propanol

Alcohol Use Disorders Identification
        Test (AUDIT) 560
aldehydes 244–6
    formula and examples 224, 244
    see also acetaldehyde;
        formaldehyde; glutaraldehyde
aldicarb 196, 208, 209
aldrin 209
    dermal biotransformation 77
    epoxidation 74
    hepatotoxicity 893
alicyclic hydrocarbons and halogenated
        derivatives, occupational
        diseases caused by (EC schedule)
        43
aliphatic amines and halogenated
        derivatives, occupational
        diseases caused by (EC schedule)
        44
aliphatic chemical compounds 221–60
    disease diagnosis 221
    formulae and examples 224
    information sources 221, 223
    poisoning
        absorption prevention 223
        elimination 223
        first aid 223
        management principles 223
    see also organic chemical compounds;
        and individual chemicals
aliphatic hydrocarbons and
        halogenated derivatives,
        occupational diseases caused by
        (EC schedule) 43
aliphatic mixtures 224, 255–6
    see also white spirits
aliphatic nitrated derivatives,
        occupational diseases caused by
        (EC schedule) 43
Alkali Acts 1863 149
alkali industry 149
alkaline phosphatase 21
alkaline phosphatase isoenzymes,
        abnormal liver function tests
        883
alkanes 224–32
    branched 225
    chemical structures 224–5
    formula and examples 224, 224–5,
        225
    halogenated, see halogenated
        alkanes
    linear 225
    nomenclature 225
    see also halogenated alkanes; n-
        hexane
alkenes 232–7
    formula and examples 224
alkyd resins 639
alkyl amine gases 157–8
alkylaryl oxides, halogenated
        derivatives of, occupational
        diseases caused by (EC schedule)
        44
alkylaryl sulphonates, halogenated
        derivatives of, occupational
        diseases caused by (EC schedule)
        44

alkylating agents
    carcinogenicity 766
    genotoxicity *777*
alkyl naphthalenes 273
alkyl sulphates 242
alkyl thiocyanate insecticides 195
alkynes **239**
    formula and examples *224*, 239
allergenicity, characteristics 640
allergens
    allergic contact dermatitis 727
    chemical tests 729
    determination of concentration 647
    identification of 643
    patch testing 728–9
    respiratory ailments caused by (EC
        schedule) *44*
    skin diseases caused by (EC schedule)
        44
    see also sensitizers
allergens/allergen mixes,
        radioallergosorbent tests (RAST)
        21, 21–2
allergic alveolitis, cases reported to
        SWORD *31*
allergic contact dermatitis, *see* contact
        dermatitis
allergic rhinitis 713
    fitness for flying and 378
    as prescribed disease *52–3*
allergy
    to complex platinum salts 640
    to enzymes 637
    laboratory animal allergy (LAA) 636,
        636
    to latex 637–8
    occupational asthma and **640–1**
    see also atopy
alloying, lead use *844*
alloys
    beryllium 101
    cobalt 105
    copper 107
    nickel 109
    osmium 110
    platinum 110
    steel, *see* iron and steel
    tellurium 112
    tin 114
    vanadium 116
    zinc 116
allyl chloride
    hepatotoxicity *884*
    neurotoxic effects 868
Aloe vera 329
alpha-chloralose 212
alpha-particle emitters 115
alpha-particles *398*, 398
alstroemeria, contact dermatitis 734
Alternaria 716
Alternaria alternata 636, 653
Alternaria tenuis 623, 643
alternobaric vertigo 348
altitudes, high **383–96**
    at-risk groups 388–9
    carbon monoxide effects 145
    on land, gender and 386
    natural radiation at 407

sleep problems 389
    see also acute mountain sickness;
        altitude sickness
altitude sickness
    affecting physically fit 386
    infection and 390
    management *394*
    prevention 390–4
    susceptibility 386
    symptoms and signs 383, 384
        'Red Alert' symptoms 393, *394*
    treatment 391–4
    types of 383
    see also acute mountain sickness
alumina (aluminium oxide), neurotoxic
        effects 99
aluminium **99–100**
    absorption 99, 99–100
    biological monitoring tests and
        guidance values *18*
    brain as target for toxicity 184
    carcinogenicity/cancers *814*
    chronic obstructive lung disease and
        699
    encephalopathy 99, 871
    granulomatous lung disease due to
        702
    Hall–Heroult process 152
    intravenous absorption 100
    neurotoxic effects 871
    pot room asthma and 152
    production/manufacture, hazards
        152
    pulmonary fibrosis due to 99
    smelting, hazards 99
    Soderberg process 152
    'stamping' 99
    transport, bound to transferrin 100
    uses 99
aluminium citrate 673
aluminium lung 701
aluminium oxide (alumina), neurotoxic
        effects 99
aluminium phosphide 163, 210–11
    exposure
        occupational and accidental
            210–11
        routes of 210
    ingestion, deliberate 211
    management of poisoning 211
    toxicity mechanism 210
aluminium powder, prophylactic
        administration to miners 99, 673
aluminium production, genotoxic
        exposures *776*
aluminium silicates 696
aluminium smelting, as prescribed
        disease, urinary tract
        malignancies due to *51*
aluminium sulphate, water
        contamination, Camelford 25,
        100
aluminium workers, bladder and lung
        cancers *815*
alveolar cells, damage in acute silicosis
        673
alveolar concentration, volatile
        compounds 71–2

alveolar hydatid disease 495
alveolar ventilation, volatile compound
        delivery 71
alveoli, macrophage clearance of
        particles 664
alveolitis, acute silicosis 673
Alzheimer's disease
    aluminium and 99, 100
    magnetic field exposure and 446
Amblyseius cucermeris,
        radioallergosorbent tests (RAST)
        21
Amchem grass killer 249
American Academy of Otolaryngology
        and Ophthalmology (AAOO) 295
American Conference of Governmental
        Industrial Hygienists (ACGIH)
        151
    Biological Exposure Indices 17
    biological monitoring tests and
        guidance values *18*
    exposure limits
        benzine 262
        lasers 428–9, 432, 437
        styrene 265
        toluene 263
        o-toluidine 267
        xylene 264
    occupational exposure
        recommendations 7
    office building recommendations
        717
    vibration standards 318–19
American National Standards Institute
        (ANSI)
    laser exposure limits 428–9
    laser eye protection 432
    non-ionizing radiation 434, 437
    vibration 317, 319
Ames test 764, 766
    benzene 262
amides 249, **250–1**
    formula and examples *224*
    see also acrylamide;
        dimethylformamide
amine hardening agents, occupational
        asthma due to *647*
aminoaciduria
    in cadmium poisoning 94
    in lead poisoning 86
aminobenzene, *see* aniline
aminobiphenyl, DNA adducts 21
4-aminobiphenyl 797, *814*
    bladder malignancies *4*, 810
    genotoxicity *776*
amino-derivatives of benzene,
        prescribed diseases due to *50*
4-aminodiphenyl 269
2-aminoethanol, in nucleic acid
        extraction *529*
aminoglycosides, in brucellosis 492
5-aminolaevulinic acid (ALA) 85
    biological effect monitoring *19*
    urinary levels 85, 87
5-aminolaevulinic acid dehydratase
        (ALAD) 85, 87, 906
5-aminolaevulinic acid synthetase
        (ALAS) 886

p-aminophenol (metol), dermatoses 735
p-aminophenol haemoglobin conjugate, biological monitoring tests and guidance values *18*
aminopterin, as tissue culture additive *528*
2-aminotoluene, *see o*-toluidine
aminotriazole 204
  as non-genotoxic carcinogen *765*
amitriptyline 330, 483
amitrole 204
ammonia **157**
  anaerobic fermentation producing 135, 136
  characteristics and sources 157
  clinical manifestations 157
  health effect levels *127*
  London Blitz incident 123
  occupational asthma due to *634*
  occupational diseases caused by (EC schedule) *43*
  uses and exposure levels 157
ammonium compounds, in nucleic acid extraction *529*
ammonium hexachloroplatinate 640, 641, 643–4
ammonium persulphate, dermatoses 734
amoebae, humidifier fever and 712
amoebiasis, EC schedule of occupational diseases *44*
amoebic colitis 513
amosite (brown asbestos) 687
amoxicillin, Lyme disease 497
amphetamines, detoxification 74
amphibole asbestos 666, 686, 687, 695
  mesothelioma due to 693, 694
  protection suits 695
  see also asbestos
ampicillin, listeriosis 496
amputation, after accidental self-injection of veterinary products 214
α-amylase
  fungal 637
  radioallergosorbent tests (RAST) *21*
amyl nitrite 146
p-amyl phenol 272
amyl phenols 271
amyotrophic lateral sclerosis, magnetic field exposure and 446
anaemia **905–7**
  aplastic, *see* aplastic anaemia
  haemolytic, *see* haemolytic anaemia
  hypoproliferative 906–7
  iron deficiency 87
  lead-induced 23, 85, 87, 904, **905–6**
  megaloblastic, in arsenic poisoning 97
  methaemoglobinaemia 905
  microcytic, normocytic, macrocytic 904, 905
anaerobic fermentation 135–6
anaesthetic agents 124–5, **167–9**
  chloroform 230
  exposure standards 168

first aid 131
general anaesthetics 167–8
nephrotoxic effects 167
nitrous oxide 168–9
reproductive hazards 167, *828*, 829
  to embryo/fetus 831
scavenging systems 167, 168
trichloroethylene 233, 234
see also solvents
anaesthetists/anaesthetic room attendants 167–8
  gaseous hazards 167–8, 168
  opiate/anaesthetic misuse 565
  reproductive hazards 167, *828*, 829
analgesics
  back pain 482, 483
  hip and knee osteoarthritis *467*
analytes, in biological monitoring *18–19*, 19
anemometers 327
aneuploidy 744, 773
angina pectoris
  carbon monoxide poisoning and 144
  high altitudes 388
  methylene chloride use 143
angiogenesis 755
angioneurotic diseases caused by vibration, EC schedule of occupational diseases *45*
angiosarcoma of the liver 754, 809, 924
  in arsenic poisoning 97
  as prescribed disease *51*
  vinyl chloride exposure 170, 803
  vinyl chloride monomer causing 732
anhydrides 249
  mixed, radioallergosorbent tests (RAST) *21*
anhydrous hydrofluoric acid, *see* hydrogen fluoride
aniline 267
  biological monitoring tests and guidance values *18*
  methaemoglobinaemia due to 267
aniline glucuronide 75
'aniline tumours' 269
animal bites 499
animal handlers 494, 512
  protein contact dermatitis 731
animal products, prescribed diseases due to *48*
animal proteins, extrinsic allergic alveolitis due to 653
animals
  diseases transmitted from (EC schedule) *44*
  laboratory animals 636
    learned helplessness 541
  occupational asthma due to contact with 636, *636*, *647*
  prescribed diseases due to contact with *48, 49, 52, 53*
  reproduction and relationship to humans *825–6*, 836
  ruminant feed ban 500, 501
  toxicity testing, pesticides 197, 198
  urine proteins, occupational asthma due to *634*
  see also rodents

animal toxicity studies 68
  1,3-butadiene 237, 238
  1,2-dichloroethane (ethylene dichloride) 230
  extrapolation of reproductive hazard data 836
  fluorinated hydrocarbons 154, 155
  formaldehyde 245
  long-term carcinogenicity tests 766
  new methods 766–7
  non-genotoxic carcinogens *765*
  trichloroacetic acid (TCA) 249
  vinyl chloride 170
  vinylidene chloride 236
  xylene 264
ankles
  annual radiation dose limits *409*
  oedema 336
ankylosing spondylitis
  as cause of back pain *479*
  clinically similar to 'poker back' 151
ankylostomiasis 924
  as prescribed disease *49*
anorexia, in decompression illness 352
anosmia, in cadmium poisoning 94
Antabuse, *see* disulfiram
anthophyllite 680, 687
  pleural plaques due to 690
anthracene 272
  skin diseases caused by (EC schedule) *44*
anthracene compounds, skin diseases caused by (EC schedule) *44*
anthrax 489, **490–1**, 735
  cutaneous 491
  early studies 924
  immunization 490, 491
  intestinal 491
  as prescribed disease *48*, 491
  pulmonary 491
antibiotics
  contact dermatitis 730
  β-lactam, allergenicity 640
  leptospirosis 496
  listeriosis 496
  Lyme disease 497
  occupational asthma due to *634*, *636*, *647*
  prescribed diseases due to *52, 53*
  radiation casualties 401
  as tissue culture additives *528*, 529
  see also specific antibiotics
anticholinesterase poisoning, *see also* organophosphate pesticides
antidepressants 549
anti-emetics *394*
  radiation casualties 414
anti-epileptic drugs, back pain 483
anti-freeze solutions, methanol in 241
antifungals 502
antigen level detection, sick building syndrome and 716
anti-G straining manoeuvre (AGSM) 366
antihelminthics 495
  accidental self-injection with 214
antihistamines 373, 627
anti-inflammatory drugs, back pain 483

anti-knock agents 83, 810, 872
  carbon tetrachloride and 228
  1,2-dibromoethane (ethylene
      dibromide) 232
  1,2-dichloroethane (ethylene
      dichloride) 230
  ethane 169
antimalarials 512–13
antimoniosis 701
antimony **100–1**, 163
  arsenic and 100
  carcinogenicity 100–1
  derivatives, occupational diseases
      caused by (EC schedule) 44
  ECG changes 100
  lung cancer and 100
  occupational diseases caused by (EC
      schedule) 44
  pneumoconiosis and 100
  toxic effects 100
  uses 100
  workers 100
antimony hydride (stibine) 101, 163
  acute lung injury due to 698, 698
antimony pentachloride, acute lung
      injury due to 698, 698
antimony pneumoconiosis 701
antimony spots 100
antimony trichloride, acute lung injury
      due to 698, 698
antimony trioxide 163
antimony trisulphide 100
antineoplastic drugs
  monitoring occupational exposure to
      774–5
  reproductive hazards to
      embryo/fetus 831
  as tissue culture additives 528
anti-oncogenes, see tumour-suppressor
      genes
anti-spasmodic drugs, back pain 483
α1-antitrypsin, non-invasive screening
      882
anti-vibration chainsaws 317
anti-vibration gloves 317
ANTU (1-naphthylthiourea) 269
  biotransformation 77
anxiety 573
  anxiety symptoms 572
  presentation 572
Apiaceae, contact dermatitis 734
aplastic anaemia 130, 210, 906–7
  agents causing 4, 906–7
    benzene 4, 262, 262–3, 906
  occupations causing 4
apoptosis, in DNA repair 746
aquamarine 101
aqueous 421, 422
arc-eye 6, 185, 434
archaeologists
  infections 515
  rabies 499
arc lamps, eye damage from 420
arc welding, see welders/welding
argon 140
  in earth's atmosphere 135
argon lasers 427, 428
  exposure limits 429

eye damage from 420
argyria 112
armed forces
  alcohol-related problems 559
  exposure to fumes 159
  leptospirosis 496
  war gases 171
  zoonoses 489
Armstrong line 362
aromatic amines (arylamines) **267–70**
  acetylation 21
  bladder cancer 267, 268, **269–70**,
      792, 815
  derivatives, occupational diseases
      caused by (EC schedule) 44
  dermatitis 270
  occupational diseases caused by (EC
      schedule) 44
  see also 2-naphthylamine; o-
      toluidine; and other organic
      amines
aromatic chemicals **261–79**
  fused ring compounds 272–3
  see also individual chemicals/groups
      of chemicals
aromatic compounds 223, **272–5**
aromatic hydrazines and derivatives,
      occupational diseases caused by
      (EC schedule) 44
aromatic hydrocarbons
  halogenated derivatives of,
      occupational diseases caused by
      (EC schedule) 43
  nitrated derivatives of, occupational
      diseases caused by (EC schedule)
      44
  see also polycyclic aromatic
      hydrocarbons; polynuclear
      aromatic hydrocarbons
aromatics, EC comparable data
      collection 41
arrhythmias, pesticide exposure and
      200
arsenic **95–7**
  antimony and 100
  biological monitoring tests and
      guidance values 18
  cancers due to 814
  carcinogenicity 700
  environmental poisoning, West
      Bengal and Bangladesh 893
  excretion 96
  genotoxicity 776
  in hair and nails 96, 97
  half-life 96
  hepatotoxicity 884, 885, 892–3
    treatment 887
  liver cancer 886
  lung and sino-nasal cancers 815
  metabolism 96
  nephrotoxicity 853
  neurotoxic effects 871
  occupational diseases caused by (EC
      schedule) 43
  peripheral neuropathy 871
  poisoning, see arsenic poisoning
  prescribed diseases due to 49, 50, 97
  sources 95

supervision of workers 97
  urine levels 97
  uses and historical uses 95–6
arsenical insecticides, lung and skin
      cancers 815
arsenical pesticide workers, lung cancer
      815
arsenical pigments 96
arsenicals, causing aplastic anaemia
      907
arsenic compounds
  carcinogenicity 814
  genotoxicity 776
  in insecticides 195
  lung and skin cancers 815
  occupational diseases caused by (EC
      schedule) 43
  prescribed diseases due to 49, 50
arsenic poisoning 96–8
  acute 96
  cancer and 96, 97, 807
  chronic 96–7
  hepatocellular toxicity 97
  neurotoxic effects 96–7
  peripheral neuropathy 96–7
  as prescribed disease 49, 50, 97
  skin cancer 96
  symptoms and signs 96, 96–7
arsine 96, 97, **162–3**, 853
  acute lung injury due to 698, 698
  Asiafreighter incident 162
  characteristics and sources 97,
      162–3
  chronic poisoning 163
  clinical features of poisoning 162–3
  hepatotoxicity 885
  organic derivatives 97
  in semi-conductor industry 162, 172
  stibine association 101
arterial concentrations, inhaled
      compounds 72
art glass manufacture, genotoxicity 777
arthralgia
  brucellosis 492
  lead poisoning 86
arthritis
  Campylobacter infection 493
  frostbite arthritis 329
  in Lyme disease 497
arthropods
  occupational asthma due to 647
  prescribed diseases due to contact
      with 52, 53
artificial respiration, hydrogen cyanide
      poisoning 131, 146
arylamines, see aromatic amines
aryl esterases 75
aryl hydrocarbon hydroxylase,
      metabolic polymorphisms with
      cancer susceptibility links 758
aryl hydrocarbon hydroxylase receptor,
      metabolic polymorphisms with
      cancer susceptibility links 758
asbestiform fibres, in talc, lung cancer
      815
asbestos 686, 817
  amosite (brown) 687
  amphiboles, see amphibole asbestos

anthophyllite 680, 687
in buildings 695
cancer sites *815, 816*
carcinogenicity *4*, 779, 802–3, *814*
  epidemiological history 802–3
  fibre dimensions and 686
  gastrointestinal cancer 694
  laryngeal cancer 691
  latent interval 665
  lung cancer, *see* lung cancer
  mesothelioma, *see* mesothelioma
chrysotile (white), *see* chrysotile
complications in the form of
    bronchial cancer, EC schedule of
    occupational diseases *44*
countries banning use of 687–8, 695
crocidolite (white), *see* crocidolite
exposure limits 695
exposure sources 686
genotoxicity *776*
industries/users, respiratory tract
    malignancies *4*
P53 gene mutations 755
prescribed diseases related to *52, 54,*
    689
research into hazards 687–8
risk to welders 182, 183, 184
smokers and 691
substitutes for 696–7
varieties 686
see also asbestosis; mesothelioma
asbestos bodies 666, 680, 688
asbestos dust
  EC comparable data collection *41*
  mesothelioma after inhalation of,
      occupational diseases caused by
      (EC schedule) *44*
  prescribed diseases due to *52, 54,*
      689
asbestos exposure 793
  peripheral NK cells and 22
  smokers and 816
asbestosis 688–9
  chest radiography 688
  clinical features 688–9
  confluent fibrosis 666
  cryptogenic fibrosing alveolitis *vs*
      660
  EC schedule of occupational diseases
      44
  imaging 596, 600–2
  malignancy 687, 689
  mortality *29*
  pathology 688
  as prescribed disease *52, 54,* 689
  see also lung cancer; pulmonary
      fibrosis
asbestos minerals 686–7
asbestos-related diseases **687–95**
  asbestos warts 688
  bilateral diffuse pleural thickening
      691
  epidemiology 695
  history 687–8
  pathogenesis 694
  pleural effusion in 601, 690–1
  pleural plaques 690
  prevention 695

pulmonary fibrosis, *see* asbestosis
  see also lung cancer; mesothelioma
asbestos substitutes
  carcinogenicity 808
  see also man-made vitreous fibres
asbestos warts 688
asbestos workers, carcinogenic risk *815*
ascites, treatment 887
ascorbic acid 112, 268
aspartate aminotransferase (AST) 226,
    251, 562
aspartate transaminase (AST), abnormal
    liver function tests 883
Aspergillus spp. 525
  radioallergosorbent tests (RAST) *21*
Aspergillus clavatus 654, 655
  spores 653, 655
Aspergillus fumigatus 711
Aspergillus niger 524, *527,* 623
Aspergillus oryzae 637
Aspergillus penicillium, ill health due
    to, in biotechnology *527*
asphyxia 136
  welders 182
asphyxiant gases 124
  chemical 124, **141–7**
  first aid for 131
  hypoxia due to 134
  oxygen treatment 131
  simple 124, **137–41**
  see also gases; *and specific gases*
Aspinall v Sterling Mansell Ltd (1981) 59
aspirin
  in decompression illnesses 355
  xylene exposure and 264
assembly line workers
  shoulder tendinitis *455*
  tension neck syndrome 457
  thoracic outlet syndrome 457
assertiveness training 544
assistive devices, hearing loss 300
AST, *see* aspartate aminotransferase;
    aspartate transaminase
asteatotic eczema 734
Asteraceae, contact dermatitis 733
asthma
  cases reported to SWORD *31*
  cobalt asthma 699
  cryptogenic 608
  definition 633
  initiators 633
  irritant-induced 633, 635, 699
    diagnostic criteria *635*
    hypersensitivity-induced *vs* 633–4
  in population at large 616
  provokers 633
  vehicle exhausts and 616
  see also asthmatics; bronchial asthma
asthma, occupational 5, **633–51**
  agents causing *634, 636,* 636–40,
      713
    acid anhydrides *634, 636,* 639–40,
        642, *647*
    cobalt 106
    colophony *634, 636,* 638–9, 641
    complex platinum salts *634, 636,*
        640, *647*
    diisocyanates 639

enzymes *634, 636,* 637
flour *634, 636,* 637, *647*
glutaraldehyde 246
grain dust *636,* 636–7
laboratory animals 636, *636*
latex *634, 636,* 637–8
methyl methacrylate 250
nickel inhalation 110
platinum 110
wood dusts 638, *647*
allergy and 640–1
biotechnology hazard *527,* 528
byssinosis as 607
chemical inducers 613–14
chronic obstructive pulmonary
    disease (COPD) and 607–8
compensation, statutory 647
definition 633
determinants/factors affecting
    641–2
  atopy 641
  exposure duration 646
  exposure intensity 641
  human leucocyte antigen (HLA)
      phenotype 642
  smoking 8, 641–2
diagnosis 642
differential diagnosis 642
duration of exposure 646
EC comparable data collection *41*
grain dust causing 613
hypersensitivity-induced 633, *634,*
    634, 642
  causes 636–40
  irritant-induced *vs* 633–4
IIAC recommendations 40
importance 634–5
incidence 634
indoor air pollution and **713**
inducers, naturally occurring
    613
initiators 633–4, *634*
investigations 643–5
  immunological 643–4
  inhalation tests 644–5
  peak expiratory flow (PEF)
      measurement 643
irritant-induced 633, *634,* 635
  diagnostic criteria *635*
  hypersensitivity-induced *vs*
      633–4
isocyanates causing 613
management 646
metal-induced 699–700
  causes 699–700
  clinical characteristics 699
outcome 645–6
pot room asthma 152, 699–700
as prescribed disease 647, *647*
  agents causing *53–4*
prevalence 634
prevention 646–7
provokers 633–4, *634*
questions about 5
welding fume exposure 182–4, 616
see also asthmatics
asthma-like condition, in aluminium
    workers 99

asthmatics
    CS gas and 172
    high altitudes 389
        treatment clinics 389
    hydrogen sulphide and 160
    nitrogen dioxide sensitivity 159
    ozone exposure affecting 158
    sulphur dioxide sensitivity 156
astronauts, nitrogen dioxide exposure
        159
ataxia telangiectasia 400, 405, 406, 746
    susceptibility and germline mutation
        750
atelectasis, round atelectasis 602
atherosclerosis 144
athletes, carbon monoxide levels 143
atmospheric monitoring, see air
        monitoring
atomic bomb radiation 403, 403–4, 405
atomic weapons, uranium in 115
atoms 397
atopy
    byssinosis and 623, 624–5
    irritant contact dermatitis
        susceptibility 728, 729
    occupational asthma development
        641
    see also allergy
atropine
    in acute carbamate poisoning 209
    in acute organophosphate poisoning
        207
    in organophosphate poisoning 873
attapulgite 696
audiograms
    4kHz notch 290, 291, 293, 295
    6kHz notch 290, 293
audiometry 298
    cortical evoked response (CERA)
        302–3
    electric response (ERA) 298, 300–3
    evoked response 300–3
    pure tone 298
    self-recording 298
    sweep frequencies 298
Audiometry in Industry 298
AUDIT (Alcohol Use Disorders
        Identification Test) 560
auditory brainstem response (ABR)
        301–2
aural disorders, see hearing loss; noise;
        occupational noise-induced
        hearing loss
auramine
    bladder cancer 4, 269, 810
        as prescribed disease 51
    manufacture
        carcinogenicity 814, 815
        genotoxic exposures 776
auramine manufacture, carcinogenic
        risk in 815
Aureobasidium pululans 711
Australia
    repetitive strain injury (RSI)
        compensation 462
        proposed clinical grading scheme,
            New South Wales 463
    workers compensation schemes 571

autoclave workers, vinyl chloride
        exposure 170
autoimmune deafness 293
autoimmune disorders, non-invasive
        screening 882
autoimmune hepatitis, non-invasive
        screening 882
autonomic function tests 867
avian chlamydiosis 492–3
    as prescribed disease 49, 493
avian excreta and bloom, extrinsic
        allergic alveolitis due to 654,
        655
avian serum proteins, bird fancier's
        lung 653, 654, 655
aviation, see entries beginning with air
aviators, see aircrew; airline pilots
avocado, latex sensitivity and 638
Avomine 373
axonal swelling
    carbon disulphide exposure 869
    n-hexane exposure 870
azacytidine, genotoxicity 777
azaperone, accidental self-injection
        with 214
azathioprine 659
    genotoxicity and 776
azodicarbonamide
    occupational asthma due to 647
    prescribed diseases due to 52, 53
azodicarbonamide workers 646
azoospermia, causes 829, 829
azotaemia 229

Babesia microti 497
bacille Calmette–Guérin (BCG) 510–11,
        675
Bacillus spp. 523
    in office buildings 717
Bacillus anthracis 490
Bacillus subtilis 524, 525, 711
Bacillus subtilis enzymes, occupational
        asthma and 637, 641, 643, 647
back pain 477–86
    acute 478, 479
    assessment 479–80
    biomechanical factors 480
    causes 478–9
    change of work 481–2
    chronic 478–9, 483–4
    chronicity 481, 482
    classification 478–9, 479, 482
    costs of 478
    disability 477–8
    disability benefits 478
    emergency referral indications 479
    ergonomic advice 481–2
    examination 479–80
    exercise for 481, 483
    fitness and 480
    functional restoration programmes
        484
    guidelines on lifting weights 481–2
    hydrotherapy 483
    imaging 479–80
    injection therapy 483
    magnitude of problem 477–8

    manipulation 482–3
    medication 482, 483
    nerve root pain/compression 479,
        479, 480, 483
    non-specific 478, 479
    OPCS survey 477
    physiotherapy 482–3, 483
    predictive factors 480
    pre-employment screening 481
    prevalence 477
    prevention 481–4
        primary 481–2
        secondary 482–4
    prevention training 481
    probability of returning to work 478
    psychosocial risk factors 480–1, 481,
        483
        yellow flag symptoms 481
    recurrent 477, 478, 483
    referred 479
    rest, benefits? 482
    risk factors 480–1
    sciatica 477, 482
    simple 479, 482
    spinal pathology, red flag symptoms
        479
    subacute 482–3
    treatment 482–4
    vibration causing 318
    work loss 477–8, 481
baclofen, back pain 483
Bacon, Francis, Lord 289
bacteria
    extrinsic allergic alveolitis 711
    humidifier fever 712
    sick building syndrome 716–17
    see also health care workers
bacterial diseases, as cause of back pain
        479
bacterial endotoxins 623
bagasse 655
    dust inhalation, EC schedule of
        occupational diseases 44
    handling, prescribed diseases due to 49
    mouldy, extrinsic allergic alveolitis
        due to 654
bagassosis 654, 654, 655
Baker, George Sir 82
bakery workers, occupational asthma
        and 634, 635, 637, 641
balanced living, training 578
BAL (British anti-lewisite), see dimercaprol
bananas, latex sensitivity and 638
banding, as varices treatment 887
Banti's syndrome 885
barbers, genotoxic exposures 777
baritosis 101, 701
barium 101
barium carbonate (witherite) 101
barium dust inhalation, EC schedule of
        occupational diseases 44
barium fumes, in welding fume 185
barium nitrite 101
barium pneumoconiosis 701
barium sulphate (barytes) 101
barley 655
barley dust
    occupational asthma due to 647

prescribed diseases due to *52, 53*
barley flour, radioallergosorbent tests
  (RAST) *21*
barometric pressure
  raised **343–60**
    see also diving; hyperbaric
      environment
  reduced **361–5**
    gas expansion 361–2
    in space flight 375–6
    see also acute mountain sickness;
      altitude sickness;
      decompression sickness;
      hypoxia
barotrauma **347–8**
  compression **347–8**
  decompression **350–6**
  as prescribed disease *46*, 355
  pulmonary, *see* decompression
    illnesses; pulmonary
    barotrauma
  see also diving; hyperbaric
    environment
Barr, Thomas 289
barrier creams 730
barytes (barium sulphate) 101
basal cell carcinoma, arsenic poisoning
  and 96
basal ganglia
  acute carbon monoxide poisoning 144
  see also Parkinson-like syndrome
basophilic granules in lead poisoning
  86
bat handlers, rabies immunization 499
bats, rabies 499
batteries
  cadmium in 849
  lead in 83
  nickel in 109
  stibine (antimony hydride) in 101
battery manufacture, lead use *844*
bauxite 152
bauxite smelting, aluminium lung and
  701
BCG, *see* bacille Calmette–Guérin
BCME, *see* bis(chloromethyl) ether
beat conditions 464
  EC comparable data collection *41*
  as prescribed diseases 464
beat elbow 464
beat hand 464
beat knee 464
Beck Depression Inventory 573
beclomethasone 627
becquerel (Bq), definition 398
beef, minced 494
beer
  arsenic in 892
  cobalt addition and effects 106
behavioural tests, *see also*
  neurobehavioural testing
Belgium, contaminated animal feed
  275
'bends' 351, 358, 364
Benefits Agency 39
bentonite(s) 681
  in paraquat poisoning treatment
    202

benz[a]anthracene 273
  genotoxicity *777*
benzalkonium chloride 713, 715
1,2-benzanthracene 272
benzenamine, *see* aniline
benzene **261–3**, 811, 817
  absorption 262
  aplastic anaemia due to 262, 262–3,
    907
  biological monitoring tests and
    guidance values *18*
  blood dyscrasias/malignancies *4*,
    262
  carcinogenicity 262, *814*
  characteristics and uses 261
  chronic poisoning 261, 262
  clinical effects 262
  confused with benzine 9, 261
  EC comparable data collection *41*
  in exhaled breath 262
  exposure limits 262
  as genotoxic carcinogen 262
  genotoxicity *775, 776*
  haematological effects 907
  hepatotoxicity *884*
  leukaemia and 32, 75, 909
  leukaemogenesis *775*
  lymphatic and haemopoietic system
    cancers *815*
  metabolism 262
  metabolites 262, 909
  monitoring 262, 263
  myelodysplasia and 910–11
  in nucleic acid extraction *529*
  occupational diseases caused by (EC
    schedule) *43*
  prescribed disease due to *50*, 263
  preventive measures 263
  reproductive hazards, to mother 830
  risk assessments 262
  sino-nasal cancer and leukaemia
    816
  as solvent 909
  toxicity, bone marrow 74–5
  see also petrol
benzene chloride 266
benzene counterparts, occupational
  diseases caused by (EC schedule)
  43
benzene derivatives **261–7**
  amino-derivatives 266
  chloro-derivatives 266
  nitro-derivatives 266
  poisoning, as prescribed disease *50*,
    263
benzene epoxide, metabolism 74
γ-benzene hexachloride, causing
  aplastic anaemia 907
benzene insecticides 209
benzidine 267, 269, 797
  bladder cancer *4*, 792, 810
  carcinogenicity *814*
  genotoxicity *776*
  hepatotoxicity *884*
  urinary tract neoplasms due to *51*
benzidine-based dyes, genotoxicity *777*
benzine 255
  confused with benzene 9, 261

benzo[a]pyrene 272, 273, 745
  carcinogenicity 272, 273
  genotoxicity *777*
  hydroxylation 75
  lung and bladder cancers *815*
benzo[a]pyrene-7,8-diol-9,10-epoxide
  75
benzoates 263
benzodiazepines 389
  addicts 563, 564
benzol, *see* benzene
benzoquinones, occupational diseases
  caused by (EC schedule) *44*
1,2-benzpyrene, *see* benzo[a]pyrene
benzyl benzoate 511
benzyl methyl ketone 74
beryl (beryllium aluminium silicate)
  101
beryllia 101
berylliosis, *see* beryllium poisoning:
  chronic beryllium disease
beryllium **101–4**, 701–2
  carcinogenicity 103, 808, *814*
  chronic obstructive lung disease and
    699
  dusts and inhalation of 102, 103
  genotoxicity *776*
  hepatotoxicity *884, 885*, 893
  lung cancer due to 700
  nephrotoxicity 853
  occupational diseases caused by (EC
    schedule) *43*
  occurrence and properties 101
  prescribed diseases due to *50*, 103
  reproductive hazards to mother 830
  thermal protection 101
  uses 101
  workers, supervision 104
beryllium alloys, hepatotoxicity *884*
beryllium aluminium silicate (beryl)
  101
Beryllium Case Register 101, 103
beryllium compounds
  carcinogenicity *814*
  genotoxicity *776*
  occupational diseases caused by (EC
    schedule) *43*
  prescribed diseases due to *50*
beryllium lung 701–2
beryllium lymphocyte proliferation test
  102
beryllium oxide, acute lung injury due
  to *698*
beryllium phosphor 101
beryllium pneumoconiosis, sarcoidosis
  vs 666
beryllium poisoning 101–3
  acute 101–2
  chronic beryllium disease 102–3,
    701–2
    beryllium sensitivity *vs* 103
    classification (groups) 102
    diagnosis 102–3
    genetic factors 702
    pathogenesis 103
    presentation and clinical course
      702
    prognosis 103–4

beryllium poisoning – *contd*
  chronic beryllium disease – *contd*
    pulmonary function 102
    radiographic changes 102
    sarcoidosis *vs* 102, 702
    symptoms 102
    treatment 103
  neighbourhood cases 103
  occupational hygiene 104
  as prescribed disease *50*, 103
  skin disease 102
beryllium sensitivity, chronic beryllium
    disease *vs* 103
beta-blockers, as varices treatment 887
beta particles (β-particles) *398*, 398
Bhopal incident 123, 165, 584
bias
  in cohort studies 801
  'healthy worker' effect 799
  infertile worker effect 835
  recall bias 799, 834
  in reproductive hazard investigations
    835
bichromates, prescribed diseases due to
    52
bicipital tendinitis *454*, 456
bilirubin, abnormal liver function tests
    883
biocides
  asthma and 713
  dermatoses 734
  sick building syndrome and 715, 716
Biojec, accidental self-injection with
    213
biological agents
  EC comparable data collection *41*
  prescribed diseases due to *48–9*
Biological Agents Directive 502
biological effect monitoring 15, 16
  analyte choice 19
  recent developments 20
biological exposure
  monitoring 16
  standards 7
Biological Exposure Indices (BEI) 7, 17,
    18
biological monitoring 15, 16
  action levels 17, *18*
  analyte choice 19
  benchmark concept 17
  benchmark guidance values 17
  of cadmium 23
  of carbon monoxide 23–4
  carcinogen exposure in the
    workplace 767–75
  of carcinogenic substances 23
  carcinogens and susceptibility 21
  confounding factors 773–4
  creatinine correction 20
  detection of renal effects 21
  diagnosing occupational and
    environmental diseases 22–5
  ethical issues 16–17
  examples in occupational cancer
    768–9
  guidance values 17, *18*
  of hand–arm vibration syndrome
    (HAVS) 22

health guidance values 17
hygiene-based benchmark value 16
interfering/confounding factors 20
inter-individual variation 773
for mercury 23
method 767–73
for multiple chemical
    hypersensitivity 24–5
of mutagenic substances 23
no-adverse effect levels 16, 17
non-specific symptoms 25
  multifactorial approach 24
non-statutory guidance 17
in occupational cancer, examples
    768–9
occupational exposure to anti-
    neoplastic drugs 774–5
pesticides 198–9
practical considerations 19–20
quality assurance 20
recent developments 20
of renal effects 21
of respiratory effects 21–2
results interpretation 17
sample choice 19
sampling time *18*, *19*, 20
setting up of programme 19
specimens 767
suspension levels 17
tests and guidance values *18*
see also monitoring of workers
biological response modifiers,
    manufacture of 522
Biologische Arbeitsstofftoleranzwerte
    (BAT) 17, *18*
biomarkers
  effects of metabolic polymorphisms
    on *770–2*
  of exposure and early effects and of
    susceptibility 774
  prediction of cancer risk? 774
  of susceptibility 15
  types 767
biomass production 524
biomechanical factors, in back pain
    480
biomonitoring, *see* biological
    monitoring; biomarkers
biopsychosocial model of health 925
biotechnology **521–35**
  cancer association in workers 528,
    532, 533
  containment levels *530*, 531, *531*
  control measures 531, *531*
  definition 521
  development 521–2
  donor organisms 523
  downstream processing *525*, 526
  environmental considerations 530
  genetic modification, *see* genetic
    modification
  hazards
    biological hazards 526–8
    biological processes and 525–6
    chemical hazards *528*, 528–9, *529*
    classification scheme 530
    communication about 531
    contamination organisms 528

ergonomic hazards 529
    guidelines on risk assessment and
      control 522
    mental stressors 529–30
    physical hazards 529
    toxic effects 528
  health surveillance 532–3
  incidents of ill-health 526, *527*
  industrial applications 521, 522, 525
  medical records/contact cards 533
  monitoring of workers 532–3
  organisms used in 523–4
  products 524–5
  regulations 522–3
  stages in 525–6
  storage of serum samples 533
  therapeutic/prophylactic products
    522
  tissue culture additives *528*
biotite 680
biotransformation
  comparative capability of organs *73*
  dermal 77
  extrahepatic sites 76
  phase 1 73, 73–5
  phase 2 73, 75–6
  pulmonary 76–7
  see also detoxification; metabolism
biphasic decompression illness, case
    history 353
biphenyls, hepatotoxicity *884*
bird fancier's lung *654*, 654, **655**
  chest radiograph 658
  management 660
  see also extrinsic allergic alveolitis
birds
  chlamydiosis 492
  Newcastle disease from 498
  prescribed diseases due to contact
    with *49*
N,N-bis(2-chloroethyl)-2-
    naphthylamine
    (Chlornaphazine), genotoxicity
    776
bischloroethyl nitrosourea (BCNU),
    genotoxicity 777
bis(chloromethyl) ether (BCME) 10, *224*,
    252
  cancers due to *814*
  carcinogenicity 28, 252, *814*
  characteristics and uses 252
  clinical manifestations 252
  genotoxicity 776
  lung cancer 4, 252, *815*
    as prescribed disease *54*, 252, 807
  metabolism/biochemical effects 252
bismuth, nephrotoxicity 853
bites
  animal 499
  see also mosquitoes; ticks
bitumen
  prescribed diseases due to *50*
  skin diseases caused by (EC schedule)
    44
black damp 137
blackheads 731
blacksmith's deafness 289
black water fever 513

bladder cancer 742, 762, 810–11
  agents causing 4
  aromatic amines causing 267, 268, 269–70
  benzidine 267
  carcinogens 269–70
    aromatic amines 792
    2-naphthylamine, see 2-naphthylamine
  in coal gas manufacturers 28
  industries/occupations associated with 815
  latent period 269–70
  4,4′-methylene bis(2-chloroaniline) (MbOCA) causing 270
  2-naphthylamine causing 268, 269
  non-genotoxic carcinogen mechanisms 765
  occupational history 794
  occupations associated with 4, 269, 810
  oncogene activation in 749
  as prescribed disease 51
  in rubber workers 27–8
  screening 818
  smoking and 269, 810, 811
  surveillance for 269–70
  o-toluidine 267, 269
bladder dysfunction, back pain and 479
blanching of fingers
  episodic, as prescribed disease 48
  in hand-arm vibration syndrome 309, 309–10
  treatment 314
blast furnace gas 142
blast injuries, underwater 349
blast trauma 294
bleach
  chlorine 148
  dermatoses 734
bleomycin, as tissue culture additive 528
blepharoconjunctivitis 426
blisters
  in frostbite 329
  mercury compounds 91
blister (vesicant) agents 171, 171–2
blood analysis, radiation casualties 415
blood-borne viruses
  health care workers 502–9
  patient testing 508
  prescribed diseases due to contact with 49
  see also hepatitis B; HIV infection
blood–brain barrier, mercury distribution 91, 92
blood dyscrasias 907
  benzene 262
  occupations/agents causing 4
  as prescribed diseases 46
blood pressure, lead exposure and 86
Bloom's syndrome 746, 757
blowroom workers 622
Blue John 150
blue light damage 424, 425
board manufacturers
  hand/wrist tendinitis 459

shoulder tendinitis 455
bobbin cleaning, prescribed diseases due to 47
body burden 69
  lead 84–5
body clock 581
body compartments 69
body fluids, biomonitoring 767
body tissues
  biomonitoring 767
  vaporization at high altitudes 362
boilermakers, hearing damage 289
boilermakers' bronchitis 698
bone
  cysts, and vibration 310
  fluoride retained in 150, 151
  necrosis 356–8
    phosphorus causing 98
bone/bonemeal handlers/processors, anthrax 490
bone changes in children, lead poisoning 87
bone lead measurement 847, 848
bone marrow
  aplasia 400
    in radiation casualties 414
  benzene toxicity 74–5
  biological monitoring tests 18
  depression, by benzene 262
  erythroid hyperplasia 906
  erythroid hypoplasia 906
  graft rejection 402
  hypoplasia 906
    and ethylene glycol mono methyl ether 907
  myelodysplasia 75
  nitrous oxide induced changes 168
  radiation damage 400, 402
  radiation-induced aplasia 907–8
  sideroblastic 906
  threshold levels of radiation dose 400
  transplantation 908
  see also aplastic anaemia
bone marrow cancer, industries/occupations associated with 815, 816
bones, prescribed diseases 46
boot and shoe industry, see shoe manufacturing industry
Bordeaux mixture (copper sulphate), hepatotoxicity 885, 892
boric acid, male fertility/sexual behaviour 829
boron hydrides 166
boron trichloride 149
boron trifluoride 152
Borrelia burgdorferi 496
borrelial lymphocytoma 497
bovine animals, working with, prescribed diseases due to contact with 48
bovine spongiform encephalopathy (BSE) 500
bovine tuberculosis 489, 490
bowel dysfunction, back pain and 479
Bowen's disease, arsenic poisoning and 96

Bowman's layer 422
Boyle's law 344–5
brain
  AChE inhibition 205
  cancer risk and germline mutations 751
  cysts 356
  swelling, in lead poisoning 871
  target for aluminium toxicity 184
brain development, in children exposed to lead 87
brain injury, hypoxic 134
brain tumours 810
  electromagnetic field exposure 441–2, 444, 445
  occupations associated with 810
bread contamination
  hexachlorobenzene contamination, Turkey 266, 267
  4,4′-methylenedianiline, Epping jaundice incident 270, 883
break-off phenomena, air pilots 372
breast cancer
  airliner cabin attendants 374
  familial, susceptibility and germline mutation 750
  incidence 794
  lindane and 210
  male/female, electromagnetic field exposure and 442–3
  oncogene activation in 749
  radiogenic 406
  risk, and germline mutations 750, 751
breast feeding, biotechnology workers 531
breast milk
  1,2-dichloroethane in 230
  fluorides and 151
  mercury in 91
  postnatal exposure via 833
breath analysis 71, 72
breathing, see inhalation
breathing apparatus
  closed-circuit 344, 346, 349
  scuba 343
  self-contained 343
  underwater 332
breathlessness 665
  in acute allergic alveolitis 657
  in asbestosis 688
  in benign pleural effusion 691
  in byssinosis 626, 626
  in chronic (active) silicosis 673
  in chronic allergic alveolitis 658
  in mesothelioma 692
  paraquat poisoning and 201
  in pneumoconiosis 665
breath sampling 19
Brenner scheme, genetically modified organism risk assessment 530, 530
brewery workers, alcohol-related problems 559
bricklayers 727
British anti-lewisite (BAL), see dimercaprol

British Association of Audiological Physicians (BAAP) 294
British Association of Audiological Scientists (BAAS) 294
British Association of Counselling (BAC) 578–9
British Association of Otolaryngologists (BAOL) 294
British Medical Association Stress Counselling Service 565
British Society of Audiologists (BSA) 294
British Standards
    audiometric reference pressure 284
    hearing threshold of disability 295
    noise-excluding helmets 298
    non-ionizing radiation 437
    vibration 317, 319
British Thoracic Society 674
    tuberculosis guidelines 510–11
broadcasters, dry throat 713
brodifacoum 212
bromelain 637
bromine, occupational diseases caused by (EC schedule) 43
bromoacetic acid 232
bromoacetone, occupational diseases caused by (EC schedule) 43
5-bromo-4-chloro-3-indolyl phosphate p-toluidine, in nucleic acid extraction 529
bromodiolone 212
bromomethane, see methyl bromide
bromotrifluoromethane (Halon 1301) 155
bromoxynil 202
bronchi
    malignant neoplasms, occupations/agents causing 4
    primary carcinoma
        as prescribed disease 50
        see also lung cancer
bronchial asthma 624, 639, **699–700**
    cobalt causing 106
    high altitudes 390
bronchial cancer, EC schedule of occupational diseases 44
bronchial carcinoma 599
    imaging 602
bronchial hyperreactivity
    byssinosis 624–5, 625
    see also airway: hyperresponsiveness
bronchial inflammation, COPD and 610
bronchial lavage, see bronchoalveolar lavage
bronchiolitis obliterans 133
    COPD and 610, 612
    methyl isocyanate 165
    nitrogen dioxide 159
bronchitic changes, inorganic dusts 664–5
bronchitis 665
    biotechnology hazard 527
    cases reported to SWORD 31
    chromium causing 105
    chronic 608, 627–8, 664
        IIAC recommendations 39–40
        phosphorus causing 99
        as prescribed disease 55, 683, 684

coalworkers 40, 682, 683, 684
cotton vs man-made-fibre workers 627–8
eosinophilic 640
industrial 608
    welding fume and 615
inhaled diisocyanates causing 639
smokers' 608
welders and 183, 184
bronchoalveolar lavage
    asbestosis 688
    extrinsic allergic alveolitis 656–7
    pneumoconiosis 666
bronchoalveolitis, in zinc smelting 186
bronchodilators 627, 629
bronchopneumonia 698
    at high altitudes 387–8
bronchopulmonary ailments, EC schedule of occupational diseases 44
bronchorrhoea, pesticide exposure and 200
bronchus, see bronchi
Brucella infection 603
    as prescribed disease 49, 492
Brucella abortus 491
Brucella maris 491
Brucella melitensis 491
Brucella suis 491
brucellosis 490, **491–2**, 603
    clinical features 491–2
    diagnosis 491, 492
    EC schedule of occupational diseases 44
    epidemiology 491
    as prescribed disease 49, 492
    treatment 492
Bruch's membrane 423
brucite 686
BSE, see bovine spongiform encephalopathy
buccal ulceration, pesticide exposure/poisoning and 200, 201
budgerigar fancier's lung 655, 659
    see also extrinsic allergic alveolitis
building industry, see construction industries; vibration
buildings, radon concentrations in 407
building sickness, see sick building syndrome
building symptom index, sick building syndrome 715, 717
bullae 132
    carbon dioxide poisoning 139
bullets, lead in 83
bullying
    children and adults 541, 542
    mobbing 540
    research studies 540, 541
    at work **539–44**
        aim 540
        case histories 539, 542–3
        categories 540
        causes 542–3
        definitions 539–40, 541, 544
        directed at women 540
        effects of 540–2

gender and 543, 544
incidence 543
National Workplace Bullying Advice Line 543
perpetrators' characteristics 542
personality clash? 543, 544
prevalence 543–4
prevention 544
psychiatric disorders resulting from 541, 543
relationships with colleagues/managers 542
risk, large vs small organizations 544
victims' characteristics 540
victims' perceptions 540
victims' reactions to 541
see also violence at work
buoyancy aids 332
buprenorphine 328
Burkitt's lymphoma, oncogene activation in 749
burnout, see also bullying
burns
    ammonia 157
    bis(chloromethyl) ether (BCME) 252
    chlorine 133
    corrosive gases 132
    in fires 130
    fluorine 150
    in gassing accidents 131, 132
    mercury compounds 91
    methyl bromide 164
    methylene chloride (dichloromethane) 227
    microwave radiation 431
    organotin compounds 114
    phenol 271
    phosphorus 98
    radiation 401, 411, 415
    selenium dioxide 111
    silver nitrate 112
    thermal, radiation casualties 415
bursitis 459
    at/about elbow/knee, as prescribed disease 46
Burtonian line (blue line) on gums 83, 86, 92, 904
bus drivers, fear of assault and work-related stress 553
busulphan, genotoxicity 776
butadiene, leukaemia 813
1,3-butadiene 224, **237–9**
    carcinogenicity 238
    characteristics and uses 237
    clinical manifestations 238
    frostbite from 239
    genotoxicity 777
    management 238–9
    metabolism/biochemical effects 237
butane 225
n-butane 170
1,4-butanediol, occupational diseases caused by (EC schedule) 43
1,4-butanediol dimethanesulphonate, genotoxicity 776
butanol 242–3

1-butanol (*n*-butyl alcohol) *224*, 242, 243
2-butanol (*sec*-butyl alcohol) *224*, 242, 243
iso-butanol (2-methylpropan-1-ol) *224*, *239*, 242, 243
n-butanol *239*
sec-butanol *239*
tert-butanol (2-methylpropan-2-ol) *224*, *239*, 242, 243
butan-2-one, biological monitoring tests and guidance values *18*
butchers
  erysipeloid 501
  hepatitis B 503
  zoonoses 489
butene 232
butoxyacetic acid, biological monitoring tests and guidance values *18*
2-butoxyethanol, biological monitoring tests and guidance values *18*
butyl alcohol, occupational diseases caused by (EC schedule) *43*
n-butyl alcohol (1-butanol) *224*, 242, 243
sec-butyl alcohol (2-butanol) *224*, 242, 243
butylated hydroxyanisole, as non-genotoxic carcinogen *765*
butylated hydroxytoluene, as non-genotoxic carcinogen *765*
butylated hydroxytoluene (BHT), lung damage 77
butyl benzyl phthalate, carcinogenicity 766
p-tert-butyl catechol 271, 272
t-butyl methyl ketone *247*
p-tert-butyl phenol 271, 272
  hepatotoxicity *884*
butyl phenols 271
1-butyne *239*
2-butyne *239*
butyric acid 249
butyrylcholinesterase 876
byssinosis **621–31**
  acute 621, 625
  atopy 623, 624–5
  bronchial hyperreactivity 624–5, 625
  'bronchitic' 624
  chronic 621, 626–7
  chronic bronchitis 627–8
  classification/grading schemes *626*, 626–7
  clinical features 625–7
  cotton dust and 607
  grades 607–8
  immunological mechanisms 622–3
  investigations 627
  lung function 623, 625, *626*, 627
  management 629
  morbidity and mortality 625
  as occupational asthma 607
  pathogenesis 622–4
  pathology 622
  pharmacological responses 627
  physical signs 627
  as prescribed disease 52
  prevalence 622
  prevention 628–9
  radiology 627
  severity, by working days 626, 627
  smoking and 8, 622, 627
  textile dust causing 621, 622

cabinet making, *see* furniture makers/manufacturers
cable covering manufacturing, lead use 844
cable makers, bladder cancer *815*
cachexia, in mercury poisoning 89
cacodylic acid 96, 97
cadmium **93–5**
  absorption 82, 93
  ageing and 20
  biological effect indicators *19*
  biological monitoring 23
    tests and guidance values *18*
  blood levels 93, 95
  carcinogenicity/cancers due to *814*
  chronic obstructive lung disease due to 698
  chronic obstructive pulmonary disease due to 614
  decomposition 9
  dusts 93
  EC comparable data collection *41*
  emphysema due to 27, 94
  excretion 93
  genotoxicity *776*
  half-life 93
  hepatotoxicity *884*, *885*, 893
  hypertension and 94
  lung cancer due to 700
  metabolism 93
  nephrotoxicity, *see* cadmium nephrotoxicity
  occupational diseases caused by (EC schedule) *43*
  permissible exposure limits (PEL) 850
  poisoning, *see* cadmium poisoning
  smoking and 20, 93
  supervision of workers 95
  toxic pneumonitis due to 698
  urine levels 95
  uses 93, 849
  in welding 186
cadmium compounds
  carcinogenicity *814*
  genotoxicity *776*
  occupational diseases caused by (EC schedule) *43*
cadmium nephrotoxicity **849–51**
  clinical syndromes 850–1
  management 850, 851
  metabolism 849
  renal tubular dysfunction in 849–50
  toxicity 849
  treatment 851
  urinary excretion 850
  urinary markers 850–1
cadmium oxide fumes, poisoning 9, 93, 94
cadmium oxides, acute lung injury due to *698*, 698

cadmium poisoning 93, 94
  acute 94
  chronic 94, 95
  critical concentration in kidney 94, 95
  diagnosis and treatment 94–5
  itai-itai disease 94
  osteomalacia 94
  as prescribed disease *50*, 94
  signs and symptoms 94
cadmium workers 94
  monitoring 95
caesium
  ionizing radiation properties *398*
  radiation contamination treatment *413*
caesium-137 397
caffeine 234
CAGE questionnaire, alcohol abuse 573
caisson-workers 343
calcific tendinitis 455–6
calcination 682
calcium, lead effect on 85
calcium chromate, lung cancer as prescribed disease due to *54*, 105
calcium cyanide 145
calcium fluoride 150
calcium phosphate 98
calcium silicates 696
calculi, urinary 849
calendering, lymphatic and haemopoietic system cancers *815*
calomel (mercurous chloride) 852
Camelford, aluminium sulphate contamination of water 25, 100
Cameroon, Lake Nyos incident 139
Campylobacter 493, 513
Canada, workers' compensation schemes 38, 571
canal workers, leptospirosis 496
cancer
  'cancer genes' 748
  clonal composition 746–7
  as genetic disorder of somatic cells 742–3, 747, 763
  genetic predisposition 746
  genotype 757, 762
  hereditary and chromosomal anomalies 746
  metabolic polymorphisms
    differences in ethnic groups 762–3
    interactions between *760–1*
    and susceptibility to cancer 757–62, *758–9*
  oral 754
  phenotype 757, 762
  sporadic 757
  susceptibility to *750–1*, 756–7, *758–61*
    environmental factors 757
    metabolic polymorphisms 757–62, *758–9*
    oncodemes and 757
  see also specific cancers/carcinogens and cancer sites

cancer, occupational *4*, 5, **739–819**
  arsenic poisoning and 96, 97
  biological mechanisms 741–89
  biological monitoring tests *18*
  burden of 793–4
  carcinogens, *see* carcinogenesis;
      carcinogenicity; carcinogens
  causes 814, *815–16*
  clinical approach **805–13**
  clinical assessment procedures
      794–6, 805–6
  costs (direct/indirect) 794
  EC schedule *44*
  electromagnetic fields, long-term
      effect 440–4
  epidemiology, *see* epidemiological
      studies
  genetic modification work associated
      with 528, 532, 533
  incidence statistics 794
  interactions between causative
      agents 814–16
  investigations 805–6
  occupational factors, difficulty in
      identifying 796
  occupational history 794–6
  presentation (earlier/younger) 805
  prevention 794, **817–18**
    difficulties 817
    primary 817
  promoting agents 742
  public attitude 793
  scientific basis for establishing
      causality 796–7
  screening 817–18
  *see also specific cancers/carcinogens
      and cancer sites*
candidiasis, oral, in AIDS/HIV infection
      507
Caplan's syndrome 674, 686
capsaicin cream *467*, 467
capsulitis
  adhesive 456
  shoulder (frozen shoulder) *454*, 456
capsulotomy, posterior 427
captafol, genotoxicity *777*
carbamate insecticides 208–9
  acute poisoning 208–9
    complications 208–9
    management 209
  detecting exposure to 207–8
    electrophysiology 207
    measurement of cholinesterase
        activity 207
    monitoring 207–8
    organophosphate metabolites
        207
  hepatotoxicity *884*
  neurotoxic effects 873–4
  pre-employment assessment 208
  routes of exposure 208
    foodborne 208
  symptoms and signs of exposure to
      200
  toxicity
    acute 208
    chronic 208
    mechanism of 208

carbamazepine, back pain 483
carbapenam 640
carbaryl
  dermal biotransformation 77
  reproductive hazards *828*
carbaryl toxicity 208
carbazole/carbazole compounds, skin
      diseases caused by (EC schedule)
      44
carbofuran toxicity 208
carbohydrate-deficient transferrin (CDT)
      562
carbolic acid, *see* phenol
carbon-14 406
carbon bisulphide poisoning, as
      prescribed disease *50*
carbon dioxide **138–40**, 346, 639
  anaerobic fermentation producing
      135, 136
  in confined spaces 136
  in earth's atmosphere *135*
  in geothermal power production 173
  health effect levels *127*
  Kyoto Protocol agreement 135
  Lake Nyos incident 139
  as measure of rate of air exchange
      125
  monitoring levels of 139, 140
  respiration changes with 139
  toxic properties 139–40
  uses 138–9
  and welder's exposure to ozone 181
  in wells 140
carbon dioxide lasers
  exposure limits *429*
  eye damage from *420*, 430
'carbon dioxide retainers' 346, 349, 356
carbon dioxide scrubbers 346, 348, 349
carbon disulphide *224*, **253–5**
  biological monitoring tests and
      guidance values *18*
  characteristics and uses 253
  clinical manifestations 254–5
  coronary heart disease and 254, 255
  EC comparable data collection *41*
  long-term exposure 869
  male fertility/behaviour 829
  management 255
  metabolism/biochemical effects
      253–4
  neurotoxic effects 254, 868–9
  occupational diseases caused by (EC
      schedule) *43*
  overexposure syndromes 254
  psychiatric disturbances 254
  reproductive hazards 254, *828*, 829
carbon fibres 696
carbonic anhydrase inhibitors 391, 392
carbon monoxide **141–5**, 227
  acute poisoning 143–4
  in ambient air 144–5
  atherosclerosis and 144
  biological effect indicators *19*
  biological monitoring 23–4
    tests and guidance values *18*
  blood levels 142–3
  characteristics 142
  concentrations in gas mixtures 142

delayed deterioration 869
  in earth's atmosphere *135*
  effects at high altitude 145
  faulty heaters producing 125
  in fires 129, 130
  formula for calculating
      carboxyhaemoglobin levels
      142–3
  ischaemic heart disease 144, 145
  mechanism of action 142
  methylene chloride and 143
  in mines 137
  neurotoxic effects 869
  occupational diseases caused by (EC
      schedule) *43*
  pregnancy and 144, 144–5
  smokers, levels in 142
  sources 125, 136, **142**, 170
  toxic hazard to embryo/fetus 830
  treatment 869
  in welding fume 182
carbon monoxide poisoning
  angina pectoris 144
  clinical features 143–4
  delayed neurological sequelae 144
  hypoxia due to 134
  neuropsychiatric damage 143, 144
  neurotoxic effects 142
  oxygen treatment 131
  skin colour 131, 143
carbon oxychloride, occupational
      diseases caused by (EC schedule)
      43
carbon tetrachloride *224*, **228–9**
  absorption and distribution in body
      228
  aplastic anaemia due to 907
  carcinogenicity 228
  centrilobular necrosis and 883
  characteristics and uses 228
  cirrhosis due to 882
  clinical manifestations 229
  hepatotoxicity 226, 228, 229, *885*,
      890–1
    mechanisms of 887–9
    treatment 887
  management 229
  metabolism/biochemical effects 228
  mortality rate 891
  nephrotoxicity 228
  as non-genotoxic carcinogen *765*
  in nucleic acid extraction *529*
  phenothiazines and 882
  prescribed disease due to *51*
  pulmonary biotransformation 76
  structural formula 228
carbonyl chloride 228, 229
carbonyl compounds **244–51**
carbonyl fluoride 152
carbonyl sulphide 161–2
carboplatin 110
carborundum 701
carboxyhaemoglobin 142, 144, 227,
      869
  affecting work capacity 144
  biological effect monitoring *19*
  biological monitoring tests and
      guidance values *18*

half-life 131, 144
  measurement 142, 167
  produced from different substances
    20
carboxyhaemoglobin levels, in blood,
    health effects 24
carboxylesterases 75
carboxylic acids **249**
  chlorinated compounds 224
  formula and examples 224
  functional derivatives 249–51
carcinogenesis
  cell cycle 747
  genes involved **748–55**
    see also oncogenes; tumour-
      suppressor genes
  genetic change, evidence **742–7**
  initiation 741, 742
  ionizing radiation
    DNA damage 405
    no-fault compensation scheme
      404
    probability of causation (PC)
      404–5
    radiation effect 403–5
    risk estimates 403
    susceptibility factors 405–6
  long-term animal tests 766
  metastases, invasion mechanisms
    755–6
  multi-step process **741–2**
  pathways in 756
  processes perturbed during 747–8
  progression 741, 742
  promotion 741, 742
  somatic mutation theory 742
  see also carcinogenicity; carcinogens;
    DNA: damage; mutations
carcinogenicity 814, **815–16**
  acetaldehyde 245
  acrylamide 250
  acrylonitrile (vinyl cyanide) 253
  alkyl sulphates 242
  animal tests
    long-term 766
    new methods 766–7
  antimony 100–1
  aromatic amines 269–70
  asbestos, see asbestos:
    carcinogenicity
  benzene 262, 814
  benzo[a]pyrene 272, 273
  beryllium 103, 808, 814
  bis(chloromethyl) ether (BCME) 28,
    252, 814
  1,3-butadiene 238
  carbon tetrachloride 228
  chloroform 230
  chromium compounds 105, 807, 814
  cobalt 106, 700
  1,2-dibromoethane (ethylene
    dibromide) 232
  dichloroacetylene 239
  1,2-dichloroethane (ethylene
    dichloride) 231
  dimethylformamide 251
  dioxin (2,3,7,8-tetrachlorodibenzo-p-
    dioxin) 274, 814

epichlorohydrin (1-chloro-2, 3-
    epoxypropane) 252
  ethylene oxide 166, 814
  formaldehyde 244, 805, 808
  IARC monographs 802
  lead 85
  methyl chloride 165
  4,4'-methylene bis(2-chloroaniline)
    (MbOCA) 270, 810
  methylene chloride
    (dichloromethane) 227
  mineral fibres 697
  nickel 109, 700
  nickel carbonyl 166
  polycyclic aromatic hydrocarbons
    (PAHs) 152, 273, 741
  prediction, tests 774
  selenium 111
  sulphur dioxide 156
  sulphuric acid 156, 814
  testing chemicals for 763–7
  2,3,7,8-tetrachlorodibenzo-p-dioxin
    (dioxin) 274, 814
  tetrachloroethylene
    (perchloroethylene) 236
  o-toluidine 267, 269
  trichloroethylene 234, 755
  trihalomethanes 148
  vinyl bromide 170
  vinylidene chloride (1,1-
    dichloroethylene) 237
  white spirits 256
  see also carcinogens; and individual
    carcinogens
carcinogens 741, 814, 815–16
  biomonitoring in workplace **767–75**
  classes 741–2
  classification by genotoxicity 776–7
  epigenetic, see carcinogens, non-
    genotoxic
  established hazards, examples 776
  features of importance to cancer
    studies 793
  first produced experimentally 741
  genotoxic 741–2, 743–5, 765
    'acceptable levels' 766
    broad-spectrum, mechanisms
      775–8
  interaction of two or more 742,
    814–16
  mutagenic and DNA-damaging
    effects 743–5
  non-genotoxic 741–2, 765, 765–6
    mitogenesis 765, 766
  'no observable effect' levels 766
  occupational
    classification by genotoxicity
      776–7
    mechanisms **775–9**
  occupational history 794–6
  presumptive hazards, examples
    777
  proximate 74
  site-specificity **742**
  susceptibility and 21
  see also carcinogenicity; and
    individual carcinogens
carcinoid syndrome 234

carcinomas, non-genotoxic carcinogen
    mechanisms 765
cardiac arrhythmias
  fluorinated hydrocarbons causing
    154
  in hypothermia 332
  in spaceflight 376
  see also tachycardia; ventricular
    fibrillation
cardiac dysrhythmias, in hypothermia
    331
cardiac output
  alveolar concentration and 71
  at high altitudes 388
    'double product' 388
cardiopulmonary decompression illness
    352
cardiopulmonary resuscitation, gassing
    accidents 131
cardiovascular diseases, shift work 583,
    588
cardiovascular shock, paraquat
    poisoning and 201
cardiovascular system, welding and
    185
cardroom workers 622, 625, 627, 628,
    629
carers, see patient carers
Carhart notch 293
car industry, hepatotoxicity in 884,
    891–2
carpal tunnel syndrome (CTS) 310, 311,
    314–16, 460–1, 468
  case-control studies 461
  clinical aspects 460–1
  epidemiology 460
  hand–arm vibration syndrome vs
    314, 315, 315
  and IIAC 40
  management 461
  median nerve entrapment and 460
  occupational studies 460
  as prescribed disease 48, 464
  risk factors 316
  treatment 315
  vibration and 316, 460, 461
  work-related 454
carriers, xenobiotics 68
cars, see motor vehicles
car workers 857, 858
case-control studies 33, 799–800
  bias in 799
  choice of controls 799
case-referent studies, see case control
    studies
case studies
  mesothelioma 795
  occupational history 11, 795–6
cash register operators, thoracic outlet
    syndrome 457
castor beans
  dust, prescribed diseases due to 52,
    53
  occupational asthma due to 636,
    647
  radioallergosorbent tests (RAST) 21
catalase 116
catalytic converters 142

cataracts 402
  definition 422
  EC schedule of occupational diseases
      45
  in glass blowers 430
  infrared-induced 430
  microwave-induced 431
  optical radiation causing 420
  photochemical damage 424
  as prescribed disease 46
  radiation levels causing 400
  from sun exposure 429
  see also heat cataract
catechol(s) 271
  leucoderma due to 272
  metabolism 74
catecholamines
  contraindication in chloroform
      exposure 230
  in trichloroethylene exposure 234
catering and hotel industry
  dermatoses in 730, 733
  see also food industry; restaurant
      trade
cattle
  Q fever 498
  vaccination and quarantine 490
cattle ringworm 733
cattle vaccines 213
cattle workers, cryptogenic fibrosing
      alveolitis and 660
cauda equina syndrome 479
CCNU (1-(2-chloroethyl)-3-cyclohexyl-1-
      nitrosourea), genotoxicity 777
cefotaxime, in Lyme disease 497
ceftriaxone, in Lyme disease 497
cefuroxime axetil 497
cell cycle 747
cell-mediated immunity, see also
      delayed hypersensitivity
cell membrane, movement of
      chemicals across 68
cells, stippled 86–7
cellular proto-oncogenes, see proto-
      oncogenes
cellulitis
  misdiagnosis of Streptococcus suis as
      500
  subcutaneous, as prescribed disease
      46
'cement hepatitis' 250
cement ulcers (cement burns) 732–3,
      734
census, occupational mortality analysis
      from 32
Central Index on Dose Information
      (CIDI), Health and Safety
      Executive 407
central nervous system (CNS)
  acrylamide effects 251, 868
  alkanes 225
  biological monitoring tests 18
  cancer risk and germline mutations
      751
  carbon disulphide exposure 254
  carbon monoxide effect 142, 869
  carbonyl sulphide 162
  cumene effect 266

1,2-dibromoethane (ethylene
      dibromide) and 232
dichlorobenzene effect 266
1,2-dichloroethane (ethylene
      dichloride) 230–1
dimethylformamide effect 251
dysfunction of, as prescribed disease
      51
ethylene oxide effect 166
n-hexane 870
in lead poisoning 86
in Lyme disease 497
mercury effect 91, 872
methanol exposure 241
methyl bromide exposure 164
methylene chloride
      (dichloromethane) effects 227
nitrobenzene effect 266
organotin poisoning 114
phenol effect 271
phosphine exposure 164
radiation damage 402
raised barometric pressure sequelae
      356
solvents 223
styrene effect 265
sulphur-containing compounds 254
tetrachloroethylene
      (perchloroethylene) effect 235
1,1,1-trichloroethane (methyl
      chloroform) effect 231
tumours, see brain tumours
vinylidene chloride (1,1-
      dichloroethylene) effect 237
welding fume exposure effects 184
xylene effect 264
centrilobular necrosis 883, 891
cephalosporins
  erysipeloid and 501
  occupational asthma due to 636
Cephalosporium spp. 711
ceramic fibres 697
cerebellar ataxia, in mercury poisoning
      92
cerebral decompression sickness, case
      history 353–4
cerebral dysfunction, decompression
      illness 352
cerebral impairment, methylene
      chloride (dichloromethane) 227
cerebral oedema
  dichloroacetylene exposure 239
  high-altitude (HACO) 383, 384, 386,
      387
  organotin poisoning 114
  treatment 392, 394, 887
  triethyltin toxicity 114
cerebral symptoms, high-altitude 'Red
      Alert' symptoms 394
cerebrovascular disease, in lead
      poisoning 86
cerium, granulomatous lung disease
      due to 702–3
cervical cancer, oncogene activation in
      749
cervical spondylosis 454, 456–7
cervical syndrome 457
cervicobrachial disorders 462

CFCs, see chlorofluorocarbons
chain saws
  anti-vibration 317
  prescribed diseases due to use of 47,
      48
Challenger space shuttle 584
charcoal, activated
  alpha-chloralose and 212
  in lindane poisoning 210
  in paraquat poisoning treatment
      202
Charles' law 345
chelation tests 847
chelation therapy 844, 848
  cadmium poisoning 95
  lead poisoning 87–8, 871
  mercury poisoning 92
  radiation exposure 410
chemical agents/chemicals 65–279
  absorption, see absorption
  aircrew exposure to 374
  aliphatic, see aliphatic chemical
      compounds
  clearance 70
  detoxification, see detoxification
  diffusion 68
  distribution 68
  EC comparable data collection 41
  elimination 69, 70, 72–7
  filtration 68
  half-life 69
  impure 9–10
  industrial, reproductive hazards 828
  information sources 221, 223
  kinetic profile 69
  kinetics of exposure 71–2
  laboratory analysis 221
  metabolism, see metabolism
  multiple, sensitivity, biological
      monitoring 24–5
  occupational diseases caused by (EC
      schedule) 43–4
  organic, see organic chemical
      compounds
  prescribed diseases due to 49–52
  testing for genotoxicity and
      carcinogenicity 763–7
    structural alerts 763–4
  toxicity, see toxicity; toxicokinetics
  transport mechanisms 68
  volume of distribution 69–70
  see also metabolism; toxicokinetics
chemical exposure, assessment 16
chemical industry
  carcinogenic risk in 815
  dermatoses 733
  hepatotoxicity in 884
chemical laboratories, reproductive
      hazards to mother 831
chemical names, confusion over 9
chemical pneumonitis, see pneumonitis
chemical processors, asthma incidence
      635
chemicals, see chemical
      agents/chemicals
chemical solvents, in nucleic acid
      extraction 529, 529
chemical weapons 171–2

organic derivatives of arsine 97
chemotherapy, genotoxicity *776*
Chernobyl incident 131, 397, 403, 584,
    908
    bone marrow transplantations 402
    thyroid cancer increase 415
chest
    gas in, *see also* pulmonary
        barotrauma
    tightness, in byssinosis 626, *626*
chestnuts, latex sensitivity and 638
chest pain 666
    in mesothelioma 692–3
    in pulmonary barotrauma 352
chest radiography 593–4
    asbestosis 688
    berylliosis *vs* sarcoidosis 702
    beryllium poisoning 101, 102
    chlamydiosis 492
    cryptogenic fibrosing alveolitis 660
    extrinsic allergic alveolitis 657
    humidifier fever 712
    IIAC criteria 40
    ILO classification 667–9
    patient variables 593–4
    pneumoconiosis 666–9
        coalworker's pneumoconiosis
            666, 683
        slate pneumoconiosis 678
    Q fever 498
    radiographic film 593
    silicotuberculosis 674
    tuberculosis 510
    ventilation pulmonitis 656
Cheyne–Stokes respiration (periodic
        breathing) at high altitude 383,
        389
Chicago, Coconut Grove disaster 548
chicken pox 510
Chikungunya 509
children
    bone changes in lead poisoning 87
    brain development and lead
        exposure 87
    cancer
        fathers exposed to electromagnetic
            fields 445
        fathers exposed to ionizing
            radiation 405
    chimney sweeps' climbing boys
        918
    effects of electromagnetic field
        exposure 440
    at high altitudes 386, 388
        sickle cell anaemia 389
    in mills 920
    in mining 921–2
    noise-induced hearing loss 290
    radiation-induced tumours 403
Children's Employment Commission
    Report 1842 921
chillers, sick building syndrome and
    715, 716
chimneys 918
    soot in 918
chimney sweeps 741, 792, 807
    bladder cancer 811
    climbing boys 918

chimney sweep's cancer, as prescribed
    disease 50
China, pyrethroid exposure incident
    211
china clay (kaolin) 679, 680
china stone 676, 679, 680
Chinese hamster ovaries *522*
chiropractice, back pain 482
Chlamydia psittaci 492, 493
    prescribed disease due to *49*
chlamydiosis 492–3
    avian 492–3
        as prescribed disease *49*, 493
    ovine 493
        as prescribed disease *49*, 493
    in pregnancy 490
chloracetaldehyde 74
chloracne 273, 274, 275, 732, 733
chloral hydrate, in nucleic acid
    extraction *529*
chlorambucil
    genotoxicity *776*
    as tissue culture additive *528*
chloramine 715
chloramine gas 148
chloramine T, radioallergosorbent tests
    (RAST) *21*
chloramphenicol 431
    genotoxicity *777*
    as tissue culture additive *528*
chlorapatite 98
chlorate pesticides
    acute poisoning, features and
        management 202
    symptoms and signs of exposure to
        200
chlordane 209, 210
    hepatotoxicity 893
chlordecone (Kepone) 209, 210
    confused with dodecane 9
    hepatotoxicity *884*, 893
        treatment 887
    male fertility/sexual behaviour 829
    neurotoxicity 874
    as non-genotoxic carcinogen 765
    reproductive hazards *828*, *829*, 829
chlorethylene oxide 889
    epoxidation 74
chlorhexidine 715
chlorinated dibenzofurans (PCDFs) 273,
    274
chlorinated dioxins (PCDDs) 273
chlorinated naphthalene(s) 273
    chloracne 273
    hepatotoxicity 892
    prescribed disease due to *50*, 273
chlorine **147–8**, 715
    characteristics and sources 147
    clinical manifestations of exposure
        147
    dose–effect relations 147
    drinking water and 148
    EC comparable data collection *41*
    emergency planning in disasters
        126–9
        casualty expectations *128*
    exposure in accidents 123, 126–8,
        147

    health effect levels *127*
    hospital management 132, *133*
    management of poisoning 147
    occupational asthma due to 633,
        634, 635
    occupational diseases caused by (EC
        schedule) *43*
    as war gas 171
chlorine dioxide 147
chlorine monoxide 154
chlorine production, use of mercury 90
chlorine trifluoride 152
Chlornaphazine (*N,N*-bis(2-chloroethyl)-
    2-naphthylamine), genotoxicity
    776
chlor[o]acetaldehyde 889
chloroacetone, occupational diseases
    caused by (EC schedule) *43*
chloroalkali industry, mercury usage
    851
chloroalkali process 90
chloroalkanes, formula and examples
    224
chloroalkenes **232–7**
    formula and examples *224*
    see also tetrachloroethylene;
        trichloroethylene; vinylidene
        chloride
chloroalkynes **239**
chloro-2 amino phenol 272
o-chlorobenzylidene malanonitrile (CS
    gas) 171–2
chloro-derivatives of benzene,
    prescribed diseases due to *50*
chlorodifluoromethane (CFC-22; Freon-
    22) 154
    in nucleic acid extraction *529*
1-chloro-2,3-epoxypropane, *see*
    epichlorohydrin
chloroethane (ethyl chloride) 169
1-(2-chloroethyl)-3-cyclohexyl-1-
    nitrosourea (CCNU), genotoxicity
    777
1-(2-chloroethyl)-3-(4-
    methylcyclohexyl)-1-nitrosourea
    (methyl-CCNU), genotoxicity
    776
chlorofluorocarbons
    fully halogenated (CFCs) 150, 154
        plans to phase out 154
        substitutes for 155
    hydrogenated partially halogenated,
        see hydrochlorofluorocarbons
chloroform (trichloromethane) 148,
    167, *224*, **229–30**
    carcinogenicity/cancers 230
    catecholamines and 230
    characteristics and uses 229
    clinical manifestations 229–30
    hepatotoxicity 229, *884*, *885*, 891
    management 230
    metabolism/biochemical effects 229
    as non-genotoxic carcinogen 765
    in nucleic acid extraction *529*
    prescribed diseases due to *51*
    'sniffers' 230
    structural formula 229
chloromethane, *see* methyl chloride

chloromethyl ether 10, 807
chloromethyl methyl ether (CMME) 10
    carcinogenicity *814*
    genotoxicity *776*
    lung cancer *815*
        as prescribed disease *54*, 807
4-chloro-2-methylphenoxyacetic acid
        (MCPA) *203*
4-(4-chloro-2-methylphenoxy) butyric
        acid (MCPB) *203*
2-(4-chloro-2-methylphenoxy) propionic
        acid (MCPP; mecoprop) *203*,
        203
chloropentafluoroethane (Genetron-
        115) 154
chlorophacinone 212
chlorophenols 271–2
chlorophenoxyacetate herbicides
        202–3, *203*
    gastric lavage 203
    ingestion, deliberate 203
    management of acute poisoning 203
    occupational exposure to 203
    sarcomas and lymphomas 203
chlorophenoxy herbicides,
        hepatotoxicity 894
chloropicrin 873
chloroplatinate salts 110
chloroprene
    male fertility/sexual behaviour 829
    reproductive hazards *828*, 829
chloroquine 379
    malaria 513
    as treatment for liver disease 887
1-chloro-1,2,2,2-tetrafluoroethane
        (HCFC 124) 155
chlorothalonil 735
p-chloro-*o*-toluidine
    bladder cancer 810
    genotoxicity *777*
chlorotrifluoromethane (Freon-13;
        Genetron-13) 154
chlorovinyldichloroarsine (lewisite) 97,
        171
chlorozotocin, genotoxicity *777*
chlorphentermine 77
chlorpromazine, carbon tetrachloride
        and 882
'chokes' 352, 364
cholestasis 882–3
    abnormal liver function tests 883
    treatment 887
cholestyramine 893
    in lindane poisoning 210
    in mercury poisoning 92
    as treatment for liver disease 887
    warfarin ingestion and 212
cholinesterase inhibition, biological
        effect monitoring *19*
cholinesterase reactivators, in acute
        organophosphate poisoning 207
chondroprotective agents 467
choroid 421, 423
chromate
    in cement 733, 734
    genotoxicity 778
    postoccupational dermatitis due to
        730

chromate industry/workers
    lung and sino-nasal cancer *815*
    lung cancer risk 700
chromate pigment production,
        carcinogenic risk in *815*
chromates
    P53 gene mutations 755
    prescribed diseases due to *52*
    respiratory tract malignancies *4*
    see also chromium compounds
chromatography 529
chrome, carcinogenicity 700
chrome dermatitis, as prescribed
        disease *52*
chrome pigment industry 105
chrome ulcers (chrome holes) 104, 732
chromic acid 104
    carcinogenicity 807
    in nucleic acid extraction *529*
    prescribed diseases due to *52*
chromic oxide 104
chromic sulphate 104
chromium **104–5**
    absorption and metabolism 104–5
    biological monitoring tests and
        guidance values *18*
    EC comparable data collection *41*
    as genotoxic carcinogen 778
    half-life 104
    hepatotoxicity *884*, *885*, 893
    hexavalent 778
    metal-induced asthma due to 699
    monitoring of workers 105
    nephrotoxicity 853
    occupational diseases caused by (EC
        schedule) *43*
    respiratory tract malignancies and *4*,
        105
    trivalent/hexavalent compounds in
        welding fume 181, 183
    urine levels 105
    uses 104
    water insoluble compounds, welding
        fume and 181
chromium compounds 104
    carcinogenicity 105, 807, *814*
    genotoxicity *776*, 778
    hexavalent 104, 105
    inhalation 105
    lung and sino-nasal cancer *815*
    occupational diseases caused by (EC
        schedule) *43*
    trivalent 104, 105
chromium platers, lung cancer *815*
chromium trichloride, in nucleic acid
        extraction *529*
chromium trioxide 104
chromophores 424, *424*–5
chromosomal aberrations
    benzene causing 262
    carcinogenesis mechanism 745
    ethylene oxide causing 166
    hereditary cancer and 746
    inversions 743
    in peripheral blood lymphocytes
        773, 774
    styrene causing 265
    translocations 743

chromosomal mutations 743
chromosome painting 773
chronic beryllium disease, *see under*
        beryllium poisoning
chronic obstructive airway disease
        (COAD)
    at high altitudes 389
    see also chronic obstructive lung
        disease; chronic obstructive
        pulmonary disease
chronic obstructive lung disease 698–9
    industries affected 699
    see also chronic obstructive airway
        disease; chronic obstructive
        pulmonary disease
chronic obstructive pulmonary disease
        (COPD) **607–19**
    agents known to induce occupational
        asthma 613–14
    agents not known to induce
        occupational asthma 614–16
    asthma and 607–8
    cadmium causing 614
    coal dust causing 614, 615
    coal miners, mortality 33
    cotton dust causing 607, 608
    cross-sectional and longitudinal data
        discrepancies 611–12
    disease mechanism 609
    disease pathways 608
    Dutch hypothesis 613
    emphysema and 609, 610
    forced expiratory volume (FEV$_1$) and
        32
    genetic factor 612
    historical background 607–8
    mineral dusts and 614–15
    'multiple hit' hypothesis 616, 617
    non-occupational factors 612–13
    pathophysiology and disease
        definitions 609–10
    in polymer fume fever 187
    in population at large 616–17
    as prescribed disease 615
    smoking and 611, 613, 617
        confounding and interactions
            608–9
        'never-smokers' 609, 614, 615
        survival bias 609
    summary 617
    uncertainties and controversies 608
    urban *vs* rural communities 616–17
    ventilatory function decline 610–13
    welding fume and 615–16
    see also byssinosis; chronic
        obstructive airway disease:
        chronic obstructive lung
        disease; ventilatory function
chronic productive cough, *see* industrial
        bronchitis
chronic wasting disease (CWD) 500
chrysanthemums, contact dermatitis
        734
chrysoberyl 101
chrysotile (white asbestos) 686–7,
        687–8, 695, 817
    carcinogenicity 694–5
    countries banning use of 687–8

exposure limits 695
fibres and fibrils 686
lung cancer and 803
mesothelioma and 694
mining 687
tremolite contaminating 687
uses 686
see also asbestosis
cigarettes, polymer contamination 187
cigarette smoking, *see* smoking
ciliary body 421, 423
CIMAH (Control of Industrial Major
    Accident Hazards) Regulations
    1984 126
cimetidine
    occupational asthma due to *647*
    prescribed diseases due to *52, 53*
cinnarizine 373
ciprofibrate, as non-genotoxic
    carcinogen *765*
ciprofloxacin
    for legionnaires' disease 711
    traveller's diarrhoea 513
circadian rhythms
    desynchronization 582, 585
    'morning and evening types' 585
    shift work and 581–2, 586
    susceptibility to chemical agents 584
    variation in urinary excretion
        lead 85
        mercury 93
circulatory disorders, hand–arm
    vibration syndrome 308
cirrhosis, hepatic
    abnormal liver function tests 883
    alcohol-related 559
    in arsenic poisoning 97
    non-invasive screening *882*
cisplatin 110, 111
    genotoxicity *777*
Civil Aviation Authority, medical
    certificates, types of *377*
Civil Evidence Act 1995 61
civil law **57–8**
Civil Procedure Rules 59, 63
CJD, *see* Creutzfeldt–Jakob disease
Cladosporium 716
Cladosporium herbarum 636, 643, 653
Clara cells 132
    proteins 22
    xenobiotic metabolism 76, 77
clarythromycin, for legionnaires'
    disease 711
clavulanic acid 640
clay mining, prescribed diseases due to
    54
clays
    fibrous 696
    non-fibrous 681–2
Clean Air Acts 664
cleaners/cleaning
    bleaches (chlorine) effect 148
    dermatoses 733
    office cleaning 713, 717
clearance, of chemicals 70
climbing boys 918
clindamycin, erysipeloid and 501
clones 746–7

somatic mutation and 747
clonidine 563
cloprostenol, accidental self-injection
    with 214
clothing, cleaning
    prescribed urinary tract neoplasms in
        51
    see also dry-cleaning industry
clotrimazole, ringworm 502
clubbing, fingers in lung cancer in
    asbestosis 691
clusters of disease, occupational 28–9
CMME, *see* chloromethyl methyl ether
coach painters, asthma incidence *635*
coagulopathy, hepatic, treatment 887
coal distillation 261
    byproducts, skin diseases caused by
        (EC schedule) *44*
    EC comparable data collection *41*
coal dust, COPD and 614, 615
coal gas 137–8
    manufacturers, bladder cancer 28
coal gasification
    carcinogenicity *814*
    genotoxic exposures *776*
coal miners' bronchitis, smoking and,
    IIAC recommendations 40
coal miners/mining
    chronic obstructive pulmonary
        disease (COPD) mortality 33
    open cast 683
    prescribed diseases *46, 55*
    progressive massive fibrosis 684–5
    respiratory diseases in 614–15
    silicosis 685
        mortality *29*
    see also coalworker's pneumoconiosis
coal mines 682–3
    radon concentrations in 407
coal oven gas 142
coal tar
    cancer and 741, 792, *814*
    genotoxicity *776*
coal tar pitch
    carcinogenicity *814*
    genotoxicity *776*
    volatiles, urinary tract neoplasms as
        prescribed disease due to *51*
coalworker's pneumoconiosis **682–6**
    chest radiography 666, 683
    compensation/benefits 684
    complicated 684–6
        imaging 599
    control measures 682
    history 682, 921
    imaging 599
    research 682
    rheumatoid 685–6
    simple 683–4
    sources of dust 682–3
cobalt **105–7**
    absorption 106
    biological monitoring tests and
        guidance values *18*
    carcinogenicity 106, 700
    chronic obstructive lung disease and
        699
    dermatitis 734

excretion 106
    inhalation 106
    ionizing radiation properties *398*
    left ventricular failure 106
    metal-induced asthma due to 699
    monitoring of workers 106–7
    pulmonary toxicity mechanism
        703–4
    radioactive 105
    in urine 106–7
    uses and properties 105
cobalt asthma 699
cobalt chloride hexahydrate, in nucleic
    acid extraction *529*
cobalt compounds, carcinogenicity
    106
cobalt dust
    exposure 703
    inhalation, EC schedule of
        occupational diseases *44*
cobalt lung 703–4
cobalt oxides, acute lung injury due to
    698
cochlea
    anatomy 286–7
    hair cells 292–3
    implantation 300
    travelling wave theory 287, 289, 292
cochlear fluids 286
cochlear otosclerosis 293
Coconut Grove disaster, Chicago 548
Code of Practice on Carcinogens, COSHH
    817
coffee beans, *see* green coffee beans
cohort studies 33, 798–9
coke oven emissions, urinary tract
    malignancies *4*
coke oven gas 142
coke oven workers
    kidney malignancies *4*
    polycyclic aromatic hydrocarbons
        (PAHs) exposure 273
    respiratory tract malignancies *4*
    skin neoplasms *4*
coke plant workers, lung cancer *815*
coke production
    carcinogenicity *814*
    genotoxic exposures *776*
colchicine, as treatment for liver disease
    887
cold **327–33**
    adaptation and habituation 328
    cold strain, assessment 327–8
    cold stress **327–33**
        assessment 327
        water immersion 330
    drowning related to 331
    effect on performance 332–3
    exposure, divers 349
    in flying 367
    hypothermia, *see* hypothermia
    local injuries
        freeze–thaw–refreeze 329
        freezing cold injuries 328–9
        freezing of tissues 328–9
        frostbite, deep and complicated
            329
        frostnip 328

cold – *contd*
  local injuries – *contd*
    non-freezing cold injury (NFCI)
        329–31
    rewarming after 328, 329, 330
    superficial frostbite 328–9
  prevention of injury/stress 337–40
    control of environment 339–40
    personal protective equipment
        339
    previous disorders affecting
        susceptibility 338
    the worker 337–8
  respiratory disease related to 332
  responses to 326
  reversed interpretation in
      decompression illnesses 352
  training in the cold 338
  working in 337–9
cold injuries, liquefied gases 132
cold sensitization 329, 330
'cold shock' 331–2
cold water humidifiers, *see*
      humidification systems
colon cancer 742
  hereditary non-polyposis,
      susceptibility and germline
      mutation *750*
  oncogene activation in *749*
  risk of, and germline mutations *750*
  see also colorectal cancer
colony forming units (CFUs) 901, 902
colophony (pinewood resin)
  dermatitis 734, 735
  occupational asthma due to *634,
      636,* 638, 641
colorectal cancer 742, 762, 809–10
  genetic model 743, 747
  see also colon cancer
colour discrimination impairment in
      carbon disulphide exposure
      254
colour manufacturing, lead use *844*
colour vision, aircrew 369
COMAH (Control of Major Accident
      Hazards) Regulations 1999 129
comedones 731, 732
Committee on the Medical Aspects of
      Radiation in the Environment
      (COMARE), UK 405
communication workers 431
compensation 11
  claims and awards 30
  coalworker's pneumoconiosis 684
  by Criminal Injuries Compensation
      Board 57
  extrinsic allergic alveolitis 660–1
  hand–arm vibration syndrome
      (HAVS) 314
  hearing disability 289, 294, 295
  mesothelioma 694
  nuclear industry no-fault scheme 404
  occupational cancer 796
  repetitive strain injury 462, *462*
  statutory, occupational asthma 647
  work-related illnesses 571
  see also compensation schemes;
      prescribed diseases

'compensationitis' 61
compensation schemes **37–55**
  adjudicating authorities 39
  employees' lack of awareness of 37
  European perspective 40–1
  future possibilities 42
  historical background 37–8
  ideal characteristics of 39
  individual proof 38, 40, 41
  industrial injuries schemes outside
      UK 38, 40–2
  information for patients 37
  moral responsibility of State 42
  no-fault schemes 37, 38, 42
  presumption element 38
  principles of 38–9
  self-employed and 38, 42
  state *vs* privatized schemes 42
  Tort System for negligence claims 42
  US perspective 38, 42
  workings of 39
  see also compensation; Industrial
      Injuries Schemes; prescribed
      diseases
complement, activation by cotton dust
      623
Compositae, contact dermatitis 733,
      734
compressed air, prescribed diseases due
      to *46*
compressed-air diving 343–4, 346
  depth limits 344, 346, 347, 348
compressed-air workers 343, 344, 345,
      347
  decompression illnesses,
      classification 350
  hearing loss 356
  musculoskeletal pain 351
compression barotrauma **347–8**
  alternobaric vertigo 348
  inner ear 348
  middle ear 347–8
  pulmonary 348
  'reversed ear' 347
  sinus, eyes, skin and teeth 348
compression illnesses/sickness, EC
      schedule of occupational
      diseases *45*
computed radiography (CR), in
      occupational lung disease
      594–5
computed tomography (CT)
  asbestos-related diseases 688
  mesothelioma 692, 693
  in occupational lung disease 595
  in pleural disease 600–1
  pneumoconiosis 669
  pulmonary fibrosis (asbestosis) 688
  see also high resolution computed
      tomography (HRCT)
computer workstations, *see*
      ergonomics; visual display unit
      (VDU) operators
conception, delay in 826
Concorde 363, 365
  radiation exposure 374
concrete industry, prescribed diseases
      in *47*

conduction velocities, *see* nerve
      conduction velocities
cones, of eye 422
confidence limits, in epidemiological
      studies 800
confined spaces
  carbon dioxide in 140
  gases in 136–7
    CS gas 172
  phosgene in 148
  physical suitability of workers 137
Confined Spaces Regulations 1997 137
congenital malformations 831
  aetiology *830*
  anaesthetic gases and drugs 831
  electromagnetic field exposure and
      444
  ionizing radiation causing 831–2
  mercury causing 831
  video display units (VDUs) and 445
  see also fetus
congreve matches 98
conjugation reactions 75–6
  carbon disulphide 254
  toluene 263
conjunctivae, transient burning of,
      pesticide exposure and *200*
conjunctival ailments, EC schedule of
      occupational diseases *45*
conjunctivitis
  biotechnology hazard *527*
  chromium causing 105
  Newcastle disease and 498
  osmium causing 110
  selenium dioxide causing 111
consciousness
  impaired, paraquat poisoning and
      201
  loss of
    carbon monoxide poisoning 143
    in decompression illnesses 352,
        353
    divers in water **348–9**
    G-induced (G-LOC) 366
    hydrogen sulphide and 160–1
    oxygen-deficient atmospheres 135
    'time of useful consciousness' 363
construction industries/workers
  alcohol-related problems 559
  carcinogenic risk in *816*
  dermatoses 734
  radiographers in 407
contact dermatitis 726
  allergic 727
    allergens 727
    causative agents 727
    corticosteroids 729
    elicitation 727
    induction 727
    occupations associated with 727
    patch testing 728–9
    sensitization 727
    treatment 729–30
  in beryllium poisoning 102
  biotechnology hazard 528
  causative mechanisms 726
  chrome compounds 104
  clinical diagnosis 727–8

differential diagnosis 726
hard metal 115
irritant **726–7**
  age at onset 726–7
  causative agents 726, 727
  exposure length 727
  occupations associated with 727
  susceptibility to 726
  treatment 729–30
nickel 110
osmium causing 110
patch testing 728–9
pre-employment assessment 730
prevention 728, 730
prick tests 729
prognosis 730–1
protein contact dermatitis 731
radioallergosorbent tests (RAST) 729
treatment 729–30
welders 184
work-relatedness 728
see also dermatitis
contact lenses
  aircrew 369
  welders 185
contact urticaria **731**
  causes 731, 733
  investigations 729
containment levels, microorganisms, genetically modified 530, 531, 531
contraceptive pills, reproductive hazards 829
contract workers 8
Control of Industrial Major Accident Hazards (CIMAH) Regulations 1984 126
Control of Major Accident Hazards (COMAH) Regulations (1999) 129
Control of Substances Hazardous to Health (COSHH) Regulations 1988/1994 7, 817
  anaesthetic gases 168
  aromatic amine exposure 269
  Biological Agents Directive 502
  laboratory work risk assessment 512
convulsions
  gassing accidents 132
  methyl bromide causing 132
  oxygen at high partial pressures 345
  paraquat poisoning and 201
cooling towers 173
  distance from, related to disease outbreaks 710
  legionnaires' disease and 709, 710, 711
  regulations and maintenance guidelines 710
  replacement by air-cooled units 710
COPD, see chronic obstructive pulmonary disease
coping skills, training 578
copper **107**
  absorption and transport 107
  characteristics and uses 107
  excretion 107
  function in body 107
  hepatotoxicity 884, 885, 892

treatment 887
  nephrotoxicity 853
  poisoning 107
copper cyanide 145
copper fumes 697
copper miners 107
copper smelters 156, 815
copper solution, accidental self-injection with 214
copper sulphate 107
  hepatotoxicity 885, 892
copper workers, lung cancer and 700
coproporphyrin 85
coproporphyrinuria 886, 889
core temperature 327
Coriolis illusions, aircrew 371
cornea
  anatomy 421, 422
  damage from optical radiation 420
  dystrophy, as prescribed disease 50
  endothelium 422
  epithelium 420, 422
  flash burns 430
  radiation absorption 424
  ulceration, as prescribed disease 50
  ulceration and opacification, osmium causing 110
corn oil, as non-genotoxic carcinogen 765
coronary heart disease
  biological monitoring tests 18
  carbon disulphide association 254, 255
  see also ischaemic heart disease; myocardial infarction
coroners' courts 58
corrosive gases 131
  burns 132
  irritant gases 124
cortical evoked response audiometry (CERA) 302–3
corticosteroids
  adhesive capsulitis 456
  allergic contact dermatitis 729
  altitude sickness 390
  beryllium poisoning 103
  chlorine poisoning 133
  in decompression illnesses 355
  extrinsic allergic alveolitis 659
  hard metal lung disease and 703
  solar retinopathy 426
cortisone therapy 458
corundum 701
Corynebacterium spp., in office buildings 717
COSHH, see Control of Substances Hazardous to Health Regulations 1988/1994
cosmic radiation 399, 406
  aircrew exposure 374, 407
cotrimoxazole, brucellosis 492
cottage industries 919
cotton
  acute effects of exposure to dust 624
  antigens and fungal contaminants 623, 624
  bracts 622, 623, 624
  dust/fibres 621, 622, 624, 629

mortality and morbidity of workers 625
  prescribed diseases due to 52
  steaming 622, 629
  see also byssinosis
cotton dust 185
  chronic obstructive pulmonary disease (COPD) due to 607, 608
  inhalation, EC schedule of occupational diseases 44
  personal exposure dust standard (UK) 629
cotton seed, radioallergosorbent tests (RAST) 21
cotton spinner's phthisis 621
cotton workers
  byssinosis and smoking 8
  smoking and 608
coughing, paraquat poisoning and 201
coumatetralyl 212
counselling 578
  British Association of Counselling (BAC) 578–9
  British Medical Association Stress Counselling Service 565
  National Counselling Service for Sick Doctors 565
  post-traumatic stress disorder 548–9
  United Kingdom Council for Psychotherapy (UKCP) 579
cow dander, radioallergosorbent tests (RAST) 21
Cowden disease, susceptibility and germline mutation 751
cowpox 490, 501
cow urine, radioallergosorbent tests (RAST) 21
Coxiella burnetii 498
craft palsy 464
cramp 336
  hand/forearm 462, 464
    as prescribed disease 46, 464
cranial nerve palsy, brucellosis 492
creatinine correction 20
'creeps' 364
creosote 271, 272
  genotoxicity 777
crepitations, paraquat poisoning and 201
Creutzfeldt–Jakob disease (CJD) 500–1
  variant (vCJD) 500–1
Crimean Congo haemorrhagic fever 509
Criminal Injuries Compensation Board 57
criminal law **57–8**
cristobalite 672, 676, 681
  limits/recommendation 677
crocidolite (blue asbestos) 687, 695
  carcinogenicity 694, 695
  mesothelioma due to 687, 693, 694, 695
  see also asbestosis
Crohn's disease, high altitudes 390
crop spraying, from the air 374
cross-coupled illusions, aircrew 371
cross-sectional studies 34

crustaceans
  occupational asthma due to *647*
  prescribed diseases due to *53, 54*
cryolite 150
cryolite workers
  dental fluorosis and breast milk 151
  osteofluorosis 151
cryptogenic asthma 608
cryptogenic fibrosing alveolitis 602,
      660
  differential diagnosis 660
cryptosporidiosis 490, 494
Cryptosporidium 493
Cryptosporidium parvum 494
Cryptostroma corticale, extrinsic
      allergic alveolitis due to *654*
crystalline silica
  carcinogenicity *814*
  nephrotoxicity 853–4
CS gas (*o*-chlorobenzylidene
      malanonitrile) 171–2
cumene 266
cumol (cumene) 266
cumulative trauma disorders, *see*
      repetitive strain injury
cupric acetoarsenite (Paris green) 96
cupric arsenite (Scheele's green) 96
curing agents, acid anhydrides and
      asthma 639
cutaneous decompression illness 351
cutaneous melanoma
  cancer risk and germline mutations
      750
  familial, susceptibility and germline
      mutation *750*
cutis marmorata 351
cutting, eye protectors *433*
cutting fluid dermatitis 730
cutting oils bacteria,
      radioallergosorbent tests (RAST)
      21
cyanide(s)
  detoxification 76
  formula and examples *224*
  occupational diseases caused by (EC
      schedule) *43*
  poisoning in acrylonitrile exposure
      253
  see also hydrogen cyanide
cyanide compounds, occupational
      diseases caused by (EC schedule)
      43
cyanide salts 145
cyanogen 145
cyanogen bromide 146
  in nucleic acid extraction 529, *529*
cyanogen chloride 145, 146
  in nucleic acid extraction *529*
cyanosis
  central 904
    gassing accidents 131
  in methaemoglobinaemia 268
  paraquat poisoning and *201*
  in sulphaemoglobinaemia 268
cyclodiene insecticides 209
cyclohexane 225
  Flixborough accident 123, 225
  insecticides 209

in nucleic acid extraction *529*
cyclohexanone *247*
cyclopentanone *247*
cyclopentolate 185, 431
cyclophosphamide 659, 895
  beryllium poisoning 103
  genotoxicity *776*
  as tissue culture additive *528*
cycloplegia 185
cyclopropane 167, 169
cyclosporin, genotoxicity *776*
cypermethrin 211
cytochrome *c* reductase 73
cytochrome P450 73, 74, 76, 744, 882,
      883, 888
  induction
    by methyl *n*-butyl ketone (M*n*BK)
      247
    by methyl ethyl ketone (MEK) 248
    by methyl isobutyl ketone (MIBK)
      248
  methyl mercury and 825
'cytogenic noise' 746
cytomegalovirus 510
Cytophaga allerginae 711
cytosine 743, 745
cytostatic agents, hepatotoxicity *884*,
      885, 895
cytotoxic drugs
  bone marrow cancer *816*
  reproductive hazards *828*, *829*, 829,
      831
cytotoxicity, in contact dermatitis 726
cytotoxins, as tissue culture additives
      528
Czech Republic, compensation schemes
      41

daffodils, contact dermatitis 734
daily personal exposure to noise (LEPd)
      296–7
dairy farmers/workers, leptospirosis
      496
Dale Committee (1947) 38
Dalton's law 345, 363
damages 60
  for injuries 60
  for loss of earnings, Social Security
      benefits and 61
  out-of-court settlements 62
  periodical payments 60
  provisional 60–1
  special and general 61
  structured settlements 60
Damages Act 1996 60
dandelion, contact dermatitis 733
Dangerous Trades committees 923
Danish painters' syndrome 264
dapsone 500
dark-room disease 156
data entry operators, *see* keyboard
      operators
Data Protection Acts 1984 and 1998
      58–9
daunorubicin, as tissue culture additive
      528
Davy, Humphrey, Sir 137, 147

DBCP, *see* 1,2-dibromo-3-chloropropane
2,4-DB (4-(2,4-dichlorophenoxy)butyric
      acid) *203*
DCPP (dichloroprop; 2-(2,4-
      dichlorophenoxy)propionic
      acid) *203*, 203
2,4-D (2,4-dichlorophenoxyacetic acid)
      202, *203*, 203
DDT (dichlorodiphenyltrichloroethane)
      209, 210, 275, 809
  half-life 198
  hepatotoxicity 882, *884*, 893
  neurotoxicity 874
  as non-genotoxic carcinogen *765*
deafness
  autoimmune 293
  occupational, industrial injury
      benefit awards 30, *30*
  as prescribed disease *46–8*
  see also hearing loss; noise;
      occupational noise-induced
      hearing loss
dealkylation 75
  tetraethyl lead 85
death, *see* mortality
death certificates 29, 30
debriefing
  psychological 549
  violence at work 553
debrisoquine, metabolizers 68
debrisoquine hydroxylase, metabolic
      polymorphisms with cancer
      susceptibility links *758*
decaborane 166
decane 225
decanting (surface decompression) 344
decatenation 745
decay, of organic matter 136
decibel scales *284*, 284–5
decipols 716
decomposition of materials 9
decompression
  diving tables and mathematical
      models 347, 351
  procedures for 344
  rapid 364–5
  surface decompression (decanting) 344
  theory 346–7
decompression chambers, air force
      training in 363
decompression computers 351
decompression illnesses **350–6**, 350
  biphasic 353
  cardiopulmonary 352
  case histories 353–5
  causes 351
  classification 350
  constitutional manifestations 352
  cutaneous 351
  decompression sickness, *see*
      decompression sickness
  diagnosis 350, 353
  EC schedule of occupational diseases
      45
  latency 353
  long-term effects **356–8**
  lymphatic 351
  musculoskeletal 351–2

neurological 352–3, 355–6
pathogenesis 350–1
prognosis 355
relapse 355
treatment 354–5
at depth 355
types of 350
see also pulmonary barotrauma
decompression sickness 350, 352, 364
in aviation 364
after diving 364
U-2 pilots 364
causes 351
clinical manifestations 351
EC schedule of occupational diseases 45
incidence 364
neurological symptoms 364
pathogenesis 351
predisposing factors 347, 364
as prescribed disease 46, 355
prevention 364
spinal 354, 355
treatment 364
visual symptoms 364
decongestants, topical 362
deep vein thrombosis
aircrew 374
airline passengers 379
deep-water blackout 348–9
deerstalkers, Lyme disease 497
defibrillators, electromagnetic fields and 185
defoliants, Agent Orange 274
'degreasers' flush' 234, 251
degreasing
machine degreasing, hepatotoxicity 884
1,1,1-trichloroethane 231
trichloroethylene 233, 234
dehumidifiers 715
dehydration, aircrew 374
delayed hypersensitivity, aromatic amines 270
deltamethrin 211
dementia 573–4
alcohol use and 558
methylene chloride (dichloromethane) causing 227
presentation 572
demolition industry/engineers
cancer sites 816
lead in 83, 844
prescribed diseases associated with 48
demyelinating sensorimotor distal polyneuropathy, methyl iso-butyl ketone (MiBK) 248
dengue 509
denitrogenation 364
Denmark, occupational diseases schedule 41
dental amalgam 851, 852
as mercury source 23
dental assistants and dentists
anaesthetic gas exposure 168
dermatoses 734
hepatitis B 502, 503

hepatitis C 503, 504
mercury vapour inhalation 90
methyl methacrylate effects 250
nitrous oxide exposure 168
reproductive hazards
anaesthetic gases 831
mercury 831
dental fluorosis 151–2
dental problems, phosphorus causing 98
dental technician's pneumoconiosis 701
dentists, cervical spondylosis 457
depigmentation of skin 732
causes 272
see also vitiligo
depression 573
risk factors 574
depressive disorders, presentation 572
de Quervain's disease 454, 459
dermal absorption 72, 77
dermal biotransformation 77
dermatitis
aromatic amines causing 270
biological monitoring tests 18
copper workers 107
EC comparable data collection 41
formaldehyde causing 244
glutaraldehyde causing 246
methyl methacrylate causing 250
nickel 110
non-infective, as prescribed disease 53
osmium causing 110
phenol derivatives causing 271
platinum causing 111
postoccupational 730
radiation-induced 792
selenium dioxide causing 111
types 726
see also chrome dermatitis; contact dermatitis
dermatoses, see skin diseases
Descemet's membrane 112, 422
desquamation 401
radiation levels causing 400
desquamative eosinophilic bronchitis 633
desquamative interstitial pneumonitis 703
detergents 637
contact dermatitis 733
detergent workers 641
detoxification 72–7
by biotransformation 73
see also metabolism
conjugation reactions 75–6
by linkage to proteins 76
in liver 73–6
see also biotransformation
deuterium 141
Deutsche Forschungsgemeinschaft (DFG)
biological monitoring tests and guidance values 18
biological tolerance values 17
Devonshire colic 82
dexamethasone 391, 392, 394

in lead poisoning 871
as tissue culture additive 528
dextroamphetamine, jet lag and 374
diabetes, diagnosis by expired air 71
diabetic neuropathy, role of solvents in 855–6
diacetone alcohol, occupational diseases caused by (EC schedule) 43
N,N'diacetylbenzidine (N,N'-DAB) 855
diagnosis, occupational and environmental diseases 22–5
Diagnostic and Statistical Manual (DSM-IV), post-traumatic stress disorder 542, 545, 547
dialysis
costs 843
as treatment for liver disease 887
dialysis fluid, aluminium encephalopathy 100
p-diaminobenzene (para-phenylenediamine) 266
diaminodiphenylmethane (4,4'-methylenedianiline) 270
biological monitoring tests and guidance values 18
hepatotoxicity 884
liver injury 883
diamond polishing
cobalt and 106
hard metal disease 703
metal-induced asthma due to 699
dianisidine 269
o-dianisidine 810–11
diarrhoea
paraquat poisoning and 201
in radiation casualties 402, 414
diarrhoeal diseases
cryptosporidiosis 494
Escherichia coli 494
in travellers 513–14
diatomite (kieselgahr) 681
diazepam
in acute carbamate poisoning 209
alcohol abuse 558, 563
in decompression illness 355
organic lead poisoning 89
dibasic lead phthalate 83
dibenz[a,h]anthracene 273, 741
genotoxicity 777
1,2,5,6-dibenzanthracene 792
dibenzodioxins 732
dibenzofurans, postnatal exposure 833
diborane 166
acute lung injury due to 698, 698
1,2-dibromethane, see 1,2-dibromoethane
dibromochloropropane (DBCP), see 1,2-dibromo-3-chloropropane
1,2-dibromo-3-chloropropane (DBCP) 232
1,2-dibromoethane (ethylene dibromide) vs 232
live birth rates and 835
male fertility/sexual behaviour 829
reproductive hazards 826, 828, 829, 829, 835

1,2-dibromoethane (ethylene
        dibromide) 195, *224*, **232**
    carcinogenicity 232
    characteristics and uses 232
    clinical manifestations 232
    1,2-dibromo-3-chloropropane *vs* 232
    genotoxicity *777*
    metabolism/biochemical effects 232
    mutagenicity 232
    reproductive hazards 232, *828*
1,2-dibromotetrafluoroethane
        (fluorocarbon-114 B2) 155
dibutyltin 114
dicamba 202
dicentric counting, radiation
        measurement 399
dichloramine 147, 148
dichloroacetylene *224*, **239**
    carcinogenicity 239
    characteristics and uses 239
    clinical manifestations 239
    metabolism/biochemical effects 239
1,2-dichlorobenzene 266
1,4-dichlorobenzene (*p*-
        dichlorobenzene) 266
    as non-genotoxic carcinogen *765*
m-dichlorobenzene 266
o-dichlorobenzene 266
p-dichlorobenzene 266
dichlorobenzidine 269
3,3′-dichlorobenzidine, bladder cancer
        810
dichlorodifluoromethane (Freon-12;
        Genetron-12) 154, 166
dichlorodiphenyltrichloroethane, *see*
        DDT
1,1-dichloroethane (ethylidene
        dichloride) 230
1,2-dichloroethane (ethylene
        dichloride) *224*, **230–1**
    animal studies 230
    carcinogenicity 231
    characteristics and uses 230
    clinical manifestations 230–1
    hepatotoxicity 230, *885*
    management 231
    metabolism/biochemical effects 230
    mutagenicity 231
1,1-dichloroethylene, *see* vinylidene
        chloride
dichlorofluoromethane (Freon-21) 154
dichloroisopropyl ether, occupational
        diseases caused by (EC schedule)
        43
dichloromethane, *see* methylene
        chloride
2,4-dichlorophenoxyacetic acid 202,
        203, 203, 274
    reproductive hazards *828*
4-(2,4-dichlorophenoxy)butyric acid
        (2,4-DB) *203*
2-(2,4-dichlorophenoxy)propionic acid
        (2,4-DP; dichloroprop) *203*,
        203
dichloroprop (DCPP; 2-(2,4-
        dichlorophenoxy)propionic
        acid) *203*, 203
dichlorosilane 149

1,2-dichlorotetrafluoroethane (Freon-
        114; Genetron-114) 154
1,1-dichloro-2,2,2-trifluoroethane
        (HCFC 123) 155
dichromates 104
diclofenac, back pain 483
dicobalt edetate 146
dicofol 210
Didymella exitialis 636
Dieffenbachia, contact dermatitis 734
dieldrin 209, 275
    aldrin epoxidation 74
    hepatotoxicity 893
dienes **237–9**
    formula and examples *224*
    see also 1,3-butadiene
diesel engine exhaust gas 142
    genotoxicity *777*
diet
    confounding variable in carcinogen
        exposure monitoring 773
    effect on biological monitoring 20
    radioactivity in 406
diethylene dioxide (dioxan) 10
    dioxin confused with dioxan 9
    prescribed diseases due to *50*
diethylene glycol, occupational diseases
        caused by (EC schedule) *43*
diethylene triamine pentoacetic acid
        (DTPA) 410
diethyl ether 167, 169
di-(2-ethyl hexyl) phthalate,
        hepatotoxicity/hepatocarcinoge
        nicity 895
diethyl ketone *247*
diethyl lead 85
diethylstilboestrol (DES), reproductive
        hazards 825, 827, *829*
diethyl sulphate, genotoxicity *777*
diethyltin compounds 114
difenacoum 212
diffusion, of chemicals 68
    facilitated 68
1,1-difluoro-1-chloroethane (Genetron-
        142B) 155
1,1-difluoroethylene (Genetron-1132A)
        155
digestive disorders, shift work 583
digestive system, *see* gastrointestinal
        tract
digital imaging 594, 595
Dignity at Work Bill (1996) 544
diiododiethyltin 114
diisocyanates
    extrinsic allergic alveolitis due to *654*
    inhaled 639
    occupational asthma due to 639
    reactions 639
diisopropylethylamine, in nucleic acid
        extraction *529*
dimenhydrinate 373
dimercaprol (BAL) 97, 852
    in arsenic poisoning 871
    in cadmium poisoning 95
    in lead poisoning 871
    in mercury poisoning 92, 93
    in organotin poisoning 115
    as treatment for liver disease 887

2,3-dimercaprol (BAL), *see* dimercaprol
dimercaptopropane sulphonate 848
2,3-dimercaptopropane sulphonate
        (DMPS) 88, 871
2,3-dimercapto-1-propane-sulphonic
        acid (sodium salt) 852
dimercaptosuccinic acid (DMSA) 88,
        848
dimercaptosulphonic acid 848
dimethoxybenzidine dihydrochloride,
        in nucleic acid extraction *529*
dimethylacetamide, hepatotoxicity *884*
N,N-dimethylacetamide, biological
        monitoring tests and guidance
        values *18*
dimethylamine 157
dimethylaminoproprionitrile (DMAPN),
        neurotoxic effects 869–70
dimethylarsine 96
7,12-dimethylbenz[a]anthracene 742
dimethyl benzene, *see* xylene
2,2′-dimethylbutane 225
2,3-dimethylbutane 225
dimethylcarbamoyl chloride,
        genotoxicity *777*
1,1′dimethyl 4,4′dipyridylium
        dichloride, *see* paraquat
dimethyl ether 169
dimethylformamide (DMF) *224*, **251**
    biological monitoring tests and
        guidance values *18*
    carcinogenicity 251
    characteristics and uses 251
    clinical manifestations 251
    hepatotoxicity *884*
    metabolism/biochemical effects 251
1,2-dimethylhydrazine
    colon cancer 742
    hepatotoxicity *885*
dimethylnitrosamine 745
    centrilobular necrosis and 883
dimethylnitrosamine *N*-dimethylase,
        metabolic polymorphisms with
        cancer susceptibility links *758*
2,2-dimethyl propane 169
dimethylselenide 111
dimethyl sulphate
    genotoxicity *777*
    in nucleic acid extraction 529
dimethyl sulphide 155, 161
1,3-dinitrobenzene, reproductive
        hazards 826
dinitro-*o*-cresol (DNOC) 271
dinitrophenol (DNP) 271
    prescribed disease due to *50*
dinitrotoluene, reproductive hazards
        826
dioctyl phthalate 639
    hepatotoxicity/hepatocarcinogenicity
        895
dioctyltin 114
diode lasers 427
diols **243–4**
    formula and examples *224*
dioxan, *see* diethylene dioxide
dioxane, *see* diethylene dioxide
dioxin, *see* 2,3,7,8-tetrachlorodibenzo-
        p-dioxin

diphacinone 212
diphenyl, substituted, urinary tract
   neoplasms due to *51*
diphenyl methane 4,4 diisocyanate
   (MDI) 9, 639
   extrinsic allergic alveolitis due to
     654
dippers' flu 873
diquat 202
   symptoms and signs of exposure to
     200
'dirty worker' phenomenon 68
disability
   hearing, *see* hearing disability
   WHO definition 294
disability allowance, *see* compensation
Disability Discrimination Act 1995 (DDA)
   571, 577
disability pensions, cotton workers 625
disablement 38–9
disacclimatization 336
disc degeneration 480, 483
disc prolapse 479
disease clusters 28–9
diseases
   effect on occupation **12–13**
   germ theory 923
   not ascribable to occupation? 32–3
   occasional surveys 31–2
   occupational, estimating extent of
     27–35
   reporting schemes
     statutory 30–1
     voluntary 31
   spread of, by air travel 379
diseases, occupational 6
   Charles Thackrah and prevention
     919–20
   defining 6
   diagnostic criteria 6–7
     differential diagnosis 7
     effect 6
     exposure 7
     time sequence 7
   European Schedule of *43–5*
   history **917–25**
   impact of war on prevention of 924
   infectious diseases **489–520**
   international collaboration 923–4
   modern industrial experience 924–5
   see also prescribed diseases; *and*
     individual diseases
dismissal, unfair 542
disodium cromoglycate 627
distribution, of chemicals **68**
disulfiram (Antabuse) 167, 563
dithiocarbamates 195, 254
diuresis 163, 223
   alkaline, in mercury poisoning 93
diuretics
   chlorine poisoning *133*
   as treatment for liver disease 887
divers 343
   'acclimatization' 347, 351
   carbon dioxide increased, effects
     346
   compression barotrauma 347–8
   decompression, *see* decompression;

decompression illnesses;
   decompression sickness
deep diving, medical emergencies
   349
   ear and skin infections **349–50**
   fitness for work 355, 358
   flying after diving, decompression
     sickness 364
   guidance documents for 13
   high-pressure neurological syndrome
     (HPNS) 346
   hypoxia 346, 349
   insidious hypothermia 332
   long-term effects on **356–8**
   nitrogen narcosis 346
   saturation, latency in decompression
     illness 353
   unconsciousness in water **348–9**
     treatment 349
   see also diving procedures;
     hyperbaric environment
diving bell 343, 344, 349
Diving Medical Advisory Committee
   (DMAC) 356
diving procedures **343–4**
   compressed air 343–4, 346
     depth limits 344, 346, 347, 348
   decompression, *see* decompression
   'no-stop' diving 346
   saturation diving 344, 346
     ear and skin infections 349–50
     latency 353
     musculoskeletal pain 351
     osteonecrosis and 358
     treatment of decompression
       illness 355
   scuba 343, 350
   see also divers
diving response 331
diving tables 347, 351
divinylbenzene, occupational diseases
   caused by (EC schedule) *43*
DIY (do-it-yourself), toxic materials used
   in 5, *6*
dizziness
   in heat 336
   lack of oxygen 135
DMF, *see* dimethylformamide
DNA
   damage 21, 743–5
     adducts, *see* DNA adducts
     by carbon tetrachloride 888
     carcinogen action 743–4
     dioxin and 890
     direct/indirect-acting agents 744
     frameshift mutations 743
     free radicals 745
     germ cell 828–9
     hydrolytic 744
     metabolic activation 744
     mutations 743–4, 744–5
     by vinyl chloride 889
   genetic modification techniques 523
   intercalation 745
   lead and 85
   methylation 744
   microchip technology 763
   repair 745–6

   strand breakage 745
   synthesis, nitrous oxide effect on 168
DNA adducts 21, 744–5
   consequences of formation 744–5
   etheno adducts 754
   formation 744–5
   protein adducts 773
DNOC, *see* dinitro-*o*-cresol
DNP, *see* dinitrophenol
doctor experts, court cases 59–60
doctor participants, in court cases
   58–9
   disclosure privilege and 58, 59
doctors
   provision of medicolegal reports
     58–60
   see also medical profession
Doctors' and Dentists' Group, Medical
   Council on Alcoholism 565
dodecane *225*
   confused with chlordecone (Kepone)
     9
Dogger Bank itch 734
dogs
   care/handling, prescribed diseases
     due to *48, 49*
   hydatid disease and 495
do-it-yourself (DIY), toxic materials used
   in 5, *6*
Doll Report 446
dopamine agonists 836
dosemeters 399
dose–response relationship 67
Down's syndrome, aluminium and 100
doxorubicin 745, 895
doxycycline 379
   brucellosis 492
   chlamydiosis 493
   leptospirosis 496
   Lyme fever 497
   Q fever 498
   traveller's diarrhoea 513
2,4-DP (2-(2,4-
   dichlorophenoxy)propionic
   acid) *203*, 203
Dramamine 373
dressers, title covering diversity of jobs
   4
dressing fungicides 212
drink, aircrew 374
drinking water
   acrylamide contamination 251
   chlorine and 148
   fluoride in 150, 151–2
   trichloroacetic acid in 249
drivers
   alcohol-related effects 558
   fitness to drive 12–13
   truck drivers, bladder cancer 811
Driving and Vehicle Licensing Authority
   (Swansea), Medical Advisory
   Branch 13
driving licences
   alcohol and drug abusers 564
   high risk offender scheme 564
drowning
   cold-related 331–2
   secondary 332

drug abuse 557
  abstinence after 563
  assessment 560
  coercion? ethics and efficacy 562–3
  consent to tests 561
  counselling 563
  deterrent medication 563
  detoxification 563
  identification 559–62
  legal and ethical pitfalls 561
  management in the workplace 562–3
    constructive coercion 562–3
  prevention 565
  prognosis 564
  successful treatment 563–4
  testing for 561
  treatment monitoring 561–2
  vocational driving licences 564
  withdrawal 563
  workplace policies 562
  workplace urine screening 561–2
drugs
  drug testing programmes 561
  objective markers 561–2
  reproductive hazards 828, 831
  see also teratogenicity; and
    individual drugs
dry bulb temperature 327, 333
dry-cleaning industry
  bladder cancer 811
  hepatotoxicity in 884, 891
  perchloroethylene exposure 857
  postnatal exposure effects 833
  tetrachloroethylene
    (perchloroethylene) in 235
duodenum, cancer risk and germline
  mutations 750
Dupuytren's contracture 316, **463–4**
  acute injury and 463
  epidemiology 463
  occupational studies 463–4
  vibration and 464
dusts
  EC comparable data collection 41
  endotoxins in 22
  inorganic **663–708**
    see also inorganic dust diseases
  lead-bearing 83
  lung defences against 663–4
  nuisance dusts 679, 681, 682
  occupational asthma due to 647
  organic, see also byssinosis; extrinsic
    allergic alveolitis (EAA)
  prescribed diseases due to 52, 53, 54
  respiratory ailments caused by
    inhalation of, EC schedule of
    occupational diseases 44
  in sick building syndrome 717
  textile **621–31**
    see also byssinosis
  see also specific dusts
Dutch hypothesis, in COPD 613
duty of care, employers' 539, 544
dye manufacturing industry
  bladder cancer 4, 815
  menstrual disturbances 830
dyes
  benzidine-based, genotoxicity 777

bladder cancer due to 815
eye damage from 420
hair 734
reactive
  occupational asthma due to 636,
    647
  prescribed diseases due to 53, 54
  radioallergosorbent tests (RAST)
    21
dye trades 266
dying back neuropathy
  acrylamide causing 250
  arsenic poisoning 96
  thallium poisoning 113
dysarthria, in mercury poisoning 92
dysbaric osteonecrosis 356–8
  as prescribed disease 355
  radiological classifications 357
dysbarism, as prescribed disease 46,
  355
dysphagia, paraquat poisoning and 201
dyspnoea, see also breathlessness
dystonia, in manganese poisoning 108

ear(s)
  anatomy and physiology 285–9
    inner ear 287–9
    middle ear 285–6
    outer ear 285
  chronic inflammatory middle ear
    disease 293
  infections, in saturation diving
    349–50
  inner, barotrauma 348
  middle
    barotrauma 347–8
    gas in 362
    protection 297–8
    welding injuries 184, 185
eardrum perforation, at high altitudes
  388
earmuffs 297
earplugs 297–8
  air passengers 368
Eastern Europe, compensation schemes
  41
Ebola haemorrhagic fever 509
Ebola virus 509
echinococcosis 495–6
Echinococcus granulosus 495
Echinococcus multilocularis 495
eczema
  asteatotic 734
  see also dermatitis
EDTA (ethylenediaminetetraacetic acid)
  847, 886
  in cadmium poisoning 95
  in chromium poisoning 104
  in manganese poisoning 108
  in nucleic acid extraction 529
education, occupational noise-induced
  hearing loss (ONIHL) prevention
  298
EEC directives on workplace carcinogens
  817
effluent, from biotechnological
  processes 530

Ehrlichia spp. 497
ejection from aircraft 370
  ejection seats 375
elbow problems 457–9
  aetiology 458
  beat elbow 464
  clinical aspects 458
  epicondylitis 454, 458, 459, 461, 462
  epidemiology 458
  management 458–9
  occupational studies 458
  work-related 454
elbows, prescribed diseases affecting
  46
electrical industry, hepatotoxicity in
  884
electrical insulation product workers,
  menstrual disturbances 830
electrical workers
  acute effects of electromagnetic
    fields 440
  brain cancers 441–2
  cancer risk 440–4
  leukaemia 813, 909
  magnetic field exposure 439
  microshocks 440
  occupational groups studied 440
  reproductive effects of
    electromagnetic fields 444
  see also electromagnetic fields
electric arc welding, see
  welders/welding
electric blankets 444
electric fields 439, 440
  exposure measurement 439, 443–4
electric fires, eye damage from 420
electric industries, carcinogenic risk in
  816
electricity 439
electricity workers, post-traumatic
  stress disorder 546, 547
electric response audiometry (ERA)
  298, 300–3
electric shock 439
electrocardiograph, abnormalities in
  antimony workers 100
electrocochleography (ECochG) 302
electrolyte movement, ionic
  dissociation and 68
electromagnetic fields (EMF), extremely
  low frequency **439–50**
  acute effects 440
  brain tumours and 810
  cancer risk 440–4, 816
  defibrillators and 185
  epidemiological studies 440, 444
  exposure guidelines 446, 447
  exposures (domestic/occupational)
    439
  gene expression 444
  laboratory research into 444
  leukaemogenic effects 909
  long-term health effects 440–6
  magnetic resonance imaging 446
  measurement 439
    electric fields 443–4
  National Academy of Science Report
    447

nature of 439
neurobehavioural/neurodegenerativ
e effects 445–6
pacemakers and 185
pulsed (PEMF) 443
reproductive effects 444–5
welders/welding apparatus 184, 185,
439
electromagnetic radiation
prescribed diseases due to *46*
see also non-ionizing radiation;
visual display unit (VDU)
operators
electromyography, in exposure to
organophosphorus insecticides
207
electronic circuits, hazards 172
electronic monitoring, at place of work,
leading to violence 552
electronics industry/workers
carcinogenic risk *816*
colophony fume and asthma 638
dermatoses 734
nickel and 109
thallium and 113
electron microscopy 700
asbestos fibres 694
electroretinogram (ERG) 242
elimination, of chemicals 69, **72–7**
rate 70
EMAS, *see* Employment Medical
Advisory Service
embalmers
blood-borne viruses 505
brain tumours 810
hepatitis B infection 503
emboli, *see* gas embolism
embryo
radiation damage/threshold dose
400, 402
toxicity of chemicals/agents 830–2
embryonal renal neoplasia, cancer risk
and germline mutations *751*
embryotoxicity, acrylonitrile (vinyl
cyanide) 253
emerald 101
emergency planning, major toxic gas
releases 126–9
casualty numbers calculation *128*
emergency services, stress and 571
emery 701
EMF, *see* electromagnetic fields
emollients, in contact dermatitis
protection 730
emphysema
byssinosis and 622
cadmium-induced 27, 94, 614
cases reported to SWORD *31*
centrilobular 665, 683
computed tomography and 669
and COPD 609, 610
IIAC recommendations 39, 40
as prescribed disease *55*
in coalworkers 683, 684
employee assistance programmes
(EAPs), mental health 578
employees
support for 578–9

work stress and support from home
572
employers
duty of care 539, 544, 570–1
impact of employee stress on
financial 571
legal 570–1
legal duties, hearing protection
298–9
responsibilities 7–8
Employment Medical Advisory Service
(EMAS) 8, 12, 82, 659
advice from 806
industrial chemicals information
223
laboratory analysis 221
Employment Protection (Consolidation)
Act 1978 544
employment tribunals 58
empty field myopia 369
Encarsia, radioallergosorbent tests
(RAST) *21*
encephalomyelitis, in Lyme disease 497
encephalopathy
acrylamide 868
aluminium 99, 871
arsenic 97
carbon disulphide 868–9
ethylene oxide 166
hepatic, treatment 887
lead poisoning 86, 87, 871
manganese fume and welders 184
solvent-induced 875
endocarditis
brucellosis 492
Q fever 498
endocrine control of reproduction 825
endolymphatic hydrops 303–4
endoplasmic reticulum (ER) 73
vinylidene chloride (1,1-
dichloroethylene) metabolism
236
endotoxins
biotechnology hazard 528
byssinosis and 623
enflurane 167
exposure standards 168
engineering industries
post-traumatic stress disorder 545,
546, 547
radiographers in 407
engineers, bone marrow and brain
cancers *816*
Entamoeba histolytica 514
Enterobacter 623
Entonox 167
environment
Agent Orange 274
arsenical pigments occurrence 96
biotechnology and 530
cadmium occurrence and poisoning
(itai-itai disease) 94
control in thermal illness prevention
339–40
DDT poisoning 275
dioxin exposures (Seveso incident)
274–5, 876, 886, 890
fires and toxic gases 129–31

gases in 135–6
see also individual gases
genetically modified organisms
release 530
'greenhouse gases' 135, 150, 154
heat exchange and 326
hexachlorobenzene contamination
(Turkey) 267
hydrogen chloride 149
mercury occurrence and poisoning
(Minamata Bay) 90, 852, 872
methyl/ethyl mercury and
reproductive hazards 830
nuclear reactor incidents 131
oxygen-deficient atmospheres 135,
136, 137
oxygen excess 135
polybrominated biphenyls (PBBs)
poisoning 275
polychlorinated biphenyls (PCBs)
exposure/incidents 273–4
polycyclic aromatic hydrocarbons
(PAHs) exposure 272
temperature, *see* temperature
thallium occurrence and poisoning
113
toxic gas releases 126–9
see also air pollution; drinking water;
indoor air; indoor air pollution;
water pollution
environmental concentration, volatile
organic compounds 71
environmental occupations,
hepatotoxicity in *884*
Environmental Protection Act 1990,
genetically modified organisms
522
enzootic abortion of ewes (EAE) 493
enzymes
expression, prenatal exposure effects
825
occupational asthma due to *634*,
636, 637
production, biotechnology
application 525
see also liver enzymes
enzymuria 852
chromium and 853
petroleum-based paints and 857
solvents and 856
eosinophilia 495
eosinophilic bronchitis 640
epichlorohydrin (1-chloro-2,3-
epoxypropane) *224*, **252–3**
carcinogenicity 252
genotoxicity *777*
leukaemia 813
in trichloroethylene 233
epicondylitis 458, 462
lateral (tennis elbow) *454*, 458, 459,
461
medial (golfer's elbow) *454*, 458
epidemiological studies 924–5
bias 801
cancer 797–8
analytical studies 798–800
electromagnetic fields and 440,
444

epidemiological studies – *contd*
  cancer – *contd*
    exploratory studies 798
    hazard identification 802–5
    interpretation 800–1
    negative studies and no effect
      thresholds 801
    chance 800
    confidence limits 800
    confounding factors 800–1
    neurotoxic effects of exposures 867–8
    solvent-induced 875
epidemiology
  biases in 801
  cancer 793, 796–7
  case-control studies 799–800
  cohort studies 798–9
  identification of occupational
    hazards, *see* hazards,
    occupational
  molecular 797
  new developments 801–2
  of occupational injuries/disease
    27–8
  reproductive hazards 834
  skin disease 725
  see also epidemiological studies;
    hazards, occupational
EPIDERM recording project for skin
  diseases 31, 725
epilepsy, alcohol-related 558
epileptiform attacks 345, 346
epoxidation 74
epoxides **252–3**
  formula and examples *224*
epoxy resins 639
  allergic contact dermatitis 734
  curing agents, prescribed diseases
    due to *52, 53*
  as hazardous DIY material *6*
  hepatotoxicity in *884*
Epping Forest jaundice incident 270,
  883
  see also methylenedianiline
Epstein–Barr virus 272
equine animals, prescribed diseases
  due to contact with *48*
erbium lasers
  exposure limits *429*
  eye damage from *420*, 430
erethism, in mercury poisoning 89, 91,
  92
ergonomic advice, back pain
  prevention 481–2
ergonomic hazards in biotechnology
  529
ergonomics, musculoskeletal disorders
  and
  risk assessment and reduction
    468–70
  risk factors 467–70
erionite 694, 696
  carcinogenicity *814*
  genotoxicity *776*
erysipeloid 501
Erysipelothrix rhusiopathiae 501
erythema
  radiation levels causing *400*

in welding 184
erythema migrans 497
erythrocyte protoporphyrin, biological
  effect monitoring *19*, 20
erythrocytes, *see* red cells
erythroid hyperplasia, bone marrow
  906
erythroid hypoplasia, bone marrow
  906
erythroleukaemia, occupations/agents
  causing *4*
erythromycin
  Campylobacter infections 493
  chlamydiosis 493
  erysipeloid and 501
  legionnaires' disease 711
  leptospirosis 496
  listeriosis 496
  ovine chlamydiosis 493
erythropoiesis, ineffective 905–6
erythropoietin, biotechnology product
  522, *522*, 524
eschars 491
Escherichia coli 522, 523, 524, 528
  enterotoxin-producing (ETEC) 513
  O157 490, 493–4
essential hypertension *390*
esterases 75
esters **249–50**
  formula and examples *224*
  see also methyl methacrylate
Estrumate, accidental self-injection
  with *213*
ethane 169, *225*
ethanol *239*
  breath analysis 71
  management of methanol poisoning
    241
  in nucleic acid extraction *529*
ethers **251–2**
  formula and examples *224*, 251
  in nucleic acid extraction *529*
ethical issues
  biological monitoring 16–17
  occupational history 11–12, *12*
  reproductive health safeguarding
    836–7
ethidium bromide 529
ethmoid sinus cancer 808
ethnicity, metabolism of solvents and
  20
2-ethoxyethanol, reproductive hazards
  828
ethoxyquin, in contact dermatitis
  733
ethyl acetate 249
ethyl alcohol, *see* alcohol; ethanol
ethyl benzene 266
ethyl chloride (chloroethane) 169
ethylene 169, 232
ethylene chloride, *see* 1,2-
  dichloroethane
ethylene chlorohydrin (EtC), neurotoxic
  effects 870
ethylenediaminetetraacetic acid, *see*
  EDTA
ethylene dibromide, *see* 1,2-
  dibromoethane

ethylene dichloride, *see* 1,2-
  dichloroethane
ethylene glycol *239*
  in nucleic acid extraction *529*
  occupational diseases caused by (EC
    schedule) *43*
ethylene glycol mono methyl ether, and
  bone marrow hypoplasia 907
ethylene oxide 165–6
  carcinogenicity 166, *814*
  characteristics, sources and uses
    165–6
  clinical manifestations of exposure
    166
  genotoxicity *776*
  leukaemia and 813, 909
  lymphatic and haemopoietic system
    cancers *816*
  peripheral neuropathy 166
  radioallergosorbent tests (RAST) *21*
ethylene oxide (EtO), neurotoxic effects
  870
ethyl ether, occupational diseases
  caused by (EC schedule) *43*
ethylidene chloride, *see* ethylidene
  dichloride
ethylidene dichloride (1,1-
  dichloroethane) 230
ethyl mercury, reproductive hazard
  830
N-ethyl-*N*-nitrosourea, genotoxicity
  777
ethylthiourea, as non-genotoxic
  carcinogen *765*
ethyltin 114
ethyne (acetylene) 169, 239
European Union/Commission
  Biological Agents Directive 502
  civil and criminal law and 58
  collaboration in pesticide evaluation
    198
  genetic modification directives 530
  health certification of psittacine
    birds, directive 492
  industrial injuries schemes 38
  Information Notices on the Diagnosis
    of Occupational Diseases 41
  Schedule of occupational diseases
    40–1, *43–5*
  shortlist of prescribed agents for
    comparable data collection
    (Euro-30) *41*
  Working Hours Directive 585–6, 588
evaporation 327
evoked response audiometry 300–3
Excimer lasers 427
  eye damage from *420*
exercise
  in acute mountain sickness (AMS) 392
  for back pain 481, 483
  hip and knee osteoarthritis 466–7,
    467
  provoking occupational asthma *634*
  strenuous, reproductive hazards to
    embryo/fetus *832*
  thermoregulation and 325–6
expert medical reports, *see* medicolegal
  reports

expert witnesses
  court proceedings 62–3
  demeanour in court 62
  doctor experts 59–60
  as independent advisers to court
    62
  legal liability 63–4
  objectivity of 62, 63
  and the Woolf reforms 63
  see also medicolegal reports
explosions/explosion hazards
  alkanes 225
  in confined spaces 136
  flammable gases 123, 125, 136
  methane 137, 138
  in mines 137
  otic blast injury and acoustic trauma
    294
  sulphide dust 155
  toxic gas accidents 123
explosives
  nitro-explosives 159
  white phosphorus in 98
explosives manufacture
  aluminium lung and 701
  blood dyscrasias/malignancies 4
exposure
  assessment
    chemical exposure 16
    in health surveillance 15–16
  to chemicals 221
  extent of 8
  to gases
    in fires 129–31
    in indoor and outdoor air 125
    in industrial accidents 126–9
    in industry 125
    see also individual gases
  kinetics of 71–2
    dermal 72
    inhalation kinetics 71–2
  monitoring, see biological effect
    monitoring; biological
    monitoring
  standards 7
extraction ratio (ER) 70
extrapyramidal signs, in manganese
  poisoning 872
extrathoracic manifestations, imaging
  602
extrinsic allergic alveolitis (EAA)
  653–61, 711
  acute 603, 657
  air trapping in 598
  biotechnology hazard 528
  causes 653–4, *654*, 711
    characteristics of 653
  chemicals causing *654*
  chronic 603, 657–8
  clinical features 657–8
  compensation, statutory 660–1
  contaminated humidifier water and
    712
  diagnosis 658–9
  differential diagnosis 659
  EC schedule of occupational diseases
    44
  farmer's lung and 634–5

hypersensitivity pneumonitis
  hard metal lung disease *vs* 703
  summer type allergic alveolitis
    711
  in welding 186
  imaging 603
  immunopathogenesis 656–7
  indoor air pollution causing 654,
    655–6
  infective pneumonias *vs* 603
  inhaled diisocyanates 639
  lung function 657, 658, 659, 660
  management 659–60
  organic dusts causing 653, *654*
  outbreaks 711
  outcome 659
  pathology 656
  as prescribed disease *49*, 660
  radionuclide studies 599
  sarcoidosis *vs* 656
  smoking and 8
  summer type allergic alveolitis 711
  T lymphocytes in 656
eye(s)
  ageing changes 425, 429–30
  anatomy 421–3
  compression barotrauma 348
  dry eyes, sick building syndrome 713
  light absorption 424–5
  light damage *420*, 425
    acute 426–9
    basic mechanisms 423–4
    chronic 429–30
    mechanical (ionization) 423, 427
    photochemical 423, 424
    protection 431–5
    spectral bands 425
    thermal 423, 423–4, 427
  non-ionizing radiation damage, *see*
    non-ionizing radiation
  radiation damage 402, *420*
    infrared 430
    microwaves 430
  radiation safety evaluation 432
  screening tests 429
  welding injuries 185
  xylene damage 264
  see also cornea; lens, of eye; retina
eye irritation
  biological monitoring tests *18*
  bis(chloromethyl) ether (BCME) 252
  dimethylformamide 251
  glutaraldehyde 246
  methanol 241
  methyl *iso*-butyl ketone (M*i*BK) 248
  tetrachloroethylene
    (perchloroethylene) 235
  trichloroethylene 234
eyelid ulceration, chromium causing
  105
eye protectors
  aircrew 370
  design and standards 431–2
  firefighters 433
  lasers 433–4
  types and selection criteria 432, *433*
  ultraviolet and infrared protection
    432

eyesight, screening tests 429

facilitated diffusion 68
factor VIII, biotechnology product *522*
factor IX, biotechnology product *522*
Factory Act 1833 922–3
factory inspectors 922–3
factory system 919–20
Faculty of Occupational Medicine, UK,
  guidelines on drug abuse testing
  561
fainting, in heat 336
falciparum malaria 513
familial medullary thyroid carcinoma,
  oncogene activation in *749*
family and social life, effect of shift
  work 582
Fanconi-like syndrome
  in cadmium workers 94
  in lead poisoning 86
Fanconi's anaemia 746
Fanconi syndrome 848
farmers/farm workers
  anthrax 490
  brucellosis 491
  Campylobacter infections 493
  erysipeloid 501
  extrinsic allergic alveolitis 711
  food-borne zoonotic infections 493
  hantavirus infection 494
  hydatid disease 495
  hydrogen sulphide exposure 160
  leptospirosis 496
  listeriosis 496
  Lyme disease 497
  nitrogen dioxide exposure 159
  non-Hodgkin's lymphoma 910
  ringworm 502
  skin and lip cancers *815*
  toxic gas exposure 135–6
  zoonoses 489
  see also agricultural
    workers/occupations
farmer's lung 653, *654*, 654, **654–5**,
  656
  extrinsic allergic alveolitis and
    634–5
  management 660
  outcome 659
  as prescribed disease *49*
  prevalence 654
  prevention 654–5
  respiratory protection 654–5, 660
  serum precipitins 659
  see also extrinsic allergic alveolitis
    (EAA)
farms, health risks to visitors 490
fat, unsaturated, as non-genotoxic
  carcinogen *765*
fatigue
  in decompression illness 352
  in lead poisoning 86
  shift work 582–3, 584
feet
  annual radiation dose limits *409*
  non-freezing cold injury (NFCI) 330
femur, osteonecrosis of head of 357

fenofibrate, as non-genotoxic
    carcinogen *765*
fenoprop (MCPA; 4-chloro-2-
    methylphenoxyacetic acid) *203*
fenvalerate 211
ferrochelatase 85
ferrochromium 853
ferrochromium workers, lung cancer
    815
ferrovanadium 116
fertility
    assessment and records 834
    factors affecting 826–7
    female *828, 830, 832*
    impaired 833–5
    male *828, 829, 832*
    see also infertility
fertilizer production, phosphates 150
fetotoxicity 830–2
    1,3-butadiene 238
    xylene 264
fettlers, silicosis prevention 676–7
fetus
    malformations, *see* congenital
        malformations
    radiation damage/threshold dose
        400, 402
    rubella and 510
    toxoplasmosis and 500
    see also fetotoxicity
FEV₁, *see* forced expiratory volume
fibreglass, *see* glass fibre
fibres 686
    fibre counting 695
    man-made, *see* man-made
        mineral/vitreous fibres
fibromyalgia 463
    as cause of back pain *479*
fibrosarcoma, cancer risk and germline
    mutations *750*
fibrosis
    in liver 885
        treatment 887
    pulmonary, *see* asbestosis;
        pulmonary fibrosis
fibrous clays 696
fibrous mineral dusts 686–97
    see also asbestos; asbestosis; glass
        fibre; rock wool
Ficus spp., radioallergosorbent tests
    (RAST) *21*
Ficus benjamina (Weeping Fig) 713
Fighter Index of Thermal Stress (FITS)
    333
figs, contact dermatitis 734
film badges 399
filter materials, protective 432–5
filtration, of chemicals 68
fingers
    prescribed diseases affecting *48, 51*
    see also vibration white finger
Finland, occupational asthma causes
    and incidence 634–5
Finnish Institute of Occupational Health
    (FIOH), biological monitoring
    tests and guidance values 17,
    18
firearms, *see* gunfire

firearms instructors/enthusiasts and
    lead absorption 83
firecracker manufacture, phosphorus
    hepatotoxicity 893
fire damp 137
fire extinguishants 155
firefighters 130–1
    diet effect on adduct levels 773
    eye protectors 433
    fitness 337
    hydrogen cyanide inhalation 145
    post-traumatic stress disorder 547,
        548
    protective equipment 337, 338
    respiratory protection 130
fires 129–31
    chemical fallout from oil-fires
        129–30
    combustion products 129
    see also smoke
fireworks manufacture
    aluminium lung and 701
    hepatotoxicity in *884*
first aid, gassing accidents 131–2, 145
fish
    mercury content 852
    occupational asthma due to *647*
    organoarsenicals in 97
    prescribed diseases due to *53, 54*
fish consumption
    arsenic levels 20
    mercury levels 20, 23
fishermen
    alcohol-related problems 559
    erysipeloid 501
fish filleters, cold adaptation 328
fish handlers, dermatoses 734
fishing
    carcinogenic risk in *815*
    using dynamite for 349
fishing industry, gas hazard from
    decaying fish 136, 157, 160
fishmongers
    erysipeloid 501
    zoonoses 489
fishmonger's finger/disease 501
Fish Odour Syndrome 157
fish tank granuloma 501
fish vaccines 213, 214
fish workers, leptospirosis 496
fitness for flight
    aircrew 362, 372, 377–8
    airline passengers 379
fitness for work 12–13
    aircrew 362, 372, 377–8
    divers 355, 358
    stress-related illness 576
Fitness for Work: the Medical Aspects
    12, 13
fitness to drive 12–13
flammable gases 123, 125, 136
Flanders foot 330
flash-blindness 434
flash burns, corneal 430
flatus 135
flavin-monooxygenases, pulmonary 77
flax, weaving, byssinosis as prescribed
    disease due to *52*

flax dust 185, 621, 622
    inhalation, EC schedule of
        occupational diseases *44*
flax workers 621, 622
Flixborough accident 123, 225
floristry, dermatoses 734
floumafen 212
flour
    contamination with thallium 113
    occupational asthma due to *634,*
        636, 637, *647*
    prescribed diseases due to *52, 53*
flours, mixed, radioallergosorbent tests
    (RAST) *21*
flow cytometry 22
fluazifop butyl, dermal
    biotransformation 77
flu-like illness
    acute allergic alveolitis 657
    in biotechnology workers *527*
    legionnaires' disease 711
    listeriosis 496
    rabies 499
flumethrine 211
fluorapatite 98, 150
fluorescence *in situ* hybridization (FISH)
    399, 764, 767, 773
fluorescent lamp manufacture,
    reproductive hazards 831
fluorescent lights/lamps
    beryllium in 101, 702
    eye damage from *420,* 429
fluoride(s)
    acute effects 150–1
    biological monitoring tests and
        guidance values *18*
    chronic toxicity 151–2
    daily intake 151
    management of systemic poisoning
        152
    nephrotoxicity 167
    occupational systemic poisoning
        152
    toxic effects 151
    see also hydrogen fluoride
fluoride salts 152
fluorinated hydrocarbons **154–7**
    see also chlorofluorocarbons
fluorine 150
    occupational diseases caused by (EC
        schedule) *43*
fluorine compounds, occupational
    diseases caused by (EC schedule)
    43
fluorocarbon-114 B2 (1,2-
    dibromotetrafluoroethane) 155
fluoroform (Freon-23) 154
fluorosis 150, 151
    dental 151–2
    skeletal 151
5-fluorouracil 895
fluorspar 150
    radon concentrations in mines 407
fluorspar miners
    lung cancers 28
    respiratory tract malignancies *4*
fluosilicic acid 150, 153
flurane 167

flushing, in trichloroethylene exposure 234
fluxes, bone marrow and brain cancer *816*
fly ash 700
flying, *see entries beginning with* air
foetor hepaticus 161
foliar fungicides 212
folinic acid 241, 242
follicle-stimulating hormone (FSH) 825, 826, 834, 835
folliculitis, in spaceflight 376
folliculogenesis 824–5
food
    aircrew 374
    containing pesticide residues 195, 196, 199
food handlers, traveller's diarrhoea 514
food industry
    prescribed diseases in *53, 54*
    see also catering and hotel industry; restaurant trade
foodstuffs, dermatitis 731
foot drop 871
footwear industry, *see* shoe manufacturing industry
forced alkaline diuresis 223
forced diuresis, arsine poisoning 163
forced expiratory volume in one second (FEV₁)
    asbestosis 689
    in byssinosis 623, 625, *626*, 627
    chronic obstructive lung disease 699
    chronic obstructive pulmonary disease (COPD) 32, 611–12
        age-related changes *612*, 612–13
    diisocyanate inhalation 639
    extrinsic allergic alveolitis 657, 658
    inorganic dust diseases 670
    loss of, and toluene diisocyanate exposure 613, 614
    occupational asthma investigation 644
    silica dust exposure 677
    see also lung function
forced vital capacity (FVC)
    asbestosis 689
    byssinosis 625
    extrinsic allergic alveolitis 657, 658
    inorganic dust diseases 670
    silica dust exposure 677
    see also lung function
forearm disorders, work-related *454*
forearms, annual radiation dose limits *409*
forestomach tumours, non-genotoxic carcinogen mechanisms *765*
forestry/forestry workers
    carcinogenic risk in *815*
    dermatoses 735
    hantavirus infection 494
    lindane and 209
    Lyme disease 497
    prescribed diseases *47, 48, 49*
forging of metal, prescribed diseases *46*
formaldehyde *224,* **244–5**

carcinogenicity 244, 805, 808
characteristics and uses 244
clinical manifestations 244
dermatoses 734, 735
genotoxicity *777*
as hazardous DIY material *6*
metabolism/biochemical effects 244–5
methanol metabolism 241
occupational diseases caused by (EC schedule) *43*
radioallergosorbent tests (RAST) *21*
reproductive hazards 830
as sterilizing agent 529
formaldehyde acetic acid 241
formalin 244
    radioallergosorbent tests (RAST) *21*
    see also formaldehyde
formic acid 249
    methanol metabolism 241
    in nucleic acid extraction *529*
formication 364
foundry work/workers
    lung cancer 700
    prescribed diseases *47*
fovea 423, 425
France
    occupational diseases schedule 41
    organotin compound poisoning incident 114
free radicals 745
    carbon tetrachloride hepatotoxicity 228
freeze–thaw–refreeze injury 329
freezing, of tissues 328–9
freezing cold injury 328–9
    long-term sequelae 329
Frenzel manoeuvre 347, 362
Freon-11 154
Freon-12 (dichlorodifluoromethane) 154, 166
Freon-13 (chlorotrifluoromethane) 154
Freon-14 (tetrafluoromethane) 154
Freon-21 (dichlorofluoromethane) 154
Freon-22 (chlorodifluoromethane) 154
Freon-23 (fluoroform) 154
Freon-113 (1,1,2-trichloro-1,2,2-trifluoroethane) 154
Freon-114 (1,2-dichlorotetrafluoroethane) 154
Freon-116 (hexafluoroethane) 154
freons 150
    see also chlorofluorocarbons
frostbite
    1,3-butadiene causing 239
    deep and complicated 329
    rewarming after 328, 329
    superficial 328–9
frostbite arthritis 329
frostnip 328
frozen shoulder (shoulder capsulitis) *454*, 456
fruit cultivation
    occupational asthma due to *647*
    prescribed diseases associated with *52, 53*
fruit juice, preventing scurvy 918
fruits, contact urticaria 731

frullania 735
frusemide 391, 392
fuel storage tanks, organic lead poisoning 89
fuller's earth 681
    in paraquat poisoning treatment 202
fume, definition 124
fumes, prescribed diseases due to *52, 53, 54*
fumigants
    hydrogen cyanide 145
    methyl bromide 164–5
    non-Hodgkin's lymphoma and 910
    phosphine (hydrogen phosphide) 163–4
'fuming sulphuric acid' (oleum) 156
'functional overlay' 61
fungal antigens 623
fungi
    contaminants of cotton dust 623, 624
    extrinsic allergic alveolitis and 711
    grain contamination and asthma 636
    humidifier fever and 712
    occupational asthma and 636
    prescribed diseases due to *49*
    ringworm due to 502
    sick building syndrome and 716–17
    spores 636
fungicides 212
    hexachlorobenzene 266
    mercurial 90
    non-Hodgkin's lymphoma and 910
fungus enzymes, in cotton dust 624
furnaces, eye damage from *420*
furniture makers/manufacturers
    cancers *814*
    ethmoid sinus cancer 808
    genotoxic exposures *776*
    nasal cancer in 28
    respiratory tract malignancies *4*
    sino-nasal cancer *816*
    1,1,1-trichloroethane (methyl chloroform) in 231
furocoumarins 734
furunculosis 213
Fusarium graminearum 524
Fusarium solani 623
fuscudic acid 431
fused ring aromatic compounds **272–3**
FVC, *see* forced vital capacity

galactic radiation, *see* cosmic radiation
galena (lead sulphide) 82, 83
gallium-67 (⁶⁷Ga) 599
gallium arsenide 172
gallium arsenide lasers, eye damage from *420*
gametogenesis 824–5
gamma-aminobutyric acid (GABA) transmission 85
gamma benzene hexachloride, *see* lindane
gamma-rays (γ-rays) *398*, 398
    terrestrial 406

Gamow Bags 392, 393, *394*
gangrene, hand–arm vibration
    syndrome 310
gardening, hepatotoxicity in *884*
garlic-like smell
  arsine 97
  on breath, hydrogen selenide 162
  dimethylselenide 111
  tellurium 112
garment workers, shoulder tendinitis
    455
gas
  definition 124
  expansion 350, **361–2**
gas appliances, faulty, deaths from 142
gas cookers, domestic 159, 160
gas embolism 353
  arterial 351, 356
    case history 353
  venous 347
gases **123–78**
  accidents and fires 123, 126–31
    acute lethality equation 126
    contours of individual risk 129
    cyclohexane, Flixborough 123
    fires 123, 129–31
    first aid 131–2, 145
    hydrogen sulphide release 161
    industrial accidents 123, 126
    investigation 134
    liquid petroleum, Mexico City 123
    London Blitz incident 123
    major toxic releases 126–9
    methyl isocyanate, Bhopal 123,
      165, 584
    nuclear reactor incidents 131
    psychological support 132, 134
    treatment 131–4
  in ambient air 135–7
    in confined spaces 136–7
    in mines 137
    oxygen deficiency 135, 136, 137
    oxygen excess 135
  anaerobic fermentation producing
    135–6
  anaesthetic, *see* anaesthetic agents
  asphyxiant, *see* asphyxiant gases
  classification by health effects 124–5
  concentration in air, ways of
    expressing 124
  in confined spaces 136–7
  corrosive 124, 131
    burns 132
  drug-like 124–5
  exposure limits 126, *127*
  flammable 123, 125, 136
  gas laws 344–5
  'greenhouse' 135, 150, 154
  hazardous, characteristics 125
  historical background 123
  industrial, definition and examples
    124
  irritant, *see* irritant gases
  liquefied petroleum gases 123, 170–1
  maximum exposure limit (MEL) 125
  mixed
    concentrations in air, formula 124
    mixed exposures 171–3

occupational exposures in industry
    125, 126–31
occupational exposure standards
    (OES) 125
partial pressures 345
prescribed diseases due to *46*
pressure and volume 344–5
pyrophoric 125
solubility and uptake 345
transfer in lungs 71–2
war and riot control 171–2
see also air pollution; environment;
    welding fume; *and individual*
    gases
gas industry workers, bladder tumours
    810
gas mask workers 695
gasoline, *see* petrol
gas retort house workers, lung and
    bladder cancer *815*
gas transfer coefficient (KCO), in
    extrinsic allergic alveolitis 657,
    658
gastroenteritis, thallium poisoning 113
gastrointestinal bleeding, pesticide
    exposure and *200*
gastrointestinal disorders
  as prescribed diseases *51*
  in radiation casualties 414
gastrointestinal tract
  biotransformation capability *73*
  digestive system malignancies
    808–10
  dimethylformamide effect 251
  metal absorption 82
  radiation damage 401
  tumours 808–10
    asbestos exposure 694
gas turbines, prescribed diseases and
    48
gas workers
  carcinogenic risk *815*
  elbow problems 458
gel electrophoresis 529
gene amplification 751
General Medical Council (GMC) 564, 565
genes
  'cancer genes' 748
  involved in carcinogenesis 748–55
  mismatch-repair genes 746, 753
  mutational spectra 754
  see also tumour-suppressor genes
genetically modified organisms 522
  classification of microorganisms 530
Genetically Modified Organisms
    (Contained Use) Regulations
    1996 522, 530
Genetically Modified Organisms
    (Deliberate Release) Regulations
    1995 522
genetic change, carcinogenesis causing
    742–7
genetic modification 523
  containment levels and control
    measures *530*, 531, *531*
  definition 521
  higher risk 532–3
  human health hazards 526–8

low risk 532
risk assessment 530, 531
risk management 530–1
safety committees 530
vectors 521
see also genetically modified
    organisms
genetic polymorphisms, chemical
    metabolism 68
genetic susceptibility
  cancer 756–63
  screening, ethical issues 763
Genetron-12 (dichlorodifluoromethane)
    154
Genetron-13 (chlorotrifluoromethane)
    154
Genetron-113 (1,1,2-trichloro-1,2,2-
    trifluoroethane) 154
Genetron-114 (1,2-dichlorotetrafluoro-
    ethane) 154
Genetron-115 (chloropentafluoro-
    ethane) 154
Genetron-142B (1,1-difluoro-1-
    chloroethane) 155
Genetron-1132A (1,1-difluoroethylene)
    155
genitourinary tract cancer, oncogene
    activation in *749*
Genklene 231
genomic instability 742, 746
genomic mutations 744
genomic stability 748
genotoxic carcinogens, *see* carcinogens:
    genotoxic
genotoxicity 743–5
  acetaldehyde 245
  acrylamide 250, *777*
  benzene 262, 775, *776*
  monitoring body fluids and tissues
    767
  occupational carcinogen
    classification by 776–7
  testing chemicals for 763–7
  see also DNA
'genotoxic noise' 773
genotypes 756–7, 762
gentamicin
  legionnaires' disease and 711
  as tissue culture additive *528*
geothermal power, emissions 172–3
germane 163
German measles 510
Germany
  MAK exposure values 7
  occupational diseases schedule 41
  pollution patterns in East and West
    616
germ cells
  DNA damage 828–9
  irradiation 405
  mutation 828–9
germicidal lamps, eye damage from
    420
germline mutation *750–1*, 752, 753
  somatic mutation *vs* 756
germ theory of disease 923
Gerstmann–Straussler–Scheinker
    syndrome (GSSS) 500

giant cell interstitial pneumonitis 703, 704

Giardia spp. 493

Giardia lamblia 513, 514

giardiasis 514

Gilbert's syndrome 881
  abnormal liver function tests 883

gilding, mercury poisoning 89

gingivae, *see* gums

gingivitis
  in mercury poisoning 91, 92
  in spaceflight 376

glanders, as prescribed disease *48*

glare, eye protectors *433*

glass 672

glass fibres 696, 697

glass manufacture
  eye damage in 430
  genotoxicity *777*
  lead use *844*
  prescribed diseases in *48, 54*

glass melt fibres, *see* glass fibres

globalization of industry 925

global warming 135, 137

globin, butadiene metabolite adducts
  with 237

glomerulonephritis 854, 855, 856, 858,
  859
  hydrocarbons and 227
  USA 843

glomerulosclerosis 845
  USA 843

gloves
  absorption increased by 221
  anti-vibration 317
  in contact dermatitis protection 730
  phenylenediamine derivatives,
    dermatitis worsened 270
  as source of sensitization 728, 731,
    733
  surgical 680
  zoonoses protection 490
  see also rubber gloves

glucinium, occupational diseases
  caused by (EC schedule) *43*

glucocorticosteroids 132, 159

glucose-6-phosphate dehydrogenase
  (G6PD) deficiency 268, 273

glucuronic acid, conjugation of
  chemicals with 75

glucuronide conjugation 75

glue sniffing 264, 891

γ-glutamyltransferase (γGT) 235, 237,
  562

γ-glutamyl transpeptidase 881, 894,
  895
  abnormal liver function tests 883

glutaraldehyde (1,5-pentanedial) *224,*
  246, 715
  occupational asthma due to *647*
  prescribed diseases due to *52, 53*
  sensitization hazard in dermatoses
    734
  in x-ray developer 715

glutathione 75, 132, 229, 744
  in pulmonary detoxification 77
  in red cell metabolism 902, 903

glutathione depletion, treatment 887

glutathione peroxidase 893

glutathione-*S*-transferases, metabolic
  polymorphisms with cancer
  susceptibility links *759*

glyceraldehyde-3-phosphate 96

glycerin *239*

glycerol derivatives, occupational
  diseases caused by (EC schedule)
  43

glyceryl thioglycolate (GTG), dermatoses
  734

glycidamide 250

glycidol, as genotoxic carcinogen 766

glycol derivatives, occupational
  diseases caused by (EC schedule)
  43

glycol ethers
  causing aplastic anaemia 907
  reproductive hazards to mother 831

glycoproteins 901–2

glycosuria
  in cadmium poisoning 94
  in lead poisoning 86

Glycyphagus domesticus 637

glyphosate-containing herbicides
  203–4
  exposure to 203
  ingestion, deliberate 203–4
  management 204

GMC (General Medical Council) 564,
  565

goats, prescribed diseases due to
  contact with *49*

goggles, night flying 370

goitre 147

gold melting 893

gold miners, and COPD 615

goldsmiths, mercury poisoning 89

golfer's elbow (medial epicondylitis)
  454, 458

gonadotrophin-releasing hormone
  (GnRH) 825, 826

gonads, radiation damage 402

Gonioma kamassi (African box wood)
  poisoning, as prescribed disease
  50

Goodpasture's antigen 857

Goodpasture's disease 855

Gore, Oklahoma, uranium processing
  plant incident 131, 150

gout 844, 847
  in lead poisoning 86
  saturnine 86

grain
  mouldy, farmer's lung *654*, 654
  occupational asthma due to *636*

grain dust 185
  asthma and COPD 613
  occupational asthma due to *636,*
    636–7
  prescribed diseases due to *52, 53*

grain fever 185

grain mites, occupational asthma due
  to *636*

grain workers/harvesters
  aluminium phosphide and 210–11
  hantavirus infection 494

Gram-negative bacteria 621, 623

granite tunnelling/quarrying,
  prescribed diseases due to *54*

granulocytes
  reduction by benzene 262
  see also agranulocytosis

granulomata
  beryllium causing 102
  copper causing 107
  dimethylselenide causing 111
  in extrinsic allergic alveolitis 656
  granulomatous lung disease 701,
    702–3
  talc causing 680

grape vine sprayers, lung disease from
  copper sulphate 107

graphite dust inhalation, EC schedule of
  occupational diseases *44*

graphite fibres 696

gravitational stress 365–6
  anti-G straining manoeuvre (AGSM)
    366
  effects 365–6
  G-induced loss of consciousness (G-
    LOC) 366
  protection 366
  Qigong manoeuvre 366

gravity, microgravity 376

Gravol 373

gray, radiation dose 398, 399

Greece, occupational diseases schedule
  41

green coffee beans
  dust, prescribed diseases due to *53,*
    54
  and occupational asthma *636, 647*
  radioallergosorbent tests (RAST) *21*

'greenhouse gases' 135, 150, 154

grey-out 366
  factors affecting *366*

grinders, silicosis prevention 675–6

grinding
  granulomatous lung disease in lens
    grinding 702
  metal-induced asthma due to 699

grip strength, hand–arm vibration
  syndrome 310

griseofulvin, ringworm 502

grog crusher, occupational history
  example 11

growth factor, oncogenes coding for
  748

growth factor receptors, oncogenes
  coding for 748

growth hormones
  biotechnology products 522, *522,*
    524
  as tissue culture additives *528*

GRP plastics manufacture,
  hepatotoxicity in *884*

grunerite 687

guaiscol, occupational diseases caused
  by (EC schedule) *43*

guanine 743, 745

Guidelines for Medicolegal Practice 294

Guillain–Barré-like syndrome, thallium
  poisoning 113

Gulf War 171
  oil well fires 129–30

Gulf War syndrome 876–7
gums
    bleeding, pesticide exposure and
        200
    blue line 83, 86, 92, 904
    see also gingivitis
gunfire
    acoustic trauma 289, 294
    impulse noise 285
    lead absorption and 83
gypsum 681–2
gypsum mines, radon concentrations in
        407

Haber's rule 126
haem
    biological monitoring tests 18
    synthesis 84, 85
        effect of lead 23
haemangioblastoma, cancer risk and
        germline mutations 751
haemangiosarcoma of liver 4
    see also angiosarcoma of the liver
haematite mining
    carcinogenicity 814
    radon and genotoxic exposures 776
haematological disorders
    anaemia, see anaemia
    clinical evaluation 903–5
    history 903–4
    laboratory investigation into 904–5
    leukaemia, see leukaemia
    myelodysplasia, see myelodysplasia
    symptoms and signs 904
    treatment
        case studies 910–11
        work-related issues 910–11
haematological screening, benzene
        exposure 263
haematopoiesis depression, radiation
        levels causing 400
haematopoietic system, radiation
        damage 400–1
haematotoxic effects, biological
        monitoring tests 18
haemochromatosis, non-invasive
        screening 882
haemodialysis
    in chemical elimination 223
    in chlorate poisoning 202
    in chlorophenoxyacetate poisoning
        203
    methanol poisoning 241, 242
haemofiltration, as treatment for liver
        disease 887
haemoglobin, in red cell metabolism
        902
haemoglobinopathies, altitude sickness
        risk 389
haemoglobinuria
    arsine poisoning 162–3
    differential diagnosis 163
haemolysis
    abnormal liver function tests 883
    arsine poisoning 97, 162, 163
    biological monitoring tests 18
    and hyperbaric oxygen 905

mechanisms of 905
    naphthalene causing 273
    oxidative 903
    phenylhydrazine causing 268
haemolytic anaemia 162, 905
    in antimony poisoning 101
    case study 911
    copper salts 107
    organic tin 114
haemolytic uraemic syndrome (HUS)
        490, 494
haemopoiesis, regulation of 901–2
haemopoietic effects of exposures
        1–13
haemopoietic system 901
    benzene effects 262
    maturation of cells 902
    red cell metabolism 902–3
    regulation of haemopoiesis 901–2
    stems cells and progenitor cells 901
    structure and function 901–3
    toluene effects 263
    tumours 811–13
        industries/occupations associated
            with 815, 816
    see also specific tumours
haemoptysis 666, 684, 686
    nitrogen dioxide poisoning 159
haemorrhagic colitis 494
haemorrhagic fevers
    Crimean Congo haemorrhagic fever
        509
    Korean haemorrhagic fever 494
    Omsk haemorrhagic fever 509
    with renal syndrome (HFRS) 494
    viral 509–10
haem synthesis disturbance 889
hair analysis, in drugs screening 561
hair bleach, dermatoses 734
hair cells 292–3
hairdressers
    dermatoses 734
    genotoxic exposures 777
    occupational asthma 647
hair dyes 734
    causing aplastic anaemia 907
hair loss, thallium poisoning 113
Haldane, J S 921
half-life
    of chemicals 20, 20, 69
    definition 398
halitosis 161
    in spaceflight 376
Hall–Heroult aluminium process 152
haloalkanes, hepatotoxicity 885, 890–2
halogenacne 732
halogenated alkanes 226–32
    epidemiological studies 226–7
    hepatotoxicity ranking 226
    renal function impairment 226
    see also carbon tetrachloride;
        chloroform; 1,2-dichloroethane;
        methylene chloride; 1,1,1-
        trichloroethane
halogens, metal, acute lung injury due
        to 698
Halon 1301 (bromotrifluoromethane)
        155

halothane 167
    exposure standards 168
Hamburg, phosgene incident 148
hand
    beat hand 464
    see also fingers; hand–arm vibration
        syndrome
hand–arm vibration syndrome (HAVS)
        308–17
    assessment 22
    carpal tunnel syndrome vs [TAB 2nd]
        314, 315, 315
    compensation 314
    definition 308
    diagnosis 310–11
    diagnostic tests 311
    drug therapy 314
    EC comparable data collection 41
    health effects 308–10
    measurement standards 317
    occupational noise-induced hearing
        loss (ONIHL) and 310
    occupations associated with 308, 309
    pathophysiology 311–14
    peripheral components 308
    as prescribed disease 48, 314
    prevention 316–17
    related conditions 314–16
    smoking and 310, 314
    sources 317
    Stockholm classification 309, 309–10
    tools associated with 308, 308, 309,
        310, 317
    treatment 314
    worker education 317
    see also vibration; vibration white
        finger
Handbook of Medical Ethics 12
handicap
    hearing 294
    WHO definition 294
handling 8–9
hands
    annual radiation dose limits 409
    contact dermatitis 726
    prescribed diseases affecting 46, 48
handwriting, prescribed diseases due to
        46
Hantaan virus 509
hantavirus infections 494–5
hantavirus pulmonary syndrome (HPS)
        494
harassment
    communication typology 541
    definition 540, 544
    sexual 540
    see also bullying; violence at work
hardening agents
    as hazardous DIY material 6
    occupational asthma due to 647
    prescribed diseases due to 52, 53
    see also acid anhydrides
hard metal 703
    chronic obstructive lung disease and
        699
hard metal disease 106, 115
    cryptogenic fibrosing alveolitis vs
        660

hard metal-induced bronchial asthma 703
hard metal lung disease 703–4
  hypersensitivity pneumonitis *vs* 703
hard metal pneumoconiosis, *see* hard metal lung disease
hard rock mining, silicosis prevention 676
hardwood dusts
  respiratory tract malignancies and *4*
  see also wood dust; woodworkers/woodworking
harvest moulds, occupational asthma due to *636*
hat makers, mercury poisoning 89, 872
'hatter's shakes' 89
HAVS, *see* hand–arm vibration syndrome
hay
  mouldy, extrinsic allergic alveolitis due to 653, *654*, 654
  silage as substitute in farmer's lung 654
hazard, definition 9, 82
hazards, occupational **27–35**
  assessing impact of 29–34
  clinical observations and investigations 27
  disease clusters 28–9
  epidemiology of occupational injuries/disease 27–8
  identification 27–9
    carcinogenic 802
  indications of, from geographical statistics 28
  mortality analyses 28
  toxicology 28
headaches
  methanol exposure 241
  methylene chloride (dichloromethane) 227
  organotin poisoning 114
  sick building syndrome 713
  trichloroethylene 234
head and neck cancer, oncogene activation in *749*
head-lice shampoos 209
health
  biopsychosocial model 925
  WHO definition 569
Health and Safety at Work Act 1974 8, 298, 570
  bullying 544
  genetically modified organisms 522
Health and Safety (Display Screen Equipment) Regulations 1992 471–2
Health and Safety Executive (HSE)
  Audiometry in Industry 298
  biological monitoring guidance values 17, *18*
  biotechnology guidelines 522
  Central Index on Dose Information (CIDI) 407
  EH40 exposure standards 7
  Employment Medical Service, *see* Employment Medical Advisory Service

exposure limits
  benzene 262
  4,4'-methylene *bis*(2-chloroaniline (MbOCA) 270
  o-toluidine 267
  xylene 262
  fitness for diving 355, 358
  Guidelines for Medicolegal Practice 294
  Noise at Work: Guidance on Regulations 298
  pesticide regulations and 197–8
  prosecutions by 57
  registering of disease 31
  Sound Solutions 297
  stress guidance 576
health-care industry, carcinogenic risk in *816*
health care workers
  CS gas and 172
  dermatoses 731, 734
  infectious diseases, *see* health care workers, infectious diseases
  microbial diseases
    HIV infections, *see* HIV infection
    Legionella pneumophila exposure 710
  nitrous oxide abuse 168
  see also anaesthetists; laboratory workers; medical/paramedical staff
health care workers, infectious diseases **502–12**
  blood-borne viruses 502–9
  clinical features 506–7
  hepatitis B 502–3
    transmission to patients 506
    vaccination 506, 508
  hepatitis C 503–4
    transmission to patients 505–6, 506
  management 507
  means of transmission 504–5
  prevention of infection 507–9
  scabies 511
  staphylococcal infections 511–12
  transmission risks 505–6
  tuberculosis 510–11
  viral haemorrhagic fevers 509–10
health promotion 565
health records, *see* medical records
health surveillance 15
  biotechnology workers 532–3
  exposure assessment 15–16
  pesticides 198–9
  see also monitoring of workers
health warning cards 490
'healthy worker effect' 799
hearing
  International Standards 295
  loss, *see* hearing loss
  measurement 298
    see also audiometry
  UK National Study of Hearing 289–90
hearing aids 299–300
  background noise 300
  compression aids 300

design and fitting 300
  distortion in 299
  environmental 300
  venting 300
hearing conservation programmes 295–9
hearing disability
  assessment 294–5
    'Blue Book' 294
    fence values 295
  compensation 289, 294, 295
  predictors 295
hearing loss
  age-related 290, 295
  children 290
  divers and compressed-air workers 356
  idiopathic 293
  non-organic (exaggerated; functional) 301
  risk 290
  risk minimization 295–9
  sensorineural 293
  in shipyards, court case 61
  see also deafness; noise; occupational noise-induced hearing loss
hearing protective devices 297–8, 298
hearing threshold
  international standards 295
  permanent shifts 290–1
  temporary shifts 289, 290
hearsay evidence, in expert reports 61
heart disease
  in firefighters 130–1
  in Lyme disease 497
  see also ischaemic heart disease; myocardial infarction
heart failure
  chloroform causing 229
  cobalt salts and heavy drinkers 106
  trichloroethylene causing 229–30
heart muscle, biotransformation capability *73*
heart rate, electromagnetic field effect 440
heat
  acclimatization 335, 337
    training in the heat 337
  balance, principles **325–7**
  effect on performance 336–7
  evaporative loss 327
  in flying 367–8
  heat equation 325, 340
  heat exchange 325, 326
  heat exhaustion 335
  heat loss 325
  heat strain
    assessment 334–5
    conditions due to 335–6
    immediate consequences 335–6
  heat stress **333–7**
    assessment 333–4
    indices 333–4
    psychrometric charts 333–4
  heat stroke 336
    cooling-management 336
  male fertility decrease 829
  prevention of illness 337–40

heat – *contd*
  prevention of illness – *contd*
    control of environment 339–40
    personal protective equipment
      338–9
    previous disorders affecting
      susceptibility 338
    the worker 337–8
    prickly heat (miliaria rubra) 336
    reproductive hazards *829*, 829
    responses to 326–7
    reversed interpretation in
      decompression illnesses 352
    working in 337–9
heat cataract
  EC comparable data collection *41*
  EC schedule of occupational diseases
    45
  as prescribed disease *46*
heavy metals, nephrotoxic effects 843
Heinz bodies 904, 905
helicopters
  escape from 375
  noise in 368
  spatial disorientation when landing
    371
  vibration in 368
    casualty evacuation and 368
helium 140–1
  for divers 344, 345
  in earth's atmosphere *135*
  and welder's exposure to ozone 181
helium-neon lasers
  exposure limits *429*
  eye damage from *420*
helmets
  aircrew 365, 368, 370
  noise-excluding 298
hematite mining, siderosis and 701
hemp dust/fibres 185, 621, 622
  inhalation, EC schedule of
    occupational diseases *44*
hemp workers 621
henna
  occupational asthma due to *647*
  as prescribed disease *52*, *53*
Henry's law 345
heparin, in decompression illness 355
hepatic angiosarcoma 74
hepatic steatosis 881, 891
  non-invasive screening *882*
hepatic vein occlusion, non-invasive
  screening *882*
hepatitis
  abnormal liver function tests 883
  acute toxic
    carbon tetrachloride 229
    4,4'-methylenedianiline (MDA)
      270
  'cement hepatitis' 250
  non-A, non-B 506
  non-invasive screening *882*
  Q fever and 498
  trichloroethylene exposure 891
  viral, *see* viral hepatitis
hepatitis A 514
  vaccine 514
hepatitis B 506

clinical features 506
  health care workers 502–3
    transmission to patients 506
    vaccination 508
  hepatoma and Kaposi's syndrome
    816
  needlestick injury 503, 505
  as prescribed disease 507
  serological markers/antigens 505,
    505
  vaccination 506, 508, 525
hepatitis B immunoglobulin (HBIG) 508
hepatitis B surface antigen,
    biotechnology product *522*, 525
hepatitis C
  clinical features 506
  health care workers 503–4
    needlestick injuries 505–6
    transmission to patients 505–6,
      506
  hepatoma and Kaposi's syndrome
    816
  post-exposure prophylaxis 508
  as prescribed disease 507
hepatocellular carcinoma 809
hepatocellular damage, paraquat
    poisoning and *201*
hepatomas
  industries/occupations associated
    with *816*
  non-genotoxic carcinogen
    mechanisms *765*
  non-invasive screening *882*
hepatomegaly
  brucellosis 492
  chloroform causing 229
  toluene exposure 263
hepatotoxic effects, biological
    monitoring tests *18*
hepatotoxicity **881–99**
  carbon tetrachloride 226, 228, 229,
    885, 887–8, 890–1
  chemically induced *882*
  chloroform (trichloromethane) 226,
    229, *884*, *885*, 891
  1,2-dichloroethane (ethylene
    dichloride) 230, *885*
  halogenated alkanes 226
  mechanisms 887–90
  methylene chloride
    (dichloromethane) 227
  occupations/agents associated with
    884–5
  tetrachloroethylene
    (perchloroethylene) 226, 235,
    884, *885*, 891
  trichloroethylene ('trike') 226, 234,
    884, 891
  vinylidene chloride (1,1-
    dichlorethylene) 236, 237
  see also hepatotoxins; liver; liver
    disease; *and specific*
    hepatotoxins
hepatotoxins *884–5*, 890–5
  haloalkanes 890–2
  liver toxicity mechanisms 887–90
  metals and metalloids 892–3
  pesticides 893–4

  see also hepatotoxicity; *and specific*
    hepatotoxins
heptachlor, hepatotoxicity 893
heptane *225*
Heptavac, accidental self-injection with
    213
Heptavac P, accidental self-injection
    with *213*
herbicides
  chlorophenoxyacetate herbicides
    203
  hepatotoxicity *885*, 893–4
  phenoxyacetic acid and non-
    Hodgkin's lymphoma 910
  poisoning with 200–4
  sclerodermatous syndrome and 732
  see also pesticides; weedkillers; *and*
    individual herbicides
hereditary effects, ionizing radiation
    405–6
herpes, dichloroacetylene exposure 239
herpes B virus 512
herpetic whitlow 510
Hevea brasiliensis 637
  radioallergosorbent tests (RAST) *21*
hevein, contact urticaria 731
hexacarbon solvents, neurotoxic effects
    870
hexachlorobenzene (perchlorobenzene)
    266–7, 886
  hepatotoxicity *884*
  mechanisms of 889
hexachlorocyclohexane, *see* lindane
γ-hexachlorocyclohexane,
    hepatotoxicity *884*
hexachloroethane 235
hexachlorophene 271
hexacyclohexane, as non-genotoxic
    carcinogen *765*
hexafluoroacetone 166
  occupational diseases caused by (EC
    schedule) *43*
hexafluoroethane (Freon-116) 154
hexahydrophthalic anhydride 639
hexamethylene diisocyanate (HDI) 639
hexane *225*
  chemical structure 225
n-hexane 224, **225–6**, *247*
  absorption 225
  biochemical effects 226
  biological monitoring tests and
    guidance values *18*
  characteristics and uses 225–6
  clinical manifestations 226
  management of exposures 226
  metabolism 226, 870
  neurotoxic effects 226, 870
  prescribed diseases due to *52*
2,5-hexanedione 247, 248
  biological monitoring tests and
    guidance values *18*
  neurotoxic effects 226, 870
n-hexanol 239
2-hexanone, *see* methyl *n*-butyl ketone
3-hexanone *247*
high-altitude cerebral oedema (HACO)
    383, 384, 386, *387*
  treatment 392, *394*

high-altitude pulmonary oedema
        (HAPO) 383, 384–6, *387*
    childrens' susceptibility to 386, 388
    mortality rate 386
    treatment 392, *394*
high-pressure neurological syndrome
        (HPNS) 346
high resolution computed tomography
        (HRCT)
    in extrinsic allergic alveolitis 603
    in occupational lung disease 595–8
    in pulmonary disease 602
    reconstruction algorithm 596–8
    section thickness 595–6
Hillsborough tragedy 571
himic anhydride 639
hip
    hip replacements, 'cement hepatitis'
        250
    osteoarthritis 466
hippocampus, acute carbon monoxide
        poisoning 144
Hippocrates 843
hippuric acid 263
histamine
    challenge tests
        byssinosis 624
        occupational asthma 644, 645
    provoking occupational asthma 633,
        634, 637
    release, byssinosis pathogenesis 622,
        623–4
history
    occupational, *see* occupational
        history
    of occupational diseases
        917–25
HIV (human immunodeficiency virus)
        infection
    clinical features 506–7
    in health care workers 504
        needlestick injuries 506
        transmission to patients 507
    Injuries Benefit and 507
    laboratory workers 512
    non-Hodgkin's lymphoma and *816*
    occupational transmission incidents
        505
    post-exposure prophylaxis 508
    serum storage and testing 533
    see also AIDS
Hodgkin's disease 909–10
    chlorophenol exposure and 272
    TCDD and 876
    woodworkers 909–10
Hodgkin's lymphoma (HL),
        chlorophenoxyacetate
        herbicides and 203
hog farmers 136
'Hohendiuresis' 391
home mist vaporizers 713
hookworm 924
hormones
    in reproduction 825
    as tissue culture additives *528*
hormone weedkillers, *see*
        chlorophenoxyacetate
        herbicides

horses, extrinsic allergic alveolitis due to 658
horticulture
    dermatoses 734
    hepatotoxicity in *884*
    prescribed diseases in *49*
    see also plants
hospitals, as ionizing radiation sources *398*
hospital workers
    hyperbaric units 343
    porters, occupational history
        example 11
    see also health care workers;
        medical/paramedical staff
hotels, legionnaires' disease 709, 710
hot water systems, legionnaires' disease
        and 709, 710
'hot work' 8
Hughes v Lloyds Bank plc (1998) 64
Human Genome Project 763
human immunodeficiency virus
        infection, *see* HIV infection
human insulin, biotechnology product
        522, *522*, 524
human leucocyte antigen (HLA)
        phenotype 642
humerus, head, osteonecrosis 357
humidification systems 655–6
    extrinsic allergic alveolitis and 711, 712
    need for, in temperate climates? 715
    organisms associated with 712
humidifier fever 656, **712**
    causes 712
    organisms associated with 712
    Pontiac fever as 711
    symptoms 711
    ventilation pneumonitis *vs* 655–6
    welding and 185
humidity
    low, dermatoses due to 734
    sick building syndrome and 715
Hunter, Donald ii, xiii, 110, 791, 923, 924
hunting reaction 326
hybridization 523
hybridomas 522, *522*, 523
hydatid disease 495–6
    alveolar 495
hydatidosis 495–6
    as prescribed disease *49*
hydrazine
    lung toxicity 77
    in nucleic acid extraction *529*
hydrides, acute lung injury due to *698*
hydrocarbons 854
    aromatic, *see* aromatic
        hydrocarbons; polycyclic
        aromatic hydrocarbons;
        polynuclear aromatic
        hydrocarbons
    fluorinated 154–7
    glomerulonephritis and 227
    reproductive hazards 829
    see also chloroalkenes;
        chloroalkynes; solvents: organic
hydrochloric acid
    compounds hydrolysing to 149
    in nucleic acid extraction *529*
hydrochlorofluorocarbons, partially
        halogenated (HCFCs) 154, 155

hydrochlorthiazide, altitude sickness
        390
hydrocyanic acid, occupational diseases
        caused by (EC schedule) 43
hydrofluoric acid
    anhydrous, *see* hydrogen fluoride
    in DNA pair sequencing 529
    gases hydrolysing to 152–4
    skin exposure 152
hydrofluorocarbons (HFCs) 150
    Kyoto Protocol agreement 135
hydrogen 135, 141
    in earth's atmosphere *135*
hydrogen bromide 149, 150
hydrogen chloride **148–9**, 150
    characteristics and sources 148, 149
    exposure levels 148–9
    health effect levels *127*
hydrogen cyanide 9, **145–7**
    antidotes 145–6
    blood levels 145
    characteristics and sources 145
    as chemical warfare agent 171
    in fires 129, 130
    health effect levels *127*
    olfactory fatigue 125, 145
    poisoning
        clinical features 145
        diagnosis 145, 146
        first aid 131, 145
        first aid, Health and Safety
            Executive advice 145–6, *146*
        hypoxia and 134
        treatment 145, 146
    uses 145
    see also cyanide
hydrogen fluoride **150–2**
    absorption and excretion 150, 151
    accidental releases 150
    acute health effects 150–1
    characteristics and sources 150
    chronic toxicity 151–2
    health effect levels *127*
    pot room asthma 152
    processes associated with 150
    tolerance levels 150
    uses 150
    see also fluorides
hydrogen-fluoride lasers, exposure
        limits *429*
hydrogen halides 149
hydrogen iodide 149
hydrogen phosphide, *see* phosphine
hydrogen selenide 111, 162
    acute lung injury due to *698*
hydrogen sulphide **160–1**
    in animal houses 136
    characteristics and sources 160
    clinical manifestations of exposure
        160–1
    geothermal fields 161, 172
    health effect levels *127*
    hypoxia and 134
    keratoconjunctivitis 136, 161
    olfactory fatigue 125, 160
    Rotorua and Poza Rica incidents 161
    uses and occupations exposed to 160
hydrogen telluride 112

hydrolases 75
hydrolysis, of chemicals 75
hydroquinone 271, 272
  as hazardous DIY material 6
  metabolism 74
  prescribed diseases due to 50, 51
hydroquinone ethers, prescribed
      diseases due to 51
hydroquinone monomethyl ether 253
hydrotherapy 467
  back pain 483
hydroxocobalamin 146
N-hydroxy-2-acetylaminofluorene 75
N-hydroxyacetylaminofluorene 75
N-hydroxyacetylaminoglucuronide 75
5-hydroxy-2-hexanone 247
hydroxylation 74–5
hydroxyl radical 745
4-hydroxy-4-methyl-2-pentanone 248
1-hydroxypyrene 273
5-hydroxytryptamine (5-HT) 401
hyoscine 373
L-hyoscine hydrobromide 373
hyperbaric chambers 364
  Gamow Bags 392, 393, 394
hyperbaric environment 343–60
  basic physics and physiology 344–7
  carbon dioxide effects 346
  compression barotrauma in 347–8
  high-pressure neurological syndrome
      (HPNS) 346
  hospital workers 343
  long-term effects 356–8
  nitrogen narcosis 346
  occupations involving 343
  toxic effects of oxygen 345–6
  wet vs dry environments 343
  see also divers; and decompression
      entries
hyperbaric oxygen 131, 144, 146
  and haemolysis 905
hyperbilirubinaemia 881
hypercalcaemia, beryllium causing
      103, 853
hypercalciuria, beryllium causing 103,
      853
hypercapnia 346
hyperhydrosis 329
hyperkalaemia 152, 223, 229
  in heat strain 336
hyperkeratosis 904
hypermagnesaemia 152
hypernatraemia 241
hyperphosphaturia, in lead poisoning
      86
hyperpigmentation, in arsenic
      poisoning 96
hyperresponsiveness, see airway:
      hyperresponsiveness; bronchial
      hyperreactivity
hypersalivation, mercury poisoning 92
hypersensitivity
  delayed, aromatic amines 270
  Type IV 727
hypersensitivity-induced asthma 633,
      642
  causes 636–40
  irritant-induced vs 633–4

hypersensitivity pneumonia, in welding
      186
hypersensitivity pneumonitis, see
      extrinsic allergic alveolitis
hypertension
  cadmium and 94
  essential hypertension, high altitude
      exposure 390
  portal 885
    non-invasive screening 882
  pulmonary, in high-altitude
      pulmonary oedema 392
hyperuricaemia, chronic beryllium
      disease 103
hyperventilation 332, 335
  in divers 346
  hypoxia and 363
  organic solvents causing 642
  vibration causing 368
hypervolaemia 241
hypnotics, jet lag and 374
hypoacusis
  EC schedule of occupational diseases
      45
  see also occupational noise-induced
      hearing loss
hypocalcaemia 152
hypochlorite 655
hypoglycaemia
  aircrew 374
  in hypothermia 331
hypophosphataemic osteomalacia in
      cadmium poisoning 94
hypoproliferative anaemia, see aplastic
      anaemia
hypothermia 325, 331–2
  in divers 332, 349
  external cardiac massage and 332
  freezing cold injury and 328
  immersion hypothermia 331–2
  insidious 332
  on land 331
  rewarming 331
  rewarming collapse 332
  threshold 327
  treatment 331
hypothyroidism 401
  radiation levels causing 400
hypoxaemia
  in altitude sickness 386
  first aid 131
  nitrogen dioxide causing 159
  during sleep at high altitudes 389
hypoxia 131, 362–4
  biological monitoring tests 18
  brain injury 134
  in divers 346, 349
  gases causing 134
  at high altitudes 363
    case history 363
    causes, in flight 363, 367
    prevention 363
  hyperventilation and 363
  oxygen provision and 363
  prevention 363
  signs and symptoms 363
  'silent hypoxia' 349
  'time of useful consciousness' 363

hyrdocortisone 211

ibuprofen
  altitude sickness 392, 394
  back pain 482, 483
ice hockey players 159
idiopathic portal hypertension 885
idiopathic pulmonary fibrosis
      (cryptogenic fibrosing alveolitis)
      602, 660
IIAC (Industrial Injuries Advisory
      Council) 38, 39, 39–40, 41
Illuminating Engineering Society of
      North America (IESNA) 431, 437
illusions, aircrew 371–2
imaging
  computed radiography (CR) 594–5
  computed tomography (CT), see
      computed tomography
  in lung diseases, see lung diseases,
      imaging
  magnetic resonance imaging (MRI)
      446, 598–9
  radionuclide studies 113, 599
  ultrasound 304, 598
  see also under individual disorders
immersion foot 330
immersion hypothermia 331–2
  after rescue 332
  rescue mode 332
  survival system 332
  see also hypothermia
immortalization, cells 748
immune complexes, extrinsic allergic
      alveolitis pathogenesis 656
immunization, see vaccination/vaccines
immunoglobulin A (IgA), bird fancier's
      lung 655
immunoglobulin E (IgE)
  byssinosis 623
  to flour 637
  occupational asthma 640
immunoglobulin G (IgG)
  byssinosis 623
  extrinsic allergic alveolitis 656, 657
  occupational asthma 640
immunological investigations, in
      occupational asthma 643–4
immunological mechanism, byssinosis
      pathogenesis 623–4
immunosuppressants 659
impact noise 285
impact vibration 310
impairment
  auditory 294
  WHO definition 294
implantation, cochlea 300
implants, and magnetic fields 446
impulse noise 285
impure chemicals 9–10
incandescent lamps, eye damage from
      420
indinavir 508
indium, nephrotoxicity 843
individual proof, compensation
      schemes and 38, 40, 41
indomethacin 458

indoor air
  air freshness 716
  carbon dioxide levels 139, 140
  carbon monoxide in 142
  exposure to gases 125
  nitrogen dioxide in 159
  oxygen excess 135
  ozone in 158
  toxic gases in 125
  see also confined spaces
indoor air pollution **709–21**
  allergic rhinitis 713
  arsenical pigment occurrence 96
  extrinsic allergic alveolitis 654,
    655–6, 711
  humidifier fever, *see* humidifier fever
  legionnaires' disease 710
  occupational asthma 713
  Pontiac fever 711
  sick building syndrome, *see* sick
    building syndrome
  smoking 714
  see also air pollution; environment
induction period for workers 471
industrial chemicals, *see* chemical
  agents/chemicals
Industrial Injuries Advisory Council
  (IIAC) 38, 39, 39–40, 41, 684
industrial injuries schemes 30, 37–8, 40
  adjudicating authorities 39
  outside UK 38, 40–2
  see also compensation schemes
Industrial Revolution 663, 919–21
industrial workers, male, shoulder
  tendinitis *455*
industry
  cottage industries 919
  factory system 919–20
  multinational companies 925
ineffective erythropoiesis 905–6
infection
  reproductive hazards *829*
  spread of, by air travel 379
  see also health care workers
infectious diseases **489–520**
  cases reported to SWORD *31*
  as cause of back pain *479*
  EC schedule *44*
  see also individual diseases
infertile worker effect 835
infertility 826
  definition 834
  investigation of complaints 833–4
  see also fertility
infiltration, abnormal liver function
  tests 883
inflammatory diseases, as cause of back
  pain *479*
inflammatory response, pathogenesis
  of inorganic dust diseases 665
information sources
  chemicals 221, 223
  toxic hazards 7–8
infrared radiation
  eye damage from *420*, 430
  eye protectors 432–3
  ocular penetration/absorption 424,
    425

  sources *420*, 430
  wavelengths 419, *420*
infrasound 304
inhalation
  accidents, cases reported to SWORD
    31
  kinetics of 71–2
  occupational diseases caused by (EC
    schedule) *44*
  tests
    byssinosis 623
    in occupational asthma 644–5
inhalation fevers 185–7
inhalation injury 698
initiation, carcinogenesis 741, 742
initiators, of occupational asthma
  633–4, *634*
injection therapy, back pain 483
injuries
  occupational, estimating extent of
    27–35
  reporting schemes
    statutory 30–1
    voluntary 31
inorganic-acid mists containing
  sulphuric acid, genotoxicity *776*
inorganic dust diseases **663–708**
  coalworker's pneumoconiosis, *see*
    coalworker's pneumoconiosis
  fibrous mineral dusts 686–97
  investigation and diagnosis 665–72
  lung damage process 665
  lung defences against 663–4
  lung disorders caused by metals
    701–4
  metal dusts **697–700**
  non-fibrous mineral dusts 672–86
    see also quartz dust; silicosis
  pathogenesis 664–5
  symptoms and signs 666
  see also clays; pneumoconiosis; *and*
    individual dusts/dust types
insecticides **11–18**
  alkyl thiocyanate insecticides 195
  arsenic 892
  arsenic-containing compounds 195
  benzene insecticides 209
  carcinogenic risk *815*
  causing aplastic anaemia 907
  cyclodiene insecticides 209
  cyclohexane insecticides 209
  neurotoxic effects 873–4
  non-arsenical, genotoxicity *777*
  non-Hodgkin's lymphoma and 910
  poisoning 204–12
  see also carbamate insecticides;
    organochlorine pesticides;
    organophosphate pesticides
insecticide sprays, hepatotoxicity *885*
insects
  occupational asthma due to *647*
  prescribed diseases due to contact
    with *52, 53*
  see also mites
insidious hypothermia 332
insomnia, at high altitudes 389
Institute of Occupational Medicine
  682, 683

insulation, man-made vitreous fibres,
  see man-made vitreous fibres
insulation workers 695
  see also asbestos
insulators, cancer sites *816*
insulin, human, biotechnology product
  522, *522*
insulin-dependent diabetes mellitus
  (IDDM), solvent exposure and
  856
interferon(s) 506, 524, 528
interferon-α, biotechnology product
  522
interferon-β, biotechnology product
  522
γ-interferon, radiation casualties 415
interleukins 524, 528
International Agency for Research on
  Cancer (IARC) 675
  benzene studies 262
  cancer biomonitoring reviews 767
  monographs 802
  welding fume carcinogenicity 181,
    184
International Animal Health Code 492
International Atomic Energy Association
  (IAEA) 404, 413
International Classification of Diseases
  (ICD-10), post-traumatic stress
  disorder 545, 547
international collaboration 923–4
International Commission on
  Radiological Protection (ICRP)
  398, 404, 408, 415
International Health Regulations 379
International Labour Office (ILO)
  chest radiography classification
    667–9
  formation of 924
  Night Work Convention and
    Recommendation 585
International Labour Organization (ILO),
  radiographic classification of
  pneumoconioses 603–4, *604*
International Standards
  audiometric reference pressure 284
  hearing 295
  heat stress/exhaustion 334, 337
  whole-body vibration 319
International Union of Pure and
  Applied Chemistry (IUPAC) 225
Inter-Society Working Group, on hearing
  disability compensation 294–5
interstitial fibrosis 665, 666
  computed tomography use 669
  talc exposure 680
interstitial nephritis
  tubular 850
  USA 843
interstitial oedema, chlorine 147
interstitial pneumonitis, chlamydiosis
  492
intervertebral disc
  degeneration 480, 483
  herniated, as cause of back pain *479*
  prolapse 479
intestinal anthrax 491
iodine 329

iodine – *contd*
  occupational diseases caused by (EC
      schedule) *43*
  radiation contamination treatment
      413, 415
iodine-131 131
iodine-azide reaction 254
ion exchange chemists/manufacture,
      respiratory tract malignancies *4*
ionic dissociation, electrolyte
      movement and 68
ionic lead 85
ionizing particles, prescribed diseases
      due to *46*
ionizing radiation **397–418**, 901
  anaemia and 907–8
  atoms 397
  blood dyscrasias/malignancies and *4*
  bone marrow cancer *816*
  brain tumours 810
  cancer and 792–3
  carcinogenesis 403–5
    DNA damage 405
  casualties, contaminated 411–13
  Central Index on Dose Information
      (CIDI) 407
  dermatitis 792
  detection of, physical/biological 399
  dose
    absorbed dose 398
    median 400
    occupational 407–8
    threshold dose [TAB 2nd] 399,
        400, *400*
    total 407–8
    units 398–9
  dose limits
    for general public 408, *409*
    in pregnancy 408, *409*, 410
    for workers (classified persons)
        408–9, *409*
    for workers (non-classified
        persons) 408, *409*
  EC comparable data collection *41*
  EC schedule of occupational diseases
      45
  effect on blood counts 908
  genotoxicity 775
  half-life of isotopes 398
  health effects of 399–406
    deterministic (early) 399–400,
        400, 400–3, 416
    hereditary 399, 405–6
    somatic 399, 399–405
    stochastic (latent) 399–400,
        403–5, 416
  health surveillance 409–13
    external contamination 410–11
    external exposure 410
    internal exposure 410
    medical records 411
    reassurance 409–10
    return to work 411
  isotopes 398
  late effects of exposure,
      carcinogenesis 792–3
  legislation 408–9
  leukaemia and 908

male fertility decrease 829
medical aspects 409, 409–13
  further reading 418
medical exposures 407, 408
monitoring of workers 407, 409
myelodysplasia and 908
natural background radiation 399
non-ionizing radiation *vs* 419
occupational exposure 407
  definition 400
  dose limits 408–9, *409*
  doses 407, *407–8*
partial body exposure, effects 403
penetration of matter 398
pregnancy and 408, *409*, 410
properties and types of *398*
protection
  external contamination 408
  external irradiation 408
  internal irradiation 408
  principles 408
radiation weighting factor 398–9
reproductive hazards *829*
  to embryo/fetus 402, 831–2, *832*
sources and magnitudes 397, 406–8
uses 407
weighting factors 398–9
whole-body radiation 402–3, *402*
  threshold 399, *400*
see also radiation accidents
Ionizing Radiations Regulations 1985
      (IRR85) 408, 413
ioxynil 202
ipecacuanha
  occupational asthma due to *647*
  prescribed diseases due to *52, 53*
4-ipomeanol, pulmonary
      biotransformation 76, 77
IQ, and blood lead 23
Iraq, organic mercurial poisoning
      incident 90
Iraq/Iran war, vesicant agents in 171
iridotomy 427
iris 421, 423
  damage from optical radiation *420*
iron
  manganese absorption and 108–9
  in porphyrin metabolism 886
iron and steel founding
  carcinogenicity *814*
  genotoxic exposures *776*
iron deficiency anaemia, cause of
      raised blood zinc
      protoporphyrin (ZPP) 87
iron dusts, imaging 603
iron founders, lung cancer *815*
iron magnesium silicate 687
iron ore miners/mining
  lung cancer *815*
  siderosis and 701
iron oxide 112
  in welding fume 181, 183
iron workers, carcinogenic risk *815*
irritable bowel syndrome 514, 541
irritant dermatitis, *see* contact
      dermatitis: irritant
irritant gases 124
  characteristics 125

first aid 131–2
health effect levels 127
localization of effects 125
primary 124, **147–62**
secondary, with systemic toxic effects
      124, **162–7**
war 171
irritant-induced asthma 633, 635, 699
  diagnostic criteria 635
  hypersensitivity-induced *vs* 633–4
  see also reactive airways dysfunction
      syndrome
irritants, biological monitoring tests *18*
irritative substances, skin diseases
      caused by (EC schedule) *44*
ischaemic heart disease
  altitude sickness/risk 388–9
  carbon monoxide poisoning 144,
      145
  see also coronary heart disease; heart
      disease; myocardial infarction
isobutane 169
isobutylene 169
isocyanates
  EC comparable data collection *41*
  as hazardous DIY material *6*
  hypersensitivity to 639
  occupational asthma due to 613,
      634, 636, 647
  occupational diseases caused by (EC
      schedule) *43*
  prescribed diseases due to *52, 53*
  smoking and isocyanate exposure
      613–14
  see also diisocyanates
isoflurane 167
  exposure standards 168
isolan, hepatotoxicity *884*
isometric exercises, abdominal muscles
      483
isoniazid 675
  hepatotoxicity 68
  neuropathy 68
isophorene, as non-genotoxic
      carcinogen *765*
isoprene 237
isopropanol *239*
isopropanol manufacture, genotoxic
      exposures *776*
isopropyl alcohol (2-propanol)
  manufacturing *814*
    paranasal sinus cancer *815*
    respiratory tract malignancies *4*
  occupational diseases caused by (EC
      schedule) *43*
isopropylbenzene (cumene) 266
4-isopropyl catechol 272
isopropyl ether, occupational diseases
      caused by (EC schedule) *43*
N-isopropyl-N'-phenyl-*p*-
      phenylenediamine (IPDD),
      dermatoses 733
isothiazolinones 715
  dermatoses 734, 735
isotopes 398
ispaghula
  occupational asthma due to *636,
      647*

prescribed diseases due to *52, 53*
   radioallergosorbent tests (RAST) *21*
itai-itai disease 94, 850
Italy, occupational diseases schedule
   41
itraconazole, ringworm 502

Jack o' Lantern 138
jacuzzis, legionnaires' disease and 710
jade polishing, silicosis prevention 676
Japan
   sarin incident, Tokyo 171
   sulphuric acid emissions 156
jaundice 833
   biological monitoring tests *18*
   Epping Forest incident 270, 883
   non-invasive screening *882*
   paraquat poisoning and *201*
Java, 'Valley of Death' 140
jaw, phossy jaw (phosphorus-induced
      necrosis) 98
jet fuel 256
jet lag 373–4, 582
   protection 373–4
jewellers' rouge 112
jewellery manufacture, lead use *844*
job rotation 471
job titles 3–5
joint pain
   decompression illness 351
   decompression sickness 364
jury trials 57, 58
jute dust inhalation, EC schedule of
      occupational diseases *44*

Kanechlor 274
kaolin (china clay) 679, 680
kaolin industry 679
kaolinite 679
kaolin pneumoconiosis 679–80
   clinical manifestations 679–80
   pathology 680
   prevention 680
kapok dust 185
Kaposi's sarcoma,
      industries/occupations
      associated with *816*
karoshi 588
Kepone, *see* chlordecone
keratectomy, photoreactive 427
keratitis, chromium causing 105
keratoconjunctivitis, hydrogen sulphide
      161
keratotomy
   photorefractive (PRK) 369
   radial, aircrew and 369
kerosene, hepatotoxicity *884*
ketoconazole, ringworm 502
ketones **246–9**
   formula and examples *224*, 246, *247*
Kevlar 696
keyboard operators
   carpal tunnel syndrome case-control
      studies *461*
   female, shoulder tendinitis *455*
   prescribed diseases *46*

repetitive strain injury/upper limb
      pain 461, 462
   tension neck syndrome 457
   see also office workers; repetitive
      strain injury; visual display unit
      operators
kibyo (Minamata disease) 90, 852, 872
kidneys
   biotransformation capability *73*
   in cadmium poisoning 94, 95
   kidney damage, as prescribed disease
      51
   in mercury poisoning 91, 92
   pains, biotechnology hazard *527*
   see also entries beginning with renal
kidney tumours
   non-genotoxic carcinogen
      mechanisms *765*
   occupations/agents causing *4*
kieselgahr (diatomite) 681
kinetic profile, of chemicals 69
kinetics
   of exposure **71–2**
   see also inhalation; toxicokinetics
knees
   beat knee 464
   meniscus lesions caused by kneeling,
      EC schedule of occupational
      diseases *45*
   osteoarthritis 465–6
   prescribed diseases affecting *46*
   replacement, 'cement hepatitis' 250
Konesta 249
Korean haemorrhagic fever 494
krypton 141
   in earth's atmosphere *135*
krypton lasers 427
   eye damage from *420*
kuru 500
Kussmaul's sign 89, 91
Kuwait, oil well fires 129–30
Kveim test 103, 666
Kwells 373
K x-ray fluorescence 848, 849
Kyanasur Forest disease 509
Kyoto Protocol agreement, 'greenhouse
      gases' 135

laboratory analysis 221
laboratory animal allergy (LAA) 636,
      636
laboratory animals
   learned helplessness 541
   occupational asthma due to 636,
      636, 647
   see also animals; animal toxicity
      studies
laboratory equipment, ergonomic
      hazards 529
laboratory techniques **15–26**
   importance of 15
   see also biological effect monitoring;
      biological monitoring
laboratory tools 15
laboratory workers 512
   brain tumours 810
   brucellosis 491

handling hazards 529
hantavirus infection 494
hepatitis A 514
hepatotoxicity in *884*
HIV infection 512
mercury vapour inhalation 90–1
occupational asthma 634, *635, 647*
prescribed diseases associated with
      52, 53
primates, work involving 512
protective equipment 508
Q fever 498
serum storage 533
viral haemorrhagic fevers 509
zoonoses 489
see also biotechnology
laboratory work risk assessment, COSHH
      regulations 512
labourers 3–4
labyrinth, osseous/membranous 287
lacquer, as hazardous DIY material *6*
β-lactam antibiotics, allergenicity 640
lactulose, as treatment for liver disease
      887
Lake Nyos, Cameroon, incident 139
laminin 857, 858
   measurement 95
lamivudine 508
lamp assemblers, tension neck
      syndrome 457
landfill gas 138
lanthanides, granulomatous lung
      disease due to 702–3
laryngeal oedema 131
   ammonia causing 131, 157
   chlorine causing 147
   hydrogen chloride causing 149
laryngeal spasm, ammonia causing
      157
laryngeal tumours
   agents causing *4*, 808
   asbestos exposure and 691
   industries/occupations associated
      with *4, 815*
laryngitis 698
laser *in situ* keratomileusis (LASIK)
      369
Laser Institute of America 434
laser printers, ozone production 158
lasers **427–8**
   accidents 427–8
   exposure limits 428–9, *429*
   eye damage from *420*
   eye protectors *433*, 433–4
      information source 434
      national and international
         standards 434, 437
      optical density (OD) 433–4
   hazard classes 427, 431
   in military flying 370
   national and international standards
      437
   safety standards 431
      information source 434
   uses 427
Lassa fever 509
   differential diagnosis 509
Lassa virus 509

lateral epicondylitis (tennis elbow) *454*, 458, 459, 461
  aetiology 458
latex
  occupational asthma due to *634*, *636*, 637–8
  radioallergosorbent tests (RAST) *21*
  recommendations for latex sensitive persons *638*
  see also rubber
latex production workers, bladder cancer *815*
lathe operators, skin neoplasms *4*
n-lauryl alcohol *239*
law, *see* medicolegal considerations; medicolegal reports; *and entries beginning with* legal
L-dopa 108
lead **82–9**
  absorption/uptake 83–4
  anaemia and 23, 85, 87, 904, **905–6**
  biochemical effects 85
  biological effect indicators *19*
  biological monitoring 23
    tests and guidance values *18*
  blood lead concentration 83, 84–5
    inorganic lead poisoning 87
    organic lead poisoning 89
  carcinogenicity 85
  compounds 83
  control regulations 17
  distribution in body 84–5
  EC comparable data collection *41*
  excretion 85
  exposure to 905–6
  half-life 84
  handling 8–9
  historical uses 82
  industries using *844*
  ingestion 84
  inhalation 84
  IQ and blood lead 23
  male fertility/sexual behaviour 829
  manufacturing 83
  metabolism 85
  nephropathy, *see* lead poisoning: nephropathy
  occupational diseases caused by (EC schedule) *43*
  organic compounds 83
  poisoning, *see* lead poisoning
  prescribed diseases due to *49*, 87
  present day exposures 83
  properties 82
  reproductive hazards *828*, *829*, 829, 830
  skeletal pool 84
  smelting 83
  solubility 83
  toxic hazard to embryo/fetus 830
  in urine and faeces 85
  uses 83, 871
lead-210 406
lead alloys, lead use *844*
lead-bearing dust 83
lead carbonates 83
lead chlorosilicate 83
lead chromate 83

lead compounds
  manufacturing, lead use *844*
  occupational diseases caused by (EC schedule) *43*
  prescribed diseases due to *49*, 87
leaded petrol 83, 89
lead-induced anaemia 904, 905–6
lead lanthanum zirconate titanate (PLZT) 370
lead oxide, absorption/inhalation 83
lead paints 83
lead poisoning 82–3, 904
  19th century work in Europe and USA 923–4
  clinical manifestations 871
  encephalopathy 871
  inorganic lead 85–8
    abdominal discomfort 86
    biochemical effects 85
    diagnosis and investigations 86–7
    encephalopathy 86
    peripheral neuropathy 86
    statutory procedure for treatment, UK 87
    subclinical 85
    symptoms and signs 86–7
    treatment 87–8
  nephropathy **844–9**
    acute 844
    bone lead measurement 847, 848
    chelation therapy 848
    chronic 844–5
    cross-sectional studies *846*
    diagnosis 847–8
    EDTA chelation tests 847
    management 848–9
    mortality 845–7, *846*
    renal failure 844, 847
    renal hypertension 844, 847
  neurotoxic effects 871
    mechanisms 871
  organic lead 88–9
    blood lead concentration 89
    case report 88
    management 89
    symptoms and signs 89
    see also tetraethyl lead
  as prescribed disease *49*, 87
  subclinical 83, 85
  treatment 871
  work of Sir Thomas Legge 923
lead sulphide (galena) 82, 83
'leans' 371, 372
learned helplessness 541
leather dust, sino-nasal cancer and leukaemia *816*
leather industry
  carcinogenic risk in *816*
  reproductive hazards to embryo/fetus 831
  respiratory cancer risk 808
Leblanc process 149
lecturers, violence to 552–3
Lee v South West Thames Regional Health Authority (1985) 59
left ventricular failure due to cobalt 106
legal aid 58

legal considerations, employers' duty of care 570–1
legal provisions 57–8
  civil and criminal law 57–8
  legal duties of employers, hearing protection 298–9
  withholding of material facts 63
  see also medicolegal considerations
legal reports, *see* medicolegal reports
Legge, Sir Thomas 923, 924
Legionella spp. 710, 711
Legionella feeleii 711
Legionella pneumophila 185, 709–11
legionellosis, *see* legionnaires' disease
legionnaires' disease **709–11**
  causes 709
  diagnosis 710–11
  incidence 709, 710
  as lobar pneumonia 710–11
  methods of acquisition 709
  outbreaks 709–10, 711
  treatment 711
Leguminosae, contact dermatitis 734
leishmaniasis, antimony in treatment of 100
leisure industries
  farmers and 490
  Lyme disease 497
lens, of eye
  anatomy 421, 422
  annual radiation dose limits *409*
  damage from optical radiation *420*
  opacities, *see* cataracts
  threshold levels of radiation dose *400*
lens grinding, granulomatous lung disease due to 702
LEPd (daily personal exposure to noise) 296–7
Leptidoglycus destructor 637, 643
leptospira infections, as prescribed diseases *48*
Leptospira interrogans 495
  serotypes 495, 496
    Li canicola 495
    Li hardjo 495, 496
    Li icterohaemorrhagiae 495, 496
leptospirosis 495–6, 734
  clinical features and management 496
  sewage workers 515
lethargy
  in lead poisoning 86
  sick building syndrome 713
leucocyanidin 623
leucocytosis
  arsine causing 163
  peripheral 697
leucoderma 272, 732
  mimicking idiopathic vitiligo 732
  as prescribed disease 732
leukaemia 811–13
  acute lymphoid 441
    occupations/agents causing *4*
  acute myeloid 441
    occupations/agents causing *4*
  acute non-lymphotic myeloblastic 262

agents causing *4*, 813
  benzene 811
  ethylene oxide 166
atomic bomb survivors 404
benzene-induced 32, 75, 262, 263,
    907, 909
biological monitoring tests *18*
cancer risk and germline mutations
    751
childhood leukaemia 440
chronic lymphocytic 441
chronic myeloid 441
electromagnetic field exposure and
    440–1, 443–4, 813
ethylene oxide exposure and 909
industries/occupations associated
    with *816*
ionizing radiation and 792, 908
    probability of causation (PC) 404
lymphoblastic, oncogene activation
    in *749*
lymphocytic, oncogene activation in
    749
myelogenous, oncogene activation in
    749
myeloid 907, 909, 910–11
non-ionizing radiation and 909
T-cell, oncogene activation in *749*
leukaemogenesis, benzene 775
lewisite (chlorovinyldichloroarsine) 97,
    171
libido, loss of 829
lichens 735
Li-Fraumeni syndrome 405, 752–3
  susceptibility and germline mutation
    751
lifting 481–2
  training and 481
light, visible
  ocular penetration/absorption 424,
    425
  sources, eye damage and absorption
    420
  wavelengths 419, *420*
limb pain, decompression illness 355
D-limonene 735
  as non-genotoxic carcinogen *765*
Lind, James 918
lindane 209, 210
  aplastic anaemia and 262–3, 907
  biological monitoring tests and
    guidance values *18*
  breast cancer and 210
  head-lice shampoos 209
  hepatotoxicity 893
linear energy transfer (LET) 398–9,
    405
linter dust 624
lipid solubility 68
lipofuscin 424
liquefied petroleum gases 170–1
  explosions 123
liquid argon 141
liquid nitrogen 136, 141
Listeria monocytogenes 496
listeriosis 496
lithium compounds, in nucleic acid
    extraction *529*

lithium hydride, acute lung injury due
    to *698*, 698
litigation 793
Littlewoods
  dignity at work policy 544
    'supporters' 544
liver
  amoebic abscess 513–14
  angiosarcoma, *see* angiosarcoma of
    the liver
  arsenic and 97
  biotransformation capability *73*
  cadmium levels in 94, 95
  cancer, *see* liver tumours
  carbon tetrachloride-induced
    damage 228
  cirrhosis, *see* cirrhosis
  cytochrome P450 in 73
  dimethylformamide exposure 251
  liver failure, treatment 887
  metabolism of chemicals in 73–6
  transplantation 887
  tumours, *see* liver tumours
  see also hepatotoxicity
liver disease 881, 895
  acute 882–3
  chronic 885
    non-invasive screening *882*
  hydrochlorofluorocarbons causing
    155
  malignant change 886
  non-invasive screening *882*
  porphyrin metabolism 886
  as prescribed disease *51*
  treatment 886–7, *887*
  vascular lesions 885–6
  see also hepatotoxicity; *and entries
    beginning with* hepatic
liver enzymes
  dimethylformamide exposure 251
  halogenated alkane toxicity 226
  tetrachloroethylene
    (perchloroethylene) 235
  vinylidene chloride (1,1-
    dichloroethylene) exposure 237
  see also γ-glutamyltransferase;
    alanine aminotransferase
liver function tests, abnormal
  disorders producing 881, 883
  screening 881, *882*
liver tumours 886
  carbon tetrachloride association 228
  dioxin association 886, 890
  haemangiosarcoma *4*
  hepatocellular carcinoma 809
  industries/occupations associated
    with *815*
  non-genotoxic carcinogen
    mechanisms *765*
  screening 818
  see also angiosarcoma of the liver
livestock handlers, ringworm 502
lobar pneumonia, *see* legionnaires'
    disease
locusts, occupational asthma due to
    636
lofexidine 563
loperamide 514

low birth weight 831
  carbon monoxide poisoning and 144
lower limb disorders, *see* osteoarthritis
lucifer match 98
lumbar spine, degenerative disease
    483
lumbar spondylosis, as cause of back
    pain *479*
lumbermen, hantavirus infection 494
luminous paint 793
lung(s)
  acute inhalation injury 698–700
  autopsy in inorganic dust diseases
    671–2
  biopsy 666
  biotransformation capability *73*,
    76–7
  cancer, *see* lung cancer
  cavitation, in coalworkers 684
  changes after raised barometric
    pressures 356
  compression barotrauma 348
  confluent fibrosis 666
  defences **663–4**
    lower airway filter 664
    lymphatics 664
    macrophage clearance 664
    upper airway filter 663–4
  eggshell calcification 673, 674, 679,
    685
  fibrosis, *see* pulmonary fibrosis
  function tests, *see* lung function
  gas transfer rates 71
  granulomatous disease, copper
    causing 107
  granulomatous inflammatory
    reaction 653, 656
  inorganic dust diseases, *see* inorganic
    dust diseases
  interstitial fibrosis 665, 666
    computed tomography use 669
    talc exposure 680
  masses, in progressive massive
    fibrosis in coalworkers 684
  metal absorption 82
  metal-induced interstitial disorders
    700–4
  nodules 665, 674
    in acute allergic alveolitis 657
  non-ciliated bronchiolar cells, *see*
    Clara cells
  radiation damage/threshold dose
    400, 401
  radiographic opacities
    asbestos-related diseases 688
    chronic silicosis 674
    coalworker's pneumoconiosis
      683
    ILO classification 603–4
    kaolin pneumoconiosis 679
    large 604, 667
    slate pneumoconiosis 678–9
    small 603–4, 667, 668–9
    talc pneumoconiosis 680
  as target organ for toxicity 76
  toxic effects of oxygen 345
  see also pneumoconiosis; *and entries
    beginning with* pulmonary

lung cancer *4*, 700–1
  acrylonitrile 253
  agents causing *4*, 806–7, 808
  antimony workers 100
  arsenic exposure and 97, 807
  asbestos exposure *4*, 687, 691, 793, 803
    prognosis 691
    smoking and 8, 691, 816
  beryllium association 103
  bis(chloromethyl) ether (BCME) *4*, 252, 815
    prescribed disease due to *54*, 252, 807
  cadmium workers 94
  cases reported to SWORD *31*
  chloromethyl ethers 807
  chromium compounds and 105
  copper 107
  early (historical) observation 792
  electromagnetic field exposure and 443
  epidemiological studies 700
  exposure circumstances 806, 808
  fluorspar miners 28
  formaldehyde exposure 805
  foundry workers 700
  hard metal exposure 106
  incidence 794
  industries/occupations associated with *4*, *815*, *816*
  nickel associated with 109, 807
  oncogene activation in *749*
  as prescribed disease *50*, *52*, *54*
  radioactive isotopes and 793
  radiogenic 406
  screening 818
  silicosis, risk in 675
  slag wool and rock wool causing 697, 805
  talc contamination with fibres causing 680
  tin miners 114–15
  uranium miners 115
  vine sprayers 107
  in welders 183
lung diseases
  imaging, *see* lung diseases, imaging
  inhalation of dust causing, EC schedule of occupational diseases *44*
  occupational **599–603**
  see also inorganic dust diseases
lung diseases, imaging **599–603**
  asbestosis 596, 600–2
  coalworker's pneumoconiosis 599
  complicated coalworker's pneumoconiosis 599
  extrathoracic manifestations 602
  extrinsic allergic alveolitis 603
  ILO radiographic classification 603–4, *604*
  imaging techniques 593–606
    chest radiography 593–4
    computed radiography (CR) 594–5
    computed tomography (CT) 595
    digital 594, 595

high resolution computed tomography (HRCT) 595–8
    magnetic resonance (MR) 598–9
    radionuclide studies 599
    ultrasound 598
  pleural disease 600–1
  pulmonary disease 601–2
  sarcoidosis 600
  siderosis 603
  silicosis 599–600
  stannosis 603
  zoonoses 603
lung disorders, occupational, SORDSA recording scheme (South Africa) 31
lung fibrosis
  biological monitoring tests *18*
  paraquat 77
lung function
  asthma and 183
  bilateral diffuse pleural thickening 691
  byssinosis 623, 625, *626*, 627
    endotoxin levels 623
  cadmium poisoning 94
  chronic beryllium disease 102
  chronic silicosis 673
  extrinsic allergic alveolitis 657, 658, 659, 660
  inhaled diisocyanates 639
  inorganic dusts 669–71
  kaolin pneumoconiosis 679–80
  monitoring in silicosis prevention 677
  occupational asthma 643, 644
  polymer fume fever 187
  progressive massive fibrosis 684
  transfer factor for carbon monoxide (TLCO), in extrinsic allergic alveolitis 657, 658, 659
  vital capacity 345, 356
  welders 183, 184
  see also forced expiratory volume in one second; forced vital capacity; peak expiratory flow
lung injury, inhaled toxicants causing 132
luteinizing hormone (LH) 825, 826, 834, 835
Lyme borreliosis, *see* Lyme disease
Lyme disease 496–8
  diagnosis 497
  treatment 497
lymphadenopathy, brucellosis 492
lymphatics
  clearance of dust via 664
  decompression illness 351
lymphatic system, tumours, industries/occupations associated with *815*, *816*
lymphocytes
  peripheral blood lymphocytes and cancer 773, 774
  after radiation damage 401
  see also T lymphocytes
lymphocytopenia 262, 266
lymphoid neoplasms, oncogene activation in *749*

lymphoma
  benzene causing 262
  oncogene activation in *749*
lymphopenia 904
lymphoreticular system, cancer risk and germline mutations *750*
Lynch syndrome, susceptibility and germline mutation *750*

McIntyre (aluminium) powder, prophylactic administration to miners 99, 673
macrophages
  clearance of dust to airways 664
  clearance of dust via lymphatics 664
  pathogenesis of inorganic dust diseases 664–5
  quartz dust effect on 672–3
macula 423
macular degeneration, age-related 424, 429–30
macular pigment 423, 424–5
magenta manufacture
  bladder malignancies *4*, 269, *814*
  genotoxic exposures *776*
  urinary tract malignancies, as prescribed diseases *51*
magnesium phosphides 210
magnetic fields 439, 440, 446
  see also electromagnetic fields
magnetic resonance imaging (MRI) **446**
  in occupational lung disease 598–9
magnetophosphenes 440
maintenance industries/staff *4*, 8
  carcinogenic risk in *816*
  prescribed diseases *51*
maize dust
  occupational asthma due to *647*
  prescribed diseases due to *52*, *53*
malaise, in decompression illness 352
malaria 512–13
  complications 513
  diagnosis 513
  falciparum malaria 513
  parasites causing 512–13
  prevention 512–13
    aircrew and passengers 379
  treatment 513
  vaccine 525
malathion 77, 511
  hepatotoxicity *884*
maleic anhydride (MA) 639
  radioallergosorbent tests (RAST) *21*
malignancies 791–2
  occupationally related *4*
  see also cancer; *and individual malignancies*
malignant melanoma 810
  electromagnetic field exposure and 443
malingering 61
maltings, mouldy, extrinsic allergic alveolitis due to *654*
malt worker's lung 653, *654*, 654, **655**
malt-working, prescribed diseases due to *49*

mammary gland tumours, non-
    genotoxic carcinogen
    mechanisms *765*
Management of Health and Safety at
    Work Regulations 1992 570
The Management of Imminent Violence
    553
mandelic acid 265
    biological monitoring tests and
        guidance values *18*
    produced from different substances
        20
Maneb (manganese ethylene-bis-
    dithiocarbamate) 108
manganese **107–9**
    absorption 108
    chronic obstructive lung disease and
        699
    EC comparable data collection *41*
    excretion 108
    function in body 108
    male fertility/behaviour 829
    prescribed diseases due to *49*, 108
    reproductive hazards *828*, 829
    supervision of workers 109
    uptake and iron interaction 107,
        108–9
    uses 108
manganese compounds
    occupational diseases caused by (EC
        schedule) *43*
    prescribed diseases due to *49*
manganese dioxide 108
manganese ethylene-bis-
    dithiocarbamate (Maneb) 108
manganese fume, welders' exposure to
    184
manganese oxides, acute lung injury
    due to *698*
manganese poisoning 108
    development stages 108
    neuropathology 108
    neurotoxic effects 108, 872
    parkinsonian features 872
    parkinsonism *vs* 108
    as prescribed disease *49*, 108
    susceptibility 108–9
    treatment 108
manganic madness 108
Manhattan project 853
manipulation, back pain 482–3
manipulative therapy 457
man-made mineral/vitreous fibres
    (MMMF/MMVF) 696–7, 804–5
    carcinogenicity 779, 805
    risks 817
mannitol, as treatment for liver disease
    887
Mantoux test 675
manual handling of loads, *see* lifting
manual labour, prescribed diseases due
    to *46*
manual metal arc welding, *see*
    welders/welding
maple bark stripper's lung *654*
marathon runners 335
Marburg virus 509
marine animals, injuries by 349

Marjolin's ulcer 329
marsh gas 138, 163
masks 8
    oronasal, in military aircraft 363
    oxygen masks 363
        drop-down 365
masons
    silicosis mortality *29*
    silicosis prevention 676
mast cells, increase in extrinsic allergic
    alveolitis 657
match making, phosphorus in 98
material safety data sheets (MSDS) 7
matrix metalloproteinases 756
Matsumoto, sarin incident 171
Mauna Kea, Hawaii 383–5, 386, 389,
    393
    medical emergencies *387–8*
MbOCA, *see* 4,4'-methylene *bis*(2-
    chloroaniline)
MCPA (4-chloro-2-methylphenoxyacetic
    acid; fenoprop) *203*
    hepatotoxicity *884*
MCPB (4-(4-chloro-2-methylphenoxy)
    butyric acid) *203*
MCPP (2-(4-chloro-2-methylphenoxy)
    propionic acid; mecoprop) *203*,
    203
MDA, *see* 4,4'-methylenedianiline
MDI, *see* methylenediphenyl
    diisocyanate
meal
    occupational asthma due to *647*
    prescribed diseases due to *52, 53*
meat carriers, cervical spondylosis
    457
meat cutters, elbow problems 458
meat wrappers' asthma 170
mebendazole 495
mechanical causes of back pain *479*
mecoprop (MCPP; 2-(4-chloro-2-
    methylphenoxy) propionic acid)
    203, 203
medial epicondylitis (golfer's elbow)
    454, 458
median nerve compression, *see* carpal
    tunnel syndrome
mediastinitis, paraquat poisoning and
    201
medical appeal tribunals (MATs) 58
Medical Aspects of Fitness to Drive 13
medical contact cards 533
Medical Council on Alcoholism, Doctors'
    and Dentists' Group 565
medical/paramedical staff
    radiation exposure 407, 408
    reproductive hazards to
        embryo/fetus 831
    see also health care workers
medical profession, alcohol and drug
    related problems 564–5
medical records
    biotechnology workers 533
    disclosure 58–9
Medical Research Council 289
    Pneumoconiosis Unit 921
medication, back pain 482, 483
medicine, genotoxic exposures *776, 777*

medicolegal considerations
    occupational cancer 796
    see also legal provisions
medicolegal reports **57–64**
    both parties relying on one report
        59, 63
    causation aspects 61
    confidentiality 58–9
    doctor experts 59–60
    doctor participants 58–9
    doctors' role in providing 58–60
    effect of disability 61–2
    form of 61–2
    hearsay evidence 61
    purpose of 60–1
    structure of 62
    see also expert witnesses
meerschaum 696
Mee's lines 904
mefloquine 379, 513
megaloblastic anaemia, arsenic
    poisoning 97
melanin 423, 424
melanoma
    cancer risk and germline mutations
        750
    malignant 810
        electromagnetic field exposure
            and 443
    oncogene activation in *749*
melanoptysis 666, 684
melatonin, jet lag and 374
melatonin secretion, electromagnetic
    field exposure and 445
melphalan, genotoxicity *776*
membranous labyrinth 286–7
memory impairment, in mercury
    poisoning 92
memory registration, in cooling 333
Ménière's disease 293, 301
meningitis
    brucellosis 492
    in Lyme disease 497
    Streptococcus suis infection 499
meningoencephalitis 496
meniscus lesions, EC schedule of
    occupational diseases *45*
menstrual function
    disturbances 830
    records 834
mental function, in cooling 333
mental health
    raising awareness 569, 576
    see also mental illness; psychiatric
        disorders
mental illness
    management at work 577–8
    rehabilitation of employees after 578
    work loss 570
    see also mental health; psychiatric
        disorders; stress
menthol 271
2-mercaptoethanol, in nucleic acid
    extraction *529*
mercaptopropionyl glycine, in organic
    mercury poisoning 93
Merchant Shipping Notice M1331 13
mercurial micro-parkinsonism 92

mercurial ptyalism 92
mercuric chloride 90, 852
  ingestion 852
mercurous chloride (calomel) 852
mercury 9, **89–93**
  absorption/uptake 90–1
  biological monitoring 23
    tests and guidance values *18*
  blood levels 91, 92, 93
  distribution in body 91
  EC comparable data collection *41*
  excretion 91, 93
  forms of 90
  gingivitis 91, 92
  in hair and nails 23
  half-life 91
  health risk assessment 23
  hepatotoxicity *885*
  historical uses 89, 872
  ingestion 90
  inhalation 90, 93
  inorganic 91
  metabolism 90–1
  nephrotoxicity **851–2**
    clinical studies 852
    nephrotic syndrome 852
    treatment after cessation of
      exposure 852
  occupational diseases caused by (EC
      schedule) *43*
  organic, fetal risk 23
  poisoning, *see* mercury poisoning
  prescribed diseases due to *49*, 92
  reproductive hazards *828*, 830,
      830–1
    inorganic mercury *828*, 831
    organic mercury 830
  skin absorption 90–1
  sources 23
  spina bifida and 831
  supervision of workers 93
  urine levels 91, 93
  uses 90, 851
mercury compounds, occupational
      diseases caused by (EC schedule)
      43
mercury fume, Smelter Disease due to
      156
mercury lamps, eye damage from *420*
mercury poisoning 91–3
  acute 91
  chelation therapy 92
  chronic 91–2
  first aid 92
  gums, blue line 92
  inorganic 92, 872
  laboratory diagnosis 92
  Minamata disease 90, 852, 872
  neurotoxic effects 92, 872
  organic 92, 872
    see also methyl mercury
  as prescribed disease *49*, 92
  treatment 92–3
mercury salts 851, 852
mercury vapour
  acute lung injury due to *698*, 698
  exposure/handling, prescribed
      disease due to *49*

hepatotoxicity *884*
  inhalation 90, 93
mesangial proliferative
    glomerulonephritis 855
mesityl oxide *247*
  occupational diseases caused by (EC
      schedule) *43*
mesothelioma 692–4
  asbestos and 687, 692–3, 695, 793,
      803
    exposure latent interval 694
  case history 795
  cases reported to SWORD *31*
  clinical features 692–4
  compensation and disability benefit
      694
  diagnosis 692, 694
  EC schedule of occupational diseases
      44
  erionite causing 696
  man-made vitreous fibres and 804
  mortality 30
  pathology 692
  peritoneal 602, 693–4
  pleural 598, 601, 692–3
    asbestos and *4*
    asbestos and, in women 27
  as prescribed disease *52*, 694
  prognosis 692
  secondaries 692
  shipbuilding and 28
  smoking and 8, 692
  talc contamination with fibres
      causing 680
  vermiculite association 681
  in welders 184
metabolic acidosis 223
  methanol poisoning 241, 242
  paraquat poisoning and *201*
metabolic disorders, as cause of back
      pain *479*
metabolic (pharmacogenetic)
      polymorphisms
  cancer susceptibility 757–62, *758–9*
  detection methods 757–62
    genotyping 762
    phenotyping 762
  differences in ethnic groups 762–3
  effects on biomarkers relevant to
      cancer *770–2*
  interactions between, related to
      cancer risk *760–1*
metabolism, 'specific dynamic effect'
      326
metabolism, of chemicals 68
  genetic polymorphisms 68
  interindividual variations 67–8
  in liver 73–6
  phase 1 reactions 73, 73–5
    dealkylation 75
    decreased toxicity 74–5
    epoxidation 74
    hydrolysis 75
    hydroxylation 74–5
    increased toxicity 74
    oxidation 75
    reduction 75
  phase 2 reactions 73, 75–6

  pulmonary 76–7
  sites *73*, 76–7
  in skin 72, 77
  species differences 77
  see also biotransformation
metabolites, production 524
metal active gas welding, *see*
      welders/welding
metaldehyde 212–13
metal dusts **697–700**
  cryptogenic fibrosing alveolitis and
      660
metal fume, pneumonia 28
metal fume fever 107, 116, 182, **185–6**,
      697
  acute toxic pneumonitis *vs* 698
  pathogenesis 186
  tumour necrosis factor 186
metal halogens, acute lung injury due
      to *698*
metal inert gas welding, *see*
      welders/welding
metalloids 81
  hepatotoxicity *885*, 892–3
  selenium 111
metallothionein 76, 849, 850, 851
  cadmium binding 93
  mercury binding 91
  zinc binding 116
metal ore mining, prescribed diseases
      due to *54*
metal oxides
  acute lung injury due to *698*, 698
  particles, in welding fume 181
metal pigments, as hazardous DIY
      material *6*
metal production/use, hepatotoxicity in
      884
metal reclamation industry, lead use
      844
metals **81–122**
  absorption 82
  carcinogenic 778
  categories 697
  'concentration windows' 81
  contaminants and welding 182
  definition 81
  diagnosis of poisoning 82
  factors affecting toxicity 81–2
  hepatotoxicity *885*, 892–3
  neurotoxic effects **871–2**
  solubility 82
  speciation 82
  surface coatings and welding 182
  susceptibility to, individual variation
      in 82
  toxic *vs* essential 81
  valency 82
  see also individual metals
metal speciation 697
metal welding, *see* welders/welding
metal workers
  asthma incidence *635*
  carcinogenic risk *815*
  dermatoses 730, 731, 734
  hearing loss as prescribed disease
      46, 47
  silicosis mortality *29*

methacholine
   airway responsiveness to 612
   challenge tests
      byssinosis 624
      occupational asthma 644
      welding fume 616
   provoking occupational asthma 633,
      634
methadone in treatment of opiate
      addicts 563, 564
methaemoglobin
   determination in nitrogen dioxide
      exposure 159–60
   in red cell metabolism 902, 903
methaemoglobinaemia 160, **268**, 826,
      902, 905
   aniline 267
   chemicals and drugs causing 268
   clinical manifestations 268
   cyanosis and hypoxia due to 131
   p-dichlorobenzene 266
   inherited disorders causing 268
   methylene blue for 202
   methyl mercaptan (methanethiol)
      162
   nitric oxide 158
   pesticide exposure and *200*
   phenylhydrazine causing 268
   o-toluidine 267
   treatment 268
methane **137–8**, *225*
   Abbeystead incident 138
   anaerobic fermentation producing
      135, 136
   characteristics and sources 137–8
   in earth's atmosphere *135*
   Kyoto Protocol agreement 135
   in mines 137
   in sewers 136
methanethiol (methyl mercaptan) 161,
      162
methanol (methyl alcohol) *224*, *239*,
      240–2
   central nervous system symptoms
      241
   characteristics and uses 240–1
   clinical manifestations 241
   management of poisoning 241–2
   metabolism/biochemical effects 241
   in nucleic acid extraction *529*
   occupational diseases caused by (EC
      schedule) *43*
methazolamide 391, 392
methicillin-resistant *Staphylococcus
      aureus* (MRSA) 511–12
methomyl 208
methotrexate 528, 895
methoxychlor, hepatotoxicity 893
methoxyethyl-mercuric chloride 212
methoxyflurane 167
8-methoxypsoralen (8-MOP) 431
N-methylacetamide, biological
      monitoring tests and guidance
      values *18*
methyl alcohol, *see* methanol
2-methylaniline, *see o*-toluidine
methylated spirits 241
7-methylbenz[a]anthracene 745

2-methylbenzenamine, *see o*-toluidine
methyl benzene, *see* toluene
methyl bromide (bromomethane)
      164–5
   characteristics, sources and uses 164
   clinical manifestations and
      management 164–5
   convulsions, treatment 132
   exposure levels 164, 165
   hepatotoxicity *884*
   neurotoxic effects 872–3
   phasing out 164
   prescribed diseases due to *50*, 165
methyl *iso*-butyl ketone (M*i*BK) 172,
      224, **247–8**, *247*
   characteristics and uses 247
   clinical manifestations 248
   metabolism/biochemical effects 248
   occupational diseases caused by (EC
      schedule) *43*
   toxicity 226, 248–9
methyl *n*-butyl ketone (M*n*BK; 2-
      hexanone) *224*, **246–7**
   biochemical effects 247
   characteristics and uses 246
   clinical manifestations 247
   exposure, prescribed disease *52*
   management 247
   metabolism 247, 870
   neurotoxic effects 870
   occupational diseases caused by (EC
      schedule) *43*
   peripheral neuropathy 247
methylcarbamates, *see* carbamate
      insecticides
methyl catechol 272
methyl-CCNU, genotoxicity *776*
methyl chloride (chloromethane) 165,
      212
   carcinogenicity 165
   prescribed diseases due to *51*
   teratogenicity 165
methyl chloride (monochloromethane),
      hepatotoxicity *885*
methyl chloroform, *see* 1,1,1-
      trichloroethane
2-methyl-4-chlorophenoxyacetic acid
      (MCPA), hepatotoxicity *884*
methyl cyanide (acetonitrile) 145
2-methylcyclohexanone, occupational
      diseases caused by (EC schedule)
      43
4,4′-methylene *bis*(2-chloroaniline)
      (MbOCA) 270, 797
   biological monitoring tests and
      guidance values *18*
   bladder cancer 270, 810
   DNA adducts 21
   genotoxicity *777*
   urinary tract malignancies, as
      prescribed diseases due to *51*
methylene blue 268
   for methaemoglobinaemia 202
methylene chloride (dichloromethane)
      143, *224*, **227**
   biological monitoring tests and
      guidance values *18*
   carcinogenicity 227

   characteristics and uses 227
   clinical manifestations 227
   as hazardous DIY material *6*
   hepatotoxicity 227
   management 227
   metabolism/biochemical effects 227
4,4′-methylenedianiline (MDA;
      diaminodiphenylmethane) 270
   biological monitoring tests and
      guidance values *18*
   hepatotoxicity *884*
   liver injury 883
methylene dichloride, hepatotoxicity
      226
methylene diphenyl diisocyanate, *see*
      diphenyl methane 4,4
      diisocyanate
methyl ether, occupational diseases
      caused by (EC schedule) *43*
methyl ether of hydroquinone (MEHQ)
      236
1-methylethyl benzene (cumene) 266
methyl ethyl ketone (MEK) *224*, *247*,
      248
   characteristics and uses 248
   clinical manifestations 248
   as hazardous DIY material *6*
   individual susceptibility factor 870
   management 248
   metabolism/biochemical effects 248
   neurotoxicity 226, 248, 248–9, 870
   occupational diseases caused by (EC
      schedule) *43*
N-methylformamide 251
   biological monitoring tests and
      guidance values *18*
methylhippuric acid 264
   biological monitoring tests and
      guidance values *18*
1-methyl-imidazole-4-acetic acid 623
methyl iodide 165
methyl isocyanate (MIC) 165
   Bhopal incident 123, 165, 584
   decomposition 9
methyl mercaptan (methanethiol) 161,
      162
methyl mercury
   distribution in body 91
   neurotoxic effects 92, 872
   poisoning 90, 852
   prenatal exposure effects 825
   reproductive hazard 825, 826, 830
   see also mercury poisoning
methyl methacrylate *224*, **249–50**
   clinical manifestations 250
   as hazardous DIY material *6*
   management 250
   metabolism/biochemical effects 250
Methylophilus methanolica, ill-health
      due to, in biotechnology *527*
Methylophilus methylotrophus 524
   ill-health due to, in biotechnology
      527
2-methylpentane, chemical structure
      225
3-methylpentane, chemical structure
      225
4-methyl-2-pentanol 248

4-methylpentan-2-one, biological monitoring tests and guidance values *18*
methylprednisolone 364
  chlorine poisoning *133*
2-methylpropan-1-ol (*iso*-butanol) *224*, *239*, 242, 243
2-methylpropan-2-ol (*tert*-butanol) *224*, *239*, 242, 243
4-methylpyrazole 241–2
N-methylthiobenzamide, biotransformation 77
methylthiourea, as non-genotoxic carcinogen *765*
methyl vinyl ether 169
methyl vinyl ketone *247*
metol (*p*-aminophenol), dermatoses 735
metolcarb (metoyl methyl carbamate) poisoning 209
metoyl methyl carbamate (metolcarb) poisoning 209
metronidazole 514
Mexico, hydrogen sulphide incident, Poza Rica 161
Mexico City, liquid petroleum gas explosion 123
mica 680–1
  kaolin contaminated by 679
mice
  occupational asthma due to *636*
  prescribed disease due to working at infested places *48*
  transgenic 767
Michigan, polybrominated biphenyls (PBBs) in animal feed 275
microbial diseases **487–535**
  health care workers, *see* health care workers
  see also individual diseases/occupations
microbial proteins, occupational asthma due to *636*
Micrococcus spp., in office buildings 717
microelectronics industry, reproductive hazards to mother 831
β2-microglobulins 95, 849
  biological effect monitoring *19*, 21
β2-microglobulinuria 94, 850
microgravity 376
micro-organisms
  genetically modified, *see* biotechnology
  see also bacteria; health care workers; *and individual micro-organisms*
Micropolyspora faeni 653, *654*, 654, 659, 711
microshocks 440
microsomal enzymes, abnormal liver function tests 883
microsomes 73
Microsporum canis 502
Microsporum gypseum 502
microwave radiation
  exposure limits 431
  eye damage from 431

eye protectors *433*
reproductive hazards to embryo/fetus 831–2, *832*
skin burns 431
sources 431
wavelengths 419
middle ear disease 293
Midland Bank, policy on bullying 544
midwives, reproductive hazards, anaesthetic gases 831
migraine headaches, at high altitudes *387*, 392
mild steel welders
  asthma in 183
  reproductive hazards 184
  welding fume 616
miliaria rubra 336
milk
  for lead workers 84
  in mercury poisoning 92
  pasteurization 494, 498, 500
mill fever 185, 621
milling, carcinogenic risk in *815*
Minamata disease 90, 852, 872
mineral dusts
  COPD and 614–15
  fibrous 686–97
  non-fibrous 672–86
mineral fibres, man-made, *see* man-made mineral/vitreous fibres
mineral oils
  carcinogenicity *814*
  genotoxicity *776*
  polycyclic aromatic hydrocarbons (PAHs) in 273
  prescribed diseases due to *50*
  skin diseases caused by (EC schedule) *44*
  skin neoplasms and *4*
minerals, occupational asthma due to *636*
mineral spirits, *see* white spirits
mineral wool 696
miners/mining
  aluminium oxide powder use 99
  carcinogenic risk in *815*
  cervical spondylosis 457
  dermatoses 732, 734
  early cancer observations 792
  gases in mines 137
  at high altitudes 383, 393–4
  history 920–1
  irradiation hazard, *see* radon
  lung cancer 700, *815*
  prescribed diseases *46*, *49*, *54*
  respiratory diseases in 614–15
  silicosis mortality *29*
  silicosis prevention 676
  uranium, lung cancer and 115
  see also specific types of mining
miners' nystagmus
  EC schedule of occupational diseases *45*
  as prescribed disease *46*
Minimental State 574
mirrors, silvering 89
miscarriage, *see* abortion
mismatch-repair genes 746, 753

missiles, exhaust gases 148
mists, particle size 72
mites, inhalation 637
mitochondria, vinylidene chloride (1,1-dichloroethylene) metabolism 236
mitogenesis 765, 766
mitral valve prolapse, high altitudes *390*
mittens 339
mobbing
  definition 540
  see also bullying
mobile telephones 793
moisturizers, in contact dermatitis protection 730
molecular epidemiology 797
molluscicides 212–13
molten/red hot material, prescribed disease due to rays from *46*
molybdenum **109**
  toxic effects 109
molybdenum trioxide 109
Mond process 110, 166, 167
monitoring
  electronic, at place of work, leading to violence 552
  see also biological monitoring
monitoring of workers
  aircrew 377–8
  aromatic amines 269–70
  arsenic 97
  asbestos exposure 695
  benzene 262, 263
  beryllium 104
  biotechnology workers 532–3
  bladder tumours 269–70
  cadmium 95
  carbon disulphide 254
  chromium 105
  coalworkers 682
  cobalt 106–7
  dimethylformamide (DMF) 251
  divers 358
  ethyl benzene 266
  ionizing radiation 407, 409
  manganese 109
  mercury 93
  organotin compounds 115
  phosphorus 99
  reproductive function 834–5
  selenium 112
  silicosis prevention 677
  silver 112
  styrene 265
  tellurium 112–13
  tetrachloroethylene (perchloroethylene) 235
  toluene 263
  1,1,1-trichloroethane 231
  trichloroethylene 234
  vanadium 116
  xylene 264
  see also biological monitoring; health surveillance; lung function; pre-employment screening
monobromoethane (methyl bromide), hepatotoxicity *884*

monochloramine 147, 148
monochloroacetic acid 889
monochlorobenzene 266
monochloromethane (methyl chloride),
   hepatotoxicity 885
monoclonal antibodies 523, 525
monomers, see acrylamide monomer
   poisoning; vinyl chloride
   monomer
monomethylamine 157
monomethyl arsonic acid 96, 97
N-monomethylcarbamic acids
   (methylcarbamates), see
   carbamate insecticides
monomethylformamide 251
mono-oxygenases 744
monosomy 744
montmorillonite 681
Montreal study, occupational history of
   cancer patients 28
Montreal Treaty, on CFCs 154
moonshine (illicitly distilled spirits) 853
MOPP
   carcinogenicity 814
   genotoxicity 776
Moraceae, contact dermatitis 734
morphine 328, 330
mortality
   alcohol-related 559
   byssinosis 625
   in cohort studies 799
   geographical relationship to industry
      28
   occupational 28
      statistics 29, 29–30
   proportional mortality ratio (PMR)
      32–3, 800
   radiation levels causing death 400
   shift work and 584
   standardized mortality ratio (SMR)
      32, 799
   trichloroethylene causing sudden
      death 234
mosquitoes
   bite prevention 512
   malaria 512–13
   viral haemorrhagic fevers 509
mothballs 272
motion sickness, space motion sickness
   376
motor disturbances, hand–arm
   vibration syndrome 308
motorists, ethanol and breath analysis
   71
motor vehicles
   engines as source of nitrogen dioxide
      159
   exhausts/emissions 123, 125, 142,
      144
      asthma and 616
      genotoxicity 777
   radiator repairs, lead use 844
   as source of vibration 317
moulders, silicosis prevention 676–7
moulding 654, 655
moulds
   occupational asthma due to 636, 637
   prescribed diseases due to 49

see also fungi
mountaineers 383
   altitude sickness
      prevention 390–1
      treatment 391–4
      see also acute mountain sickness
   'Red Alert' symptoms 393, 394
      see also acute mountain sickness;
         barometric pressure: reduced
mucochloric acid, hepatotoxicity 884
muconic acid 74
mucus gland hyperplasia, in byssinosis
   622
mucus hypersecretion 608, 627, 628,
   664
Muir–Torre syndrome, susceptibility
   and germline mutation 750
mullite 676
multiple endocrine neoplasia,
   oncogene activation in 749
multiple myeloma, benzene causing
   262
mumps, reproductive hazards 829
munitions, see explosives
munitions work, hepatotoxicity in 884,
   892
muscle
   biotransformation capability 73
   weakness, in lead poisoning 86
muscle fasciculation, pesticide
   exposure and 200
muscovite 680
muscular insertions, overstraining, EC
   schedule of occupational
   diseases 45
muscular problems, see also back pain;
   repetitive movement disorders;
   repetitive strain injury
musculoskeletal disorders, work-related
   453–75
   disease clustering 470–1
   identification 470–1
   management 471–2
   prevention 471–2
   risk factors 467–70
   work association, definitions 453–4
musculoskeletal system
   decompression illness 351–2
   disorders due to vibration 308
   welding injuries 184
mushroom cultivation 655
mushroom worker's lung 654, 654, 655
mustard gas (sulphur mustard) 171
   cancers due to 814
   genotoxicity 776
   lung cancer 815
   manufacture, respiratory tract
      malignancies 4
mutagenesis 522, 523
mutagenicity
   acrylamide 250
   1,2-dibromoethane (ethylene
      dibromide) 232
   ethidium bromide 529
   methyl bromide 165
   methyl chloride 165
   4,4′-methylene bis(2-chloroaniline)
      (MbOCA) 270

methyl iodide 165
styrene 265
1,1,1-trichloroethane (methyl
   chloroform) 231
vinyl bromide 170
mutagens 742
mutations 743–4
   biomethylation effect 753–4
   carcinogenesis 743
   chromosomal 743
   DNA damage 743–4, 744–5
   frameshift mutations 743
   genetic modification 523
   genomic 744
   germ cell 828–9
   'hotspots' 745, 753
   mutational screening 767
   mutational spectra of genes 754
   point mutations 744
      P53 gene 753
      transitions/transversions 743
   serial accumulation 747
   somatic 742, 752
      clonal evolution and 747
      germline mutation vs 756
   in von Hippel–Lindau tumour-
      suppressor gene 755
mutator phenotypes 753
myalgic encephalomyelitis (ME) 541
mycetoma 684
Mycobacterium marinum 501, 734
Mycobacterium tuberculosis 507, 511
   multidrug-resistant 511
mycotoxins, pulmonary
   biotransformation 76
myelodysplasia 903, 907
   benzene exposure 910–11
   bone marrow and benzene toxicity
      75
   ionizing radiation and 908
myeloid leukaemia, benzene-induced
   907, 909, 910–11
Myleran, genotoxicity 776
myocardial infarction
   methylene chloride use 143, 227
   see also ischaemic heart disease
myocardium, 'sensitization of the
   myocardium' 229
myopia, empty field myopia 369

nafenopin, as non-genotoxic carcinogen
   765
NAG, see N-acetyl-β-D-glucosaminidase
nails, metal, cutting/shaping/cleaning,
   prescribed diseases due to 47
naltrexone 563
napalm 98
naphthacene 272
naphthalene(s) 272–3
   chlorinated, see chlorinated
      naphthalene(s)
   in nucleic acid extraction 529
   occupational diseases caused by (EC
      schedule) 43
naphthalene counterparts,
   occupational diseases caused by
   (EC schedule) 43

naphthalene diisocyanate (NDI) 639
naphthols and halogenated derivatives,
	occupational diseases caused by
	(EC schedule) 43
1-naphthylamine 269
	bladder malignancies and 4
	urinary tract malignancies as
		prescribed diseases due to 51
2-naphthylamine 268, 269, 797
	bladder tumours 4, 268, 269, 742,
		792, 810
	cancer prevention 817
	carcinogenicity 814
		rubber production 28
	genotoxicity 776
	hepatotoxicity 884
	as prohibited carcinogenic substance
		269
	urinary tract malignancies as
		prescribed diseases due to 51
α-naphthylamine, see 1-naphthylamine
β-naphthylamine, see 2-naphthylamine
naphthylamines, as carcinogenic risk
	815
1-naphthylthiourea (ANTU) 269
	biotransformation 77
α-naphthylthiourea, see 1-
	naphthylthiourea
narcissi, contact dermatitis 734
Narcotics Anonymous (NA) 563
nasal cancer
	formaldehyde 805
	in furniture manufacturers 28
	industries/occupations associated
		with 815, 816
	nasal sinus cancer 808, 815, 816
	nickel associated with 109
	nickel compounds 807
	as prescribed disease 50, 53
nasal cartilaginous septum, perforation
	97, 100, 105
nasal cavities, malignant neoplasms,
	occupation/agents causing 4
nasal irritation, trichloroethylene 234
nasal sinus cancer 808, 815, 816
	see also nasal cancer
nasal symptoms, sick building
	syndrome and 713
nasopharyngitis, in acute beryllium
	poisoning 101
National Academy of Science, USA 447
National Arrangements for Incidents
	involving Radioactivity (NAIR)
	413–14
National Counselling Service for Sick
	Doctors 565
National Health Service, risk of violence
	at work 551, 553
National Institute of Abuse and
	Alcoholism (NIAAA), USA 578
National Institute of Occupational
	Safety and Health (NIOSH), USA
	82, 336
	acrylamide exposure levels 868
	benzene threshold limit 262
	1,3-butadiene carcinogenicity 238
	hand–arm vibration syndrome
		(HAVS) 316

industrial chemicals information 223
	recommended exposure limits 7
	SENSOR reporting scheme 31
National Insurance (Industrial Injuries)
	Act 1946 38
National Morbidity Surveys in General
	Practice in England and Wales
	454
National Poisons Information Service
	advice from 199
	information on locations of
		pralidoxime supplies 207
	telephone numbers 200
National Radiological Protection Board
	(NRPB), UK 400–1, 407
National Registry of Radiation Workers,
	UK 404
National Toxicology Program (NTP), USA
	766
	1,3-butadeine carcinogenicity 238
	methylene chloride carcinogenicity
		227
National Workplace Bullying Advice
	Line 543
natural gas 137, 159, 161
	odourants 161
nausea and vomiting
	arsine poisoning 162
	dichloroacetylene exposure 239
	1,2-dichloroethane (ethylene
		dichloride) 230
	paraquat poisoning and 201
	pesticide exposure and 200
	radiation casualties 402
Naylor v Preston Area Health Authority
	(1987) 60
NDI (naphthalene diisocyanate) 639
neck pain 456
	as risk factor in back pain 480
neck problems 456–7
	cervical spondylosis 454, 456–7
	cervical syndrome 457
	epidemiology 456
	management 457
	occupational studies 456–7
	tension neck syndrome 454, 457
	thoracic outlet syndrome 454, 457
	work-related 454
necrosis, radiation levels causing 400
needlestick injuries 504–5
	hepatitis B infection 503, 505
	hepatitis C infection 505–6
	HIV infection 506
	malaria 512
	underreporting 505
	veterinarians 213
negligence, claims under Tort 42
neighbourhood cases, beryllium
	poisoning 103
neodymium YAG lasers 428
	exposure limits 429
	eye damage from 420
neomycin 895
	as treatment for liver disease 887
neon 141
	in earth's atmosphere 135
neoplastic disorders, as cause of back
	pain 479

neoprene applications, hepatotoxicity
	in 884
nephritis, chronic 844
nephropathy, tetrachloroethylene
	(perchloroethylene) workers
	235–6
nephrotic syndrome 852
nephrotoxic effects of exposures
	843–66
	biological monitoring tests 18
nephrotoxicity
	fluoride compounds 167
	trichloroethylene ('trike') 234
nerve conduction tests 867
nerve conduction velocities, reduced
	acrylamide 868
	arsenic poisoning 96–7
	carbon disulphide 254
	carpal tunnel syndrome 461
	n-hexane 226, 870
	lead poisoning 85
	mercury poisoning 92
	methyl methacrylate causing 250
	styrene causing 265
	trichloroethylene exposure 234
nerve entrapment, carpal tunnel 460
nerve gases, in war 171
nerve paralysis, EC schedule of
	occupational diseases 45
nerve pressure, EC comparable data
	collection 41
nerve root compression 480
nerve root pain 479, 479, 483
nervous system, see central nervous
	system; peripheral neuropathy
Netherlands, disability benefit scheme
	38
neurasthenic syndrome 264
neurobehavioural effects
	benzene exposure 262
	electromagnetic field exposure 445–6
	styrene exposure 265
	toluene exposure 263
neurobehavioural testing 867–8
neuroblastoma 746
	parental exposure to electromagnetic
		fields 445
neurodegenerative effects,
	electromagnetic field exposure
	445–6
neurofibromatosis, peripheral,
	susceptibility and germline
	mutation 750
neurofilament accumulations,
	paranodal 226
neurological manifestations
	biological monitoring tests 18
	decompression illness 352–3, 355–6
	decompression sickness 364
neurological sequelae
	delayed, carbon monoxide poisoning
		144
	fires 130
	hydrogen sulphide poisoning 161
	of raised barometric pressure 356
neuropathic syndrome, in
	dimethylaminoproprionitrile
	exposure 869–70

neuropathy target esterase (NTE)
873–4, 876
neuropsychiatric damage, carbon
monoxide 144
neuropsychiatric disease, *see*
psychiatric disorders
neurotic illness
management at work 577
see also anxiety; depression
neurotoxic effects of exposures **867–80**
acrylamide 868
allyl chloride 868
assessment 867
biological monitoring tests *18*
carbon disulphide 868–9
carbon monoxide 869
dimethylaminoproprionitrile
869–70
epidemiological studies 867–8
ethylene oxide 870
hexacarbon solvents 870
metals 871–2
methyl bromide 872
pesticides 873–4
pyrethroids 874
solvent mixtures 875
styrene 874–5
toluene 875
trichloroethylene 875–6
wartime exposure 876–7
see also individual chemicals/metals
neurotoxicity, oxygen at high partial
pressures 345
neutron activation analysis 95, 850
neutrons 397–8, *398*
neutropenia
occupations/agents causing *4*
symptoms and signs 904
Newcastle disease 490, 498
Newcastle Scale 574
New Zealand
Accident Compensation scheme 38
hydrogen sulphide pollution,
Rotorua 161
nickel **109–10**
carcinogenicity 109, 700
dermatitis 110, 734
EC comparable data collection *41*
as genotoxic carcinogen 778–9
hepatotoxicity *884, 885*
lung cancer associated with *4*, 109,
807
metal-induced asthma due to 699
nasal cancer associated with *4*, 109,
807, 808
occupational diseases caused by (EC
schedule) *43*
prescribed diseases due to *50*
refineries 109
smelting/refining, respiratory tract
malignancies *4*
soluble 109
uses 109
in welding fume 181
nickel arsenide 807
nickel carbonyl 110, 166–7
acute lung injury due to *698*, 698
clinical manifestations 166, 167

poisoning, as prescribed disease *50*,
110
prescribed diseases due to 167
welding fume and 181
nickel compounds
cancers *814*
carcinogenicity 28
genotoxicity *776*
occupational diseases caused by (EC
schedule) *43*
sino-nasal and lung cancers *815*
nickel itch 110
nickel oxides 109
acute lung injury due to *698*
nickel refining
nasal sinus cancer 808
sino-nasal and lung cancers *815*
nickel silver 109
nickel subsulphide 109
nickel sulphate 109, 807
nickel sulphides 109
nickel tetracarbonyl 109
nifedipine 330, 391, 392, *394*
night vision
flying 370
goggles 370
night work 581–2, *582*
ILO Convention and
Recommendation 585
see also shift work; work hours
Nipah virus infection 498
nitric acid, occupational diseases
caused by (EC schedule) *43*
nitric oxide 158, 159
in welding fume 181–2
nitriles **253**
nitrilotriacetates, as non-genotoxic
carcinogens *765*
nitroaromatics, hepatotoxicity *885*, 892
nitrobenzene 266
hepatotoxicity *885*
nitrochlorbenzene, prescribed disease
due to *50*
nitro-derivatives of benzene, prescribed
diseases due to *50*
4-nitrodiphenyl 269
nitroethane, hepatotoxicity *885, 891*
nitro-explosives 159
nitrogen 135, 141, 344
in earth's atmosphere *135*
narcosis 346
nitrogen dioxide 125, **158–60**
bronchiolitis obliterans caused by
133
characteristics and sources 158–9
clinical manifestations of exposure
159
health effect levels *127*
management of exposures 159–60
treatment 159–60
uses and occurrences 158–9
nitrogen mustard 171
genotoxicity *777*
nitrogen oxides 158–60
occupational diseases caused by (EC
schedule) *43*
poisoning 159
prescribed diseases due to *50*, 159

in welding fume 181–2
see also nitric oxide; nitrogen dioxide
nitrogen tetroxide 376
nitrogen trichloride 147
nitrogen trifluoride 153
nitromethane, hepatotoxicity *885*, 891
1-nitronaphthalene 76
nitroparaffins, hepatotoxicity *885*, 891
nitropropane, hepatotoxicity *885*
1-nitropropane, hepatotoxicity 891
2-nitropropane, hepatotoxicity *884,
885*, 891
nitroreductases 75
nitrosamines, stomach cancer 808
N-nitroso compounds 742
nitrosyl chloride 149
nitrous oxide 168–9
abuse 168–9
anaesthetists' exposure to 167, 168
changes in bone marrow 168
discovery and early use 167
in earth's atmosphere *135*
Kyoto Protocol agreement 135
levels in delivery rooms 167
neuropathy 168
neurotoxic effects 168
reproductive hazards 168, 169
to embryo/fetus 831
nitrous oxide analgesia, decompression
illnesses and 355
Noble v Robert Thompson (1979) 59
noise 285
action levels 296–7, 299
active cancellation 297
in biotechnology plants 529
classification 285
daily personal exposure to noise
(LEPd) calculation 296–7
in flying 368
active noise reduction (ANR) 368
protection 368
hearing loss relationship to exposure
296–7
impact noise 285
impulse noise 285
measurement 296–7
noise control 297
recreational 299
reduction 297–8
regulations and legal provisions
298–9
reproductive hazards to
embryo/fetus 832, *832*
steady-state 285
see also hearing loss; occupational
noise-induced hearing loss;
sound
Noise at Work: Guidance on Regulations
298
Noise at Work Regulations 1989 298–9
noise-induced hearing loss (NIHL), *see*
occupational noise-induced
hearing loss
nonane *225*
non-fibrous clays 681–2
non-fibrous mineral dusts, diseases due
to **672–86**
non-freezing cold injury (NFCI) 329–31

non-freezing cold injury (NFCI) – *contd*
  late consequences 330
  presentation and management
    330–1
non-genotoxic carcinogens, *see*
    carcinogens: non-genotoxic
non-hepatic disorders, abnormal liver
    function tests 883
non-Hodgkin's lymphoma 811, 909–10
  chlorophenol exposure and 272
  chlorophenoxyacetate herbicides and
    203
  farm workers 910
  industries/occupations associated
    with *816*
  skin cancer and 810
  2,3,7,8-tetrachlorodibenzo-*p*-dioxin
    (TCDD) and 876
non-ionizing radiation 419, 832
  and the eye **419–37**
    eye protection *433*
    health and safety directives 437
    human exposure limits 432
    ionizing radiation *vs* 419
    optical radiation safety evaluation
      432
    sources, eye damage and
      absorption *420*
    see also cataracts; ultraviolet
      radiation
    wavelengths 419
non-specific symptoms 25
  multifactorial approach to biological
    monitoring 24
non-steroidal anti-inflammatory drugs
    (NSAIDs), hip and knee
    osteoarthritis 467
Nordic questionnaire 471
Norway, COPD survey 616–17
Norwegian scabies 511
nose, *see entries beginning with* nasal
nuclear explosions, fireball, eye
    damage 370
nuclear power industry/workers,
    radiation doses 407
nuclear power plants/reactors
  incidents 131
  uranium in 115
  see also Chernobyl incident
nuclear reactor accidents, casualty
    handling plan 413–15
  clinical treatment/care 414–15
    combined injury 415
    cutaneous 414–15
    gastrointestinal conditions 414
    general 414
    laboratory samples *415*
    marrow aplasia 414
    sepsis 414
    treatment categories 414
  hospitals 413–14
  reception centre 413
  see also radiation accidents
Nuclear Regulatory Commission
    (NUREG), USA 400–1
nuclear weapons, whole body radiation
    403
nucleic acid extraction 529

extractants and precipitating agents
    529
nuisance dusts 679, 681, 682
numbness, methyl *n*-butyl ketone
    causing 247
nurses/nursing
  bone marrow cancer *816*
  genotoxic exposures *776, 777*
  hepatotoxicity in *884*
  and workplace violence 551, 553
nylon 697
nystagmus, *see* miners' nystagmus

oat flour, radioallergosorbent tests
    (RAST) *21*
oats dust
  occupational asthma due to *647*
  prescribed diseases due to *52, 53*
obesity
  fitness for flying and 378
  hip and knee osteoarthritis 467
obsessional personalities 572, 574
obstructive bronchiolitis, *see*
    bronchiolitis obliterans
occupation
  as cause of/contributor to illness 3
  change of, due to occupational
    asthma 646
  effect of disease on **12–13**
  simple questions on **3–6**
  see also individual occupations
occupational asthma, *see* asthma,
    occupational
occupational cancer, *see* cancer,
    occupational; *and individual
    cancers*
Occupational Deafness 293
'occupational deafness', *see* deafness;
    occupational noise-induced
    hearing loss
occupational diseases, *see* diseases,
    occupational
Occupational Exposure Standards (UK)
    17
occupational hazards, *see* hazards,
    occupational
Occupational Health and Safety
    Administration (OSHA), USA 82
  benzene exposure limits 262
occupational history **3–13**, 794–6
  from cancer patients 795–6
  case studies/examples 11, 795–6
  confusion over chemicals in 9–10
  detailed history 10
  ethical considerations 11–12, *12*
  exposure extent 8
  importance of 3
  information sources, *see* information
    sources
  in inorganic dust diseases 665–6
  occupation as cause/contributor of
    illness 3, *4, 6*
  questionnaire 796
  reliability and validity scores 10–11
  simple questions 3–6
occupational noise-induced hearing
    loss (ONIHL) **289–94**

4kHz notch 290, 291, 293, 295
6kHz notch 290, 293
adaptation 290
in developing countries 290
diagnosis 293–4
divers and compressed-air workers
    356
EC comparable data collection *41*
EC schedule of occupational diseases
    45
epidemiology 289–90
hand–arm vibration syndrome
    (HAVS) and 310
hazardous noise effect 290–1
hearing thresholds, international
    standards 295
historical aspects 289
information and education 298
legal provisions/aspects 298–9
management 299–300
middle ear disease and 293
noise exposure relationship 296–7
occupations associated with *46–8*
pathology 291–3
permanent threshold shifts 290–1
post-stimulatory fatigue 290
as prescribed disease *46–8*
pre-stimulatory fatigue 290
prevention 297–8, 298–9
sensorineural hearing loss and 293,
    299
sound stimulation effect 290–1
temporary threshold shifts 289,
    290
welding injuries 185
occupational noise-induced tinnitus
    303
occupational noise-induced vertigo
    303–4
occupational physician role 579
Occupational Physicians Reporting
    Activity (OPRA) surveillance
    scheme, reports to 725
Occupational Safety and Health
    Administration (OSHA), USA
  exposure limits 7
  material safety data sheet format 7
occupational therapy, hip and knee
    osteoarthritis *467*
octane *225*
oedema
  ankle 336
  pulmonary, *see* pulmonary oedema
oesophageal perforation, paraquat
    poisoning and *201*
oestrogenic steroids, as non-genotoxic
    carcinogens *765*
oestrogens
  environmental contamination and
    275
  male fertility/sexual behaviour 829
  male fetus and 825
  as non-genotoxic carcinogens *765*
office buildings, control of environment
    of 716–17
offices
  cleaning, *see* cleaners/cleaning
  radon concentrations in 407

office workers
  dermatoses 734
  ozone effects 158
  sick building syndrome, *see* sick
      building syndrome
  ventilation pneumonitis (indoor
      extrinsic allergic alveolitis) *654,
      654, 655–6*
  see also keyboard operators; visual
      display unit operators
ofloxacin, for legionnaires' disease 711
oil acne (oil folliculitis) 731
oil folliculitis (oil acne) 731
oil refinery workers, hydrocarbon
      exposure 856
oil rigs
  Piper Alpha disaster 546, 547
  workers' epilepsy and alcohol
      dependence 558
oils
  skin diseases caused by (EC schedule)
      44
  soluble, dermatoses 734
oil warts 733
oil well fires 129–30
olefins, *see* alkenes
oleum ('fuming sulphuric acid') 156
olfactory fatigue 125, 145, 160
olfs 716
oligospermia 824, *829*, 829
oliguria, carbon tetrachloride causing
      229
Oliver, Thomas 254
Omsk haemorrhagic fever 509
oncodemes, susceptibility to cancer 757
oncogenes 528, 748–52
  activation *749*
oncology unit workers 895
ondansetron 414
oocysts 494
oocytes 824–5
open cast coal mining 683
ophthalmic instruments 426
opiate abuse
  clinical features 561
  detoxification 563
  maintenance methadone 564
  see also drug abuse
OPRA (occupational physician reporting
      activity) scheme 31
optical atrophy
  bis(chloromethyl) ether 252
  methanol 241
optical density (OD) 433–4
optic atrophy, methyl bromide causing
      164
optic disc oedema 241
optic neuritis 241
oral cancer 754
oral candidiasis (thrush), in AIDS/HIV
      infection 507
orchitis, in brucellosis 492
orf 490, 501–2, 733
  as prescribed disease *49*
organic acids, occupational diseases
      caused by (EC schedule) *43*
organic brain syndrome 875
organic chemical compounds 223

aliphatic **223–60**, *224*
aromatic 223, **261–79**
volatile, *see* volatile organic
      compounds
see also individual compounds
organic dusts
  extrinsic allergic alveolitis due to
      653, *654*
  see also byssinosis
organic dust syndromes 136, 185
organic psychosis, *see* toxic organic
      psychosis
organic solvents, *see* solvents, organic
organizational changes, and violence at
      work 552
organoarsenicals, in fish 97
organochlorine pesticides 209–10
  in breast milk 833
  clinical features of acute poisoning
      210
  management of acute poisoning 210
  neurotoxic effects 874
  occupational and chronic exposure
      209–10
  routes of exposure 209
  toxicity mechanisms 209
organ of Corti 287, 288
organomercurial fungicides 212
organomercury 92
organomercury compounds 91
organophosphate pesticides
  acute poisoning 205, 206–7
    features of 206–7
    intermediate syndrome 206
    management 206–7
    organophosphate-induced delayed
      neuropathy 206
  chronic poisoning 205–6
    behavioural and psychological
      effects 205
    management principles 205–6
    neurological sequelae 205
  cognitive impairment syndrome due
      to 25
  detecting exposure to 207–8
    electrophysiology 207
    measurement of cholinesterase
      activity 207
    monitoring 207–8
    organophosphate metabolites 207
  neurotoxic effects 873–4
  and non-Hodgkin's lymphoma 910
  pre-employment assessment 208
  subclinical poisoning 206
  symptoms and signs of exposure to
      200
  toxicity mechanisms 204–5
  treatment of poisoning 873
organophosphorous esters,
      occupational diseases caused by
      (EC schedule) *43*
organophosphorus compounds (OPs)
      204–8
  biological effect indicators *19*
  war 171
organotin compounds 114, 735
  absorption and metabolism 114
  poisoning outbreak (France) 114

supervision of workers 115
  toxicity 114
  treatment of poisoning 115
organotropy 742
Orlon, acrylonitrile fibre 253
ornithosis 492
osmic acid (osmium tetroxide) 110
osmiridium 110
osmium **110**
osmium oxides, acute lung injury due
      to *698*
osmium tetroxide (osmic acid) 110
osseous labyrinth 286–7
ossicular fixation 293
osteitis, in brucellosis 492
osteoarthritis **464–7**
  clinical features 464–5
  epidemiology 464–5
  hip 33, 466
  knee 465–6
  management 466–7
    exercise 466–7
    hydrotherapy 467
    non-pharmacological therapy *467*
    pharmacological therapy *467*
    surgery 467
  occupational studies 465–6
osteoarticular diseases of hands and
      wrists, EC schedule of
      occupational diseases *45*
osteofluorosis 151–2
osteolysis, phalangeal, as prescribed
      disease *51*
osteomalacia
  abnormal liver function tests 883
  cadmium-induced renal calcium
      wasting and 850
  in cadmium workers 94
osteonecrosis
  dysbaric 356–8
  as prescribed disease *46*, 355
osteopathy, back pain 482
osteoporosis, as cause of back pain
      479, 480
osteosarcoma, cancer risk and germline
      mutations *751*
OSWAS (Ovako Working Posture
      Analysing System) 468
otic blast injury 294
otitic barotrauma 362
otitis externa 350
otosclerosis 293
ouch-ouch, *see* itai-itai disease
outdoor air pollution, legionnaires'
      disease 709
Ovako Working Posture Analysing
      System (OSWAS) 468
ovarian cancer
  familial, susceptibility and germline
      mutation *750*
  oncogene activation in *749*
  risk of, and germline mutations *750*
ovaries, threshold levels of radiation
      dose *400*
overbreathing, *see also* hyperventilation
overhead work, shoulder problems 455
ovine chlamydiosis, as prescribed
      disease *49*, 493

ovine enzootic abortion (OEA) 493
Ovivac P, accidental self-injection with
        213
Owen, Robert 919
oxidase enzymes 73
oxidation, of chemicals in
        biotransformation 75
oxidative haemolysis 903
oxidative phosphorylation 271, 272
oximes, in acute carbamate poisoning
        209
oxygen
    atmospheres deficient in 135, 136
    in carbon monoxide poisoning 131
    in diving, lack of 346, 349
    diving procedures using 343–4
    in earth's atmosphere 135
    excess 135
    in hydrogen cyanide poisoning 145
    hyperbaric 131, 144
    low concentrations, effects 135
    masks 363
    minimum content in air 124
    neurotoxicity 345
    oxygen tension, and unconsciousness
        in water 348–9
    partial pressure 363
    pre-oxygenation 364, 376
    pulmonary toxicity 345
    therapy, altitude sickness 392
    toxicity at high pressures 345
    see also hypoxia
oxygen cylinders, high altitude
        transportation problems 392
oxygen difluoride 153
oxygen ear 363
oxygen radicals, see free radicals
oxygen systems, in flying, risks in
        extreme cold 367
oxy-helium, for divers 344, 345
oxy-nitrogen 344
oxyprenolol, altitude sickness 390
ozone 157–8
    depletion by CFCs 154
    in earth's atmosphere 135
    exposure levels and effects 158
    lung injury from inhalation 132
    sources 158
    uses 158
    in welding fume 181

P53 gene 745, 752–3
    function and involvement 751
    germline mutations 752
    point mutations 753
    specific carcinogenic exposures 754–5
pacemakers
    electromagnetic fields and 185
    magnetic fields and 446
packers
    elbow problems 458
    hand/wrist tendinitis 459
    shoulder tendinitis 455
paddy foot 330
Paget's disease 151
    abnormal liver function tests 883
    as cause of back pain 479

pain
    neck pain 456
    shoulder pain 455
paint
    as hazardous DIY material 6
    lead in 83
painters/painting
    cancers 814
        bladder cancer 815
        carcinogenic risk 815
        lung cancer 803–4, 815, 816
    genotoxic exposures 776
    hepatotoxicity in 885
    lead use 844
    solvent-induced encephalopathies
        875
    toxic DIY materials 6
    see also spray painting
paint manufacturers/industries
    dermatoses 735
    xylene exposure 264
paint removers
    benzene in 261
    carbon monoxide poisoning 143
paint sprayers 857
paint strippers
    as hazardous DIY materials 6
    methylene chloride
        (dichloromethane) in 227
palladium, metal-induced asthma due
        to 699
pallidum, manganese poisoning 108
pallor, in lead poisoning 86
palygorskite 696
pancreatic cancer 809
    non-genotoxic carcinogen
        mechanisms 765
    oncogene activation in 749
    risk of, and germline mutations 750
pancreatitis, in hypothermia 331
pancytopenia 907, 908
    case study 910–11
    symptoms and signs 904
papain 637
paper, sick building syndrome and 714
paper industry, carcinogenic risk in 816
papillary necrosis, in mercury
        poisoning 91
papillary thyroid carcinoma, oncogene
        activation in 749
papilloedema, in high altitude cerebral
        oedema 386
papillomas, non-genotoxic carcinogen
        mechanisms 765
Paracelsus 920, 921
paracentesis, as treatment for liver
        disease 887
paracetamol
    altitude sickness 392, 394
    back pain 482, 483
    hip and knee osteoarthritis 467, 467
    as non-genotoxic carcinogen 765
paraesthesia
    arsenic exposure 96
    n-hexane exposure 226
    mercury poisoning 92
paraffin
    prescribed diseases due to 50

skin diseases caused by (EC schedule)
        44
paraformaldehyde, in nucleic acid
        extraction 529
parahydroxyamphetamines 74
parahydroxyphenobarbitone 74
paraldehyde 245
paramedical staff, see health care
        workers; medical/paramedical
        staff
paramyl-phenol, prescribed disease due
        to 51
paranasal sinuses, gas in 362
paraoxon, parathion metabolized to
        74, 75
paraphenylene diamine derivatives, as
        hazardous DIY material 6
paraplegia, decompression sickness
        352, 355
paraquat 200–2
    exposure consequences 200–1
    hepatotoxicity 884, 894
    ingestion, deliberate 197, 201
    lung fibrosis 77
    symptoms and signs of exposure 200
    toxicokinetics and toxicity
        mechanism 200
    transport into lung cells 68
paraquat poisoning
    diagnosis 201
    features of 201
    gastric lavage 202
    lethal dose 201
    management 201–2
    outcome 201
    oxygen and 202
    time course 201
    treatment 202
parasitic diseases, EC schedule 44
para-tertiary-butylcatechol, prescribed
        disease due to 51
para-tertiary-butylphenol, prescribed
        disease due to 51
parathion
    metabolism 74
    oxidation 75
paratoluenediamine, causing aplastic
        anaemia 907
parenchymal fibrosis, in welders 183,
        184
parental radiation exposure, see
        children
Paris green (cupric acetoarsenite) 96
parkinsonian features, manganese
        poisoning 872
parkinsonism 108
    manganese poisoning vs 108
Parkinson-like syndrome
    methanol exposure 241
    see also carbon monoxide: acute
        poisoning
Parkinson's disease, magnetic field
        exposure and 446
paronychia 510, 733
partial body radiation exposure 403
partial pressure 345, 363
    volatile compounds 71
particle radiation 398, 398

parvovirus 510
parvovirus vaccine 214
passenger transport systems, drug
    screening tests for operational
    staff 561
patch testing **728–9**
    berylliosis 702
    dilution for 728–9
pathologists, phosphine hazard 163
patient carers, carcinogenic risk *816*
PBB, *see* polybrominated biphenyls
PCB, *see* polychlorinated biphenyls
PCDD, *see* chlorinated dioxins
PCDF, *see* chlorinated dibenzofurans
peak expiratory flow (PEF)
    in byssinosis 627, 628
    occupational asthma investigation
        643
    see also lung function
peas, contact dermatitis and 734
peau d'orange 351
pectinase, radioallergosorbent tests
    (RAST) *21*
pediculosis, treatment 210
PEF, *see* peak expiratory flow
peliosis hepatis 885, 894
pelvic disorders, as cause of back pain
    479
pemoline, jet lag and 374
penicillamine 892
    copper poisoning 107
    lead poisoning 87–8
    mercury poisoning 92, 93
    as treatment for liver disease 887
penicillin
    anthrax 491
    erysipeloid 501
    leptospirosis 496
    listeriosis 496
    Lyme disease 497
    occupational asthma due to *636*
    Streptococcus suis infection 500
Penicillium spp. 711
Penicillium chrysogenum 711
Penicillium cyclopium 711
pentaborane 166
pentachlorophenol (PCP) 212, 271, 272,
    275
    aplastic anaemia and 262–3
pentane *225*
1,5-pentanedial, *see* glutaraldehyde
peptide hormones, in reproduction 825
peptides 524
perchlorate, as non-genotoxic
    carcinogen *765*
perchloric acid, in nucleic acid
    extraction 529
perchlorobenzene, *see*
    hexachlorobenzene
perchloroethylene, *see*
    tetrachloroethylene
perchloryl fluoride 153
percussive tools, prescribed diseases
    due to *46, 48*
perfluorocarbons, Kyoto Protocol
    agreement 135
performance efficiency, shift work 582,
    583–4, 588

perhexiline neuropathy 68
periarticular sacs, EC schedule of
    occupational diseases *45*
periodic breathing, (Cheyne–Stokes
    respiration) at high altitude
    383, 389
peripheral nerve function, assessment
    867
peripheral nervous system, effects of
    exposure to welding fume 182
peripheral neuropathy
    arsenic exposure 96, 871, 904
    carbon disulphide exposure 254
    carbon monoxide poisoning 869
    ethylene oxide 166
    n-hexane 226
    ketones causing 248–9
    lead poisoning 86, 87, 871, 904
    in Lyme disease 497
    mercury poisoning 92
    methyl *n*-butyl ketone exposure 247
    methyl ethyl ketone 248, 249
    methyl isobutyl ketone 249
    methyl methacrylate causing 250
    as prescribed disease *52*
    thallium poisoning 113
peripheral neurotoxins, biological
    monitoring tests *18*
periportal fibrosis, vinyl chloride
    exposure 170
peritendineum, overstraining, EC
    schedule of occupational
    diseases *45*
peritendinitis 459–60
peritoneal mesothelioma 602, 693–4
peritoneal tumours,
    industries/occupations
    associated with *815, 816*
'perk' (perchloroethylene), *see*
    tetrachloroethylene
Permanent Commission for
    Occupational Health 924
permethrin 211, 511
    pesticides, symptoms and signs of
        exposure to *200*
personality changes, in mercury
    poisoning 872
personal protective equipment, *see*
    protective equipment, personal
Perspex 249–50
persulphate salts
    occupational asthma due to *647*
    prescribed diseases due to *52, 53*
pest control
    occupational asthma due to *647*
    prescribed diseases associated with
        52, 53
pesticide exposure
    bystanders 196
    in dilution and application 196
    in harvesting and packing 196
    management
        immediate responses 199
        principles 199–200
        reassurance 200
        unknown pesticides 200
    in manufacturing 196
    symptoms and signs *200*

pesticide industry
    carcinogenic risk in *815*
    hepatotoxicity in *884*, 892
pesticide poisoning
    classification *196*
    epidemiology 197
    suicide 199
pesticides **195–219**
    Advisory Committee on Pesticides
        197
    arsenical, lung cancer and 700
    biological monitoring 198–9
    in breast milk 833
    chlorate *200, 212*
    contact dermatitis 733
    definitions 195
    dermal biotransformation 77
    dose–exposure relationship 198
    education of operators 196, 199
    European collaboration in evaluation
        198
    exposure to, *see* pesticide exposure
    food contamination? 195
    health surveillance 198–9
    hepatotoxicity *884, 885*, 892, 893–4
    increased toxicity by
        biotransformation 74
    ingestion
        accidental 196
        deliberate 197, 199
        factors influencing 198
    major disasters 197
    manufacturing regulations 197
    neurotoxic effects **873–4**
    non-Hodgkin's lymphoma and 910
    organochlorines, *see* organochlorine
        pesticides
    organophosphates, *see*
        organophosphate pesticides
    personal protective equipment 198
    poisoning, *see* pesticide poisoning
    prevention of health impairment by
        197–9
    regulation 197–8
    reproductive hazards *828*
        to mother 830
    residue monitoring 199
    residues on food 195, 196
    skin contamination 196
    synthetic 195
    see also fungicides; herbicides;
        insecticides; molluscicides;
        National Poisons Information
        Service; rodenticides
pesticide workers, carcinogenic risk
    815
petrochemical plant workers, brain
    tumours 810
petrol 142, 255
    leaded 83, 89
    occupational diseases caused by (EC
        schedule) *43*
    sniffing 83
    unleaded 261, *765*
    see also anti-knock agents; benzine;
        tetraethyl lead
petroleum, as source of aromatic
    compounds 261

petroleum ether 255
petroleum industry, carcinogenic risk in
    815
petroleum oils, folliculitis due to 731
petroleum products,
    glomerulonephritis and 227
petroleum refining
    genotoxic exposures *777*
    skin neoplasms *4*
petroleum solvents **255–6**
    see also white spirits
petroleum spirit, occupational diseases
    caused by (EC schedule) *43*
pet shop workers
    chlamydiosis 492
    Newcastle disease 498
phagocytosis 68
phalanges, *see* fingers
Phalen's test 461
pharmaceutical industries
    bone marrow cancer *816*
    dermatoses 733
    hepatotoxicity in *885*
pharmaceutical laboratories,
    reproductive hazards to mother
    831
pharmacists
    bone marrow cancer *816*
    drug misuse 565
pharmacogenetic polymorphisms, *see*
    metabolic (pharmacogenetic)
    polymorphisms
pharmacogenetics, application to
    occupational cancer 762–3
pharmacokinetic analysis 69
pharmacokinetics, animal and human
    differences 826
phenanthrene 272, 273
Phenergan 373
phenobarbitone
    cirrhosis due to 882
    detoxification 74
    as non-genotoxic carcinogen *765*
phenol (carbolic acid) **271**
    acute/chronic systemic poisoning
        271
    benzene epoxide metabolism 74
    benzene exposure monitoring 262
    characteristics and uses 271
    splashes 271
phenol derivatives **271–2**
    halogenated, occupational diseases
        caused by (EC schedule) *43*
    leucoderma due to 272
    nitrated derivatives, occupational
        diseases caused by (EC schedule)
        44
    see also catechol(s); hydroquinone;
        and other specific derivatives
phenol-formaldehyde resin 696
phenol glucuronide 76
phenols, occupational diseases caused
    by (EC schedule) *43*
phenothiazides, eye damage and 431
phenothiazines, carbon tetrachloride
    and 882
phenotypes 756–7, 762
    mutator phenotypes 753

phenoxyacetic acid herbicides, and
    non-Hodgkin's lymphoma 910
phenoxy acid herbicides, lymphomas
    associated with 811
phenylamine, *see* aniline
m-phenylenediamine 270
p-phenylenediamine 266, 270
    dermatoses 734
phenylethane (ethyl benzene) 266
phenylethylene, *see* styrene
phenylglyoxylic acid 265
phenylhydrazine 267, 268
    in nucleic acid extraction *529*
S-phenylmercapturic acid 262
    biological monitoring tests and
        guidance values *18*
phenylmercuric acetate 212
o-phenylphenol 272
2-phenylpropane (cumene) 266
pheochromocytoma, cancer risk and
    germline mutations *750, 751*
phlebotomists 504–5
phlogopite 680
phorbol esters 742
phosgene **148**, 229
    Hamburg incident 148
    as war gas 131, 171
phosphate fertilizers 150
phosphate rock 98
phosphaturia, in cadmium poisoning
    94
phosphine (hydrogen phosphide) 99,
    163–4, 210
    acute lung injury due to *698*, 698
    characteristics and sources 163
    clinical manifestations 164
    exposure levels 164
    as fermentation product 138
    in ships' cargoes 164
    symptoms of exposure to 164
    uses 163–4
phosphoric acid 98
phosphoric sulphides 98
phosphorus **97–9**
    allotropes 98
    hepatotoxicity *884, 885,* 893
    occupational diseases caused by (EC
        schedule) *43*
    occurrence 98
    poisoning, necrosis of jaw 98
    prescribed diseases due to *49*
    supervision of workers 99
    uses and historical uses 98
    white, in matches 98
    yellow 98, 99
phosphorus compounds
    occupational diseases caused by (EC
        schedule) *43*
    prescribed diseases due to *49,* 99
phosphorus-induced necrosis (phossy
    jaw) 98
phosphorus pentachloride 99
phosphorus pentafluoride 153
phosphorus trichloride 99
phosphorus trifluoride 153
phossy jaw (phosphorus-induced
    necrosis) 98
photic retinopathy 426

photoconjunctivitis 426
photodamage, *see* non-ionizing
    radiation
photodermatitis, welders 184
photoengraving 703
photographic processing, dermatoses
    735
photography, toxic DIY materials *6*
photokeratitis *420,* 426, 434
photophthalmia 426
photoreactive keratectomy 427
photoreceptors, retinal 422, 423
photosensitizers, eye damage and 431
phototransduction 423
phthalate esters, hepatotoxicity *885,*
    895
phthalic anhydride (PA) 639
    prescribed diseases due to *52, 53*
    radioallergosorbent tests (RAST) *21*
physical agents **281–450**
    EC comparable data collection *41*
    occupational diseases caused by (EC
        schedule) *45*
    prescribed diseases due to *46–8*
physical factors, reproductive hazards
    to embryo/fetus 832, *832*
physiotherapists, reproductive hazards
    to embryo/fetus 831–2
physiotherapy
    back pain 482–3, *483*
    hip and knee osteoarthritis *467*
phytomenadione, warfarin ingestion
    and 212
phytophotodermatitis 734
Phytoseiulus persimilis,
    radioallergosorbent tests (RAST)
    21
pickling workers, laryngeal and lung
    cancers *815*
picrotoxin 209
picture archiving and communication
    system (PACS) 594
pigeon breeders/fanciers/racers 655,
    656, 657, 659, 660
pig farming 136, 157
pigmentation changes
    depigmentation 272, 732
    hyperpigmentation 96
    raindrop 96
    silver causing 112
    vitiligo, *see* vitiligo
    welding injuries 184
pigment manufacturing, lead use *844*
pigs
    Brucella suis infection 491
    Nipah virus infection 498
    prescribed disease due to contact *48,*
        49
pig urine, radioallergosorbent tests
    (RAST) *21*
pig workers
    leptospirosis 496
    Streptococcus suis infection 499
piloerection 326
pinewood resin, *see* colophony
pink disease 852
pinocytosis 68
Piper Alpha oil rig disaster 547

case history 546
pitch
  prescribed diseases due to *50*
  skin cancer 733
  skin diseases caused by (EC schedule)
    44
  see also coal tar pitch
pituitary gland cancer, electromagnetic
    field exposure and 443
pituitary tumours, non-genotoxic
    carcinogen mechanisms *765*
Planches, Tanquerel des 83, 923
planning authorities, land development
    near major hazard sites 128–9
plant cell fusion 522
plants
  dermatitis from 734
  indoor 713
  phytophotodermatitis 734
  see also horticulture
plasma, as treatment for liver disease 887
plasmapheresis 202
plasma spray guns, prescribed diseases
    due to use of *47*
Plasmodium falciparum 512, 513
Plasmodium malariae 512, 513
Plasmodium ovale 512, 513
Plasmodium vivax 512, 513
plaster of Paris 681–2
plastics
  polyvinyl chloride (PVC), lead
    compounds in 83
  toxic DIY materials *6*
plastics industry/workers
  asthma incidence *635*
  hepatotoxicity in *884*, *885*
  reproductive hazards to mother 831
platelet transfusion, radiation
    casualties 401, 414
plate workers
  shoulder tendinitis *455*
  thoracic outlet syndrome 457
platinum **110–11**
  uses 110
platinum salts
  metal-induced asthma due to 699
  occupational asthma due to 110,
    634, *636*, 640, *647*
  prescribed diseases due to *52*, *53*
platinum workers, occupational asthma
    in 642
pleura
  bilateral diffuse thickening, in
    asbestos exposure 691
    as prescribed disease *54*, 691
  calcification 667
    ILO classification *604*, 604
  mesothelioma, *see* mesothelioma
  plaques 687, 690
    in asbestos exposure 600
  thickening 600–1, 667, 668
    ILO classification *604*, 604
    as prescribed disease *54*, 691
  ultrasound and 598
pleural disease
  imaging 600–1
  non-malignant, cases reported to
    SWORD *31*

pleural effusion
  in asbestos exposure 601
  benign, in asbestos exposure 690–1
  in mesothelioma 601
pleural mesothelioma
  asbestos and *4*
  in women 27
pleural tumours,
    industries/occupations
    associated with *815*, *816*
pleurocentesis 352
plicatic acid, occupational asthma due
    to *634*, *636*, 638
plumbers 4
  hantavirus infection 494
plutonium
  ionizing radiation properties *398*
  radiation contamination treatment
    413
PMRs (proportional mortality ratios)
    32–3
pneumatic tools
  hand–arm vibration syndrome 308,
    310
  prescribed diseases due to use of *46*
pneumoconiosis
  antimony workers 100
  asbestosis, *see* asbestosis
  cases reported to SWORD *31*
  coalworker's, *see* coalworker's
    pneumoconiosis
  'complicated' 666, 684–6
  definition 665
  diatomite (kieselgahr) 681
  dust silicates causing, EC schedule of
    occupational diseases *44*
  fibrous clays 696
  gypsum 682
  hard-metal pneumoconiosis (hard
    metal disease) 703–4
  investigation and diagnosis 665–72
  kaolin 679–80
  metal-induced 700–4
  mica 681
  mortality in coal mining areas 40
  nodular, in talc mining 680
  non-fibrous clays 681
  occupational history 665–6
  as prescribed disease *52*
  rheumatoid 685–6
  silicate dust pneumoconiosis 672
  silicosis, *see* silicosis
  silver polishers' lung 112
  slateworker's, *see* slateworker's
    pneumoconiosis
  smoking and 8
  stannosis 114
  symptoms and signs 666
  talc 680
  time lapse in developing 5
  see also inorganic dust diseases;
    interstitial fibrosis; pulmonary
    fibrosis
Pneumoconiosis Field Research scheme
    683
Pneumocystis carinii 507
pneumonia
  extrinsic allergic alveolitis *vs* 659

hypersensitivity pneumonia, in
    welding 186
  legionnaires' disease 709, 710, 711
  in manganese workers 108
  metal fume exposure 28
  Q fever 498
pneumonitis
  acute toxic, metal fume fever *vs* 698
  cadmium causing 698
  chemical 132, 698
    acute beryllium poisoning 101,
      101–2
    mercury poisoning 91, 93
  hypersensitivity pneumonitis
    hard metal lung disease *vs* 703
    summer type allergic alveolitis
      711
  in welding 186
  paraquat poisoning and *201*
  radiation levels causing *400*
  radiation pneumonitis 401
  space crew 376
  toxic, in welding 186
  ventilation, *see* ventilation
    pneumonitis
Pneumonocystis carinii 659
pneumonoencephalitis 498
pneumothorax 352
  case history 354
poison gas manufacture, lung cancer
    815
poisons, *see* National Poisons
    Information Service
'poker back' 151
police, post-traumatic stress disorder
    546, 547
Police and Criminal Evidence Act 1984
    60
polishers, silicosis prevention 676
polishing, *see also* diamond polishing;
    jade polishing
pollution, *see* air pollution;
    environment; soil pollution;
    water pollution
polonium 115
polonium-210 406
polyacrylamide gel 529
polyamines, occupational asthma due
    to *636*
polybrominated biphenyls (PBBs) 275
polycarbonate laser protective lenses
    434
polychlorinated biphenyls (PCBs)
    273–4
  in breast milk 833
  genotoxicity *777*
  hepatotoxicity *884*, *885*, 894
  as non-genotoxic carcinogens *765*
  prenatal exposure effects 825
  reproductive hazards *828*
  Yusho and Taiwan incidents 274
polychlorinated quarterphenyls (PCQs)
    273, 274
polychloroprene, hepatotoxicity *884*
polychromasia 905
polycyclic aromatic hydrocarbons 272,
    273
  carcinogenicity 152, 273, 741

polycyclic aromatic hydrocarbons – *contd*
  lung toxicity 77
  see also polynuclear aromatic
      hydrocarbons
polycythaemia, cobalt causing 106
polyethylene 171
polymerase chain reaction 767
polymer fume fever (polymer
      inhalation fever) 185, 187
  symptoms 187
polymerization 170
polymorphisms 757
  see also metabolic (pharmacogenetic)
      polymorphisms
polyneuropathy, methyl ethyl ketone
      (MEK) causing 248
polynuclear aromatic hydrocarbons
  cancer 792
      bladder cancer 811, *815*
      lung cancer *815*
      scrotal cancer *815*
      skin cancer 810
  EC comparable data collection *41*
  see also polycyclic aromatic
      hydrocarbons
polyolefin plastics 171
polyploidy 744
polypropylene 171
polytetrafluoroethylene (PTFE) 187
polyurethane 639
polyurethane foam, extrinsic allergic
      alveolitis due to *654*
polyvinyl chloride (PVC) 170–1, 803
  as benzene source 262
  combustion in fires 129
  lead compounds in 83
  production, hepatotoxicity in *885*
Pontiac fever 185, 711
porphobilinogen (PBG) 85
porphyria
  hepatotoxicity treatment 887
  lead-induced 85
porphyria cutanea tarda (PCT) 267, 886,
      889
  urinary/faecal content 886
porphyrias
  acquired hepatic, causes 267
  classification 267
  hexachlorobenzene causing 267
porphyrin metabolism, hepatic,
      disturbances 886
porphyrinogens 85
porphyrins 85, 267
portal fibrosis, non-cirrhotic, as
      prescribed disease *51*
portal hypertension
  idiopathic 885
  non-cirrhotic 885
  non-invasive screening *882*
  vinyl chloride exposure 170
portal vein occlusion, non-invasive
      screening *882*
portering staff
  hepatitis B infection 505
  see also health care workers
postnatal development 825
postnatal exposures, workplace agents
      832–3

post-traumatic stress disorder **544–50**,
      571
  advice to victims and families 549
  bullying causing 542
  case histories 545–6, 548
  counsellors 548–9
  description 544–5
  diagnostic labels 544
  effects of trauma 550
  gassing accidents causing 132
  information leaflet 549, 550
  neuroendocrine basis of 548
  predisposing factors 547–8
  presentation 572
  prognosis, long-term 546
  psychological debriefing 549
  reactions to traumatic event 550
  rehabilitation programme 549
  treatment 548–9
potassium, thallium poisoning and 113
potassium-40 406
potassium chlorate poisoning 202
potassium cyanide 145
potassium ferrihexacyanoferrate
      (Prussian blue) 113
potassium iodate 412
potassium permanganate 108, 211
potency, loss of 829
Pott, Percival 741, 792, 918
pot room asthma 152, 699–700
pot room workers, bladder cancer 811
pottery industry
  kaolin pneumoconiosis 679
  lead use *844*
  lung carcinoma as prescribed disease
      54
  silicosis prevention 676
  stillbirth after lead poisoning 82
poultry workers
  Campylobacter infections 493
  chlamydiosis 492
  erysipeloid 501
  Newcastle disease 498
  zoonoses 489
povidone 329
power stations
  as source of nitrogen dioxide 159
  see also nuclear power
      plants/reactors
power tools, prescribed diseases due to
      46
Poza Rica, Mexico, hydrogen sulphide
      incident 161
P-postlabelling 767, 773
pralidoxime 207
  in organophosphate poisoning 873
  side-effects 207
precipitins, serum, in extrinsic allergic
      alveolitis 656, 659
predicted 4-hour sweat rate (P4SR) 334
Predicted Mean Vote (PMV) thermal
      stress index 334
Predicted Percentage of Dissatisfied
      (PPD), thermal stress index 334
prednisolone 167, 659
prednisolone acetate 431
prednisone, as tissue culture additive
      528

pre-employment screening
  back pain prevention 481
  dermatitis prevention 730
  tuberculosis 510–11
  see also monitoring of workers
pre-excitation syndrome, high altitudes
      390
pregnancy
  biotechnology workers 531
  carbon monoxide and 144, 144–5
  chlamydiosis 490
  counselling after exposures 837
  cytomegalovirus 510
  exposure to sheep 493
  ionizing radiation and 408, *409*, 410
  listeriosis 496
  magnetic resonance imaging and
      446
  methylene chloride and 145
  outcomes 826–7
      electromagnetic field exposure
          and 445
  ovine chlamydiosis and 493
  rubella 510
  success, likelihood of 826–7
  surveillance systems 835
      records 834
  toxic hazards
      to embryo/fetus 830–2
      to mother 830
  toxoplasmosis 490, 500
  see also reproductive function;
      reproductive hazards
pre-oxygenation 364, 376
Prescott v Bulldog Tools (1981) 59
prescribed diseases *46–55*
  biological agents causing *48–9*
  chemical agents causing *49–52*
  claims for, *see* compensation;
      damages
  criteria for 38
  IIAC role 38, 39–40
  individual proof 38, 40, 41
  miscellaneous conditions *52–5*
  physical agents causing *46–8*
  see also diseases, occupational; *and
      individual diseases/disorders*
pressure
  barometric, *see* barometric pressure
  as stimulus 570
pressure breathing 363–4
pressure changes, *see* barometric
      pressure
*Prevention of Damage to Hearing from
      Noise at Work* 297
prickly heat 336
prick tests, *see* skin prick tests
primaquine 513
primates, laboratory work involving
      512
Primula obconica, contact dermatitis
      734
printing industry/workers
  dermatoses 735
  extrinsic allergic alveolitis 711
  humidifier fever 712
  leukaemia risk 909
prion diseases 500

procarbazine hydrochloride,
     genotoxicity 777
prodromal syndrome, radiation levels
     causing 400
producer gas 142
professions, at higher risk of alcohol-
     related problems 559
progenitor cells 901
progestagens, as non-genotoxic
     carcinogens 765
progesterone, and altitude sickness
     386
progression, carcinogenesis 741, 742
progressive massive fibrosis (PMF)
   coalworkers 684–5
   in kaolin pneumoconiosis 679
   occupational history example 12
proguanil 379
   malaria 513
prolonged duress stress disorder 545
promazine, carbon tetrachloride and
     882
promethazine 373
   carbon tetrachloride and 882
propacetamol 734
propane 170, 225
propane-1,2-diol (1,2-propylene glycol)
     224, 243
propane-fuelled equipment 142
propanol 242
2-propanol, see isopropyl alcohol
n-propanol 239, 242
propionic acid
   in prevention of bagasse moulding
     655
   in prevention of grain moulding 654
proportional mortality ratio (PMR)
     32–3, 800
proportional mortality studies 800
propoxur 208
propranolol, altitude sickness 390
PROPULSE recording project for
     occupational respiratory disease
     (Quebec) 31
propylene 170, 232
1,2-propylene glycol (propane-1,2-diol)
     224, 243
propyne 239
prosecution 57
prostacycline 891
   as treatment for liver disease 887
prostaglandin H-synthase 77
prostatic cancer
   acrylonitrile and 253
   in cadmium workers 94
   electromagnetic field exposure and
     443
   risk of, and germline mutations 750
protective equipment, personal 8, 221,
     338–9
   amphiboles and 695
   anti-G suits 366
   blood-borne viruses 508
   cold environments 339
   cold immersion 332
   contact dermatitis 730
   1,2-dibromethane penetration of
     clothing 232

eyes, see eye protectors
firefighters 130, 337–8
   in handling primates 512
hearing loss prevention 297–8, 298,
     299
hot environments 338–9
masks 8
medical staff handling radiation
     casualties 413
military aircraft crew 367
   disadvantages 367
occupational asthma 646
pesticides 198
spacesuits 376
thermal stress prevention 337, 338
zoonoses 490
see also gloves; rubber gloves
protein contact dermatitis 731
proteins, occupational asthma due to
     634
proteinuria 857
   cadmium causing 94, 849
   chromium causing 853
   mercury causing 852
   petroleum-based paints 857
   solvents causing 856
proteolytic enzymes
   occupational asthma due to 637,
     647
   prescribed diseases due to 52, 53
protons 397
proto-oncogenes
   activation 749, 751, 752
   cellular 748–9, 749
   occurrence in cancer 749
protoplast fusion 523
protoporphyrin 85
provokers, of occupational asthma
     633–4, 634
pruritus 734
Prussian blue (potassium
     ferrihexacyanoferrate) 113
Pruteen 524
'pseudo-clubbing' 170
pseudofractures 850
Pseudomonas spp., in office buildings
     717
Pseudomonas aeruginosa, ill-health
     due to, in biotechnology 527
Pseudomonas pyocynea 350
pseudosulphaemoglobin 269
psittacosis 492
   imaging 603
psoralen plus UV-A therapy (PUV-A) 431
psoralens 734
   eye damage and 431
psoriasis 725
psychiatric disorders
   bullying at work causing 541, 543
   clinical assessment 573
   'not coping' situation, assessment of
     573–6
   presentation 572–3
   referrals 572
     self-referral 572
     by a third party 572
   see also mental health; mental
     illness; stress

psychiatric symptoms
   carbon disulphide exposure 254
   lead poisoning 86
   white spirit exposure 256
psychological debriefing 549
psychoneurotic troubles, shift work
     582–3
psychoorganic syndrome 264, 266
psychosocial factors, in back pain
     480–1, 481, 483
psychotherapy, United Kingdom
     Council for Psychotherapy
     (UKCP) 579
psychrometric charts, heat stress
     assessment 333–4
PTFE (polytetrafluoroethylene) 187
Public Health (Aircraft) Regulations
     1979 379
pulmonary anthrax 491
pulmonary barotrauma 352
   clinical manifestations 352
   pathogenesis 350–1
   prognosis 356
   see also decompression illnesses;
     decompression sickness
pulmonary biotransformation 76–7
pulmonary disease
   effects of exposure to welding fume
     182
   imaging 601–2
pulmonary fibrosis
   in aluminium workers 99
   asbestos causing, see asbestosis
   beryllium causing 853
   cobalt inhalation 106
   in extrinsic allergic alveolitis 656,
     657, 658, 659, 660
   ventilation pneumonitis causing 655
   see also interstitial fibrosis;
     pneumoconiosis
pulmonary function, see lung function
pulmonary haemorrhage–haemolytic
     anaemia syndrome 640
pulmonary infiltrations,
     paraquat/diquat exposure and
     200
pulmonary oedema
   causative agents
     ammonia 157
     cadmium 94
     chlorine 147, 148
     diborane 166
     1,2-dibromethane (ethylene
       dibromide) 232
     hydrogen chloride 149
     hydrogen cyanide 146
     hydrogen fluoride 151
     hydrogen selenide 162
     hydrogen sulphide 161
     irritant gases 131
     mercury 91
     methyl bromide 164
     methyl isocyanate 165
     methyl mercaptan 162
     1-naphthylthiourea (ANTU) 77
     nickel carbonyl 166
     nitric oxide 158
     nitrogen dioxide 159

pulmonary oedema – *contd*
  causative agents – *contd*
    ozone 158
    phosgene 148
    phosphine (hydrogen phosphide)
      164
    selenium dioxide 111
    sulphur dioxide 155
    tellurium hexafluoride 112
  haemorrhagic 698
  high-altitude (HAPO) 383, 384–6,
    387
    treatment 392, *394*
  investigation into gassing accidents
    134
  non-cardiogenic 131, 149, 161, 698
  silicosis 673
  in welders 186
pulmonary oxygen toxicity, at high
    partial pressures 345
pulmonary pseudotumour 602
pulmonary thrombosis, high altitudes
    391
pulmonary tuberculosis, EC schedule of
    occupational diseases *44*
pulp mill workers, sulphur compounds
    exposure 156, 161
pulsed electromagnetic fields (PEMF)
    443
pulse oximetry, in carbon monoxide
    poisoning 131
pumping stations, methane accident
    138
puna, *see* altitude sickness
pure tone audiometry 298
purines 743
purpura, phosphine causing 164
putamen, methanol effect 241
putrescine 68
PVC, *see* polyvinyl chloride
pyramin, hepatotoxicity *884*
pyrethroids 211–12
  chronic poisoning 211
  exposure, accidental and
    occupational 211
  ingestion 211–12
  management of poisoning 212
  neurotoxic effects 874
  toxicity mechanisms 211
pyrethrum 211–12
N-3-pyridomethyl-*N*-*p*-nitrophenylurea
    (PNU) 876
pyridostigmine 374
pyrimethamine 500
pyrimidines 743
pyrocatechol 272
pyrolysis 129
pyruvate diphosphoglycerate 96

Q fever 498–9
  endocarditis 498
  imaging 603
  meningoencephalitis 498
  as prescribed disease *49*
  treatment 498
  vaccine 498–9
Qigong manoeuvre 366

quantum, *see* damages
quarantine 490
Quarivexin, accidental self-injection
    with *213*
quarrying, prescribed diseases
    associated with *46*, *48*
quarry workers, silicosis mortality *29*
quartz 672
  coalworkers' progressive massive
    fibrosis 685
  kaolin contaminated by 679, 680
  metal oxides with 673
  pulmonary tuberculosis and 677
  in slate 678
quartz dust 672–7
  limits/recommendations 677
  mixed dust containing 677–82
  silicosis and 672–3
  toxicity mechanism 672–3
  see also silicosis
quicksilver mines 89
quinine 330
quinolone compounds, Q fever
    meningoencephalitis 498
quinone, corneal dystrophy as
    prescribed disease due to *50*
quinone oxido-reductase, metabolic
    polymorphisms with cancer
    susceptibility links *759*
quinoxaline, in contact dermatitis
    733
Quorn 524

rabies 499
  control measures 499
  vaccine 490, 499, 525
radar workers 431
radiation
  cosmic 399, 406
    aircrew exposure 374, 407
  ionizing, *see* electromagnetic
    radiation; ionizing radiation
  non-ionizing, *see* non-ionizing
    radiation
  radiofrequency radiation, brain
    cancer and 441
  spaceflight 376
  thermal, flying and 367
  uranium hazards 115
  from welding 179
radiation accidents
  casualty treatment 411
  contaminated casualties 411–13
    external exposure 411, *412*
    internal exposure 411–13, *413*
  designated treatment areas 413
  nuclear reactor accidents, casualty
    handling plan 413–15
  protective measures 415
    medical staff 413
  see also nuclear power
    plants/reactors
radiation burns 401, 411, 415
Radiation Emergency Medical
    Preparedness Assistance
    Network (REMPAN) (WHO) 414
radiation pneumonitis 401

radiation syndrome
  acute *401*, 401
  chronic 403
radiation thyroiditis 401
radiation weighting factor 398–9
radiculoneuritis, in Lyme disease 497
radioactive decay 398
radioactivity 398
radioallergosorbent tests (RAST) *21*,
    21–2
  contact dermatitis 729
  contact urticaria 729, 731
radiofrequency radiation, brain cancer
    and 441
radiographers 407
  bone marrow cancer *816*
  eye and respiratory inflammation
    156
  glutaraldehyde causing asthma 246
  sick building syndrome 714, 715
radiographic film 593
radiographic opacities, *see* lung(s):
    radiographic opacities
radiographic silicosis 675
radiography
  chemicals 714, 715
  chest 593–4
  industrial 407
  in lead poisoning 87
  see also chest radiography; imaging;
    x-rays
radiologists 397
  bone marrow cancer *816*
radionuclide, definition 398
radionuclide imaging, thallium used in
    113
radionuclide studies, in occupational
    lung disease 599
radium, in uranium ores 115
radon 406, 407
  cancers due to *814*
  in earth's atmosphere *135*
  genotoxic exposures *776*
  lung cancer 700, 792
    in tin miners 115
  respiratory tract malignancies and *4*
  underground exposure 792
  in uranium ores 115
radon decay products, lung and bone
    marrow cancers *815*
railway workers, *see* train drivers
raindrop pigmentation 96
Ramazzini, Bernardino 3, 792, 917–18
rapid decompression 364–5
Rapid Upper Limb Assessment (RULA)
    technique 468
rare earths, granulomatous lung
    disease due to 702–3
rarefied air, prescribed diseases due to
    46
rashes
  decompression illness 351
  in scabies 511
  visual display unit operators 713,
    714
rats
  occupational asthma due to *636*
  poisons, *see* rodenticides

prescribed diseases due to working at infested places *48*
rat urine protein 636, 641, 644, 647
'ray burn', in welding 184
Raynaud's disease 314
Raynaud's phenomenon 170, 312, 314, 316
  cold-induced *309*, 309
RB1 gene 752, 753
  function and involvement *751*
reactive airways dysfunction syndrome (RADS) 134, 147, 152, 155, 612
  see also irritant-induced asthma
reactive dyes, radioallergosorbent tests (RAST) *21*
reactive dye screen, radioallergosorbent tests (RAST) *21*
Read test 346
recall bias 799, 834
recombinant DNA technology 524–5
recombinant pharmaceutical products 524–5
recompression 353
  osteonecrosis and 358
  rash and 351
  tables and algorithms 354
recompression chamber 355
records
  on reproductive function/hazards 834
  see also medical records
recreational inhalation 870
recruitment, in hearing loss 299
red cells
  basophilic stippling 904, 906
  damage to 905
  Heinz bodies 904, 905
  in lead poisoning 87
  metabolism 902–3
redeployment 471
red spider mites (*Tetranychus urticae*), radioallergosorbent tests (RAST) *21*
Reduced Earnings Allowance 39
reduction, of xenobiotics 75
reference pressures, audiometric 284
referral, psychiatric disorders 572
referred pain, back pain *479*
refineries, nickel, *see* nickel
refining, lead use *844*
refractory ceramic fibres 697
refractory making, silicosis prevention 676
refrigerants 154, 157, 169, 170
refrigeration, hepatotoxicity in *885*
registers, of occupational diseases/injuries 30–1
rehabilitation 471
  employees returning to work after mental illness 578
rehydration 336
rehydration solutions, in traveller's diarrhoea 513
renal calculi
  in beryllium disease 103
  space flight and 376
renal cell cancer, risk of, and germline mutations *751*

renal damage
  cadmium poisoning 94
  carbon tetrachloride 229
  chromium 105
  1,2-dichloroethane (ethylene dichloride) 230
  lead poisoning 86, 87
  mercury poisoning 91, 92
  as prescribed disease *51*
  tetrachloroethylene (perchloroethylene) exposure 236
  thallium poisoning 113
  uranium 116
  see also kidneys
renal dialysis, copper poisoning 107
renal disease
  lead exposure and, mortality *846*
  mercury-induced 852
renal effects
  biological monitoring tests *18*
  detection of 21
renal failure
  arsine poisoning 162, 163
  glomerulonephritis after hydrocarbon exposure 226–7
  paraquat/diquat exposure and *200*
  paraquat poisoning and *201*
  role of lead in 844, 847
  tetrachloroethylene (perchloroethylene) exposure 236
  treatment 887
renal function
  assessment, in cadmium workers 95
  impairment, halogenated alkanes 226
renal hypertension 844, 847
renal interstitial fibrosis 844, 845, 848
renal replacement therapy (RRT) 843
renal tubular damage, paraquat poisoning and *201*
renal tubular dysfunction
  in cadmium nephrotoxicity 849–50
  lead poisoning 86
renal tubular necrosis
  acute
    arsenic causing 853
    bismuth causing 853
    chromium causing 853
    copper sulphate causing 853
    mercuric chloride causing 852
  in mercury poisoning 92
renal tubular proteinuria, in cadmium poisoning 94
repetitive movement disorders, prescribed diseases due to *46*
repetitive strain injury (RSI) 461–2
  clinical aspects 463
  compensation 462, *462*
  incidence *462*
  management 463
  proposed clinical grading scheme, New South Wales 463
  work-related 462
  see also upper limb disorders
reporting, *see* registers

Reporting of Injuries, Diseases and Dangerous Occurrences Regulations (RIDDOR) 31
  benzene poisoning 263
reproduction, normal **823–5**
  animals *vs* humans **825–6**, 836
  gametogenesis 824–5
  uncertainties and vulnerable stages **826–7**
reproductive cycle 823, 824
reproductive function
  epidemiological investigation 833–4, 834
    end point reliability 834–5
  investigation of complaints of effects on 833–4
  monitoring 834–5
    data collection difficulties 834–5
  records 834
  women and shift work 584
reproductive hazards **821–40**
  agents *828*
  anaesthetic gases 167, *828*, 829, 831
  carbon disulphide exposure 254, *828*, 829
  cytomegalovirus 510
  1,2-dibromoethane (ethylene dibromide) 232, *828*
  drugs *828*, 831
  electromagnetic fields 444–5
  endocrine control process susceptibility 825
  ethylene oxide 166
  experimental data extrapolation 836
  female fertility *828*, 830, *832*
  germ cell mutations 828–9
  immediate or late effects 824, 827
  ionizing radiation *829*, 829, 831–2
    hazards to embryo/fetus 402
  male sexual behaviour and fertility *828*, 829, *832*
  mercury *828*, 830–1
  nitrous oxide 168, 169
  physical factors 832, *832*
  possible harmful effects 827
  postnatal exposures 832–3
  in pregnancy 830–2
  prenatal exposure effects 825, 830–2
  prevention responsibilities and ethics 836–7
  records 834
  rubella 510
  semiconductor industry 172
  solvents *828*, 831
  toxicity of chemical agents
    to embryo/fetus 830–2
    to mother 830
  toxoplasmosis 500
  visual display units and 832
  whole-body vibration 318
  xylene 264
  see also abortion; congenital malformations; infertility; pregnancy
reproductive system, effects of exposure to welding fume 184
research workers, *see* laboratory workers

resins
    formaldehyde use in 244
    see also colophony; epoxy resins
respiration, *see* inhalation
respiratory alkalosis 391
respiratory damage, paraquat
        poisoning and *201*
respiratory depression,
        tetrachloroethylene
        (perchloroethylene) 235
respiratory diseases
    altitude sickness risk 389
    biological monitoring tests *18*
    cold related 332
    EC schedule *44*
    effects of exposure to welding fume
        182–4
    in gold miners given aluminium 99
    registers 31, *31*
respiratory distress syndrome 698
respiratory dysfunction, biological
        monitoring tests *18*
respiratory effects
    biological monitoring tests *18*, 21–2
    decompression sickness 364
    radioallergosorbent tests (RAST) *21*,
        21–2
respiratory failure
    chlorine causing 147
    hydrogen cyanide causing 146
    paraquat poisoning and *201*
    pesticide exposure and *200*
respiratory illnesses, extrinsic allergic
        alveolitis *vs* 659
respiratory paralysis
    carbonyl sulphide causing 162
    methyl mercaptan causing 162
respiratory symptoms
    biotechnology hazard *527*
    high-altitude 'Red Alert' symptoms
        394
respiratory system, effects of exposure
        to welding fume 182–4
respiratory tract
    defences against dusts 663–4
    effect of gases on
        ammonia 157
        chlorine 147
        in fires 130
        hydrogen fluoride 151
        hydrogen sulphide 160–1
        irritant gases 125, 131
        methyl isocyanate release, Bhopal
            123, 165
        nitrogen dioxide 159
        ozone 158
        sulphur dioxide 155, 156
        sulphur trioxide 156
    irritation
        1,3-butadiene 238
        byssinosis *626*, 626–7
        cumene causing 266
        1,2-dibromoethane (ethylene
            dibromide) 232
        1,2-dichloroethane (ethylene
            dichloride) 230
        formaldehyde 244
        glutaraldehyde 246

vinylidene chloride (1,1-
        dichloroethylene) 237
    xylene causing 264
malignancies 806–8
    in firefighters 131
    occupations/agents causing *4*
    see also lung cancer
mucociliary lining 664
see also airway; lung(s); *and entries
        beginning with* pulmonary
responsibilities, employers' 7–8
restaurant trade
    nitrous oxide abuse 168–9
    see also catering and hotel industry;
        food industry
rest breaks 471
resuscitation, cardiopulmonary, gassing
        accidents 131
reticulocytosis, arsine causing 163
retina
    anatomy 421, 422
    blue light damage 424
    chromophores 424, 424–5
    damage from optical radiation *420*
    hazard region wavelengths 428
    layers 422
    methanol-induced changes 241
    neural 422
    photic retinopathy 426
    photochemical damage,
        classification 424
    photoreceptors 422, 423
    phototransduction 423
    retinal pigment epithelium *420*,
        422–3, 424
    solar retinopathy 426
retinal scatter photocoagulation 427
retinoblastoma 746, 752, 757
    cancer risk and germline mutations
        751
    familial, susceptibility and germline
        mutation 751
retinol-binding protein (RBP) *19*, 21,
        23, 94, 95, 849
retinopathy
    photic 426
    solar 426
retirement
    early, mental health problems 571
    premature, after bullying 542,
        543
'reversed ear' 347
rhabdomyolysis 336
rheumatoid arthritis, as cause of back
        pain *479*
rheumatoid pneumoconiosis 685–6
rhinitis 698
    allergic **713**
        as prescribed disease *52–3*
    chromium causing 105
    platinum causing 110
    sick building syndrome and 713
    wood dusts 638
rhodopsin 422, 423
Rhodotorula 713
ribavirin 495
riboflavine deficiency, thallium
        poisoning resembling 113

rice oil contamination, Yusho and
        Taiwan incidents 274, *884*, 894
rice oil disease 274
rickets, vitamin D resistant 844
rickettsial infections, Q fever 498
RIDDOR (Reporting of Injuries, Diseases
        and Dangerous Occurrences
        Regulations) 31
rifampicin
    brucellosis 492
    for legionnaires' disease 711
    Q fever 498
    as tissue culture additive *528*
Rift valley fever 509
rigidity, in manganese poisoning 108
Ringer–Locke solution, administration
        in mercury poisoning 93
ringworm 502
    in cattle 733
riot control gases 171–2
risk, definition 9, 82
risks, comparative *415*
RNA, lead and 85
road construction, prescribed diseases
        associated with *48*
road traffic accidents 512
rocket industry, hepatotoxicity in *885*
rock wool 696, 805
    carcinogenicity 805
rock work, in coal mines 682–3
rodent control, hepatotoxicity in *885*
rodenticides 212
    phosphine (hydrogen phosphide)
        163
    thallium-containing 113
rodents
    hantavirus infection and 494
    non-genotoxic carcinogens *765*
    reproductive processes 826, 836
rodent studies, non-genotoxic
        carcinogens *765*
rodent trappers, zoonoses 489
rods, of eye 422
'rose eye' 111
rosin fumes
    occupational asthma due to *647*
    prescribed diseases due to *52*, *53*
rotary tools, prescribed disease due to
        use of *48*
rotator cuff tendinitis *454*, 455
    definition 455
    treatment 456
rotogravure industry, hepatotoxicity in
        885
Rotorua, New Zealand, hydrogen
        sulphide pollution 161
round atelectasis 602
Royal Air Force, post-traumatic stress
        disorder rehabilitation
        programme 549
RSI, *see* repetitive strain injury
rubber 237
    ABS rubber/plastics 237, 253, 264
    synthetic 237
    vulcanization, carbon disulphide
        exposure 254
    see also latex
rubber chemicals, dermatitis 734, 735

rubber gloves 638
  contact urticaria 731
  see also gloves
rubber industry/workers
  benzene use 261, 909
  bladder cancer *4*, 27–8
  blood dyscrasias/malignancies *4*
  1,3-butadiene exposure 237
  cancers *814*
  carcinogenic risk *815*
  genotoxic exposures *776*
  leukaemia risk 909
  lymphatic and haemopoietic system
    cancers *815*
  menstrual disturbances 830
  reproductive hazards 830, 831
  see also 4-aminobiphenyl; auramine;
    magenta; 2-naphthylamine;
    styrene
rubella 510
'rum fits' 558
ruminant feed ban 500, 501
Russian hogweed, contact dermatitis
    734
Rutaceae, contact dermatitis 734
R v Turner (1975) 59
rye dust
  occupational asthma due to *647*
  prescribed diseases due to *52, 53*
rye flour, radioallergosorbent tests
    (RAST) *21*

Saccharomyces cerevisiae 522, 523, 524
safety lamp, miners' 137
Sahara dusts 673
salbutamol 627
  chlorine poisoning *133*
Salem sarcoid 101
salicylic acid, metabolization 76
salivation, excessive in mercury
    poisoning 89, 92
salmon, radioallergosorbent tests
    (RAST) *21*
Salmonella 493, 496, 513
Salmonella test, *see* Ames test
salmonellosis 512
salt
  depletion, in heat strain 336
  retention, heat acclimatization 335
  thallium in table salt 113
sand-hogs 343
sandstone tunnelling/quarrying,
    prescribed diseases due to *54*
sarcoidosis
  beryllium disease *vs* 103, 666, 702
  CD4:CD8 T lymphocytes ratio 656
  extrinsic allergic alveolitis *vs* 656
  imaging 600
sarcomas
  beryllium association 103
  cancer risk and germline mutations
    751
  chlorophenoxyacetate herbicides and
    203
Sarcoptes scabiei 511
sarin 171
saturation diving 344, 346

ear and skin infections 349–50
  latency 353
  musculoskeletal pain 351
  osteonecrosis and 358
  treatment of decompression illness
    355
saturnine gout 86
sausage makers
  elbow problems 458
  hand/wrist tendinitis 459
saws, prescribed diseases due to use of
    47, 48
SBR (standardized birth ratio) 835
scabies 511
  mimicking contact dermatitis 725
  treatment 210
Scandinavia, disease data and national
    identity numbers 33
Scheele's green (cupric arsenite) 96
schistosomiasis, antimony in 100
schizophrenia, management at work
    577–8
Schlumbergera cacti, contact urticaria
    734
Schwannoma, cancer risk and germline
    mutations *750*
sciatica 477, 482
scissor makers, tension neck syndrome
    457
sclera 421, 423
scleroderma **170**
  occupational 314, 316
scleroderma-like diseases 732, 734
sclerotherapy, as varices treatment
    887
L-scopolamine hydrobromide 373
Scopulariopsis brevicaulis 96
scrapie 500
scrap industry, lead use *844*
screening
  cancers 817–18
  pre-employment, *see* pre-
    employment screening
  see also monitoring of workers
scrotal cancer 741, 792
  case histories 795
  chimney sweeps' climbing boys 918
  industries/occupations associated
    with *815*
  mineral-oil-induced 795
  occupations/agents causing *4*
scrubbers, *see* carbon dioxide scrubbers
'scuba' divers 343
  arbitrary stops 350
scurvy 918
seafarers, guidance documents for 13
seamen
  alcohol-related problems 559
  hepatitis B 503
  skin and lip cancers *815*
seawater, freezing point 330
  see also immersion hypothermia
selenium **111–12**
  absorption 111
  carcinogenicity 111
  chronic poisoning 111
  excretion 111
  function in body 111

hepatotoxicity *884, 885,* 893
  supervision of workers 112
  uses 111
selenium compounds 111
selenium diethyldithiocarbamate 111
selenium dioxide 111
  dusts 111
selenium hexafluoride 111
self-injection of veterinary products,
    accidental, *see* veterinary
    products
self-referral, psychiatric disorders 572
Sellafield nuclear reprocessing plant
    405
semen, characteristics and assessment
    835
semiconductor industry 172
  arsine in 162, 172
  diborane in 166
  dichlorosilane in 149
  hydrogen selenide in 162
  phosphine (hydrogen phosphide) in
    163
  silane in 162
  toxic gases and hazards in 172
semustine, genotoxicity *776*
senescence 748
'sensitization of the myocardium' 229
sensitizers
  asthma as prescribed disease due to
    53–4
  beryllium 102
  chromium compounds 104
  ethylene oxide 166
  methyl methacrylate 250
  nickel 109–10
  platinum 110
  respiratory, in disinfectants 136
  see also allergens
sensorimotor neuropathy, acrylamide
    exposure 868
sensorineural hearing loss 292
  loss of discrimination 299
  as prescribed disease *46–8*
SENSOR (Sentinel Event Notification
    Scheme for Occupational Risks),
    USA 31
sensory disturbances, hand–arm
    vibration syndrome (HAVS) 308
sensory function tests 867
sensory polyneuropathy, *see* peripheral
    neuropathy
Sentinel Event Notification Scheme for
    Occupational Risks (SENSOR),
    USA 31
sepiolite 696
sepsis, in radiation casualties 414
septicaemia 496
serotonin antagonists, back pain 483
serotonin reuptake inhibitors 549
serum glutamic-oxaloacetic
    transaminase (SGOT) 226, 235,
    237
serum glutamic-pyruvic transaminase
    (SGPT) 226, 235, 237
serum samples storage 533
settlements
  out-of-court 62

settlements – *contd*
    structured 60
    see also damages
Seveso, EU directive 126
Seveso incident 274–5, 876, 886, 890
sewage workers 514–15
    leptospirosis 496
sewer workers 135, 136, 137
    Aberdeen incident 137
sewing workers
    elbow problems 458
    hand/wrist tendinitis 459
    shoulder tendinitis *455*
sex, effect on biological monitoring 20
sexual behaviour, male, and agents
        affecting 829
sexual harassment 540
sex workers 514
SFR (standardized fertility ratio) 835
shale oils
    cancers *814*
    genotoxicity *776*
shallow-water blackout 348
shampoos
    dermatitis from 734
    head-lice 209
sharps injuries 504, 504–5, 508, 509
Shaver's disease 701
sheep
    enzootic abortion of ewes (EAE) 493
    hydatid disease and 495
    orf 501–2
    ovine enzootic abortion (OEA) 493
    prescribed diseases due to contact
        with *49*
    Q fever 498
sheep dippers/dipping
    arsenic exposure and 96, 97
    cognitive impairment syndrome 25
    organophosphate exposure and
        neurotoxicity 873
sheep handlers, *Chlamydia* infection
        493
shellfish, organoarsenicals in 97
shelter limb 330
shepherds
    hydatid disease 495
    Lyme disease 497
shift work **581–9**
    absenteeism 584
    accidents 583–4
    biological and social interference
        581–2
    cardiovascular diseases 583, 588
    circadian rhythms 581–2, 584, 585,
        586
    contraindication 586–7
    definition 581
    digestive disorders 583
    disorders affecting suitability for
        586–7
    family and social life 582
    fatigue 582–3, 584
    flexibility in social life 582
    health effects 582–3
    health reviews 587
    measures for counteracting effects of
        587

medical surveillance and preventive
        measures 585–7
    mortality and 584
    performance efficiency 582, 583–4,
        588
    positive aspects 582
    progressive increase in 581
    psychoneurotic troubles 582–3
    psychophysical conditions 581–2
    rotational systems 582, 586
    shift system design criteria 586
    sleep 582–3, 585, 586
    social factors 585
    social marginalization 582
    tolerance factors 584–5
    toxicological risk 584
    women's reproductive function 584
    see also night work; work hours
shigellae 513
shingles 510
shipbuilding
    lead use *844*
    mesothelioma and 28
ship cargoes/holds
    arsine poisoning 162
    phosgene exposure 148
    phosphine exposure 163, 164
ships' engine room workers, prescribed
        diseases and *48*
shipyard welders, asbestos risk 183
shipyard workers
    cancer sites *815*
    chronic obstructive lung disease and
        699
    shoulder tendinitis *455*
    welding fume and 615
shivering 326
    in hypothermia 331
shoe manufacturing industry
    benzene exposure 261
    carcinogenicity and cancers *814*
    genotoxic exposure *776*
    hepatotoxicity in *885*
    n-hexane neurotoxicity 226
    menstrual disturbances 830
    prescribed diseases *48*, *53*
    respiratory cancer risk 808
    respiratory tract malignancies *4*
    sino-nasal cancer and leukaemia
        816
shoes, hip and knee osteoarthritis 467
shoulder capsulitis (frozen shoulder)
        454, 456
shoulder disorders 454–6
    age-related 454
    capsulitis 456
    clinical aspects 455–6
    epidemiology 454–5
    incidence 454–5
    management 456
    occupational studies 455
    tendinitis *454*, *455*, 455–6
    work-related *454*
shoulder pain 454–5
    welders 184
showers, *Legionella* infection from 710
sick building syndrome **713–18**
    air-conditioning systems and 715

allergic rhinitis 713
    causes 713–17
    economic consequences 717–18
    gender and 714
    public *vs* private sector buildings
        714
    symptoms 713
sick leave 571
sickle cell anaemia 389
sickle cell trait 389
sickness, long-term, resulting from
        bullying 541
sickness absence, sick building
        syndrome 717–18
siderosilicosis 701
siderosis 701
    EC schedule of occupational diseases
        44
    imaging 603
    welders 183, 184
sieverts 399
silage 136, 159
    substitution for hay to prevent
        farmer's lung 654
silane 162
'silent hypoxia' 349
silica
    carcinogenicity *814*
    COPD and 615
    crystalline, nephrotoxicity 853–4
    kidney damage 672
    lung cancer due to 675
    see also quartz; silicosis
silica crystalline, genotoxicity *776*
silica dust
    crystalline 672, 701
    EC comparable data collection *41*
    non-crystalline 672
    prescribed diseases due to *54*
silica exposure, copper miners 107
silica flour 673, 676
silica sand 672, 676
    see also quartz; silicosis
silicate dust pneumoconiosis 672
silicates, dust *44*
    EC comparable data collection *41*
    occupational diseases caused by (EC
        schedule) *44*
silicatosis 672
siliceous materials, prescribed disease
        due to *54*
silicic acid 162, 672
silicon carbide 701
silicon carbide dust 675–6
silicon carbide fibres 696, 697
silicon chips 172
silicon dioxide, *see* silica
silicon tetrafluoride 150, 153
silicosis 672, 672–7
    accelerated 673, 674
    acute 673
    aluminium powder prophylaxis 673
    chronic (active) 673–4
    chronic (inactive) 674
    in coalworkers 682, 685
    dust monitoring 677
    EC schedule of occupational diseases
        44

history 921
imaging 599–600
lung cancer risk 675, 808
medical monitoring of workers 677
mortality *29*
no treatment for 673
as prescribed disease *52, 54*
prevention 675–7
quartz dust toxicity 672–3
radiographic 675
tuberculosis risk 675
see also quartz dust; silica
silicotic alveolar proteinosis
(lipoproteinosis) 673
silicotuberculosis 674–5
prevention 675
silk (Bombix mori), radioallergosorbent
tests (RAST) *21*
silk waste, radioallergosorbent tests
(RAST) *21*
silo fillers' disease 159
silver **112**
accumulation (argyria) 112
lead sulphide in 82
uses 112
workers, monitoring 112
silvering, of mirrors 89
silver mines 82, 792
silver nitrate 112
silver polishers' lung 112
single-cell protein production 524
single-cell proteins 528
sintering 703
sinus
compression barotrauma 348
see also nasal sinus cancer
sinus barotrauma 362
sinus cancer, industries/occupations
associated with *815, 816*
sinuses, carcinoma of, as prescribed
disease *50, 53*
sisal dust/fibres 622
sisal dust inhalation, EC schedule of
occupational diseases *44*
situational awareness 371
skeletal fluorosis 151
biological monitoring tests *18*
skeletal muscle, biotransformation
capability *73*
skid transfer banks, prescribed diseases
associated with *47*
skin
absorption of chemicals 72
see also specific chemicals
biotransformation capability *73*
bullae formation 132, 139
burns, *see* burns
cancer, *see* skin cancer
compression barotrauma 348
decompression illness 351
decompression sickness 364
depigmentation 272
dimethylformamide (DMF) effect
251
diseases, *see* skin diseases
dryness, sick building syndrome and
713
epichlorohydrin (1-chloro-2,3-

epoxypropane) 252
infections, in saturation diving
349–50
irritation
ethyl benzene causing 266
xylene causing 264
metabolism of xenobiotics 72, 77
radiation casualties 414–15
radiation damage/threshold doses
400, 401, *403*
transient burning of, pesticide
exposure and *200*
trichloroacetic acid effect 249
welding injuries 184–5
see also dermatitis
skin burns, microwave radiation 431
skin cancer 733, 810
agents causing *4*
arsenic poisoning and 96
chemical carcinogens 792
EC schedule of occupational diseases
44
industries/occupations associated
with *4, 815*
non-Hodgkin's lymphoma and 810
screening 818
squamous cell carcinoma, *see*
squamous cell carcinoma
see also melanoma, malignant
skin diseases **725–37**
beryllium poisoning 102
clinical range 725
costs 725
EC schedule of occupational diseases
44
epidemiology 725
EPIDERM recording project 31
localized new growth as prescribed
disease *50*
non-eczematous 731
occupations causing 733–5
pigmentation and, *see* pigmentation
changes
prevalence 725
zoonotic diseases 501–2
see also contact dermatitis; contact
urticaria; *and individual skin
diseases*
skin effects, biological monitoring tests
18
skin prick tests
allergens 641
availability of resuscitation
equipment 731
contact dermatitis 729
contact urticaria 729, 731
enzymes 637
platinum exposure 110
platinum salts 643–4
skin tests
byssinosis 622, 624
occupational asthma 640, 643–4
slag wool 696, 805
carcinogenicity 805
slate industry 677–8
prescribed diseases in *54*
slate pencils 679
slates, for roofing 678–9

slateworker's pneumoconiosis 677–9
clinical manifestations and
pathology 678–9
exposure 678
prevention 679
tuberculosis confusion 678
tuberculosis risk 679
slaughterhouse workers, *see* abattoir
workers
sleep
disturbances, at high altitudes 389
jet lag and 373
shift work 582–3, 586
truncation 582, 585, 586
sleep apnoea 389
small intestine, radiation sensitivity
401
smallpox
archaeologists and 515
vaccination 533
smaltite 105
smells, assessment and units 716
Smelter Disease 156
smelting
aluminium 99
lead and 83, *844*
sulphur dioxide exposure 156
smog 124, 156, 664
photochemical 158
smoke
constituents 129
from domestic fires 918
exposure effects 130
see also fires
smoke bombs, acute lung injury due to
698, 698
smoke hoods, airline passengers 375
smokers' bronchitis 608
smoking 8
antigen expression affected by 657
asbestos exposure and 691, 816
as benzene source 262
bladder tumours and 269, 811
byssinosis and 622, 627
cadmium and 614
cancer and 762–3
cancer due to, prevalence 794
carbon monoxide levels 142
chronic obstructive pulmonary
disease (COPD) and 611, 613,
617
confounding and interactions
608–9
'never-smokers' 609, 614, 615
survival bias 609
coal miners' bronchitis and, IIAC
recommendations 40
coalworker's pneumoconiosis 683
as confounding factor 800–1
in carcinogen exposure monitoring
773
and COPD 32
cotton workers and 608
hand–arm vibration syndrome
(HAVS) and 310, 314
hypoxia at high altitudes 389
indoor air pollution 714
inorganic dust diseases and 665, 666

smoking – *contd*
  interaction effect 742
  interactions with carcinogenic agents
    816
  and isocyanate exposure 613–14
  lung cancer
    after asbestos exposure 8, 691,
      816
    risk of 77
    in uranium miners 115
  lung changes 671
  mesothelioma and 692
  miners 614–15
  occupational asthma development
    641–2
  occupational exposure groups and
    609
  occupational lung disease and 665
  passive, sick building syndrome and
    714
  platinum sensitization and 110
  polymer contamination and welding
    187
  promotion phase of cancer 406
  welders 182, 183
    and lung cancer 183–4
  welding fume and 615
  workers' and apprentice school
    leavers' habits *609*
smooth muscle hypertrophy, in
    byssinosis 622
SMRs (standardized mortality ratios) 32
sniffing
  chloroform (trichloromethane) 230
  glue sniffing 264, 891
  petrol sniffing 83
  trained sniffers 716
  1,1,1-trichloroethane (methyl
    chloroform) 231
snowblindness 426
snow crab processing workers,
    occupational asthma and 642,
    645–6
snuff 792
social life, effect of shift work 582
Social Security Act 1989 61
Social Security benefits, deductions
    from damages for loss of
    earnings 61
Social Security Contributions and
    Benefits Act 1992 38
Social Security (Industrial Injuries)
    (Prescribed Diseases)
    Regulations 1985 *52*
Soderberg aluminium process 152
  urinary tract neoplasms as prescribed
    disease due to *51*
sodium-23 398
sodium azide, as tissue culture additive
    528, 529
sodium bicarbonate, in hypothermia
    331
sodium calcium edetate
  in lead poisoning 87, 88
  in mercury poisoning 92
sodium chlorate poisoning 202
sodium cromoglycate 646
sodium cyanide 145

sodium fluoride 152
sodium nitrilotriacetate, as non-
    genotoxic carcinogen *765*
sodium para-aminosalicylic acid 108
sodium salt (2,3-dimercapto-1-propane-
    sulphonic acid) 852
sodium sulphate, in mercury poisoning
    92
sodium thiosulphate 146
sodium trichloroacetate 249
sodium valproate, back pain 483
soil fungicides 212
soil gas 140
soil pollution
  cadmium occurrence/poisoning (itai-
    itai disease) 94
  see also environment
solar radiation, genotoxicity *776*
solar retinopathy 426
soldering, eye protectors *433*
soldering fluxes 638–9
  occupational asthma due to 638–9,
    647, 700
  prescribed diseases from use of *52, 53*
  see also colophony
solubility, of metals 82
soluble oils, dermatoses 734
solvent naphtha, *see* white spirits
solvents 221–3
  chemical, in nucleic acid extraction
    529, *529*
  as hazardous DIY material *6*
  hepatotoxicity 890, 891
  metabolism and ethnic groups 20
  organic
    in breast milk 833
    causing hyperventilation 642
    hexacarbon solvents, neurotoxic
      effects 870
    neurotoxic effects 870, 875
    reproductive hazards *828*, 831
    see also hydrocarbons
  organic, and renal disease **854–9**
    case-control studies 855–6
    case reports and experimental
      studies 855–8
    cohort studies 857–8
    cross-sectional studies 856–7
    mechanisms of solvent-induced
      nephrotoxicity 858–9
    progression of renal failure 856
  petroleum solvents 255–6
  see also nitroparaffins; *and
    individual solvents*
soman 171
somatic cells, cancer as genetic disorder
    of 747
somatic mutation 742, 752
  clonal evolution and 747
  germline mutation *vs* 756
somatic mutation theory of
    carcinogenesis 742
somatogravic illusions, aircrew 371
somatogyral illusions, aircrew 371
somatostatin, biotechnology product
    522, 524
soot
  cancers due to *4, 814*

in chimneys 918
  genotoxicity *776*
  laryngeal oedema and 131
  prescribed diseases due to *50*
  skin diseases caused by (EC schedule)
    44
soot warts 918
SORDSA recording scheme for lung
    disorders (South Africa) 31
sound **283–306**
  decibel scales *284*, 284–5
  physics of 283–5
  reference pressures 284
  sound wave frequency 285
  sound wave intensity 283–5
  see also noise
sound pressure level (SPL) 284
Sound Solutions 297
South Africa, gold miners and COPD
    615
soya beans
  occupational asthma due to *647*
  prescribed diseases due to *53, 54*
soya flour, as non-genotoxic carcinogen
    765
spaceflight 375–7
  medical problems 376
  protection 376–7
  radiation exposure 376
  re-entry 375, 377
  risks 375–6
  space motion sickness 376
  toxic contamination incidents 376
space motion sickness 376
Space Shuttle, medications carried 376
spacesuits 376
Spain
  occupational diseases schedule 41
  toxic oil syndrome, hepatotoxicity
    884
spathe flowers (*Spathiphyllum walisii*)
    713
Spathiphyllum walisii (spathe flowers)
    713
spatial disorientation, aircrew 371–2
  causes 371
  as factor in military aircraft crashes
    375
  illusions, types of 371
  incidence 372
  protection 372
  training in prevention of 372
spatter 181, 184
special boiling point mixtures (SBPs)
    225, 255
speciation, of metals 82
species susceptibility differences 68, 77
'specific dynamic effect' 326
spectacles, aircrew 369
sperm
  carbon disulphide effect 254
  count/motility/morphology, agents
    affecting 829
  development and environmental
    sensitivity 824
  DNA mutation 828–9
  epichlorohydrin (1-chloro-2,3-
    epoxypropane) effect 253

quality, lead poisoning and 87
spermatogenesis 824, 835
   agents affecting 829
spermiogenesis 824
Sphaeropsidales spp. 711
spina bifida, mercury and 831
'spinal bends' 352
spinal cord
   decompression sickness 354, 355
   subacute combined degeneration
      168
spinal disease, in brucellosis 492
spinal stenosis, as cause of back pain
      479
spiramicin, toxoplasmosis 500
spirits, home-distilled 86
spirochaetal infections
   leptospirosis 495–6
   Lyme disease 496–8
spirometric tests 669–71
spironolactone 391
spleen, biotransformation capability
      73
splenomegaly
   benzene causing 262
   brucellosis 492
spondylarthropathies, as cause of back
      pain 479
spondylolisthesis, as cause of back pain
      479
spondylosis, cervical 454, 456–7
spongiform encephalopathies 500–1,
      532
spores
   fungal
      inhalation 636
      see also fungi
   microbial, extrinsic allergic alveolitis
      due to 653, 654, 654, 655
spray guns, prescribed diseases due to
      use of 47
spraying, genotoxicity 777
spray painting
   asthma and 634, 635
   diisocyanates and asthma 639
   extrinsic allergic alveolitis due to
      654
sprays, particle size 72
spurges, contact dermatitis 734
sputum, examination 666, 674–5
squamous cell carcinoma 733
   arsenic poisoning and 96
   formaldehyde association 244
   of skin, as prescribed disease 50
squatting, meniscus lesions caused by,
      EC schedule of occupational
      diseases 45
stable workers, ringworm 502
'staggers' 352
stainless steel welders/welding
   asthma in 183
   carcinogenicity of chrome salts 105
   fumes from, prescribed diseases due
      to 53, 54
   occupational asthma due to 647
   reproductive hazards 184
   welding fume 616
standardized birth ratio (SBR) 835

standardized fertility ratio (SFR) 835
standardized mortality ratio (SMR) 32,
      799
stannosis 114, 701
   imaging 603
stannous chloride 114
staphylococcal infections 511–12
Staphylococcus spp., in office buildings
      717
Staphylococcus aureus, methicillin-
      resistant (MRSA) 511–12
starch powder 680
state compensation, *see* compensation
steatorrhoea 514
steatosis
   hepatic 881, 891
      non-invasive screening 882
steel welders/welding 699
   bronchitis and 699
   chronic obstructive lung disease and
      699
   welding fume 616
   see also stainless steel
      welders/welding
steel workers
   lung cancer 815
   see also iron and steel founding
stem cells 901
sterility, radiation levels causing 400,
      402
sterilization unit workers, lymphatic
      and haemopoietic system
      cancers 816
sterilizing agents
   ethylene oxide 165–6
   glutaraldehyde (1,5-pentanedial)
      246
steroid hormones, in reproduction 825
steroids, hip and knee osteoarthritis
      467
stibine (antimony hydride) 101, 163
   acute lung injury due to 698, 698
stibnite 100
stilboestrol, reproductive hazards 828
stillbirth 831
   lead poisoning 82
stippled cells 86–7
Stockholm Workshop Scales 22
   hand–arm vibration syndrome
      (HAVS) 309, 309–10
Stoddard solvent, *see* white spirits
stokers 4
stomach cancer 808–9
   incidence 794
   oncogene activation in 749
stomach pains, biotechnology hazard
      527
stone cutting/cutters
   prescribed disease due to 54
   silicosis mortality 29
stool analysis, radiation casualties 415
storage mites 637
   mixed, radioallergosorbent tests
      (RAST) 21
strain, definition 325
stratum corneum 72
straw, mouldy, extrinsic allergic
      alveolitis due to 654

Streptococcus spp., in office buildings
      717
Streptococcus suis 499–500
   infection, as prescribed disease 49
   misdiagnosis as cellulitis 500
Streptococcus zooepidemicus 500
Streptomyces spp. 523
   ill-health due to, in biotechnology
      527
streptomycin
   brucellosis 492
   as tissue culture additive 528
Stresnil, accidental self-injection with
      213
stress 569–70
   British Medical Association Stress
      Counselling Service 565
   declining performance at work
      574–6
   definition 325, 570
   high-stress jobs 575
   at home 574
   home/work interaction 574–5
   impact on employers
      financial 571
      legal 570–1
   pressure as stimulus 570
   risk to employees 576–7
      job-type level 576–7
      organizational level 576
      personal level 577
   sick building syndrome 717, 718
   support as factor in coping with 572
   at work 574
   see also bullying; psychiatric
      disorders
stress-related illness
   definition 570
   fitness to work assessment 576
   healthy-worker effect 570
   incidence 570
   risk factors 571–2
   work loss 570
striatum, manganese poisoning 108
stroma 422
strontium 807
strontium chromate, lung cancer as
      prescribed disease due to 54,
      105
structured settlements 60
Stugeron 373
styrene (vinyl benzene; phenylethylene)
      264–5
   absorption and metabolism 265
   biological monitoring tests and
      guidance values 18
   characteristics and uses 264
   clinical effects 265
   cumene in styrene production 266
   exposure, and urinary albumin
      concentration 856
   exposure limits 265
   hepatotoxicity 884
   leukaemia and 813
   lymphocyte subsets and 22
   neurotoxic effects 874–5
   occupational diseases caused by (EC
      schedule) 43

styrene (vinyl benzene; phenylethylene)
    – contd
    polymerization, hepatotoxicity in
        885
    reproductive hazards to mother 830,
        831
styrene butadiene rubber 237, 264
styrene-7,8-oxide, genotoxicity 777
subcutaneous cellulitis, see cellulitis
subcutaneous tissues, prescribed
        diseases 46
submarine-escape training 351, 352
substance abuse **557–67**
    constructive coercion 562–3
    definitions 557
    motivation to change 562–3
    see also alcohol abuse; drug abuse
substantia nigra, manganese poisoning
        108
sudden death, trichloroethylene 234
sugar, bagassosis 655
suicide
    aluminium phosphide 163
    anaesthetists 167–8
    bullying and 540
    copper ingestion 107
    depression and 573
    electromagnetic field exposure
        445
    hydrogen cyanide 146
    on railway lines 547
sulphadiazine 500
sulphaemoglobinaemia 161, **268–9**
sulphasalazine, altitude sickness 390
sulphate, conjugates 76
sulphur, historical uses 195
sulphur-containing compounds **253–5**
    formula and examples 224
    see also carbon disulphide
sulphur dioxide **155–6**
    characteristics and sources 155
    exposure levels 155–6
    health effect levels 127
    initiating and provoking
        occupational asthma 633, 634
    odour threshold 156
    uses 155
sulphur hexafluoride 153
    Kyoto Protocol agreement 135
sulphuric acid
    aerosols 156
    anhydride (sulphur trioxide) 156
    carcinogenicity 156, 814
    emissions, Japan 156
    genotoxicity 776
    laryngeal and lung cancer 815
    occupational diseases caused by (EC
        schedule) 43
sulphur mines, high altitudes 393–4
sulphur mustard, see mustard gas
sulphur oxides, occupational diseases
        caused by (EC schedule) 43
sulphur tetrafluoride 153
sulphur trioxide 156
sulphuryl difluoride 154
sulphuryl fluoride 154
sulphydryl groups, lead affinity for 85
sumatriptan, altitude sickness 392

summer type allergic alveolitis
        (hypersensitivity pneumonitis)
        711
sun beds, eye damage from 420
sunflower seed, radioallergosorbent
        tests (RAST) 21
sunglasses, aircrew 370
sun lamps, eye damage from 420
sunlight
    dermatitis as exposure risks 734
    eye damage from 420, 429
    P53 gene mutations 754
    skin cancers and 810
    wavelengths 419
supervision of workers, see monitoring
        of workers
superwarfarins 212
    symptoms and signs of exposure to
        200
support
    for employees 578–9
        work stress and support from
            home 572
supraspinatus tendinitis 455
Supreme Court Act 1991 58
surface decompression (decanting) 344
surgeons
    hepatitis B infection 502, 503
    hepatitis C infection 504
    HIV infection 504
    sharps injuries 504
    see also health care workers
surgery, flying after 361–2
surgical gloves, and talc 680
Surveillance of work-related and
        occupational respiratory
        disease, see SWORD
survivor guilt 545, 546, 547
susceptibility, carcinogens and 21
sweating 326, 333, 335
    required sweat rate 334
swimming failure, in hypothermia 332
swimming pools, chlorine hazard 147,
        148
SWORD (Surveillance of work-related
        and occupational respiratory
        disease) 31, 31, 634
    gas-related incident reports 123
    inhalation accidents reported to 635
    non-fibrous mineral dusts 672
    occupational asthma reported to 637
symptoms, non-specific 25
synovitis 459
    in brucellosis 492
synthetic mineral fibres 696–7
syphilis, treatment with mercury 89
systemic sclerosis, see scleroderma

2,4,5-T, see 2,4,5-
        trichlorophenoxyacetic acid
tabun 171
tachycardia, high altitudes 390
Taiwan incident 274
talc 680
    asbestiform fibres in
        genotoxicity 776
        lung cancer 815

    disease prevention 680
    lung cancer and mesothelioma 680
    mining and uses of 680
    pneumoconiosis 680
tanning industry
    dermatoses 735
    zoonoses 489
tantalum, nephrotoxicity 843
Taq enzyme 523
tar
    prescribed diseases due to 50
    skin cancer 4, 733
    skin diseases caused by (EC schedule)
        44
tar distillers, skin neoplasms 4
task optimization 471
taxidermists, chlamydiosis 492
TCDD, see 2,3,7,8-tetrachlorodibenzo-p-
        dioxin
TCP, see 2,4,5-trichlorophenol
TCPA, see tetrachlorophthalic anhydride
TDI, see toluene diisocyanate
teachers, and workplace violence
        552–3, 553
tea dust
    occupational asthma due to 647
    prescribed diseases due to 53, 54
teasing 540
technetium-99 408
technetium-99m diethylenetriamine
        penta-acetic acid (Tc^{99}m DTPA)
        599
teeth
    compression barotrauma 348
    erosion
        by hydrogen chloride 149
        by sulphuric acid mists 156
    loss, in mercury poisoning 89, 92
    phosphorus necrosis and 98
Teflon 187
telegraphist's cramp 464
telephones, mobile 793
telephone workers, repetitive strain
        injury 462
telephonists, dry throat 713
tellurium **112–13**
    metabolism and absorption 112
    neurotoxic effects 872
    supervision of workers 112–13
    toxicity 112
    in urine 112–13
    uses 112
tellurium compounds 112
tellurium dioxide 112
tellurium hexafluoride 112
telomerase 748
telomeres 748
temazepam
    altitude sickness 389, 392
    jet lag and 374
temperature
    in aviation 366–8
        cold 367
        heat 367–8
    core body 327
    dry bulb 327, 333
    oral 327
    rectal 327

sick building syndrome and 715
skin 326, 327–8
wet bulb 333
wind chill equivalent 327, *327*
tendinitis
calcific 455–6
prescribed disease status and 40
shoulder *454*
bicipital tendinitis *454*, 456
calcific tendinitis 455–6
occupational studies *455*
rotator cuff tendinitis *454*, 455, 456
supraspinatus 455
tendonous insertions, overstraining, EC schedule of occupational diseases *45*
tendons, traumatic inflammation as prescribed disease *46*
tendon sheaths
overstraining, EC schedule of occupational diseases *45*
see also tenosynovitis
tennis elbow (lateral epicondylitis) *454*, 458, 459, 461
aetiology 458
tenosynovitis 459–60, 461–2
clinical aspects 459
de Quervain's disease *454*, 459
epidemiology 459
occupational studies 459
as prescribed disease *46*
trigger finger 459–60
of the wrist *454*, 459
tension neck syndrome *454*, 457
TENS (transcutaneous electrical nerve stimulation) 457, 483
teratogenesis 826
radiation levels causing *400*
teratogenicity 836
dioxin (2,3,7,8-tetrachlorodibenzo-*p*-dioxin (TCDD)) 274
methyl chloride 165
no observed effect level (NOEL) 836
tellurium 112
terbinafine, ringworm 502
terbutaline, chlorine poisoning *133*
testes
biotransformation capability *73*
damage, tellurium 112
function impairment by 1,2-dibromoethane (ethylene dibromide) 232
threshold levels of radiation dose *400*
tumours, dimethylformamide causing 251
testicular cancer, electromagnetic field exposure and 443
testosterone 835
tetanus, EC schedule of occupational diseases *44*
tetanus prophylaxis, superficial frostbite 329
tetraalkyltin compounds, biotransformation 114
tetracarbonylnickel, *see* nickel carbonyl

2,3,7,8-tetrachlorodibenzo-*p*-dioxin (TCDD; dioxin) 10, 203, **274–5**, **889–90**
carcinogenicity 274, *814*
dioxan confused with dioxin 9
genotoxicity *776*
as hepatocarcinogen 886, 890
hepatotoxicity 894
mechanisms 889–90
treatment 887
Seveso incident 274–5, 876, 886, 890
toxicity 198
in Vietnam War 274, 876
tetrachloroethane
hepatotoxicity 226, *885*, 891
mortality rate 891
poisoning, as prescribed disease *50*
for treating wartime aircraft wings 924
tetrachloroethylene (perchloroethylene) 224, **234–7**, *765*
biological monitoring tests and guidance values *18*
in breast milk 833
carcinogenicity 236
characteristics and uses 234–5
clinical manifestations 235–6
cross-sectional studies 857
genotoxicity *777*
hepatotoxicity 235, *884*, 891
long-term exposures 236
management 236
metabolism/biochemical effects 235
as non-genotoxic carcinogen *765*
reproductive hazards 830, 831
tetrachloromethane, *see* carbon tetrachloride
tetrachlorophthalic anhydride (TCPA) 639, 641, 645, 646
prescribed diseases due to *52*, *53*
radioallergosorbent tests (RAST) *21*
tetracycline
anthrax 491
brucellosis 492
chlamydiosis 493
erysipeloid and 501
Lyme disease 497
Q fever 498
tetraethyl lead 83, 88–9, 810
absorption 89
dealkylation 85
inhalation and skin contact 89
see also lead poisoning
1,1,1,2-tetrafluoroethane (HCFC134a) 155
tetrafluorohydrazine 153
tetrafluoromethane (Freon-14) 154
tetramethyl lead 83
tetramine platinum dichloride 110
Tetranychus urticae, radioallergosorbent tests (RAST) *21*
textile dusts 621–31
see also byssinosis; cotton
textile industry
asbestos exposure 687
prescribed diseases in *47*

tetrachloroethylene in 235
see also byssinosis; cotton; cotton dust
textile workers
elbow pain 458
owners' attitudes to 919–20
Thackrah, Charles Turner 919–20
thalidomide 830
thallium **113**
absorption and excretion 113
acute intoxication 113
chronic poisoning 113
half-life 113
mechanisms of action 113
in radionuclide imaging 113
in table salt 113
treatment of poisoning 113
in urine 113
uses 113
thallium sulphate 113
theatrical fogging machines, *see* 1,2-propylene glycol
thermal injuries, in fires 130
thermal radiation, flying and 367
thermal strain, reduction **337–40**
thermal stress
Fighter Index of Thermal Stress (FITS) 333
training and acclimatization 337–8
see also cold; heat
Thermoactinomyces sacchari 654, 655
Thermoactinomyces vulgaris 654, 654, 659, 711
thermogenesis 326
thermophilic actinomycetes 654, 654, 655, 659
Thermophilus aquaticus 523
thermoregulation 325, 326, 333
thiocyanate 145, 146–7
thiol groups, mercury affinity for 91
thiosulphate 146
thiotepa, genotoxicity *776*
thiothiazolidine-4-carboxylic acid, biological monitoring tests and guidance values *18*
2-thiothiazolidine-4-carboxylic acid (TTCA) 254
thistle, contact dermatitis 733
Thompson v Smiths Shiprepairers (1984) 61
thoracic outlet syndrome *454*, 457
thoracoscopy 666
thoracotomy 666
thorium 183–4
thorium dioxide (Thorotrast) 809
Three Mile Island 131, 584
threshold shifts (hearing)
permanent 290–1
temporary 289, 290
throat, dry, sick building syndrome and 713
throat pain, paraquat poisoning and *201*
thrombocytopenia 262, 266, 400, 908
thrombosis, *see* deep vein thrombosis
thrombotic thrombocytopenic purpura (TTP) 494
thromboxane 329

thrush (oral candidiasis), in AIDS/HIV
    infection 507
Thuja plicata (Western Red Cedar),
    occupational asthma due to
    634, *636*, *638*, 646
thumb, episodic blanching as
    prescribed disease *48*
thymine 743
thymol 271
thymoxamine 330
thyroid
    cancer
        oncogene activation in *749*
        risk of, and germline mutations
            751
    cobalt effect on function 106
    radiation damage, in children 401,
        403
    radiation damage/threshold dose
        400, 401
    tumours, non-genotoxic carcinogen
        mechanisms *765*
thyroiditis, radiation 401
ticks 497, 509
    Lyme disease transmission 496, 497
tilmicosin, accidental self-injection with
        214
'time of useful consciousness' 363
tin **113–15**
    absorption and excretion 114
    inorganic, toxicity 114
    metabolism 114
    occurrence and forms of 114
    organic, *see* organotin compounds
    uses 113–14
tin dust
    imaging 603
    inhalation, EC schedule of
        occupational diseases *44*
tinea pedis 734
Tinel's test 461
tingling
    decompression illnesses 352
    methyl *n*-butyl ketone causing 247
tinidazole 514
tin miners/mining
    bone marrow cancers *815*
    lung cancer 114–15, *815*
        as prescribed disease due to *54*
    radon concentrations in mines 407
tinnitus 291
    occupational noise-induced 303
tin pneumoconiosis 701
tissue culture additives, biotechnology
        528
tissue plasminogen activator,
        biotechnology product 522,
        522, 524
titanium, granulomatous lung disease
        due to 702
titanium dioxide, chronic obstructive
        lung disease and 699
titanium tetrachloride, acute lung
        injury due to *698*, 698
T lymphocytes
    allergic contact dermatitis 727
    CD4:CD8 ratio 656
    extrinsic allergic alveolitis 656–7

in occupational asthma 640
    TH₂ lymphocytes 640
    in sarcoidosis 656
TMA, *see* trimellitic anhydride
TMTD, *see* tetramethyl thiuram
        disulphide
TNT, *see* trinitrotoluene
tobacco
    P53 gene mutations 754
    see also smoke; smoking
tobacco snuff 792
tobramycin, as tissue culture additive
        528
Tokyo, sarin incident 171
toluene 261, **263**, 854
    characteristics and uses 263
    clinical effects 263
    exposure limits 263
    as hazardous DIY material 6
    hepatotoxicity *885*, 891–2
    impurity 9–10
    metabolism 263
    monitoring 263
    neurotoxic effects 263, 875
    in nucleic acid extraction 529
    reproductive hazards to mother 831
toluene diisocyanate (TDI) 9
    extrinsic allergic alveolitis due to
        654
    FEV₁ loss and TDI exposure 613, 614
    neurological symptoms after fire 130
    occupational asthma and 639, 641,
        645, 646
m-toluidine 269
o-toluidine 267, 269
    exposure limits 267
p-toluidine 269
toluol, *see* toluene
2,4-tolylene diisocyanate, *see* toluene
        diisocyanate
tolylmercuric acetate 212
tools
    associated with hand–arm vibration
        syndrome (TAB 2nd) *308*, 308,
        309, 310, *317*
    prescribed disease due to vibration
        48
    vibratory, carpal tunnel syndrome
        (CTS) 316
tooth cavity, gas in 362
topoisomerases 745
torch brazing, eye protectors *433*
torch soldering
    eye protectors *433*
    see also soldering
Tort system for negligence claims 42
tourist industries
    farmers and 490
    Lyme disease 497
toxic gases, *see* gases
toxic hazards, information sources 7–8
toxicity, of chemicals 67–8
    animal toxicity tests 68
    decreased 74
    dose–response relationship 67
    increased 74
    ratings *67*
    susceptibility 68, 77

toxic oil syndrome (Spain),
        hepatotoxicity *884*
toxicokinetics **68–70**
    analysis 69
    clearance 70
    compartmental models 69
    concepts 69–70
    definition 69
    extraction ratio 70
    first order kinetics 69
    half-life 69
    kinetics of exposure 71–2
    reproductive hazards and 836
    volume of distribution 69–70
    zero order (saturation) kinetics 69
    see also absorption; chemical
        agents/chemicals;
        detoxification; elimination;
        metabolism
toxicological research 28
toxicology 67
toxic organic psychosis
    lead poisoning 88–9
    mercury poisoning 92
toxic substances, information on risks
        and safety procedures 911
Toxoplasma gondii 500
toxoplasmosis 500
    cerebral 500
    congenital 500
    in pregnancy 490, 500
Toynbee manoeuvre 347
2,4,5-TP (2-(2,4,5-trichlorophenoxy)
        propionic acid) *203*
trachea
    irritation, in pulmonary oxygen
        poisoning 345
    malignant neoplasms,
        occupations/agents causing *4*
tracheobronchitis 698
    in acute beryllium poisoning 101
    in smoke exposure 130
traction 457
train drivers, post-traumatic stress
        disorder 546, 547
training
    back pain prevention 481
    balanced living 578
    coping skills 578
    management of change 578
    zoonoses prevention and control 490
transcutaneous electrical nerve
        stimulation (TENS) 457, 483
transfection 523
transfer factor for carbon monoxide
        (TLCO), in extrinsic allergic
        alveolitis 657, 658, 659
transferrin 849
    aluminium transport 100
    carbohydrate-deficient transferrin
        (CDT) 562
    genetic defect 100
    zinc binding 116
transformation processes,
        biotechnology application 525
transitional epithelium tumours, non-
        genotoxic carcinogen
        mechanisms *765*

transitions, point mutations 743
transjugular intrahepatic portal-
        systemic shunt (TIPS), as varices
        treatment 887
transmissible mink encephalopathy
        (TME) 500
transmissible spongiform
        encephalopathies (TSEs) 500–1
transport
    carcinogenic risk in 815
    of chemicals 68
    drug screening tests for passenger
        transport operational staff 561
    see also travel
Transport and Works Act 1992 561
transversions, point mutations 743
travel
    by air, spread of disease 379
    infections associated with 512–14
    malaria 512–13
    traveller's diarrhoea, see traveller's
        diarrhoea
    zoonoses 489
    see also transport
traveller's diarrhoea 513–14
    management 513–14
    prevention 513
trekkers, high altitude, cerebral
        oedema 386
tremolite 680, 687
    chrysotile contamination by 687
    mesothelioma/lung cancer and 680,
        695
    pleural plaques due to 690
    pneumoconiosis and 680
    talc contamination by 680
    vermiculite contamination by 681
tremor
    in manganese poisoning 108
    in mercury poisoning 89, 91, 92, 872
trench foot 330
treosulfan, genotoxicity 776
Trialeurodes vaporarorium,
        radioallergosorbent tests (RAST)
        21
trialkylphosphorothioates, lung
        damage 77
trialkyltin 114
triazine herbicides 204
tribavirin 509
tribunals 58
    see also Medical Appeal Tribunals
tributyltin 114
trichloroacetic acid (TCA) 224, **249**
    biological monitoring tests and
        guidance values 18
    characteristics and uses 249
    clinical manifestations of exposure
        249
    metabolism/biochemical effects 249
    as metabolite of other compounds
        231, 233
    in nucleic acid extraction 529
1,1,1-trichloroethane (methyl
        chloroform) 154, 224, **231–2**
    characteristics and uses 231
    clinical manifestations 231
    hepatotoxicity 226, 884, 885, 891

management 232
    metabolism/biochemical effects 231
    mutagenicity 231
    'sniffing' 231
1,1,2-trichloroethane, hepatotoxicity
        226
trichloroethanol 233
2,2,2-trichloroethanol 231
trichloroethene, see trichloroethylene
trichloroethylene ('trike') 167, 224,
        232–4
    biological monitoring tests and
        guidance values 18
    carcinogenicity 234, 755
    characteristics and uses 232–3
    clinical manifestations 234
    decomposition 9
    genotoxicity 777
    heart failure 229–30
    hepatotoxicity 226, 234, 884, 891
    management 234
    metabolism/biochemical effects
        233–4
    nephrotoxicity 234
    neurotoxic effects 875–6
    reproductive hazards 830
trichloromethane, see chloroform
trichlorophenol 10
2,4,5-trichlorophenol (TCP)
    hepatotoxicity 884
    TCDD production and 274
2,4,5-trichlorophenoxyacetic acid
        (2,4,5-T) 10, 203
    hepatotoxicity 894
    neurotoxicity 876
    in Vietnam War 274, 876
2-(2,4,5-trichlorophenoxy) propionic
        acid (2,4,5-TP) 203
1,2,3-trichloropropane, genotoxicity
        777
1,1,2-trichloro-1,2,2-trifluoroethane
        (Freon-113; Genetron-113) 154
Trichophyton mentagrophytes 502
Trichophyton verrucosum 502
Trichosporon cutaneum 711
tricyclic antidepressants 549
tridymite 672
    limits/recommendations 677
triethylene-tetramine, prescribed
        diseases due to 52, 53
triethyltin 114
trigeminal nerve, in trichloroethylene
        exposure 876
trigger finger 459–60
triglycidyl isocyanurate (TGIC), contact
        dermatitis 735
trihalomethanes 148
1,2,4-trihydroxybenzene, metabolism
        74
'trike', see trichloroethylene
trimellitic anhydride (TMA) 639–40
    prescribed diseases due to 52, 53
    radioallergosorbent tests (RAST) 21
trimethoprim, traveller's diarrhoea 513
trimethylamine 157
2,2,4-trimethyl pentane, as non-
        genotoxic carcinogen 765
trinitrotoluene (TNT)

blood dyscrasias/malignancies and 4
    hepatotoxicity 884, 885, 892
    wartime production 924
triorthocresyl phosphate,
        hepatotoxicity 884
triphenyltin 114
tris(2,3-dibromopropyl)phosphate,
        genotoxicity 777
tris(2-ethylhexyl)phosphate,
        carcinogenicity 766
trisomy 744
tritium, radiation contamination
        treatment 413
Trivexin T, accidental self-injection with
        213
trout, radioallergosorbent tests (RAST)
        21
truck drivers, bladder cancer 811
trypsin inhibitors, as non-genotoxic
        carcinogens 765
tuberculin test 666
tuberculosis
    as cause of back pain 479
    EC comparable data collection 41
    EC schedule of occupational diseases
        44
    health care workers 510–11
    inorganic dust diseases and 665
    multidrug-resistant 511
    as prescribed disease 49, 511
    risk
        in coalworkers 684
        in silicosis 674
        in slateworker's pneumoconiosis
            679
    screening 510–11, 677
    slateworker's pneumoconiosis,
        confusion with 678
tubulo-interstitial disease 855, 856
tulips, contact dermatitis 734
Tullio phenomenon 303
tumour necrosis factor, metal fume
        fever 186
tumours, see cancer; and specific
        cancers
tumour-suppressor genes 752–3
    functions and involvement 750–1
    von Hippel–Lindau gene 755
tungsten **115**
    toxicity 115–14
    uses 115
tungsten carbide 115
tungsten inert gas welding, see
        welders/welding
tuning fork tests, of hearing 285
tunnel workers 343
    silicosis 673, 676
Turkey
    contaminated bread incident 266,
        267
    porphyria cutanea tarda outbreak
        886
turpentine 735
turpentine substitute, see white spirits
twister's cramp 464
tympanic membrane, rupture 348
typhoid fever 509
typing, prescribed diseases due to 46

typists
    occupational risk factors 468
    see also keyboard operators
tyre workers, lymphatic and
            haemopoietic system cancers
            815
tyrosine iodinase, inhibition 106

U-2 aircraft 364
UDP-glucuronyltransferase 76
UK National Study of Hearing 289–90
ulceration 732–3
    from freezing cold injuries 329
    pesticide exposure/poisoning and
            200, 201
ultrasound 304
    in occupational lung disease 598
ultraviolet radiation
    acute light damage 426
    conjunctival ailments from exposure
            to (EC schedule) 45
    eye protectors 432, 433
    genotoxicity 777
    lip cancers 815
    ocular penetration/absorption 424,
            425
    P53 gene mutations 754
    skin cancers 810, 815
    sources, eye damage and absorption
            420
    wavelengths 419, 420
Umbelliferae, contact dermatitis 734
unconsciousness, see consciousness:
            loss of
undecane 225
unfair dismissal 542
United Kingdom Council for
            Psychotherapy (UKCP) 579
United Nations Scientific Committee on
            the Effects of Atomic Radiations
            (UNSCEAR) 400, 402–3, 404
Unit Pulmonary Toxic Dose (UPTD) of
            oxygen 345
universal precautions 508
unleaded petrol
    benzene in 261
    as non-genotoxic carcinogen 765
unsaturated fat, as non-genotoxic
            carcinogen 765
upholstery industry, 1,1,1-
            trichloroethane (methyl
            chloroform) in 231
upper limb disorders
    carpal tunnel syndrome, see carpal
            tunnel syndrome
    chronic pain 461–3
    clinical aspects 463
    elbow disorders 454, 457–9
    epidemiology 462–3
    forearm disorders 454
    identification checklist 470
    management 463
    neck disorders 454, 456–7
    peritendinitis 459–60
    prescribed disease status and 40
    shoulder disorders 454, 454–6
    tenosynovitis 459–60, 461–2

wrist disorders 454, 459, 461
    see also repetitive strain injury
uraemia, diagnosis by expired air 71
uranium 115–16
    chemical toxicity 116
    mineworkers
        lung cancer and smoking 8
        respiratory tract malignancies 4,
            115
    nephrotoxicity 853
    processing plant incidents 131, 150
    radiation hazards 115
    uses 115
uranium hexafluoride, acute lung
            injury due to 698, 698
uranium miners, lung cancer 700, 815
uranium oxide 115
    urban pollution, see air pollution;
            environment
urethane reaction 639
urinary bladder, see entries beginning
            with bladder
urinary calculi 849
urinary tract malignancies
    occupations/agents causing 4
    as prescribed diseases 51
    see also bladder cancer
urine
    analysis, radiation casualties 415
    screening in workplace, substance
            abuse 561–2
urobilinogen 231, 235
uroporphyrinogen decarboxylase
            (UROD) 886
uroporphyrinuria 886, 889
urothelial tumours 269
    as prescribed disease 269
urothelium, cancer risk and germline
            mutations 750
ursodeoxycholic acid, as treatment for
            liver disease 887
urticaria, see contact urticaria
USA
    biotechnology regulations/control
            522–3
    costs of back pain 478
    industrial injuries/workers'
            compensation schemes 38, 42,
            571
    proportional mortality statistics 33
    registering of diseases 30–1
uterus, cancer risk and germline
            mutations 750
utility workers, see electrical workers

vaccination/vaccines 490
    aircrew and passengers 379
    anthrax 490, 491
    bacille Calmette–Guérin 511
    hepatitis A 514
    hepatitis B 508
    Lyme disease 498
    orf 502
    Q fever 498–9
    rabies 490, 499
vaccinia virus 533
Vacor, neurotoxic effects 876

vaginal bleeding 830
valency, of metals 82
'Valley of Death', Java 140
Valsalva manoeuvre 348, 362
vanadium 116
    half-life 116
    occupational diseases caused by (EC
            schedule) 43
    supervision of workers 116
    toxicity 116
    uses 116
vanadium compounds, occupational
            diseases caused by (EC schedule)
            43
vanadium oxides, acute lung injury due
            to 698
vanadium pentoxide 116
    acute lung injury due to 698
    occupational asthma due to 700
vapour-permeable materials 339
vapours 124–5
    definition 124
varicella zoster 510
varices, treatment 887
Varitox 249
varnish, as hazardous DIY material 6
vasoconstriction, in cold 326, 330
vasodilatation
    cold-induced 326
    nitric oxide effect 158
VCM, see vinyl chloride monomer
vegetable matter, mouldy, prescribed
            diseases due to 49
vegetable proteins, occupational
            asthma due to 636
vegetables, contact urticaria 731
vehicles, see motor vehicles
ventilation, sick building syndrome and
            715
ventilation pneumonitis 654, 654,
            655–6
    humidifier fever vs 655–6
    see also extrinsic allergic alveolitis
ventilatory function
    age-related changes 612
    decline of, in COPD 610–13
    influences on 611, 612
    see also chronic obstructive
            pulmonary disease
ventricular fibrillation
    cold-related hazards and cold
            weather, in hypothermia 331,
            332
    trichloroethylene and 234
vermiculite 681
Vernon v Bosley (No 2) (1997) 63
vertigo
    air pilots 371
    alternobaric 348
    occupational noise-induced 303–4
vesicant (blister) agents 171, 171–2
veterinarians
    anaesthetic gas exposure 168
    anthrax 490
    brucellosis 491
    chlamydiosis 492
    dermatoses 735
    drug misuse 565

erysipeloid 501
leptospirosis 496
listeriosis 496
needlestick injuries 213
Newcastle disease 498
pustular dermatitis 496
rabies 499
ringworm 502
scabies 511
toxoplasmosis 500
zoonoses 489
veterinary products, accidental self-
injection with 213, 213–14
amputation after 214
clinical sequelae 213–14
epidemiology 213
management 214
vibration 307–23
in aircraft 368–9
effect on crew 368
protection 369
carpal tunnel syndrome case-control
studies 460, 461
diseases caused by, EC schedule of
occupational diseases 45
Dupuytren's contracture and 464
EC comparable data collection 41
frequency and acceleration 307
impact vibration 310
measurement 307–8
median nerve neuropathy 461
reproductive hazards to
embryo/fetus 832, 832
vibrating tools, prescribed disease
due to 48
wave form analysis 307
whole body, back pain and 480
see also hand–arm vibration
syndrome; whole-body
vibration
vibration sense, loss of, in arsenic
poisoning 96
vibration white finger 22, 309
as prescribed disease 48
see also hand–arm vibration
syndrome
Vietnam War 876
vincristine 895
as tissue culture additive 528
vinegar (acetic acid) 249
vine sprayers' lung 107
vineyard workers/vintners 885, 892
skin and lip cancers 815
vinyl benzene, see styrene
vinyl bromide 170
genotoxicity 777
vinyl chloride 170, 236
cancers 814
carcinogenicity 74
epoxidation 74
genotoxicity 776
hepatotoxicity 884, 885, 886, 894–5
mechanisms 888, 889
liver angiosarcoma 170, 803
liver cancer 886
liver haemangiosarcoma 4
P53 gene mutations 754
poisoning as prescribed disease 803

production, liver cancer 815
reproductive hazards 829
scleroderma 732
vinyl chloride monomer (VCM) 170,
817, 924
liver cancer 815
prescribed disease due to work in
and around 51
see also vinyl chloride
vinyl cyanide, see acrylonitrile
vinyl ether, occupational diseases
caused by (EC schedule) 43
vinyl fluoride 171
genotoxicity 777
vinylidene chloride (1,1-
dichloroethylene) 224, 236–7
carcinogenicity 237
characteristics and uses 236
clinical effects 237
hepatotoxicity 236, 237
management 237
metabolism/biochemical effects
236–7
violence at work 550–4
antecedents of 554
case histories 550–1, 552–3
causes 551–2
debriefing 553
effects of 552–3
feelings of injustice 551, 552
management 553–4
The Management of Imminent
Violence 553
in the NHS 551
outcomes 553
prevalence 551
psychological vs physical 551
reducing the impact of 553–4
see also bullying
viral haemorrhagic fevers 509–10
clinical manifestations 509
in health care workers 509–10
management guidelines 509–10
mortality rates 509
viral hepatitis
EC comparable data collection 41
EC schedule of occupational diseases
44
as prescribed disease 49, 502
viral oncogenes 748
viral warts 733
visible light, see light
vision
basic principles 419–23
in flying 369–70
night vision 370
visors, aircrew 370
visual acuity
and aircraft vibration 369
fitness for flying and 378
visual display unit (VDU) operators
ergonomic factors 832
eye damage 430
Health and Safety (Display Screen
Equipment) Regulations 1992
471–2
musculoskeletal disorders 461, 471
pregnancy outcomes 445

rashes 713, 714
reproductive hazards to
embryo/fetus 832
sick building syndrome and 714
spontaneous abortions and 445, 832
see also keyboard operators
visual symptoms, decompression
sickness 364
vital capacity 345, 356
see also lung function
vitamins
vitamin B12 146
inactivation of, by nitrous oxide
168
vitamin C deficiency 918
vitamin D
cadmium poisoning and 94
malignant melanoma and 810
'vitamin F' 114
vitamin K, warfarin ingestion and
212
vitiligo
catechols causing, see styrene
leucoderma mimicking 732
as prescribed disease 51, 272
vitreous 421, 422
vitreous fibres, man-made, see man-
made mineral/vitreous fibres
volatile liquids, see solvents
volatile organic compounds 71–2
alveolar concentration 71–2
alveolar ventilation 71
breath analysis 71, 72
environmental concentration 71
as gas mixture 71
inhalation kinetics 71–2
partial pressures 71
rate of delivery 71
solubility effect on alveolar
concentration 71–2
volcanic ash 696
volcanoes
hydrogen chloride 149
hydrogen sulphide 160
voles, prescribed disease due to working
at infested places 48
volume of distribution, of chemicals
69–70
vomiting
arsine poisoning 162
dichloroacetylene exposure 239
1,2-dichloroethane (ethylene
dichloride) 230
paraquat poisoning and 201
pesticide exposure and 200
in radiation casualties 402, 414
radiation levels causing 400
von Hippel–Lindau disease,
susceptibility and germline
mutation 751
von Hippel–Lindau tumour-suppressor
gene 755
von Recklinghausen's
neurofibromatosis,
susceptibility and germline
mutation 750
vulcanization of rubber, carbon
disulphide exposure 254

Vulcano Island, Italy
  carbon dioxide in wells 140
  hydrogen sulphide 160

*Walker v Northumberland County
    Council* (1994) 570–1, 578
walking sticks, hip and knee
    osteoarthritis 467
wallpaper contaminants, arsenic
    poisoning 96
war
  chemical weapons, organic
    derivatives of arsine 97
  gases used in 171
  impact of, on prevention of
    occupational diseases 924
warfarin 212
  ingestion 212
  symptoms and signs of exposure to
    200
warts
  oil warts 733
  viral 733
water
  drinking water, *see* drinking water
  in earth's atmosphere *135*
water gas 142
water immersion 330
  cold, survival 332
  intake and acclimatization 335
  partial 327
  seawater 330
water jetting industry, prescribed
    diseases in *47*
water pollution
  aluminium contamination
    (Camelford) 100
  aluminium sulphate contamination,
    Camelford 25
  cadmium poisoning (itai-itai disease)
    94
  mercury poisoning (Minamata Bay)
    90, 852, 872
  see also drinking water; environment
water workers, elbow problems 458
Watson v M'Ewan (1905) 63
Waugh v British Rail (1980) 59
wax pressmen, scrotal cancer *815*
weakness, pesticide exposure and *200*
Weavers' Bottom 6
weaving, prescribed diseases due to *47,
  52*
weedkillers
  hormone weedkillers, *see*
    chlorophenoxyacetate
    herbicides
  sodium trichloroacetate 249
  see also herbicides; phenoxy acid
    herbicides; 2,4,5-
    trichlorophenoxyacetic acid
weeds, contact dermatitis 733, 734
Weeping Fig (*Ficus benjamina*) 713
Wegener's granulomatosis 853
weight loss
  extrinsic allergic alveolitis 657, 658
  hip and knee osteoarthritis *467*, 467
Weil's disease 495

welders/welding **179–94**
  arc welding, safety standards 431
  asbestos risk 182, 183, 184
  asphyxia 182
  asthma 182–3, 700
  barium exposure 101
  bronchitis 699
  carcinogenicity of chrome salts 105
  chronic obstructive lung disease and
    699
  consumable electrodes 180
  contact lenses and spectacles 185
  definition of welding 179
  electric arc welding 179–80
  electrodes 180
  electromagnetic fields 184, 185
  emissions from welding, *see* welding
    fume
  eye protectors *433, 434*
  gas shield 180, 181
  health hazards 179
  injuries, physical 184–5
    ears 184, 185
    eyes 185
    musculoskeletal system 184
    noise-induced hearing loss 185
    penetrating 184–5
    skin 184–5
  lung cancer 183
  magnetic field exposure 439
  manual metal arc welding 180
  mesothelioma 184
  metal active gas welding 180
  metal inert gas welding 180
  nitrogen dioxide released 159
  phosgene poisoning 148
  pneumonia 28, 186
  prescribed diseases due to *53, 54*
  protective lenses 185
  respiratory tract malignancies 807
  tungsten inert gas welding 180
  zinc oxide fumes 116
  see also stainless steel
    welders/welding; steel
    welders/welding
welder's flash 434
welder's pneumoconiosis 701
welding arc maculopathy 426
welding arcs 426
  eye damage from *420*
welding filters **434–5**
  autodarkening **434–5**
welding fume 179, 180–2, **615–16**
  airway responsiveness 616
  asthma and 616
  carcinogenicity 183–4
  cardiovascular system and 185
  composition 180–1
  COPD and 615–16
  gaseous emissions 181–2
  health effects of exposure to 182–5
    central and peripheral nervous
      systems 184
    reproductive system 184
    respiratory system 182–4
  influence of coatings and
    contaminants 182
  inhalation fevers 185–7

  inhaled fumes 181
  methacholine tests 616
  oxygen enrichment and fires 182
  particulate emissions 181
  shipyard workers and 615
  and smoking 615
  spatter 181, 184
Welding Institute 179
well-being, model of 575, 576
wells
  carbon dioxide in 140
  geothermal steam 172–3
  oil well fires 129–30
Western Red Cedar (*Thuja plicata*),
    occupational asthma due to
    634, 636, 638, 646
wet bulb globe temperature (WBGT)
    index 333, 334
wheal-and-flare reaction 731
wheat dust
  occupational asthma due to *647*
  prescribed diseases due to *52, 53*
wheat flour, radioallergosorbent tests
    (RAST) *21*
whisky distilleries, malt worker's lung
    655
white finger attacks, *see* hand–arm
    vibration syndrome: vibration
    white finger
white-fly (*Trialeurodes vaporariorum*),
    radioallergosorbent tests (RAST)
    21
Whitehouse v Jordan (1981) 62
white lead pigment industry 923
white spirits *224*, **255–6**
  carcinogenicity 256
  characteristics and uses 255
  chemical composition 255, *256*
  clinical manifestations 255–6
  as hazardous DIY material *6*
  management 256
  metabolism/biochemical effects 255
  psychiatric symptoms 256
Whitfield's ointment, ringworm 502
whole-body radiation exposure
  acute/chronic 402–3
  annual dose limits *409*
  signs and symptoms *402*
  threshold levels of dose 399, *400*
whole-body vibration (WBV) 317–19
  acceptable values *318*
  definition 308
  epidemiology 318
  health effects 317–18
  occupations associated with 317
  prevention 318
  sources *317*
  standards 318–19
Will o' the Wisp 138
Willson v Ministry of Defence (1991) 61
Wilms' tumour 746, 752, 757
  susceptibility and germline mutation
    751
Wilson's disease 892
  non-invasive screening *882*
wind chill equivalent temperature 327,
    327
wind speed 327

wine, adulteration with lead 82
wine industry, hepatotoxicity in *885*
witherite (barium carbonate) 101
Wolff–Parkinson–Wright syndrome *390*
wollastonite 696
women
    exposure to lead in ceramics industry
        923
    in mining 921–2
    noise-induced hearing loss 290
    shift work and reproductive function
        584
wood dust 185
    asthma and COPD 613
    cryptogenic fibrosing alveolitis and
        660
    genotoxicity *776*
    as hazardous DIY material *6*
    inhalation of, EC schedule of
        occupational diseases *44*
    occupational asthma due to 638,
        647
    prescribed diseases due to *52, 53*
    sino-nasal cancer *816*
    see also hardwood dusts;
        woodworkers/woodworking
wood industry, formaldehyde resins
    244
wood pulp industry, carcinogenic risk in
    816
woodworkers/woodworking
    cancer and 794
    dermatoses 735
    Hodgkin's disease 909–10
    prescribed diseases *47, 53*
    respiratory tract malignancies *4*
    toxic DIY materials *6*
Woolf Report/reforms 62, 63
wool handlers, Q fever 498
wool sorter's disease, *see* anthrax
workers
    monitoring/supervision of, *see*
        monitoring of workers
    see also specific occupations
workers' compensation schemes,
        outside UK 38, 571
work hours
    European Union Directive 585–6,
        588
    extended
        definition 581
        health effects 587–8
    see also night work; shift work
work loss, back pain and 477–8, 481
Workman's Compensation Act 1897
    37–8
work-related upper limb disorder, *see*
    repetitive strain injury

Worksafe Australia, material safety data
    sheet format 7
World Health Organization (WHO)
    Alcohol Use Disorders Identification
        Test (AUDIT) 560
    byssinosis classification *626*, 627
    carbon disulphide exposure
        symptoms 254
    definition of health 569
    hydrogen sulphide guideline
        concentration limit 161
    impairment/disability/handicap
        definitions 294–5
    office building guidelines 716–17
    Radiation Emergency Medical
        Preparedness Assistance
        Network (REMPAN) 414
    zoonosis list 489
wrist(s)
    carpal tunnel syndrome case-control
        studies *461*
    prescribed diseases affecting *46*
    splints 458
    tenosynovitis *454*, 459
    work-related conditions 454
wrist drop, in lead poisoning 86, 871
writer's cramp 462, 464
    prescribed disease status and 40
writing, prescribed diseases due to *46*
W v Edgell (1990) 60

xanthophyll 423, 424
xenobiotics 68
    biotransformation, *see also*
        metabolism
    detoxification and elimination of
        72–7
    shift workers' susceptibility to 584
    see also biotransformation; chemical
        agents/chemicals; metabolism
xenon 141
    in earth's atmosphere *135*
xenon-chloride lasers, exposure limits
    429
xeroderma pigmentosum 746
x-ray chemicals 714
x-rays *398*, 398
    discovery of 397
    reproductive hazards to
        embryo/fetus 829, *832*
xylene (dimethyl benzene) **263–4**,
    854
    absorption 264
    biological monitoring tests and
        guidance values *18*
    characteristics and uses 263
    clinical effects 264

    as hazardous DIY material *6*
    hepatotoxicity *885*
    isomers 263
    metabolism 264
    monitoring 264
    reproductive hazards to mother
        831
o-xylene 261
xylol, *see* xylene

yeasts, ill-health due to, in
        biotechnology *527*
yellow fever 509
yellow phosphorus
    hepatotoxicity *885*
    steatosis 883
Yusho incident 274, *884*, 894

zeolites 696
zidovudine 508
zinc **116–17**
    absorption and distribution 116
    function in body 116
    in welding 186
zinc chloride
    acute lung injury due to *698*
    toxicity 116
zinc chromate 807
    lung cancer as prescribed disease *54*,
        105
zinc fumes 697
zinc oxide
    fumes 697
    inhalation 185–6
    toxicity 116
    see also metal fume fever
zinc protoporphyrin (ZPP) 85, 87, 88
zirconium **117**
    granulomatous lung disease due to
        702
zirconium tetrachloride, acute lung
        injury due to *698*, 698
zoologists
    rabies 499
    zoonoses 489
zoonoses 214, **489–502**
    EC comparable data collection *41*
    food-borne infections 493–4
    imaging 603
    occupational infections 490–3
    prevention and control 490
    skin diseases 501–2
    workers at risk 489
    see also animals; *individual zoonotic*
        infections; and specific diseases